Physician's Guide to the Diagnosis, Treatment, and Follow-Up of Inherited Metabolic Diseases

Nenad Blau • Carlo Dionisi Vici
Carlos R. Ferreira • Christine Vianey-Saban
Clara D. M. van Karnebeek
Editors

# Physician's Guide to the Diagnosis, Treatment, and Follow-Up of Inherited Metabolic Diseases

Second Edition

Volume I

Springer

*Editors*
Nenad Blau
Division of Metabolism
University Children's Hospital
Zürich
Switzerland

Carlos R. Ferreira
Division of Genetics and Metabolism
Children's National Health System
Washington, DC
USA

Clara D. M. van Karnebeek
Departments of Pediatrics and Human Genetics
Emma Children's Hospital, Amsterdam
University Medical Centers
Amsterdam
The Netherlands

Carlo Dionisi Vici
Division of Metabolic Disease, Department
of Pediatric Subspecialties
Bambino Gesù Children's Hospital-IRCCS
Rome
Italy

Christine Vianey-Saban
Department of Inborn Errors of Metabolism
and Newborn Screening
CHU Lyon, Centre de Biologie et de Pathologie
Est
Bron Cedex
France

ISBN 978-3-030-67729-9 ISBN 978-3-030-67727-5 (eBook)
https://doi.org/10.1007/978-3-030-67727-5



This Springer imprint is published by the registered company Springer Nature Switzerland AG
The registered company address is: Gewerbestrasse 11, 6330 Cham, Switzerland

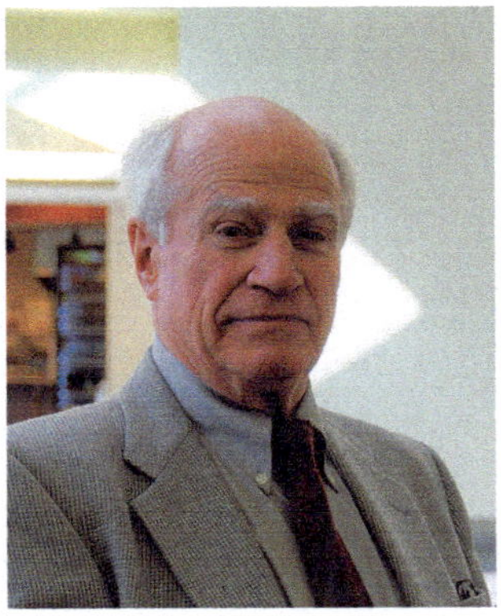

**Stephen Irwin Goodman (1938–2020)**

*The Editors take this opportunity to acknowledge Stephen Irwin Goodman, MD—one of the pioneers in the field of diagnosis and treatment of inborn errors of metabolism, who passed away while this book was in press, on October 30, 2020—for his longstanding efforts and contributions to our series Physician's Guide in Inherited Metabolic Disease. A founding member of both the Society for Inherited Metabolic Disorders and the American College of Medical Genetics (and Genomics), Steve spent his entire professional career at the University of Colorado in Denver with his wife, Patricia, their daughters Michelle and Karen, and their families.*

*Steve is remembered for his role in establishing the diagnostic methods for organic acidemias, for writing a seminal text on use of GC-MS for analysis of organic acids (with Sanford Markey), defining and characterizing glutaric acidurias type I and II, and contributing knowledge to the diagnosis and management of many other inborn errors of metabolism.*

*In recognition of his constant guidance and valuable contributions (see Chap. 71), we wish to dedicate this edition of the Physician's Guide to the Diagnosis, Treatment, and Follow-Up of Inherited Metabolic Diseases to his memory.*

*Nenad Blau*
*Carlo Dionisi Vici*
*Carlos R. Ferreira*
*Christine Vianey-Saban*
*Clara D.M. van Karnebeek*

# Foreword

A new edition for an old subject

The study of inborn errors of metabolism arguably began with Garrod's seminal 1902 paper on alkaptonuria (Garrod 1902). At the time, the diagnosis of this disorder was achieved using state-of-the-art technology: visual inspection of recently voided urine. Garrod's genius was to use this method to identify and collect a large number of individuals with this rare disorder and to recognize, with input from Bateson, that the familial clustering and distribution of affected individuals (19 affected of 48 individuals in 9 sibships) was consistent with observations made by Gregor Mendel in pea plants some 37 years earlier. An additional feature of alkaptonuria, crucial for Garrod's study, is that, at the phenotypic level, it is a relatively mild disorder with minimal, if any, effect on life span. To quote Garrod, "an alternative course of metabolism, harmless and usually congenital and lifelong." Thus, it was possible for Garrod to collect affected individuals, many of whom were adults at the time of diagnosis.

From this modest beginning, Garrod not only demonstrated that Mendelism held true in humans, but also suggested that alkaptonuria and a handful of similar disorders (cystinuria, pentosuria, and albinism) were "merely extreme examples of variations in chemical behavior which are probably everywhere present in minor degree" so that "just as no two individuals of a species are absolutely identical in bodily structure neither are their chemical processes carried out on exactly the same lines." First stated in 1902, these ideas lead to Garrod's definition in 1931 (Garrod 1931) of "chemical individuality" as genetically determined biochemical characteristics and capabilities which confer "predisposition to and immunities from the various mishaps which are spoken of as diseases." We are only now beginning to put meat on the bones of these prescient predictions.

From Garrod's time to the present, progress in identifying specific inborn errors of metabolism has been dependent on technological advances. Thus, in the early 1950s following the development of the first amino acid analyzer, a host of "new" (really "newly recognized") disorders were described on the basis of abnormal patterns of amino acids in plasma and/or urine. Similarly, the development of GC/MS technology leads to the recognition of many organic acidemias, and the development of tissue culture and somatic cell genetic techniques leads to a burst of newly recognized lysosomal storage diseases.

Currently, we are experiencing at least two technologic revolutions: genomic sequencing methods that began with the seminal 2009 paper of Ng et al. (2009) showing that the cause of rare Mendelian disorders could be identified by applying genomic methods to well-phenotyped patients and, more recently, the development of unstructured metabolomic methods that measure thousands of metabolites not previously examined by classical biochemical methods. Application of genomic methods has already had a profound effect on our identification and diagnosis of patients with inborn errors (Posey et al. 2019; Bamshad et al. 2019). Advances and widespread application of metabolomics seems likely to have a similar effect (Burrage et al. 2019; Miller et al. 2015). Moreover, the two technologies are synergistic in their power to identify newly recognized monogenic disorders and to expose their pathophysiology.

While exciting and gratifying, this rapid expansion of the number of recognizable inborn errors is a daunting challenge to the beleaguered clinicians who take care of these patients; one can never know what the next patient who comes to clinic will have: a defect in purine metabolism; a problem in lysosomal function; a peroxisome biogenesis disorder; or some tRNA charging abnormality impairing translation. The possibilities are as broad as all biology and hence justify newly revised editions of this text and associated online resources.

A salient challenge derived from the rapid expansion of our field and any such effort to describe it, is how to modernize the definition of inborn errors of metabolism, a term, after all, that has been in use since 1908 when Garrod coined it in his Croonian lectures (Garrod 1908). Recent efforts to update the definition have included inclusion of phenotypic features, diagnostic technologies, and limitations to specific biological systems (Morava et al. 2015; Ferreira et al. 2019). While useful, phenotypic features for any disorder are always variable and typically overlap with those of other disorders. Diagnostic technology changes over time and will continue to do so. A focus on biologic systems is useful for understanding pathophysiology, but the margins of any particular system often overlap with those of others and, currently, we do not have a well-defined list of all biological systems.

Based on these considerations, I argue that we consider all monogenic disorders as Garrodian inborn errors of metabolism. This gene-based definition is enriched by a foundation built on genetic principles and emphasizes the discrete monogenic cause of these disorders. It also benefits from the fact that it is easier to enumerate and designate all the genes in the genome than all the phenotypes that bring patients to our clinics. For example, at the time I write this (25 November 2020), OMIM lists 4355 genes with variants that cause monogenic disease (OMIM® n.d.). This number is increasing steadily with no asymptote in sight (Posey et al. 2019; Bamshad et al. 2019). Moreover, all monogenic disorders have an associated biochemical phenotype increasingly recognized by standard or newly developed technologies such as metabolomics or proteomics. Identification of the biochemical abnormalities associated with each monogenic disease is sometimes challenging but feasible and leads to improved understanding of the pathophysiology of each disorder, a necessary step on the path to rational development of treatment.

One possible concern of a gene-based definition of IEM is that for some genes, allelic heterogeneity produces phenotypic variation which in some instances is so extreme that we do not a priori expect variants in the same gene to underlie the apparently discrete phenotypes. For example, variants in *FBN1* can cause either Marfan syndrome (OMIM 154700) with tall stature, arachnodactyly, loose joints, ectopia lentis and aortic root aneurysms or stiff skin syndrome (OMIM 184900) with short stature, no arachnodactyly, limited range of joint mobility, and no ocular nor aortic symptoms. In fact, about a third of disease genes listed in OMIM are responsible for two or more clinically discrete phenotypes (OMIM® n.d.). A gene-based definition of IEM would, however, anticipate this biologic complexity and incorporate it so that each gene would be linked to a specific phenotype or set of phenotypes, with the benefit that we would expect these genotype–phenotype relationships as a part of disease biology and use them to inform our understanding of the disorders and the function of the protein(s) encoded by each gene.

Using this definition, the ultimate number of IEMs depends on how many genes are found to house variants of major effect, sufficient to produce a phenotype. The fact that evolution seems to care about (conserve) the vast majority of protein-coding genes in the genome suggests that certain variants in nearly all protein-coding genes will ultimately be found to be capable of producing a monogenic phenotype (and thus, by this definition, be considered an inborn error of metabolism or, perhaps better, simply an inborn error). This logic suggests that long non-coding RNA genes, which are less well conserved, may play a much smaller role in monogenic disease. How this will end up in the future is an uncertain but exciting prospect.

One thing for sure is that new resources for clinicians and investigators such as this new edition of a *Physician's Guide to the Diagnosis, Treatment, and Follow-Up of Inherited Metabolic Diseases* will be much needed and appreciated.

David Valle
McKusick-Nathans Department of Genetic Medicine
The Johns Hopkins University School of Medicine
Baltimore, MD, USA

## References

Bamshad MJ, et al. Mendelian gene discovery: fast and furious with no end in sight. Am J Hum Genet. 2019;105:448–55.

Burrage LC, et al. Untargeted metabolomic profiling reveals multiple pathway perturbations and new clinical biomarkers in urea cycle disorders. Genet Med. 2019;21:1977–86.

Ferreira CR, et al. A proposed nosology of inborn errors of metabolism. Genet Med. 2019;21:102–6.

Garrod AE. The incidence of alkaptonuria: a study in chemical individuality. The Lancet. 1902;2:1616–20.

Garrod AE. The Croonian Lectures on inborn errors of metabolism. The Lancet. 1908;2:1–7, 73–9, 142–8, 214–20.

Garrod AE. Inborn factors in disease. Oxford University Press; 1931.

Miller MJ, et al. Untargeted metabolomic analysis for the clinical screening of inborn errors of metabolism. J Inherit Metab Dis. 2015;38:1029–39.

Morava E, et al. Quo vadis: the re-definition of inborn metabolic diseases. J Inherit Metab Dis. 2015;38:1003–6.

Ng SB, et al. Targeted capture and massively parallel sequencing of 12 human exomes. Nature. 2009;461:272–6.

Online Mendelian Inheritance in Man, OMIM®. McKusick-Nathans Department of Genetic Medicine, Johns Hopkins University (Baltimore, MD), 24 November 2020. https://omim.org/

Posey JE, et al., Insights into genetics, human biology, and disease gleaned from family based genomic studies. Genet Med. 2019;21:798–812.

# Preface

Our expert faculty of more than 170 recognized authorities has broadened the scope and content of this book, the fourth edition of the Physician's Guide series. We overhauled the structure of the book to accommodate 18 new chapters: 73 chapters now address almost 1200 inherited metabolic disorders. The original edition, published in 1996, focused on diagnosis only and was translated into Chinese in 2001. Today, along with a comprehensive update to this vital aspect of care, the current edition presents the state of the art on the treatment and follow-up, providing insight into the full clinical course of these rare diseases.

Based upon their experience, our expert faculty have created flowcharts and diagnostic algorithms for each disorder. Initially, recommendations on confirmatory tests and initial treatment regimens are provided for practitioners who lack extensive experience in the management of inborn errors of metabolism. The second part of each chapter describes the treatment of groups of disorders in more detail. The book presents the signs and symptoms of most of the recognized inborn errors of metabolism in relation to age, with a chronological sequence of signs and symptoms from infancy through childhood, adolescence, and adulthood. In addition, reference and pathological values are provided for each of the disorders to simplify and facilitate the interpretation of the results of laboratory tests.

The guide will also be available in an eBook format that will allow the user to locate a disorder rapidly, using standard searches with keywords. Additionally, the entire content of this edition is stored in a single database, IEMbase (http://www.iembase.org). This comprehensive online resource provides the foundation for the current and future knowledge base of inborn errors of metabolism.

While the major goals of this edition remain comparable to those of earlier editions, we, the Editors, feel that this new edition takes clinical practice in rare metabolic disorders to the next level. We hope that our readers will find this edition helpful, both now and in the future, for the treatment and care of patients with inborn errors of metabolism.

Finally, we acknowledge the former Editors, Dr. Marinus Duran and Dr. K. Michael Gibson in supporting this book project.


| | |
|---|---|
| Zürich, Switzerland | Nenad Blau |
| Rome, Italy | Carlo Dionisi Vici |
| Washington, DC, USA | Carlos R. Ferreira |
| Lyon, France | Christine Vianey-Saban |
| Amsterdam, The Netherlands | Clara D. M. van Karnebeek |


The original version of this book has been updated: fifth Editor Dr. Clara D. M. van Karnebeek's affiliation has been updated. A Correction to this book is available at https://doi.org/10.1007/978-3-030-67727-5_74

# How to Use This Book

This book is meant to supply clinicians and clinical biochemists with data that should facilitate the diagnosis of an inherited metabolic disorder. No information about detailed laboratory methods is given; rather, the relationship between laboratory data and clinical signs and symptoms is highlighted. Furthermore the current knowledge on the immediate emergency intervention, standard treatment, and experimental options is given. Entry to the book is achieved by scanning either of the indices, i.e., the signs and symptoms index, the tests index, or the disorders index. Due to the great clinical variability of inherited metabolic diseases, one should not restrict oneself to one disorder when observing a given symptom or sign. Most chapters have a uniform layout as given below. In a few chapters, however, this was not possible, and information is given for the entire related group of disorders in the chapter.

## Introduction

The introduction gives a brief overview of the clinical conditions described in the chapter and relates them to the biochemical abnormalities. Key references for further reading are provided.

## Nomenclature

Disorders in each chapter are numbered in accordance with the corresponding OMIM number, gene symbols and gene products, and chromosomal localization if known.

## Metabolic Pathway

Disorders are identified by corresponding reference numbers at the step where the defect is localized. Pathological metabolites ("markers") are given in most chapters.

## Signs and Symptoms

The tables describe most, if not all, of the signs and symptoms for each disorder, including its reference number, and the most important laboratory tests, in relation to age. In all instances, the signs and symptoms are found in the untreated patients. The signs written in **bold** represent characteristic features of the particular disease.

± indicates that a sign or symptom *may* occur but is not inevitably present.

+ indicates that a sign or symptom is always or nearly always present. If there are significant clinical signs and symptoms which exceed the usual, or if changes occur, this is indicated with + to + + +, etc.

n (normal) is used only when it is significant and may be useful in distinguishing one condition from another.

Relative increases or decreases of substances, compounds, metabolites, etc., are indicated with the use of arrows; for example, metabolite X ↑ to ↓↓↓. Where metabolite X *may* change, it would be indicated by n-↑ for a possible increase or ↓-n for a possible decrease, whichever the case.

In all tables, the test substance, material, compound, metabolite, etc., are listed and the source—(U), (B), (CSF), (P), (RBC), etc.—is given in parentheses, with an arrow or arrows indicating increase/decrease or relative increase/decrease.

Body fluids, cells, tissues, etc., are defined as:

| | | | |
|---|---|---|---|
| P | Plasma | CV | Chorionic villi |
| S | Serum | AF | Amniotic fluid |
| B | Blood | AFC | Amniocytes |
| U | Urine | CCV | Cultured chorionic villi |
| CSF | Cerebrospinal fluid | PLT | Platelets |
| RBC | Red blood cells | WBC | White blood cells |
| LYM | Lymphocytes | Hb | Hemoglobin |
| FB | Fibroblasts | creat | Creatinine |
| BM | Bone marrow | | |

Age groups are defined as:

| | |
|---|---|
| Neonatal | Birth to 1 month |
| Infancy | 1–18 months |
| Childhood | 1.5–11 years |
| Adolescence | 11–16 years |
| Adulthood | >16 years |

## Reference Values/Pathological Values/Differential Diagnosis

Reference and pathological values are listed for all parameters relevant to the diagnosis according to the specimen (e.g., P, U, CSF) and age. For some parameters, reference values depend on methodology and may differ from chapter to chapter. Methods are specified where necessary.

Pathological values are listed either as absolute values or with symbols (e.g., ↑, ↓) according to the disorder. Values are limited to the analyses which can be performed in a laboratory experienced in selective screening. Data on enzyme studies are not given in most cases, but can be found in the pertinent literature.

## Loading Tests

There is a brief description of the tests, with a table or figure to illustrate the interpretation.

## Diagnostic Flow Chart

The flow charts use simple yes/no algorithms to demonstrate the sequence for differential diagnosis, starting with clinical symptoms or general tests and proceeding to specific tests and a final diagnosis.

## Specimen Collection

This table lists preconditions, material, handling, and pitfalls for each parameter used in the diagnosis.

## Prenatal Diagnosis

This table lists the tissue or specimen, timing, and pitfalls for each disorder.

## DNA Analysis

This table lists the tissue or specimen and methodology for each disorder.

## Treatment and Follow-Up

This section outlines urgent treatment to consider before a definitive diagnosis is established for each (or each group of) disorder(s). Long-term treatment and alternative therapeutic options are highlighted in this book.

## Indices

Three indices are included: (1) disorders, (2) signs and symptoms, and (3) tests and medications. Each entry is linked to the corresponding disorder or page.

# Contents

# Contributors

**Cécile Acquaviva** CHU de Lyon, Department of Biochemistry & Molecular Biology, Division of Inborn Errors of Metabolism, Lyon University Hospital Centre, Bron, France

**Majid Alfadhel** King Abdullah International Medical Research Centre, King Saud bin Abdulaziz University for Health Sciences, Riyadh, Saudi Arabia

**Anna Ardissone** Unit of Child Neurology, Fondazione IRCCS Istituto Neurologico Carlo Besta, Milan, Italy

**Jean-Baptiste Arnoux** French Metabolic Network G2M, Necker-Enfants Malades Hospital, APHP, Paris, France

**Rafael Artuch** CIBERER, Instituto de Salud Carlos III, Madrid, Spain

Clinical Chemistry Department, Institut de Recerca Sant Joan de Déu, Barcelona, Spain

Pathology Department, Institut de Recerca Sant Joan de Déu, Barcelona, Spain

**Tamar V. Av-Shalom** Department of Medical Genetics, Centre for Molecular Medicine and Therapeutics, BC Children's Hospital Research Institute, University of British Columbia, Vancouver, BC, Canada

**Ivo Barić** Division for Genetics and Metabolic Diseases, Department of Pediatrics, University Hospital Center Zagreb and University of Zagreb, School of Medicine, Zagreb, Croatia

**Bruce A. Barshop** Department of Pediatrics, University of California San Diego, La Jolla, CA, USA

**Matthias R. Baumgartner** Division of Metabolism and Children's Research Center, University Children's Hospital Zürich, University of Zürich, Zürich, Switzerland

**Bodo B. Beck** Department of Human Genetics, University Hospital Cologne, Cologne, Germany

**Michael Beck** SphinCS GmbH–Clinical Science for LSD, Hochheim, Germany

**Cinzia Maria Bellettato** Regional Coordinating Center for Rare Diseases, Udine University Hospital, Udine, Italy

**Jean-François Benoist** APHP, Reference Center for Inborn Error of Metabolism and Filiere G2M, Pediatrics Department, Necker Univ Hospital, Paris, France

**Anna Biason-Lauber** Division of Medicine, University of Fribourg, Fribourg, Switzerland

**Jörgen Bierau** Department of Clinical Genetics, Erasmus MC, Rotterdam, The Netherlands

**Nenad Blau** Division of Metabolism, University Children's Hospital, Zürich, Switzerland

**Annet M. Bosch** Department of Pediatrics, Emma Children's Hospital, Amsterdam University Medical Centers, Amsterdam, The Netherlands

**Olivier Braissant** Service of Clinical Chemistry, Department of Laboratories, University Hospital and University of Lausanne, Lausanne, Switzerland

**Anaïs Brassier** APHP, Reference Center for Inborn Error of Metabolism and Filiere G2M, Pediatrics Department, Necker Univ Hospital, Paris, France

**Stefan Bröer** Research School of Biology, The Australian National University, Canberra, ACT, Australia

**Alberto Burlina** Division of Inherited Metabolic Diseases, Reference Centre Expanded Newborn Screening, Department of Woman's and Child's Health, University Hospital, Padova, Italy

**John R. Burnett** Department of Clinical Biochemistry, Royal Perth Hospital and Fiona Stanley Hospital, PathWest Laboratory Medicine WA, Perth, WA, Australia

School of Medicine, University of Western Australia, Perth, WA, Australia

**Maria Domenica Cappellini** Fondazione Ca Granda Policlinico IRCCS, Università di Milano, Milan, Spain

**Rosalba Carrozzo** Molecular Genetic, Bambino Gesù Children's Hospital, Rome, Italy

**Rita Carsetti** Diagnostic Immunology Clinical Unit, Bambino Gesù Children's Hospital IRCCS, Rome, Italy

**David Cassiman** Center for Metabolic Diseases, University of Leuven, Leuven, Belgium

**Peter T. Clayton** UCL GOS Institute of Child Health, University College, London, UK

**Karlien L. M. Coene** Translational Metabolic Laboratory, Department Laboratory Medicine, Radboud University Medical Centre, Nijmegen, The Netherlands

**Curtis R. Coughlin II** Section of Clinical Genetics and Metabolism, Department of Pediatrics, University of Colorado, Children's Hospital Colorado, Aurora, CO, USA

**James Davison** Metabolic Unit, Great Ormond Street Hospital for Children, NHS Foundation Trust and Institute for Child Health, London, UK

**Lonneke de Boer** Department of Pediatrics, Radboud Center for Mitochondrial Medicine, Radboud University Medical Centre (Radboudumc), Nijmegen, The Netherlands

**Tom J. de Koning** Department of Clinical Sciences, Lund University, Lund, Sweden

**Pascale de Lonlay** French Metabolic Network G2M, Necker-Enfants Malades Hospital, APHP, Paris, France

**Linda de Meirleir** Department of Pediatric Neurology, UZ-Brussel, Brussels, Belgium

**Terry G. J. Derks** Section of Metabolic Diseases, Beatrix Children's Hospital, University Medical Center Groningen, Groningen, The Netherlands

**Maaike C. de Vries** Department of Pediatrics, Radboud Center for Mitochondrial Medicine, Radboud University Medical Centre (Radboudumc), Nijmegen, The Netherlands

**Ivano Di Meo** Unit of Medical Genetics and Neurogenetics, Fondazione IRCCS Istituto Neurologico Carlo Besta, Milan, Italy

**Daria Diodato** Neuromuscular and Neurodegenerative Disease Unit, Children Hospital Bambino Gesù, Rome, Italy

**Carlo Dionisi Vici** Division of Metabolism, Department of Pediatric Medicine, Bambino Gesù Children's Research Hospital, IRCCS, Rome, Italy

**Katrina M. Dipple** Division of Genetic Medicine, Department of Pediatrics, University of Washington School of Medicine and Seattle Children's Hospital, Seattle, WA, USA

**Francesco Emma** Department of Pediatric Subspecialties, Division of Nephrology and Dialysis, Bambino Gesù Children's Hospital, IRCCS, Rome, Italy

**Marc Engelen** Departments of Pediatric Neurology, Emma Children's Hospital, Amsterdam University Medical Centers, Academic Medical Center, Amsterdam, The Netherlands

**Udo F. H. Engelke** Translational Metabolic Laboratory, Department Laboratory Medicine, Radboud University Medical Centre, Nijmegen, The Netherlands

**Sacha Ferdinandusse** Laboratory Genetic Metabolic Diseases, Amsterdam UMC, Amsterdam, The Netherlands

**Carlos R. Ferreira** Division of Genetics and Metabolism, Children's National Health System, Washington, DC, USA

**Ralph Fingerhut** SYNLAB MVZ Weiden, Weiden, Germany

**Janice Fletcher** SA Pathology (at Women's and Children's Hospital), Adelaide, SA, Australia

**Brian Fowler** Division for Metabolic Diseases, University Children's Hospital, Zürich, Switzerland

**D. Sean Froese** Division of Metabolism and Children's Research Center, University Children's Hospital Zürich, University of Zürich, Zürich, Switzerland

**Silvia Funghini** Newborn Screening, Clinical Chemistry and Pharmacology Lab, Meyer Children's University Hospital, Florence, Italy

**Roberto Giugliani** Department of Genetics, Federal University of Rio Grande do Sul, Porto Alegre, RS, Brazil

Medical Genetics Service, Hospital de Clinicas de Porto Alegre, Porto Alegre, RS, Brazil

**Stephen I. Goodman** University of Colorado Denver School of Medicine, Aurora, CO, USA

**Andrea Gropman** Department of Neurology, Children's National Health System, Washington, DC, USA

**Sarah C. Grünert** Zentrum für Kinder- und Jugendmedizin, Universitätsklinikum Freiburg, Freiburg, Germany

**Stephanie Grünewald** Metabolic Unit, Great Ormond Street Hospital for Children, NHS Foundation Trust and Institute for Child Health, London, UK

**Chandan Guha** Marion Bessin Liver Research Center, Albert Einstein College of Medicine, Bronx, NY, USA

Departments of Radiation Oncology and Pathology, Albert Einstein College of Medicine, Bronx, NY, USA

**Johannes Häberle** Division of Metabolism and Children's Research Center, University Children's Hospital, Zürich, Switzerland

**Robert A. Hegele** Schulich School of Medicine and Dentistry, University of Western Ontario, London, ON, Canada

**Georg F. Hoffmann** University Children's Hospital, Heidelberg, Germany

**Carla Hollak** Division of Endocrinology and Metabolism, Department of Internal Medicine, Academic Medical Center, University of Amsterdam, Amsterdam, The Netherlands

**Ian J. Holt** Biodonostia Health Research Institute, San Sebastián, Spain

IKERBASQUE, Basque Foundation for Science, Bilbao, Spain

CIBERNED (Center for Networked Biomedical Research on Neurodegenerative Diseases, Ministry of Economy and Competitiveness Institute Carlos III), Madrid, Spain

**Amanda J. Hooper** Department of Clinical Biochemistry, Royal Perth Hospital and Fiona Stanley Hospital, PathWest Laboratory Medicine WA, Perth, WA, Australia

School of Medicine, University of Western Australia, Perth, WA, Australia

**Bernd Hoppe** Hyperoxaluria Center, German Hyperoxaluria Center, Bonn, Germany

**Hidde H. Huidekoper** Center for Lysosomal and Metabolic diseases, Department of Pediatrics, Erasmus MC University Medical Center, Rotterdam, The Netherlands

**Jaak Jaeken** Center for Metabolic Disease, University Hospital Gasthuisberg, Leuven, Belgium

**Judith J. M. Jans** Translational Metabolic Laboratory, Department Laboratory Medicine, Radboud University Medical Centre, Nijmegen, The Netherlands

**Mirian C. H. Janssen** Department of Internal Medicine, Radboud Center for Mitochondrial Medicine, Nijmegen, The Netherlands

**Heinz Jungbluth** Department of Paediatric Neurology, Evelina Children's Hospital, Guy's and St Thomas' Hospital NHS Foundation Trust, London, UK

**Richard I. Kelley** Central Pennsylvania Clinic, Belleville, PA, USA

**Femke C. C. Klouwer** Departments of Neurology and Pediatric Neurology, Emma Children's Hospital, Amsterdam University Medical Centers, Amsterdam, The Netherlands

**Stefan Kölker** Division of Pediatric Neurology and Metabolic Medicine, Clinic I, Center for Pediatric and Adolescent Medicine, Heidelberg, Germany

**Werner J. H. Koopman** Department of Biochemistry, Radboud Institute for Molecular Life Sciences (RIMLS), Radboud Center for Mitochondrial Medicine, Radboud University Medical Centre (Radboudumc), Nijmegen, The Netherlands

**Viktor Kožich** Department of Pediatrics and Inherited Metabolic Diseases, Charles University-First Faculty of Medicine and General University Hospital in Prague, Praha, Czech Republic

**Lisa E. Kratz** Department of Neurogenetics, Kennedy Krieger Institute, Baltimore, MD, USA

**Ilja Kubisch** Center of Internal Medicine II, Gastroenterology, Hepatology, Endocrinology, Metabolic Disorders, Oncology, Saxony Porphyria Center, Klinikum Chemnitz gGmbH, Chemnitz, Germany

**Martina Kutmon** Department of Bioinformatics—BiGCaT, NUTRIM, Maastricht University, Maastricht, The Netherlands

Maastricht Centre for Systems Biology—MaCSBio, Maastricht University, Maastricht, The Netherlands

**Giancarlo la Marca** Newborn Screening, Clinical Chemistry and Pharmacology Lab, Meyer Children's University Hospital, Florence, Italy

Department of Experimental and Clinical Biomedical Sciences, University of Florence, Florence, Italy

**Jessica J. Y. Lee** Department of Medical Genetics, Centre for Molecular Medicine and Therapeutics, BC Children's Hospital Research Institute, University of British Columbia, Vancouver, BC, Canada

**Min Ae Lee-Kirsch** Department of Pediatrics, Medizinische Fakultät Carl Gustav Carus, Technische Universität Dresden, Dresden, Germany

**Elena Levtchenko** Department of Pediatric Nephrology, University Hospitals Leuven, Catholic University of Leuven, Leuven, Belgium

**Nicola Longo** University of Utah and ARUP Laboratories, Salt Lake City, UT, USA

**Charlotte M. A. Lubout** Section of Metabolic Diseases, Beatrix Children's Hospital, University Medical Center Groningen, Groningen, The Netherlands

**Zoltan Lukacs** Newborn Screening and Metabolic Diagnostics Unit, Hamburg University Medical Center, Hamburg, Germany

**Arianna Maiorana** Division of Metabolism, Department of Pediatric Subspecialties, Bambino Gesù Children's Hospital, Rome, Italy

**Sabrina Malvagia** Newborn Screening, Clinical Chemistry and Pharmacology Lab, Meyer Children's University Hospital, Florence, Italy

**Diego Martinelli** Division of Metabolism, Department of Pediatric Medicine, Bambino Gesù Children's Research Hospital, Rome, Italy

Division of Metabolic Diseases, Bambino Gesù Children's Hospital, IRCCS, Rome, Italy

**Cristina Martin-Higueras** Department of Pediatrics, Division of Pediatric Nephrology, University Hospital Bonn, Bonn, Germany

Department of Basic Medical Science, Faculty of Medicine, University of La Laguna, La Laguna, Spain

**Dietrich Matern** Biochemical Genetics Laboratory, Department of Laboratory Medicine and Pathology, Mayo Clinic, Rochester, MN, USA

**Ertan Mayatepek** Department of General Pediatrics, Neonatology and Pediatric Cardiology, University Children's Hospital, Heinrich-Heine University Düsseldorf, Düsseldorf, Germany

**Johannes A. Mayr** University Children's Hospital, Paracelsus Medical University, Salzburg, Austria

**Philippa B. Mills** UCL GOS Institute of Child Health, University College, London, UK

**Fanny Mochel** Reference Center for Adult Neurometabolic diseases, La Pitié-Salpêtrière University Hospital, Paris, France

**Eva Morava** Department of Medical Genetics, Mayo Clinic, Rochester, MN, USA

**Marwan Nashabat** King Abdulaziz Medical City, Riyadh, Saudi Arabia

**Gaia Novarino** Institute of Science and Technology (IST) Austria, Klosterneuburg, Austria

**Thomas Opladen** Division of Neuropediatrics and Metabolic Medicine, Department of Pediatrics, University Children's Hospital, Heidelberg, Germany

**Simona Orcesi** Unit of Child Neurology and Psychiatry, IRCCS Mondino Foundation, Pavia, Italy

**Esmee Oussoren** Center for Lysosomal and Metabolic diseases, Department of Pediatrics, Erasmus MC University Medical Center, Rotterdam, The Netherlands

**Manuel Palacín** Institute for Research in Biomedicine (IRB Barcelona), Barcelona Institute of Science and Technology, Barcelona, Spain

Barcelona, Centro de Investigación Biomédica en Red de Enfermedades Raras (CIBERER), Spain

Department of Biochemistry and Molecular Biomedicine, Faculty of Biology, University of Barcelona, Barcelona, Spain

**Giancarlo Parenti** Department of Translational Medical Sciences, Federico II University, Naples, Italy

Telethon Institute of Genetics and Medicine, Pozzuoli, Italy

**Marzia Pasquali** University of Utah and ARUP Laboratories, Salt Lake City, UT, USA

**Phillip L. Pearl** Department of Neurology, Boston Children's Hospital, Harvard Medical School, Boston, MA, USA

**Verena Peters** Centre for Pediatric and Adolescent Medicine, University of Heidelberg, Heidelberg, Germany

**Barbara Plecko** Department of Pediatrics and Adolescent Medicine, Division of General Pediatrics, Medical University of Graz, Graz, Austria

**Giulia Polo** Division of Inherited Metabolic Diseases, Department of Women and Children's Health, Regional Center for Expanded Neonatal Screening, University Hospital of Padova, Padova, Italy

**Holger Prokisch** Institute of Human Genetics, Technische Universität München, Munich, Germany

Institute of Neurogenomics, Helmholtz Zentrum München, Munich, Germany

**Enzo Ranieri** SA Pathology (at Women's and Children's Hospital), Adelaide, SA, Australia

**Antonia Ribes** Section of Inborn Errors of Metabolism, Department of Biochemistry and Molecular Genetics, Hospital Clinic de Barcelona, IDIBAPS, CIBERER, Barcelona, Spain

**Marlène Rio** Genetic Department, Necker-Enfants Malades Hospital, APHP, Paris, France

**Lance Rodan** Department of Neurology, Boston Children's Hospital, Harvard Medical School, Boston, MA, USA

**Richard J. Rodenburg** Department of Paediatrics, Translational Metabolic Laboratory, Radboud Center for Mitochondrial Medicine, Nijmegen, The Netherlands

**Jayanta Roy-Chowdhury** Depatments of Medicine and Genetics, Albert Einstein College of Medicine, Bronx, NY, USA

Marion Bessin Liver Research Center, Albert Einstein College of Medicine, Bronx, NY, USA

**Namita Roy-Chowdhury** Depatments of Medicine and Genetics, Albert Einstein College of Medicine, Bronx, NY, USA

Marion Bessin Liver Research Center, Albert Einstein College of Medicine, Bronx, NY, USA

**Vicente Rubio** Structural Enzymopathology Unit, Department of Genomics and Proteomics, Instituto de Biomedicina de Valencia of the Spanish National Research Council (CSIC) and Centre for Biomedical Network Research on Rare Diseases (CIBERER-ISCIII), Valencia, Spain

**Frans G. M. Russel** Department of Pharmacology and Toxicology, Radboud Center for Mitochondrial Medicine, Radboud Institute for Molecular Life Sciences, Radboud University Medical Center, Nijmegen, The Netherlands

**Gajja Salomons** Department of Genetic Metabolic Diseases, Amsterdam University Medical Centers, Amsterdam, The Netherlands

**Leonardo Salviati** Clinical Genetics Unit, Department of Women and Children's Health, University of Padova and IRP Città della Speranza, Padova, Italy

**René Santer** Department of Paediatrics, University Medical Center Eppendorf, Hamburg, Germany

**Jörn Oliver Sass** Research Group Inborn Errors of Metabolism, Department of Natural Sciences & Institute for Functional Gene Analytics (IFGA), Bonn-Rhein-Sieg University of Applied Sciences, Rheinbach, Germany

**Maurizio Scarpa** Regional Coordinating Center for Rare Diseases, Udine University Hospital, Udine, Italy

**Manuel Schiff** APHP, Reference Center for Inborn Error of Metabolism and Filière G2M, Pediatrics Department, Necker Univ Hospital, Paris, France

**Tom J. J. Schirris** Department of Pharmacology and Toxicology, Radboud Center for Mitochondrial Medicine, Radboud Institute for Molecular Life Sciences, Radboud University Medical Center, Nijmegen, The Netherlands

**Andreas Schulze** Division of Clinical and Metabolic Genetics, The Hospital for Sick Children, Toronto, ON, Canada

Departments of Pediatrics and Biochemistry, University of Toronto, Toronto, ON, Canada

**Detlef Schuppan** Institute of Translational Immunology and Research Center for Immune Therapy, University Medical Center, Johannes Gutenberg University, Mainz, Germany

Division of Gastroenterology, Beth Israel Deaconess Medical Center, Harvard Medical School, Boston, MA, USA

**Bernd C. Schwahn** Willink Metabolic Unit, Manchester Centre for Genomic Medicine, Manchester University Hospitals NHS Foundation Trust, Saint Mary's Hospital, Manchester, UK

**Guenter Schwarz** Department of Chemistry, Center for Molecular Medicine, Institute of Biochemistry, University of Cologne, Koeln, Germany

**Ivan Šebesta** Institute of Medical Biochemistry and Laboratory Medicine, Institute of Inherited Metabolic Disorders, First Faculty of Medicine, Charles University, Prague 2, Czech Republic

**Annalisa Sechi** Regional Coordinating Center for Rare Diseases, Udine University Hospital, Udine, Italy

**Denise N. Slenter** Department of Bioinformatics—BiGCaT, NUTRIM, Maastricht University, Maastricht, The Netherlands

**Jan A. M. Smeitink** Department of Pediatrics, Radboud Center for Mitochondrial Medicine, Radboud University Medical Center, Nijmegen, The Netherlands

**Johannes N. Spelbrink** Department of Paediatrics, Radboud Center for Mitochondrial Medicine, Nijmegen, The Netherlands

**Ute Spiekerkoetter** Department of Pediatrics and Adolescent Medicine, University Children's Hospital, Albert Ludwigs University, Freiburg, Germany

**Antonella Spinazzola** MRC Centre for Neuromuscular Diseases, UCL Queen Square Institute of Neurology and National Hospital for Neurology and Neurosurgery, London, UK

Department of Clinical and Movement Neurosciences, UCL Queen Square Institute of Neurology, London, UK

**Thomas Stauch** Department of Clinical Chemistry and Toxicology, German Competence Center for Porphyria Diagnosis and Consultation, MVZ Labor PD Dr. Volkmann und Kollegen GbR, Karlsruhe, Germany

**Robert Steinfeld** Division of Pediatric Neurology, University Children's Hospital Zürich, Zürich, Switzerland

**Sarah L. Stenton** Institute of Human Genetics, Technische Universität München, Munich, Germany

Institute of Neurogenomics, Helmholtz Zentrum München, Munich, Germany

**Sylvia Stöckler-Ipsiroglu** Division of Biochemical Genetics, BC Children's Hospital, Vancouver, BC, Canada

Department of Pediatrics, University of British Columbia, Vancouver, BC, Canada

**Ulrich Stölzel** Center of Internal Medicine II, Gastroenterology, Hepatology, Endocrinology, Metabolic Disorders, Oncology, Saxony Porphyria Center, Klinikum Chemnitz gGmbH, Chemnitz, Germany

**Eduard A. Struys** Metabolic Unit, Clinical Chemistry, VUmc Medical Center, Amsterdam, The Netherlands

**Michael A. Swanson** Section of Clinical Genetics and Metabolism, Department of Pediatrics, University of Colorado, Children's Hospital Colorado, Aurora, CO, USA

**Isabel Tavares de Almeida** Metabolism and Genetics, iMed.UL, Faculdade de Farmácia da Universidade de Lisboa, Lisboa, Portugal

**Valeria Tiranti** Unit of Medical Genetics and Neurogenetics, Fondazione IRCCS Istituto Neurologico Carlo Besta, Milan, Italy

**Davide Tonduti** Child Neurology Unit, COALA (Center for Diagnosis and Treatment of Leukodystrophy)—V. Buzzi Children's Hospital, Milano, Italy

**Frederic Tort** Section of Inborn Errors of Metabolism-IBC, Department of Biochemistry and Molecular Genetics, Hospital Clínic de Barcelona, CIBERER, Barcelona, Spain

**Victoria Tüngler** Department of Pediatrics, Medizinische Fakultät Carl Gustav Carus, Technische Universität Dresden, Dresden, Germany

**Karin Tuschl** Department of Developmental Neurobiology, Kings College, London, UK

Department of Cell and Developmental Biology, University College, London, UK

UCL GOS Institute of Child Health, University College, London, UK

**Lambert van den Heuvel** Institute for Genetic and Metabolic Disease, Nijmegen Medical Centre, Radboud University, Nijmegen, The Netherlands

**Johan L. K. Van Hove** Section of Clinical Genetics and Metabolism, Department of Pediatrics, University of Colorado, Children's Hospital Colorado, Aurora, CO, USA

**Clara D. M. van Karnebeek** Departments of Pediatrics and Human Genetics, Emma Children's Hospital, Amsterdam University Medical Centers, Amsterdam, The Netherlands

**Francjan J. van Spronsen** Division of Metabolic Diseases, University of Groningen, University Medical Center Groningen, Beatrix Children's Hospital, Groningen, The Netherlands

**Frédéric M. Vaz** Laboratory Genetic Metabolic Diseases, Amsterdam UMC, Amsterdam, The Netherlands

**Nanda Verhoeven-Duif** Section Metabolic Diagnostics, Department of Genetics, University Medical Center Utrecht, Utrecht, The Netherlands

**Christine Vianey-Saban** CHU de Lyon, Department of Biochemistry & Molecular Biology, Division of Inborn Errors of Metabolism, Lyon University Hospital Centre, Bron, France

**Jerry Vockley** Children's Hospital of Pittsburgh, University of Pittsburgh Medical Center, University of Pittsburgh, Pittsburgh, PA, USA

**Mirjam M. C. Wamelink** Metabolic Unit, Department of Clinical Chemistry, Amsterdam UMC, Vrije Universiteit Amsterdam, Amsterdam, The Netherlands

**Ronald J. A. Wanders** Departments of Pediatrics, Emma Children's Hospital, and Laboratory Medicine, Amsterdam University Medical Centers, Academic Medical Center, Amsterdam, The Netherlands

**Wyeth W. Wasserman** Department of Medical Genetics, Centre for Molecular Medicine and Therapeutics, BC Children's Hospital Research Institute, University of British Columbia, Vancouver, BC, Canada

**Hans R. Waterham** Departments of Pediatrics, Emma Children's Hospital, and Laboratory Medicine, Amsterdam University Medical Centers, Academic Medical Center, Amsterdam, The Netherlands

**Ron A. Wevers** Translational Metabolic Laboratory, Department Laboratory Medicine, Radboud University Medical Centre, Nijmegen, The Netherlands

**Matthew T. Whitehead** Department of Radiology, Children's National Health System, Washington, DC, USA

**Monique Williams** Metabolic Unit, Department of Clinical Chemistry, Amsterdam UMC, Vrije Universiteit Amsterdam, Amsterdam, The Netherlands

**Egon L. Willighagen** Department of Bioinformatics—BiGCaT, NUTRIM, Maastricht University, Maastricht, The Netherlands

**Mathias Woidy** Department of Paediatrics, University Medical Center Eppendorf, Hamburg, Germany

**Saskia B. Wortmann** Institute of Human Genetics, Academic Medical Center, Munich, Germany

Institute of Neurogenomics, Helmholtz Zentrum München, Munich, Germany

University Children's Hospital, Paracelsus Medical University, Salzburg, Austria

Radboud Centre for Mitochondrial Medicine, Amalia Children's Hospital, Radboudumc, Nijmegen, The Netherlands

**Johannes Zschocke** Institute of Human Genetics, Medical University Innsbruck, Innsbruck, Austria

# Part I

# General Subjects and Profiles

# Newborn Screening for Inborn Errors of Metabolism

1

Ralph Fingerhut, Janice Fletcher, and Enzo Ranieri

## Contents



**Abstract**

Newborn screening (NBS) is a public health measure for the early detection of inborn errors of metabolism (IEM), endocrinopathies, and a variety of other disorders, where early presymptomatic detection and treatment can prevent mental retardation, disabilities, or death, or at least can improve the quality of life and extend the life span of affected patients. Newborn screening started in the early 1960s, however there are still countries around the world, that do not have a newborn screening program. Newborn screening has evolved over the years and has become a program, that goes far beyond the laboratory test alone. However, long-term follow-up is still very often neglected by stakeholders, health insurance companies, and governmental authorities. Although this chapter focuses on the laboratory tests, which use whole blood, taken by heel prick, dried on special blood collection devices, the so-called dried blood samples (DBS), it also touches additional topics.

R. Fingerhut (✉)
SYNLAB MVZ Weiden, Weiden, Germany
e-mail: ralph.fingerhut@synlab.com

J. Fletcher · E. Ranieri
SA Pathology (at Women's and Children's Hospital), Adelaide, SA, Australia
e-mail: janice.fletcher@sa.gov.au

## Introduction

Newborn screening (NBS) is a public health measure for the early detection inborn errors of metabolism (IEM), endocrinopathies, and a variety of other disorders, where early presymptomtic detection and treatment can prevent mental retardation, disabilities, or death, or at least can improve the quality of life and extend the life span of affected patients. This chapter focuses on the laboratory tests, which use whole blood, taken by heel prick, dried on a special blood collection device, the so-called dried blood samples (DBS). During the last 20 years, other genetic conditions, like hemoglobinopathies, cystic fibrosis, infectious disease like HIV and CMV, immunodeficiencies like SCID, or muscular dystrophies like Duchenne muscular dystrophy (DMD), or spinal muscular atrophy (SMA), were added to the NBS panel. In



N. Blau et al. (eds.), *Physician's Guide to the Diagnosis, Treatment, and Follow-Up of Inherited Metabolic Diseases*,
https://doi.org/10.1007/978-3-030-67727-5_1

addition, there are also conditions that use point-of-care testing, which are not lab-based tests, like newborn hearing screening, using otoacoustic testing, or screening for critical congenital heart defects (CCHD) using pulse oximetry. This chapter also provides an overview of the history of NBS, principles, goals, and some pitfalls.

## History of Newborn Screening

Newborn screening as a laboratory test started with the invention of the bacterial inhibition assay for the detection of phenylketonuria (PKU) in 1963 by Robert Guthrie (Guthrie and Susi 1963; Guthrie 1996). However, sometimes forgotten, at least three mothers of mentally retarded children should be mentioned, who pushed scientists on, because they would not just accept the disability of their children as fate, but wanted a diagnosis or treatment. The first is Pearl S. Buck. Although she was not successful, she wrote down the story of her child in a touching book: *The Child Who Never Grew*. The second are Harry and Borgny Egeland from Oslo who got in touch with Dr. Ivar Asbjørn Følling, who finally could isolate phenylpyruvic acid from the urine of their two disabled children, which also gave the name, phenylketonuria, to the disorder (Fölling 1934). Then in 1951 again there was a mother, Mrs. Jones, who had a diagnosis for her daughter Sheila (PKU), who now insisted that the pediatrician, Dr. Horst Bickel, should look for a possible treatment. Maybe the persistency of Mrs. Jones, lead Horst Bickel to introduce a phenylalanine-free diet (Bickel et al. 1953), which has been proposed a few years before by Woolf et al. (Woolf and Vulliamy 1951; Woolf et al. 1955). The initiation of treatment and the proof of effectiveness have been very well documented also on Super 8 films and can be found at https://www.youtube.com/watch?v=OqZ7QHO5_hs. Sheila Jones' diagnosis was made at the age 2 years with the ferric chloride test, or the Følling-Test as it is called in some countries. But although the treatment with the phenylalanine-free diet could improve the clinical situation of the patient, it could not reverse mental retardation. However, with the introduction of a treatment option for PKU and a simple urine test, all newborn siblings of PKU patients could be tested and treated early, from birth on. The next step was the introduction of the so-called diaper test by Dr. Centerwall et al. (1960). They adopted the ferric chloride test for newborns by just pouring ferric chloride solution onto the wet diapers of newborns to detect excreted phenylpyruvic acid. The test worked in principle, only the sensitivity was poor. With the diaper test only the very severe cases of PKU could be detected, who already had a very high concentration of phenylpyruvate in urine. And again, it was a father of a child with PKU who approached Robert Guthrie at a meeting of families with disabled children, whether he could not try to develop a more sensitive test, so that all children with PKU could be treated early enough to prevent mental retardation. This was the start of NBS for PKU in the USA in 1963, and many countries followed in the following years. And still today, the NBS test, using whole blood taken by heel prick and dried on a special blood collection device, is often called the "Guthrie Test."

**Table 1.1** Wilson and Jungner classic screening criteria

| | |
|---|---|
| 1. | The condition sought should be an important health problem |
| 2. | There should be an accepted treatment for patients with recognized disease |
| 3. | Facilities for diagnosis and treatment should be available |
| 4. | There should be a recognizable latent or early symptomatic stage |
| 5. | There should be a suitable test or examination |
| 6. | The test should be acceptable to the population |
| 7. | The natural history of the condition, including development from latent to declared disease, should be adequately understood |
| 8. | There should be an agreed policy on whom to treat as patients |
| 9. | The cost of case finding (including diagnosis and treatment of patients diagnosed) should be economically balanced in relation to possible expenditure on medical care as a whole |
| 10. | Case finding should be a continuing process and not a "once and for all" project |

Then step by step new tests for other disorders were developed and included into NBS in several countries, like galactosemia (Paigen et al. 1982), biotinidase deficiency (Heard et al. 1984), maple syrup urine disease, MSUD (Naylor and Guthrie 1978), homocystinuria (Whiteman et al. 1979), congenital hypothyroidism (Larsen and Broskin 1975; Dussault et al. 1976), and congenital adrenal hyperplasia (Cacciari et al. 1982).

In 1968, the World Health Organization (WHO) had initiated a study to define criteria for the introduction of population screening, which had been accomplished by Wilson and Jungner (Wilson and Jungner 1968; Jungner et al. 2017).

The introduction of tandem mass spectrometry (TMS) has somehow revolutionized NBS. It changed the paradigm from one disorder—one test, to one technology—multiple disorders. This changed the interpretation of criteria no. 9 from the Wilson and Jungner criteria totally. Once TMS was introduced, the cost of adding another disorder, which could be detected in the profile of amino acids or acylcarnitines was more or less zero. Therefore, it was necessary to revise the Wilson and Jungner criteria the new situation (Andermann et al. 2008) (Table 1.1).

Three points of these criteria should be especially discussed. First, criteria no. 7, "The natural history of the condition, including development from latent to declared disease, should be adequately understood." This works easily, while screening an adult population for a certain disease. Medical history of the patients (or probands) are normally available, repeat testing can be easily done, and normally there are well-defined criteria, who should be declared as a patient (criteria no. 8). For conditions that are included in NBS, the knowledge of the natural history is not always well understood, due to several reasons. First of all, it has to be beared in mind that scientific and medical knowledge expands over time. For example, before NBS for PKU was started, variant hyperphenylalaninemias were more or less unknown, and also disorders of the cofactor metabolism of the phenylalanine hydroxylase, tetrahydrobiopterine, were unknown or not well understood (see Chap. xx). The introduction of NBS for PKU also developed a new "condition": Maternal PKU, which could not be anticipated beforehand. Another example is NBS for galactosemia. It started with the measurement of total galactose in DBS (Paigen et al. 1982), which was accomplished by the so-called Beutler test (Beutler et al. 1964), which was a qualitative or semiquantitative test to measure the activity of the galactose-1-phosphate uridyltransferase, the enzyme deficient in classical galactosemia. The introduction of the Beutler test led to the detection of a variant form of galactosemia, the so-called Duarte-2 galactosemia. At the beginning, the patients with the Duarte-2 variant were treated the same way as patients with classical galactosemia, and it was only in the 1990s, when increasing knowledge about the natural history of galactosemia showed that these Duarte-2 variant patients normally do not need any treatment at all. And just recently, a fourth disorder in the galactose metabolism has been described, galactose mutarotase (GALM) deficiency (Iwasawa et al. 2019). Other examples are histidinemia, which was introduced in several countries, probably after a single case report (Garvey and Gordon 1969) and a method paper, which afterwards proved that elevated histidine in blood is a condition without clinical significance (Brosco et al. 2010). There are also other conditions, where the clinical relevance or the clinical penetrance of the disorder is unclear or very low, like SCADD, and 3-MCC deficiency. A last example are pilot urine newborn screening programs for neuroblastoma in Quebec, Austria, Germany, the UK, and Japan. But, although early treatment with a combination of surgery and chemotherapy seemed to work well, the death rate from neuroblastoma tumors did not change. Therefore, it was suspected that NBS for neuroblastoma had detected previously unrecognized mild tumors that would have spontaneously regressed, also without any therapy (Riley et al. 2003; Maris and Woods 2008). Secondly, criteria no. 3, "Facilities for diagnosis and treatment should be available" in connection with criteria no. 8 again. A "facility for the diagnosis," together with an "agreed policy on whom to treat," should be interpreted as: ***After a positive NBS test, there should be a definite diagnostic test available to decide directly after the diagnostic test, whether a child has a condition, and needs immediate treatment, or whether the child is not affected, and can be released as healthy.*** There are some disorders that do not fulfill this criteria, for example, VLCADD, where acylcarnitine profiles can be totally normal when the patients are in an anabolic status (Spiekerkoetter et al. 2010), or several of the lysosomal storage disorders, where the residual enzyme activity alone, cannot predict 100% whether the disease will progress, and also genetic analysis is not 100% helpful, and often there is no other metabolic marker available to determine the progression, or normalization. And the third point directly emerges from this problem, it is criteria no. 6, "The test should be acceptable to the population." Different stakeholders of NBS programs can have totally different opinions about it. Pediatricians and patient organizations for a certain disorder can be extremely in favor for NBS, even if there is a long time of uncertainty, whether treatment is necessary or not. At the other end, there may be a big number of parents who rather not want to have this particular disorder included because of this uncertainty. However, informed consent, although it is nowadays included in most countries is not an easy task, and the burden of false-positive NBS results have been described by several groups (Morrison and Clayton 2011; Schmidt et al. 2012; Johnson et al. 2019).

Decision-making for NBS programs is not an easy task. In many countries, it is formalized like in the USA (DHHS 2013), Germany, Switzerland, the UK, for example, but although many countries have celebrated their 50th anniversary of NBS during the last years, there are still a lot of countries around the world that have not started any newborn screening, or just had some pilot programs (Pandey et al. 2019), and sometimes NBS is only available for a small part of the population, who can afford to pay for NBS by themselves.

## Newborn Screening: A Public Health Program

Newborn screening is not just a laboratory test; it should be recognized as a whole program. It includes midwives, nurses, gynecologists, neonatologists, the laboratory, special diagnostic centers, and specialized treatment centers. NBS programs should include information material about the extent of the program for parents and midwives, nurses, gynecologists, and neonatologists, for the latter especially also information how a positive NBS result will be communicated. Ideally, there should also be designated specialized centers for the final diagnostic test, and specialized centers for the treatment. And there must be a feedback about the outcome of the diagnostic test, back to the newborn screening laboratory, in order to generate reliable statistical data: Number of newborns screened, and for each disorder, recall rate, positive predictive value (ppv), negative predictive value (npv), and incidence.

The structure of NBS programs is quite diverse worldwide and also the way how new disorders are integrated into existing NBS programs is diverse. A helpful guideline for countries that have no legitimate guideline, the Recommended Uniform Screening Panel (RUSP) of the US Advisory Committee on Heritable Disorders in Newborns and Children could be a helpful guide for decision-making. The latest update can always be found at https://www.hrsa.gov/advisory-committees/heritable-disorders/rusp/index.html.

In addition, the Clinical and Laboratory Standards Institute (CLSI) has published several guidelines (https://clsi.org/standards/products/newborn-screening/) for the implementation of NBS.

One problem that NBS programs are faced with is often the lack of financial support for those parts of the NBS program that are not directly related to the laboratory test, and often there is no connection between the DBS-NBS, and newborn hearing screening, and screening for CCHD. One example is the state of Bavaria in Germany, where a public health screening center coordinates tracking of all NBS tests statewide. This includes checking of completeness, follow-up of positive NBS results, and diagnostic tests, and also whether the patients with a definite diagnosis have been admitted to a specialized center (https://www.lgl.bayern.de/gesundheit/praevention/kindergesundheit/neugeborenenscreening/index.htm). Another issue is often the enormous costs of new therapies, for so far untreatable disorders, like enzyme replacement therapy for LSDs, or the treament for SMA.

## Principles and Practice in the NBS Laboratory

It should be kept in mind that every NBS test, whether immunoassay, enzymatic assay, metabolite determination by tandem mass spectrometry, determination of profiles by HPLC, IEF, or determination of copy numbers by rtPCR, is ONLY a SCREENING TEST, and not a diagnostic test. A definition of screening (not only NBS) has been published by Wald (1994): "Screening is the systematic application of a test or enquiry **to identify individuals at sufficient risk** of a specific disorder to benefit from further investigations or treatment, among persons who have not sought medical attention on account of symptoms of that disorder." This definition implements three things: (a) Newborn screening is not a diagnostic test, (b) it needs further investigations to confirm a positive screening test, (c) among the screened population there can be individuals that have a low risk of having a certain condition, according to the screening result, but still can have or develop the disease.

Improvements in instrumentation and methodology have continuously improved the detection limits of analytes, and the sensitivity and specificity of laboratory tests. Still every newborn screening laboratory has to define cut-offs for their primary screening test, which will effect sensitivity, specificity, ppv, and npv.

### Sensitivity and Specificity

Ideally, the distribution of metabolite concentrations or enzyme activities shows a normal distribution. Ideally, the affected and unaffected individuals are completely seperated from each other (Fig. 1.1a). However, normally there is always on overlap between these two groups (Fig. 1.1b). The cut-off is normally choosen in a way that there are no fn results.

However, this would for some disorders (like CF) result in an enormous number of fp results. In these cases, a second-tier test can improve the situation (Fig. 1.2). But sometimes it has to be accepted that a screening test is not able to pick up all cases. However, sometimes the combination of marker metabolites can result in 100% sensitivity and 100% specificity, like in CPT-I deficiency (Fingerhut et al. 2001) (Fig. 1.3).

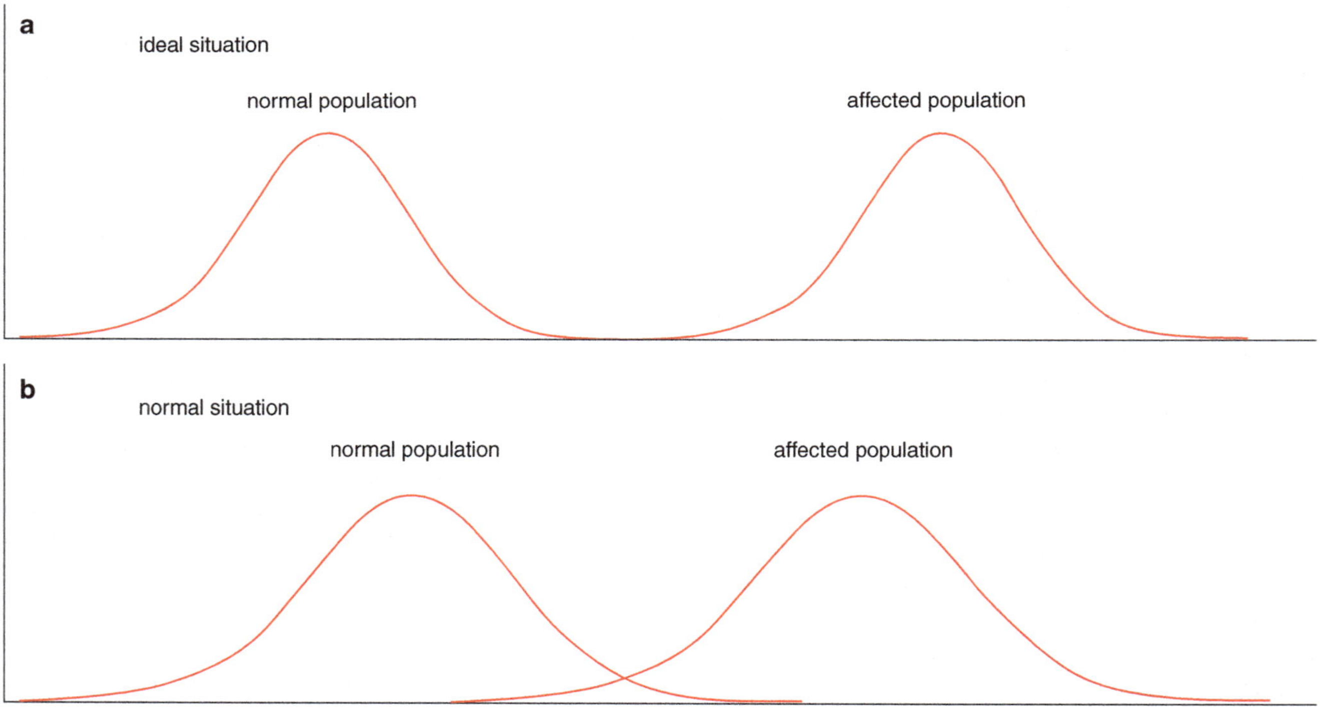


**Fig. 1.1** Frequency distributions between normal and affected population

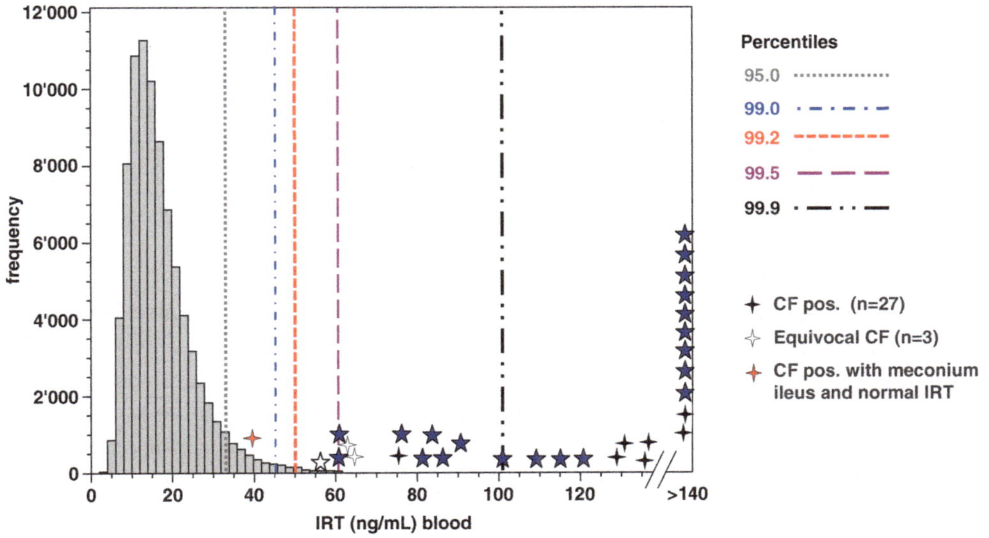


**Fig. 1.2** Distribution of IRT values from normal newborns and newborns with CF

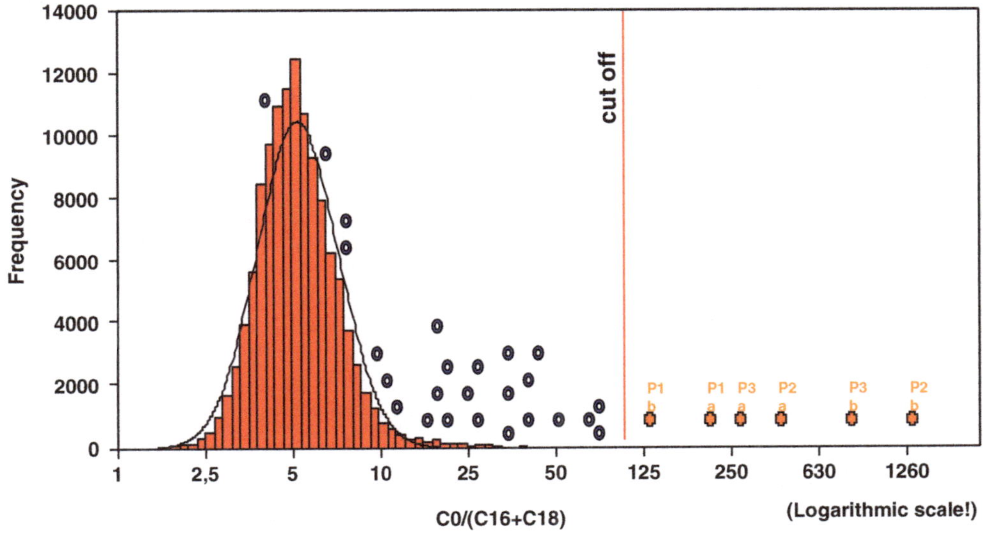


**Fig. 1.3** Distribution of the ratio of C0/(C16 + C18) from normal newborns (red bars), newborns on carnitine supplementation (blue circle) and newborns with CPT-I deficiency (orange crosses)

Sensitivity is the percentage of affected individuals that are detected with the respective test.

Specificity is the percentage of unaffected individuals that are correctly detected as unaffected.

$$\text{Sensitivity} = rp / rp + fn, \text{Specificity} = rn / fp + rn$$

(rp = right positive; rn = right negative; fp = false positive; fn = false negative)

## What Is a "False-Positive" Result?

Different NBS programs often use different terminology. In this chapter, we will use "abnormal" result and "normal" result, which are ultimately defined by the choosen cut-off for each laboratory test. If the first measurement from a specific NBS card is "abnormal," the test should always be repeated from the same NBS card in duplicate. This will eliminate a laboratory error. If two results are not plausible, the laboratory should search for an explanation. Since every test has also a certain uncertainty of measurement, this needs to be included into the cut-off consideration. If the repeat testing is again "abnormal," this will result in a "Positive Screening Result" for a specific disorder. If then, either a second DBS is taken, or a specific diagnostic test is made, and this second test results in a "normal" test result, or the diagnostic test excludes the condition, for which the initial screening test was "positive," then the initial screening will be called a "False-Positive" result.

False-positive results (fp) are expected in NBS because the major goal is not to miss a patient that has the respective condition. There are several reasons for a false-positive screening result. (a) Screening tests with a high uncertainty of measurement also tend to have a higher fp rate. (b) Higher biological variation of the disease marker will also lead to a higher fp rate. (c) If the marker metabolite is not specific for a certain disorder. (d) The metabolite level is influenced by nutrition and diet. (e) The metabolite levels are influence by the mother, for example, free carnitine levels in CUD, or Vitamin B12 levels in disorders of cobalamin metabolism.

Fp result can be effectively reduced, when it is possible to use not only one primary disease markers, but several markers or additional ratios. Even more effective are second-tier tests which are more specific than the primary test, but too expensive or labor intensive to apply them directly to all DBS. For example, second-tier genetic testing in CF screening, or the determination of allo-isoleucine by HPLC or UPLC in MSUD screening (Fig. 1.4). Major causes of fp results are summarized in Table 1.2 (Table 46.2 from the previous edition of this book).

When comparing fp rates between different NBS programs and published data, it is important that a clear definition has been given for fp results. For example, a DBS of a newborn with a complete glucose-6-phosphate dehydrogenase deficiency will give an abnormal screening result for classical galactosemia, if only the Beutler test is used. This could be counted as a fp result for galactosemia screening, however from the design of the Beutler test, which uses four different enzymes that are present in the DBS, galactose-1-phosphate uridyltransferase (GALT), phosphoglucomutase (PGM), glucose-6-phosphate dehydrogenase (G6PD), and 6-phosphogluconate dehydrogenase, it is an expected finding, and therefore it could be as well defined as a true positive result.

## What Is a "False-Negative" Result?

False-negative results (fn) in screening are unwanted, but it is important to keep in mind that a screening test can never be 100% sensitive. There are several examples, where biological variability will result in fn results. One example is homocystinuria. The primary marker is methionine because the determination of total homocysteine is not feasible as a primary test. However, with methionine as a marker only patients with classical homocystinuria (cystathionine synthase deficiency) can be detected. In addition, earlier sampling due to improved sensitivity, earlier discharge from

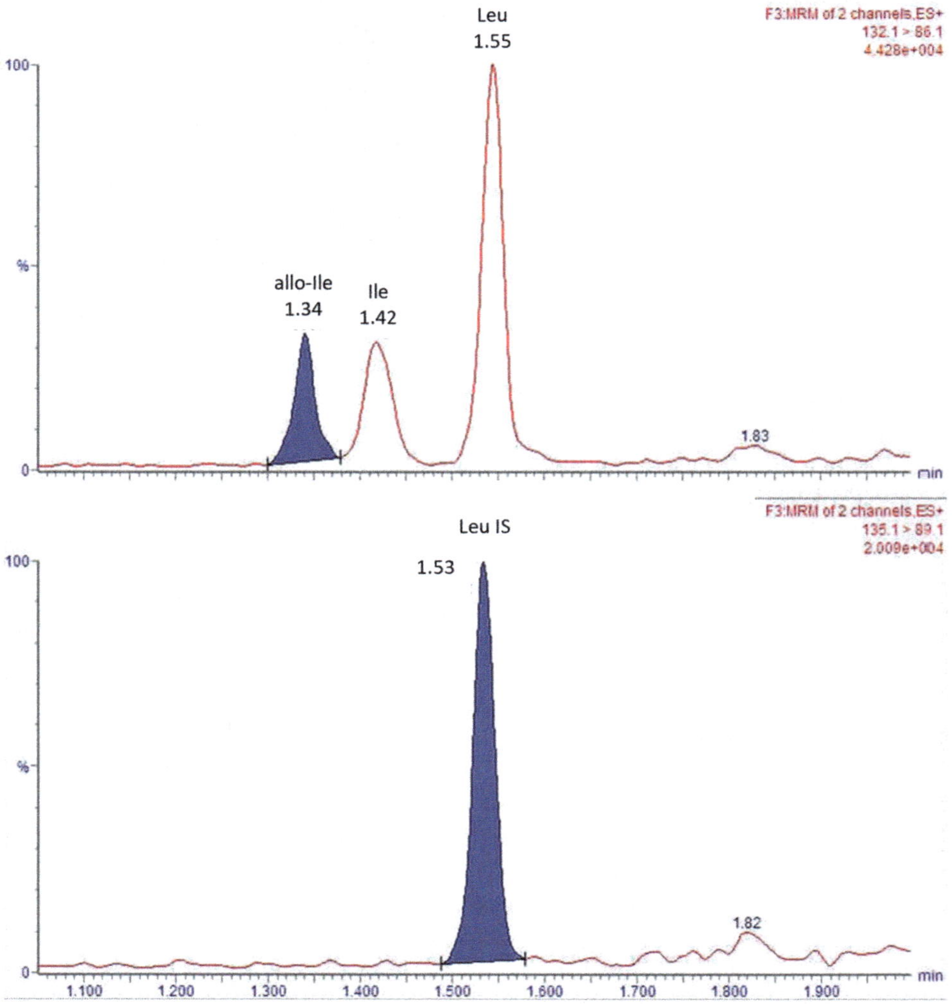


**Fig. 1.4** Separation of leucine, isoleucine, and allo-isoleucine by UPLC-MS/MS

**Table 1.2** Commonly[a] used methods in bloodspot NBS (historic or currently used)

| | Principle | False positives | False negative | Uses and comments |
|---|---|---|---|---|
| Bacterial inhibition assay | Measures analyte by effect of analyte level on growth of bacteria selected for dependence on analyte | Physiologic variations of analyte levels, effect of other medical conditions, effect of intake (feeding, hyperalimentation) | Physiologic variations of analyte levels, effects of antibiotics | The original method of screening for PKU and other IEM as designed by R. Guthrie and used until replaced by fluorescence and/or MS/MS |
| Fluorescent or other colorimetric | Measures analyte by the amount of fluorescence or color compared with standard | Physiologic variations and effect of other medical conditions, effect of intake (feeding, hyperalimentation) | Physiologic variations of analyte levels, effects of dietary intake of analytes | PKU, maple syrup urine disease, homocystinuria, galactosemia |
| Immune assay | Measures the presence of protein based on interaction with an antibody against the protein; various markers for levels, e.g., radioactivity for radioimmunoassay (RIA) | Physiologic variation | Physiologic variation; for CF it is notable that immunoreactive trypsinogen (IRT), the marker for CF, is not elevated in babies with meconium ileus | Thyroid and thyroid-stimulating hormone (for hypothyroidism); immunoreactive trypsinogen (IRT) for cystic fibrosis; steroid hormone analytes for congenital adrenal hyperplasia |
| Electrophoresis | Measures the presence or absence of protein with specific mass and charge | Transfusion | Transfusion | Hemoglobinopathies; method in use for decades also identifies carrier status |
| Enzyme assay | Measures the ability of enzyme in sample to transform substrate to product; semiquantitative or quantitative determination | Heat inactivation of enzyme in transport; deficiency of other pathway required for generation of marker for product (Beutler assay for galactosemia depends on integrity of the enzyme G6PD); pseudodeficiency | Transfusion | Galactosemia (by assay called "Beutler"), biotinidase deficiency, some lysosomal enzymes. Can identify carriers, identifies healthy individuals with pseudodeficient states, and (especially for lysosomal disorders) identifies affected individuals who may have adult-onset phenotype |
| MS/MS | Tandem mass spectrometry, inferring levels of metabolites based on amounts of (and ratios of) molecular fragments compared against isotopically labeled standards | Physiologic variations and effect of other medical conditions, effect of intake (feeding, hyperalimentation), effect of some medications | Physiologic variations of analyte levels, effects of dietary intake of analytes | PKU and other amino acidopathies, methylmalonic acidemia, and other organic acidemias, MCADD, and other disorders of fatty acid oxidation and carnitine metabolism, some urea cycle disorders. The accuracy of levels and the ability to examine ratios dramatically improve sensitivity and specificity compared with bacterial inhibition and fluorescence |
| DNA mutation analyses | Analyzes the presence or absence of specific sequence changes or specific known deletions or duplications | Unless method identifies all mutations (see false-negative column), it may be necessary to perform diagnostic testing on those identified by screening as having one mutation<br>Two mutations may be present in cis in an individual who is carrier but not affected | For virtually all conditions, there will be false negatives if DNA is the primary screen or required to be positive as a second-tier test in screening. The number of cases missed depends on the number of mutations for which the sample is screened and the frequency with which individuals in the screened population have disease caused by mutation(s) not on the panel | Occasionally used as primary screen but more often used as second-tier test for cystic fibrosis, medium-chain acyl-CoA dehydrogenase deficiency and galactosemia<br>Will identify carriers<br>To screen for spinal muscular atrophy, DNA testing must be used as primary method |
| DNA repeat size | Analyzes the length of triplet repeat segments | Hypothetically none | Mosaicism for repeat size | Fragile X; should also identify carriers |
| DNA—TREC | Quantifies fragments of DNA (cell receptor excision circles) generated in T-cell function maturation | Physiologic | Some cases of adenosine deaminase (ADA) deficiency | Severe combined immune deficiency, including several conditions which can present with immune deficiency, such as T-cell deficiency due to deletion of 22q |

[a]Includes methods used for IEM and for other (including nongenetic as well as non-metabolic) conditions. Less commonly used methodologies, e.g., HPLC, are not included here

hospital, and inclusion of more severe disorders with earlier onset, like MSUD, will lead to more fn results because methionine rises rather slowly, even in classical homocystinuria. A second example is tyrosinemia type I. Again using tyrosine as the primary marker will lead to fn results because in case of tyrosinemia type I it is not the enzyme block that will lead to the elevation of tyrosine, it is the liver damage that produces the elevation of tyrosine, together with elevated phenylalanine, methionine, and the branched chain amino acids. The third example is glutaric aciduria type I (GA-I). In GA-I, it is well known that the so-called non-excretors, patients with clinically and genetically proven GA-I that do not excrete 3-hydroxyglutaric or glutaric acid in the urine, are missed by NBS (Gallagher et al. 2005). Also for CF it is well known that the sensitivity is only around 95–96%, meaning that 4–5% of cases are missed by NBS (Heidendael et al. 2014).

## Positive and Negative Predictive Values

The positive predictive value (ppv) and the negative predictive value (npv) are necessary measures, when communicating a NBS result.

$$npv = rn / rn + fn, ppv = rp / rp + fp$$

The npv and ppv describe, how reliable a test result is, related to the disease state of the respective newborn. If the npv is 100%, it means the risk for a newborn with a normal test result to have this respective disorder is zero. On the other hand, a ppv of 100% means that the chance for newborn with a positive test result, not to have the respective disorder is also zero. In reality, neither npv nor ppv reach 100%. However, the npv is normally >99.9%, but it still means that there is still a chance that a newborn with a normal test result can have the respective disease. The ppv is quite variable, and as already discussed above, dependent on the choosen cut-off. However, very often the ppv can also be dependent on the test value. For example, a TSH value of >100 mU/L has probably a ppv of 100%, while a TSH value of 21 mU/L has probably a ppv of only 1–5%. Or when we look at CF screening with second-tier genetic testing: if second-tier testing finds two disease causing mutations, the ppv is 100%, irrespective of the initial IRT value. However, if no mutation is found, then the ppv is most likely again dependent on the IRT level.

## Methodology

Since this book deals with inborn errors of metabolism, the description of methodology focuses on detection of amino acids and acylcarnitines by flow injection tandem mass spectrometry (FI-MS/MS). For the determination of amino acids and acylcarnitines by FI-MS/MS, there are two different methods in use. Extraction into an organic phase either (a) after derivatization to the respective butyl esters, or (b) without derivatization. The method with butylation results in higher signal intensities than the method without derivatization; however, the modern tandem MS instruments tend to be so sensitive that this has no effect on the sensitivity of the test results. It only has to be kept in mind that same isobaric compounds are not isobaric anymore after butylation, e.g., C4DC and C5OH. Dicarboxylic acid will add two butyl ester groups, while the hydroxyacids will only have one butyl group.

Table 1.3 provides an update from Fingerhut (2009) of target diseases for NBS, which can be compared with the RUSP.

Table 1.4 provides a list of the primary marker metabolites that can be detected by FI-MS/MS, and possible secondary markers.

## The Newborn Screening Process

The primary responsibility for the whole NBS process is very often in the hands of the newborn screening laboratory, unless it is embedded in a clearly defined NBS program. The integration of non-laboratory screenings, like newborn hearing screening and screening for CCHD, is even more complex and will not be discussed in detail here.

### Blood Sampling

The standard specimen for NBS is capillary whole blood dried on a special blood collection device, the so-called dried blood spots (DBS). The test cards should be distributed by the screening laboratory to their customers, midwives, hospitals, pediatricians, and general physicians, and they should include all necessary information that are needed for the correct interpretation of test results. The blood collection device must have a special quality and should (ideally) by approved by FDA, or a comparable national institution (Hall 2017).

Since the number of people involved in blood sampling is normally quite high, it is necessary to provide regular information and education to the customers (Evans et al. 2019).

### Laboratory Test

The number of tests, and the methodology used for NBS varies between different countries (Loeber et al. 2021). A summary is given in Table 1.3.

### Confirmatory Testing

Confirmatory testing is often not performed in the screening laboratory, but it is a crucial part of the NBS program. It is already mentioned by Wilson and Jungner (criteria no. 8):

**Table 1.3** Target diseases for newborn screening

| Disease | Methods | Relevance ranking | Screening programs | Test[a] available | Therapy available | Benefit from early detection | Remarks |
|---|---|---|---|---|---|---|---|
| Aminoacidopathies | | | | | | | |
| Phenylketonuria | TMS | ++ | a | y | y | y | Alternative therapies for mild phenylketonuria have been introduced, and further new therapies are under investigation |
| Maple syrup urine disease | TMS | ++ | m | y | y | y | Early blood collection is necessary |
| Homocystinuria | TMS | + | m | n | y | y | Sensitivity and specificity low with methionine as primary marker; determination of homocysteine would improve NBS |
| Tyrosinemia type I | TMS | ++ | m | y | y | y | |
| Citrullinemia | TMS | + | m | y | | | Positive effect on outcome is not yet certain; patients with a mild biochemical phenotype might never develop symptoms |
| Argininosuccinic acidemia | TMS | + | m | y | | | Positive effect on outcome is not yet certain |
| Arginase deficiency | TMS | + | m | y | | | Very rare; first results of NBS and early treatment seem promising |
| Hyperornithinemia (OAT deficiency and HHH syndrome) | TMS | | m | n | | | Normal ornithine levels during the first weeks of life |
| Nonketotic hyperglycinemia | TMS | - - | m | n | n | n | No therapy available |
| Histidinemia | TLC | - - | d | - - | - - | n | Benign, does not require treatment |
| Hydroxyprolinemia | TLC | - - | d | - - | - - | n | Benign, does not require treatment |
| Serin | TMS | | | | y | | No prospective data available |
| Organic acidemias | | | | | | | |
| Glutaric aciduria type I | TMS | ++ | m | y | y | y | The so-called non-excretors can be missed by NBS |
| Isovaleric acidemia | TMS | ++ | m | y | y | y | NBS also detects unaffected patients with mild variants |
| Propionic acidemia | TMS | + | m | y | y | | Acylcarnitine profile in PA and MMA are indistinguishable |
| Methylmalonic acidemia (mutase) | TMS | + | m | y | y | | Acylcarnitine profile in PA and MMA are indistinguishable |
| Methylmalonic acidemia (disorders of cobalamin metabolism A-D,F) | TMS | + | m | y | y | y | Sensitivity unclear; propionylcarnitine level is soften only slightly elevated |
| Cobalamin E/G defect | TMS | - - | | | | | Low methionine level is the only marker; sensitivity and specificity unknown, but presumably low; determination of homocysteine would improve NBS |
| Malonyl-CoA decarboxylase deficiency | TMS | + | m | y | y | y | Very rare; no prospective data |
| 3-MCC deficiency | TMS | – | m | y | y | | Low clinical expressivity and penetrance |
| 3-Hydroxymethylglutaryl-CoA lyase deficiency | TMS | | m | y | y | y | Reliable discrimination from 3-MCC deficiency not possible |
| Holocarboxylase synthase deficiency | TMS | | m | y | y | y | Very rare, but easily treatable with biotin; Reliable discrimination from 3-MCC deficiency not possible |
| ß-Ketothiolase deficiency | TMS | + | m | y | y | y | Sensitivity and specificity presumably low |
| Disorders of glutathione metabolism | TMS | | m | | | | No prospective data |
| ß-Oxidation defects/disorders of carnitine metabolism | | | | | | | |
| SCAD deficiency | TMS | - - | a | y | y | y | Causality between enzyme defect and clinical outcome is not proven |

(continued)

**Table 1.3** (continued)

| Disease | Methods | Relevance ranking | Screening programs | Test[a] available | Therapy available | Benefit from early detection | Remarks |
|---|---|---|---|---|---|---|---|
| MCAD deficiency | TMS | ++ | m | y | y | y | Positive effect unquestioned; however patients that might never become symptomatic are also detected |
| MCHAD deficiency | TMS | | m | y | y | | Very rare; no prospective data |
| VLCAD deficiency | TMS | + | m | y | y | y | Mild variants might be missed when the samples are taken under anabolic conditions |
| LCHAD/TFP deficiency | TMS | + | m | y | y | y | Information on long-term outcome are rare; prognosis for TFP is rather bad |
| Carnitine transporter deficiency | TMS | + | m | | y | y | Sensitivity unclear; free carnitine level can be normal postpartum, depending on maternal supply and renal loss |
| CPT-I deficiency | TMS | ++ | m | y | y | y | Ratio of free carnitine to the sum of palmitoylcarnitine and stearylcarnitine is sensitive and highly specific |
| CPT-II deficiency | TMS | + | m | y | y | y | Neonatal onset form with bad prognosis despite early diagnosis; in the late-onset form mainly skeletal muscle is involved, seems to have normal levels of acylcarnitines in the neonatal period |
| Translocase deficiency | TMS | + | m | y | y | y | Bad prognosis despite early diagnosis |
| Endocrinopathies | | | | | | | |
| Congenital hypothyroidism | ELISA | ++ | a | y | y | y | |
| Congenital adrenal hyperplasia | ELISA | ++ | a | y | y | y | Sensitivity for the salt-wasting form is good, for simple virilizing congenital adrenal hyperplasia approximately 50% |
| Hemoglobinopathies | | | | | | | |
| Sickle cell anemia | IEF/HPLC | ++ | e | y | y | y | |
| Hemoglobin S/ß-thalassemia | IEF/HPLC | ++ | e | y | y | y | |
| Hemoglobin SC disease | IEF/HPLC | ++ | e | y | y | y | |
| Hemoglobin H | IEF/HPLC | ++ | e | y | y | y | |
| Other inborn errors of metabolism | | | | | | | |
| Biotinidase deficiency | Enzyme assay | ++ | a | y | y | y | |
| Galactosemia | Substrate and/or enzyme assay | ++ | a | y | y | y | Long-term outcome not as favorable as initially thought in the 1970s |
| Glucose-6-phosphate dehydrogenase deficiency | Enzyme assay | | e | y | y | y | High genetic variability |
| Phosphoglucomutase deficiency | Enzyme assay | | | y | y | y | Very rare, no prospective data available |
| Disorders of creatine metabolism | TMS | | p | y | y | | Feasibility has been demonstrated, results on long-term outcome not yet available |
| Lysosomal storage disorders | Enzyme assay (TMS/fluorimetric) | | p | y | y | | Long delay/uncertainty between the positive NBS result and a clear confirmation of the disease; age of onset extremely variable and not predictable |
| Cystic fibrosis | IRT/DNA | ++ | m | y | y | y | |
| Diabetes mellitus type I | DNA | | p | | y | y | "Genetic risk" screening |
| Other diseases | | | | | | | |

| | | | | | | | |
|---|---|---|---|---|---|---|---|
| Hearing screening | Otoacoustic | + + | m | y | y | y | POCT |
| Congenital CMV infection | CMV viral load | + | p | y | y | y | |
| Congenital toxoplasmosis infection | Toxoplasmosis viral load | - - | mat | - - | - - | - - | Not recommended, (prenatal care) |
| Congenital syphilis infection | Nontreponemal antibodies | - - | mat/epd | - - | - - | - - | Not recommended, (prenatal care) |
| Neuroblastoma screening[b] | HPLC | - - | d | y | y | n | Not recommended |
| Duchenne muscular dystrophy | Creatine kinase activity | - - | p | y | n | n | New therapies in development |
| Spinal muscular atrophy | DNA | + | p | y | y | | First outcome studies are promising; however, the observation time is only 4–5 years so far |
| Severe combined immunodeficiency | TREC/KREC copy numbers | + + | m | y | y | y | |
| HIV | ELISA | | epd | - - | - - | - - | Not recommended |
| Hepatitis C | ELISA | | epd | - - | - - | - - | Not recommended, (prenatal care) |
| Hepatitis B | HBsAg | | epd | - - | - - | - - | Not recommended, (prenatal care) |

*CPT-I* carnitine palmitoyl transferase I, *CPT-II* carnitine palmitoyl transferase II, *HBsAg* hepatitis B surface antigen, *HHH* hyperornithinemia–hyperammonemia–homocitrullinuria, *HPLC* high performance liquid chromatography, *IEF* isoelectric focusing, *IRT* immunoreactive trypsin, *LCHAD* long-chain hydroxyacyl-CoA dehydrogenase, *MCAD* medium-chain acyl-CoA dehydrogenase, *MCHAD* medium-chain hydroxyacyl-CoA dehydrogenase, *3-MCC* 3-methylcrotonyl-CoA carboxylase, *NBS* newborn screening, *OAT* ornithine aminotransferase, *SCAD* short-chain acyl-CoA dehydrogenase, *SCID* severe combined immunodeficiency, *TFP* trifunctional protein, *TLC* thin-layer chromatography, *TMS* tandem mass spectrometry, *VLCAD* very long-chain acyl-CoA dehydrogenase, *a* all, *d* discontinued, *e* ethnic, *epd* epidemiologic, *m* most, *mat* recommended as a prenatal screening test, *n* no, pilot, *y* yes, + + unquestioned, + favorable, - unfavorable, - - not recommended

[a]With sufficient sensitivity and specificity, economically justifiable

[b]Specimen for screening is urine dried on filter paper

**Table 1.4** Primary markers, and secondary markers and/or ratios for FI-MS/MS

| Metabolite (primary) | | Disorder | Secondary markers/ratios |
|---|---|---|---|
| Free carnitine (C0) | N, ↓ | Carnitine transporter deficiency | Total carnitine ↓ |
| Free carnitine (C0) | N, ↓ | All OAs, FAO disorders | |
| Free carnitine (C0) | N, ↑ | CPT-I deficiency | C0/(C16 + C18) ↑ |
| Acetyl carnitine (C2) | | Unspecific | |
| Propionylcarnitine (C3) | ↑ | PA, MMA | C3/C2, C3/C4, C3/C16 |
| | ↑ | Disorders of cobalamin metabolism | C3/C2, C3/C4, C3/C16 ↑ Met N, ↓ |
| Malonylcarnitine (C3DC)* | ↑ | Malonyl-CoA decarboxylase deficiency | C3DC/C5DC |
| Butyrylcarnitine (C4) | ↑ | MADD | C5DC, C5, C12, C14, C14:1 |
| Methylmalonylcarnitine/Succinylcarnitine (C4DC)* | ↑ | MMA (mut 0) | |
| Isovalerylcarnitine (C5) | ↑ | IVA | C5/C4, C5/C8 |
| Glutarylcarnitine (C5DC)* | | | C5DC/C4, C5DC/C12, C5DC/C8, C5DC/C3DC |
| Hydroxyisovalerylcarnitine (C5-OH)* | ↑ | 3-MCC def./3-HMG-CoA lyase def./ß-Ketothiolase | C5-OH/C3, C5:1, C6DC |
| Pentenoylcarnitine (C5:1) | ↑ | ß-Ketothiolase | C5-OH; C5-OH/C3 |
| Methylglutarylcarnitine (C6DC)* | ↑ | HMG-CoA lyase def. | C5-OH; C5-OH/C3 |
| Hexanoylcarnitine (C6) | ↑ | MCADD | |
| Octanoylcarnitine (C8) | ↑ | MCADD | C8/C12, C8/C6, C8/C10, (C6OH) |
| Decanoylcarnitine (C10) | ↑ | MCADD | |
| Decenoylcarnitine (C10:1) | ↑ | MCADD | |
| Hydroxyhexanoylcarnitine (C6OH)* | N, ↑ | MCADD | |
| Dodecanoylcarnitine (C12) | ↑ | VLCADD, LCHADD, MADD | |
| Tetradecanoylcarnitine (C14) | ↑ | VLCADD, LCHADD, MADD, CPT-II, Translocase | |
| Tetradecenoylcarnitine (C14:1) | ↑ | VLCADD, LCHADD, MADD, CPT-II, Translocase | C14:1/C4 |
| Tetradecadienoylcarnitine (C14:2) | ↑ | VLCADD, LCHADD, MADD, CPT-II, Translocase | |
| Hydoxytetradecanoylcarnitine (C14-OH) | ↑ | LCHADD, CPT-II, Translocase | |
| Hydroxypalmitoylcarnitine (C16-OH) | ↑ | LCHADD, CPT-II, Translocase | |
| Hydroxyhexadecenoylcarnitine (C16:1-OH) | ↑ | LCHADD, CPT-II, Translocase | |
| Hydroxyoctadecenoylcarnitine (C18:1-OH) | ↑ | LCHADD, CPT-II, Translocase | |
| Palmitoylcarnitine (C16) | ↑ | CPT-II, Translocase | |
| Palmitoylcarnitine (C16) | ↓ | CPT-I deficiency | C0/(C16 + C18) ↑ |
| Stearylcarnitine (C18) | ↑ | CPT-II, Translocase | |
| Stearylcarnitine (C18) | ↓ | CPT-I deficiency | C0/(C16 + C18) ↑ |
| Phenylalanine (Phe) | ↑ | PKU, liver disease | Phe/Tyr |
| Tyrosine (Tyr) | ↓ | PKU | Phe/Tyr |
| Tyrosine (Tyr) | ↑ | Tyrosinemia Type I, II, and III | Tyr/Ser |
| Methionine (Met) | ↑ | Homocystinuria, MAT | Met/Leu, Met/Phe |
| Methionine (Met) | ↓ | Disorders of cobalamin metabolism | C3, C3/C2, C3/C4, C3/C16 ↑ |
| Leucine (Leu)* | ↑ | MSUD, liver disease, hydroxyprolinemia | Leu/Phe, Leu/Ala, FQ |
| Valine (Val) | ↑ | MSUD, liver disease | Val/Phe, Val/Ala, FQ |
| Citrulline (Cit) | ↑ | Citrullinemia | Cit/Phe, Cit/Tyr |
| Citrulline (Cit) | ↓ | UCDs | |
| Arginine (Arg) | ↓ | UCDs | |
| Arginine (Arg) | ↑ | Arginase def. | Arg/Phe |
| Ornithine (Orn) | ↑ | Hyperornithinemia | Orn/Phe, Orn/Ser |
| Alanine (Ala) | ↑ | Lactic acidosis | |
| Alanine (Ala) | ↓ | MSUD | |
| Gly (Gly) | ↑ | NKH | Gly/Ala |
| 5-Oxoproline/Pyroglutamate (PyrGlu) | ↑ | 5-Oxoprolinemia, Glutathionsynthase def. | PyrGlu/Phe |

Metabolites marked with an asterix (*) have isobaric compounds, that cannot be destinguished from each other with the screening method.

"There should be an agreed policy on whom to treat as patients." That means there must be a well-defined testing for the confirmation of the so far "suspicion" that an abnormal NBS result represents. Without a definite positive confirmatory test, no screening program should count an abnormal NBS result as a detected case. Unfortunately, this is often neglected, which can be seen from a lot of publications on screening for CH during the last years that can be summarized under the title: "Increasing incidence for CH by lowering the cut-off for TSH."

**Treatment and Follow-up**

The last part of the NBS process is the referral of newborns with a positive screening test to a specialized center, initiation of treatment, and follow-up. While the quality of the ***NBS tests*** can be measured by the number of correctly detected cases (e.g., ppv, fp rate, fn), the quality and success of the ***NBS program*** will be measured by the outcome of detected cases. Therefore, long-term outcome studies are extremely important for the evaluation of NBS programs (Badawi et al. 2019). Unfortunately, the costs for this quality assessment are mostly neither covered by the health insurance, within the reimbursement for NBS, nor by the health authorities. This is absolutely incomprehensible in these times of quality control, where nearly everything is certified, or accredited by any "*ISO-XXXX*."

## Perspective

Newborn screening will steadily improve and the number of disorders will increase. This will be driven either by improved methods and technology, which makes screening possible, when marker metabolites get measurable, or by new treatment option, when sofar untreatable disorders get treatable by the invention of new therapeutics, like SMA.

And last but not least, the decrease in cost for next-generation sequencing (NGS), whole exome sequencing, or whole genome sequencing, have started the debate, whether this will be the future of NBS (Yang et al. 2019; Phornphutkul and Padbury 2019).

## Conclusion

Newborn screening is surely one of the most effective preventive health care programs in the world. It has a history of more than 50 years (in some regions), not to forget those countries, where they just start to think about introducing NBS. During the last 50 years, NBS has evolved from a laboratory test, to a public health care program, still there is work to do to improve. In addition, new technologies will continuously challenge the newborn screening laboratories.

## References


Andermann A, Blancquaert I, Beauchamp S, Dery V. Revisiting Wilson and Jungner in the genomic age: a review of screening criteria over the past 40 years. Bull World Health Organ. 2008;86(4):317–9.

Badawi D, Bisordi K, Timmel MJ, Sorongon S, Strovel E. Newborn screening long term follow-up in the medical home. Int J Neonatal Screen. 2019;5(3):25.

Beutler E, Baluda M, Donnell GN. A new method for the detection of galactoxemia and its carrier state. J Lab Clin Med. 1964;64:694–705.

Bickel H, Gerrard J, Hickmans EM. Influence of phenylalanine intake on phenylketonuria. Lancet. 1953;265(6790):812–3.

Brosco JP, Sanders LM, Dharia R, Guez G, Feudtner C. The lure of treatment: expanded newborn screening and the curious case of histidinemia. Pediatrics. 2010;125(3):417–9.

Cacciari E, Balsamo A, Piazzi S, Salardi S, Pirazili P, Capelli M, Cassio A, Bernardi F, Cicognani A, Zappulla F, Paolini M. Neonatal screening for congenital adrenal hyperplasia. Lancet. 1982;1(8280):1069.

Centerwall WR, Chinnock RF, Pusavat A. Phenylketonuria: screening programs and testing methods. Am J Public Health Nations Health. 1960;50:1667–77.

Dussault JH, Parlow A, Letarte J, Guyda H, Laberge C. TSH measurements from blood spots on filter paper: a confirmatory screening test for neonatal hypothyroidism. J Pediatr. 1976;89:550–2.

Evans A, LeBlanc K, Bonhomme N, Shone SM, Gaviglio A, Freedenberg D, Penn J, Johnson C, Vogel B, Dolan AM, Goldenberg AJ. A newborn screening education best practices framework: development and adoption. Int J Neonatal Screen. 2019;5(2):22.

Fingerhut R, Röschinger W, Muntau AC, Dame T, Kreischer J, Arnecke R, Superti-Furga A, Troxler H, Liebl B, Olgemöller B, Roscher AA. Hepatic carnitine palmitoyltransferase I deficiency: acylcarnitine profiles in blood spots are highly specific. Clin Chem. 2001;47(10):1763–8.

Fingerhut R, Olgemöller B. Newborn screening for inborn errors of metabolism and endocrinopathies: an update. Anal Bioanal Chem. 2009;393(5):1481–97.

Fölling A. Über Ausscheidung von Phenylbrenztraubensäure in den Harn als Stoffwechselanomalie in Verbindung mit Imbezillität. Zt Physiol Chem. 1934;227:169–76.

Gallagher RC, Cowan TM, Goodman SI, Enns GM. Glutaryl-CoA dehydrogenase deficiency and newborn screening: retrospective analysis of a low excretor provides further evidence that some cases may be missed. Mol Genet Metab. 2005;86(3):417–20.

Garvey AM, Gordon N. Histidinaemia and speech disorders. Br J Disord Commun. 1969;4:146–50.

Guthrie R. The introduction of newborn screening for phenylketonuria. A personal history. Eur J Pediatr. 1996;155(Suppl 1):4–5.

Guthrie R, Susi A. A simple phenylalanine method for detecting phenylketonuria in large populations of newborn infants. Pediatrics. 1963;32:338–43.

Hall K. Suitable specimen types for newborn biochemical screening: a summary. Int J Neonatal Screen. 2017;3(3):17.

Heard GS, Secor McVoy JR, Wolf B. A screening method for biotinidase deficiency in newborns. Clin Chem. 1984;30(1):125–7.

Heidendael JF, Tabbers MM, De Vreede I. False negative newborn screen and neonatal cholestasis in a premature child with cystic fibrosis. Eur J Pediatr. 2014;173(12):1581–3.

Iwasawa S, Kikuchi A, Wada Y, Arai-Ichinoi N, Sakamoto O, Tamiya G, Kure S. The prevalence of GALM mutations that cause galactosemia: a database of functionally evaluated variants. Mol Genet Metab. 2019;126(4):362–7.

Johnson F, Southern KW, Ulph F. Psychological impact on parents of an inconclusive diagnosis following newborn bloodspot screening for cystic fibrosis: a qualitative study. Int J Neonatal Screen. 2019;5(2):23.

Jungner L, Jungner I, Engvall M, von Döbeln U. Gunnar Jungner and the principles and practice of screening for disease. Int J Neonatal Screen. 2017;3(3):23.

Larsen PR, Broskin K. Thyroxine (T4) immunoassay using a filter paper blood samples for screening of neonates for hypothyroidism. Pediatr Res. 1975;9:604–9.

Loeber JG, Platis D, Zetterström RH, et al. Neonatal Screening in Europe Revisited: An ISNS Perspective on the Current State and Developments Since 2010. Int J Neonatal Screen. 2021;7:15

Maris JM, Woods WG. Screening for neuroblastoma: a resurrected idea? Lancet. 2008;371(9619):1142–3.

Morrison DR, Clayton EW. False positive newborn screening results are not always benign. Public Health Genomics. 2011;14:173–7.

Naylor EW, Guthrie R. Newborn screening for maple syrup urine disease (branched-chain ketoaciduria). Pediatrics. 1978;61(2):262–6.

Paigen K, Pacholec F, Levy HL. A new method of screening for inherited disorders of galactose metabolism. J Lab Clin Med. 1982;99(6):895–907.

Pandey AS, Joshi S, Rajbhandari R, Kansakar P, Dhakal S, Fingerhut R. Newborn screening for selected disorders in Nepal: a pilot study. Int J Neonatal Screen. 2019;5(2):18.

Phornphutkul C, Padbury J. Large scale next generation sequencing and newborn screening: are we ready? J Pediatr. 2019;209:9–10.

Riley RD, Burchill SA, Abrams KR, et al. A systematic review and evaluation of the use of tumour markers in paediatric oncology: Ewing's sarcoma and neuroblastoma. Health Technol Assess. 2003;7(5):1–162.

Schmidt JL, Castellanos-Brown K, Childress S, Bonhomme N, Oktay JS, Terry SF, Kyler P, Davidoff A, Greene C. The impact of false-positive newborn screening results on families: a qualitative study. Genet Med. 2012;14(1):76–80.

Spiekerkoetter U, Haussmann U, Mueller M, et al. Tandem mass spectroscopy screening for very long-chain acyl-CoA dehydrogenase deficiency: the value of second-tier enzyme testing. J Pediatr. 2010;157(4):668–73.

Wald NJ. Editorial J Med Screen. 1994;1:1–2.

Whiteman PD, Clayton BE, Ersser RS, Lilly P, Seakins JWT. Changing incidence of neonatal hypermethioninaemia: implications for the detection of homocystinuria. Arch Dis Child. 1979;54:593–8.

Wilson JMG, Jungner G. Principles and practice of screening for disease. Geneva: World Health Organisation. 1968.

Woolf LI, Vulliamy DG. Phenylketonuria with a study of the effect upon it of glutamic acid. Arch Dis Child. 1951;26(130):487–94.

Woolf LI, Griffiths R, Moncrieff A. Treatment of phenylketonuria with a diet low in phenylalanine. Br Med J. 1955;1(4905):57–64.

Yang Y, Wang L, Wang B, Liu S, Yu B, Wang T. Application of next-generation sequencing following tandem mass spectrometry to expand newborn screening for inborn errors of metabolism: a multi-center study. Front Genet. 2019;10:86.

# Simple Tests and Routine Chemistry

# 2

Carlos R. Ferreira and Nenad Blau

## Content



**Abstract**

A variety of routine chemistry tests are useful in both specialist and non-specialist laboratories to assist in the differential diagnosis of inherited metabolic disorders. We provide a list of metabolic diseases associated with abnormalities in urine tests (color, odor, ferric chloride, reducing substances, DNPH, Acetest, nitroprusside test) and routine blood chemistry (hypoglycemia, hyperglycemia, hyperammonemia, hyperlactatemia, low and high creatinine, acidosis, alkalosis, hypocholesterolemia, hypercholesterolemia, hypertriglyceridemia, increased liver transaminases, increased creatine kinase, increased lactate dehydrogenase, hyperphosphatasemia, hypophosphatasemia, decreased and increased urea nitrogen, hyperuricemia and hypouricemia, hyperferritinemia and hypoferritinemia, myoglobinuria, anemia, thrombocytopenia, neutropenia, and reticulocytosis). Although some of these tests are considered obsolete in modern metabolic laboratories, we decided to include them in this chapter from the historic point of view and to maintain the information for laboratories in developing countries.

This chapter draws substantially from previous chapter by Duran M and Gibson KM (Duran and Gibson 2014), which the authors gratefully acknowledge.

C. R. Ferreira
Division of Genetics and Metabolism, Children's National Health System, Washington, DC, USA
e-mail: carlos121180@gmail.com

N. Blau (✉)
Division of Metabolism, University Children's Hospital, Zürich, Switzerland
e-mail: Nenad.Blau@kispi.uzh.ch


N. Blau et al. (eds.), *Physician's Guide to the Diagnosis, Treatment, and Follow-Up of Inherited Metabolic Diseases*,
https://doi.org/10.1007/978-3-030-67727-5_2

A variety of rapid qualitative tests (colorimetric, dipstick, precipitate, color and smell, etc.) are useful in both specialist and non-specialist laboratories to assist in the differential diagnosis of inherited metabolic disorders. Most are limited by some level of interference; yet these tests still have important utility, especially in emergency situations.

The color and odor of a patient's urine may be a valuable analysis for initial testing (Tables 2.1 and 2.2). Odor can only be reliably interpreted when the urine is preserved in an adequate way (pH 5–7, no signs of bacterial contamination as evidenced by a negative nitrite dipstick). Alkaptonuria patients show a rapid blackening of the urine upon standing; this process can be accelerated by adding a few drops of an ammonia solution to the urine test tube.

Although most of the following simple tests are considered to be obsolete in modern metabolic laboratories, we decided to include them in this book from the historic point of view and to maintain the information for laboratories in third world counties.

The ferric chloride test (Table 2.3) is employed to look for the presence of oxo-acids (formed by transamination or oxidation-reduction reactions). This test has been routinely used in the identification of classical phenylketonuria, but several other species (in addition to the intermediates of phenylalanine metabolism) react with ferric chloride to form a number of colored complexes. An alternative for the ferric chloride test is the Phenistix dipstick.

Reducing substances in urine (see Table 2.4; also commonly referred to as Benedict test or Clinitest®, Bayer Corporation) reacts with a broad spectrum of reducing sugars in urine with the formation of colored complexes (green to orange). It is commonly used for the detection of urine galactose on the suspicion of galactosemia in neonates with severe liver disease and renal Fanconi syndrome. One should

**Table 2.1** Color (urine)

| Color | Compound | Disorder—source |
|---|---|---|
| Black | Homogentisic acid | Alkaptonuria |
| Black | Melanin | Metastatic melanoma; levodopa or alpha-methyldopa in alkaline urine |
| Black | Ferrous sulfide | Iron sorbitol citrate |
| Black | Cresol | Intoxication (household disinfectant) |
| Purple | Indirubin + indigo | Purple urine bag syndrome |
| Blue | Indican | Hartnup disorder; Drummond syndrome; severe intestinal malabsorption |
| Green | Pyocyanin | Pseudomonas infection |
| Green | Biliverdin | Hyperbiliverdinemia |
| Green | Amitriptyline, indomethacin, metoclopramide, promethazine, cimetidine, methocarbamol, propofol, triamterene, carbolic acid (phenol), methylene blue, mitoxantrone, zaleplon | Drugs |
| Green | Thymol | Listerine mouthwash |
| | Chlorophyll | Clorets mints |
| Green | Imazosulfuron, mefenacet | Herbicide intoxication |
| Brown | Methemoglobin | Methemoglobinemia |
| Brown | Myoglobin | Myoglobinuria |
| Brown | Metronidazole, nitrofurantoin, chloroquine, primaquine | Drugs |
| Red-brown | Hb/methemoglobin | Hemoglobinuria |
| Red | Erythrocytes/lysate | Hematuria |
| Red | Porphyrins | Porphyria |
| Red | Pyrazolones, phenothiazines (chlorpromazine, thioridazine), deferoxamine, hydroxycobalamin (Cyanokit, ≥5 g IV) | Drugs |
| Red | Doxorubicin, senna, cascara | Anthraquinone |
| Red | Phenolphthalein, phenolsulfonphthalein | Chemicals |
| Light red/pink | Urates | Hyperuricosuria |
| Red | Beets, rhubarb, blackberries | Nutritional |
| Orange | Carotene | Nutritional (carrots) |
| Orange | Rifampin, phenazopyridine, warfarin | Drugs |
| Orange-yellow | Sulfasalazine | Drugs |
| Orange-yellow | Fluorescein | Retinal angiography |
| Yellow | Riboflavin | Vitamins |
| Yellow | Bilirubin | Hyperbilirubinemia (jaundice) |
| White[a] | Chyle | Chyluria; filariasis; schistosomiasis |
| White[a] | Caseous material | Urinary tuberculosis |
| White[a] | White blood cells | Pyuria |
| White[a] | Calcium | Hypercalciuria |
| White[a] | Oxalate | Hyperoxaluria |
| White[a] | Phosphate | Phosphaturia |
| White[a] | Fat | Lipiduria |

[a]Sediment

be aware that the Fanconi syndrome includes renal glucosuria; hence the presence of galactose cannot be deduced from the positive Clinitest.

Dinitrophenylhydrazine (DNPH, Brady's reagent) reacts with α-ketoacids to produce insoluble hydrazones, forming precipitates in urine samples (Table 2.5); it is seldom used nowadays, partly due to its explosive hazard. Conversely, Acetest analysis in urine (Bayer Corporation) complexes with urinary ketones (Table 2.5). Parallel use of DNPH and Acetest provides slightly more diagnostic capacity. A positive result of either test will always be followed up by an immediate analysis of urine organic acids. Acetest is also frequently used for the home monitoring of patients with MSUD and propionic and methylmalonic acidurias; it will give a good indication for the catabolic state of the patient, necessitating dietary intervention. This test will be of use in establishing hypoketotic hypoglycemia although the degree of ketonuria in several fatty acid oxidation disorders may be marked, especially MCAD.

The cyanide nitroprusside test (or Brand reaction) identifies sulfur-containing amino acids, with the formation of brightly colored complexes (Table 2.6). It will find its primary use in the detection of homocystinuria (both homocysteine and the cysteine-homocysteine disulfide react positively) and cystinuria. Arginine—and at a slower rate argininosuccinic acid—will react by forming a differently colored product (blue/green). A concern with the Brand test is the use of toxic cyanide.

Additional colorimetric tests can be employed for more selective identification. The Ehrlich's test employs 4-dimethylaminobenzaldehyde to assess the presence of uri-

**Table 2.2** Odor (urine)

| Odor | Compound | Disorder—source |
|---|---|---|
| Musty, mousey | Phenylacetic acid | Classical PKU; treatment of urea cycle disorders with phenylacetate |
| Maple syrup or burnt sugar | Sotolone (4,5-dimethyl-3-hydroxy-2[5*H*]-furanone) | MSUD; fenugreek; lovage |
| Sweaty feet | Isovaleric acid | Isovaleric acidemia |
| | | 3-Hydroxy-3-methylglutaric aciduria |
| | Idem + butyric + isobutyric acid | MADD (Glutaric aciduria type 2) |
| Cat urine | 3-Hydroxyisovaleric acid/3-methylcrotonic acid | 3-Methylcrotonylglycinuria |
| | | Multiple carboxylase deficiency |
| Cabbage-like | Dimethylsulfide | Methionine adenosyltransferase deficiency (Mudd disease); methanethiol oxidase deficiency; DMSO cryoprotectant (HSCT) |
| | Methanethiol | Methanethiol oxidase deficiency |
| | 2-Oxo-4-methylthiolbutyric acid | Tyrosinemia type 1 |
| Rancid butter | 2-Oxo-4-methylthiolbutyric acid | Tyrosinemia type 1 |
| Rotten eggs | Sulfur | Cystinuria, cysteamine administration |
| Fish | Trimethylamine | Trimethylaminuria; carnitine supplementation |
| | Dimethylglycine | Dimethylglycinuria |
| Dried malt or hops, celery or yeast | Alpha-hydroxybutyric acid | Oasthouse syndrome (methionine malabsorption) |
| Swimming pool, chlorine | 4-Hydroxyphenylpyruvic acid (?) | Hawkinsinuria |

*HSCT* hematopoietic stem cell transplantation

**Table 2.3** Ferric chloride test (urine)

| Color | Compound | Disorder—source |
|---|---|---|
| Blue-green | Phenylpyruvic acid | Classical PKU |
| | Imidazolepyruvic acid | Histidinemia |
| | Catecholamines | Pheochromocytoma; neuroblastoma |
| | Xanthurenic acid | Xanthurenic aciduria (B6 def.) |
| Transient blue-green | Homogentisic acid | Alkaptonuria |
| Greenish-gray | Branched chain oxoacids | MSUD |
| Green | 4-Hydroxyphenylpyruvic acid | Tyrosinemia types 1 and 2 |
| Yellow | Lactic acid | Lactic acidosis |
| Gray-black | Melanin | Melanoma |
| Deep green | Bilirubins | Conjugated hyperbilirubinuria |
| Cherry red | Acetoacetic acid | Diabetic ketoacidosis; 3-oxothiolase def. + other organic acids |
| Purple red-brown | 2-Oxobutyric acid | Methionine malabsorption |
| Purple | Ketones | 3-Oxothiolase deficiency |
| | Salicylates | Drug treatment |
| Purple or green | Phenothiazines | Drug treatment |

**Table 2.4** Reducing substances (urine)

| Compound | Disorder—source |
|---|---|
| Galactose | Galactosemia |
| | Galactokinase deficiency |
| | Fanconi-Bickel syndrome |
| | Citrin deficiency |
| Fructose | Hereditary fructose intolerance |
| | Essential fructosuria |
| 4-Hydroxyphenylpyruvic acid | Tyrosinemia types 1 and 2 |
| Homogentisic acid | Alkaptonuria |
| Xylose | Pentosuria |
| Glucose | Diabetes mellitus |
| | Renal Fanconi syndrome; cystinosis; etc. |
| Oxalic acid | Hyperoxaluria |
| Salicylates, levodopa, cephalosporins, tetracyclines, isoniazid, probenecid, nalidixic acid, nicotinic acid | Drug treatment |
| Uric acid | Hyperuricosuria |
| Hippuric acid | Treatment with sodium benzoate; severe malabsorption |
| Ascorbic acid | Excessive vitamin use |
| Contrast agents | Radiographic evaluation |

nary porphobilinogen and urobilinogen, markers for the heritable porphyrias, but it will also react with substances such as hydroxyproline, tryptophan, citrulline, and homocitrulline. The nitrosonaphthol test represents a colorimetric analysis of 4-hydroxylated phenol acids and metabolites of tyrosine metabolism (e.g., 4-hydroxyphenylpyruvate, 4-hydroxyphenyllactate, and 4-hydroxyphenylacetate). Artefactual results with nitrosonaphthol are common in patients with liver disease and severe intestinal malabsorption and those receiving parenteral nutrition. The sulfite dipstick qualitatively assesses urine sulfite, indicative of sulfite oxidase and molybdenum cofactor deficiencies. It is reputedly performed in fresh urine samples, and only few false-positive test results have been reported, a well-known one being the use of 2-mercaptoethanesulfonate (Mesna), which can also cause false-positive results to the nitroprusside reaction. Every faint positive sulfite test result should be verified by *S*-sulfocysteine measurement.

Routine blood chemistry provides a plethora of diagnostic insights (e.g., glucose, ammonia, blood gases, creatinine, urea, uric acid, liver enzymes, etc.) (Table 2.7). Table 2.7

**Table 2.5** Dinitrophenylhydrazine (DNPH) and Acetest (urine)

| DNPH | Acetest | Positive compound | Disorder—source |
|---|---|---|---|
| + | – | Phenylpyruvic acid | Classical PKU |
| + | – | 2-Oxoisocaproic acid | MSUD |
| + | – | 2-Oxo-3-methylvaleric acid | MSUD |
| (+) | – | Imidazolepyruvic acid | Histidinemia |
| + | + | Acetone | 3-Oxothiolase def.; ketosis; Succinyl-CoA:3-ketoacid-CoA-transferase deficiency |
| – | + | 2-Methylacetoacetate | 3-Oxothiolase deficiency |
| – | + | 2-Butanone | 3-Oxothiolase deficiency |
| + | + | Acetoacetate | Succinyl-CoA:3-ketoacid-CoA-transferase deficiency; ketosis |
| + | – | 4-Hydroxyphenylpyruvic acid | Liver disease; Tyrosinemia types 1 and 2 |
| + | – | 2-Oxobutyric acid | Methionine malabsorption |
| + | + | Pyruvate | Lactic acidosis |

**Table 2.6** Nitroprusside test (urine)

| Positive compound | Disorder—source |
|---|---|
| Cystine | Cystinuria |
| Cystine | Generalized aminoaciduria |
| Cystine | Fanconi syndrome |
| 3-Mercaptolactatecysteine-disulfide | 3-Mercaptolactatecysteine-disulfiduria |
| Homocystine, cysteine-homocysteine mixed disulfide | Homocystinuria |
| | B 12 def. and cobalamin C, D, E, G |
| | Methylene tetrahydrofolate reductase def. |
| | Cystathioninuria (bacterial formation of Hcy) |
| Glutathione | Glutathionuria |
| Ketones + high creatinine | Dehydration |

**Table 2.7** Routine chemistry in blood (plasma or serum)

| **Glucose ↓ (hypoglycemia)** | |
|---|---|
| Name | Gene |
| **Disorders of nitrogen-containing compounds** | |
| Carbonic anhydrase VA deficiency | *CA5A* |
| Dopamine beta-hydroxylase deficiency | *DBH* |
| Adenosine kinase deficiency | *ADK* |
| Maple syrup urine disease | *BCKDHA, BCKDHB, DBT* |
| Isovaleryl-CoA dehydrogenase deficiency | *IVD* |
| 2-Methylbutyryl-CoA dehydrogenase deficiency | *ACADSB* |
| 3-Methylcrotonyl-CoA carboxylase 1 and 2 deficiency | *MCCC1* |
| 3-Methylglutaconyl-CoA hydratase deficiency | *AUH* |
| HSD10 disease | *HSD17B10* |
| 3-Hydroxy-3-methylglutaryl-CoA lyase deficiency | *HMGCL* |
| Propionyl-CoA-carboxylase deficiency | *PCCA, PCCB* |
| Methylmalonyl-CoA mutase deficiency | *MMUT* |
| Combined MMA and MA | *ACSF3* |
| Malonyl-CoA decarboxylase deficiency | *MLYCD* |
| Alpha-amino adipic semialdehyde (AASA) dehydrogenase deficiency | *ALDH7A1* |
| 2-Ketoadipic aciduria | *DHTKD1* |
| **Disorders of vitamins, cofactors, metals, and minerals** | |
| NFS1 deficiency | *NFS1* |
| Multiple acyl-CoA dehydrogenase deficiency | *ETFDH, ETFA, ETFB* |
| Nicotinamide nucleotide transhydrogenase deficiency | *NNT* |
| Pyridox(am)ine 5′-phosphate oxidase deficiency | *PNPO* |
| **Disorders of carbohydrates** | |
| Fanconi-Bickel syndrome[a] | *SLC2A2* |
| Fructose-1-phosphate aldolase deficiency | *ALDOB* |
| Transaldolase deficiency | *TALDO1* |
| ATP-sensitive potassium channel regulatory subunit deficiency | *ABCC8* |
| ATP-sensitive potassium channel pore-forming subunit deficiency | *KCNJ11* |
| Glutamate dehydrogenase superactivity | *GLUD1* |
| HNF4-alpha deficiency | *HNF4A* |
| HNF1-alpha deficiency | *HNF1A* |
| Uncoupling protein 2 deficiency | *UCP2* |
| Hyperinsulinemic hypoglycemia 5 | *INSR* |

**Table 2.7** (continued)

| Name | Gene |
|---|---|
| AKT2 superactivity | *AKT2* |
| Glucose-6-phosphate translocase deficiency | *SLC37A4* |
| Glycogen storage disease type III | *AGL* |
| Liver glycogen phosphorylase deficiency | *PYGL* |
| Liver glycogen synthase deficiency[a] | *GYS2* |
| Hepatic phosphorylase kinase α2 subunit deficiency | *PHKA2* |
| Phosphorylase kinase β subunit deficiency | *PHKB* |
| Hepatic phosphorylase kinase γ2 subunit deficiency | *PHKG2* |
| Constitutional AMP-activated protein kinase activation | *PRKAG2* |
| Glycogen storage disease type I a | *G6PC* |
| Fructose-1,6-bisphosphatase deficiency | *FBP1* |
| Pyruvate carboxylase deficiency | *PC* |
| Mitochondrial phosphoenolpyruvate carboxykinase deficiency | *PCK2* |
| Glucokinase superactivity | *GCK* |
| **Mitochondrial disorders of energy metabolism** | |
| 2-Oxoglutarate dehydrogenase deficiency | *OGDH* |
| Acyl-CoA Dehydrogenase 9 deficiency | *ACAD9* |
| Mitochondrial complex III subunit deficiency (UQCRB) | *UQCRB* |
| Mitochondrial complex III assembly deficiency (UQCRC2) | *UQCRC2* |
| Mitochondrial complex III assembly deficiency (TTC19) | *TTC19* |
| Mitochondrial complex III assembly deficiency (UQCC3) | *UQCC3* |
| Mitochondrial ATP synthase F1 subunit δ deficiency | *ATP5F1D* |
| Mitochondrial cytochrome beta deficiency | *MTCYB* |
| Mitochondrial deoxyguanosine kinase deficiency | *DGUOK* |
| MPV17 deficiency | *MPV17* |
| tRNA 5-carboxymethylaminomethyl transferase deficiency | *MTO1* |
| Mitochondrial transcription factor A deficiency | *TFAM* |
| Mitochondrial ribosomal small subunit 2, 7,23 and 28 deficiency | *MRPS2* |
| Mitochondrial tryptophanyl-tRNA synthetase deficiency | *WARS2* |
| Mitochondrial glutamyl-tRNA(Gln) amidotransferase subunit B deficiency | *GATB* |
| MEGDEL Syndrome | *SERAC1* |
| Barth syndrome | *TAZ* |
| MICOS complex subunit MIC13 deficiency | *MICOS13* |
| **Disorders of lipids** | |
| Organic cation carnitine transporter 2 deficiency | *SLC22A5* |
| Carnitine palmitoyltransferase 1 deficiency | *CPT1A* |
| Carnitine palmitoyltransferase 2 deficiency | *CPT2* |
| Carnitine acylcarnitine translocase deficiency | *SLC25A20* |
| Short-chain acyl-CoA dehydrogenase deficiency | *ACADS* |
| Medium-chain acyl-CoA dehydrogenase deficiency | *ACADM* |
| Very long-chain acyl-CoA dehydrogenase deficiency | *ACADVL* |
| Short-chain L-3-hydroxyacyl-CoA dehydrogenase deficiency | *HADH* |
| Long-chain 3-hydroxyacyl-CoA dehydrogenase deficiency | *HADHA* |
| Trifunctional protein deficiency | *HADHB* |
| TANGO2 deficiency | *TANGO2* |
| 3-Hydroxy-3-methylglutaryl-CoA synthase deficiency | *HMGCS2* |
| Succinyl-CoA:3-oxoacid CoA transferase deficiency | *OXCT1* |
| Monocarboxylate transporter gain-of-function | *SLC16A1* |
| Methylacetoacetyl-CoA thiolase deficiency | *ACAT1* |
| Glycerol kinase deficiency, isolated | *GK* |
| Catalytic phosphatidylinositol 3-kinase α subunit superactivity | *PIK3CA* |
| **Congenital disorders of glycosylation** | |
| Phosphomannomutase 2 deficiency PMM2-CDG | *PMM2* |
| Phosphomannose isomerase deficiency MPI-CDG | *MPI* |
| Mannosyltransferase 6 deficiency ALG3-CDG | *ALG3* |

(continued)

Table 2.7 (continued)

| Name | Gene |
|---|---|
| Mannosyltransferase 8 deficiency ALG12-CDG | *ALG12* |
| Phosphoglucomutase 1 deficiency PGM1-CDG | *PGM1* |
| **Glucose ↑** | |
| **Disorders of nitrogen-containing compounds** | |
| Pterin carbinolamine-4a-dehydratase deficiency | *PCBD1* |
| **Disorders of vitamins, cofactors, metals, and minerals** | |
| Thiamine-responsive megaloblastic anemia syndrome (SLC19A2) | *SLC19A2* |
| Hereditary hemochromatosis (type 1) | *HFE* |
| Hereditary hemochromatosis (type 2a) | *HFE2* |
| Hereditary hemochromatosis (type 2b) | *HAMP* |
| Hereditary hemochromatosis (type 3) | *TFR2* |
| **Disorders of carbohydrates** | |
| Fanconi-Bickel syndrome[a] | *SLC2A2* |
| Galactose-1-phosphate uridyltransferase deficiency[b] | *GALT* |
| Uridine diphosphate galactose-4-epimerase deficiency[b] | *GALE* |
| ATP-sensitive potassium channel regulatory subunit superactivity | *ABCC8* |
| ATP-sensitive potassium channel pore-forming subunit superactivity | *KCNJ11* |
| Glucokinase deficiency | *GCK* |
| Liver glycogen synthase deficiency[a] | *GYS2* |
| **Mitochondrial disorders of energy metabolism** | |
| Mitochondrial tRNA(Ser) 2 deficiency | *MTTS2* |
| **Disorders of lipids** | |
| 3-Oxothiolase deficiency | *ACAT1* |
| Estrogen resistance | *ESR1* |
| **Storage disorders** | |
| Nephropathic cystinosis | *CTNS* |
| **Ammonia ↑ (Hyperammonemia)** | |
| **Disorders of nitrogen-containing compounds** | |
| *N*-Acetylglutamate synthase deficiency | *NAGS* |
| Carbamoyl phosphate synthetase I deficiency | *CPS1* |
| Ornithine transcarbamylase deficiency | *OTC* |
| Argininosuccinate synthetase deficiency | *ASS1* |
| Argininosuccinate lyase deficiency | *ASL* |
| Arginase 1 deficiency | *ARG1* |
| Mitochondrial ornithine transporter deficiency | *SLC25A15* |
| Citrin deficiency | *SLC25A13* |
| Carbonic anhydrase VA deficiency | *CA5A* |
| Lysinuric protein intolerance | *SLC7A7* |
| Isovaleryl-CoA dehydrogenase deficiency | *IVD* |
| 3-Hydroxy-3-methylglutaryl-CoA lyase deficiency | *HMGCL* |
| Propionyl-CoA-carboxylase deficiency | *PCCA, PCCB* |
| Methylmalonyl-CoA mutase deficiency | *MMUT* |
| Pyrroline-5-carboxylate synthetase deficiency | *ALDH18A1* |
| Ornithine aminotransferase deficiency | *OAT* |
| Glutamate dehydrogenase superactivity | *GLUD1* |
| Glutamine synthetase deficiency | *GLUL* |
| **Disorders of vitamins, cofactors, metals, and minerals** | |
| Adenosylcobalamin synthesis defect—cblD-MMA | *MMADHC* |
| Adenosylcobalamin synthesis defect—cbl A/B | *MMAA/B* |
| Mitochondrial coenzyme A transporter deficiency | *SLC25A42* |
| **Disorders of carbohydrates** | |
| Pyruvate carboxylase deficiency | *PC* |
| **Mitochondrial disorders of energy metabolism** | |
| Acyl-CoA Dehydrogenase 9 deficiency | *ACAD9* |
| Mitochondrial complex III assembly deficiency (UQCRC2) | *UQCRC2* |
| Mitochondrial ATP synthase F1 subunit δ deficiency | *ATP5F1D* |
| Transmembrane protein 70 deficiency | *TMEM70* |

**Table 2.7** (continued)

| Name | Gene |
|---|---|
| Mitochondrial cytochrome c1 deficiency | *CYC1* |
| FBXL4 deficiency | *FBXL4* |
| Combined Oxidative Phosphorylation Defect 5 | *MRPS22* |
| **Disorders of lipids** | |
| Carnitine-acylcarnitine translocase deficiency | *SLC25A20* |
| Carnitine palmitoyltransferase 2 deficiency, severe | *CPT2* |
| Long-chain 3-hydroxyacyl-CoA dehydrogenase deficiency | *HADHA* |
| Trifunctional protein deficiency | *HADHB* |
| TANGO2 deficiency | *TANGO2* |
| Alpha-methylacetoacetic aciduria | *ACAT1* |
| **Lactate ↑** | |
| **Disorders of nitrogen-containing compounds** | |
| Glutathione synthetase deficiency, severe | *GSS* |
| Carbonic anhydrase VA deficiency | *CA5A* |
| Mitochondrial sulfur dioxygenase deficiency | *ETHE1* |
| Isovaleric acidemia | *IVD* |
| Mitochondrial short-chain enoyl-CoA hydratase 1 deficiency | *ECHS1* |
| HSD10 disease | *HSD17B10* |
| 3-Hydroxy-3-methylglutaryl-CoA lyase deficiency | *HMGCL* |
| Methylmalonate semialdehyde dehydrogenase deficiency | *ALDH6A1* |
| Propionyl-CoA-carboxylase deficiency | *PCCA, PCCB* |
| Methylmalonyl-CoA mutase deficiency | *MMUT* |
| Combined MMA and MA | *ACSF3* |
| Malonyl-CoA decarboxylase deficiency | *MLYCD* |
| 3-Hydroxyisobutyrate dehydrogenase deficiency | *HIBADH* |
| **Disorders of vitamins, cofactors, metals, and minerals** | |
| Lipoyltransferase 2 deficiency | *LIPT2* |
| Lipoic acid synthase deficiency | *LIAS* |
| Lipoyltransferase 1 deficiency | *LIPT1* |
| NFU1 deficiency | *NFU1* |
| BOLA3 deficiency | *BOLA3* |
| Glutaredoxin 5 deficiency | *GLRX5* |
| IBA57 deficiency | *IBA57* |
| ISCA1 deficiency | *ISCA1* |
| ISCA2 deficiency | *ISCA2* |
| ISCU deficiency | *ISCU* |
| NFS1 deficiency | *NFS1* |
| ISD11 deficiency | *LYRM4* |
| Ferredoxin 2 deficiency | *FDX2* |
| Biotinidase deficiency | *BTD* |
| Holocarboxylase synthetase deficiency | *HLCS* |
| Biotin and thiamine basal ganglia disease | *SLC19A3* |
| Thiamine metabolism dysfunction syndrome 5 | *TPK1* |
| Mitochondrial NAD kinase 2 deficiency | *NADK2* |
| Phosphopantothenoylcysteine synthetase deficiency | *PPCS* |
| Mitochondrial coenzyme A transporter deficiency | *SLC25A42* |
| PROSC-deficient B6-dependent epilepsy | *PLPBP* |
| **Disorders of carbohydrates** | |
| Glucose-6-phosphatase deficiency | *G6PC* |
| Glucose-6-phosphate translocase deficiency | *SLC37A4* |
| Fructose-1,6-bisphosphatase deficiency | *FBP1* |
| Pyruvate carboxylase deficiency | *PC* |
| D-lactate dehydrogenase deficiency | *LDHD* |
| **Mitochondrial disorders of energy metabolism** | |
| Pyruvate dehydrogenase complex deficiency E1a | *PDHA1* |

(continued)

**Table 2.7** (continued)

| Name | Gene |
|---|---|
| Pyruvate dehydrogenase complex deficiency E1b | *PDHB* |
| Dihydrolipoyl transacetylase deficiency | *DLAT* |
| Pyruvate dehydrogenase complex deficiency E3 X | *PDHX* |
| Pyruvate dehydrogenase complex deficiency PDHP | *PDP1* |
| ATP-specific succinyl-CoA ligase β subunit deficiency | *SUCLA2* |
| GTP-specific succinyl-CoA ligase α subunit deficiency | *SUCLG1* |
| Fumarase deficiency | *FH* |
| Mitochondrial malate dehydrogenase deficiency | *MDH2* |
| 2-Oxoglutarate dehydrogenase deficiency | *OGDH* |
| L-2-hydroxyglutarate dehydrogenase deficiency | *L2HGDH* |
| Adenine nucleotide translocator deficiency AR | *SLC25A4* |
| Mitochondrial phosphate carrier deficiency | *SLC25A3* |
| Aspartate-glutamate carrier 1 deficiency | *SLC25A12* |
| Mitochondrial complex I subunit deficiency (NDUFV1) | *NDUFV1* |
| Mitochondrial complex I subunit deficiency (NDUFV2) | *NDUFV2* |
| Mitochondrial complex I subunit deficiency (NDUFS1) | *NDUFS1* |
| Mitochondrial complex I subunit deficiency (NDUFS2) | *NDUFS2* |
| Mitochondrial complex I subunit deficiency (NDUFS3) | *NDUFS3* |
| Mitochondrial complex I subunit deficiency (NDUFS7) | *NDUFS7* |
| Mitochondrial complex I subunit deficiency (NDUFS4) | *NDUFS4* |
| Mitochondrial complex I subunit deficiency (NDUFS6) | *NDUFS6* |
| Mitochondrial complex I subunit deficiency (NDUFA1) | *NDUFA1* |
| Mitochondrial complex I subunit deficiency (NDUFA2) | *NDUFA2* |
| Mitochondrial complex I subunit deficiency (NDUFA9) | *NDUFA9* |
| Mitochondrial complex I subunit deficiency (NDUFA10) | *NDUFA10* |
| Mitochondrial complex I subunit deficiency (NDUFB3) | *NDUFB3* |
| NADH dehydrogenase β subcomplex subunit 8 deficiency | *NDUFB8* |
| Mitochondrial complex I subunit deficiency (NDUFB11) | *NDUFB11* |
| Mitochondrial complex I subunit deficiency (MTND2) | *MTND2* |
| Mitochondrial complex I subunit deficiency (MTND3) | *MTND3* |
| Mitochondrial complex I subunit deficiency (MTND4) | *MTND4* |
| Mitochondrial complex I subunit deficiency (MTND5) | *MTND5* |
| Mitochondrial complex I subunit deficiency (MTND6) | *MTND6* |
| NADH dehydrogenase α subcomplex subunit 6 deficiency | *NDUFA6* |
| Mitochondrial complex I subunit deficiency (NDUFB9) | *NDUFB9* |
| Mitochondrial complex I subunit deficiency (NDUFA13) | *NDUFA13* |
| Mitochondrial complex I subunit deficiency (NDUFA11) | *NDUFA11* |
| NADH dehydrogenase β subcomplex subunit 10 deficiency | *NDUFB10* |
| Mitochondrial complex I assembly deficiency (NDUFAF1) | *NDUFAF1* |
| Mitochondrial complex I assembly deficiency (NDUFAF2) | *NDUFAF2* |
| Mitochondrial complex I assembly deficiency (NDUFAF2) | *NDUFAF2* |
| Mitochondrial complex I assembly deficiency (NDUFAF3) | *NDUFAF3* |
| Mitochondrial complex I assembly deficiency (NDUFAF4) | *NDUFAF4* |
| Mitochondrial complex I assembly deficiency (NDUFAF5) | *NDUFAF5* |
| Mitochondrial complex I assembly deficiency (NDUFAF6) | *NDUFAF6* |
| Mitochondrial complex I assembly deficiency (FOXRED1) | *FOXRED1* |
| NUBPL deficiency | *NUBPL* |
| Acyl-CoA Dehydrogenase 9 deficiency | *ACAD9* |
| TIMMDC1 deficiency | *TIMMDC1* |
| Mitochondrial complex III subunit deficiency (UQCRB) | *UQCRB* |
| Mitochondrial complex III assembly deficiency (UQCRC2) | *UQCRC2* |
| Mitochondrial complex III subunit deficiency (UQCRQ) | *UQCRQ* |
| GRACILE syndrome | *BCS1L* |
| Mitochondrial complex III assembly deficiency (TTC19) | *TTC19* |
| Mitochondrial complex III assembly deficiency (LYRM7) | *LYRM7* |
| UQCC2 deficiency | *UQCC2* |
| Mitochondrial complex III assembly deficiency (UQCC3) | *UQCC3* |

**Table 2.7** (continued)

| Name | Gene |
|---|---|
| Mitochondrial complex IV subunit deficiency (MTCO1) | *MTCO1* |
| Mitochondrial complex IV subunit deficiency (MTCO2) | *MTCO2* |
| Mitochondrial complex IV subunit deficiency (MTCO3) | *MTCO3* |
| Mitochondrial complex IV subunit deficiency (COX6B1) | *COX6B1* |
| Mitochondrial complex IV subunit deficiency (COX7B) | *COX7B* |
| Cytochrome c oxidase subunit 5A deficiency | *COX5A* |
| Mitochondrial complex IV assembly deficiency (COA6) | *COA6* |
| Mitochondrial complex IV assembly deficiency (COX10) | *COX10* |
| Mitochondrial complex IV assembly deficiency (COX15) | *COX15* |
| Mitochondrial complex IV assembly deficiency (COX20) | *COX20* |
| Mitochondrial complex IV assembly deficiency (SCO1) | *SCO1* |
| Mitochondrial complex IV assembly deficiency (SCO2) | *SCO2* |
| Mitochondrial complex IV assembly deficiency (SURF1) | *SURF1* |
| Leigh Syndrome with French-Canadian Ethnicity | *LRPPRC* |
| TACO1 deficiency | *TACO1* |
| PET100 deficiency | *PET100* |
| FASTKD2 deficiency | *FASTKD2* |
| CEP89 deficiency | *CEP89* |
| Mitochondrial complex IV assembly deficiency (COX14) | *COX14* |
| Mitochondrial complex I subunit deficiency (NDUFA4) | *NDUFA4* |
| Mitochondrial ATP synthase F1 subunit a deficiency | *ATP5F1A* |
| Mitochondrial ATP synthase F1 subunit δ deficiency | *ATP5F1D* |
| Mitochondrial ATP synthase F1 subunit e deficiency | *ATP5F1E* |
| Mitochondrial complex V subunit deficiency (MTATP6) | *MTATP6* |
| DAPIT deficiency | *ATP5MD* |
| Transmembrane protein 70 deficiency | *TMEM70* |
| Mitochondrial complex V assembly deficiency (ATPAF2) | *ATPAF2* |
| Mitochondrial cytochrome b deficiency | *MTCYB* |
| Mitochondrial cytochrome c1 deficiency | *CYC1* |
| Mitochondrial Depletion Syndrome 4A | *POLG* |
| Mitochondrial DNA polymerase g accessory subunit deficiency | *POLG2* |
| Mitochondrial deoxyguanosine kinase deficiency | *DGUOK* |
| MPV17 deficiency | *MPV17* |
| Mitochondrial thymidine kinase 2 deficiency | *TK2* |
| Mitochondrial ribonucelotide reductase subunit 2 deficiency | *RRM2B* |
| Thymidine phosphorylase deficiency | *TYMP* |
| Mitochondrial ribonuclease H1 deficiency | *RNASEH1* |
| FBXL4 deficiency | *FBXL4* |
| Mitochondrial RNA import protein deficiency | *PNPT1* |
| Ribonuclease P 5′ tRNA processing enzyme deficiency | *TRMT10C* |
| Ribonuclease Z 3′ tRNA processing enzyme deficiency | *ELAC2* |
| Mitochondrial methionyl-tRNA formyltransferase deficiency | *MTFMT* |
| tRNA 5-taurinomethyluridine modifier deficiency | *GTPBP3* |
| tRNA 5-carboxymethylaminomethyl transferase deficiency | *MTO1* |
| Pseudouridine synthase 1 deficiency | *PUS1* |
| tRNA methyltransferase 5 deficiency | *TRMT5* |
| Mitochondrial poly(A) exoribonuclease deficiency | *PDE12* |
| Mitochondrial ribosomal large subunit 3 deficiency | *MRPL3* |
| Mitochondrial ribosomal small subunit 2 deficiency | *MRPS2* |
| Combined Oxidative Phosphorylation Defect 2 | *MRPS16* |
| Combined Oxidative Phosphorylation Defect 5 | *MRPS22* |
| Mitochondrial ribosomal small subunit 14 deficiency | *MRPS14* |
| Mitochondrial ribosomal small subunit 7 deficiency | *MRPS7* |
| Mitochondrial ribosomal large subunit 12 deficiency | *MRPL12* |
| Mitochondrial ribosomal small subunit 28 deficiency | *MRPS28* |

(continued)

**Table 2.7** (continued)

| Name | Gene |
|---|---|
| RMND1 deficiency | *RMND1* |
| Combined Oxidative Phosphorylation Defect 1 | *GFM1* |
| Combined Oxidative Phosphorylation Defect 3 | *TSFM* |
| Combined Oxidative Phosphorylation Defect 4 | *TUFM* |
| Combined Oxidative Phosphorylation Defect 7 | *C12ORF65* |
| Mitochondrial tRNA(Arg) deficiency | *MTTR* |
| Mitochondrial tRNA(Asn) deficiency | *MTTN* |
| Mitochondrial tRNA(Cys) deficiency | *MTTC* |
| Mitochondrial tRNA(Glu) deficiency | *MTTE* |
| Mitochondrial tRNA(Gly) deficiency | *MTTG* |
| Mitochondrial tRNA(Ile) deficiency | *MTTI* |
| Mitochondrial tRNA(Leu) 1 deficiency | *MTTL1* |
| Mitochondrial tRNA(Lys) deficiency | *MTTK* |
| Mitochondrial tRNA(Met) deficiency | *MTTM* |
| Mitochondrial tRNA(Phe) deficiency | *MTTF* |
| Mitochondrial tRNA(Thr) deficiency | *MTTT* |
| Mitochondrial tRNA(Trp) deficiency | *MTTW* |
| Mitochondrial arginine-tRNA synthetase deficiency | *RARS2* |
| Mitochondrial asparaginyl-tRNA synthetase deficiency | *NARS2* |
| Leukoencephalopathy with brainstem and spinal cord involvement and lactate elevation | *DARS2* |
| Mitochondrial cysteinyl-tRNA synthetase deficiency | *CARS2* |
| Mitochondrial glutamyl-tRNA synthetase deficiency | *EARS2* |
| Mitochondrial leucyl-tRNA synthetase deficiency | *LARS2* |
| Mitochondrial phenylalanyl-tRNA synthetase deficiency | *FARS2* |
| Mitochondrial seryl-tRNA synthetase deficiency | *SARS2* |
| Mitochondrial tyrosyl-tRNA synthetase deficiency | *YARS2* |
| Mitochondrial tryptophanyl-tRNA synthetase deficiency | *WARS2* |
| Mitochondrial glutamyl-tRNA(Gln) amidotransferase subunit A deficiency | *QRSL1* |
| Mitochondrial glutamyl-tRNA(Gln) amidotransferase subunit C deficiency | *GATC* |
| Mitochondrial glutamyl-tRNA(Gln) amidotransferase subunit B deficiency | *GATB* |
| Mitochondrial threonyl-tRNA synthetase deficiency | *TARS2* |
| Peroxisomal and mitochondrial fission defect | *DNM1L* |
| Mitochondrial fission factor deficiency | *MFF* |
| STAT2 deficiency | *STAT2* |
| Optic Atrophy 1 and Deafness | *OPA1* |
| Acylglycerol kinase deficiency | *AGK* |
| MEGDEL Syndrome | *SERAC1* |
| Tafazzin deficiency | *TAZ* |
| TIMM50 deficiency | *TIMM50* |
| GFER deficiency | *GFER* |
| Mitochondrial processing peptidase β deficiency | *PMPCB* |
| Mitochondrial intermediate peptidase deficiency | *MIPEP* |
| CLPB deficiency | *CLPB* |
| HSP60 deficiency | *HSPD1* |
| HTRA2 deficiency | *HTRA2* |
| Pitrilysin metallopeptidase 1 deficiency | *PITRM1* |
| YME1L1 deficiency | *YMEL1* |
| Mitochondrial inorganic pyrophosphatase 2 deficiency | *PPA2* |
| Sideroflexin 4 deficiency | *SFXN4* |
| Combined Oxidative Phosphorylation Defect 6 | *AIFM1* |
| C1q binding protein deficiency | *C1QBP* |
| MICOS complex subunit MIC13 deficiency | *MICOS13* |
| Mitochondrial thioredoxin 2 deficiency | *TXN2* |
| CoQ2 deficiency | *COQ2* |
| CABC1/ADCK3 deficiency | *COQ8A* |
| CoQ9 deficiency | *COQ9* |

**Table 2.7** (continued)

| Name | Gene |
|---|---|
| **Disorders of lipids** | |
| Carnitine acylcarnitine translocase deficiency | *SLC25A20* |
| Long-chain 3-hydroxyacyl-CoA dehydrogenase deficiency | *HADHA* |
| Trifunctional protein deficiency | *HADHB* |
| TANGO2 deficiency | *TANGO2* |
| Cytosolic acetoacetyl-CoA thiolase deficiency | *ACAT2* |
| Mitochondrial acetyl-CoA carboxylase 2 deficiency | *ACACB* |
| **Congenital disorders of glycosylation** | |
| Heparan sulfate 6-*O*-sulfotransferase 2 deficiency | *HS6ST2* |
| COG6-CDG | *COG6* |
| **Creatinine ↓** | |
| **Disorders of nitrogen-containing compounds** | |
| Arginine:glycine amidinotransferase deficiency | *GATM* |
| Guanidinoacetate methyltransferase deficiency | *GAMT* |
| Ornithine aminotransferase deficiency | *OAT* |
| **Creatinine ↑** | |
| **Disorders of nitrogen-containing compounds** | |
| Lysinuric protein intolerance | *SLC7A7* |
| Prolidase deficiency | *PEPD* |
| Sarcosine oxidase deficiency[c] | *SDH* |
| **Disorders of vitamins, cofactors, metals, and minerals** | |
| Methylmalonic aciduria due to methylmalonyl-CoA mutase deficiency | *MMUT* |
| Methylmalonic aciduria, cblB type | *MMAB* |
| Methylmalonic aciduria and homocystinuria, cblC type | *MMACHC* |
| **Disorders of carbohydrates** | |
| Transaldolase deficiency | *TALDO* |
| **Disorders of lipids** | |
| Lecithin cholesterol acyl transferase deficiency | *LCAT* |
| Lipoprotein glomerulopathy | *APOE* |
| **Storage disorders** | |
| Fabry disease | *GLA* |
| Galactosialidosis | *CTSA* |
| Nephropathic cystinosis | *CTNS* |
| **Disorders of peroxisomes and oxalate** | |
| Alanine-glyoxylate aminotransferase deficiency | *AGXT* |
| Glyoxylate reductase/hydroxypyruvate reductase deficiency | *GRHPR* |
| 4-hydroxy-2-oxoglutarate aldolase deficiency | *HOGA1* |
| **Acidosis (inc. ketoacidosis and lactic acidosis)** | |
| **Disorders of nitrogen-containing compounds** | |
| Glutathione synthetase deficiency, severe | *GSS* |
| 5-Oxoprolinase deficiency | *OPLAH* |
| Mitochondrial sulfur dioxygenase deficiency | *ETHE1* |
| Maple syrup urine disease | *BCKDHA, BCKDHB, DBT* |
| Isovaleryl-CoA dehydrogenase deficiency | *IVD* |
| 3-Methylcrotonyl-CoA carboxylase 1 and 2 deficiency | *MCCC1/2* |
| 3-Methylglutaconyl-CoA hydratase deficiency | *AUH* |
| 3-Hydroxyisobutyryl-CoA deacylase deficiency | *HIBCH* |
| HSD10 disease | *HSD17B10* |
| 3-Hydroxy-3-methylglutaryl-CoA lyase deficiency | *HMGCL* |
| Propionyl-CoA-carboxylase deficiency | *PCCA, PCCB* |
| Methylmalonyl-CoA mutase deficiency | *MMUT* |
| Combined MMA and MA | *ACSF3* |
| Malonyl-CoA decarboxylase deficiency | *MLYCD* |
| 3-Hydroxyisobutyrate dehydrogenase deficiency | *HIBADH* |
| 2-Aminoadipic 2-oxoadipic aciduria | *DHTKD1* |

(continued)

Table 2.7 (continued)

| Name | Gene |
|---|---|
| **Disorders of vitamins, cofactors, metals, and minerals** | |
| Adenosylcobalamin synthesis defect—cblD-MMA | *MMADHC* |
| Adenosylcobalamin synthesis defect—cbl A/B | *MMAA/B* |
| Multiple acyl-CoA dehydrogenase deficiency DH | *ETFA, ETFB, ETFDH* |
| 2,4-dienoyl-CoA reductase deficiency with hyperlysinemia | *NADK2* |
| Mitochondrial coenzyme A transporter deficiency | *SLC25A42* |
| **Mitochondrial disorders of energy metabolism** | |
| Pyruvate dehydrogenase complex deficiency E1a | *PDHA1* |
| Pyruvate dehydrogenase complex deficiency E1b | *PDHB* |
| Pyruvate dehydrogenase complex deficiency E2 | *DLAT* |
| Pyruvate dehydrogenase complex deficiency E3 X | *PDHX* |
| Pyruvate dehydrogenase complex deficiency PDHP | *PDP1* |
| ATP-specific succinyl-CoA ligase β subunit deficiency | *SUCLA2* |
| GTP-specific succinyl-CoA ligase α subunit deficiency | *SUCLG1* |
| Fumarase deficiency | *FH* |
| 2-Oxoglutarate dehydrogenase deficiency | *OGDH* |
| SAM transporter deficiency | *SLC25A26* |
| Mitochondrial complex I subunit deficiency (NDUFV2) | *NDUFV2* |
| Mitochondrial complex I subunit deficiency (NDUFS1) | *NDUFS1* |
| Mitochondrial complex I subunit deficiency (NDUFS4) | *NDUFS4* |
| Mitochondrial complex I subunit deficiency (NDUFS6) | *NDUFS6* |
| Mitochondrial complex I subunit deficiency (NDUFA1) | *NDUFA1* |
| Mitochondrial complex I subunit deficiency (NDUFA9) | *NDUFA9* |
| Mitochondrial complex I subunit deficiency (NDUFB3) | *NDUFB3* |
| NADH dehydrogenase β subcomplex subunit 8 deficiency | *NDUFB8* |
| Mitochondrial complex I subunit deficiency (NDUFB11) | *NDUFB11* |
| Mitochondrial complex I subunit deficiency (MTND6) | *MTND6* |
| NADH dehydrogenase α subcomplex subunit 6 deficiency | *NDUFA6* |
| Mitochondrial complex I subunit deficiency (NDUFB9) | *NDUFB9* |
| Mitochondrial complex I subunit deficiency (NDUFA11) | *NDUFA11* |
| Mitochondrial complex I assembly deficiency (NDUFAF1) | *NDUFAF1* |
| Mitochondrial complex I assembly deficiency (NDUFAF4) | *NDUFAF4* |
| Mitochondrial complex I assembly deficiency (NDUFAF5) | *NDUFAF5* |
| Mitochondrial complex I assembly deficiency (NDUFAF6) | *NDUFAF6* |
| Mitochondrial complex I assembly deficiency (FOXRED1) | *FOXRED1* |
| Mitochondrial complex III subunit deficiency (UQCRB) | *UQCRB* |
| Mitochondrial complex III assembly deficiency (UQCRC2) | *UQCRC2* |
| GRACILE syndrome | *BCS1L* |
| Mitochondrial complex III assembly deficiency (UQCC3) | *UQCC3* |
| Mitochondrial ATP synthase F1 subunit δ and e deficiency | *ATP5F1D/E* |
| Transmembrane protein 70 deficiency | *TMEM70* |
| Mitochondrial cytochrome c1 deficiency | *CYC1* |
| FBXL4 deficiency | *FBXL4* |
| tRNA 5-carboxymethylaminomethyl transferase deficiency | *MTO1* |
| tRNA methyltransferase 5 deficiency | *TRMT5* |
| Mitochondrial poly(A) exoribonuclease deficiency | *PDE12* |
| Mitochondrial ribosomal small subunit 28 deficiency | *MRPS28* |
| RMND1 deficiency | *RMND1* |
| Mitochondrial tRNA(Cys) deficiency | *MTTC* |
| Mitochondrial tRNA(Met) deficiency | *MTTM* |
| Mitochondrial leucyl-tRNA synthetase deficiency | *LARS2* |
| Mitochondrial phenylalanyl-tRNA synthetase deficiency | *FARS2* |
| Mitochondrial tryptophanyl-tRNA synthetase deficiency | *WARS2* |
| Mitochondrial glutamyl-tRNA(Gln) amidotransferase subunit C deficiency | *GATC* |
| UGO-1 like protein deficiency | *SLC25A46* |
| Tafazzin deficiency | *TAZ* |
| Mitochondrial intermediate peptidase deficiency | *MIPEP* |

Table 2.7 (continued)

| Name | Gene |
|---|---|
| Mitochondrial inorganic pyrophosphatase 2 deficiency | *PPA2* |
| Sideroflexin 4 deficiency | *SFXN4* |
| CoQ9 deficiency | *COQ9* |
| **Disorders of lipids** | |
| Long-chain 3-hydroxyacyl-CoA dehydrogenase deficiency | *HADHA* |
| Trifunctional protein deficiency | *HADHB* |
| Succinyl-CoA:3-oxoacid CoA transferase deficiency | *OXCT1* |
| Beta-Ketothiolase deficiency | *ACAT1* |
| Monocarboxylate transporter-1 deficiency | *SLC16A1* |
| Mitochondrial acetyl-CoA carboxylase 2 deficiency | *ACACB* |
| **Alkalosis** | |
| **Disorders of nitrogen-containing compounds** | |
| Urea cycle disorders | Several |
| **Mitochondrial disorders of energy metabolism** | |
| Mitochondrial seryl-tRNA synthetase deficiency | *SARS2* |
| **Disorders of lipids** | |
| Glucocorticoid receptor deficiency | *NR3C1* |
| Congenital adrenal hyperplasia, 17-alpha-hydroxylase def. | *CYP17A1* |
| Congenital adrenal hyperplasia, 11-β-hydroxylase deficiency | *CYP11B1* |
| 11-β-hydroxysteroid dehydrogenase type 2 deficiency | *HSD11B2* |
| **Total cholesterol ↓** | |
| **Disorders of nitrogen-containing compounds** | |
| Malonyl-CoA decarboxylase deficiency | *MLYCD* |
| **Mitochondrial disorders of energy metabolism** | |
| Tafazzin deficiency | *TAZ* |
| **Disorders of lipids** | |
| Microsomal triglyceride transfer protein deficiency | *MTTP* |
| Chylomicron retention disease | *SAR1B* |
| Familial hypobetalipoproteinemia type 1 | *APOB* |
| Familial hypobetalipoproteinemia type 2 | *ANGPTL3* |
| Mevalonate kinase deficiency | *MVK* |
| Squalene synthase deficiencyl | *FDFT1* |
| Smith-Lemli-Opitz syndrome | *DHCR7* |
| 3β-Hydroxy-Δ5-C27-steroid dehydrogenase/isomerase deficiency | *HSD3B7* |
| Peroxisomal branched-chain acyl-CoA oxidase deficiency | *ACOX2* |
| **Storage disorders** | |
| Gaucher disease | *GBA* |
| **Congenital disorders of glycosylation** | |
| PMM2-CDG | *PMM2* |
| MPI-CDG | *MPI* |
| ALG9-CDG | *ALG9* |
| ALG12-CDG | *ALG12* |
| ALG6-CDG | *ALG6* |
| B4GALT1-CDG | *B4GALT1* |
| **Total cholesterol ↑** | |
| **Disorders of carbohydrates** | |
| Glucose-6-phosphatase deficiency | *G6PC* |
| Glucose-6-phosphate transporter deficiency | *SLC37A4* |
| Liver glycogen phosphorylase deficiency | *PYGL* |
| Hepatic phosphorylase kinase α2 subunit deficiency | *PHKA2* |
| **Disorders of lipids** | |
| LDL receptor deficiency | *LDLR* |
| LDL receptor adaptor protein 1 deficiency | *LDLRAP1* |
| Hypercholesterolemia due to ligand-defective apoB | *APOB* |
| PCSK9 superactivity | *PCSK9* |
| STAP1 deficiency | *STAP1* |

(continued)

**Table 2.7** (continued)

| Name | Gene |
|---|---|
| Sitosterolemia due to ABCG5 deficiency | *ABCG5* |
| Sitosterolemia due to ABCG8 deficiency | *ABCG8* |
| Apolipoprotein E deficiency | *APOE* |
| Hepatic lipase deficiency | *LIPC* |
| Cholesterol 7 alpha-hydroxylase deficiency | *CYP7A1* |
| **Storage disorders** | |
| Acid sphingomyelinase deficiency | *SMPD1* |
| Lysosomal acid lipase deficiency | *LIPA* |
| **Congenital disorders of glycosylation** | |
| TMEM199-CDG | *TMEM199* |
| CCDC115-CDG | *CCDC115* |
| ATP6AP1-CDG | *ATP6AP1* |
| **Triglycerides ↑** | |
| **Disorders of carbohydrates** | |
| Fanconi-Bickel syndrome | *SLC2A2* |
| Fructose-1-phosphate aldolase deficiency | *ALDOB* |
| Glucose-6-phosphate translocase deficiency | *SLC37A4* |
| Glycogen storage disease type III | *AGL* |
| Liver glycogen phosphorylase deficiency | *PYGL* |
| Hepatic phosphorylase kinase α2 subunit deficiency | *PHKA2* |
| Phosphorylase kinase β subunit deficiency | *PHKB* |
| Hepatic phosphorylase kinase γ2 subunit deficiency | *PHKG2* |
| Glucose-6-phosphatase deficiency | *G6PC* |
| Fructose-1,6-bisphosphatase deficiency | *FBP1* |
| **Disorders of lipids** | |
| Angiopoietin-like 3 deficiency | *ANGPTL3* |
| Chylomicron retention disease | *SAR1B* |
| Apolipoprotein E deficiency | *APOE* |
| Apolipoprotein E superactivity | *APOE* |
| Lipoprotein glomerulopathy | *APOE* |
| Lipoprotein lipase deficiency | *LPL* |
| Apolipoprotein C2 deficiency | *APOC2* |
| GPIHBP1 deficiency | *GPIHBP1* |
| Hepatic lipase deficiency | *LIPC* |
| Lipase maturation factor 1 deficiency | *LMF1* |
| Apolipoprotein A5 deficiency | *APOA5* |
| Familial LCAT deficiency (complete) | *LCAT* |
| Tangier disease | *ABCA1* |
| **Storage disorders** | |
| Lysosomal acid lipase deficiency | *LIPA* |
| **Congenital disorders of glycosylation** | |
| PIGA-CDG | *PIGA* |
| **ASAT and ALAT (transaminases) ↑** | |
| **Disorders of nitrogen-containing compounds** | |
| Carbamoylphosphate synthetase 1 deficiency | *CPS1* |
| Ornithine transcarbamylase deficiency | *OTC* |
| Argininosuccinate synthetase deficiency | *ASS1* |
| Argininosuccinate lyase deficiency | *ASL* |
| Arginase 1 deficiency | *ARG1* |
| Mitochondrial ornithine transporter deficiency | *SLC25A15* |
| Citrin deficiency | *SLC25A13* |
| Lysinuric protein intolerance | *SLC7A7* |
| Tyrosinemia type 1 | *FAH* |
| Glycine *N*-methyltransferase deficiency | *GNMT* |
| *S*-adenosylhomocysteine hydrolase deficiency | *AHCY* |
| Adenosine kinase deficiency | *ADK* |
| 3-Hydroxy-3-methylglutaryl-CoA lyase deficiency | *HMGCL* |

Table 2.7 (continued)

| Name | Gene |
|---|---|
| **Disorders of vitamins, cofactors, metals, and minerals** | |
| ISD11 deficiency | *LYRM4* |
| Multiple acyl-CoA dehydrogenase deficiency | *ETFDH, ETFA, ETFB* |
| Wilson disease | *ATP7B* |
| MEDNIK syndrome | *AP1S1* |
| Hereditary hemochromatosis (type 1) | *HFE* |
| Hypermanganesemia with dystonia type 1 | *SLC30A10* |
| **Disorders of carbohydrates** | |
| Fanconi-Bickel syndrome | *SLC2A2* |
| Galactose-1-phosphate uridyltransferase deficiency | *GALT* |
| Uridine diphosphate galactose-4-epimerase deficiency | *GALE* |
| Fructose-1-phosphate aldolase deficiency | *ALDOB* |
| Transaldolase deficiency | *TALDO1* |
| Amylo-1,6-glucosidase (debrancher) deficiency | *AGL* |
| Glycogen branching enzyme deficiency | *GBE1* |
| Liver glycogen phosphorylase deficiency | *PYGL* |
| Hepatic phosphorylase kinase α2 subunit deficiency | *PHKA2* |
| Phosphorylase kinase β subunit deficiency | *PHKB* |
| Hepatic phosphorylase kinase γ2 subunit deficiency | *PHKG2* |
| Glycogen storage disease type II b | *LAMP2* |
| Glucose-6-phosphatase deficiency | *G6PC* |
| **Mitochondrial disorders of energy metabolism** | |
| GTP-specific succinyl-CoA ligase α subunit deficiency | *SUCLG1* |
| Mitochondrial complex III assembly deficiency (UQCRC2) | *UQCRC2* |
| Mitochondrial deoxyguanosine kinase deficiency | *DGUOK* |
| Mitochondrial transcription factor A deficiency | *TFAM* |
| Mitochondrial ribosomal small subunit 2 deficiency | *MRPS2* |
| Mitochondrial ribosomal small subunit 16 deficiency | *MRPS16* |
| Mitochondrial ribosomal small subunit 28 deficiency | *MRPS28* |
| Mitochondrial ribosomal large subunit 3 deficiency | *MRPL3* |
| Mitochondrial valyl-tRNA synthetase deficiency | *VARS* |
| **Disorders of lipids** | |
| Trifunctional protein β subunit deficiency | *HADHB* |
| 3-Hydroxy-3-methylglutaryl-CoA synthase deficiency | *HMGCS2* |
| Chanarin-Dorfman syndrome | *ABHD5* |
| 3β-Hydroxy-Δ5-C27-steroid dehydrogenase/isomerase deficiency | *HSD3B7* |
| Δ4-3-Oxosteroid-5β-reductase deficiency | *AKR1D1* |
| Oxysterol 7α-hydroxylase deficiency | *CYP7B1* |
| Congenital bile acid synthesis defect | *ABCD3* |
| **Disorders of peroxisomes and oxalate** | |
| Zellweger spectrum disorders | *PEX1* and other PEX genes |
| **Congenital disorders of glycosylation** | |
| PMM2-CDG | *PMM2* |
| MPI-CDG | *MPI* |
| ALG3-CDG | *ALG3* |
| Dolichol-*P*-mannose synthase-2 deficiency DPM2-CDG | *DPM2* |
| Phosphoglucomutase 1 deficiency PGM1-CDG | *PGM1* |
| COG4-CDG | *COG4* |
| ATP6AP1-CDG | *ATP6AP1* |
| TMEM199-CDG | *TMEM199* |
| CCDC115-CDG | *CCDC115* |
| Congenital disorder of glycosylation TMEM165-CDG | *TMEM165* |
| *N*-glycanase 1 deficiency | *NGLY1* |

(continued)

Table 2.7 (continued)

| Name | Gene |
|---|---|
| **Creatine kinase (CK) ↑** | |
| **Disorders of nitrogen-containing compounds** | |
| Adenosine monophosphate deaminase deficiency | *AMPD1* |
| *S*-adenosylhomocysteine hydrolase deficiency | *AHCY* |
| Adenosine kinase deficiency | *ADK* |
| 3-Methylglutaconyl-CoA hydratase deficiency | *AUH* |
| **Disorders of vitamins, cofactors, metals, and minerals** | |
| ISCA1 deficiency | *ISCA1* |
| ISCU deficiency | *ISCU* |
| NFS1 deficiency | *NFS1* |
| Ferredoxin 2 deficiency | *FDX2* |
| Multiple acyl-CoA dehydrogenase deficiency | *ETFDH, ETFA, ETFB* |
| Mitochondrial coenzyme A transporter deficiency | *SLC25A42* |
| **Disorders of carbohydrates** | |
| Lysosomal alpha-1,4-glucosidase deficiency | *GAA* |
| Amylo-1,6-glucosidase (debrancher) deficiency | *AGL* |
| Muscle phosphorylase deficiency | *PYGM* |
| Muscle phosphorylase kinase deficiency | *PHKA1* |
| Constitutional AMP-activated protein kinase activation | *PRKAG2* |
| LAMP2 deficiency | *LAMP2* |
| Muscle phosphofructokinase deficiency | *PFKM* |
| Aldolase A deficiency | *ALDOA* |
| Muscle phosphoglycerate kinase deficiency | *PGK1* |
| Muscle phosphoglycerate mutase deficiency | *PGAM2* |
| Beta-enolase deficiency | *ENO3* |
| Lactate dehydrogenase A deficiency | *LDHA* |
| **Mitochondrial disorders of energy metabolism** | |
| Mitochondrial complex I subunit deficiency (NDUFS6) | *NDUFS6* |
| Acyl-CoA Dehydrogenase 9 deficiency | *ACAD9* |
| Transmembrane protein 70 deficiency | *TMEM70* |
| Mitochondrial cytochrome b deficiency | *MTCYB* |
| Mitochondrial DNA polymerase gamma accessory subunit deficiency | *POLG2* |
| Mitochondrial thymidine kinase 2 deficiency | *TK2* |
| DNA2 helicase deficiency | *DNA2* |
| Mitochondrial ribonuclease H1 deficiency | *RNASEH1* |
| Mitochondrial elongation factor Ts deficiency | *TSFM* |
| Mitochondrial tRNA(Ala) deficiency | *MTTA* |
| Mitochondrial tRNA(Asp) deficiency | *MTTD* |
| Mitochondrial tRNA(Glu) deficiency | *MTTE* |
| Mitochondrial tRNA(Gly) deficiency | *MTTG* |
| Mitochondrial tRNA(Leu) 1 deficiency | *MTTL1* |
| Mitochondrial glutamyl-tRNA(Gln) amidotransferase subunit A deficiency | *QRSL1* |
| Mitochondrial glutamyl-tRNA(Gln) amidotransferase subunit C deficiency | *GATC* |
| MSTO1 deficiency | *MSTO1* |
| Tafazzin deficiency | *TAZ* |
| Valosin-containing protein superactivity | *VCP* |
| Pitrilysin metallopeptidase 1 deficiency | *PITRM1* |
| C1q binding protein deficiency | *C1QBP* |
| Mitochondrial calcium uniporter deficiency | *MICU1* |
| CHCHD10 deficiency | *CHCHD10* |
| CoQ2 deficiency | *COQ2* |
| **Disorders of lipids** | |
| Primary carnitine deficiency | *SLC22A5* |
| Carnitine palmitoyltransferase 2 deficiency | *CPT2* |
| Carnitine acylcarnitine translocase deficiency | *SLC25A20* |
| Very long-chain acyl CoA dehydrogenase deficiency | *ACADVL* |
| Long-chain 3-hydroxyacyl-CoA dehydrogenase deficiency | *HADHA* |

**Table 2.7** (continued)

| Name | Gene |
|---|---|
| Trifunctional protein deficiency | *HADHB* |
| TANGO2 deficiency | *TANGO2* |
| Lipin 1 deficiency | *LPIN1* |
| Chanarin-Dorfman syndrome | *ABHD5* |
| Adipose triglyceride lipase deficiency | *PNPLA2* |
| Chylomicron retention disease | *SAR1B* |
| Mevalonate kinase deficiency | *MVK* |
| X-linked spinal and bulbar muscular atrophy, Kennedy disease | *AR* |
| **Congenital disorders of glycosylation** | |
| DPAGT1-CDG | *DPAGT1* |
| ALG14-CDG | *ALG14* |
| ALG2-CDG | *ALG2* |
| RFT1-CDG | *RFT1* |
| B4GALT1-CDG | *B4GALT1* |
| POMT1-CDG | *POMT1* |
| POMT2-CDG | *POMT2* |
| POMGNT1-CDG | *POMGNT1* |
| B3GALNT2-CDG | *B3GALNT2* |
| POMK-CDG | *POMK* |
| ISPD-CDG | *ISPD* |
| FKRP-CDG | *FKRP* |
| FKTN-CDG | *FKTN* |
| RXYLT1-CDG | *RXYLT1* |
| B4GAT1-CDG | *B4GAT1* |
| LARGE1-CDG | *LARGE1* |
| DPM1-CDG | *DPM1* |
| DPM2-CDG | *DPM2* |
| DPM3-CDG | *DPM3* |
| MPDU1-CDG | *MPDU1* |
| GNE myopathy | *GNE* |
| GFPT1-CDG | *GFPT1* |
| PGM1-CDG | *PGM1* |
| GMPPB-CDG | *GMPPB* |
| COG6-CDG | *COG6* |
| COG7-CDG | *COG7* |
| COG8-CDG | *COG8* |
| TRAPPC11-CDG | *TRAPPC11* |
| TMEM165-CDG | *TMEM165* |
| **Lactate dehydrogenase (LDH) ↑** | |
| **Disorders of nitrogen-containing compounds** | |
| Lysinuric protein intolerance | *SLC7A7* |
| **Disorders of vitamins, cofactors, metals, and minerals** | |
| Dihydrofolate reductase deficiency | *DHFR* |
| **Disorders of carbohydrates** | |
| Glucose-6-phosphate dehydrogenase deficiency | *G6PD* |
| **Mitochondrial disorders of energy metabolism** | |
| Pitrilysin metallopeptidase 1 deficiency | *PITRM1* |
| **Alkaline phosphatase (ALP) ↑** | |
| **Disorders of nitrogen-containing compounds** | |
| Sodium-dependent multivitamin transporter deficiency | *SLC5A6* |
| **Disorders of carbohydrates** | |
| Transaldolase deficiency | TALDO1 |
| **Mitochondrial disorders of energy metabolism** | |
| Valosin-containing protein superactivity | *VCP* |

(continued)

**Table 2.7** (continued)

| Name | Gene |
|---|---|
| **Disorders of lipids** | |
| 3β-Hydroxy-Δ5-C27-steroid dehydrogenase/isomerase deficiency | *HSD3B7* |
| Δ4-3-Oxosteroid-5β-reductase deficiency | *AKR1D1* |
| Oxysterol 7α-hydroxylase deficiency | *CYP7B1* |
| Peroxisomal branched-chain acyl-CoA oxidase deficiency | *ACOX2* |
| Bile acid-CoA:aminoacid *N*-acyl transferase deficiency | *BAAT* |
| **Congenital disorders of glycosylation** | |
| PIGA-CDG | *PIGA* |
| PIGH-CDG | *PIGH* |
| PIGW-CDG | *PIGW* |
| PIGN-CDG | *PIGN* |
| PIGO-CDG | *PIGO* |
| PIGT-CDG | *PIGT* |
| GPAA1-CDG | *GPAA1* |
| PGAP1-CDG | *PGAP1* |
| PGAP3-CDG | *PGAP3* |
| PGAP2-CDG | *PGAP2* |
| PIGB-CDG | *PIGB* |
| PIGY-CDG | *PIGY* |
| Component of COG complex 4 deficiency COG4-CDG | *COG4* |
| ATP6AP1-CDG | *ATP6AP1* |
| TMEM199-CDG | *TMEM199* |
| CCDC115-CDG | *CCDC115* |
| **Alkaline phosphatase (ALP) ↓** | |
| **Disorders of vitamins, cofactors, metals, and minerals** | |
| Congenital hypophosphatasia | *ALPL* |
| Acrodermatitis enteropathica | *SLC39A4* |
| **Urea ↓** | |
| **Disorders of nitrogen-containing compounds** | |
| Ornithine transcarbamylase deficiency | *OTC* |
| Argininosuccinate synthetase deficiency | *ASS1* |
| Argininosuccinate lyase deficiency | *ASL* |
| Arginase 1 deficiency | *ARG1* |
| Mitochondrial ornithine transporter deficiency | *SLC25A15* |
| **Urea ↑** | |
| **Disorders of vitamins, cofactors, metals, and minerals** | |
| Methylmalonic aciduria due to methylmalonyl-CoA mutase deficiency | *MMUT* |
| Methylmalonic aciduria, cblB type | *MMAB* |
| Methylmalonic aciduria and homocystinuria, cblC type | *MMACHC* |
| **Disorders of carbohydrates** | |
| Transaldolase deficiency | *TALDO* |
| **Disorders of lipids** | |
| Lecithin cholesterol acyl transferase deficiency | *LCAT* |
| **Disorders of peroxisomes and oxalate** | |
| Peroxisomal alanine-glyoxylate aminotransferase deficiency | *AGXT* |
| Glyoxylate reductase/hydroxypyruvate reductase deficiency | *GRHPR* |
| Mitochondrial 4-hydroxy-2-oxoglutarate aldolase deficiency | *HOGA1* |
| **Uric acid ↑** | |
| **Disorders of nitrogen-containing compounds** | |
| Phosphoribosyl pyrophosphate synthetase 1 superactivity | *PRPS1* |
| Hypoxanthine guanine phosphoribosyltransferase deficiency | *HPRT1* |
| Methylmalonyl-CoA mutase deficiency | *MMUT* |
| **Disorders of carbohydrates** | |
| Fanconi-Bickel syndrome | *SLC2A2* |
| Fructose-1-phosphate aldolase deficiency | *ALDOB* |
| Glucose-6-phosphate translocase deficiency | *SLC37A4* |

Table 2.7 (continued)

| Name | Gene |
|---|---|
| Amylo-1,6-glucosidase (debrancher) deficiency | *AGL* |
| Muscle phosphorylase deficiency | *PYGM* |
| Liver glycogen phosphorylase deficiency | *PYGL* |
| Muscle phosphorylase kinase deficiency | *PHKA1* |
| Glucose-6-phosphatase deficiency | *G6PC* |
| Fructose-1,6-bisphosphatase deficiency | *FBP1* |
| Muscle phosphofructokinase deficiency | *PFKM* |
| Muscle phosphoglycerate mutase deficiency | *PGAM2* |
| Lactate dehydrogenase A deficiency | *LDHA* |
| **Mitochondrial disorders of energy metabolism** | |
| Mitochondrial seryl-tRNA synthetase deficiency | *SARS2* |
| **Uric acid ↓** | |
| **Disorders of nitrogen-containing compounds** | |
| Pyrimidine 5′-nucleotidase superactivity | *NT5C3A* |
| Purine nucleoside phosphorylase deficiency | *PNP* |
| Xanthine oxidase deficiency | *XDH* |
| Urate transporter 1 deficiency | *SLC22A12* |
| Urate voltage-driven efflux transporter 1 deficiency | *SLC2A9* |
| **Disorders of vitamins, cofactors, metals, and minerals** | |
| Molybdenum cofactor deficiency A | *MOCS1* |
| Molybdenum cofactor deficiency B | *MOCS2* |
| Molybdenum cofactor deficiency C | *GPHN* |
| Molybdenum cofactor sulfurase deficiency | *MOCOS* |
| **Storage disorders** | |
| Nephropathic cystinosis | *CTNS* |
| **Ferritin ↑** | |
| **Disorders of nitrogen-containing compounds** | |
| Lysinuric protein intolerance | *SLC7A7* |
| Mitochondrial glycine transporter deficiency | *SLC25A38* |
| **Disorders of vitamins, cofactors, metals, and minerals** | |
| Glutaredoxin 5 deficiency | *GLRX5* |
| Hereditary hemochromatosis | *HFE, HFE2, HAMP, TFR2* |
| Aceruloplasminemia | *CP* |
| Hyperferritinemia-cataract syndrome | *FTL* |
| **Mitochondrial disorders of energy metabolism** | |
| GRACILE syndrome | *BCS1L* |
| Mitochondrial deoxyguanosine kinase deficiency | *DGUOK* |
| **Storage disorders** | |
| Gaucher disease | *GBA* |
| **Disorders of tetrapyrroles** | |
| Erythroid 5-aminolevulinate synthase deficiency | *ALAS2* |
| **Ferritin ↓** | |
| **Disorders of vitamins, cofactors, metals, and minerals** | |
| Hypermanganesemia with dystonia type 1 | *SLC30A10* |
| **Disorders of tetrapyrroles** | |
| Ferrochelatase deficiency | *FECH* |
| Erythroid 5-aminolevulinate synthase superactivity | *ALAS2* |
| **Myoglobin (urine) ↑** | |
| **Disorders of vitamins, cofactors, metals, and minerals** | |
| ISCU deficiency | *ISCU* |
| Ferredoxin 2 deficiency | *FDX2* |
| **Disorders of carbohydrates** | |
| Muscle phosphorylase deficiency | *PYGM* |
| Muscle phosphorylase kinase deficiency | *PHKA1* |
| Muscle phosphofructokinase deficiency | *PFKM* |

(continued)

Table 2.7 (continued)

| Name | Gene |
|---|---|
| Muscle phosphoglycerate kinase deficiency | *PGK1* |
| Muscle phosphoglycerate mutase deficiency | *PGAM2* |
| Beta-enolase deficiency | *ENO3* |
| Lactate dehydrogenase A deficiency | *LDHA* |
| **Mitochondrial disorders of energy metabolism** | |
| Mitochondrial cytochrome B deficiency | *MT-CYB* |
| **Disorders of lipids** | |
| Carnitine palmitoyltransferase 2 deficiency | *CPT2* |
| Carnitine acylcarnitine translocase deficiency | *SLC25A20* |
| Very long-chain acyl CoA dehydrogenase deficiency | *ACADVL* |
| Long-chain 3-hydroxyacyl-CoA dehydrogenase deficiency | *HADHA* |
| Trifunctional protein deficiency | *HADHB* |
| TANGO2 deficiency | *TANGO2* |
| Lipin 1 deficiency | *LPIN1* |
| **Congenital disorders of glycosylation** | |
| PGM1-CDG | *PGM1* |
| GMPPB-CDG | *GMPPB* |
| **Hemoglobin ↓ (anemia)** | |
| **Disorders of nitrogen-containing compounds** | |
| CAD trifunctional protein deficiency 50 CAD-CDG | *CAD* |
| Orotate phosphoribosyltransferase deficiency | *UMPS* |
| Pyrimidine-5′-nucleotidase I deficiency | *NT5C3A* |
| Adenylate kinase 1 deficiency | *AK1* |
| Gamma-glutamylcysteine synthetase deficiency | *GCLC* |
| Glutathione synthetase deficiency | *GSS* |
| Lysinuric protein intolerance | *SLC7A7* |
| Isobutyryl-CoA dehydrogenase deficiency | *ACAD8* |
| Propionyl-CoA-carboxylase deficiency PCCA | *PCCA, PPCB* |
| Methylmalonic aciduria due to methylmalonyl-CoA mutase deficiency | *MMUT* |
| Prolidase deficiency | *PEPD* |
| Mitochondrial glycine transporter deficiency | *SLC25A38* |
| **Disorders of vitamins, cofactors, metals, and minerals** | |
| Glutaredoxin 5 deficiency | *GLRX5* |
| ABCB7 deficiency | *ABCB7* |
| Ferredoxin 2 deficiency | *FDX2* |
| Intrinsic factor deficiency | *CBLIF* |
| Cubilin deficiency | *CUBN* |
| Amnionless deficiency | *AMN* |
| Transcobalamin II deficiency | *TCN2* |
| Methylmalonic aciduria and homocystinuria, cblF type | *LMBRD1* |
| Methylmalonic aciduria and homocystinuria, cblJ type | *ABCD4* |
| Methylmalonic aciduria and homocystinuria, cblC type | *MMACHC* |
| Epi-cblC | *MMACHC + PRDX1* |
| cblD disease | *MMADHC* |
| Methionine synthase reductase deficiency | *MTRR* |
| Methionine synthase deficiency | *MTR* |
| Proton-coupled folate transporter (PCFT) deficiency | *SLC46A1* |
| 5,10-Methylene-tetrahydrofolate dehydrogenase deficiency | *MTHFD1* |
| Dihydrofolate reductase deficiency | *DHFR* |
| Thiamine-responsive megaloblastic anemia syndrome | *SLC19A2* |
| Wilson disease | *ATP7B* |
| Atransferrinemia | *TF* |
| **Disorders of carbohydrates** | |
| Glucose transporter 1 deficiency | *SLC2A1* |
| Galactose-1-phosphate uridyltransferase deficiency | *GALT* |
| Glucose-6-phosphate dehydrogenase deficiency | *G6PD* |
| Transaldolase deficiency | *TALDO1* |

Table 2.7 (continued)

| Name | Gene |
|---|---|
| HOIL1 interacting protein deficiency | *RNF31* |
| Muscle phosphofructokinase deficiency | *PFKM* |
| Aldolase A deficiency | *ALDOA* |
| Triosephosphate isomerase deficiency | *TPI1* |
| Muscle phosphoglycerate kinase deficiency | *PGK1* |
| Pyruvate kinase deficiency | *PKLR* |
| **Mitochondrial disorders of energy metabolism** | |
| Mitochondrial dicarboxylate transporter deficiency | *SLC25A10* |
| NADH dehydrogenase beta subcomplex subunit 11 deficiency | *NDUFB11* |
| TMEM126B deficiency | *TMEM126B* |
| COX10 deficiency | *COX10* |
| Mitochondrial ATP synthase F0 subunit 6 deficiency | *MTATP6* |
| CCA-adding tRNA-nucleotidyltransferase deficiency | *TRNT1* |
| Pseudouridine synthase 1 deficiency | *PUS1* |
| Mitochondrial oxodicarboxylate carrier deficiency | *SLC25A21* |
| Mitochondrial leucyl-tRNA synthetase deficiency | *LARS2* |
| Mitochondrial phenylalanyl-tRNA synthetase deficiency | *FARS2* |
| Mitochondrial seryl-tRNA synthetase deficiency | *SARS2* |
| Mitochondrial tyrosyl-tRNA synthetase deficiency | *YARS2* |
| Mitochondrial glutamyl-tRNA(Gln) amidotransferase subunit A deficiency | *QRSL1* |
| Mitochondrial glutamyl-tRNA(Gln) amidotransferase subunit C deficiency | *GATC* |
| Mitochondrial glutamyl-tRNA(Gln) amidotransferase subunit B deficiency | *GATB* |
| DNAJC19 deficiency | *DNAJC19* |
| HSPA9 deficiency | *HSPA9* |
| Sideroflexin 4 deficiency | *SFXN4* |
| **Disorders of lipids** | |
| Thromboxane synthase deficiency | *TBXAS1* |
| Prostaglandin transporter deficiency | *SLCO2A1* |
| Cytosolic phospholipase A2α deficiency | *PLA2G4A* |
| Mevalonate kinase deficiency | *MVK* |
| PMP70 deficiency | *ABCD3* |
| **Disorders of tetrapyrroles** | |
| Erythroid 5-aminolevulinate synthase deficiency | *ALAS2* |
| Uroporphyrinogen cosynthase deficiency | *UROS* |
| Ferrochelatase deficiency | *FECH* |
| GATA1 deficiency | *GATA1* |
| Heme oxygenase 1 deficiency | *HMOX1* |
| Erythropoietic protoporphyria type 2 | *CLPX* |
| **Storage disorders** | |
| Gaucher disease | *GBA* |
| Saposin C deficiency | *PSAP* |
| Lysosomal acid lipase deficiency, severe | *LIPA* |
| Mucopolysaccharidosis-plus | *VPS33A* |
| **Congenital disorders of glycosylation** | |
| ALG8-CDG | *ALG8* |
| Glucose-6-phosphatase catalytic subunit 3 deficiency | *G6PC3* |
| SEC23B-CDG | *SEC23B* |
| **Thrombocytopenia** | |
| **Disorders of nitrogen-containing compounds** | |
| Lysinuric protein intolerance | *SLC7A7* |
| Isovaleryl-CoA dehydrogenase deficiency | *IVD* |
| Propionyl-CoA-carboxylase deficiency | *PCCA, PCCB* |
| Methylmalonyl-CoA mutase deficiency | *MMUT* |
| Prolidase deficiency | *PEPD* |
| **Disorders of vitamins, cofactors, metals, and minerals** | |
| 5,10-Methylene-tetrahydrofolate dehydrogenase deficiency | *MTHFD1* |

(continued)

**Table 2.7** (continued)

| Name | Gene |
|---|---|
| Thiamine-responsive megaloblastic anemia syndrome | *SLC19A2* |
| Wilson disease | *ATP7B* |
| **Disorders of carbohydrates** | |
| Transaldolase deficiency | *TALDO1* |
| **Mitochondrial disorders of energy metabolism** | |
| Mitochondrial cytochrome c deficiency | *CYCS* |
| Mitochondrial leucyl-tRNA synthetase deficiency | *LARS2* |
| Mitochondrial seryl-tRNA synthetase deficiency | *SARS2* |
| **Disorders of lipids** | |
| 3-Oxothiolase deficiency | *ACAT1* |
| Thromboxane synthase deficiency | *TBXAS1* |
| Apolipoprotein E superactivity | *APOE* |
| Mevalonate kinase deficiency | *MVK* |
| **Disorders of tetrapyrroles** | |
| GATA1 deficiency | *GATA1* |
| **Storage disorders** | |
| Gaucher disease | *GBA* |
| Saposin C deficiency | *PSAP* |
| Acid sphingomyelinase deficiency | *SMPD1* |
| **Congenital disorders of glycosylation** | |
| ALG8-CDG | *ALG8* |
| STT3B-CDG | *STT3B* |
| Glucose-6-phosphatase catalytic subunit 3 deficiency | *G6PC3* |
| SLC35A1-CDG | *SLC35A1* |
| **Neutropenia** | |
| **Disorders of nitrogen-containing compounds** | |
| Lysinuric protein intolerance | *SLC7A7* |
| Isovaleryl-CoA dehydrogenase deficiency | *IVD* |
| Propionyl-CoA-carboxylase deficiency | *PCCA, PCCB* |
| Methylmalonyl-CoA mutase deficiency | *MMUT* |
| **Disorders of carbohydrates** | |
| Glucose-6-phosphate translocase deficiency | *SLC37A4* |
| **Mitochondrial disorders of energy metabolism** | |
| Fumarase deficiency | *FH* |
| FBXL4 deficiency | *FBXL4* |
| Tafazzin deficiency | *TAZ* |
| CLPB deficiency | *CLPB* |
| HTRA2 deficiency | *HTRA2* |
| **Disorders of lipids** | |
| 3-Oxothiolase deficiency | *ACAT1* |
| **Disorders of tetrapyrroles** | |
| GATA1 deficiency | *GATA1* |
| **Congenital disorders of glycosylation** | |
| PGM3-CDG | *PGM3* |
| Glucose-6-phosphatase catalytic subunit 3 deficiency | *G6PC3* |
| Jagunal 1 deficiency | *JAGN1* |
| Cohen syndrome | *VPS13B* |
| **Reticulocytosis** | |
| **Disorders of nitrogen-containing compounds** | |
| Gamma-glutamylcysteine synthetase deficiency | *GCLC* |
| Glutathione synthetase deficiency | *GSS* |
| **Disorders of carbohydrates** | |
| Glucose-6-phosphate dehydrogenase deficiency | *G6PD* |
| Muscle phosphofructokinase deficiency | *PFKM* |

**Table 2.7** (continued)

| Name | Gene |
|---|---|
| Aldolase A deficiency | *ALDOA* |
| Triosephosphate isomerase deficiency | *TPI1* |
| Muscle phosphoglycerate kinase deficiency | *PGK1* |
| Pyruvate kinase deficiency | *PKLR* |
| **Disorders of vitamins, cofactors, metals, and minerals** | |
| Wilson disease | *ATP7B* |
| **Disorders of tetrapyrroles** | |
| GATA1 deficiency | *GATA1* |

[a]Causes fasting hypoglycemia with postprandial hyperglycemia
[b]Causes pseudohyperglycemia, as some point-of-care glucometers will falsely read galactose as glucose (discrepancy between capillary bedside glucose and venous glucose)
[c]False elevation with the enzymatic method but not with Jaffé method

is structured according to the proposed nosology of IEMs (Ferreira et al. 2019), and information on diseases and corresponding laboratory tests was obtained from the knowledgebase of IEMs (Lee et al. 2018). The same information can be found in most chapters of this book. Care should be taken to not only interpret one clinical chemistry test result but also always review the other test results which may guide the diagnostic algorithm in a logical direction. As an example, low blood glucose together with low plasma free fatty acids and the absence of ketones will most likely be the result of endocrine anomalies (hyperinsulinism), whereas sharply increased levels of the free fatty acids generally indicate defects of the mitochondrial fatty acid beta-oxidation.

## References

Duran M, Gibson KM. Simple tests. In: Blau N, Duran M, Gibson KM, Dionisi-Vici C, editors. Physician's guide to the diagnosis, treatment, and follow-up of inherited metabolic diseases. Berlin-Heidelberg: Springer; 2014. p. 743–7.

Ferreira CR, van Karnebeek CDM, Vockley J, Blau N. A proposed nosology of inborn errors of metabolism. Genet Med. 2019;21:102–6.

Lee JJY, Wasserman WW, Hoffmann GF, van Karnebeek CDM, Blau N. Knowledge base and mini-expert platform for the diagnosis of inborn errors of metabolism. Genet Med. 2018;20:151–8.

# Amino Acids

3

Marzia Pasquali and Nicola Longo

## Contents



**Summary**

The measurement of amino acids in the blood, plasma, urine, and cerebrospinal fluid is essential for the diagnosis and monitoring of patients with different inherited metabolic diseases, including disorders of amino acid metabolism and transport, organic acidemias, and urea cycle defects. Measurement of amino acids in whole blood spotted on filter paper screens for many amino acidopathies and urea cycle defects in newborns. Plasma amino acids can identify patients with a suspected disorder of amino acid metabolism and/or aid in monitoring treatment. Urinary amino acids screen for disorders of amino acid transport (cystinuria, lysinuric protein intolerance, or Hartnup disease) or for generalized renal tubular dysfunction. The analysis of cerebrospinal fluid, usually in addition to plasma amino acids, is necessary in the evaluation of patients with neurometabolic disorders, such as glycine encephalopathy or disorders of serine metabolism. Traditionally, amino acids in biological fluids have been quantified by ion exchange chromatography using post-column derivatization with ninhydrin and spectrophotometric detection. Newer methodologies are based on liquid chromatographic separation with detection by mass spectrometry or spectrophotometry. Liquid chromatography/tandem mass spectrometry (LC-MS/MS) analysis of amino acids is becoming the method of choice by more and more laboratories because of its speed, sensitivity, and increased specificity. The interpretation of the results of plasma amino acid analysis requires the knowledge of metabolic disorders, availability of age-specific reference ranges, and consideration of physiological factors or medications affecting levels of individual or multiple amino acids.

M. Pasquali · N. Longo (✉)
University of Utah and ARUP Laboratories,
Salt Lake City, UT, USA
e-mail: pasquam@aruplab.com; Nicola.Longo@hsc.utah.edu

## Introduction

Amino acids are the building block of all proteins and are therefore of vital importance for the integrity of the organism. In addition, some amino acids play an additional important role as neurotransmitters (or their precursors), modulators of neurotransmitter action, precursors of hormones, cofactors, purine, and pyrimidines. Amino



N. Blau et al. (eds.), *Physician's Guide to the Diagnosis, Treatment, and Follow-Up of Inherited Metabolic Diseases*,
https://doi.org/10.1007/978-3-030-67727-5_3

acids, with a few exceptions, are water soluble due to the presence of both an amino and a carboxylic group that in water become ionized. Amino acids are filtered by the kidney and could be easily lost in urine in the absence of an efficient renal tubular reabsorption mechanism. There are several amino acid transporters whose deficiency can result in urinary loss of one or a group of amino acids and specific clinical manifestations. Excess amino acids are degraded by specific sets of enzymes, thereby generating energy and urea from the nitrogen group during catabolism. Defects in these enzymes cause inborn errors of amino acid metabolism, almost all of which are transmitted as autosomal recessive traits. This leads to either the buildup of the parent amino acid or its byproducts or of the catabolic products (organic acids) depending on the location of the enzyme block. The nitrogen group of the amino acid upon degradation will result in the formation of ammonia which is then removed by the urea cycle in the liver. The lack of an enzyme or transporter in this cycle will result in hyperammonemia. Accurate measurement of amino acids is essential to diagnose disorders of amino acid metabolism and to follow treatment in patients affected by aminoacidopathies, urea cycle disorders, organic acidemias, or disorders of amino acid transport. This chapter will discuss how amino acids are analyzed in biological fluids and the main alterations encountered in common disorders.

**Table 3.1** Amino acid concentrations in plasma (μmol/L). The values represent the central 95% range of normal results by LC-MS/MS. Number of observations for each age group is indicated in parenthesis

| Amino acid | <1 month ($n$ = 600) | 1–12 months ($n$ = 1300) | >1 year ($n$ = 4000) |
|---|---|---|---|
| Alanine | 140–480 | 150–520 | 160–530 |
| α-Aminoadipate | ≤4 | ≤4 | ≤4 |
| α-Aminobutyrate | ≤40 | ≤40 | ≤40 |
| Arginine | 16–140 | 35–140 | 35–125 |
| Asparagine | 20–80 | 20–80 | 20–80 |
| Aspartic acid | ≤45 | ≤30 | ≤15 |
| Citrulline | 7–40 | 7–40 | 10–45 |
| Cystine | 10–60 | 10–50 | 10–65 |
| Glutamic acid | 30–240 | 30–210 | 15–130 |
| Glutamine | 295–900 | 400–850 | 380–680 |
| Glycine | 160–470 | 120–375 | 140–420 |
| Histidine | 50–130 | 50–130 | 50–130 |
| Hydroxyproline | 15–90 | 10–70 | 5–40 |
| Isoleucine | 20–110 | 30–120 | 30–120 |
| Leucine | 50–180 | 50–180 | 60–180 |
| Lysine | 70–270 | 80–260 | 85–230 |
| Methionine | 15–55 | 15–55 | 15–40 |
| Ornithine | 30–180 | 30–140 | 25–110 |
| Phenylalanine | 30–95 | 30–90 | 30–82 |
| Proline | 110–340 | 100–320 | 90–350 |
| Sarcosine | ≤5 | ≤5 | ≤5 |
| Serine | 90–340 | 90–275 | 60–170 |
| Taurine | 30–250 | 30–170 | 30–130 |
| Threonine | 60–400 | 60–310 | 60–190 |
| Tryptophan | 15–75 | 20–85 | 25–80 |
| Tyrosine | 30–140 | 30–130 | 35–110 |
| Valine | 80–270 | 90–310 | 120–320 |

## Preanalytical Conditions

### Specimens

Amino acids can be measured in different sample types (whole blood, plasma, cerebrospinal fluid, urine) depending upon the reason for the amino acids analysis. Whole blood spotted on filter paper is used almost universally for neonatal screening of inherited disorders of metabolism. Analysis of amino acids in plasma represents the first approach to the study of a patient with a suspected disorder of amino acid metabolism (Table 3.1) (Held et al. 2011; Gregory et al. 1986; Applegarth et al. 1979; Armstrong et al. 2007). This will identify elevated phenylalanine in phenylketonuria, elevated branched-chain amino acids, and the presence of alloisoleucine in maple syrup urine disease, abnormalities of citrulline, and glutamine in different urea cycle defects. The study of urinary amino acids is performed to screen for disorders of amino acids transport, such as cystinuria, lysinuric protein intolerance, or Hartnup disease (Table 3.2) (Parvy et al. 1988). In addition, it is a useful test for renal tubular capacity that becomes abnormal in most cases of renal Fanconi syndrome. The analysis of cerebrospinal fluid (CSF), usually in addition to plasma amino acids, is necessary in the evaluation of patients with neurometabolic disorders, such as glycine encephalopathy or disorders of serine metabolism (Table 3.3) (Applegarth et al. 1979).

Amino acids can be measured also in other biological specimens, such as vitreous fluid (Table 3.4) (Honkanen et al. 2003; Bertram et al. 2008), especially in post-mortem samples, when urine is often not available and blood is unsuitable. However, this type of analysis should be limited to laboratories with experience in these studies, since post-mortem changes rapidly occur even in vitreous fluid. Amniotic fluid has limited value in prenatal diagnosis for aminoacidopathies. Unlike the organic acid disorders, in most amino acid disorders the metabolites do not accumulate before birth. Abnormal amino acid patterns in amniotic fluid have only been found in two of the urea cycle disorders, namely, argininosuccinate lyase deficiency (argininosuccinic acidemia) and argininosuccinate synthetase deficiency (citrullinemia type 1). Tables 3.1, 3.2, 3.3, and 3.4 (Held et al. 2011; Gregory et al. 1986; Applegarth et al. 1979; Armstrong et al. 2007; Parvy et al. 1988; Honkanen et al. 2003; Bertram et al. 2008) list amino acid reference ranges in the blood, urine, CSF, and vitreous fluid and are included as examples. However, it should be noted that, even when using the same

**Table 3.2** Amino acid concentrations in urine expressed in μmol/g creatinine. The values represent the central 95% range of normal results by LC-MS/MS. Number of observations for each age group is indicated in parenthesis

| Amino acid | 0–3 months ($n = 133$) | 3–12 months ($n = 85$) | 1–3 years ($n = 82$) | 3–6 years ($n = 67$) | 6–12 years ($n = 81$) | ≥12 years ($n = 445$) |
|---|---|---|---|---|---|---|
| Alanine | 475–3330 | 270–3020 | 170–1750 | 100–1000 | 80–930 | 60–500 |
| *a*-Aminoadipate | ≤700 | ≤520 | ≤470 | ≤200 | ≤125 | ≤100 |
| *a*-Aminobutyrate | ≤120 | ≤80 | ≤70 | ≤60 | ≤50 | ≤25 |
| *β*-Aminoisobutyrate | ≤6680 | ≤6000 | ≤5500 | ≤3490 | ≤1720 | ≤1200 |
| Arginine | ≤470 | ≤340 | ≤390 | ≤270 | ≤160 | ≤100 |
| Asparagine | 55–1445 | 45–910 | 80–675 | 50–345 | 40–390 | 25–180 |
| Aspartic acid | ≤370 | ≤160 | ≤65 | ≤25 | ≤25 | ≤25 |
| Citrulline | ≤145 | ≤75 | ≤40 | ≤15 | ≤15 | ≤15 |
| Cystine | ≤870 | ≤300 | ≤150 | ≤125 | ≤100 | ≤150 |
| Glutamic acid | ≤560 | ≤360 | ≤190 | ≤80 | ≤70 | ≤52 |
| Glutamine | 380–3860 | 310–3240 | 340–2225 | 300–1525 | 165–1530 | 100–665 |
| Glycine | 1620–19,725 | 915–10,220 | 775–6600 | 600–4600 | 310–5700 | 230–3510 |
| Histidine | 325–4940 | 290–4850 | 340–4420 | 315–2460 | 160–2380 | 80–1130 |
| Homocitrulline | ≤675 | ≤220 | ≤150 | ≤100 | ≤70 | ≤40 |
| Hydroxyproline | ≤6100 | ≤1270 | ≤100 | ≤35 | ≤20 | ≤30 |
| Isoleucine | ≤360 | ≤140 | ≤100 | ≤70 | ≤60 | ≤45 |
| Leucine | 20–420 | 20–195 | 20–190 | 20–110 | 20–100 | ≤45 |
| Lysine | 120–2270 | 55–1260 | 45–930 | 40–475 | 25–440 | ≤355 |
| Methionine | ≤100 | ≤60 | ≤50 | ≤30 | ≤30 | ≤20 |
| 3-Methylhistidine | 160–665 | 155–390 | 150–555 | 130–540 | 120–440 | 100–340 |
| Ornithine | ≤475 | ≤150 | ≤70 | ≤30 | ≤30 | ≤30 |
| Phenylalanine | 45–360 | 65–370 | 50–350 | 35–170 | 30–140 | 1 |
| Phosphoethanolamine | ≤370 | ≤485 | ≤440 | ≤235 | ≤150 | ≤60 |
| Proline | 130–2340 | ≤1190 | ≤170 | ≤60 | ≤40 | ≤35 |
| Sarcosine | ≤300 | ≤75 | ≤25 | ≤25 | ≤25 | ≤25 |
| Serine | 70–4125 | 275–2730 | 390–1890 | 260–990 | 130–1100 | 90–470 |
| Taurine | 95–9800 | ≤7400 | ≤9000 | ≤4400 | ≤3800 | ≤3200 |
| Threonine | 125–2890 | 50–1300 | 85–910 | 50–380 | 40–470 | 25–250 |
| Thryptophan | 25–395 | 45–390 | 45–325 | 35–150 | 20–180 | 15–95 |
| Tyrosine | 50–870 | 70–700 | 65–560 | 40–300 | 40–280 | 15–150 |
| Valine | 40–425 | 30–250 | 40–280 | 30–160 | 20–120 | ≤55 |

method and instrumentation, reference values may vary from laboratory to laboratory. Each laboratory should establish its own reference ranges.

## Patient Status/Patient Information

Clinical information is a necessary element for the accurate interpretation of amino acid profiles and to correctly diagnose patients with disorders of amino acid metabolism. Several common clinical features should prompt an investigation for a metabolic disorder. These include symptoms related to the CNS (lethargy, seizures, coma); GI tract (vomiting, poor feeding, failure to thrive); liver (hepatomegaly); cardiovascular, respiratory, and renal (kidney stones) systems; eye (lens dislocation, retinitis pigmentosa, optic atrophy); skeletal system; and skin. A positive family history (consanguineous parents, affected sibling or family member) and/or a positive newborn screen result should also initiate a diagnostic metabolic work-up. One should keep in mind that the same disease may present with different symptoms at different ages and that inherited disorders of metabolism are not limited to infants and children, with late-onset diseases presenting in adulthood as well. In other words, a metabolic disorder should not be dismissed because of age. Routine chemistry laboratory tests, such as blood gases, pH, electrolytes, anion gap, glucose, and ammonia, provide clues to the kind of metabolic disorder and guide the testing. These laboratory data, along with a brief clinical history, should be made available to the metabolic laboratory for better interpretation of the results. The physiological status of the patient is also important, since significant variations can be seen in post-prandial specimen, after prolonged fasting, and during catabolism. A list of medications taken at the time of specimen collection should also be provided, since some may interfere with the analysis or may cause alterations in the concentration of some amino acids, such as increased glycine levels secondary to valproate therapy.

**Table 3.3** Normal range of amino acid concentrations in CSF, expressed in μmol/L, obtained by LC-MS/MS. The values represent the central 95% range of normal results by LC-MS/MS. Number of observations is indicated in parenthesis

| Amino acid | μmol/L (*n* = 921) |
|---|---|
| Alanine | 16–46 |
| Arginine | 8–31 |
| Asparagine | 4–13 |
| Aspartate | ≤5 |
| Citrulline | ≤5 |
| Cystine | ≤5 |
| Glutamine | 330–630 |
| Glutamic acid | ≤5 |
| Glycine | 5–20 |
| Histidine | 7–24 |
| Hydroxyproline | ≤4 |
| Isoleucine | ≤12 |
| Leucine | 5–22 |
| Lysine | 10–36 |
| Methionine | 2–7 |
| Ornithine | ≤10 |
| Phenylalanine | 6–20 |
| Proline | ≤5 |
| Serine | 18–66 |
| Taurine | ≤13 |
| Threonine | 14–59 |
| Tryptophan | ≤5 |
| Tyrosine | 5–23 |
| Valine | 8–30 |

**Table 3.4** Concentrations of amino acids in vitreous fluid (average ± SD, μmol/L). Modified from Honkanen et al. (2003); Bertram et al. (2008)

| Amino acid | μmol/L (*n* = 17) |
|---|---|
| Alanine | 159.5 ± 54.9 |
| Arginine | 39.4 ± 16.3 |
| Asparagine | 35.8 ± 11.6 |
| Aspartate | 1.4 ± 1.0 |
| GABA | 0.6 ± 0.2 |
| Glutamate | 5.2 ± 2.3 |
| Glutamine | 1192.9 ± 404.4 |
| Glycine | 8.5 ± 2.5 |
| Histidine | 38.4 ± 10.0 |
| Isoleucine | 37.9 ± 11.6 |
| Leucine | 89.7 ± 28.4 |
| Lysine | 115.4 ± 33.7 |
| Methionine | 22.3 ± 8.1 |
| Phenylalanine | 44.4 ± 14.2 |
| Serine | 103.9 ± 24.4 |
| Threonine | 85.5 ± 28.4 |
| Tyrosine | 58.2 ± 18.8 |
| Valine | 112.0 ± 4.4 |

## Specimen Collection

The timing of the specimen collection is important in the detection of metabolic disorders. In acutely ill patients, the blood and urine specimens on admission are likely to be most revealing and most appropriate for metabolic screening. It is good practice to save these specimens from all patients in whom the diagnosis is unclear. For the detection of aminoacidopathies, this is not as critical as it is for other metabolic disorders. For amino acid analysis, the volume of specimen required depends on the methodology used, typically 100–500 μL of plasma or CSF are required. The volume of urine required varies depending on creatinine concentration; each laboratory should list the minimum volumes acceptable for each analysis.

For the diagnosis of most amino acid disorders, blood specimens collected after an overnight fast are preferred or, alternatively, at least 3 h after a meal. Samples from young infants should be collected immediately before the next scheduled feeding (at least 2–3 h after the last feeding). For hyperammonemia screening, postprandial samples are more suited since elevation of blood ammonia may be intermittent and present only in the fed state. It is not uncommon for a laboratory to receive a sample for amino acid analysis collected while the patient is receiving intravenous hyperalimentation. These samples are often uninterpretable as they show elevations in all the amino acids present in the IV solution. If it is possible, intravenous hyperalimentation should be discontinued for at least 2–3 h prior to specimen collection. If intravenous hyperalimentation cannot be discontinued, appropriate care should be taken in drawing the sample away from the site of entry of the solution.

The concentration of the majority of the physiological amino acids is the same in red blood cells and in plasma, with exception of taurine, glutamate, aspartate, and argininosuccinate. Thus, hemolyzed samples may show an increased concentration of these amino acids. The enzyme arginase converts arginine into ornithine and urea and is expressed in red blood cells. Hemolysis will release arginase in the plasma causing hydrolysis of arginine. Therefore, a decrease in arginine with an increase in ornithine is often seen in hemolyzed samples.

Whole blood collected for amino acids analysis should be spun down as soon as possible; the plasma should be kept frozen during transport and until analysis is performed. Refrigerated conditions may be acceptable for a short period of time. Improper handling of specimens can result in artifactual changes in the amino acid contents. Table 3.5 lists possible artifacts due to collection, handling, and storage of samples.

**Table 3.5** Collection, handling, and storage artifacts

| Factor/condition | Source | Amino acid(s) affected | Value |
|---|---|---|---|
| Contamination, bacterial | U | Ala, Gly, Pro | ↑ H |
| Contamination, bacterial | U | Trp, aromatic amino acids, Ser | ↓ L |
| Contamination, fecal | U | Pro, Glu, Leu, Ile, Val, OH-pro-line | ↑ H |
| Contamination, protein | U | Cys | ↓ L |
| Contamination, RBC | U | Orn | ↑ H |
| Contamination, unwashed skin | B | Most amino acids | ↑ H |
| Contamination, WBC | U | Tau | ↑ H |
| Contamination, WBC | B | Asp, Glu, Tau | ↑ H |
| Hemolysis | B | Asp, Glu, Gly, Orn | ↑ H |
| Hemolysis | B | Arg, Gln | ↓ L |
| Serum vs. plasma | B | Serum Tau > plasma Tau | |
| Storage | U | Glu, Asp, GABA | ↑ H |
| Storage | U | Gln, Asn, phosphoethanolamine | ↓ L |
| Storage | B | Gln, Cys, homocystine | ↓ L |
| Storage | B | Glu | ↑ H |
| Tube artifact, thrombin | B | Gly | ↑ H |
| Tube artifact, EDTA | B | Ninhydrin positive artifact | |
| Tube artifact, metasulfite | B | *S*-sulfocysteine | ↑ H |
| Unspun blood left at rm. temp. | B | Orn, total homocysteine | ↑ H |
| Unspun blood left at rm. temp. | B | Arg, Cys, homocystine | ↓ L |

**Table 3.6** Nutritional status and amino acid values

| Factor/condition | Source | Amino acid(s) affected | Value |
|---|---|---|---|
| Diet, canned formula or milk | U | Homocitrulline | ↑ H |
| Diet, gelatin | U | Gly | ↑ H |
| Diet, high protein (infants) | B | Met, Tyr | ↑ H |
| Diet, shellfish | U | Taurine | ↑ H |
| Diet, white meat from fowl | U | Anserine, 1-methylhistidine, carnosine | ↑ H |
| Folate deficiency | B | Total Homocyst(e)ine | ↑ H |
| Kwashiorkor | B | Pro, Ser, Gly, Phe | ↑ H |
| Kwashiorkor | B | Leu, Ile, Val, Trp, Met, Thr, Arg | ↓ L |
| Obesity | B | Branched chain amino acids, Phe,Tyr | ↑ H |
| Obesity | B | Gly | ↓ L |
| Starvation, 1–2 days (with or without vomiting) | B | Branched chain amino acids, Gly | ↑ H |
| Starvation, 1–2 days (with or without vomiting) | B | Alanine | ↓ L |
| Vitamin B12 deficiency | B | Total homocyst(e)ine | ↑ H |
| Vitamin B6 deficiency | U | Cystathionine | ↑ H |

*B* blood, *U* urine, *H* increased, *L* decreased

The conversion of arginine into ornithine by arginase can be observed even in unspun samples left at room temperature, even without obvious hemolysis. Free cystine and homocystine bind to protein and will be lost in samples that are not spun immediately and/or are stored for a prolonged period of time. The loss of cystine and homocystine is evident even when samples are stored at −20 °C, while storage at −70 °C prevents this effect. Glutamine is unstable and breaks down with prolonged storage resulting in increased glutamate.

If serum is used for amino acids analysis, depending on how it has been obtained, all the artifacts listed above could be present. Low serine in urine may be due to bacterial contamination, and the presence of hydroxyproline can be due to fecal contamination. Urine is not the fluid of choice in the diagnostic investigation of an aminoacidopathy (phenylketonuria, maple syrup urine disease, homocystinuria, etc.) as plasma is a better sample type. Urine amino acids analysis is, instead, the diagnostic test when disorders of amino acid transport are investigated (cystinuria, lysinuric protein intolerance, Hartnup) or in prolidase deficiency. Although a random specimen is usually sufficient for diagnostic purposes, a timed urine collection may be required for reabsorption studies in conjunction with a plasma sample collected at mid-point. Results of urine amino acids analysis are usually reported in reference to creatinine; however for samples very diluted or very concentrated, this correction may not be very accurate. The interpretation of urine amino acids relies on patterns of amino acids more than on absolute values; therefore, a careful examination of the profile should lead to a correct diagnosis. Tables 3.5, 3.6, 3.7, and 3.8 list artifacts due to specimen collection as well as the effect of nutritional status, illnesses, and medications on amino acids values.

## Analysis

Amino acids studies are performed for (1) diagnostic purposes and (2) monitoring of therapy in patients with a known metabolic disorder. Methods for amino acids analysis should be sensitive (to identify even very low concentration of

**Table 3.7** Effects of illness/disease on amino acid values

| Factor/condition | Source | Amino acid(s) affected | Value |
|---|---|---|---|
| Burn >20% of surface area (0–7 days after injury) | B | Phe | ↑ H |
| Burn >20% of surface area (0–7 days after injury) | U | Ala, Gly, Thr, Ser, Glu, Gln, Orn, Pro | ↓ L |
| Diabetes | B | Leu, Ile, Val | ↑ H |
| Hepatic disease | B | Tyr, Phe, Met, Orn, GABA | ↑ H |
| Hepatic disease | B | Branched chain amino acids | ↓ L |
| Hepatoblastoma | U | Cystathionine | ↑ H |
| Hyperinsulinism | B | Leu, Ile, Val | ↓ L |
| Hypoparathyroidism, primary | U | All amino acids | ↑ H |
| Infection | B | All amino acids | ↓ L |
| Infection | B | Phe/Tyr ratio | ↑ H |
| Infection | U | All amino acids | ↑ H |
| Ketosis | B | Leu, Ile, Val | ↑ H |
| Ketotic hypoglycemia | B | Ala | ↓ L |
| Leukemia, acute | U | Advanced disease: all amino acids | ↑ H |
| Leukemia, acute | U | On therapy: gly, asp, thr, ser | ↑ H |
| Neuroblastoma | U | Cystathionine | ↑ H |
| Renal failure | U | Phe, Val | ↓ L |
| Renal failure | U | His | ↑ H |
| Renal failure | B | Phe, Cit, Cys, Gln, homocyst(e)ine | ↑ H |
| Renal failure | B | Leu, Val, Ile, Glu, Ser | ↓ L |
| Respiratory distress on oxygen | B | Cystine | ↓ L |
| Rickets | U | Gly | ↑ H |

*B* blood, *U* urine, *H* increased, *L* decreased

**Table 3.8** Effect of medications on amino acid values

| Factor/condition | Source | Amino acid(s) affected | Value |
|---|---|---|---|
| Arginine infusion | B | Arg | ↑ H |
| Arginine infusion | U | Arg, Lys, Orn, Cys | ↑ H |
| Bile acid sequestrants (colestipol, niacin) | B | Homocyst(e)ine | ↑ H |
| Cyclosporin A | B | Total homocysteine | ↑ H |
| 2-Deoxycoformycin | B | Homocyst(e)ine | ↓ L |
| Lysine aspirin | U | Lys | ↑ H |
| Methotrexate therapy | B | Homocyst(e)ine | ↑ H |
| Methotrexate therapy | B | Phe/Tyr ratio | ↑ H |
| Nitrous oxide anesthesia | B | Homocyst(e)ine | ↑ H |
| Oral contraceptives | B | Pro, Gly, Ala, Val, Leu, Tyr | ↓ L |
| D-Phenylalanine | U | Phe | ↑ H |
| Tamoxifen | B | Homocyst(e)ine | ↓ L |
| Tetracycline, renal toxicity | U | All amino acids | ↑ H |
| Valproate | B,U | Gly | ↑ H |
| Vigabatrin/vinyl-GABA | U | $\beta$-alanine, $\beta$-aminoisobutyrate, GABA | ↑ H |
| Vigabatrin/vinyl-GABA | CSF | GABA, $\beta$-alanine | ↑ H |
| Vigabatrin/vinyl-GABA | B,U | 2-Aminoadipic acid | ↑ H |

*B* blood, *U* urine, *H* increased, *L* decreased

amino acids), specific (to separate isomeric species), and accurate (to enable monitoring of dietary therapy).

Paper chromatography, thin-layer chromatography, and two-dimensional chromatography by high-voltage electrophoresis for amino acids screening have been used in the past, but are now obsolete and should not be used for amino acids screening.

Quantitative analysis of amino acids in physiological fluids can be performed by ion-exchange chromatography (IEC), reverse-phase high-performance liquid chromatography (HPLC), gas-chromatography (GC), and liquid chromatography/tandem mass spectrometry (LC-MS/MS).

**IEC** has been the most widely used method in clinical laboratories, and it is still considered the gold standard for amino acid analysis. With this technique, amino acids are separated using a cation-exchange column and a lithium buffer system. The detection is performed by colorimetry after post-column derivatization with ninhydrin. The adduct between ninhydrin and primary amines has a maximum absorbance at wavelength $\lambda_{max}$ = 570 nm, while the adduct between ninhydrin and secondary amines (hydroxyproline, proline) has a $\lambda_{max}$ = 440 nm. The samples are monitored at both wavelengths to allow quantification of all physiological amino acids. This method is highly reproducible, with a wide dynamic range and excellent linearity range (5–3000 μmol/L). The disadvantage of the method is the long analysis time (90–150 min) and the lack of specificity. In fact several metabolites other than amino acids, including medications and dietary supplements, react with ninhydrin and coelute with amino acids. This is particularly challenging when evaluating urine samples. Depending on the methodology used, special processing of the sample is required to identify and quantify certain amino acids. A classic example is argininosuccinic acid. With IEC the free acid elutes in the region of neutral amino acids, often coeluting with tyrosine or leucine, depending on the buffer system and column used. Conversion of the free acid into anhydrides by boiling the deproteinized sample increases sensitivity and allows more accurate results.

**HPLC**-based methods usually require a pre-column derivatization step with chemicals that react with the primary or secondary amino group of amino acids to form derivatives detectable with fluorescent, UV, or electrochemical detectors. The analysis time of these methods is shorter than ion-exchange chromatography, but sample preparation is more laborious and the derivatives may be instable. In addition, the sensitivity for some critical amino acids, such as alloisoleucine (the diagnostic amino acid for maple syrup urine disease), argininosuccinic acid (the diagnostic amino acid for argininosuccinic acid lyase deficiency), and homocystine may not be sufficient to identify mild elevations of these amino acids and some patients can be missed.

**Tandem mass spectrometry** analysis of amino acids by flow injection is routinely used for neonatal screening using whole blood spotted on filter paper. Amino acids are extracted from the blood spot using an organic solvent (methanol) containing stable-isotope-labeled amino acids. The limitation of this method is that isomers and isobars cannot be separated; however, the speed of the analysis makes it a superb screening method. For diagnostic and/or monitoring purposes, similar methods can be used, and to increase the specificity, a liquid chromatographic separation is performed prior to MS/MS detection. **Liquid chromatography/tandem mass spectrometry** (LC-MS/MS) analysis of amino acids in physiological fluids is now the method of choice by more and more laboratories, because of its speed, sensitivity, and increased specificity. Accurate quantitation by MS/MS requires the use of stable-isotope-labeled internal standards; ideally each amino acid quantified should have its internal standard. The detection of amino acids by MS/MS is usually done using selective reaction monitoring (SRM); therefore, the analysis is targeted. This method will not detect unusual amino acids, such as cystinylglycine (characteristic of gamma glutamyltranspeptidase deficiency), unless they are included in the method. As a consequence, amino acids analysis methods available for clinical diagnostic application are not suitable for new discovery. With the use of MS/MS for neonatal screening, milder variants of metabolic disorders are now identified, and the biochemical phenotype may be more subtle. Good communication between the testing laboratory and the physicians helps in clarifying these cases.

The method used for quantifying amino acids in physiological fluids should also have a wide dynamic range, high sensitivity, sufficient to measure concentrations as low as a few micromoles/liter, and high upper limit of linearity, to accurately quantify high concentrations of amino acids for diet/therapy monitoring. Citrulline, alloisoleucine, argininosuccinic acid, and free homocystine are examples of amino acids requiring high sensitivity, with citrulline and argininosuccinic acid requiring also high upper limit of linearity. It is important to be able to detect even trace amounts of these amino acids to reach a correct diagnosis. LC-MS/MS-based methods are usually highly sensitive and specific; however, their dynamic range may not be as good as IEC.

## Interpretation of Amino Acids Results and Reference Values

Clinical information, age of the patient, diet, and medications are critical to provide an accurate interpretation for metabolic testing in general, including amino acids analysis. The interpretation of amino acid profiles relies on pattern recognition; therefore, laboratories should be familiar with metabolic disorders and the changes observed in presence of a metabolic block. In the past when most laboratories used similar methods, amino acids were reported in the order of chromatographic separation. With the advent of different methodologies, many laboratories report amino acids in alphabetical order to facilitate their reading and personal interpretation by referring physicians. All of our tables now report them in alphabetical order.

**Age**. The normal concentration range of most amino acids changes with age, and appropriate reference ranges are essential for accurate interpretation. Renal tubular function is not mature in many infants who can have generalized aminoaciduria until several months of age. Homocitrulline in the urine of infants is usually derived from diet and is only rarely due to a metabolic disorder. Taurine is normally excreted in large amounts in the first week of life and decreases thereafter. However, the urine from infants less than 1 year of age often contains taurine from breast milk and/or taurine-supplemented formula, and the amount can fluctuate widely depending on the time of urine collection in relation to the time of feeding. Taurine is not detected in urine from infants fed unsupplemented formulas. Taurine is a constituent of several energy drinks and can increase in adolescents and young adults consuming these products. Administration of parenteral amino acid solutions can also cause altered blood amino acid patterns.

The urinary excretion of glycine is quite variable. It can be of dietary origin (e.g., gelatin) as well as secondary to medication (e.g., valproate). Persistent isolated hyperglycinuria with normal plasma glycine levels suggests familial iminoglycinuria that is usually a benign variant. Urine histidine is increased during pregnancy. The concentration of plasma amino acids is low compared to normal controls during pregnancy, especially in the last trimester, due to hemodilution.

In young infants, particularly in preterm infants, the quantity and quality of protein feeding has a direct effect on the plasma amino acid concentrations. The postprandial rise of total amino acids is more pronounced in infants on higher protein feeding. Transient hypertyrosinemia and hypermethioninemia can result from excessive protein load such as with the use of non-infant milk. The same pattern of elevation can be seen in premature infants or infants with immature hepatocellular function. Table 3.6 lists the most common effects of diet and nutritional status on amino acid values.

**Circadian rhythm** is a physiological basis for higher amino acid concentrations, up to 10–15%, in the blood in the afternoon. A mild generalized increase in urine amino acids is a relatively common finding in hospitalized children. Branched-chain amino acids are elevated in blood of patients with maple syrup urine disease; however, in these patients the presence of alloisoleucine allows the correct interpretation of the results. Vomiting and poor oral intake for 1–2 days may cause mild elevations (two- to threefold) of the plasma branched-chain amino acids, and this should not be mistaken as a disease pattern. In a patient with MSUD and metabolic decompensation, the pattern of branched-chain amino acids will show a disproportionately high leucine compared to isoleucine and valine and a markedly reduced alanine in addition to the presence of alloisoleucine. With ion-exchange chromatography, alloisoleucine coelutes with cystathionine, and laboratories using this method should develop protocols to distinguish the two amino acids, such as the evaluation of the ratio of the absorbance at 570 nm and 440 nm, which is much lower for cystathionine as compared to alloisoleucine.

**Secondary amino acid changes** can be a clue to other types of metabolic disorders such as galactosemia, organic acidemias, and disorders of pyruvate metabolism.

Gross elevations of many amino acids, particularly glutamine and alanine in blood, have been reported in moribund children; however, elevations of the branched-chain amino acids, citrulline, and arginine can be secondary to hypoxia and liver failure. Post-mortem blood shows similar but more pronounced amino acid changes (Table 3.7).

**Citrulline** is the amino acid critical in identifying disorders of the urea cycle. It is absent or markedly reduced in proximal blocks of the urea cycle (NAGS, CPS1, OTC deficiencies); it is markedly elevated in citrullinemia type I (argininosuccinate synthase deficiency) and, to a lower extent, in argininosuccinic aciduria (argininosuccinate lyase deficiency); and it is moderately but variably elevated in citrullinemia type II (citrin deficiency). Citrulline can also be used to assess functional enterocyte mass in patients with necrotizing enterocolitis, short bowel syndrome, and intestinal transplant. Very low levels of citrulline can be seen in these patients, usually with a completely normal concentration of all other amino acids, including glutamine.

**Several medications** can affect the levels or interfere with quantitation of amino acids in blood and urine (Table 3.8). The use of disulfide agents, such as penicillamine, can result in the formation of unusual amino acids whose quantitation can help in determining compliance with therapy.

Table 3.9 lists the amino acids and the disorders in which the amino acid level is abnormal. An abnormal concentration of an amino acid may be suggestive of several different inborn errors. Conversely, some disorders are characterized by abnormalities in several different amino acids, and analysis of the pattern of variation is more important than analysis of a single amino acid level in establishing a diagnosis. This table serves as a quick guide to more detailed information found in other chapters in this book.

**Table 3.9** Pathologic conditions associated with abnormal amino acids concentrations

| Amino acid | Source | Disorder(s) | Value |
|---|---|---|---|
| All amino acids | U | Classic galactosemia, Renal Fanconi syndrome, Lowe syndrome | ↑ H |
| All amino acids | U | Tyrosinemia type 1, hereditary fructose intolerance | ↑ H |
| All amino acids | U | Vitamin D-dependent rickets, mitochondrial disorders | ↑ H |
| Neutral amino acids | U | Hartnup disorder | ↑ H |
| Alanine | P | Lactic acidosis, disorders of pyruvate metabolism, mitochondrial disorders, hyperammonemic syndromes, glucagon receptor defect | ↑ H |
| Alanine | P | Maple syrup urine disease | ↓ L |
| β-Alanine | P/U | β-Alaninemia | ↑ H |
| β-Alanine | CSF | GABA-transaminase deficiency | ↑ H |
| β-Alanine | U | Pyrimidine disorders, methylmalonate semialdehyde dehydrogenase deficiency | ↑ H |
| Allo-isoleucine | P/U/ CSF | Maple syrup urine disease, $E_3$ deficiency | ↑ H |
| α-Aminoadipic | U | α-Aminoadipic/α-Ketoadipic aciduria | ↑ H |
| β-Aminoisobutyric acid | U | β-Alaninemia, β-Aminoisobutyric acid aminotransferase deficiency (benign) | ↑ H |
| δ-Aminolevulinic acid | U | Tyrosinemia type I, porphyria | ↑ H |
| Arginine | U | Cystinuria, dibasic aminoaciduria, lysinuric protein intolerance | ↑ H |
| Arginine | P | Arginase deficiency, glucagon receptor defect | ↑ H |
| Arginine | P | HHH syndrome, ornithine aminotransferase deficiency, urea cycle defects (except arginase deficiency) | ↓ L |
| Argininosuccinate | P/U/ CSF | Argininosuccinate lyase deficiency | ↑ H |
| Asparagine | P/CSF | Asparagine synthase deficiency | ↓ L |
| Aspartic acid | U | Dicarboxylic aminoaciduria | ↑ H |
| Aspartic acid | U | Pyruvate carboxylase deficiency type B | ↓ L |
| Aspartylglucosamine | P/U | Aspartylglucosamidase deficiency | ↑ H |
| Carnosine | U | Carnosinemia | ↑ H |
| Citrulline | P | Citrullinemia type I (argininosuccinate synthase deficiency), Citrullinemia type II (citrin deficiency), argininosuccinate lyase deficiency, pyruvate carboxylase deficiency type B | ↑ H |

Table 3.9 (continued)

| Amino acid | Source | Disorder(s) | Value |
|---|---|---|---|
| Citrulline | P | Δ-pyrroline-5-carboxylate synthase deficiency, lysinuric protein intolerance, NAGS, CPS, OTC deficiencies, mitochondrial disorders | ↓ L |
| Cystathionine | P/U | Cystathionase deficiency | ↑ H |
| Cystine | U | Cystinuria, hyperlysinemia, hyperornithinemia | ↑ H |
| Cystine | P | Molybdenum cofactor deficiency, sulfite oxidase deficiency | ↓ L |
| Formiminoglutamic acid (FIGLU) | U | Formiminoglutamic aciduria | ↑ H |
| GABA | P/U | β-Alaninemia | ↑ H |
| GABA | P/U/CSF | GABA transaminase deficiency | ↑ H |
| Glutamic acid | U | Dicarboxylic aminoaciduria | ↑ H |
| Glutamic acid | P | Glutamic acidemia, glutamine synthase deficiency | ↑ H |
| Glutamine | P/U/CSF | Urea cycle defects | ↑ H |
| Glutamine | P | Glutaminase deficiency (normal ammonia) | ↑ H |
| Glutamine | P | Glutamine synthase deficiency, propionic acidemia, methylmalonic acidemia, maple syrup urine disease, pyruvate carboxylase deficiency | ↓ L |
| Glycine | P/U/CSF | Glycine encephalopathy, glycine transporter deficiency, propionic acidemia, methylmalonic acidemia, D-Glyceric aciduria | ↑ H |
| Glycine | U | Familial renal iminoglycinuria, hyperprolinemia type I and II | ↑ H |
| Glycine | P/CSF | Serine deficiency disorders | ↓ L |
| Glycylproline | U | Prolidase deficiency | ↑ H |
| Hawkinsin | U | Hawkinsinuria | ↑ H |
| Histidine | P/U | Histidinemia | ↑ H |
| Homoarginine | P/U | Hyperlysinemia | ↑ H |
| Homocarnosine | CSF | Homocarnosinosis | ↑ H |
| Homocitrulline | P/U | HHH syndrome, saccharopinuria | ↑ H |
| Homocyst(e)ine | P/U | Cystathionine-β-synthase deficiency, cobalamin disorders, folate disorders, methionine synthase (MS) and MS reductase deficiency | ↑ H |
| Homocyst(e)ine | P | Methionine adenosyltransferase deficiency, *S*-Adenosylhomocysteine hydrolase deficiency, glycine-*N*-methyltransferase deficiency, adenosine kinase deficiency | ↑ H |
| Homocysteine-cysteine disulfide | P | Cystathionine-β-synthase deficiency | ↑ H |
| Total Homocysteine | P | Molybdenum cofactor deficiency, sulfite oxidase deficiency | ↓ L |
| Hydroxylysine | U | Hydroxylysinuria | ↑ H |
| Hydroxyproline | U | Familial renal iminoglycinuria, hyperprolinemia type I and II | ↑ H |
| Hydroxyproline | P/U | Hydroxyprolinemia | ↑ H |
| Imidodipeptides | U | Prolidase deficiency | ↑ H |
| Isoleucine | P/U | Maple syrup urine disease, E3 deficiency | ↑ H |
| Leucine | P/U | Maple syrup urine disease, E3 deficiency | ↑ H |
| Lysine | U | Cystinuria, lysinuric protein intolerance, dibasic aminoaciduria | ↑ H |
| Lysine | P/U | Hyperlysinemia, saccharopinuria | ↑ H |
| Lysine | P | HHH syndrome, ornithine aminotransferase deficiency, lysinuric protein intolerance | ↓ L |
| Lysine | P | Urea cycle defects, pyruvate carboxylase deficiency type B | ↑ H |
| Methionine | P/CSF | Homocysteine remethylation disorders | ↓ L |
| Methionine | P/U | Cystathionine-β-synthase deficiency, hypermethioninemias | ↑ H |
| Methionine sulfoxide | P | Cystathionine-β-synthase deficiency, hypermethioninemias | ↑ H |
| Ornithine | U | Cystinuria, dibasic aminoaciduria, hyperlysinemia, lysinuric protein intolerance | ↑ H |
| Ornithine | P | HHH syndrome, ornithine aminotransferase deficiency | ↑ H |
| Ornithine | P | Δ-pyrroline-5-carboxylate synthase deficiency | ↓ L |
| Phenylalanine | P/U | Phenylketonuria, hyperphenylalaninemias, pterin disorders | ↑ H |
| Phenylalanine | P | Tyrosinemia type I | ↑ H |
| Phosphoethanolamine | U | Hypophosphatasia | ↑ H |
| Pipecolic acid | P | Hyperlysinemia, antiquitin deficiency (pyridoxine responsive seizures) | ↑ H |
| Pipecolic acid | U | Hyperprolinemia type II | ↑ H |
| Pipecolic acid | P/U | Peroxisomal disorders | ↑ H |
| Proline | P | Δ-pyrroline-5-carboxylate synthase deficiency | ↓ L |

(continued)

**Table 3.9** (continued)

| Amino acid | Source | Disorder(s) | Value |
|---|---|---|---|
| Proline | U | Familial renal iminoglycinuria | ↑ H |
| Proline | P/U | Hyperprolinemia type I and II, lactic acidosis, multiple acyl-CoA dehydrogenase deficiency | ↑ H |
| Saccharopine | P/U | Saccharopinuria | ↑ H |
| Sarcosine | P/U | Sarcosinemia, mitochondrial disorders, glutaric acidemia type II, Betaine therapy | ↑ H |
| Serine | P/CSF | Serine deficiency disorders | ↓ L |
| *S*-Sulfocysteine | P/U | Molybdenum cofactor deficiency, sulfite oxidase deficiency | ↑ H |
| Taurine | U | Molybdenum cofactor deficiency, sulfite oxidase deficiency, β-Alaninemia | ↑ H |
| Threonine | P/CSF | Pyridoxal phosphate-dependent seizures, citrullinemia type II (citrin deficiency) | ↑ H |
| Tryptophan | U | Tryptophanuria | ↑ H |
| Tyrosine | P/U | Tyrosinemia type I, II, III, transient tyrosinemia of the newborn | ↑ H |
| Tyrosine | P | Phenylketonuria, pterin disorders | ↓ L |
| Valine | P/U | Maple syrup urine disease, E3 deficiency, branched chain amino transferase 2 deficiency | ↑ H |

*P* plasma, *U* urine, *CSF* cerebrospinal fluid, *H* high, *L* low

## References


Applegarth DA, Edelstein AD, Wong LT, Morrison BJ. Observed range of assay values for plasma and cerebrospinal fluid amino acid levels in infants and children aged 3 months to 10 years. Clin Biochem. 1979;12:173–8.

Armstrong M, Jonscher K, Reisdorph NA. Analysis of 25 underivatized amino acids in human plasma using ion-pairing reversed-phase liquid chromatography/time-of-flight mass spectrometry. Rapid Commun Mass Spectrom. 2007;21:2717–26.

Bertram KM, Bula DV, Pulido JS, Shippy SA, Gautam S, Lu MJ, Hatfield RM, Kim JH, Quirk MT, Arroyo JG. Amino-acid levels in subretinal and vitreous fluid of patients with retinal detachment. Eye. 2008;22:582–9.

Gregory DM, Sovetts D, Clow CL, Scriver CR. Plasma free amino acid values in normal children and adolescents. Metab Clin Exp. 1986;35:967–9.

Held PK, White L, Pasquali M. Quantitative urine amino acid analysis using liquid chromatography tandem mass spectrometry and aTRAQ reagents. J Chromatogr B Analyt Technol Biomed Life Sci. 2011;879:2695–703.

Honkanen RA, Baruah S, Zimmerman MB, Khanna CL, Weaver YK, Narkiewicz J, Waziri R, Gehrs KM, Weingeist TA, Boldt HC, Folk JC, Russell SR, Kwon YH. Vitreous amino acid concentrations in patients with glaucoma undergoing vitrectomy. Arch Ophthalmol. 2003;121:183–8.

Parvy PR, Bardet JI, Rabier DM, Kamoun PP. Age-related reference values for free amino acids in first morning urine specimens. Clin Chem. 1988;34:2092–5.

# Organic Acids

# 4

Isabel Tavares de Almeida and Antonia Ribes

## Contents



**Abstract**

Organic acid disorders (OAD) are a relevant group of inborn errors of metabolism (IEM), not only in severely ill children but in adults as well, namely, with neurological symptoms. OAD are due to defect in intermediary metabolic pathways of carbohydrate, amino acids, lipids, Krebs cycle, vitamins, and nucleic acids, leading to the accumulation in the body fluids of the so-called organic acids, the metabolic pathways' intermediates. Analysis of organic acids profiles is a powerful tool for the IEM differential diagnosis. Herein, an updated reference guide in OAD is presented, incorporating the affected protein, the altered gene, and the organic acids with diagnostic value. Valuable clues for the correct interpretation of an organic acids profile are discussed with focus on some puzzling organic acids and on the artefacts arising from diet, gut bacterial action, drugs, and sample bacterial contamination.

I. Tavares de Almeida (✉)
Metabolism and Genetics, iMed.UL, Faculdade de Farmácia da Universidade de Lisboa, Avenida Prof. Gama Pinto, Lisboa, Portugal
e-mail: italmeida@ff.ul.pt

A. Ribes
Section of Inborn Errors of Metabolism, Department of Biochemistry and Molecular Genetics, Hospital Clinic de Barcelona, IDIBAPS, CIBERER, Barcelona, Spain
e-mail: aribes@clinic.cat

## Introduction

Organic acid disorders (OAD) are a relevant group of inborn errors of metabolism (IEM), not only in severely-ill children but as well in adults, namely, with neurological symptoms.

OAD are due to defects in intermediary metabolism of various cellular components, such as amino acids, lipids, carbohydrates, Krebs cycle, vitamins, nucleic acids, and steroids. It gives rise to the accumulation, in tissues and body fluids, of diverse metabolic pathways' intermediates: the organic acids. More than 65 organic acidurias have been described; the incidence varies, individually, from 1 out of 10,000 to >1 out of 1,000,000 live births. Collectively, their incidence approximates 1 out of 3000 live births (Villani et al. 2017).

Organic acids are low-molecular weight (mass < 300) organic substances, with one or more carboxylic acid groups, and may have keto or hydroxy groups, making them polar compounds. Over all, the physiological organic acids are weak acids, which implies that they are fully ionized at $pH > 4$, i.e., values observed in plasma or urine. Consequently, accumulation of organic acids in the blood ("acidemia") will lead to a shift in blood pH to lower values with the emerging of the so-called metabolic acidosis, which is accompanied by a negative base excess as well as an increased anion gap. The organic acids are strongly hydrophilic compounds enabling their rapid excretion into the urine ("aciduria"), the preferably biological fluid for the analysis of organic acids. Fatty




N. Blau et al. (eds.), *Physician's Guide to the Diagnosis, Treatment, and Follow-Up of Inherited Metabolic Diseases*,
https://doi.org/10.1007/978-3-030-67727-5_4

acids with chain length > $C_8$ such as lauric, palmitic, and oleic acids are non-polar organic acids, which are bound to plasma proteins and are not excreted into the urine.

Physiologically, organic acids are often present as their coenzyme A esters; good examples are propionyl-CoA and isovaleryl-CoA. To facilitate its excretion, the metabolites are conjugated with carnitine or glycine, a process similar to the one leading to the production of acylglucuronides. Formation of acylcarnitines and acylglycines can be regarded as a process aimed at restoring the coenzyme A homeostasis, being at the same time a process of detoxification of the harmful organic acids.

From a biochemical point of view, OAD are characterized by the accumulated organic acids, in body fluids, which may display a panel of organic acids, more or less specific, incorporating primary and unusual secondary metabolites, the by-products of alternative metabolic pathways, as well as specific acylcarnitines and/or acylglycines, often crucial in the unequivocal characterization of the OAD and a single pathognomonic metabolite (cf. *N*-acetylaspartic acid in Canavan disease) or the "normal" physiological metabolites in enhanced concentration (cf. methylmalonic acid in Vit$B_{12}$ deficiency).

Organic acid analysis is a key diagnostic hint for the achievement of the differential diagnosis in systemic intoxication, in unexplained metabolic crisis, or in the presence of inexplicable routine biochemical findings such as metabolic acidosis, altered anion gap, and hypoglycemia among others. Amino acids and lipid intermediary metabolic defects, namely, branched chain amino acids and fatty acids catabolic pathways, are the leading causes of organic acidurias. Nevertheless, several hundreds of other organic acids or similar structural compounds with diagnostic value can be identified in a single run; typical examples are orotic acid, thymine, and uracil and their respectively di-hydro derivatives, glycerol, and several others derived from medication or diet. Key metabolites reference guide that may allow the biochemical diagnosis or raise the suspicion of an organic aciduria is shown in Table 4.1, which is organized, whenever possible, according the IEM-adopted classification in this book.

Organic acid analysis by gas chromatography-mass spectrometry (GC/MS) is a powerful methodology providing the identification of normal and abnormal acids, which have allowed for the discovery of new disorders and the biochemical characterization of a great set of diseases. The complementation with acylcarnitine analysis becomes the basis of the expanded newborn screening by tandem mass spectrometry (MS/MS) (McHugh et al. 2011).

## Preanalytical Conditions

Organic acids are, in general, highly water-soluble compounds and, thus, efficiently excreted by the kidney leading to their accumulation in urine. Therefore, urine is the biological fluid of choice for the evaluation of organic acid profiles. Other biological fluids such as plasma, CSF, or vitreous humor may be used when urine is not available.

A random urine sample is usually used for the organic acid analysis. The timing of the urine collection is not really important. If the sample collection is planned, the first morning specimen is requested. The chance to detect metabolites with low concentration will be higher as well as the probability to detect key metabolites in patients with fasting intolerance. Whenever an organic acid profile is unclear and does not allow a solid diagnosis, the use of in vivo loading tests is advocated because these tests have proven to substantially enhance the organic acid excretion (Garcia-Villoria et al. 2009). A 24-h urine collection may be requested in special occasions in the follow-up of patients, e.g., in the process of treatment monitoring. For post-mortem screening of organic aciduria, urine should be obtained via bladder puncture. In order avoid as much as possible artefactual alterations, the samples should be kept at −20 °C and shipped frozen. The more unstable organic acids (cf. ketoacids) may be degraded, and several organic acids, namely, the tricarboxylic acids, may be decreased and/or enhanced by bacterial contamination activity.

Diet and drugs are the main disturbing factors of the organic acid profile and may cause serious interpretative difficulties. The best known dietary disturbances are those caused by the use of medium-chain triglyceride containing diets giving rise to the excretion of $C_6$-$C_{10}$ dicarboxylic acids as well as (ω-1)-hydroxy acids. Also partially hydrolyzed protein sources in infant formula may pose problems due to the interfering components/additives, e.g., dioctyl phthalate, which appears in the organic acid chromatogram. Various dietary carbohydrates do not survive the food processing steps and may give rise to artefacts such as furane-2,5-dicarboxylic acid, 2,4-dihydroxybutyric acid, or glucosan (Table 4.2).

For the correct evaluation of the organic acid profiles, it is mandatory to have precise information concerning the type of diet; the drugs, including vitamers; and the natural supplements under which the patients are submitted or have been, at least 48 h before sample collection.

## Analysis/Methods

The gold standard method for the analysis of organic acids in a biological matrix is gas-chromatography coupled with a mass spectrometry detector (GC-MS). Accordingly, the compounds of interest must be isolated from the sample's matrix and further transformed in derivatives suitable for GC-MS analysis.

The extraction of the organic acids is accomplished by solid-phase or liquid-liquid extraction, the latter one being the most widely used. For standardization of the method and internal quality control, one or two internal standards (non-physiological organic acid), such as 2-phenylbutyric acid or pentadecanoic acid, are added to the sample prior the extraction procedure.

**Table 4.1** Key metabolite reference guide in organic acids analysis. Symbol (#) shows the corresponding chapter number where the disorder is presented according the classification used throughout this book

| Disorder | Affected protein | Altered gene | Key metabolites/profiles | Ch. # |
|---|---|---|---|---|
| Organic acid disorders in aromatic amino acid metabolism | | | | |
| Phenylketonuria (PKU) | Phenylalanine hydroxylase | *PAH* | 2-Hydroxyphenylacetic acid<br>Phenyllactic acid<br>Phenylacetic acid<br>Phenylpyruvic acid<br>Mandelic acid | 20 |
| Tyrosinemia Type I | Fumarylacetoacetase | *FAH* | 4,6-Diketoheptanoic acid<br>(=succinylacetone)<br>*N*-Acetyl-tyrosine<br>4-Hydroxyphenyllactic acid<br>4-Hydroxyphenylpyruvic acid<br>4-Hydroxyphenylacetic acid | 21 |
| Tyrosinemia Type II<br>Tyrosinemia Type III | Tyrosine aminotransferase<br>4-Hydroxyphenylpyruvate dioxygenase | *TAT*<br>*HPD* | 4-Hydroxyphenyllactic acid<br>4-Hydroxyphenylpyruvic acid<br>4-Hydroxyphenylacetic acid<br>*N*-Acetyl-tyrosine | 21 |
| Hawkinsinuria | 4-hydroxyphenylpyruvate dioxygenase | *HPD* | 4-Hydroxycyclohexylacetic acid | 21 |
| Alkaptonuria | Homogentisic acid oxidase | *HGD* | Homogentisic acid | 21 |
| Organic acid disorders in branched-chain amino acid metabolism | | | | |
| Maple Syrup Urine Disease (MSUD):<br>MSUD Type 1a<br>MSUD Type 1b<br>MSUD Type 2<br>BCKDC (PDHC/α-KDHC) deficiency | Branched-chain 2-ketoacid dehydrogenase complex (BCKDC):<br>E1α subunit deficiency/BC ketoacid dehydrogenase<br>E1β subunit deficiency/BC ketoacid dehydrogenase<br>E2 subunit deficiency/Dihydrolipoyl transacylase<br>E3 subunit deficiency/Dihydrolipoyl dehydrogenase | *BCKDHA*<br>*BCKDHB*<br>*DBT*<br>*DLD* | 2-Ketoisocaproic acid<br>2-Ketoisovaleric acid<br>2-Keto-3-methylvaleric acid<br>2-Hydroxyisocaproic acid<br>2-Hydroxyisovaleric acid<br>2-Hydroxy-3-methylvaleric acid<br>(lactic and ketoglutaric acids) | 23 |
| Isovaleric acidemia | Isovaleryl-CoA dehydrogenase | *IVD* | Isovalerylglycine<br>3-Hydroxyisovaleric acid<br>Isovalerylglutamic acid | 23 |
| 3-Methylcrotonylglycinuria | 3-Methylcrotonyl-CoA carboxylase | *MCCC1*<br>*MCCC2* | 3-Methylcrotonylglycine<br>3-Hydroxyisovaleric acid | 23 |
| 3-Methylglutaconic aciduria Type 1 | 3-Methylglutaconyl-CoA hydratase | *AUH* | 3-Methylglutaconic acid<br>3-Methylglutaric acid<br>3-Hydroxyisovaleric acid | 23 |
| 3-Hydroxy-3-methylglutaric aciduria | 3-Hydroxy-3-methyl-glutaryl-CoA lyase | *HMGCL* | 3-Hydroxy-3-methylglutaric acid<br>3-Methylglutaconic acid<br>3-Methylglutaric acid<br>3-Hydroxyisovaleric acid<br>Glutaric acid<br>3-Methylcrotonylglycine<br>C6-C10 Dicarboxylic acids | 23 |

(continued)

**Table 4.1** (continued)

| Disorder | Affected protein | Altered gene | Key metabolites/profiles | Ch. # |
|---|---|---|---|---|
| 2-Methylbutyrylglycinuria | 2-Methylbutyryl-CoA dehydrogenase | *ACADSB* | 2-Methylbutyrylglycine | 23 |
| 2-Methyl-3-hidroxybutyric acidúria/HSD10 disease | 2-Methyl-3-hydroxybutyryl-CoA dehydrogenase | *HSD17B10* | 2-Methyl-3-hydroxybutyric acid Tiglylglycine<br>Ethylhydracrylic acid | 23 |
| 2-Methylacetoacetic aciduria/β-Ketothiolase deficiency | 3-Oxothiolase (mitochondrial) | *ACAT1* | 2-Methyl-3-ketobutyric acid<br>2-Methyl-3-hydroxybutyric acid Tiglylglycine<br>2-Ethylhydracrylic acid | 23 |
| Isobutyrylglycinuria | Isobutyryl-CoA dehydrogenase | *ACAD8* | Isobutrylglycine | 23 |
| Mitochondrial short-chain enoyl-CoA hydratase 1 deficiency | Mitochondrial short-chain enoyl-CoA hydratase (Crotonase) | *ECHS1* | 2-Methyl-2-3-dihydroxy-butyrate<br>3-Methylglutaconic acid | 23 |
| Methacrylic aciduria | 3-Hydroxyisobutyryl-CoA deacylase | *HIBADH* | NONE, cf. 3-hydroxyisobutyryl-carnitine | 23 |
| 3-Hydroxyisobutyric aciduria | 3-Hydroxyisobutyrate dehydrogenase | *HIBCH* | 3-Hydroxyisobutyric acid<br>3-Hydroxypropionic acid<br>2-Ethyl-3-hydroxy-<br>propionic acid<br>Isobutyrylglycine | 23 |
| Methylmalonic semialdehyde dehydrogenase deficiency | Methylmalonic semialdehyde dehydrogenase | *ALDH6A1* | Methylmalonic acid<br>3-Hydroxyisobutyric acid<br>3-Hydroxypropionic acid | 23 |
| Propionic aciduria | Propionyl-CoA carboxylase α-subunit<br>Propionyl-CoA carboxylase β-subunit | *PCCA*<br>*PCCB* | 3-Hydroxypropionic acid<br>Methylcitric acid<br>2-Methyl-3-hydroxybutyric acid<br>3-Hydroxyvaleric acid<br>Propionylglycine | 23 |
| Isolated methylmalonic aciduria | Methylmalonyl-CoA epimerase<br>Methylmalonyl-CoA mutase<br>Mitochondrial Cbl transporter, CblA type<br>Cobalamin adenosyltranferase, CblB type<br>Cobalamin D-MMA type<br>SUCLA2; SUCLG1 (*vd.*Krebs cycle) | *MCEE*<br>*MUT*<br>*MMAA*<br>*MMAB*<br>*MMADHC* | Methylmalonic acid<br>3-Hydroxypropionic acid<br>Methylcitric acid<br>2-Methyl-3-hydroxybutyric acid<br>3-Hydroxy-valeric acid | 23 |
| Malonic aciduria | Malonyl-CoA decarboxylase | *MLYCD* | Malonic acid | 23 |
| Combined methylmalonic and malonic aciduria | Acetyl-CoA synthase (family member 3) | *ACSF3* | Methylmalonic acid<br>Malonic acid | 23 |
| Ethylmalonic aciduria (SCAD deficiency and ETHE1 encephalopathy) | Ethylmalonyl-CoA decarboxylase | *ECHDC1* | Ethylmalonic acid | – |
| Organic acid disorders in lysine and hydroxylysine metabolism | | | | |
| 2-Amioadipic and 2-ketoadipic aciduria | 2-Ketoadipic acid dehydrogenase (?) | *DHTKD1* | 2-Ketoadipic acid<br>2-Hydroxyadipic acid<br>Dicarboxylic acids | – |
| Glutaric aciduria Type I | Glutaryl-CoA dehydrogenase | *GCDH* | Glutaric acid<br>3-Hydroxyglutaric acid<br>Glutaconic acid | 69 |
| Glutaric aciduria Type III | Succinyl-CoA:glutarate-CoA transferase | *SUGCT (C7orf10)* | Glutaric acid | – |

| | | | | |
|---|---|---|---|---|
| Organic acid disorders in (mitochondrial) fatty acid oxidation metabolism | | | | |
| Short-chain acyl-CoA dehydrogenase deficiency (Ethylmalonic aciduria) | Short-chain acyl-CoA dehydrogenase (SCAD) | *ACADS* | Ethylmalonic acid<br>Methylsuccinic acid | 48 |
| Medium-chain acyl-CoA dehydrogenase deficiency | Medium-chain acyl-CoA dehydrogenase (MCAD) | *ACADM* | Dicarboxylic acids (sat/unsat.)<br>Hexanoylglycine<br>Suberylglycine<br>5-Hydroxyhexanoic acid<br>3-Hydroxysebacic acid<br>Phenylpropionylglycine | 48 |
| Very long-chain acyl-CoA dehydrogenase deficiency | Very long-chain acyl-CoA dehydrogenase (VLCAD) | *ACADVL* | Dicarboxylic acids (sat/unsat) | 48 |
| Long-chain 3-hydroxyacyl-CoA dehydrogenase deficiency<br>Mitochondrial trifunctional protein deficiency | Long-chain 3-hydroxyacyl-CoA dehydrogenase (LCHAD)<br>Mitochondrial trifunctional protein (MTP) | *HADHA*<br>*HADHB* | 3-Hydroxyadipic acid + lactone<br>3-Hydroxydicarboxylic acids<br>Dicarboxylic acids (sat/unsat) | 48 |
| Short-chain 3-hydroxyacyl-CoA dehydrogenase deficiency | Short-chain 3-hydroxyacyl-CoA dehydrogenase (SCHAD) | *HADHSC* | L-3-Hydroxybutyric acid<br>3-Hydroxyglutaric acid | 48 |
| Multiple acyl-CoA dehydrogenase deficiency | (*vd.* riboflavin metabolism) | – | | 32 |
| Organic acid disorders in ketones bodies metabolism | | | | |
| Succinyl-CoA:3-ketoacid-CoA transferase deficiency<br>Monocarboxylate transporter1 deficiency | Succinyl-CoA:3-ketoacid transferase (SCOT)<br>Monocarboxylate transporter1 (MCT1) | *SCOT*<br>*MCT1* | 3-Hidroxybutyric acid<br>2-Hydroxybutyric acid<br>Acetoacetic acid | 50 |
| Organic acid disorders in Krebs cycle | | | | |
| 2-Ketoglutarate dehydrogenase complex (KGDHC):<br>2-Ketoglutarate dehydrogenase deficiency KGDHC (plus BCKDC/PDHC) | 2-Ketoglutarate dehydrogenase (KGDHC-E1 subunit)<br>Dihydrolipoyl succinyltransferase (KGDHC-E2 subunit)<br>Dihydrolipoyl dehydrogenase (KGDHC-E3 subunit) | *OGDH*<br>*DLST*<br>*DLD* | 2-Ketoglutaric acid<br>Lactic acid<br>Plus branched chain keto acids/2-hydroxy-keto acids | 42 |
| ATP-specific succinyl-CoA ligase β subunit deficiency<br>GTP-specific succinyl-CoA ligase α subunit deficiency | Succinyl-CoA ligase β subunit (SUCLA2)<br>Succinyl-CoA ligase α subunit (SUCLG1) | *SUCLA2*<br>*SUCLG1* | Methylmalonic acid<br>Succinic acid | 42 |
| Fumaric aciduria | Fumarase | *FH* | Fumaric acid | 42 |
| Malate dehydrogenase deficiency | Malate dehydrogenase | *MDH2* | Citric acid<br>Fumaric acid<br>Malic acid<br>Succinic acid | 42 |
| Organic acid disorders in oxalate metabolism | | | | |
| Primary hyperoxaluria type I | Alanine-glyoxylate amino-transferase | *AGXT* | Oxalic acid<br>Glycolic acid<br>Glyoxylic acid | 67 |
| Primary hyperoxaluria type II | Glyoxylate reductase | *GRHPR* | Oxalic acid<br>l-Glyceric acid | 67 |
| Primary hyperoxaluria type III | 4-Hydroxy-2-oxoglutarato aldolase, mitochondrial | *HOGA1* | Oxalic acid<br>Glycolic acid | 67 |

(continued)

**Table 4.1** (continued)

| Disorder | Affected protein | Altered gene | Key metabolites/profiles | Ch. # |
|---|---|---|---|---|
| Organic acid disorders in pyruvate metabolism | | | | |
| Pyruvate carboxylase deficiency | Pyruvate carboxylase (PC) | *PC* | Lactic acid; Pyruvic acid<br>3-Hydroxybutyric acid; acetoacetic acid<br>2-ketoglutaric acid;<br>Succinic acid<br>Malic acid; Fumaric acid | 42 |
| Pyruvate dehydrogenase complex (PDHC):<br>Pyruvate dehydrogenase deficiency<br>PDHC (plus BCKDC / KDHC) deficiency | Pyruvate dehydrogenase (E1α–subunit)<br>Pyruvate dehydrogenase (E1β–subunit)<br>Dihydrolipoyl acetyltransferase (E2-subunit)<br>PDH- componente X<br>Dihydrolipoamide dehydrogenase (PDHC-E3 subunit) | *PDHA*<br>*PDHB*<br>*DLAT*<br>*PDHX*<br>*DLD* | Lactic acid<br>Pyruvic acid<br>Plus branched chain keto acids/2-hydroxy-keto acids | 42 |
| D-Lactic aciduria[a] | D-Lactate Dehydrogenase | *LDHD* | D-Lactic acid | – |
| Diverse organic acid disorders | | | | |
| Aromatic L-amino acid descarboxylase deficiency | Aromatic L-amino acid descarboxylase (AADC) | *AADC* | 3-Methoxy-4-hydroxyphenyl-lactic acid (Vanillactic acid) | 19 |
| Canavan disease | Aspartoacylase | *ASPA* | *N*-acetylaspartic acid | 69 |
| Ethylmalonic encephalopathy (ETHE) | Mitochondrial sulfur dioxygenase (ETHE1 protein) | *ETHE1* | Ethylmalonic acid<br>Isobutyryl/Isovaleryl-glycine | – |
| D-Glyceric aciduria | Glycerate kinase | *GLYCTK* | D-Glyceric acid | 49 |
| Glycerol kinase deficiency | Glycerol kinase | *GK* | Glycerol | 49/46 |
| 4-Hydroxybutyric aciduria | Succinic-semialdehyde dehydrogenase | *ALDH5A1* | 4-Hydroxybutyric acid + lactone<br>Erythro-/threo- 4,5-dihydroxy-octanoic acids<br>2,4-dihydroxybutyric acid | 24 |
| L-2-Hydroxyglutaric aciduria | L-2-Hydroxyglutaric acid dehydrogenase | *L2HGDH* | L-2-Hydroxyglutaric acid + lactone | 69 |
| D-2-Hydroxyglutaric aciduria type I<br>D-2-Hydroxyglutaric aciduria type II | D-2-Hydroxyglutaric acid dehydrogenase<br>Isocitrate dehydrogenase 2 | *D2HGD*<br>*IDH2* | D-2-Hydroxyglutaric acid +<br>Lactone | 69 |
| Methylglutaconic acidurias (MGA)–secondary:<br>Barth syndrome<br>Costeff syndrome<br>MEGDEL syndrome<br>Others | Mitochondrial dysfunction | *TAZ*<br>*OPA3*<br>*SERAC1*<br>*DNAJ19;CLPB;*<br>*HTRA2;TIMM50;*<br>*TMEM70;ATPAF2;*<br>*QIL1;AGK;ATP5FID* | 3-Methylglutaconic acid<br>3-Methylglutaric acid | 70/51 |
| Mevalonic aciduria/Hyper-IgD syndrome | Mevalonate kinase | *MVK* | Mevalonic acid + lactone | 54 |
| Disorders of protein lipoilation | Protein lipoilation defects | *NFU1;ISCU;LIPT1;*<br>*LIPT2; BOLA3;LIAS;*<br>*IBA57;ISCA2;*<br>*GLRX5;FSDX2;*<br>*LYRM4;NFS1* | 2-Hydroxyadipic acid<br>2-Ketoadipic acid<br>Glutaric acid<br>2-Ketoglutaric acid<br>Isobutyryl/Isovaleryl/2-methyl-butyryl-glycine | 27 |

| | | | | |
|---|---|---|---|---|
| Pyroglutamic aciduria | Glutathione synthase<br>5-oxoprolinase | *GSS*<br>*OPLAH* | Pyroglutamic acid | 16 |
| Reversible leukoencephalopathy | Plasma membrane $Na^+$/dicarboxylate cotransporter 3 | *SLC13A3* | 2-Ketoglutaric and succinic acid<br>Fumaric acid<br>*N*-acetylaspartic acid | 43 |
| Organic acidurias in vitamin metabolism | | | | |
| *Biotin metabolism* | | | | |
| Multiple carboxylase deficiency | Biotinidase<br>Holocarboxylase synthetase | *BTD*<br>*HLCS* | 3-Methylcrotonylglycine<br>3-Hydroxyisovaleric acid<br>3-Hydroxypropionic acid<br>2-Methylcitric acid<br>Lactic and Pyruvic acids | 30 |
| *Cobalamin metabolism* | | | | |
| GIF, CUBN/AMN, HC, TCbl, TCblR, CblF, CblJ, CblC, CblD, CblD-MMAtype, CblA, CblB and CblX deficiencies | Uptake, intracellular transport, Cbl metabolism deficiencies | *GIF/TCNIII;CUBN;*<br>*AMN;TCNI;TCNII;*<br>*CD320;LMBRD1;*<br>*ABCD4;MMACHC;*<br>*MMADCH;MMAA;*<br>*MMAB; HCFC1* | Methylmalonic acid (and homocystinuria) | 28 |
| *Folate metabolism* | | | | |
| Formiminoglutamic aciduria (FIGLURIA) | Glutamateformimino-transferase | *FTCD* | Hidantoin-5-propionic acid | 29 |
| *Pyridoxine metabolism* | | | | |
| Pyridox(am)ine-5-phosphate oxidase deficiency<br>Vit 6 dependent epilepsy | Pyridox(am)ine-5-phosphate oxidase (PNPO)<br>Pyridoxal phosphate binding protein | *PNPO*<br>*PROSC* | 3-Methoxy-4-hydroxyphenyl-lactic acid (vanillactic acid) | 34 |
| *Riboflavin metabolism* | | | | |
| Multiple acyl-CoA dehydrogenase (MADD) deficiency/Glutaric aciduria Type II (ETF-Type 2A /2B)<br>Riboflavin-responsive MADD (ETF)<br>MADD (ETF-DH) | Electron transfer flavoprotein (ETF: α or β subunit)<br>Electron transfer flavoprotein (ETF)<br>Electron transfer flavoprotein dehydrogenase (ETF-DH) | *ETFA*<br>*ETFB*<br>*ETFDH*<br>*ETFDH* | Short-chain acylglycines (C4–C8)<br>C5–C10 Dicarboxylic acids<br>3-Hydroxy-sebacic acid<br>Ethylmalonic acid<br>D-2-Hydroxyglutaric acid<br>Glutaric acid | 32 |
| Riboflavin transporter 1 deficiency<br>Brownn-Vialetto-Van Laere Syndrome Type I/Type II; Fazio-Londe Syndrome<br>Flavin adenine dinucleotide synthetase deficiency | Riboflavin transporter 1-RFVT1<br>Riboflavin transporter 2-RFVT2<br>Riboflavin transporter 3-RFVT3<br>Flavin adenine dinucleotide synthetase (FADS) | *SLC52A1*<br>*SLC52A2*<br>*SLC52A3*<br>*FLAD1* | Ethylmalonic acid<br>Glutaric acid<br>C5–C10 Dicarboxylic acids<br>Short- and medium-chain acyl-Glycines (C4–C8) (can be normal) | 32 |

(continued)

**Table 4.1** (continued)

| Disorder | Affected protein | Altered gene | Key metabolites/profiles | Ch. # |
|---|---|---|---|---|
| Other alterations detectable through the organic acid profile | | | | |
| Ammonia detoxification disorders:<br>Ornithine transcarbamylase deficiency<br>Citrullinemia<br>Argininosuccinic acidúria<br>Arginemia<br>HHH syndrome<br>Lysinuric protein intolerance | Ornithine transcarbamylase (OTC)<br>Argininosuccinate synthase (ASS)<br>Argininosuccinate lyase (ASL)<br>Arginase<br>Mitochondrial Ornithine transporter<br>Amino acid transport system γ+L | *OTC*<br>*ASS*<br>*ASL*<br>*ARG1*<br>*SLC25A1*<br>*SLC7A7* | Orotic acid; (occasionally plus Uracil)<br>4,5-dihydroformamida-2-pyrrole carboxylic acid (cyclic derivative of citrulline) | 17 |
| Dihydropyrimidinuria | Dihydropyrimidinase | *DPYS* | Dihydrothymine<br>Dihydrouracil<br>Thymine<br>Uracil | 24 |
| Hyperprolinaemia Type II | Δ-pyrroline-carboxylate dehydrogenase | *ALDH4A1* | $\Delta^1$-Pyrroline-5-carboxyl-glycine | 25 |
| Mitochondrial Neurogastrointestinal encephalomyopathy (MNGIE) | Thymidine phosphorylase | *TYMP* | Thymine<br>Uracil | 24 |
| Orotic aciduria | Bifunctional enzyme: orotate phosphoribosyltransferase (OPRT) and orotidylic decarboxylase (ODC) | *UMPS* | Orotic acid | 24 |
| Refsum disease | Phytanoyl-CoA hydroxylase | *PHYH* | 3-Methyl-adipic acid<br>2,6-dimethylsuberic acid | 66 |
| Thymine-uraciluria | Dihydropyrimidine dehydrogenase | *DPYD* | Thymine<br>Uracil | 24 |
| Zellweger disease | Peroxisomal biogenesis | *PEX1* | 2-Hydroxysebacic acid<br>Epoxydicarboxylic acids | 66 |

[a]Monroe et al. (2019)

Abbreviations: *CUBN* cubilin, *AMN* amnionless, *CblA, CblB, CblC, CblD CblF, CblJ, CblX* cobalamin A,B,C,D, F,J,X; *CblD-MMAtype* cobalamin D-Methylmalonic type, *GIF* gastric intrinsic factor, *HC* haptocorrin, *TCbl* transcobalamin, *TCblR* transcobalamin receptor, *HHH syndrome* hyperornithinemia-hyperammonemia-homocitrulinuria syndrome, *MEDGEL syndrome* 3-methylglutaconic aciduria with deafness-encephalopathy-Leigh-like syndrome

**Table 4.2** Dietary, drug, non-IEM disorders and bacterial artefacts in organic acid analysis

| Compound | Condition |
|---|---|
| *N*-Acetyltyrosine | Parenteral feeding |
| Aromatic acids (4-hydroxyphenyl) | Gut bacterial action |
| | Liver diseases |
| Benzoic acid | Benzoate sodium therapy |
| | Bacterial contamination |
| Cyclohexanediol | Medication |
| $C_{10} > C_8 > C_6$ dicarboxylic acids | MCT-diet |
| Dicarboxylic acids | Valproate therapy |
| Ethosuximide metabolites | Antiepileptic therapy |
| Di-(2-ethylhexyl)phthalate | Nutramigen feeding |
| | Pregestimil feeding |
| Ethylmalonic acid | *ACADS* polymorphisms |
| Furane-2,5-dicarboxylic acid | Heated sugars |
| Furoylglycine | Heated sugars |
| Glucosan | Heated sugar |
| Glutaric acid | Gut bacterial action, 2-ketoadipic decarboxylation |
| Glycerol | Balm contamination |
| Glycolic acid | Ethylene glycol poisoning |
| Hippuric acid | Benzoate sodium therapy |
| Homovanillic acid | Neuroblastoma |
| 4-Hydroxybutyric acid | Gamma-hydroxyanesthesia |
| | Illegal use of 4-hydroxybutyrate |
| 2,4-Di-hydroxybutyric acid | Heated sugar |
| 4-Hydroxycyclohexanecarboxylic acid | Food processing |
| 3-Hydroxydicarboxylic acids | Coeliac disease |
| | Long fasting |
| | MCT supplementation |
| 2-Hydroxyglutaric acid | 2-ketoadipate decomposition (bacterial contamination) |
| 5-Hydroxyhexanoic | MCT-diet |
| 2-Hydroxyhippuric acid | Salicylate ingestion |
| 5-Hydroxyindoleacetic acid | Carcinoid syndrome |
| D-2-Hydroxyisocaproic acid | Short-bowel syndrome |
| 3-Hydroxyisovaleric acid | Valproate medication |
| 7-Hydroxyoctanoic acid | MCT-diet |
| 3-Hydroxypropionic acid | Gut bacterial action |
| | Colon rectal cancer |
| Keppra metabolites | Antiepileptic therapy |
| D-Lactic acid | Short-bowel syndrome |
| Mandelic acid | Albumin infusion |
| Methylmalonic acid | Vitamin $B_{12}$-deficiency (vegans, vegetarian diet) |
| D-Phenyllactic acid | Short-bowel syndrome |
| Phenytoin metabolites | Antiepileptic therapy |
| Pyroglutamic acid | Glutamine decomposition |
| | Flucloxacillin toxicity |
| | Severe denutrition |
| | Renal disease |
| Suberylglycine (trace amounts) | MCT-diet |
| Succinic acid | 2-Ketoglutarate decomposition |
| Valproate metabolites | Depakine therapy |
| Vanillactic acid | Dopa therapy |
| Vanilmandelic acid | Neuroblastoma, pheochromocytoma |

In native urine (pH 5–7), the acids are present as salts ($Na^+$, $K^+$). Therefore, the urine should be acidified (pH 1–2) to promote the protonation of the acids, which turns them suitable to be extracted by an organic solvent of intermediate polarity. Ethyl acetate or di-ethyl ether is the most widely used. Extraction recoveries depend on the polarity of the acid: the more hydroxyl-groups, the less recovery.

For an accurate analysis, some precautions are necessary to be taken prior the extraction procedure. Keto acids deserve special attention due to the fact of being unstable compounds, thus the keto group must be protected by formation of an oxime derivative through reaction with hydroxylamine or methoxyamine; an example is succinylacetone (4,6-diketo-heptanoic acid), the key tyrosinemia type 1 metabolite.

The analysis by GC-MS obliges volatile analytes. Organic acids do not fulfil this requirement and must be transformed in volatile derivatives. Derivatization of the acid (COOH), the hydroxy (C-OH), and the keto (C=O) groups increases their volatility. The most widely used derivatization procedure is the formation of a trimethylsilylated (TMS) derivative. This transforms the molecule into a more balloon-like structure which can easily be volatilized upon the injection and move faster along the column. The larger the molecule, the later it elutes having higher retention times that may vary slightly depending on the column and on the instrument.

The derivatives are separated in the GC-capillary column, and the detection is accomplished by MS which allows the unequivocal identification of the detected metabolites. All separated compounds enter the ion source. They are ionized (obtain a positive electric charge) and fragmented and then deflected in an electromagnetic field. Variation of the electromagnetic field will cause the passage of ions with increasing mass to pass the ion exit slit and hit the ion collector (detector). The fragments of any given compound are like a fingerprint and give the unique identification of the compound. Every modern GC-MS instrument has library search facilities. This gives for each peak the most likely structure. Nevertheless, the interpretation of the library data should be done with care and the predicted structure should be cross examined with the determined retention times, i.e., the position in the total ion chromatogram. Unknown compounds with different chromatographic properties may have great similarity with fragmentation spectrum of known compounds. There are even sophisticated methods for the simultaneous deconvolution, identification, and quantitation of organic acids using a dedicated library of mass spectra and a list of retention indices (Halket et al. 1999). Several experienced laboratories have developed search routines in which the mass spectrometer automatically checks for the presence of all diagnostic organic acids listed in Table 4.1.

An organic acid chromatogram may display hundreds of tiny small peaks, and a full quantitative analysis can be really time-consuming. Therefore, urinary organic acids analysis, in general, is run in a qualitative or semi-quantitative mode. In order achieve a visual comparison of the organic acid total ion chromatograms, the starting volume of urine used in the assay should correspond to a fixed amount of creatinine present in the sample.

Precise quantification of specific metabolites, in particular cases, for differential diagnosis purposes or for the monitoring of treatment may be required. Therefore, accuracy of the organic acid analysis in the lower concentration range can be improved by using a stable isotope dilution assay. This is based on the addition of a stable isotope-labeled ($^{13}C$ or $^{2}H$) internal standard which behaves identically in all steps of the analysis, i.e., extraction, derivatization, and chromatographic separation. A range of applications has been developed, for example, succinylacetone for the follow-up of tyrosinemia type 1 patients (Sander et al. 2006), mevalonic acid for hyper IgD patients (Houten et al. 1999), and methylmalonic acid for vitamin $B_{12}$-related disorders (Blom et al. 2007), among others.

The recent availability of electrospray tandem mass spectrometers (MS/MS) together with a high range of isotope-labeled internal standards has resulted in the introduction of quantitative organic acid analysis in many labs by means of selective mass spectrometric detection and quantification via multiple reaction monitoring (MRM). This targeted analysis is of great value for some applications, particularly for the follow-up of some organic acidurias. However, the untargeted added value of GC-MS for the analysis of organic acids is still difficult to overcome. Recently, quantitative organic acid analysis by LC-QTOF/MS has been revealed as a technique that should be taken into account in the near future, particularly when urine is analyzed as a front-line specimen including also amino acids, acylcarnitines, purine and pyrimidines, and other metabolites in a unique run (Körver-Keularts et al. 2018).

## Interpretation/Reference Values

Interpretation of organic acid profiles is a demanding and complex issue. Besides the organic acids with diagnostic value, hundreds of substances are excreted into the urine of healthy and diseased subjects and are also detected in the organic acid chromatogram. It is therefore essential to gain experience in pattern recognition, in order to provide a reliable descriptive interpretation of the organic acid profile. This is one of the major tasks of the Biochemical Genetics Laboratory.

The recognition of a normal excretion profile is the starting point. It is necessary to be aware that the excretion profile depends on the age of the individual, the diet, the use of dietary supplements or vitamers, the intake of drugs, and the physical condition (fasting, exercise, etc.). A set of organic acids will always be detectable essentially in all urine samples of healthy individuals (Table 4.3). Due to differences in

**Table 4.3** Organic acids detectable essentially in all urines. Reference values of control individuals on a normal diet, without any medication and without signs of intestinal disease

| Compound | Reference values (mmol/mol creat) | | | |
|---|---|---|---|---|
| | 0–4 months | 4 months–2 years | 2–10 years | >10 years |
| Glycolic acid | 13–129 | 32–162 | 48–164 | 23–146 |
| Lactic acid | – | <200 | <85 | <50 |
| Oxalic acid | 140–360 | <160 | <125 | <70 |
| 3-Hydroxypropionic acid | 0–38 | 10–44 | 4–30 | 4–23 |
| 3-Hydroxy(iso)butyric acid | 0–38 | 20–118 | | 4–19 |
| 3-Hydroxyisovaleric acid | 2–47 | 10,154 | 10–66 | 6–49 |
| Methylmalonic acid | 1–11 | 2–13 | 1–4 | 0–4 |
| Ethylmalonic acid | 0–15 | 0–15 | 0–9 | 2–10 |
| Succinic acid | 40–125 | 44–79 | 5–81 | <16 |
| Phosphoric acid | Var. | – | – | – |
| Glutaric acid | 0–11 | 2–15 | 1–10 | 1–4 |
| Adipic acid | 2–27 | 0–25 | 2–10 | 1–7 |
| 2-Hydroxyglutaric acid | 6–67 | 11–49 | 6–35 | 4–16 |
| 3-Hydroxy-3-methylglutaric acid | 15–105 | 13–49 | 6–27 | 3–11 |
| 2-Ketoglutaric acid | 100–500 | 60–120 | <80 | <80 |
| 4-Hydroxyphenylacetic acid | – | – | – | <60 |
| Homovanillic acid | 3–20 | 2–19 | 1–14 | 1–5 |
| *N*-Acetylaspartic acid | 0–92 | 0–56 | 0–39 | 0–11 |
| Suberic acid | 1–15 | 2–15 | 1–10 | 1–6 |
| *cis*-Aconitic acid | Var. | 40–80 | – | – |
| Citric acid | Var. | 140–500 | – | – |
| Hippuric acid | Var. | – | – | – |

*Var.* variable
The lower and upper reference values represent the 5th and 95th percentiles

methodologies approaches for the sample analytical procedures among laboratories as well as equipment sensitivity, reference values between laboratories are usually not comparable, and available published data (Hoffmann et al. 1989) should be used as guidance only.

Therefore, each laboratory must have its own reference values, since distortions of relative concentrations may be informative. For this reason, ERNDIM (www.erndim.org) has launched a program for quantitative analysis of organic acids in urine, which is expected to be useful for the comparison of interlaboratory results. Moreover, sharing of true patients samples between laboratories will be of great value for the trainee. Organic acid acidurias are a huge group of disorders; some of them are quite rare, and it is easy to miss a diagnosis if one has not seen it before. Participation in the qualitative ERNDIM programs will eventually result in the collection of a series of study rare cases.

The easiest diagnoses rely on the massive excretion of one or a few pathognomonic metabolites. Good examples are $mut^0$ methylmalonic acidemia and 3-hydroxy-3-methylglutaryl-CoA (HMG-CoA) lyase deficiency (*vd.* Table 4.1). On the other hand, there are many defects showing only marginally increased organic acids. Well-known examples are 2-methyl-3-hydroxybutyryl-CoA dehydrogenase deficiency (Ofman et al. 2003; Garcia-Villoria et al. 2009), mevalonate kinase deficiency (Houten et al. 1999), and glutaric acidemia type 1 (Baric et al. 1999; Busquets et al. 2000). In those cases, it is of great importance to have an accurate quantitative organic acid analysis with one's own well-defined normal ranges. Sometimes even a trace amount of a key metabolite may be diagnostic as evidenced by some cases of tyrosinemia type I having only traces of succinylacetone in their urine (Haagen and Duran 1987). Patients with episodic fever and the hyper-IgD syndrome may have urinary mevalonic acid levels which are just twice the upper reference level of 0.8 mmol/mol creatinine (Houten et al. 1999).

As already emphasized, the here described analytical method does not exclusively detect organic acids; other low molecular compounds with diagnostic value may also be picked up. Important findings are the pyrimidines (uracil, thymine, dihydrothymine, dihydrouracil) associated with inborn errors of the pyrimidine breakdown pathway, and orotic acid, a marker of urea cycle defects (Table 4.1).

It is necessary to be aware that not all elevated organic acids may be related to an inherited disorder (Kumps et al. 2002); the primary accumulating organic acid may be the diagnostic hallmark by itself, as exemplified by pyroglutamic acid in oxoprolinase deficiency (Larsson et al. 1981), but it should be noted that pyroglutamic acid can arise from glutamine as an artefact during storage, and it can also be present in the urine of critically ill patients who are being treated with flucloxacillin and paracetamol.

**Table 4.4** Impact of acylcarnitines in the diagnosis of organic acidurias

| Organic aciduria | Acylcarnitines (P; DBS) |
|---|---|
| Methylmalonic | C3; C3/C2; C3/C16; C4DC; C16:1OH |
| Propionic | C3; C3/C2; C3/C16; C16:1OH |
| Isovaleric | C5; C5/C0; C5/C3; C5/C2 |
| 3-Methylcrotonylglycinuria | C5OH; C5OH/C0; C5OH/C8; C5:1 |
| HMG-CoA Lyase deficiency | C5OH; C5OH/C0; C5OH/C8; C6DC |
| Glutaric type I | C5DC; C5DC/C3DC; C5DC/C5OH; C5DC/C16; C5DC/C8, C5DC/C10 |
| Ketothiolase deficiency | C5OH; C5OH/C0; C5OH/C8; C5:1 |
| Biotinidase deficiency/ HCS deficiency | C5OH; C5OH/C0; C5OH/C8; C3; C3/C2; C3/C16 |
| 2-Methylbutyrylglycinuria | C5; C5/C0; C5/C3; C5/C2 |

Abbreviations: *P* plasma, *DBS* dried blood spot, *HMG-CoA* 3-Hydroxy-3-methyl-glutaryl-CoA, *HCS* Holocarboxilase synthetase

The most important non-genetic anomalies currently observed in the organic acid profiling are summarized in Table 4.2. The contribution of the diet, the gut bacterial action, and the anti-epileptic medication is most pronounced and should always be taken in mind.

A number of the organic acid coenzyme A esters will readily form carnitine esters as a mechanism for replenishing free CoA stores and as a tool for detoxifying the potential toxic acyl-CoA's. Table 4.4 shows the acylcarnitine accumulation in the most common organic acidemias in the metabolism of amino acids. Therefore, several organic acidemias may reliably be diagnosed by acylcarnitine analysis, either in plasma or in a dried blood spot (DBS), thereby enabling the large-scale newborn screening of these disorders (McHugh et al. 2011). Due to the diagnostic value of acylcarnitines, namely, for mitochondrial fatty acid oxidation defects (*vd.* acylcarnitines Chap. 5 in this book), it has become good laboratory practice to perform simultaneous GC/MS of urine organic acids and MS/MS of plasma or DBS acylcarnitines in any acutely sick patient in whom an organic acidemia is suspected.

Over the years, experience has been gained about multiple secondary enzyme reactions using the accumulating organic acid as a substrate and giving rise to characteristic diagnostic secondary metabolites (Table 4.5). Knowledge of biochemical pathways as well as enzyme biochemistry will be of great help in putting the identities of the secondary metabolites into place. Sometimes the production of secondary metabolites masks the presence of the primary metabolite such as observed in methylmalonic acidemia (Tavares de Almeida et al. 1991). In this respect, both propionic acidemia (Przyrembel et al. 1979) and isovaleric acidemia (Loots 2009) are notorious for their wealth of secondary metabolites. It is still a matter of debate whether the occurrence of potential toxic secondary metabolites plays a role in the development of specific symptoms in individual patients. Metabolomics studies of groups of patients may be helpful in answering these queries (Reinecke et al. 2012).

**Table 4.5** Examples of secondary metabolites derived from key metabolites in the organic acidurias

| Key metabolite | Biochemical process | Secondary metabolite |
|---|---|---|
| Ethylmalonyl-CoA | Mutase reaction | Methylsuccinicacid |
| Hexanoyl-CoA | (ω-1)-Hydroxylation | 5-Hydroxyhexanoic acid |
| 4-Hydroxybutyric acid | β-Oxidation | 3,4-Di-Hydroxybutyric acid |
| 2-Hydroxyglutaric acid | Lactone formation | 2-Hydroxyglutaric acid lactone |
| Isovaleryl-CoA | β-Oxidation | 3-Hydroxyisovaleric acid |
| Isovaleryl-CoA | ω-Oxidation | 4-Hydroxyisovaleric acid |
| Isovaleryl-CoA | Glutamic acid conjugation | *N*-Isovalerylglutamic acid |
| 2-Ketoadipic acid | Decarboxylation | Glutaric acid |
| 3-Methylcrotonyl-CoA | Glycine conjugation | 3-Methylcrotonylglycine |
| 3-Methylglutaconyl-CoA | Reduction | 3-Methylglutaric acid |
| Octanoic acid | Glucuronic acid conjugation | Octanoylglucuronide |
| Propionyl-CoA | Carnitine conjugation | Propionylcarnitine |
| Propionyl-CoA | Ketone formation | 3-Keto-n-valeric acid |
| Propionyl-CoA | Citrate synthase reaction | Methylcitric acid |
| Tiglyl-CoA | Carboxylation | 2-Methylglutaconic acid |

## Differential Diagnosis

The interpretation of an organic acid analysis can be a complex task. As already emphasized, for a comprehensive evaluation of the obtained profile, and in order not get lost by the nondiagnostic compounds, it is necessary to have in mind that multiple factors may have influence on the observed pattern, such as the clinical status of the patient, diet plus dietary supplementations, and medication. Moreover, in an emergency situation sample, collection timing may also have impact in the excreted pattern of organic acids. Therefore, detailed clinical and therapeutic information should be provided with the request for organic acid analysis. In these cases, it is mandatory to integrate all the information available. For example, in general, mitochondrial fatty acid beta-oxidation defects are associated with hypoketotic hypoglycemia, a finding that will be useful to differentiate a dicarboxylic acid pattern induced by a physiologic fasting which is accompanied by a gross excretion of ketones. The finding of moderately elevated C6-C12 (hydroxyl) dicarboxylic acids, especially in the absence of excessive amounts of ketones, may indicate mitochondria malfunction, and a mitochondrial beta-oxidation defect should be suspected.

Several key organic acids may be observed in multiple different organic acidurias or, simply, as an artefact from gut bacterial action, drug interactions in metabolic pathways, or sample bacterial contamination.

3-Methylglutaconic acid is a hallmark of 3-methylglutaconic aciduria type I, but it also appears, isolated or in combination with 3-mehylglutaric acid, in multiple conditions without a plausible biochemical support. However, it has been associated with mitochondrial membrane disruption and defective phospholipid remodeling (Wortmann et al. 2015); thus it should be monitored, and a persistent high level must be regarded as a signal for further investigation by molecular genetic analysis (Tort et al. 2019).

Another puzzling organic acid is ethylmalonic acid (EMA) (Duran et al. 1983), which is formed by the catalytic action of acetyl-CoA carboxylase and propionyl-CoA carboxylase upon butyryl-CoA, the substrate for short-chain acyl-CoA dehydrogenase, a member of the ACADs family (van Maldegem et al. 2006). It is a hallmark for SCAD deficiency, but it is also present in ethylmalonic encephalopathy (*ETHE1*) (Tiranti et al. 2004), multiple acyl-CoA dehydrogenase (MAD), respiratory chain, and possibly ethylmalonyl-CoA decarboxylase (ECHDC1) (Linster et al. 2011) disorders. Due to the high incidence of the ACADs-polymorphisms, EMA may be seen in multiple genetic defects.

In the organic acid analysis, low-molecular compounds other than organic acids with diagnostic informative value are detected. These key compounds allow to pursue the investigation through an oriented differential diagnosis flowchart procedure. It is the case of orotic acid, which is associated with urea cycle disorders, lysinuric protein intolerance, and HHH syndrome as well as that of pyrimidine compounds—thymine, uracil, dihydrothymine, and dihydrouracil—allowing the diagnosis of pyrimidine metabolism defects. The extraction recovery of these compounds from the urine matrix is quite low, and an accurate quantitative analysis is recommended or the use of an analytical dedicated method for further evaluation.

Other interesting compounds are the epoxydicarboxylic acids (Korman et al. 2000) suggestive of peroxisomal biogenesis defects, cf. Zellweger syndrome, as well as 3-methyladipic acid and 2,6-dimethylsuberic acid which have been detected in adults with Refsum disease (Greter et al. 1983; Wierzbicki et al. 2003). Therefore, plasma phytanic acid should be evaluated.

In some cases, the pathological excretion levels of the disorders' hallmark may be quite low, and a sensitive quantitative method using isotope dilution analysis will be demanded for an accurate diagnosis in selected cases.

Moreover, one must have in consideration the high informative level of acylglycines, detected in the organic acid run, in the differential diagnosis, as well as in that of acylcarnitines, which will be discussed in Chap. 5 of this book. The organism uses alternative pathways to get rid of the accumulated organic acids, and these metabolites in the form of CoA esters are further conjugated with the amino acid glycine to form the so-called acylglycines. Acylglycines are an important diagnostic tool in branched-chain amino acid breakdown pathways and in fatty acid oxidation defects (Table 4.1).

*Finally one should realize that organic acid analysis as a tool for diagnosing inborn errors will always be carried out in conjunction with complementary analyses such as those of acylcarnitines and amino acids. Only an integrated view of the disturbed metabolism will enable the assessment of a presumptive diagnosis, which will then be confirmed by molecular or enzyme studies* (Tavares de Almeida and Duran 2014).

**Acknowledgments** The authors deeply acknowledge the contribution of Dr. Marinus Duran to the Organic Acids chapter in the previous edition (2014, pp 761–773) of this book, on which this chapter is based.

## References

Baric I, Wagner L, Feyh P, et al. Sensitivity and specificity of free and total glutaric acid and 3-hydroxyglutaric acid measurements by stable-isotope dilution assays for the diagnosis of glutaric aciduria type I. J Inherit Metab Dis. 1999;22(8):867–82.

Blom HJ, van Rooij A, Hogeveen M. A simple high-throughput method for the determination of plasma methylmalonic acid by liquid chromatography-tandem mass spectrometry. Clin Chem Lab Med. 2007;45:645–50.

Busquets C, Merinero B, Christensen E, et al. Glutaryl-CoA dehydrogenase deficiency in Spain: evidence of two groups of patients, genetically, and biochemically distinct. Pediatr Res. 2000;48(3):315–22.

Duran M, Walther FJ, Bruinvis L, Wadman SK. The urinary excretion of ethylmalonic acid: what level requires further attention? Biochem Med. 1983;29:171–5.

Garcia-Villoria J, Navarro-Sastre A, Fons C, Pérez-Cerdá C, Baldellou A, Fuentes-Castelló MA, González I, Hernández-Gonzalez A, Fernández C, Campistol J, Delpiccolo C, Cortés N, Messeguer A, Briones P, Ribes A. Study of patients and carriers with 2-methyl-3-hydroxybutyryl-CoA dehydrogenase (MHBD) deficiency: difficulties in the diagnosis. Clin Biochem. 2009;42(1–2):27–33.

Greter J, Lindstedt S, Steen G. 2,6-Dimethyloctanedioic acid—a metabolite of phytanic acid in Refsum's disease. Clin Chem. 1983;29:434–7.

Haagen AAM, Duran M. Absence of increased succinylacetone in the urine of a child with hereditary tyrosinemia type I. J Inherit Metab Dis. 1987;10:323–5.

Halket JM, Przyborowska A, Stein SE, Mallard WG, Down S, Chalmers RA. Deconvolution gas chromatography/mass spectrometry of urinary organic acids—potential for pattern recognition and automated identification of metabolic disorders. Rapid Commun Mass Spectrom. 1999;13:279–84.

Hoffmann G, Aramaki S, Blum-Hoffmann E, Nyhan WL, Sweetman L. Quantitative analysis for organic acids in biological samples: batch isolation followed by gas chromatographic-mass spectrometric analysis. Clin Chem. 1989;35(4):587–95.

Houten SM, Kuis W, Duran M, de Koning TJ, van Royen-Kerkhof A, Romeijn GJ, Frenkel J, Dorland L, de Barse MM, Huijbers WA, Rijkers GT, Waterham HR, Wanders RJ, Poll-The BT. Mutations in MVK, encoding mevalonate kinase, cause hyperimmunoglobulinaemia D and periodic fever syndrome. Nat Genet. 1999;22:175–7.

Korman SH, Mandel H, Gutman A. Characteristic urine organic acid profile in peroxisomal biogenesis disorders. J Inherit Metab Dis. 2000;23:425–8.

Körver-Keularts IMLW, Wang P, Waterval HWAH. Fast and accurate quantitative organic acid analysis with LC-QTOF/MS facilitates screening of patients for inborn errors of metabolism. J Inherit Metab Dis. 2018;41(3):415–24.

Kumps A, Duez P, Mardens Y. Metabolic, nutritional, iatrogenic, and artifactual sources of urinary organic acids: a comprehensive table. Clin Chem. 2002;48:708–17.

Larsson A, Mattsson B, Wauters EAK, van Gool JD, Duran M, Wadman SK. 5-oxoprolinuria due to hereditary 5-oxoprolinase deficiency in two brothers—a new inborn error of the gamma-glutamyl cycle. Acta Paediatr Scand. 1981;70:301–8.

Linster CL, Noël G, Stroobant V, Vertommen D, Vincent MF, Bommer GT, Veiga-da-Cunha M, Van Schaftingen E. Ethylmalonyl-CoA decarboxylase, a new enzyme involved in metabolite proofreading. J Biol Chem. 2011;286(50):42992–3003.

Loots DT. Abnormal tricarboxylic acid cycle metabolites in isovaleric acidemia. J Inherit Metab Dis. 2009;32:403–11.

McHugh D, Cameron CA, Abdenur JE, et al. Clinical validation of cut-off ranges in newborn screening of metabolic disorders by tandem mass spectrometry: a worldwide collaborative project. Genet Med. 2011;13:230–54.

Monroe GR, van Eerde AM, Tessadori F, et al. Identification of human D-lactate dehydrogenase deficiency. Nat Commun. 2019;10:1477.

Ofman R, Ruiter JPN, Feenstra M, Duran M, Poll-The BT, Zschocke J, Ensenauer R, Lehnert W, Sass JO, Sperl W, Wanders RJ. 2-Methyl-3-hydroxybutyryl-CoA dehydrogenase deficiency is caused by mutations in the *HADH2* gene. Am J Hum Genet. 2003;72:1300–7.

Przyrembel H, Bremer HJ, Duran M, Bruinvis L, Ketting D, Wadman SK, Baumgartner R, Irle U, Bachmann C. Propionyl-CoA carboxylase deficiency with overflow of metabolites of isoleucine catabolism at all levels. Eur J Pediatr. 1979;130:1–14.

Reinecke CJ, Koekemoer G, van der Westhuizen FH. Metabolomics of urinary organic acids in respiratory chain deficiencies in children. Metabolomics. 2012;8:264–83.

Sander J, Janzen N, Peter M, Sander S, Steuerwald U, Holtkamp U, Schwahn B, Mayatepek E, Trefz FK, Das AM. Newborn screening for hepatorenal tyrosinemia: tandem mass spectrometric quantification of succinylacetone. Clin Chem. 2006;52:482–7.

Tavares de Almeida I, Duran M. Organic acids. In: Blau N, Duran M, Gibson KM, Dionisi-Vici C, editors. Physician's guide to the diagnosis, treatment, and follow-up of inherited metabolic diseases; 2014. p. 761–73.

Tavares de Almeida I, Duran M, Silva MF, Portela R, Cabral A, Tasso T, Eusébio F, Silveira C. Mild form of methylmalonic aciduria misdiagnosed as propionic acidaemia during a ketotic crisis. J Inherit Metab Dis. 1991;14:259–62.

Tiranti V, D'Adamo P, Briem E, Ferrari G, Mineri R, Lamantea E, Mandel H, Balestri P, Garcia-Silva MT, Vollmer B, Rinaldo P, Hahn SH, Leonard J, Rahman S, Dionisi-Vici C, Garavaglia B, Gasparini P, Zeviani M. Ethylmalonic encephalopathy is caused by mutations in *ETHE1*, a gene encoding a mitochondrial matrix protein. Am J Hum Genet. 2004;74:239–52.

Tort F, Ugarteburu O, Texidó L, Gea-Sorlí S, García-Villoria J, Ferrer-Cortès X, Arias Á, Matalonga L, Gort L, Ferrer I, Guitart-Mampel M, Garrabou G, Vaz FM, Pristoupilova A, Rodríguez MIE, Beltran S, Cardellach F, Wanders RJ, Fillat C, García-Silva MT, Ribes A. Mutations in TIMM50 cause severe mitochondrial dysfunction by targeting key aspects of mitochondrial physiology. Hum Mutat. 2019;40(10):1700–12.

van Maldegem BT, Duran M, Wanders RJA, Niezen-Koning KE, Hogeveen M, Ijlst L, Waterham HR, Wijburg FA. Clinical, biochemical, and genetic heterogeneity in short-chain acyl-coenzyme A dehydrogenase deficiency. JAMA. 2006;23:943–52.

Villani GRD, Gallo G, Sclolamiero E, Salvatore F, Ruoppolo M. "Classical organic acidurias": diagnosis and pathogenesis. Clin Exp Med. 2017;17(3):305–23.

Wierzbicki AS, Mayne PD, Lloyd MD, Burston D, Mei G, Sidey MC, Feher MD, Gibberd FB. Metabolism of phytanic acid and 3-methyl-adipic acid excretion in patients with adult Refsum disease J Lipid. Research. 2003;44:1481–8.

Wortmann SB, Espeel M, Almeida L, Reimer A, Bosboom D, Roels F, de Brouwer AP, Wevers RA. Inborn errors of metabolism in the biosynthesis and remodelling of phospholipids. J Inherit Metab Dis. 2015;38:99–110.

# Acylcarnitines

# 5

Dietrich Matern

## Contents



**Abstract**

Carnitine and its esters (acylcarnitines) are physiologically present in all biological fluids, but carnitine is most abundant in tissues with high energy requirements, particularly skeletal and cardiac muscle. Acylcarnitine analysis is a useful tool in the evaluation of patients at risk for inborn errors of mitochondrial fatty acid oxidation and for organic acidemias primarily due to defects in branched-chain amino acid metabolism. Given the diverse clinical presentation of these conditions, acylcarnitine analysis has become an integral part of the biochemical genetic laboratory investigation of a large number of patients. With the additional application to newborn screening, acylcarnitine analysis is the most widely used biochemical genetic laboratory test. Aside from clinical and newborn screening indications, a relevant family and/or prenatal history, and sudden unexpected death also represent valid reasons to pursue an acylcarnitine analysis. However, several preanalytical and analytical pitfalls must be considered when interpreting acylcarnitine profiles.

D. Matern (✉)
Biochemical Genetics Laboratory, Department of Laboratory Medicine and Pathology, Mayo Clinic, Rochester, MN, USA
e-mail: matern@mayo.edu

## Introduction

Carnitine and its esters are physiologically present in all biological fluids, but carnitine is most abundant in tissues with high energy requirements, particularly skeletal and cardiac muscle. In 1973, the first two clinically relevant disorders affecting this pathway were described: primary carnitine deficiency and carnitine palmitoyl transferase type II deficiency (DiMauro and DiMauro 1973; Engel and Angelini 1973). To date, more than 20 different enzyme deficiency states affecting fatty acid transport and mitochondrial β-oxidation (FAO) are known, and additional enzymes involved in this pathway are still being discovered (Bosch et al. 2011; Knottnerus et al. 2018; Rinaldo et al. 2002).

Carnitine is involved as a detoxifying agent in branched-chain amino acid metabolism. Most of the classic organic acidurias are associated with secondary carnitine deficiency.


N. Blau et al. (eds.), *Physician's Guide to the Diagnosis, Treatment, and Follow-Up of Inherited Metabolic Diseases*,
https://doi.org/10.1007/978-3-030-67727-5_5

In fact, the clinical utility of acylcarnitine analysis was first identified for several organoacidopathies, and urine was the preferred specimen. However, plasma became the specimen of choice because acylcarnitine profiles are less complex in plasma than in urine and because the sensitivity of acylcarnitine analysis is higher when plasma is analyzed, especially for the diagnosis of long-chain FAO disorders (Millington et al. 1992). Today, urine acylcarnitine analysis is limited to specific analytes where diagnostic value is added to the metabolic work up of patients with organic acidemias but inconclusive or borderline abnormal urine organic acid and plasma acylcarnitine profiles (Ensenauer et al. 2004; Oglesbee et al. 2007; Tortorelli et al. 2005). Blood dried on filter paper is analyzed for newborn screening and, together with bile, in the postmortem evaluation of cases of sudden and unexpected death (Rinaldo et al. 2004). Cell-free supernatant of amniotic fluid can be used for the prenatal diagnosis of selected inborn errors of metabolism (Rinaldo et al. 2001).

Cultured fibroblasts or amniocytes can be probed with FAO substrates and carnitine. Cell cultures deficient of an FAO enzyme will accumulate specific acylcarnitine species when incubated with substrates such as palmitate, allowing for the diagnosis of FAO disorders (Roe et al. 2001; Shen et al. 2000; Young et al. 2003). Modifications of this assay system have also been developed for the diagnosis of defects affecting the metabolism of branched chain amino acids and for the study of peripheral blood mononuclear cells (Schulze-Bergkamen et al. 2005).

Acylcarnitine analysis is almost exclusively performed by tandem mass spectrometry (MS/MS) using stable isotope-labeled internal standards that allow quantitation of acylcarnitine species. However, to provide meaningful results to referring healthcare providers, it is critical to complement analytical proficiency with in-depth interpretation of results as is true for many other examples of complex metabolic profiles.

## Carnitine and Acylcarnitines

Carnitine, L-3-hydroxy-4-(trimethylammonium)butyrate, is a water-soluble, trimethylammonium derivative of γ-amino-β-hydroxybutyric acid which is formed from trimethyllysine via γ-butyrobetaine (Vaz and Wanders 2002) (Fig. 5.1). Carnitine originates to about 75% from dietary intake of meat, fish, and dairy products containing proteins with trimethyllysine residues. Under normal conditions, endogenous synthesis from lysine and methionine plays a minor role. Carnitine is excreted in urine and bile as free carnitine or as conjugated carnitine esters. Adequate intracellular levels of carnitine depend on diet, endogenous synthesis, reabsorption, and cellular uptake.

Under physiologic conditions, carnitine is primarily required to shuttle long-chain fatty acids across the inner mitochondrial membrane for fatty acid β-oxidation and products of peroxisomal β-oxidation to the mitochondria for further metabolism in the citric acid cycle (Vaz and Wanders 2002). Acylcarnitines (the carnitine esters) are formed by conjugating acyl-CoA moieties to carnitine which for activated long-chain fatty acids is accomplished by carnitine palmitoyl transferase type I (CPT-I) (Fig. 5.1). The acyl-group of the activated fatty acid (fatty acyl-CoA) is transferred by CPT-I from the sulfur atom of CoA to the hydroxyl group of carnitine (Knottnerus et al. 2018). Carnitine acylcarnitine translocase (CACT) then transfers the long-chain acylcarnitines across the inner mitochondrial membrane, where CPT-II reverses the action of CPT-I by formation of acyl-CoA and release of free carnitine.

In pathologic conditions, such as FAO disorders or organic acidemias due to acyl-CoA dehydrogenase deficiencies, the functions of carnitine as regulator of substrate flux and energy balance across cell membranes and as modulator of intracellular concentrations of free CoA become crucial. In such conditions, acyl-CoAs accumulate inside the mitochondrial matrix, and carnitine is utilized to shuttle

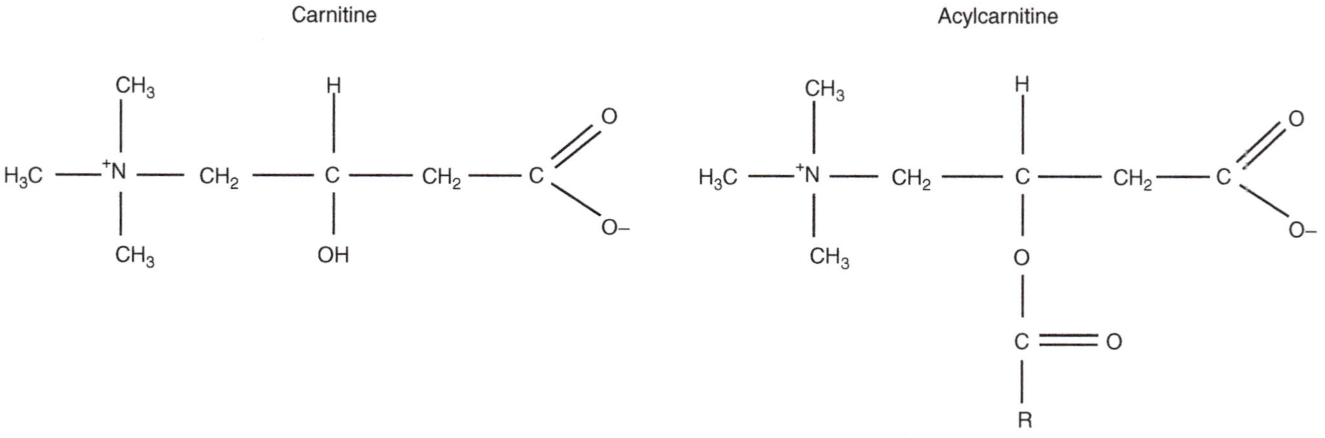


**Fig. 5.1** Structures of carnitine and acylcarnitine. The R represents the acylcarnitine species with up to 18 carbons which are typically the aim of an acylcarnitine analysis

these compounds out of the mitochondria as acylcarnitines, thereby restoring free CoA.

Carnitine and its esters are present in all biological fluids albeit very low in the CSF, and depending on the enzyme defect, a particular acylcarnitine pattern becomes apparent where those acylcarnitine species serving as direct substrates for the defective enzyme accumulate disproportionately to the down- and upstream metabolites (Table 5.1).

**Table 5.1** Clinically relevant acylcarnitine species (as butylesters) included in a typical acylcarnitine analysis and their relevance when abnormally elevated (unless otherwise noted)

| Acylcarnitine species | | Disorder |
|---|---|---|
| C0 | Free carnitine | Carnitine supplementation (deficiency if low) |
| C2 | Acetyl- | Carnitine supplementation or ketosis (deficiency if low) |
| C3 | Propionyl- | PA, MCD, MMA, SUCLA2 (Carrozzo et al. 2007), treatment with heptanoic acid |
| m/z 287 | FIGLU (Malvagia et al. 2006) | Glutamate formimino-transferase deficiency |
| C4 | Butyrl-/isobutyryl- | SCAD, IBDH, MADD, EE |
| C5:1 | Tiglyl- | MAT, MCC, MHBD, MCD |
| C5 | Isovaleryl-/2-methylbutyryl-/Pivaloyl- | IVA, SBCAD, MADD, EE, antibiotics derived artifact (Abdenur et al. 1998), treatment with heptanoic acid |
| C4-OH | 3-hydroxybutyryl- | SCHAD, ketosis |
| C6:1 | 3-methylglutaconyl- | MGA |
| C6 | Hexanoyl- | MCAD, MKAT, MADD |
| C5-OH | 3-hydroxyisovaleryl- | BIOT[a], HMG, MCC, MCD, MGA |
| | 2-methyl-3-hydroxybutyryl- | MAT, MHBD |
| m/z 322 | Benzoyl- | Treatment with Na-benzoate |
| m/z 325 | Dextrose (fragment) | Sample contamination with dextrose |
| C7 | Heptanoyl- | Treatment with heptanoic acid |
| m/z 336 | Phenylacetyl- | Treatment with phenylacetic acid |
| m/z 338 | Salicylyl- | Treatment with salicylic acid |
| C8 | Octanoyl- | MCAD, M/SCHAD, MKAT, MADD |
| C3-DC | Malonyl- | Malonic aciduria |
| C8-OH | 3-hydroxyoctanoyl- | MKAT |
| C10:2 | Decadienoyl- | DCR (Houten et al. 2014) |
| C10:1 | Decenoyl- | MCAD |
| C10 | Decanoyl- | MCAD, MADD |
| C4-DC | Methylmalonyl-/succinyl- | MMA[a], SUCLA2 (Carrozzo et al. 2007) |
| C5-DC | Glutaryl- | GA-1 |
| C10-OH | 3-hydroxydecanoyl- | M/SCHAD, MKAT |
| m/z 399 | Dextrose (fragment) | Sample contamination with dextrose |
| C12 | Dodecanoyl- | MADD |
| C6-DC | 3-methylglutaryl- | HMG |
| C12-OH | 3-hydroxydodecanoyl- | LCHAD/TFP |
| C14:1 | Tetradecenoyl- | MADD, VLCAD, LCHAD/TFP |
| C14 | Tetradecanoyl- (myristoyl-) | CACT, CPT-II, MADD, VLCAD, LCHAD/TFP |
| C14-OH | 3-hydroxytetradecanoyl- | LCHAD/TFP |
| C16 | Hexadecanoyl- (palmitoyl-) | CACT, CPT-II, MADD, VLCAD, LCHAD/TFP; CPT-I[b] |
| C16:1-OH | 3-hydroxyhexadecenoyl- | Antibiotics derived artifact (Vianey-Saban et al. 2004) |
| C16-OH | 3-hydroxyhexadecanoyl- | LCHAD/TFP |
| m/z 473 | Dextrose (fragment) | Sample contamination with dextrose |
| C18:2 | Octadecadienoyl- (linolyl-) | CACT, CPT-II, MADD, VLCAD, LCHAD/TFP |
| C18:1 | Octadecenoyl- (oleyl-) | CACT, CPT-II, MADD, VLCAD, LCHAD/TFP; CPT-I[b] |
| C18 | Octadecanoyl- (stearyl-) | CACT, CPT-II, MADD, VLCAD, LCHAD/TFP |
| C18:1-OH | 3-hydroxyoctadecenoyl- | LCHAD/TFP |
| C18-OH | 3-hydroxy octadecanoyl- | LCHAD/TFP deficiency |

[a]Respective analyte is not consistently elevated in this disorder

[b]CPT type I is suggested by low concentrations of long-chain acylcarnitine species and relatively high free carnitine; *BIOT* biotinidase deficiency, *CACT* carnitine-acylcarnitine translocase deficiency, *CPT* carnitine palmitoyl transferase deficiency, *DCR* 2,4-dienoyl-CoA reductase deficiency, *EE* ethylmalonic encephalopathy, *FIGLU* formininoglutamate, *GA-1* glutaric acidemia type I (glutaryl-CoA dehydrogenase deficiency), *HMG* 3-hydroxy 3-methylglutaryl-CoA lyase deficiency, *IBDH* isobutyryl-CoA dehydrogenase deficiency, *IVA* isovaleric acidemia (isovaleryl-CoA dehydrogenase deficiency), *LCHAD* long-chain 3-hydroxy acyl-CoA dehydrogenase deficiency, *MADD* multiple acyl-CoA dehydrogenase deficiency, *MAT* mitochondrial acetoacetyl-CoA thiolase (β-ketothiolase) deficiency, *MCAD* medium-chain acyl-CoA dehydrogenase deficiency, *MCC* 3-methylcrotonyl-CoA carboxylase deficiency, *MCD* multiple carboxylase (holocarboxylase synthetase and biotinidase) deficiency, *MGA* 3-methylglutaconic aciduria type I (3-methylglutaconyl-CoA hydratase deficiency), *MHBD* 2-methyl 3-hydroxy butyryl-CoA dehydrogenase deficiency, *MMA* methylmalonic acidemias, *PA* propionic acidemia (propionyl-CoA carboxylase deficiency), *SCAD* short-chain acyl-CoA dehydrogenase deficiency, *SCHAD* short-chain 3-hydroxy acyl-CoA dehydrogenase deficiency, *SUCLA2* succinate-CoA ligase ADP-forming beta subunit, *TFP* mitochondrial trifunctional protein deficiency, *VLCAD* very long-chain acyl-CoA dehydrogenase deficiency

## Indications for an Acylcarnitine Analysis

Acylcarnitine analysis has proven a useful tool in the evaluation of patients at risk for inborn errors of mitochondrial fatty acid oxidation and for organic acidemias that are primarily due to defects in branched-chain amino acid metabolism. Given the diverse clinical presentation of these conditions, acylcarnitine analysis has become an integral part of the biochemical genetic laboratory investigation of a large number of patients. Other laboratory studies that should be considered in such patient evaluations include urine organic acid and acylglycine, as well as plasma free fatty acid analyses. With the additional application to newborn screening, among esoteric tests acylcarnitine analysis has the highest sample throughput. Aside from clinical and newborn screening indications, a relevant family and/or prenatal history and sudden unexpected death also represent valid reasons to pursue an acylcarnitine analysis (Table 5.2). An unequivocal indication as a test to monitor treated patients has not yet been established, although it is frequently being performed for this purpose.

Especially since newborn screening for X-Adrenoleukodystrophy was proposed, attempts have been made to expand the typical acylcarnitine profile (see Table 5.1) to include acylcarnitine species with chain lengths greater than 18 carbons (up to C26) in order to identify patients with this and other peroxisomal disorders. However, this approach was found to have less sensitivity and specificity than the traditional analyses of very long chain fatty acids and corresponding lysophosphatidylcholines described in "Chap. 66" (Herzog et al. 2017; Huffnagel et al. 2017).

**Table 5.2** Indications for acylcarnitine analysis

| Clinical signs and symptoms | Routine laboratory findings |
|---|---|
| Respiratory distress | Acidosis |
| Lethargy | Ketosis |
| Coma | Hypoglycemia |
| Recurrent vomiting | Hyperammonemia |
| Failure to thrive | Elevated liver enzymes |
| Feeding difficulty | Elevated creatine kinase |
| Apnea | |
| Hypotonia | |
| Bradycardia | **Other abnormal laboratory findings** |
| Ventricular arrhythmias | Dicarboxylic aciduria (excluding dietary MCT) |
| Cardiomyopathy | Hydroxydicarboxylic aciduria |
| Hepatic steatosis | Abnormal acylcarnitines by newborn screening |
| Hepatomegaly | Fatty acid profile suggestive of a FAO disorder |
| Encephalopathy | |
| Seizures | |
| Dystonia | **Family history of** |
| Myopathy | Affected sibling(s) |
| Rhabdomyolysis | Sudden unexplained death or SIDS in sibling(s) |
| Renal tubular acidosis | Maternal pregnancy complications (AFLP, HELLP) |
| Polycystic kidneys | |
| Reye or Reye-like syndrome | |
| Apparent life-threatening event/"near-miss" SIDS | |

## Methods

Several techniques have been described to differentiate and eventually quantify specific carnitine esters. These include gas chromatography-mass spectrometry (GC-MS), thin layer chromatography (TLC) and radioisotopic exchange/HPLC, liquid-chromatography (LC) MS, and LC-MS/MS. However, the predominant method applied is flow injection analysis (FIA) MS/MS using triple quadrupole analyzers combined with electrospray ionization (ESI). The advantage of this approach is its sensitivity that allows for simple, but efficient preparation procedures of small sample volumes and fast analytical times, therefore providing for a rapid throughput of large numbers of samples. The disadvantage is that a few isomeric acylcarnitine species are not distinguishable by FIA-MS/MS (see Sect. 5.11 Pitfalls) which is why some laboratories opt for methods based on chromatographic separation by LC-MS/MS analysis with longer analytical times and at higher cost (Minkler et al. 2015). In a typical set up, acylcarnitines are extracted from the sample by mixing with methanol or an acidified acetonitrile solution containing isotopically labeled acylcarnitines of various chain lengths at defined concentrations as internal standards. Following centrifugation the supernatant is evaporated, and the residue is usually derivatized with either *n*-butanol HCl or *n*-methanol HCl yielding the acylcarnitines for analysis by flow injection ESI-MS/MS. Of note, some laboratories, in particular, newborn screening laboratories, omit the derivatization step, although problems may arise with the identification particularly of dicarboxylic species at the decision level due to lower ionization efficiency (De Jesús et al. 2010). Following analysis, a graphical acylcarnitine profile is generated which can be interpreted qualitatively. (Semi-)quantitative calculation of the concentration of each individual acylcarnitine species is based on the abundance of the assigned internal standard (Smith and Matern 2010).

## Specimen

A variety of body fluids can be used for acylcarnitine analysis, but testing of plasma or whole blood spotted on filter paper is most common. All sample types, except for dried blood and bile spots and fibroblast cultures which can be sent at room temperature, should be kept frozen until analysis. Reliable results, particularly for short-chain acylcarnitine species, for any sample, liquid or dried on filter paper, cannot be achieved following long-term storage at ambient temperatures (Matern et al. 1999).

## Plasma and Serum

Heparinized plasma is the preferred specimen for acylcarnitine analysis, but EDTA plasma and serum are also acceptable. Hemolyzed or lipemic specimens can also be analyzed without negative impact on sensitivity or specificity as long as the laboratory considers the effect of hemolysis on the abundance of long-chain acylcarnitine species when interpreting results. An amount of 100 μL is typically sufficient material to conduct the analysis and repeat it at least once if necessary. Most informative results are generally achieved when samples are obtained during acute illness. Because inborn errors of metabolism are traditionally not entered early into differential diagnostic considerations, sample collection should alternatively be timed before a meal, preferably after an overnight fast. A prolonged fasting challenge, however, should not routinely be undertaken as these require close surveillance typically not possible in an outpatient setting.

## Dried Blood and Dried Bile Spots

Acylcarnitine analysis has been introduced into newborn screening laboratories in the late 1990s and is now part of almost all newborn screening programs. Because newborn screening tests make use of dried blood spots (DBS) collected after a heel prick on the second to fifth day of life, the DBS is the most common specimen used for acylcarnitine analysis. In addition, many biochemical genetics laboratories offer clinical testing of acylcarnitines in DBS for patients at any age. As is true for plasma samples, the most informative results are obtained when blood samples are collected during acute illness or at least prior to a meal. Blood should be obtained by capillary stick of well perfused skin (heels in young infants or fingers) and free dripping of a few drops of blood directly on the filter paper card. For postmortem analysis, blood and bile are collected at the latest at the time of autopsy.

Following complete drying at room temperature for at least 3 h, the sample can be sent ambient. While diagnostic results can be obtained in most cases of medium- and long-chain FAO defects even after prolonged storage time at room temperature, samples should be stored frozen (with desiccant) because particularly short-chain acylcarnitine species are not reliably measurable several months after collection (Matern et al. 1999). At least one blood or bile spot with a diameter of 1 cm should be collected to allow for any necessary repeat testing which usually requires only a DBS punch of 3 mm in diameter.

## Urine

While initially the favored specimen, urine acylcarnitine analysis is the least appropriate when a FAO disorder is under diagnostic consideration. Long-chain acylcarnitines are typically bound to plasma albumin and are not excreted by the kidney. Urine is collected from patients suspected to have an organic acidemia preferably during an acute metabolic decompensation. As this is often not possible, an early morning specimen should be collected. The minimum volume of urine is 1 mL which allows for acylcarnitine and creatinine analysis; the latter is essential to normalize quantitative acylcarnitine results. The sample should be sent frozen and without preservatives.

## Fibroblast Culture Medium

Most FAO disorders present similarly, and their biochemical diagnosis can be difficult because common metabolite screens, such as urine organic acids, plasma acylcarnitines, and fatty acids, are influenced by dietary factors and the clinical status of the patient (Van Hove et al. 2000) leading to incomplete diagnostic information or even false-negative results (Browning et al. 2005). Enzyme assays are limited to one enzyme per assay, and molecular genetic analysis of a relevant gene or gene panels can be complicated by the discovery of genotypes of uncertain significance. The in vitro probe assay offers screening for several defects of FAO and organic acid metabolism under controlled laboratory conditions using fibroblast cultures (Table 5.3). The principle of this assay relies on the assumption that skin fibroblasts of patients affected with relevant conditions will accumulate certain acylcarnitine species reflecting the metabolic defect when the cell medium is supplemented with a long-chain fatty acid, branched-chain amino acids, and L-carnitine. An acylcarnitine analysis can be performed in the post-incubation cell medium by tandem mass spectrometry as for the other sample types (Smith and Matern 2010).

Fibroblasts are typically grown from a small skin biopsy collected during an outpatient visit or as part of a planned surgical procedure following routine culturing techniques. Cell cultures may also derive from umbilical cord or, for prenatal diagnostic purposes, from amniocytes obtained by amniocentesis. Samples should be sent at ambient temperatures.

**Table 5.3** Disorders detectable by the in vitro probe assay

| | |
|---|---|
| Fatty acid β-oxidation disorders | Short-chain acyl-CoA dehydrogenase (SCAD) deficiency |
| | Medium-chain acyl-CoA dehydrogenase (MCAD) deficiency |
| | Long-chain 3-hydroxyacyl-CoA dehydrogenase (LCHAD) deficiency |
| | Mitochondrial trifunctional protein (TFP) deficiency |
| | Very long-chain acyl-CoA dehydrogenase (VLCAD) deficiency |
| | Carnitine palmitoyl transferase type II (CPT-II) deficiency |
| | Carnitine-acylcarnitine translocase (CACT) deficiency |
| Organic acid disorders | Electron transfer flavoprotein (ETF) deficiency, ETF-dehydrogenase deficiency (multiple acyl-CoA dehydrogenase deficiency, MADD; glutaric acidemia type II) |
| | Isovaleric Acidemia |
| | Short-branched-chain acyl-CoA dehydrogenase deficiency (SBCAD deficiency; 2-methylbutyrylglycinuria) |
| | Isobutyryl-CoA dehydrogenase (IBD) deficiency |

**Table 5.4** Reference range for acylcarnitine species (as butylesters) in plasma (nmol/mL)

| | ≤7 days (*n* = 1551) | | | 8 days–7 years (*n* = 26,701) | | | >7 years (*n* = 12,783) | | |
|---|---|---|---|---|---|---|---|---|---|
| Acylcarnitine species | 1st %ile | | 99th %ile | 1st %ile | | 99th %ile | 1st %ile | | 99th %ile |
| C0 | 4.82 | – | 24.28 | 6.13 | – | 32.30 | 5.92 | – | 30.61 |
| C2 | 1.86 | – | 17.50 | 2.40 | – | 27.62 | 1.77 | – | 24.10 |
| C3 | | < | 1.17 | | < | 1.60 | | < | 1.46 |
| FIGLU | | < | 0.10 | | < | 0.04 | | < | 0.04 |
| C4 | | < | 0.81 | | < | 0.81 | | < | 0.78 |
| C5:1 | | < | 0.05 | | < | 0.04 | | < | 0.05 |
| C5 | | < | 0.71 | | < | 0.54 | | < | 0.39 |
| C4-OH | | < | 0.16 | | < | 0.30 | | < | 0.27 |
| C6:1 | | < | 0.05 | | < | 0.05 | | < | 0.05 |
| C6 | | < | 0.17 | | < | 0.22 | | < | 0.19 |
| C5-OH | | < | 0.21 | | < | 0.15 | | < | 0.08 |
| C7 | | < | 0.05 | | < | 0.05 | | < | 0.05 |
| C6-OH | | < | 0.06 | | < | 0.07 | | < | 0.05 |
| C8:1 | | < | 0.73 | | < | 0.75 | | < | 0.70 |
| C8 | | < | 0.41 | | < | 0.41 | | < | 0.45 |
| C3-DC/ C8-OH | | < | 0.11 | | < | 0.13 | | < | 0.16 |
| C10:2 | | < | 0.10 | | < | 0.10 | | < | 0.10 |
| C10:1 | | < | 0.34 | | < | 0.43 | | < | 0.46 |
| C10 | | < | 0.50 | | < | 0.56 | | < | 0.67 |
| C4-DC | | < | 0.07 | | < | 0.06 | | < | 0.07 |
| C10:1-OH | | < | 0.06 | | < | 0.04 | | < | 0.05 |
| C5-DC/ C10-OH | | < | 0.10 | | < | 0.08 | | < | 0.10 |
| C12:1 | | < | 0.15 | | < | 0.18 | | < | 0.19 |
| C12 | | < | 0.21 | | < | 0.20 | | < | 0.19 |
| C6-DC | | < | 0.13 | | < | 0.13 | | | 0.13 |
| C12:1-OH | | < | 0.05 | | < | 0.06 | | < | 0.07 |
| C12-OH | | < | 0.07 | | < | 0.08 | | < | 0.11 |
| C14:2 | | < | 0.10 | | < | 0.13 | | < | 0.13 |
| C14:1 | | < | 0.19 | | < | 0.25 | | < | 0.24 |
| C14 | | < | 0.12 | | < | 0.12 | | < | 0.11 |
| C14:1-OH | | < | 0.03 | | < | 0.04 | | < | 0.04 |
| C14-OH | | < | 0.03 | | < | 0.02 | | < | 0.03 |
| C16:1 | | < | 0.09 | | < | 0.08 | | < | 0.09 |
| C16 | | < | 0.29 | | < | 0.24 | | < | 0.22 |
| C16:1-OH | | < | 0.37 | | < | 0.04 | | < | 0.03 |
| C16-OH | | < | 0.05 | | < | 0.03 | | < | 0.03 |
| C18:2 | | < | 0.16 | | < | 0.17 | | < | 0.19 |
| C18:1 | | < | 0.29 | | < | 0.32 | | < | 0.35 |
| C18 | | < | 0.11 | | < | 0.11 | | < | 0.12 |
| C18:2-OH | | < | 0.02 | | < | 0.02 | | < | 0.03 |
| C18:1-OH | | < | 0.02 | | < | 0.03 | | < | 0.03 |
| C18-OH | | < | 0.02 | | < | 0.02 | | < | 0.02 |

## Interpretation and Reference Ranges

The laboratory director, typically a board certified Clinical Biochemical Geneticist or equivalent, reviews all profiles and provides an interpretation based on pattern recognition and not on single abnormal values (Tables 5.1, 5.4, 5.5, 5.6, and 5.7). Simple reporting of numeric results is not appropriate because most physicians are not familiar with pattern recognition. A comprehensive interpretation takes into consideration any available clinical and dietary information and other laboratory results and provides possible differential diagnoses, recommendations for additional biochemical testing, and confirmatory studies if indicated, as well as contact information for the laboratory director in case the referring physician has additional questions.

## Pitfalls

The ordering physician must be aware of the limitations of a laboratory test and should consider involving the biochemical genetics laboratory in discussions regarding the most appropriate diagnostic work up of patients.

### Pitfalls in Acylcarnitine Analysis of Plasma, Serum, Blood Spots, and Bile Spots

Acylcarnitine profiles are dependent on the clinical status of the patient at the time of sample collection (Van Hove et al. 2000). Accordingly, all samples should be submitted to the biochemical genetics laboratory with information regarding the clinical context during which the sample was collected. The laboratory must be aware of the fact that carnitine deficiency states can cause seemingly normal acylcarnitine profiles due to the lack of carnitine as substrate for carnitine palmitoyl transferases. Accordingly, it is crucial to review the complete profile and to initiate follow-up when even bor-

**Table 5.5** Reference range of acylcarnitine species (as butylesters) in dried blood spots of adult controls (in nmol/mL)

| | Blood spots | | |
|---|---|---|---|
| | ($n = 99$) | | |
| Acylcarnitine species | 1st percentile | | 99th percentile |
| C0 | 11.16 | – | 40.08 |
| C2 | 5.77 | – | 20.23 |
| C3 | | < | 2.82 |
| C4 | | < | 0.43 |
| C5:1 | | < | 0.05 |
| C5 | | < | 0.30 |
| C4-OH | | < | 0.11 |
| C6 | | < | 0.14 |
| C5-OH | | < | 0.61 |
| C6-OH | | < | 0.06 |
| C8:1 | | < | 0.26 |
| C8 | | < | 0.25 |
| C3-DC | | < | 0.06 |
| C10:2 | | < | 0.04 |
| C10:1 | | < | 0.47 |
| C10 | | < | 0.35 |
| C4-DC | | < | 0.66 |
| C5-DC | | < | 0.07 |
| C12:1 | | < | 0.30 |
| C12 | | < | 0.28 |
| C12:1-OH | | < | 0.06 |
| C12-OH | | < | 0.03 |
| C14:2 | | < | 0.14 |
| C14:1 | | < | 0.31 |
| C14 | | < | 0.41 |
| C14-OH | | < | 0.12 |
| C16:1 | | < | 0.10 |
| C16 | | < | 1.72 |
| C16:1-OH | | < | 0.05 |
| C16-OH | | < | 0.04 |
| C18:2 | | < | 0.48 |
| C18:1 | | < | 1.49 |
| C18 | | < | 0.93 |
| C18:2-OH | | < | 0.07 |
| C18:1-OH | | < | 0.06 |
| C18-OH | | < | 0.02 |

derline elevated acylcarnitines are noted in the presence of abnormally low free and acetylcarnitine. If clinically indicated, a repeat sample should be collected as early as 24 h after L-carnitine supplementation.

The laboratory must also note when specimens are hemolyzed because it will lead to an increase in long-chain acylcarnitines which needs to be considered when interpreting the acylcarnitine profile to avoid unnecessary follow-up investigations to rule out a long-chain FAO disorder (Mancinelli et al. 2007).

While FIA-MS/MS allows for unequivocal identification of most metabolites, there are a few exceptions (Table 5.1). In particular, the short-chain acylcarnitines of 4 and 5 carbons represent more than one analyte. $C_4$-Acylcarnitine is known to be a mixture of butyrylcarnitine derived from fatty acid metabolism and isobutyrylcarnitine derived from the metabolism of valine (Oglesbee et al. 2007). $C_4$-OH acylcarnitine can be a mixture of the D-3-OH-butyrylcarnitine, associated with ketosis; L-3-OH-butyrylcarnitine, associated with SCHAD-deficiency; or 3-OH-isobutyrylcarnitine, characteristic of the valine degradation defect 3-OH-isobutyryl-CoA hydrolase deficiency. $C_5$-Acylcarnitine is a mixture of isovalerylcarnitine and 2-methylbutyrylcarnitine derived from leucine and isoleucine degradation, respectively (Ensenauer et al. 2004; Matern et al. 2003). Samples of patients treated with antibiotics containing pivalic acid (trimethylacetic acid) such as pivampicillin, may contain pivaloylcarnitine, another C5 species. Several other metabolites are also nonspecific markers for several disorders. For example, $C_5$-OH acylcarnitine, which represents 3-hydroxyisovalerylcarnitine and 2-methyl-3-hydroxybutyrylcarnitine, can be elevated in seven different organic acidemias. The interpretation of elevated $C_5$-OH acylcarnitine in newborns or breast-fed infants is further complicated by the fact that it can indicate maternal 3-methylcrotonylglycinuria while the infant is only an unaffected carrier (Gibson et al. 1998). Differentiation is of clinical importance and most efficiently achieved by urine acylglycine and organic acid analyses, or by plasma acylcarnitine analysis by LC-MS/MS.

CPT-I deficiency, characterized by high free carnitine and relatively low long-chain acylcarnitine species, is more challenging to detect in plasma than in DBS because of already lower abundance of long-chain acylcarnitines in plasma. The long-chain FAO disorders of CACT deficiency and CPT-II deficiency cannot be differentiated because both cause accumulation of the same long-chain acylcarnitine species which is explained by the fact that neither enzyme is involved in the chain-shortening action of FAO. Isolated LCHAD deficiency and complete mitochondrial TFP deficiency also cannot be differentiated by routine acylcarnitine analysis (Van Hove et al. 2000). When such profiles are encountered, delineation of the correct defect is only possible by either specific enzyme assay in cell cultures or molecular genetic analysis of the relevant genes. MCAD and multiple acyl-CoA dehydrogenase (MAD) defects require the identification of medium-chain acylcarnitines. In this respect, it is important to realize that patients on a medium-chain triglyceride containing diet may accumulate C8 and C10 carnitine, potentially obscuring the diagnosis.

Isolated elevations of propionylcarnitine ($C_3$) are not specific for propionic acidemia but also observed in methylmalonic acidemias of various etiologies. Because methylmalonylcarnitine ($C_4$-DC) is not consistently elevated in methylmalonic acidemias, elucidation of the correct diagnosis requires at a minimum urine organic acid analysis.

Another antibiotic that may cause problems in the interpretation of butylated acylcarnitines is cefotaxime

**Table 5.6** Percentile ranks of acylcarnitine species (as butylesters) in postmortem dried blood and bile spots (in nmol/mL)

| | Blood spots ($n = 9788$) | | | Bile spots ($n = 8848$) | | |
|---|---|---|---|---|---|---|
| Acylcarnitine species | 5th percentile | | 95th percentile | 5th percentile | | 95th percentile |
| C0 | 29 | – | 203 | 57 | – | 371 |
| C2 | 26.8 | – | 194 | 36 | – | 311 |
| C3 | | < | 10.9 | | < | 11.6 |
| C4 | | < | 17.2 | | < | 7.5 |
| C5:1 | | < | 0.23 | | < | 0.71 |
| C5 | | < | 2.10 | | < | 3.13 |
| C4-OH | | < | 7.36 | | < | 3.05 |
| C6 | | < | 2.19 | | < | 2.64 |
| C5-OH | | < | 0.96 | | < | 1.24 |
| C7 | | < | 0.16 | | < | 0.92 |
| C6-OH | | < | 0.56 | | < | 1.22 |
| C8:1 | | < | 0.77 | | < | 26.1 |
| C8 | | < | 0.78 | | < | 5.20 |
| C3-DC | | < | 0.45 | | < | 1.35 |
| C10:2 | | < | 0.11 | | < | 2.53 |
| C10:1 | | < | 0.17 | | < | 6.66 |
| C10 | | < | 0.52 | | < | 4.33 |
| C4-DC | | < | 1.10 | | < | 1.21 |
| C10:1-OH | | < | 0.15 | | < | 1.36 |
| C5-DC | | < | 0.30 | | < | 1.13 |
| C12:1 | | < | 0.11 | | < | 5.19 |
| C12 | | < | 0.54 | | < | 5.47 |
| C12:1-OH | | < | 0.13 | | < | 1.96 |
| C12-OH | | < | 0.17 | | < | 1.00 |
| C14:2 | | < | 0.56 | | < | 4.31 |
| C14:1 | | < | 0.24 | | < | 5.26 |
| C14 | | < | 0.46 | | < | 2.28 |
| C14:1-OH | | < | 0.09 | | < | 1.34 |
| C14-OH | | < | 0.09 | | < | 0.57 |
| C16:1 | | < | 0.27 | | < | 1.76 |
| C16 | | < | 2.04 | | < | 3.07 |
| C16:1-OH | | < | 0.11 | | < | 1.21 |
| C16-OH | | < | 0.11 | | < | 0.68 |
| C18:2 | | < | 0.69 | | < | 2.15 |
| C18:1 | | < | 1.98 | | < | 3.38 |
| C18 | | < | 1.54 | | < | 3.58 |
| C18:2-OH | | < | 0.13 | | < | 0.58 |
| C18:1-OH | | < | 0.14 | | < | 0.70 |
| C18-OH | | < | 0.11 | | < | 0.61 |

(Vianey-Saban et al. 2004). This antibiotic or metabolites thereof reveals itself by acylcarnitine analysis (following derivatization to butylesters) at m/z 470 which otherwise represents monounsaturated 3-hydoxyhexadecenoylcarnitine ($C_{16:1}$-OH). In poorly resolved scans, this may be difficult to differentiate from m/z 472 which is a marker for LCHAD and TFP deficiencies. However, whereas m/z 472 ($C_{16}$-OH) is more abundant than $C_{16:1}$-OH in these FAO disorders, the profile of a patient treated with cefotaxime usually reveals an m/z 470 to m/z 472 ratio that is greater than 1. Furthermore and in contrast to cefotaxime treatment, both LCHAD and TFP deficiencies are usually accompanied by elevations of other long-chain species (Table 5.1) (Van Hove et al. 2000).

Formiminoglutamate (FIGLU), a marker for glutamate formimino-transferase deficiency, is revealed in acylcarnitine profiles by a peak with m/z 287 (Malvagia et al. 2006). In poorly resolved acylcarnitine profiles, this peak may be confused with iso-/butyrylcarnitine (m/z 288). To avoid the incorrect interpretation of acylcarnitine profiles, the analysis is best performed in product scan mode as opposed to multiple reaction monitoring (MRM) mode.

**Table 5.7** Reference range for urine acylcarnitines (as butylesters) based on samples with normal organic acid results ($n = 40$)

| Acylcarnitine species | (mmol/mol creatinine) | | |
|---|---|---|---|
| C0 | 0.35 | – | 31.60 |
| C2 | | < | 16.46 |
| C3 | | < | 1.20 |
| C4 | | < | 2.74 |
| C5:1 | | < | 0.34 |
| C5 | | < | 1.53 |
| C4-OH | | < | 0.26 |
| C6 | | < | 0.16 |
| C5-OH | | < | 0.52 |
| C6-OH | | < | 0.32 |
| C8:1 | | < | 4.30 |
| C8 | | < | 0.61 |
| C3-DC | | < | 0.50 |
| C10:2 | | < | 0.48 |
| C10:1 | | < | 0.65 |
| C10 | | < | 0.21 |
| C4-DC | | < | 0.57 |
| C10:1-OH | | < | 0.26 |
| C5-DC (C10-OH) | | < | 0.37 |
| C12:1 | | < | 0.07 |
| C12 | | < | 0.19 |
| C6-DC | | < | 0.81 |
| C12:1-OH | | < | 0.27 |
| C12-OH | | < | 0.16 |
| C14:2 | | < | 0.02 |
| C14:1 | | < | 0.21 |
| C14 | | < | 0.39 |
| C14:1-OH | | < | 0.14 |
| C14-OH | | < | 0.09 |
| C16:1 | | < | 0.04 |
| C16 | | < | 0.18 |
| C16:1-OH | | < | 0.02 |
| C16-OH | | < | 0.05 |
| C18:2 | | < | 0.02 |
| C18:1 | | < | 0.02 |
| C18 | | < | 0.05 |
| C18:2-OH | | < | 0.01 |
| C18:1-OH | | < | 0.03 |
| C18-OH | | < | 0.02 |

### Pitfalls in Acylcarnitine Analysis of Urine

Aside from the abovementioned potential problems (see D.7.1) such as the inability to discriminate isomers and interfering metabolites of antibiotics, urine also often contains a variety of non-identified substances. This makes the interpretation of urine acylcarnitine profiles inherently more complex, and overinterpretation must be avoided. Therefore, urine acylcarnitine analysis should not be included in the first line of screening investigations but be targeted to specific diagnostic considerations, in particular, organic acidemias. A role of urine acylcarnitine analysis for the diagnosis of FAO disorders has not been established.

### Pitfalls in Acylcarnitine Analysis of Post-incubation Fibroblast Culture Medium

The in vitro probe assay is performed under standardized conditions and is independent of the patient's status at the time the skin biopsy is obtained. The accumulation of acylcarnitines in this assay system appears to be dependent on potentially present residual enzyme activity and therefore provides information regarding the severity of an enzyme deficiency state for some disorders such as VLCAD and SCAD deficiencies. Furthermore, as is true for acylcarnitine analysis of other sample types, TFP and isolated LCHAD deficiencies as well as CPT-II and CACT deficiencies cannot be differentiated. The analysis of fibroblasts also does not allow for the diagnosis of enzyme deficiency states that are not expressed in this tissue (e.g., the liver-specific SCHAD deficiency). Finally, conditions not associated with an abnormal accumulation of acylcarnitines, such as CPT-I or primary carnitine deficiencies, are not identified by this assay.

## References


Abdenur JE, Chamoles NA, Guinle AE, Schenone AB, Fuertes AN. Diagnosis of isovaleric acidaemia by tandem mass spectrometry: false positive result due to pivaloylcarnitine in a newborn screening programme. J Inherit Metab Dis. 1998;21:624–30.

Bosch AM, Abeling NG, Ijlst L, Knoester H, van der Pol WL, Stroomer AE, Wanders RJ, Visser G, Wijburg FA, Duran M, Waterham HR. Brown-Vialetto-Van Laere and Fazio Londe syndrome is associated with a riboflavin transporter defect mimicking mild MADD: a new inborn error of metabolism with potential treatment. J Inherit Metab Dis. 2011;34:159–64.

Browning MF, Larson C, Strauss A, Marsden DL. Normal acylcarnitine levels during confirmation of abnormal newborn screening in long-chain fatty acid oxidation defects. J Inherit Metab Dis. 2005;28:545–50.

Carrozzo R, Dionisi-Vici C, Steuerwald U, Lucioli S, Deodato F, Di Giandomenico S, Bertini E, Franke B, Kluijtmans LA, Meschini MC, Rizzo C, Piemonte F, Rodenburg R, Santer R, Santorelli FM, van Rooij A, Vermunt-de Koning D, Morava E, Wevers RA. SUCLA2 mutations are associated with mild methylmalonic aciduria, Leigh-like encephalomyopathy, dystonia and deafness. Brain. 2007;130:862–74.

De Jesús VR, Chace DH, Lim TH, Mei JV, Hannon WH. Comparison of amino acids and acylcarnitines assay methods used in newborn screening assays by tandem mass spectrometry. Clin Chim Acta. 2010;411:684–9.

DiMauro S, DiMauro PM. Muscle carnitine palmityltransferase deficiency and myoglobinuria. Science. 1973;182:929–31.

Engel AG, Angelini C. Carnitine deficiency of human skeletal muscle with associated lipid storage myopathy: a new syndrome. Science. 1973;179:899–902.

Ensenauer R, Vockley J, Willard JM, Huey JC, Sass JO, Edland SD, Burton BK, Berry SA, Santer R, Grunert S, Koch HG, Marquardt I, Rinaldo P, Hahn S, Matern D. A common mutation is associated with a mild, potentially asymptomatic phenotype in patients with isovaleric acidemia diagnosed by newborn screening. Am J Hum Genet. 2004;75:1136–42.

Gibson KM, Bennett MJ, Naylor EW, Morton DH. 3-methylcrotonyl-coenzyme a carboxylase deficiency in amish/mennonite adults identified by detection of increased acylcarnitines in blood spots of their children. J Pediatr. 1998;132:519–23.

Herzog K, van Lenthe H, Wanders RJA, Vaz FM, Waterham HR, Ferdinandusse S. Identification and diagnostic value of phytanoyl- and pristanoyl-carnitine in plasma from patients with peroxisomal disorders. Mol Genet Metab. 2017;121:279–82.

Houten SM, Denis S, Te Brinke H, Jongejan A, van Kampen AH, Bradley EJ, Baas F, Hennekam RC, Millington DS, Young SP, Frazier DM, Gucsavas-Calikoglu M, Wanders RJ. Mitochondrial NADP(H) deficiency due to a mutation in NADK2 causes dienoyl-CoA reductase deficiency with hyperlysinemia. Hum Mol Genet. 2014;23:5009–16.

Huffnagel IC, van de Beek MC, Showers AL, Orsini JJ, Klouwer FCC, Dijkstra IME, Schielen PC, van Lenthe H, Wanders RJA, Vaz FM, Morrissey MA, Engelen M, Kemp S. Comparison of C26:0-carnitine and C26:0-lysophosphatidylcholine as diagnostic markers in dried blood spots from newborns and patients with adrenoleukodystrophy. Mol Genet Metab. 2017;122:209–15.

Knottnerus SJG, Bleeker JC, Wüst RCI, Ferdinandusse S, IJlst L, Wijburg FA, Wanders RJA, Visser G, Houtkooper RH. Disorders of mitochondrial long-chain fatty acid oxidation and the carnitine shuttle. Rev Endocr Metab Disord. 2018;19:93–106.

Malvagia S, La Marca G, Casetta B, Gasperini S, Pasquini E, Donati MA, Zammarchi E. Falsely elevated C4-carnitine as expression of glutamate formiminotransferase deficiency in tandem mass spectrometry newborn screening. J Mass Spectrom. 2006;41:263–5.

Mancinelli A, Iannoni E, Calvani M, Duran M. Effect of temperature on the stability of long-chain acylcarnitines in human blood prior to plasma separation. Clin Chim Acta. 2007;375:169–70.

Matern D, Strauss AW, Hillman SL, Mayatepek E, Millington DS, Trefz FK. Diagnosis of mitochondrial trifunctional protein deficiency in a blood spot from the newborn screening card by tandem mass spectrometry and DNA analysis. Pediatr Res. 1999;46:45–9.

Matern D, He M, Berry SA, Rinaldo P, Whitley CB, Madsen PP, Van Calcar SC, Lussky RC, Andresen BS, Wolff JA, Vockley J. Prospective diagnosis of 2-methylbutyryl-CoA dehydrogenase deficiency in the Hmong population by newborn screening using tandem mass spectrometry. Pediatrics. 2003;112:74–8.

Millington DS, Terada N, Chace DH, Chen YT, Ding JH, Kodo N, Roe CR. The role of tandem mass spectrometry in the diagnosis of fatty acid oxidation disorders. Prog Clin Biol Res. 1992;375:339–54.

Minkler PE, Stoll MS, Ingalls ST, Kerner J, Hoppel CL. Quantitative acylcarnitine determination by UHPLC-MS/MS—going beyond tandem MS acylcarnitine "profiles". Mol Genet Metab. 2015;116:231–41.

Oglesbee D, He M, Majumder N, Vockley J, Ahmad A, Angle B, Burton B, Charrow J, Ensenauer R, Ficicioglu CH, Keppen LD, Marsden D, Tortorelli S, Hahn SH, Matern D. Development of a newborn screening follow-up algorithm for the diagnosis of isobutyryl-CoA dehydrogenase deficiency. Genet Med. 2007;9:108–16.

Rinaldo P, Studinski AL, Matern D. Prenatal diagnosis of disorders of fatty acid transport and mitochondrial oxidation. Prenat Diagn. 2001;21:52–4.

Rinaldo P, Matern D, Bennett MJ. Fatty acid oxidation disorders. Annu Rev Physiol. 2002;64:477–502.

Rinaldo P, Hahn S, Matern D. Clinical biochemical genetics in the twenty-first century. Acta Paediatr. 2004;93:22–6.

Roe DS, Vianey-Saban C, Sharma S, Zabot MT, Roe CR. Oxidation of unsaturated fatty acids by human fibroblasts with very-long-chain acyl-CoA dehydrogenase deficiency: aspects of substrate specificity and correlation with clinical phenotype. Clin Chim Acta. 2001;312:55–67.

Schulze-Bergkamen A, Okun JG, Spiekerkotter U, Linder M, Haas D, Kohlmuller D, Mayatepek E, Schulze-Bergkamen H, Greenberg CR, Zschocke J, Hoffmann GF, Kolker S. Quantitative acylcarnitine profiling in peripheral blood mononuclear cells using in vitro loading with palmitic and 2-oxoadipic acids: biochemical confirmation of fatty acid oxidation and organic acid disorders. Pediatr Res. 2005;58:873.

Shen JJ, Matern D, Millington DS, Hillman S, Feezor MD, Bennett MJ, Qumsiyeh M, Kahler SG, Chen YT, Van Hove JL. Acylcarnitines in fibroblasts of patients with long-chain 3-hydroxyacyl-CoA dehydrogenase deficiency and other fatty acid oxidation disorders. J Inherit Metab Dis. 2000;23:27–44.

Smith EH, Matern D. Acylcarnitine analysis by tandem mass spectrometry. Curr Protoc Hum Genet. 2010;Chapter 17: Unit 17.8.1–20.

Tortorelli S, Hahn SH, Cowan TM, Brewster TG, Rinaldo P, Matern D. The urinary excretion of glutarylcarnitine is an informative tool in the biochemical diagnosis of glutaric acidemia type I. Mol Genet Metab. 2005;84:137–43.

Van Hove JL, Kahler SG, Feezor MD, Ramakrishna JP, Hart P, Treem WR, Shen JJ, Matern D, Millington DS. Acylcarnitines in plasma and blood spots of patients with long-chain 3-hydroxyacyl-coenzyme A dehydrogenase defiency. J Inherit Metab Dis. 2000;23:571–82.

Vaz FM, Wanders RJ. Carnitine biosynthesis in mammals. Biochem J. 2002;361:417–29.

Vianey-Saban C, Boyer S, Levrat V, Cheillan D, Piraud M, Guffon N, Maire I. Interference of Cefotaxime in plasma acylcarnitine profile mimicking an increase of 3-hydroxypalmitoleylcarnitine (C16:1-OH) using butyl esters. J Inherit Metab Dis. 2004;27(Suppl 1):94.

Young SP, Matern D, Gregersen N, Stevens RD, Bali D, Liu HM, Koeberl DD, Millington DS. A comparison of in vitro acylcarnitine profiling methods for the diagnosis of classical and variant short chain acyl-CoA dehydrogenase deficiency. Clin Chim Acta. 2003;337:103–13.

# Lysosomals

6

Silvia Funghini, Sabrina Malvagia, Giulia Polo, and Giancarlo la Marca

## Contents



**Abstract**

Lysosomal storage diseases (LSDs) are a group of inherited metabolic disorders that result from lysosomal dysfunction. Most LSDs are autosomal recessively inherited disorders, with only three exceptions that are X-linked. The overall incidence is about 1 in 5000 live births. Mutations in genes encoding lysosomal proteins cause lysosomal malfunction with the gradual accumulation of substrates leading to cell dysfunction and cell death. LSDs are generally classified based on the biochemical type of accumulated substrate that leads to a heterogeneous spectrum of clinical manifestations. The diagnostic suspicion of LSDs is based on clinical symptoms, and the measurement of the abnormal accumulation of substrates in biological fluids. The diagnosis is confirmed by enzymatic and/or genetic analysis, including next-generation sequencing and whole exome sequencing. In the last years, many efficient therapies have been developed. New treatments and the evidence that the early treatment shortly after birth can permit a better outcome have led to the development of several pilot newborn screening programs for some LSDs. Early detection in a presymptomatic state and prompt treatment can modify the natural history of LSD disease preventing irreversible damage of the involved key organs.

S. Funghini · S. Malvagia
Newborn Screening, Clinical Chemistry and Pharmacology Lab, Meyer Children's University Hospital, Florence, Italy
e-mail: s.funghini@meyer.it; s.malvagia@meyer.it

G. Polo
Division of Inherited Metabolic Diseases, Department of Women and Children's Health, Regional Center for Expanded Neonatal Screening, University Hospital of Padova, Padova, Italy
e-mail: giulia.polo@aopd.veneto.it

G. la Marca (✉)
Newborn Screening, Clinical Chemistry and Pharmacology Lab, Meyer Children's University Hospital, Florence, Italy

Department of Experimental and Clinical Biomedical Sciences, University of Florence, Florence, Italy
e-mail: g.lamarca@meyer.it

## Introduction

Lysosomal storage diseases (LSDs) are a group of more than 70 inherited metabolic disorders that result from lysosomal dysfunction. Most LSDs are autosomal recessively inherited disorders, with only three exceptions that are X-linked. These disorders are individually rare, but collectively the incidence is about 1 in 5000 live births (Platt et al. 2018). Mutations in genes encoding lysosomal proteins, such as proteases, transporters, or integral membrane proteins,


N. Blau et al. (eds.), *Physician's Guide to the Diagnosis, Treatment, and Follow-Up of Inherited Metabolic Diseases*,
https://doi.org/10.1007/978-3-030-67727-5_6

cause lysosomal malfunction with the gradual accumulation of substrates that lead to cell dysfunction and cell death. LSDs are classified based on the biochemical type of accumulated substrate, or on whether disorders involve integral membrane proteins or lipofuscin production (Table 6.1). The storage process leads to a heterogeneous spectrum of clinical manifestations depending on the specific substrate and site of accumulation. Age at onset can range from newborns to adults, and these disorders are progressive. The diagnostic suspicion of LSDs is based on clinical symptoms, and the valuation of the abnormal accumulation of substrates in biological fluids (mostly urine) is the first step in the diagnos-

**Table 6.1** Classification of lysosomal storage disorders

| Disease | Alternative titles | Primary defect | OMIM |
|---|---|---|---|
| ***Mucopolysaccharidoses*** | | | |
| MPS type I | Hurler syndrome, Hurler-Scheie syndrome, Scheie syndrome | Alpha-L-iduronidase | 252800 |
| MPS type II | Hunter syndrome | Iduronate 2-sulfatase | 309900 |
| MPS type IIIA | Sanfilippo syndrome A | *N*-Sulfoglucosamine sulfohydrolase | 252900 |
| MPS type IIIB | Sanfilippo syndrome B | *N*-Alpha-acetylglucosaminidase | 252920 |
| MPS type IIIC | Sanfilippo syndrome C | Heparan acetyl-CoA:alpha-glucosaminide *N*-acetyltransferase | 252930 |
| MPS type IIID | Sanfilippo syndrome D | *N*-Acetylglucosamine-6-sulfatase | 252940 |
| MPS type IVA | Morquio syndrome A | *N*-Acetylgalactosamine-6-sulfatase | 253000 |
| MPS type IVB | Morquio syndrome B | Beta-galactosidase | 253010 |
| MPS type VI | Maroteaux-Lamy syndrome | Arylsulfatase B | 253200 |
| MPS type VII | Sly syndrome | Beta-glucuronidase | 253220 |
| MPS type IX | Natowicz syndrome | Hyaluronidase 1 | 601492 |
| ***Glycoproteinoses*** | | | |
| Aspartylglucosaminuria | | Glycosylasparaginase | 208400 |
| Fucosidosis | | Alpha-L-fucosidase | 230000 |
| Galactosialidosis | Goldberg syndrome | Protective protein cathepsin A, secondary deficiency in beta-galactosidase and neuraminidase 1 | 256540 |
| α-Mannosidosis | | Alpha-mannosidase | 248500 |
| β-Mannosidosis | | Beta-mannosidase | 248510 |
| Mucolipidosis I | Sialidosis type II | Neuraminidase 1 | 256550 |
| Schindler disease | Neuroaxonal dystrophy, Schindler type | Alpha-*N*-acetylgalactosaminidase | 609241 |
| ***Sphingolipidoses*** | | | |
| Fabry disease | Anderson-Fabry disease | Alpha-galactosidase A | 301500 |
| Farber disease | Farber lipogranulomatosis | *N*-Acylsphingosine amidohydrolase | 613468 |
| Gaucher disease | | Beta-glucosidase (beta-glucocerebrosidase) | 230800 |
| GM1 Gangliosidosis | | Beta-galactosidase-1 | 230500 |
| GM2 Gangliosidosis type I | Tay-Sachs disease | Beta-hexosaminidase A | 272800 |
| GM2 Gangliosidosis type II | Sandhoff disease | Beta-hexosaminidase A + B | 268800 |
| GM2 activator deficiency | AB variant | GM2 ganglioside activator | 613109 |
| Krabbe disease | Globoid cell leukodistrophy | Galactosylceramidase | 245200 |
| Metachromatic leukodystrophy | | Arylsulfatase A, prosaposin, saposin B | 250100 |
| Niemann-Pick disease type A | | Acid sphingomyelinase | 257200 |
| Niemann-Pick disease type B | | Acid sphingomyelinase | 607616 |
| ***Glycogen storage disease*** | | | |
| Glycogen storage disorder type II | Pompe disease | Acid-alpha-glucosidase | 232300 |
| ***Lipid storage diseases*** | | | |
| Lysosomal acid lipase deficiency | Wolman disease | Lysosomal acid lipase | 278000 |
| ***Post-translational modification defects*** | | | |
| Multiple sulfatase deficiency | Mucosulfatidosis | Family of sulfatase enzymes | 272200 |
| Mucolipidosis II | I-cell disease | *N*-acetylglucosamine-1-phosphotransferase | 252500 |
| Mucolipidosis III | Pseudo-Hurler polydystrophy | *N*-acetylglucosamine-1-phosphotransferase | 252600 |
| ***Integral membrane protein disorders*** | | | |
| Cystinosis | | Cystinosin | 219800 |
| Glycogen storage disorder type IIb | Danon disease | LAMP-2 | 300257 |
| Sialuria | Salla disease | Vesicular excitatory amino acid transporter (VEAT) | 604369 |
| Niemann-Pick disease type C1 | Niemann-Pick disease type C | NPC intracellular cholesterol transporter 1 | 257220 |
| Niemann-Pick disease type C2[a] | | Niemann-Pick disease type C2 protein | 607625 |
| Mucolipidosis IV | Sialolipidosis | Mucolipin 1 | 252650 |

**Table 6.1** (continued)

| Disease | Alternative titles | Primary defect | OMIM |
|---|---|---|---|
| ***Neuronal ceroid lipofuscinoses*** | | | |
| CLN1 | Santavuori-Haltia disease | Palmitoyl-protein thioesterase 1 | 256730 |
| CLN2 | Jansky-Bielshowsky disease | Tripeptidyl-peptidase 1 | 204500 |
| CLN3 | Batten disease | Battenin | 204200 |
| CLN4A | Kufs disease type A | Ceroid-lipofuscinosis neuronal protein 6 | 204300 |
| CLN4B | Kufs disease type B | DnaJ homolog subfamily C member 5 | 162350 |
| CLN5 | | Ceroid-lipofuscinosis neuronal protein 5 | 608102 |
| CLN6 | | Ceroid-lipofuscinosis neuronal protein 6 | 601780 |
| CLN7 | Turkish variant | Major facilitator superfamily domain-containing protein 8 | 610951 |
| CLN8 | | Protein CLN8 | 600143 |
| CLN9 | | Unknown | |
| CLN10 | | Cathepsin D | 610127 |
| CLN11 | | Progranulin | 614706 |
| CLN12 | Kufor-rakeb syndrome | Cation-transporting ATPase 13A2 | 606693 |
| CLN13 | Kufs disease type B | Cathepsin F | 615362 |
| CLN14 | | BTB/POZ domain-containing protein KCTD7 | 611726 |

[a]Although NPC1 is an integral membrane protein, NPC2 is an intralysosomal soluble protein

tic flow chart. Although in very recent years many papers have been published with very high potentiality, there is no single instrument platform/analytical technique that currently can analyze all metabolites involved in LSDs, and the metabolomics approach is still not widely available. LSD analysis is generally performed on a single category of molecules with classical biochemical tests ranging from thin layer chromatography, liquid chromatography, or electrophoresis. The diagnosis must be confirmed by enzymatic and/or genetic analysis, including next-generation sequencing and whole exome sequencing. In the last years, many therapeutic options, such as enzyme replacement therapy (ERT), hematopoietic stem cell transplantation, substrate reduction therapy, pharmacological chaperone therapy, and gene therapy, have been developed. New treatments and the evidence that the early treatment shortly after birth often leads to a better outcome have led to the development of several pilot newborn screening programs for some LSDs (Gelb 2018). Early detection in a presymptomatic state and prompt treatment can modify the natural history of LSD disease preventing irreversible damage of the involved key organs.

## Preanalytical Conditions

### Glycosaminoglycans in Urine

Urine samples should be collected for 24 h, when possible. But considering that prolonged urine collections are quite difficult especially in newborns or very young babies, a random sample, preferably the first morning voiding, is acceptable (not less than 15–20 mL). Storage temperature must be −20 °C until analysis. No preservatives are required.

### Oligosaccharides in Urine

Urine samples collected for 24 h are mandatory. The minimum volume of urine is 5 mL, and the storage temperature must be −20 °C until analysis. No preservatives are required.

### Free and Total Sialic Acid

Urine samples collected for 24 h are mandatory. The minimum volume of urine is 5 mL, and the storage temperature must be −20 °C until analysis. No preservatives are required.

### Enzymatic Assays on Dried Blood Spot

1. Newborn screening: dried blood spot is collected by neonatal heel prick. It is important to apply single drops of blood only on one side of the filter paper (not apply multiple drops of blood in the same circle or in front and behind the filter). Avoid touching the area within the circles on the filter paper section before, during, and after collection of the specimen. Cards with blood spots must be dried at room temperature, far from heat sources, for not less than 90 min. Most enzymes are stable at room temperature for the first 20 days, but storage temperature between +4 °C and −20 °C is advised for greater stability.
2. Venous blood collection: dried venous blood spot is collected by finger prick. For the collection and storage, follow the previous indications.
3. Venous blood collection from tubes: apply 20 μL of blood from heparin/EDTA tubes and follow the previous indications.

### Chitotriosidase in Plasma

For this analysis, 1–2 mL of blood in heparinized tube is needed. Plasma must be separated from blood within 1 h, and it can be stored at −20 °C until the assay.

**Enzymatic Assays on Leukocytes**

For most assays, 6–10 mL of blood in heparinized/EDTA tube at room temperature is needed. It is important to use a needle with less chance of hemolysis. The separation of leukocytes from whole blood must be performed within 24 h from the collection. Leukocyte pellets can be stored at −20 °C until the assay.

**Enzymatic Assays on Fibroblasts**

Fibroblast cultures are generally derived from forearm skin biopsies. For most testing, two 75 $cm^2$ flasks are sufficient. Fibroblast pellets can be stored at −20 °C until the assay.

### Other Specimens

Amniotic fluid, tear fluid, chorionic villi, and amniocytes can be used in some isolated cases.

## Analysis

### Glycosaminoglycans Assay

The mucopolysaccharidoses are a group of LSDs characterized by an accumulation of mucopolysaccharides, also known as glycosaminoglycans (GAGs), causing dysfunction of cells, tissues, and organs. Each disorder results from a specific lysosomal enzyme defect that affects the normal degradation pathway of glycosaminoglycans. Undegraded or partially degraded GAGs are accumulated in lysosomes and then excreted in the urine. The correlation between biochemical findings and enzymatic defect is reported in Table 6.2, and the correlation between structure and catabolism is reported and shown in Fig. 6.1.

**Total Glycosaminoglycans Analysis in Urine**

An initial screening test to check for an elevation in total GAGs concentration can be a useful tool when a MPS disorder is suspected. Several methods have been developed for GAGs quantification in urine. One first approach is an Alcian blue (tetravalent cationic dye) spot test, which semi-quantitatively estimates the amount of total GAGs present. Even if the complex formation with Alcian blue depends on the sulfation patterns and keratan sulfate fragments with low degree of sulfation may not be detected, patients with Morquio syndrome can be equally detected due to excretion of chondroitin 6-sulfate. Cetylpyridinium chloride (CPC) is generally used to extract urinary GAGs prior to analysis. Quantitation can be performed by carbazole method determining uronic acid formation. Another simple test is based on the modification of dimethylmethylene blue (DMB) assay (de Jong et al. 1992). It allows the measurement of all GAGs without response difference among urinary metabolites. By using all methods, false-negative results may occur especially in MPS-I, MPS-III, MPS-IV, MPS-VI, and MPS-VII. Many cases of false-positive results have been reported in literature. Some of these concerned other LSD non-mucopolysaccharidoses with normal total concentrations of urinary GAGs but isolated increment such as in multiple sulphatase deficiency (HS), $GM_1$ (KS), Morquio IV A and B (KS), and fucosidosis (KS). A new DMB-based method named GAG-Test® has been recently reported with a referred sensitivity of 100% (Lage et al. 2011). In addition, total GAGs can be quantified and analyzed by HPLC (Studelska et al. 2006) and capillary electrophoresis (Ucakturk et al. 2014).

Total urinary GAGs show significant age-related difference: infants tend to have higher average GAG levels than adults. Reference values of urine GAGs are reported in Table 6.3.

**Qualitative and Quantitative Glycosaminoglycan Analysis in Urine**

Eleven enzymes are involved in the catabolic pathways of GAGs. Deficiencies in each of these enzymes result in specific GAG accumulation: chondroitin sulfate (CS), dermatan sulfate (DS), heparan sulfate (HS), keratan sulfate (KS), or hyaluronan.

**Table 6.2** Classification of the mucopolysaccharidoses

| Mucopolysaccharidoses | Glycosaminoglycans excreted in urine | Defective enzyme | Inheritance |
|---|---|---|---|
| MPS-I H/S | DS; HS | Alpha-L-iduronidase | AR |
| MPS-II | DS; HS | Iduronate sulfatase | XR |
| MPS-IIIA | HS | Heparan *N*-sulfatase | AR |
| MPS-IIIB | HS | Alpha-*N*-acetylglucosaminidase | AR |
| MPS-IIIC | HS | Acetyl CoA:alpha-glucosaminide acetyltransferase | AR |
| MPS-IIID | HS | *N*-acetylglucosamine-6-sulfatase | AR |
| MPS-IVA | KS; C 6-S | *N*-acetylgalactosamine-6-sulfate sulfatase | AR |
| MPS-IVB | KS | Beta-galactosidase | AR |
| MPS-VI | DS | *N*-acetylgalactosamine-4-sulfatase | AR |
| MPS-VII | DS; HS; C 4,6-S | Beta-glucuronidase | AR |
| MPS-IX | Hyaluronan | Hyaluronidase | AR |

*DS* Dermatan sulfate, *HS* heparan sulfate, *KS* keratan sulfate, *C 6-S* chondroitin 6-sulfate, *C 4,6-S* chondroitin 4,6-sulfate, *AR* autosomal recessive, *XR* X-linked recessive

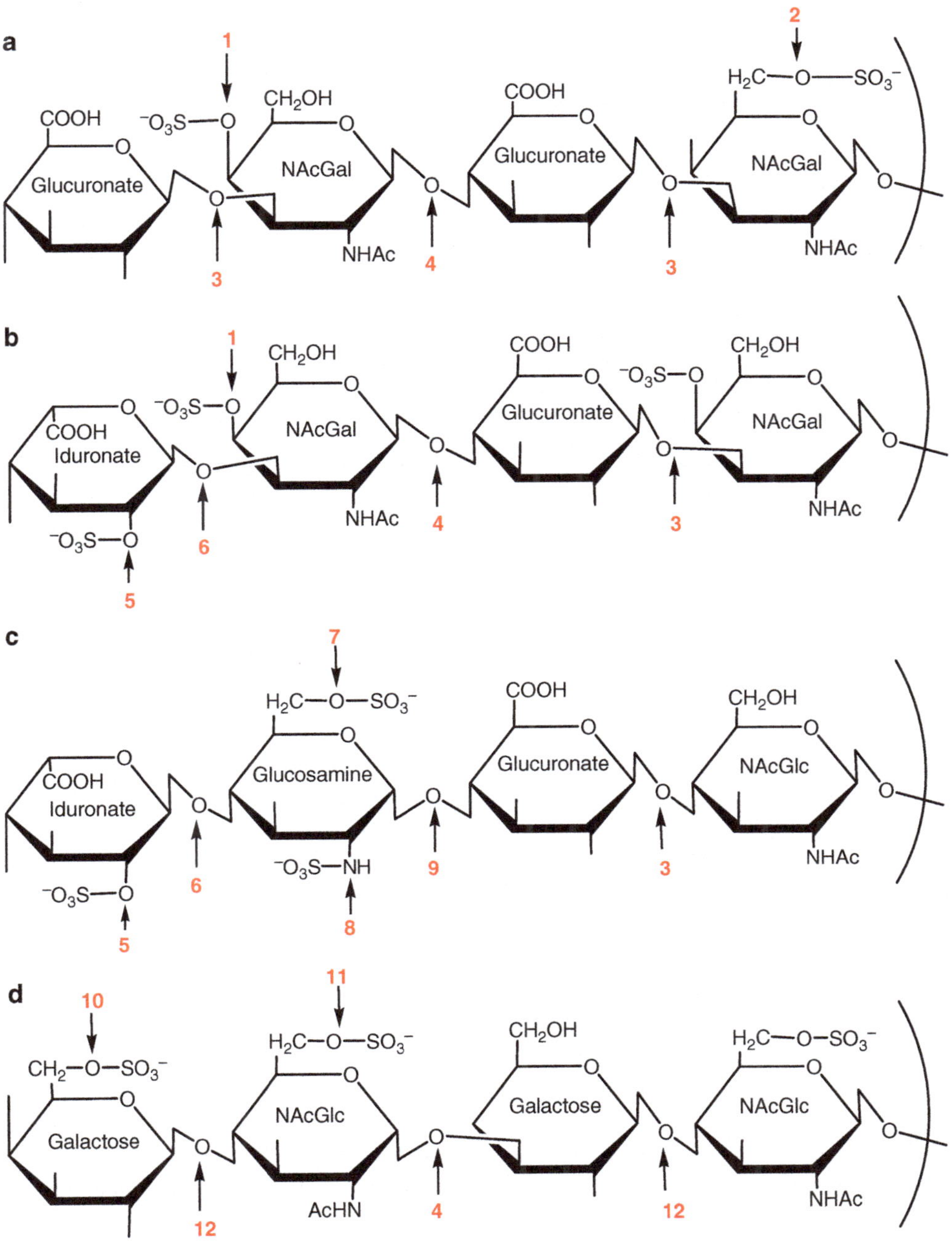


**Fig. 6.1** NAcGlc: *N*-acetylglucosamine; NAcGal: *N*-acetylgalactosamine. (**a**) Chondroitin 4,6-sulfate; (**b**) Dermatan sulfate; (**c**) Heparan sulfate; (**d**) Keratan sulfate. 1: *N*-acetylgalactosamine-4-sulfatase (VI); 2: *N*-acetylgalactosamine 6-sulfatase (IVA); 3: β-glucuronidase (VII); 4: β-hexosaminidase ($GM_2$-Sandhoff disease); 5: Iduronate 2-sulfatase (II); 6: α-L-iduronidase (I); 7: *N*-acetylglucosamine 6-sulfatase (IIID); 8: Heparan *N*-sulfatase (IIIA) followed by Acetyl-CoA:α-glucosaminide *N*-acetyltransferase (IIIC); 9: α-*N*-acetyl-glucosaminidase (IIIB); 10: *N*-acetyl-galactosamine-6-sulfatase (IVA); 11: *N*-acetylglucosamine-6-sulfatase (IIID); 12: β-galactosidase-1 ($GM_1$ gangliosidosis, IVB)

Several methods have been proposed for quantitative analysis of specific GAGs (Kubaski et al. 2017). Paper or thin layer chromatography, gas-liquid chromatography, capillary electrophoresis, and high performance liquid chromatography were reported to be able to identify and separate different GAGs.

Mass spectrometry has been used in recent years for its high sensitivity and accuracy. A limitation of MS-based technologies is that large molecules such as GAGs need to be broken down into sulfated disaccharide fragments before analysis. An alternative method to enzymatic digestion for GAG identification by mass spectrometry is based on chemical cleavage. A fast test able to quantify glycosaminoglycans in urine by a LC-MS/MS method has been recently developed for selective MPS-I, MPS-II, and MPS-VI mucopolysaccharidoses (Auray-Blais et al. 2011). The test is performed on random urine samples and the concentration expressed as a ratio to creatinine for normalization purposes. Dermatan sulfate (DS) and heparan sulfate (HS) are measured as derivatives by using calibration curve in urine, after a chemical degradation step (methanolysis). The authors reported glycosaminoglycan quantification on 28 patients and 55 controls. Besides DS and HS, chondroitin sulfate was measured in all samples and confirmed it was not a useful marker for the diagnosis of MPS due to the fact that it is normally excreted in urine. No DS and HS were found in control urines, while DS and in most cases HS were quantified in MPS-I, MPS-II, or MPS-VI patients. Based on the

**Table 6.3** GAGs reference ranges in urine

| Age (year) | Alcian blue[a] (mg/mmol creatinine) | DMB-Tris (mg/mmol creatinine) | CPC/Carbazole (µmol uronic acid/mmol creatinine) | GAG-Test® (mg/mmol creatinine) |
|---|---|---|---|---|
| <0.1 | 10–40 | | | 26.1 ± 8.1 |
| <0.3 | 10–35 | | | |
| <0.5 | 10–30 | 33.6 ± 9.2 | | |
| <1 | 5–25 | 23.3 ± 4.1 | 17.8 ± 8.2 | 17.1 ± 7.7 |
| <2 | | 19.5 ± 5.2 | 14.6 ± 6.1 | |
| <3 | 5–20 | 14.5 ± 3.4 | | 12.0 ± 4.2 |
| <5 | 2–15 | 11.0 ± 1.7 | 10.7 ± 6.7 | |
| <6 | | | 8.3 ± 2.2 | 10.3 ± 3.7 |
| <7 | | 9.3 ± 1.8 | | |
| <9 | | 8.4 ± 1.6 | | |
| <10 | | | 6.2 ± 1.9 | |
| <14 | | 7.0 ± 1.8 | | 4.6 ± 2.6 |
| <15 | 2–12 | | 7.0 ± 4.4 | |
| <18–20 | | 4.1 ± 1.3 | 3.2 ± 1.6 | |
| >18–20 | 1–5 | 3.3 ± 0.9 | 1.6 ± 1.2 | 3.2 ± 1.6 |

[a]These data were supplied by E. Young, Institute of Child Health, London

**Table 6.4** Source material for MPS enzymatic assays

| Disorder | Enzyme defect | Material: Postnatal | Material: Prenatal |
|---|---|---|---|
| MPS-I | Alpha-L-iduronidase | P, WBC, FB, LYM | CV, CCV, CAFC |
| MPS-II | Iduronate sulfatase | P, WBC, FB, LYM | CV, CCV, CAFC |
| MPS-IIIA | Heparan *N*-sulfatase | WBC, FB, LYM | CV, CCV, CAFC |
| MPS-IIIB | Alpha-*N*-acetylglucosaminidase | P, WBC, FB, LYM | CV, CCV, CAFC |
| MPS-IIIC | Acetyl CoA:alpha-glucosaminide acetyltransferase | WBC, FB, LYM | CV, CCV, CAFC |
| MPS-IIID | *N*-acetylglucosamine 6-sulfatase | WBC, FB, LYM | CV, CCV, CAFC |
| MPS-IVA | *N*-acetylgalactosamine-6-sulfate sulfatase | WBC, FB, LYM | CV, CCV, CAFC |
| MPS-IVB | Beta-galactosidase | P, WBC, FB, LYM | CV, CCV, CAFC |
| MPS-VI | *N*-acetylgalactosamine-4-sulfatase | WBC, FB, LYM | CV, CCV, CAFC |
| MPS-VII | Beta-glucuronidase | P, WBC, FB, LYM | CV, CCV, CAFC |
| MPS-IX | Hyaluronidase | WBC, FB, LYM | CV, CCV, CAFC |

*P* plasma, *WBC* white blood cells, *LYM* lymphocytes, *FB* fibroblasts, *CV* chorionic villi, *CAFC* cultured amniotic fluid cells, *CCV* cultured chorionic villi

consideration that residual glycosaminoglycans are present in patient urine even after treatment, this test is also useful for monitoring therapeutic enzyme replacement treatment.

An MS-based method using butanolysis to quantify HS showed higher signal responses compared to those generated by using methanolysis (Trim et al. 2015). Recently, Forni and colleagues have developed a new fast LC–MS/MS assay for the simultaneous quantification of HS and DS using small amounts of urine. This method requires an easy sample preparation by using butanolysis, and it is less time consuming if compared with enzyme-digestion process (Forni et al. 2019).

For the definitive diagnosis, enzyme activity test is needed. Appropriate enzyme sources are summarized in Table 6.4. Considering that no homogeneous data of the different enzyme activity are present in literature, normal values are not referred.

## Oligosaccharide Assay

Oligosaccharidoses/glycoproteinoses are lysosomal storage disorders due to lost activity of one of the lysosomal hydrolases involved in the degradation of oligosaccharide components of glycoproteins.

Oligosaccharides are molecules containing a small number (3 to approximately 10) of monosaccharide residues connected by glycosidic linkages. Small amounts of carbohydrates and oligosaccharides are present in normal urine depending on different factors (diet, medication, blood group type, etc.). Oligosaccharides can be studied by thin-layer chromatography of urine samples (Palo and Savolainen 1972; Humbel and Collart 1975; Friedman et al. 1978; Sewell 1981; Tsai and Marshall 1979).

One-dimensional thin layer chromatography is performed on 20 × 20 silica gel plate. Urine samples containing about 15 µg of creatinine are applied directly on silica gel plate. Lactose, maltotetraose, and sialic acid at concentration of 1 mg/mL are used as reference standards.

The plate is developed overnight in a freshly prepared mobile phase containing *n*-butanol–glacial acetic acid–distilled water (10:5:5 v/v/v). The plate is then removed, dried at room temperature (about 1 h), and sprayed with freshly prepared solution containing 3,5-dihydroxytoluene (orcinol) 400 mg/dL in sulfuric acid 10%. Spots corresponding to oligosaccharides develop by heating the plate at 130 °C for about 10 min and are looked by transparency. The excretion of oligosaccharides is identified by the presence of colored bands. This method is suitable for screening purposes. Interpretation can be difficult and requires experience. Specific oligosaccharide patterns are indicative of diagnostic suspicion of a specific disease (Sewell 1991). Neonatal urine samples could present many bands, mimicking an α-mannosidosis pattern, due to parenteral nutrition. This fact is not indicative of disease. In this case, it is recommended to repeat the assay after the age of 6 months. Alternatively, the combination of two one-dimensional TLC systems proposed

**Table 6.5** Source material for oligosacchariduria enzymatic assays

| Disorder | Enzyme defect | Material | |
|---|---|---|---|
| | | Postnatal | Prenatal |
| Aspartylglucosaminuria | Glycosylasparaginase | WBC, FB | CV, CAFC |
| Fucosidosis | Alpha-L-fucosidase | P, WBC, FB | CV, CAFC |
| Galactosialidosis | Cathepsin A/beta-galactosidase/neuraminidase | WBC, FB | CV, CAFC |
| α-Mannosidosis | Alpha-mannosidase | P, WBC, FB | CV, CAFC |
| β-Mannosidosis | Beta-mannosidase | P, WBC, FB | CV, CAFC |
| Mucolipidosis I | Alpha-neuraminidase | FB, WBC[a] | CV, CCV, CAFC |
| Mucolipidosis II | *N*-acetylglucosamine-1-phosphotransferase | FB | CV, CCV, CAFC |
| Mucolipidosis III | *N*-acetylglucosamine-1-phosphotransferase | FB | CCV, CAFC |
| Schindler disease | Alpha-*N*-acetylgalactosaminidase | WBC, FB | CV, CAFC |
| GM1 Gangliosidosis | Beta-galactosidase-1 | WBC, FB | CV, CAFC |
| Krabbe disease | Galactosylceramidase | WBC, FB | CV, CAFC |
| GM2 Gangliosidosis type I | Beta-hexosaminidase A | P, WBC, FB | CV, CAFC |
| GM2 Gangliosidosis type II | Beta-hexosaminidase A + B | P, WBC, FB | CV, CAFC |

[a]Fresh material, not frozen; *P* plasma, *WBC* white blood cells, *FB* fibroblasts, *CV* chorionic villi, *CAFC* cultured amniotic fluid cells, *CCV* cultured chorionic villi

by Abeling and collaborators (Abeling et al. 1996) can be performed to distinguish urine of breastfed newborns from that of α-mannosidosis patients.

Some authors reported a new useful semiquantitative method based on tandem mass spectrometry for the diagnosis of the oligosaccharidurias (Ramsay et al. 2005). It is a 1-phenyl-3-methyl-5-pyrazolone (PNP) in ammonia derivatization-based method, followed by a liquid/liquid extraction with $CHCl_3$ and solid-phase extraction on a C18 column. The mass spectra were acquired on a triple quadrupole mass spectrometer operating in both precursor ion scan and multiple reaction monitoring (MRM) modes, in positive ionization. Patients with I-cell disease, mucolipidoses type II and III, alpha–mannosidosis, Pompe disease, $GM_1$ gangliosidosis, $GM_2$ type II, sialidosis, alpha-fucosidosis, Gaucher disease, and SADS (sialic acid storage disorders) have been analyzed and differentiated from controls. This new procedure seems to be sensitive, robust, automatable, and faster than classical TLC ones. When stable isotope labeled internal standards will become commercially available, this method will be considered a powerful tool for quantitative determination of oligosaccharides in urine.

To date, in any case, a confirmatory enzyme assay must be performed in serum, fibroblasts, or leucocytes for the definitive diagnosis. Appropriate enzyme sources are summarized in Table 6.5.

## Analysis of Free and Total Sialic Acid in Urine

Sialic acid (SA) represents the *N*- or *O*-substituted derivatives of monosaccharide neuraminic acid. It is a major component of complex glycoproteins and glycolipids, in which it commonly forms the terminal constituent of sugar side chains. Many forms of sialic acid exist in every tissue, but *N*-acetylneuraminic acid (NANA) is the predominant one in humans. Sialic acids often represent part of antigenic determinants of glycolipids or glycoproteins. Urine total SA is increased in some lysosomal disorders such as sialidosis, galactosialidosis, Kanzaki disease, and mucolipidosis II and III. Heterozygotes do not excrete increased amounts of bound sialic acid. It has been reported that an increase in urine total SA is also found in individuals with chronic glomerulonephritis and rheumatoid arthritis, in lupus erythematosus, in pseudohypoparathyroidism, and in diabetic patients. In all these diseases, the excretion of bound SA is lower than in conditions involving the neuraminidase enzyme. About 40% of SA is in a free form although the majority of urine SA is bound to glycoproteins and oligosaccharides. Urine SA also can be increased (predominantly as free SA) in other inborn errors of metabolism such as infantile sialic acid storage disease (ISSD), sialuria, and Salla disease. The excretion of free SA is tenfold higher in patients with Salla disease and with ISSD than normal subjects, while patients with sialuria display free SA levels about 100-fold higher than those in the healthy population. However, only few patients have been reported in the literature; therefore, a distinction among these forms of sialuria cannot be made on the basis of the sialic acid excretion. Many methods have been described for the determination of both free and bound SA. In many laboratories, the measurement of urinary SA is performed by using a modified colorimetric assay (thiobarbituric acid test) developed to eliminate the ubiquitary interferent 2-deoxyribose. As an alternative method, Okamura-Oho et al. (1984) proposed an enzymatic procedure based on cleavage of NANA by aldolase to *N*-acetylmannosamine and pyruvic acid with following spectrophotometric determination (340 nm) with NADH and lactic dehydrogenase. For the measurement of free sialic acid, an incubation step with neuraminidase is

**Table 6.6** Free and total sialic acid reference ranges in urine

| Free sialic acid (mmol/mol creatine) | | Total sialic acid (mmol/mol creatine) | |
|---|---|---|---|
| Age (year) | Mean ± 2SD | Age (year) | Mean ± 2SD |
| <0.5 | 45 ± 38 | <0.5 | 156 ± 120 |
| <1 | 32 ± 28 | <1 | 100 ± 70 |
| 1–3 | 29 ± 21 | 1–3 | 90 ± 70 |
| 3–5 | 21 ± 13 | 3–5 | 63 ± 40 |
| 5–10 | 15 ± 12 | 5–10 | 51 ± 37 |
| 10–20 | 9 ± 8 | 10–20 | 34 ± 30 |
| >20 | 7 ± 6 | >20 | 31 ± 25 |

Modified from van der Ham et al. (2007)

performed. Many kits are now commercially available based on this modified method. Free sialic acid is oxidized by an enzyme reaction and in the presence of a chromogenic probe develops a red complex. The content of sialic acid can be calculated by measuring the OD value at 560 nm. Some authors (van der Ham et al. 2007) have proposed an LC-MS/MS-based method for the assay of total and free sialic acid. For free SA assay, the procedure required a filtration step followed by a dilution. Quantitative results were obtained by using isotope dilution technique and an eight-point calibration curve. Total SA analysis was performed after a hydrolytic step in sulfuric acid 63 mmol at 80 °C per 1 h. MS data were obtained in a triple quadrupole system operating in MRM mode in negative ionization. The method is rapid (6 min), semi-automatic, specific, robust, and sensitive and therefore could be considered suitable for high-throughput analysis. Reference ranges of urinary free and total sialic acid are reported in Table 6.6.

## Enzymatic Tests in Dried Blood Spots

For the majority of LSD, the measurement of the specific enzyme activity in white cells (leukocytes, lymphocytes) or fibroblast is still considered the gold standard for the diagnosis. Chamoles et al. (2001) introduced for the first time the use of the whole blood dried spot (DBS), the traditional NBS sample, to determine enzymatic activity for several LSDs using a commercially available fluorogenic substrate (4-methlyumbelliferone).

Successively, the use of a DBS for the enzymatic determination has been proposed as alternative for a rapid detection of LSDs, mainly in newborn screening and in high-risk population screening. Experimental approaches on DBS were adopted for pilot studies on Fabry disease and/or Pompe disease in Italy, Taiwan, and Japan (Spada et al. 2006; Chien et al. 2008; Oda et al. 2011).

However, conventional methods for quantifying enzymatic activity have the limitations of specificity and limited capacity for multiplexing. Moreover, not all lysosomal enzymes can be assayed by traditional methods because the incorporation of a chromophore or fluorophore into the substrate can cause false-negative results.

The use of mass spectrometric techniques has shown advantages over fluorometric or spectrophotometric assays in the simultaneous quantification of several enzyme activity (Gelb et al. 2006). In fact, based on the studies of Chamoles, the group of Gelb and coworkers used tandem mass spectrometry (MS/MS) and internal standards to detect multiple enzymatic products in a multiplex analysis for Fabry, Gaucher, Krabbe, mucopolysaccharidosis-I (MPS-I), Niemann-Pick-A/B, and Pompe diseases.

Since the first description of the flow injection analysis (FIA) MS/MS assay, modifications including the number of enzymes, sample preparation steps, and the addition of liquid chromatography (LC) have been reported in order to simplify the analysis (Zhang et al. 2008; la Marca et al. 2009; Metz et al. 2011).

More recently, Gelb and coworkers developed a UHPLC-MS/MS multiplex assay with up to 9 LSD (the above-described 6-plex plus MPS-II, MPS-IVA, and MPS-VI) using a single 3 mm DBS punch incubated with 9 substrates and internal standards in a single buffer (Spacil et al. 2013). The MS/MS has been adopted in LSD newborn screening programs worldwide including in Taiwan (Chiang et al. 2018), Italy (Burlina et al. 2018), and the USA (Burton et al. 2017).

The entire assay comprises a 2-day process. On day 1, incubation cocktail containing buffers, substrates, and internal standards for the six enzymes was added to a 3.2 mm DBS and incubated overnight. On day 2, the reaction was stopped and a liquid-liquid extraction was performed. For the quantitation measurements, the tandem mass spectrometer was operated in MRM mode.

The activities of GAA, ABG, GLA, ASM, GALC, and IDUA enzymes in newborns (<7 days of life) and non-newborns tested by multiplex MS/MS are reported in Table 6.7.

The median enzyme activity in non-newborns was lower than in newborns due to lower leukocyte counts on older patient's dried blood spots. Since correction for white blood cell count was not possible on DBS, it is necessary to establish age-matched reference values. All samples collected from affected patients (newborn and non-newborns) had low enzyme activities that could be clearly distinguished from those of age-matched healthy controls, with the exception of female patients tested for Fabry disease, for whom the enzyme activity assay does not reliably discern heterozygosity. The screening panel for LSDs was expanded and includes MS/MS assays for MPS-II, MPS-IVA, and MPS-VI. The activities of IDS, ASB, and GALNS are reported in Table 6.8.

Recently, the group of Gelb described a new 7-plex assay by MS/MS for the mucopolysaccharidoses (MPS-I, MPS-II, MPS-IIIB, MPS-IVA, MPS-VI, and MPS-VII) and type 2 neuronal ceroid lipofuscinosis (LINCL) (Liu et al. 2017). Another analytical multiplex approach to NBS for

**Table 6.7** Enzyme activities from dried blood spot measured by MS/MS

| | Healthy newborns $n = 40{,}000$ | | | Affected newborns | | | Non-newborns $n = 500$ | | | Affected non-newborns | | | Heterozygous | | |
|---|---|---|---|---|---|---|---|---|---|---|---|---|---|---|---|
| Enzyme | Median | 0.1 ile | 99.9 ile | Mean (*n*) | Min | Max | Median | 2.5ile | 97.5 ile | Mean (*n*) | Min | MAX | Mean (*n*) | Min | Max |
| ABG | 9.09 | 2.1 | 40.43 | 1.05 (7) | 0.44 | 2.01 | 3.88 | 1.37 | 9.74 | 0.4 (21) | 0.09 | 1.08 | – | – | – |
| ASM | 5.37 | 1.52 | 21.34 | 0.53 (1) | – | – | 2.90 | 1.23 | 8.95 | 0.16 (4) | 0.04 | 0.23 | – | – | – |
| GAA | 13.98 | 3.57 | 39.69 | 0.99 (8) | 0.2 | 1.94 | 5.79 | 2.34 | 13.19 | 0.60 (9) | 0.35 | 1.13 | – | – | – |
| GALC | 3.52 | 0.49 | 21.66 | na | na | na | 1.84 | 0.59 | 4.70 | 0.08 (3) | 0.06 | 0.10 | – | – | – |
| GLA | 9.56 | 3.03 | 41.67 | 0.96 (8) | 0.6 | 1.51 | 4.15 | 1.48 | 9.54 | 0.37 (14) | 0.17 | 0.86 | 2.05 (17) | 0.67 | 4.04 |
| IDUA | 10.1 | 2.47 | 26.87 | 0.2 (2) | 0.17 | 0.22 | 5.45 | 2.32 | 11.36 | 0.19 (3) | 0.06 | 0.43 | – | – | – |

*GAA* acid-alpha-glucosidase, *ABG* acid beta-glucosidase, *GLA* alpha-galactosidase A, *GALC* galactosylceramidase, *IDUA* alpha-L-iduronidase

**Table 6.8** Enzyme activities from dried blood spot

| Enzyme | Control newborns (*n*) | | | Patients (*n*) | | |
|---|---|---|---|---|---|---|
| | Median | High value | Low value | Median | High value | Low value |
| IDS | 9.10 (75) | 16 | 4.8 | 0.29 (14) | 0.52 | 0.17 |
| ASB | 7.40 (89) | 16.9 | 1.4 | 0.12 (1) | 0.12 | 0.12 |
| GALNS | 1.84 (30) | 4.37 | 0.64 | 0.014 (9) | 0.26 | 0.006 |

*IDS* iduronate 2-sulfatase, *ASB* *N*-acetylgalactosamine-6-sulfatase, *GALNS* *N*-acetylgalactosamine-4-sulfatase

LSDs, also based on Chamoles' fluorometric enzyme activity assays, was developed by Advanced Liquid Logic, Inc. (ALL; now called Baebies Inc.) (Sista et al. 2011). Their procedure has the ability to simultaneously perform up to five different enzyme assays on a single DBS. The method utilized minimal sample (DBS extract, 3.4 μL) and reagent volumes that are applied on disposable cartridges for 48 samples and analyzed on a small table-top instrument. Sub-microliter droplets of sample are moved by electrowetting on an electrode-plate chip under a layer of oil to prevent evaporation. Since 2013, the Missouri state was using the method for the newborn screening of MPS-I, Fabry, Gaucher, and Pompe diseases (Hopkins et al. 2015). The latest version of this "digital microfluidics" (DMF) that include these four diseases obtained the approval from the US FDA for its use as a medical device in 2017.

The literature highlights the fact that either method, MS/MS or DMF, can be used for efficient LSD newborn screening. Both platforms are liable to false-positive results due to the presence of pseudo-deficiency alleles that exhibit low enzyme activity in an individual with no disease phenotype and normal endogenous enzyme function. These false-positives have complicated the implementation of LSD NBS, especially for Pompe and Hurler diseases (Donati et al. 2018; Chuang et al. 2018). Second-tier testing for some LSDs has recently become available and may also be effective, especially in Pompe and MPS-I diseases (Tortorelli et al. 2018; de Ruijter et al. 2012).

## References


Abeling NG, Rusch H, van Gennip AH. Improved selectivity of urinary oligosaccharide screening using two one-dimensional TLC systems. J Inherit Metab Dis. 1996;19:260–2.

Auray-Blais C, Bhérer P, Gagnon R, Young SP, Zhang HH, An Y, Clarke JT, Millington DS. Efficient analysis of urinary glycosaminoglycans by LC-MS/MS in mucopolysaccharidoses type I, II and VI. Mol Genet Metab. 2011;102:49–56.

Burlina AB, Polo G, Salviati L, Duro G, Zizzo C, Dardis A, Bembi B, Cazzorla C, Rubert L, Zordan R, Desnick RJ, Burlina AP. Newborn screening for lysosomal storage disorders by tandem mass spectrometry in North East Italy. J Inherit Metab Dis. 2018;41:209–19.

Burton BK, Charrow J, Hoganson GE, Waggoner D, Tinkle B, Braddock SR, Schneider M, Grange DK, Nash C, Shryock H, Barnett R, Shao R, Basheeruddin K, Dizikes G. Newborn screening for lysosomal storage disorders in Illinois: the initial 15-month experience. J Pediatr. 2017;190:130–5.

Chamoles NA, Blanco M, Gaggioli D. Diagnosis of alpha-L-iduronidase deficiency in dried blood spots on filter paper: the possibility of newborn diagnosis. Clin Chem. 2001;47:780–1.

Chiang SC, Chen PW, Hwu WL, Lee AJ, Chen LC, Lee NC, Chiou LY, Chien YH. Performance of the four-plex tandem mass spectrometry lysosomal storage disease newborn screening test: the necessity of adding a 2nd tier test for Pompe disease. Int J Neonatal Screen. 2018;4:41.

Chien YH, Chiang SC, Zhang XK, Keutzer J, Lee NC, Huang AC, Chen CA, Wu MH, Huang PH, Tsai FJ, Chen YT, Hwu WL. Early detection of Pompe disease by newborn screening is feasible: results from the Taiwan screening program. Pediatrics. 2008;122:e39–45.

Chuang CK, Lin HY, Wang TJ, Huang YH, Chan MJ, Liao HC, Lo YT, Wang LY, Tu RY, Fang YY, Chen TL, Ho HC, Chiang CC, Lin SP. Status of newborn screening and follow up investigations for Mucopolysaccharidoses I and II in Taiwan. Orphanet J Rare Dis. 2018;13:84.

de Jong JG, Wevers RA, Liebrand-van Sambeek R. Measuring urinary glycosaminoglycans in the presence of protein: an improved screening procedure for mucopolysaccharidoses based on dimethylmethylene blue. Clin Chem. 1992;38:803–7.

de Ruijter J, de Ru MH, Wagemans T, Ijlst L, Lund AM, Orchard PJ, Schaefer GB, Wijburg FA, van Vlies N. Heparan sulfate and dermatan sulfate derived disaccharides are sensitive markers for newborn screening for mucopolysaccharidoses types I, II and III. Mol Genet Metab. 2012;107:705–10.

Donati MA, Pasquini E, Spada M, Polo G, Burlina A. Newborn screening in mucopolysaccharidoses. Ital J Pediatr. 2018;44(S2):126.

Forni G, Malvagia S, Funghini S, Scolamiero E, Mura M, Della Bona M, Villanelli F, Damiano R, la Marca G. LC-MS/MS method for simultaneous quantification of heparan sulfate and dermatan

sulfate in urine by butanolysis derivatization. Clin Chim Acta. 2019;488:98–103.
Friedman RB, Williams MA, Moser HW, Kolodny EH. Improved thin-layer chromatographic method in the diagnosis of mannosidosis. Clin Chem. 1978;24:1576–7.
Gelb MH. Newborn screening for lysosomal storage diseases: methodologies, screen positive rates, normalization of datasets, second-tier tests, and post-analysis tools. Int J Neonatal Screen. 2018;4:23.
Gelb MH, Turecek F, Scott CR, Chamoles NA. Direct multiplex assay of enzymes in dried blood spots by tandem mass spectrometry for the newborn screening of lysosomal storage disorders. J Inherit Metab Dis. 2006;29:397–404.
Hopkins PV, Campbell C, Klug T, Rogers S, Raburn-Miller J, Kiesling J. Lysosomal storage disorder screening implementation: findings from the first six months of full population pilot testing in Missouri. J Pediatr. 2015;166:172–7.
Humbel R, Collart M. Oligosaccharides in urine of patients with glycoprotein storage diseases. I. Rapid detection by thin-layer chromatography. Clin Chim Acta. 1975;60:143–5.
Kubaski F, Osago H, Mason RW, Yamaguchi S, Kobayashi H, Tsuchiya M, Orii T, Tomatsu S. Glycosaminoglycans detection methods: applications of mass spectrometry. Mol Genet Metab. 2017;120:67–77.
la Marca G, Casetta B, Malvagia S, Guerrini R, Zammarchi E. New strategy for the screening of lysosomal storage disorders: the use of the online trapping-and-cleanup liquid chromatography/mass spectrometry. Anal Chem. 2009;81:6113–21.
Lage S, Prieto JA, Andrade F, Sojo A, Sanjurjo P, Aldámiz-Echevarría LJ. Reliability of a visual test for the rapid detection of mucopolysaccharidoses: GAG-test(®). J Clin Lab Anal. 2011;25:179–84.
Liu Y, Yi F, Kumar AB, Kumar Chennamaneni N, Hong X, Scott CR, Gelb MH, Turecek F. Multiplex tandem mass spectrometry enzymatic activity assay for newborn screening of the mucopolysaccharidoses and type 2 neuronal ceroid lipofuscinosis. Clin Chem. 2017;63:1118–26.
Metz TF, Mechtler TP, Orsini JJ, Martin M, Shushan B, Herman JL, Ratschmann R, Item CB, Streubel B, Herkner KR, Kasper DC. Simplified newborn screening protocol for lysosomal storage disorders. Clin Chem. 2011;57:1286–94.
Oda E, Tanaka T, Migita O, Kosuga M, Fukushi M, Okumiya T, Osawa M, Okuyama T. Newborn screening for Pompe disease in Japan. Mol Genet Metab. 2011;104:560–5.
Okamura-Oho Y, Yamanaka T, Suzuki Y, Akagi M, Kobayashi T. A simple enzymatic determination of urinary sialic acid—its significance in the diagnosis of disorders of sialic acid metabolism. Clin Chim Acta. 1984;144:263–7.
Palo J, Savolainen H. Thin-layer chromatographic demonstration of aspartylglycosylamine and a novel acidic carbohydrate in human tissues. J Chromatogr. 1972;65:447–50.
Platt FM, d'Azzo A, Davidson BL, Neufeld EF, Tifft CJ. Lysosomal storage diseases. Nat Rev Dis Primers. 2018;4:27.
Ramsay SL, Meikle PJ, Hopwood JJ, Clements PR. Profiling oligosaccharidurias by electrospray tandem mass spectrometry: quantifying reducing oligosaccharides. Anal Biochem. 2005;345:30–46.
Sewell AC. Simple laboratory determination of excess oligosacchariduria. Clin Chem. 1981;27:243–5.
Sewell AC. Urinary oligosaccharides. In: Hommes FA, editor. Techniques in diagnostic human biochemical genetics. 1st ed. New York: Wiley-Liss; 1991. p. 219–31.
Sista RS, Eckhardt AE, Wang T, Graham C, Rouse JL, Norton SM, Srinivasan V, Pollack MG, Tolun AA, Bali D, Millington DS, Pamula VK. Digital microfluidic platform for multiplexing enzyme assays: implications for lysosomal storage disease screening in newborns. Clin Chem. 2011;57:1444–51.
Spacil Z, Tatipaka H, Barcenas M, Scott CR, Turecek F, Gelb MH. High-throughput assay of 9 lysosomal enzymes for newborn screening. Clin Chem. 2013;59:502–11.
Spada M, Pagliardini S, Yasuda M, Tukel T, Thiagarajan G, Sakuraba H, Ponzone A, Desnick RJ. High incidence of later-onset fabry disease revealed by newborn screening. Am J Hum Genet. 2006;79:31–40.
Studelska DR, Giljum K, McDowell LM, Zhang L. Quantification of glycosaminoglycans by reversed-phase HPLC separation of fluorescent isoindole derivatives. Glycobiology. 2006;16:65–72.
Tortorelli S, Eckerman JS, Orsini JJ, Stevens C, Hart J, Hall PL, Alexander JJ, Gavrilov D, Oglesbee D, Raymond K, Matern D, Rinaldo P. Moonlighting newborn screening markers: the incidental discovery of a second-tier test for Pompe disease. Genet Med. 2018;20:840–6.
Trim PJ, Hopwood JJ, Snel MF. Butanolysis derivatization: improved sensitivity in LC-MS/MS quantitation of heparan sulfate in urine from mucopolysaccharidosis patients. Anal Chem. 2015;87:9243–50.
Tsai MY, Marshall JG. Screening for urinary oligosaccharides and simple sugars by thin-layer chromatography. Med Lab Sci. 1979;36:85–90.
Ucakturk E, Cai C, Li L, Zhang F, Linhardt RJ. Capillary electrophoresis for total glycosaminoglycan analysis. Anal Bioanal Chem. 2014;406:4617–26.
van der Ham M, Prinsen BH, Huijmans JG, Abeling NG, Dorland B, Berger R, de Koning TJ, de Sain-van der Velden MG. Quantification of free and total sialic acid excretion by LC-MS/MS. J Chromatogr B Analyt Technol Biomed Life Sci. 2007;848:251–7.
Zhang XK, Elbin CS, Chuang WL, Cooper SK, Marashio CA, Beauregard C, Keutzer JM. Multiplex enzyme assay screening of dried blood spots for lysosomal storage disorders by using tandem mass spectrometry. Clin Chem. 2008;54:1725–8.

# Untargeted Metabolomics: Next-Generation Metabolic Screening

# 7

Karlien L. M. Coene, Judith J. M. Jans, Udo F. H. Engelke, and Ron A. Wevers

## Contents



**Summary**

This chapter paints a picture of a new dawn for clinicians and laboratory specialists in the metabolic field that arises from the clinical application of untargeted metabolomics. This technology offers unprecedented opportunities to diagnose patients with inborn errors of metabolism and to gain insight in disease mechanisms at the molecular level. The most recent generation of untargeted metabolomics analyses relies on the use of high-resolution mass spectrometry technology, which can be successfully applied to body fluids to reveal known as well as yet unknown IEMs in an individual patient. As such, the technique holds the capacity to replace a large number of current targeted diagnostic techniques. Additionally, it can be applied for the discovery of novel biomarkers for long-known metabolic diseases, which may provide further insight into the pathophysiology of such IEMs. Typically, the analysis of a single sample results in over 10,000 metabolite-related signals (referred to as "features"). It requires a sophisticated bioinformatic pipeline to extract the clinically relevant features from the "big data" that is generated and ignore features from diet- or medication-derived molecules. The application of untargeted metabolomics for IEM diagnostics has been coined next-generation metabolic screening (NGMS). This chapter describes four different ways of applying NGMS in the clinical diagnostic setting and briefly touches on clinical indications for requesting NGMS.

## Introduction

Traditionally, the laboratory diagnosis of inborn errors of metabolism has largely relied on targeted hypothesis-driven measurements of metabolites in body fluids. The hypothesis is usually based on the phenotypic characteristics of the patient, defined through deep clinical phenotyping. The biochemical phenotype, or rather the "metabolite profile," reflects both endogenous factors such as genotype(s), gene expression, the different chemical reactions taking place in the body, as well

K. L. M. Coene · U. F. H. Engelke · R. A. Wevers (✉)
Translational Metabolic Laboratory, Department Laboratory Medicine, Radboud University Medical Centre, Nijmegen, The Netherlands
e-mail: Karlien.Coene@radboudumc.nl; udo.engelke@radboudumc.nl; Ron.Wevers@radboudumc.nl

J. J. M. Jans
Section Metabolic Diagnostics, Department of Genetics, University Medical Center Utrecht, Utrecht, The Netherlands
e-mail: j.j.m.jans@umcutrecht.nl


N. Blau et al. (eds.), *Physician's Guide to the Diagnosis, Treatment, and Follow-Up of Inherited Metabolic Diseases*, https://doi.org/10.1007/978-3-030-67727-5_7

as exogenous factors such as dietary habits, drug metabolism, and products from the microbiome. The last decade has seen the emergence of untargeted, hypothesis-free measurements of the human metabolome in body fluids. Nuclear magnetic resonance (NMR) spectroscopy is well-known as an untargeted metabolomics technique to analyze body fluids. In the last couple of years, mass spectrometry (MS) techniques have entered the stage of untargeted metabolomics with the advantage of being a factor of roughly thousand times more sensitive than NMR. Mass spectrometry with or without prior separation techniques paves the way to an important next step in our understanding of inborn errors of metabolism.

In this era of increasing use of whole exome sequencing (WES) techniques, an unmet need for functional proof supporting pathogenicity of unknown variants in the genomic DNA comes forward. The metabolic laboratory may help interpreting variants of unknown significance (VUS) found in WES analysis when these occur in genes encoding enzymes or transporters. The diagnostic future may be that WES/WGS and untargeted omics techniques are applied in parallel for patient diagnostics, which further integrates the functional genomics and metabolic laboratories.

The aim of untargeted metabolomics is to capture the complete metabolic profile or fingerprint in a patient's body fluid, including yet unknown metabolites, in order to unravel genetically determined metabolic defects. Typically, untargeted MS-based metabolomics techniques show more than 10,000 "features" in a single body fluid sample. Bioinformatic and chemometric techniques are required to reveal the relevant diagnostic features and filter out dietary- and medication-derived signals. This is essential to find the specific biomarkers for the metabolic derangement in the individual patient. This approach is rather different from classical metabolomics studies that usually describe the comparison between a patient group and a control group. NGMS techniques now enable the use of untargeted metabolomics for diagnostics in a clinical setting. Examples from NMR spectroscopy and untargeted MS analyses have already been described that unravel the identity of hitherto unknown inborn errors of metabolism or uncover novel biomarkers for long-known metabolic diseases.

## NMR-Based Metabolomics

Proton NMR spectroscopy is considered the cornerstone of classical untargeted metabolomics. It provides an overview of proton-containing metabolites in the micromolar and higher concentration range. All metabolites in the NMR spectrum can be quantitatively evaluated without the use of individual internal standards. The signal from a particular proton or group of equivalent protons may consist of one or more peaks under the influence of its chemical environment. These can be singlet, doublet, triplet, quartet, and multiplet resonances. Figure 7.1a gives the NMR spectra of lactate and alanine to illustrate that molecules with a high degree of similarity can be observed as separate resonances in the spectrum. The methyl groups of lactate and alanine show as doublet resonances. The proton from their methylene group gives a quartet in the spectrum.

Body fluid NMR spectroscopy can detect a vast array of IEMs, including most organic acidurias, aminoacidurias, and diseases in purine and pyrimidine metabolism. Figure 7.1b shows the accumulation of dimethylglycine in dimethylglycine dehydrogenase deficiency. This example also shows that metabolites that usually are not detected in conventional targeted metabolic screening techniques can also be seen in the NMR spectrum. This has contributed to the discovery of seven novel diseases with the use of NMR. The discovery of squalene synthase deficiency may serve as the most recent example (Coman et al. 2018). A comprehensive overview of the diagnostic potential including the spectral characteristics of over 100 IEMs is available in book form and online (Engelke et al. 2014).

## MS-Based Metabolomics

In the field of inborn errors of metabolism, targeted MS-based metabolomics methods, mostly on triple quadrupole (QqQ) instruments, have been well established in clinical diagnostics. These targeted methods are focused at quantitative determination of a predefined set of known metabolites, such as acylcarnitines or purines and pyrimidines. However, to uncover yet unknown metabolic diseases, an unbiased, holistic screening of the metabolite profile, or metabolome, is required. Technological innovations in high-resolution mass spectrometry (HRMS) now allow for the simultaneous detection (and semi-quantification) of as many individual metabolites as possible in a very small volume of biological sample (Fig. 7.2). This ability relies on the unprecedented mass accuracy that can be achieved by HRMS instruments, which reaches the parts per million (ppm) range. Based on this very accurate mass, which is up to four digits precise, the elemental composition of a metabolite can be deduced, which enables metabolite identification without the need for previous knowledge on which metabolites are expected to be present in the sample. Additionally, HRMS methods offer high sensitivity, reaching the low nanomolar range. These characteristics of HRMS make it a powerful tool to identify yet unknown metabolic derangements in patients suspected of an inborn error of metabolism.

HRMS-based metabolomics can be either performed by direct injection into a mass spectrometer such as direct infusion mass spectrometry (DI-HRMS; (Haijes et al. 2019a); Fig. 7.2) or preceded by chromatographic separation of metabolites on a column in liquid (LC; Fig. 7.2) or gas phase (GC), capillary electrophoresis (CE), or using ion mobility (Coene et al. 2018; Tebani et al. 2018). DI-HRMS and LC-HRMS are currently applied in clinical diagnostics for IEM and will be discussed in more detail below.

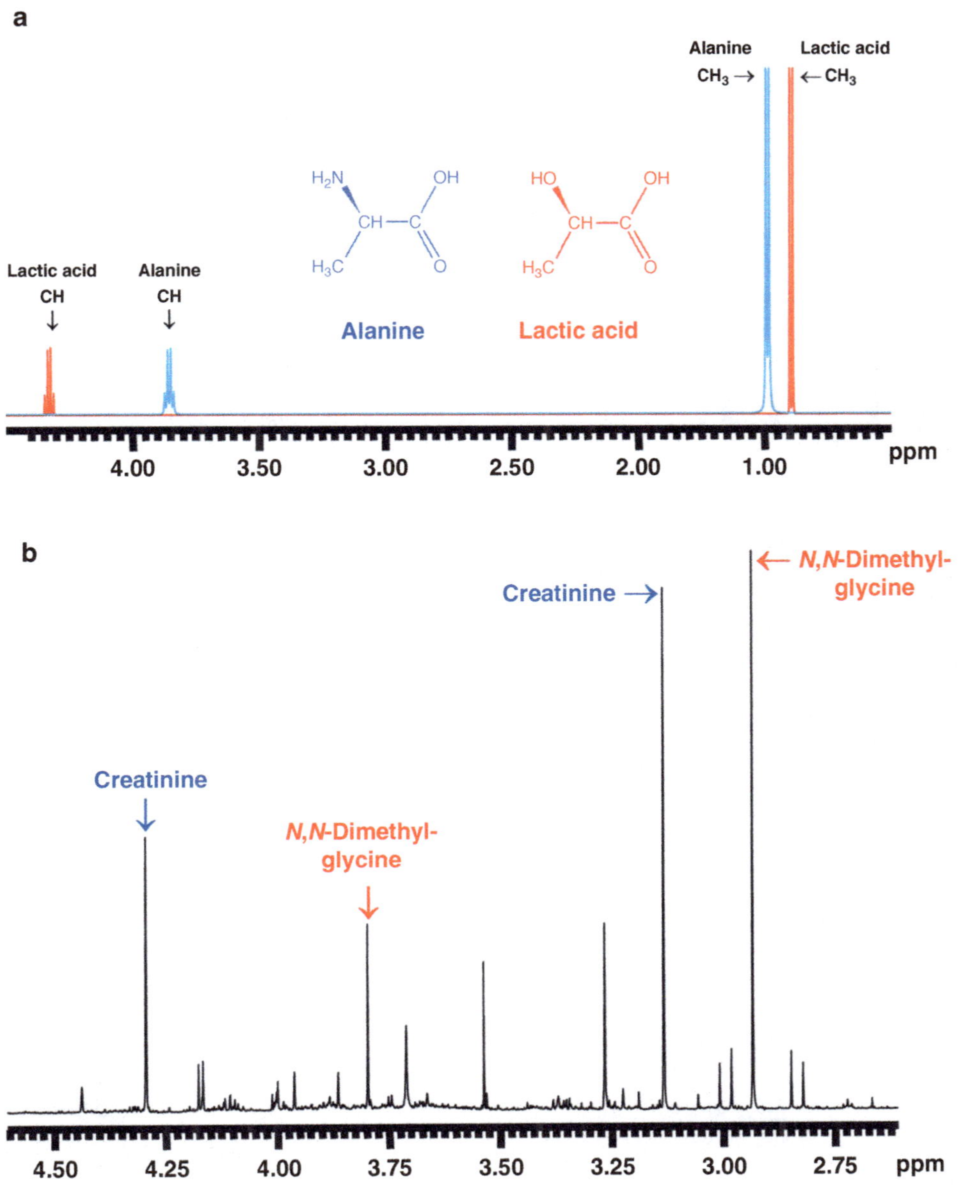


**Fig. 7.1** Typical examples of proton NMR spectra. (**a**) NMR spectrum of chemically similar molecules: lactate and alanine. The doublet resonance derives from the methyl group protons (–$CH_3$) and the quartet from the methylene protons (–CH). (**b**) The two singlet resonances in the NMR spectrum of this urine sample both derive from dimethylglycine. The increased concentration of this metabolite is the biomarker for the diagnosis dimethylglycinuria (# 605850) in this patient

– Direct infusion mass spectrometry (DI-HRMS)

In DI-HRMS, no chromatographic separation is performed (Fig. 7.2). Sample preparation is technically uncomplicated, and only a very small sample volume is needed (20 μL plasma, one 3 mm punch from a dried blood spot (DBS), 10 μL cerebrospinal fluid). Features measured through DI-HRMS contain two dimensions of metabolite information: accurate mass to charge ratios (m/z) and signal intensity. Subsequent annotation and putative identification of detected metabolites are solely based on accurate mass. As a consequence, metabolites with an identical mass (e.g., leucine and isoleucine) cannot be distinguished by DI-HRMS. DI-HRMS circumvents the need to create an experimental library containing metabolite masses and retention times, and no alignment of chromatographic peaks is necessary (Haijes et al. 2019a, b; de Sain-van der Velden et al. 2017).

– *Ultra high performance liquid chromatography–high-resolution mass spectrometry* based metabolomics (UHPLC-HRMS)

By performing chromatographic separation before MS analysis, the complex composition of a biological sample can be reduced, as it enables sequential MS analysis of the different metabolites (Fig. 7.2). In this way, matrix effects on ionization efficiency are minimized. Importantly, the retention time of a metabolite adds an additional layer of information for metabolite identification: potential isomers with similar masses can be resolved based on their retention time, and also retention time provides insight in general chemical properties of a metabolite. Ions or "features" measured through UHPLC MS therefore contain

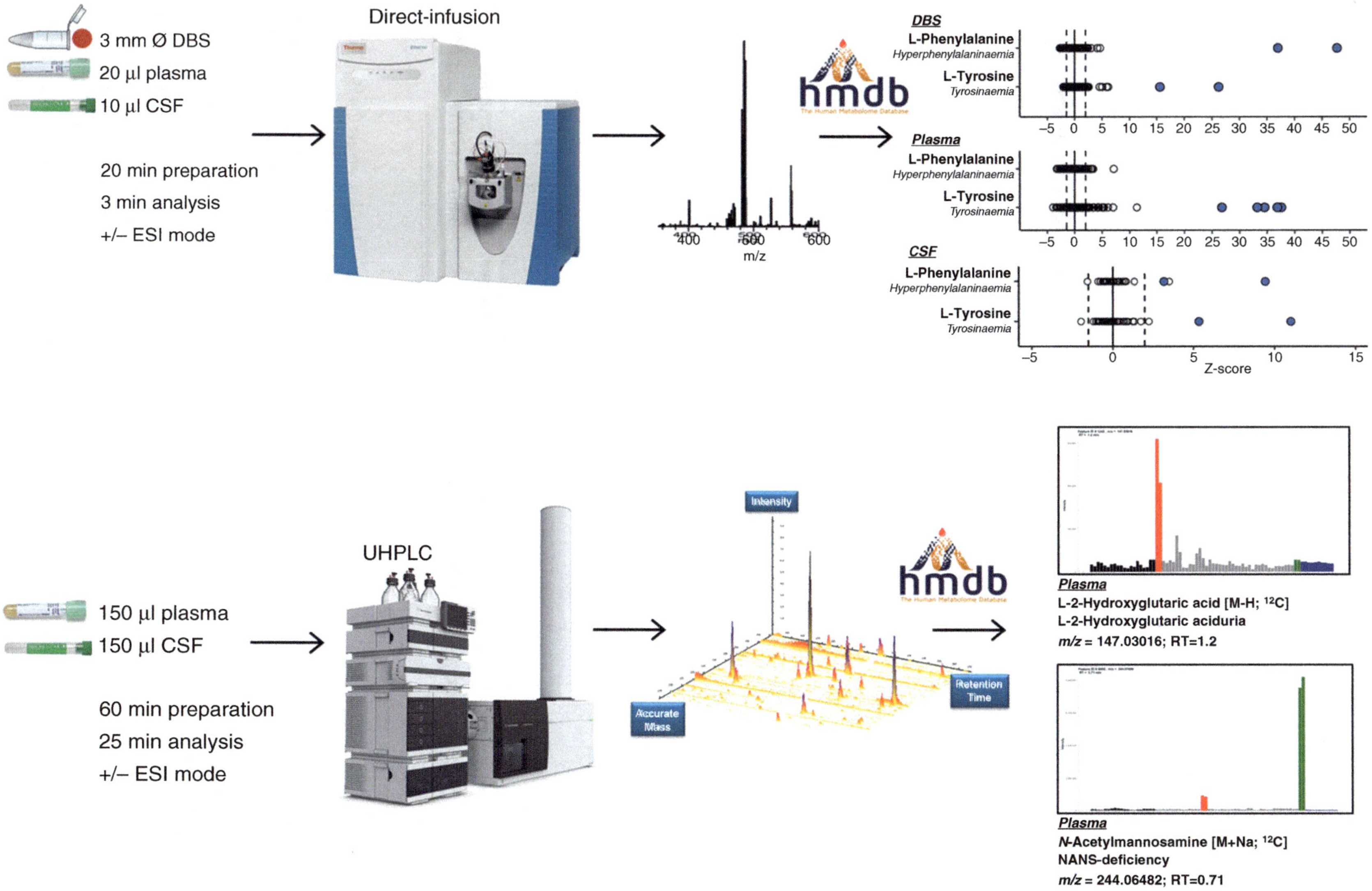


**Fig. 7.2** Next-generation metabolic screening: Schematic representation of untargeted metabolomics workflows. The upper workflow shows a direct infusion HRMS strategy, which provides two-dimensional (m/z and intensity) information on detected features. The human metabolome database (HMDB) is used to annotate features for putative identification. Significantly disrupted metabolites can be evaluated and visualized using *Z*-scores. Examples of increased phenylalanine and tyrosine in plasma, DBS, and CSF for hyperphenylalaninaemia and tyrosinaemia are shown, with patients depicted as blue circles and controls as white circles. The lower workflow depicts an ultrahigh pressure liquid chromatography (UHPLC) HRMS approach, which provides three-dimensional (m/z, retention time and intensity) information on detected features. Features can be aligned through XCMS and subsequently annotated using HMDB. Significantly disrupted metabolites can be evaluated based on Bonferroni-corrected *p*-values and visualized in bar plots. To illustrate this, bar plots of L-2-hydroxyglutaric acid in L-2-hydroxyglutaric aciduria and *N*-acetylmannosamine in NANS-deficiency are shown. In red, the patient signal is shown (two bars represent duplicate measurement), black signals represent control individuals; gray signals other patients in the analytical run; blue signals the control plasma, used for analytical quality control purposes; and in green the validation plasma, used for data analysis quality control purposes. The validation plasma is a plasma pool to which different diagnostic metabolites were spiked, including *N*-acetylmannosamine

three dimensions of metabolite information: accurate m/z, retention time, and signal intensity. When using UHPLC-HRMS metabolomics, a minimal volume of 150 μL of a body fluid sample (plasma, urine or cerebrospinal fluid) is required for a single measurement; however, the analyzing laboratory prefers to receive an amount of 500 μL to be able to perform additional measurements or further feature identification.

Different column types exist, which vary in their separation performance for polar metabolites. For untargeted metabolomics, reversed-phase (RP) chromatography can be used, which provides optimal separation for nonpolar and weakly polar metabolites with highly reproducible retention times. Hydrophilic interaction liquid chromatography (HILIC) may provide more optimal separation of polar compounds.

For analysis of UHPLC-HRMS data, typical processing of the raw data involves nonlinear alignment of feature peaks between the different samples in an analytical batch. Several commercial, open-access tools are available for feature alignment, including XCMS (Forsberg et al. 2018). This processing step results in a feature matrix output that contains the m/z ratios, retention time, and intensities of all features identified for each sample analyzed in an analytical batch. This matrix can be used as input for subsequent annotation of metabolites and statistical comparison of metabolites between patients and controls.

## Interpretation and Data Statistics

The interpretation of the features detected, whether they come from a DI-HRMS or UHPLC-HRMS experiment, begins with annotation of the exact feature masses to metabolites. The exact masses of features can be queried in open-access databases such as HMDB or Metlin, which contain information on metabolites matching these exact masses for putative identification.

The initial application of untargeted metabolomics has covered comparative analysis of predefined patient groups to controls, both outside and inside the field of inborn errors. The aim of this kind of experiment is to identify a metabolic fingerprint that can make a clear distinction between the disease and control group. For comparing metabolomics data of a disease group versus an unrelated control group, two popular multivariate analysis methods are principal component analysis (PCA) and partial least squares projection–discriminant analysis (PLS-DA). It is beyond the scope of this chapter to further discuss these methods.

To unlock the full clinical potential of untargeted metabolomics for diagnostics in inborn errors of metabolism, however, the focus should be on the analysis of the individual patient suspected of a metabolic disease. Features that are significantly perturbed in a patient sample compared to controls or other patient samples should be identified from the data. Since untargeted metabolomics methods render semi-quantitative results on feature intensity, no reference concentration ranges for individual features can be defined. Absolute intensities can vary between analytical runs; therefore, in general, evaluation of altered metabolite concentrations is based on comparison to a within-run average intensity. The magnitude of the feature alteration can be expressed as fold change or *Z*-score. Statistical testing to assess the significance of individual features can be performed, by a student T-test (if data is normally distributed) or a Mann-Whitney test (no normal distribution). Since the number of univariate comparisons made in such statistical analysis will be equal to the number of features detected (>10,000), there will be a large number of false positives, which is undesirable. Therefore, the *p*-value assigning significance to a finding should be corrected for multiple testing. Two commonly used approaches include the Bonferroni and the False Discovery Rate corrections. Subsequently, metabolites identified as aberrant should be further assessed for clinical relevance.

## Examples of Diagnostic and Research Applications of Untargeted Metabolomics/Next-Generation Metabolic Screening

Three consecutive steps in the diagnostic application of untargeted metabolomics data can be recognized. As a first step, the laboratory specialists can focus the interpretation of the untargeted metabolomics data of an individual patient on known biomarkers for known IEMs. In a second interpretation step, candidate genes that derive from exome or genome sequencing can be taken into account to specifically evaluate biochemical signatures of possibly pathogenic gene variants. In a third step, the full untargeted metabolomics data is available to "open the metabolome." This means that the more than 10,000 features that typically result from a single sample are taken into account. The laboratory will use a strategy to prioritize relevant aberrant metabolites for further study. The remaining list of aberrant metabolites may contain features that seldom or never occur in controls and features that are always present but have an abnormally high or low concentration in the specific patient sample. These features may represent the metabolic signature of a genetic disease, but they also may be the result of exogenous factors such as medication, diet, or the microbiome. A fourth application of untargeted metabolomics in IEM is the discovery of novel biomarkers for known diseases, which can provide further insight in the molecular mechanism of a disease or can predict the clinical status of the patient. The four different applications of untargeted metabolomics in IEMs are further discussed below, and specific examples of the four applications are given.

1. **Analysis of a selection of metabolites known to be associated with IEMs (IEM panel)**

   Analogous to disease gene panel analysis for whole exome sequencing data (WES), a predefined selection of metabolites can be extracted from untargeted metabolomics data as a first step in diagnostic evaluation. This strategy minimizes the risk of missing a diagnosis because a specific targeted assay was not performed based on clinical information. This metabolite panel approach has been shown to be successful in the diagnosis of a broad range of known IEMs in plasma (Coene et al. 2018). For patients with a complex, nonspecific IEM-suspected phenotype, showing clinical signs of neurological dysfunction, energy deficiency, intoxication and/or aberrant storage, a holistic metabolic screening starting with an IEM panel analysis is highly relevant. Figure 7.3a gives an example of the diagnosis in a patient with renal stones due to xanthinuria.

   It should be noted that at present, there is no single metabolomics method which can cover all diagnostically relevant metabolites in one analytical run, due to the diverse chemical nature of different classes of metabolites. The laboratory performing IEM panel analysis from untargeted metabolomics data should be able to provide information on which metabolites and diseases are covered (also comparable to sharing the composition of exome panels) and should perform complementary targeted assays to provide optimal metabolite coverage if indicated based on the clinical phenotype.

2. **Targeted evaluation of metabolites putatively linked to a variant of uncertain significance (VUS) in a metabolically active gene**

   The clinical application of whole exome sequencing techniques generates an unmet need for functional evidence on the pathogenicity of genomic DNA variants (variants of uncertain diagnostic significance, VUS). When these variants occur in metabolically active genes, the untargeted metabolomics data can be mined for the presence of a specific biochemical signature of the variant, which can provide insight in its pathogenicity (e.g., see (Haijes et al. 2019a; Coene et al. 2018; Van Karnebeek et al. 2016; Tarailo-Graovac et al. 2016)). This approach also prevents the need to develop separate targeted assays to evaluate functional consequences of VUS identified in open exome data in metabolically active genes that have not yet been associated with human disease. Based on combining information from the KEGG database with the IEMbase (Lee et al. 2018), it is estimated that over 1200 genes have a function in human metabolism, but have not yet been linked to a known IEM.

   Additionally, upon identification of a heterozygous variant that is known to be pathogenic for an autosomal recessive IEM, functional information can provide the answer whether a second variant may have been missed in the exome data, or whether there could be allelic expression imbalance of the pathogenic variant (Falkenberg et al. 2017). Figure 7.3b shows an example of a patient with a homozygous VUS in the *ASPA* gene in WES analysis. The untargeted metabolomics data show that this VUS is nonpathogenic.

   To assure that a diagnostic link can be made between metabolomics and exome data, the metabolic and genetic laboratory should be tightly connected to discuss patient results and integrate genetic and functional data when reporting to the clinician.

3. **Unbiased analysis of untargeted metabolomics data ("open the metabolome")**

   When no diagnostic leads have been found in IEM panel analysis and clinical suspicion of an IEM remains high, a patient's untargeted metabolomics data can be investigated beyond known IEM-associated metabolites, thereby venturing into the unknown areas of the human metabolome. This is still a challenging endeavor, as the majority of metabolites detected in an untargeted setting are of unknown or uncertain identity. Especially when exome data did not render clear metabolic leads or is not available, the diagnostic interpretation of the untargeted metabolome can be difficult and time-consuming. A combined approach of exome sequencing and MS-based untargeted metabolomics in an individual patient is the discovery of NANS-deficiency (Fig. 7.3c). This was the first example of the ability of this combined approach to find as yet unknown IEMs (Van Karnebeek et al. 2016). To select clinically relevant metabolites and prioritize unknown features for further identification, it is advisable to collect at least two samples of an individual patient at different timepoints to eliminate dietary effects on the metabolome. Also, an accurate overview of the patient's medication should be provided to the laboratory performing untargeted metabolomics, as features arising from medication can obscure the metabolomic profile. Valproic acid, for example, is notorious for this.

4. **Identification of novel biomarkers for known IEMs**

   For the diagnosis and follow-up of therapy of an IEM, current methods often rely on single biomarkers, usually the substrate of the defective enzyme. This may work very well to delineate the diagnosis; however, metabolites further down- or upstream of the metabolic block may prove to be more relevant when it comes to reflecting the clinical signs and symptoms, as is known for neurotransmit-

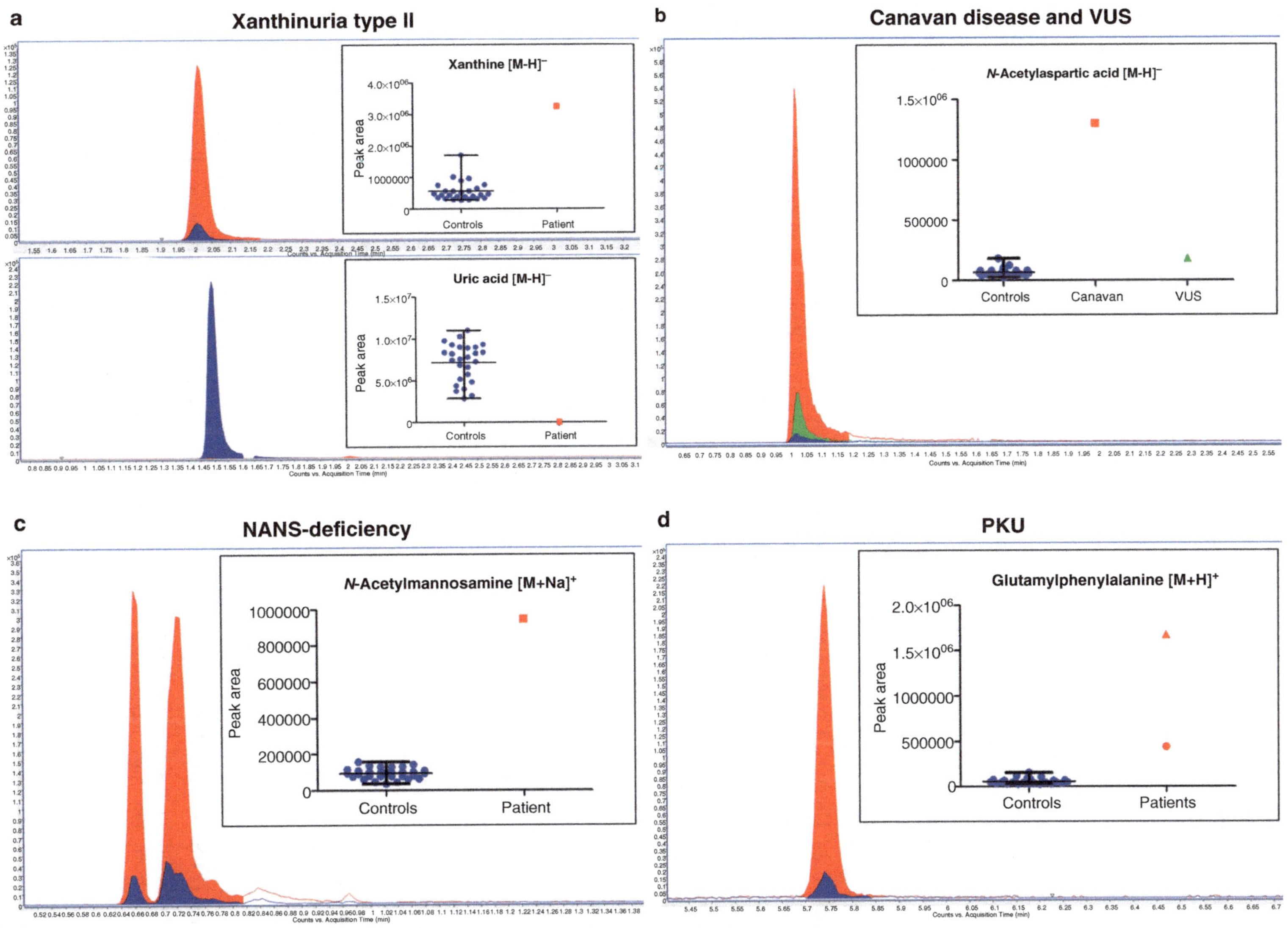


**Fig. 7.3** Four different applications of untargeted plasma metabolomics in IEM. (**a**) Extracted ion chromatogram (EIC) of masses 151.0261 and 167.0211 from xanthine [M-H]⁻ and uric acid [M-H]⁻, respectively, in plasma of a patient with xanthinuria type II and one representative control (blue). The insets show the feature intensity distribution in a scatter plot of xanthine and uric acid (blue, controls $n = 26$; red, patient $n = 1$). (**b**) EIC of mass 174.0408 from *N*-acetylaspartic acid [M-H]⁻ in plasma of patient with Canavan disease (red), a patient with a VUS in the Canavan-associated *ASPA* gene (green) and one representative control (blue). The inset shows the feature intensity distribution in a scatter plot of *N*-acetylaspartic acid (blue, controls $n = 26$; red, Canavan patient $n = 1$; green VUS patient $n = 1$). The profile allows the conclusion that the VUS is nonpathogenic and the patient does not suffer from classical Canavan disease. (**c**) EIC of mass 244.0792 from *N*-acetylmannosamine [M + Na]⁺ in plasma of patient with NANS-deficiency (red) and one representative control (blue). The inset shows the feature intensity distribution in a scatter plot *N*-acetylmannosamine (blue, controls $n = 31$; red, NANS patient $n = 1$). (**d**) EIC of mass 295.1289 from glutamylphenylalanine [M + H]⁺ in plasma of patient with PKU (red) and one representative control (blue). The inset shows the feature intensity distribution in a scatter plot of glutamylphenylalanine (blue, controls $n = 28$; red, PKU patients $n = 2$) (*red triangle* untreated, *red circle* treated)

ter defects. Additionally, alternative metabolism of the accumulating substrate may be pivotal for our understanding of the pathophysiology of a disease. The untargeted metabolomics technology may provide us with a window of opportunity for this. Because of the holistic and highly sensitive character of this approach, it will enable us to simultaneously evaluate an array of relevant metabolites from the affected pathway and from other pathways that maybe are influenced by the defect. The paper of Václavík et al. nicely illustrates this for PKU (Václavík et al. 2018). In a group of seven clinically stable PKU patients under adequate treatment, six novel biomarkers for PKU were discovered (in Fig. 7.3d the novel biomarker glutamyl-phenylalanine, a dipeptide with m/z 295.1289, is shown as an example) (Václavík et al. 2018). Such additional metabolic disturbances that now come to light will inspire investigators to do future studies on the pathophysiology of PKU. Another example concerns Snyder-Robinson syndrome (SRS). At the metabolite level, this disease was hitherto diagnosed by analysis of the spermine/spermidine ratio in lymphoblasts. Untargeted plasma metabolome analysis revealed significantly elevated levels of N8-acetylspermidine, a precursor of spermine biosynthesis, as an easy plasma biomarker for SRS (Abela et al. 2016). These studies illustrate the potential of metabolomics in clinical practice and research.

## Features of Unknown Significance

A significant percentage of features in MS-based untargeted metabolomics data cannot be easily identified using the existing knowledge stored in public databases like HMDB. They are features of unknown identity. These may be "known unknowns" that are commonly occurring in the population, which are not clinically relevant when their concentration is not unusual. In that case the bioinformatic pipeline may be able to filter these out. Potentially more interesting are the "unknown unknowns" that are specifically abundant in the patient under investigation and not in controls. Biomarkers of an IEM of that patient may be among them. Collectively, the features in this latter group are coined as **Features of Unknown Significance (FUS).** Further they reflect known intermediates of primary human metabolism, metabolites from secondary metabolism, but also metabolites from uncharted metabolic pathways. Additionally, they may derive from the diet, the microbiome, or the medication that the patient uses. For the metabolic laboratories, it is therefore of utmost importance to have the information about medication used when interpreting an untargeted metabolomics profile. These unknowns may warrant additional strategies to identify the metabolite behind that feature. To identify a feature of unknown significance, the University of Alberta offers a web-based program, "My Compound ID" (http://mcid.chem.ualberta.ca/) that allows a user to search a query mass to generate a list of possible matches with metabolites in an evidence-based metabolome library. This library is composed of 8021 known human endogenous metabolites and their predicted metabolic products (375,809 compounds from one metabolic reaction and 10,583,901 from two reactions). If the MS/MS spectrum of the query mass ion is available, this program also allows the user to interpret the MS/MS spectral pattern against the list of metabolite candidates generated from the mass search to narrow down the list into one or a few unique structures.

Currently, there are four other options that may help to identify the so-called FUS: (1) First there are the in-source fragments that are formed in the MS-detector from the feature at stake. (2) Multistep fragmentation techniques (so-called $MS^n$) as used in the paper by Václavík (Václavík et al. 2018). (3) NMR spectroscopy as illustrated in the paper of van Karnebeek et al. (Van Karnebeek et al. 2016). (4) LC-infrared ion spectroscopy as explained and shown in the paper of Martens et al. (2018).

When more groups around the world will be using untargeted metabolomics techniques and start sharing their data, the issue of the substantial amount of features that cannot be identified will gradually diminish.

## Future Perspectives and Challenges

HRMS-based untargeted metabolomics methods now offer an unprecedented opportunity to fully dissect the human metabolome, down to metabolites in the low nanomolar concentration range. Whereas the use of untargeted metabolomics in diagnostic practice for IEM is currently limited to a few clinical laboratories, we anticipate that its application will increase exponentially in the near future. More laboratories will gain access to HRMS set-ups, and bioinformatics solutions will allow for the integration of NGMS data with WES or WGS data in a combined diagnostic report.

However, several challenges in the application of untargeted metabolomics in clinical practice still exist. A major challenge is formed by the detection of features of unknown clinical significance or even of unknown identity in the vast amount of untargeted metabolomics data.

For building knowledge on clinical significance, many factors need to be taken into account including genomic variation as well as exogenous factors such as medication, food intake, age, microbiotic composition, etc. This daunting amount of information that we cannot judge appropriately yet can only be addressed by recording as much information as possible and sharing the information on these big data internationally. The multifactorial nature of the metabolome is also partially represented in "The Virtual Metabolic Human"

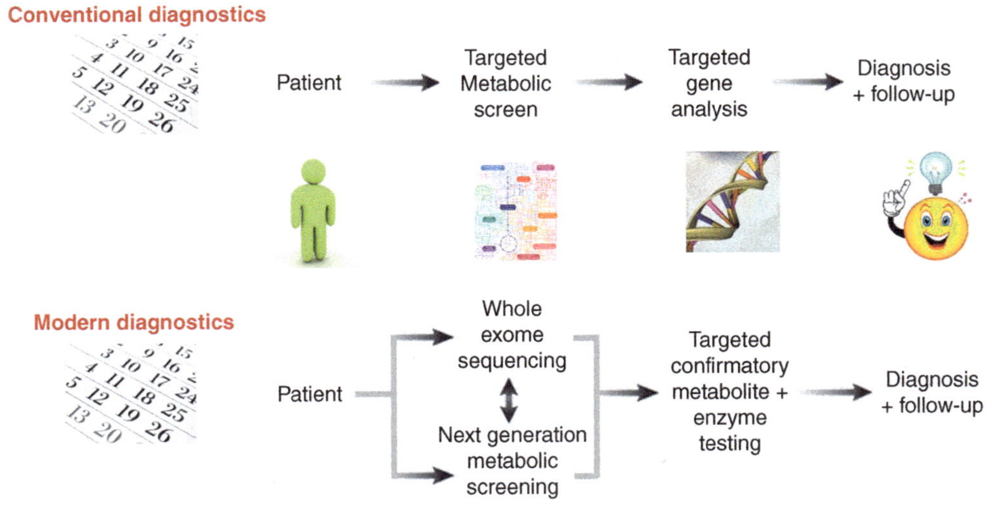


**Fig. 7.4** NGMS and WES/WGS in concert. The conventional method of finding the diagnosis of an IEM compared to the proposed contemporary approach where WES/WGS is used in parallel with NGMS to obtain an optimal diagnostic efficacy

(VMH, www.vmh.life), a database capturing information on human and gut microbial metabolism and linking this information to diseases and nutritional data. The VMH at the time of writing this chapter captures 5180 unique metabolites, 17,730 unique reactions, 3695 human genes, 255 Mendelian diseases, 818 microbes, 632,685 microbial genes, and 8790 food items (Noronha et al. 2019).

Public databases like the Human Metabolome Database (HMDB) and Metlin are essential in the interpretation of the large amount of features in the untargeted metabolomics data. It will be a major effort, requiring the input of many colleagues and laboratories, to identify all small molecule features occurring in human body fluids. Analogous to deciphering the significance of genetic variants of unknown significance, national and international collaboration in the metabolic community will be pivotal to bring our understanding of human metabolism to the next level. Databases such as the HMDB are a perfect vehicle to store new metabolic knowledge and share it with the IEM and broader scientific community. Although there is progress, it is at the same time clear that we are far from understanding the full complexity of the many metabolites in our body fluids.

In addition to expanding our knowledge on interpreting the metabolome of an individual, efforts will be directed toward making untargeted metabolomics accessible and integrating it smoothly in diagnostic practice. An integrated diagnostic report of WES/WGS and metabolomics results report should be feasible within the near future by combining the various existing databases with genetic and metabolic information using bioinformatics (Fig. 7.4). Despite the multifaceted functions, untargeted metabolomics can serve in diagnostics of IEMs, an important role of targeted metabolomics in patient care will remain in the foreseeable future. MS-based untargeted metabolomics provides semi-quantitative data. For patients with a known disease, requiring quantitative assessment of specific metabolites for therapy follow-up, a dedicated quantitative analysis may be desired.

Unfortunately, no single analytical technique will be able to reveal the complete spectrum of metabolites in body fluids or cell extracts. The untargeted metabolomics techniques in this chapter are not suited for holistic analysis of lipids, which requires dedicated lipidomics techniques. Metabolic workup of a patient traditionally relies on metabolite analysis in body fluids. This also means that metabolites that cannot escape the cellular surroundings will generally not be detected when assessing plasma. Examples are phosphorylated metabolites and again the lipids. This stresses the relevance of analyzing the intracellular metabolome for future diagnostic purposes.

## References

Abela L, Simmons L, Steindl K, Schmitt B, Mastrangelo M, Joset P, Papuc M, Sticht H, Baumer A, Crowther LM, Mathis D, Rauch A, Plecko B. N(8)-acetylspermidine as a potential plasma biomarker for Snyder-Robinson syndrome identified by clinical metabolomics. J Inherit Metab Dis. 2016;39(1):131–7. PubMed PMID:26174906.

Coene KLM, Kluijtmans LAJ, van der Heeft E, Engelke UFH, de Boer S, Hoegen B, Kwast HJT, van de Vorst M, Huigen MCDG, Keularts IMLW, Schreuder MF, van Karnebeek CDM, Wortmann SB, de Vries MC, Janssen MCH, Gilissen C, Engel J, Wevers RA. Next-generation metabolic screening: targeted and untargeted metabolomics for the diagnosis of inborn errors of metabolism in individual patients. J Inherit Metab Dis. 2018;41(3):337–53. PubMed PMID: 29453510; PubMed Central PMCID: PMC5959972.

Coman D, Vissers LELM, Riley LG, Kwint MP, Hauck R, Koster J, Geuer S, Hopkins S, Hallinan B, Sweetman L, Engelke UFH, Burrow TA, Cardinal J, McGill J, Inwood A, Gurnsey C, Waterham HR, Christodoulou J, Wevers RA, Pitt J. Squalene synthase deficiency: clinical, biochemical, and molecular characterization of a defect in cholesterol biosynthesis. Am J Hum Genet. 2018;103(1):125–30. PubMed PMID: 29909962; PubMed Central PMCID: PMC6037199.

de Sain-van der Velden MGM, van der Ham M, Gerrits J, Prinsen HCMT, Willemsen M, Pras-Raves ML, Jans JJ, Verhoeven-Duif

NM. Quantification of metabolites in dried blood spots by direct infusion high resolution mass spectrometry. Anal Chim Acta. 2017;979:45–50. PubMed PMID: 28599708.

Engelke U, Kluijtmans L, Huigen M, Goudswaard A, van der Graaf M, Heerschap A, Morava-Kozicz E, Wortmann-Hagemann S, Wevers RA. Handbook NMR spectroscopy and brain MR spectroscopy. 3rd ed. 2014. ISBN 978-90-9028358-6. www.bodyfluidnmr.nl.

Falkenberg KD, Braverman NE, Moser AB, Steinberg SJ, Klouwer FCC, Schlüter A, Ruiz M, Pujol A, Engvall M, Naess K, van Spronsen F, Körver-Keularts I, Rubio-Gozalbo ME, Ferdinandusse S, Wanders RJA, Waterham HR. Allelic expression imbalance promoting a mutant PEX6 allele causes Zellweger spectrum disorder. Am J Hum Genet. 2017;101(6):965–76. PubMed PMID: 29220678; PubMed Central PMCID: PMC5812895.

Forsberg EM, Huan T, Rinehart D, Benton HP, Warth B, Hilmers B, Siuzdak G. Data processing, multi-omic pathway mapping, and metabolite activity analysis using XCMS Online. Nat Protoc. 2018;13(4):633–51. PubMed PMID: 29494574; PubMed Central PMCID: PMC5937130.

Haijes HA, Willemsen M, Van der Ham M, Gerrits J, Pras-Raves ML, Prinsen HCMT, Van Hasselt PM, De Sain-van der Velden MGM, Verhoeven-Duif NM, Jans JJM. Direct infusion based metabolomics identifies metabolic disease in patients' dried blood spots and plasma. Metabolites. 2019a;9(1). pii: E12. PubMed PMID: 30641898; PubMed Central PMCID: PMC6359237.

Haijes HA, van der Ham M, Gerrits J, van Hasselt PM, Prinsen HCMT, de Sain-van der Velden MGM, Verhoeven-Duif NM, Jans JJM. Direct-infusion based metabolomics unveils biochemical profiles of inborn errors of metabolism in cerebrospinal fluid. Mol Genet Metab. 2019b. S1096-7192(19)30035-6. PubMed PMID: 30926434.

Lee JJY, Wasserman WW, Hoffmann GF, van Karnebeek CDM, Blau N. Knowledge base and mini-expert platform for the diagnosis of inborn errors of metabolism. Genet Med. 2018;20(1):151–8. PubMed PMID: 28726811; PubMed Central PMCID: PMC5763153.

Martens J, Berden G, Bentlage H, Coene KLM, Engelke UF, Wishart D, van Scherpenzeel M, Kluijtmans LAJ, Wevers RA, Oomens J. Unraveling the unknown areas of the human metabolome: the role of infrared ion spectroscopy. J Inherit Metab Dis. 2018;41(3):367–77. PubMed PMID: 29556837; PubMed Central PMCID: PMC5959965.

Noronha A, Modamio J, Jarosz Y, Guerard E, Sompairac N, Preciat G, Daníelsdóttir AD, Krecke M, Merten D, Haraldsdóttir HS, Heinken A, Heirendt L, Magnúsdóttir S, Ravcheev DA, Sahoo S, Gawron P, Frisciomi L, Garcia B, Prendergast M, Puente A, Rodrigues M, Roy A, Rouquaya M, Wiltgen L, Žagare A, John E, Krueger M, Kuperstein I, Zinovyev A, Schneider R, Fleming RMT, Thiele I. The Virtual Metabolic Human database: integrating human and gut microbiome metabolism with nutrition and disease. Nucleic Acids Res. 2019;47(D1):D614–24. PubMed PMID: 30371894; PubMed Central PMCID: PMC6323901.

Tarailo-Graovac M, Shyr C, Ross CJ, Horvath GA, Salvarinova R, Ye XC, Zhang LH, Bhavsar AP, Lee JJ, Drögemöller BI, Abdelsayed M, Alfadhel M, Armstrong L, Baumgartner MR, Burda P, Connolly MB, Cameron J, Demos M, Dewan T, Dionne J, Evans AM, Friedman JM, Garber I, Lewis S, Ling J, Mandal R, Mattman A, McKinnon M, Michoulas A, Metzger D, Ogunbayo OA, Rakic B, Rozmus J, Ruben P, Sayson B, Santra S, Schultz KR, Selby K, Shekel P, Sirrs S, Skrypnyk C, Superti-Furga A, Turvey SE, Van Allen MI, Wishart D, Wu J, Wu J, Zafeiriou D, Kluijtmans L, Wevers RA, Eydoux P, Lehman AM, Vallance H, Stockler-Ipsiroglu S, Sinclair G, Wasserman WW, van Karnebeek CD. Exome sequencing and the management of neurometabolic disorders. N Engl J Med. 2016;374(23):2246–55. PubMed PMID: 27276562; PubMed Central PMCID: PMC4983272.

Tebani A, Afonso C, Bekri S. Advances in metabolome information retrieval: turning chemistry into biology. Part I: analytical chemistry of the metabolome. J Inherit Metab Dis. 2018;41(3):379–91. PubMed PMID: 28840392; PubMed Central PMCID: PMC5959978.

Václavík J, Coene KLM, Vrobel I, Najdekr L, Friedecký D, Karlíková R, Mádrová L, Petsalo A, Engelke UFH, van Wegberg A, Kluijtmans LAJ, Adam T, Wevers RA. Structural elucidation of novel biomarkers of known metabolic disorders based on multistage fragmentation mass spectra. J Inherit Metab Dis. 2018;41(3):407–14. PubMed PMID:29139026.

Van Karnebeek CD, Bonafé L, Wen XY, Tarailo-Graovac M, Balzano S, Royer-Bertrand B, Ashikov A, Garavelli L, Mammi I, Turolla L, Breen C, Donnai D, Cormier-Daire V, Heron D, Nishimura G, Uchikawa S, Campos-Xavier B, Rossi A, Hennet T, Brand-Arzamendi K, Rozmus J, Harshman K, Stevenson BJ, Girardi E, Superti-Furga G, Dewan T, Collingridge A, Halparin J, Ross CJ, Van Allen MI, Rossi A, Engelke UF, Kluijtmans LA, van der Heeft E, Renkema H, de Brouwer A, Huijben K, Zijlstra F, Heise T, Boltje T, Wasserman WW, Rivolta C, Unger S, Lefeber DJ, Wevers RA, Superti-Furga A. NANS-mediated synthesis of sialic acid is required for brain and skeletal development. Nat Genet. 2016;48(7):777–84;49(6):969. PubMed PMID: 27213289.

# MRI and In Vivo Spectroscopy of the Brain

8

Matthew T. Whitehead and Andrea Gropman

## Contents



M. T. Whitehead (✉)
Department of Radiology, Children's National Health System,
Washington, DC, USA
e-mail: MWhitehe@childrensnational.org

A. Gropman
Department of Neurology, Children's National Health System,
Washington, DC, USA
e-mail: agropman@childrensnational.org


N. Blau et al. (eds.), *Physician's Guide to the Diagnosis, Treatment, and Follow-Up of Inherited Metabolic Diseases*,
https://doi.org/10.1007/978-3-030-67727-5_8

**Summary**

Most inborn errors of metabolism (IEMs) have a potential for central nervous system (CNS) injury resulting in chronic encephalopathy. IEMs may affect CNS structures in a manner dependent upon disorder type, stage of brain development, severity, and/or duration. Several of the disorders share a final common pathway to brain dysfunction such as disruption of astrocyte function, excitotoxicity, and/or energy failure.

Neuroimaging has emerged as a powerful clinical tool to study the brain in a noninvasive manner in order to assist in distinguishing disorders from one another, despite very similar clinical manifestations. As there are limited ways in which the CNS can respond to insults, imaging manifestations are often nonspecific. Nonetheless, there is a striking anatomical pattern of vulnerability in many IEMs. Some IEMs cause reasonably predictable disease patterns that can be suggestive or diagnostic. Specific neuroimaging patterns of inborn metabolic errors are the focus of this chapter.

## Introduction

It is important to alert the radiologist or neuroradiologist whenever there is clinical concern for a metabolic abnormality affecting the CNS. The MRI armamentarium contains numerous sequences that can be chosen to identify alterations in brain structure, texture, water movement, metabolism, and mineralization and to detect hemorrhage. Time constraints limit sequence selection to only those most necessary and relevant. Therefore, the provided history should be as specific as possible to ensure that the imaging exam will be tailored using an appropriate pulse-sequence prescription most likely to determine the IEM type and/or answer the clinical question. "New onset generalized seizures and developmental regression" is an example of an adequate history, while "encephalopathy" is more nonspecific and "rule out pathology" is simply unacceptable. "Rule out x" is never appropriate in isolation, but welcomed after explaining *why* x needs to be excluded. Pertinent lab values and head circumference are useful to include in the neuroimaging order request in some cases. A history of prematurely and estimated gestational age should always be disclosed as the expected normal appearance of the brain changes over time, especially with regard to myelination. This concept is best captured by the idiom "garbage in, garbage out." Inadequate exam indications have a higher chance of yielding the unsavory phrase, "correlate clinically."

Dominant factors influencing modality selection and examination protocols include patient age, past medical history (especially contraindications to contrast material and/or MRI), signs, symptoms, and the history of present illness. Head ultrasound is often the initial imaging exam in the neonatal setting given its near universal access, portability, ease of acquisition, and lack of ionizing radiation. Drawbacks of ultrasound include a relative insensitivity and poor specificity for brain pathology. CT excels in the detection of calcifications and hemorrhage. It can also be useful in the acute setting to quickly identify actionable intracranial abnormalities and when sonographic findings require clarification. However, MRI is the reigning gold standard in the neuroimaging assessment of the CNS. In addition to its ability to demonstrate multiplanar fine structural details, it exploits inherent and acquired differences in tissue properties to reveal changes in disease states. Therefore, the sensitivity and specificity of MRI generally exceed those of ultrasound and CT.

A typical brain MR protocol for suspected metabolic abnormalities should include both conventional sequences (i.e., T1WI, T2WI) and advanced imaging techniques such as diffusion tensor imaging, perfusion, and proton magnetic resonance spectroscopy (1H MRS). A magnetization transfer sequence is also useful in the evaluation of leukodystrophies to determine the type of white matter disturbance. Intravenous gadolinium-based contrast agents (GBCAs) may be useful when the specific diagnosis is uncertain as these add specificity to some IEMs and help exclude mimics such as infection and subacute infarction. Spine MR imaging can also be useful in some disorders to improve diagnostic specificity.

1H MRS has great utility in the initial work-up and subsequent follow-up of metabolic disturbances/disorders. Although a nonspecific pattern (elevated choline, depressed NAA) is common in many types of brain disease, short echo 1H MRS (TE < 40 ms) can reveal more specific metabolic signatures. Furthermore, temporal changes on subsequent exams can support or refute the benefit of ongoing therapeutic measures. A simple single voxel technique boasts better signal-to-noise ratios and allows shorter TE options when compared with multivoxel technique (Bluml and Panigrahy 2013). Voxel size is a balance between signal-to-noise (SNR) and tissue specificity; ideally, it should be as large as possible to achieve satisfactory SNR but small enough to target the area of interest. Generally, a 2 × 2 × 2 cm voxel is used; voxels smaller than 1 $cm^3$ are unlikely to be worthy of the acquisition time it would require to achieve reasonable SNR. Voxel location and echo times should be selected based on the suspected and/or discovered disease patterns. Hemorrhage, iron, and calcification hamper 1H MRS quality and impact SNR; these should be avoided, and if unavoidable, 1H MRS should not be performed as misleading information could be returned. In our experience, two acquisitions using two different echo (short and longer) are more useful and preferable to one whenever feasible. The reasons are multifactorial, but some notable issues relate to the fact that metabolites in small concentrations tend to be more visible using short echo times, metabolic peak overlap may be more or less apparent at different echo times, J coupling and J modulation are altered at different echo times, longer echo times have less inherent noise, and metabolites have different T2 properties. We typically perform ultrashort (TE 14, TR 1500; STEAM technique), short (TE 35, TR 1500–2000; PRESS technique), and intermediate (TE 144, TR 1500–2000; PRESS) or long (TE 288, TR 1500–2000; PRESS) echo time sequences. Magnetic field strength dictates the choice of the longest echo time; because lactate detection is unreliable at 144 ms TE at 3 T field strength, we use a 288 ms TE at 3 T instead (Lange et al. 2006).

The vast majority of inborn errors of metabolism (IEM) have a nonspecific neuroimaging phenotype. Imaging manifestations often overlap among IEMs and more broadly with other CNS diseases. This is especially true at the extremes of the disease time course where normal exams may be found early on and in presymptomatic individuals, and diffuse chronic brain changes are often present in the end-stage patient. However, some IEMs tend to be more specific, and others can be diagnostic using MRI and/or MRS. After a deviation from the age-expected normal appearance is recognized, the next step in interpretation is to determine the disease pattern, if present, using images from all available modalities and time points. Several imaging features raise concern for the possibility of an IEM: symmetric abnormalities in brain signal/density/echogenicity, disease patterns atypical for ischemic and infectious insults, mixed aged lesions, temporal variability inconsistent with the expected evolution of a static encephalopathy, and unexpected spectroscopic abnormalities. Of course, the imaging results should always be interpreted in the context of the clinical picture. Metabolic disorders with suggestive or diagnostic neuroimaging appearances in the therapeutic naive state are discussed in the following paragraphs with associated figures.

## Intoxication Type Disorders/Acute Metabolic Encephalopathy

**The disorders typically defined as intoxication type share a similar clinical presentation. Several groups of IEM including the organic acidemias, urea cycle disorders, and certain disorders of amino acid metabolism typically present with acute life-threatening symptoms and a rapidly evolving encephalopathy. These symptoms are the result of a toxic accumulation of metabolites in the CNS. Symptoms may include seizures, apnea, respiratory distress, and lethargy progressing to coma due in part to ensuing brain edema. While nonspecific in nature and clinically difficult to differentiate the underlying diagnosis, several of these diseases have characteristic imaging patterns, some of which are illustrated below.**

## Maple Syrup Urine Disease (MSUD)

Neonatal encephalopathy is the most common presentation of this aminoacidopathy. Marked, extensive brain edema is typical, comprised of mixed subtypes: vasogenic edema in unmyelinated white matter and intramyelinic edema in myelinating white matter (Whitehead and Gropman 2018; Jan et al. 2003; Sakai et al. 2005; Terek et al. 2013; Ha et al. 2004). White matter reduced diffusion is usually quite profound, especially in the projectional fibers, thalami, globus pallidus, pontocerebellar fibers, and deep cerebellar nuclei (Whitehead and Gropman 2018; Jan et al. 2003; Ha et al. 2004; Barkovich and Patay 2019) (Fig. 8.1). Diffusion abnormalities may in part reflect spongiotic dysmyelination with intramyelinic edema rather than demyelination given the lack of magnetization transfer signal, prolonged persistence in patients under dietary control, and the presence in presymptomatic patients (Terek et al. 2013; Ha et al. 2004; Sener 2002; Myers et al. 2012). Diffusion abnormalities in more maturely myelinated brains may be more widespread (Sakai et al. 2005). Milder phenotypes may show only hypomyelination and mild atrophy, T2 prolongation in the globus pallidus, and/or deep cerebral white matter hyperintensity (Ishikawa et al. 1991; Li et al. 1997; Muller et al. 1993). In adolescent and adults, extensive cerebral cortical restricted can occur during metabolic decompensation (Jan et al. 2003). Central spinal cord T2 prolongation has been shown in a sibling pair with MSUD (Bhat et al. 2013).

MRS shows multiple enlarged macromolecular peaks corresponding to branched chain amino acids (BCAAs), branched chain ketoacids (BCKAs), lipid, and lactate along with elevated choline and myoinositol and depressed *N*-acetylaspartate (NAA) (Bluml and Panigrahy 2013; Jan et al. 2003; Terek et al. 2013) (Fig. 8.1). Notably, longer echo times improve diagnostic specificity in MSUD by eliminating the normal background macromolecular signal that can hide BCAA/BCKA peaks (Jan et al. 2003).

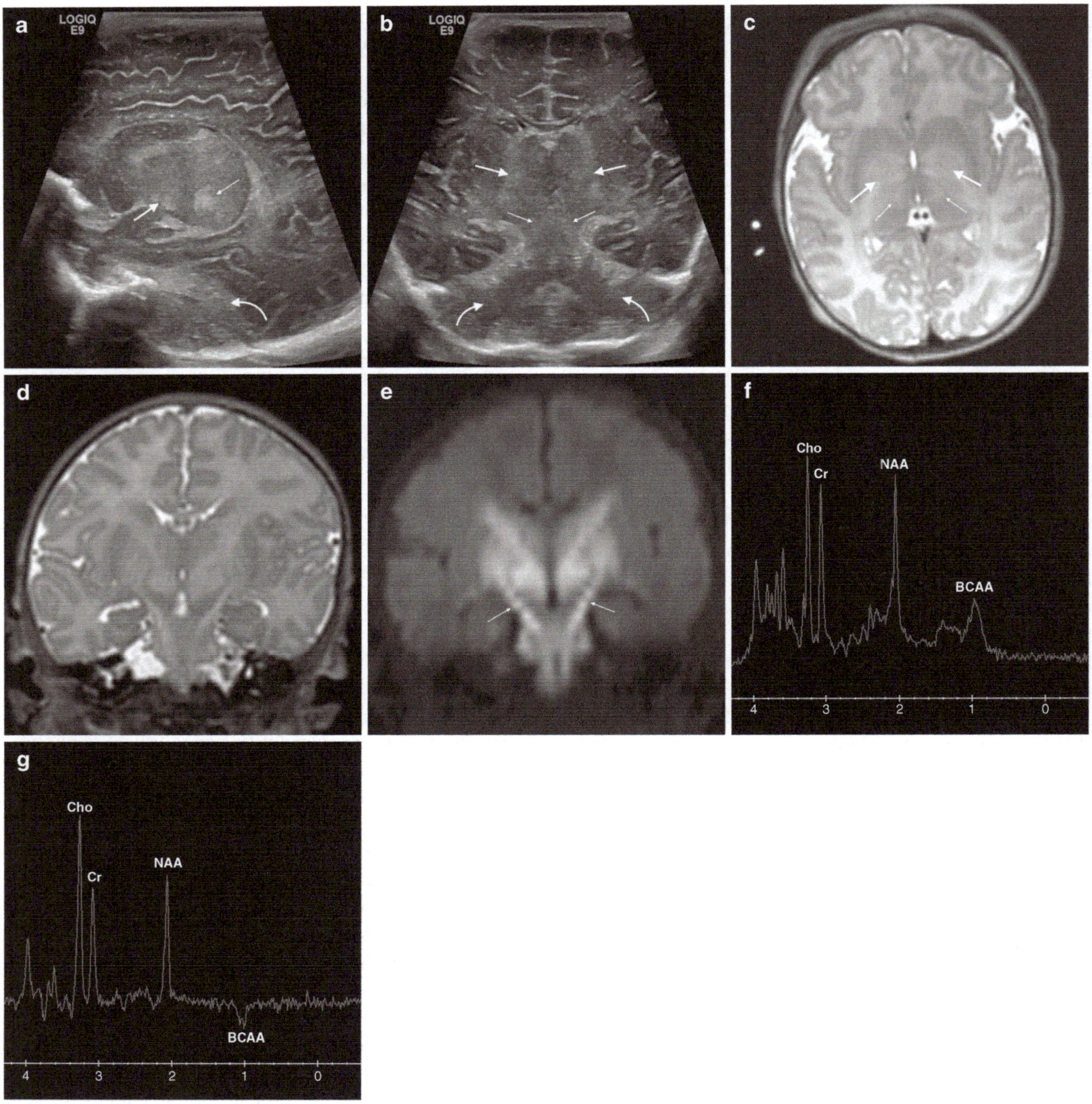


**Fig. 8.1** Neonatal female with maple syrup urine disease (MSUD). (**a**) Parasagittal gray-scale ultrasound image of the brain shows abnormal hyperechogenicity in the cerebral white matter, lentiform nuclei (thick arrow), thalamus (thin arrow), and imaged cerebellum representing edema (curved arrow). (**b**) Coronal gray-scale ultrasound image of the brain shows thalamic (thick arrows), brainstem (thin arrow), and cerebellar (curved arrow) hyperechogenicity representing edema. (**c**) Axial T2-weighted MR image (TR/TE msec, 2500/65) through the basal ganglia depicts abnormal hyperintense signal in parts of the globi pallidi (thick arrows), thalami (thin arrows), and white matter. Coronal T2WI (TR/TE msec, 2500/65) (**d**) and corresponding diffusion weighted image (TR/TE msec, 8000/84) (**e**) in a similar plane to (**b**) show signal abnormality and reduced diffusion representing intramyelinic edema in the basal ganglia, thalamus, and brainstem with notable involvement of projectional fibers representing intramyelinic edema (arrows, **e**). Single voxel MRS over the left basal ganglia (TR/TE msec, 1500/35) (**f**) and (TR/TE msec, 1500/144) (**g**) reveal a broadened metabolic peak at 0.9–1.1 ppm that inverts on the longer echo time MRS (arrows), representing branch chain amino acids/branch chain keto acids (BCAA)

## Nonketotic Hyperglycinemia (NKH)

NKH is an amino acidopathy that typically presents in the neonatal period with encephalopathy, seizures, and hypotonia. Neuroimaging features can be quite specific when MRI and 1H MRS are obtained and interpreted in parallel. Namely, intramyelinic edema manifested by reduced diffusion can be seen in the myelinating fibers of the cerebrum, cerebellum, and brainstem, with excessive hyperintense signal on T2WI in the unmyelinated white matter either representing undermyelination and/or vasogenic edema (Whitehead and Gropman 2018; Whitehead et al. 2015; Stence et al. 2019) (Fig. 8.2). These changes occur in similar locations as those found in maple syrup urine disease (MSUD), but are typically much less severe and extensive. The corpus callosum is often hypogenetic and the total brain volume small (Whitehead and Gropman 2018; Whitehead et al. 2015; Stence et al. 2019) (Fig. 8.2). Wei and colleagues reported a case of long tract hyperintensity on T2WI spanning from the dorsal medulla into the cervical and thoracic dorsomedial spinal cord (Wei et al. 2011).

1H MRS reveals elevated glycine at 3.55 ppm that correlates more reliably with the clinical status than plasma and CSF glycine concentrations (Bluml and Panigrahy 2013; Whitehead and Gropman 2018; Whitehead et al. 2015; Heindel et al. 1993) (Fig. 8.2). It is necessary to obtain at least one 1H MRS data point using an intermediate (i.e., 144 ms) or long (i.e., 288 ms) echo time to remove the spectral contamination of MI around 3.5 ppm.

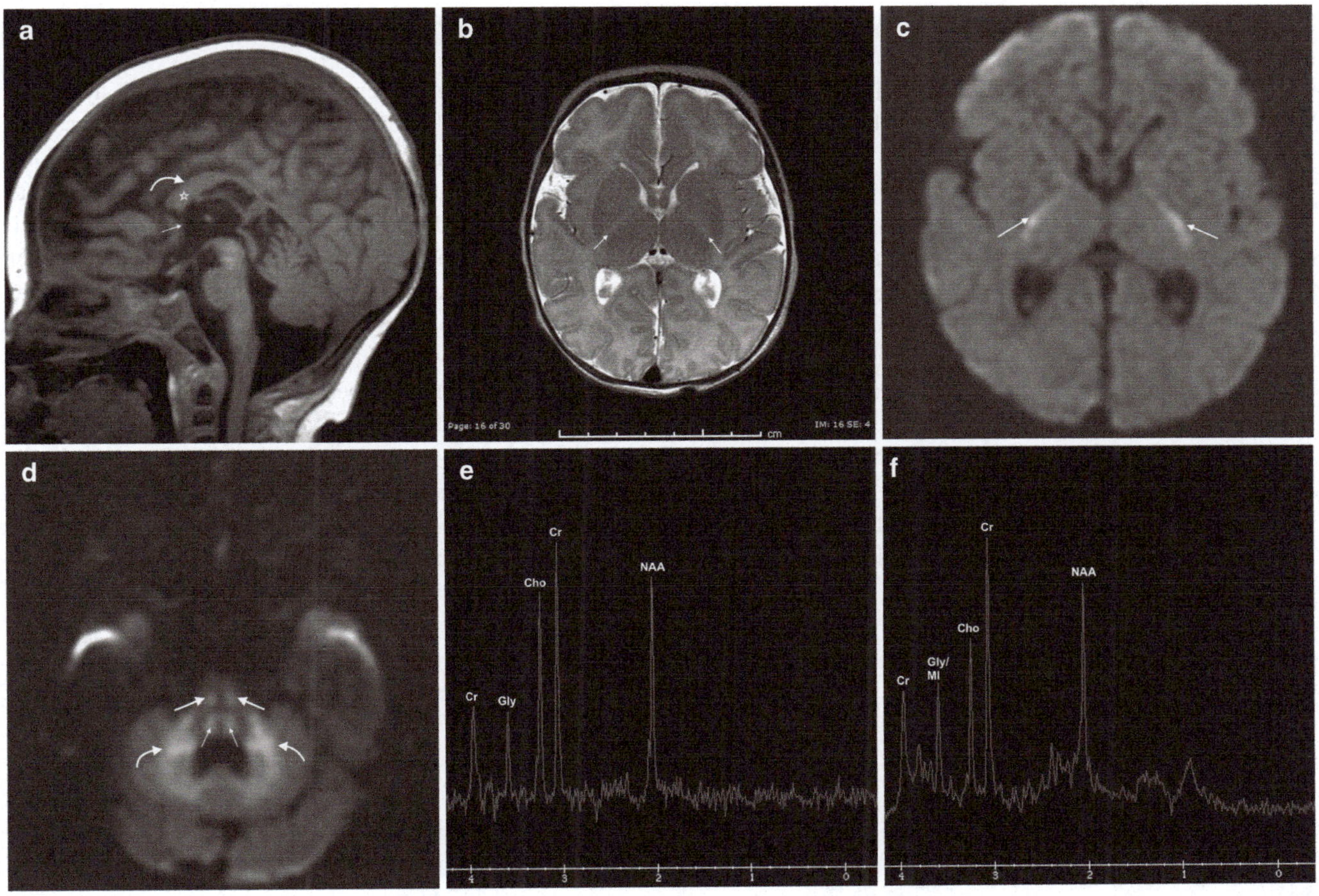


**Fig. 8.2** Neonatal female with nonketotic hyperglycinemia. (**a**) Sagittal midline T1WI (TR/TE msec, 7/2) demonstrates multiple structural midline abnormalities including a thin, shortened hypogenetic corpus callosum (curved arrow), marked hypoplasia of the anterior commissure (thin arrow), hypoplasia of the septum pellucidum (star), and mild pontine hypoplasia. (**b**) Axial T2WI (TR/TE msec, 3183/96) at the level of the basal ganglia shows lack of normal myelination-related hypointensity of the posterior limb of the internal capsule (PLIC) (arrows). Axial DWI (TR/TE msec, 80,000/85) through the basal ganglia (**c**) and posterior fossa (**d**) shows increased signal/reduced diffusion in the PLIC (arrows, **c**), corticospinal tracts (thick arrows, **d**), central tegmental tracts (thin arrows, **d**), and middle cerebellar peduncles/deep cerebellar white matter (curved arrows, **d**). Single voxel MRS over the left basal ganglia (TR/TE msec, 1500/144) (**e**) and (TR/TE msec, 1500/35) (**f**) reveals an abnormal metabolic peak at 3.6 ppm that overlaps with myoinositol on the short echo MRS consistent with glycine (gly). Creatine (Cr) is elevated, while choline (Cho) is mildly depressed, altering the normal ratios of NAA, Cr, and Cho

## Methylmalonic Aciduria (MMA)

Typical presentation of metabolic acidosis and coma is not enough to differentiate this clinically from other intoxication disorders. In MMA, the basal ganglia are commonly affected with or without concurrent involvement of the substantia nigra and dentate nuclei. In particular, the globus pallidi are involved dominantly or in isolation (Whitehead and Gropman 2018). In decompensation, reduced diffusion is present in the basal ganglia, and chronic injury leads to regional volume loss and hyperintense signal on T2WI with facilitated diffusion (Fig. 8.3). Lactic acidosis is often shown on 1H MRS (Bluml and Panigrahy 2013).

## Glutaric Aciduria Type I

This IEM may be differentiated clinically due to movement disorders that may present acutely and may have associated macrocrania. On MRI, hyperintense basal ganglia signal on T2WI with restricted diffusion sparing the thalami may be found in acute symptomatic patients (Whitehead and Gropman 2018; Barkovich and Patay 2019; Whitehead et al. 2015) (Fig. 8.4). Cerebral white matter hyperintensity and cerebellar deep gray nuclear involvement may also be present. Important structural features that help distinguish glutaric aciduria from other IEMs include underopercularization and enlarged extra-axial spaces in the middle cranial fossae (Whitehead and Gropman 2018; Barkovich and Patay 2019; Whitehead et al. 2015) (Fig. 8.4). Progressive atrophy often leads to development of nontraumatic subdural hemorrhage. Glutaric acid has been found using 1H MRS, along with reduced NAA and creatine, elevated choline, and lactate (Bluml and Panigrahy 2013; Harting et al. 2015).

## L-2-Hydroxyglutaric Aciduria

In this rare IEM, clinical symptoms overlap with those of other intoxicating disorders. Conversely, neuroimaging features are quite suggestive when present, as this is one of the few disorders that manifests a centropedal cerebral lesion severity gradient from superficial to central (Barkovich and Patay 2019; Fourati et al. 2016) (Fig. 8.5). Thus, subcortical precedes deep white matter involvement, and external and extreme capsules are affected prior to the deep gray structures. Cerebellar deep gray nuclei are also quite commonly affected (Barkovich and Patay 2019; Fourati et al. 2016). In addition to decreased NAA and choline concentrations, L-2-hydroxyglutaric acid elevation has been suggested on MRS at 2.5 ppm (Fourati et al. 2016; Anghileri et al. 2016).

## Urea Cycle Disorders (UCD)

Acute metabolic decompensation associated with hyperammonemia (HA) and intermediate metabolite toxicity causes brain swelling, edema, and variable injury, especially in the neonatal period and more commonly in complete proximal urea cycle defects (Helman et al. 2014; Pacheco-Colon et al. 2013). Patients may have mild (partial deficiencies, later onset) to severe HA (infant onset). There is a metabolic alkalosis that can, for example, help distinguish UCD from MMA that can have lower levels of HA. Disease patterns may vary based on the specific enzymatic or transporter defect, though phenotypic similarities are common among UCD subtypes (Barkovich and Patay 2019). The most familiar imaging patterns are "diffuse" and "central" with the latter isolated to the insular/peri-insular, perisylvian, perirolandic, internal capsular, and/or basal ganglia regions

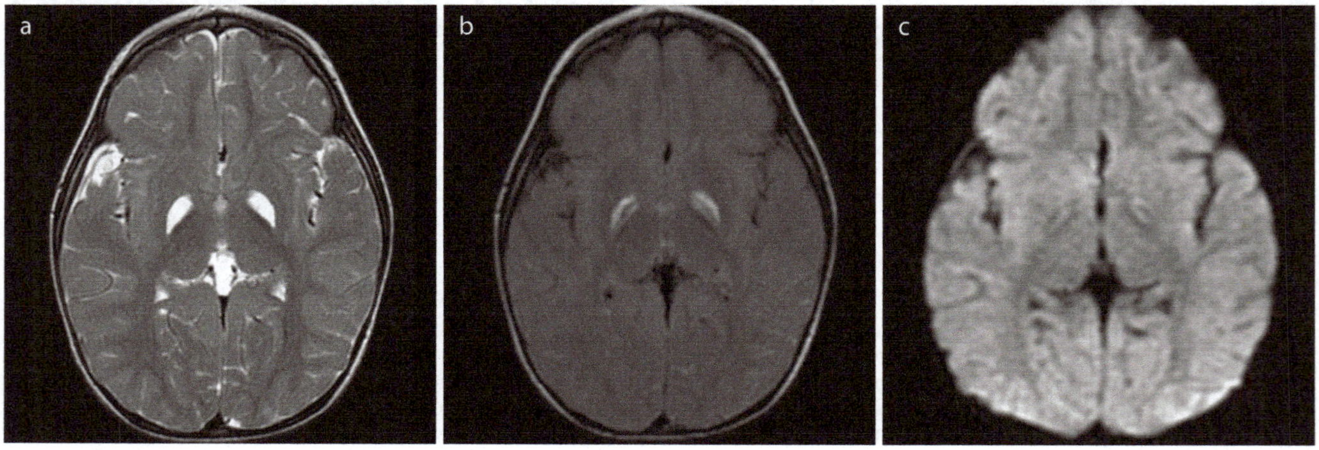


**Fig. 8.3** A 15-year-old female with methylmalonic aciduria. (**a**) Axial T2WI (TR/TE msec, 4217/101) through the basal ganglia shows hyperintense globi pallidi. The corresponding T2/FLAIR sequence (TR/TE/TI msec, 10,000/136/2200) (**b**) and diffusion-weighted sequence (TR/TE msec, 9300/93) (**c**) demonstrate mixed globi pallidi signal changes with central suppression/necrosis and peripherally reduced diffusion, representing acute on chronic metabolic injury

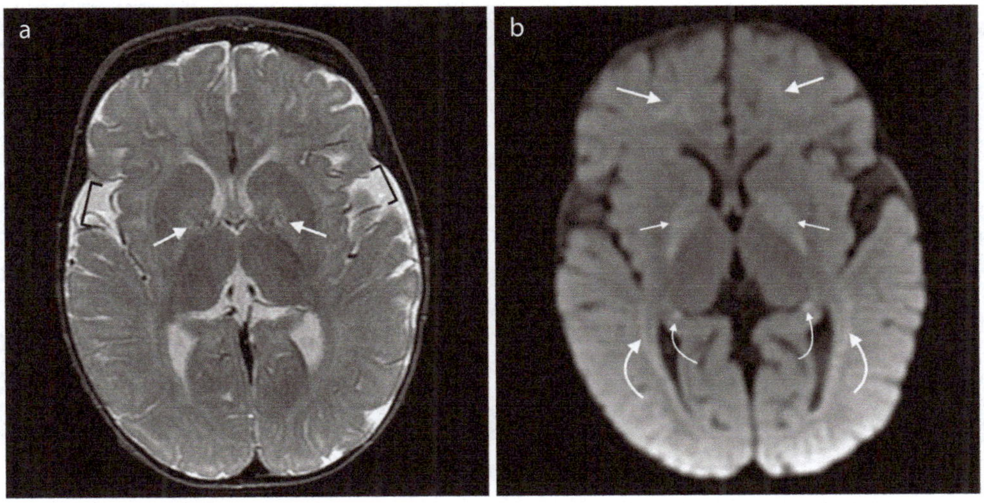


**Fig. 8.4** A 9-month-old female with glutaric aciduria type I. (**a**) Axial T2WI (TR/TE msec, 3200/90) through the basal ganglia reveals hyperintense signal in the globi pallidi (arrows) and underopercularization (brackets). (**b**) The corresponding axial diffusion-weighted image (TR/TE msec, 10,000/91) shows hyperintense signal in the globi pallidi (small straight arrows), frontal subcortical white matter (large straight arrows), sagittal stratum (large curved arrows), and hippocampal tails (small curved arrows) representing reduced diffusion/white matter intramyelinic edema and seizure-related changes in the hippocampi

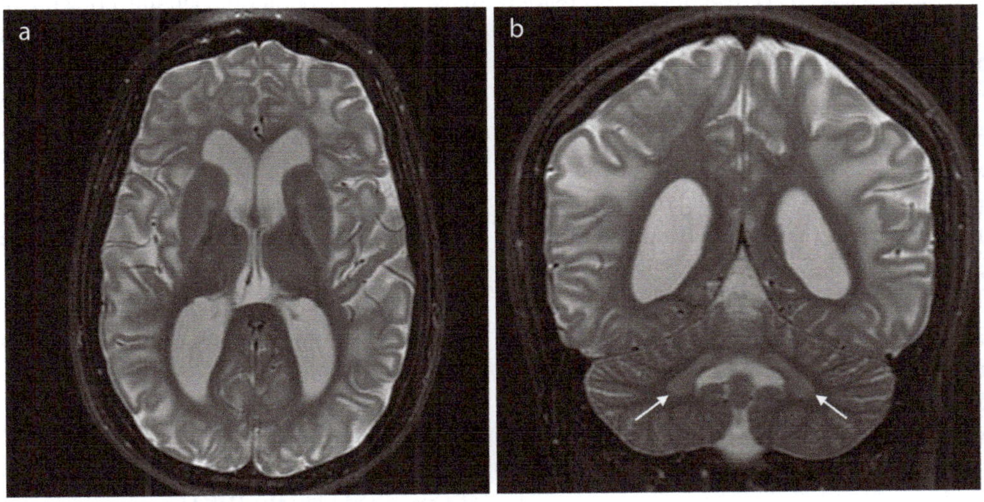


**Fig. 8.5** A 2-year-old female with L-2-hydroxyglutaric aciduria. (**a**) Axial T2WI (TR/TE msec, 5347/101) at level of the basal ganglia shows a centropedal pattern of white matter hyperintensity affecting the superficial more than deep white matter with relative sparing of the corpus callosum. (**b**) Coronal T2WI (TR/TE msec, 5347/101) redemonstrates the centropedal pattern of white matter hyperintensity and shows abnormal hyperintensity of the cerebral deep gray nuclei (arrows). Ventriculomegaly reflects white matter volume loss

(Barkovich and Patay 2019; Gunz et al. 2013; Takanashi et al. 2003; Bireley et al. 2012) (Fig. 8.6). An unsolicited imaging diagnosis can be tricky as UCD disease patterns overlap considerably with that of the far more common hypoxic ischemic encephalopathy (HIE) (Whitehead and Gropman 2018; Pacheco-Colon et al. 2013).

UCD brain edema is often mixed; vasogenic (facilitated diffusion), cytotoxic (gray matter, restricted diffusion), and/or intramyelinic (white matter, restricted diffusion) edema may be present depending on the imaging timing and disease activity. Diffusion abnormalities evolve quickly toward hyperintense signal on T1WI, representing laminar, deep gray, and white matter necrosis with associated volume loss. In all but the most severe cases, the thalami and brainstem are spared, which may help distinguish it from HIE (Whitehead and Gropman 2018; Barkovich and Patay 2019; Pacheco-Colon et al. 2013; Bireley et al. 2012). Also, a peri-insular and cingulate predilection can be a clue, but these structures may also be involved in HIE as well (Whitehead and Gropman 2018; Barkovich and Patay 2019). In distal UCD subtypes, later onset cases, and/or milder phenotypes, brain lesions and volume deficits tend to be less severe and

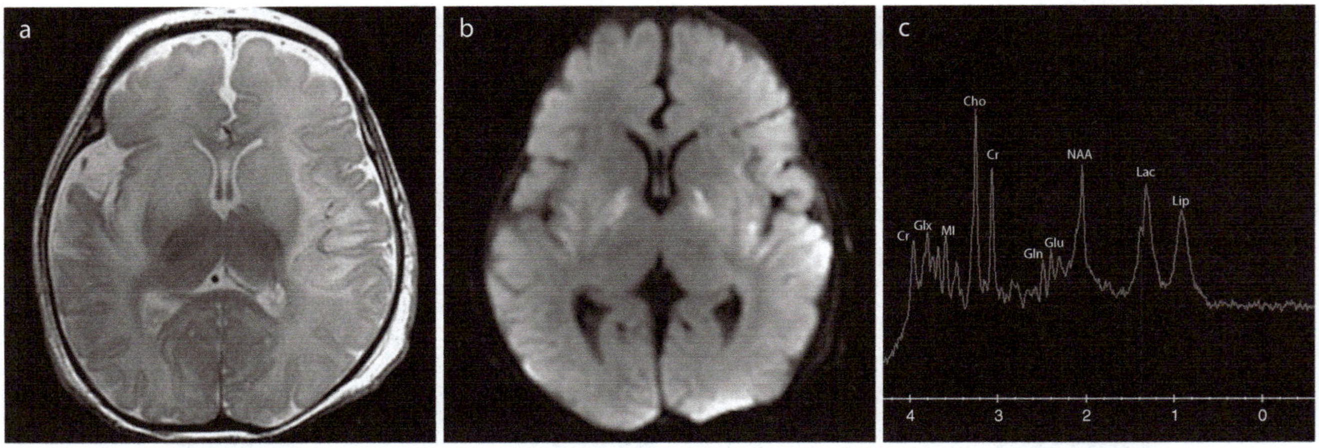


**Fig. 8.6** A 10-day-old male with citrullinemia (argininosuccinate synthetase deficiency). (**a**) Axial T2WI (TR/TE msec, 5725/78) at the level of the basal ganglia shows cortical/subcortical temporo-insular/perisylvian predominant and striatal hyperintensity consistent with edema; note thalamic sparing. The corresponding DWI (TR/TE msec, 10,000/95) (**b**) shows reduced diffusion in the same regions representing cytotoxic and intramyelinic edema. Short echo single voxel MRS over the left basal ganglia (TR/TE msec, 1500/35) (**c**) shows elevated glutamine (Gln), glutamate (Glu), lipids (Lip), and lactate (Lac) with reduced myoinositol (MI). Elevated alpha proton-associated metabolic peak at 1.8 ppm confirms glutamine and glutamate elevation (Glx)

less extensive. In these cases, DTI can reveal decreased microstructural integrity in otherwise normal appearing white matter (Pacheco-Colon et al. 2013; Gropman et al. 2008a, b).

1H MRS can reveal elevated brain glutamine and glutamate in presymptomatic, symptomatic, convalescent, and asymptomatic phases (Pacheco-Colon et al. 2013; Gropman et al. 2008a, b) (Fig. 8.6). Myoinositol, an osmotic buffer, is typically depressed prior to and is inversely correlated with glutamine concentration (Pacheco-Colon et al. 2013; Gropman et al. 2008a, b). Accumulated guanidinoacetate has been shown in arginosuccinate lyase deficiency (Sijens et al. 2006). Arginine elevation has been described in arginase deficiency (Gungor et al. 2008).

## Molybdenum Cofactor Deficiency

A devastating neonatal IEM, molybdenum cofactor deficiency results in massive destructive changes throughout the cerebral white matter and deep gray structures with progression to cystic necrosis and marked volume loss (Whitehead and Gropman 2018; Barkovich and Patay 2019; Schuierer et al. 1995; Stence et al. 2013) (Fig. 8.7). Lesional hemorrhages and deep gray nuclear and/or cerebral white matter calcifications may also be present. Widespread cortical restricted diffusion has also been described, especially affecting sulcal depths and leading to ulegyria (Stence et al. 2013). Changes can mimic HIE, but the pattern is less typical, often sparing the thalami, and destruction more severe in the majority of cases. Mixed aged lesions, pontocerebellar hypoplasia, and enlarged cisterna magna are additional features that favor molybdenum cofactor deficiency over HIE. Disease onset can be either pre- or postnatal; cystic necrosis encountered in the first week of life is most indicative of a prenatal onset. MRS may show elevated lipid and lactate in the active phase of disease (Salvan et al. 1999).

## Chronic Metabolic Encephalopathies

**Several of the IEMs do not typically present initially with an acute decompensation, but rather with ongoing brain injury in recognizable patterns. These are discussed below.**

## Phenylketonuria (PKU)

Phenylketonuria, an autosomal recessive condition, is characterized by deficiency in phenylalanine hydroxylase, an essential precursor to an array of neurotransmitters, notably dopamine which is critically involved in higher order cognition. The majority of patients have extensive white matter damage, in both untreated and early treated PKU cases. Classic MR imaging features include posterior predominant cerebral periventricular hyperintensity on T2WI with or without reduced diffusion, usually sparing the juxtacortical white matter, cortex, brainstem, and cerebellum (Whitehead and Gropman 2018; Anderson and Leuzzi 2010; Kono et al. 2005) (Fig. 8.8). White matter diffusion restriction reflecting intramyelinic edema tends to occur when plasma phenylalanine levels exceed 8.5 mg/dL (Kono et al. 2005).

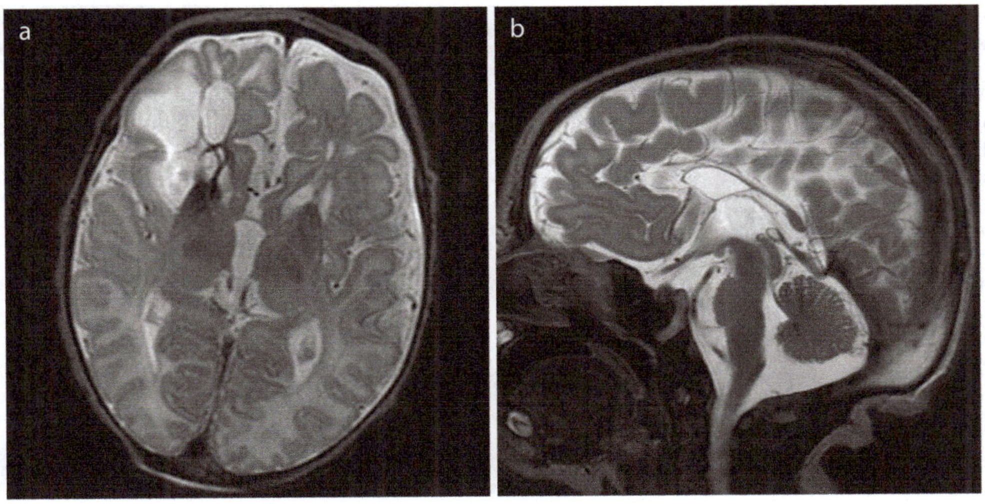


**Fig. 8.7** A 3-day-old female with molybdenum cofactor deficiency. (**a**) Axial T2WI (TR/TE msec, 3500/126) at the level of the basal ganglia demonstrates frontal volume loss and heterogenous, mixed hyperintense and hypointense signal in the basal ganglia and frontal white matter, right more than left, consistent with chronic sequela of prior hemorrhages and infarctions with resultant cystic/necrotic encephalomalacia. (**b**) Sagittal midline T2WI (TR/TE msec, 3500/126) shows marked thinning of the corpus callosum most pronounced anteriorly reflecting the cerebral white matter volume loss

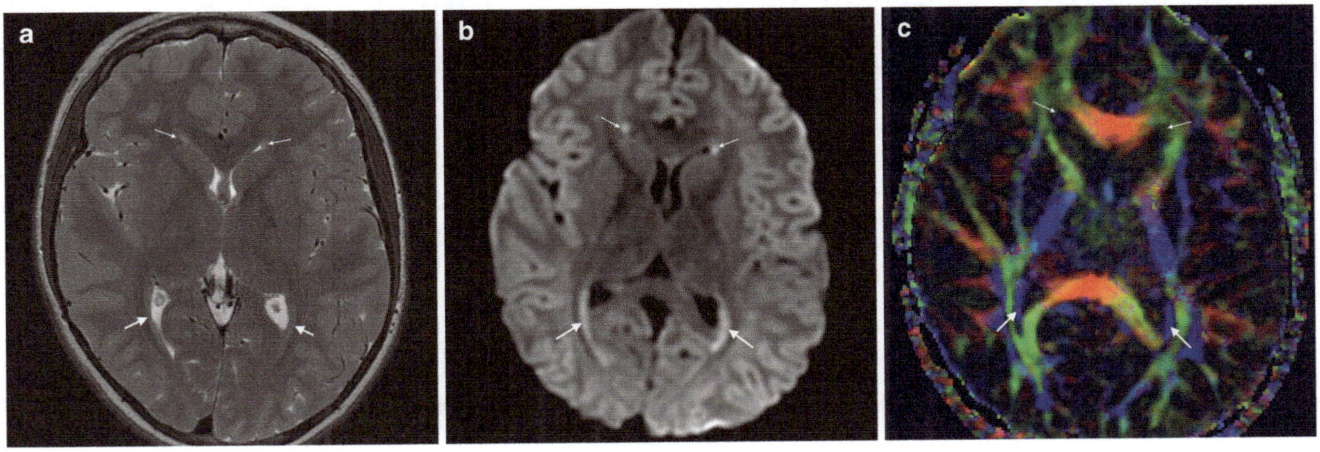


**Fig. 8.8** A 9-year-old male with phenylketonuria (PKU). Axial T2WI (TR/TE msec, 3350/102) (**a**) and corresponding DWI (TR/TE msec, 10,000/82) (**b**) at the level of the basal ganglia show hyperintense signal in the paraventricular frontal and temporo-occipital tissues; in correlation with the directionally encoded DTI color map (**c**), the signal changes correspond to myelin edema in the frontal subependymal white matter fibers (small arrows) and temporo-occipital tapetum (large arrows), typical sites of PKU-associated intramyelinic edema

1H MRS in isolation or in combination with MRI is specific to the diagnosis when correctly performed using a specialized short-echo sequence and postprocessing to identify the generally small phenylalanine peak at 7.3–7.4 ppm downstream beyond the suppressed water peak (Bluml and Panigrahy 2013). The alpha proton associated with elevated phenylalanine can be seen at 3.8 ppm; however, there is considerable overlap with other metabolites at this same location (Sener 2003). NAA, creatine, choline, and other conventional metabolites tend to be normal.

## Pantothenate Kinase-Associated Neurodegeneration (PKAN)

A form of neurodegeneration with brain iron accumulation (NBAI), PKAN is classically known for its "eye of the tiger sign" on MRI (Fig. 8.9). Dark iron deposition in the globus pallidus and bright central necrosis contribute to this appearance. Accelerated iron deposition is also common in the substantia nigra, while the dentate nucleus is rarely affected (Hayflick et al. 2018). These features help distinguish PKAN

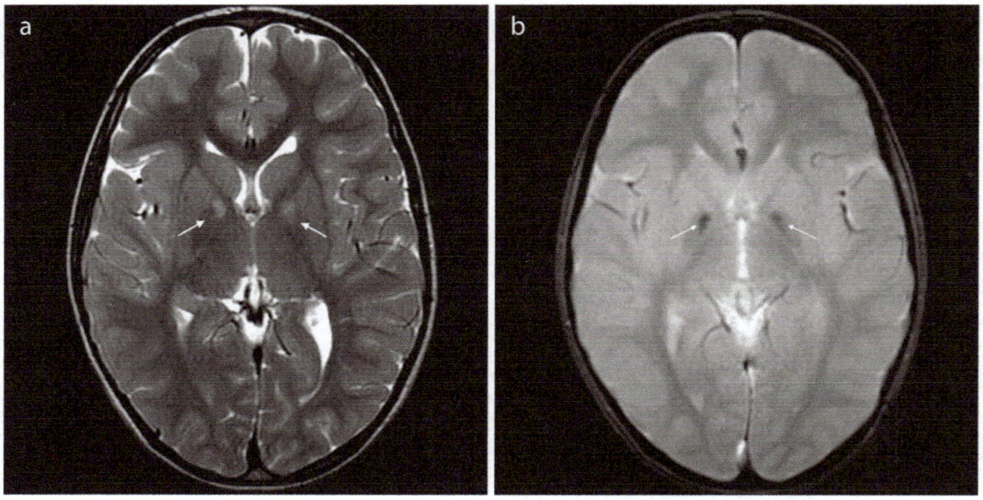


**Fig. 8.9** A 5-year-old male with pantothenate kinase-associated neurodegeneration (PKAN). Axial T2WI (TR/TE msec, 6350/97) (**a**) through the basal ganglia shows globi pallidi signal abnormality with peripheral hypointensity and central hyperintensity representing accelerated iron deposition and central necrosis, the "eye of the tiger" sign of PKAN (arrows). The corresponding axial gradient echo sequence (**b**) confirms increased iron deposits with dark susceptibility effect (arrows)

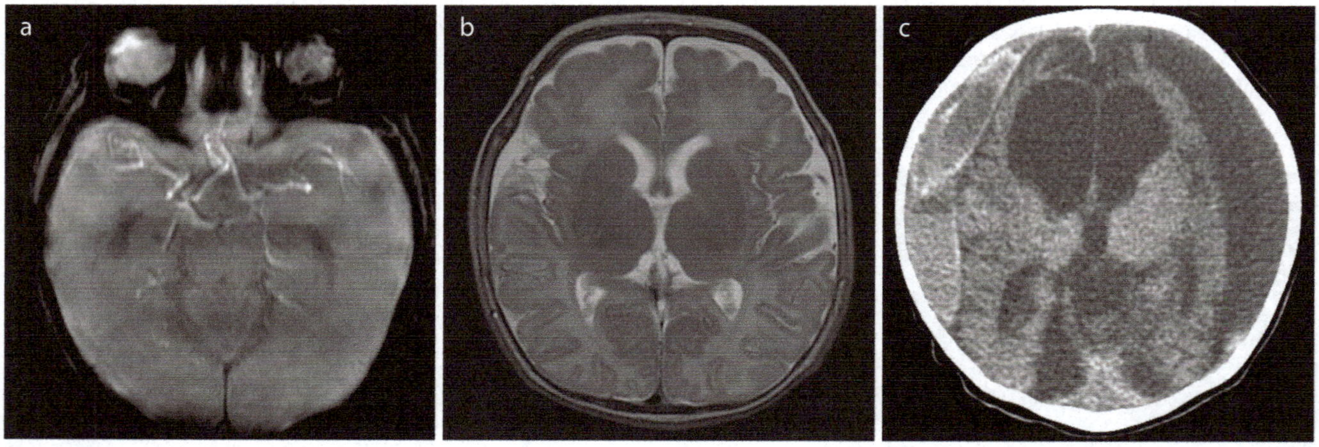


**Fig. 8.10** Menkes disease in a male child performed at 3 months (**a, b**) and 12 years (**c**) of age. (**a**) Axial susceptibility weighted angiography (SWAN; TR/TE msec, 68/24) at the level of the circle of Willis shows multiple tortuous, elongated intracranial arteries. (**b**) Axial T2WI (TR/TE msec, 5900/91) of the cerebrum at the level of the basal ganglia is normal for age. (**c**) Follow-up head CT at age 12 years reveals interval development of bilateral subdural hemorrhages of varying age, marked parenchymal atrophy, and bilateral cerebral encephalomalacia

from other forms of NBAI, such as infantile neuroaxonal dystrophy that lacks "eye of the tiger sign," beta-propellar protein-associated neurodegeneration (BPAN) with dominant subtantia nigra involvement showing a hyperintense "halo", and neuroferritonopathy and aceruloplasminemia where iron deposition is more widespread to name a few (Hayflick et al. 2018).

## Menkes Disease

Deficient tissue copper results in various vascular and brain abnormalities. Elongated, tortuous intracranial arteries have a disorganized, spaghetti-like appearance (Whitehead et al. 2015; Manara et al. 2017a, b) (Fig. 8.10). Cerebral white matter disease with delayed myelination and basal ganglia lesions are characteristic (Manara et al. 2017a, b). Transient tumefactive temporal lobe vasogenic edema is reasonably common in the infantile period (Whitehead et al. 2015). Progressive volume loss and subdural hemorrhages are frequent features in the chronic disease stage (Manara et al. 2017a, b) (Fig. 8.10). MRS reveals lactate, reduced NAA, and/or increased choline in some cases (Ito et al. 2011; Munakata et al. 2005).

## Congenital Disorders of Glycosylation (CDG)

Reduced brain volume and variable signal changes are common in CDG. There are now over 30 subtypes of CDG. The prototypical subtype, CDG Type Ia, commonly shows pontocerebellar hypoplasia and superimposed cerebellar volume loss with cortical hyperintensity, referred to as the "shrunken, bright cerebellar sign" (Whitehead et al.

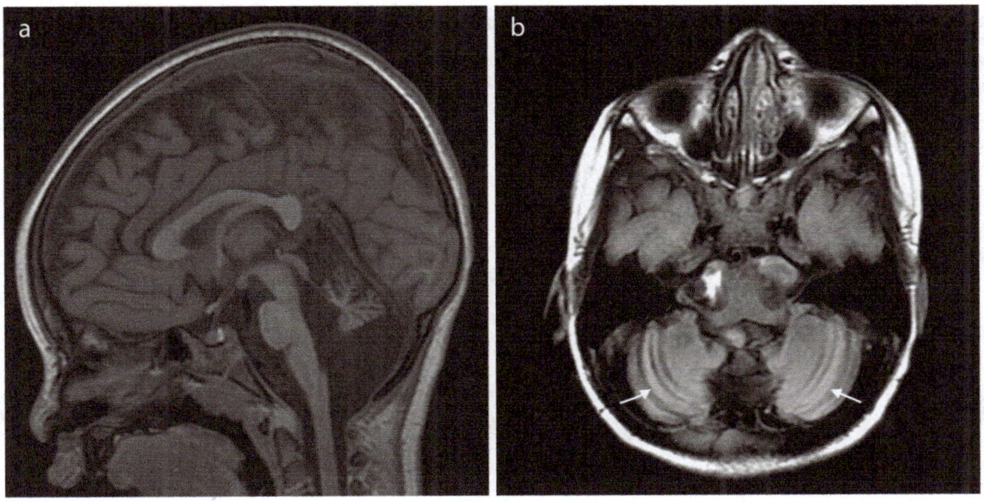


**Fig. 8.11** A 3-year-old male with congenital disorder of glycosylation type Ia. (**a**) Sagittal midline T1WI (TR/TE msec, 11/5) shows a markedly small cerebellum that is shortened with widened fissures representing combined volume loss and hypoplasia. Mild pontine hypoplasia is also present. The fourth ventricle and posterior fossa cisterna spaces are enlarged secondary to the rhombencephalic volume deficit. (**b**) Axial T2 FLAIR image (TR/TE/TI msec, 10,000/126/2250) through the cerebellum shows volume loss and cortical hyperintensity, the "shrunken, bright cerebellar sign" consistent with CDGIa (arrows)

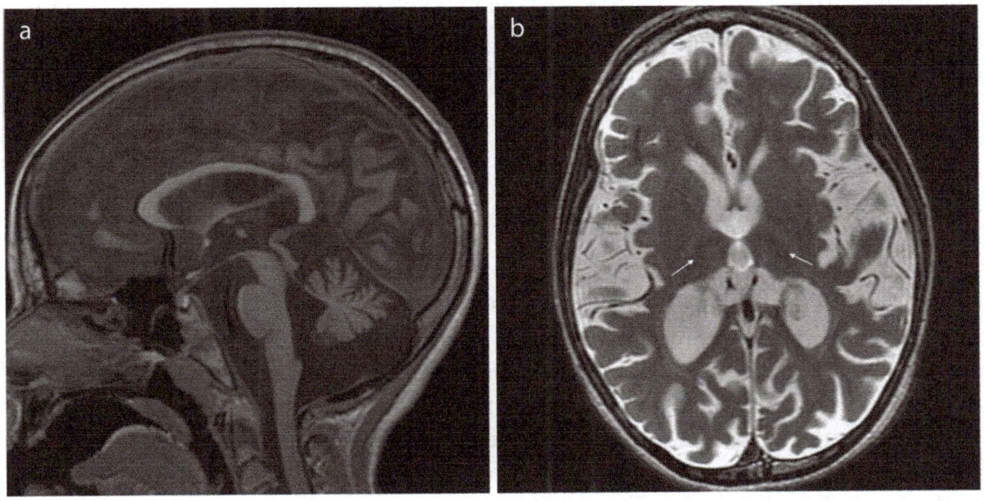


**Fig. 8.12** A 5-year-old female with neuronal ceroid lipofuscinosis. (**a**) Sagittal midline T1WI (TR/TE msec, 11/5) demonstrates diffuse moderate cerebral and cerebellar cortical volume loss with enlarged sulci, cerebellar fissures, and cisternal spaces. (**b**) Axial T2WI (TR/TE msec, 4250/97) also shows the moderate diffuse gray matter predominate cerebral volume loss and relative hypointensity of the thalami (arrows)

2015; Feraco et al. 2012) (Fig. 8.11). Vasculopathy and/or hemorrhages may occur at some point in the disease course, occasionally as the presenting symptom (Stefanits et al. 2014; Cohn et al. 2006). MRS shows decreased NAA, decreased choline, increased myoinositol, and/or increased glutamine and glutamate (Takeuchi et al. 2003; Holzbach et al. 1995).

## Neuronal Ceroid Lipofuscinosis (NCL)

This group of neurodegenerative disorders causes progressive cerebral and cerebellar cortical gray matter brain volume loss and white matter signal alteration (Whitehead and Gropman 2018) (Fig. 8.12). As with other lysosomal storage disorders, thalamic hypointensity is also common, but an often overlooked feature (Autti et al. 2007). NAA may be decreased in keeping with neuronal loss (Bluml and Panigrahy 2013; Whitehead and Gropman 2018).

## Mucopolysacharidoses (MPS)

Concurrent brain and bone abnormalities are key diagnostic features in MPS. Leukoencephalopathy with enlarged perivascular spaces is the most common brain manifestations (Barkovich and Patay 2019; Whitehead et al. 2015; Zafeiriou and Batzios 2013) (Fig. 8.13). Hydrocephalus is another frequent disease attribute. Dysostosis multiplex is found in the spine, commonly with craniocervical junction abnormalities

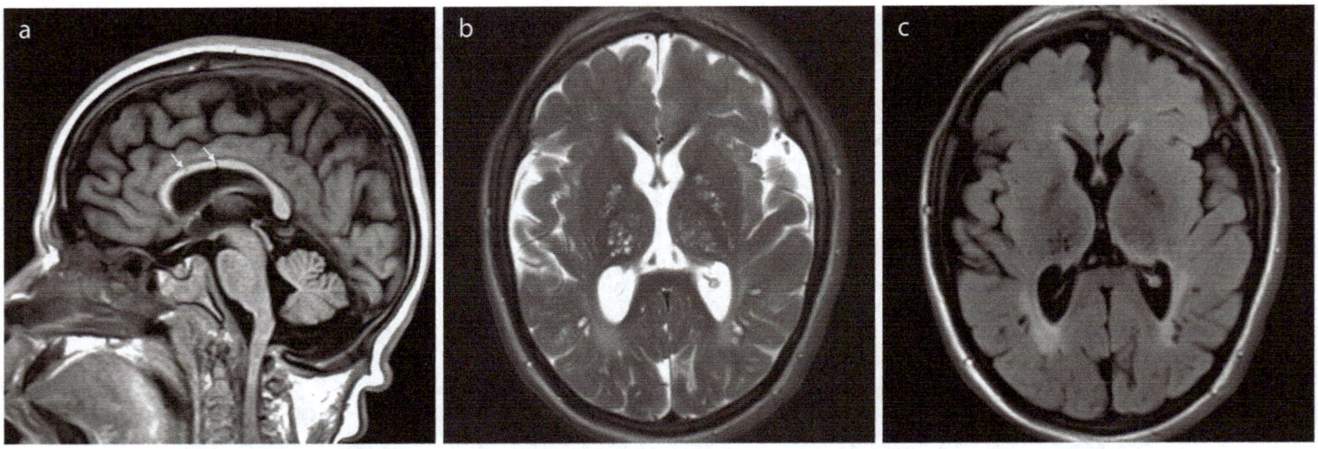


**Fig. 8.13** A 19-year-old male with mucopolysacharidosis (Hunter syndrome). (**a**) Sagittal midline T1WI (TR/TE msec, 15/7) demonstrates skullbase and spinal hypopoplasia/dysplasia with underdevelopment of the clivus, dysmorphic cervical vertebrae, and spinal/foramen magnum stenosis. The callosal genu and body are thin with small foci of hypointensity representing perivascular space enlargement (arrows). Hazy hypointense signal in the brainstem represents enlarged perivascular spaces. Axial T2WI (TR/TE msec, 3500/120) (**b**) and T2/FLAIR sequence (TR/TE/TI msec, 8000/82/2200) (**c**) reveal multiple prominent perivascular spaces in the white and deep gray matter (T2 hyperintense, FLAIR hypointense) on the background of FLAIR hyperintense white matter signal

and skull base dysplasia (Whitehead et al. 2015; Zafeiriou and Batzios 2013) (Fig. 8.13). MRS may demonstrate elevated myoinositol, increased glutamate, increased or decreased choline, decreased NAA, and/or abnormal lactate (Zafeiriou and Batzios 2013).

## Mitochondrial Disorders

**The mitochondrial respiratory chain disorders have a multisystem presentation and genetic origin. The combination of any symptom, organ or tissues, compounded with any age of presentation accounts for the challenge in diagnosing these conditions. From a neuroimaging standpoint, there are several hallmark features that when taken together with the clinical history should alert one to the possibility of these conditions. The more common disorders with characteristic imaging features are discussed below.**

## Leigh Disease

Leigh disease may be caused by a mitochondrial defect in a nuclear or mitochondrial gene and may have multiple organ system involvement. The most common presentation is the early infancy onset associated with severe neurodegeneration with encephalopathy, seizures, blindness, and progressive psychomotor regression typically resulting in death within 2–3 years, usually due to respiratory failure (Thorburn et al. 2003). MRI results in a distinctive brain disease characterized by variable signal changes in the basal ganglia, thalami, brainstem, and/or cerebellum with restricted diffusion ultimately evolving to combination of gliosis and necrosis (Whitehead and Gropman 2018; Whitehead et al. 2016) (Fig. 8.14). Arterial spin-labeling (ASL) perfusion sequence can show hyperperfusion in regions of active brain disease that may correspond to small vessel proliferation described on pathology (Whitehead et al. 2016) (Fig. 8.14). $^{1}$H MRS demonstrates elevated lactate in many cases; however, its absence does not exclude the disease.

## MELAS Syndrome

Mitochondrial encephalopathy with lactate acidosis and stroke-like episodes (MELAS) syndrome is typically of childhood onset characterized by stroke-like episodes, migraine, hearing loss, diabetes, and seizures. In those patients that survive into the late teens and early twenties, a severe gastroparesis is seen (Gagliardi et al. 2019). Characteristic brain lesions involve overlapping large vascular territories that help distinguish it from a non-metabolic thromboembolic infarction (Whitehead and Gropman 2018) (Fig. 8.15). Posterior predominant cortical and subcortical disease is typical, with progressive atrophy. The "black toenail sign" corresponding to gyral necrosis is a common neuroimaging finding associated with cerebral lesions of sufficient severity and chronicity (Whitehead et al. 2017a) (Fig. 8.15). Abnormal T2 FLAIR hyperintensity in and along cortical veins may predict disease severity and future development of brain lesions (Whitehead et al. 2017b) (Fig. 8.15). Deep gray nuclear mineralization is often present, though these structures may be spared of significant volume loss and focal lesions unlike in other mitochondrial diseases. MR spectroscopy shows elevated lactate most commonly at times of metabolic decompensation and may show reduced NAA in the setting of neuronal loss.

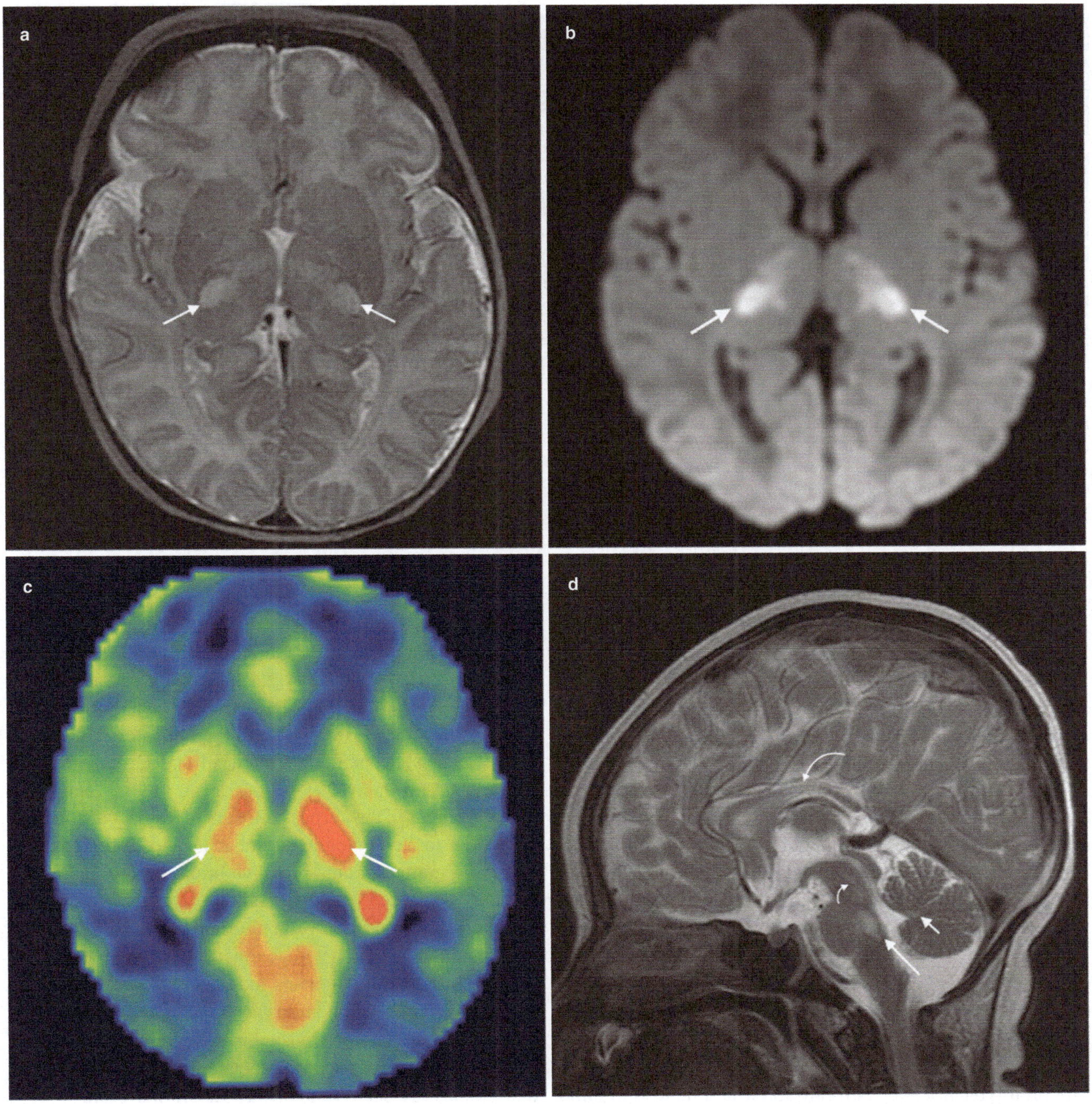


**Fig. 8.14** A 2-month-old female with Leigh disease due to a TRMU gene defect. (**a**) Axial T2WI (TR/TE msec, 3500/120) and (**b**) diffusion weighted image (TR/TE msec, 8000/85) at the level of the basal ganglia demonstrate T2 prolongation and reduced diffusion in the thalami (arrows). (**c**) The corresponding arterial spin labeling (ASL) perfusion sequence shows thalamic hyperperfusion (arrows). (**d**) Sagittal midline T2WI (TR/TE msec, 3500/156) shows hyperintense lesions in the callosal body (long curved arrow), midbrain tegmentum (short curved arrow) pontine tegmentum (long straight arrow), and central vermis (short straight arrow). There is mild pontine hypoplasia and thinning of the corpus callosum

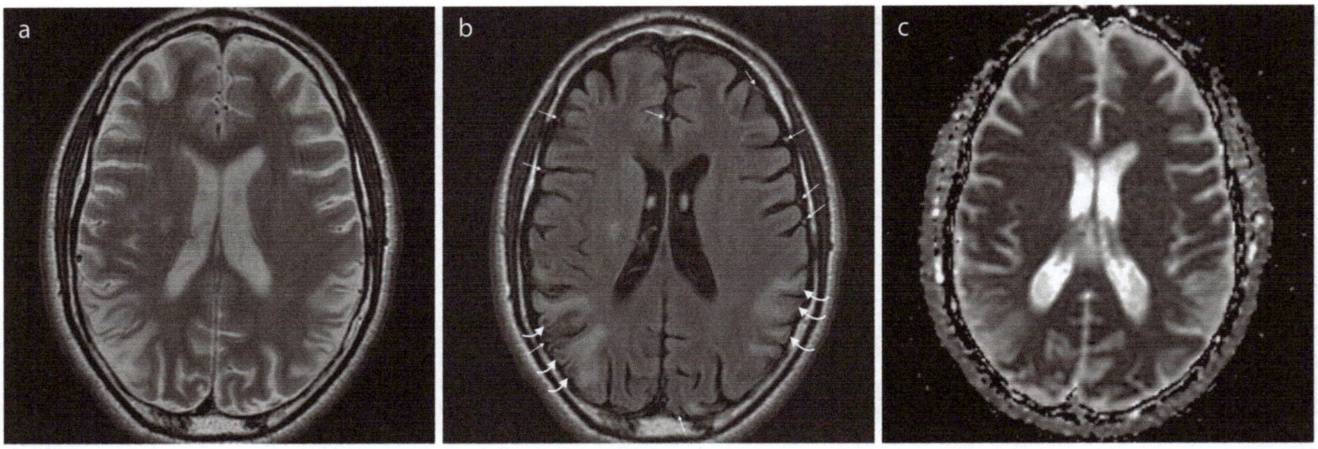


Fig. 8.15 A 19-year-old male with MELAS. Axial T2WI (TR/TE msec, 3543/98) (**a**), T2 FLAIR (TR/TE/TI msec, 10,000/124/2200) (**b**), and apparent diffusion coefficient map (TR/TE msec, 10,000/95) (**c**) at the level of the lateral ventricles show bilateral parieto-occipital cortical/subcortical hyperintensity not confined to large arterial territories with partial signal suppression superficially consistent with necrosis and the "black toenail" sign compatible with chronic MELAS-related brain injury (curved arrows, **b**). Note several cortical veins show FLAIR hyperintensity that may represent venopathy (straight arrows, **b**)

## White Matter Disorders/Leukodystrophies

**Leukodystrophy is one of a group of disorders characterized by degeneration of the white matter in the brain. Many are of genetic etiology due to IEMs (van der Knaap and Bugiani** 2017**). Leukodystrophies are often degenerative in nature, but some only impair white matter function. The clinical course may be static or progressive, but may also improve with time. Progressive leukodystrophies are often fatal. There has been a large increase in the number of genetically defined leukodystrophies in recent years due to recognition of magnetic resonance imaging patterns coupled with next-generation and whole exome sequencing (van der Knaap and Bugiani** 2017**).**

## X-linked Adrenoleukodystrophy (X-ALD)

The prototypical leukodystrophy for which there is significant MRI literature is X-ALD. The three recognizable clinical phenotypes are childhood cerebral disease, adrenomyeloneuropathy (AMN), and Addison disease. AMN manifests most commonly in an individual in his twenties or middle age with progressive lower extremity spastic weakness, sphincter disturbances, sexual dysfunction, and, often, impaired adrenocortical function. Addison disease only presents with primary adrenocortical insufficiency between age 2 years and adulthood and most commonly by age 7.5 years, usually without neurologic abnormality (Raymond et al. 1999). All are associated with elevation of very long chain fatty acids due to a mutation in the ABCD1 gene, which encodes for a peroxisomal very long chain fatty acid transporter.

The callosal splenium is usually the earliest and most commonly affected part of the brain in X-ALD (Barkovich and Patay 2019) (Fig. 8.16). Lesions quickly spread to the forceps major and, in worse cases, involve the projectional white matter fibers extending into the brainstem along with other brain white matter (Whitehead and Gropman 2018; Barkovich and Patay 2019; Loes et al. 1994). Laminated signal changes in the corpus callosum and adjacent commissural fibers are common in the subacute and chronic phases, reflecting multiple bouts of active brain disease and representing combined edema, inflammatory changes, and destructive changes (demyelination and necrosis). Therefore, the signal intensity is heterogenous and variable, often with mixed restricted diffusion and facilitated diffusion and variable contrast enhancement in the areas of active inflammation. Corticospinal tracts, visual, and auditory pathways are often involved. Loes score associated with lesion location and extent has been validated to determine brain disease severity and transplant candidacy (Loes et al. 1994). MRS is nonspecific, often depicting lactate, increased lipids, decreased NAA, and elevated choline (Bluml and Panigrahy 2013). However, an NAA:Cho less than 5 has been shown to predict clinical decline (Barkovich and Patay 2019).

## Zellweger Syndrome

Another peroxisomal-based disorder, Zellweger syndrome is a severe IEM with multisystemic manifestations. From a neurological standpoint, there is both gray and white matter

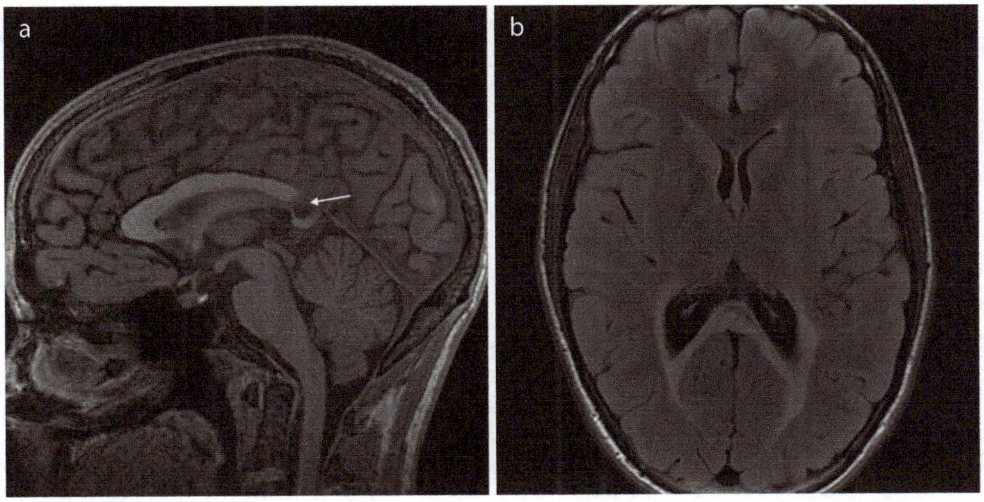


**Fig. 8.16** A 16-year-old male with X-linked adrenoleukodystrophy. (**a**) Sagittal midline T1WI (TR/TE msec, 8/3) demonstrates marked hypointensity within a mildly thinned callosal splenium (arrow). (**b**) Axial T2/FLAIR (TR/TE/TI msec, 10,000/144/2250) shows signal abnormality in the callosal splenium and forceps major with partial signal suppression in the splenium representing chronic demyelination/gliosis and necrosis

involvement. Neuroimaging findings are typified by cerebral polymicrogyria, often perisylvian predominant, caudothalamic groove germinolytic cysts, and white matter hyperintensity on T2WI (Whitehead et al. 2015) (Fig. 8.17). Germinolytic cysts carry a differential diagnosis of prior germinal matrix hemorrhage, TORCH infection, genetic, and toxic/metabolic disturbances (Herini et al. 2003). Significant hydrocephalus is unusual, unlike in the dystroglycanopathies. MRS can show elevated lipids associated with hepatic disease and decreased NAA (Bluml and Panigrahy 2013).

## Aicardi-Goutieres Syndrome (AGS)

Imaging manifestations in AGS are typified by leukoencephalopathy (diffuse or displaying an anteroposterior severity gradient), frontotemporal white matter rarefaction, reduced brain volume, and, importantly, parenchymal calcifications collectively overlapping with the appearance of some TORCH infections (La Piana et al. 2016; Vanderver et al. 2015) (Fig. 8.18). Brain malformations may include dysgenesis of the corpus callosum and/or cerebellar hypoplasia; however, malformations of cortical development are typically absent unlike in many cases of congenital CMV. Calcifications, a cornerstone feature, are generally detectable using certain gradient echo sequences; however, CT is more sensitive and may be required if the diagnosis is suspected, but no calcifications are found using MRI (La Piana et al. 2016). Central spinal cord signal hyperintensity has been described (Samanta and Ramakrishnaiah 2019). 1H MRS demonstrates reduced NAA and elevated MI (Robertson et al. 2004).

## Krabbe Disease

There are two main age-specific neuroimaging manifestations of Krabbe disease. In the infantile period, dentate hilar and basal ganglia signal abnormalities are present, whereas in later onset forms, a cerebral leukodystrophy with a posteroanterior (PA) and centrifugal gradient predominates often manifesting a "tigroid" pattern of signal alteration (Whitehead and Gropman 2018; Whitehead et al. 2015) (Fig. 8.19). The cerebral corticospinal tracts are often affected from the corona radiata to the cerebral peduncles. Cauda equina and cranial nerves (especially the optic pathway) may be thickened and show abnormal contrast enhancement. Deep cerebral white and gray matter mineralization is common; CT is useful for confirmation (Whitehead and Gropman 2018; Whitehead et al. 2015). MRS shows variable metabolic changes that may include elevated myo-inositol and/or glutamate, increased or decreased choline, decreased NAA, and/or abnormal lactate (Bluml and Panigrahy 2013; Whitehead and Gropman 2018; Whitehead et al. 2015).

## Metachromatic Leukodystrophy (MLD)

Metachromatic leukodystrophy is an inherited disorder characterized by the accumulation of sulfatides. Sulfatide accumulation in myelin-producing cells causes progressive destruction of white matter throughout the nervous system, including the brain, spinal cord, and peripheral nerves. Imaging features of MLD are similar to Krabbe in

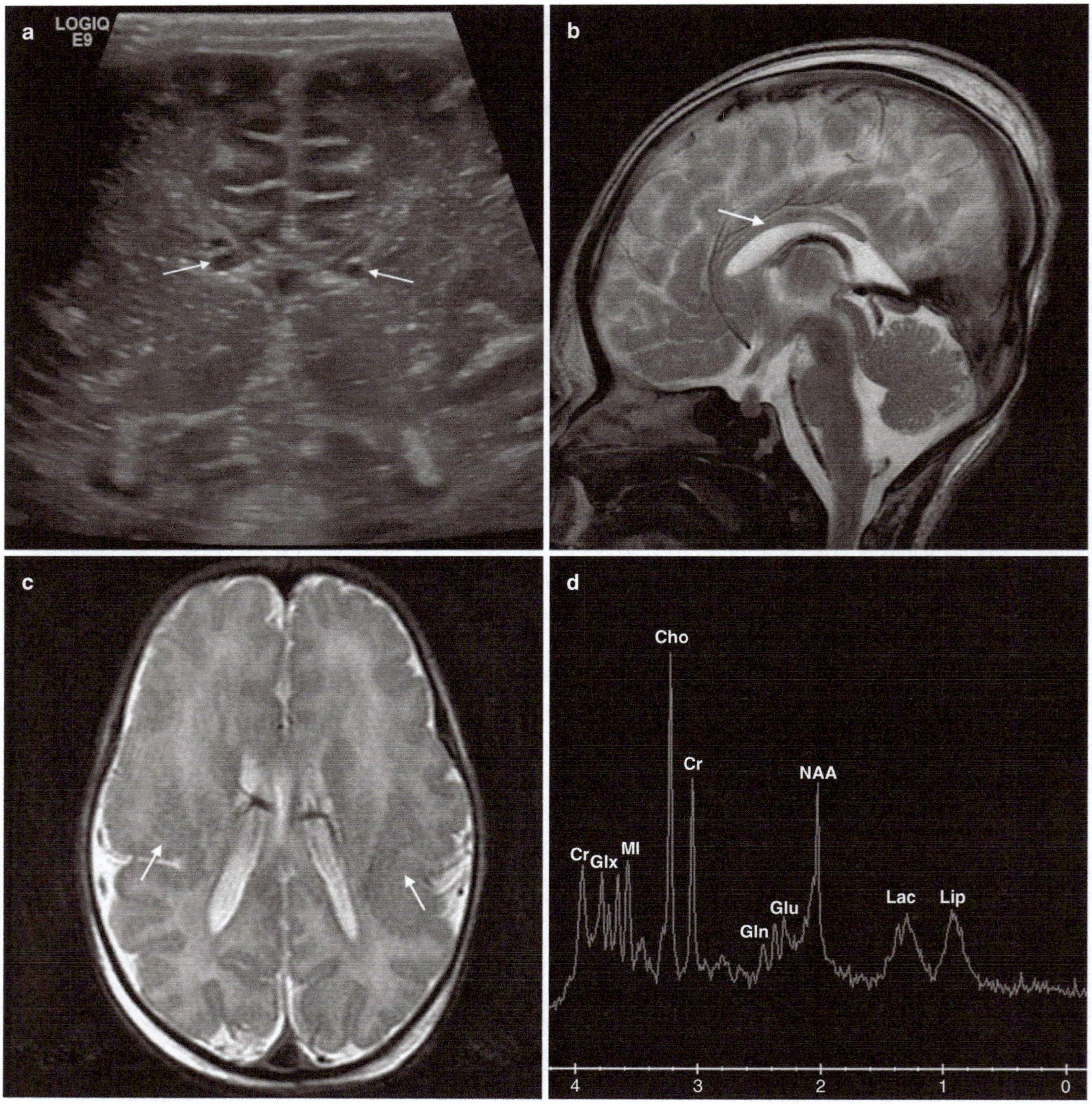


**Fig. 8.17** Neonatal female with Zellweger syndrome. (**a**) Coronal gray-scale head ultrasound shows bilateral caudothalamic groove germinolytic cysts (arrows). (**b**) Sagittal midline T2WI (TR/TE msec, 3500/158) shows mild thinning/dysmorphia of the corpus callosum consistent with hypogenesis/dysgenesis (arrow) and pontine hypoplasia. (**c**) Axial T2WI (TR/TE msec, 3500/120) through the lateral ventricles depicts perisylvian predominant polymicrogyria (arrows). Short echo single voxel MRS over the left basal ganglia (TR/TE msce, 1500/35) (**d**) shows elevated lipids (Lip) and lactate (Lac), increased glutamine (Gln; Glx), and glutamate (Glu; Glx). NAA, Cr, and Cho ratios are borderline but within normal range

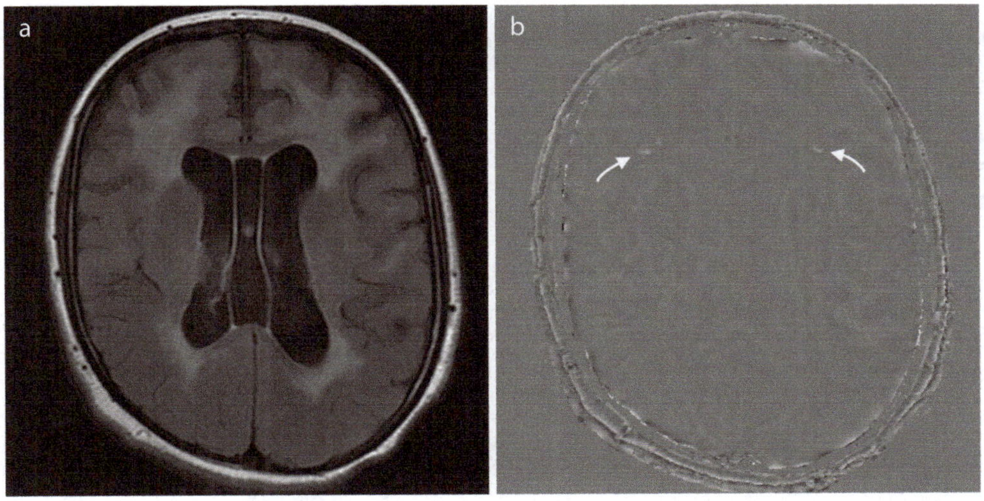


**Fig. 8.18** A 12-year-old female with Aicardi-Goutieres syndrome. (**a**) Axial T2 FLAIR (TR/TE/TI msec, 10,000/149/2200) MR image through the lateral ventricles shows anterior predominant white matter signal hyperintensity and ventriculomegaly reflecting cerebral volume loss. (**b**) The corresponding phase map from a susceptibility weighted sequence (SWAN; TR/TE msec, 38/23) shows bright dystrophic calcifications in the frontal subcortical white matter (arrows)

many ways including the tigroid cerebral white matter pattern, a PA and centrifugal gradient (in children), cranial nerve and cauda equina involvement, and elevated myo-inositol (Whitehead and Gropman 2018) (Fig. 8.20). Dentate nuclei tend to be spared and calcifications are absent, however.

## Canavan Disease

Aspartoacylase deficiency induced dysmyelination in Canavan disease causes diffuse spongiform thickening of the cerebral, cerebellar, and brainstem white matter with resultant macrocephaly in the infant brain (McAdams et al. 1990; Brismar et al. 1990). Neuroimaging shows swelling and widespread hyperintense white matter signal on T2WI often involving the thalami, globus pallidus, and cerebellar deep gray nuclei with relative sparing of the striatum (McAdams et al. 1990; Brismar et al. 1990) (Fig. 8.21). Sometimes the capsules, corpus callosum, and deep cerebellar white matter are also spared with more pronounced subcortical white matter involvement unlike in Krabbe and MLD. The absence of contrast enhancement and presence of restricted diffusion thought to represent water trapping associated with vacuolization helps distinguish Canavan from Alexander disease (Brismar et al. 1990; Sener 2004). Parenchymal volume loss may be present at diagnosis or develop over time; therefore macrocephaly is not universal (Brismar et al. 1990). MRS shows abnormally accumulated/elevated NAA, characteristic to the disease (Bluml and Panigrahy 2013) (Fig. 8.21). Milder juvenile forms of the disease have differing imaging changes including mild or absent leukodystrophy, striatum signal changes, and lack of NAA elevation (Toft et al. 1993; Nguyen and Ishak 2015).

## tRNA Synthetase Disorders

Brain disease in tRNA synthetase disorders includes leukodystrophy, hypomyelination, Leigh-like, and/or MELAS-like patterns with metabolic strokes; lactate may be present on MRS. AARS2, DARS2, and EARS2 are three of the most well-described gene defects with fairly specific imaging manifestations. In AARS2, a deep anterior frontal and posterior parietal leukodystrophy develops, relatively sparing frontoparietal junctional tissue but involving the corticospinal tracts, frontopontine, and parietooccipital pontine fibers (Dallabona et al. 2014). DARS2 genetic abnormalities cause leukoencephalopathy with brainstem and spinal cord involvement and lactate elevation (LBSL); the deep cerebral white matter is involved with or without a PA severity gradient, multiple brainstem white matter tracts are affected (corticospinal, spinocerebellar, medial lemniscus, cerebellar peduncles, and intraparenchymal trigeminal nerve fibers), and spinal cord signal changes are present (Kassem et al. 2014). In EARS2, neuroimaging patterns may include hypomyelination, deep cerebral leukodystrophy with relative periventricular sparing, and Leigh-like involvement of the thalamus, dentate nucleus, and dorsal brainstem (Steenweg et al. 2012).

## Substrate Depletion Disorders

**The more common disorders with substrate depletion are discussed below.**

## Creatine Deficiency Syndromes

The cerebral creatine deficiency syndromes are inborn errors of creatine metabolism that include the creatine biosynthesis disorders, guanidinoacetate methyltransferase (GAMT) defi-

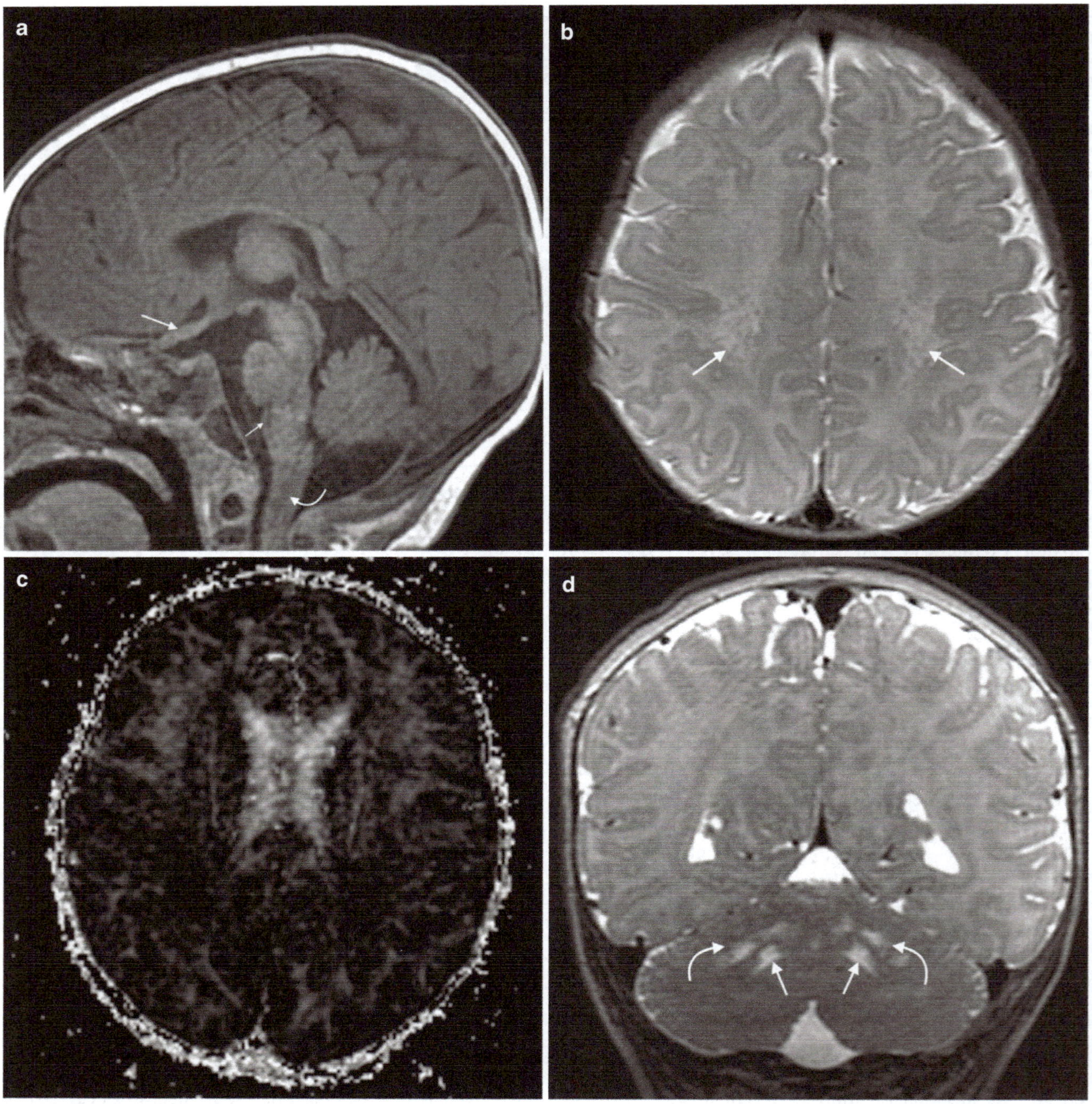


**Fig. 8.19** A 4-month-old male with Krabbe disease. (**a**) Sagittal midline T1WI (TR/TE msec, 8/3) shows thickening of the optic chiasm (large arrow), thickening of the medulla oblongata and hypointensity of the pyramidal tracts (small arrow), and thickening of the upper cervical spinal cord with abnormal hypointense signal (curved arrow). (**b**) Axial T2WI (TR/TE msec, 3500/90) at the level of the corona radiata depicts striated/tigroid deep frontoparietal white matter signal (arrows). (**c**) DTI image (TR/TE msec, 10,000/92) at a slightly lower section of the cerebrum demonstrates a posterior to anterior gradient of diffused anisotropy with hypointense white matter. (**d**) Coronal T2WI (TR/TE msec, 3500/90) through the cerebellum shows abnormally increased signal in the dentate hila (straight arrows) and cerebellar white matter (curved arrows)

ciency, and L-arginine:glycine amidinotransferase (AGAT or GATM) deficiency, as well as the creatine transporter (SLC6A8) deficiency. All three are characterized by clinical presentation including seizures and intellectual disability, although behavioral difficulties such as autism spectrum and an extrapyramidal movement disorder may be seen. Onset is between ages 3 months and 3 years. The phenotype of SLC6A8 deficiency in affected males ranges from mild intellectual disability and speech delay to significant intellectual disability, seizures, and behavioral disorder. GAMT and

AGAT deficiency are autosomal recessive conditions, whereas the transport defect is an X-linked disorder (Gropman 2012). Apart from occasional periventricular white matter signal hyperintensity, structural imaging fails to disclose significant abnormalities. MR spectroscopy is critical for the diagnosis and useful in follow-up by demonstrating reduced concentration of creatine compounds at 3 and 3.9 ppm (Whitehead and Gropman 2018) (Fig. 8.22) (Table 8.1).

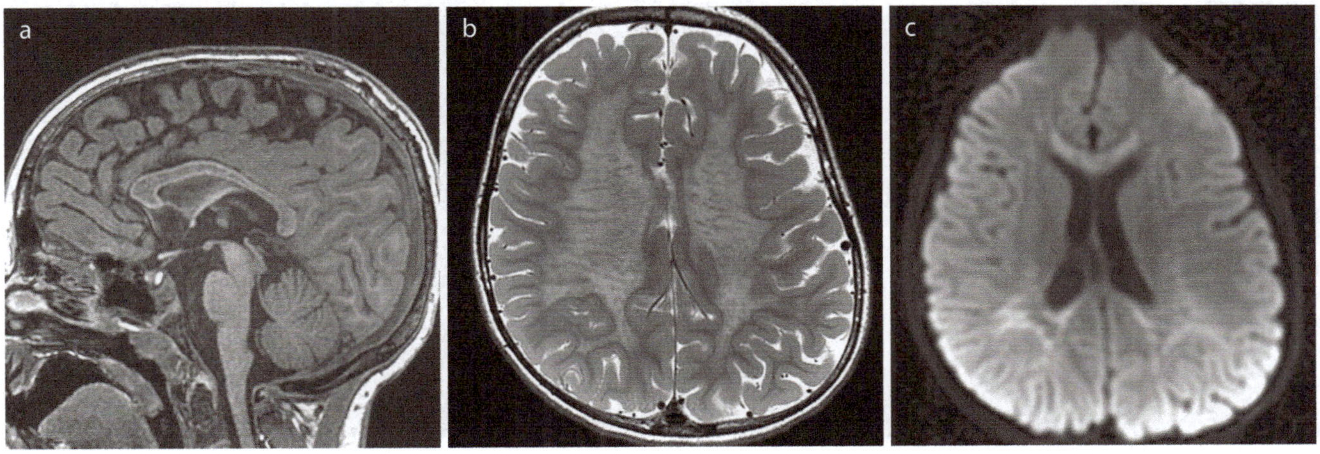


**Fig. 8.20** A 6-year-old female with metachromatic leukodystrophy. (**a**) Sagittal midline T1WI (TR/TE msec, 8/3) demonstrates extensive hypointense signal throughout most of the corpus callosum, sparing peripheral most fibers and some central fibers with a stippled appearance; the posterior fossa structures are normal. (**b**) Axial T2WI (TR/TE msec, 3205/102) at the level of the corona radiata depicts striated/tigroid deep frontoparietal white matter signal. (**c**) Axial diffusion weighted image (TR/TE msec, 10,000/70) at a slightly lower section of the cerebrum demonstrates striated and confluent deep and periventricular white matter reduced diffusion consistent with intramyelinic edema

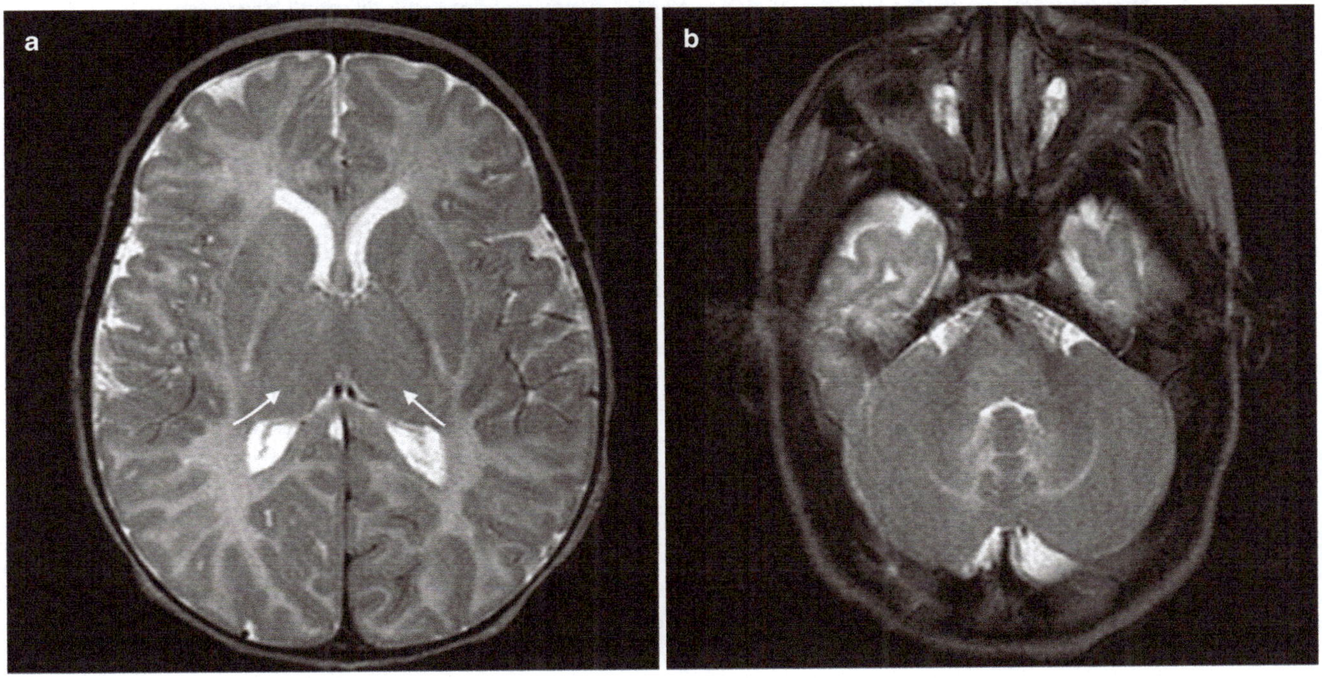


**Fig. 8.21** A 2-month-old female with Canavan disease. Axial T2WI (TR/TE msec, 3500/10) through the basal ganglia (**a**) and cerebellum (**b**) reveals generalized mild cerebral, cerebellar, and brainstem white matter hyperintensity for age and subtle increased signal in the thalami (arrows, **a**). (**c**) Axial diffusion weighted image (TR/TE msec, 7500/61) through the basal ganglia hyperintense signal of the cerebral white matter and thalami representing reduced diffusion/intramyelinic edema; note sparing of the striatum. (**d**) Single voxel MRS over the left basal ganglia (TR/TE msec, 1500/35) shows abnormal NAA elevation (NAA), diagnostic of Canavan disease

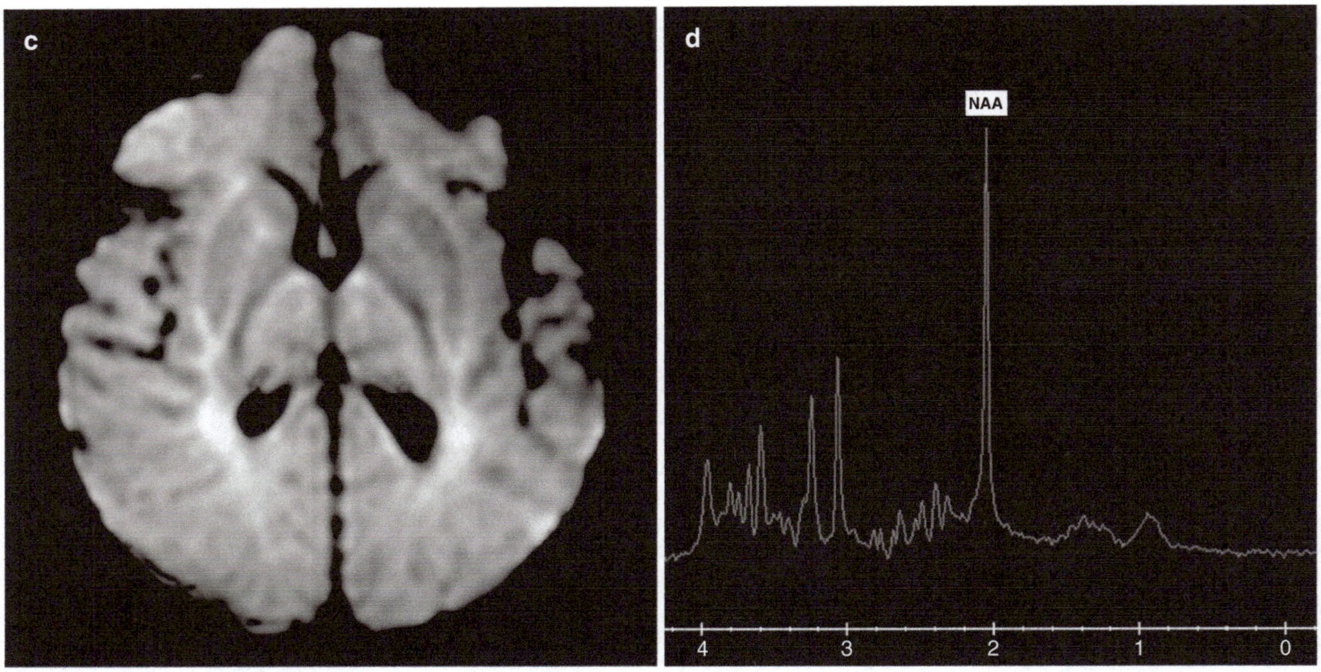


**Fig. 8.21** (continued)

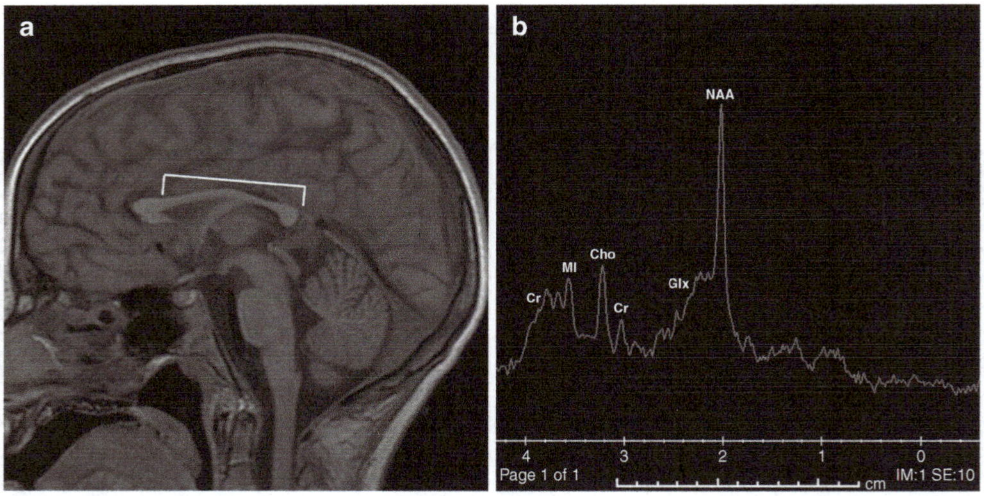


**Fig. 8.22** An 11-year-old male with X-linked creatine transporter deficiency secondary to a SLC6A8 gene defect. (**a**) Sagittal midline T1WI (TR/TE msec, 11/5) shows thinning of the body, isthmus, and genu of the corpus callosum representing mild posterior predominant cerebral white matter volume loss without signal alterations (bracket). (**b**) Single voxel MRS over the left basal ganglia (TR/TE msec, 1500/35) shows marked reduction of creatine compounds (Cr) at 3 and 3.9 ppm; other metabolites including *N*-acetylaspartate (NAA), glutamine and glutamate (Glx), choline (Cho), and myoinositol (MI) are normal

**Table 8.1** This table was constructed after a thorough review of existing medical literature and is arranged consecutively by chapter. Brain/spine MR imaging patterns were compiled based on lesion location within the cerebrum, cerebellum, brainstem, and/or spinal cord, texture (signal changes on different sequences), volume, concurrent malformations, and other manifestations for each disease process. The range of reported brain MRS alterations was also documented. Diseases with normal or nonspecific imaging patterns were excluded. We emphasize that the current medical literature does not accurately reflect the entire imaging spectrum of all metabolic disease phenotypes. Therefore, the information in this table should be considered dynamic and no more than a loose guideline. We hope that this information will be elaborated upon and altered when it becomes necessary to enhance specificity as new data comes to light in the future

| | | | Cerebrum | | | Cerebellum | | | Brainstem | | | | | |
|---|---|---|---|---|---|---|---|---|---|---|---|---|---|---|
| Chapter | Disease | Prevailing pattern(s) | Location | Texture | Volume | Location | Texture | Volume | Location | Texture | Volume | Spinal cord | Malformations and other findings | MRS (ppm) |
| 13.11 | Adenylosuccinate lyase deficiency | Hypomyelination | cortex: n<br>wmsc: + | DWI:?<br>T2: ↑ | ↓-n | cortex: n<br>wmsc: + | DWI:?<br>T2: ↑ | ↓-n | mb: n<br>pons: n | DWI:?<br>T2: ↑ | ↓-n | ? | – | Succinyladenosine (8.3)<br>Succinylaminoimidazole carboxamide riboside (7.5) |
| | | | wmd: +<br>BG: n<br>Thal: n | myelin: ↓<br>Nec: –<br>Ca: –<br>CE:? | | wmd: +<br>DN: n | myelin: ↓<br>Nec: –<br>Ca: –<br>CE:? | | med: + | myelin: ↓<br>Nec: –<br>Ca: –<br>CE:? | | | | |
| 13.14 | Adenosine monophosphate deaminase 2 deficiency | PCH<br>CCD<br>Midbrain "figure of 8" sign | n | n | ↓ | n | n | ↓-↓↓ | n | n | ↓↓-↓↓↓ | ? | ACC, HCC, CCD<br>PCH | ? |
| 13.17 | Adenosine deaminase 2 deficiency | Lacunar infarcts<br>Vasculopathy | cortex: +/–<br>wmsc: +/–<br>wmd: +/– | DWI: +/–<br>T2: ↑-n<br>myelin: n | ↓-n | n | n | n | mb: +/–<br>pons: +/–<br>med: +/– | DWI: +/–<br>T2: ↑-n<br>myelin: n | n | ? | SDH +/–<br>IVH +/–<br>COW stenoses/ occlusions +/– | |
| | | | BG: +/–<br>Thal: +/– | Nec: –<br>Ca: –<br>CE: +/–<br>Hem: +/– | | | | | | Nec: –<br>Ca: –<br>CE: +/– | | | | |
| 14.1–14.11 | Aicardi-Goutières syndrome (ACG) and ACG-like (Shared features) | Calcifications<br>Leukoencephalopathy (diffuse or anteroposterior gradient with frontotemporal white matter rarefaction) | cortex: n<br>wmsc: ++ | DWI: –<br>T2: ↑-↑↑↑ | n-↓↓↓ | cortex: n<br>wmsc: + | DWI: +/–<br>T2: ↑ | n-↓↓↓ | mb: +/–<br>pons: +/– | DWI: +/–<br>T2: ↑ | n-↓↓ | ↑T2 central +/–<br>Patchy enhancement+/– | Cerebellarhypoplasia+/–<br>HCC +/– | NAA ↓<br>MI ↑ |
| | | Atrophy | wmd: ++<br>BG: ++<br>Thal: + | myelin: ↓<br>Nec: +/–<br>Ca: +++<br>CE: – | | wmd: +<br>DN: +/– | myelin: ↓<br>Nec: –<br>Ca: +/–<br>CE: +/– | | med: +/– | myelin: ↓<br>Nec: –<br>Ca: +/–<br>CE: +/– | | | | |
| 15.2 | Guanidinoacetate methyltransferase deficiency (cerebral Cr deficiency syndrome type 2) | MRS: Cr reduction<br>Globus pallidus hyperintensity | cortex: n<br>wmsc: n | DWI: –<br>T2: ↑-n | ↓-n | n | n | n | mb: +/–<br>pons: +/– | DWI: +/–<br>T2: ↑-n | n | ? | – | Cr ↓ to absent<br>Guanadinoacetate (3.8) |
| | | | wmd: n<br>BG: ++<br>Thal: n | myelin: n<br>Nec: –<br>Ca: –<br>CE:? | | | | | med: +/– | myelin: n<br>Nec: –<br>Ca: –<br>CE:? | | | | |
| 15.3 | Creatine transporter deficiency (cerebral Cr deficiency syndrome type 1) | MRS: Cr reduction<br>PVWM hyperintensity | cortex: n<br>wmsc: n<br>wmd: +/–<br>BG: n<br>Thal: n | DWI: –<br>T2: ↑-n<br>myelin: n<br>Nec: –<br>Ca: –<br>CE:? | ↓-n | n | n | n | n | n | n | ? | – | Cr ↓ to absent |

(continued)

**Table 8.1** (continued)

| Chapter | Disease | Prevailing pattern(s) | Cerebrum | | | Cerebellum | | | Brainstem | | | Spinal cord | Malformations and other findings | MRS (ppm) |
|---|---|---|---|---|---|---|---|---|---|---|---|---|---|---|
| | | | Location | Texture | Volume | Location | Texture | Volume | Location | Texture | Volume | | | |
| 17.2 | Carbamoylphosphate synthetase I deficiency | Diffuse cerebral edema/injury | cortex: ++ | DWI: +/– | n-↓↓↓ | n | n | n | n | n | n | ? | – | Glx ↑ |
| | | Central cerebral predominant injury pattern sparing thalami | wmsc: ++ | T2: ↑-↑↑↑ | | | | | | | | | | Lactate |
| | | Metabolic stroke | wmd: ++ | myelin: n | | | | | | | | | | NAA n-↓ |
| | | | BG: ++ | Nec: +/– | | | | | | | | | | |
| | | | Thal: +/– | Ca: – | | | | | | | | | | |
| | | | | CE:? | | | | | | | | | | |
| 17.3 | Ornithine transcarbamylase deficiency | Diffuse cerebral edema/injury | cortex: ++ | DWI: +/– | n-↓↓↓ | n | n | n-↓ | n | n | n | ? | – | Glx ↑ |
| | | Central cerebral predominant injury pattern sparing thalami | wmsc: ++ | T2: ↑-↑↑↑ | | | | | | | | | | Cho ↓ |
| | | Metabolic stroke | wmd: ++ | myelin: n | | | | | | | | | | MI ↓ |
| | | | BG: ++ | Nec: +/– | | | | | | | | | | NAA n-↓ |
| | | | Thal: +/– | Ca: – | | | | | | | | | | |
| | | | | CE: – | | | | | | | | | | |
| 17.4 | Argininosuccinate synthetase deficiency | Central cerebral predominant injury pattern sparing thalami | cortex: ++ | DWI: +/– | n-↓↓↓ | n | n | n-↓ | mb: +/– | DWI: +/– | n | ? | – | Glx ↑ |
| | | Diffuse cerebral edema/injury | wmsc: ++ | T2: ↑-↑↑↑ | | | | | pons: +/– | T2: ↑-n | | | | Cho ↓ |
| | | Metabolic stroke | wmd: ++ | myelin: n | | | | | med: n | myelin: n | | | | MI ↓ |
| | | | BG: ++ | Nec: – | | | | | | Nec: – | | | | Lactate +/– |
| | | | Thal: +/– | Ca: – | | | | | | Ca: – | | | | |
| | | | | CE:? | | | | | | CE:? | | | | |
| 17.5 | Argininosuccinate lyase deficiency | Central cerebral predominant injury pattern sparing thalami | cortex: +/– | DWI: +/– | ↓-n | n | n | n | n | n | n | ? | Heterotopia | Guanadinoacetate (3.8) |
| | | | wmsc: +/– | T2: n-↑↑ | | | | | | | | | | Cr n-↓ |
| | | | wmd: +/– | myelin: n | | | | | | | | | | |
| | | | BG: +/– | Nec: – | | | | | | | | | | |
| | | | Thal: n | Ca: – | | | | | | | | | | |
| | | | | CE:? | | | | | | | | | | |
| 17.6 | Arginase deficiency | MRS: arginine | cortex: +/– | DWI: +/– | ↓-n | n | n | ↓-n | n | n | n | ? | – | Arginine (3.8) |
| | | | wmsc: +/– | T2: n-↑↑ | | | | | | | | | | NAA n-↓ |
| | | | wmd: +/– | myelin: n | | | | | | | | | | Cho n-↓ |
| | | | BG: +/– | Nec: – | | | | | | | | | | Glx n-↑ |
| | | | Thal: n | Ca: – | | | | | | | | | | |
| | | | | CE:? | | | | | | | | | | |

| | | | | | | | | | | | | | | |
|---|---|---|---|---|---|---|---|---|---|---|---|---|---|---|
| 17.17 | Pyruvate carboxylase deficiency | Periventricular cysts/ cystic necrosis | cortex: n | DWI:? | n-↓↓ | cortex: n | DWI:? | n | mb: +/– | DWI:? | n | ? | SDH +/– | Lactate |
| | | Temporopolar white matter rarefaction | wmsc: +/– | T2: ↑↑ | | wmsc: +/– | T2: ↑-n | | pons: +/– | T2: ↑-n | | | | NAA ↓ |
| | | | wmd: +/– | myelin: ↓ | | wmd: +/– | myelin: ↓-n | | med: +/– | myelin: ↓-n | | | | Cho ↑ |
| | | | BG: n | Nec: ++ | | DN: n | Nec: – | | | Nec: – | | | | |
| | | | Thal: n | Ca: – | | | Ca:– | | | Ca: – | | | | |
| | | | | CE:? | | | CE:? | | | CE:? | | | | |
| | | | | hem: +/– | | | hem: +/– | | | hem: – | | | | |
| 20.1 | Phenylalanine hydroxylase deficiency | PVWM involvement | cortex: n | hem: +/– | n | n | n | n | n | n | n | ? | – | Phe (7.3–7.4) |
| | | MRS: Phe | wmsc: +/– | T2: ↑-↑↑ | | | | | | | | | | |
| | | | wmd:+++ | myelin: n | | | | | | | | | | |
| | | | BG: n | Nec: – | | | | | | | | | | |
| | | | Thal: n | Ca: +/– | | | | | | | | | | |
| | | | | CE:? | | | | | | | | | | |
| 20.4 | Dihydropteridine reductase deficiency | Leukodystrophy, cerebrum | Cortex: +/– | DWI:? | n-↓↓ | n | n | ↓-n | – | n | n | ? | – | ? |
| | | | wmsc: +++ | T2: ↑↑↑ | | | | | | | | | | |
| | | | wmd:+++ | Myelin: n | | | | | | | | | | |
| | | | BG: +/– | Nec: + | | | | | | | | | | |
| | | | Thal: n | Ca: ++ | | | | | | | | | | |
| | | | | CE:? | | | | | | | | | | |
| 21.2, 21.3 | Tyrosinemia | Globus pallidus lesions | cortex: n | DWI: ++ | n | n | n | n | n | n | n | ? | – | ? |
| | | Intramyelinic edema | wmsc:+/– | T2: ↑ | | | | | | | | | | |
| | | | wmd:+/– | Myelin: n | | | | | | | | | | |
| | | | BG: ++ | Nec: – | | | | | | | | | | |
| | | | Thal: n | Ca: – | | | | | | | | | | |
| | | | | CE:? | | | | | | | | | | |
| 22.6 | Cystathionine β-synthase deficiency (classic homocystinuria) | Transient intramyelinic edema diffuse cerebral white matter | cortex: +/– | DWI:+/– | n-↓↓↓ | n | n | n-↓ | n | n | n | n | Sinus thrombosis +/– | Cho ↓-n-↑ |
| | | Venous thromboses +/– venous infarct | wmsc:+/– | T2: ↑ | | | | | | | | | Arterial thrombosis +/– | |
| | | Arterial thrombosis +/– arterial infarct | wmd:+/– | Myelin: n | | | | | | | | | Ectopic lens +/– | |
| | | | BG: n | Nec: – | | | | | | | | | Hydrocephalus +/– | |
| | | | Thal: n | Ca: – | | | | | | | | | | |
| | | | | CE:? | | | | | | | | | | |
| | | | | Hem: +/– | | | | | | | | | | |

(continued)

**Table 8.1** (continued)

| Chapter | Disease | Prevailing pattern(s) | Cerebrum | | | Cerebellum | | | Brainstem | | | Spinal cord | Malformations and other findings | MRS (ppm) |
|---|---|---|---|---|---|---|---|---|---|---|---|---|---|---|
| | | | Location | Texture | Volume | Location | Texture | Volume | Location | Texture | Volume | | | |
| 22.9 | Isolated sulfite oxidase deficiency | Cavitating leukodystrophy, cerebrum | cortex: +/– | DWI: +/– | n-↓↓↓ | cortex: n | DWI: +/– | n-↓ | mb: +/– | DWI: +/– | n-↓↓ | Cervical cord volume ↓ | Ectopic lens +/– | Lactate |
| | | Progressive cerebral atrophy | wmsc:+/– | T2: ↑↑ | | wmsc:+/– | T2: ↑-n | | pons: +/– | T2: ↑-n | | | SDH +/– | NAA n-↓ |
| | | Decreased brainstem/cerebellar volume | wmd:+/– | Myelin: n | | wmd: +/– | myelin: n | | med: +/– | myelin: n | | | Ectatic arteries +/– | Cho n-↑ |
| | | | BG: ++ | Nec: ++ | | DN: +/– | Nec: – | | | Nec: – | | | Ulegyria +/– | |
| | | | Thal: +/– | Ca: +/– | | | Ca: – | | | Ca: +/– | | | | |
| | | | | CE:? | | | CE:? | | | CE:? | | | | |
| 23.1 | Branched-chain aminotransferase 2 deficiency | Cerebral white matter intramyelinic edema | cortex: n | DWI: ++ | n | n | n | n | n | n | n | n | – | n |
| | | | wmsc:++ | T2: ↑↑ | | | | | | | | | | |
| | | | wmd:++ | Myelin: n | | | | | | | | | | |
| | | | BG: n | Nec: – | | | | | | | | | | |
| | | | Thal: n | Ca: – | | | | | | | | | | |
| | | | | CE: – | | | CE:? | | | | | | | |
| 23.2 | Branched-chain ketoacid dehydrogenase E1α deficiency (MSUD type 1a) | Leukodystrophy, cerebrum without edema | cortex: n | DWI: – | n | cortex: n | DWI: – | n | mb: n | DWI: – | n | ? | – | BCAA |
| | | | wmsc:+/– | T2: ↑-n | | wmsc:+/– | T2: ↑-n | | pons: +/– | T2: ↑-n | | | | BCKA |
| | | | wmd:+/– | Myelin: n | | wmd: +/– | myelin: n | | med: n | myelin: n | | | | Lac |
| | | | BG: n | Nec: – | | DN: n | Nec: – | | | Nec: – | | | | NAA↓ |
| | | | Thal: n | Ca: – | | | Ca:– | | | Ca: – | | | | Cho↑ |
| | | | | CE:? | | | CE:? | | | CE:? | | | | MI↑ |
| 23.2 | Branched-chain ketoacid dehydrogenase E1β deficiency (MSUD type1b) | Intramyelinic edema myelinating white matter | cortex: +/– | DWI: +++ | ↑-n-↓ | cortex: n | DWI: +++ | ↑-n-↓ | mb:+++ | DWI: +++ | ↑-n-↓ | ↑T2 central +/– | – | BCAA |
| | | Vasogenic edema unmyelinated white matter | wmsc:+++ | T2: ↑↑ | | wmsc: ++ | T2: ↑↑ | | p:+++ | T2: ↑↑ | | | | BCKA |
| | | | wmd:+++ | Myelin: ↓ | | wmd:+++ | Myelin: ↓ | | m:+++ | Myelin: ↓ | | | | Lac |
| | | | BG: +++ | Nec: – | | D:+++ | Nec: – | | | Nec: -– | | | | NAA↓ |
| | | | Thal: +++ | Ca: – | | | Ca: – | | | Ca: – | | | | Cho↑ |
| | | | | CE:? | | | CE:? | | | CE:? | | | | MI↑ |
| 23.10 | 3-methylglutaconyl-CoA hydratase deficiency (3-methylglutaconic aciduria type I) | MRS: 3-HIVA | cortex: n | DWI: -– | n-↓ | cortex: n | DWI: – | n | mb: n | DWI: – | n | n | – | 3-HIVA (1.28) |
| | | | wmsc: +/– | T2: ↑↑ | | wmsc: n | T2: ↑↑ | | p: + | T2: ↑↑ | | | | |
| | | | wmd: +/– | Myelin: n | | wmd: + | Myelin: n | | m: n | Myelin: n | | | | |
| | | | BG: +/– | Nec: – | | D: n | Nec: – | | | Nec: – | | | | |
| | | | Thal: – | Ca: – | | | Ca: – | | | Ca: – | | | | |
| | | | | CE: – | | | CE: – | | | CE: – | | | | |

| | | | | | | | | | | | | | | |
|---|---|---|---|---|---|---|---|---|---|---|---|---|---|---|
| 23.17 | Propionic acidemia due to propionyl-CoA carboxylase deficiency | Leigh-like | cortex: n | DWI: +/– | n-↓↓ | cortex: n | DWI: – | n | n | n | n | ? | Optic neuropathy +/– | Lactate +/– |
| | | GP often spared | wmsc: n | T2: n-↑↑↑ | | wmsc: n | T2: n-↑ | | | | | | ACC +/– | Glx ↓-n-↑ |
| | | Thalamus and brainstem spared | wmd: +/– | Myelin: n-↓ | | wmd: n | Myelin: n | | | | | | MTS +/– | NAA n-↓ |
| | | | BG: +/– | Nec: +/– | | D: n | Nec: – | | | | | | | MI n-↓ |
| | | | Thal: n | Ca: – | | | Ca: – | | | | | | | |
| | | | | CE:? | | | CE:? | | | | | | | |
| 23.19 | Methylmalonic aciduria due to methylmalonyl-CoA mutase deficiency | Leigh-like | cortex: n | DWI: – | n-↓ | n | n | n-↓ | mb: +/– | DWI: – | n-↓ | SA | – | Lactate +/– |
| | | | wmsc: +/– | T2: n-↑↑ | | | | | p: n | T2: n-↑ | | | | |
| | | | wmd: +/– | Myelin: n-↓ | | | | | m: n | Myelin: n | | | | |
| | | | BG: +/– | Nec: – | | | | | | Nec: – | | | | |
| | | | Thal: n | Ca: – | | | | | | Ca: – | | | | |
| | | | | CE:? | | | | | | CE:? | | | | |
| 26.1–26.2 | Nonketotic hyperglycinemia | Intramyelinic edema myelinating white matter | cortex: +/– | DWI: + | n-↓↓↓ | cortex: n | DWI: + | n-↓↓↓ | mb: + | DWI: + | n-↓↓ | Dorsal paramedian cervicothoracic lesions +/– | CCH | Glycine (3.55) |
| | | Hypomyelination | wmsc: + | T2: ↑ | | wmsc: +/– | T2: ↑ | | p: + | T2: ↑ | | | BS hypoplasia | Cho n-↓ |
| | | HCC | wmd: + | Myelin: ↓ | | wmd: +/– | Myelin: n-↓ | | m: + | Myelin: n-↓ | | | Vermis hypoplasia +/– | Glx n-↑ |
| | | MRS: glycine | BG: +/– | Nec: – | | D: +/– | Nec: – | | | Nec: – | | | Hydrocephalus +/– | Cr n-↑ |
| | | | Thal: + | Ca: – | | | Ca: – | | | Ca: – | | | Delayed gyration +/– | |
| | | | | CE:? | | | CE:? | | | CE:? | | | Retrocerebellarcyst+/– | |
| 27.4 | NFU1 deficiency | Cavitating leukodystrophy, cerebrum | cortex: n | DWI: +/– | ↓-↓↓ | n | n | n | mb: +/– | DWI: +/– | n | Cervical SA | – | Lactate |
| | | | wmsc: ++ | T2: ↑↑ | | | | | p: +/– | T2: n-↑ | | | | NAA n-↓ |
| | | | wmd: +++ | Myelin: ↓ | | | | | m: +/– | Myelin: n | | | | |
| | | | BG: +/– | Nec: ++ | | | | | | Nec: – | | | | |
| | | | Thal: n | Ca: – | | | | | | Ca: – | | | | |
| | | | | CE:? | | | | | | CE:? | | | | |
| 27.5 | BOLA3 deficiency | Cavitating leukodystrophy, cerebrum | cortex: +/– | DWI: +/– | n | cortex:+/– | DWI: +/– | n | mb: +/– | DWI: +/– | n | Diffuse cord SA; DWI +/– | Optic neuritis +/– | Lactate |
| | | | wmsc: ++ | T2: ↑↑ | | wmsc:+/– | T2: n-↑ | | p: +/– | T2: n-↑ | | Cervical cord DC SA; CE +/– | | |
| | | | wmd: +++ | Myelin: n | | wmd: +/– | Myelin: n | | m: +/– | Myelin: n | | | | |
| | | | BG: +/– | Nec: + | | D: n | Nec: – | | | Nec: – | | | | |
| | | | Thal: +/– | Ca: – | | | Ca: – | | | Ca: – | | | | |
| | | | | CE: + | | | CE: – | | | CE: – | | | | |

(continued)

**Table 8.1** (continued)

| Chapter | Disease | Prevailing pattern(s) | Cerebrum | | | Cerebellum | | | Brainstem | | | Spinal cord | Malformations and other findings | MRS (ppm) |
|---|---|---|---|---|---|---|---|---|---|---|---|---|---|---|
| | | | Location | Texture | Volume | Location | Texture | Volume | Location | Texture | Volume | | | |
| 27.6 | Glutaredoxin 5 deficiency | Cavitating leukodystrophy, cerebrum | cortex: n | DWI: + | ↓↓ | n | n | n | n | n | n | Central cervical cord SA | – | ? |
| | | | wmsc: ++ | T2: ↑↑ | | | | | | | | | | |
| | | | wmd: +++ | Myelin: n | | | | | | | | | | |
| | | | BG: n | Nec: + | | | | | | | | | | |
| | | | Thal: n | Ca: – | | | | | | | | | | |
| | | | | CE:? | | | | | | | | | | |
| 27.7 | IBA57 deficiency | Cavitating leukodystrophy, cerebrum +/– cerebellum | cortex: +/– | DWI: + | n-↓↓ | cortex: n | DWI: – | n-↓ | mb: +/– | DWI: – | n-↓↓ | ? | PMG +/– | Lactate |
| | | | wmsc: ++ | T2: ↑↑ | | wmsc: +/– | T2: n-↑ | | p: +/– | T2: n-↑ | | | | cho ↑ |
| | | | wmd: +++ | Myelin: n-↓ | | wmd: +/– | Myelin: n | | m: +/– | Myelin: n | | | | NAA ↓ |
| | | | BG: n | Nec: + | | D: +/– | Nec: +/– | | | Nec: – | | | | |
| | | | Thal: n | Ca: – | | | Ca: – | | | Ca: – | | | | |
| | | | | CE:? | | | CE: – | | | CE: – | | | | |
| 27.8–27.9 | ISCA1 deficiency | Leukodystrophy | cortex: n | DWI:? | n | cortex: n | DWI:? | n | n | n | n | ? | – | ? |
| | | | wmsc: +++ | T2: ↑↑ | | wmsc: n | T2: ↑↑ | | | | | | | |
| | | | wmd: +++ | Myelin: ↓ | | wmd: + | Myelin: n | | | | | | | |
| | | | BG: n | Nec: – | | D: n | Nec: – | | | | | | | |
| | | | Thal: n | Ca: – | | | Ca: – | | | | | | | |
| | | | | CE:? | | | CE: – | | | | | | | |
| 27.16 | Frataxin deficiency (Friedreich ataxia) | Spinal cord atrophy | n | n | n-↓ | cortex: n | DWI: – | n-↓ | n | n | n | Atrophy | – | ? |
| | | Accelerated iron deposition dentate nucleus | | | | wmsc: n | T2: ↓ | | | | | | | |
| | | | | | | wmd: n | Myelin: n | | | | | | | |
| | | | | | | D: ++ | Nec: – | | | | | | | |
| | | | | | | | Ca: – | | | | | | | |
| | | | | | | | CE: – | | | | | | | |
| 28.5 | Transcobalamin II deficiency | Cerebellar cortical encephalomalacia | cortex: n | DWI: +/– | n | cortex: n | DWI: – | n-↓ | n | n | n | ? | – | Lactate |
| | | GP infarction/necrosis | wmsc: n | T2: n-↑ | | wmsc: n | T2: ↓ | | | | | | | |
| | | | wmd: n | Myelin: n-↓ | | wmd: n | Myelin: n-↓ | | | | | | | |
| | | | BG(gp):+/– | Nec: +/– | | D: ++ | Nec: – | | | | | | | |
| | | | Thal: n | Ca: – | | | Ca: – | | | | | | | |
| | | | | CE:? | | | CE: – | | | | | | | |

| | | | | | | | | | | | | | | |
|---|---|---|---|---|---|---|---|---|---|---|---|---|---|---|
| 28.7–28.9 | Methylmalonic aciduria and homocystinuria | Leigh-like | cortex: +/– | DWI: +/– | ↑-n-↓↓↓ | n | n | n-↓↓ | n | n | n-↓↓ | ? | Hydrocephalus +/– | Lactate +/– |
| | | | wmsc: +/– | T2: n-↑ | | | | | | | | | SE hemorrhage +/– | |
| | | | wmd: +/– | Myelin: n-↓ | | | | | | | | | PH | |
| | | | BG: +/– | Nec: +/– | | | | | | | | | | |
| | | | Thal: n | Ca: – | | | | | | | | | | |
| | | | | CE: +/– | | | | | | | | | | |
| 28.14–28.15 | Methylmalonic aciduria | Leigh-like | cortex: +/– | DWI: +/– | n-↓↓↓ | n | n | n-↓ | mb: +/– | DWI: +/– | n | ? | PF cyst +/– | Lactate |
| | | GP infarction | wmsc: +/– | T2: n-↑ | | | | | p: n | T2: n-↑ | | | Chiari I +/– | Glx n-↑ |
| | | | wmd: +/– | Myelin: n-↓ | | | | | m: n | Myelin: n | | | Optic neuritis +/– | NAA n-↓ |
| | | | BG: ++ | Nec: +/– | | | | | | Nec: –– | | | | MI n-↓ |
| | | | Thal: – | Ca: +/– | | | | | | Ca: – | | | | |
| | | | | CE: +/– | | | | | | CE: – | | | | |
| 29.2 | Folate receptor α deficiency | Hypomyelination | cortex: +/– | DWI:? | n-↓ | n | n | ↓-↓↓ | n | n | n-↓ | ? | – | Cho n-↓ |
| | | Cerebellar atrophy | wmsc: + | T2: ↑ | | | | | | | | | | MI n-↓ |
| | | MRS: reduced choline | wmd: + | Myelin: ↓↓ | | | | | | | | | | NAA n-↓ |
| | | BG and/or white matter calcificaitons | BG: +/– | Nec: – | | | | | | | | | | |
| | | | Thal: n | Ca: +/– | | | | | | | | | | |
| | | | | CE:? | | | | | | | | | | |
| 29.3 | 5,10-methylenetetrahydrofolate reductase deficiency | Stroke | cortex: +/– | DWI: +/– | n-↓↓↓ | cortex:+/– | DWI: +/– | n-↓ | mb: +/– | DWI: +/– | n-↓ | ? | Arterial thrombosis +/– | NAA n-↓ |
| | | Vascular thromboses | wmsc: +/– | T2: n-↑↑ | | wmsc:+/– | T2: n-↑ | | p: +/– | T2: n-↑ | | | Venous thrombosis +/– | |
| | | Leukoencephalopathy | wmd: +/– | Myelin: n-↓ | | wmd: +/– | Myelin: n | | m: +/– | Myelin: n | | | Hydrocephalus +/– | |
| | | | BG: +/– | Nec: +/– | | D: n | Nec: – | | | Nec: – | | | Vermis hypoplasia +/– | |
| | | | Thal: +/– | Ca: +/– | | | Ca: – | | | Ca: – | | | BS hypoplasia +/– | |
| | | | | CE:? | | | CE:? | | | CE:? | | | | |
| | | | | Hem: +/– | | | | | | | | | | |
| 29.5 | Dihydrofolate reductase deficiency | Delayed myelination | cortex: n | DWI:? | ↓ | n | n | ↓↓ | n | n | ↓ | ? | Vermis hypoplasia | ? |
| | | Decreased brain volume | wmsc: + | T2: ↑ | | | | | | | | | PH | |
| | | | wmd: + | Myelin: ↓ | | | | | | | | | | |
| | | | BG: n | Nec: – | | | | | | | | | | |
| | | | Thal: n | Ca: – | | | | | | | | | | |
| | | | | CE:? | | | | | | | | | | |
| 30.1 | Biotinidase deficiency | NMO-mimic | cortex: +/– | DWI: +/– | n-↓ | cortex: n | DWI: +/– | n-↓ | mb: +/– | DWI: +/– | n | Cervical cord T2 ↑;CE+/– | Optic neuritis | Lactate +/– |
| | | | wmsc: +/– | T2: n-↑ | | wmsc:+/– | T2: n-↑ | | p: +/– | T2: n-↑ | | Thoracicl cord T2 ↑;CE+/– | SDH +/– | NAA n-↓ |
| | | | wmd: +/– | Myelin: n-↓ | | wmd: +/– | Myelin: n | | m: +/– | Myelin: n | | | | |
| | | | BG: n | Nec: – | | D: n | Nec: – | | | Nec: – | | | | |
| | | | Thal: +/– | Ca: – | | | Ca: – | | | Ca: – | | | | |
| | | | | CE: +/– | | | CE: +/– | | | CE: +/– | | | | |

(continued)

**Table 8.1** (continued)

| Chapter | Disease | Prevailing pattern(s) | Cerebrum Location | Cerebrum Texture | Cerebrum Volume | Cerebellum Location | Cerebellum Texture | Cerebellum Volume | Brainstem Location | Brainstem Texture | Brainstem Volume | Spinal cord | Malformations and other findings | MRS (ppm) |
|---|---|---|---|---|---|---|---|---|---|---|---|---|---|---|
| 31.1 | Thiamine transporter 2 deficiency (biotine and thiamine responsive basal ganglia disease) | Leigh-like | cortex: +/– | DWI: +/– | ↑-n-↓↓↓ | cortex:+/– | DWI: +/– | ↑-n-↓↓ | mb: +/– | DWI: +/– | ↑-n-↓↓ | Cervical cord SA | – | Lactate +/– |
| | | Wernicke encephalopathy-mimic | wmsc: +/– | T2: ↑-↑↑ | | wmsc:+/– | T2: n-↑ | | p: +/– | T2: n-↑ | | | | Pyruvate (2.4) +/– |
| | | | wmd: +/– | Myelin: n | | wmd: +/– | Myelin: n | | m: +/– | Myelin: n | | | | NAA n-↓ |
| | | | BG: +/– | Nec: +/– | | D: +/– | Nec: – | | | Nec: – | | | | Cho n-↑ |
| | | | Thal: +/– | Ca: – | | | Ca: – | | | Ca: – | | | | |
| | | | | CE:? | | | CE:? | | | CE:? | | | | |
| 31.3 | Thiamine pyrophosphokinase deficiency | Leigh-like | cortex: n | DWI:? | n-↓ | cortex: n | DWI:? | n | mb: +/– | DWI:? | n | ? | – | ? |
| | | | wmsc: +/– | T2: ↑ | | wmsc:+/– | T2: ↑ | | p: +/– | T2: n-↑ | | | | |
| | | | wmd: +/– | Myelin: ↓ | | wmd: +/– | Myelin: n | | m: +/– | Myelin: n | | | | |
| | | | BG: ++ | Nec: +/– | | D: ++ | Nec: – | | | Nec: – | | | | |
| | | | Thal: n | Ca: – | | | Ca: – | | | Ca: – | | | | |
| | | | | CE:? | | | CE:? | | | CE:? | | | | |
| 31.4 | Mitochondrial thiamine pyrophosphate transporter deficiency | Severe brain hypoplasia and pachygyria/ lisencephaly (amish lethal microcephaly) | n | n | ↓↓↓ | n | n | ↓↓-↓↓↓ | n | n | ↓↓↓ | ? | Brain hypoplasia; pachygyria/ lisencephaly; malformed deep gray nuclei | |
| 32.1–32.2 | Riboflavin transporter deficiency (Brown-Vialetto-van Laere syndrome) | Medullary and/or MCP lesions | n | n | n | n | n | n | mb: n | DWI: – | n-↓ | Cervical cord DC T2↑ | Optic atrophy +/– | ? |
| | | DC spinal cord SA | | | | | | | p: +/– | T2: n-↑ | | Thoracic cord DC T2↑ | Optic nerve hyperintense T2 +/– | |
| | | | | | | | | | m: +/– | Myelin: n | | Thick C4 nervesandCE+/– | MCPhyperintensity+/– | |
| | | | | | | | | | | Nec: – | | Ventral cauda equina CE +/– | Thick CC +/– | |
| | | | | | | | | | | Ca: – | | | | |
| | | | | | | | | | | CE: – | | | | |
| 32.6–32.7 | Electron transfer flavoprotein subunit or dehydrogenase deficiency (glutaric aciduria type 2) | Intramyelinic edema cerebrum and/or cerebellum | cortex: n | DWI: +/– | n-↓↓ | cortex: n | DWI: +/– | n | n | n | n | n | Temporalhypoplasia+/– | Lactate |
| | | Temporal hypoplasia | wmsc: +/– | T2: n-↑ | | wmsc:+/– | T2: n-↑ | | | | | | Frontal hypoplasia +/– | NAA ↓ |
| | | | wmd: +/– | Myelin: +/– | | wmd: +/– | Myelin: n | | | | | | CCH +/– | Cho ↑ |
| | | | BG: +/– | Nec: – | | D: n | Nec: – | | | | | | MCPhyperintensity+/– | |
| | | | Thal: n | Ca: – | | | Ca: – | | | | | | | |
| | | | | CE: – | | | CE: – | | | | | | | |

| | | | | | | | | | | | | | | |
|---|---|---|---|---|---|---|---|---|---|---|---|---|---|---|
| 33.9 | Pantothenate kinase 2 deficiency | "Eye of the tiger" sign | cortex: n | DWI: – | n-↓↓ | cortex: n | DWI: +/– | n-↓↓↓ | mb: +/– | DWI: – | n-↓↓↓ | ? | Optic atrophy +/– | NAA ↓ |
| | | | wmsc: +/– | T2: ↓;↑ | | wmsc: +/– | T2:↓- n-↑ | | p: n | T2: n-↓ | | | | MI ↑ |
| | | | wmd: +/– | Myelin: n-↓ | | wmd: +/– | Myelin: n | | m: n | Myelin: n | | | | |
| | | | BG(gp): +++ | Nec: + | | D: +/– | Nec: – | | | Nec: – | | | | |
| | | | Thal: n | Ca: +/– | | | Ca: – | | | Ca: – | | | | |
| | | | | CE: – | | | CE: – | | | CE: – | | | | |
| 33.11 | Coenzyme A synthase deficiency | "Eye of the tiger" sign | cortex: n | DWI: – | n-↓ | n | n | n | n | n | n | ? | – | ? |
| | | | wmsc: +/– | T2: ↑ | | | | | | | | | | |
| | | | wmd: +/– | Myelin: n | | | | | | | | | | |
| | | | BG: +++ | Nec: +/– | | | | | | | | | | |
| | | | Thal: + | Ca: +/– | | | | | | | | | | |
| | | | | CE: – | | | | | | | | | | |
| 34.1 | α-aminoadipic semialdehyde dehydrogenase deficiency | CC malformation | cortex: +/– | DWI: +/– | n-↓↓↓ | n | n | n-↓↓↓ | n | n | n-↓↓↓ | ? | ACC, CCD, HCC +/– | ? |
| | | Brain underdevelopment or malformation | wmsc: +/– | T2: n-↑ | | | | | | | | | MCD, heterotopia +/– | |
| | | | wmd: +/– | Myelin: n-↓ | | | | | | | | | Thalamic union +/– | |
| | | | BG: +/– | Nec: +/– | | | | | | | | | Brain hypoplasia +/– | |
| | | | Thal: +/– | Ca: – | | | | | | | | | MCM +/– | |
| | | | | CE:? | | | | | | | | | Chiari I +/– | |
| | | | | Hem: +/– | | | | | | | | | Germinolytic cysts +/– | |
| 35.1–35.3 | Molybdenum cofactor deficiency | Cystic encephalomalacia | cortex: +/– | DWI: +/– | n-↓↓↓ | cortex: n | DWI: – | n-↓↓ | mb: +/– | DWI: +/– | n-↓↓↓ | ? | SDH +/– | Lactate |
| | | PCH | wmsc: +/– | T2: n-↑↑ | | wmsc: +/– | T2: n-↑ | | p: n | T2: n-↑ | | | PF cyst +/– | NAA n-↓ |
| | | | wmd: +/– | Myelin: n-↓ | | wmd: +/– | Myelin: n | | m: n | Myelin: n | | | MCM +/– | Cho n-↑ |
| | | | BG: ++ | Nec: ++ | | D: +/– | Nec: – | | | Nec: – | | | Brainstemhypoplasia+/– | MI n-↓ |
| | | | Thal: +/– | Ca: +/– | | | Ca: – | | | Ca: – | | | Cerebellarhypoplasia+/– | Cr n-↓ |
| | | | | CE: – | | | CE: – | | | CE: – | | | Lens subluxation +/– | |
| | | | | Hem: +/– | | | | | | | | | HCC, CCD +/– | |
| 36.1 | Copper-transporting ATPase β subunit deficiency (Wilson disease) | Mixed T2 signal cerebral deep gray and midbrain | cortex: +/– | DWI: +/– | n-↓↓↓ | cortex: n | DWI: – | n-↓↓ | mb: +/– | DWI: +/– | n-↓↓ | "Bullet shaped" vertebral dysplasia +/– | Claustum lesions +/– | Lactate +/– |
| | | Dentorubrothalamic tract involvement | wmsc: +/– | T2: ↓-n-↑ | | wmsc: n | T2: ↓-n-↑ | | p: +/– | T2: ↓-n-↑ | | | | NAA n-↓ |
| | | T1 shortening BG +/– midbrain | wmd: +/– | T1: ↓-n-↑ | | wmd: +/– | T1: ↓-n | | m: +/– | T1: ↓-n-↑ | | | | Cho ↓-n-↑ |
| | | Claustrum T2 hyperintesity | BG: +/– | Myelin: n | | D: +/– | Myelin: n | | | Myelin: n | | | | MI n-↓ |
| | | | Thal: +/– | Nec: +/– | | | Nec: – | | | Nec: – | | | | Lipids n-↑ |
| | | | | Ca: +/– | | | Ca: +/– | | | Ca: – | | | | Cr n-↓ |
| | | | | CE: +/– | | | CE: – | | | CE: – | | | | |

(continued)

**Table 8.1** (continued)

| | | | Cerebrum | | | Cerebellum | | | Brainstem | | | | Malformations and | |
|---|---|---|---|---|---|---|---|---|---|---|---|---|---|---|
| Chapter | Disease | Prevailing pattern(s) | Location | Texture | Volume | Location | Texture | Volume | Location | Texture | Volume | Spinal cord | other findings | MRS (ppm) |
| 36.2 | Copper-transporting ATPase α subunit deficiency (Menke disease) | Tortuous, elongated arteries | cortex: +/– | DWI: +/– | ↑-n-↓↓↓ | cortex: n | DWI: – | n-↓↓ | mb: +/– | DWI: – | n-↓↓ | C2 posterior arch defects +/– | Tortuous, elongated arteries | Lactate +/– |
| | | Delayed myelination | wmsc: +/– | T2: n-↑↑ | | wmsc: n | T2: n-↑ | | p: +/– | T2: n-↑ | | | Dural sinus ectasia +/– | Glx n-↑ |
| | | Basal ganglia lesions | wmd: +/– | Myelin: n-↓ | | wmd: +/– | Myelin: n | | m: +/– | Myelin: n | | | SDH +/– | NAA n-↓ |
| | | Infantile transient temporal lobe tumafactive edema | BG: +/– | Nec: +/– | | D: n | Nec: – | | | Nec: – | | | Wormian bones +/– | |
| | | SDH | Thal: +/– | Ca: – | | | Ca: – | | | Ca: – | | | | |
| | | | | CE:? | | | CE:? | | | CE:? | | | | |
| | | | | Hem: +/– | | | | | | | | | | |
| 37.1–37.5 | Heredetary hemachromatosis | Deep gray nuclear iron depostion | cortex: n | DWI: n | n-↓ | cortex: n | DWI: – | n-↓ | mb: +/– | DWI: – | n | ? | Pituitary iron deposition | ? |
| | | | wmsc: +/– | T2: ↓-↑ | | wmsc: n | T2: ↓ | | p: n | T2: n-↓ | | | | |
| | | | wmd: +/– | T1: n-↑ | | wmd: n | T1: n-↑ | | m: n | Myelin: n | | | | |
| | | | BG: +++ | Myelin: n | | D: ++ | Myelin: n | | | Nec: – | | | | |
| | | | Thal: +/– | Nec: – | | | Nec: – | | | Ca: – | | | | |
| | | | | Ca: – | | | Ca: – | | | CE: – | | | | |
| | | | | CE: – | | | CE: – | | | | | | | |
| 37.7 | Ferritin light chain superactivity (neuroferritinopathy) | Widespread gray matter iron deposition +/– necrosis | cortex: + | DWI: n | n-↓ | cortex:+/– | DWI: – | n-↓ | mb: +/– | DWI: – | n-↓ | ? | – | ? |
| | | "Eye of the tiger" sign | wmsc: n | T2: ↓-↑ | | wmsc: n | T2: ↓-↑ | | p: n | T2: n-↓ | | | | |
| | | | wmd: n | T1: n-↑ | | wmd: n | T1: n | | m: n | Myelin: n | | | | |
| | | | BG: +++ | Myelin: n | | D: ++ | Myelin: n | | | Nec: +/– | | | | |
| | | | Thal: +/– | Nec: +/– | | | Nec: +/– | | | Ca: – | | | | |
| | | | | Ca: – | | | Ca: – | | | CE: – | | | | |
| | | | | CE: – | | | CE: – | | | | | | | |
| 37.8 | Hereditary ceruloplasmin deficiency | Widespread homogeneous gray matter iron deposition | cortex: + | DWI: n | n-↓ | cortex:+/– | DWI: – | n-↓↓ | mb: + | DWI: – | n-↓↓ | ? | – | ? |
| | | Necrosis unusual | wmsc: n | T2: ↓ | | wmsc: n | T2: ↓ | | p: n | T2: ↓ | | | | |
| | | | wmd: n | T1: n | | wmd: n | T1: n | | m: n | Myelin: n | | | | |
| | | | BG: ++ | Myelin: n | | D: ++ | Myelin: n | | | Nec: – | | | | |
| | | | Thal: +/– | Nec(thal):+/– | | | Nec: – | | | Ca: – | | | | |
| | | | | Ca: – | | | Ca: – | | | CE: – | | | | |
| | | | | CE: – | | | CE: – | | | | | | | |

| | | | | | | | | | | | | | | |
|---|---|---|---|---|---|---|---|---|---|---|---|---|---|---|
| 38.1 | Hypermanganesemia with dystonia type 1 | T1 ↑ BG, BS, deep cerebellum | cortex: n<br>wmsc: n<br>wmd: n<br>BG: +++<br>Thal: +/– | DWI: n<br>T2: ↓<br>T1: ↑↑<br>Myelin: n<br>Nec: –<br>Ca: –<br>CE: – | n | cortex: n<br>wmsc: n<br>wmd: +/–<br>D: + | DWI: –<br>T2: n<br>T1: ↑<br>Myelin: n<br>Nec: –<br>Ca: –<br>CE: – | n | mb: +<br>p: +/–<br>m: n | DWI: –<br>T2: n<br>T1: ↑<br>Myelin: n<br>Nec: –<br>Ca: –<br>CE: – | n-↓ | ? | Pituitary T1↑ +/– | ? |
| 38.2 | SLC39A14 deficiency | T1 ↑ BG and brain white matter | cortex: n<br>wmsc: +<br>wmd: +<br>BG: ++<br>Thal: n | DWI: n<br>T2: ↓<br>T1: ↑↑<br>Myelin: n<br>Nec: –<br>Ca: –<br>CE: – | n-↓ | cortex: n<br>wmsc: +<br>wmd: +<br>D: + | DWI: –<br>T2: ↓<br>T1: ↑<br>Myelin: n<br>Nec: –<br>Ca: –<br>CE: – | n-↓ | mb: +<br>p: +<br>m: n | DWI: –<br>T2: n<br>T1: ↑<br>Myelin: n<br>Nec: –<br>Ca: –<br>CE: – | n-↓ | T1 ↑ | Pituitary T1↑ +/– | ? |
| 38.3 | SLC39A8 deficiency | Leigh-like | cortex: n<br>wmsc: n<br>wmd: n<br>BG: ++<br>Thal: +/– | DWI: +/–<br>T2: ↑-↑↑<br>Myelin: n<br>Nec: +/–<br>Ca: –<br>CE:? | n-↓ | n | n | n-↓ | n | n | n | ? | – | ? |
| 39.11–39.13 | Galactosemia | MRS: Galactitol | cortex: +/–<br>wmsc: +/–<br>wmd: +/–<br>BG: +/–<br>Thal: n | DWI: +/–<br>T2: n-↑<br>T1: ↓-n-↑<br>Myelin: n-↓<br>Nec: –<br>Ca: –<br>CE: – | n-↓↓ | cortex: n<br>wmsc: +/–<br>wmd: +/–<br>D: +/– | DWI: –<br>T2: n-↑<br>Myelin: n-↓<br>Nec: –<br>Ca: –<br>CE: – | n-↓↓ | mb: +/–<br>p: +/–<br>m: +/– | DWI: –<br>T2: n-↑<br>Myelin: n<br>Nec: –<br>Ca: –<br>CE: – | n | ? | AC +/– | Galactitol (3.7)<br>NAA n-↓<br>MI n-↓<br>cho n-↓ |
| 39.18 | Glucose-6-phosphate transporter deficiency | Hypoglycemic brain injury pattern<br>Moyamoya | cortex: +/–<br>wmsc: +/–<br>wmd: +/–<br>BG: n<br>Thal: n | DWI: +/–<br>T2: n-↑<br>Myelin: n<br>Nec: +/–<br>Ca: –<br>CE:? | n-↓↓ | n | n | n | n | n | n | ? | Moyamoya +/– | ? |
| 39.21 | Glycogen branching enzyme deficiency | Leukodystrophy<br>CST and ML SA<br>SC atrophy | cortex: n<br>wmsc: +<br>wmd: ++<br>BG: n<br>Thal: n | DWI: +/–<br>T2: ↑<br>Myelin: n-↓<br>Nec: –<br>Ca: –<br>CE: – | ↓ | cortex:+/–<br>wmsc:+/–<br>wmd: +/–<br>D: +/– | DWI: –<br>T2: n-↑<br>Myelin: n<br>Nec: –<br>Ca: –<br>CE: – | ↓↓ | mb: +<br>p: +<br>m: + | DWI: –<br>T2: ↑<br>Myelin: n<br>Nec: –<br>Ca: –<br>CE: – | ↓↓ | Marked diffuse atrophy<br>DC T2↑ +/– | | NAA ↓<br>Lactate |

(continued)

**Table 8.1** (continued)

| Chapter | Disease | Prevailing pattern(s) | Cerebrum | | | Cerebellum | | | Brainstem | | | Spinal cord | Malformations and other findings | MRS (ppm) |
|---|---|---|---|---|---|---|---|---|---|---|---|---|---|---|
| | | | Location | Texture | Volume | Location | Texture | Volume | Location | Texture | Volume | | | |
| 41.15 | Catalytic phosphatidylinositol 3-kinase α subunit superactivity | MCD and MEG or hemi-MEG | cortex: + | DWI: – | ↑-↑↑ | n | n | n-↑ | n | n | n-↑ | ? | AC +/– | ? |
| | | PVWM hyperintensity | wmsc: + | T2: n-↑ | | | | | | | | | Chiari I +/– | |
| | | | wmd: +/– | Myelin: n | | | | | | | | | | |
| | | | BG: n | Nec: – | | | | | | | | | | |
| | | | Thal: n | Ca: – | | | | | | | | | | |
| | | | | CE: – | | | | | | | | | | |
| 41.16 | Phosphomannomutase 2 deficiency (PMM2-CDG; CDG Type 1a) | Cerebellar hypoplasia and atrophy with cortical hyperintensity | cortex: +/– | DWI: +/– | n-↓↓ | cortex:+/– | DWI: – | n-↓↓↓ | mb: +/– | DWI: – | n-↓↓ | ? | OPCH +/– | NAA n-↓ |
| | | OPCH | wmsc: +/– | T2: ↓- n-↑ | | wmsc: n | T2: n-↑ | | p: +/– | T2: n-↑ | | | SDH or IVH +/– | Glx n-↑ |
| | | Hemorrhage +/– | wmd: +/– | Myelin: n-↓ | | wmd: n | Myelin: n | | m: n | Myelin: n | | | Cerebralhemorrhage+/– | MI n-↑ |
| | | | BG: +/– | Nec: – | | D: n | Nec: – | | | Nec: – | | | Vasculopathy +/– | Cho n-↓ |
| | | | Thal: n | Ca: – | | | Ca: – | | | Ca: – | | | | |
| | | | | CE:? | | | CE:? | | | CE: – | | | | |
| | | | | Hem: +/– | | | | | | | | | | |
| 42.2–42.3 | Pyruvate dehydrogenase E1-α or E1-β deficiency | CCD | cortex: n | DWI: +/– | n-↓↓↓ | cortex: n | DWI: – | n-↓↓ | mb: +/– | DWI: – | n-↓↓ | ? | ACC, CCD, HCC +/– | Lactate |
| | | Cavitating leukodystrophy, deep cerebrum | wmsc: +/– | T2: n-↑ | | wmsc: n | T2: n-↑ | | p: +/– | T2: n-↑ | | | Germinolytic cysts +/– | Pyruvate (2.4) +/– |
| | | | wmd: +/– | Myelin: n-↓ | | wmd: n | Myelin: n | | m: n | Myelin: n | | | Ventricularseptations+/– | |
| | | | BG: +/– | Nec: +/– | | D: +/– | Nec: – | | | Nec: – | | | Hippocampal underrotation +/– | |
| | | | Thal: +/– | Ca: – | | | Ca: – | | | Ca: – | | | Vermianhypoplasia+/– | |
| | | | | CE:? | | | CE:? | | | CE: – | | | MCD, PMG +/– | |
| 42.4 | Dihydrolipoamide acetyltransferase deficiency | GP lesions | BG(gp): ++ | T2: ↑-↑↑ | n | n | n | n | n | n | n | ? | – | n |
| 42.5 | Pyruvate dehydrogenase E3-binding protein deficiency | Leigh-like | cortex: +/– | DWI: +/– | n-↓↓ | n | n | n | n | n | n | ? | Germinolytic cysts +/– | ? |
| | | Cavitating leukodystrophy, deep cerebrum | wmsc: +/– | T2: n-↑ | | | | | | | | | Ventricularseptations+/– | |
| | | | wmd: +/– | Myelin: n-↓ | | | | | | | | | MCD +/– | |
| | | | BG: +/– | Nec: +/– | | | | | | | | | | |
| | | | Thal: +/– | Ca: – | | | | | | | | | | |
| | | | | CE:? | | | | | | | | | | |
| 42.14 | ATP-specific succinyl-CoA ligase β subunit deficiency | Leigh-like | cortex: n | DWI:? | n-↓↓ | n | n | n-↓ | n | n | n-↓ | ? | Retinoblastoma +/– | Lactate |
| | | | wmsc: +/– | T2: n-↑ | | | | | | | | | | |
| | | | wmd: +/– | Myelin: n | | | | | | | | | | |
| | | | BG: +/– | Nec: – | | | | | | | | | | |
| | | | Thal: n | Ca: – | | | | | | | | | | |
| | | | | CE:? | | | | | | | | | | |

| | | | | | | | | | | | | | | |
|---|---|---|---|---|---|---|---|---|---|---|---|---|---|---|
| 42.15 | GTP-specific succinyl-CoA ligase α subunit deficiency | Leigh-like | cortex: n | DWI: +/– | n-↓↓ | n | n | n-↓ | n | n | n | ? | – | Lactate |
| | | | wmsc: +/– | T2: n-↑ | | | | | | | | | | NAA ↓ |
| | | | wmd: +/– | Myelin: n | | | | | | | | | | |
| | | | BG: +/– | Nec: +/– | | | | | | | | | | |
| | | | Thal: n | Ca: – | | | | | | | | | | |
| | | | | CE:? | | | | | | | | | | |
| 42.16–42.17 | Succinate dehydrogenase subunit A and/or B deficiency | Cavitating leukodystrophy, involving CST, sparing U-fibers and CC outer blade | cortex: n | DWI: +/– | n-↓↓ | cortex: n | DWI: – | n-↓ | mb: +/– | DWI: – | n-↓ | Cervical SC graymatterT2↑+/– | Paraganglioma +/– | Succinate (2.4) +/– |
| | | Thalamic nuclei involvement | wmsc: +/– | T2: n-↑ | | wmsc: n | T2: n-↑ | | p: +/– | T2: n-↑ | | | Pheochromocytoma+/– | Lactate +/– |
| | | Cervical SC gray matter SA | wmd: +/– | Myelin: n-↓ | | wmd: +/– | Myelin: n | | m: +/– | Myelin: n | | | | |
| | | MRS: succinate | BG: +/– | Nec: +/– | | D: n | Nec: – | | | Nec: – | | | | |
| | | | Thal: +/– | Ca: – | | | Ca: – | | | Ca: – | | | | |
| | | | | CE: +/– | | | CE: – | | | CE: – | | | | |
| 44.1–44.4 | NADH dehydrogenase flavoprotein 1 and/or 2 deficiency; NADH dehydrogenase iron-sulfur protein 1 and/or 2 deficiency | Cavitating leukodystrophy, deep cerebrum, sparing CC inner/outer blades | cortex: n | DWI: +/– | n-↓↓ | cortex: n | DWI: +/– | n | mb: +/– | DWI: +/– | n | Cervical cord T2↑ anterolaterally+/– | – | Lactate +/– |
| | | | wmsc: +/– | T2: ↑-↑↑ | | wmsc: +/– | T2: n-↑ | | p: +/– | T2: n-↑ | | | | NAA n-↓ |
| | | | wmd: +/– | Myelin: n | | wmd: +/– | Myelin: n | | m: +/– | Myelin: n | | | | MI n-↑ |
| | | | BG: +/– | Nec: + | | D: n | Nec: +/– | | | Nec: – | | | | |
| | | | Thal: +/– | Ca: – | | | Ca: – | | | Ca: – | | | | |
| | | | | CE: – | | | CE: – | | | CE: – | | | | |
| 44.5 | NADH dehydrogenase iron-sulfur protein 3 deficiency | Cavitating leukodystrophy, deep cerebrum, sparing CC inner/outer blades | cortex: n | DWI: + | n-↓ | n | n | n | mb: + | DWI: + | n | ? | – | ? |
| | | Leigh-like | wmsc: + | T2: ↑-↑↑ | | | | | p: n | T2: ↑ | | | | |
| | | | wmd: ++ | Myelin: n | | | | | m: n | Myelin: n | | | | |
| | | | BG: ++ | Nec: + | | | | | | Nec: – | | | | |
| | | | Thal: ++ | Ca: – | | | | | | Ca: – | | | | |
| | | | | CE:? | | | | | | CE:? | | | | |
| 44.10 | NADH dehydrogenase α subcomplex subunit 1 deficiency | Leigh-like | cortex: n | DWI: – | n | n | n | n-↓ | mb: + | DWI: – | n | Cervical SC T2↑ | – | ? |
| | | Spinal cord anterior horn SA | wmsc: n | T2: n-↑ | | | | | p: n | T2: ↑ | | | | |
| | | | wmd: n | Myelin: n | | | | | m: +/– | Myelin: n | | | | |
| | | | BG: +/– | Nec: – | | | | | | Nec: – | | | | |
| | | | Thal: n | Ca: – | | | | | | Ca: – | | | | |
| | | | | CE:? | | | | | | CE: – | | | | |

(continued)

**Table 8.1** (continued)

| Chapter | Disease | Prevailing pattern(s) | Cerebrum | | | Cerebellum | | | Brainstem | | | Spinal cord | Malformations and other findings | MRS (ppm) |
|---|---|---|---|---|---|---|---|---|---|---|---|---|---|---|
| | | | Location | Texture | Volume | Location | Texture | Volume | Location | Texture | Volume | | | |
| 44.11 | NADH dehydrogenase α subcomplex subunit 9 deficiency | Leigh-like | cortex: n | DWI: – | ↓ | n | n | ↓ | n | n | ↓ | ? | – | ? |
| | | | wmsc: n | T2: ↑ | | | | | | | | | | |
| | | | wmd: n | Myelin: n | | | | | | | | | | |
| | | | BG: + | Nec: + | | | | | | | | | | |
| | | | Thal: + | Ca: – | | | | | | | | | | |
| | | | | CE:? | | | | | | | | | | |
| 44.15 | NADH dehydrogenase α subcomplex subunit 12 deficiency | Leigh-like | BG(gp): + | T2: ↑ | n | n | n | n | n | n | n | ? | – | Lactate |
| 44.18 | NADH dehydrogenase β subcomplex subunit 8 deficiency | Leigh-like | cortex: +/– | DWI: +/– | ↓-↓↓↓ | n | n | n | mb: +/– | DWI: +/– | n-↓↓↓ | ? | SDH +/– | ? |
| | | Cavitating leukodystrophy, deep cerebrum | wmsc: +/– | T2: ↑-↑↑ | | | | | p: n | T2: n-↑ | | | | |
| | | | wmd: +/– | Myelin: n | | | | | m: n | Myelin: n | | | | |
| | | | BG: +/– | Nec: +/– | | | | | | Nec: – | | | | |
| | | | Thal: +/– | Ca: – | | | | | | Ca: – | | | | |
| | | | | CE: +/– | | | | | | CE: – | | | | |
| 44.21, 44.23, 44.25–44.27 | NADH dehydrogenase core subunit deficiency 1,3,4L, 5, 6 | Leigh-like | cortex: +/– | DWI: +/– | n-↓↓↓ | cortex:+/– | DWI: – | n-↓ | mb: +/– | DWI: +/– | n-↓ | CervicalT2↑+/– | Optic neuritis +/– | Lactate |
| | | MELAS | wmsc: +/– | T2: ↑-↑↑ | | wmsc:+/– | T2: n-↑ | | p: +/– | T2: n-↑ | | | | NAA n-↓ |
| | | Optic neuritis | wmd: +/– | Myelin: n | | wmd: +/– | Myelin: n | | m: +/– | Myelin: n | | | | |
| | | | BG: +/– | Nec: +/– | | D: +/– | Nec: – | | | Nec: – | | | | |
| | | | Thal: +/– | Ca: +/– | | | Ca: – | | | Ca: – | | | | |
| | | | | CE: +/– | | | CE: – | | | CE: – | | | | |
| 44.21 | NADH dehydrogenase core subunit 1 deficiency | Leigh-like | cortex: +/– | DWI: +/– | n-↓↓ | n | n | n | mb: +/– | DWI: +/– | n | ? | Optic neuritis +/– | ? |
| | | Optic neuritis | wmsc: +/– | T2: n-↑↑ | | | | | p: +/– | T2: n-↑ | | | | |
| | | Vestibular nuclei lesions | wmd: n | Myelin: n | | | | | m: n | Myelin: n | | | | |
| | | Inferior collicular lesions | BG: +/– | Nec: +/– | | | | | | Nec: – | | | | |
| | | | Thal: +/– | Ca: – | | | | | | Ca: – | | | | |
| | | | | CE: +/– | | | | | | CE: – | | | | |
| 44.29 | NADH dehydrogenase α subcomplex assembly factor 2 deficiency | Leigh-like; basal ganglia spared | cortex: n | DWI: – | n-↓ | cortex: n | DWI: – | n | mb: +/– | DWI: +/– | n | CervicalT2↑+/– | – | ? |
| | | | wmsc: n | T2: n-↑ | | wmsc:+/– | T2: n-↑ | | p: +/– | T2: ↑-↑↑ | | | | |
| | | | wmd: +/– | Myelin: n | | wmd: +/– | Myelin: n | | m: +/– | Myelin: n | | | | |
| | | | BG: n | Nec: – | | D: n | Nec: – | | | Nec: +/– | | | | |
| | | | Thal: n | Ca: – | | | Ca: – | | | Ca: – | | | | |
| | | | | CE:? | | | CE:? | | | CE: – | | | | |

| | | | | | | | | | | | | | | |
|---|---|---|---|---|---|---|---|---|---|---|---|---|---|---|
| 44.30 | NADH dehydrogenase α subcomplex assembly factor 3 deficiency | Leigh-like | cortex: n | DWI: +/– | n | n | n | n | mb: + | DWI: +/– | n | ? | – | Lactate |
| | | Cavitating leukodystrophy, patchy cerebral WM lesions; CC involved outer blades spared | wmsc: + | T2: ↑-↑↑ | | | | | p: n | T2: ↑ | | | | |
| | | | wmd: + | Myelin: n | | | | | m: n | Myelin: n | | | | |
| | | | BG: + | Nec: + | | | | | | Nec: – | | | | |
| | | | Thal: + | Ca: – | | | | | | Ca: – | | | | |
| | | | | CE:? | | | | | | CE:? | | | | |
| 44.32 | NADH dehydrogenase α subcomplex assembly factor 5 deficiency | Leigh-like | cortex: +/– | DWI: +/– | n | n | n | n | mb: + | DWI: +/– | n | ? | – | ? |
| | | Cavitating leukodystrophy, patchy cerebral WM lesions | wmsc: + | T2: ↑-↑↑ | | | | | p: n | T2: ↑ | | | | |
| | | | wmd: + | Myelin: n | | | | | m: n | Myelin: n | | | | |
| | | | BG: + | Nec: + | | | | | | Nec: – | | | | |
| | | | Thal: + | Ca: – | | | | | | Ca: – | | | | |
| | | | | CE:? | | | | | | CE:? | | | | |
| 44.33 | NADH dehydrogenase α subcomplex assembly factor 6 deficiency | Leigh-like | cortex: n | DWI: n | n | cortex: n | DWI: – | n-↓ | mb: + | DWI: n | n | ? | – | ? |
| | | | wmsc: n | T2: n-↑ | | wmsc: n | T2: ↑ | | p: n | T2: ↑ | | | | |
| | | | wmd: n | Myelin: n | | wmd: n | Myelin: n | | m: n | Myelin: n | | | | |
| | | | BG: +/– | Nec: – | | D: ++ | Nec: – | | | Nec: – | | | | |
| | | | Thal: n | Ca: – | | | Ca: – | | | Ca: – | | | | |
| | | | | CE:? | | | CE:? | | | CE:? | | | | |
| 44.35 | NUBPL deficiency | Cavitating leukodystrophy, deep cerebrum frontal predominant; CC involved outer blades spared | cortex: n | DWI: +/– | ↑-n-↓↓ | cortex: ++ | DWI: – | n-↓↓ | mb: n | DWI: – | n-↓↓↓ | ? | – | ? |
| | | Cerebellar cortical/ subcortical diffuse SA | wmsc: +/– | T2: ↑-↑↑ | | wmsc: ++ | T2: ↑-↑↑↑ | | p: + | T2: ↑ | | | | |
| | | | wmd: ++ | Myelin: n | | wmd: +/– | Myelin: n | | m: + | Myelin: n | | | | |
| | | | BG: n | Nec: + | | D: n | Nec: +/– | | | Nec: – | | | | |
| | | | Thal: n | Ca: – | | | Ca: – | | | Ca: – | | | | |
| | | | | CE: +/– | | | CE: +/– | | | CE: +/– | | | | |
| 44.45 | Succinate dehydrogenase complex assembly factor 1 deficiency | Cavitating leukodystrophy, deep cerebrum | cortex: n | DWI:? | n-↓ | cortex: n | DWI:? | n | mb: n | DWI:? | n | ? | – | Succinate (2.4) +/– |
| | | MRS: succinate | wmsc: n | T2: n-↑ | | wmsc:+/– | T2: n-↑ | | p: +/– | T2: n-↑ | | | | |
| | | | wmd: +/– | Myelin: n | | wmd: +/– | Myelin: n | | m: n | Myelin: n | | | | |
| | | | BG: n | Nec: +/– | | D: n | Nec: – | | | Nec: – | | | | |
| | | | Thal: n | Ca: – | | | Ca: – | | | Ca: – | | | | |
| | | | | CE:? | | | CE:? | | | CE:? | | | | |

(continued)

**Table 8.1** (continued)

| Chapter | Disease | Prevailing pattern(s) | Cerebrum Location | Cerebrum Texture | Cerebrum Volume | Cerebellum Location | Cerebellum Texture | Cerebellum Volume | Brainstem Location | Brainstem Texture | Brainstem Volume | Spinal cord | Malformations and other findings | MRS (ppm) |
|---|---|---|---|---|---|---|---|---|---|---|---|---|---|---|
| 44.49 | UQCRQ deficiency | Leigh-like | cortex: n | DWI:? | ↓ | n | n | n | n | n | n | ? | – | ? |
| | | | wmsc: n | T2: ↑↑ | | | | | | | | | | |
| | | | wmd: n | Myelin: n | | | | | | | | | | |
| | | | BG: ++ | Nec: + | | | | | | | | | | |
| | | | Thal: n | Ca: – | | | | | | | | | | |
| | | | | CE:? | | | | | | | | | | |
| 44.52 | TTC19 deficiency | Leigh-like | cortex: n | DWI: +/– | n-↓ | n | n | n-↓ | mb: +/– | DWI:? | n | n | Vermianhypoplasia+/– | Lactate +/– |
| | | | wmsc: n | T2: n-↑↑ | | | | | p: n | T2: n-↑ | | | | |
| | | | wmd: n | Myelin: n | | | | | m: +/– | Myelin: n | | | | |
| | | | BG: +/– | Nec: +/– | | | | | | Nec: – | | | | |
| | | | Thal: n | Ca: – | | | | | | Ca: – | | | | |
| | | | | CE:? | | | | | | CE:? | | | | |
| 44.54 | LYRM7 deficiency | Cavitating leukodystrophy, patchy cerebral wm lesions | cortex: n | DWI: +/– | n-↓↓ | cortex: n | DWI:? | n-↓↓ | mb: +/– | DWI:? | n-↓↓ | SC SA +/– | Optic chiasm T2 hyperintensity | ? |
| | | Spinal cord SA | wmsc: +/– | T2: ↑-↑↑ | | wmsc: +/– | T2: n-↑ | | p: +/– | T2: ↑-↑↑ | | | | |
| | | | wmd: ++ | Myelin: n-↓ | | wmd: +/– | Myelin: n | | m: ++ | Myelin: n | | | | |
| | | | BG: n | Nec: + | | D: n | Nec: – | | | Nec: – | | | | |
| | | | Thal: +/– | Ca: – | | | Ca: – | | | Ca: – | | | | |
| | | | | CE: +/– | | | CE:? | | | CE: – | | | | |
| 44.55 | Cytochrome c oxidase subunit 1 deficiency | Leigh-like | cortex: n | DWI: +/– | n | n | n | n | n | n | n | ? | – | ? |
| | | | wmsc: n | T2: ↑↑ | | | | | | | | | | |
| | | | wmd: n | Myelin: n | | | | | | | | | | |
| | | | BG: ++ | Nec: + | | | | | | | | | | |
| | | | Thal: n | Ca: – | | | | | | | | | | |
| | | | | CE:? | | | | | | | | | | |
| 44.60 | Cytochrome c oxidase subunit 6B1 deficiency | Cavitating leukodystrophy, deep cerebrum | cortex: n | DWI: +/– | ↓-↓↓ | n | n | n | n | n | n | ? | – | ? |
| | | | wmsc: +/– | T2: ↑↑ | | | | | | | | | | |
| | | | wmd: +++ | Myelin: n | | | | | | | | | | |
| | | | BG: n | Nec: + | | | | | | | | | | |
| | | | Thal: n | Ca: – | | | | | | | | | | |
| | | | | CE:? | | | | | | | | | | |
| 44.75 | SURF1 deficiency | Leigh-like | cortex: n | DWI: +/– | n-↓↓ | cortex: n | DWI:? | n-↓↓↓ | mb: +/– | DWI: +/– | n-↓ | Cervical T2↑ | HOD +/– | ? |
| | | HOD | wmsc: n | T2: n-↑↑ | | wmsc: +/– | T2: n-↑↑ | | p: +/– | T2: n-↑↑↑ | | | | |
| | | STN lesions, cerebral deep gray nuclei often spared | wmd: +/– | Myelin: n-↓ | | wmd: +/– | Myelin: n | | m: +/– | Myelin: n | | | | |
| | | | BG: +/– | Nec: +/– | | D: +/– | Nec: +/– | | | Nec: +/– | | | | |
| | | | Thal: +/– | Ca: – | | | Ca: – | | | Ca: – | | | | |
| | | | | CE: – | | | CE: – | | | CE: – | | | | |

| | | | | | | | | | | | | | | |
|---|---|---|---|---|---|---|---|---|---|---|---|---|---|---|
| 44.76 | LRPPRC deficiency | Cavitating leukodystrophy, deep cerebrum | cortex: n | DWI: +/– | n-↓↓ | cortex: n | DWI: +/– | n-↓↓ | mb: +/– | DWI: +/– | n | ? | MCD | Lactate |
| | | | wmsc: +/– | T2: n-↑↑ | | wmsc: n | T2: n-↑ | | p: n | T2: n-↑ | | | PMG | |
| | | | wmd: +/– | Myelin: n | | wmd: +/– | Myelin: n | | m: +/– | Myelin: n | | | Pachygyria | |
| | | | BG: +/– | Nec: – | | D: +/– | Nec: – | | | Nec: – | | | CCD/HCC | |
| | | | Thal: n | Ca: – | | | Ca: – | | | Ca: – | | | Hippocampal malformation | |
| | | | | CE:? | | | CE:? | | | CE:? | | | Cerebellar hypoplasia | |
| 44.77 | TACO1 deficiency | Leigh-like | cortex: n | DWI: +/– | ↓-↓↓ | n | n | n | n | n | n | ? | – | ? |
| | | | wmsc: +/– | T2: ↑-↑↑ | | | | | | | | | | |
| | | | wmd: +/– | Myelin: n | | | | | | | | | | |
| | | | BG: ++ | Nec: + | | | | | | | | | | |
| | | | Thal: n | Ca: – | | | | | | | | | | |
| | | | | CE:? | | | | | | | | | | |
| 44.80 | APOPT1 deficiency | Cavitating leukodystrophy, deep cerebrum | cortex: n | DWI: + | n-↓↓↓ | n | n | n | mb: +/– | DWI: – | n | ? | – | Lactate +/– |
| | | | wmsc: +/– | T2: ↑-↑↑ | | | | | p: +/– | T2: n-↑ | | | | |
| | | | wmd: ++ | Myelin: n | | | | | m: +/– | Myelin: n | | | | |
| | | | BG: n | Nec: + | | | | | | Nec: – | | | | |
| | | | Thal: n | Ca: – | | | | | | Ca: – | | | | |
| | | | | CE:? | | | | | | CE:? | | | | |
| 44.85 | Mitochondrial ATP synthase F0 subunit 6 deficiency | Leigh-like | cortex: +/– | DWI: +/– | n-↓ | cortex:+/– | DWI: – | n-↓↓ | mb: +/– | DWI: – | n-↓↓ | ? | – | Lactate +/– |
| | | | wmsc: +/– | T2: ↑-↑↑ | | wmsc:+/– | T2: n-↑ | | p: +/– | T2: n-↑ | | | | NAA n-↓ |
| | | | wmd: +/– | Myelin: n | | wmd: +/– | Myelin: n | | m: +/– | Myelin: n | | | | |
| | | | BG: +/– | Nec: +/– | | D: n | Nec: – | | | Nec: – | | | | |
| | | | Thal: +/– | Ca: – | | | Ca: – | | | Ca: – | | | | |
| | | | | CE:? | | | CE:? | | | CE:? | | | | |
| 45.01, 45.03–45.07, 45.11–45.12 | Mitochondrial DNA depletion syndromes | Occpital cortex, thalamus, inferior olives, deep cerebellar lesions | cortex: +/– | DWI: +/– | n-↓↓↓ | cortex:+/– | DWI: – | n-↓↓ | mb: +/– | DWI: – | n-↓ | RST T2↑ +/– | Germinolytic cysts +/– | Lactate |
| | | MELAS | wmsc: +/– | T2: n-↑ | | wmsc: + | T2: ↑ | | p: +/– | T2: n-↑ | | | Periventricularcysts+/– | NAA n-↓ |
| | | Leigh-like | wmd: +/– | Myelin: n-↓ | | wmd: + | Myelin: n | | m: +/– | Myelin: n | | | | Cho n-↓ |
| | | | BG: +/– | Nec: +/– | | D: +/– | Nec: – | | | Nec: – | | | | |
| | | | Thal: +/– | Ca: – | | | Ca: – | | | Ca: – | | | | |
| | | | | CE:? | | | CE:? | | | CE:? | | | | |
| 45.17 | Mitochondrial RNA import protein deficiency | Striatum lesions | BG: + | T2: ↑ | ↓ | n | n | n | n | n | n | ? | – | ? |

(continued)

**Table 8.1** (continued)

| | | | Cerebrum | | | Cerebellum | | | Brainstem | | | | Malformations and | |
|---|---|---|---|---|---|---|---|---|---|---|---|---|---|---|
| Chapter | Disease | Prevailing pattern(s) | Location | Texture | Volume | Location | Texture | Volume | Location | Texture | Volume | Spinal cord | other findings | MRS (ppm) |
| 45.24 | Mitochondrial methionyl-tRNA formyltransferase deficiency | Leigh-like | cortex: n | DWI: +/– | n-↓ | cortex:+/– | DWI: – | n | mb: +/– | DWI: – | n | ? | – | ? |
| | | Multiple scelrosis mimic | wmsc: +/– | T2: ↑ | | wmsc:+/– | T2: n-↑ | | p: +/– | T2: n-↑ | | | | |
| | | | wmd: +/– | Myelin: n | | wmd: n | Myelin: n | | m: +/– | Myelin: n | | | | |
| | | | BG: +/– | Nec: +/– | | D: n | Nec: – | | | Nec: – | | | | |
| | | | Thal: +/– | Ca: – | | | Ca: – | | | Ca: – | | | | |
| | | | | CE: +/– | | | CE: +/– | | | CE: +/– | | | | |
| 45.50–45.71 | Mitochondrial tRNA deficiencies | Leukodystrophy | cortex: +/– | DWI: +/– | n-↓ | cortex: n | DWI: – | n | mb: +/– | DWI: – | n | ? | Optic atrophy +/– | Lactate +/– |
| | | MELAS | wmsc: +/– | T2: n-↑ | | wmsc:+/– | T2: n-↑ | | p: +/– | T2: n-↑ | | | Aneurysms +/– | |
| | | Leigh-like | wmd: +/– | Myelin: n | | wmd: +/– | Myelin: n | | m: +/– | Myelin: n | | | | |
| | | | BG: +/– | Nec: – | | D: +/– | Nec: – | | | Nec: – | | | | |
| | | | Thal: +/– | Ca: +/– | | | Ca: – | | | Ca: – | | | | |
| | | | | CE:? | | | CE:? | | | CE:? | | | | |
| 45.72 | Mitochondrial arginine-tRNA synthetase deficiency (AARS2) | Leukodystrophy, frontal and parietal dominant, relative sparing of frontoparietal junction | cortex: n | DWI: +/– | n-↓↓↓ | n | n | n-↓↓↓ | mb: +/– | DWI: – | n-↓ | ? | – | Cr ↑ |
| | | White matter tract involvement: CC, FP, POP, CST | wmsc: +/– | T2: ↑-↑↑ | | | | | p: +/– | T2: n-↑ | | | | Citrate (2.6) |
| | | | wmd: ++ | Myelin: n-↓ | | | | | m: +/– | Myelin: n | | | | Glycine (3.5) |
| | | | BG: n | Nec: + | | | | | | Nec: – | | | | |
| | | | Thal: n | Ca: – | | | | | | Ca: – | | | | |
| | | | | CE: – | | | | | | CE: – | | | | |
| 45.75 | Mitochondrial aspartyl-tRNA synthetase deficiency (DARS2) | Leukodystrophy, deep cerebrum (+/– PA gradient), CST, ASCT, ML, TGNF, cerebellar peduncles, DC, LCST | cortex: n | DWI: – | n-↓ | cortex: n | DWI: – | n | mb: n | DWI: – | n | Diffuse T2↑ LCT and DC | – | Lactate |
| | | MRS: lactate | wmsc: +/– | T2: ↑↑ | | wmsc: n | T2: ↑-↑↑ | | p: + | T2: ↑ | | | | |
| | | | wmd: ++ | Myelin: n | | wmd: + | Myelin: n | | m: + | Myelin: n | | | | |
| | | | BG: +/– | Nec: +/– | | D: n | Nec: – | | | Nec: – | | | | |
| | | | Thal: n | Ca: – | | | Ca: – | | | Ca: – | | | | |
| | | | | CE:? | | | CE:? | | | CE:? | | | | |

| | | | | | | | | | | | | | | |
|---|---|---|---|---|---|---|---|---|---|---|---|---|---|---|
| 45.77 | Mitochondrial glutamyl-tRNA synthetase deficiency (EARS2) | Leukodystrophy, deep cerebrum, periventricular sparing or hypomyelinating leukodystrophy | cortex: n | DWI: – | n | cortex: n | DWI: – | n | mb: + | DWI: – | n | ? | HCC/CCD +/– | Lactate +/– |
| | | Leigh-like; thalamus, dentate, dorsal BS lesions | wmsc: +/– | T2: ↑-↑↑ | | wmsc: + | T2: ↑ | | p: + | T2: ↑ | | | | |
| | | MRS: lactate | wmd: + | Myelin: ↓ | | wmd: + | Myelin: ↓ | | m: + | Myelin: ↓ | | | | |
| | | HCC | BG: n | Nec: – | | D: ++ | Nec: – | | | Nec: – | | | | |
| | | | Thal: + | Ca: – | | | Ca: – | | | Ca: – | | | | |
| | | | | CE:? | | | CE:? | | | CE:? | | | | |
| 45.85 | Mitochondrial phenylalanyl-tRNA synthetase deficiency (FARS2) | Necrotizing leukodystrophy, cerebrum SCWM | cortex: +/– | DWI: +/– | n-↓↓↓ | cortex: n | DWI: – | n-↓ | mb: n | DWI: + | n | Atrophy +/– | – | Lactate +/– |
| | | | wmsc: ++ | T2: ↑-↑↑↑ | | wmsc: n | T2: ↑ | | p: +/– | T2: n-↑ | | | | |
| | | | wmd: +/– | Myelin: n-↓ | | wmd: + | Myelin: n | | m: n | Myelin: n | | | | |
| | | | BG: n | Nec: + | | D: +/– | Nec: – | | | Nec: – | | | | |
| | | | Thal: +/– | Ca: – | | | Ca: – | | | Ca: – | | | | |
| | | | | CE:? | | | CE:? | | | CE:? | | | | |
| 45.92 | Mitochondrial and cytoplasmic lysyl-tRNA synthetase deficiency (KARS) | Leukodystrophy | cortex: +/– | DWI: – | n-↓↓↓ | cortex: n | DWI: – | n-↓ | mb: +/– | DWI: – | n-↓↓ | Track-like spinal cord calcifications+/– | – | Lactate |
| | | IC calcifications “boomerang sign” | wmsc: +/– | T2: ↑ | | wmsc:+/– | T2: n-↑ | | p: +/– | T2: n-↑ | | DC T2↑ +/– | | |
| | | Track-like spinal cord calcifications | wmd: +/– | Myelin: n-↓ | | wmd: +/– | Myelin: n | | m: +/– | Myelin: n | | | | |
| | | | BG: n | Nec: – | | D: +/– | Nec: – | | | Nec: – | | | | |
| | | | Thal: +/– | Ca: +/– | | | Ca: +/– | | | Ca: +/– | | | | |
| | | | | CE: – | | | CE: – | | | CE: – | | | | |
| 46.2 | Mitochondrial fission factor deficiency | Leigh-like | cortex: n | DWI: +/– | ↓-↓↓ | cortex: n | DWI: – | ↓-↓↓ | mb: +/– | DWI: – | n-↓ | ? | – | ? |
| | | | wmsc: n | T2: ↑-↑↑ | | wmsc: n | T2: n-↑ | | p: n | T2: n-↑ | | | | |
| | | | wmd: +/– | Myelin: n | | wmd: n | Myelin: n | | m: n | Myelin: n | | | | |
| | | | BG: ++ | Nec: + | | D: +/– | Nec: – | | | Nec: – | | | | |
| | | | Thal: +/– | Ca: – | | | Ca: +/– | | | Ca: – | | | | |
| | | | | CE:? | | | CE:? | | | CE:? | | | | |
| 46.3 | GDAP1 deficiency | Deep cerebellar and MCP leukoencephalopathy | n | n | n | wmd: ++ | T2: ↑↑ | ↓ | n | n | n | ? | – | ? |

(continued)

**Table 8.1** (continued)

| Chapter | Disease | Prevailing pattern(s) | Cerebrum Location | Cerebrum Texture | Cerebrum Volume | Cerebellum Location | Cerebellum Texture | Cerebellum Volume | Brainstem Location | Brainstem Texture | Brainstem Volume | Spinal cord | Malformations and other findings | MRS (ppm) |
|---|---|---|---|---|---|---|---|---|---|---|---|---|---|---|
| 46.9 | MSTO1 deficiency | Cerebellar atrophy +/– cortical hyperintensity | cortex: n | DWI: – | n-↓ | cortex:+/– | DWI: – | ↓-↓↓↓ | n | n | n-↓ | ? | – | ? |
| | | | wmsc: n | T2: n-↑ | | wmsc: n | T2: n-↑ | | | | | | | |
| | | | wmd: +/– | Myelin: n | | wmd: n | Myelin: n | | | | | | | |
| | | | BG: n | Nec: – | | D: n | Nec: – | | | | | | | |
| | | | Thal: n | Ca: – | | | Ca: – | | | | | | | |
| | | | | CE:? | | | CE:? | | | | | | | |
| 46.17–46.18 | Mitochondrial processing peptidase alpha or beta deficiency | Cerebellar atrophy +/– cortical hyperintensity | cortex: n | DWI: – | n-↓↓↓ | cortex:+/– | DWI: – | ↓↓-↓↓↓ | n | n | n-↓ | ? | – | Lactate +/– |
| | | Leigh-like | wmsc: n | T2: n-↑ | | wmsc: n | T2: n-↑ | | | | | | | |
| | | | wmd: n | Myelin: n | | wmd: n | Myelin: n | | | | | | | |
| | | | BG: +/– | Nec: – | | D: n | Nec: – | | | | | | | |
| | | | Thal: n | Ca: – | | | Ca: – | | | | | | | |
| | | | | CE:? | | | CE:? | | | | | | | |
| 46.24 | HSP60 deficiency | Hypomyelinating leukodystrophy | cortex: n | DWI: +/– | ↓-↓↓ | cortex: n | DWI: – | n | mb: + | DWI: – | n-↓ | ? | – | ? |
| | | | wmsc: + | T2: ↑ | | wmsc: + | T2: ↑ | | p: + | T2: ↑ | | | | |
| | | | wmd: + | Myelin: ↓ | | wmd: + | Myelin: ↓ | | m: + | Myelin: ↓ | | | | |
| | | | BG: n | Nec: – | | D: n | Nec: – | | | Nec: – | | | | |
| | | | Thal: n | Ca: – | | | Ca: – | | | Ca: – | | | | |
| | | | | CE:? | | | CE:? | | | CE:? | | | | |
| 47.1–47.4; 47.6–47.8 | Primary coenzyme Q10 deficiency | Cerebellar atrophy | cortex: +/– | DWI: +/– | n-↓ | n | n | ↓↓-↓↓↓ | mb: n | DWI: – | n-↓↓ | ? | ACC +/– | ? |
| | | Leigh-like | wmsc: +/– | T2: n-↑ | | | | | p: n | T2: n-↑ | | | | |
| | | MELAS | wmd: +/– | Myelin: n | | | | | m: +/– | Myelin: n | | | | |
| | | | BG: +/– | Nec: – | | | | | | Nec: – | | | | |
| | | | Thal: +/– | Ca: – | | | | | | Ca: – | | | | |
| | | | | CE:? | | | | | | CE:? | | | | |
| 48.1 | Primary carnitine deficiency | Cerebral infarctions | cortex: +/– | DWI: + | n-↓ | cortex: n | DWI: + | n | mb: +/– | DWI: +/– | n | ? | – | ? |
| | | Arterial stenoses | wmsc: + | T2: ↑ | | wmsc:+/– | T2: ↑ | | p: +/– | T2: n-↑ | | | | |
| | | Cerebral white matter intramyelinic edema | wmd: +/– | Myelin: n | | wmd: + | Myelin: n | | m: +/– | Myelin: n | | | | |
| | | Hypoglycemic brain injury pattern | BG: +/– | Nec: – | | D: n | Nec: – | | | Nec: – | | | | |
| | | | Thal: n | Ca: – | | | Ca: – | | | Ca: – | | | | |
| | | | | CE: – | | | CE: – | | | CE: – | | | | |
| 48.2 | Carnitine palmitoyltransferase 1A deficiency | MRS: lipids | n | n | n | n | n | n | n | n | n | ? | – | Lipids ↑ |
| | | | | | | | | | | | | | | NAA ↑ |
| | | | | | | | | | | | | | | Glx ↑ |

| | | | | | | | | | | | | | | |
|---|---|---|---|---|---|---|---|---|---|---|---|---|---|---|
| 48.4 | Carnitine palmitoyltransferase 2 deficiency | MRS: lipids<br>Brain malformations | cortex: +/–<br>wmsc: +/–<br>wmd: +/–<br>BG: n<br>Thal: n | DWI: –<br>T2: n-↑<br>Myelin: n<br>Nec: +/–<br>Ca: +/–<br>CE: – | n-↓ | n | n | n-↓ | n | n | n-↓ | ? | MCD: PMG, dysplasia,heterotopia+/–<br>DWM +/–<br>ACC +/–<br>Vermianhypoplasia+/–<br>Hemorrhages +/–<br>Hydrocephalus +/– | Lipids ↑ |
| 48.5 | Carnitine-acylcarnitine translocase deficiency | Cerebral infarcts<br>Arterial stenoses<br>MRS: lipids | cortex: +/–<br>wmsc: +<br>wmd: +/–<br>BG: +/–<br>Thal: n | DWI: +<br>T2: ↑<br>Myelin: n<br>Nec: –<br>Ca: –<br>CE: – | n-↓ | n | n | n | n | n | n | ? | Arterial stenoses +/– | Lipids ↑ |
| 48.9 | Short-chain acyl-CoA dehydrogenase deficiency | Cavitating leukodystrophy, cerebrum anteroposterior gradient<br>Leigh-like | cortex: +/–<br>wmsc: +/–<br>wmd: +/–<br>BG: +/–<br>Thal: +/– | DWI: +/–<br>T2: ↑<br>Myelin: n<br>Nec: +/–<br>Ca: –<br>CE:? | n-↓↓↓ | cortex: n<br>wmsc: n<br>wmd: +/–<br>D: + | DWI: –<br>T2: ↑<br>Myelin: n<br>Nec: –<br>Ca: –<br>CE:? | n | n | n | n | ? | PMG +/– | ? |
| 48.10 | Medium-chain acyl-CoA dehydrogenase deficiency | Leigh-like | cortex: n<br>wmsc: n<br>wmd: +<br>BG: ++<br>Thal: +/– | DWI: +/–<br>T2: ↑<br>Myelin: n<br>Nec: +/–<br>Ca: –<br>CE:? | n-↓↓ | n | n | n | n | n | n | ? | – | Glx n-↑<br>GABA (1.9) n-↑<br>Cr n-↑<br>MI n-↓ |
| 48.23 | Fatty aldehyde dehydrogenase deficiency (Sjögren-Larsson syndrome) | Leukodystrophy<br>MRS: lipids | cortex: n<br>wmsc: +/–<br>wmd: ++<br>BG: n<br>Thal: n | DWI: –<br>T2: ↑<br>Myelin: n-↓<br>Nec: –<br>Ca: –<br>CE: – | n-↓ | n | n | n | mb: +/–<br>p: +/–<br>m: +/– | DWI: –<br>T2: n-↑<br>Myelin: n<br>Nec: –<br>Ca: –<br>CE: – | n | ? | – | Lipids ↑<br>NAA n-↓<br>MI n-↑<br>Cr n-↑<br>Cho n-↑ |
| 50.3 | Mitochondrial acetoacetyl-CoA thiolase deficiency (β-ketothiolase deficiency) | Leigh-like | cortex: n<br>wmsc: n<br>wmd: n<br>BG: ++<br>Thal: n | DWI: +/–<br>T2: ↑-↑↑↑<br>Myelin: n-↓<br>Nec: +/–<br>Ca: –<br>CE: – | n | n | n | n | n | n | n | ? | – | ? |

(continued)

**Table 8.1** (continued)

| Chapter | Disease | Prevailing pattern(s) | Cerebrum | | | Cerebellum | | | Brainstem | | | Spinal cord | Malformations and other findings | MRS (ppm) |
|---|---|---|---|---|---|---|---|---|---|---|---|---|---|---|
| | | | Location | Texture | Volume | Location | Texture | Volume | Location | Texture | Volume | | | |
| 51.2 | SERAC1 deficiency (MEGDEL syndrome) | Leigh-like; spares posterior putamen "putamen eye sign" | cortex: n | DWI: +/– | n-↓↓↓ | n | n | n | mb: +/– | DWI: – | n | ? | – | ? |
| | | | wmsc: n | T2: ↑-↑↑ | | | | | p: +/– | T2: n-↑ | | | | |
| | | | wmd: n | Myelin: n | | | | | m: +/– | Myelin: n | | | | |
| | | | BG: ++ | Nec: +/– | | | | | | Nec: – | | | | |
| | | | Thal: n | Ca: – | | | | | | Ca: – | | | | |
| | | | | CE: – | | | | | | CE: – | | | | |
| 51.10 | Mitochondrial enoyl-CoA reductase deficiency | Leigh-like | cortex: n | DWI: +/– | n-↓ | n | n | n | n | n | n | ? | – | Lactate |
| | | | wmsc: n | T2: ↑-↑↑↑ | | | | | | | | | | |
| | | | wmd: n | Myelin: n | | | | | | | | | | |
| | | | BG: ++ | Nec: +/– | | | | | | | | | | |
| | | | Thal: n | Ca: – | | | | | | | | | | |
| | | | | CE: – | | | | | | | | | | |
| 51.11 | Very long-chain fatty acid elongase 1 deficiency | Hypomyelinating leukodystrophy, diffuse | cortex: n | DWI: – | n-↓ | cortex: n | DWI: – | n | mb: + | DWI: – | n | ? | – | ? |
| | | | wmsc: + | T2: ↑ | | wmsc: + | T2: ↑ | | p: + | T2: ↑ | | | | |
| | | | wmd: + | Myelin: ↓ | | wmd: + | Myelin: ↓ | | m: + | Myelin: ↓ | | | | |
| | | | BG: n | Nec: – | | D: n | Nec: – | | | Nec: – | | | | |
| | | | Thal: n | Ca: – | | | Ca: – | | | Ca: – | | | | |
| | | | | CE: – | | | CE: – | | | CE: – | | | | |
| 51.30 | Phospholipase A2 group 6 deficiency (INAD) | NBAI, GP +/– STN lesions; "eye of the tiger sign" +/– (usually absent) | cortex: n | DWI: – | n-↓ | cortex:+/– | DWI: – | n-↓↓ | mb: n | DWI: – | n | ? | Clava hypertrophy | ? |
| | | Cerebellar atrophy and cortical hyperintensity | wmsc: n | T2: ↓; n-↑ | | wmsc: n | T2: n-↑ | | p: n | T2: n-↑ | | | | |
| | | Clava hypertrophy | wmd: +/– | Myelin: n | | wmd: n | Myelin: n | | m: +/– | Myelin: n | | | | |
| | | | BG: ++ | Nec: – | | D: n | Nec: – | | | Nec: – | | | | |
| | | | Thal: n | Ca: – | | | Ca: – | | | Ca: – | | | | |
| | | | | CE: – | | | CE: – | | | CE: – | | | | |
| 51.47 | Fatty acid 2-hydroxylase deficiency | Leukodystophy, cerebrum | cortex: n | DWI: – | n-↓ | n | n | n-↓ | n | n | n-↓ | ? | – | ? |
| | | NBAI, GP | wmsc: +/– | T2: ↑-n-↓ | | | | | | | | | | |
| | | | wmd: + | Myelin: n-↓ | | | | | | | | | | |
| | | | BG: + | Nec: – | | | | | | | | | | |
| | | | Thal: n | Ca: – | | | | | | | | | | |
| | | | | CE: – | | | | | | | | | | |

| | | | | | | | | | | | | | | |
|---|---|---|---|---|---|---|---|---|---|---|---|---|---|---|
| 53.8, 53.9 | Sitosterolemia | Spinal and/or cerebellomedullary angle xanthogranulomas | n | n | n | n | n | n | n | n | n | Intradural extramedullary enhancing masses | – | ? |
| 53.17 | Apolipoprotein C2 deficiency | Perivascular, intradural, and vitreous fat deposition | cortex: + | DWI: – | n-↓↓↓ | n | n | n | n | n | n | ? | – | ? |
| | | | wmsc: + | T2: ↑ | | | | | | | | | | |
| | | | wmd: + | T1: ↑ | | | | | | | | | | |
| | | | BG: + | Myelin: n | | | | | | | | | | |
| | | | Thal: + | Nec: – | | | | | | | | | | |
| | | | | Ca: – | | | | | | | | | | |
| | | | | CE: – | | | | | | | | | | |
| 53.26 | Tangier disease | Cerebral infarction | cortex: n | DWI: +/– | n | n | n | n | n | n | n | Cervical cord atrophy | – | ? |
| | | Cervical SC atrophy | wmsc: n | T2: ↑ | | | | | | | | | | |
| | | | wmd: + | Myelin: n | | | | | | | | | | |
| | | | BG: ++ | Nec: – | | | | | | | | | | |
| | | | Thal: n | Ca: – | | | | | | | | | | |
| | | | | CE: – | | | | | | | | | | |
| 54.17 | 7-dehydrocholesterol reductase deficiency (Smith-Lemli-Opitz syndrome) | Midline structural abnormalities | cortex: n | DWI: – | n-↓ | n | n | n-↓ | n | n | n | ? | HPE +/– | Lipids ↑ |
| | | MRS: lipids | wmsc: +/– | T2: n-↑ | | | | | | | | | CSP +/– | Cho ↑ |
| | | | wmd: +/– | Myelin: n | | | | | | | | | ACC/CCD/HCC +/– | |
| | | | BG: +/– | Nec: – | | | | | | | | | AC +/– | |
| | | | Thal: n | Ca: – | | | | | | | | | Vermis hypoplasia +/– | |
| | | | | CE: – | | | | | | | | | Thick TMI +/– | |
| | | | | | | | | | | | | | DWM+/– | |
| | | | | | | | | | | | | | GCT +/– | |
| | | | | | | | | | | | | | Pituitary lipoma +/– | |
| 55.01 | 21-hydroxylase deficiency | Leukoencephalopathy, cerebrum and cerebellum | cortex: +/– | DWI: +/– | n-↓ | cortex: n | DWI: – | n-↓ | n | n | n-↓ | ? | ACC/CCD/HCC +/– | Cho ↓ |
| | | Cerebral infarctions | wmsc: +/– | T2: n-↑↑ | | wmsc:+/– | T2: n-↑ | | | | | | Hippocampal dysgensis or volume loss +/– | |
| | | Midline malformations | wmd: +/– | Myelin: n | | wmd: +/– | Myelin: n | | | | | | Hypothalamic hamartoma +/– | |
| | | | BG: n | Nec: +/– | | D: n | Nec: – | | | | | | Germinoma +/– | |
| | | | Thal: n | Ca: – | | | Ca: – | | | | | | | |
| | | | | CE: – | | | CE: – | | | | | | | |
| 55.28 | X-linked spinal and bulbar muscular atrophy (Kennedy syndrome) | SC hyperintensity and volume loss | n | n | n | n | n | n | n | n | n | Cervical cord T2↑ +/– | Pituitary hyperplasia | |
| | | | | | | | | | | | | Spinal cord atrophy +/– | White matter microstructural defects | |
| 55.29 | Steroid sulfatase deficiency | MCD | n | n | n-↓ | n | n | n-↓ | n | n | n-↓ | ? | PMG +/– | ? |
| | | Olfactory hypoplasia | | | | | | | | | | | Heterotopia +/– | |
| | | | | | | | | | | | | | Olfactoryhypoplasia+/– | |

(continued)

**Table 8.1** (continued)

| | | | Cerebrum | | | Cerebellum | | | Brainstem | | | | | |
|---|---|---|---|---|---|---|---|---|---|---|---|---|---|---|
| Chapter | Disease | Prevailing pattern(s) | Location | Texture | Volume | Location | Texture | Volume | Location | Texture | Volume | Spinal cord | Malformations and other findings | MRS (ppm) |
| 56.5 | Sterol 27-hydroxylase deficiency (cerebrotendinous xanthomatosis) | Dentate calcifications +/– necrosis | cortex: n | DWI: – | n-↓ | cortex: n | DWI: – | n | mb: +/– | DWI: – | n | Lateral and DC T2↑ +/– | – | ? |
| | | Leukoencephalopathy, cerebrum and cerebellum | wmsc: +/– | T2: n-↑ | | wmsc: +/– | T2: ↓-n-↑ | | p: +/– | T2: n-↑ | | | | |
| | | | wmd: +/– | Myelin: n | | wmd: + | Myelin: n | | m: +/– | Myelin: n | | | | |
| | | | BG: n | Nec: – | | D: ++ | Nec: +/– | | | Nec: – | | | | |
| | | | Thal: n | Ca: – | | | Ca: +/– | | | Ca: – | | | | |
| | | | | CE: – | | | CE: – | | | CE: – | | | | |
| 56.7 | α-methylacyl-CoA racemase deficiency | Dentatorubrothalamic tract involvement without HOD | cortex: +/– | DWI: +/– | n-↓ | cortex: n | DWI: – | n-↓ | mb: +/– | DWI: – | n-↓ | ? | – | ? |
| | | | wmsc: +/– | T2: n-↑ | | wmsc: n | T2: n-↑ | | p: +/– | T2: n-↑ | | | | |
| | | | wmd: n | Myelin: n | | wmd: +/– | Myelin: n | | m: n | Myelin: n | | | | |
| | | | BG: n | Nec: – | | D: +/– | Nec: – | | | Nec: – | | | | |
| | | | Thal: +/– | Ca: – | | | Ca: – | | | Ca: – | | | | |
| | | | | CE: – | | | CE: – | | | CE: – | | | | |
| 57.4 | Porphobilinogen deaminase deficiency (acute intermittent porphyria) | PRESS | cortex: +/– | DWI: – | n-↓↓ | cortex: +/– | DWI: +/– | n-↓↓ | n | n | n-↓ | ? | Transientvasospasm+/– | ? |
| | | Leukoencephalopathy, deep cerebrum (IC, CC, BG spared), thalami, and central pons | wmsc: +/– | T2: n-↑ | | wmsc: +/– | T2: n-↑ | | | | | | | |
| | | Cortical infarction | wmd: +/– | Myelin: n | | wmd: n | Myelin: n | | | | | | | |
| | | | BG: n | Nec: – | | D: n | Nec: – | | | | | | | |
| | | | Thal: +/– | Ca: – | | | Ca: – | | | | | | | |
| | | | | CE: +/– | | | CE: – | | | | | | | |
| 59.1 | EPG5 deficiency | ACC/HCC | cortex: n | DWI: – | n-↓ | n | n | n-↓↓↓ | n | n | n-↓↓↓ | ? | ACC/HCC +/– | ? |
| | | MCD | wmsc: n | T2: n-↑ | | | | | | | | | Absent TMI +/– | |
| | | Hypomyelination | wmd: +/– | Myelin: n-↓ | | | | | | | | | PMG +/– | |
| | | | BG: n | Nec: – | | | | | | | | | | |
| | | | Thal: n | Ca: – | | | | | | | | | | |
| | | | | CE:? | | | | | | | | | | |
| 59.2 | WDR45 deficiency (BPAN) | NBAI (SN > GP iron deposition) | cortex: n | DWI: – | n-↓↓↓ | n | n | n | mb: ++ | DWI: – | n-↓ | ? | Hippocampal dysgensis +/– | ? |
| | | T1↑ halo CP/SN | wmsc: n | T2: ↓-↓↓ | | | | | p: n | T2: ↓-↓↓ | | | | |
| | | | wmd: n | Myelin: n-↓ | | | | | m: n | Myelin: n | | | | |
| | | | BG: + | Nec: – | | | | | | Nec: – | | | | |
| | | | Thal: n | Ca: +/– | | | | | | Ca: – | | | | |
| | | | | CE:? | | | | | | CE: – | | | | |

| | | | | | | | | | | | | | | |
|---|---|---|---|---|---|---|---|---|---|---|---|---|---|---|
| 59.22 | Cohen syndrome | Thick CC, microcephaly | n | n | ↓ | n | n | ↓ | n | n | ↓ | ? | Thick CC | ? |
| | | | | | | | | | | | | | Vermis and BS hypoplasia | |
| | | | | | | | | | | | | | PMG +/– | |
| 60.1–60.9; 60.13 | Neuronal ceroid lipofuscinosis | Cerebral and cerebellar atrophy | cortex: n | DWI: – | n-↓↓↓ | cortex: n | DWI: – | ↓-↓↓↓ | n | n | n-↓ | ? | Cerebellarhypoplasia+/– | NAA ↓ |
| | | Thalamic hypointensity | wmsc: n | T2: n-↑ | | wmsc: n | T2: n-↑ | | | | | | | |
| | | | wmd: +/– | Myelin: n | | wmd: n | Myelin: n | | | | | | | |
| | | | BG: n | Nec: – | | D: +/– | Nec: – | | | | | | | |
| | | | Thal: n | Ca: – | | | Ca: – | | | | | | | |
| | | | | CE: – | | | CE: – | | | | | | | |
| 60.17–60.20 | GM1 and/or GM2 gangliosidoses | Thalamic and dentate SA | cortex: n | DWI: – | ↑-n-↓ | cortex: n | DWI: – | n-↓↓↓ | mb: +/ | DWI: – | n | ? | – | MI n-↑ |
| | | | wmsc: n | T2:↑;↓(DGN) | | wmsc: n | T2: n-↑ | | p: +/– | T2: n-↑ | | | | NAA n-↓ |
| | | | wmd: +/– | Myelin: n-↓ | | wmd: +/– | Myelin: n | | m: n | Myelin: n | | | | Cho n-↑ |
| | | | BG: +/– | Nec: – | | D: n | Nec: – | | | Nec: – | | | | |
| | | | Thal: +/– | Ca: +/– | | | Ca: – | | | Ca: – | | | | |
| | | | | CE: – | | | CE: – | | | CE: – | | | | |
| 60.21 | β-galactosylceramidase deficiency (Krabbe disease) | Leukodystrophy, deep cerebrum; PA gradient | cortex: n | DWI: +/– | n-↓ | cortex: n | DWI: – | n | mb: +/– | DWI: – | n | Cauda equina thickening/CE+/– | Optic nerve enlargement +/– | MI ↑ |
| | | CST involvement, corona radiata to cerebral peduncles | wmsc: +/– | T2:↑;↓(thl) | | wmsc: n | T2: n-↑ | | p: +/– | T2: n-↑ | | Atrophy +/– | | NAA n-↓ |
| | | Tigroid white matter signal | wmd: ++ | Myelin: n-↓ | | wmd: +/– | Myelin: n | | m: +/– | Myelin: n | | | | Cho ↓-n-↑ |
| | | Cranial and/or spinal nerve enhancement | BG: +/– | Nec: – | | D(hila):+/– | Nec: – | | | Nec: – | | | | Glu n-↑ |
| | | Deep cerebral mineralization | Thal: +/– | Ca: +/– | | | Ca: – | | | Ca: – | | | | Lactate +/– |
| | | | | CE(CN): +/– | | | CE: – | | | CE: – | | | | |
| 60.22 | Arylsulfatase A deficiency (metachromatic leukodystrophy) | Leukodystrophy, deep cerebral white matter; PA gradient (pediatrics), AP gradient (adults) | cortex: n | DWI: +/– | n-↓↓ | cortex: n | DWI: – | n-↓ | mb: +/– | DWI: – | n-↓ | Cauda equina thickening/ enhancement+/– | Optic nerve enlargement +/– | MI ↑ |
| | | Tigroid white matter signal | wmsc: +/– | T2:↑;↓(thl) | | wmsc: n | T2: n-↑ | | p: +/– | T2: n-↑ | | | | NAA n-↓ |
| | | Cranial and/or spinal nerve enhancement | wmd: ++ | Myelin: n-↓ | | wmd: +/– | Myelin: n | | m: n | Myelin: n | | | | cho n-↑ |
| | | Thalamic hypointensity | BG: n | Nec: – | | D: n | Nec: – | | | Nec: – | | | | Lactate +/– |
| | | | Thal: +/– | Ca: – | | | Ca: – | | | Ca: – | | | | Glu n-↓ |
| | | | | CE(CN): +/– | | | CE: – | | | CE: – | | | | |

(continued)

**Table 8.1** (continued)

| Chapter | Disease | Prevailing pattern(s) | Cerebrum Location | Cerebrum Texture | Cerebrum Volume | Cerebellum Location | Cerebellum Texture | Cerebellum Volume | Brainstem Location | Brainstem Texture | Brainstem Volume | Spinal cord | Malformations and other findings | MRS (ppm) |
|---|---|---|---|---|---|---|---|---|---|---|---|---|---|---|
| 60.24 | α-Galactosidase A deficiency (Fabry disease) | Strokes | cortex: +/– | DWI: +/– | n-↓ | cortex:+/– | DWI: +/– | n-↓ | mb: +/– | DWI: +/– | n-↓ | ? | Vasculopathy | NAA n-↓ |
| | | Leukoencephalopathy | wmsc: + | T2: ↑- ↑↑ | | wmsc:+/– | T2: n-↑ | | p: +/– | T2: n-↑ | | | Basilar artery ectasia | Cho n-↑ |
| | | Pulvinar T1↑ ("pulvinar sign") | wmd: + | T1: n-↑ | | wmd: +/– | Myelin: n | | m: +/– | Myelin: n | | | | |
| | | Microhemorrhages | BG: +/– | Myelin: n | | D: n | Nec: +/– | | | Nec: +/– | | | | |
| | | Basilar ecasia | Thal: +/– | Nec: +/– | | | Ca: – | | | Ca: – | | | | |
| | | | | Ca: +/– | | | CE:? | | | CE: – | | | | |
| | | | | CE:? | | | Hem: +/– | | | Hem: +/– | | | | |
| | | | | Hem: +/– | | | | | | | | | | |
| 60.27, 60.29 | Mucolipin 1 deficiency (mucolipidosis type IV) | Hypomyelination | cortex: n | DWI: – | n-↓↓ | n | n | n-↓↓ | n | n | n-↓↓ | ? | HCC | Cho n-↓ |
| | | Deep cerebral gray nuclei iron deposition | wmsc: +/– | T2: ↓(thl)-n-↑ | | | | | | | | | | |
| | | Hypoplastic corpus callosum | wmd: +/– | Myelin: ↓ | | | | | | | | | | |
| | | | BG: +/– | Nec: – | | | | | | | | | | |
| | | | Thal: +/– | Ca: – | | | | | | | | | | |
| | | | | CE: – | | | | | | | | | | |
| 60.30–60.31 | Niemann-Pick disease type C | Hypomyelination, cerebrum sparing CC and PLIC | cortex: n | DWI: – | n-↓↓ | n | n | n-↓↓↓ | n | n | n | ? | – | Lipids ↑ |
| | | | wmsc: + | T2: ↑ | | | | | | | | | | Cho n-↑ |
| | | | wmd: + | Myelin: ↓ | | | | | | | | | | NAA n-↓ |
| | | | BG: +/– | Nec: – | | | | | | | | | | |
| | | | Thal: n | Ca: – | | | | | | | | | | |
| | | | | CE: – | | | | | | | | | | |
| 60.37 | Cathepsin A deficiency | Leukoencephalopathy, cerebrum, brainstem, and cerebellum | cortex: n | DWI: +/– | n-↓ | cortex: n | DWI: – | n | mb: + | DWI: – | n | ? | – | ? |
| | | | wmsc: +/– | T2: ↑-↑↑ | | wmsc: n | T2: ↑-↑↑ | | p: + | T2:↑-↑↑ | | | | |
| | | | wmd: ++ | Myelin: n | | wmd: + | Myelin: n | | m: n | Myelin: n | | | | |
| | | | BG: + | Nec: – | | D: + | Nec: – | | | Nec: – | | | | |
| | | | Thal: + | Ca: – | | | Ca: – | | | Ca: – | | | | |
| | | | | CE: – | | | CE: – | | | CE: – | | | | |
| | | | | Hem: +/– | | | Hem: – | | | Hem: – | | | | |
| 61.3 | α-mannosidase deficiency | Leukoencephalopathy, cerebrum | cortex: n | DWI: – | n-↓ | n | n | n-↓↓ | n | n | n | Cervicalsyrinx+/– | Cerebellarhypoplasia+/– | Oligosacharides (3.7) |
| | | DGN hypointensity | wmsc: +/– | T2:↓(DGN); n-↑ | | | | | | | | | Skull diploic space thickening | |
| | | MRS: oligosacharides | wmd: +/– | Myelin: n-↓ | | | | | | | | | | |
| | | | BG: +/– | Nec: – | | | | | | | | | | |
| | | | Thal: +/– | Ca: – | | | | | | | | | | |
| | | | | CE: – | | | | | | | | | | |

| | | | | | | | | | | | | | | |
|---|---|---|---|---|---|---|---|---|---|---|---|---|---|---|
| 61.6 | α-fucosidase deficiency (fucosidosis) | Leukonecephalopathy, cerebrum | cortex: n | DWI: – | n-↓↓ | cortex: n | DWI: – | ↑-n-↓ | mb: +/– | DWI: – | n | Dysostosis multiplex | Hypothalamic involvement +/– | Oligosacharides and/or glycolipids (3.8) |
| | | DGN hypointensity | wmsc: +/– | T2:↓(DGN); n-↑ | | wmsc: +/– | T2: n-↑ | | p: n | T2: n-↓ | | | | Fructose (1.2) |
| | | Thalamic and globus pallidus GP internal medullary lamina T2↑ | wmd: +/– | T1(DGN): n-↑ | | wmd: +/– | Myelin: n-↓ | | m: n | Myelin: n-↓ | | | | |
| | | MRS: oligosacharides and fructose | BG: +/– | Myelin: n-↓ | | D: n | Nec: – | | | Nec: – | | | | |
| | | Dysostosis multiplex | Thal: +/– | Nec: – | | | Ca: – | | | Ca: – | | | | |
| | | | | Ca: – | | | CE: – | | | CE: – | | | | |
| | | | | CE: – | | | Hem: – | | | | | | | |
| 61.7 | Aspartylglucosaminidase deficiency | Leukonecephalopathy, cerebrum | cortex: n | DWI: – | n-↓↓↓ | n | n | n-↓↓ | n | n | n-↓↓↓ | ? | – | ? |
| | | DGN hypointensity | wmsc: + | T2:↓(DGN); n-↑ | | | | | | | | | | |
| | | Pulvinar T2↓ | wmd: + | T1(DGN): n-↑ | | | | | | | | | | |
| | | | BG: +/– | Myelin: ↓ | | | | | | | | | | |
| | | | Thal: + | Nec: – | | | | | | | | | | |
| | | | | Ca: – | | | | | | | | | | |
| | | | | CE: – | | | | | | | | | | |
| 61.8 | Sialin deficiency; Infantile sialic acid storage disease (severe); Salla disease (milder) | Hypomyelination, cerebrum +/– cerebellum | cortex: n | DWI: – | n | n | n | n-↓↓ | n | n | n | ? | HCC +/– | NAA n-↑ |
| | | Cerebellar atrophy | wmsc: + | T2:↓(GP); n-↑ | | | | | | | | | | MI n-↑ |
| | | | wmd: + | T1(DGN): n-↑ | | | | | | | | | | Lactate +/– |
| | | | BG: +/– | Myelin: ↓ | | | | | | | | | | |
| | | | Thal: n | Nec: – | | | | | | | | | | |
| | | | | Ca: – | | | | | | | | | | |
| | | | | CE: – | | | | | | | | | | |
| 62.1–62.4, 62.9 | Mucopolysacharidoses I, II, IIIa, IIIb, VI | Enlarged PVS | cortex: n | DWI: – | n-↓↓ | n | n | n-↓ | n | n | n | Dysostosis multiplex | Enlarged PVS | MI n-↑ |
| | | Leukoencephalopathy, cerebrum | wmsc: +/– | T2: n-↑ | | | | | | | | Myleopathy+/– | Hydrocephalus +/– | NAA n-↓ |
| | | Hydrocephalus | wmd: + | Myelin: ↓ | | | | | | | | | MCM +/– | Cho ↓- n-↑ |
| | | Dysostosis multiplex | BG: +/– | Nec: – | | | | | | | | | Sellar malfomation | Glu n-↓ |
| | | | Thal: +/– | Ca: – | | | | | | | | | Chiari I +/– | |
| | | | | CE: – | | | | | | | | | | |
| 64.6 | X-linked adrenoleukodystrophy | Leukodystrophy, deep cerebrum, PA gradient >AP gradient | cortex: n | DWI: +/– | n-↓ | cortex: n | DWI: – | n-↓ | mb: +/– | DWI: – | n | Atrophy +/– | – | Cho n-↑ |
| | | Visual, auditory, and corticospinal tract involvement | wmsc: +/– | T2: ↑- ↑↑ | | wmsc: n | T2: n-↑ | | p: +/– | T2: n-↑ | | | | NAA n-↓ |
| | | CE and/or restricted diffusion in areas of demyelination | wmd: + | Myelin: n-↓ | | wmd: +/– | Myelin: n | | m: +/– | Myelin: n | | | | MI n-↑ |
| | | | BG: +/– | Nec: +/– | | D: n | Nec: – | | | Nec: – | | | | Lactate +/– |
| | | | Thal: n | Ca: +/– | | | Ca: – | | | Ca: – | | | | |
| | | | | CE: +/– | | | CE: – | | | CE: – | | | | |

(continued)

**Table 8.1** (continued)

| Chapter | Disease | Prevailing pattern(s) | Cerebrum | | | Cerebellum | | | Brainstem | | | Spinal cord | Malformations and other findings | MRS (ppm) |
|---|---|---|---|---|---|---|---|---|---|---|---|---|---|---|
| | | | Location | Texture | Volume | Location | Texture | Volume | Location | Texture | Volume | | | |
| 64.13–64.25 | Peroxisomal Biosynthesis disorders | Leukodystrophy, cerebrum (PA gradient or diffuse), brainstem, cerebellum | cortex: n | DWI: – | n-↓↓ | cortex: n | DWI: – | n | mb: +/– | DWI: – | n | ? | MDC; perisylvian polymicrogyria +/– | Lipids n-↑ |
| | | CST, ML, dentatorubrothalamic tract involvement | wmsc: +/– | T2: ↑- ↑↑ | | wmsc: n | T2: ↑ | | p: +/– | T2: n-↑ | | | Germinolytic cysts +/– | NAA ↓ |
| | | | wmd: ++ | Myelin: ↓ | | wmd: + | Myelin: n | | m: +/– | Myelin: n | | | | Cho ↑ |
| | | | BG: n | Nec: – | | D(hilus): + | Nec: – | | | Nec: – | | | | |
| | | | Thal: +/– | Ca: –<br>CE: +/– | | | Ca: –<br>CE: – | | | Ca: –<br>CE: +/– | | | | |
| 64.14 | Peroxin 1 deficiency (Zellwegger Syndrome) | Abnormal myelination | cortex: n | DWI: n | n-↓↓ | cortex: n | DWI: – | n-↓ | n | n | n-↓ | ? | Germinolytic cysts +/– | Lipids n-↑ |
| | | MCD; polymicrogyria, perisylvian | wmsc: + | T2: ↑ | | wmsc: n | T2: n-↑ | | | | | | MDC; perisylvian polymicrogyria or pachygyria +/– | NAA ↓ |
| | | Germinolytic cysts | wmd: + | T1(BG): n-↑ | | wmd: +/– | Myelin: n | | | | | | HCC +/– | Cho ↑ |
| | | | BG: +/– | Myelin: ↓ | | D: n | Nec: – | | | | | | | Lactate +/– |
| | | | Thal: n | Nec: –<br>Ca: –<br>CE: – | | | Ca: –<br>CE: – | | | | | | | |
| 66.29–66.37, 66.40 | Alpha dystroglycanopathies (WWS, MEB, Fukayama muscular dystrophy, etc.) | Variable diffuse brain malformation/ hypoplasia | cortex: + | DWI: n | ↓-↓↓↓ | cortex: + | DWI: – | ↓-↓↓↓ | mb: +/– | DWI: – | ↓-↓↓↓ | ? | MCD; cobblestone complex, PMG, pachygyria, dysplasia | NAA n-↓ |
| | | Cobblestone complex | wmsc: +/– | T2: ↑ | | wmsc: + | T2: ↑ | | p: +/– | T2: n-↑ | | | Cerebellar hypoplasia/ dysplasia +/– cysts | Cho n-↑ |
| | | Brainstem and cerebellum hypoplasia/dysplasia | wmd: + | Myelin: ↓ | | wmd: + | Myelin: n-↓ | | m: +/– | Myelin: n-↓ | | | Brainstem hypoplasia/ dysplasia; Z-shape +/–, AP patterning defects +/–, pontine cleft +/– | |
| | | Z-shaped brainstem, pontine cleft, and/or AP patterning defects | BG: n | Nec: – | | D: n | Nec: – | | | Nec: – | | | CCD +/– | |
| | | Cerebellar cysts | Thal: n | Ca: – | | | Ca: – | | | Ca: – | | | Hydrocephalus +/– | |
| | | Hypomyelination and leukoencephalopathy | | CE: – | | | CE: – | | | CE: +/– | | | Ocularmalformations+/– | |

| | | | | | | | | | | | | | | |
|---|---|---|---|---|---|---|---|---|---|---|---|---|---|---|
| 69.1 | Aspartoacylase deficiency (Canavan disease) | Leukodystrophy, cerebrum (striatum spared, thalamus involved), brainstem, cerebellum; myelin edema, no CE | cortex: n | DWI: +/– | ↑-n-↓↓ | cortex: n | DWI: +/– | ↑-n-↓ | mb: + | DWI: +/– | ↑-n-↓ | ? | Enlarged PVS +/– | NAA ↑ |
| | | MRS: Increased NAA | wmsc: ++ | T2: ↑ | | wmsc: n | T2: ↑ | | p: + | T2: ↑ | | | | Gu n-↑ |
| | | Enlarged PVS ("beaded white matter sign)" +/– | wmd: + | Myelin: ↓ | | wmd: + | Myelin: ↓ | | m: + | Myelin: ↓ | | | | MI n-↑ |
| | | | BG: +/– | Nec: – | | D: + | Nec: – | | | Nec: – | | | | |
| | | | Thal: + | Ca: – | | | Ca: – | | | Ca: – | | | | |
| | | | | CE: – | | | CE: – | | | CE: – | | | | |
| 69.2 | Glutaryl-CoA dehydrogenase deficiency (Glutaric aciduria Type I) | BG lesions initiating in the lentiform nucleus, reduced diffusion in acute lesions | cortex: n | DWI: +/– | n-↓↓ | cortex: n | DWI: – | n | mb: +/– | DWI: – | n | ? | Underopercularization | Glutaric acid (2.1–2.3) |
| | | Underopercularization | wmsc: +/– | T2: ↑ | | wmsc: n | T2: n-↑ | | p: +/– | T2: n-↑ | | | Enlarged MCF fluid spaces | NAA n-↓ |
| | | Enlarged MCF fluid spaces | wmd: +/– | Myelin: n | | wmd: +/– | Myelin: n | | m: +/– | Myelin: n | | | SDH +/– | Cho n-↑ |
| | | MRS: glutaric acid | BG: ++ | Nec: – | | D: +/– | Nec: – | | | Nec: – | | | | Cr n-↓ |
| | | | Thal: +/– | Ca: – | | | Ca: – | | | Ca: – | | | | Lactate +/– |
| | | | | CE: – | | | CE: – | | | CE: – | | | | |
| 69.4 | l-2-hydroxyglutarate dehydrogenase deficiency (L2-hydroxyglutaric aciduria) | Leukodystrophy, cerebrum, centropedal gradient | cortex: +/– | DWI: – | ↑-n-↓↓ | cortex: n | DWI: – | n-↓ | mb: +/– | DWI: – | n | | Cerebral neoplasm +/– | NAA ↓ |
| | | Dentate and basal ganglia lesions | wmsc: ++ | T2: ↑ | | wmsc: n | T2: ↑ | | p: n | T2: n-↑ | | | | MI n-↑ |
| | | MRS: l-2-hydroxyglutaric acid | wmd: +/– | Myelin: n | | wmd: n | Myelin: n | | m: n | Myelin: n | | | | Cho ↓- n-↑ |
| | | | BG: +/– | Nec: +/– | | D: ++ | Nec: +/– | | | Nec: – | | | | Glx n-↑ |
| | | | Thal: +/– | Ca: – | | | Ca: – | | | Ca: – | | | | l-2-hydroxyglutaric acid (2.5) |
| | | | | CE: – | | | CE: – | | | CE: – | | | | Lactate +/– |

*3-HIVA* 3-hydroxyisovaleric acid, *AC* arachnoid cyst, *ACC* agenesis of the corpus callosum, *AP* anteroposterior, *ASCT* anterior spinocerebellar tract, *BCAA* branched-chain amino acids, *BCKA* branched-chain keto-acids, *BG* basal ganglia, *BS* brainstem, *Ca* calcifications, *CC* corpus callosum, *CCD* corpus callosum dysgenesis, *CE* contrast enhancement, *Cho* choline, *CN* cranial nerves, *COW* circle of Willis, *CP* cerebral peduncle, *Cr* Creatine, *CSP* cavum septum pellucidum, *CST* corticospinal tract, *D* dentate nucleus, *DC* dorsal column, *DGN* deep gray nuclei, *DWI* diffusion weighted-imaging signal (increase = restricted/reduced diffusion), *DWM* Dandy-Walker malformation, *FP* frontopontine fibers, *GCT* germ cell tumor, *Gln* glutamine, *Glu* glutamate, *Glx* glutamine and/or glutamate, *GP* globus pallidus, *HCC* hypogenesis of the corpus callosum, *Hem* hemorrhage, *HOD* hypertrophic olivary degeneration, *HPE* holoprosencephaly, *IC* internal capsule, *IVH* intraventricular hemorrhage, *mb* midbrain, *med* medulla, *MEG* megalencephaly, *LCST* lateral cortical spinal tracts, *Leigh-like* Leigh or Leigh-like disease pattern, *MCD* malformation of cortical development, *MCF* middle cranial fossa, *MCM* mega cisterna magna, *MCP* middle cerebellar peduncle(s), *MI* myoinositol, *ML* medial lemniscus, *MRS* proton magnetic resonance spectroscopy, *MTS* mesial temporal sclerosis, *myelin* myelinization, *n* normal, *NAA N*-acetylaspartate, *NBAI* neurodegeneration with brain iron accumulation, *Nec* necrosis, *ppm* parts per million, *NMO* neuromyelitis optica, *OPCH* olivopontocerebellar hypoplasia, *PA* posteroanterior, *PCH* pontocerebellar hypoplasia, *PF* posterior fossa, *PH* pontine hypoplasia, *Phe* phenylalanine, *PLIC* posterior limb internal capsule, *PMG* polymicorgyria, *POP* parieto-occipital pontine fibers, *PVS* perivascular spaces, *PVWM* periventricular white matter, *RST* reticulospinal tract, *SA* unspecified signal abnormality, *SC* spinal cord, *SDH* subdural hemorrhage, *SE* subependymal, *SN* substantia nigra, *STN* subthalamic nucleus, *T1* T1-weighted image signal, *T2* T2-weighted image signal, *Thal* thalamus, *TGNF* trigeminal nerve fibers, *TMI* thalamic massa intermedia, *wm* white matter, *wmsc* subcortical white matter, *wmd* deep white matter,? unknown/no known literature, – absent, +/– may be affected, + almost always affected (+ to +++), ↑ increase in signal, volume, or metabolite (↑-↑↑↑), ↓ decrease in signal, volume, or metabolite (↓-↓↓↓), n-↑ normal to increase in signal, volume, or metabolite (n-↑↑↑), n-↓ normal to decrease in signal, volume or metabolite (n-↓↓↓)

## References

Anderson PJ, Leuzzi V. White matter pathology in phenylketonuria. Mol Genet Metab. 2010;99(Suppl 1):S3–9.

Anghileri E, Bertolino N, Salsano E, Antelmi L, Carpinelli P, Castellotti B, Zucca I, Gellera C, Bisogno R, Caccia C, Cuccarini V. In-vivo brain H1-MR-Spectrocopy identification and quantification of 2-hydroxyglutarate in L-2-Hydroxyglutaric aciduria. Brain Res. 2016;1648(Pt A):506–11.

Autti T, Joensuu R, Aberg L. Decreased T2 signal in the thalami may be a sign of lysosomal storage disease. Neuroradiology. 2007;49(7):571–8.

Barkovich JA, Patay Z. Metabolic, toxic, and autoimmune/inflammatory brain disorders. In: Barkovich AJ, Raybaud C, editors. Pediatric neuroimaging. 6th ed. Philadelphia: Lippincott Williams & Wilkins; 2019.

Bhat M, Prasad C, Bindu PS, Aziz Z, Christopher R, Saini J. Unusual imaging findings in brain and spinal cord in two siblings with maple syrup urine disease. J Neuroimaging. 2013;23(4):540–2.

Bireley WR, Van Hove JL, Gallagher RC, Fenton LZ. Urea cycle disorders: brain MRI and neurological outcome. Pediatr Radiol. 2012;42(4):455–62.

Bluml S, Panigrahy A. MR spectroscopy of pediatric brain disorders. New York: Springer Publishing; 2013.

Brismar J, Brismar G, Gascon G, Ozand P. Canavan disease: CT and MR imaging of the brain. AJNR Am J Neuroradiol. 1990;11(4):805–10.

Cohn RD, Eklund E, Bergner AL, Casella JF, Woods SL, et al. Intracranial hemorrhage as the initial manifestation of a congenital disorder of glycosylation. Pediatrics. 2006;118(2):e514–21.

Dallabona C, Diodato D, Kevelam SH, Haack TB, Wong LJ, et al. Novel (ovario) leukodystrophy related to AARS2 mutations. Neurology. 2014;82(23):2063–71.

Feraco P, Mirabelli-Badenier M, Severino M, Alpigiani MG, Di Rocco M, Biancheri R, Rossi A. The shrunken, bright cerebellum: a characteristic MRI finding in congenital disorders of glycosylation type Ia. AJNR Am J Neuroradiol. 2012;33(11):2062–7.

Fourati H, Ellouze E, Ahmadi M, Chaari D, Kamoun F, Hsairi I, Triki C, Mnif Z. MRI features in 17 patients with l2 hydroxyglutaric aciduria. Eur J Radiol Open. 2016;3:245–50.

Gagliardi D, Mauri E, Magri F, Velardo D, Meneri M, et al. Can intestinal pseudo-obstruction drive recurrent stroke-like episodes in late-onset MELAS syndrome? A case report and review of the literature. Front Neurol. 2019;10:38.

Gropman AL. Patterns of brain injury in inborn errors of metabolism. Semin Pediatr Neurol. 2012;19(4):203–10.

Gropman AL, Seltzer RR, Yudkoff M, Sawyer A, VanMeter J, Fricke ST. 1H MRS allows brain phenotype differentiation in sisters with late onset ornithine transcarbamylase deficiency (OTCD) and discordant clinical presentations. Mol Genet Metab. 2008a;94(1):52–60.

Gropman AL, Fricke ST, Seltzer RR, Hailu A, Adeyemo A, Sawyer A, van Meter J, Gaillard WD, McCarter R, Tuchman M, Batshaw M, Urea Cycle Disorders Consortium. 1H MRS identifies symptomatic and asymptomatic subjects with partial ornithine transcarbamylase deficiency. Mol Genet Metab. 2008b;95(1–2):21–30.

Gungor S, Akinci A, Firat AK, Tabel Y, Alkan A. Neuroimaging findings in hyperargininemia. J Neuroimaging. 2008;18(4):457–62.

Gunz AC, Choong K, Potter M, Miller E. Magnetic resonance imaging findings and neurodevelopmental outcomes in neonates with urea-cycle defects. Int Med Case Rep J. 2013;6:41–8.

Ha JS, Kim TK, Eun BL, Lee HS, Lee KY, Seol HY, Cha SH. Maple syrup urine disease encephalopathy: a follow-up study in the acute stage using diffusion-weighted MRI. Pediatr Radiol. 2004;34(2):163–6.

Harting I, Boy N, Heringer J, Seitz A, Bendszus M, Pouwels PJ, Kolker S. (1)H-MRS in glutaric aciduria type 1: impact of biochemical phenotype and age on the cerebral accumulation of neurotoxic metabolites. J Inherit Metab Dis. 2015;38(5):829–38.

Hayflick SJ, Kurian MA, Hogarth P. Neurodegeneration with brain iron accumulation. Handb Clin Neurol. 2018;147:293–305.

Heindel W, Kugel H, Roth B. Noninvasive detection of increased glycine content by proton MR spectroscopy in the brains of two infants with nonketotic hyperglycinemia. AJNR Am J Neuroradiol. 1993;14(3):629–35.

Helman G, Pacheco-Colon I, Gropman AL. The urea cycle disorders. Semin Neurol. 2014;34(3):341–9.

Herini E, Tsuneishi S, Takada S, Sunarini, Nakamura H. Clinical features of infants with subependymal germinolysis and choroid plexus cysts. Pediatr Int. 2003;45(6):692–6.

Holzbach U, Hanefeld F, Helms G, Hanicke W, Frahm J. Localized proton magnetic resonance spectroscopy of cerebral abnormalities in children with carbohydrate-deficient glycoprotein syndrome. Acta Paediatr. 1995;84(7):781–6.

Ishikawa A, Okayasu T, Miyasak K, Fukushima N, Takase A, Wagatsuma Y. A mild variant case of maple syrup urine disease. No To Hattatsu. 1991;23(1):71–4.

Ito H, Mori K, Sakata M, Naito E, Harada M, Kagami S. Transient left temporal lobe lesion in Menkes disease may influence the generation of tonic spasms. Brain Dev. 2011;33(4):345–8.

Jan W, Zimmerman RA, Wang ZJ, Berry GT, Kaplan PB, Kaye EM. MR diffusion imaging and MR spectroscopy of maple syrup urine disease during acute metabolic decompensation. Neuroradiology. 2003;45(6):393–9.

Kassem H, Wafaie A, Abdelfattah S, Farid T. Leukoencephalopathy with brainstem and spinal cord involvement and lactate elevations (LBSL): assessment of the involved white matter tracts by MRI. Eur J Radiol. 2014;83(1):191–6.

Kono K, Okano Y, Nakayama K, Hase Y, Minamikawa S, Ozawa N, Yokote H, Inoue Y. Diffusion-weighted MR imaging in patients with phenylketonuria: relationship between serum phenylalanine levels and ADC values in cerebral white matter. Radiology. 2005;236(2):630–6.

La Piana R, Uggetti C, Roncarolo F, Vanderver A, Olivieri I, et al. Neuroradiologic patterns and novel imaging findings in Aicardi-Goutieres syndrome. Neurology. 2016;86(1):28–35.

Lange T, Dydak U, Roberts TPL, Rowley HA, Bjeljac M, Boesinger P. Pitfalls in lactate measurements at 3T. AJNR Am J Neuroradiol. 2006;27:895–901.

Li PH, Ma JS, Chi CS, Mak SC. Intermittent form of maple syrup urine disease: report of one case. Zhonghua Min Guo Xiao Er Ke Yi Xue Hui Za Zhi. 1997;38(6):468–71.

Loes DJ, Hite S, Moser H, Stillman AE, Shapiro E, Lockman L, Latchaw RE, Krivit W. AJNR Am J Neuroradiol. 1994;15(9):1761–6.

Manara R, D'Agata L, Rocco MC, Cusmaj R, Freri E, et al. Menkes Working Group in the Italian Neuroimaging Network for Rare Diseases. Neuroimaging changes in Menkes disease, part 1. AJNR Am J Neuroradiol. 2017a;38(10):1850–7.

Manara R, D'Agata L, Rocco MC, Cusmaj R, Freri E, et al. Menkes Working Group in the Italian Neuroimaging Network for Rare Diseases. Neuroimaging changes in Menkes disease, part 2. AJNR Am J Neuroradiol. 2017b;38(10):1858–65.

McAdams HP, Geyer CA, Done SL, Deigh D, Mitchell M, Ghaed VN. CT and MR imaging of Canavan disease. AJNR Am J Neuroradiol. 1990;11(2):397–9.

Muller K, Kahn T, Wendel U. Is demyelination a feature of maple syrup urine disease. Pediatr Neurol. 1993;9(5):375–82.

Munakata M, Sakamoto O, Kitamura T, Ishitobi M, Yokoyama H, et al. The effects of copper-histidine therapy on brain metabolism in a patient with Menkes disease: a proton magnetic resonance spectroscopic study. Brain Dev. 2005;27(4):297–300.

Myers KA, Reeves M, Wei XC, Khan A. Cerebral edema in maple syrup urine disease despite newborn screening diagnosis and early initiation of treatment. JIMD Rep. 2012;3:103–6.

Nguyen HV, Ishak GE. Canavan disease—unusual imaging features in a child with mild clinical presentation. Pediatr Radiol. 2015;45(3):457–60.

Pacheco-Colon I, Fricke S, VanMeter J, Gropman AL. Advances in urea cycle neuroimaging: proceedings from the 4th International Symposium on urea cycle disorders, Barcelona, Spain. Mol Genet Metab. 2013;113(1–2):118–26.

Raymond GV, Moser AB, Fatemi A. X-linked adrenoleukodystrophy. In: Adam MP, Ardinger HH, Pagon RA, Wallace SE, Bean LJH, Stephens K, Amemiya A, editors. GeneReviews® [Internet]. Seattle: University of Washington, Seattle; 1993–2019; 1999. [Updated 2018 Feb 15].

Robertson NJ, Stafler P, Battini R, Cheong J, Tosetti M, Bianchi MC, Cox IJ, Cowan FM, Cioni G. Brain lactic alkalosis in Aicardi-Goutieres syndrome. Neuropediatrics. 2004;35(1):20–6.

Sakai M, Inoue Y, Oba H, Ishiguro A, Sekiguchi K, Tsukune Y, Mitomo M, Nakamura H. Age dependence of diffusion-weighted magnetic resonance imaging findings in maple syrup urine disease encephalopathy. J Comput Assist Tomogr. 2005;29(4):524–7.

Salvan AM, Chabrol B, Lamoureux S, Confort-Gouny S, Cozzone PJ, Vion-Dury J. In vivo brain proton MR spectroscopy in a case of molybdenum cofactor deficiency. Pediatr Radiol. 1999;29(11):846–8.

Samanta D, Ramakrishnaiah R. Recurrent encephalopathy with spinal cord involvement: an atypical manifestation of Aicardi-Goutieres syndrome. Ann Indian Acad Neurol. 2019;22(1):111–5.

Schuierer G, Kurlemann G, Bick U, Stephani U. Molybdenum-cofactor deficiency: CT and MR findings. Neuropediatrics. 1995;26(1):51–4.

Sener RN. Diffusion magnetic resonance imaging in intermediate form of maple syrup urine disease. J Neuroimaging. 2002;12(4):368–70.

Sener RN. Phenylketonuria: diffusion magnetic resonance imaging and proton magnetic resonance spectroscopy. J Comput Assist Tomogr. 2003;27(4):541–3.

Sener RN. Diffusion magnetic resonance imaging patterns in metabolic and toxic brain disorders. Acta Radiol. 2004;45(5):561–70.

Sijens PE, Reijngoud DJ, Soorani-Lunsing RJ, Oudkerk M, van Spronsen FJ. Cerebral 1H MR spectroscopy showing elevation of brain guanidinoacetate in argininosuccinate lyase deficiency. Mol Genet Metab. 2006;88(1):100–2.

Steenweg ME, Ghezzi D, Haack T, Abbink TE, Martinelli D, et al. Leukoencephalopathy with thalamus and brainstem involvement and high lactate 'LTBL' caused by EARS2 mutations. Brain. 2012;135(Pt 5):1387–94.

Stefanits H, Konstantopoulou V, Kuess M, Milenkovic I, Matula C. Initial diagnosis of the congenital disorder of glycosylation PMM2-CDG (CDG1a) n a 4-year-old girl after neurosurgical intervention for cerebral hemorrhage. J Neurosurg Pediatr. 2014;14(5):546–9.

Stence NV, Coughlin CR, Fenton LZ, Thomas JA. Distinctive pattern of restricted diffusion in a neonate with molybdenum cofactor deficiency. Pediatr Radiol. 2013;43(7):882–5.

Stence NV, Fenton LZ, Levek C, Tong S, Coughlin CR 2nd, Hennermann JB, Wortmann SB, Van Hove JLK. Brain imaging in classic nonketotic hyperglycinemia: quantitative analysis and relation to phenotype. J Inherit Metab Dis. 2019;42(3):438–50.

Takanashi J, Barkovich AJ, Cheng SF, Weisiger K, Zlatunich CO, Mudge C, Rosenthal P, Tuchman M, Packman S. Brain MR imaging in neonatal hyperammonemic encephalopathy resulting from proximal urea cycle disorders. AJNR Am J Neuroradiol. 2003;24(6):1184–7.

Takeuchi M, Harada M, Hisaoka S, Nishitani H, Mori K, Sakama M. Magnetic resonance imaging and proton MR spectroscopy of the brain in a patient with carbohydrate-deficient glycoprotein syndrome type I. J Magn Reson Imaging. 2003;17(6):722–5.

Terek D, Koroglu O, Yalaz M, Gokben S, Calli C, Coker M, Kultursay N. Diagnostic tools of early brain disturbances in an asymptomatic neonate with maple syrup urine disease. Neuropediatrics. 2013;44(4):208–12.

Thorburn DR, Rahman J, Rahman S. In: Adam MP, Ardinger HH, Pagon RA, Wallace SE, Bean LJH, Stephens K, Amemiya A, editors. Mitochondrial DNA-associated Leigh syndrome and NARP. GeneReviews® [Internet]. Seattle: University of Washington, Seattle; 1993–2019; 2003. [Updated 2017 Sept 28].

Toft PB, Geiss-Holtorff R, Rolland MO, Pryds O, Muller-Forell W, et al. Magnetic resonance imaging in juvenile Canavan disease. Eur J Pediatr. 1993;152(9):750–3.

van der Knaap MS, Bugiani M. Leukodystrophies: a proposed classification system based on pathologic changes and pathogenetic mechanisms. Acta Neuropathol. 2017;134(3):351–82.

Vanderver A, Prust M, Kadom N, Demarest S, Crow YJ, et al. Early-onset Aicardi-Goutieres syndrome: magnetic resonance imaging (MRI) patterns recognition. J Child Neurol. 2015;30(10):1343–8.

Wei SH, Weng WC, Lee NC, Hwu WL, Lee WT. Unusual spinal cord lesions in late-onset non-ketotic hyperglycinemia. J Child Neurol. 2011;26(7):900–3.

Whitehead MT, Gropman AL. Other metabolic syndromes. In: Lewis J, Keshari K, editors. Imaging and metabolism. Cham: Springer; 2018.

Whitehead MT, Fricke ST, Gropman AL. Structural brain defects. Clin Perinatol. 2015;42(2):337–361, ix.

Whitehead MT, Lee B, Gropman A. Lesional perfusion abnormalities in Leigh disease demonstrated by arterial spin labeling correlate with disease activity. Pediatr Radiol. 2016;46(9):1309–16.

Whitehead MT, Wien M, Lee B, Bass N, Gropman A. Black toenail sign in MELAS syndrome. Pediatr Neurol. 2017a;75:61–5.

Whitehead MT, Wien M, Lee B, Bass N, Gropman A. Cortical venous disease severity in MELAS syndrome correlates with brain lesion development. Neuroradiology. 2017b;59(8):813–8.

Zafeiriou DI, Batzios SP. Brain and spinal MR imaging findings in mucopolysacharidoses: a review. AJNR Am J Neuroradiol. 2013;34(1):5–13.

# Genomic Approaches for the Diagnosis of Inborn Errors of Metabolism

9

Sarah L. Stenton, Johannes A. Mayr, Saskia B. Wortmann, and Holger Prokisch

## Contents




S. L. Stenton · H. Prokisch (✉)
Institute of Human Genetics, Technische Universität München, Munich, Germany

Institute of Neurogenomics, Helmholtz Zentrum München, Munich, Germany
e-mail: sarah.stenton@helmholtz-muenchen.de; prokisch@helmholtz-muenchen.de

J. A. Mayr
University Children's Hospital, Paracelsus Medical University, Salzburg, Austria
e-mail: h.mayr@salk.at

S. B. Wortmann
Institute of Human Genetics, Technische Universität München, Munich, Germany

Institute of Neurogenomics, Helmholtz Zentrum München, Munich, Germany

University Children's Hospital, Paracelsus Medical University, Salzburg, Austria
e-mail: saskia.wortmann@helmholtz-muenchen.de




N. Blau et al. (eds.), *Physician's Guide to the Diagnosis, Treatment, and Follow-Up of Inherited Metabolic Diseases*,
https://doi.org/10.1007/978-3-030-67727-5_9

**Summary**

The implementation of whole-exome sequencing (WES) in molecular diagnostics has resulted in increased understanding of the genetic basis of inborn errors of metabolism (IEM) and genotype-phenotype relationships. As a consequence, there has been acceleration in the implementation of genomics in clinical medicine. Though whole-genome sequencing (WGS) is not yet well established in routine clinical practice, increasing evidence of clinical validity and utility is moving WGS towards integration in the near future.

## Introduction

Inborn errors of metabolism (IEM) are a heterogeneous group of more than 1000 genetic disorders, where genetic variation leads to deficient activity of an enzyme or structural protein involved in a cellular biochemical pathway, resulting in one or a combination of energy deficiency, intolerably low essential products, and toxic substance accumulation (Ferreira et al. 2019). Mutations in a growing number of more than 900 nuclear encoded genes and 37 mitochondrial DNA (mtDNA) encoded genes are known to cause IEM, with further novel disease causative genes recognised year on year (Ferreira et al. 2019; Schlieben and Prokisch 2020; Gusic and Prokisch 2021). The increase in our knowledge of the genetic landscape of IEM is predominantly due to the advent of the unbiased genomic approaches: whole-exome sequencing (WES) and whole-genome sequencing (WGS).

Querying genome-wide, for rare variants predicted to be damaging, allows a swift and precise diagnosis to be pursued. This is of great importance: firstly, in establishing the genetic aetiology and inheritance pattern of the disease, which in turn informs genetic counselling, provides insight into the prognosis, allows estimation of the recurrence risk, and informs future family planning; secondly, in circumventing the need for invasive diagnostic procedures, such as a muscle biopsy; and thirdly, in allowing initiation of personalised disease surveillance for genotype-specific complications and exploration of defect-specific treatment options (Ouwehand 2019; Distelmaier et al. 2016).

### "Functional and Metabolite Tests First"

The routine diagnostic workup in IEM includes biochemical and metabolic investigations of the blood, urine, and cerebrospinal fluid (CSF), enzyme analyses, radiological investigations such as magnetic resonance imaging (MRI) of the brain, electroencephalography (EEG), and where appropriate invasive muscle biopsy or biopsy of the affected organ for biochemical and histochemical study. Having formed a clearer picture of the patient's disease manifestation, these investigations have conventionally informed the decision on which individual candidate gene(s) to test via Sanger sequencing. This diagnostic workup can encompass consultations with multiple medical specialists and is referred to as a "diagnostic odyssey" (Vissers et al. 2017). Moreover, despite all efforts, it can result in an inconclusive outcome. The diagnostic yield of each individual test is low, leaving ample room for improvement.

### Challenges in the Diagnosis of IEM

The IEM disease subsets can be encoded by a single gene to vast collections of genes (Fig. 9.1) (Ferreira et al. 2019). The largest subsets of disease are the congenital disorders of glycosylation (CDG), accounting for over 10% of IEM, where more than 75 genes are involved, and mitochondrial diseases, accounting for over 30% of IEM, where variants in more than 300 genes, represented within 24 disease subsets in Fig. 9.1, result in defects in energy production at the mitochondrial level, rarely with defect-specific biomarkers (Stenton and Prokisch 2018; Ferreira et al. 2019). Given that no single gene accounts for more than a few per cent of IEM as a whole, the conventional gene-by-gene approach to diagnosis in the "functional and metabolite tests first" approach is often laborious, expensive, and time-consuming.

Furthermore, the genetic heterogeneity in IEM is mirrored by phenotypic heterogeneity. IEM manifest with a broad range of phenotypes from non-specific global developmental delay to acute decompensation and premature death with multi-organ failure and severe metabolic acidosis. The clinical phenotype and metabolic profile can vary within individual genetic defects, and conversely, with the exception of a small number of IEM, such as in phenylketonuria (PKU), one clinical phenotype can result from a vast number of different genetic defects, such as in Leigh syndrome, a clinical presentation due to defects in over 75 different disease genes (Lake et al. 2016). Though clinical criteria are established to assist in their diagnosis, misdiagnosis and delayed diagnosis in IEM are commonplace, predisposing to irreversible organ damage and early demise.

Due to their heterogeneity, the vast number of different diseases involved, and the capability to prove a genetic diagnosis, IEM are most effectively characterised by the underlying genetic defect (Wanders et al. 2019). This paves the way for the successful application of genomic sequencing (WES and WGS) as the first-tier diagnostic test, to provide a conclusive genetic diagnosis without incurring higher costs (Farnaes et al. 2018; Vissers et al. 2017 Tan et al. 2017).

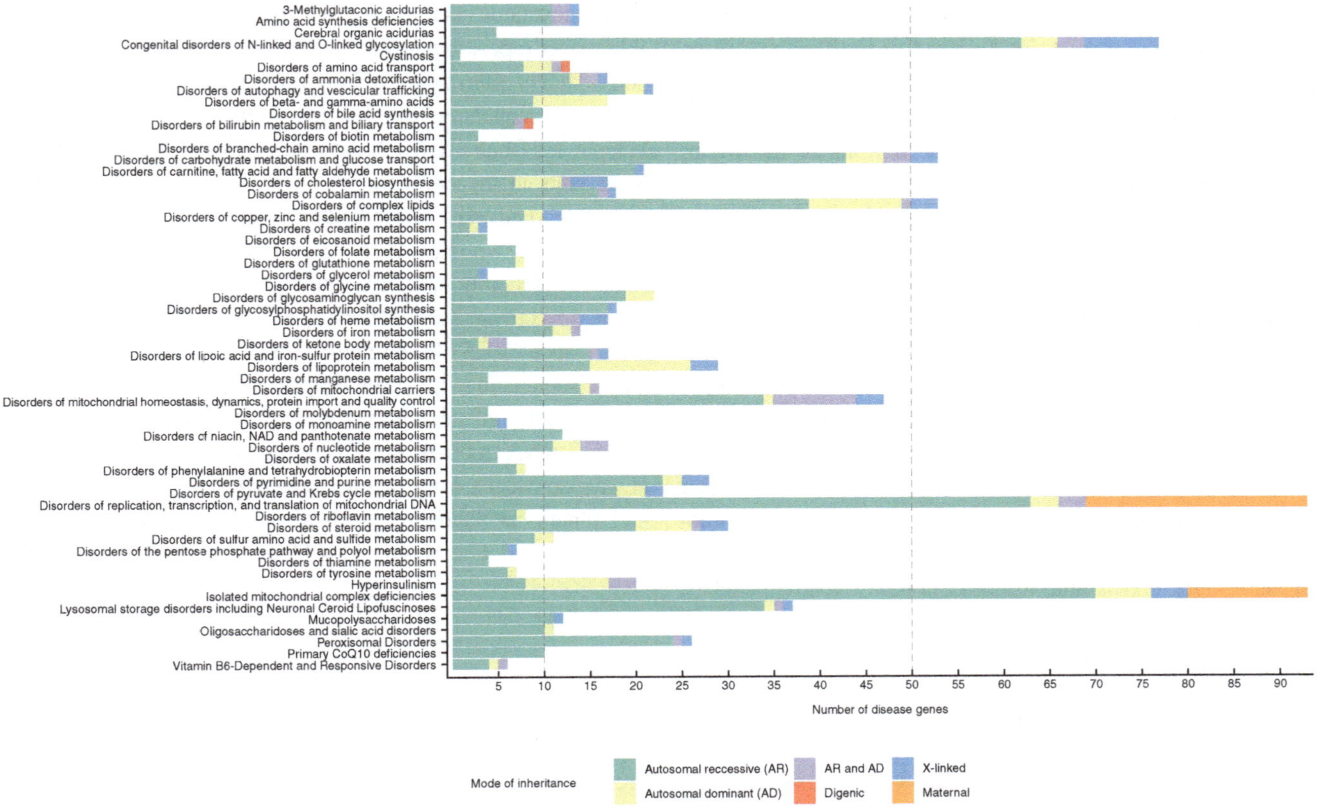


**Fig. 9.1** IEM is an umbrella term for subsets of disease encoded by a single gene to vast collections of genes. The number of genes, and mode of inheritance by gene, per disease subset is depicted

### "Genetics First"

Next-generation sequencing (NGS) is a term encompassing technologies for the rapid sequencing of a large number of DNA segments, up to and including the entire exome (WES) and genome (WGS). At the beginning of the NGS era, a full low-pass genome with low coverage and a base error rate of around 1% would cost 20,000 Euro. However, in recent years, this price has decreased tenfold, allowing a high-coverage genome to be sequenced for around 1–2000 Euro with a base error rate lower than 0.1%. Given the rapidly decreasing costs, we foresee WES and WGS reaching the affordable level of just a few 100 Euro in the near future.

WES and WGS have an immense advantage over other genetic investigations, by providing one assay for all genetic diseases, with the potential to be automated from collection of the blood sample to genotype. Digital phenotyping allows further automated support in variant interpretation by the integration of available genotype-phenotype associations. By sequencing genome-wide, these approaches maintain the power to detect the underlying variants in genes not known to be associated with IEM, however presenting clinically as such, in known disease genes where the patient is presenting atypically, and in novel disease genes. This is helpful in bridging the diagnostic gap left by candidate gene sequencing by eliminating the need for a priori assumptions (Stenton and Prokisch 2020). Therefore, with the exception of a strong genotype-phenotype correlation, which can suitably direct selection of a candidate gene(s) for sequencing or where the gene panel of interest is small and the diagnostic rate high (Fig. 9.1), genome-wide sequencing is in many ways the diagnosis tool of choice.

The ever-increasing availability and decreasing cost have led to the adoption of NGS in clinical laboratories. These tests can be divided into two fundamentally different approaches: the unbiased techniques of WES and WGS and the targeted technique of gene panels. In the setting of IEM, the advantage of these approaches has been illustrated by achieving diagnostic yields of around 45% and subsequently enabling change in management in over 30% of cases (Tarailo-Graovac et al. 2016).

## Whole-Exome Sequencing (WES) and Whole-Genome Sequencing (WGS)

### Whole-Exome Sequencing

WES describes sequencing of the protein-coding regions of the genome, the exons. Exons account for ~2% of the genome. These protein-coding regions are the most likely components of the genome to contain mutations resulting in a clinical phenotype and are reported to harbour ~85% of known monogenic disease-causing mutations. In a standard WES protocol, over 95% of bases are covered reliably on average at least 20 times, with some regions of far higher coverage (Van Hout et al. 2019). This is in the range of sensitivity achieved by Sanger sequencing.

### Whole-Genome Sequencing

WGS describes sequencing of the entire genome, providing a comprehensive overview of all variants in the coding and non-coding regions. The principal advantages and limitations of WGS are displayed in Table 9.1. Technically, WGS has higher sensitivity than WES for certain coding variants, indels, chromosomal rearrangements, copy number variants, and short-tandem repeats (STR), and is able to detect complex rearrangements, such as inversions and transposons. It is however unable to reliably detect repeat expansions, some insertions, and some deletions. This is a limitation of WGS which may be overcome by long-read sequencing in the near future (Ouwehand 2019; Valente and Bhatia 2018). Moreover, WGS enables the detection of variants in the non-coding regions such as regulatory and intronic variants. Our understanding of the non-coding regions is incomplete in comparison to the protein-coding regions, which results in difficulty in interpretation of the detected variants. To further investigate and functionally validate variants of uncertain significance (VUS) in the non-coding regions, transcriptomics (RNA sequencing) has been employed (please see Sect. 9.6). Theoretically, all laboratories with NGS established can also provide RNA sequencing. Therefore, it is recommended to always consider taking biological samples for RNA extraction and functional validation, such as a skin biopsy to establish a fibroblast cell line, when taking blood samples from patients.

**Table 9.1** The principal advantages and limitations of whole-genome sequencing (WGS)

| | Advantages | Limitations and requirements |
|---|---|---|
| Comprehensive | WGS (and WES) analysis provide knowledge of all variants in all genes; therefore we learn about allele frequency of all (non) pathogenic variation<br>If the patient does not have an IEM the diagnosis can still be found<br>All medically actionable genes can be investigated<br>There is complete capture of the mtDNA.<br>Aggregated genome-wide data will allow the search for modifiers in regulatory regions in the affected gene in addition to other genes | WES is limited to the detection of pathogenic intronic variants close to the exon-intron boundaries<br>The coverage of mtDNA is lower than for targeted mtDNA sequencing<br>The more comprehensive the assay, the more variants of uncertain significance (VUS) are detected.<br>With functional follow-up studies, the diagnostic yield but also the workload is increasing |
| Time | Provides one assay for all genetic diseases and allows automation from blood to genotype<br>While WES requires enrichment of the target region, WGS can be undertaken in <50 h and even <21 h which is faster than Sanger sequencing (Clark et al. 2019; Saunders et al. 2012)<br>WGS can meet the need for an urgent diagnosis, for treatment initiation, and for optimisation | High computational power and storage is required in the analysis of the vast amount of data generated<br>While finding the clear diagnosis may save considerable time and effort, the time for clinical interpretation will increase with the number of candidate genes |
| Technical | PCR-free genome amplifies GC-rich regions which are problematic in Sanger, WES, and gene panel approaches<br>WGS has higher sensitivity than WES and gene panels for certain coding variants, indels, copy number variants, and chromosomal rearrangements, and can define breakpoints | Currently repeat expansions and certain indels are not detected reliably |
| Cost | The cost of WES/WGS is rapidly decreasing and may reach a few 100 Euro in the near future<br>WES/WGS is cost-effective as it reduces the number of other investigations needed in the diagnostic workup | There are barriers to funding WES, WGS, and RNA sequencing which are currently rarely covered by health insurance |
| Availability | WGS is gradually becoming more accessible, including through national programmes such as Genomics England (Turnbull 2018) and Genomic Medicine France (Lethimonnier and Levy 2018) | WGS is established in very few centres to date |
| Automation and reanalysis | Potential to automate workflow, such as in prioritisation of genes for manual curation<br>Reanalysis of negative cases periodically, with increasing bioinformatic capabilities and genetic discoveries implicating novel genes in IEM, can reach a conclusive diagnosis in an additional 15% of cases (Nambot et al. 2018) | Assays for functional validation of variants of uncertain significance (VUS) are rarely established or are only established for a specific subset of diseases in diagnostic genetic departments<br>A global registry and funding for functional validation of specific genetic defects is missing |

## Targeted Gene Panel Sequencing

Gene panels allow the targeted sequencing of a selection of genes specific to suspected disease. The panels vary in size and selection of genes, based on the choices of the individual lab. Panels can be custom designed or a commercially available panel can be chosen. If variants in a small number of genes explain nearly all cases in a disease subset (Fig. 9.1), panel sequencing is a cost-effective strategy. When optimised, gene panels cover 100% of the targeted regions and provide the highest sensitivity for variant detection within those regions.

The diagnostic success of a gene panel is subject to the selection of genes and to the stringency of patient selection, such as paediatric, biochemically confirmed cases in suspected mitochondrial disease. In IEM, published gene panels achieve diagnostic rates of 10–50% (Ponzi et al. 2018; Legati et al. 2016; DaRe et al. 2013). Phenotypic mimicry is of particular importance in large heterogenous IEM subsets such as congenital disorder of glycosylation (CDG) and mitochondrial disease, where the diagnosis might fall outside of the genes captured, allowing the diagnosis to evade detection. Furthermore, the shelf-life of the gene panel is limited, and as the molecular genetic underpinning of the disease group is further elucidated, it becomes nearly impossible to keep up-to-date.

An intermediate option between targeted gene panel sequencing and WES or WGS, or an initial step in exome investigation, is the virtual gene panel. Here, WES or WGS data is filtered to focus the analysis to a virtual panel of genes. This approach, however, combines the disadvantages of both the panel and WES or WGS approaches concerning comprehensibility and sensitivity (coverage), respectively, and is restricted to known disease genes selected according to the clinical presentation. However, it has the advantage of reduced time needed for the clinical interpreation.

## Variant Calling

The development of WES and WGS has been reflected by a synergistic improvement of bioinformatic pipelines in terms of sequence alignment and variant calling capabilities. Sequencing reads are aligned to the reference genome in order to call variants encompassing single-nucleotide variants (SNV), deletions, insertions, and copy number variants (CNV), in addition to structural variants such as translocations and inversions (Fig. 9.2) (Pfundt et al. 2017). Around 80% of known pathogenic variants are missense, stop gain, stop loss, and small insertions or deletions, all well covered with current sequencing approaches. Larger deletions and variants affecting splicing (accounting for ~15% of pathogenic variants) are more difficult to detect and can be missed by exon-based methods. Complex rearrangements and repeat variations are more likely to be discovered by WGS than any other sequencing method. Disease variation database are therefore biased by exon targetted methods.

WES reveals an estimated 50,000 variants per individual, of which 20,000 are coding variants (Van Hout et al. 2019; Kremer et al. 2017). Of these variants, 9000 are predicted to alter the protein, 400–500 of which are rare with a minor allele frequency (MAF) <1% (Van Hout et al. 2019; Kremer et al. 2017). As an expected consequence of expanding the genomic space sampled, WGS reveals an estimated 3–5 million variants per individual, 30,000 of which are rare and predominantly non-exomic (Ouwehand 2019). With such vast numbers of intronic variants called in WGS, variant prioritisation to distinguish pathogenic and clinically relevant variants from benign variants present in the healthy individual becomes the primary challenge without the availability of complementary functional data (Fig. 9.3).

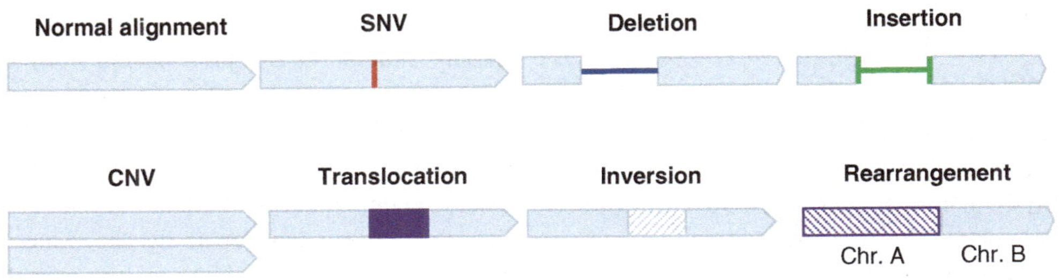


Fig. 9.2 Once aligned to the reference genome, sequencing reads are used to analyse genomic sequence and copy number to call variants. These variants encompass single-nucleotide variants (SNV), deletions, insertions, copy number variants (CNV), and structural variants such as translocations, inversions, and chromosome rearrangements

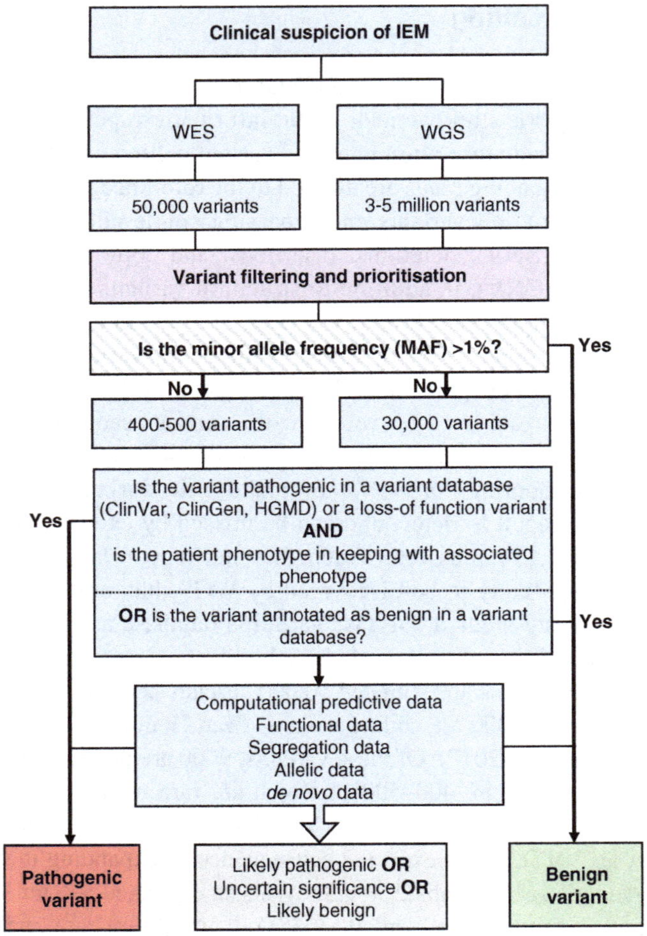


**Fig. 9.3** Variants called from whole-exome sequencing (WES) and whole-genome sequencing (WGS) are filtered and prioritised. A minor allele frequency (MAF) filter of >1% removes the vast majority of variants from the analysis as presumably benign. Variants with known pathogenic status and in keeping with the patient's phenotype or variants with known benign status in variant databases such as ClinVar, ClinGen, and HGMD can be identified and prioritised accordingly. The remaining variants require further exploration to determine pathogenicity. These steps allow allocation of variant pathogenicity to the classification benign (class 1), likely benign (class 2), uncertain significance (class 3), likely pathogenic (class 4), and pathogenic (class 5)

**mtDNA Sequencing**

mtDNA is a circular genome of 16.5 kb encoding two rRNAs, 22 tRNAs, and 13 polypeptides. Disease-causing variation in the mtDNA encompasses copy number alterations (mtDNA depletion, single or multiple mtDNA deletion(s)) and mtDNA point mutations. Sanger sequencing or targeted massive parallel sequencing of mtDNA (mtDNA-NGS) can be applied in detection of such variants, and long-range PCR can be applied for deletions with Southern blot for quantification, as a first-line approach in clinically suspected mitochondrial disease cases.

The extraction and annotation of the mitochondrial genome from WES is now recognised as a highly precise method for the discovery of variants in mtDNA-encoded disease genes, reducing the cost and duration of investigating both the nuclear and mtDNA by separate methods (Wagner et al. 2019; Griffin et al. 2014; Diroma et al. 2014). The validity of this approach has been investigated by direct comparison of WES with both complete mtDNA Sanger sequencing and the gold standard targeted mtDNA-NGS, showing high sensitivity and precision (96.2% and 99.5%, respectively). This implies that WES can be reliably used in the diagnostic setting as a single test to identify pathogenic variants in both nuclear DNA-encoded and mtDNA-encoded genes. The naturally high abundance of the mtDNA molecules (100–10,000) in each cell allows the off-target capture of mtDNA variants as contaminants together with the reliable quantification of mitochondrial heteroplasmy, crucial for the clinical interpretation of mtDNA variants.

Tissue specificity plays an important role in the discovery of mtDNA variants. The absence of pathogenic mtDNA mutations in WES from DNA derived from peripheral blood does not exclude the possibility of a pathogenic mtDNA point mutation in the primary affected tissue such as skeletal muscle, together with somatic mutations. This argues in favour of conducting WES analysis on DNA extracted from the clinically affected tissue. Furthermore, single and multiple deletions and depletion of the mtDNA are problematic to detect by WES. It therefore remains inferior to targeted mtDNA-NGS of affected (and other) tissues.

## Variant Prioritisation

Variant annotation and prioritisation play a central role in clinical sequencing (Fig. 9.3). Prioritisation is defined as the process of determining which of the called variants have the potential to damage function and manifest with the patient's disease phenotype. Comprehensive, clearly structured guidelines have been developed by the American College of Medical Genetics (ACMG), a workgroup formed with the goal of ensuring unambiguous designation of variant pathogenicity status, for the interpretation of genetic variants (Richards et al. 2015). The objective framework allows classification of variants into a five-tier system: "pathogenic", "likely pathogenic", "uncertain significance", "likely benign", and "benign". This designation takes into consideration population, computational and predictive, functional, segregation, de novo, and allelic data, amongst others. Of note, WES and WGS, as holistic approaches, also include copy number variant (CNV) analysis.

To optimise analysis, WES and WGS should ideally be carried out by familial "trio" sequencing, by sequencing the parents of the affected individual, for the following reasons: (1) trio sequencing provides quality control, for example, in sample swapping, (2) it provides validation of variants seen in the affected individual, (3) it allows phasing of variants and ensures the variants segregate with the phenotype in the family, (4) mtDNA variants can be contextualised by comparison to the mutational load in the mother, and (5) autosomal dominant (AD) and de novo variants can be detected. As a consequence, it significantly improves the diagnostic rate (Clark et al. 2018). Together, these advantages argue for "trio" sequencing as a cost-effective approach. Of note, though "trio" sequencing allows optimal analysis, AD and de novo variants can be prioritised also in "index-only" WES by consideration of the pLI score, a score indicating the probability that a gene is intolerant to loss-of-function, and common prediction algorithms.

Most benign variants are easily identified by allele frequency. A minor allele frequency (MAF) >1% accounts for the vast majority of called variants which are presumably common benign polymorphisms (Van Hout et al. 2019). Filtering by MAF keeps only rare variants, statistically more likely to be pathogenic in nature. The frequency of the disease determines the selection of the MAF threshold. Assuming complete penetrance, everything above this threshold is designated as benign. MAF data is readily available in population variation databases such as the Exome Aggregation Consortium (ExAC) database (exac.broadinstitute.org), containing the sequence data of over 60,000 individuals, and the Genome Aggregation Database (gnomAD) (gnomad.broadinstitute.org), containing over 125,000 exomes and 15,000 genomes. ExAC and gnomAD provide information on allele frequency from the general "healthy" population. However, these individuals may be presymptomatic of a disease at the time of inclusion, and indeed almost 3% of the ExAC population has been found to carry "likely pathogenic" or "pathogenic" variants reported in ClinVar (Tarailo-Graovac et al. 2017). Presence of a variant in this database does not therefore automatically exclude it as pathogenic.

Pathogenic variants can be identified as those confirmed to be disease-causing in curated databases, such as ClinVar (ncbi.nlm.nih.gov/clinvar), ClinGen (clinicalgenome.org), and HGMD (hgmd.cf.ac.uk), and those which are loss-of-function in nature, identified within a known disease gene, and in keeping with the patient's clinical phenotype. Loss-of-function variants encompass (1) nonsense variants, where a single-nucleotide variant introduces a premature stop codon; (2) splice-site variants, disrupting the canonical splicing of the gene; and (3) frameshift variants, insertions or deletions involving a number of base pairs that are not a multiple of three, consequently disrupting the reading frame of the coding sequencing and often resulting in a truncated protein due to introduction of a premature stop codon. However, not all annotations are correct, and not all protein truncation variants cause loss-of-function. These variants therefore still need clinical interpretation and in certain cases functional validation.

For all other variants, interpretation of pathogenicity is more challenging and is managed by enforcing a number of criteria. The challenge is referred to as identifying the "needle in the haystack" and requires the expertise of, and discussion amongst, medical physicians, geneticists, and bioinformaticians. The resultant evidence must be considered in aggregate in the context of the patient's phenotype to make a clinical assertion. The analysis can be guided by metabolic profiles, clinical signs and symptoms, the identification of one established pathogenic variant in a recessive disorder, or a candidate gene list.

Computational and predictive data arises from in silico tools developed to predict the potential impact of a variant on the protein. These tools can predict the following:

1. Whether a missense variant, a single-nucleotide variant changing the encoded amino acid, is damaging to the resultant protein function or structure (this depends on criteria such as evolutionary conservation, location within the protein sequence, and consequence of the amino acid substitution); such in silico prediction tools include VEP, CADD, MutationTaster2, PolyPhen-2, and SIFT.
2. Whether the variant has an effect on splicing (given that these predictions are highly sensitive and poorly specific, they result in a high number of false-positive and should be interpreted with caution and in combination).

There is currently no single point of contact for comprehensive functional data on all genetic variants. Functional validation provides evidence for pathogenicity of variants and helps to delineate novel pathways underlying disease, providing a basis for the development of novel defect-specific therapy (Distelmaier et al. 2016). In the field of inborn errors of metabolism (IEM), the underlying pathophysiology is often measurable in the metabolome and on the cellular level giving rise to many possibilities for functional validation, such as to be modelled in vitro in personalised and patient-derived cellular model and in vivo in a wide range of animal models. Furthermore, when validating variants in a novel disease gene, identification of multiple cases with a similar phenotype is enabled by collaborative platforms such as GeneMatcher and Matchmaker Exchange for all genes and networks for specific diseases such as GENOMIT for mitochondrial diseases, amongst others (Bruel et al. 2019; Philippakis et al. 2015).

The variant(s) should segregate with the disease phenotype in the pedigree. Assuming autosomal recessive inheritance, variant must be homozygous or compound heterozygous. Where "trio" sequencing is not available, biallelic inheritance of compound heterozygous variants can be determined by manual inspection of the sequencing data in Integrative Genomics Viewer (IGV) (when the variants are of close proximity), by long-range PCR of DNA or reverse transcribed mRNA and allele-specific sequencing, or by Sanger sequencing of the parents. The latter is most convenient, if parental DNA is available. Where a variant is observed to have arisen de novo, parental samples should be confirmed to be negative, and consideration must be made for germ-line mosaicism with regard to recurrence risks.

Movement has been made towards standardisation of phenotypic data collection to increase interpretive capacity. HPO ("Human Phenotype Ontology") terms describe over 13,000 clinical abnormalities with 156,000 annotations to hereditary diseases mapped into an ontological multitiered structure (HPO.jax.org). Such standardisation of data promotes the inclusion of clinical information into computational development to assist clinical interpretation and increase sensitivity of variant discoveries which have a known genotype-phenotype correlation.

In unsolved cases, with or without candidate variants, complementary "multi-omics" such as transcriptomics (RNA sequencing) may be incorporated into the analysis.

## Challenges in Interpretation

Penetrance, variability of clinical phenotype, and genetic modifiers present future challenges to be overcome in variant interpretation. This will require the accumulation of large databases, as opposed to case-by-case analyses.

### Incomplete Penetrance and Phenotype Variability

Incomplete penetrance is well documented in IEM and creates difficulty in accurately determining the risk of having a symptomatic child and predictions of disease progression in order to determine the necessity for intervention. Penetrance describes whether individuals with a given genotype express a phenotype. Incomplete penetrance means that not all individuals with a given genotype express the phenotype. It is associated primarily with autosomal dominant and maternal inheritance, however was recently also demonstrated for an autosomal recessive mitochondrial disease gene *DNAJC30* (Stenton et al. 2021). The phenomenon of variable penetrance describes the degree to which individuals express the corresponding phenotype, and substantial difference in clinical phenotype can be observed. This explains why genetic diseases are occasionally transmitted through seemingly "unaffected" parents and, conversely, why healthy individuals can harbour numerous variants of pathogenic effect without manifestation of a disease. Many variables are proposed to be involved in penetrance such as differential allelic expression; copy number variation; the modulating influence of additional genetic variants in cis or in trans, termed "genetic modifiers"; epigenetic changes; and environmental factors, amongst others.

### Genetic Modifiers

The aforementioned WES and WGS analysis pipelines consider Mendelian inheritance of autosomal recessive (AR), autosomal dominant (AD), de novo, genetic mosaic, X-linked, and mitochondrial nature in a "one-gene one-disease" manner. However, the ultimate aim should be to understand how an individual's phenotype arises given their primary disease-causing mutation on the background of the sum of variation within their entire genome. The concept of such "genetic modifiers" is particularly poignant in IEM as patients often present with a spectrum of disease phenotypes showing poor correlation with the underlying pathogenic mutation.

This phenomenon was recognised early in IEM in phenylketonuria (PKU), a typical monogenic autosomal recessive disease. In PKU, genetic variation in *PAH* leads to the enzymatic phenotype of impaired function of phenylalanine hydroxylase. However, PKU is further characterised by cognitive and metabolic phenotypes, beyond the control of the *PAH* gene itself. This gives rise to the idea of a major locus in determining certain parameters of phenotype, but additionally a role for further modifier genes accounting for the complexities of, variation in, and additions to, the phenotype, not entirely unlike complex genetic traits. The identification of genetic modifiers may not only aid in prediction of variant pathogenicity and penetrance but also aid in the discovery of novel therapeutic targets in a movement towards personalised precision medicine.

### Multiple Diagnoses

Almost 5% of solved cases have a diagnosis involving two or more disease genes (Posey et al. 2017). These diseases can be distinct or overlap in phenotype, resulting in phenotype blending. This is a challenge for genotype-phenotype driven searches and also indicates that the analysis should not be prematurely stopped when a pathogenic variant is found as this may not provide the complete picture.

## Transcriptomics

The end of the twentieth century marked the dawn of the "multi-omics" era, most importantly to IEM, in transcriptomics, proteomics, and metabolomics (Stenton et al. 2020; Wanders et al. 2019; Graham et al. 2018; Alston et al. 2021). In "multi-omics", thousands of variables can be measured simultaneously, be it transcript, protein, or metabolite, and can complement genomic sequencing data by the parallel detection and functional annotation of variants. These approaches have the power to track the impact of a variant from RNA abundance and form to protein level and the influence on metabolite level given the function of the respective gene products, and vice versa, tracing the abnormal metabolite level, aberrant expression, and splicing pattern back to the responsible variants. The comprehensive capture of the functional consequence of variants can bridge the evidence gap in support of a definitive IEM diagnosis, thereby reducing our reliance on individually tailored, sophisticated, and often time-consuming functional validation experiments.

Here, we focus on transcriptomics as it is also based on NGS and therefore likely available in the same laboratory. Transcriptomics can be applied in two settings: (1) in validation of variants of uncertain significance (VUS) prioritised in the analysis of WES and WGS and (2) in reprioritisation and validation of variants eluding the WES/WGS analysis pipelines, where it can step into a discovery role. Transcriptomics (RNA sequencing) describes the comprehensive, systematic identification and quantification of messenger RNA transcripts (and also other facultative RNA species) in a given sample. Around 10,000 transcribed protein-coding genes are reliably detected in most tissues, providing insight into the pathogenicity of genetic variants, both exonic and intronic, that result in changes in mRNA expression level and form (Fig. 9.4) (Kremer et al. 2017; Cummings et al. 2017; Frésard et al. 2019; Gonorazky et al. 2019).

Pathogenic variants are detected by (1) loss or reduced expression of a given gene; (2) mono-allelic expression (MAE) of a heterozygous pathogenic variant, eluding prioritisation in WES and WGS due to absence of a second pathogenic allele for biallelic inheritance; and (3) aberrant splice patterns, frequently resulting in a frameshift, a premature stop codon, and provoking nonsense-mediated decay (NMD) of the transcript (Fig. 9.4). The complementation of WES with transcriptomics allows a further 10–35% of inconclusive cases to be solved (Kremer et al. 2017; Cummings et al. 2017).

Aberrant expression results in expression outliers (Yépez 2021). These statistically significant deviations from normal physiological range result from coding variants, from noncoding variants in regulatory regions, such as promoters, enhancers, and suppressors, and from RNA degradation by NMD. Mono-allelic expression (MAE) describes the silencing of one allele (Gonorazky et al. 2019; Kremer et al. 2017; Cummings et al. 2017). It allows reprioritisation of rare heterozygous SNVs, mimicking homozygosity and thereby fitting the recessive mode of inheritance (most commonly seen in IEM). Aberrant splicing is an important phenomenon in Mendelian disease genetics, accounting for at least 10% of pathogenic variants (Soemedi et al. 2017; Lee et al. 2017) and readily detectable by RNA sequencing (Mertes et al. 2021). It results from variation in splice sites, near splice sites,

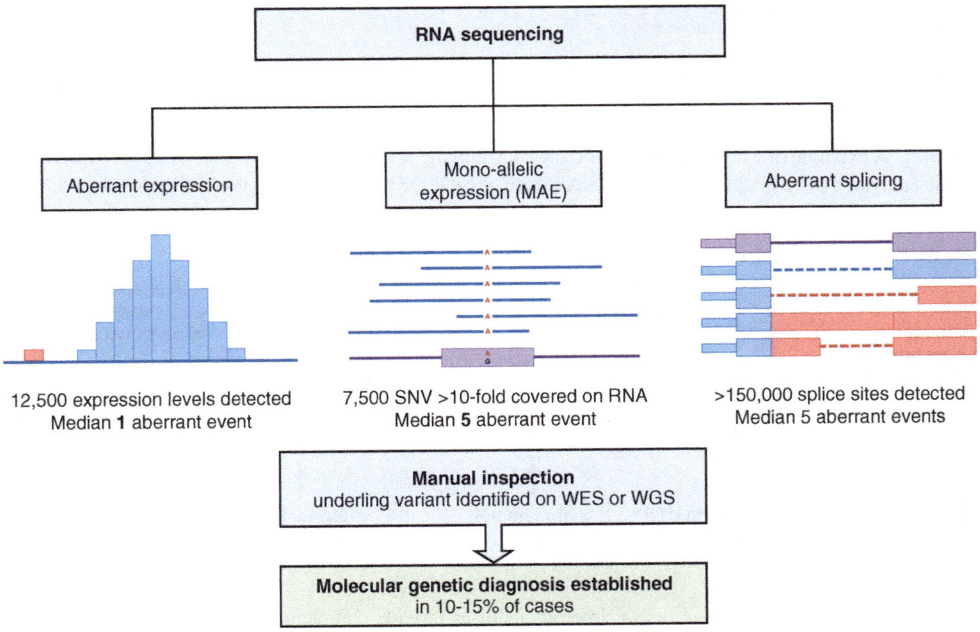


**Fig. 9.4** The transcriptomic (RNA-sequencing) analysis pipeline. Pathogenic variants are detected by aberrant expression, mono-allelic expression, and aberrant splice pattern. This results in a manageable number of candidates for manual inspection and typically achieves diagnostic rates of 10–15% when applied as a complementary analysis tool to unsolved WES cases

splicing regulatory elements, and activation of cryptic splice sites deep within the intronic regions. The variants can result in a plethora of aberrant splice isoforms, ranging from exon creation, skipping, extension, and truncation, to intron inclusion. The subsequent splice isoforms can be quantified (Fig. 9.5) to determine the percentage of functional transcript and thereby gene product in the patient. For the discovery of aberrantly expressed genes, in all three analyses, stringent filtering must be applied for rare events with strong effect size. This typically results in a median of one aberrant expression, six MAE, and five aberrant splicing events per sample when searching genome-wide for aberration (Kremer et al. 2017). This is a feasible number of candidates for manual inspection to identify the responsible pathogenic coding and non-coding variants within the WES and WGS data, in order to provide a definitive diagnosis to the patient.

Notably, RNA sequencing can both prove the pathogenicity of seemingly benign variants, such as synonymous variants creating novel splice sites, and disprove the pathogenicity of a seemingly loss-of-function variants resulting in a normal transcript (Fig. 9.6). With regard to synonymous variants, defined as single-nucleotide variants (SNVs) which do not cause a change in the encoded amino acid, the variants are typically filtered out as "benign" in the WES and WGS analysis pipeline; however, evidence for pathogenicity can be brought to light by transcriptomics and may lead to synonymous variants being reprioritised in inconclusive cases. With regard to nonsense variants, those arising early in the transcript mark the termination of translation, however, it is feasible for post-termination ribosomes to reinitiate translation at a downstream AUG codon, the RNA equivalent to the DNA-encoded ATG start codon. This can lead to the expression of a truncated, yet functional, protein. And equally, nonsense variants late in the transcript, also resulting in expression of a truncated protein, may result in normal function, especially when the C-terminus is poorly conserved. Moreover, most genes have several transcripts and clinical interpretation needs to consider the affected subset of transcripts. This highlights the need to take care when assuming the pathogenicity of seemingly loss-of-function variants. Moreover, by the quantification of aberrant expression and splice isoforms, the impact of a given patient's phenotypic severity may be queried. Again, highlighting that though splice variants are typically deemed to be loss-of-function in nature, they do not strictly lead to complete loss of the native transcript, and thus the phenotype may be dependent on the

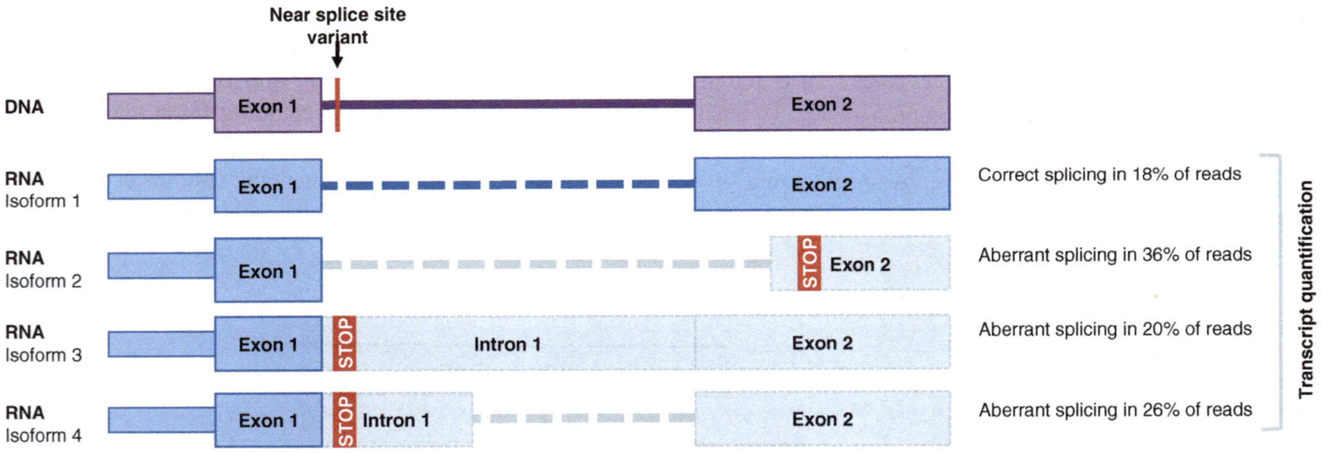


**Fig. 9.5** A example of a complex pattern of aberrant splicing due to a near splice site variant in *MRPL44*. Each isoform detected in the transcriptomic analysis can be quantified, and the percentage of functional transcript and thereby gene product, can be determined

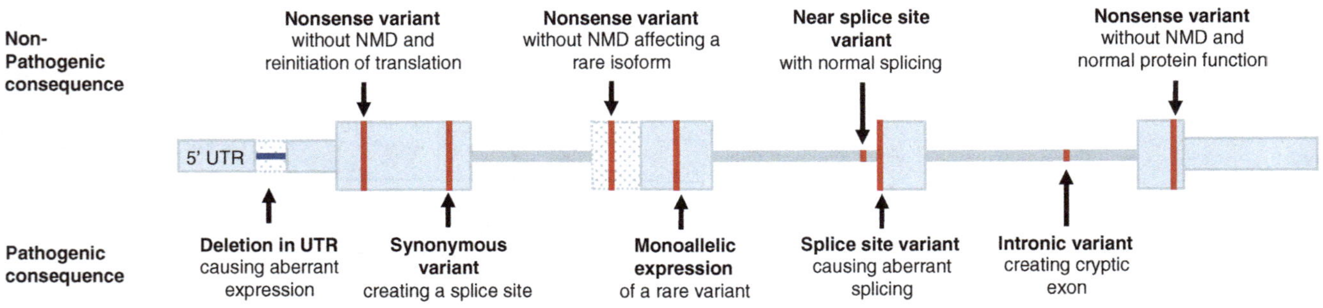


**Fig. 9.6** Select examples where transcriptomic analyses provide complementary information to genomic sequencing to prove or disprove the pathogenicity of a given variant

balance between aberrantly and normally spliced transcripts.

The principal limitation of RNA sequencing is the choice of tissue for interrogation. Easily accessible tissues such as blood and fibroblasts, from a minimally invasive punch biopsy of the skin, reliably detect over 65% and 70% of known IEM disease genes, respectively (Stenton et al. 2020; Ferreira et al. 2019). The primary affected tissue provides a further option. However, it is often inaccessible to minimally invasive sampling, such as heart, brain, and liver. Moreover, tissue-specific physiological consequences of the underlying variant are likely to cause further aberrations in expression of a number of genes and cloud the detection of the underlying causative aberrant event. Selection of the optimal surrogate tissue for RNA sequencing, in which the disease genes of interest are optimally expressed, can be guided by gene expression databases, such as GTEx comprising approximately 11,500 RNA-sequencing samples across more than 50 tissues (gtexportal.org/home/).

## The Value of a Molecular Genetic Diagnosis

Knowledge of the molecular genetic defect and inheritance pattern is essential for provision of counselling for the patient and their family. This includes the implication for family members of presymptomatic testing, only permitted in children where there is a therapeutic consequence, and for future family planning such as in recurrence risks and the possibility for preimplantation and prenatal diagnostics. Furthermore, prognostic counselling can be provided when the natural history of the disease is well established and may allow for the prevision of a targeted precision therapy (Zhou et al. 2020; Zhou et al. 2020), such as for one of the increasing number of recognised cofactor metabolism defects, amongst others (Distelmaier et al. 2016). However, for many IEM, effective defect-targeted treatment options are still sough-after.

Given the vast spectrum of IEM, the mode of inheritance of a given defect can be autosomal recessive, autosomal dominant, de novo, genetic mosaic, digenic, X-linked, or maternal, by mitochondrial DNA (mtDNA) (as seen in Fig. 9.1). The majority (80%) are inherited in an autosomal recessive (AR) manner with onset in childhood, whereby one disease allele is typically inherited from each parent of carrier status (Ferreira et al. 2019). The recurrence risk is 25% in future offspring. Siblings of the affected child may be presymptomatic, asymptomatic carrier of the variant, or unaffected. Following genetic counselling, their status can be confirmed by targeted sequencing of the disease gene. Where carrier status is known, unrelated partners of carriers can choose to undergo testing to determine whether they are also a carrier of a pathogenic variant in the same gene.

Autosomal dominant (AD) inheritance occurs in over 15% of IEM (Ferreira et al. 2019). The disease allele is inherited from one affected parent and a healthy "wild-type" allele from the second parent. The recurrence risk is 50% in future offspring of the affected parent. Siblings of the affected child may be presymptomatic (depending on the age of onset of the disease), affected, or unaffected. Following genetic counselling, their status can be confirmed by targeted sequencing of the disease gene. Complexities in genetic counselling arise in AD disease due to incomplete or variable penetrance, such as in PEO due to *POLG* or *TWNK* defects, whereby inheritance of the disease allele does not mean with absolute certainty that the individual will be symptomatic.

De novo inheritance describes the occurrence of a variant in the child which is present in neither of the parents and therefore arose "de novo". The recurrence risk for de novo defects in future offspring is on average low, at ~1%, due to gonadal mosaicism but may vary from case to case. If the de novo mutation arose on the paternal allele, the actual risk may be determined by genotyping of sperm cells. Recurrence risk in the offspring of the affected individual increases to 50% as per AD inheritance. In IEM, de novo mutations are a rare, yet present, disease-causing mechanism. Moreover, in a number of genes, de novo mutations occur with higher frequency termed "recurrent de novo". Such examples include early-onset mitochondrial depletion syndrome due to recurrent de novo variants in *SLC25A4* and X-linked adrenoleukodystrophy due to recurrent de novo variants in *ABCD1* (Thompson et al. 2016; Wang et al. 2011).

In X-linked inheritance, the causal variant harbours on the X chromosome. This accounts for ~5% of IEM (Ferreira et al. 2019). Typically, males are more severely affected than females as they have only one X chromosome (46XY). As females have two X chromosomes (46XX), they can either be affected, usually to a lesser severity, or unaffected. This is dependent on the phenomenon of X-inactivation, a random process in each female cell where the expression of one X chromosome is inactivated. Skewed X-inactivation towards inactivation of the healthy "wild-type" allele may result in manifestation (or increase in severity) of the disease phenotype. The male offspring of a female X-linked disease carrier has a 50% chance of being affected and the female offspring a 50% chance of being a carrier. Where a male is affected, the X-linked condition cannot be transmitted to his male offspring as he will pass on only the Y chromosome; however, he will transmit the defect to all of his female offspring. Examples of X-linked inheritance in IEM include Barth syndrome due to *TAZ* defects and pyruvate dehydrogenase deficiency due to *PDHA1* defects.

Digenic inheritance requires defects in two genes for the syndrome to manifest. Two digenic IEM are described, Rotor syndrome, a disorder of bilirubin metabolism and biliary transport resulting in hyperbilirubinemia due to AR defects in both the *SLCO1B1* and *SLCO1B3* genes, and iminoglycinuria, inherited in either an AR or digenic pattern in *SLC36A2* (±*SLC6A20*).

**Maternal Inheritance of IEM**

Maternal inheritance of mtDNA defects is common in adult-onset mitochondrial disease. mtDNA is exclusively inherited from the mother as mtDNA from sperm is actively excluded upon fertilisation of the oocyte. The disease phenotype is expressed when the level of heteroplasmy, the "mutational load", crosses a specific threshold. This threshold is typically dependent on the minimum percentage of healthy mtDNA required to support the energy demand, and therefore healthy functioning, of a given tissue. For this reason, the most frequently affected organs in mitochondrial disease are the high-energy demanding organs such as the brain, heart, muscle, and liver. In both homoplasmic and heteroplasmic mtDNA defects, it is difficult to predict with certainty whether the offspring will express the phenotype. Variable penetrance occurs in homoplasmic mtDNA defects such as in LHON, where only 50% of males of 10% of females express the phenotype. With regard to heteroplasmic mtDNA defects, a higher heteroplasmy level may result in an affected individual as compared to a lower heteroplasmy level resulting in an asymptomatic individual. Accurate annotation of the level of heteroplasmy, tissue-specific threshold, and influence of mitochondrial haplogroup are currently not reported in publicly available databases; this would be of great value to aid genetic counselling in the future. Furthermore, as with nuclear DNA defects, variants can arise de novo in the mtDNA. The recurrence risk of de novo mtDNA mutations is ~1% based on the possibility of gonadal (oocyte) mosaicism.

## Possibility for Prevention

Predictive testing can be used to determine whether an embryo or foetus carries a given genetic defect. This can be undertaken in the preimplantation setting by testing of the embryo or in the prenatal setting by testing of the foetus and helps to guide clinician and parental decisions for further evaluation and management of the pregnancy.

Preimplantation genetic diagnosis (PIGD) requires harvesting of the gametes and in vitro fertilisation (IVF) to generate multiple zygotes. The embryo is allowed to divide until reaching a multicellular stage at ~3–5 days. At this stage, one to two cells are removed for genetic testing of the specific pathogenic mutation(s) identified in the family. The unaffected embryo(s), where available, can subsequently be implanted and additional unaffected embryos frozen for future cycles. It is recommended that further prenatal testing is undertaken during the pregnancy to form an accurate picture of the genotype—options available include chorionic villus sampling (CVS) and amniocentesis. PIGD can be problematic, as a chromosomally normal, mutation-free embryo for transfer may not be generated in the cycle, or damage may occur to the embryo while removing the cells for testing. Furthermore, in mtDNA defects, from the mutational load in the embryo at 3–5 days, it is difficult to extrapolate the mutational load for different tissues in the future child, and it is unlikely to generate an embryo with an absent mutational load, creating limitations in predictive accuracy.

## Prenatal Diagnosis

Chorionic villus sampling (CVS) can be offered at 10–12 weeks of gestation. Chorionic villi cells, surrounding the foetus and later developing into the placenta, are sampled transabdominally or transcervically. The cells are cultured and subsequently tested to determine the genetic status. The chorionic villi cells are genetically identical to the foetus, with the rare exception of confined placental mosaicism, where the genetic abnormality occurs in the placenta and not the foetus. Results from CVS are typically available within 2 weeks and can therefore guide the decision on continuation of the pregnancy.

Amniocentesis can be offered at 14–16 weeks of gestation. Amniotic fluid surrounding the foetus is removed by a needle biopsy transabdominally. The amniotic fluid contains cells from the foetus which are subsequently tested to determine the genetic status. Results from amniocentesis are typically available within 2–6 weeks and can guide the decision on continuation of the pregnancy.

While CVS and amniocentesis in combination with advances in cytogenetics and molecular technologies have expanding and improved prenatal diagnostic, the small risk of miscarriage is a deterrent to their acceptance by the patient.

## Noninvasive Testing of Foetal DNA in Maternal Circulation

Noninvasive prenatal testing relies on distinguishing the foetal and maternal genomes by identification of the minor proportion of cell-free foetal DNA (cfDNA) in the maternal circulation. This can be detected earlier in the pregnancy and with significantly less risk than conventional approaches. The cfDNA molecules are tagged, followed by enrichment and next-generation sequencing (NGS). The approach is currently targeted towards the detection of foetal aneuploidies and chromosomal abnormalities, such as trisomy 13, 18, or 21, sex chromosome aneuploidies, and microdeletions, with high sensitivity and specificity. Promise is now emerging in the detection of de novo and paternally inherited disease-causing variants in monogenic diseases (Zhang et al. 2019). However, at this time, the approach cannot reliably identify recessive conditions and maternally inherited monogenic diseases.

**Specific Considerations in Mitochondrial Disease**

Recent advancements in the mitochondrial disease field have led to the opportunity for mitochondrial donation including pronuclear transfer, metaphase II spindle transfer, and polar body transfer with the hope to prevent transmission of the mtDNA defect from mother to child. Mitochondrial donation is currently permitted in the UK in licenced centres under the regulation of the Human Fertilisation and Embryology Authority (HFEA). Although some studies suggest good safety and efficacy profiles of these techniques, an international consensus is needed on the regulation of these approaches.

## The Concern with the Genomic Approach

### Secondary Findings

As capabilities in the era of genomic medicine increase, so do the incidence of secondary findings. This has arisen as a key issue in recent years, catalysed by the American College of Medical Genetics and Genomics (ACMG), who in 2013 first released recommendations for reporting of secondary findings in exome and genome sequencing (Green et al. 2013). In the years following, at national-, European-, and global-level, debates on the development of recommendations for handling such findings, encompassing ethical commentaries, guidelines, and diverse policies, have ensued. The principal areas of debate regard the suitability of terminology, application of opportunistic screening, informed consent and genetic counselling procedures, opt-out possibilities, reporting in minors, and values surrounding professional duty, patient autonomy, and actionability (Fig. 9.7) (Saelaert et al. 2018; Mackley and Capps 2017).

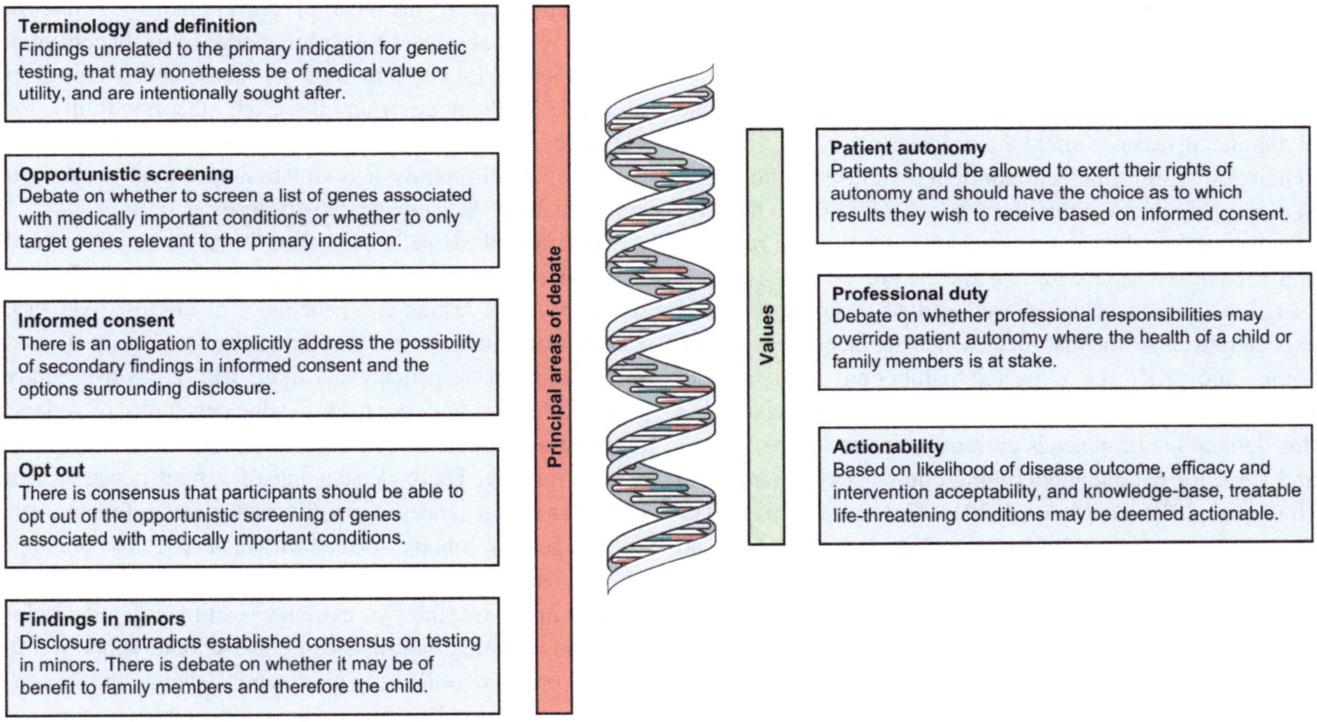


| Disclosure | Non-disclosure |
|---|---|
| • Findings impact medical management leading to better clinical outcome<br>• Findings allows informed reproductive choices<br>• Findings promote patient well-being<br>• Benefits potentially extend to members of the patient's family | • Findings for which there is absence of clinical utility and intervention<br>• Incomplete certainly of the predictive value of testing and of penetrance<br>• Possibility to cause psychological harm<br>• Unnecessary investigation and surveillance of false-positive findings<br>• Harms potentially extend to members of the patient's family |

**Fig. 9.7** Exploration of the principal areas of debate and values surrounding the key issue of secondary findings in exome and genome sequencings

Secondary findings are defined as pathogenic alterations in genes unrelated to the primary diagnostic indication for sequencing, which may nevertheless be of significant medical value to the patient and the clinician. The findings are termed "secondary findings" as opposed to "incidental findings", the first term applied to such findings, as they result from the deliberate search for pathogenic alterations. The term "secondary" is, however, not without objection as it may minimise the significance of the result, relative to the "primary" finding.

The distinction between clearly focussed diagnostic testing and opportunistic screening loses much of its sharpness in the context of genome sequencing, and there is much debate on the genes in which opportunistic screening for pathogenic variants should be conducted, if at all. The term "actionability" is frequently used here to describe genes in which there is a high likelihood of disease outcome (high penetrance) and there is efficient and acceptable intervention and a robust knowledge-base, thereby impacting on the clinical management and reproductive choices. The ACMG defines a list of medically actionable genes which are regularly refined and updated (ncbi.nlm.nih.gov/clinvar/docs/acmg/), selected due to strong evidence of high probability of severe adverse medical outcome, the possibility for verifiability by other diagnostic methods, and early intervention likely to prevent or ameliorate serious morbidity or early mortality. Of note, only one metabolic disease is included in this list, X-linked OTC deficiency (ornithine carbamoyltransferase deficiency). Secondary findings within these genes fall into two descriptive categories: "sequence variation previously reported and recognised as a cause of the disorder" or "sequence variation previously unreported and of the type which is expected to cause the disorder" which are labelled as known pathogenic (KP) and expected pathogenic (EP), respectively. The rate of discovery of secondary findings within this defined list of genes is currently reported as between 1 and 3.5% for patients undergoing clinical sequencing (Van Hout et al. 2019; Dewey et al. 2016; Green et al. 2013). The European Society of Human Genetics (ESHG) and Canadian College of Medical Genetics (CCMG) take a more cautious approach to "actionability" and its implication in disclosure, acknowledging the current lack of empiric knowledge on their utility, and do not endorse the intentional analysis of all "actionable" genes, preferring to use a targeted approach to the primary clinical question in order to minimise secondary findings.

Though challenging, the informed consent procedure, inclusive of a level of information and counselling required to realise a truly informed consent and an acceptable understanding of secondary findings and their implications, is essential. This includes decisions on whether to "opt out" of intentional opportunistic screening and decisions on disclosure. There is also discussion of the potential role for dynamic or staged consent procedures, in which the validity of patient preferences is not limited to a single moment prior to testing. Regarding the screening and reporting of results in minors, guidelines are widely disputed, and the ACMG argues that disclosure of findings for adult-onset conditions may be clinically useful to the parents and, in turn, benefit the child themselves. However, this argument departs from well-established paediatric genetic testing practice recommendations and is therefore not unanimously supported.

Many challenges surrounding secondary findings are grounded in difference in prioritisation of values. It is widely agreed that patients should be allowed to exert their rights of autonomy and have the choice as to which results they wish to receive, defined in the informed consent, with the decision to "opt out" of opportunistic screening. Debate arises in the duty of the doctor in beneficence and non-maleficence, such as in disclosing information on potentially treatable life-threatening conditions, and whether professional responsibilities may override patient autonomy where the health of the patient or their family members is at stake. Non-disclosure of a clinically actionable variant conveying with near certainty an adverse, yet potentially preventable, medical outcome, in order to uphold patient autonomy, requires convincing ethical justification and remains of intense debate. While absence of a strong evidence for benefit may justify the disinclination to disclose, "actionability" is not an objective medical criterion; therefore, the possibility for dynamic or staged consent would further allow weighing of these values differently and situation-specifically, to reach contextualised decisions on the disclose.

To harness the benefits of genomic medicine, policies need to be evidence-based. Important considerations arise in the predictive value of testing and penetrance of disclosed variants. Current knowledge of variant penetrance is largely derived from symptomatic patients and those with a positive family history. Plentiful evidence regarding the penetrance of variants amongst asymptomatic carriers with absence of a family history is missing. For understanding of variant penetrance to evolve and to generate informative penetrance estimates, it is encouraged for cohorts of cases in which secondary findings are disclosed, to be followed longitudinally (Green et al. 2013).

To summarise, the two extreme positions of full disclosure and complete non-disclosure are seldom supported in clinical practice. Balance in disclosure decisions should consider the potential benefits to the patient and their family of optimised medical management, reproductive choices, and well-being, versus the risk of the psychological burden, the potential exposure to iatrogenic harm due to unnecessary diagnostic investigation, and the clinical surveillance of a false-positive findings, amongst others. Given the complexity of the issue, regarding the integration and alignment of terminology, policy, and values, international disagreement remains, and the pursuit of consensus on future well-grounded practice is yet to be established.

## A Perspective for WGS in Newborn Screening

The need for early recognition and initiation of rational therapeutics, also in presymptomatic stages of disease, has led to the inclusion of many IEM in newborn screening programmes. This has been pivotal in initiating therapy before the onset of progressive irreversible organ damage. The era of newborn screening has been greatly influenced by Wilson and Junger, whom in 1969 formulated a report commissioned by the World Health Organization, defining a number of screening criteria to guide the selection of medical conditions suitable for screening. These standards, considered the gold standard in making screening test decisions, covered the concept of disease importance, natural history, detectability at an early stage, treatability, the associated risk benefit, and cost-effectiveness.

Newborn screening aims to achieve presymptomatic diagnosis of treatable diseases for which timely intervention proves vital in preventing disability or death. With recent advancement of genomic sequencing technology, the rate at which novel disease genes are identified is out-pacing the ability of professionals and policy-makers to assess the potential benefits and pitfalls of introducing or expanding genetic screening programmes, propelling WGS into discussion as a first-tier test in newborn screening programmes. This would also allow screening for disorders for which no other biomarker is known or is difficult to be implemented in current screening procedures, including, for example, a number of cofactor deficiencies.

Genomic screening has a number of positives over conventional newborn screening: Firstly, WGS is time-independent and can be performed from birth, a limitation of biochemical profiling, allowing earlier intervention. Secondly, as a global approach, WGS hold to potential to reveal all actionable disease variants, inclusive of far rarer conditions often not included in routine screening in a "one-test-fits-all" manner, providing a comprehensive picture of future disease status, unachievable by a targeted screen as discussed earlier in diagnostics in general.

Interpretation of genetic variants prior to symptomatic onset requires confidence in prior knowledge of function and genotype-phenotype correlation. A further consideration is treatment requirement. This becomes particularly problematic when the proposed treatment is not curative, has significant complications, or is inherently not without risk itself. In diseases where the natural history is well documented, to reach a balance in variant disclosure, information could be provided to the individual at the age when treatment should be started or specific tests should be performed.

Genetic screening is therefore an area of growing importance and controversy, arising as a potential player in translating genomic advances into improvement in population health. However, prior to implementation, we must have the knowledge to clearly distinguish affected from unaffected newborns.

## Conclusion

In conclusion, advances in molecular genetics in the last decade have revolutionised the field of IEM and are challenging our long-standing, stepwise approach, to the diagnosis of IEM in clinical practice. The unbiased and reliable manner in which genomic sequencing can pinpoint the underlying cause of a patient disease is propelling WES and WGS into the first tier of diagnostics in suspected IEM, which is now well established in routine clinical practice. Further consideration is required of the role of WES and WGS in prenatal testing and newborn screening. Furthermore, as the interpretation of "multi-omics" data evolves, we are likely to see increased integration of these comprehensive functional data into analysis of the ever-growing number of variants of uncertain significance (VUS) detected by genomic sequencing and of inconclusive cases in the near future. High-throughput functional validation studies will therefore play a pivotal role in the years to come.

## References


Alston CL, Stenton SL, Hudson G, Prokisch H, Taylor RW. The genetics of mitochondrial disease: dissecting mitochondrial pathology using multi-omic pipelines. J Pathol. 2021.

Bruel AL, Vitobello A, Mau-Them FT, et al. 2.5 years' experience of GeneMatcher data-sharing: a powerful tool for identifying new genes responsible for rare diseases. Genet Med. 2019;21(7):1657–61.

Clark MM, Stark Z, Farnaes L, et al. Meta-analysis of the diagnostic and clinical utility of genome and exome sequencing and chromosomal microarray in children with suspected genetic diseases. NPJ Genom Med. 2018;3:16.

Clark MM, Hildreth A, Batalov S, et al. Diagnosis of genetic diseases in seriously ill children by rapid whole-genome sequencing and automated phenotyping and interpretation. Sci Transl Med. 2019;11(489):eaat6177.

Cummings BB, Marshall JL, Tukiainen T, et al. Improving genetic diagnosis in Mendelian disease with transcriptome sequencing. Sci Transl Med. 2017;9(386):eaal5209.

DaRe JT, Vasta V, Penn J, et al. Targeted exome sequencing for mitochondrial disorders reveals high genetic heterogeneity. BMC Med Genet. 2013;14(1):118.

Dewey FE, Murray MF, Overton JD, et al. Distribution and clinical impact of functional variants in 50,726 whole-exome sequences from the DiscovEHR study. Science. 2016;354(6319):aaf6814.

Diroma MA, Calabrese C, Simone D, et al. Extraction and annotation of human mitochondrial genomes from 1000 Genomes Whole Exome Sequencing data. BMC Genomics. 2014;15(3):S2.

Distelmaier F, Haack TB, Wortmann SB, et al. Treatable mitochondrial diseases: cofactor metabolism and beyond. Brain. 2016;140(2):e11.

Farnaes L, Hildreth A, Sweeney NM, et al. Rapid whole-genome sequencing decreases infant morbidity and cost of hospitalization. NPJ Genom Med. 2018;3(1):10.

Ferreira CR, van Karnebeek CD, Vockley J, et al. A proposed nosology of inborn errors of metabolism. Genet Med. 2019;21(1):102.

Frésard L, Smail C, Ferraro NM, Teran NA, Li X, Smith KS, et al. Identification of raredisease genes using blood transcriptome sequencing and large control cohorts. Nat Med. 2019;25(6):911–9.

Gonorazky HD, Naumenko S, Ramani AK, Nelakuditi V, Mashouri P, Wang P, et al. Expanding the boundaries of RNA sequencing as a diagnostic tool for rare Mendelian disease. Am J Hum Genet. 2019;104(3):466–83.

Graham E, Lee J, Price M, et al. Integration of genomics and metabolomics for prioritization of rare disease variants: a 2018 literature review. J Inherit Metab Dis. 2018;41(3):435–45.

Green RC, Berg JS, Grody WW, et al. ACMG recommendations for reporting of incidental findings in clinical exome and genome sequencing. Genet Med. 2013;15(7):565.

Griffin HR, Pyle A, Blakely EL, et al. Accurate mitochondrial DNA sequencing using off-target reads provides a single test to identify pathogenic point mutations. Genet Med. 2014;16(12):962.

Gusic M, Prokisch H. Genetic basis of mitochondrial diseases. FEBS Letters. 2021. https://doi.org/10.1002/1873-3468.14068.

Kremer LS, Bader DM, Mertes C, et al. Genetic diagnosis of Mendelian disorders via RNA sequencing. Nat Commun. 2017;8:15824.

Lake NJ, Compton AG, Rahman S, Thorburn DR. Leigh syndrome: one disorder, more than 75 monogenic causes. Ann Neurol. 2016;79(2):190–203.

Lee M, Roos P, Sharma N, et al. Systematic computational identification of variants that activate exonic and intronic cryptic splice sites. Am J Hum Genet. 2017;100(5):751–65.

Legati A, Reyes A, Nasca A, et al. New genes and pathomechanisms in mitochondrial disorders unraveled by NGS technologies. Biochim Biophys Acta. 2016;1857(8):1326–35.

Lethimonnier F, Levy Y. Genomic medicine France 2025. Ann Oncol. 2018;29(4):783–4.

Mackley MP, Capps B. Expect the unexpected: screening for secondary findings in clinical genomics research. Br Med Bull. 2017;122(1):109–22.

Mertes C, Scheller IF, Yépez VA, Çelik, MH, Liang Y, Kremer LS, et al. Detection of aberrant splicing events in RNA-seq data using FRASER. Nat Commun. 2021;12(1):1–13.

Nambot S, Thevenon J, Kuentz P, et al. Clinical whole-exome sequencing for the diagnosis of rare disorders with congenital anomalies and/or intellectual disability: substantial interest of prospective annual reanalysis. Genet Med. 2018;20(6):645.

Ouwehand WH. Whole-genome sequencing of rare disease patients in a national healthcare system. bioRxiv. 2019;507244.

Pfundt R, Del Rosario M, Vissers LE, et al. Detection of clinically relevant copy-number variants by exome sequencing in a large cohort of genetic disorders. Genet Med. 2017;19(6):667.

Philippakis AA, Azzariti DR, Beltran S, et al. The Matchmaker Exchange: a platform for rare disease gene discovery. Hum Mutat. 2015;36(10):915–21.

Ponzi E, Maiorana A, Lepri FR, et al. Persistent hypoglycemia in children: targeted gene panel improves the diagnosis of hypoglycemia due to inborn errors of metabolism. J Pediatr. 2018;202:272–8.

Posey JE, Harel T, Liu P, et al. Resolution of disease phenotypes resulting from multilocus genomic variation. N Engl J Med. 2017;376(1):21–31.

Richards S, Aziz N, Bale S, et al. Standards and guidelines for the interpretation of sequence variants: a joint consensus recommendation of the American College of Medical Genetics and Genomics and the Association for Molecular Pathology. Genet Med. 2015; 17(5):405.

Saelaert M, Mertes H, De Baere E, Devisch I. Incidental or secondary findings: an integrative and patient-inclusive approach to the current debate. Eur J Hum Genet. 2018;26(10):1424.

Saunders CJ, Miller NA, Soden SE, et al. Rapid whole-genome sequencing for genetic disease diagnosis in neonatal intensive care units. Sci Transl Med. 2012;4(154):154ra135.

Schlieben LD, Prokisch H. The dimensions of primary mitochondrial disorders. Front Cell Dev Biol. 2020;8.

Soemedi R, Cygan KJ, Rhine CL, et al. Pathogenic variants that alter protein code often disrupt splicing. Nat Genet. 2017;49(6):848.

Stenton SL, Prokisch H. Advancing genomic approaches to the molecular diagnosis of mitochondrial disease. Essays Biochem. 2018;62(3):399–408.

Stenton SL, Prokisch H. Genetics of mitochondrial diseases: Identifying mutations to help diagnosis. EBioMedicine. 2020;56:102784.

Stenton SL, Sheremet NL, Catarino CB, Andreeva N, Assouline Z, Barboni P, et al. Impaired complex I repair causes recessive Leber's hereditary optic neuropathy. J Clin Investig. 2021.

Stenton SL, Kremer LS, Kopajtich R, et al. The diagnosis of inborn errors of metabolism by an integrative "multi-omics" approach: a perspective encompassing genomics, transcriptomics and proteomics. J Inherit Metab Dis. 2020;43(1):25–35.

Tan TY, Dillon OJ, Stark Z, et al. Diagnostic impact and cost-effectiveness of whole-exome sequencing for ambulant children with suspected monogenic conditions. JAMA Pediatr. 2017;171(9):855–62.

Tarailo-Graovac M, Shyr C, Ross CJ, et al. Exome sequencing and the management of neurometabolic disorders. N Engl J Med. 2016;374(23):2246–55.

Tarailo-Graovac M, Wasserman WW, Van Karnebeek CD. Impact of next-generation sequencing on diagnosis and management of neurometabolic disorders: current advances and future perspectives. Expert Rev Mol Diagn. 2017;17(4):307–9.

Thompson K, Majd H, Dallabona C, et al. Recurrent de novo dominant mutations in SLC25A4 cause severe early-onset mitochondrial disease and loss of mitochondrial DNA copy number. Am J Hum Genet. 2016;99(4):860–76.

Turnbull C. Introducing whole-genome sequencing into routine cancer care: the Genomics England 100 000 Genomes Project. Ann Oncol. 2018;29(4):784–7.

Valente EM, Bhatia KP. Solving Mendelian mysteries: the non-coding genome may hold the key. Cell. 2018;172(5):889–91.

Van Hout CV, Tachmazidou I, Backman JD, et al. Whole exome sequencing and characterization of coding variation in 49,960 individuals in the UK Biobank. bioRxiv. 2019;572347.

Vissers LE, Van Nimwegen KJ, Schieving JH, et al. A clinical utility study of exome sequencing versus conventional genetic testing in pediatric neurology. Genet Med. 2017;19(9):1055–63.

Wagner M, Berutti R, Lorenz-Depiereux B, et al. Mitochondrial DNA mutation analysis from exome sequencing—a more holistic approach in diagnostics of suspected mitochondrial disease. J Inherit Metab Dis. 2019;42:909.

Wanders RJ, Vaz FM, Ferdinandusse S, et al. Translational metabolism: a multidisciplinary approach towards precision diagnosis of inborn errors of metabolism in the omics era. J Inherit Metab Dis. 2019;42(2):197–208.

Wang Y, Busin R, Reeves C, et al. X-linked adrenoleukodystrophy: ABCD1 de novo mutations and mosaicism. Mol Genet Metab. 2011;104(1–2):160–6.

Yépez VA, Mertes C, Müller MF, Klaproth-Andrade D, Wachutka L, Frésard L, et al. Detection of aberrant gene expression events in RNA sequencing data. Nat Protoc. 2021;1–21.

Zhang J, Li J, Saucier JB, et al. Non-invasive prenatal sequencing for multiple Mendelian monogenic disorders using circulating cell-free fetal DNA. Nat Med. 2019;25(3):439.

Zhou L, Deng J, Stenton SL, Zhou J, Li H, Chen C, Fang F. case report: rapid treatment of uridine-responsive epileptic encephalopathy caused by cad deficiency. Front Pharmacol. 2020;11:1956.

Zhou J, Li J, Stenton SL, Ren X, Gong S, Fang F, Prokisch H. NAD (P) HX dehydratase (NAXD) deficiency: a novel neurodegenerative disorder exacerbated by febrile illnesses. Brain. 2020;143(2):e8.

# Other -omics Approaches and Their Integration for the Diagnosis and Treatment of Inborn Errors of Metabolism

10

Clara D. M. van Karnebeek and Nanda Verhoeven-Duif

## Contents



**Summary**

Here we provide an overview of the different -omics approaches and their application and integration for the purpose of improving diagnosis and treatment of patients with inborn errors of metabolism. Given the molecular diversity of biomarkers, the high-throughput -omics technologies offer an amazing opportunity for holistic investigation and contextual pathophysiologic understanding of disease, as well as their identification and management. Phenomics, genomics, metabolomics, lipidomics, glycomics, proteomics, and transcriptomics are each important to systems medicine, but some are clear more mature than others, reflected in the varying applications as a clinically reimbursed test versus a research tool only. Generation of big data is relatively easy; the challenge lies in the integration and interpretation of these systems biology data and functional characterization and translation of the results into something clinically meaningful for our patients. Partnerships with patients and families and multidisciplinary collaboration between clinicians and researchers are essential for success in the -omics era.

C. D. M. van Karnebeek (✉)
Department of Pediatrics, Emma Children's Hospital, Amsterdam University Medical Centres, Amsterdam, The Netherlands
e-mail: c.d.vankarnebeek@amsterdamumc.nl

N. Verhoeven-Duif
Section Metabolic Diagnostics, Department of Genetics, University Medical Center Utrecht, Utrecht, The Netherlands
e-mail: n.verhoeven@umcutrecht.nl

## Introduction

The era of big data promises to accelerate the diagnostic and treatment process dramatically. Given the molecular diversity of biomarkers, the high-throughput -omics technologies offer


N. Blau et al. (eds.), *Physician's Guide to the Diagnosis, Treatment, and Follow-Up of Inherited Metabolic Diseases*,
https://doi.org/10.1007/978-3-030-67727-5_10

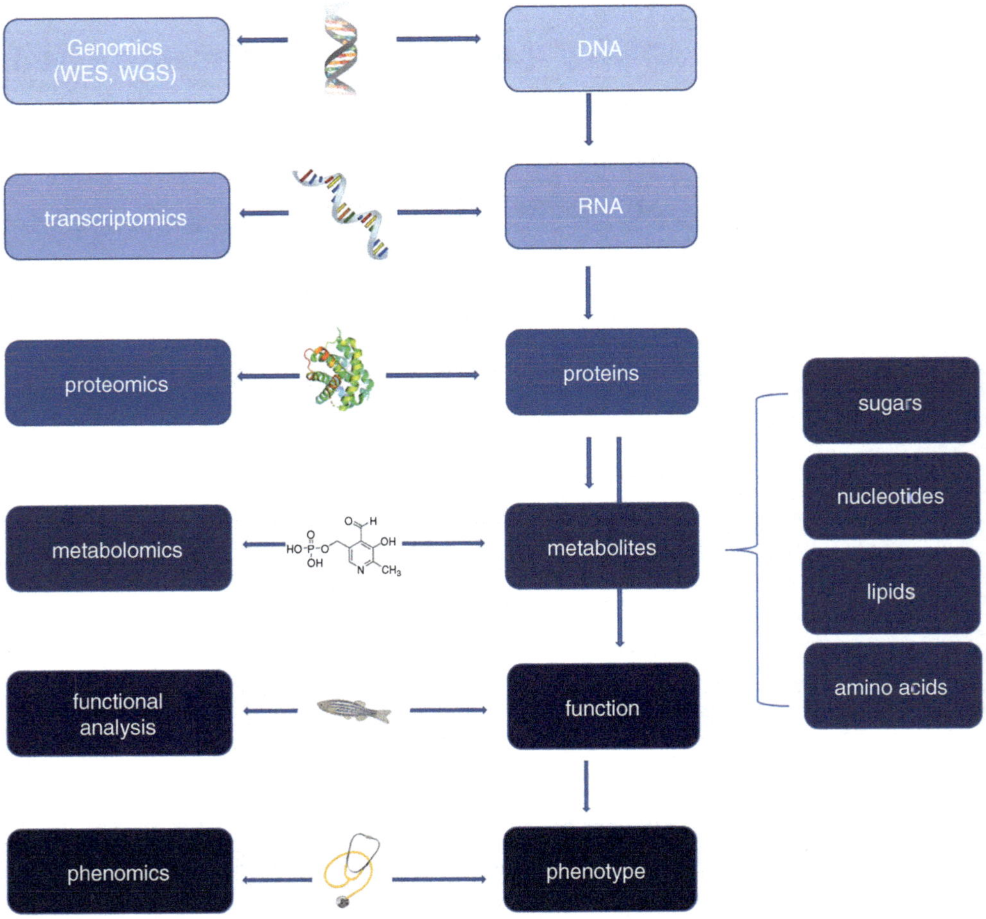


**Fig. 10.1** -Omics refers to the study of biological processes by analysing pools of biological molecules: DNA molecules by genomics (WES and WGS), RNA expression by transcriptomics, proteins by proteomics, and metabolites by metabolomics, including the subgroups of glycoproteins (glycomics) and lipids (lipidomics). Altogether, these molecules define function (as can be tested by functional analyses, e.g. in model systems) and phenotype (phenomics)

an amazing opportunity for holistic investigation (Benson 2016) and contextual pathophysiologic understanding of disease for better diagnosis and treatment (Alyass et al. 2015; Ahn et al. 2006; Tebani et al. 2016). While each of the -omics technologies depicted in Fig. 10.1 is important to systems medicine, some are clearly more mature than others (Julkowska et al. 2017). WES is slowly emerging as a reimbursed test in clinics around the world, while epigenomics and exposomics (the environmental effects ranging from exposures to toxic substances or drugs to diet) are applied mainly in research settings. Of the mass spectrometry (MS)-based technologies, metabolomics is much closer to being introduced into clinical practice than proteomics, because targeted MS-based metabolite analyses to improve pathophysiologic understanding and enhance accurate diagnostics and tailored care have already been adopted in clinical chemistry laboratories. Whether in the research or clinical setting, the challenge lies in the integration and interpretation of these systems biology data and translation of the results into something clinically meaningful for our patients. A daunting task, this challenge can only be overcome through partnership with the patients and families and close collaboration between clinicians and researchers in the basic, computer, and clinical sciences (van Karnebeek et al. 2018).

## Phenomics

Phenomics is the acquisition of detailed phenotypic data on an organism-wide scale. In practice, this includes the dysmorphologic, neurologic, and systemic characterization of the patient, as well as in vivo technologies such as neuroimaging/spectroscopy, and electrophysiologic, biochemical, and other functional studies. The dimensionality of phenomes is high, and so analyses of phenomic data call for new concepts and techniques. To integrate phenomic information, non-linear models that integrate information across the phenotypic hierarchy are necessary (Rahman and Rahman 2019).

Phenomic data allow a better understanding of the pathways that connect genotypes to phenotypes. Caveat of WGS or WES outputs are the variants of unknown significance (VUS), which can number in the thousands. It is often difficult to disentangle pathogenic variants from variants caused by genetic variation in the population and naturally occurring individual mutations (an average of ~100 naturally occurring loss-of-function variants per genome). The annotation of phenotypic abnormalities and their integration into the diagnostic pipeline can identify functional groups of

**Table 10.1** Online databases and knowledge bases

| Name | Abbreviation | Description | URL |
|---|---|---|---|
| ClinVar | – | An archival database that aggregates information about genomic variation and its relationship to human health | www.ncbi.nlm.nih.gov/clinvar/ |
| Clinical genome resource | ClinGen | An authoritative central resource that defines the clinical relevance of genes and variants, for use in precision medicine and research | www.clinicalgenome.org |
| The Leigh map | – | A novel gene-to-phenotype interaction network which can be used as a diagnostic resource for Leigh syndrome | vmh.uni.lu/#leighmap |
| Phenomizer | – | A web-based application for clinical diagnostics in human genetics, using semantic similarity searches in ontology | compbio.charite.de/phenomizer_orphanet |
| Human phenotype ontology | HPO | A standardized vocabulary of phenotypic abnormalities encountered in human disease | www.human-phenotype-ontology.org |
| Inborn errors of metabolism knowledge base | IEMbase | An online knowledge base and smart system (artificial intelligence) for curation and diagnosis support of inborn errors of metabolism | www.iembase.org |

genes, which can help to pinpoint truly pathogenic variants and obtain definitive genetic diagnoses.

In recent years, several gene-to-phenotype databases and knowledge bases have emerged (Table 10.1), including large-scale international expert-curated knowledge bases such as ClinVar and ClinGen. In addition, there are several niche phenomic resources (e.g. Leigh Map) which were developed by experts within a specific disease field to enhance diagnosis and clinical management (Rahman et al. 2017). Other tools can be integrated within the bioinformatic pipeline of WES/WGS and use machine learning and data mining of several clinical and biological knowledge bases to enhance prediction. One example resource is Phenomizer, which automatically consults several rare disease knowledge bases and, based on text inputs from the user, provides a candidate gene list based on both known gene-phenotype associations and alternative genes within the same gene family.

The increasing availability of phenomic repositories is an exciting addition to the field of -omics, yet has its challenges. Phenomic resources are supplements to, and not replacements for, clinical and genetic expertises. If a particular genetic defect is associated with a pathognomonic clinical presentation well-known to clinicians, it is unlikely that there will be a need to consult a phenomic resource. Conversely, some resources generate hundreds of outputs that may be too large to be manageable or interpreted meaningfully. Critical to the success are computer-readable patient descriptions; the Human Phenotype Ontology project (HPO) has been developed to meet this need (Table 10.1). Its main components are phenotype vocabulary, disease-phenotype annotations, and algorithms that operate on these. However, there are still several phenotypes, for example, some biochemical phenotypes, which do not yet have an HPO number and cannot be integrated in resources linked with HPO. Efforts to standardize the collection, annotation, and storage of phenotypic data are crucial for the interoperability between different resources and geographical regions. An internationally recognized nosology for the increasing numbers of IMDs is equally important and currently in the last phase of development (Ferreira et al. 2019).

IEMbase meets many of these needs (Table 10.1, (Lee et al. 2018)). It is an expert-generated and continuously updated database on IMDs, which accepts an array of biochemical and clinical symptoms from a user, maps these to HPO terms, and returns a ranked list of possible IMDs that match the input profile. In addition, the system can explain the rationale of its results, suggest possible tests that would assist in narrowing down the differential diagnosis, and provide access to its database of biochemical, molecular, and clinical information if more evidence is desired.

We emphasize that contributions by the IMD clinical and research community to the curation and updating of biochemical data are urgently needed to fully enable the application of text-based phenomics to facilitate data-sharing for IMD patients (Maiella et al. 2018). Expert curation, crowdsourcing, and automated machine learning methods can facilitate the process and should be a priority for funding.

## Exome and Genome Sequencing

The exome is the collection of all protein-encoding parts, exons, of the genome. It is estimated that 85% of mutations that have a large impact on disease are within the exome. Diagnostic whole exome sequencing (WES) aims to identify genetic variants that alter proteins and thus will identify mutations in genes encoding enzymes and transporters. WES consists of two steps: selection of all 180,000 exons and sequencing of this exonic DNA by high-throughput sequencing technology followed by bioinformatic data analysis. In whole genome sequencing (WGS), the entire genomic DNA of an organism is sequenced. WGS has technical advantages over WES, as no selection step is needed and sensitivity (coverage) is higher. Furthermore, disease-related variants in intronic DNA and regulatory domains can be detected, as well as copy number variants. The percentage of WES-solved cases is with 30% still quite low, which is likely caused by either the lack of sequence coverage of the variant, by disease causes outside the coding sequences, or the misinterpretation of "variants of unknown significance". WGS is therefore postulated as a superior tool to identify unsolved IMD (Gilissen et al. 2014; Belkadi et al. 2015; Stavropoulos et al. 2016; Lionel et al. 2018). Convincing examples of the added value of WGS in IMD disease discovery is the description of glutaminase deficiency in ataxia patients caused by short tandem repeat expansions in *GLS* (van Kuilenburg et al. 2019) and the discovery of a coenzyme Q10 biosynthesis defect (Malicdan et al. 2018). WGS may reveal multiple genetic conditions in a single patient, as recently demonstrated by the discovery of a new defect in pyrimidine metabolism in a patient with an additional known genetic disease, probably leading to a blended phenotype (Perez-Torras et al. 2019) as well as a novel sialic catabolism disorder in a patient with skeletal and cardiomyopathy due to recessive *NPL* mutations, as well as deafness caused by *GJB2* mutations (Wen et al. 2018).

Both in WES and WGS, interpretation of variants often has to be based on *in silico* prediction with an accurate prediction score of only 60–70%. Five different classes of sequence variants are distinguished, of which only the extremes, "clearly not pathogenic" and "clearly pathogenic", are consequential in clinical practice. Thus, additional -omics techniques and functional studies are valuable in making a definite diagnosis. The *in vivo* treatment response should also be taken into consideration when classifying variants (Shen et al. 2021).

## Proteomics

Proteomics gives insight into the composition, structure, and function of the proteome, the entire set of proteins that is produced in a specific state of an organism or a cell population. Interrogation of proteomic data is a powerful approach to reveal impaired protein synthesis, folding, stability, and degradation, by detecting reduced protein levels and by detection of specific proteomic signatures (Stenton et al. 2020). There are many approaches to characterizing the human proteome, which is estimated to contain between 20,000 and 25,000 nonredundant proteins. Most currently used methods are mass spectrometry-based and involve separation by capillary electrophoresis or liquid chromatography.

Quantification is a real challenge in proteomics, and several approaches, including incorporation of stable isotopes, chemical derivatization, and label-free strategies have been reported (McAlister et al. 2014). Proteins frequently function in dynamic and labile multiprotein complexes, the function and stability of which depend on the availability of all constituents. Thus, one can look not only for aberrant expression of an isolated protein but also for all constituents of a protein complex. This may add evidence for the characterization of VUS (Kremer et al. 2017; Lake et al. 2017; Stroud et al. 2016). Complexome analysis, specifically developed to yield insight into the size, composition, and stability of protein complexes, is a powerful method to study the impact of VUS on protein complex assembly. Complexome analysis separates native intact proteins and protein complexes, indicating the composition of functional complexes by the identification of co-migrating proteins (Heide and Wittig 2013). Prokisch and colleagues illustrated that over 4500 proteins can be detected in total, around 50% of which appear within protein complexes (Prokisch 2018). Indeed, complexome analysis has proven fruitful in novel disease gene validation (Heide et al. 2012).

Similar to RNA-seq, outliers can be detected in the proteomic data. Strongly reduced protein level in one sample compared to other samples or to controls provides robust evidence for pathogenicity of underlying variants in autosomal recessive traits. Indeed, although proteomics has not single-handedly uncovered an IMD, it certainly contributes to the diagnostic and validation process. A proteome-wide screen for expression outliers provides valuable information—by inferring the protein-encoding gene(s) in which pathogenic variants may harbour—and paves the way for proteomics, above and beyond functional validation, as a routine test in the diagnostic pipeline (Ferreira et al. 2019; Kremer et al. 2017).

## Transcriptomics

The transcriptome is a quantitative snapshot of all (m)RNAs present in a specific cell population, in time, and under specific circumstances, thus reflecting gene expression. The study of the transcriptome by high-throughput methods is known as transcriptomics. RNA sequencing (RNA-seq), the state-of-the-art technique for transcriptomics, starts with the isolation of RNA from the target tissue or cells, after which it is enzymatically copied to complementary DNA (cDNA). The cDNA is sequenced, after which a transcriptome is assembled using bioinformatic tools.

RNA-seq requires the availability of disease-relevant tissue as the source of RNA. Genetic disorders usually show specificity to some tissues, most of which require invasive methods to obtain or cannot be obtained at all. For disorders in which biopsy of the target tissue is unfeasible, analyses are possible through identification of proxy tissues. In a recent study, the use of whole-blood RNA-seq transcriptomics was investigated in 94 individuals with undiagnosed rare disease, comparing data from these individuals with large sets of RNA-seq data from controls. Across this cohort, transcriptomics yielded a 7.5% diagnostic rate and an additional 16.7% with improved candidate gene resolution (Fresard et al. 2019). Another study demonstrated a 10% diagnostic yield, using dermal fibroblasts, taken during muscle biopsy in patients suspected of a mitochondriopathy (Kremer et al. 2017). A study in muscle biopsies in 50 patients with rare muscle disorders showed splice-altering variants in 35% (Cummings et al. 2017). Alternative to the use of blood or tissue biopsies, patient cells can be reprogrammed into induced pluripotent stem cells and differentiated into disease-relevant cells of interest.

RNA-seq reveals gene expression patterns, indicating which cellular processes are active and which are dormant. In genetic disease, the disease gene may show normal expression when mutations in the coding region affect the function of the gene without affecting its expression level. RNA-seq, however, can also expose coding and noncoding variants, aberrant splicing, allelic expression imbalance, post-transcriptional modifications, and gene fusion, all relevant for diagnosing genetic diseases (Gonorazky et al. 2019). Allelic expression imbalance is especially important to detect, as heterozygous pathogenic variants not prioritized after WES or WGS may have a dominant effect in case the unaffected gene is not expressed. Kremer et al. (2018) reviewed how transcriptomics led to a molecular diagnosis in 10–35% of patients in whom whole exome sequencing failed to do so (Kremer et al. 2018). Recent advances in RNA-seq include direct RNA sequencing, single-cell sequencing, and in situ sequencing of fixed tissue.

## Metabolomics

Metabolomics is described in Chap. 7.

## Lipidomics

Lipids are highly diverse molecules which are traditionally best known for their role in the formation of biological membranes in cellular systems and as a way to store energy. They were traditionally analysed by thin-layer chromatography, gas chromatography, and mass spectrometry. Technical advances in mass spectrometry have paved the way for the realization of a new type of metabolomics: lipidomics. Lipidomics aims to study the pathways and networks of cellular lipids by characterization and quantitation of all lipids present in a biological system. Especially the development of "soft" ionization techniques as electrospray ionization (ESI) and exact mass resolution, high-resolution mass spectrometers have greatly propelled the field of lipidomics. In addition, new bioinformatic tools have been developed to cope with the increasing amounts of raw data and extract relevant information to yield biological insight. The association of lipidomic data with gene expression and sequencing of lipid-specific proteins/enzymes should be furthermore clarified (Zhang et al. 2018).

State-of-the-art lipidomic platforms can annotate about 2000 lipid species in cellular systems, and in plasma about 900 species can be identified (Vaz et al. 2015). The cellular lipidome includes organelle-specific lipids that are not present in extracellular media such as plasma, which is important for the identification and elucidation of organelle-related and other metabolic disorders (Herzog et al. 2018).

Lipidomics is being applied to find biomarkers suitable for diagnosis, follow-up, and ideally prognosis in order to characterize the course of the patient's disorder. Also it can play a central role in the discovery of novel IMDs as underlying cause of phenotypes such as complex hereditary spastic paraplegias ((Vaz et al. 2019), currently under review).

In addition to validating new monogenetic inborn errors of lipid metabolism, there are a growing number of links being uncovered between lipid metabolism and complex genetic traits as obesity, diabetes, atherosclerosis, and cancer (Hyotylainen and Oresic 2014). The corresponding research communities increasingly use lipidomics underscoring the broad application of this technique for research in general.

## Glycomics

Glycosylation is considered the most common post-translational modification of proteins. In the biological process of protein glycosylation, many genes are involved. These genes encode not only the enzymes of N- and O-glycosylation steps but also nucleotide sugar transporters, vesicular transport, and dolichol biosynthesis, which influence protein glycosylation. Clinical glycomics is an approach to gain insight into protein glycosylation and includes diverse analytical methodologies for the analysis of protein-bound, protein-derived, or free glycans.

In general, the methods include the enzymatic or chemical cleavage of N- or O-linked glycans from a single purified protein like transferrin or from multiple proteins present in a biological sample. Then, glycans are separated by electrophoresis or chromatography, after which they are detected by mass spectrometry (Van Scherpenzeel et al. 2016). This approach can be quantitative, which is of high relevance as some type II congenital disorders of glycosylation subtypes are associated with specific N-glycan structures, but others only produce changes in relative levels (Barbosa et al. 2019). In addition to the analysis of protein-released glycans, advances in technology allow the analysis of intact glycoproteins, which obviates the need for enzymatic cleavage of N-glycans, is fast and robust, and enables high-throughput analysis (Van Scherpenzeel et al. 2016; Abu Bakar et al. 2018).

As a source of protein, plasma, serum, urine, and cerebrospinal fluid are all suitable. A recent study used mass spectrometry to identify abnormalities of N-linked and O-linked glycans in plasma and free oligosaccharides in the urine of

207 undiagnosed patients. Sixty percent of these patients had a glycome profile that differed from control values in at least one of the body fluids. Whole exome sequencing revealed some patients with CDGs, along with several others having disorders indirectly altering glycosylation. Thus, glycomics not only is of diagnostic relevance to CDGs but also adds to the pathogenic knowledge in a much larger group of IEMs (Davids et al. 2019). Furthermore, glycomics reflects environmental influences on glycosylation, which makes it of interest for application in monitoring therapeutic interventions.

## Function First

Even with the application of big data technologies, additional functional work is often required, setting the stage for a functional genomics laboratory (Thompson et al. 2019). Model organisms including flies, yeast, worms, zebrafish, rodents, and other mammals are indispensable for the functional investigation of novel genes and variants as well as for delineation of pathophysiology and treatment strategies (Wangler et al. 2017). To accelerate rare disease discovery, the Rare Disease Model Organisms and Mechanisms was established in 2013 and demonstrates success in the connection between clinicians and model organism researchers for a large number of diseases including IMDs (Wangler et al. 2017; Foley 2015).

## Integration: "-omics in Concert"

Diagnosing IMDs should, with some exceptions, not be based on a single approach. Especially when a new inborn error is encountered, the diverse platforms should be combined to generate a solid diagnosis that can form the base for intervention and family counselling.

Phenomics, the thorough description of the patient's phenotype, should always be part of integrated approaches. Furthermore, WES or WGS will give a definite answer to a diagnostic question in case a gene with known function is mutated with a proven pathogenic mutation. In all other cases, additional, functional studies are warranted.

An example of genomics and metabolomics in concert is the discovery of NANS deficiency in patients with intellectual disability, dysmorphisms, and skeletal dysplasia (van Karnebeek et al. 2016). WES in one of the patients, a 3-year-old boy, yielded variants in 19 different genes, whereas untargeted metabolomics performed at the same time led to the discovery of elevated levels of the metabolite *N*-acetylmannosamine, which could only be caused by two enzymatic deficiencies in the de novo sialic acid synthesis pathway. Putting the data sets together facilitated the disease gene (NANS) identification, validation of the deleterious impact of the recessive variants through accumulation of the substrate of the enzyme (*N*-acetylmannosamine), which also serves as a new biomarker with which multiple patients around the world have been subsequently diagnosed. Importantly, knockdown zebrafish recapitulated the human phenotype which was rescued with early sialic acid supplementation, opening up avenues for treatments similar to what is in trial for GNE myopathy, a rare muscle disease resulting from the upstream enzymatic defect (Argov et al. 2016).

The combination of using WES/WGS and transcriptomics and, potentially, proteomics has recently be reviewed (Stenton et al. 2020). Depending on the part of metabolism that is presumably affected, metabolomics, glycomics, and lipidomics may have added value. However, no established strategy is available yet, as these techniques are still evaluated for general diagnostic purposes. Their values, however, have been illustrated by small studies.

Bioinformatic-based integration of technologies is easier said than done. Currently, a combined pipeline for WES and metabolomic data is under construction in some laboratories. This approach prioritizes the genes with potential disease-causing mutations based on alterations in the metabolome of the patient. In cases of inborn errors, this will improve the interpretation of WES and will elucidate defects that may be missed by prediction software.

Clinical caution in the -omics era: Ultimately, the optimal approach to an undiagnosed patient with a suspected IMD remains embedded in clinical expertise and laboratory tests available in a given jurisdiction; however, we expect these broad assessment technologies will merge in the future as a single test for a patient with a suspected IMD. At the same time, proper interpretation of these big data will require functional assays, and the clinician must be cautious in assigning etiologic diagnoses based on -omics findings alone. Also, blended phenotypes caused by two distinct genetic conditions are more frequent than previously assumed (Posey et al. 2017) and should motivate us to perform a complete analysis yielding an explanation for the full phenotype observed.

The combined "omics" technologies will, by elucidating new disease-causing genes, allow the identification of novel points of therapeutic intervention, like splice variants amenable to antisense oligonucleotide treatment. Antisense oligonucleotides are single strands of nucleic acid, 20–25 bases in length, that can bind to a specific RNA sequence, altering splicing. This approach is currently used in spinal muscular atrophy (SMA) and Duchenne muscular dystrophy (DMD) (Bergsma et al. 2018).

**Acknowledgements** We are grateful to the patients and families for inspiring us, to our clinical and research colleagues for teaching us and collaborating with us, and finally to Ms E Ferreira (Amsterdam UMC) for her writing support.

## References


Abu Bakar N, Voermans NC, Marquardt T, Thiel C, Janssen MCH, Hansikova H, et al. Intact transferrin and total plasma glycoprofiling for diagnosis and therapy monitoring in phosphoglucomutase-I deficiency. Transl Res. 2018;199:62–76.

Ahn AC, Tewari M, Poon CS, Phillips RS. The limits of reductionism in medicine: could systems biology offer an alternative? PLoS Med. 2006;3(6):e208.

Alyass A, Turcotte M, Meyre D. From big data analysis to personalized medicine for all: challenges and opportunities. BMC Med Genomics. 2015;8:33.

Argov Z, Caraco Y, Lau H, Pestronk A, Shieh PB, Skrinar A, et al. Aceneuramic acid extended release administration maintains upper limb muscle strength in a 48-week study of subjects with GNE myopathy: results from a phase 2, randomized, controlled study. J Neuromuscul Dis. 2016;3(1):49–66.

Barbosa EA, Fontes NDC, Santos SCL, Lefeber DJ, Bloch C, Brum JM, et al. Relative quantification of plasma N-glycans in type II congenital disorder of glycosylation patients by mass spectrometry. Clin Chim Acta. 2019;492:102–13.

Belkadi A, Bolze A, Itan Y, Cobat A, Vincent QB, Antipenko A, et al. Whole-genome sequencing is more powerful than whole-exome sequencing for detecting exome variants. Proc Natl Acad Sci U S A. 2015;112(17):5473–8.

Benson M. Clinical implications of omics and systems medicine: focus on predictive and individualized treatment. J Intern Med. 2016;279(3):229–40.

Bergsma AJ, van der Wal E, Broeders M, van der Ploeg AT, Pim Pijnappel WWM. Alternative splicing in genetic diseases: improved diagnosis and novel treatment options. Int Rev Cell Mol Biol. 2018;335:85–141.

Cummings BB, Marshall JL, Tukiainen T, Lek M, Donkervoort S, Foley AR, et al. Improving genetic diagnosis in Mendelian disease with transcriptome sequencing. Sci Transl Med. 2017;9(386):eaal5209.

Davids M, Kane MS, Wolfe LA, Toro C, Tifft CJ, Adams D, et al. Glycomics in rare diseases: from diagnosis to mechanism. Transl Res. 2019;206:5–17.

Ferreira CR, van Karnebeek CDM, Vockley J, Blau N. A proposed nosology of inborn errors of metabolism. Genet Med. 2019;21(1):102–6.

Foley KE. Model network: Canadian program aims to generate models for rare disease. Nat Med. 2015;21(11):1242–3.

Fresard L, Smail C, Ferraro NM, Teran NA, Li X, Smith KS, et al. Identification of rare-disease genes using blood transcriptome sequencing and large control cohorts. Nat Med. 2019;25(6):911–9.

Gilissen C, Hehir-Kwa JY, Thung DT, van de Vorst M, van Bon BW, Willemsen MH, et al. Genome sequencing identifies major causes of severe intellectual disability. Nature. 2014;511(7509):344–7.

Gonorazky HD, Naumenko S, Ramani AK, Nelakuditi V, Mashouri P, Wang P, et al. Expanding the boundaries of RNA sequencing as a diagnostic tool for rare Mendelian disease. Am J Hum Genet. 2019;104(3):466–83.

Heide H, Wittig I. Methods to analyse composition and dynamics of macromolecular complexes. Biochem Soc Trans. 2013;41(5):1235–41.

Heide H, Bleier L, Steger M, Ackermann J, Drose S, Schwamb B, et al. Complexome profiling identifies TMEM126B as a component of the mitochondrial complex I assembly complex. Cell Metab. 2012;16(4):538–49.

Herzog K, Pras-Raves ML, Ferdinandusse S, Vervaart MAT, Luyf ACM, van Kampen AHC, et al. Plasma lipidomics as a diagnostic tool for peroxisomal disorders. J Inherit Metab Dis. 2018;41(3):489–98.

Hyotylainen T, Oresic M. Systems biology strategies to study lipidomes in health and disease. Prog Lipid Res. 2014;55:43–60.

Julkowska D, Austin CP, Cutillo CM, Gancberg D, Hager C, Halftermeyer J, et al. The importance of international collaboration for rare diseases research: a European perspective. Gene Ther. 2017;24(9):562–71.

Kremer LS, Bader DM, Mertes C, Kopajtich R, Pichler G, Iuso A, et al. Genetic diagnosis of Mendelian disorders via RNA sequencing. Nat Commun. 2017;8:15824.

Kremer LS, Wortmann SB, Prokisch H. "Transcriptomics": molecular diagnosis of inborn errors of metabolism via RNA-sequencing. J Inherit Metab Dis. 2018;41(3):525–32.

Lake NJ, Webb BD, Stroud DA, Richman TR, Ruzzenente B, Compton AG, et al. Biallelic mutations in MRPS34 lead to instability of the small mitoribosomal subunit and Leigh syndrome. Am J Hum Genet. 2017;101(2):239–54.

Lee JJY, Wasserman WW, Hoffmann GF, van Karnebeek CDM, Blau N. Knowledge base and mini-expert platform for the diagnosis of inborn errors of metabolism. Genet Med. 2018;20(1):151–8.

Lionel AC, Costain G, Monfared N, Walker S, Reuter MS, Hosseini SM, et al. Improved diagnostic yield compared with targeted gene sequencing panels suggests a role for whole-genome sequencing as a first-tier genetic test. Genet Med. 2018;20(4):435–43.

Maiella S, Olry A, Hanauer M, Lanneau V, Lourghi H, Donadille B, et al. Harmonising phenomics information for a better interoperability in the rare disease field. Eur J Med Genet. 2018;61(11):706–14.

Malicdan MCV, Vilboux T, Ben-Zeev B, Guo J, Eliyahu A, Pode-Shakked B, et al. A novel inborn error of the coenzyme Q10 biosynthesis pathway: cerebellar ataxia and static encephalomyopathy due to COQ5 C-methyltransferase deficiency. Hum Mutat. 2018;39(1):69–79.

McAlister GC, Nusinow DP, Jedrychowski MP, Wuhr M, Huttlin EL, Erickson BK, et al. MultiNotch MS3 enables accurate, sensitive, and multiplexed detection of differential expression across cancer cell line proteomes. Anal Chem. 2014;86(14):7150–8.

Perez-Torras S, Mata-Ventosa A, Drogemoller B, Tarailo-Graovac M, Meijer J, Meinsma R, et al. Deficiency of perforin and hCNT1, a novel inborn error of pyrimidine metabolism, associated with a rapidly developing lethal phenotype due to multi-organ failure. Biochim Biophys Acta Mol Basis Dis. 2019;1865(6):1182–91.

Posey JE, Harel T, Liu P, Rosenfeld JA, James RA, Coban Akdemir ZH, et al. Resolution of disease phenotypes resulting from multilocus genomic variation. N Engl J Med. 2017;376(1):21–31.

Prokisch H. Transcriptomics in rare disease diagnosis. Society for the study of inborn errors of metabolism (SSIEM). 2018. Athens, Greece, 4–7 Sept 2018.

Rahman J, Rahman S. The utility of phenomics in diagnosis of inherited metabolic disorders. Clin Med (Lond). 2019;19(1):30–6.

Rahman J, Noronha A, Thiele I, Rahman S. Leigh map: a novel computational diagnostic resource for mitochondrial disease. Ann Neurol. 2017;81(1):9–16.

Shen JJ, Wortmann SB, de Boer L, Kluijtmans LAJ. The role of clinical response to treatment in determining pathogenicity of genomic variants. Genet Med. 2021;23(3):581–5.

Stavropoulos DJ, Merico D, Jobling R, Bowdin S, Monfared N, Thiruvahindrapuram B, et al. Whole genome sequencing expands diagnostic utility and improves clinical management in pediatric medicine. NPJ Genom Med. 2016;1:15012.

Stenton SL, Kremer LS, Kopajtich R, Ludwig C, Prokisch H. The diagnosis of inborn errors of metabolism by an integrative "multi-omics" approach: a perspective encompassing genomics, transcriptomics and proteomics. J Inherit Metab Dis. 2020;43(1):25–35.

Stroud DA, Surgenor EE, Formosa LE, Reljic B, Frazier AE, Dibley MG, et al. Accessory subunits are integral for assembly and function of human mitochondrial complex I. Nature. 2016;538(7623):123–6.

Tebani A, Afonso C, Marret S, Bekri S. Omics-based strategies in precision medicine: toward a paradigm shift in inborn errors of metabolism investigations. Int J Mol Sci. 2016;17(9):1555.

Thompson K, Collier JJ, Glasgow RIC, Robertson FM, Pyle A, Blakely EL, et al. Recent advances in understanding the molecu-

lar genetic basis of mitochondrial disease. J Inherit Metab Dis. 2019;43(1):36–50.
van Karnebeek CD, Bonafe L, Wen XY, Tarailo-Graovac M, Balzano S, Royer-Bertrand B, et al. NANS-mediated synthesis of sialic acid is required for brain and skeletal development. Nat Genet. 2016;48(7):777–84.
van Karnebeek CDM, Wortmann SB, Tarailo-Graovac M, Langeveld M, Ferreira CR, van de Kamp JM, et al. The role of the clinician in the multi-omics era: are you ready? J Inherit Metab Dis. 2018;41(3):571–82.
van Kuilenburg ABP, Tarailo-Graovac M, Richmond PA, Drogemoller BI, Pouladi MA, Leen R, et al. Glutaminase deficiency caused by short tandem repeat expansion in GLS. N Engl J Med. 2019;380(15):1433–41.
Van Scherpenzeel M, Willems E, Lefeber DJ. Clinical diagnostics and therapy monitoring in the congenital disorders of glycosylation. Glycoconj J. 2016;33(3):345–58.
Vaz FM, Pras-Raves M, Bootsma AH, van Kampen AH. Principles and practice of lipidomics. J Inherit Metab Dis. 2015;38(1):41–52.
Vaz F, McDermott J, Alders M. Hypomorphic PCYT2 variants disrupt ether(phospho)lipid biosynthesis causing complex hereditary spastic paraplegia with intellectual disability and epilepsy. (Under review). Brain. 2019;142(11):3382–97.
Wangler MF, Yamamoto S, Chao HT, Posey JE, Westerfield M, Postlethwait J, et al. Model organisms facilitate rare disease diagnosis and therapeutic research. Genetics. 2017;207(1):9–27.
Wen XY, Tarailo-Graovac M, Brand-Arzamendi K, Willems A, Rakic B, Huijben K, et al. Sialic acid catabolism by N-acetylneuraminate pyruvate lyase is essential for muscle function. JCI Insight. 2018;3(24):e122373.
Zhang L, Han X, Wang X. Is the clinical lipidomics a potential goldmine? Cell Biol Toxicol. 2018;34(6):421–3.

# Emergency Diagnostic Procedures and Emergency Treatment

# 11

Stephanie Grünewald, James Davison, Diego Martinelli, and Carlo Dionisi Vici

## Contents



Summary

Metabolic emergencies need to be recognized promptly, and effective treatment needs to be initiated immediately to optimize clinical outcomes. A significant proportion of patients with inborn errors of metabolism are at risk of developing a metabolic emergency at some time of their life, particularly those children affected by an inborn error of metabolism that manifests as an acute intoxication or energy deficiency. These patients usually present as a neonate—typically after an initial symptom-free interval of some days—in an emergency situation. Treatment needs to be initiated immediately even without having arrived at the exact diagnosis.

S. Grünewald (✉) · J. Davison
Metabolic Unit, Great Ormond Street Hospital for Children, NHS Foundation Trust and Institute for Child Health, London, UK
e-mail: stephanie.grunewald@gosh.nhs.uk; james.davison@gosh.nhs.uk

D. Martinelli · C. Dionisi Vici
Division of Metabolism, Department of Pediatric Medicine, Bambino Gesù Children's Research Hospital, Rome, Italy
e-mail: diego.martinelli@opbg.net; carlo.dionisivici@opbg.net

## Introduction

Inborn errors of metabolism, especially those causing acute biochemical intoxication, can present with metabolic emergencies that require prompt recognition and early initiation of appropriate treatment. Many such patients present in the neonatal period, typically after an initial symptom-free interval, although later-onset forms of the conditions can present for the first time at any age including in adulthood. Furthermore, in patients with an established diagnosis and who are on appropriate treatment, acute "decompensation episodes" can occur.

Metabolic crises potentially leading to catabolism can be triggered by infections, vomiting, fasting, or strenuous exercise. Other exogenous triggers include exposure to inappropriate dietary protein in a patient with an aminoacidopathy (AA), organic aciduria (OA), or urea cycle disorder (UCD), exposure to dairy products in patients with galactosemia, or long-chain fat in those with fatty acid oxidation (FAO) disorders. Drugs including valproic acid can result in deterioration in those with mitochondrial disorders.

Although there are numerous metabolic conditions, the acute manifestations share common biochemical and clinical features, and there are a limited number of immediate thera-


N. Blau et al. (eds.), *Physician's Guide to the Diagnosis, Treatment, and Follow-Up of Inherited Metabolic Diseases*,
https://doi.org/10.1007/978-3-030-67727-5_11

peutic measures that are needed. They should be available in any clinical setting (Saudubray 2012; Dionisi-Vici and Ogier de Baulny 2012; Häberle et al. 2019; Baumgartner et al. 2014). Frequent biochemical presentations include hypoglycemia, hyperammonemia, and metabolic acidosis (including lactic acidosis and ketosis). Emergency treatment should proceed in parallel with specific diagnostic tests to correct the abnormal biochemistry even before the underlying diagnosis is known.

### The Acutely Unwell Neonate

The differential diagnosis for an acutely unwell neonate will include sepsis, peripartum hypoxic-ischemic encephalopathy (HIE), intraventricular hemorrhage, congenital viral infection, congenital cardiac disease, and inborn errors of metabolism. Thus as part of the initial assessment of a neonate in an emergency situation, information needs to be gathered about the preceding pregnancy, delivery and neonatal resuscitation, family history (including consanguinity and unexplained sibling deaths), feeding history, presence of symptom-free period, and progression of symptoms. Typically, neonates with an inborn error of metabolism will present after an initial "well period" with progressive refusal of feeds, weight loss, hypotonia, and lethargy progressing to coma.

Initial examination and baseline clinical chemistry will identify the key clinical and biochemical features: encephalopathy manifesting as hypotonia, decreased feeding, irritability, seizures, lethargy, or coma, hepatopathy with coagulopathy and increased transaminases/hepatomegaly, cardiac failure, respiratory distress or failure as compensation for metabolic acidosis, and tachypnea due to the respiratory stimulant effect of hyperammonemia.

*Neurological deterioration*: Toxic encephalopathy is the commonest presentation and most often associated with urea cycle disorders (UCDs); "classical" branched-chain organic acidemias (BCOAs) such as propionic, methylmalonic, or isovaleric acidemia; and maple syrup urine disease (MSUD). Toxicity in UCDs is caused by hyperammonemia and hyperglutaminemia, in BCOAs by metabolic acidosis with/without hyperammonemia, and in MSUD by accumulating leucine and isocaproic acid. Intractable convulsions are associated with amino acid disorders (particularly nonketotic hyperglycinemia (NKH), vitamin B6 deficiency) or purine disorders (adenylosuccinate lyase (ADSL) deficiency or molybdenum cofactor or sulfite oxidase deficiency).

*Liver failure*: Hepatic manifestation of galactosemia, hereditary fructose intolerance, and tyrosinemia type I usually manifest with some delay in the first weeks of life and are amenable to emergency treatment. Some mitochondrial cytopathies can present with early liver failure, as can neonatal hemochromatosis.

*Cardiac failure*: In neonates, fatty acid oxidation defects and mitochondrial trifunctional protein deficiency can present with cardiac failure. Pompe disease presents with hypertrophic cardiomyopathy and hypotonia.

### Later-Onset Patients

Older children, adolescents, or even adults may encounter any of the abovementioned clinical threats. Any type of coma or acute psychiatric symptom can be the presenting sign of a metabolic disorder. In addition, patients may suffer from recurrent attacks of unexplained dehydration, abdominal pain, muscle pain and rhabdomyolysis, or peripheral neuropathy.

A summary of the most characteristic acute signs and differential diagnoses is listed in Table 11.1.

## Emergency Diagnostic Procedures

Basic biochemical tests should be obtained in any acutely unwell neonate or child and will help guide immediate therapeutic decision-making. Basic tests should include full blood count, liver and kidney function tests, electrolytes, blood gas, and calculation of anion gap [($Na^+ + K^+$) − ($Cl^-$ + bicarbonate)], lactate, glucose, ammonia, and urine or blood ketones. Creatine kinase (CK) and uric acid should also be tested. These basic laboratory investigations should be available in any hospital offering emergency treatment at any time.

If the basic biochemical tests raise the possibility of a metabolic disorder, second-line metabolic investigations should be obtained, including:

- Acylcarnitine profile (blood spot or plasma)
- Plasma amino acids
- Urine organic acids and orotic acid
- Hypoglycemia screen if low blood glucose (see below)

These results should be available within 24–48 h.

Depending on the differential diagnosis, additional specific tests will be required as directed by discussion with a metabolic expert clinical team.

## Emergency Scenarios

The most frequently observed metabolic emergencies present biochemically as hyperammonemia, metabolic acidosis, or hypoglycemia.

**Table 11.1** Characteristic acute signs, symptoms, and metabolic differential diagnoses

| Sign | Disease |
|---|---|
| Acute cardiorespiratory signs | |
| Cardiomyopathy | FAO, carnitine transporter def., OXPHOS, Fabry, GSD III, GSD II, BCOAs, MPS-LYSO, Barth syndrome, TMEM70 |
| Arrhythmia | FAO, Kearns-Sayre, Danon, cardiac glycogenosis, triose phosphate isomerase, D-2-hydroxyglutaric aciduria, thiamine deficiency/dependency |
| Pulmonary hypertension | MTHFR, OXPHOS, NFU1, LYSO, Cbl-C, TMEM70 |
| Stridor | Biotinidase, PDH, OXPHOS, Gaucher II, Krabbe |
| Acute neurological signs | |
| Coma | UCDs, BCOAs, MSUD, multiple carboxylase, GA-1, MADD, OXPHOS, FAO, ketolysis, hyperinsulinism, gluconeogenesis |
| Seizures | UCDs, BCOAs, hyperinsulinism, NKH, SO-XO def., PEROX, pyridoxine-dependent epilepsy, pyridoxal phosphate-dependent epilepsy, biotinidase def., cerebral folate receptor-alpha, creatine transporter, GAMT, AGAT, holocarboxylase synthetase, Menkes disease/occipital horn syndrome, PGDH, phosphoserine phosphatase, phosphoserine aminotransferase, OXPHOS, LYSO (Gaucher III, NP disease type C, MLD, GM1, GM2), NCL, GABA transaminase, PDH, ADSL, GS, GLUT1, homocystinuria and remethylation disorders, CDGs |
| Oculogyric crisis | Neurotransmitter disorders, DGUOK def., PUS1, COQ2, KARS |
| Dystonia | BCOAs and vitamin B12 metabolism disorders, GA-1, MEGDEL, OXHPHOS, Wilson disease, aceruloplasminemia, biotin-responsive basal ganglia disease, neurotransmitter disorders, GAMT, homocystinuria, MHBD, HMG-CoA lyase, HMG-CoA synthetase, LSD, NKH, beta-ketothiolase, Lesch-Nyhan, P5CS deficiency |
| Stroke-like episode | OXPHOS (MELAS), OTC, CDGs, homocystinuria, BCOAs, MSUD, Fabry, beta-ketothiolase |
| Ataxia | MSUD, PDH, multiple carboxylase, UCDs, BCOAs and inborn errors of cobalamin metabolism, GLUT1, Hartnup, CoQ10, CTX, LYSO (NP disease type C), NKH, SSADH, thiamine-responsive encephalopathy |
| Dementia | Aceruloplasminemia, Wilson disease, alpha-mannosidosis, X-ALD, CTX, Gaucher disease type III, MPS I, MPS II, MPS III, NP disease type C, MLD, MHBD, MELAS |
| Psychiatric signs | UCDs, citrin def., porphyria, MPS VII, MTHFR, Hartnup, creatine transporter, GAMT, homocystinuria, cobalamin and remethylation disorders, metabolism, MSUD (variant), MELAS, MLD, BCOAs, NP disease type C, SSADH, Wilson disease |
| Sudden visual loss | MELAS, LEBER, MMA, PA, homocystinurias, X-ALD, porphyria, biotinidase def. |
| Sudden hearing loss | MELAS, biotinidase def. |
| Pain | Fabry, Gaucher, Krabbe, prolidase deficiency |
| Acute peripheral neuropathy | PDH, biotinidase, porphyria, MSUD (variant), MLD, tyrosinemia type I, LCHAD/MTP |
| Basal ganglia lesions | OXPHOS, BCOAs, MSUD, beta-ketothiolase, GA I, MADD, HMG-CoA lyase, HMG-CoA synthetase, MHBD SCOT, biotin-responsive T1 transporter, Wilson disease, aceruloplasminemia, GAMT, sulfite oxidase def., MOCO def. |
| Hydrocephalus | MPS I, MPS II, MPS VI, Cbl-C, Cbl-D, MTHFR, Gaucher, NKH, mannosidosis |
| Myoglobinuria | FAO, muscle GSD, OXPHOS, LIPIN1, LIPIN2, porphyria, Wilson disease |
| Cramps | FAO, muscle GSD |
| Acute hematological and vascular signs | |
| Hemolytic anemia | GSH synthetase, gamma-glutamylcysteine synthetase, Wilson disease, Cbl-C |
| Nonhemolytic anemia | Orotic aciduria, inborn errors of cobalamin metabolism, methionine synthetase, inborn errors of folate metabolism, MK, Pearson syndrome, OXPHOS, BCOAs, thiamine-responsive megaloblastic anemia |
| Non-macrocytic and hemolytic anemia or anemia due to combined mechanisms | Abetalipoproteinemia, adenylate kinase, adenosine triphosphatase carnitine uptake, porphyria, di-metal transporter 1, porphyria, galactosemia, glycolytic and pentose-phosphate enzyme, hemochromatosis, IRIDA, LCAT, MK, mitochondrial tyrosyl-tRNA synthetase, MLASA syndrome, pyroglutamic aciduria, pyrimidine 5-nucleotidase, red blood cell glycolysis defects, TALDO, Wilson disease, Wolman disease, X-linked sideroblastic anemia, pyridoxine-responsive epilepsy |
| Neutropenia | GSD1b, Barth syndrome, CLPB, BCOAs |
| Thrombocytopenia | BCOAs, CDGs |
| Pancytopenia | Pearson syndrome, BCOAs, Gaucher types I and III, NP types A and B, OXPHOS, adenylate kinase 2, TALDO |
| Macrophage activation syndrome, HLH | LPI, Cbl-C, Wolman disease, Gaucher disease, NP disease |
| Coagulopathy | CDGs, HHH |
| Subdural hematoma | HHH, GA-I, Menkes disease |
| Thromboembolism | CDGs, homocystinurias |
| Acute liver and digestive signs | |
| Fetal hydrops | LYSO (GM1 gangliosidosis; sialidosis type II; I-cell disease; Niemann-Pick type A/C; MPS I, IV, VI, VII; galactosialidosis; mannosidosis; Farber; Austin; Wolman), TALDO, CDGs, mevalonic aciduria, Smith-Lemli-Opitz, PEROX |

(continued)

**Table 11.1** (continued)

| Sign | Disease |
|---|---|
| Acute liver failure | Tyrosinemia type I, UCDs, citrin def., OXPHOS, CDGs, HFI, FAOD, galactosemia, TALDO, HHH, Wilson disease, neonatal hemochromatosis, Wolman disease, NBAS, SCYL1, RINT2 |
| Cholestatic jaundice | Arginase, bile acid synthesis, CDGs, CTX, cholesterol synthesis defects, citrin, galactosemia, LCHAD/MTP, MK, Niemann-Pick type A/C, Gaucher, PEROX, TALDO, tyrosinemia type I, ADK, ARC syndrome |
| Pancreatitis | FAOD, BCOAs, GSD1, CBS, OXPHOS (MELAS), Pearson syndrome, LPL |
| Intestinal pseudo-obstruction | MNGIE, MK def., MELAS, NARS2 def. |
| Recurrent vomiting | UCDs, OAs, HFI, LPI |
| Acute endocrinological signs | |
| Adrenal insufficiency | SLO, ALD, OXPHOS |
| Hyperinsulinemic hypoglycemia | HI, HI/HA, SCHAD, CDGs, ADK |
| Diabetes | Abnormal proinsulin cleavage, diabetes, deafness and TRMA Kir 6.2, glucokinase, MMA, PA, IVA, ketolytic, OXPHOS, Wolfram syndrome, Pearson and Kearns-Sayre syndrome |
| Acute nephrological signs | |
| Hemolytic uremic syndrome | Cbl-C, MTHFR |
| Fanconi syndrome and renal tubular acidosis | Tyrosinemia type I, galactosemia, OXPHOS, cystinosis, HFI, Fanconi-Bickel, Wilson disease, LPI, CPT1, EHHADH, ARC syndrome, HNF4A |
| Acute renal failure | Oxalosis, FAOD |
| Nephrotic syndrome | CoQ10, CDGs |
| Acute dermatological signs | |
| Skin rash | Biotinidase, MK, holocarboxylase synthetase, Hartnup, porphyria, steroid sulfatase, MEDNIK |
| Orthostatic cyanosis, petechiae | ETHE1 def. |
| Abnormal urine and sweat odor | |
| Sweaty feet odor | IVA, 3-methylcrotonylglycinuria, MADD |
| Maple syrup odor | MSUD |
| Musty odor | PKU |
| Fish odor | Trimethylaminuria, dimethylglycine dehydrogenase |
| Other | |
| Febrile episodes | MK |
| Maternal disease of pregnancy/HELLP | LCHAD/MTP |

## Supportive Care

There is an extensive group of metabolic disorders with acute life-threatening presentation. Long-term outcome is often poorer in patients with early onset of symptoms and/or where initiation of treatment is delayed.

Many acutely sick patients, especially newborn infants, will require circulatory and ventilatory support. Most of them will need rehydration and correction of mineral and/or electrolyte imbalances ($Ca^{2+}$, $PO_4$, $Mg^{2+}$). Given their importance, such treatment should be started immediately and should not delay the initiation of more specific therapeutic measures. Patients with a metabolic crisis might suffer from infections and septicemia, which can result in catabolism and lead to therapeutic failure. Consequently, infections must be prevented, thoroughly investigated for, and, if present, treated aggressively.

In disorders of the intoxication type, such as OAs, AAs, UCDs, FAOs, galactosemia, or fructose intolerance, the oral intake of toxic precursors must be stopped immediately.

## Hyperammonemia

Hyperammonemia should be considered in any unexplained encephalopathy. Hyperammonemia is a major contributor to the pathophysiology of protein catabolism disorders (urea cycle disorders and organic acidurias). Early initiation of treatment is of utmost importance to provide the best possible outcome, since the neurological sequelae depend on the extent and duration of hyperammonemia.

Table 11.2 lists inborn errors of metabolism leading to hyperammonemia, guiding the differential diagnosis.

**Table 11.2** Bedside differential diagnosis of hyperammonemia

| | Urea cycle enzyme defect | Urea cycle intermediate transporter defects | Organic aciduria | Fatty acid oxidation defect | HIHA | PC | HMG-CoA lyase def. | Carbonic anhydrase Va def. | TMEM70/SERAC | PEPCK |
|---|---|---|---|---|---|---|---|---|---|---|
| Hyperammonemia | ↑↑ | ↑ | ↑↑ | ↑ | ↑ | ↑ | ↑ | ↑ | ↑ | ↑ |
| Acidosis | n-↑ | n-↑ | ↑↑ | n-↑ | – | ↑↑ | ↑ | ↑ | ↑ | ↑ |
| Ketonuria | – | – | ↑↑ | -(↓) | – | ↑ | – | ↑ | – | – |
| Glycemia | n | n-↓ | n-↑-↓ | ↓ | ↓↓ | n-↓ | ↓ | ↓ | ↓ | ↓ |
| Lactate | – | – | n-↑ | n-↑ | – | ↑↑ | n-↑ | ↑ | ↑ | ↑ |
| ASAT-ALAT | n-↑ | n-↑ | – | ↑↑ | – | n-↑ | n-↑ | n | n-↑ | |
| Glutamine | ↑ | n | n-↓ | n | n | n | n | n | n | n |
| CK | – | – | – | n-↑↑ | – | – | n-↑ | n | n | |
| Uric acid | – | – | n-↑ | n-↑ | – | n-↑ | ↑ | n | n | |
| WBC/RBC/Plt | – | – | ↓ | – | – | – | n-↓ | n | n | |
| Weight loss | – | – | ↑ | – | – | n-↑ | ↑/– | – | | |
| Other | | | | | | | | | 3-methylglutaconic acid (U) | |

↑ elevated, ↓ decreased, n-↑ normal to elevated, n-↓ normal to decreased, ↑↑ very elevated, (↓) inappropriately low, – no

[a]Only in neonates

Secondary (acquired) disorders can also be associated with hyperammonemia, and these should be considered in the history, examination, and investigations of a child with unexplained hyperammonemia. These include the so-called transient hyperammonemia of the newborn, liver failure from any cause, valproate therapy, and systemic herpes simplex in neonates (Häberle et al. 2019).

### Diagnostic Tests

Hyperammonemia in a newborn patient should trigger investigations to exclude or confirm differential diagnosis such as urea cycle disorders, organic acidemias, and fatty acid oxidation disorders, as well as the more common neonatal septicemias, liver failure, and congenital infections. In late-onset cases, hyperammonemia and metabolic decompensation can be triggered by infection, catabolism, excessive protein intake, medication, and other stressing events, both physiological and psychological (Broomfield and Grunewald 2012; Häberle et al. 2019). Therapy must not be delayed and should proceed simultaneously with the diagnostic workup. Specific metabolic investigations required are:

- Ammonia level (urgent confirmatory sample)
- Liver function tests and clotting profile
- Plasma amino acids
- Urinary organic acids (and orotic acid)
- Blood/plasma acylcarnitine profile
- Urinary amino acids (for transporter defects)
- DNA (for confirmation of diagnosis)

Hyperammonemia is an acute toxic event. It is particularly harmful to the brain as hyperammonemia and the associated hyperglutaminemia lead to astrocyte swelling and brain edema, resulting in irreversible brain damage (Albrecht and Norenberg 2006; Rama Rao and Norenberg 2014). The prognosis of any hyperammonemic patient is strongly influenced by the extent and duration of hyperammonemia, and therefore treatment should not be delayed.

### Acute Management

#### Stop Protein Intake and Promote Anabolism

All protein intake (oral feeds and any parenteral nutrition) need to be stopped immediately, and intravenous glucose commenced to stop catabolism (see table). At least 110% of daily energy demand should be provided.

*To promote anabolism give*:

| Age (years) | Weight | Glucose to provide (mg/kg/min) | Glucose 10% (mL/kg/day) |
|---|---|---|---|
| 0–2 | | 10 | 150 |
| 2–6 | | 8 | 120 |
| >6 | <30 kg | 6 | 90 |
| >6 | 30–50 | 4.5 | 67 |
| >6 | >50 | 3 | 45 |

Hyperglycemia may occur, but glucose infusion should not be reduced. Insulin infusion following local protocols should be given if necessary.

#### Nitrogen Alternative Pathway Therapy

Nitrogen scavenger therapies provide an alternative pathway to the urea cycle for the removal of nitrogen and hence lower ammonia. It is useful to start with a combination of different drugs. The use of these ammonia scavengers represents the mainstay of therapy for detoxification of ammonia in UCDs (Feillet and Leonard 1998; Batshaw et al. 2001; Summar 2001; Häberle et al. 2019). Their use is still debated in BCOAs because of the potential risk of increasing intramitochondrial accumulation of CoA esters and of further depleting free CoA pools (Griffith et al. 1989; Baumgartner et al. 2014). However, sodium benzoate has been reported to be safe (Walter et al. 1995), and most metabolic centers regularly use this drug in organic acidurias. The use of sodium phenylbutyrate in organic acidurias raises further concern because in these diseases hyperammonemia is usually associated with decreased levels of glutamine, with a risk of further depletion of the glutamine/glutamate pool (Filipowicz et al. 2006; Baumgartner et al. 2014).

Recently published UCD guidelines (Häberle et al. 2019) suggest an IV equimolar solution of sodium benzoate and sodium phenylacetate can be used: 250 mg/kg as intravenous bolus over 90–120 min and then 250 mg/kg as continuous IV infusion over 24 h. The combination of sodium benzoate and sodium phenylacetate is available as a drug, registered by the FDA (available in the EU on named patient basis), and can be used as an adjunctive therapy for the treatment of acute hyperammonemia and associated encephalopathy in patients with UCDs.

*Benzoate* is conjugated with glycine to form hippurate, which is then rapidly excreted into the urine. Approximately 1 mole of nitrogen (=ammonia) is then lost for each mole of benzoate administered.

An intravenous loading dose (if the child is not on the drug already) of 250 mg/kg can be administered over 90–120 min followed by 250 mg/kg/day as a continuous infusion. The infusion may be increased to 500 mg/kg/day if required. Subsequent oral dosing is given in 4–6 divided doses.

If patient's weight is >20 kg, the suggested dose for benzoate is 5.5 g/m$^2$/day (up to 12 g/day).

*Phenylbutyrate* is first oxidized to phenylacetate and then conjugated with glutamine to form phenylacetylglutamine. This is excreted into the urine, and theoretically 2 moles of nitrogen are removed for each mole of phenylbutyrate given. An intravenous loading dose (if the child is not on the drug already) of 250 mg/kg can be administered over 90 min followed by 250 mg/kg/day as a continuous infusion. The infusion may be increased to 500 mg/kg/day if required. Subsequent oral dosing is given in 4–6 divided doses. If patient's weight is >20 kg, the suggested dose for phenylbutyrate is 5.5 g/m$^2$/day (up to 12 g/day).

If the patient is undergoing extracorporeal detoxification, maintenance dose for sodium benzoate and phenylbutyrate/phenylacetate should be adjusted.

#### Other Drugs

L-*arginine* is normally synthesized in the urea cycle, but in urea cycle, disorders may become a semi-essential amino acid, especially in ornithine transcarbamylase (OTC) and carbamoyl phosphate synthetase (CPS) deficiency. In citrullinemia and argininosuccinic aciduria, the arginine additionally replaces ornithine that is not reformed in the cycle and thereby facilitates the removal of ammonia in the form of citrulline or ASA.

An intravenous loading dose (if the child is not on the drug already) of 250–400 mg/kg can be administered over 90–120 min followed by 250 mg/kg/day as a continuous infusion. Suggested maximal dose for arginine is 12 g/day. Subsequent oral dosing is given in 4–6 divided doses. Arginine is to be avoided in patients known to have arginase deficiency.

*N-carbamylglutamate* is an alternative activator of carbamoyl phosphate synthetase, the first enzyme in the urea cycle. *N*-carbamylglutamate can be used to treat *N*-acetylglutamate synthetase deficiency or CPS deficiency. It has been shown to be helpful as an adjunctive medication in the treatment of hyperammonemic crises secondary to organic acidemias (Daniotti et al. 2001). A loading dose (100 mg/kg, enteral route), followed by 25–62.5 mg/kg every 6 h can be considered in a neonate with unexplained hyperammonemia or in known patient with NAGS deficiency (Häberle et al. 2019).

l-*carnitine*: (See below for details.) In a child with unexplained hyperammonemia, L-carnitine may be given as an organic aciduria may be the cause. An intravenous loading dose (if the child is not on the drug already) of 100 mg/kg can be administered over 90 min followed by 100 mg/kg/day as a continuous infusion. The infusion may be increased to 300 mg/kg/day if required. Subsequent oral dosing is given in 3–4 divided doses. Carnitine should *not* be given if there is evidence of a cardiomyopathy and any cardiac arrhythmia or if a long-chain fatty acid oxidation disorder is suspected.

L-Arginine, sodium benzoate, and sodium phenylbutyrate should be made up separately in 10% glucose in 50 mL syringes or 500 mL bags (maximum concentration 2.5 g in 50 mL or 25 g in 500 mL bag) and given by a syringe pump or by an infusion pump. They can be infused via Y-connectors into a single venous line running with the 10% glucose infusion as close to the entry site as possible.

#### Extracorporeal Detoxification

In neonates and children, the response to emergency pharmacological treatment should be evaluated after 4 h; if considered inadequate, extracorporeal detoxification should be started (Häberle et al. 2019). Even patients receiving efficient extracorporeal detoxification may still have a poor cognitive prognosis (Kido et al. 2012; Hediger et al. 2018). As a prompt start of acute management is crucial to improve outcome in UCDs, recent publications suggest that dialysis should be initiated as early as possible (Hediger et al. 2018) and that patients with a peak ammonia level >180 µmol/L at the onset should be immediately considered hemodialysis to improve prognosis (Kido et al. 2012).

Of the available techniques, continuous venovenous hemodiafiltration (CVVHDF) and hemodialysis (HD) are far more efficient than peritoneal dialysis (PD) (Picca et al. 2001). PD should therefore only be used if no other form of dialysis is feasible and the patient cannot be rapidly transferred (Picca et al. 2001, 2015). Since the modality of dialysis is dependent on the local facilities, a rapid referral of patients to centers with expert metabolic clinicians and full dialysis facilities is the main determinant for the success of treatment.

### Monitoring

Ammonia levels should be monitored every 3–4 h. Electrolyte should be added to IV fluids as needed, and electrolyte supplementation needs monitoring, taking into account sodium is already given (sodium benzoate (7 mmol sodium per 1 g) or sodium phenylbutyrate (5.4 mmol sodium per 1 g)).

Subsequently the aim is to restart protein by no later than 24–48 h, and monitoring of ammonia should be performed every 12 h. Reintroducing feeds might necessitate a nasogastric or other enteral feeding tube.

## Metabolic Acidosis

Metabolic acidosis (low blood pH, low bicarbonate, base deficit) may be due to either loss of bicarbonate (renal or gastrointestinal losses) causing a normal anion gap acidosis or accumulation of acids such as keto acids (3-hydroxybutyrate and acetoacetate), lactic acid, or other organic acids resulting in an increased anion gap metabolic acidosis. Lactic acidemia (lactate >4 mmol/L) is seen in organic aciduria, gluconeogenesis disorders, or disorders of the oxidative phosphorylation (OXPHOS) system.

Table 11.3 provides a list of inborn errors of metabolism leading to metabolic acidosis. Lactic acidosis is also seen in any acutely unwell infant or child especially where there is circulatory insufficiency, ischemia, bleeding or shock, sepsis, or cardiac disease.

### Diagnostic Tests

The tests described above (Sect. 11.2) will identify the patient with metabolic acidosis and determine the anion gap. Further specific metabolic tests will aid in the differential diagnosis.

### Acute Management

Attention should be paid to identifying and treating secondary causes of acidosis, including circulatory insufficiency and sepsis. These factors should be assessed also in patients with a known diagnosis of an inborn error of metabolism as they may precipitate or worsen the metabolic acidosis.

**Table 11.3** Metabolic acidosis

| Disease | Organic acidurias | MSUD | GSDs (Ia–Ib) GSD III | Ketolysis defects | OXPHOS defects | PC def. | PDH def. | FAO defects | Ketotic hypoglycemia | Fructose 1,6 bisphosphatase deficiency | Multiple carboxylase deficiencies |
|---|---|---|---|---|---|---|---|---|---|---|---|
| Lactate | n-↑ | n-↑ | n-↑↑ | n-↑ | ↑↑ | ↑↑ | ↑↑ | n-↑ | n | n-↑ | ↑ |
| Ketone bodies | ↑↑ | ↑↑ | n-↑ | ↑↑ | n-↑ | ↑ | n | (↓) | ↑↑ | ↑ | ↑ |
| Anion gap | ↑↑ | ↑ | ↑ | ↑ | ↑↑ | ↑↑ | ↑↑ | n-↑ | ↑ | ↑ | ↑ |
| Glucose | n-↓-↑ | n-↓ | ↓↓ | n-↓ | n-↓ | n-↓ | n-↓ | ↓ | ↓ | ↓ | n-↓ |
| Ammonia | ↑↑ | n-↑ | N | n-↑ | n-↑ | n-↑ | n | n-↑ | n | | n-↑ |
| ASAT-ALAT | | | ↑ | | n-↑ | | n-↑ | ↑↑ | | ↑↑ | |
| CK | | | ↑ GSD III | | n-↑ | | | ↑↑ | | | |
| WBC | ↓ | | ↓ GSD Ib | | | | | | | | n-↓ |
| Uric acid | ↑ | ↑ | ↑ | n-↑ | n-↑ | n-↑ | n-↑ | ↑ | n-↑ | n-↑ | n-↑ |
| Abnormal organic acids | + | + | +/– | + | + | + | + | + | – | +/– | + |
| Abnormal amino acids | +/– | + | – | – | + | + | + | – | +/– | – | – |
| Abnormal acylcarnitines | + | – | – | +/– | – | – | – | + | +/– | – | + |

↑ elevated, ↓ decreased, n-↑ normal to elevated, n-↓ normal to decreased, ↑↑ very elevated, (↓) inappropriately low, + yes, – no

#### Fluid Resuscitation

*If the child is clinically shocked with poor perfusion, give normal saline (0.9% sodium chloride) 20 mL/kg* immediately, and repeat the saline bolus if poor circulation persists as for a shocked non-metabolic patient.

*Give glucose 200 mg/kg at once* (2 mL/kg of 10% glucose or 1 mL/kg of 20% glucose) over a few minutes. This promotes anabolism and stops catabolism.

Continue with i.v. infusion of glucose 10%/sodium chloride 0.45% at full maintenance rates (if this is not immediately available, continue with normal saline or 5% dextrose/saline fluids until it is ready).

If there is a strong suspicion of an underlying mitochondriopathy resulting in disturbed energy supply, correcting the metabolic acidosis is the major goal; glucose supply may need to be reduced to maintenance 5% dextrose to restrict the lactic acidosis.

#### Acid-Base Correction Therapy

If acidosis is not improved after correction of circulatory status, treatment with sodium bicarbonate will be required. Prolonged acidosis will impair cellular function and adversely affect cardiac contractility.

*Give sodium bicarbonate 8.4%* as half correction (calculated as [0.15 × weight × base deficit (mmol/L)]) over 20–30 min diluted with i.v. fluids. One milliliter of sodium bicarbonate 8.4% contains 1 mmol of sodium bicarbonate and must be diluted with *at least* 5 mL of 5% glucose for peripheral infusion. Repeat blood gases 30 min after the first dose. Consider continuous bicarbonate infusion if the bicarbonate requirement remains high.

If significant hypernatremia occurs, trometamol (THAM, tris(hydroxymethyl)aminomethane) may be considered as an alternative base therapy.

Other electrolyte imbalances, in particular hypokalemia and hypocalcaemia, must also be concurrently corrected as there is a risk of cardiac arrhythmia as the acidosis is corrected.

#### Promote Anabolism

See above.

#### Other Drugs

*Carnitine*: In organic acidurias, such as PA and MMA, the intramitochondrial accumulation of CoA esters results in the inhibition of various pathways of intermediary metabolism, as well as in depletion of free CoA and in increased levels of acylcarnitines (particularly propionylcarnitine) resulting in a depletion of the carnitine pool. Carnitine is therefore given to compensate for secondary carnitine deficiency caused by urinary excretion of carnitine-bound organic acids. As a rule, L-carnitine supplementation is never contraindicated in these disorders (Baumgartner et al. 2014). Only if a long-chain fatty acid oxidation defect is suspected, the administration of carnitine should be avoided, at least as a bolus, because of the acute accumulation of toxic long-chain acylcarnitines and the potential risk of a fatal cardiac arrhythmia (Bonnet et al. 1999).

*Vitamin therapy*: Patients with isolated methylmalonic acidemia might respond to vitamin B12 treatment. Pharmacological doses of specific vitamins should be systematically tested in each case. Vitamin responsiveness is more likely in late-onset forms than in patients presenting in the newborn period:

- Hydroxocobalamin, the cofactor of methylmalonyl-CoA mutase (and of methionine synthetase), should be tried in all suspected cases; the recommended dose is 1 mg/day given parenterally (Deodato et al. 2006; Baumgartner et al. 2014). Cyanocobalamin is less efficient but may be used temporarily until hydroxocobalamin is available.
- Biotin is the treatment of choice in both holocarboxylase synthetase and biotinidase deficiency, while there are doubts whether biotin-responsive forms of PA really exist; the recommended dose is 10 mg/day given either orally or i.v. (Grünewald et al. 2004).
- Some patients with lactic acidosis due to primary or secondary thiamine deficiency may benefit from thiamine administration (Mayatepek and Schulze 1999; Pérez-Dueñas et al. 2013).
- Riboflavin is the vitamin of choice for treating new patients with MADD, as well as patients with the riboflavin transporter defect, who may have acute paralysis of the diaphragm necessitating ventilation (Bosch et al. 2012).

### Hypoglycemia

Hypoglycemia is a common biochemical disturbance seen in children who are unwell and is also frequently seen in neonates. Specific disorders that shorten fasting tolerance include disorders of glucose homeostasis (glycogen storage disorders, disorders of gluconeogenesis, galactosemia, and congenital hyperinsulinism), disorders of inappropriate ketone synthesis (fatty acid oxidation disorders (FAO)), or inappropriate ketone utilization (ketolysis defects). In disorders of FAOD and hyperinsulinism, hypoglycemia will be combined with decreased ketone body production ("hypoketotic hypoglycemia"). Affected patients become symptomatic with hypoglycemia, particularly after prolonged fasting. Hypoglycemia can also be observed in disorders of amino acid metabolism (MSUD, tyrosinemia type 1). Glucose administration needs to meet at least the rate of hepatic glucose production.

**Table 11.4** Hypoglycemia

| Disease | GSD 1 | GSD 3 | HFI | F 1,6 DP | GALT | HI-HA | HI | Adrenal insuff. | FAO defects | HMG lyase | KH | OHPHOS | HTy1 | MSUD |
|---|---|---|---|---|---|---|---|---|---|---|---|---|---|---|
| Lactate | ↑ | n-↑ | | ↑ | | | | | n-↑ | n-↑ | | ↑↑ | | n-↑ |
| ASAT-ALAT | ↑ | ↑ | ↑ | n-↑ | ↑ | | | n-↑ | ↑ | n-↑ | | n-↑ | ↑ | |
| CK | | ↑ | | | | | | | n-↑ | | | n-↑ | | |
| Uric acid | ↑ | | n-↑ | n-↑ | | | | | ↑ | n-↑ | n-↑ | n-↑ | (↓) | n-↑ |
| FFA | | | | | | (↓) | (↓) | (↓) | ↑ | ↑ | ↑ | ↑ | | |
| Triglycerides | ↑ | | | | | | | | | | | | | |
| Ketone bodies | | ↑ | n-↑ | ↑ | | (↓) | (↓) | (↓) | (↓) | (↓) | ↑ | ↑ | | ↑ |
| Ammonia | | | | | | ↑ | | | n-↑ | n-↑ | | n-↑ | – | n-↑ |
| Anion gap | ↑ | | n-↑ | ↑ | n-↑ | | | n-↑ | n-↑ | ↑ | n-↑ | ↑ | ↑ | n-↑ |
| Coagulation | n-↓ | | n-↓ | | ↓ | | | | n-↓ | | | n-↓ | ↓ | |
| WBC | ↓ (1b) | | | | | | | | | n-↓ | | | | |
| Abnormal organic acids | | | | ± | | ± | | | + | + | + | + | + | + |
| Abnormal amino acids | | | | | ± | | | | | ± | ± | ± | + | + |
| Abnormal acylcarnitines | | | | | | | n/+ | | + | + | (+) | | | |
| Fasting hypoglycemia | + | + | | + | | | | + | + | + | + | + | | |
| Post-meal hypoglycemia | | | + fructose | | + galactose | + protein | | | | | | | | |

↑ elevated, ↓ decreased, n-↑ normal to elevated, n-↓ normal to decreased, (↓) inappropriately low, + yes, – no

Table 11.4 provides a list of inborn errors of metabolism leading to hypoglycemia.

The definition of hypoglycemia is debated, but in general a blood glucose <2.6 mmol/L (46.8 mg/dL) is considered abnormal. Neonates may tolerate lower blood glucose asymptomatically, and a neonate who is otherwise well and in whom hypoglycemia resolves promptly with feeding may not need detailed investigation. Conversely the neonate with resistant hypoglycemia requiring high glucose infusion rates may have congenital hyperinsulinism.

### Diagnostic Samples

Diagnostic samples should be collected (when clinically safe) before correction of the hypoglycemia. Critical samples include:

- Glucose and lactate
- Blood gas
- Free fatty acids (nonesterified fatty acids)
- 3-hydroxybutyrate
- Bloodspot acylcarnitine profile
- Insulin and C-peptide
- Cortisol

Urine for ketones (bedside test) and urine organic acids (the first urine passed after the hypoglycemic episode should be collected for this, but correction of hypoglycemia should not be delayed waiting for the urine sample).

Additional samples for urate, creatine kinase, liver function tests, and plasma amino acids should also be collected but do not have necessarily to be during the hypoglycemia.

### Hypoglycemia: Emergency Treatment

Hypoglycemia should be corrected. Oral/buccal glucose gel can be administered. Intravenous glucose can be given as 2 mL/kg 10% dextrose bolus. This should be followed with an infusion of 10% dextrose-containing fluids (there may be rebound hyperinsulinism and secondary hypoglycemia after the bolus).

In a child with a suspected IEM, promote anabolism (see above). Supplement sodium, potassium, and phosphate as required.

Blood glucose should be monitored and glucose infusion rate escalated to maintain normoglycemia. This may necessitate the use of higher concentrations of dextrose infusion which may require central venous access. Glucose infusion requirements of >10 mg/kg/min are suggestive of hyperinsulinism.

## Seizures

If intractable seizures dominate the clinical picture, pyridoxine (B6)-responsive, pyridoxal phosphate-responsive, and folinic acid-responsive seizures and congenital hypophosphatasia should be considered (Mills et al. 2005; Stockler et al. 2011; Rahman et al. 2013). In the case of a positive response, the therapeutic trials might be diagnostic. Many intracellular enzymes require pyridoxal phosphate as a cofactor.

Low uric acid in a neonate with intractable seizures should raise the suspicion of molybdenum cofactor or multiple sulfite oxidase deficiency. In urine, sulfocysteine and elevated levels of AASA are measured.

Metabolic investigations should be undertaken simultaneously in parallel with therapeutic interventions. Initial seizure management should follow standard protocols. Severe infantile epileptic encephalopathy is one indication for CSF analyses testing neurotransmitter and glycine CSF/plasma ratio, allowing the diagnosis of defects in the metabolism of biogenic amines and GABA transaminase deficiency and nonketotic hyperglycinemia (Hoffmann et al. 1998; Ng et al. 2015; Coughlin 2nd and Swanson 2017).

#### Pyridoxine

Pyridoxine is administered i.v. Start with a single dose of 100 mg of pyridoxine, and if the patient is nonresponsive within 10 min, the dose should be increased and repeated up to 200 mg total before concluding about pyridoxine nonresponsiveness. High doses of pyridoxine can cause severe apnea so it is recommended to be administered in an ICU setting (Bass et al. 1996; Grillo et al. 2001). If there is uncertainty about at least a partial response, pyridoxine should be continued with 5–15 mg/kg/day (up to 30 mg/kg/day) for 7 days before final conclusions are made. Patients with mutations in antiquitin (*ALDH7A1*) encoding aminoadipic acid semialdehyde dehydrogenase accumulate piperideine-6-carboxylate which inactivates pyridoxal phosphate. They have elevated urine aminoadipic semialdehyde and elevated pipecolic acid in blood, CSF, and urine. If antiquitin deficiency is confirmed, dietary lysine restriction combined with arginine supplementation should be considered (Coughlin et al. 2015).

#### Pyridoxal Phosphate

Pyridoxal phosphate 30 mg/kg/day in 3 doses orally for 3 days can be tried and is effective for patients with pyridoxamine 5′-phosphate oxidase (*PNPO*) deficiency. These patients cannot convert pyridoxine or pyridoxamine to pyridoxal phosphate and so develop intracellular pyridoxal phosphate deficiency treatable only with pyridoxal phosphate.

Patients with congenital hypophosphatasia (*TNSALP*) with characteristic biochemical abnormalities including low alkaline phosphatase and phosphate and high calcium respond to either pyridoxine or pyridoxal phosphate.

#### Folinic Acid

If the response to pyridoxine is negative or doubtful, folinic acid can be administered with 5 mg/kg/day in 3 doses intravenously or orally for 3 days. Primary cerebral folate deficiency results from defects of the blood-brain barrier folate transporter systems and inborn errors of folate metabolism. Secondary cerebral folate deficiency is frequently observed in other IEMs including mitochondrial cytopathies (Pope et al. 2019).

## Postmortem Investigations

In the event of death when metabolic disease is suspected, it is important to store adequate amounts of biological fluids and tissues for further diagnostic workup. In the case of sudden infant death syndrome (SIDS), it is important to recognize that defects of fatty acid β-oxidation may be responsible. In most cases, autopsy reveals an excess of fat droplets in the liver or heart, even in the absence of steatosis.

Should there be the suspicion of an underlying metabolic disease in a deceased child, it is critical to collect the following samples (Marín-Valencia et al. 2010):

| Sample/storage |
|---|
| Urine (−20°) |
| Amino acids, organic acids, tubulopathy markers |
| Blood (−20°) |
| DNA, uric acid, amino acids |
| Dried blood spots (room temperature) |
| Acylcarnitine profile |
| CSF sample (−70°) |
| Neurotransmitters, amino acids |
| Skin biopsy (fibroblasts, culture medium at room temperature) |
| Enzyme analysis, DNA |

Liver or muscle biopsies need to be considered in special circumstances, for example, if there is the suspicion of an underlying mitochondrial disorder. Those samples (and this also applies for plasma amino acid samples) must be taken as soon as possible postmortem to ensure reliable results. The samples need to be stored at −70 °C immediately.

## References


Albrecht J, Norenberg MD. Glutamine: a Trojan horse in ammonia neurotoxicity. Hepatology. 2006;44:788–94.

Bass NE, Wyllie E, Cohen B, Joseph SA. Pyridoxine-dependent epilepsy: the need for repeated pyridoxine trials and the risk of severe electrocerebral suppression with intravenous pyridoxine infusion. J Child Neurol. 1996;11(5):422–4.

Batshaw ML, MacArthur RB, Tuchman M. Alternative pathway therapy for urea cycle disorders: twenty years later. J Pediatr. 2001;138:S46–54; discussion S54–45.

Baumgartner MR, Hörster F, Dionisi-Vici C, et al. Proposed guidelines for the diagnosis and management of methylmalonic and propionic acidemia. Orphanet J Rare Dis. 2014;9:130.

Bonnet D, Martin D, De Lonlay P, et al. Arrhythmias and conduction defects as presenting symptoms of fatty acid oxidation disorders in children. Circulation. 1999;100:2248–53.

Bosch AM, Stroek K, Abeling NG, et al. The Brown-Vialetto-Van Laere and Fazio Londe syndrome revisited: natural history, genetics, treatment and future perspectives. Orphanet J Rare Dis. 2012;7:83.

Broomfield A, Grunewald S. How to use serum ammonia. Arch Dis Child Educ Pract Ed. 2012;97(2):72–7.

Coughlin CR 2nd, Swanson MA. The genetic basis of classic nonketotic hyperglycinemia due to mutations in GLDC and AMT. Genet Med. 2017;19(1):104–11.

Coughlin CR, van Karnebeek CD, Al-Hertani W, et al. Triple therapy with pyridoxine, arginine supplementation and dietary lysine restriction in pyridoxine-dependent epilepsy: neurodevelopmental outcome. Mol Genet Metab. 2015;116:35–43.

Daniotti M, la Marca G, Fiorini P, et al. New developments in the treatment of hyperammonemia: emerging use of carglumic acid. Int J Gen Med. 2001;4:21–8.

Deodato F, Boenzi S, Santorelli FM, et al. Methylmalonic and propionic aciduria. Am J Med Genet C Semin Med Genet. 2006;142:104–12.

Dionisi-Vici C, Ogier de Baulny H. Emergency treatment. In: Saudubray JM, van den Berge G, Walter J, editors. Inborn metabolic diseases: diagnosis and treatment. 5th ed. Heidelberg: Springer; 2012. p. 103–11.

Feillet F, Leonard JV. Alternative pathway therapy for urea cycle disorders. J Inherit Metab Dis. 1998;21(Suppl 1):101–11.

Filipowicz HR, Ernst SL, Ashurst CL, et al. Metabolic changes associated with hyperammonemia in patients with propionic acidemia. Mol Genet Metab. 2006;88:123–30.

Griffith AD, Cyr DM, Egan SG, et al. Inhibition of pyruvate carboxylase by sequestration of coenzyme A with sodium benzoate. Arch Biochem Biophys. 1989;269(1):201–7.

Grillo E, da Silva RJ, Barbato JH Jr. Pyridoxine-dependent seizures responding to extremely low-dose pyridoxine. Dev Med Child Neurol. 2001;43(6):413–5.

Grünewald S, Champion MP, Leonard JV, et al. Biotinidase deficiency: a treatable leukoencephalopathy. Neuropediatrics. 2004;35:211–6.

Häberle J, Burlina A, Chakrapani A, et al. Suggested guidelines for the diagnosis and management of urea cycle disorders: first revision. J Inherit Metab Dis. 2019;42(6):1192–230.

Hediger N, Landolt MA, Diez-Fernandez C, et al. The impact of ammonia levels and dialysis on outcome in 202 patients with neonatal onset urea cycle disorders. J Inherit Metab Dis. 2018;41:689–98.

Hoffmann GF, Surtees RA, Wevers RA. Cerebrospinal fluid investigations for neurometabolic disorders. Neuropediatrics. 1998;29:59–71.

Kido J, Nakamura K, Mitsubuchi H, et al. Long-term outcome and intervention of urea cycle disorders in Japan. J Inherit Metab Dis. 2012;35:777–85.

Marín-Valencia I, Vilaseca MA, Thió M, et al. Assessment of the perimortem protocol in neonates for the diagnosis of inborn errors of metabolism. Eur J Paediatr Neurol. 2010;14:125–30.

Mayatepek E, Schulze A. Metabolic decompensation and lactic acidosis in propionic acidaemia complicated by thiamine deficiency. J Inherit Metab Dis. 1999;22:189–90.

Mills PB, Surtees RA, Champion MP, et al. Neonatal epileptic encephalopathy caused by mutations in the PNPO gene encoding pyridox(am)ine 5′-phosphate oxidase. Hum Mol Genet. 2005;14:1077–86.

Ng J, et al. Monoamine neurotransmitter disorders—clinical advances and future perspectives. Nat Rev Neurol. 2015;11(10):567–84.

Pérez-Dueñas B, Serrano M, Rebollo M, et al. Reversible lactic acidosis in a newborn with thiamine transporter-2 deficiency. Pediatrics. 2013;131(5):1670–5.

Picca S, Dionisi-Vici C, Abeni D, et al. Extracorporeal dialysis in neonatal hyperammonemia: modalities and prognostic indicators. Pediatr Nephrol. 2001;16:862–7.

Picca S, Dionisi-Vici C, Bartuli A, et al. Short-term survival of hyperammonemic neonates treated with dialysis. Pediatr Nephrol. 2015;30:839–47.

Pope S, et al. Cerebral folate deficiency: analytical tests and differential diagnosis. J Inherit Metab Dis. 2019;42(4):655–72.

Rahman S, Footitt E, Varadkar S, et al. Inborn errors of metabolism causing encephalopathy. Dev Med Child Neurol. 2013;55:23–36.

Rama Rao KV, Norenberg MD. Glutamine in the pathogenesis of hepatic encephalopathy: the Trojan horse hypothesis revisited. Neurochem Res. 2014;39:593–8.

Saudubray JM. Clinical approach to inborn errors of metabolism in paediatrics. In: Saudubray JM, van den Berge G, Walter J, editors. Inborn metabolic diseases: diagnosis and treatment. 5th ed. Heidelberg: Springer; 2012. p. 3–52.

Stockler S, Plecko B, Gospe SM Jr, et al. Pyridoxine dependent epilepsy and antiquitin deficiency: clinical and molecular characteristics and recommendations for diagnosis, treatment and follow-up. Mol Genet Metab. 2011;104:48–60.

Summar M. Current strategies for the management of neonatal urea cycle disorders. J Pediatr. 2001;138(1 Suppl):S30–9.

Walter JH, Wraith JE, Cleary MA. Absence of acidosis in the initial presentation of propionic acidaemia. Arch Dis Child Fetal Neonatal Ed. 1995;72:197–9.

# Nosology of Inborn Errors of Metabolism

12

Carlos R. Ferreira

## Contents



**Abstract**

Inborn errors of metabolism (IEMs) have existed since prehistoric times. As an example, a mummy named Harwa, dating from approximately 1,500 B.C. and currently exhibited at the Field Museum of Natural History in Chicago, was found to have arthropathy, black articular surfaces, and accumulation of homogentisic acid, consistent with alkaptonuria. Alkaptonuria also became the first condition identified as a metabolic disease, in 1902. This chapter briefly traces the historical development of classification systems for IEMs, starting with Garrod's tetrad in 1908, and culminating with the establishment of the International Classification of Inherited Metabolic Disorders (ICIMD), a global effort to unify classification systems of metabolic disease, in 2021.

Inborn errors of metabolism (IEMs) have existed since prehistoric times. As an example, a mummy named Harwa, dating from approximately 1500 B.C. and currently exhibited at the Field Museum of Natural History in Chicago, was found to have arthropathy, black articular surfaces, and accumulation of homogentisic acid, consistent with alkaptonuria (Stenn et al. 1977). Alkaptonuria also represents the first human disease to which Mendel's concepts of heredity were applied and the first condition identified as a metabolic disease (Garrod 1902). In the words of Sir Archibald Garrod in his classic 1902 paper, alkaptonuria "is rather of the nature of an alternative course of metabolism"; he went on to write that this view of alkaptonuria as "an alternative mode of metabolism will obviously gain considerably in weight if it can be shown that it is not an isolated example of a chemical abnormality, but that there are other conditions which may reasonably be placed in the same category." Indeed, by the time of his seminal Croonian Lectures delivered to the Royal College of Physicians in 1908, he had identified four conditions (alkaptonuria, albinism, cystinuria, and pentosuria, now known as Garrod's tetrad) that were explained by this alternative mode of metabolism (Garrod 1908a, b, c, d). He coined the term "inborn errors of metabolism" to describe this altered metabolic course; his Croonian lectures were in fact collected as a book in 1909 under the title *Inborn Errors of Metabolism* (Garrod 1909). By the time the second edition of his book appeared in 1923, he included two additional IEMs, congenital porphyrinuria and congenital steatorrhea (Garrod 1923), for a total of six IEMs (or what could be named "Garrod's hexad").

Various IEMs were described over the next several decades, but it wasn't perhaps until the appearance of the first edition of *The Metabolic Basis of Inherited Disease* in 1960 that a formal classification of IEMs was attempted. In that book, the following classifications were outlined (Stanbury et al. 1960):

- Disorders of carbohydrate metabolism: diabetes mellitus, glycogen deposition diseases, pentosuria, galactosemia, fructosuria, and hyperbilirubinemia
- Disorders of amino acid metabolism: familial goiter, alkaptonuria, phenylketonuria, albinism, tyrosinosis, primary hyperoxaluria and oxalosis, and maple syrup urine disease

C. R. Ferreira (✉)
Division of Genetics and Metabolism, Children's National Health System, Washington, DC, USA
e-mail: carlos121180@gmail.com


N. Blau et al. (eds.), *Physician's Guide to the Diagnosis, Treatment, and Follow-Up of Inherited Metabolic Diseases*,
https://doi.org/10.1007/978-3-030-67727-5_12

- Disorders of lipid metabolism: essential familial hyperlipidemia, Niemann-Pick disease, Tay-Sachs disease, and Gaucher disease
- Disorders of steroid metabolism: the adrenogenital syndrome
- Diseases of purine and pyrimidine metabolism: gout, orotic aciduria, xanthinuria, and beta-aminoisobutyric aciduria
- Disorders of metal metabolism: Wilson disease, hemochromatosis, periodic paralysis, adynamia episodica hereditaria, and pseudohypoparathyroidism
- Disorders of porphyrin metabolism: the porphyrias
- Disorders blood and blood-forming tissues: hereditary spherocytosis, hemoglobinopathies and thalassemia, drug-induced hemolytic anemia (primaquine sensitivity), hereditary methemoglobinemias, and disorders of blood-clotting factors
- Disorders of renal tubular transport: familial hypophosphatemia and vitamin D-resistant rickets, Fanconi syndrome, renal glycosuria, glycinuria, renal tubular acidosis, vasopressin-resistant diabetes insipidus, and Hartnup disease
- Disorders of plasma enzymes or proteins: hypophosphatasia, acatalasia, and hereditary hypoproteinemias

Other classification systems were developed over the next following decades, including one dividing IEMs into four main groups according to mechanism of disease: disorders of transport; disorders of storage, scavenge, and secretion; disorders of synthesis; and disorders of intermediary metabolism (Sinclair 1982). A clinical classification of IEMs has also been established, dividing them into two large categories: category 1, including disorders involving only one system, presenting uniform symptoms (such as a bleeding tendency in coagulation factor defects or hemolytic anemia in defects of glycolysis), and category 2, including diseases with systemic consequences, which in turn can be subdivided into three groups—(1) disorders of complex molecules, such as lysosomal disorders, peroxisomal disorders, or congenital disorders of glycosylation; (2) intoxication disorders, such as urea cycle defects, organic acidemias, or aminoacidopathies; and (3) energy deficiency disorders, such as disorders of gluconeogenesis, glycogen storage disorders, and fatty acid oxidation defects (Saudubray and Charpentier 2014).

One of the most comprehensive attempts at a classification of IEMs was established by the Society for the Study of Inborn Errors of Metabolism (SSIEM) and is accessible via their website (http://www.ssiem.org/resources/IEC.asp). This hierarchical classification was last updated in 2012 and appeared in print in 2014 in the prior edition of this book (Zschocke 2014). It includes 487 IEMs in 86 disease groups and classifies IEMs according to the specific biochemical pathway involved.

A recently proposed nosology was published in March 2018, including 1015 well-established IEMs in 130 groups (Ferreira et al. 2019). Additionally, it included 111 IEMs described as provisional, either because their molecular basis had not been elucidated, because only a few patients had been described in decades-old reports, or because only individual families had been reported. There is a precedent for including such provisional disorders in a classification system; for example, by the time of the publication of the first edition of *The Metabolic Basis of Inherited Disease*, orotic aciduria and tyrosinosis had only been described in one patient each but were considered plausible IEMs (Stanbury et al. 1960). Just as these two conditions were eventually found to represent bona fide IEMs, it is very likely that the majority of IEMs currently considered provisional will be well-established in the future.

The current book will follow the classification system established in the aforementioned nosology. An overview of the 9 categories and 130 groups represented in the nosology is outlined in Table 12.1.

**Table 12.1** Overview of the nosology of IEMs

| | |
|---|---|
| (A) | **Disorders of nitrogen-containing compounds** |
| 1. | Disorders of pyrimidine metabolism |
| 2. | Disorders of purine metabolism |
| 3. | Disorders of nucleotide metabolism |
| 4. | Disorders of creatine metabolism |
| 5. | Disorders of choline metabolism |
| 6. | Disorders of glutathione metabolism |
| 7. | Disorders of ammonia detoxification |
| 8. | Disorders of amino acid transport |
| 9. | Aminoacylase deficiencies |
| 10. | Disorders of monoamine metabolism |
| 11. | Disorders of phenylalanine and tetrahydrobiopterin metabolism |
| 12. | Disorders of tyrosine metabolism |
| 13. | Disorders of sulfur amino acid and sulfide metabolism |
| 14. | Disorders of branched-chain amino acid metabolism |
| 15. | Disorders of lysine metabolism |
| 16. | Disorders of proline and ornithine metabolism |
| 17. | Disorders of β- and γ-amino acids |
| 18. | Disorders of histidine metabolism |
| 19. | Disorders of tryptophan metabolism |
| 20. | Disorders of glutamate metabolism |
| 21. | Disorder of glutamine metabolism |
| 22. | Disorder of asparagine metabolism |
| 23. | Disorders of serine metabolism |
| 24. | Disorders of glycine metabolism |
| (B) | **Disorders of vitamins, cofactors, metals, and minerals** |
| 25. | Disorders of lipoic acid and iron-sulfur metabolism |
| 26. | Disorders of cobalamin metabolism |
| 27. | Disorders of folate metabolism |
| 28. | Disorders of biotin metabolism |
| 29. | Disorders of thiamine metabolism |
| 30. | Disorders of riboflavin metabolism |
| 31. | Disorders of niacin and NAD metabolism |
| 32. | Disorders of pantothenate metabolism |
| 33. | Disorders of pyridoxine metabolism |

**Table 12.1** (continued)

| | |
|---|---|
| 34. | Disorder of vitamin C metabolism |
| 35. | Disorders of vitamin A metabolism |
| 36. | Disorders of vitamin D metabolism |
| 37. | Disorder of vitamin E metabolism |
| 38. | Disorders of vitamin K metabolism |
| 39. | Disorders of molybdenum metabolism |
| 40. | Disorders of copper metabolism |
| 41. | Disorders of iron metabolism |
| 42. | Disorders of manganese metabolism |
| 43. | Disorders of zinc metabolism |
| 44. | Disorders of selenium metabolism |
| 45. | Disorders of magnesium metabolism |
| (C) | **Disorders of carbohydrates** |
| 46. | Disorders of carbohydrate transport and absorption |
| 47. | Disorders of galactose metabolism |
| 48. | Disorders of fructose metabolism |
| 49. | Disorders of the pentose phosphate pathway and polyol metabolism |
| 50. | Disorders of insulin secretion and signaling |
| 51. | Glycogen storage diseases |
| 52. | Disorders of gluconeogenesis |
| 53. | Disorders of glycolysis |
| (D) | **Mitochondrial disorders of energy metabolism** |
| 54. | Disorders of pyruvate metabolism |
| 55. | Disorders of the Krebs cycle |
| 56. | Disorders of metabolite repair |
| 57. | Disorders of mitochondrial carriers |
| 58. | Disorders of complex I subunits |
| 59. | Disorders of complex I assembly |
| 60. | Disorders of complex II subunits |
| 61. | Disorders of complex II assembly |
| 62. | Disorders of complex III subunits |
| 63. | Disorders of complex III assembly |
| 64. | Disorders of complex IV subunits |
| 65. | Disorders of complex IV assembly and ancillary proteins |
| 66. | Disorders of complex V subunits |
| 67. | Disorders of complex V assembly |
| 68. | Disorders of mitochondrial cytochrome synthesis and incorporation |
| 69. | Disorders of mitochondrial DNA depletion, multiple deletion, or intergenomic communication |
| 70. | Disorders of mitochondrial transcription and RNA transcript processing |
| 71. | Mitochondrial ribosomopathies |
| 72. | Disorders of mitochondrial translation factors |
| 73. | Disorders of mitochondrial tRNA |
| 74. | Disorders of mitochondrial tRNA incorporation and recycling |
| 75. | Disorders of mitochondrial fission |
| 76. | Disorders of mitochondrial fusion |
| 77. | Disorders of mitochondrial phospholipid metabolism |
| 78. | Disorders of mitochondrial protein import |
| 79. | Disorders of mitochondrial protein quality control |
| 80. | Other disorders of mitochondrial homeostasis |
| 81. | Primary CoQ10 deficiencies |
| (E) | **Disorders of lipids** |
| 82. | Disorders of carnitine metabolism |
| 83. | Disorders of fatty acid oxidation and transport |
| 84. | Disorders of ketone body metabolism |
| 85. | Disorders of fatty acid synthesis and elongation |
| 86. | Disorder of fatty aldehyde metabolism |
| 87. | Disorders of glycerol metabolism |
| 88. | Disorders of cytoplasmic triglyceride metabolism |
| 89. | Disorders of non-mitochondrial phospholipid metabolism |
| 90. | Disorders of non-lysosomal sphingolipid metabolism |
| 91. | Disorders of eicosanoid metabolism |
| 92. | Disorders of palmitoylation |
| 93. | Disorders of phosphoinositide metabolism |
| 94. | Disorders of lipoprotein metabolism |
| 95. | Disorders of cholesterol biosynthesis |
| 96. | Disorders of steroid metabolism |
| 97. | Disorders of bile acid synthesis |
| (F) | **Disorders of tetrapyrroles** |
| 98. | Disorders of heme metabolism |
| 99. | Disorders of bilirubin metabolism and biliary transport |
| (G) | **Storage disorders** |
| 100. | Disorders of autophagy |
| 101. | Neuronal ceroid lipofuscinosis |
| 102. | Sphingolipidoses |
| 103. | Oligosaccharidoses |
| 104. | Mucolipidoses |
| 105. | Mucopolysaccharidoses |
| 106. | Disorders of lysosomal cholesterol metabolism |
| 107. | Disorders of lysosomal transport or sorting |
| 108. | Disorders of lysosomal protein degradation |
| (H) | **Disorders of peroxisomes and oxalate** |
| 109. | Disorders of plasmalogen synthesis |
| 110. | Disorders of peroxisomal β-oxidation |
| 111. | Disorder of peroxisomal α-oxidation |
| 112. | Disorders of peroxisomal biogenesis |
| 113. | Peroxisomal disorders not involving lipid metabolism |
| 114. | Disorders of oxalate metabolism |
| (I) | **Congenital disorders of glycosylation** |
| 115. | Disorders of N-linked glycosylation |
| 116. | Disorders of *O*-mannosylation |
| 117. | Disorders of *O*-xylosylation and glycosaminoglycan synthesis |
| 118. | Disorders of *O*-GalNAcylation |
| 119. | Disorders of *O*-GlcNAcylation |
| 120. | Disorder of *O*-glucosylation |
| 121. | Disorders of *O*-fucosylation |
| 122. | Disorders of glycosylphosphatidylinositol biosynthesis |
| 123. | Disorders of glycolipid glycosylation |
| 124. | Disorders of dolichol metabolism |
| 125. | Disorders of monosaccharide synthesis and interconversion |
| 126. | Disorders of nucleotide-sugar synthesis |
| 127. | Disorders of Golgi transport |
| 128. | Glycosylation disorders of vesicular trafficking |
| 129. | Disorders of Golgi homeostasis |
| 130. | Disorder of deglycosylation |
| (J) | **Miscellaneous disorders** |

The nosology of IEMs is regularly updated via IEMbase, a knowledgebase of IEMs (www.iembase.org/nosology) (Lee et al. 2018). In 14 months since the publication of this nosology, there have been 74 novel IEMs added, plus 30 new provisional IEMs (Fig. 12.1). Table 12.2 summarizes the current number of IEMs according to category, while Table 12.3 summarizes the inheritance pattern of well-established IEMs.

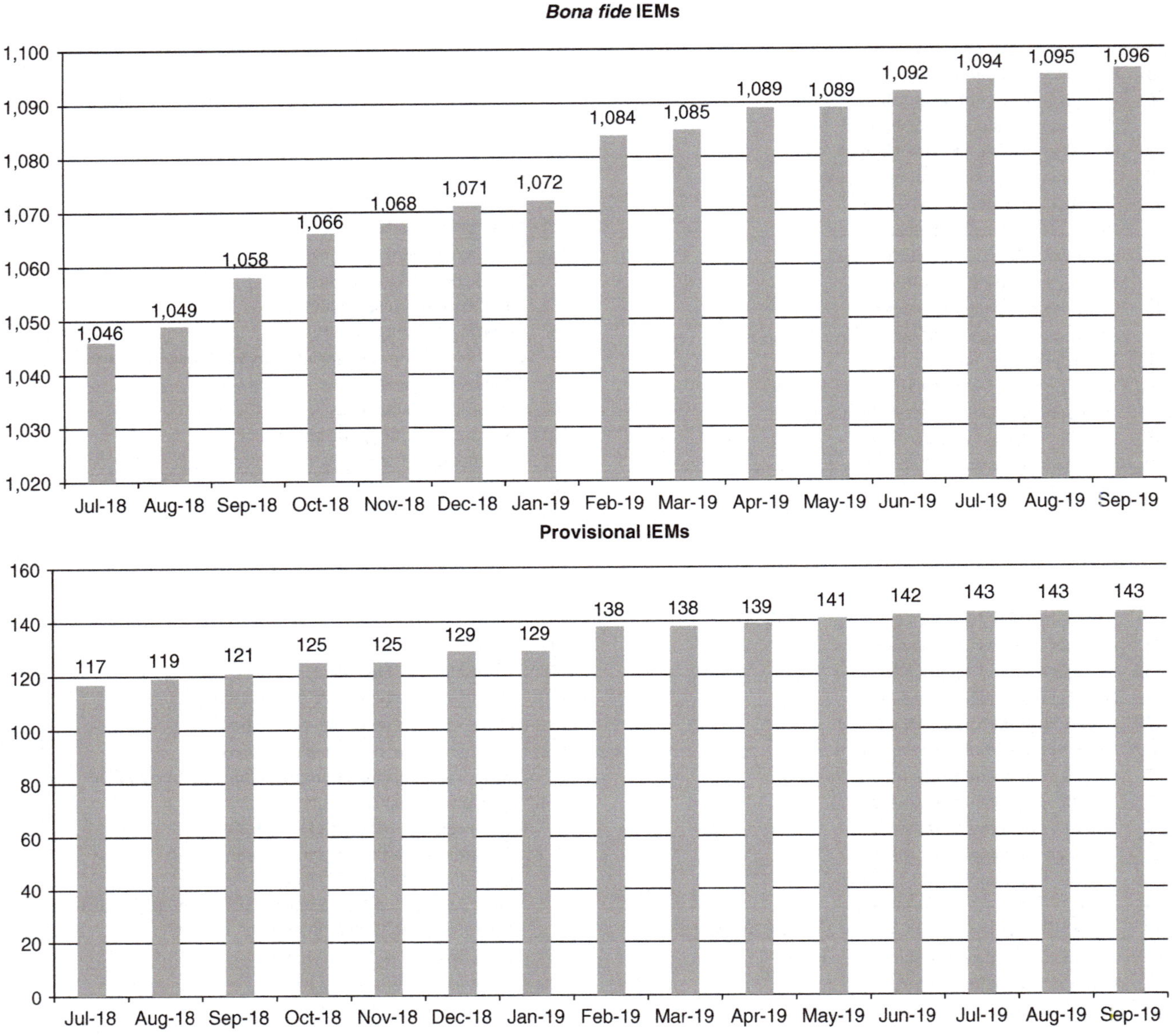


**Fig. 12.1** IEMs added since inception of the nosology

**Table 12.2** IEMs by the number

| Category | Bona fide | Provisional | Count |
|---|---|---|---|
| (A) Disorders of nitrogen-containing compounds | 200 | 30 | 230 |
| (B) Disorders of vitamins, cofactors, and minerals | 127 | 14 | 141 |
| (C) Disorders of carbohydrates | 77 | 6 | 83 |
| (D) Mitochondrial disorders of energy metabolism | 244 | 43 | 287 |
| (E) Disorders of lipids | 188 | 33 | 221 |
| (F) Disorders of tetrapyrroles | 25 | 1 | 26 |
| (G) Storage disorders | 69 | 3 | 72 |
| (H) Disorders of peroxisomes and oxalate | 30 | 1 | 31 |
| (I) Congenital disorders of glycosylation | 136 | 11 | 147 |
| (J) Miscellaneous disorders | 0 | 1 | 1 |
| **Final total** | **1096** | **143** | **1239** |

**Table 12.3** Inheritance of bona fide IEMs

| Inheritance | Count |
|---|---|
| Autosomal dominant | 184 |
| Autosomal recessive | 878 |
| X-linked | 57 |
| Digenic | 2 |
| Mitochondrial | 37 |
| Somatic | 3 |

A simplification of the nosology of IEMs has been proposed since the time of its publication, with the explicit purpose of making it more useful from a clinical diagnostic perspective. This simplified classification divides IEMs as follows: (1) disorders of small molecules (accumulation and deficiency), (2) disorders of complex molecules (accumulation, deficiency, and cell processing/trafficking defects), and (3) energy defects (membrane carriers, cytoplasmic energy defects, and mitochondrial defects) (Saudubray et al. 2019).

Finally, given the presence of more than one classification approach currently in place, a unified approach was being actively developed at the time of writing of this book by a group of several experts in their respective IEM groups. This unified system was named the "International Classification of Inherited Metabolic Diseases" (ICIMD) and sought the ratification of the different metabolic societies worldwide prior to its implementation. At the time of publication in January 2021, the ICIMD included 1450 IEMs (Ferreira et al. 2021). As with the prior nosology of IEMs, the ICIMD will be continuously updated via IEMbase and a dedicated website (www.icimd.org). Thus, the classification of IEMs has been dynamic since its origins and represents an area of active development that will benefit from regular curation and updates via electronic databases.

## References

Ferreira CR, van Karnebeek CDM, Vockley J, Blau N. A proposed nosology of inborn errors of metabolism. Genet Med. 2019;21:102–6.

Ferreira CR, Rahman S, Keller M, Zschocke J, ICIMD Advisory Group. An international classification of inherited metabolic disorders (ICIMD). J Inherit Metab Dis. 2021;44:164–77.

Garrod AE. The incidence of alkaptonuria: a study in chemical individuality. Lancet. 1902;160:1616–20.

Garrod AE. The Croonian lectures on inborn errors of metabolism. Lecture I: general and introductory. Lancet. 1908a;172:1–7.

Garrod AE. The Croonian lectures on inborn errors of metabolism. Lecture II: alkaptonuria. Lancet. 1908b;172:73–9.

Garrod AE. The Croonian lectures on inborn errors of metabolism. Lecture III: cystinuria. Lancet. 1908c;172:142–8.

Garrod AE. The Croonian lectures on inborn errors of metabolism. Lecture IV: cystinuria (continued). Lancet. 1908d;172:214–30.

Garrod AE. Inborn errors of metabolism. London: Henry Frowde; 1909.

Garrod AE. Inborn errors of metabolism. 2nd ed. London: Henry Frowde and Hodder & Stoughton; 1923.

Lee JJY, Wasserman WW, Hoffmann GF, van Karnebeek CDM, Blau N. Knowledge base and mini-expert platform for the diagnosis of inborn errors of metabolism. Genet Med. 2018;20:151–8.

Saudubray J-M, Charpentier C. Clinical phenotypes: diagnosis/algorithms. In: Beaudet AL, Vogelstein B, Kinzler KW, Antonarakis S, Ballabio A, Gibson KM, Mitchell G, editors. The online metabolic and molecular bases of inherited disease; 2014.

Saudubray J-M, Mochel F, Lamari F, Garcia-Cazorla A. Proposal for a simplified classification of IMD based on a pathophysiological approach: a practical guide for clinicians. J Inherit Metab Dis. 2019;42(4):706–27.

Sinclair L. A new look at the inborn errors of metabolism. Ann Clin Biochem. 1982;19(Pt 4):314–21.

Stanbury JB, Frederickson DS, Wyngaarden JB. The metabolic basis of inherited disease. New York: McGraw-Hill Book Company; 1960.

Stenn FF, Milgram JW, Lee SL, Weigand RJ, Veis A. Biochemical identification of homogentisic acid pigment in an ochronotic Egyptian mummy. Science. 1977;197:566–8.

Zschocke J. SSIEM classification of inborn errors of metabolism. In: Blau N, Duran M, Gibson KM, Dionisi Vici C, editors. Physician's guide to the diagnosis, treatment, and follow-up of inherited metabolic diseases. Berlin, Heidelberg: Springer; 2014. p. 817–30.

# Part II

# Disorders of Nitrogen-Containing Compounds

# Purine and Pyrimidine Disorders

# 13

Jörgen Bierau and Ivan Šebesta

## Contents



**Summary**

Genetic defects of purine and pyrimidine metabolism represent a diverse group of disorders with serious or life-threatening symptoms. Compared to other groups of disorders, the identification of these disorders had a late and slow start. Xanthinuria was the first genetic metabolic purine disorder recognised and was described as the cause of renal stones in 1954, and the genetic basis for the Lesch-Nyhan syndrome accompanied by gout in childhood and adolescence with serious neurological impairment was recognised in 1967. The number of enzyme defects identified since then has increased rapidly and now totals 33. Not surprisingly, knowledge at the clinical level has been unable to keep the pace, a problem compounded by the broad spectrum of presentation and genetic heterogeneity. Clinical presentations may involve renal, musculoskeletal, neurological, immunological and haematological systems. Although these disorders are generally paediatric problems, some disorders can manifest themselves in patients at any age from birth to advanced adulthood. These disorders are frequently misdiagnosed, not because the diagnosis is complicated and difficult to establish, but rather because of a lack of awareness, particularly in adults where such defects are increas-

J. Bierau (✉)
Department of Clinical Genetics, Erasmus MC, Rotterdam, The Netherlands
e-mail: j.bierau@erasmusmc.nl

I. Šebesta
Institute of Medical Biochemistry and Laboratory Medicine, Institute of Inherited Metabolic Disorders, First Faculty of Medicine, Charles University, Prague 2, Czech Republic
e-mail: isebes@lf1.cuni.cz


N. Blau et al. (eds.), *Physician's Guide to the Diagnosis, Treatment, and Follow-Up of Inherited Metabolic Diseases*,
https://doi.org/10.1007/978-3-030-67727-5_13

ingly being recognised. Although some conditions are relatively benign, others can have serious consequences. The fact that approximately 50% of the subjects remain asymptomatic in some disorders such as hereditary xanthinuria and hereditary hypouricaemia poses an additional serious problem for effective diagnosis and causes inaccuracy in incidence estimation of these conditions. Currently, there appear to be few laboratories worldwide providing the necessary comprehensive diagnostic services for detailed purine and pyrimidine investigations. Recent advances alert physicians to the broad spectrum of clinical presentation. The proper identification and detection of new cases will not only help a number of (un)fortunate patients but will almost certainly lead to the illumination of the still unknown pathogenesis of these disorders.

## Introduction

Purines and pyrimidines are closely related heterocyclic compounds, consisting of a single six-membered ring for pyrimidines or a nine-membered imidazole-pyrimidine for purines. The purine and pyrimidine ring structures are called bases. When the base is covalently bound to a ribose or 2-deoxyribose, the structure is called a nucleoside, and when the ribose moiety is phosphorylated, it is called a nucleotide. As far as our knowledge extends, purines and pyrimidines are present in all living creatures. Not only are they the building blocks of the genetic code in the form of DNA and RNA, they also fulfil numerous roles in biological processes, including energy transport, glycan synthesis and lipid biosynthesis, cofactor biosynthesis, signal transduction and cell cycle progression both in the intracellular and extracellular matrices. Considering this, purine and pyrimidine metabolism can be regarded to be the central connecting hub for many metabolic routes. The regulation and cellular organisation of purine and pyrimidine metabolism are complex and governed, among other factors, by the cell cycle, DNA damage and higher organisational protein structures such as the purinosome and replisome. It is therefore easy to comprehend that the metabolism of these compounds is a complex and tightly regulated interplay of numerous processes and that any disturbance herein may have a wide array of clinical consequences.

The disorders covered in this chapter are the defects in de novo biosynthesis, interconversion, breakdown and salvage (reutilisation) of purine and pyrimidine bases, nucleosides and nucleotides. Disorders of nucleic acid editing and signal transduction are outside the scope of this chapter. Some disorders that are defects of purine and pyrimidine metabolism are covered in other chapters and from a clinical perspective better at their place in that chapter. These disorders include molybdenum cofactor deficiency, adenosine kinase deficiency (ADK) and mitochondrial DNA depletion syndromes caused by deoxyguanosine kinase (DGUOK), ribonucleotide reductase (RRM2B) and thymidine kinase 2 (TK2) deficiencies. More often than not, these disorders have no (or not yet known) biomarkers directly identifying them as defects of purine and pyrimidine metabolism. Other undeniable disorders of purine and pyrimidine metabolism disorders are covered in other chapters as well as in this chapter. These disorders include thymidine phosphorylase deficiency and the pyrimidine degradation defects.

At present, approximately 33 inborn errors of metabolism giving rise to a clinical presentation or which are of pharmacogenetic consequence are known. Since the last revision of this book (Bierau and Sebesta 2014), new defects have been discovered, i.e. CAD deficiency (Koch et al. 2017), dihydroorotate dehydrogenase deficiency (DHODH) (Rainger et al. 2012), adenosine kinase deficiency (Bjursell et al. 2011) and ITPA encephalopathy (Kevelam et al. 2015). Two excellent comprehensive reviews separately covering purine and pyrimidine disorders have been published (Balasubramaniam et al. 2014a, b).

As purines and pyrimidines play many important roles in cell metabolism, the clinical presentation of these disorders is extremely diverse. There are two important conditions for the early and effective diagnosis of these genetic defects: The first one is availability of proper analytical methods (as mentioned in the next paragraph), and the second one is the appropriate identification which is closely related to the awareness of these conditions. There is no fear of misdiagnosis in newborn screening because all patients are investigated. However, in the so called selective screening (for purine and pyrimidine disorders), where the indication is in many cases based on positive family history and suspicious clinical signs, it is still possible that some patients will not be investigated as they are not sent to specialised laboratories because of the lack of awareness. Therefore diagnostic flowcharts will help for proper diagnosis. In general, there is not one presenting clinical sign that irrefutably makes a clinical diagnosis (Simmonds and Van Gennip 2003; van Gennip et al. 2006). However, some conditions have clear clinical signs, and, when present, they are very clear indications for analysis of purines and pyrimidines. Examples hereof are signs such as self-mutilation (Micheli et al. 2011), severe combined immunodeficiency disease, hereditary urolithiasis and juvenile gout particularly in women (Sebesta 2012). Additional clear indications for assessment of purine metabolism are the findings of hyperuricaemia or hypouricaemia in a routine laboratory workup. Our experience shows that purine metabolic workup is effective in subjects with the so-called 'unexplained hyperuricaemia or hypouricaemia', which means that frequent secondary causes of high or low levels of uric acid in blood were excluded. This selection, made in particular by general practitioners, helps quite a lot for effective diagnosis. The most frequent secondary causes of hyperuricaemia include excessive dietary purine intake, decreased renal function and myeloproliferative diseases. It is important to emphasise that secondary causes of hypouricaemia such as Wilson's disease, Fanconi syndrome, syndrome of inappropriate secretion of antidiuretic hormone (SIADH), heavy metal poisoning, liver diseases, medication with uricosuric agents, etc. should be excluded before sending samples or subjects for laboratory tests of purine metabolism (Sebesta et al. 2018). In most other cases, the constellation of symptoms is not very conclusive (Assmann et al. 2006), and one should have a liberal policy concerning selective screening purine and pyrimidine metabolites in body fluids. Adult medicine is also of considerable importance. An example hereof is MNGIE syndrome caused by deficiency of thymidine phosphorylase (Hirano et al. 2006). Another example is the pharmacogenetic significance of the pyrimidine degradation defects, in general, and dihydropyrimidine dehydrogenase, in particular (van Kuilenburg 2004), and the purine-metabolising enzymes thiopurine methyltransferase (Weinshilboum et al. 1999).

The laboratory approach to detect defect in purine and pyrimidine metabolism is rapidly changing with current rate technological advances. There is a clear shift towards holistic genomic approaches, which has the advantage that whereas previously these defects were often ignored, they are now included in gene panels and packages. Confirmation and classical selective metabolic screening still rely on the quantification of purines and pyrimidines in body fluids and enzymology. State of the art is LC-MS/MS analysis, which allows comprehensive screening of purines and pyrimidines and is far more powerful than (U)HPLC-UV-based methodology (Monostori et al. 2019). Urine is the preferred body fluid, as all biomarkers can be excreted in the urine. In plasma, levels are much lower than urine, and this matrix is extremely sensitive to artefacts and misguiding shifts in metabolite levels. The arrival of metabolomics adds to the holistic approach of genomics and will play a role in the near future diagnostics of purine and pyrimidine defects. Undoubtedly, new biomarkers will be identified broadening diagnostic possibilities.

## Nomenclature

| | Disease name | Alternative disease name | Disease abbreviation | Gene symbol | Chromosomal localisation | Mode of inheritance | Affected protein | Disease OMIM# |
|---|---|---|---|---|---|---|---|---|
| 13.1 | CAD trifunctional protein deficiency | Epileptic encephalopathy, early infantile, 50 | CAD-CDG | *CAD* | 2p23.3 | AR | Carbamoyl phosphate synthetase, aspartate transcarbamoylase and dihydroorotase trifunctional protein (CPSase/ATCase/DHOase) | 114010 |
| 13.2 | Dihydroorotate dehydrogenase deficiency | Postaxial acrofacial dysostosis<br>Miller syndrome<br>Genée-Wiedemann syndrome | POADS | *DHODH* | 16q22 | AR | Dihydroorotate dehydrogenase | 12664 |
| 13.3 | Uridine monophosphate synthase deficiency | Hereditary orotic aciduria | | *UMPS* | 3q21.2 | AR | Uridine monophosphate synthase | 613891 |
| 13.4 | Cytosolic pyrimidine 5′-nucleotidase deficiency | Uridine 5′-monophosphate hydrolase 1 deficiency | | *NT5C3A* | 7p14.3 | AR | Pyrimidine 5′-nucleotidase I | 606224 |
| 13.5 | Thymidine phosphorylase deficiency | Mitochondrial neurogastrointestinal encephalopathy syndrome | MNGIE | *TYMP* | 22q13.32 | AR | Thymidine phosphorylase | 131222 |
| 13.6 | Dihydropyrimidine dehydrogenase deficiency | Thymine-uraciluria | DPD | *DPYD* | 1p21 | AR | Dihydropyrimidine dehydrogenase | 612779 |
| 13.7 | Dihydropyrimidinase deficiency | Dihydropyrimidinuria | | *DPYS* | 8q22.3 | AR | Dihydropyrimidinase | 613326 |

(continued)

| | Disease name | Alternative disease name | Disease abbreviation | Gene symbol | Chromosomal localisation | Mode of inheritance | Affected protein | Disease OMIM# |
|---|---|---|---|---|---|---|---|---|
| 13.8 | β-ureidopropionase deficiency | | | *UPB1* | 22q11.23 | AR | Beta-ureidopropionase | 606673 |
| 13.9 | Phosphoribosylpyrophosphate synthetase superactivity | | PRPS1S uperactivity | *PRPS1* | Xq22-q24 | XLR | Phosphoribosyl pyrophosphate synthetase 1 | 311850 |
| 13.10 | Phosphoribosylpyrophosphate synthetase deficiency | Arts syndrome (severe)<br>X-linked Charcot-Marie-Tooth disease type 5 (intermediate)<br>X-linked deafness type 1 (milder) | PRPS1 | *PRPS1* | Xq21.32-q24 | XLR | Phosphoribosyl pyrophosphate synthetase | 311850 |
| 13.11 | Adenylosuccinate lyase deficiency | Adenylosuccinase deficiency | ADSLD | *ADSL* | 22q13.1 | AR | Adenylosuccinate lyase | 608222 |
| 13.12 | AICAR transformylase/IMP cyclohydrolase deficiency | AICA-ribosiduria | ATIC | *ATIC* | 2q35 | AR | AICAR transformylase/IMP cyclohydrolase | 601731 |
| 13.13 | Muscle adenosine monophosphate deaminase 1 deficiency | Myoadenylate deaminase deficiency | AMPD | *AMPD1* | 1p13.2 | AR | Adenosine monophosphate deaminase 1 | 102770 |
| 13.14 | Adenosine monophosphate deaminase 2 deficiency | Pontocerebellar hypoplasia type 9 (severe)<br>Autosomal recessive spastic paraplegia type 63 (milder) | PCH9, SPG63 | *AMPD2* | 1p13.3 | AR | Adenosine monophosphate deaminase 2 | 102771 |
| 13.15 | Erythrocyte adenosine monophosphate deaminase 3 deficiency | | EAMPD3 | *AMPD3* | 11p15.4 | AR | Adenosine monophosphate deaminase 3 | 102772 |
| 13.16 | Adenosine deaminase 1 deficiency | Severe combined immunodeficiency (SCID) | ADA | *ADA* | 20q13.12 | AR | Adenosine deaminase 1 | 608958 |
| 13.17 | Adenosine deaminase 2 deficiency | Polyarteritis nodosa, childhood-onset | CECR1 | *ADA2* | 22q11.1 | AR | Adenosine deaminase 2 | 607575 |
| 13.18 | Purine nucleoside phosphorylase deficiency | T-cell immunodeficiency | PNP | *PNP* | 14q11.2 | AR | Purine nucleoside phosphorylase | 164050 |
| 13.19 | Xanthine oxidase deficiency | Xanthinuria type 1 | XDH | *XDH* | 2p23.1 | AR | Xanthine dehydrogenase (oxidase) | 607633 |
| 13.20 | Hypoxanthine guanine phosphoribosyltransferase deficiency | Lesch-Nyhan syndrome (severe)<br>Kelley-Seegmiller syndrome (milder) | HGPRT | *HPRT1* | Xq26.2-q26.3 | XLR | Hypoxanthine guanine phosphoribosyltransferase | 308000 |
| 13.21 | Adenine phosphoribosyltransferase deficiency | 2,8-dihydroxyadenine urolithiasis | APRTD | *APRT* | 16q24.3 | AR | Adenine phosphoribosyl transferase | 102600 |
| 13.22 | Adenylate kinase 1 deficiency | Haemolytic anaemia due to adenylate kinase deficiency | AK1D | *AK1* | 9q34.11 | AR | Adenylate kinase 1 | 103000 |
| 13.23 | Adenylate kinase 2 deficiency | Reticular dysgenesis | AK2D | *AK2* | 1p35.1 | AR | Adenylate kinase 2, mitochondrial | 103020 |
| 13.24 | Inosine 5′-monophosphate dehydrogenase deficiency | Retinitis pigmentosa type 10<br>Leber congenital amaurosis type 11 | PR10, LCA11 | *IMPDH1* | 7q32.1 | AD | Inosine monophosphate dehydrogenase | 146690 |
| 13.25 | Inosine triphosphatase deficiency | Early infantile epileptic encephalopathy type 35 | EIEE35 | *ITPA* | 20p13 | AR | Inosine 5′-triphosphate pyrophosphohydrolase | 147520 |

| | Disease name | Alternative disease name | Disease abbreviation | Gene symbol | Chromosomal localisation | Mode of inheritance | Affected protein | Disease OMIM# |
|---|---|---|---|---|---|---|---|---|
| 13.26 | Inosine triphosphatase deficiency | Erythrocyte ITPase deficiency | | *ITPA* | 20p13 | AR | Inosine 5′-triphosphate pyrophosphohydrolase | 147520 |
| 13.27 | Thiopurine methyltransferase deficiency | Poor metabolism of thiopurines 1 | THPM1 | *TPMT* | 6p22.3 | AR | Thiopurine *S*-methyltransferase | 187680 |
| 13.28 | Hyperuricaemic nephropathy, familial juvenile 1 | Hyperuricaemic nephropathy, familial juvenile 1 | FJHN1 | UMOD | 16p12.3 | AD | Uromodulin | 162000 |
| 13.29 | Urate transporter 1 deficiency | Hereditary renal hypouricaemia type 1 | RHUC1 | *SLC22A12* | 11q13.1 | AR | Urate transporter 1 (OAT4L) | 607096 |
| 13.30 | Urate voltage-driven efflux transporter 1 deficiency | Hereditary renal hypouricaemia type 2 | RHUC2 | *SLC2A9* | 4p16.1 | AR | High-affinity urate transporter | 606142 |

## Metabolic Pathways

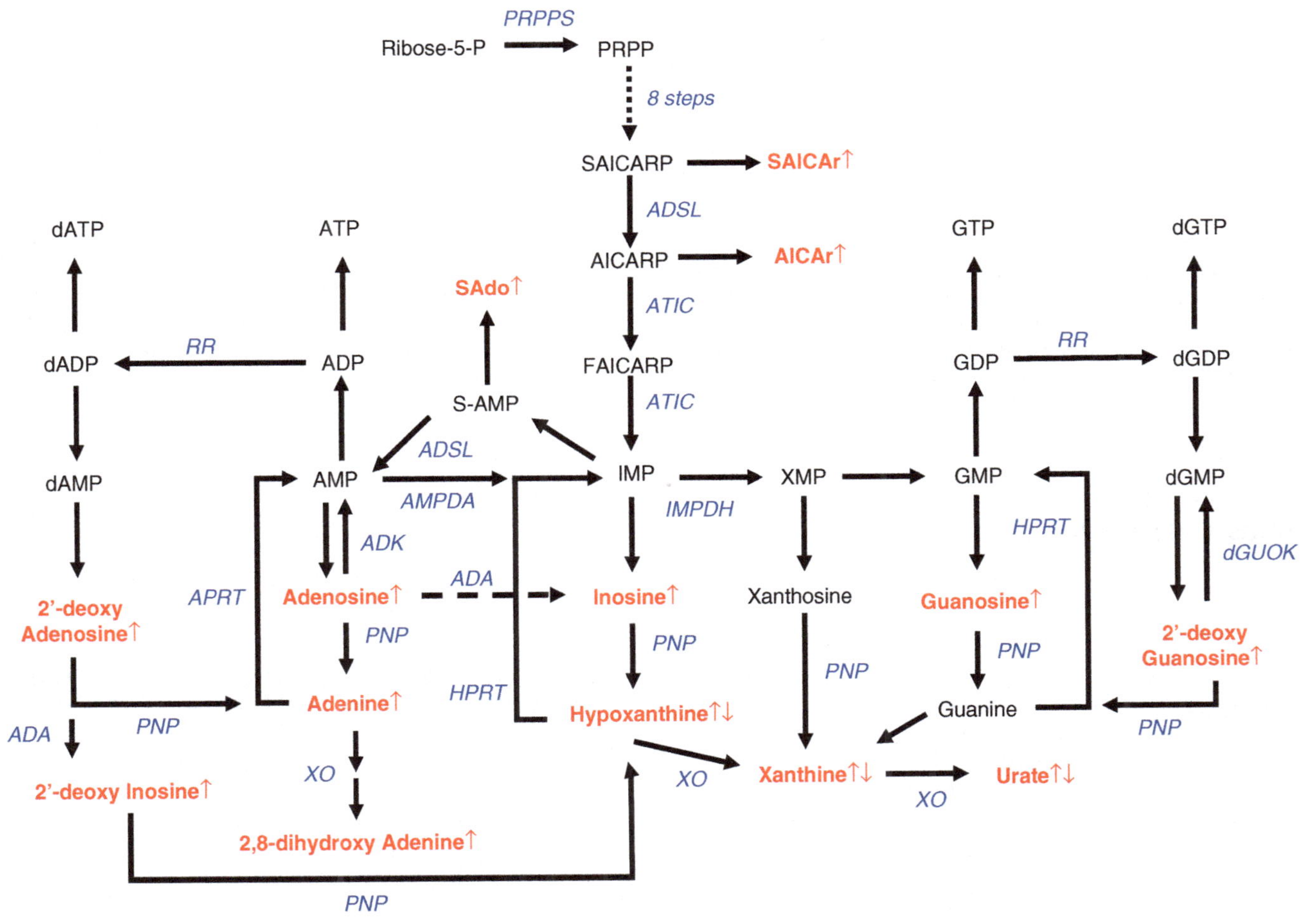


**Fig. 13.1** Overview of purine metabolism. Metabolites printed in red indicate marker metabolites, the arrow indicating the directionality. Only enzymes with disorders are mentioned. Enzyme abbreviations: *PRPPS* phosphoribosyl pyrophosphate synthetase, *ADSL* adenylosuccinate lyase, *ATIC,* AICAR transformylase/IMP cyclohydrolase, *IMPDH* inosine 5′-monophosphate dehydrogenase, *RR* ribonucleotide reductase, *HPRT* hypoxanthine-guanine phosphoribosyltransferase, *DGUOK* deoxyguanosine kinase, *PNP* purine nucleoside phosphorylase, *XO* xanthine oxidase (dehydrogenase), *AMPDA* adenosine 5′-monophosphate deaminase, *APRT* adenine phosphoribosyltransferase, *ADA* adenosine deaminase

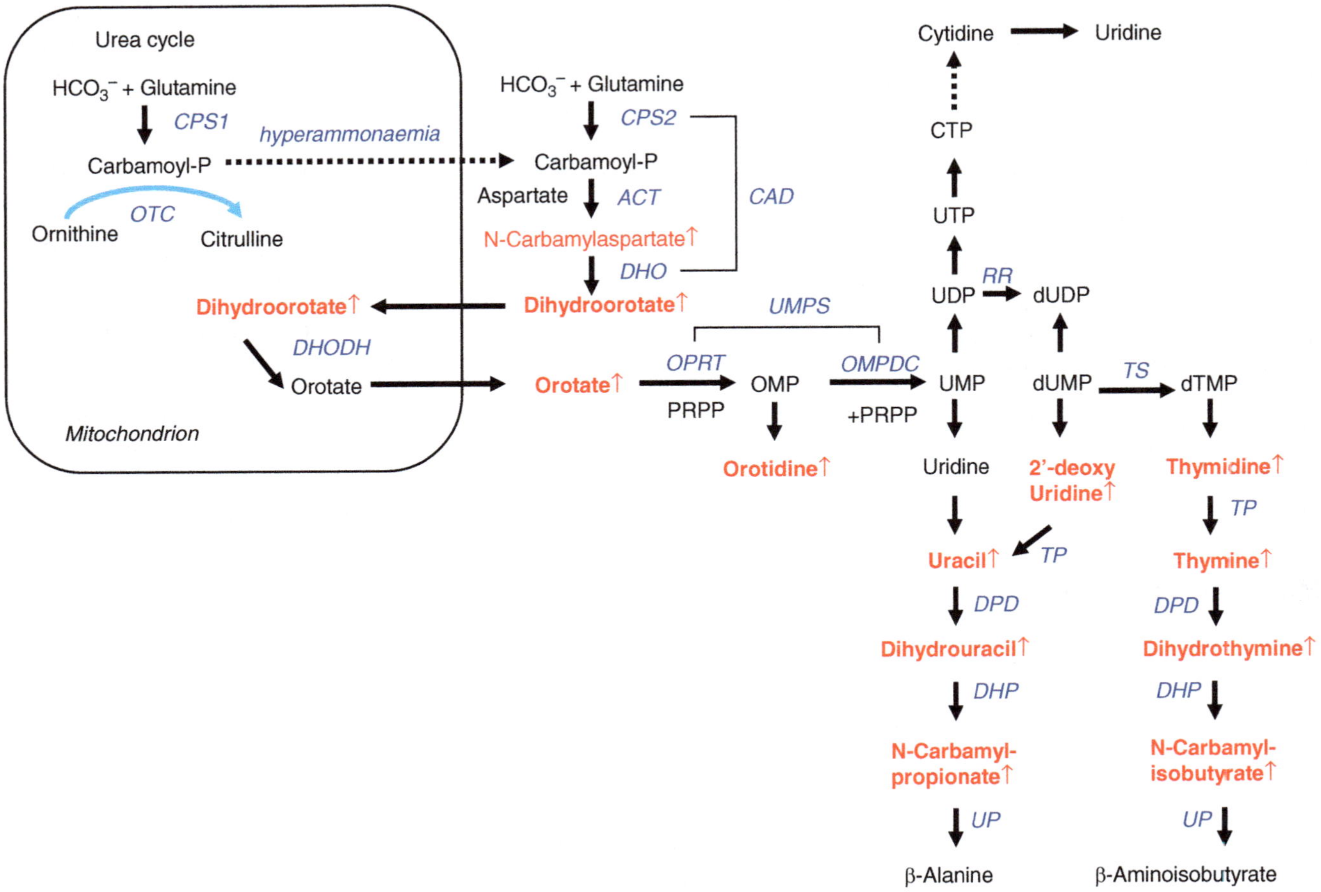


**Fig. 13.2** Overview of pyrimidine metabolism. Metabolites printed in red indicate marker metabolites, the arrow indicating the directionality. Only pyrimidine key enzymes and enzymes with known disorders are mentioned. For clarity, the link with the urea cycle is also depicted. Enzyme abbreviations: *CAD* complex of carbamoyl phosphate synthetase 2 (CPS2), aspartate carbamoyltransferase (ACT) and dihydroorotase (DHO), *CPS1* carbamoyl phosphate synthetase 1, *OTC* ornithine transcarbamylase, *DHODH* dihydroorotate dehydrogenase, *UMPS* UMP synthase complex consisting of orotate phosphoribosyltransferase (OPRT) and OMP decarboxylase (OMPDC), *RR* ribonucleotide reductase, *TS* thymidylate synthase, *TP* thymidine phosphorylase, *DPD* dihydropyrimidine dehydrogenase, *DHP* dihydropyrimidinase, *UP* ß-ureidopropionase

## Signs and Symptoms

**Table 13.1** Epileptic encephalopathy, early infantile, 50 (CAD-CDG)

| System | Symptoms and biomarkers | Neonatal (birth–1 month) | Infancy (1–18 months) | Childhood (1.5–11 years) | Adolescence (11–16 years) | Adulthood (>16 years) |
|---|---|---|---|---|---|---|
| CNS | **Developmental arrest** | | + | + | | |
| | **Epilepsy** | | + | + | | |
| | Swallowing difficulties | | ± | ± | | |
| Haematological | **Anaemia** | | + | + | | |
| | **Anisocytosis** | | + | + | | |
| | **Poikilocytosis** | | + | + | | |
| Laboratory findings | Orotic acid (urine) | | n | n | | |

**Table 13.2** Dihydroorotate dehydrogenase deficiency

| System | Symptoms and biomarkers | Neonatal (birth–1 month) | Infancy (1–18 months) | Childhood (1.5–11 years) | Adolescence (11–16 years) | Adulthood (>16 years) |
|---|---|---|---|---|---|---|
| Ear | **Coloboma** | ± | ± | ± | ± | ± |
| | Deafness, conductive | | ± | ± | ± | ± |
| Genitourinary | Cryptorchidism | + | + | + | | |
| | Micropenis | + | + | + | + | + |
| Musculoskeletal | **Absence of fifth digit in hands and feet** | + | + | + | + | + |
| | Accessory nipples | + | + | + | + | + |
| | Choanal atresia | + | + | | | |
| | Cleft lip | + | + | + | + | + |
| | Cleft palate | + | + | + | + | + |
| | **Congenital hip dislocation** | + | + | + | + | + |
| | Conical teeth | | | + | + | + |
| | **Cup-shaped ears** | + | + | + | + | + |
| | **Dysmorphic features** | + | + | + | + | + |
| | **Hypoplasia of limbs** | + | + | + | + | + |
| | **In-curving forearms** | + | + | | | |
| | **Low-set ears** | + | + | + | + | + |
| | **Malar hypoplasia** | + | + | + | + | + |
| | Micrognathia | + | + | + | + | + |
| | Midgut malrotation | + | + | ? | | |
| | Pectus excavatum | + | + | + | + | + |
| | Pyloric stenosis | + | + | + | + | + |
| | **Radioulnar synostosis** | + | + | | | |
| | Rib defects | + | + | + | + | + |
| | Supernumerary vertebrae | + | + | + | + | + |
| | **Syndactyly** | + | + | + | + | + |
| | Thumb hypoplasia | | | | | |
| Renal | Renal anomalies | + | + | + | | |
| Other | **Miller syndrome** | + | + | + | + | + |
| Laboratory findings | Dihydroorotic acid (urine) | ↑ | ↑ | ↑ | | |
| | *N*-Carbamoyl asparate | ↑↑ | ↑↑ | | | |
| | Orotic acid (urine) | ↑ | ↑ | ↑ | | |
| | Orotidine (urine) | ↑ | ↑ | | | |

**Table 13.3** Uridine monophosphate synthase deficiency

| System | Symptoms and biomarkers | Neonatal (birth–1 month) | Infancy (1–18 months) | Childhood (1.5–11 years) | Adolescence (11–16 years) | Adulthood (>16 years) |
|---|---|---|---|---|---|---|
| CNS | Development delay | ± | ± | ± | | |
| Digestive | Diarrhoea | ± | ± | ± | ± | ± |
| Haematological | **Anaemia, megaloblastic unresponsive to therapy** | +++ | +++ | +++ | +++ | +++ |
| | **Anisocytosis** | + | + | + | + | + |
| | **Hypochromia** | + | + | + | + | + |
| | Immunodeficiency, T-cell | ± | ± | ± | ± | ± |
| | Low to normal reticulocyte count | + | + | + | + | + |
| | **Poikilocytosis** | + | + | + | + | + |

(continued)

**Table 13.3** (continued)

| System | Symptoms and biomarkers | Neonatal (birth–1 month) | Infancy (1–18 months) | Childhood (1.5–11 years) | Adolescence (11–16 years) | Adulthood (>16 years) |
|---|---|---|---|---|---|---|
| Renal | **Haematuria** | + | + | + | + | + |
| | **Urolithiasis, orotic acid crystalluria** | + | + | + | + | + |
| Other | Failure to thrive | ± | ± | ± | | |
| | Recurrent infections | ± | ± | ± | ± | ± |
| Laboratory findings | Orotic acid (plasma) | ↑↑ | ↑↑ | ↑↑ | ↑↑ | ↑↑ |
| | Orotic acid (urine) | ↑↑↑ | ↑↑↑ | ↑↑↑ | ↑↑↑ | ↑↑↑ |
| | Uridine monophosphate synthase (OPRT) (red blood cells) | ↓ | ↓ | ↓ | ↓ | ↓ |

**Table 13.4** Cytosolic pyrimidine 5′-nucleotidase deficiency

| System | Symptoms and biomarkers | Neonatal (birth–1 month) | Infancy (1–18 months) | Childhood (1.5–11 years) | Adolescence (11–16 years) | Adulthood (>16 years) |
|---|---|---|---|---|---|---|
| Digestive | **Splenomegaly** | | + | + | + | + |
| Haematological | **Anaemia, non-spherocytic, haemolytic with basophilic stippling** | + | + | + | + | + |
| Musculoskeletal | **Myoglobinuria** | ± | ± | ± | ± | ± |
| Laboratory findings | Glutathione (red blood cells) | ↓-n | ↓-n | ↓-n | ↓-n | ↓-n |
| | Pyrimidine 5′-nucleotidase I (red blood cells) | ↓↓↓ | ↓↓ | ↓↓↓ | ↓↓↓ | ↓↓↓ |
| | Pyrimidine nucleotides (red blood cells) | ↑↑↑ | ↑↑↑ | ↑↑↑ | ↑↑↑ | ↑↑↑ |

**Table 13.5** Thymidine phosphorylase deficiency

| System | Symptoms and biomarkers | Neonatal (birth–1 month) | Infancy (1–18 months) | Childhood (1.5–11 years) | Adolescence (11–16 years) | Adulthood (>16 years) |
|---|---|---|---|---|---|---|
| CNS | Areflexia | | | | + | + |
| | Hypodense white matter | | | | + | + |
| | Leukoencephalopathy | | | | + | + |
| | **Neuropathy, myelinating** | | | | + | + |
| Digestive | Abdominal pain | | | | + | + |
| | Anorexia | | | | + | + |
| | Diarrhoea | | | | + | + |
| | **Gastrointestinal dysmotility** | | | | + | + |
| | **Gastroparesis** | | | | + | + |
| | Intestinal pseudo obstruction | | | | + | + |
| | **Malabsorption** | | | | + | + |
| | **Malnutrition, chronic** | | | | + | + |
| | Vomiting | | | | + | + |

**Table 13.5** (continued)

| System | Symptoms and biomarkers | Neonatal (birth–1 month) | Infancy (1–18 months) | Childhood (1.5–11 years) | Adolescence (11–16 years) | Adulthood (>16 years) |
|---|---|---|---|---|---|---|
| Metabolic | **Ragged red fibres** | | | | + | + |
| Musculoskeletal | **Muscle weakness** | | | | + | + |
| | **Myopathy** | | | | + | + |
| Laboratory findings | Deoxyuridine (plasma) | | | | ↑ | ↑ |
| | Deoxyuridine (urine) | | | | ↑↑ | ↑↑ |
| | Lactate (plasma) | | | | ↑↑ | ↑↑ |
| | Thymidine (plasma) | | | | ↑ | ↑ |
| | Thymidine (urine) | | | | ↑↑ | ↑↑ |
| | Thymidine phosphorylase (white blood cells) | | | | ↓↓↓ | ↓↓↓ |

**Table 13.6** Dihydropyrimidine dehydrogenase deficiency

| System | Symptoms and biomarkers | Neonatal (birth–1 month) | Infancy (1–18 months) | Childhood (1.5–11 years) | Adolescence (11–16 years) | Adulthood (>16 years) |
|---|---|---|---|---|---|---|
| CNS | **Autism** | | ± | ± | ± | ± |
| | Cerebral atrophy (MRI) | ± | ± | ± | ± | ± |
| | **Epilepsy** | ± | ± | ± | ± | ± |
| | Hypertonia | ± | ± | ± | ± | ± |
| | Hypotonia | ± | ± | ± | ± | ± |
| | Intellectual disability | | ± | ± | ± | ± |
| | Retardation, motor | | ± | ± | ± | ± |
| | Seizures | ± | ± | ± | ± | ± |
| | White matter abnormalities (MRI) | | ± | ± | ± | ± |
| Musculoskeletal | Microcephaly | | ± | ± | ± | ± |
| Digestive | Feeding difficulties | ± | | | | |
| Other | Failure to thrive | ± | | | | |
| Eye | Coloboma | | ± | ± | ± | ± |
| | **Eye movements, abnormal** | ± | ± | ± | ± | ± |
| | Nystagmus | | ± | ± | ± | ± |
| | Optic atrophy | | ± | ± | ± | ± |
| Psychiatric | **Hyperactivity** | ± | ± | ± | ± | ± |
| Other | Severe 5-fluorouracil toxicity, heterozygotes | | | | | +++ |
| | Severe 5-fluorouracil toxicity, homozygotes | | | | | +++ |
| Laboratory findings | Dihydropyrimidine dehydrogenase (white blood cells) | ↓ | ↓ | ↓ | ↓ | ↓ |
| | 5-OH-methyluracil | ↑↑ | ↑↑ | ↑↑ | ↑↑ | ↑↑ |
| | Thymine (plasma) | ↑↑ | ↑↑ | ↑↑ | ↑↑ | ↑↑ |
| | Thymine (urine) | ↑↑↑ | ↑↑↑ | ↑↑↑ | ↑↑↑ | ↑↑↑ |
| | Uracil (plasma) | ↑↑ | ↑↑ | ↑↑ | ↑↑ | ↑↑ |
| | Uracil (urine) | ↑↑↑ | ↑↑↑ | ↑↑↑ | ↑↑↑ | ↑↑↑ |

**Table 13.7** Dihydropyrimidinase deficiency

| System | Symptoms and biomarkers | Neonatal (birth–1 month) | Infancy (1–18 months) | Childhood (1.5–11 years) | Adolescence (11–16 years) | Adulthood (>16 years) |
|---|---|---|---|---|---|---|
| CNS | **Intellectual disability** | | ± | ± | ± | ± |
| | **Seizures** | ± | ± | ± | ± | ± |
| Musculoskeletal | **Dysmorphic features** | ± | ± | ± | ± | ± |
| Laboratory findings | Dihydrothymine (plasma) | ↑↑ | ↑↑ | ↑↑ | ↑↑ | ↑↑ |
| | Dihydrothymine (urine) | ↑↑↑ | ↑↑↑ | ↑↑↑ | ↑↑↑ | ↑↑↑ |
| | Dihydrouracil (plasma) | ↑↑ | ↑↑ | ↑↑ | ↑↑ | ↑↑ |
| | Dihydrouracil (urine) | ↑↑↑ | ↑↑↑ | ↑↑↑ | ↑↑↑ | ↑↑↑ |

**Table 13.8** Beta-ureidopropionase deficiency

| System | Symptoms and biomarkers | Neonatal (birth–1 month) | Infancy (1–18 months) | Childhood (1.5–11 years) | Adolescence (11–16 years) | Adulthood (>16 years) |
|---|---|---|---|---|---|---|
| CNS | Dystonia | ± | ± | ± | ± | ± |
| | **Hypotonia** | + | + | | | |
| | Retardation, psychomotor | ± | ± | ± | ± | ± |
| | Seizures | ± | ± | ± | ± | ± |
| | **Speech disturbances** | | | ± | ± | ± |
| Musculoskeletal | Dysmorphic features | ± | ± | ± | ± | ± |
| Laboratory findings | Dihydrothymine (plasma) | ↑ | ↑ | ↑ | ↑ | ↑ |
| | Dihydrothymine (urine) | ↑ | ↑ | ↑ | ↑ | ↑ |
| | Dihydrouracil (plasma) | ↑ | ↑ | ↑ | ↑ | ↑ |
| | Dihydrouracil (urine) | ↑ | ↑ | ↑ | ↑ | ↑ |
| | *N*-Carbamyl-β-alanine (plasma) | ↑↑ | ↑↑ | ↑↑ | ↑↑ | ↑↑ |
| | *N*-Carbamyl-β-alanine (urine) | ↑↑↑ | ↑↑↑ | ↑↑↑ | ↑↑↑ | ↑↑↑ |
| | *N*-Carbamyl-β-aminoisobutyric acid (plasma) | ↑↑ | ↑↑ | ↑↑ | ↑↑ | ↑↑ |

**Table 13.9** Phosphoribosyl pyrophosphate synthetase 1 superactivity

| System | Symptoms and biomarkers | Neonatal (birth–1 month) | Infancy (1–18 months) | Childhood (1.5–11 years) | Adolescence (11–16 years) | Adulthood (>16 years) |
|---|---|---|---|---|---|---|
| CNS | Ataxia | ± | ± | ± | | |
| | Developmental delay | ± | ± | ± | | |
| | Intellectual disability | | ± | ± | | |
| Ear | **Deafness, sensorineural** | | + | + | + | + |
| Musculoskeletal | **Dysmorphic features** | ± | ± | ± | | |
| | **Gout** | | | + | + | + |
| Renal | Urolithiasis | | | ± | ± | ± |

**Table 13.9** (continued)

| System | Symptoms and biomarkers | Neonatal (birth–1 month) | Infancy (1–18 months) | Childhood (1.5–11 years) | Adolescence (11–16 years) | Adulthood (>16 years) |
|---|---|---|---|---|---|---|
| Laboratory findings | Hypoxanthine (urine) | ↑ | ↑ | ↑ | ↑ | ↑ |
| | Phosphoribose pyrophosphate (red blood cells) | ↑ | ↑ | ↑ | ↑ | ↑ |
| | PRPP synthase activity (fibroblasts) | ↑ | ↑ | ↑ | ↑ | ↑ |
| | PRPP synthase activity (red blood cells) | ↑ | ↑ | ↑ | ↑ | ↑ |
| | Uric acid (plasma) | n-↑ | n-↑ | n-↑ | ↑↑ | ↑↑ |
| | Uric acid (urine) | ↑↑ | ↑↑ | ↑↑ | ↑↑ | ↑↑ |

**Table 13.10** Phosphoribosyl pyrophosphate synthetase 1 deficiency

| System | Symptoms and biomarkers | Neonatal (birth–1 month) | Infancy (1–18 months) | Childhood (1.5–11 years) | Adolescence (11–16 years) | Adulthood (>16 years) |
|---|---|---|---|---|---|---|
| CNS | **Ataxia** | + | | | | |
| | **Hypotonia** | + | + | | | |
| | **Intellectual disability** | ± | ± | ± | ± | ± |
| | **Neuropathy, peripheral** | | | + | + | + |
| | Retardation, motor | | + | + | + | |
| | Tetraplegia | | + | | | |
| Ear | **Deafness, sensorineural** | + | + | + | + | + |
| | **Hearing loss** | + | + | + | + | + |
| Eye | **Optic atrophy** | | + | + | + | |
| | **Vision, progressive loss** | | + | + | + | |
| Other | **Recurrent infections** | + | + | + | | |
| Laboratory findings | Phosphoribosyl pyrophosphate synthetase activity | ↓-↓↓↓ | ↓-↓↓↓ | ↓-↓↓↓ | ↓-↓↓↓ | ↓-↓↓↓ |

**Table 13.11** Adenylosuccinate lyase deficiency

| System | Symptoms and biomarkers | Neonatal (birth–1 month) | Infancy (1–18 months) | Childhood (1.5–11 years) | Adolescence (11–16 years) | Adulthood (>16 years) |
|---|---|---|---|---|---|---|
| CNS | Autism | ± | ± | ± | ± | ± |
| | Cerebellar hypoplasia | ± | ± | ± | ± | ± |
| | Epilepsy | ± | ± | ± | ± | ± |
| | Hypotonia | ± | ± | | | |
| | **Retardation, psychomotor** | + | + | + | + | + |
| Laboratory findings | Adenylosuccinate lyase (red blood cells) | ↓↓↓ | ↓↓↓ | ↓↓↓ | ↓↓↓ | ↓↓↓ |
| | SAICA riboside (cerebrospinal fluid) | ↑↑ | ↑↑ | ↑↑ | ↑↑ | ↑↑ |
| | SAICA riboside (plasma) | ↑ | ↑ | ↑ | ↑ | ↑ |
| | SAICA riboside (urine) | ↑↑ | ↑↑ | ↑↑ | ↑↑ | ↑↑ |
| | Succinyladenosine (cerebrospinal fluid) | ↑↑ | ↑↑ | ↑↑ | ↑↑ | ↑↑ |
| | Succinyladenosine (plasma) | ↑↑ | ↑↑ | ↑↑ | ↑↑ | ↑↑ |
| | Succinyladenosine (urine) | ↑↑ | ↑↑ | ↑↑ | ↑↑ | ↑↑ |

**Table 13.12** AICAR transformylase/IMP cyclohydrolase deficiency

| System | Symptoms and biomarkers | Neonatal (birth–1 month) | Infancy (1–18 months) | Childhood (1.5–11 years) | Adolescence (11–16 years) | Adulthood (>16 years) |
|---|---|---|---|---|---|---|
| CNS | **Intellectual disability** | +++ | +++ | +++ | | |
| Eye | **Blindness** | +++ | ++ | +++ | | |
| Musculoskeletal | **Dysmorphic features** | ++ | ++ | ++ | | |
| Laboratory findings | AICA riboside (urine) | ↑↑↑ | ↑↑↑ | ↑↑↑ | | |
| | AICAR transformylase/ IMP cyclohydrolase (fibroblasts) | ↓↓↓ | ↓↓↓ | ↓↓↓ | ↓↓↓ | ↓↓↓ |

**Table 13.13** Adenosine monophosphate deaminase deficiency

| System | Symptoms and biomarkers | Neonatal (birth–1 month) | Infancy (1–18 months) | Childhood (1.5–11 years) | Adolescence (11–16 years) | Adulthood (>16 years) |
|---|---|---|---|---|---|---|
| Musculoskeletal | Exercise Intolerance | | | ± | ± | ± |
| | Muscle cramps | | | ± | ± | ± |
| Other | Acquired, associated with neuromuscular rheumatological disorders | | | | | + |
| Laboratory findings | Adenosine monophosphate deaminase (muscle biopsy) | | | ↓ | ↓ | ↓ |
| | Creatine kinase (plasma) | | | ↑ | ↑ | ↑ |
| | Ischaemic muscle exercise tolerance test (plasma NH3) | | | ↓ | ↓ | ↓ |

**Table 13.14** Adenosine monophosphate deaminase 2 deficiency

| System | Symptoms and biomarkers | Neonatal (birth–1 month) | Infancy (1–18 months) | Childhood (1.5–11 years) | Adolescence (11–16 years) | Adulthood (>16 years) |
|---|---|---|---|---|---|---|
| CNS | Retardation, motor | | + | + | | + |
| | Retardation, psychomotor | ± | ± | | | |
| | **Seizures** | + | + | + | + | + |
| Musculoskeletal | **Dysmorphic features** | + | + | + | + | + |
| | **Microcephaly** | + | + | + | + | + |

**Table 13.15** Erythrocyte adenosine monophosphate deaminase 3 deficiency (reported as nondisease)

| System | Symptoms and biomarkers | Neonatal (birth–1 month) | Infancy (1–18 months) | Childhood (1.5–11 years) | Adolescence (11–16 years) | Adulthood (>16 years) |
|---|---|---|---|---|---|---|
| | No clinical significance | + | + | + | + | + |

**Table 13.16** Adenosine deaminase deficiency

| System | Symptoms and biomarkers | Neonatal (birth–1 month) | Infancy (1–18 months) | Childhood (1.5–11 years) | Adolescence (11–16 years) | Adulthood (>16 years) |
|---|---|---|---|---|---|---|
| Digestive | **Splenomegaly** | + | + | | | |
| Haematological | **Lymphopaenia** | +++ | ++ | + | + | + |
| | **Severe combined immunodeficiency (SCID)** | +++ | ++ | + | + | + |
| Other | Failure to thrive | ± | ± | | | |
| | **Recurrent infections** | +++ | +++ | +++ | +++ | +++ |
| Laboratory findings | Adenosine deaminase (red blood cells) | ↓↓↓ | ↓↓↓ | ↓↓↓ | ↓↓↓ | ↓↓↓ |
| | Deoxyadenosine (urine) | ↑↑ | ↑↑ | ↑↑ | ↑↑ | ↑ |
| | Deoxyadenosine triphosphate, dATP (red blood cells) | ↑↑↑ | ↑↑ | ↑↑ | ↑↑ | ↑ |
| | Immunoglobulins | ↓↓↓ | ↓↓ | ↓ | ↓ | ↓ |

**Table 13.17** Adenosine deaminase 2 deficiency

| System | Symptoms and biomarkers | Neonatal (birth–1 month) | Infancy (1–18 months) | Childhood (1.5–11 years) | Adolescence (11–16 years) | Adulthood (>16 years) |
|---|---|---|---|---|---|---|
| Other | **Polyarteritis nodosa** | + | + | + | + | + |
| | **Sneddon syndrome** | | | | | + |
| Laboratory findings | (Deoxy)adenosine deaminase (plasma) | | | | | ↓↓↓ |

**Table 13.18** Purine nucleoside phosphorylase deficiency

| System | Symptoms and biomarkers | Neonatal (birth–1 month) | Infancy (1–18 months) | Childhood (1.5–11 years) | Adolescence (11–16 years) | Adulthood (>16 yeears) |
|---|---|---|---|---|---|---|
| CNS | Developmental delay | + | + | + | | |
| | **Spastic diplegia** | ++ | ++ | ++ | | |
| | **Tetraparesis** | ++ | ++ | ++ | | |
| Haematological | CD4+ cells | ↓-n | ↓-n | ↓-n | | |
| | **Immunodeficiency, T-cell** | + | + | + | + | + |
| Other | **Recurrent infections** | ++ | ++ | ++ | | |
| Laboratory findings | Deoxyguanosine, dGuo (plasma) | ↑ | ↑ | ↑ | ↑ | ↑ |
| | Deoxyguanosine, dGuo (urine) | ↑↑ | ↑↑ | ↑↑ | ↑ | ↑ |
| | Deoxyinosine, dIno (plasma) | ↑ | ↑ | ↑ | ↑ | ↑ |
| | Deoxyinosine, dIno (urine) | ↑↑ | ↑↑ | ↑↑ | ↑ | ↑ |
| | Purine nucleoside phosphorylase (red blood cells) | ↓↓↓ | ↓↓ | ↓↓↓ | ↓↓↓ | ↓↓↓ |
| | Uric acid (plasma) | ↓-↓↓ | ↓-↓↓ | ↓-↓↓ | ↓ | ↓ |
| | Uric acid (urine) | ↓-↓↓ | ↓-↓↓ | ↓-↓↓ | ↓ | ↓ |

**Table 13.19** Xanthine dehydrogenase deficiency

| System | Symptoms and biomarkers | Neonatal (birth–1 month) | Infancy (1–18 months) | Childhood (1.5–11 years) | Adolescence (11–16 years) | Adulthood (>16 years) |
|---|---|---|---|---|---|---|
| Musculoskeletal | Myopathy | | | | + | + |
| Renal | **Renal failure, acute** | ± | ± | ± | ± | ± |
| | **Urolithiasis** | ± | ± | ± | ± | ± |
| | **Urolithiasis, xanthine stones** | ± | ± | ± | ± | ± |
| Other | Allopurinol to oxypurinol conversion | + | + | + | + | + |
| Laboratory findings | Hypoxanthine (plasma) | ↑ | ↑ | ↑ | ↑ | ↑ |
| | Hypoxanthine (urine) | ↑↑ | ↑↑ | ↑↑ | ↑↑ | ↑↑ |
| | Uric acid (plasma) | ↓-↓↓ | ↓-↓↓ | ↓-↓↓ | ↓-↓↓ | ↓-↓↓ |
| | Uric acid (urine) | ↓-↓↓ | ↓-↓↓ | ↓-↓↓ | ↓-↓↓ | ↓-↓↓ |
| | Xanthine (plasma) | ↑ | ↑ | ↑ | ↑ | ↑ |
| | Xanthine (urine) | ↑↑ | ↑↑ | ↑↑ | ↑↑ | ↑↑ |

**Table 13.20** Hypoxanthine guanine phosphoribosyltransferase deficiency

| System | Symptoms and biomarkers | Neonatal (birth–1 month) | Infancy (1–18 months) | Childhood (1.5–11 years) | Adolescence (11–16 years) | Adulthood (>16 years) |
|---|---|---|---|---|---|---|
| CNS | **Cerebral palsy** | + | + | + | + | + |
| | **Choreoathetosis** | | | + | + | + |
| | Intellectual disability | | ± | ± | ± | ± |
| | **Pyramidal signs** | + | + | + | + | + |
| | **Self-mutilation** | + | + | + | + | + |
| | Spasticity | + | + | + | + | + |
| Metabolic | Hematuria | | | + | + | + |
| Renal | Renal failure, acute | ± | ± | ± | ± | ± |
| | Renal stones | | | ± | ± | ± |
| | Urinary Infections | | | + | + | + |
| | **Urolithiasis** | + | + | + | + | + |
| Other | Gouty arthritis | | | | | ± |
| Laboratory findings | AICA riboside (urine) | | ↑ | ↑ | ↑ | ↑ |
| | Hypoxanthine (plasma) | ↑ | ↑ | ↑ | ↑ | ↑ |
| | Hypoxanthine (urine) | ↑↑ | ↑↑ | ↑↑ | ↑↑ | ↑↑ |
| | Hypoxanthine guanine phosphoribosyltransferase (red blood cells) | ↓↓↓ | ↓↓↓ | ↓↓↓ | ↓↓↓ | ↓↓↓ |
| | Uric acid (plasma) | ↑↑ | ↑↑ | ↑↑ | ↑↑ | ↑↑ |
| | Uric acid (urine) | ↑↑↑ | ↑↑↑ | ↑↑↑ | ↑↑ | ↑↑ |
| | Xanthine (urine) | ↑ | ↑ | ↑ | ↑ | ↑ |

**Table 13.21** Adenine phosphoribosyl transferase deficiency

| System | Symptoms and biomarkers | Neonatal (birth–1 month) | Infancy (1–18 months) | Childhood (1.5–11 years) | Adolescence (11–16 years) | Adulthood (>16 years) |
|---|---|---|---|---|---|---|
| Metabolic | **Hematuria** | + | + | + | + | + |
| Renal | **Renal colic** | + | + | + | + | + |
| | Renal failure, acute | ± | ± | ± | ± | ± |
| | **Renal failure, chronic** | | + | + | + | + |
| | **Urolithiasis** | ± | ± | ± | ± | ± |
| Laboratory findings | 2,8-Dihydroxyadenine (urine) | ↑↑ | ↑↑ | ↑↑ | ↑↑ | ↑↑ |
| | Adenine (urine) | ↑ | ↑ | ↑ | ↑ | ↑ |
| | Adenine phosphoribosyl transferase (red blood cells) | ↓↓ | ↓↓ | ↓↓ | ↓↓ | ↓↓ |

**Table 13.22** Adenylate kinase 1 deficiency

| System | Symptoms and biomarkers | Neonatal (birth–1 month) | Infancy (1–18 months) | Childhood (1.5–11 years) | Adolescence (11–16 years) | Adulthood (>16 years) |
|---|---|---|---|---|---|---|
| CNS | Retardation, psychomotor | ± | ± | ± | ± | ± |
| Haematological | **Anaemia, non-spherocytic, haemolytic with basophilic stippling** | + | + | + | + | + |
| Laboratory findings | Adenylate kinase activity (erythrocytes) | ↓↓↓ | ↓↓↓ | ↓↓↓ | ↓↓↓ | ↓↓↓ |

**Table 13.23** Adenylate kinase 2 deficiency

| System | Symptoms and biomarkers | Neonatal (birth–1 month) | Infancy (1–18 months) | Childhood (1.5–11 years) | Adolescence (11–16 years) | Adulthood (>16 years) |
|---|---|---|---|---|---|---|
| Haematological | **Congenital agranulocytosis** | + | | | | |
| | Leukopenia | + | | | | |
| | Lymphopaenia | + | | | | |
| Other | **Death in the first few weeks of life** | + | | | | |

**Table 13.24** Inosine monophosphate dehydrogenase deficiency

| System | Symptoms and biomarkers | Neonatal (birth–1 month) | Infancy (1–18 months) | Childhood (1.5–11 years) | Adolescence (11–16 years) | Adulthood (>16 years) |
|---|---|---|---|---|---|---|
| Eye | **Constricted visual fields** | | | | + | + |
| | **Leber amaurosis-like** | | + | + | | + |
| | Night blindness | | | | + | + |
| | Nystagmus | + | | | | |
| | **Pigmentary retinopathy** | | + | + | | |
| | **Retinal 'bone corpuscle; pigmentation'** | | | | + | + |
| | **Retinal dysfunction** | + | | | | |
| | **Retinal dystrophy** | + | | | | |
| | **Retinitis pigmentosa** | | | + | + | + |
| | **Vision loss** | + | | | | |

**Table 13.25** Inosine triphosphatase deficiency

| System | Symptoms and biomarkers | Neonatal (birth–1 month) | Infancy (1–18 months) | Childhood (1.5–11 years) | Adolescence (11–16 years) | Adulthood (>16 years) |
|---|---|---|---|---|---|---|
| Cardiovascular | Cardiomyopathy | ± | ± | ± | | |
| | Electrocardiogram abnormalities | ± | ± | ± | | |
| CNS | **Cerebral atrophy (MRI)** | + | + | + | | |
| | **Delayed myelination** | + | + | + | | |
| | **Encephalopathy** | + | + | + | | |
| | **Hypotonia, severe** | + | + | + | | |
| | **Retardation, psychomotor** | + | + | + | | |
| | **Seizures** | + | + | + | | |
| Digestive | **Feeding difficulties** | + | + | + | | |
| Eye | Cataract | ± | ± | ± | | |
| Haematological | Erythrocyte ITP accumulation | ↑↑↑ | ↑↑↑ | ↑↑↑ | ↑↑↑ | ↑↑↑ |
| Musculoskeletal | **Microcephaly** | + | + | + | | |
| Other | Childhood death | ± | ± | ± | | |
| Laboratory findings | Enzyme activity (FB) | ↓↓ | ↓↓ | ↓↓ | ↓↓ | ↓↓ |

**Table 13.26** Inosine triphosphatase deficiency (erythrocyte)

| System | Symptoms and biomarkers | Neonatal (birth–1 month) | Infancy (1–18 months) | Childhood (1.5–11 years) | Adolescence (11–16 years) | Adulthood (>16 years) |
|---|---|---|---|---|---|---|
| Haematological | Anaemia, protection against ribavirin-induced | | | | ± | ± |
| | Erythrocyte ITP accumulation | n-↑↑↑ | n-↑↑↑ | n-↑↑↑ | n-↑↑↑ | n-↑↑↑ |
| Other | Thiopurines, decreased tolerance | | | ± | ± | ± |
| Laboratory findings | Enzyme activity (RBC) | n-↓↓ | n-↓↓ | n-↓↓ | n-↓↓ | n-↓↓ |

**Table 13.27** Thiopurine *S*-methyltransferase deficiency

| System | Symptoms and biomarkers | Neonatal (birth–1 month) | Infancy (1–18 months) | Childhood (1.5–11 years) | Adolescence (11–16 years) | Adulthood (>16 years) |
|---|---|---|---|---|---|---|
| Other | Thiopurines, decreased tolerance | | + | + | + | + |

**Table 13.28** Hyperuricaemic nephropathy, familial juvenile 1

| System | Symptoms and biomarkers | Neonatal (birth–1 month) | Infancy (1–18 months) | Childhood (1.5–11 years) | Adolescence (11–16 years) | Adulthood (>16 years) |
|---|---|---|---|---|---|---|
| Musculoskeletal | **Gout** | | | | + | + |
| Renal | **Chronic interstitial nephritis** | | | | + | + |
| | **Nephropathy** | | | | + | + |
| | **Renal failure** | | | | + | + |
| | **Small medullary cysts** | | | | + | + |
| | **Tubular atrophy** | | | | + | + |
| Laboratory findings | Fractional excretion of uric acid | ↓ | ↓ | ↓ | ↓ | ↓ |
| | Uric acid (plasma) | | | ↑↑ | ↑↑ | ↑↑ |

**Table 13.29** Urate transporter 1 deficiency

| System | Symptoms and biomarkers | Neonatal (birth–1 month) | Infancy (1–18 months) | Childhood (1.5–11 years) | Adolescence (11–16 years) | Adulthood (>16 years) |
|---|---|---|---|---|---|---|
| Renal | Exercise-induced acute renal failure with acute tubular necrosis | | | | ± | ± |
| | Urolithiasis | | | ± | ± | ± |
| Laboratory findings | Uric acid (plasma) | | | ↓-n | ↓-n | ↓-n |
| | Uric acid (urine) | | | n-↑ | n-↑ | n-↑ |

**Table 13.30** Urate voltage-driven efflux transporter 1 deficiency

| System | Symptoms and biomarkers | Neonatal (birth–1 month) | Infancy (1–18 months) | Childhood (1.5–11 years) | Adolescence (11–16 years) | Adulthood (>16 years) |
|---|---|---|---|---|---|---|
| Renal | Exercise-induced acute renal failure | | | | | ± |
| Laboratory findings | Uric acid (plasma) | | | ↓ | ↓ | ↓ |

## Reference and Pathological Values

| | mmol/mol creatinine | | | | | | | | | | | | | |
|---|---|---|---|---|---|---|---|---|---|---|---|---|---|---|
| | Urate | 2,8-di-OH-Adenine | Ade | Ado | AICAr | dAdo | dGuo | dIno | Guo | Hyp | Ino | Sado | SAICAr | Xan |
| 0–1 month | 569–2605 | | | 0.0–2.0 | 0.0–3.3 | | | | 0.0–2.0 | 2.0–33.4 | 0.0–4.0 | 0.0–19.0 | | 2.0–37.0 |
| 1 month–2 years | 419–1963 | | | 0.0–1.0 | 0.0–3.0 | | | | 0.0–1.0 | 4.0–61.0 | 0.0–4.0 | 0.0–18.8 | | 4.0–50.8 |
| 2–4 years | 295–1508 | | | 0.0–1.0 | 0.0–2.0 | | | | 0.0–1.0 | 4.0–63.0 | 0.0–2.0 | 0.0–13.0 | | 6.0–40.0 |
| 4–10 years | 214–895 | | | 0.0 | 0.0–2.0 | | | | 0.0 | 3.0–33.0 | 0.0–1.0 | 0.0–8.0 | | 4.0–23.0 |
| 10–18 years | 132–619 | | | 0.0 | 0.0–2.0 | | | | 0.0 | 1.0–20.7 | 0.0–1.0 | 0.0–5.0 | | 1.0–19.4 |
| 18–55 years | 99–578 | | | 0.0 | 0.0–1.0 | | | | 0.0 | 1.0–12.8 | 0.0–1.0 | 0.0–4.0 | | 0.0–10.0 |
| >55 | 73–668 | | | 0.0–1.0 | 0.0–2.0 | | | | 0.0–1.0 | 0.0–18.0 | 0.0–1.0 | 0.0–4.0 | | 0.0–24.5 |

| | mmol/mol creatinine | | | | | | | | | | | | | |
|---|---|---|---|---|---|---|---|---|---|---|---|---|---|---|
| All age groups combined ($n \geq 2600$) | 135–1666 | 0.0–3.0 | 0.0–4.0 | 0.0–2.0 | 0.0–2.0 | 0.0 | 0.0 | 0.0–1.0 | 0.0–1.0 | 1.0–45.8 | 0.0–3.0 | 0.0–13.0 | 0.0–1.0 | 1.0–39.0 |
| ADA | | | | | | 10–266 | | | | | | | | |
| PNP | 21–160 | | | | | | 100–400 | 100–650 | 286–405 | 0–53[a] | 500–1900 | | | |
| XDH | | | | | | | | | | 20–660 | | | | 134–2900 |
| HPRT | 1370–6298 | | | | 2–21 | | | | | 90–270 | | | | 25–109 |
| APRT | | 23–32 | 8–41 | | | | | | | | | | | |
| ADSL | | | | | | | | | | | | 69–2603 | 9–802 | |
| PRPP superactivity | 1910–8300 | | | | | | | | | | | | | |
| ATIC ($n = 1$) | | | | | 280 | | | | | | | | | |

[a]May be within reference range to spontaneous degradation of nucleosides

| | mmol/mol creatinine | | | | | | | | | | | | | | |
|---|---|---|---|---|---|---|---|---|---|---|---|---|---|---|---|
| | NC-Aspartate | DHO | Oro (OA) | Ord | Ura | Thy | DHU | DHT | NC-BAIB | NC-BALA | dUrd | dThd | Ps-Urd | Urd | 5-OH-Me Ura |
| 0–1 month | | | 0.0–5.0 | 0.0–18.4 | 0.0–10.5 | | 0.0–15.0 | 0.0–9.0 | 0.0–23.7 | 0.0–57.2 | | | 58.8–280 | 0.0–6.0 | |
| 1 month–2 years | | | 0.0–6.0 | 0.0–9.0 | 0.0–47.5 | | 0.0–20.0 | 0.0–7.0 | 0.0–11.0 | 0.0–31.2 | | | 34.0–218 | 0.0–4.0 | |
| 2–4 years | | | 0.0–4.0 | 0.0–6.0 | 0.0–33.0 | | 0.0–7.0 | 0.0–4.0 | 0.0–7.0 | 0.0–15.0 | | | 35.0–146 | 0.0–3.0 | |
| 4–10 years | | | 0.0–3.1 | 0.0–4.0 | 0.0–20.1 | | 0.0–6.0 | 0.0–3.0 | 0.0–3.1 | 0.0–13.1 | | | 19.8–93.9 | 0.0–2.1 | |
| 10–18 years | | | 0.0–2.7 | 0.0–3.0 | 0.0–15.0 | | 0.0–5.5 | 0.0–3.0 | 0.0–2.0 | 0.0–8.5 | | | 13.0–74.4 | 0.0–2.0 | |
| 18–55 years | | | 0.0–2.0 | 0.0–2.0 | 0.0–15.0 | | 0.0–7.0 | 0.0–3.0 | 0.0–2.0 | 0.0–7.0 | | | 11.0–60.4 | 0.0–2.0 | |
| >55 | | | 0.0–3.8 | 0.0–12.0 | 0.0–18.6 | | 0.0–8.5 | 0.0–2.3 | 0.0–4.3 | 0.0–8.5 | | | 10.5–79.0 | 0.0–3.0 | |
| All age groups combined ($n \geq 2600$) | | 0.0–4.0 | 0.0–4.0 | 0.0–8.0 | 0.0–29.0 | 0.0–3.0 | 0.0–10.8 | 0.0–5.0 | 0.0–9.0 | 0.0–21.0 | 0.0–1.0 | 0.0–1.0 | 16.0–182 | 0.0–3.0 | 0.0–4.0 |
| DHODH | 149 ($n = 1$) | 39–87 | 1.0–78 | 0.0–38 | | | | | | | | | | | |
| UMPS (OPRT) | | | 180–9600 | 40–465 | | | | | | | | | | | |
| UMPS, partial deficiency (OPRT) | | | 7–53 | | | | | | | | | | | | |
| TP | | | | | 50–77 | 23–48 | | | | | 51–150 | 29–125 | | | |
| DPD | | | | | 60–680 | 9–476 | | | | | | | | | 24–140 |
| DHP | | | | | 9–144 | 12–230 | 150–804 | 10–490 | | | | | | | |
| UP | | | | | | | 13–94 | 47–201 | 187–801 | 236–1116 | | | | | |

## Diagnostic Flowchart

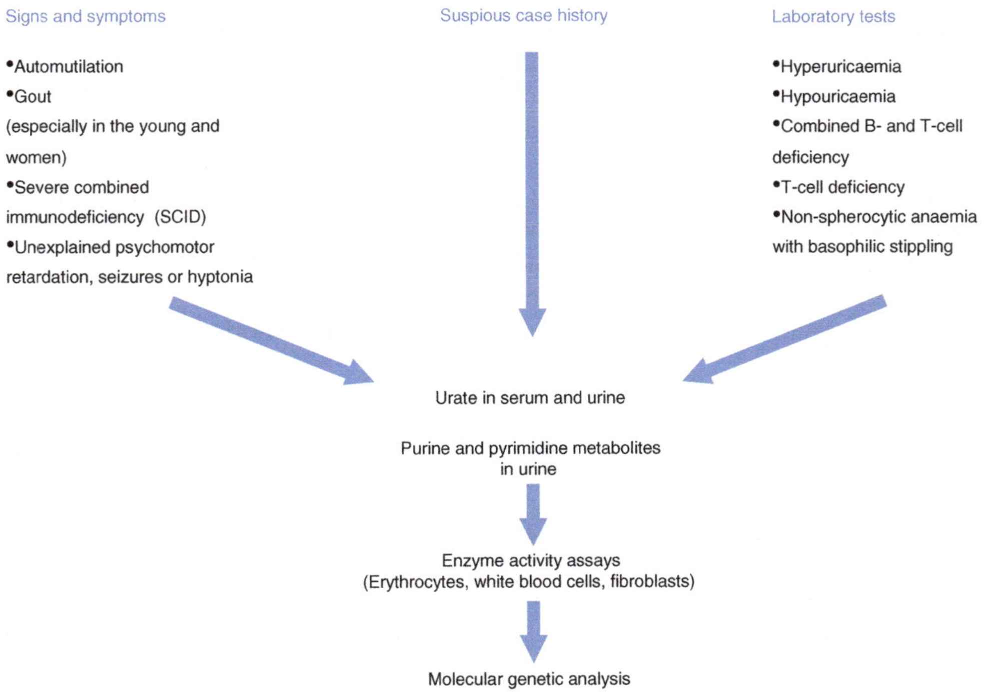


**Fig. 13.3** The justification for detailed purine and pyrimidine investigations includes three aspects: (**a**) clinical signs and symptoms (some are very characteristic such as self-mutilation or gout in young people and women or SCID (severe combined immunodeficiency) syndrome; others are shown in the information of the specific diseases), (**b**) a case history suspicious of an inborn error of metabolism and (**c**) characteristic laboratory tests. If a patient meets these criteria, the first steps are measurement of uric acid in body fluid and purine and pyrimidine metabolites in urine. It is highly recommended to estimate both plasma and urine concentrations at once to be able to assess the excretion and confirm or exclude overproduction/hypoexcretion of uric acid. The exclusion of secondary causes of hyperuricaemia/hypouricaemia (such as nephropathy, tissue breakdown, Fanconi syndrome and uricosuric drugs) is very important. Confirmation of diagnosis consists of enzyme assay and finally molecular genetic analysis

## Specimen Collection

This section is taken from the ERNDIM advisory document for the analysis of purines and pyrimidines (see Online Databases and Resources section for reference).

### Urine

Many laboratories use urine portions for diagnostic purposes, and the traditionally 24-h urine collection or overnight collection has more or less become obsolete. No preservatives are added to the urine sample; freezing the sample as soon as possible is often enough.

If a 24-h urine collection is desired, proceed as follows: during the collection period, the urine aliquots are kept refrigerated (4 °C), and after completion, the urine is sent to the laboratory in a well-isolated package and stored in the refrigerator for max. 1 week at 4 °C until analysis or stored frozen at −20 °C when analysis is carried out after more than 1 week but within 2 months. For longer periods, storage at −80 °C is recommended.

Dipstick tests for nitrite and pH should be carried out directly after receipt of the urine in order to check for bacterial contamination. In addition, qualitative tests for glucose, reducing substances, sulphite and ketone bodies should be performed. Analysis should not be performed in severely bacterially contaminated samples (pH > 7 and/or nitrite is positive).

### Plasma

The analysis of purines and pyrimidine can be performed in plasma obtained from blood anticoagulated with heparin as well as EDTA. This can be adjusted according to local protocols. In the case of capillary blood, clean and disinfect the skin thoroughly before taking the blood sample to avoid contamination from the skin surface. An absolute prerequisite is that the sample is absolutely fresh, and there should preferably be no or as little delay as possible between drawing of the blood and freezing the plasma sample. Plasma samples should be stored at −20 °C or at −80 °C if stored for a prolonged period. Plasma samples should be deproteinised before most types of analysis.

### CSF

Please refer to your own hospital protocol for the lumbar puncture procedure.

CSF samples should be deproteinised before analysis. CSF samples should be stored at −80 °C.

## Prenatal Diagnosis and DNA Analysis

Providing a table listing all disorders and materials in which molecular analysis can be performed is obsolete because of the modern sequencing techniques. All genes and their chromosomal localisations are listed above. In essence, any material from which DNA can be extracted is suitable for molecular analysis. There are good and reliable databases to be found on the Internet.

## Treatment Summary

### The Management of Purine and Pyrimidine Disorders

In the treatment of purine and pyrimidine disorders, patients and physicians need to be aware of several precautions: the dosage of allopurinol in overproduction hyperuricaemia (HPRT, PRPS) is higher than in primary gout and therefore should be reduced in the cases of renal insufficiency (risk of xanthine nephropathy!) (van Gennip et al. 2006). There is a risk of myopathy and neurotoxicity with colchicine prophylaxis in gouty patients with renal impairment and in patients receiving statins, so renal function should be assessed before prescribing colchicine or nonsteroidal anti-inflammatory drugs (NSAIDs) (Nuki et al. 2017).

Administration of fluorinated pyrimidine analogues in dihydropyrimidine dehydrogenase deficiency can be catastrophic; in thiopurine methyltransferase deficiency, there may be enhanced toxicity of mercaptopurines.

Specific treatment is available for a small number of other purine and pyrimidine disorders at present. The reason is that, in many cases, our understanding of pathogenesis how a particular point defect in a gene produces these relatively new disorders is still incomplete and requires further studies.

### The Management of Hyperuricaemia

Genetic defects with hyperuricaemia and gout represent the most frequent disorders of purine metabolism (Becker 2001). The incidence of hyperuricaemia and gout is increasing. Population-based studies have estimated an incidence of up to 21% for hyperuricaemia and 1–4% for gout (Kuo et al. 2015).

#### The Importance of Controlling Hyperuricaemia

Hyperuricaemia is the main underlying cause of gout. In addition, several studies suggest that chronic hyperuricaemia is related to the pathogenesis of multifactorial disorders such as hypertension, metabolic syndrome, chronic heart failure and chronic kidney disease (Mazzali et al. 2010; Teng et al. 2012). A recent study revealed that hyperuricaemia was a strong independent risk factor for major cardiovascular events and should be included in cardiovascular prevention strategies. Whether hypouricaemic drugs can reduce cardiovascular disease risk warrants further studies (Capuano et al. 2017). Therefore, it is important to emphasise rapid diagnosis and treatment of asymptomatic hyperuricaemia, considered as a multifactorial pathological condition very closely related to cardiovascular and renal complications. Control of hyperuricaemia should be more important to paediatricians than formerly thought. It is important to raise awareness among general practitioners to test uric acid concentrations in blood and urine more often, especially in patients with one or more risk factors for cardiovascular and renal impairment (Bove et al. 2017).

#### The Management of Gout

Recent updated recommendations of European League Against Rheumatism (EULAR) emphasise three main principles for the efficient management of gout: Firstly, every patient with gout should be fully informed about the pathophysiology of the disease, effective treatments and associated comorbidities. Secondly, every patient with gout should receive advice regarding lifestyle changes. Alcohol, especially beer, spirits and sugar-sweetened drinks, should be excluded. Avoidance of excessive intake of meat, legumes, seafood and fructose-containing foods should be recommended. Low-fat dairy products and diets high in dietary fibre should be encouraged. Weight reduction and regular exercise should be advised. Thirdly, every patient with gout should be systematically examined for associated comorbidities including hyperlipidaemia, hypertension, obesity, coronary heart disease, peripheral artery disease and renal impairment. Detection of chronic kidney disease is notably required. The measurement of the estimated glomerular filtration rate (eGFR) at the time of diagnosis of gout is recommended. The subsequent monitoring of eGFR should follow in parallel with measurements of uric acid concentrations in blood and urine (Richette et al. 2017; Nuki et al. 2017).

The main principle of the management of gout with pharmacotherapy is the need to reduce serum uric acid concentrations to below a target of 0.30 or 0.36 mmol/L depending on whether it is tophaceous or non-tophaceous, respectively (Robinson PC 2018). Urate-lowering therapy (ULT) should be discussed from the first presentation of the disease. Allopurinol is recommended as the first choice of ULT. Its dosage should be adjusted according to renal function. If it is not possible to achieve uric acid target concentration in blood, then febuxostat, uricosuric or combining a xanthine oxidase inhibitor with a uricosuric should be recommended (Richette et al. 2017; Nuki et al. 2017). Febuxostat has an excellent safety and tolerability profile also in patients with moderate renal impairment, because of its hepatic metabolism. It was also shown that its serum uric acid-lowering efficacy is greater than of allopurinol in patients with hyperuricaemia with or without chronic kidney disease (Bove et al. 2017). The use of xanthine oxidase inhibitors is recommended for the overproduction-type hyperuricaemia, while uricosuric agents are recommended for the underexcretion type. However, when uricosuric drugs are used, urinary output must be sustained, and, in addition, alkalinisation of the urine to prevent urolithiasis must be considered (Becker 2001).

It is important to note that all uric acid-lowering therapies should be started at low dose and titrated upwards until the target value is achieved. The recommendations for the treatment of flare are colchicine, nonsteroidal anti-inflammatory drugs (NSAIDs), oral or intra-articular steroids or a combination. In patients with flare and contraindications to colchicine, NSAIDs and corticosteroids, an interleukin-1 blocker should be considered. For patients with refractory gout, pegloticase is recommended (Richette et al. 2017; Nuki et al. 2017).

Recent study suggests that febuxostat may positively affect cardiovascular mortality in comparison with allopurinol in elderly patients with mild-to-moderate heart failure. This finding deserves further evaluation in the future (Cicero et al. 2019).

## Online Resources

ERNDIM offers a range of advisory documents on laboratory analyses including purines and pyrimidines (website: www.erndim.org under the header Training and Education).

The Purine and Pyrimidine Society. Scientific forum for biomedical scientists and physicians interested in purines and pyrimidines around the world (website: www.ppsociety.org).

## References


Assmann B, Gohlich G, Baethmann M, Wevers RA, Van Gennip AH, Van Kuilenburg AB, et al. Clinical findings and a therapeutic trial in the first patient with beta-ureidopropionase deficiency. Neuropediatrics. 2006;37(1):20–5.

Balasubramaniam S, Duley JA, Christodoulou J. Inborn errors of purine metabolism: clinical update and therapies. J Inherit Metab Dis. 2014a;37(5):669–86.

Balasubramaniam S, Duley JA, Christodoulou J. Inborn errors of pyrimidine metabolism: clinical update and therapy. J Inherit Metab Dis. 2014b;37(5):687–98.

Becker MA. Hyperuricemia and gout. In: Scriver CR, Beaudet AL, Sly WS, Valle D, editors. The metabolic and molecular bases of inherited disease, vol. 2. New York: McGraw-Hill; 2001.

Bierau J, Sebesta I. Purine and pyrimidine disorders. In: Blau N, Duran M, Blaskovics ME, Gibson KM, Dionisi-Vici C, editors. Physician's guide to the diagnosis, treatment, and follow-up of inherited metabolic diseases. Berlin Heidelberg: Springer; 2014. p. 641–60.

Bjursell MK, Blom HJ, Cayuela JA, Engvall ML, Lesko N, Balasubramaniam S, et al. Adenosine kinase deficiency disrupts the methionine cycle and causes hypermethioninemia, encephalopathy, and abnormal liver function. Am J Hum Genet. 2011;89(4):507–15.

Bove M, Cicero AF, Veronesi M, Borghi C. An evidence-based review on urate-lowering treatments: implications for optimal treatment of chronic hyperuricemia. Vasc Health Risk Manag. 2017;13:23–8.

Capuano V, Marchese F, Capuano R, et al. Hyperuricemia as an independent risk factor for major cardiovascular events: a 10-year cohort study from Southern Italy. J Cardiovasc Med (Hagerstown). 2017;18:159–64.

Cicero AFG, Cosentino ER, Kuwabara M, Degli Esposti D, Borghi C. Effects of allopurinol and febuxostat on cardiovascular mortality in elderly heart failure patients. Intern Emerg Med. 2019;14(6):949–56.

Hirano M, Nishino I, Nishigaki Y, Marti R. Thymidine phosphorylase gene mutations cause mitochondrial neurogastrointestinal encephalomyopathy (MNGIE). Intern Med. 2006;45(19):1103.

Kevelam SH, Bierau J, Salvarinova R, Agrawal S, Honzik T, Visser D, et al. Recessive ITPA mutations cause an early infantile encephalopathy. Ann Neurol. 2015;78(4):649–58.

Koch J, Mayr JA, Alhaddad B, Rauscher C, Bierau J, Kovacs-Nagy R, et al. CAD mutations and uridine-responsive epileptic encephalopathy. Brain. 2017;140(2):279–86.

Kuo CF, Grainge MJ, Mallen C, Zhang W, Doherty M. Rising burden of gout in the UK but continuing suboptimal management: a nationwide population study. Ann Rheum Dis. 2015;74(4):661–7.

Mazzali M, Kanbay M, Segal MS, Shafiu M, Jalal D, Feig DI, et al. Uric acid and hypertension: cause or effect? Curr Rheumatol Rep. 2010;12(2):108–17.

Micheli V, Camici M, Tozzi MG, Ipata PL, Sestini S, Bertelli M, et al. Neurological disorders of purine and pyrimidine metabolism. Curr Top Med Chem. 2011;11(8):923–47.

Monostori P, Klinke G, Hauke J, Richter S, Bierau J, Garbade SF, et al. Extended diagnosis of purine and pyrimidine disorders from urine: LC MS/MS assay development and clinical validation. PLoS One. 2019;14(2):e0212458.

Nuki G, Doherty M, Richette P. Current management of gout: practical messages from 2016 EULAR guidelines. Pol Arch Intern Med. 2017;127(4):267–77.

Rainger J, Bengani H, Campbell L, Anderson E, Sokhi K, Lam W, et al. Miller (Genee-Wiedemann) syndrome represents a clinically and biochemically distinct subgroup of postaxial acrofacial dysostosis associated with partial deficiency of DHODH. Hum Mol Genet. 2012;21(18):3969–83.

Richette P, Doherty M, Pascual E, Barskova V, Becce F, Castaneda-Sanabria J, et al. 2016 updated EULAR evidence-based recommendations for the management of gout. Ann Rheum Dis. 2017;76(1):29–42.

Robinson PC. Gout-An update of aetiology, genetics, co-morbidities and management. Maturitas. 2018;118:67–73.

Sebesta I. Genetic disorders resulting in hyper- or hypouricemia. Adv Chronic Kidney Dis. 2012;19(6):398–403.

Sebesta I, Stiburkova B, Krijt J. Hereditary xanthinuria is not so rare disorder of purine metabolism. Nucleosides Nucleotides Nucleic Acids. 2018;37(6):324–8.

Simmonds HA, Van Gennip AH. Purine and pyrimidine disorders. In: Blau ND, Duran M, Blaskovics ME, Gibson KM, editors. Physician's guide to the laboratory diagnosis of metabolic diseases. 2nd ed. Berlin: Springer; 2003.

Teng GG, Ang LW, Saag KG, Yu MC, Yuan JM, Koh WP. Mortality due to coronary heart disease and kidney disease among middle-aged and elderly men and women with gout in the Singapore Chinese Health Study. Ann Rheum Dis. 2012;71(6):924–8.

van Gennip AH, Bierau J, Nyhan WL. Inborn errors of purine and pyrimidine metabolism. In: Blau N, Hoffmann GF, Leonard J, Clarke JTR, editors. Physician's guide to the treatment and follow-up of metabolic diseases. Berlin: Springer; 2006.

van Kuilenburg AB. Dihydropyrimidine dehydrogenase and the efficacy and toxicity of 5-fluorouracil. Eur J Cancer. 2004;40(7):939–50.

Weinshilboum RM, Otterness DM, Szumlanski CL. Methylation pharmacogenetics: catechol O-methyltransferase, thiopurine methyltransferase, and histamine N-methyltransferase. Annu Rev Pharmacol Toxicol. 1999;39:19–52.

# Disorders of Nucleotide Metabolism

# 14

Min Ae Lee-Kirsch, Victoria Tüngler, Simona Orcesi, and Davide Tonduti

## Contents



**Summary**

Nucleotides are the building blocks of nucleic acids including deoxyribonucleic acid (DNA) and ribonucleic acid (RNA), both of which are essential biomolecules within virtually all forms of life. While DNA carries the genetic information required for building and maintaining an organism, RNA serves as an intermediary template for protein translation. Nucleic acids derived from pathogens, such as viruses, also represent important molecular patterns that can be sensed by pattern recognition receptors of the innate immune system as danger signals. Engagement of these nucleic acid-sensing receptors initiates activation of signaling cascades in the host immune cells leading to production and secretion of type I interferon (IFN) and other cytokines. The aim of the ensuing antiviral immune response is to eliminate infected cells and to restrict viral spread. As nucleic acid sensors have only limited capacity to differentiate between nonself- and self-DNA or RNA, a type I IFN response can also be initiated by endogenous nucleic acids. Such inappropriate activation of type I IFN can be detrimental to the host by promoting autoinflammation and a loss of immune tolerance leading to autoimmunity. Type I IFN activation induced by immune recognition of self-nucleic acids represents a central pathogenetic mechanism underlying disorders of nucleic acid metabolism and nucleic acid-sensing also referred to as type I interferonopathies.

Nucleotides play fundamental roles in cell metabolism. They provide energy in the form of nucleoside triphosphates, function as second messenger in cell signaling, and act as cofactors of enzymatic reactions. Perturbations in

M. A. Lee-Kirsch (✉) · V. Tüngler
Department of Pediatrics, Medizinische Fakultät Carl Gustav Carus, Technische Universität Dresden, Dresden, Germany
e-mail: minae.lee-kirsch@uniklinikum-dresden.de

S. Orcesi
Unit of Child Neurology and Psychiatry, IRCCS Mondino Foundation, Pavia, Italy
e-mail: simona.orcesi@mondino.it

D. Tonduti
Child Neurology Unit, COALA (Center for Diagnosis and Treatment of Leukodystrophy) - V. Buzzi Children's Hospital, Milano, Italy
e-mail: davidetondu@hotmail.com



N. Blau et al. (eds.), *Physician's Guide to the Diagnosis, Treatment, and Follow-Up of Inherited Metabolic Diseases*,
https://doi.org/10.1007/978-3-030-67727-5_14

adenosine homeostasis leading to downregulation of pyrophosphate (PPi), a key inhibitor of hydroxyapatite growth, underlie disorders of early arterial calcification. The lysosomal equilibrative nucleoside transporter 3 (ENT3) regulates intracellular nucleoside pools and thereby influences the availability of ATP and GTP, synthesis of DNA and RNA, and other metabolic pathways. Its general role in cell homeostasis likely accounts for the pleiotropy of ENT3 deficiency. Activation-induced cytidine deaminase (AID) and uracil-DNA glycosylase (UNG) mediate somatic hypermutation and class-switch recombination at the immunoglobulin gene loci, which represent key events during formation of protective antibodies by B cells. Malfunction of these pathways impedes antibody formation resulting in profound susceptibility to bacterial infections.

## Introduction

Disorders of nucleotide metabolisms can be broadly divided into disorders of nucleic acid metabolism and nucleic acid-sensing, disorders relating to nucleotide transport and metabolism, and disorders of immunoglobulin hypermutation and class-switching. Given the extraordinary functional diversity of pathways regulating nucleotide metabolism, the phenotypes of the associated disorders comprise a broad and diverse spectrum of clinical presentations.

### Disorders of Nucleic Acid Metabolism and Nucleic Acid-Sensing

#### Aicardi-Goutières Syndrome

Aicardi-Goutières syndrome (AGS) is a systemic inflammatory disorder primarily affecting the brain and skin. It is characterized by inappropriate activation of the antiviral type I IFN axis and represents the prototypic type I interferonopathy (Lee-Kirsch 2017). Type I interferonopathies comprise a heterogenous group of disorders caused by perturbations of the innate immune system associated with an abnormal activation of type I IFN.

AGS is caused by mutations in seven distinct genes encoding 3′ repair exonuclease (*TREX1*, AGS1), the three subunits of ribonuclease H2 (*RNASEH2B*, AGS2; *RNASEH2C*, AGS3; *RNASEH2A*, AGS4), sterile alpha motif (SAM) and HD-domain containing protein (*SAMHD1*, AGS5); RNA-specific adenosine deaminase (*ADAR*, AGS6), and interferon-induced helicase C domain-containing protein 1 (*IFIH1*, AGS7). All AGS-causing genes function in pathways affecting the metabolism or the immune recognition of intracellular nucleic acids including DNA and RNA (Lee-Kirsch 2017; Schlee and Hartmann 2016) (Fig. 14.1). Inheritance of AGS1 to AGS6 is predominantly autosomal recessive resulting in a loss of function of the underlying gene, although rare cases of heterozygous de novo mutations with presumably dominant negative effect have been described for *TREX1* and *ADAR*. In contrast, AGS7 is caused by heterozygous gain-of-function mutations in *IFIH1* that either occur de novo or are inherited as autosomal dominant trait with reduced penetrance (Crow et al. 2015).

AGS usually begins during the first year of life with a peak between the third and sixth month. Following a period of normal psychomotor development, infants commonly present with a subacute encephalitic-like phase characterized by irritability, unexplained fevers, dystonic movements, truncal hypotonia, as well as sleeping and feeding difficulties. After a few weeks to months, the clinical picture enters a plateau phase characterized by progressive microcephaly, spastic-dystonic tetraplegia with exaggerated startle reactions, and severe developmental delay. Children frequently present abnormal eye movements or poor visual performance, and some patients experience epilepsy. Both a neonatal and a late onset of symptoms beyond the first year of life have been described. Likewise, intrafamilial phenotypic variability can be high with one sibling presenting with severe neurological impairment and the other with only mild spasticity and normal intellect (Vogt et al. 2013; Tüngler et al. 2014). The major neuroradiological findings include leukoencephalopathy, basal ganglia calcification, and cerebral atrophy. Thus, the clinical phenotype of AGS resembles congenital viral infection. In addition, some patients develop signs that are also observed in patients with the autoimmune disorder systemic lupus erythematosus including arthritis, hepatic disease, thrombocytopenia, lymphopenia, antinuclear antibodies, as well as cold-induced erythematous skin lesions, also referred to as chilblain lesions (Ramantani et al. 2010, 2011; Cuadrado et al. 2015). Elevated liver function tests and thrombocytopenia occur more commonly in cases with neonatal onset.

Cerebrospinal fluid (CSF) lymphocytosis and increased levels of IFN-α in CSF are observed during the encephalitic phase but tend to gradually decrease over time (Goutieres et al. 1998). In the absence of lymphocytosis or IFN-α in CSF, elevated CSF pterins may be a less specific sign of CNS inflammation (Blau et al. 2003). In contrast, chronic upregulation of interferon-stimulated genes in peripheral blood cells, the so-called interferon signature, can be measured in most patients persistently throughout the course of the disease and reflects the underlying intrinsic systemic inflammation (Rice et al. 2013). The interferon signature therefore represents a more robust diagnostic tool.

#### Other AGS-Related Phenotypes

In general, the different AGS subtypes cannot be distinguished based on clinical grounds alone. However, certain clinical signs appear to be more specific for distinct AGS subtypes. Cerebral vasculopathy with early-onset strokes has been described in patients with AGS1 (*TREX1*) and AGS5 (*SAMHD1*); the latter may also present with a moyamoya-like phenotype (Xin et al. 2011; Yamashiro et al. 2013). Bilateral striatal degeneration has been observed in patients with AGS6 (*ADAR*) (Livingston et al. 2014). Magnetic resonance imaging (MRI) shows symmetrical signal changes with swelling followed by shrinkage of the corpus striatum. Patients present with subacute onset of dystonia, commonly triggered by infections. Dyschromatosis symmetrica hereditaria is a rare manifestation of autosomal dominant *ADAR* mutations found in the Japanese population. It is characterized by childhood onset of hypopigmented and hyperpigmented lesions, particularly on the extremities and not associated with AGS (Hayashi and Suzuki 2013). Isolated spastic paraparesis has been observed in patients with AGS2 (*RNASEH2B*), AGS6 (*ADAR1*), and AGS7 (*IFIH1*) who present with slowly progressive lower limb spasticity, normal cognitive function, and normal head growth. Usually, brain MRI is unremarkable (Crow et al. 2014). Overall, there is emerging evidence for a phenotypic continuum between AGS and other AGS-related phenotypes and other type I interferonopathies.

**Familial Chilblain Lupus**

Familial chilblain lupus is a monogenic form of cutaneous lupus erythematosus with onset in early childhood. It is characterized by cold-induced bluish-red skin lesions in acral locations such as fingers, toes, nose, cheeks, and ears (Lee-Kirsch et al. 2006). Patients exhibit an interferon signature in blood indicating constitutive type I IFN activation. Some patients develop arthralgia, antinuclear antibodies, immune complexes, or lymphopenia. Histological findings include perivascular inflammatory infiltrates with increased mucin, deposits of immunoglobulins or complement, and increased expression of type I IFN-induced myxovirus resistance protein 1 (Mx1) (Gunther et al. 2013). Familial chilblain lupus is caused by heterozygous *TREX* mutations (CHBL1) (Rice et al. 2007; Lee-Kirsch et al. 2007). In addition, two families with familial chilblain lupus each segregating a heterozygous mutation in *SAMHD1* (CHBL2) or in *STING* have been reported (Ravenscroft et al. 2011; König et al. 2017).

**Retinal Vasculopathy with Leukodystrophy**

Retinal vasculopathy with cerebral leukodystrophy (RVCL) is an autosomal dominant disorder with onset in adolescence or early adulthood. Patients present with progressive loss of vision, cerebrovascular disease, and dementia. Some patients also develop migraine, glomerulopathy, or Raynaud's disease. RVCL is caused by heterozygous *TREX1* mutations that lead to C-terminal truncations of TREX1 with preservation of the N-terminal DNase domain (Richards et al. 2007).

**Singleton-Merten Syndrome Type 1 and Type 2**

Singleton-Merten syndrome (SGMRT) is characterized by progressive calcifications of large vessels, dental anomalies with periodontal disease and alveolar bone loss, as well as skeletal abnormalities. Patients may also suffer from psoriasis, glaucoma, and recurrent infections. Singleton-Merten syndrome is caused by heterozygous gain-of-function mutations in interferon-induced helicase C domain-containing protein 1 (*IFIH1*, SGMRT1) or dead box polypeptide 58 (*DDX58*, SGMRT2) which encode the cytosolic dsRNA sensors, melanoma differentiation-associated gene 5 (MDA5), and retinoic acid-inducible gene I (RIGI), respectively (Rutsch et al. 2015; Jang et al. 2015).

**STING-Associated Vasculopathy with Onset in Infancy**

STING-associated vasculopathy with onset in infancy (SAVI) is an autoinflammatory vasculopathy characterized by ulcerating acral skin lesions, recurrent fever, and interstitial lung disease (Liu et al. 2014). Similar to patients with AGS or chilblain lupus, skin lesions in SAVI patients are aggravated by cold. Some patients demonstrate variable or transient autoantibody titers. SAVI is caused by heterozygous de novo mutations in transmembrane protein 173 (*TMEM173*), encoding stimulator of interferon genes (STING), the key adaptor signaling molecule of the cyclic GMP-AMP synthase (cGAS)-dependent DNA-sensing pathway (Fig. 14.1). Mutations result in a gain of function leading to constitutive activation of type I IFN. In addition, a family with SAVI and lupus-like features segregating a dominant *STING* mutation was reported (Jeremiah et al. 2014).

**RNASET2 Deficiency**

Cystic leukoencephalopathy without megalencephaly is caused by biallelic mutations in ribonuclease T2 (*RNASET2*), which has been implicated in the degradation of ribosomal self RNA, thereby modulating host immune responses (Henneke et al. 2009; Haud et al. 2011). It is characterized by bilateral anterior temporal cysts and white matter disease, a phenotype overlapping with congenital cytomegalovirus infection and AGS.

**OAS1 Deficiency**

Deficiency in 2′,5′-oligoadenylate synthetase 1 (OAS1) causes infantile-onset pulmonary alveolar proteinosis with hypogammaglobulinemia, which is characterized by progressive respiratory failure with consolidations on lung imaging and recurrent respiratory viral infection. On bronchoalveolar lavage, small and non-foamy alveolar macrophages are seen. OAS1 is a member of the 2–5A synthetase family essential for innate immune responses to viral infection. Reported heterozygous *OAS1* mutations occurred de novo or were transmitted to offspring by a mother who carried the mutation as mosaic (Cho et al. 2018).

## Disorders of Nucleotide Transport and Metabolism

### Pseudoxanthoma Elasticum

Pseudoxanthoma elasticum (PXE) is a connective tissue disorder characterized by progressive calcification of elastic fibers involving the skin, the eye, and the cardiovascular system. Typical skin lesions are yellowish papules on flexural surfaces. Retinal changes include peau d'orange and angioid streaks caused by calcification and dehiscence of Bruch's membrane, resulting in neovascularization with subsequent visual impairment. Adult patients may develop cardiovascular disease due to premature atherosclerosis. PXE is caused by autosomal recessive mutations in *ABCC6* (ATP-binding cassette, subfamily C, member 6) which belongs to the multidrug resistance-associated protein subfamily of ATP-binding cassette transmembrane transporters (Bergen et al. 2000; Struk et al. 2000). In rare cases, autosomal dominant inheritance has been described.

### Generalized Arterial Calcification of Infancy Type 1 and Type 2

General arterial calcification of infancy (GACI) is characterized by calcification of the internal elastic lamina and fibrotic myointimal proliferation of muscular arteries resulting in arterial stenosis (Nitschke et al. 2012). It is often fatal within the first 6 months of life because of myocardial ischemia leading to heart failure. Radiographic findings include diffuse vascular and periarticular soft tissue calcification. Some patients also develop hypophosphatemic rickets due to reduced renal tubular phosphate reabsorption (Rutsch et al. 2008). The majority of cases is caused by autosomal recessive mutations in *ENPP1* (ectonucleotide pyrophosphatase/phosphodiesterase 1, GACI type 1), which converts ATP to AMP and pyrophosphate, an essential physiologic inhibitor of calcification (Fig. 14.2). GACI type 2 is due to biallelic mutations in *ABCC6*. It is usually not associated with pseudoxanthoma due to early death caused by cardiovascular disease. However, GACI patients with *ENPP1* mutations who survive early childhood may develop signs of pseudoxanthoma. It is thought that ABCC6 interferes with ENPP1-associated metabolic pathways, possibly by modulating extracellular ATP concentrations.

### Cole Disease

Cole disease is characterized by congenital or early-onset punctate palmoplantar keratoderma with hypopigmented macules over the arms and legs. Some patients develop calcific tendinopathy. An autosomal dominant form due to mutations in *ENPP1*, which affect cysteine residues in the somatomedin B-like 2 domain, has been described in three families (Eytan et al. 2013). In addition, a recessive and more severe form of Cole disease due to homozygosity of the p.Cys120Arg allele has been reported in three families (Chourabi et al. 2018).

### NT5E Deficiency

Deficiency of ecto-5′-nucleotidase (NT5E) has been described in three families (St Hilaire et al. 2011). This autosomal recessive disorder is characterized by arterial and periarticular calcifications with onset in early adulthood.

### SLC29A1 Deficiency

Lack of the equilibrative nucleoside transporter 1 (ENT1, SLC29A1) results in the Augustine-null blood type and ectopic mineralization (Daniels et al. 2015). It represents an ill-defined clinical entity.

### SLC29A3 Deficiency

Autosomal recessive deficiency of the equilibrative nucleoside transporter 3 (ENT3, SLC29A3) underlies histiocytosis-lymphadenopathy plus syndrome, which encompasses a spectrum of disorders previously thought to be distinct: Faisalabad histiocytosis, sinus histiocytosis with massive lymphadenopathy, Rosai-Dorfman disease, H syndrome, and pigmented hypertrichosis with insulin-dependent diabetes mellitus syndrome (Molho-Pessach et al. 2014). In addition to histiocytosis and lymphadenopathy, recurrent fever, hepatosplenomegaly, skin manifestations, hormone deficiencies, joint contractures, or deafness can occur. Lysosomal ENT3 regulates cell homeostasis by controlling nucleoside availability and is required for T-cell survival upon activation (Wei et al. 2018).

## Disorders of Immunoglobulin Class-Switching and Hypermutation

### Hyper-IgM Syndrome Type 2 and Type 5

Deficiencies in the nucleic acid-modifying enzymes, activation-induced cytidine deaminase (AID), and uracil-DNA glycosylase (UNG) cause the primary immunodeficiency disorders hyper-IgM syndrome type 2 and type 5 (Revy et al. 2000; Imai et al. 2003). Both enzymes play a central role in B cells, which function in the humoral arm of the adaptive immune system by secreting antibodies or immunoglobulin (Ig). Production of protective antibodies by activated B cells is accomplished by two processes of diversification, somatic hypermutation (SHM) and class-switch recombination (CSR) (Lee et al. 2004; Stavnezer et al. 2008). SHM introduces mutations into the variable region of Ig genes, which encodes the antigen-binding site of the Ig receptor. Repeated rounds of mutation and selection generate high-affinity antibodies. CSR, on the other hand, involves the constant region of the Ig locus and replaces the constant region of the primary IgM antibody with the constant region of other isotypes including IgA, IgG, or IgE via deletional DNA recombination. Recombination occurs between DNA double-strand breaks introduced at defined regions (switch region) upstream of the sequences encoding the constant regions of IgA, IgG, and IgE, respectively. This process improves the ability of an Ig to remove a pathogen by augmenting its effector functions without changing its antigen specificity. SHM and CSR are initiated by AID, which converts cytosines within Ig variable regions or switch regions to uracil by deamination (Fig. 14.3). Subsequent removal of uracil by UNG and nicking by apurinic endonuclease (APE) result in DNA single-strand breaks. These DNA lesions are either processed by error-prone DNA repair, to yield mutations during SHR, or converted to DNA double-strand breaks, to initiate CSR (Lee et al. 2004; Stavnezer et al. 2008; Fear 2013). Deficiencies in AID or UNG abrogate SHM and CSR, leading to recurrent bacterial infections due to the inability to mount efficient antibody responses (Revy et al. 2000; Imai et al. 2003). Patients typically exhibit normal to increased IgM; absent IgG, IgA, and IgE; as well as lymphoid hyperplasia caused by the presence of giant germinal centers.

## Nomenclature

| | Disease name | Alternative disease name | Disease abbreviation | Gene symbol | Chromosomal localization | Mode of inheritance | Affected protein | Disease OMIM# |
|---|---|---|---|---|---|---|---|---|
| 14.1 | 3′ Repair exonuclease 1 deficiency | Aicardi-Goutières syndrome type 1 | AGS1 | *TREX1* | 3p21.31 | AR[a] | 3-prime repair exonuclease 1 | 225750 |
| 14.2 | 3′ Repair exonuclease 1 deficiency | Familial chilblain lupus type 1 | CHBL1 | *TREX1* | 3p21.31 | AD | 3-prime repair exonuclease 1 | 610448 |
| 14.3 | 3′ Repair exonuclease 1 deficiency | Retinal vasculopathy with cerebral leukodystrophy | RVCL | *TREX1* | 3p21.31 | AD | 3-prime repair exonuclease 1 | 192315 |
| 14.4 | Ribonuclease H2 subunit B deficiency | Aicardi-Goutières syndrome type 2 | AGS2 | *RNASEH2B* | 13q14.3 | AR | Ribonuclease H2, subunit B | 610181 |
| 14.4 | Ribonuclease H2 subunit C deficiency | Aicardi-Goutières syndrome type 3 | AGS3 | *RNASEH2C* | 11q13.1 | AR | Ribonuclease H2, subunit C | 610329 |
| 14.4 | Ribonuclease H2 subunit A deficiency | Aicardi-Goutières syndrome type 4 | AGS4 | *RNASEH2A* | 19p13.13 | AR | Ribonuclease H2, subunit A | 610333 |
| 14.5 | SAMHD1 deficiency | Aicardi-Goutières syndrome type 5 | AGS5 | *SAMHD1* | 20q11.23 | AR | SAM domain- and HD domain-containing protein 1 | 612952 |
| 14.6 | SAMHD1 deficiency | Familial chilblain lupus type 2 | CHBL2 | *SAMHD1* | 20q11.23 | AD | SAM domain- and HD domain-containing protein 1 | 614415 |
| 14.7 | RNA-specific adenosine deaminase deficiency | Aicardi-Goutières syndrome type 6 | AGS6 | *ADAR* | 1q21.3 | AR[b] | Adenosine deaminase, RNA-specific | 615010 |
| 14.8 | RNA-specific adenosine deaminase deficiency | Dyschromatosis symmetrica hereditaria | DSH1 | *ADAR* | 1q21.3 | AD | Adenosine deaminase, RNA-specific | 127400 |
| 14.9 | MDA5 superactivity | Aicardi-Goutières syndrome type 7 | AGS7 | *IFIH1* | 2q24.2 | de novo[c] | Interferon-induced helicase C domain-containing protein 1, melanoma differentiation-associated gene 5 | 615846 |
| 14.10 | MDA5 superactivity | Singleton-Merten syndrome type 1 | SGMRT1 | *IFIH1* | 2q24.2 | AD | Interferon-induced helicase C domain-containing protein 1. melanoma differentiation-associated gene 5 | 182250 |

(continued)

| | Disease name | Alternative disease name | Disease abbreviation | Gene symbol | Chromosomal localization | Mode of inheritance | Affected protein | Disease OMIM# |
|---|---|---|---|---|---|---|---|---|
| 14.11 | DDX58 superactivity | Singleton-Merten syndrome type 2 | SGMRT2 | *DDX58* | 9p21.1 | AD | Retinoic acid-inducible gene I | 616298 |
| 14.12 | STING superactivity | STING-associated vasculopathy with onset in infancy (SAVI, de novo) familial chilblain lupus type (dominant) | SAVI, CHBL3 | *TMEM173* | 5q31.2 | De novo[d], AD | Transmembrane protein 173; Stimulator of interferon genes | 615934 |
| 14.13 | Ribonuclease T2 deficiency | Cystic leukoencephalopathy without megalencephaly | | *RNASET2* | 6q27 | AR | Ribonuclease T2 | 612951 |
| 14.14 | 2′,5′-oligoadenylate synthetase 1 deficiency | Infantile-onset pulmonary alveolar proteinosis with hypogammaglobulinemia | PAPHG | *OAS1* | 12q24.13 | De novo, AD[e] | 2′,5′-oligoadenylate synthetase 1 | 618042 |
| 14.15 | ABCC6 deficiency | Generalized arterial calcification of infancy type 2 (severe) | GACI2 | *ABCC6* | 16p13.11 | AR[f] | ATP-binding cassette, subfamily C, member 6 | 614473 |
| 14.16 | ABCC6 deficiency | Pseudoxanthoma elasticum (milder) | PXE | *ABCC6* | 16p13.11 | AR[f] | ATP-binding cassette, subfamily C, member 6 | 264800 |
| 14.17 | Ectonucleotide pyrophosphatase/ phosphodiesterase 1 deficiency | Generalized arterial calcification of infancy type 1, autosomal recessive hypophosphatemic rickets type 2 | GACI1, ARHR2 | *ENPP1* | 6q23.2 | AR | Ectonucleotide pyrophosphatase/ phosphodiesterase | 208000, 613312 |
| 14.18 | Ectonucleotide pyrophosphatase/ phosphodiesterase 1 dimerization deficiency | Cole disease | COLED | *ENPP1* | 6q23.2 | AD, AR | Ectonucleotide pyrophosphatase/ phosphodiesterase | 615522 |
| 14.19 | Ecto-5′-nucleotidase deficiency | Arterial calcification due to deficiency of CD73 | ACDC | *NT5E* | 6q14.3 | AR | Ecto-5-prime nucleotidase | 211800 |
| 14.20 | Equilibrative nucleoside transporter 1 deficiency | Augustine-null blood type and ectopic mineralization[g] | | *SLC29A1* | 6p21.1 | AR | Equilibrative nucleoside transporter 1 | |
| 14.21 | Equilibrative nucleoside transporter 3 deficiency | Histiocytosis-lymphadenopathy plus syndrome, H syndrome, familial Rosai-Dorfman disease, Faisalabad histiocytosis | | *SLC29A3* | 10q22.1 | AR | Equilibrative nucleoside transporter 3 | 602782 |
| 14.22 | Activation-induced cytidine deaminase deficiency | Hyper-IgM syndrome type 2 | HIGM2 | *AICDA* | 12p13.31 | AR | Activation-induced cytidine deaminase | 605258 |
| 14.23 | Uracil-DNA glycosylase deficiency | Hyper-IgM syndrome type 5 | HIGM5 | *UNG* | 12q24.11 | AR | Uracil-DNA glycosylase | 608106 |

[a]Heterozygous de novo mutations described in very few patients with AGS1
[b]Heterozygous de novo mutations described in few patients with AGS6
[c]Autosomal dominant mutations with reduced penetrance described in patients with AGS7
[d]Autosomal dominant mutation in family with lupus-like disease and SAVI described
[e]Autosomal-dominant inheritance due to maternal mosaic described in one family with PAPHG
[f]Heterozygous carriers may express mild pseudoxanthoma elasticum
[g]Ill-defined clinical entity

## Metabolic Pathways

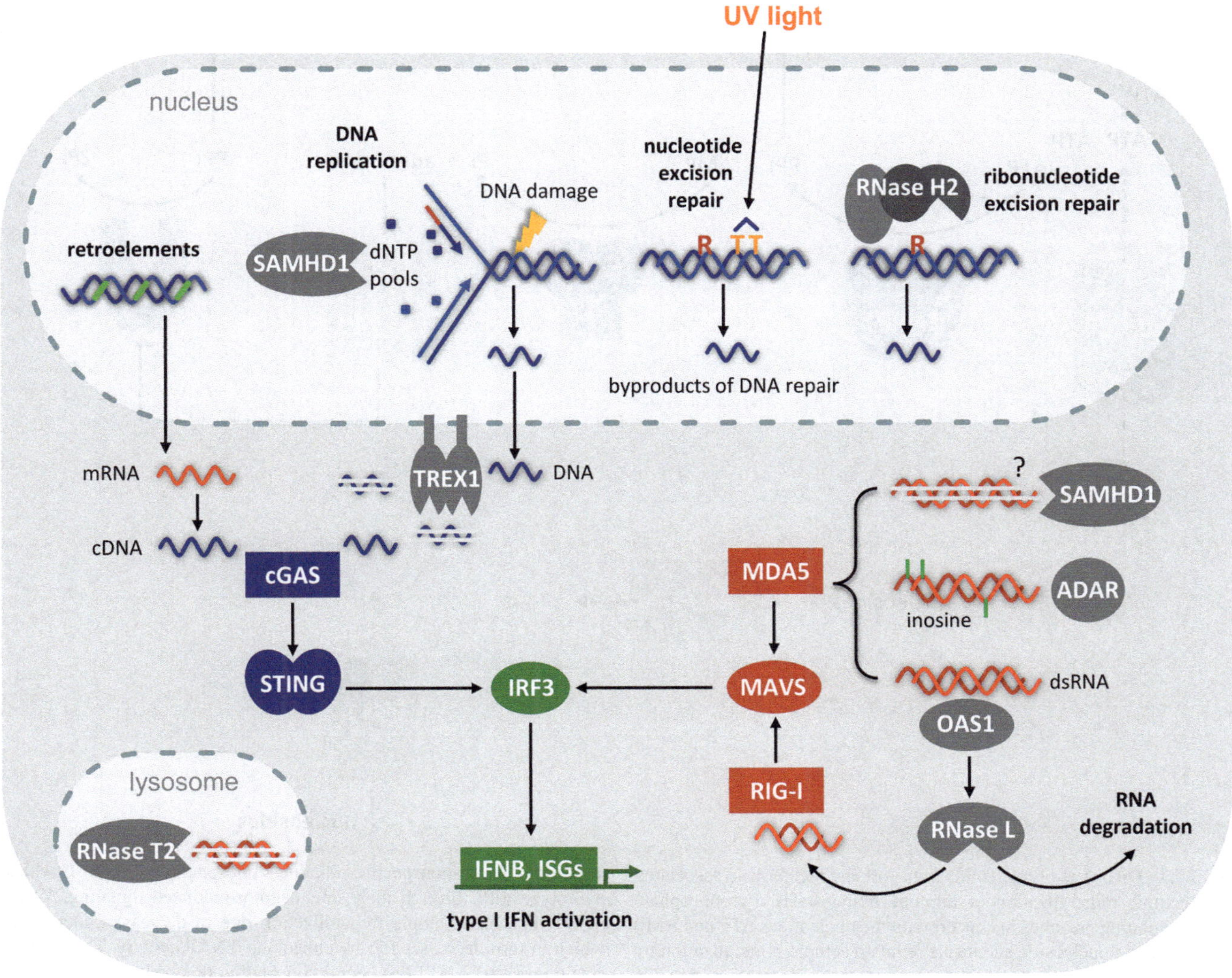


**Fig. 14.1** Pathways of nucleic acid metabolism and innate immune sensing. TREX1 is a cytosolic deoxyribonuclease anchored in the outer nuclear membrane that degrades ssDNA derived from DNA repair or reverse transcription of endogenous retroelements. A lack of TREX1 causes DNA accumulation, within both the nucleus and the cytosol. Within the cytosol, ssDNA metabolites with stem loops or dsDNA are sensed by the DNA sensor cGAS which signals via STING (encoded by *TMEM173*) to induce type I IFN production. Activating mutations in STING cause constitutive type I IFN signaling in the absence of cGAS activation. The heterotrimeric RNase H2 maintains genome integrity by removing ribonucleotides misincorporated during DNA replication. The presence of ribonucleotides in genomic DNA enhances photodimerization of adjacent pyrimidines, which are repaired by nucleotide excision repair. A lack of RNase H2 promotes DNA damage, leading to enhanced formation of DNA repair metabolites. SAMHD1 degrades deoxynucleoside triphosphates (dNTP), thereby controlling the dNTP pool required for DNA synthesis. Loss of SAMHD1 function induces cell cycle arrest and DNA damage. DNA byproducts derived from DNA repair cause cGAS-mediated type I IFN activation. SAMHD1 has also ribonuclease activity, suggesting that a loss of SAMHD1 may lead to RNA accumulation. ADAR modifies dsRNA through deamination of adenosine to inosine, thereby preventing recognition of dsRNA by the RNA sensor MDA5 (encoded by *IFIH1*). Upon binding to dsRNA, OAS1 synthesizes 2′–5′-linked oligoadenylates using ATP as substrate, which in turn activate RNase L. This leads to RNA degradation and formation of short RNA fragments that act as ligand for RIG-I (encoded by *DDX58*), another cytosolic RNA sensor. Both RNA sensors, MDA5 and RIG-I, signal via mitochondrial antiviral signaling (MAVS) to activate type I IFN. Activation of either the DNA-sensing pathway led by cGAS or the RNA-sensing pathways led by MDA5 and RIG-I result in phosphorylation of the transcription factor interferon regulatory factor 3 (IRF3) which induces expression of the *IFNB* gene and numerous interferon-stimulated genes (ISG). Activating mutations in RIG-I and MDA5 increases receptor affinity resulting in constitutive type I IFN signaling. RNase T2 degrades ribosomal RNA in lysosomes. A lack of RNase T2 causes RNA accumulation which may activate RNA sensors

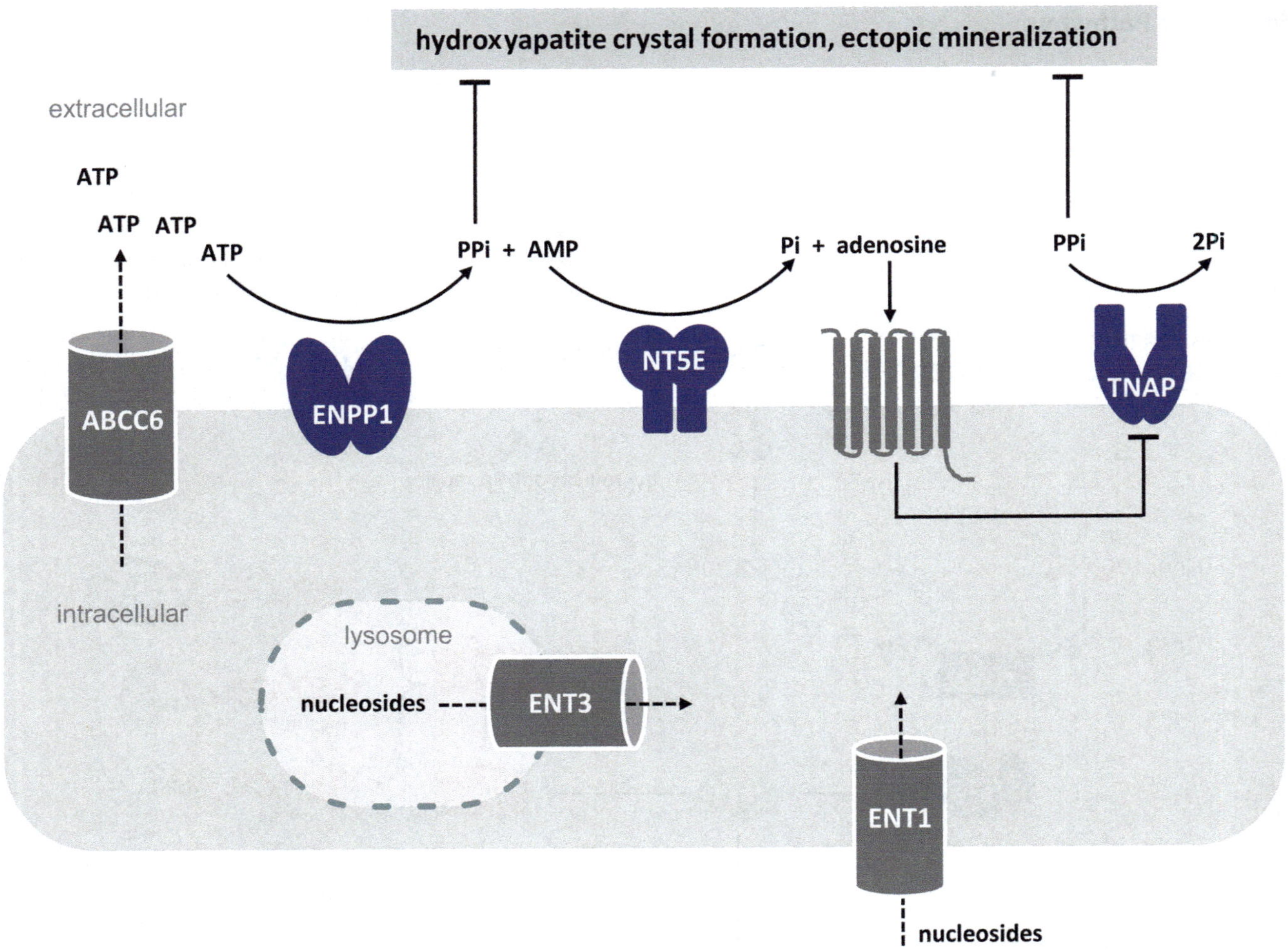


**Fig. 14.2** Disorders of nucleotide transport and metabolism associated with ectopic mineralization or immune homeostasis. Pyrophosphate (PPi)-regulating enzymes in concert with the nucleotides ATP and AMP along with the nucleoside adenosine regulate ectopic mineralization by inhibition of PPi-dependent hydroxyapatite crystal formation. ABCC6 mediates the release of ATP from the liver into the extracellular space. In the periphery, ATP is converted into the mineralization inhibitor pyrophosphate (PPi) and AMP by ENPP1. Loss of function of either ABCC6 or ENPP1 results in reduced PPi formation, leading to unabated ectopic mineralization. AMP is converted to adenosine and inorganic phosphate (Pi) by NT5E. Adenosine maintains adequate PPi levels by inhibiting tissue-nonspecific alkaline phosphatase (TNAP) which hydrolyzes PPi, through adenosine receptor-mediated signaling. A lack of NT5E causes ectopic mineralization due to decreased adenosine, which in turn decreases PPi by enhancing TNAP activity. The nucleoside transporter ENT1 has been implicated in this pathway by interfering with extracellular adenosine availability. In contrast, ENT3 regulates cell homeostasis by coordinating lysosomal function with intracellular nucleoside availability, particularly in T cells. The clinical presentation of ENT3 deficiency is highly variable and involves multiple organ systems with signs of immune dysregulation

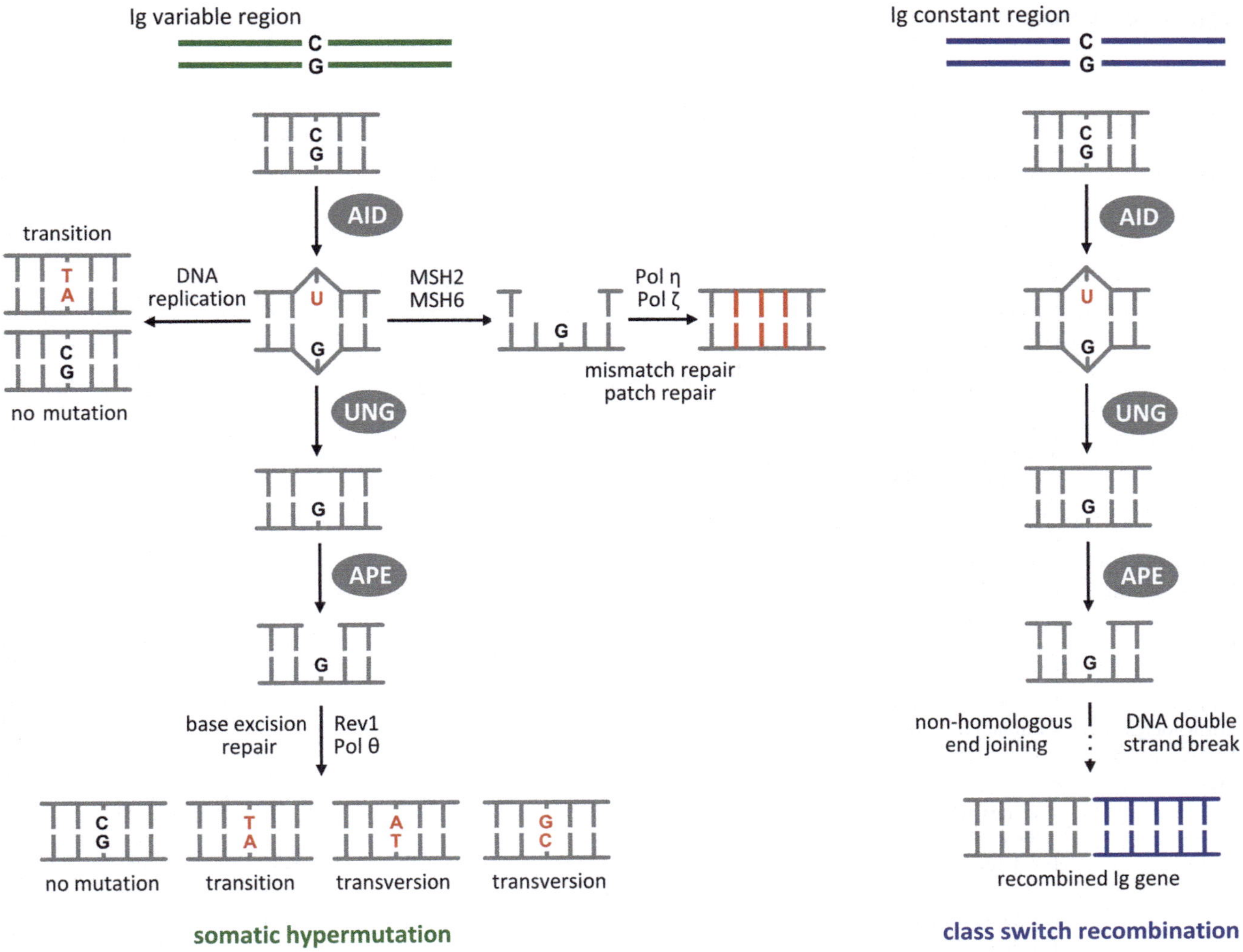


**Fig. 14.3** Somatic hypermutation and class-switch recombination of immunoglobulin genes. AID initiates SHR (left) by deamination of cytosine (C) to uracil (U) within the variable region of the Ig genes which determines antigen specificity and affinity of the Ig receptor. Different DNA repair pathways are then utilized in the resolution of AID-mediated DNA lesions. If DNA replication occurs before resolution of the C/U mismatch, uracil is used as template resulting in a C to T transition in one daughter cell, or the mismatch is repaired. Alternatively, uracil is recognized by UNG which creates an abasic site that is subsequently converted into a nick by apurinic endonuclease (APE) as the first step of base excision repair (BER). Following replication by error-prone translesion synthesis polymerases (Rev1 or Pol θ), transitions or transversions can occur. Resolution of the uracil mismatch may also occur via the mismatch repair pathway. Bases surrounding the initial U lesion are removed and replaced in an error-prone manner through the action of Pol η and Pol ζ, leading to the spreading of mutations away from the initial site of AID action. CSR (right) also begins with AID creating a uracil at specific G-rich tandem repeated DNA sequences, the so-called switch regions, which direct deletional DNA recombination within the Ig constant regions. Following UNG-mediated uracil removal and nicking by APE, DNA double-strand breaks occur through factors of the BER pathway. Directed recombination is completed by nonhomologous end joining

## Signs and Symptoms

**Table 14.1** 3′ Repair exonuclease 1 deficiency: Aicardi-Goutières syndrome type 1

| System | Symptoms and biomarkers | Neonatal (birth–1 month) | Infancy (1–18 months) | Childhood (1.5–11 years) | Adolescence (11–16 years) | Adulthood (>16 years) |
|---|---|---|---|---|---|---|
| CNS | **Cerebral atrophy** | ± | +++ | +++ | +++ | +++ |
| | Cerebrovascular disease | ± | ± | ± | ± | ± |
| | Cognitive impairment | | ++ | ++ | ++ | ++ |
| | **Dystonia** | ± | ++ | ++ | ++ | ++ |
| | Epileptic seizures | ± | ± | ± | ± | ± |
| | **Exaggerated startle reaction** | ± | +++ | +++ | ++ | |
| | Feeding difficulties | ± | ++ | ++ | + | + |
| | **Intracerebral calcifications** | ± | +++ | +++ | +++ | +++ |
| | **Irritability** | ± | +++ | +++ | ± | |
| | **Leukodystrophy** | ± | +++ | +++ | +++ | +++ |
| | **Microcephaly** | ± | +++ | +++ | +++ | +++ |
| | **Sleep disturbances** | | ++ | ++ | ± | |
| | **Spasticity** | ± | +++ | +++ | +++ | +++ |
| | Sterile pyrexia | ± | ++ | ++ | ++ | |
| Digestive | Hepatosplenomegaly | ± | ++ | ± | ± | ± |
| Immune system | Autoantibodies | | ± | ± | ± | ± |
| | Autoimmunity | | ± | ± | ± | ± |
| Cardiovascular | Hypertrophic cardiomyopathy | | ± | ± | ± | ± |
| Eye | Glaucoma | | ± | ± | ± | ± |
| Respiratory | Pulmonary hypertension | | ± | ± | ± | ± |
| Dermatological | **Chilblain lesions** | | + | + | + | + |
| Laboratory findings | ASAT, ALAT (serum) | n-↑ | n-↑ | n-↑ | n-↑ | n-↑ |
| | C26:0 fatty acid (dried blot spot) | n-↑ | | | | |
| | **Interferon-stimulated genes or interferon signature (PBMC)** | n-↑ | ↑↑↑ | ↑↑↑ | ↑↑↑ | ↑↑↑ |
| | Interferon-α (CSF) | n-↑ | ↑↑ | n-↑ | n-↑ | n-↑ |
| | Lymphocytes (CSF) | n-↑ | ↑ | ↑ | n-↑ | n-↑ |
| | Neopterin (CSF) | n-↑ | ↑ | n-↑ | n-↑ | n-↑ |
| | Platelets (EDTA blood) | ↓-n | ↓-n | n | n | n |

**Table 14.2** 3′ Repair exonuclease 1 deficiency: familial chilblain lupus type 1

| System | Symptoms and biomarkers | Neonatal (birth–1 month) | Infancy (1–18 months) | Childhood (1.5–11 years) | Adolescence (11–16 years) | Adulthood (>16 years) |
|---|---|---|---|---|---|---|
| Dermatological | **Acral violaceous plaques and nodules** | | ++ | +++ | +++ | +++ |
| | **Chilblain lesions** | | ++ | +++ | +++ | +++ |
| | **Nail dystrophy or loss** | | ± | ± | ± | ± |
| | Photosensitivity | | ± | ± | ± | ± |
| | **Ulcerative lesions with infarcts with gangrene** | | ± | ± | ± | ± |
| Musculoskeletal | Arthralgia | | ± | ± | ± | ± |
| Immune system | Autoimmunity | | ± | ± | ± | ± |
| Laboratory findings | Antinuclear antibodies (serum) | | ± | ± | ± | ± |
| | **Interferon-stimulated genes or interferon signature (PBMC)** | | ↑ | ↑↑ | ↑↑ | ↑↑ |

**Table 14.3** 3′ Repair exonuclease 1 deficiency: retinal vasculopathy with cerebral leukodystrophy

| System | Symptoms and biomarkers | Neonatal (birth–1 month) | Infancy (1–18 months) | Childhood (1.5–11 years) | Adolescence (11–16 years) | Adulthood (>16 years) |
|---|---|---|---|---|---|---|
| Autonomic system | Hypertension | | | | | ± |
| Cardiovascular | Raynaud phenomenon | | | | | ± |
| CNS | **Cerebral calcifications** | | | | | ++ |
| | **Cognitive decline** | | | | | ++ |
| | Epileptic seizures | | | | | ± |
| | **Migraine** | | | | | + |
| | **Stroke** | | | | | ++ |
| Digestive | Gastrointestinal bleeding | | | | | ± |
| Eye | **Vascular retinopathy** | | | | | + |
| Psychiatric | **Psychiatric disturbances** | | | | | ++ |
| Renal | Nephropathy | | | | | ± |
| Laboratory findings | ASAT/ALAT (serum) | | | | | n-↑ |

**Table 14.4** Ribonuclease H2 subunit B, C, and A deficiency

| System | Symptoms and biomarkers | Neonatal (birth–1 month) | Infancy (1–18 months) | Childhood (1.5–11 years) | Adolescence (11–16 years) | Adulthood (>16 years) |
|---|---|---|---|---|---|---|
| CNS | **Cerebral atrophy** | ± | +++ | +++ | +++ | +++ |
| | Cerebrovascular disease | ± | ± | ± | ± | ± |
| | Cognitive impairment | | ++ | ++ | ++ | ++ |
| | **Dystonia** | ± | ++ | ++ | ++ | ++ |
| | Epileptic seizures | ± | ± | ± | ± | ± |
| | **Exaggerated startle reaction** | ± | +++ | +++ | ++ | |
| | Feeding difficulties | ± | ++ | ++ | + | + |
| | **Intracerebral calcifications** | ± | +++ | +++ | +++ | +++ |
| | **Irritability** | ± | +++ | +++ | ± | |
| | **Leukodystrophy** | ± | +++ | +++ | +++ | +++ |
| | **Microcephaly** | ± | +++ | +++ | +++ | +++ |
| | **Sleep disturbances** | | ++ | ++ | ± | |
| | **Spasticity** | ± | +++ | +++ | +++ | +++ |
| | Sterile pyrexia | ± | ++ | ++ | ++ | |
| Gastrointestinal | Hepatosplenomegaly | ± | ++ | ± | ± | ± |
| Immune system | Autoantibodies | | ± | ± | ± | ± |
| | Autoimmunity | | ± | ± | ± | ± |
| Cardiovascular | Hypertrophic cardiomyopathy | | ± | ± | ± | ± |
| Eye | Glaucoma | | ± | ± | ± | ± |
| Respiratory | Pulmonary hypertension | | ± | ± | ± | ± |
| Dermatological | **Chilblain lesions** | | + | + | + | + |
| Laboratory findings | ASAT, ALAT (serum) | n-↑ | n-↑ | n-↑ | n-↑ | n-↑ |
| | C26:0 fatty acid (dried blood spot) | n-↑ | | | | |
| | **Interferon-stimulated genes or interferon signature (PBMC)** | n-↑ | ↑↑ | ↑↑ | ↑↑ | ↑↑ |
| | Interferon-α (CSF) | n-↑ | ↑↑ | n-↑ | n-↑ | n-↑ |
| | Lymphocytes (CSF) | n-↑ | ↑ | ↑ | n-↑ | n-↑ |
| | Neopterin (CSF) | n-↑ | ↑ | n-↑ | n-↑ | n-↑ |
| | Platelets (EDTA blood) | ↓-n | ↓-n | n | n | n |

**Table 14.5** SAMHD1 deficiency: Aicardi-Goutières syndrome type 5

| System | Symptoms and biomarkers | Neonatal (birth–1 month) | Infancy (1–18 months) | Childhood (1.5–11 years) | Adolescence (11–16 years) | Adulthood (>16 years) |
|---|---|---|---|---|---|---|
| CNS | **Cerebral atrophy** | ± | +++ | +++ | +++ | +++ |
| | **Cerebrovascular disease (stenosis, aneurysm, moyamoya-like, stroke)** | ± | ± | ± | ± | ± |
| | Cognitive impairment | | ++ | ++ | ++ | ++ |
| | **Dystonia** | ± | ++ | ++ | ++ | ++ |
| | Epileptic seizures | ± | ± | ± | ± | ± |
| | **Exaggerated startle reaction** | ± | +++ | +++ | ++ | |
| | Feeding difficulties | ± | ++ | ++ | + | + |
| | **Intracerebral calcifications** | ± | +++ | +++ | +++ | +++ |
| | **Irritability** | ± | +++ | +++ | ± | |
| | **Leukodystrophy** | ± | +++ | +++ | +++ | +++ |
| | **Microcephaly** | ± | +++ | +++ | +++ | +++ |
| | **Sleep disturbances** | | ++ | ++ | ± | |
| | **Spasticity** | ± | +++ | +++ | +++ | +++ |
| | Sterile pyrexia | ± | ++ | ++ | ++ | |
| Gastrointestinal | Hepatosplenomegaly | ± | ++ | ± | ± | ± |
| Immune system | Autoantibodies | | ± | ± | ± | ± |
| | Autoimmunity | | ± | ± | ± | ± |
| Cardiovascular | Hypertrophic cardiomyopathy | | ± | ± | ± | ± |
| Eye | Glaucoma | | ± | ± | ± | ± |
| Respiratory | Pulmonary hypertension | | ± | ± | ± | ± |
| Dermatological | **Chilblain lesions** | | + | + | + | + |
| Laboratory findings | ASAT, ALAT (serum) | n-↑ | n-↑ | n-↑ | n-↑ | n-↑ |
| | C26:0 fatty acid (dried blood spot) | n-↑ | | | | |
| | **Interferon-stimulated genes or interferon signature (PBMC)** | n-↑ | ↑↑↑ | ↑↑↑ | ↑↑↑ | ↑↑↑ |
| | Interferon-α (CSF) | n-↑ | ↑↑ | n-↑ | n-↑ | n-↑ |
| | Lymphocytes (CSF) | n-↑ | ↑ | ↑ | n-↑ | n-↑ |
| | Neopterin (CSF) | n-↑ | ↑ | n-↑ | n-↑ | n-↑ |
| | Platelets (EDTA blood) | ↓-n | ↓-n | n | n | n |

**Table 14.6** SAMHD1 deficiency: familial chilblain lupus type 2 (dominant)[a]

| System | Symptoms and biomarkers | Neonatal (birth–1 month) | Infancy (1–18 months) | Childhood (1.5-11 years) | Adolescence (11–16 years) | Adulthood (>16 years) |
|---|---|---|---|---|---|---|
| Skin | **Chilblain lesions** | | +++ | +++ | +++ | +++ |
| | Photosensitivity | | ± | ± | ± | ± |

[a]One patient described

**Table 14.7** RNA-specific adenosine deaminase deficiency: Aicardi-Goutières syndrome type 6

| System | Symptoms and biomarkers | Neonatal (birth–1 month) | Infancy (1–18 months) | Childhood (1.5–11 years) | Adolescence (11–16 years) | Adulthood (>16 years) |
|---|---|---|---|---|---|---|
| CNS | **Bilateral striatal degeneration** | ± | ± | ± | ± | ± |
| | **Cerebral atrophy** | ± | +++ | +++ | +++ | +++ |
| | Cognitive impairment | | ++ | ++ | ++ | ++ |
| | **Dystonia** | ± | ++ | ++ | ++ | ++ |
| | Epileptic seizures | ± | ± | ± | ± | ± |
| | **Exaggerated startle reaction** | ± | +++ | +++ | ++ | |
| | Feeding difficulties | ± | ++ | ++ | + | + |
| | **Intracerebral calcifications** | ± | +++ | +++ | +++ | +++ |
| | **Irritability** | ± | +++ | +++ | ± | |
| | **Leukodystrophy** | ± | +++ | +++ | +++ | +++ |
| | **Microcephaly** | ± | +++ | +++ | +++ | +++ |
| | **Sleep disturbances** | | ++ | ++ | ± | |
| | **Spasticity** | ± | +++ | +++ | +++ | +++ |
| | Sterile pyrexia | ± | ++ | ++ | ++ | |
| Gastrointestinal | Hepatosplenomegaly | ± | ++ | ± | ± | ± |
| Immune system | Autoantibodies | | ± | ± | ± | ± |
| | Autoimmunity | | ± | ± | ± | ± |
| Cardiovascular | Hypertrophic cardiomyopathy | | ± | ± | ± | ± |
| Eye | Glaucoma | | ± | ± | ± | ± |
| Respiratory | Pulmonary hypertension | | ± | ± | ± | ± |
| Dermatological | **Chilblain lesions** | | + | + | + | + |
| Routine laboratory | ASAT, ALAT (serum) | n-↑ | n-↑ | n-↑ | n-↑ | n-↑ |
| | **Lymphocytes (CSF)** | n-↑ | ↑ | ↑ | n-↑ | n-↑ |
| | Platelets (EDTA blood) | ↓-n | ↓-n | n | n | n |
| Special laboratory | **Interferon-stimulated genes or interferon signature (PBMC)** | n-↑ | ↑↑↑ | ↑↑↑ | ↑↑↑ | ↑↑↑ |
| | **Interferon-α (CSF)** | n-↑ | ↑↑ | n-↑ | n-↑ | n-↑ |
| | Neopterin (CSF) | n-↑ | ↑ | n-↑ | n-↑ | n-↑ |

**Table 14.8** RNA-specific adenosine deaminase deficiency: dyschromatosis symmetrica hereditaria (dominant)

| System | Symptoms and biomarkers | Neonatal (birth–1 month) | Infancy (1–18 months) | Childhood (1.5–11 years) | Adolescence (11–16 years) | Adulthood (>16 years) |
|---|---|---|---|---|---|---|
| Dermatological | **Hyperpigmented and hypopigmented macules (face, dorsum hands, and feet)** | + | + | + | + | |

**Table 14.9** MDA5 superactivity: Aicardi-Goutières syndrome type 7

| System | Symptoms and biomarkers | Neonatal (birth–1 month) | Infancy (1–18 months) | Childhood (1.5–11 years) | Adolescence (11–16 years) | Adulthood (>16 years) |
|---|---|---|---|---|---|---|
| CNS | **Cerebral atrophy** | ± | +++ | +++ | +++ | +++ |
| | Cognitive impairment | | ++ | ++ | ++ | ++ |
| | **Dystonia** | ± | ++ | ++ | ++ | ++ |
| | Epileptic seizures | ± | ± | ± | ± | ± |
| | **Exaggerated startle reaction** | ± | +++ | +++ | ++ | |
| | Feeding difficulties | ± | ++ | ++ | + | + |
| | **Intracerebral calcifications** | ± | +++ | +++ | +++ | +++ |
| | **Irritability** | ± | +++ | +++ | ± | |
| | **Isolated spastic paraparesis** | ± | ± | ± | ± | ± |
| | **Leukodystrophy** | ± | +++ | +++ | +++ | +++ |
| | **Microcephaly** | ± | +++ | +++ | +++ | +++ |
| | **Sleep disturbances** | | ++ | ++ | ± | |
| | **Spasticity** | ± | +++ | +++ | +++ | +++ |
| | Sterile pyrexia | ± | ++ | ++ | ++ | |
| Gastrointestinal | Hepatosplenomegaly | ± | ++ | ± | ± | ± |
| Immune system | Autoantibodies | | ± | ± | ± | ± |
| | Autoimmunity | | ± | ± | ± | ± |
| Cardiovascular | Hypertrophic cardiomyopathy | | ± | ± | ± | ± |
| Eye | Glaucoma | | ± | ± | ± | ± |
| Respiratory | Pulmonary hypertension | | ± | ± | ± | ± |
| Dermatological | **Chilblain lesions** | | + | + | + | + |
| Laboratory findings | ASAT, ALAT (serum) | n-↑ | n-↑ | n-↑ | n-↑ | n-↑ |
| | C26:0 fatty acid (dried blot spot) | n-↑ | | | | |
| | **Interferon-stimulated genes or interferon signature (PBMC)** | n-↑ | ↑↑↑ | ↑↑↑ | ↑↑↑ | ↑↑↑ |
| | Interferon-α (CSF) | n-↑ | ↑↑ | n-↑ | n-↑ | n-↑ |
| | Lymphocytes (CSF) | n-↑ | ↑ | ↑ | n-↑ | n-↑ |
| | Neopterin (CSF) | n-↑ | ↑ | n-↑ | n-↑ | n-↑ |
| | Platelets (EDTA blood) | ↓-n | ↓-n | n | n | n |

**Table 14.10** MDA5 superactivity: Singleton-Merten syndrome type 1

| System | Symptoms and biomarkers | Neonatal (birth–1 month) | Infancy (1–18 months) | Childhood (1.5–11 years) | Adolescence (11–16 years) | Adulthood (>16 years) |
|---|---|---|---|---|---|---|
| Cardiovascular | **Aortic and mitral valve calcification** | | ++ | ++ | ++ | ++ |
| | Cardiac failure | | ± | ± | ± | ± |
| Teeth | **Abnormal dentition** | | + | + | + | + |
| | **Alveolar bone loss** | | | + | + | + |
| | **Mineralization abnormalities** | | + | + | + | + |
| | **Periodontal disease** | | | + | + | + |
| Musculoskeletal | Acro-osteolysis | | + | + | + | + |
| | **Osteopenia, osteoporosis** | | + | + | + | + |
| | Short stature | | ± | ± | ± | ± |
| Immune system | Recurrent infections | | ± | ± | ± | ± |
| Eye | Glaucoma | | ± | ± | ± | ± |
| Dermatological | **Psoriasis-like** | | ++ | ++ | ++ | ++ |
| Laboratory findings | **Interferon-stimulated genes or interferon signature (PBMC)** | | ↑↑ | ↑↑ | ↑↑ | ↑↑ |

**Table 14.11** DDX58 superactivity: Singleton-Merten syndrome type 2

| System | Symptoms and biomarkers | Neonatal (birth–1 month) | Infancy (1–18 months) | Childhood (1.5–11 years) | Adolescence (11–16 years) | Adulthood (>16 years) |
|---|---|---|---|---|---|---|
| Cardiovascular | **Aortic and mitral valve calcification** | | ++ | ++ | + | + |
| | Cardiac failure | | ± | ± | ± | ± |
| Musculoskeletal | Acro-osteolysis | | + | + | + | + |
| | Phalangeal osteo-arthropathy, contractures | | + | + | + | + |
| | Short stature | | ± | ± | ± | ± |
| Teeth | Dental anomalies | | ± | ± | ± | ± |
| Eye | Glaucoma | | ± | ± | ± | ± |
| Dermatological | Psoriasis-like | | ++ | ++ | ++ | ++ |
| Laboratory findings | **Interferon-stimulated genes or interferon signature (PBMC)** | | ↑↑ | ↑↑ | ↑↑ | ↑↑ |

**Table 14.12** STING superactivity

| System | Symptoms and biomarkers | Neonatal (birth–1 month) | Infancy (1–18 months) | Childhood (1.5–11 years) | Adolescence (11–16 years) | Adulthood (>16 years) |
|---|---|---|---|---|---|---|
| Dermatological | **Acral violaceous plaques and nodules** | +++ | +++ | +++ | +++ | ++ |
| | **Chilblain lesions** | ++ | ++ | ++ | ++ | ++ |
| | Malar rash | ± | ± | ± | ± | ± |
| | **Nail dystrophy or loss** | ++ | ++ | ++ | ++ | ± |
| | **Nasal septum perforation** | ± | ± | ± | ± | ± |
| | **Ulcerative lesions with infarcts with gangrene** | +++ | +++ | +++ | +++ | ± |
| Respiratory | **Interstitial lung disease** | ++ | ++ | ++ | ++ | ± |
| Musculoskeletal | Arthralgia | + | + | + | + | + |
| | Fever | +++ | +++ | +++ | +++ | ± |
| Immunology | Recurrent infections | +++ | +++ | +++ | +++ | ± |
| | Lymphadenopathy | ++ | ++ | ++ | ++ | + |
| | Arterial hypertension | ± | ± | ± | ± | ± |
| Cardiovascular | Pulmonary hypertension | ± | ± | ± | ± | ± |
| Laboratory findings | Autoantibodies (pANCA, cANCA, anti-cardiolipin antibodies) (serum) | ↑ | ↑ | ↑ | ↑ | ↑ |
| | C-reactive protein, CRP (plasma) | ↑↑↑ | ↑↑↑ | ↑↑ | ↑↑ | ↑ |
| | Erythrocyte sedimentation rate (blood) | ↑↑↑ | ↑↑↑ | ↑↑ | ↑↑ | ↑ |
| | Gamma globulin (serum) | ↑↑ | ↑↑ | ↑↑ | ↑↑ | ↑ |
| | **Interferon-stimulated genes or interferon signature (PBMC)** | ↑↑↑ | ↑↑↑ | ↑↑↑ | ↑↑↑ | ↑↑ |
| | Lymphopenia (blood) | ↑↑ | ↑↑ | ↑↑ | ↑↑ | ↑ |

**Table 14.13** Ribonuclease T2 deficiency

| System | Symptoms and biomarkers | Neonatal (birth–1 month) | Infancy (1–18 months) | Childhood (1.5–11 years) | Adolescence (11–16 years) | Adulthood (>16 years) |
|---|---|---|---|---|---|---|
| CNS | Athetosis | ± | ± | ± | | |
| | **Cerebral atrophy** | +++ | +++ | +++ | | |
| | **Cystic leukoencephalopathy without megalencephaly** | +++ | +++ | +++ | | |
| | Dystonia | ± | ± | ± | | |
| | Epileptic seizures | ± | ± | ± | | |
| | Intracerebral calcifications | + | + | + | | |
| | **Microcephaly** | + | + | + | | |
| | Nystagmus | ± | ± | ± | | |
| | Psychomotor retardation | ++ | ++ | ++ | | |
| | Spasticity | +++ | +++ | +++ | | |
| Ear | Deafness, sensorineural | ± | ± | ± | | |
| Laboratory findings | Interferon-stimulated genes or interferon signature (PBMC) | n-↑ | n-↑ | n-↑ | | |
| | Lymphocytes (CSF) | n-↑ | n-↑ | n-↑ | | |

**Table 14.14** 2′,5′-Oligoadenylate synthetase 1 deficiency

| System | Symptoms and biomarkers | Neonatal (birth–1 month) | Infancy (1–18 months) | Childhood (1.5–11 years) | Adolescence (11–16 years) | Adulthood (>16 years) |
|---|---|---|---|---|---|---|
| Respiratory | **Pulmonary alveolar proteinosis** | + | +++ | +++ | | |
| | **Recurrent respiratory infection** | + | +++ | +++ | | |
| | **Respiratory failure** | + | +++ | +++ | | |
| Digestive | **Splenomegaly** | + | +++ | ++ | | |
| Other | **Early death** | + | ++ | ++ | | |
| | Failure to thrive | + | + | + | | |
| | Increased susceptibility to viral infection | + | ++ | ++ | | |
| Laboratory findings | Gamma globulin (serum) | ↓ | ↓↓↓ | ↓↓↓ | | |
| | Immunoglobulins (serum) | ↓↓ | ↓↓ | ↓↓ | | |
| | Leukocytes (blood) | ↓↓ | ↓↓ | ↓↓ | | |
| | Leukocytosis without abnormal distribution | + | +++ | +++ | | |
| | Small and non-foamy alveolar macrophages at bronchoalveolar lavage | + | +++ | +++ | | |

**Table 14.15** ABCC6 deficiency: generalized arterial calcification of infancy type 2

| System | Symptoms and biomarkers | Neonatal (birth–1 month) | Infancy (1–18 months) | Childhood (1.5–11 years) | Adolescence (11–16 years) | Adulthood (>16 years) |
|---|---|---|---|---|---|---|
| Cardiovascular | **Calcification of arteries** | | +++ | +++ | ++ | |
| | **Calcification of cardiac valves** | | ++ | ++ | ++ | |
| | **Cardiac failure** | | +++ | + | ± | |
| | **Coronary artery disease** | | +++ | + | ± | |
| | **Hypertension** | | +++ | + | ± | |
| | **Myocardial infarction** | | +++ | + | ± | |
| Musculoskeletal | **Joint calcifications** | | | + | + | |
| Renal | Nephrocalcinosis | | | ± | ± | |
| | Renal artery calcification | | + | + | + | |
| Other | **Early death** | | ++ | + | | |

**Table 14.16** ABCC6 deficiency: pseudoxanthoma elasticum

| System | Symptoms and biomarkers | Neonatal (birth–1 mth) | Infancy (1–18 months) | Childhood (1.5–11 years) | Adolescence (11–16 years) | Adulthood (>16 years) |
|---|---|---|---|---|---|---|
| Eye | **Angioid streaks of the retina** | | | | ± | +++ |
| | Macular degeneration | | | | ± | ± |
| | **Peau d'orange retinal changes** | | | | ± | +++ |
| | Retinal hemorrhage | | | | ± | ± |
| | **Visual impairment** | | | | ± | ++ |
| Dermatological | Redundant skin folds | | | | ± | + |
| | **Yellowish, flat papules and plaques (lateral neck, flexural areas)** | | | | ± | +++ |
| Cardiovascular | **Premature atherosclerosis, coronary artery disease, stroke** | | | | | ++ |
| Other | Gastrointestinal hemorrhage | | | | | ± |
| | Intermittent claudication | | | | | ± |
| Laboratory findings | Hematoxylin-eosin stains[a] | | | | | |
| | Skin biopsy (elastic fiber fragmentation, calcification) | | | | | +++ |

[a]Verhoeff-Gieson (for elastin) and von Kossa (for calcium deposits)

**Table 14.17** Ectonucleotide pyrophosphatase/phosphodiesterase 1 deficiency

| System | Symptoms and biomarkers | Neonatal (birth–1 month) | Infancy (1–18 months) | Childhood (1.5–11 years) | Adolescence (11–16 years) | Adulthood (>16 years) |
|---|---|---|---|---|---|---|
| Cardiovascular | **Calcification of arteries** | +++ | +++ | +++ | ++ | |
| | **Calcification of cardiac valves** | ++ | ++ | ++ | ++ | |
| | **Cardiac failure** | +++ | +++ | + | ± | |
| | **Coronary artery disease** | +++ | +++ | + | ± | |
| | **Hypertension** | +++ | +++ | + | ± | |
| | **Myocardial infarction** | +++ | +++ | + | ± | |
| Musculoskeletal | **Joint calcifications** | | | + | + | |
| Renal | Hypophosphatemic rickets[a] | | | ± | ± | |
| | Renal artery calcification | | + | + | + | |
| Dermatological | Pseudoxanthomatous skin lesions | | | ± | ± | |
| Eye | Angioid streaks, mild retinopathy | | | ± | ± | |
| Teeth | Infraocclusion, ankylosis, hypercementosis | | | ± | ± | |
| Other | **Early death** | ++ | ++ | + | | |
| | **Hyperphosphaturia** | | | + | + | |
| | **Hypophosphatemia** | | | + | + | |
| | Prenatal signs (fetal distress, polyhydramnios, pericardial effusion) | ± | | | | |
| Laboratory findings | Phosphate (plasma) | | | n-↓ | ↓↓ | |
| | Phosphate (urine) | | | n-↑ | ↑↑ | |

[a]Patients with ARHR2 show only hypophosphatemic rickets with short stature

**Table 14.18** Ectonucleotide pyrophosphatase/phosphodiesterase 1 dimerization deficiency

| System | Symptoms and biomarkers | Neonatal (birth–1 month) | Infancy (1–18 months) | Childhood (1.5–11 years) | Adolescence (11–16 years) | Adulthood (>16 years) |
|---|---|---|---|---|---|---|
| Dermatological | Calcinosis cutis | | ± | ± | ± | ± |
| | Hyperkeratotic papules | | | | | |
| | Hypopigmented macules | ± | ± | + | ++ | ++ |
| | Punctate palmoplantar keratoderma | ± | ± | + | ++ | ++ |
| Musculoskeletal | Calcific tendinopathy | | ± | ± | ± | ± |

**Table 14.19** Ecto-5′-nucleotidase deficiency

| System | Symptoms and biomarkers | Neonatal (birth–1 month) | Infancy (1–18 months) | Childhood (1.5–11 years) | Adolescence (11–16 years) | Adulthood (>16 years) |
|---|---|---|---|---|---|---|
| Cardiovascular | **Calcification of arteries (iliac, femoral, tibial)** | | | | | +++ |
| | Calcification of cardiac valve rings, aorta | | | | | ± |
| | **Intermittent claudication** | | | | | ++ |
| Musculoskeletal | Calcifications of tendons | | | | | ++ |
| | **Periarticular calcifications** | | | | | ++ |

**Table 14.20** Equilibrative nucleoside transporter 1 deficiency

| System | Symptoms and biomarkers | Neonatal (birth–1 month) | Infancy (1–18 months) | Childhood (1.5–11 years) | Adolescence (11–16 years) | Adulthood (>16 years) |
|---|---|---|---|---|---|---|
| Musculoskeletal | **Periarticular calcification** | | | | | + |
| | Pseudogout | | | | | + |
| Hematological | **Augustine-null blood type** | | | | | + |

**Table 14.21** Equilibrative nucleoside transporter 3 deficiency

| System | Symptoms and biomarkers | Neonatal (birth–1 month) | Infancy (1–18 months) | Childhood (1.5–11 years) | Adolescence (11–16 years) | Adulthood (>16 years) |
|---|---|---|---|---|---|---|
| Immune system | Antinuclear antibodies | | | ± | ± | ± |
| | Hepatosplenomegaly | | | ± | ± | ± |
| | **Histiocytosis (salivary glands, orbit, eyelid, spleen. testes)** | | | ++ | ++ | ++ |
| | **Hypergammaglobulinemia** | | | + | + | + |
| | Leukocytosis | | | ± | ± | ± |
| | **Lymphadenopathy** | | | ++ | ++ | ++ |
| | Recurrent fever | | | + | + | + |
| Musculoskeletal | Bone deformities | ± | ± | ± | ± | ± |
| | Intrauterine fractures | ± | | | | |
| | **Joint contractures** | | | ± | ± | ± |
| Dermatological | **Hyperpigmentation** | | | ± | ± | ± |
| | **Hypertrichosis** | | | ± | ± | ± |
| | Panniculitis | | | ± | ± | ± |
| Ears | **Sensorineural deafness** | | | ± | ± | ± |
| Endocrine system | Growth hormone deficiency | | | ± | ± | ± |
| | Hypergonadotropic hypogonadism | | | | ± | ± |
| | Insulin-dependent diabetes mellitus | | | | ± | ± |
| Laboratory findings | Antinuclear antibodies (serum) | | | n-↑ | n-↑ | n-↑ |
| | Erythrocyte sedimentation rate | | | ↑ | ↑ | ↑ |
| | Gamma globulin (serum) | | | ↑ | ↑ | ↑ |
| | Leukocytes (blood) | | | n-↑ | n-↑ | n-↑ |

**Table 14.22** Activation-induced cytidine deaminase deficiency

| System | Symptoms and biomarkers | Neonatal (birth–1 month) | Infancy (1–18 months) | Childhood (1.5–11 years) | Adolescence (11–16 years) | Adulthood (>16 years) |
|---|---|---|---|---|---|---|
| Immune system | **Lymphoid hyperplasia** | | +++ | +++ | +++ | |
| | **Recurrent bacterial infections** | | +++ | +++ | +++ | |
| Laboratory findings | Defective generation of somatic hypermutations | | ++ | ++ | ++ | |
| | Giant germinal centers in lymph nodes | | ++ | ++ | ++ | |
| | **IgG, IgA, IgE (serum)** | | ↓↓ | ↓↓ | ↓↓ | |
| | **IgM (serum)** | | ↑-n | ↑-n | ↑-n | |
| | Impaired Ig class-switch recombination | | ++ | ++ | ++ | |
| | Normal B-cell (CD19+) count | | ++ | ++ | ++ | |

**Table 14.23** Uracil-DNA glycosylase deficiency

| System | Symptoms and biomarkers | Neonatal (birth–1 month) | Infancy (1–18 months) | Childhood (1.5–11 years) | Adolescence (11–16 years) | Adulthood (>16 years) |
|---|---|---|---|---|---|---|
| Immune system | **Lymphoid hyperplasia** | | | +++ | +++ | +++ |
| | **Recurrent bacterial infections** | | | +++ | +++ | +++ |
| Laboratory findings | Defective generation of somatic hypermutations | | | ++ | ++ | ++ |
| | Giant germinal centers in lymph nodes | | | ++ | ++ | ++ |
| | **IgG, IgA, IgE (serum)** | | | ↓↓ | ↓↓ | ↓↓ |
| | **IgM (serum)** | | | ↑-n | ↑-n | ↑-n |
| | Impaired Ig class switch recombination | | | ++ | ++ | ++ |
| | Normal B-cell (CD19+) count | | | ++ | ++ | ++ |

## Diagnosis

### Genetic Testing

Genetic testing by symptom-driven sequencing of a larger group of genes (panel sequencing) or by whole-exome sequencing based on next-generation sequencing has facilitated the diagnosis of rare genetic disorders. This approach is particularly useful in patients presenting with leukodystrophy, autoinflammation, or immunodeficiency, all of which comprise a broad range of differential diagnoses. While both routine and special laboratory testing (Table 14.24) may aid in the differential diagnosis, generally for all diseases discussed in this chapter, the definite diagnosis is made by providing evidence for causative mutations in a specific gene by molecular genetic analysis. Confirmation of a specific diagnosis by genetic testing will also allow prenatal diagnosis.

### Specific Laboratory Investigations

**Table 14.24** Specific laboratory tests, which are helpful in the diagnostic workup of a patient suspected of a given disorder

| Disorder | Test | Material | Preconditions, handling |
|---|---|---|---|
| AGS, CHBL, SAVI | Interferon signature, upregulation of IFN-stimulated genes | Blood drawn into heparin tubes or PAX tubes | If heparin blood is used, samples should be processed within 24 h |
| AGS | IFN-α in CSF | CSF | CSF must be shipped on dry ice to special laboratory |
| AGS | Pterins in CSF | CSF | CSF must be shipped on dry ice to special laboratory |
| OAS1 deficiency | Alveolar macrophage morphology | Bronchoalveolar lavage | |
| PXE | Elastin fibers in skin with Verhoeff-van Gieson staining | Skin biopsy | Formalin-fixed, paraffin-embedded sections |
| PXE | Calcium deposits in skin with von Kossa staining | Skin biopsy | Formalin-fixed, paraffin-embedded sections |

## Treatment

### Familial Chilblain Lupus, STING-Associated Vasculopathy, and Aicardi-Goutières Syndrome

Emerging evidence indicates that an immunomodulatory intervention targeting the type I IFN axis using Janus kinase (JAK) inhibitors might be of therapeutic value (Bienias et al. 2018). JAK inhibitors such as ruxolitinib, baricitinib, and tofacitinib block signaling at the IFN receptor. Clinical improvement and suppression of the interferon signature have been demonstrated in patients with TREX1- and STING-associated familial chilblain lupus (König et al. 2017; Zimmermann et al. 2019). Improvement of skin lesion has also been observed in children with SAVI treated with ruxolitinib, tofacitinib, or baricitinib (Seo et al. 2017; Frémond et al. 2016; Sanchez et al. 2018). However, pulmonary symptoms did not consistently respond to treatment. While patients with AGS treated with ruxolitinib or baricitinib also respond with suppression of type I IFN activation and some clinical amelioration (Tüngler et al. 2016; Vanderver et al. 2020), improvement of neurological function depends on preexisting neurological damage. Given the progressive nature of AGS, a timely diagnosis is important as early therapeutic intervention can possibly ameliorate or prevent further brain damage. Although JAK inhibition represents an effective therapeutic strategy in patients with type I interferonopathies, future controlled clinical trials are required to fully assess the therapeutic effects as well as the side effects of JAK inhibitors in these patients.

### OAS1 Deficiency

Immunoglobulin replacement therapy can improve pulmonary function. Hematopoietic stem cell transplantation is considered curative treatment (Cho et al. 2018).

### Generalized Arterial Calcification of Infancy Type 1 and Type 2

In addition to symptomatic treatment with angiotensin-converting enzyme inhibitors and hydralazine, treatment with bisphosphonates can improve survival (Rutsch et al. 2008).

### Hyper-IgM Syndrome Type 2 and Type 5

Regular treatment with immunoglobulin replacement therapy markedly reduces the frequency of bacterial infections and the likelihood of developing lymphoid hyperplasia. Sometimes prophylactic antibiotic therapy will be recommended for individuals who develop complications of chronic infection such as bronchiectasis.

## References


Bergen AA, Plomp AS, Schuurman EJ, et al. Mutations in ABCC6 cause pseudoxanthoma elasticum. Nat Genet. 2000;25:228–31.

Bienias M, Brück N, Griep C, Wolf C, Kretschmer S, Kind B, Tüngler V, Berner R, Lee-Kirsch MA. Therapeutic approaches to type I interferonopathies. Curr Rheumatol Rep. 2018;20:32.

Blau N, Bonafé L, Krägeloh-Mann I, Thöny B, Kierat L, Häusler M, Ramaekers V. Cerebrospinal fluid pterins and folates in Aicardi-Goutières syndrome: a new phenotype. Neurology. 2003;61: 642–7.

Cho K, Yamada M, Agematsu K, et al. Heterozygous mutations in OAS1 cause infantile-onset pulmonary alveolar proteinosis with hypogammaglobulinemia. Am J Hum Genet. 2018;102:480–6.

Chourabi M, Liew MS, Lim S, et al. ENPP1 mutation causes recessive Cole disease by altering melanogenesis. J Invest Dermatol. 2018;138:291–300.

Crow YJ, Zaki MS, Abdel-Hamid MS, et al. Mutations in ADAR1, IFIH1, and RNASEH2B presenting as spastic paraplegia. Neuropediatrics. 2014;45:386–93.

Crow YJ, Chase DS, Lowenstein Schmidt J, et al. Characterization of human disease phenotypes associated with mutations in TREX1, RNASEH2A, RNASEH2B, RNASEH2C, SAMHD1, ADAR, and IFIH1. Am J Med Genet A. 2015;167A:296–312.

Cuadrado E, Vanderver A, Brown KJ, et al. Aicardi–Goutières syndrome harbours abundant systemic and brain-reactive autoantibodies. Ann Rheum Dis. 2015;74(10):1931–9.

Daniels G, Ballif BA, Helias V, et al. Lack of the nucleoside transporter ENT1 results in the Augustine-null blood type and ectopic mineralization. Blood. 2015;125:3651–4.

Eytan O, Morice-Picard F, Sarig O, et al. Cole disease results from mutations in ENPP1. Am J Hum Genet. 2013;93:752–7.

Fear DJ. Mechanisms regulating the targeting and activity of activation induced cytidine deaminase. Curr Opin Immunol. 2013;25: 619–28.

Frémond M-L, Rodero MP, Jeremiah N, et al. Efficacy of the Janus kinase 1/2 inhibitor ruxolitinib in the treatment of vasculopathy associated with TMEM173-activating mutations in 3 children. J Allergy Clin Immunol. 2016;138:1752–5.

Goutieres F, Aicardi J, Barth PG, Lebon P. Aicardi-Goutieres syndrome: an update and results of interferon-alpha studies. Ann Neurol. 1998;44:900–7.

Gunther C, Hillebrand M, Brunk J, Lee-Kirsch MA. Systemic involvement in TREX1-associated familial chilblain lupus. J Am Acad Dermatol. 2013;69:e179–81.

Haud N, Kara F, Diekmann S, et al. rnaset2 mutant zebrafish model familial cystic leukoencephalopathy and reveal a role for RNase T2 in degrading ribosomal RNA. PNAS. 2011;108:1099–103.

Hayashi M, Suzuki T. Dyschromatosis symmetrica hereditaria. J Dermatol. 2013;40:336–43.

Henneke M, Diekmann S, Ohlenbusch A, et al. RNASET2-deficient cystic leukoencephalopathy resembles congenital cytomegalovirus brain infection. Nat Genet. 2009;41:773–5.

Imai K, Slupphaug G, Lee W-I, et al. Human uracil-DNA glycosylase deficiency associated with profoundly impaired immunoglobulin class-switch recombination. Nat Immunol. 2003;4:1023–8.

Jang MA, Kim EK, Now H, et al. Mutations in DDX58, which encodes RIG-I, cause atypical Singleton-Merten syndrome. Am J Hum Genet. 2015;96:266–74.

Jeremiah N, Neven B, Gentili M, et al. Inherited STING-activating mutation underlies a familial inflammatory syndrome with lupus-like manifestations. J Clin Invest. 2014;124:5516–20.

König N, Fiehn C, Wolf C, et al. Familial chilblain lupus due to a gain-of-function mutation in STING. Ann Rheum Dis. 2017;76(2):468–72.

Lee GS, Brandt VL, Roth DB. B cell development leads off with a base hit: dU:dG mismatches in class switching and hypermutation. Mol Cell. 2004;16:505–8.

Lee-Kirsch MA. The type I interferonopathies. Annu Rev Med. 2017;68:297–315.

Lee-Kirsch MA, Gong M, Schulz H, Ruschendorf F, Stein A, Pfeiffer C, Ballarini A, Gahr M, Hubner N, Linne M. Familial chilblain lupus, a monogenic form of cutaneous lupus erythematosus, maps to chromosome 3p. Am J Hum Genet. 2006;79:731–7.

Lee-Kirsch MA, Chowdhury D, Harvey S, et al. A mutation in TREX1 that impairs susceptibility to granzyme A-mediated cell death underlies familial chilblain lupus. J Mol Med. 2007;85:531–7.

Liu Y, Jesus AA, Marrero B, et al. Activated STING in a vascular and pulmonary syndrome. N Engl J Med. 2014;371:507–18.

Livingston JH, Lin J-P, Dale RC, et al. A type I interferon signature identifies bilateral striatal necrosis due to mutations in ADAR1. J Med Genet. 2014;51:76–82.

Molho-Pessach V, Ramot Y, Camille F, Doviner V, Babay S, Luis SJ, Broshtilova V, Zlotogorski A. H syndrome: the first 79 patients. J Am Acad Dermatol. 2014;70:80–8.

Nitschke Y, Baujat G, Botschen U, et al. Generalized arterial calcification of infancy and pseudoxanthoma elasticum can be caused by mutations in either ENPP1 or ABCC6. Am J Hum Genet. 2012;90:25–39.

Ramantani G, Kohlhase J, Hertzberg C, et al. Expanding the phenotypic spectrum of lupus erythematosus in Aicardi-Goutieres syndrome. Arthritis Rheum. 2010;62:1469–77.

Ramantani G, Hausler M, Niggemann P, Wessling B, Guttmann H, Mull M, Tenbrock K, Lee-Kirsch MA. Aicardi-Goutieres syndrome and systemic lupus erythematosus (SLE) in a 12-year-old boy with SAMHD1 mutations. J Child Neurol. 2011;26:1425–8.

Ravenscroft JC, Suri M, Rice GI, Szynkiewicz M, Crow YJ. Autosomal dominant inheritance of a heterozygous mutation in SAMHD1 causing familial chilblain lupus. Am J Med Genet A. 2011;155A:235–7.

Revy P, Muto T, Levy Y, et al. Activation-induced cytidine deaminase (AID) deficiency causes the autosomal recessive form of the Hyper-IgM syndrome (HIGM2). Cell. 2000;102:565–75.

Rice G, Newman WG, Dean J, et al. Heterozygous mutations in TREX1 cause familial chilblain lupus and dominant Aicardi-Goutieres syndrome. Am J Hum Genet. 2007;80:811–5.

Rice GI, Forte GM, Szynkiewicz M, et al. Assessment of interferon-related biomarkers in Aicardi-Goutieres syndrome associated with mutations in TREX1, RNASEH2A, RNASEH2B, RNASEH2C, SAMHD1, and ADAR: a case-control study. Lancet Neurol. 2013;12:1159–69.

Richards A, van den Maagdenberg AM, Jen JC, et al. C-terminal truncations in human 3'-5' DNA exonuclease TREX1 cause autosomal dominant retinal vasculopathy with cerebral leukodystrophy. Nat Genet. 2007;39:1068–70.

Rutsch F, Böyer P, Nitschke Y, et al. Hypophosphatemia, hyperphosphaturia, and bisphosphonate treatment are associated with survival beyond infancy in generalized arterial calcification of infancy. Circ Cardiovasc Genet. 2008;1:133–40.

Rutsch F, MacDougall M, Lu C, et al. A specific IFIH1 gain-of-function mutation causes Singleton-Merten syndrome. Am J Hum Genet. 2015;96:275–82.

Sanchez GAM, Reinhardt A, Ramsey S, et al. JAK1/2 inhibition with baricitinib in the treatment of autoinflammatory interferonopathies. J Clin Invest. 2018;128(7):3041–52.

Schlee M, Hartmann G. Discriminating self from non-self in nucleic acid sensing. Nat Rev Immunol. 2016;16:566–80.

Seo J, Kang J-A, Suh DI, et al. Tofacitinib relieves symptoms of stimulator of interferon genes (STING)-associated vasculopathy with onset in infancy caused by 2 de novo variants in TMEM173. J Allergy Clin Immunol. 2017;139:1396–1399.e12.

St Hilaire C, Ziegler SG, Markello TC, et al. NT5E mutations and arterial calcifications. N Engl J Med. 2011;364:432–42.

Stavnezer J, Guikema JEJ, Schrader CE. Mechanism and regulation of class switch recombination. Annu Rev Immunol. 2008;26:261–92.

Struk B, Cai L, Zäch S, et al. Mutations of the gene encoding the transmembrane transporter protein ABC-C6 cause pseudoxanthoma elasticum. J Mol Med. 2000;78:282–6.

Tüngler V, Schmidt F, Hieronimus S, Reyes-Velasco C, Lee-Kirsch M. Phenotypic variability in a family with Aicardi-Goutières syndrome due to the common A177T RNASEH2B mutation. Case Rep Clin Med. 2014;3:153–6.

Tüngler V, König N, Günther C, Engel K, Fiehn C, Smitka M, von der Hagen M, Berner R, Lee-Kirsch MA. Response to: "JAK inhibition in STING-associated interferonopathy" by Crow et al. Ann Rheum Dis. 2016;75:e76.

Vanderver A, Adang L, Gavazzi F, et al. Janus kinase inhibition in the Aicardi-Goutières syndrome. N Engl J Med. 2020;383:986–9.

Vogt J, Agrawal S, Ibrahim Z, Southwood TR, Philip S, Macpherson L, Bhole MV, Crow YJ, Oley C. Striking intrafamilial phenotypic variability in Aicardi-Goutieres syndrome associated with the recurrent Asian founder mutation in RNASEH2C. Am J Med Genet A. 2013;161A:338–42.

Wei C-W, Lee C-Y, Lee D-J, et al. Equilibrative nucleoside transporter 3 regulates T cell homeostasis by coordinating lysosomal function with nucleoside availability. Cell Rep. 2018;23:2330–41.

Xin B, Jones S, Puffenberger EG, et al. Homozygous mutation in SAMHD1 gene causes cerebral vasculopathy and early onset stroke. Proc Natl Acad Sci U S A. 2011;108:5372–7.

Yamashiro K, Tanaka R, Li Y, Mikasa M, Hattori N. A TREX1 mutation causing cerebral vasculopathy in a patient with familial chilblain lupus. J Neurol. 2013;260:2653–5.

Zimmermann N, Wolf C, Schwenke R, Lüth A, Schmidt F, Engel K, Lee-Kirsch MA, Günther C. Assessment of clinical response to Janus kinase inhibition in patients with familial chilblain lupus and TREX1 mutation. JAMA Dermatol. 2019;155(3):342–6.

# Disorders of Creatine Metabolism

15

Sylvia Stöckler-Ipsiroglu, Olivier Braissant, and Andreas Schulze

## Contents



S. Stöckler-Ipsiroglu (✉)
Division of Biochemical Genetics, BC Children's Hospital, Vancouver, BC, Canada

Department of Pediatrics, University of British Columbia, Vancouver, BC, Canada
e-mail: sstockler@cw.bc.ca

O. Braissant
Service of Clinical Chemistry, Department of Laboratories, University Hospital and University of Lausanne, Lausanne, Switzerland
e-mail: Olivier.Braissant@chuv.ch

A. Schulze
Division of Clinical and Metabolic Genetics, The Hospital for Sick Children, Toronto, ON, Canada

Departments of Pediatrics and Biochemistry, University of Toronto, Toronto, ON, Canada
e-mail: andreas.schulze@sickkids.ca


N. Blau et al. (eds.), *Physician's Guide to the Diagnosis, Treatment, and Follow-Up of Inherited Metabolic Diseases*,
https://doi.org/10.1007/978-3-030-67727-5_15

**Summary**

Reduced creatine levels in the brain and in body fluids/tissues are the common denominator of primary creatine disorders (cerebral creatine deficiency syndromes types 1–3: X-linked creatine transporter (CrT/*SLC6A8*) deficiency, GAMT/*GAMT* deficiency, AGAT/*GATM* deficiency). Characteristic clinical features include developmental delay/intellectual disability; speech impairment and behavioral problems, combined with epilepsy; and movement disorders. Arginine:glycine amidinotransferase aggregation syndrome is a newly described genetic cause of renal Fanconi syndrome and kidney failure caused by aggregation of certain fully penetrant heterozygous *GATM* missense variants. OAT/*OAT* deficiency is a secondary creatine deficiency syndrome leading to chorioretinal degeneration. Diagnostic markers, besides brain creatine deficiency, include high or low levels of guanidinoacetate for GAMT and AGAT deficiency, a high urinary creatine excretion for CrT deficiency, and high plasma ornithine levels for OAT deficiency. Treatments comprise substitution of creatine (AGAT deficiency) combined with L-ornithine (GAMT deficiency) and arginine restricted diet (GAMT and OAT deficiency). Creatine and substrates for intracerebral creatine synthesis (L-arginine and L-glycine) have limited therapeutic effects in CrT deficiency. Improved outcomes after early recognition have prompted the implementation of GAMT newborn screening in various juridictions.

## Introduction

Creatine is synthesized by two enzymatic reactions: (1) the formation of guanidinoacetate (GAA) from arginine and glycine by L-arginine:glycine amidinotransferase (AGAT/*GATM*) and (2) the methylation of GAA by *S*-adenosyl-L-methionine:*N*-guanidinoacetate methyltransferase (GAMT/*GAMT*). The liver, pancreas, and kidney are the main sites of creatine synthesis. Creatine is transported into cells via an X-linked $Na^+/Cl^-$-dependent creatine transporter, CrT/*SLC6A8*. While blood-brain barrier expresses CrT allowing the brain to take up creatine, this transport from periphery has a low efficacy, and CNS must supply parts of its needs in creatine through endogenous synthesis, by expression of AGAT and GAMT (Hanna-El-Daher and Braissant 2016). Creatine plays a major role in storage and transmission of high-energy phosphates (ATP), via reversible conversion into phosphocreatine, catalyzed by creatine kinases. Creatine may also play a role in neurotransmission. Intracellular creatine and phosphocreatine are nonenzymatically converted into creatinine, which is excreted in urine. The daily creatinine excretion is directly proportional to total body creatine content. Creatine synthesis is regulated via AGAT activity. Because AGAT is inhibited by high concentrations of L-ornithine, the hyperornithinemia in ornithine aminotransferase (OAT) deficiency is associated with secondary creatine deficiency.

## Nomenclature

| No. | Disorder name | Alternative disorder names | Disorder abbreviation | Gene symbol | Chromosomal localization | Affected protein | OMIM # |
|---|---|---|---|---|---|---|---|
| 15.1 | Arginine:glycine amidinotransferase deficiency | Glycine amidinotransferase deficiency | AGAT | *GATM* | 15q15.3 | Arginine:glycine amidinotransferase | 612718 |
| 15.2 | Guanidinoacetate methyltransferase deficiency | – | GAMT | *GAMT* | 19p13.3 | Guanidinoacetate methyltransferase | 612736 |
| 15.3 | Creatine transporter deficiency | X-linked creatine deficiency syndrome, CrT, or SLC6A8 deficiency | CrT, SLC6A8, CTD | *SLC6A8* | Xp28 | SLC6A8 transporter (CrT, creatine transporter) | 300352 |
| 15.4 | Arginine:glycine amidinotransferase aggregation syndrome | AD GATM renal Fanconi syndrome | AGAT AS | *GATM* | 15q15.3 | Arginine:glycine amidinotransferase | |
| 15.5 | Ornithine aminotransferase deficiency | Gyrate atrophy of the choroid and retina | OAT, GACR | *OAT* | 10q26.13 | Ornithine aminotransferase | 258870 |

## Primary Creatine Deficiencies/AGAT, GAMT, and CrT Deficiencies

Primary creatine deficiencies comprise two autosomal recessive inborn errors of creatine synthesis, AGAT (**15.1**) and GAMT (**15.2**) deficiencies, and one X-linked defect of creatine transport, CrT (**15.3**) deficiency (Mercimek-Mahmutoglu and Salomons 2009). The main affected tissue in primary creatine deficiencies is the brain, which presents as a strongly decreased or absent peak of creatine as measured by proton magnetic resonance spectroscopy ($^{1}$H-MRS). Developmental delay and intellectual disability are their common clinical presentation. Speech impairment is most prominent even in patients with mild/moderate intellectual disability. Many patients have autistic behavior and/or various degrees of epilepsy ranging from occasional to pharmaco-resistant seizures. Additional manifestations include failure to thrive, low muscular mass, muscular hypotonia, and movement disorders (mainly extrapyramidal). Myopathy and proximal muscle weakness are an additional feature in AGAT deficiency. Pathological signal intensities of the basal ganglia have mainly been described in patients with GAMT deficiency. Approximately 120 patients are known with GAMT deficiency, and less than 20 patients are known with AGAT deficiency. CrT deficiency may represent a major cause of X-linked intellectual disability accounting for 1–2% in males with intellectual disabilities (Rosenberg et al. 2004). Detailed clinical features are described in series of cases with AGAT, GAMT, and CrT (Stöckler-Ipsiroglu et al. 2014, 2015; van de Kamp et al. 2013).

**Table 15.1** Arginine:glycine amidinotransferase deficiency

| System | Symptoms and biomarkers | Neonatal (birth–1 month) | Infancy (1–18 months) | Childhood (1.5–11 years) | Adolescence (11–16 years) | Adulthood (>16 years) |
|---|---|---|---|---|---|---|
| CNS | **Autism** | | + | + | + | + |
| | **Cerebral creatine deficiency** | +++ | +++ | +++ | +++ | +++ |
| | **Developmental delay** | | +++ | +++ | +++ | +++ |
| | **Epilepsy** | | + | + | + | + |
| | **Myopathy** | | + | + | + | + |
| | **Speech delay** | | +++ | +++ | +++ | +++ |
| Other | **Failure to thrive** | | + | + | + | + |
| Laboratory findings | Creatine (MRS) | ↓↓↓ | ↓↓↓ | ↓↓↓ | ↓↓↓ | ↓↓↓ |
| | Creatine/creatinine ratio (urine) | ↓-n | ↓-n | ↓-n | ↓-n | ↓-n |
| | Creatinine (plasma) | ↓-n | ↓-n | ↓-n | ↓-n | ↓-n |
| | Creatinine (urine) | ↓-n | ↓-n | ↓-n | ↓-n | ↓-n |
| | Guanidinoacetate (cerebrospinal fluid) | ↓↓↓ | ↓↓↓ | ↓↓↓ | ↓↓↓ | ↓↓↓ |
| | Guanidinoacetate (plasma) | ↓↓↓ | ↓↓↓ | ↓↓↓ | ↓↓↓ | ↓↓↓ |
| | Guanidinoacetate (urine) | ↓↓↓ | ↓↓↓ | ↓↓↓ | ↓↓↓ | ↓↓↓ |

**Table 15.2** Guanidinoacetate methyltransferase deficiency

| System | Symptoms and biomarkers | Neonatal (birth–1 month) | Infancy (1–18 months) | Childhood (1.5–11 years) | Adolescence (11–16 years) | Adulthood (>16 years) |
|---|---|---|---|---|---|---|
| CNS | **Autism** | | +++ | +++ | +++ | +++ |
| | **Basal ganglia abnormalities (MRI)** | | + | + | + | + |
| | **Cerebral creatine deficiency** | +++ | +++ | +++ | +++ | +++ |
| | **Developmental delay** | | +++ | +++ | +++ | +++ |
| | **Epilepsy** | | ++ | ++ | ++ | ++ |
| | **Movement disorder** | | + | + | + | + |
| | **Speech delay** | | +++ | +++ | +++ | +++ |
| Musculoskeletal | Osteoporosis | | | | ± | |

(continued)

**Table 15.2** (continued)

| System | Symptoms and biomarkers | Neonatal (birth–1 month) | Infancy (1–18 months) | Childhood (1.5–11 years) | Adolescence (11–16 years) | Adulthood (>16 years) |
|---|---|---|---|---|---|---|
| Laboratory findings | Creatine (cerebrospinal fluid) | ↓-n | ↓↓ | ↓↓ | ↓↓ | ↓↓ |
| | Creatine (plasma) | ↓-n | ↓↓ | ↓↓ | ↓↓ | ↓↓ |
| | Creatine (urine) | ↓-n | ↓↓ | ↓↓ | ↓↓ | ↓↓ |
| | Creatinine (plasma) | ↓-n | ↓ | ↓ | ↓ | ↓ |
| | Creatinine (urine) | ↓-n | ↓ | ↓ | ↓ | ↓ |
| | Guanidinoacetate (cerebrospinal fluid) | ↑↑↑ | ↑↑↑ | ↑↑↑ | ↑↑↑ | ↑↑↑ |
| | Guanidinoacetate (plasma) | ↑↑↑ | ↑↑↑ | ↑↑↑ | ↑↑↑ | ↑↑↑ |
| | Guanidinoacetate (urine) | ↑↑↑ | ↑↑↑ | ↑↑↑ | ↑↑↑ | ↑↑↑ |

**Table 15.3** Creatine transporter deficiency

| System | Symptoms and biomarkers | Neonatal (birth–1 month) | Infancy (1–18 months) | Childhood (1.5–11 years) | Adolescence (11–16 years) | Adulthood (>16 years) |
|---|---|---|---|---|---|---|
| CNS | **Autism** | | +++ | +++ | +++ | +++ |
| | **Cerebral creatine deficiency** | | +++ | +++ | +++ | +++ |
| | **Developmental delay** | | +++ | +++ | +++ | +++ |
| | **Epilepsy** | | + | + | + | + |
| | **Speech delay** | | +++ | +++ | +++ | +++ |
| Digestive | Constipation | | ± | ± | ± | ± |
| Musculoskeletal | Muscle mass, low | | ± | + | + | + |
| Laboratory findings | Creatine/creatinine ratio (urine) | | ↑↑ | ↑↑ | ↑↑ | ↑↑ |

## Arginine: Glycine Amidinotransferase Aggregation Syndrome

AGAT aggregation syndrome is a newly described genetic cause of renal Fanconi syndrome and kidney failure caused by mitochondrial aggregation of fully penetrant heterozygous *GATM* missense variants (Fanconi renotubular syndrome type 1). Four previously unreported heterozygous missense variants of evolutionary conserved amino acid residues in *GATM* (p.P320S, p.T336A, p.T336I, p.P341L) have been identified in these patients. Patients with this autosomal dominant disorders develop renal Fanconi syndrome with glucosuria, hyperphosphaturia, generalized hyperaminoaciduria, low molecular weight proteinuria, and metabolic acidosis. Debilitating rickets or bone deformities have not been described in these patients (Reichold et al. 2018).

## OAT Deficiency

OAT deficiency is a secondary creatine deficiency. Hyperornithinemia-associated gyrate atrophy of the choroid and retina is an inherited metabolic eye disease, caused by autosomal recessive deficiency of the L-ornithine:2-oxoacid aminotransferase (OAT) (**15.5**) (Valle and Simell 1995). Clinical features include progressive chorioretinal degeneration with myopia, night blindness, and loss of peripheral vision starting late in the first decade, proceeding to tunnel vision and eventually leading to blindness in the third and fourth decade. In addition to the ocular findings, some patients present systemic abnormalities. Most patients have normal intelligence. MRI findings include degenerative lesions in the white matter and premature atrophic changes. Tubular aggregates and selected atrophy of the type II fibers of skeletal muscle do not cause muscle weakness, although muscle performance of affected patients may be impaired when speed or acute strength is required.

OAT is a mitochondrial matrix enzyme that requires pyridoxal phosphate (vitamin $B_6$) for the reversible conversion of ornithine and 2-oxoglutarate to Δ1-pyrroline-5-carboxylate and glutamate. In its deficiency, the accumulation of ornithine causes secondary creatine deficiency through inhibition of AGAT activity, the rate-limiting step in endogenous creatine synthesis (Näntö-Salonen et al. 1999).

The pathways of creatine synthesis and transport are shown in Fig. 15.1.

**Table 15.4** Arginine:glycine amidinotransferase aggregation syndrome

| System | Symptoms and biomarkers | Neonatal (birth–1 month) | Infancy (1–18 months) | Childhood (1.5–11 years) | Adolescence (11–16 years) | Adulthood (>16 years) |
|---|---|---|---|---|---|---|
| Musculoskeletal | Hypophosphatemic rickets | | ↑ | ↑ | ↑ | ↑ |
| | Muscle weakness, progressive | | | + | + | + |
| | Osteomalacia | | | + | + | + |
| Renal | Aminoaciduria | + | + | + | + | + |
| | Renal failure | | | | | + |
| | **Renal tubular acidosis** | | | + | + | + |
| Laboratory findings | Amino acids (urine) | + | + | + | + | + |
| | Amino acids (urine), all | ↑ | ↑ | ↑ | ↑ | ↑ |
| | Creatinine (serum) | | | | | ↑ |
| | Cystine (urine) | | | n | n | n |
| | Glucose (urine) | ↑ | ↑ | ↑ | ↑ | ↑ |
| | Phosphate (plasma) | | | ↓ | ↓ | ↓ |
| | Phosphate (urine) | ↑ | ↑ | ↑ | ↑ | ↑ |
| | Potassium (plasma) | | | ↓ | ↓ | ↓ |
| | Proteins, low molecular weight (urine) | ↑ | ↑ | ↑ | ↑ | ↑ |

**Table 15.5** Ornithine aminotransferase deficiency

| System | Symptoms and biomarkers | Neonatal (birth–1 month) | Infancy (1–18 months) | Childhood (1.5–11 years) | Adolescence (11–16 years) | Adulthood (>16 years) |
|---|---|---|---|---|---|---|
| CNS | Cortical atrophy (MRI) | | | | ± | ± |
| | Intellectual disability | | | ± | ± | ± |
| | Neuropathy, sensory | | | ± | ± | ± |
| | Seizures | | | | ± | ± |
| | White matter abnormalities (MRI) | | | | ± | ± |
| Digestive | EM, abnormal mitochondria (liver) | | | | ± | ± |
| Eye | **Atrophy, gyrate of the choroid and retina** | | | + | ++ | +++ |
| | **Blindness** | | | | | +++[a] |
| | **Cataract, posterior subcapsular** | | | | ± | +++ |
| | **Chorioretinal degeneration** | | | + | ++ | +++ |
| | **Myopia** | | ± | + | ++ | +++ |
| | **Night blindness** | | ± | ++ | 0 | +++ |
| | Retinal detachment | | | ± | ± | ± |
| | **Vision, tunnel** | | | | + | +++ |
| Metabolic | Hyperammonemia (symptomatic) | ± | | | | |
| Musculoskeletal | EM, abnormal mitochondria (muscle) | | | ± | ± | ± |
| | EM, type 2 fiber atrophy (muscle) | | | ± | ± | ± |
| | **EM, type 2 fiber tubular aggregates (muscle)** | | | + | + | ++ |
| | Muscle weakness (mild proximal) | | | ± | ± | ± |

(continued)

**Table 15.5** (continued)

| System | Symptoms and biomarkers | Neonatal (birth–1 month) | Infancy (1–18 months) | Childhood (1.5–11 years) | Adolescence (11–16 years) | Adulthood (>16 years) |
|---|---|---|---|---|---|---|
| Laboratory findings | 3-Amino-2-piperidone (urine) | n | ↑ | ↑ | ↑ | ↑ |
| | Ammonia (blood and plasma) | n-↑↑ | n | n | n | n |
| | Arginine (urine) | n | ↑ | ↑ | ↑ | ↑ |
| | Creatine (cerebrospinal fluid) | n | ↓↓ | ↓↓ | ↓↓↓ | ↓↓↓ |
| | Creatine (plasma) | n | ↓↓ | ↓↓ | ↓↓↓ | ↓↓↓ |
| | Creatine (urine) | n | ↓↓ | ↓↓ | ↓↓↓ | ↓↓↓ |
| | Creatine/phosphocreatine ratio (brain) (MRS) | n | ↓-n | ↓ | ↓ | ↓ |
| | Creatine/phosphocreatine ratio (muscle) (MRS) | n | ↓-n | ↓ | ↓ | ↓ |
| | Creatinine (plasma) | n | ↓-n | ↓-n | ↓-n | ↓-n |
| | Guanidinoacetate (cerebrospinal fluid) | n | ↓↓ | ↓↓ | ↓↓↓ | ↓↓↓ |
| | Guanidinoacetate (plasma) | n | ↓↓ | ↓↓ | ↓↓↓ | ↓↓↓ |
| | Guanidinoacetate (urine) | n | ↓↓ | ↓↓ | ↓↓↓ | ↓↓↓ |
| | Histology and EM, type 2 fiber atrophy (muscle) | | | + | + | ++-+++ |
| | Lysine (urine) | n | ↑ | ↑ | ↑ | ↑ |
| | Ornithine (plasma) | n | ↑↑↑ | ↑↑↑ | ↑↑↑ | ↑↑↑ |
| | Ornithine (urine) | n | ↑↑↑ | ↑↑↑ | ↑↑↑ | ↑↑↑ |
| | Proline/citrulline ratio | ↑ | n | n | n | n |

[a]>30 years

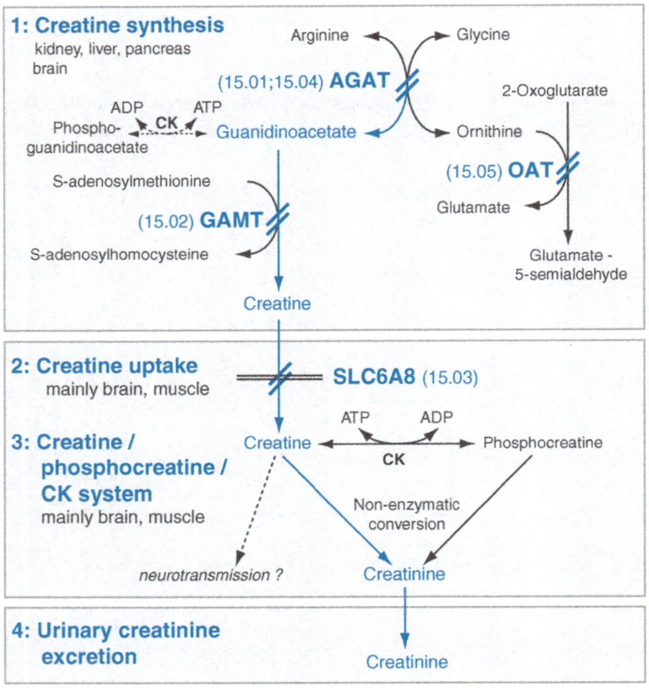


**Fig. 15.1** Pathways of creatine synthesis and transport

## Diagnosis

### AGAT, GAMT, CrT Deficiencies

Primary creatine disorders may account for a high proportion of undiagnosed and potentially treatable genetic intellectual disability syndromes in children and adults (Stöckler-Ipsiroglu and van Karnebeek 2014). Therefore, selective screening for these disorders should be included in the investigation of this population. Cerebral creatine deficiency as detected by $^1$H-MRS is the common biochemical hallmark of AGAT, GAMT, and CrT deficiencies. Biochemical indicators include the following metabolites in urine, blood, and CSF. Increased levels of GAA in body fluids are pathognomonic for GAMT deficiency, whereas GAA levels are reduced in AGAT deficiency. Increased urinary creatine and decreased creatinine excretion, resulting in an increased urinary creatine-to-creatinine ratio, are associated with CrT deficiency (Sharer et al. 2017). Heterozygous females may also be affected clinically, but it appears that urinary creatine/creatinine ratio and cerebral creatine levels are not reliable diagnostic markers in females (van de Kamp et al. 2011). Diagnosis of AGAT deficiency is particularly challenging as determination of urinary GAA excretion is lacking sensitivity. Determination of GAA in blood seems to be more sensitive (Stöckler-Ipsiroglu et al. 2015). In an increasing number of cases, next-generation sequencing has provided the primary diagnosis, while determination of characteristic metabolites and enzyme activities is used for disease confirmation. Assays have been developed for the determination of AGAT, GAMT, and CrT activities in fibroblasts and white blood cells (Verhoeven et al. 2003; Berends et al. 2017; Joncquel-Chevalier Curt et al. 2018).

Based on most favorable outcomes in early-diagnosed patients, newborn screening for GAMT deficiency has been implemented in several legislations (Sinclair et al. 2016; Pasquali et al. 2014). A second-tier LC-MS/MS assay for guanidinoacetate quantification from bloodspots removes the interference seen in the first-tier standard flow injection assay, thus greatly improving the performance of the assay.

Functional and in silico analyses of *GAMT* variants reported in public databases revealed *GAMT* carrier estimates of 1 in 372 and 1 in 812, respectively, and a calculated disease frequency of 1 in 550,000 and 1 in 2,640,000 (Desroches et al. 2015). The rarity of the condition may explain why, after screening of over one million newborns world-wide, the 1st case has only been identified this beginning of 2021.

## Arginine: Glycine Amidinotransferase Aggregation Syndrome

Extrarenal metabolic abnormalities such as creatine and GAA deficiency are not expected to occur in this condition. The diagnosis is confined to *GATM* DNA testing. Electron microscopy and immunofluorescence staining showing intramitochondrial filaments formed by AGAT aggregates may give a first hint (Reichold et al. 2018).

## OAT Deficiency

The biochemical hallmark of OAT deficiency is marked hyperornithinemia. The most important laboratory test in this disease is therefore the amino acid analysis in plasma. In patients, plasma ornithine ranges from 400 to 1400 μmol/L (normal less than 80 to 90 μmol/L). The combination of elevated plasma ornithine and characteristic ocular findings is highly specific for the disease. Ornithine is also increased in the CSF and urine. Pathologic urinary excretion of ornithine and other dibasic amino acids (arginine, lysine, cystine) typically occurs at plasma ornithine concentrations greater than 600 μmol/L. In plasma, lysine and creatine may be decreased. In urine, creatine, creatinine, and GAA are usually decreased. Investigation by in vivo $^{1}$H-MRS reveals a decreased concentration of creatine and phosphocreatine in the brain and muscle. DNA testing can be performed to confirm the diagnosis. Enzyme analysis is feasible in stimulated lymphocytes but provides only sparse additional information and is not offered for routine analysis by clinical laboratories. Prenatal diagnosis is potentially possible by ornithine aminotransferase activity measurement in amniotic fluid cells or chorionic villi or by DNA testing if the genetic variant is known in the index case.

The differential diagnosis of disorders of creatine metabolism is shown in Fig. 15.2.

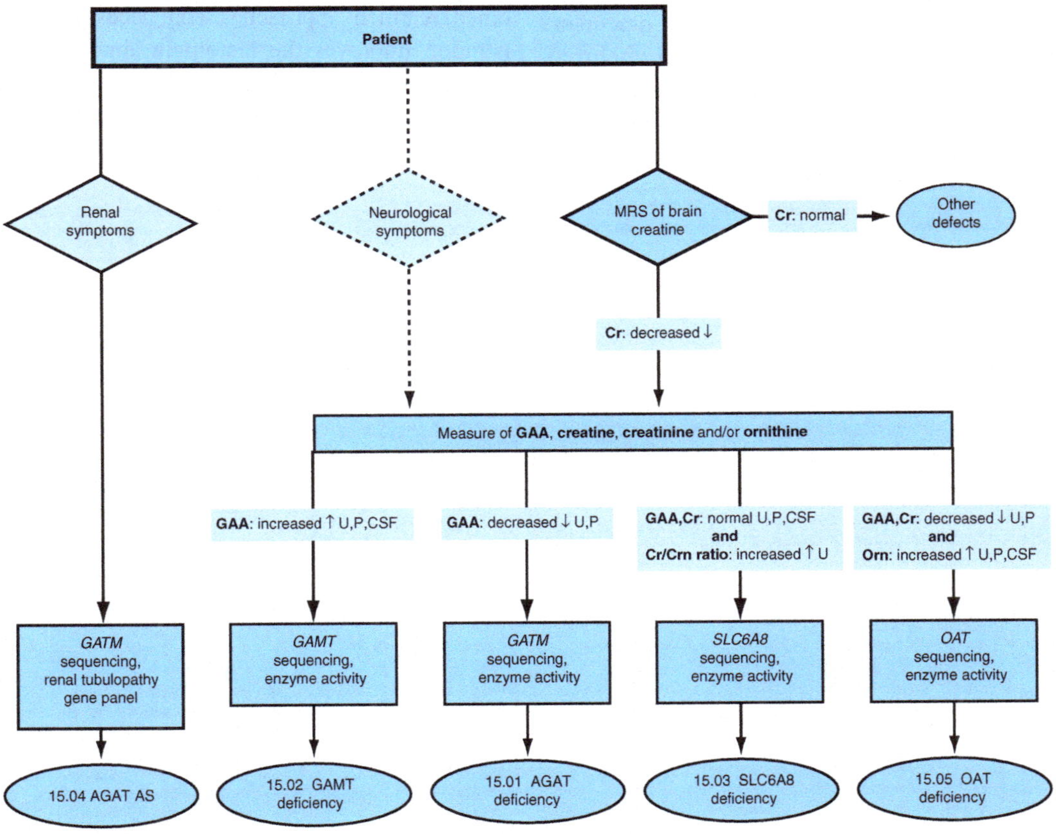


**Fig. 15.2** Differential diagnosis of disorders of creatine metabolism

## Treatments

### GAMT, AGAT, CrT Deficiencies

In GAMT and AGAT deficiencies, correction of cerebral creatine deficiency is achieved via long-term supplementation of high dosages of creatine (given as creatine monohydrate). Clinically in AGAT deficiency, this is associated with significant improvement of myopathy, limited improvement of cognitive function in older patients, and normal development in patients treated at an early age (Stöckler-Ipsiroglu et al. 2015). In GAMT deficiency, creatine supplementation is combined with pharmacological doses of L-ornithine and/or dietary arginine restriction with the aim to reduce guanidinoacetate accumulation (Schulze et al. 2001). Treatment results in improvement of seizures and movement disorders but has limited effects on cognition and behaviors in late-treated patients, while presymptomatic/early treatment appears to completely prevent all these manifestations (Stöckler-Ipsiroglu et al. 2014; Khaikin et al. 2018). Sodium benzoate has been proposed as an additional approach to reduce the production of GAA via conjugation with glycine to form hippuric acid; however, its clinical efficacy is inconclusive (Viau et al. 2013; Mercimek-Mahmutoglu et al. 2014).

In CrT deficiency, while females may benefit from creatine supplementation, treatment of male patients even with high dosages of creatine is not effective due to the absence of functional CrT. Various combinations of L-arginine, L-glycine, and *S*-adenosyl-methionine (serving as precursors for intracerebral creatine synthesis) have also been employed. While some neurological and behavioral improvements associated with these treatments were observed in a few cases, in many others, the clinical benefit was inconclusive (Bruun et al. 2018; Dunbar et al. 2014; Valayannopoulos et al. 2012; van de Kamp et al. 2012). Creatine analogues and small molecule chaperone therapies are currently under preclinical investigation as treatment options.

### Arginine: Glycine Amidinotransferase Aggregation Syndrome

It has been proposed that reduction of renal *GATM* mRNA expression via creatine supplementation may retard the formation of deleterious mitochondrial deposits (Reichold et al. 2018).

### OAT Deficiency

Permanent reduction of plasma ornithine below 200 μmol/L slows or stops the chorioretinal degeneration. A small proportion of patients respond to pharmacological doses of vitamin $B_6$. Mainstay of treatment is substrate deprivation with a diet that consists of arginine restriction and arginine-free amino acid supplements. Additional experimental approaches include augmentation of renal ornithine excretion by administration of pharmacological doses of L-lysine (Elpeleg and Korman 2001) or the non-metabolizable amino acid α-aminoisobutyric acid and proline supplementation. Since no form of therapy is unequivocally effective, combined treatment approaches seem necessary. Creatine administration improves the histologic abnormalities in muscle, but does not halt the progress of chorioretinal degeneration.

An algorithm for the assessment of Vitamin B6 responsiveness is shown in Fig. 15.3.

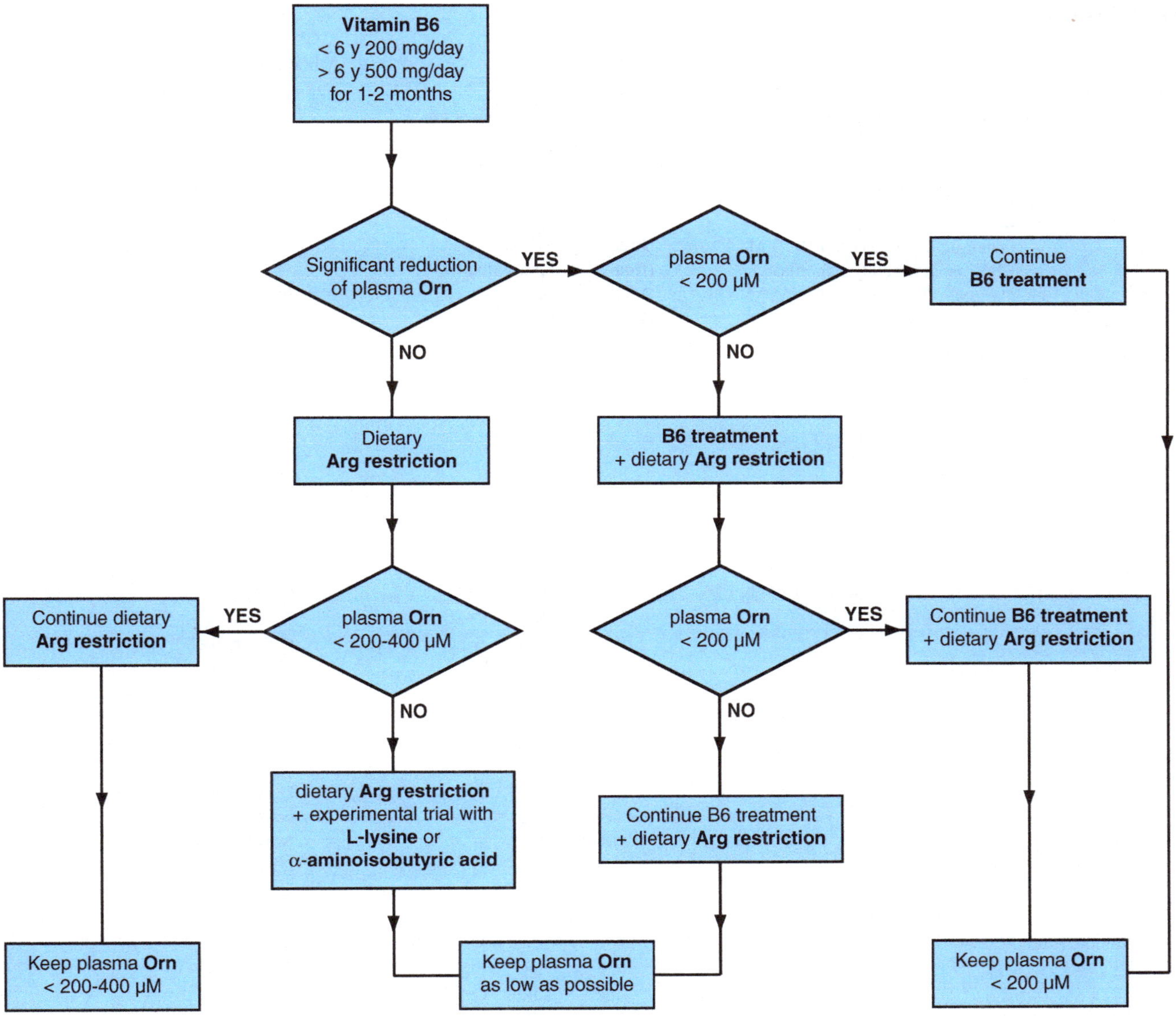


**Fig. 15.3** Algorithm for the assessment of vitamin B6 responsiveness in OAT deficiency

## Prenatal Diagnosis

| Disorder | Method/analytes | Material | Timing semester |
|---|---|---|---|
| 15.1 | AGAT/GATM activity | Cultured amniotic cells | II |
| | DNA testing | Chorionic villi, cultured amniotic cells | I, II |
| 15.2 | GAMT activity | Cultured amniotic cells | II |
| | DNA testing | Chorionic villi, cultured amniotic cells | I, II |
| | | Amniotic fluid | II |
| 15.3 | CrT/SLC6A8 activity | Cultured amniotic cells | II |
| | DNA testing | Chorionic villi, cultured amniotic cells | I, II |
| 15.4 | AGAT/GATM | Cultured amniotic cells | II |
| | DNA testing | Chorionic villi, cultured amniotic cells | I,II |
| 15.5 | OAT activity | Cultured amniotic cells | II |
| | DNA testing | Chorionic villi, cultured amniotic cells | I, II |

So far, prenatal diagnosis has been documented for disorders 15.1, 15.2, and 15.5, but not for 15.3 and 15.4

## DNA Testing

| Disorder | Tissue | Methodology | Mutations |
|---|---|---|---|
| 15.1 | Genomic DNA (blood, FB, LYM, EBV-transformed lymphoblasts) | Direct sequencing, High-throughput sequencing | http://www.LOVD.nl/GATM |
| 15.2 | Genomic DNA (blood, FB, LYM, EBV-transformed lymphoblasts) | Direct sequencing, High-throughput sequencing | http://www.LOVD.nl/GAMT |
| 15.3 | Genomic DNA (blood, FB, LYM, EBV-transformed lymphoblasts) | Direct sequencing, High-throughput sequencing | http://www.LOVD.nl/SLC6A8 |
| 15.4 | Genomic DNA (blood, FB, LYM, EBV-transformed lymphoblasts) | Direct sequencing, High-throughput sequencing | |
| 15.5 | Genomic DNA (blood, FB, LYM, EBV-transformed lymphoblasts) | Direct sequencing, High-throughput sequencing | http://www.LOVD.nl/OAT |

*FB* cultured fibroblasts, *LYM* lymphocytes

## Specimen Collection

| Test | Preconditions | Material | Handling | Pitfalls |
|---|---|---|---|---|
| Creatine | Before creatine supplementation | U | 24-h urine or spot, store at −20 °C | U: false positives in high-protein diet |
| | | CSF | Store at −20 °C | |
| | | P | EDTA or heparinate, store at −20 °C | P: probably not diagnostic in neonates |
| Creatinine | Before creatine supplementation | U | 24-h urine or spot, store at −20 °C | U: low in patients with reduced muscle mass |
| | | CSF | Store at −20 °C | U: false positives in high-protein diet |
| | | P | EDTA or heparinate, store at −20 °C | P: probably not diagnostic in neonates |
| Creatine/creatinine ratio to test CrT/SLC6A8 deficiency | | U | | Not sensitive in heterozygous females<br>Can be normal in symptomatic patients |
| Guanidinoacetate | | U | 24-h urine or spot, store at −20 °C | |
| | | CSF | Store at −20 °C | |
| | | P | EDTA or heparinate, store at −20 °C | |
| | | DBS | Room temperature | |
| Ornithine | | U | 24-h urine or spot, store at −20 °C | |
| | | CSF | Store at −20 °C | |
| | | P | EDTA or heparinate, store at −20 °C | |
| GAMT, AGAT, CrT/SLC6A8, OAT activities | | Liver | Store at −80 °C | |
| | | FB | Cultured skin cells | |
| | | LYM | EBV-transformed lymphoblasts | |

*DBS* dry blood spot, *FB* cultured fibroblasts, *LYM* lymphoblasts

## Reference Values

| | Age range | Urine [mmol/mol creatinine] | Plasma [µmol/L] | CSF [µmol/L] | Amniotic fluid [µmol/L] |
|---|---|---|---|---|---|
| Guanidinoacetate[a] | 1 week–2 years<br>1 month–2 years<br>2 years–puberty<br>Men<br>Women<br>No age range established | 28–180<br>11–40<br>11–40 | 0.20–1.46<br>0.56–1.88<br>1.58–3.64<br>0.87–3.15 | 0.015–0.100 | |
| Guanidinoacetate[b] | <10 years<br>10–15 years<br>>15 years<br><4 years<br>4–15 years<br>Male >15 years<br>Female >15 years | 20–208<br>15–152<br>5–78<br>9–128 | 0.6–2.4<br>0.9–3.0<br>1.2–3.6 | | |
| Guanidinoacetate[c] | 0–15 years<br>>15 years<br>No age range established | 4–220<br>3–78 | 0.35–1.8<br>1.0–3.5 | 0.02–0.56 | |
| Guanidinoacetate[d] | No age range established | | | 0.036–0.22 | |
| Guanidinoacetate[e] | | | | | 1.6–4.4 |
| Creatine[a] | 1 week–2 years<br>1 month–2 years<br>2 years–puberty<br>Men<br>Women<br>No age range established | 28–1700<br>3.4–191<br>3.4–360 | 50–124<br>24–109<br>5.5–54.7<br>12.8–96.8 | 35–90 | |
| Creatine[b] | <10 years<br>10–15 years<br>>15 years<br><4 years<br>4–15 years<br>Male >15 years<br>Female >15 years | 29–1551<br>19–1046<br>7–492<br>12–682 | 34–124<br>28–104<br>12–99 | | |
| Creatine[c] | 0–4 years<br>4–12 years<br>>12 years<br>0–10 years<br>>10 years<br>No age range established | 6–1208<br>17,721<br>11–244 | 17–109<br>6–50 | 17–87 | |
| Creatine[d] | 0–10 years<br>>10 years | | | 24–53<br>38–66 | |
| Creatine[e] | | | | | 28–88 |
| Ornithine[f] | 0–1 month<br>1–6 months<br>6–12 months<br>1–2 years<br>2–4 years<br>4–7 years<br>7–13 years<br>>13 years<br><3 months<br><12 months<br>Children<br>Adolescents<br>Men<br>Women | 0–19<br>0–13<br>0–8<br>0–8<br>0–7<br>0–7<br>0–6<br>0–5 | 41–129<br>20–136<br>47–195<br>55–135<br>36–96 | 0.7–15.7<br>2.0–5.9<br>3–9<br>1.7–8.1 | |

[a]*Method*: HPLC, fluorescence. *Reference*: Marescau B. Unpublished, personal communication
[b]*Method*: LC-MS/MS. Reference values modified from Joncquel et al. (2011)
[c]*Method*: GC-MS. *Reference*: Almeida et al. (2004)
[d]*Method*: LC-MS/MS. *Reference*: Young et al. (2007)
[e]*Method*: LC-/MS/MS. *Reference*: Cheillan et al. (2006)
[f]*Method*: HPLC (amino acid analyzer). *Reference:* Shih (2003)

## Pathological Values

| | | | | | | |
|---|---|---|---|---|---|---|
| Guanidinoacetate | Disorder | Urine [mmol/mol creatinine] | Plasma magnitude of change compared to normal | CSF magnitude of change compared to normal | Brain $^1$H-MRS | Amniotic fluid magnitude of change compared to normal |
| | 15.1 AGAT | <0.3[a] | <0.1× | No data available/ presumably low | No data available/ presumably not detectable | No data available/ presumably low |
| | 15.2 GAMT | >500[a] | >10× | >100× | Elevated | >3×[b] |
| | 15.3 CrT | Normal | Normal | No data available/ presumably normal | No data available/may be elevated | No data available/ presumably normal |
| | 15.4 AGAT AS | No data available/ presumably normal | No data available/ presumably normal | No data available/ presumably normal | No data available/ presumably normal | No data available/ presumably normal |
| | 15.5 OAT | Low | Low | No data available/ presumably normal | No data available/ presumably not detectable | No data available/ presumably normal |
| Creatine | Disorder | Urine [mmol/mol creatinine] | Plasma [μmol/L] | CSF [μmol/L] | Brain $^1$H-MRS | Amniotic fluid [μmol/L] |
| | 15.1 AGAT | Low | Low | No data available/ presumably low | Absent/very low | No data available/ presumably normal |
| | 15.2 GAMT | Low | <7 | 1.4–19[c] | Absent/very low | Normal[b] |
| | 15.3 CrT | High (>1400[a]) | Normal | May be normal | Very low | No data available/ presumably normal |
| | 15.4 AGAT AS | No data available/ presumably normal | No data available/ presumably normal | No data available/ presumably normal | Normal (data from 1 patient) | No data available/ presumably normal |
| | 15.5 OAT | Low | Low | No data available/ presumably low | Low | No data available/ presumably normal |
| Ornithine | Disorder | | Plasma [μmol/L] | | | |
| | 15.5 OAT | | 600–1400[d] | | | |

*AGAT AS* AGAT aggregation syndrome

[a]*Method*: GC-MS. *Reference*: Struys et al. (2008)

[b]*Method*: LC-MS/MS. *Reference*: Cheillan et al. (2006)

[c]*Method*: HPLC, fluorescence. *Reference*: Schulze A. Own observation in three patients

[d]Please note: Plasma ornithine may not be elevated in neonates and in the first months of life

## Standard Treatment

| No./symbol | Age | Medication/diet | Dosage [mg/kg per day] | Doses per day |
|---|---|---|---|---|
| 15.1 AGAT | All ages | Creatine monohydrate | 200–400[a] | 3–6 |
| 15.2 GAMT | All ages | Creatine monohydrate | 400 | 3–6 |
| | | L-Ornithine aspartate | | 3–6 |
| | All ages | Low dose | 100[b] | |
| | Children<br>Adults | High dose | 800[b]<br>400[b] | |
| | All ages | Sodium benzoate | 100 | 3 |
| | | L-Arginine intake | 15–25[c] | 3–5 daily meals |
| | | Essential amino acid mixture (arginine free) | 0.2–0.7 g essential amino acids/kg | 3–5 daily meals |
| 15.5 OAT<br>Vitamin B6 responsive form[d] | <14 years<br>>14 years | Pyridoxine hydrochloride<br>Diet (see below)<br>Pyridoxine hydrochloride<br>Diet (see below) | 40–200[e]<br>40–500[e] | 2<br>2 |
| 15.5 OAT<br>Vitamin B6 nonresponsive form[d] | All ages | Arginine-restricted diet (see below) | | |

[a]Lower dosages of creatine monohydrate might be sufficient for restoration of the cerebral creatine pool in AGAT deficiency due to the absence of GAA accumulation and no subsequent competitive inhibition of creatine uptake

[b]Aim of low-dose substitution is to provide sufficient amounts of ornithine to the urea cycle (target plasma ornithine concentration 100–200 μmol/L) in case of an arginine-restricted diet. Aim of high-dose substitution is the competitive AGAT inhibition with high intracellular ornithine concentrations ($K_m$ = 300 μmol/L)

[c]Corresponds to 0.4–0.7 g/kg natural protein. Essential amino acid mixture supplement is necessary in order to meet age-dependent physiological amino acid/protein requirements

[d]Target plasma ornithine concentration <200 μmol/L

[e]15–20 mg/day might be as effective in some patients as higher dosage (Weleber and Kennaway 1981)

**Beware/Pitfalls**

- In individuals supplemented with creatine, intake of high doses (20 g/day in adults) has been associated with weight gain (due to intracellular edema), muscle cramps, and impairment of renal function.
- Creatine monohydrate is freely available in drug stores, and attention has to be paid to the purity of the various products. In particular, after chemical synthesis from sarcosine and cyanamide, contamination with dicyanamide, which liberates HCN in the acidic conditions of the stomach, may occur as a result of incomplete purification.
- Higher doses of ornithine are preferably given as a formulation of ornithine aspartate, rather than ornithine HCl since the latter can lead to metabolic acidosis.
- Acute respiratory failure after institution of vitamin B6 is reported in a few neonates with severe seizure disorder.
- Peripheral neuropathy is associated with long-term ingestion of high-dosage vitamin B6 (>1000 mg/day).

## Dietary Treatment

| Age | Protein requirement [g/kg/day] | Natural protein [g/kg/day][a] | Arginine-free essential AAM<br>Type[b] | Arginine-free essential AAM<br>Protein equivalent[c] [g/day] |
|---|---|---|---|---|
| Infants | 1.1–2.7 | 0.4 | 1 | 2–5 |
| Children | 1.0–1.7 | 0.3–0.5 | 2 | 10–25 |
| Adults | 0.8 | 0.25 | 2 | 30–75 |

[a]According to Dewey et al. (1996)

[b]Type 1, infantile formula; type 2, childhood formula

[c]Spread as evenly as possible through the 24 h

**Beware/Pitfalls**

Overtreatment through protein restriction.

## Alternative Therapies/Experimental Trials

| No./ symbol | Age | Medication/ diet | Dosage mg/kg per day | Dosages per day | Literature |
|---|---|---|---|---|---|
| 15.3 CrT | All ages | Creatine monohydrate | 100–400 | 3–6 | Valayannopoulos et al. (2012); van de Kamp et al. (2012); Mercimek-Mahmutoglu et al. (2010); Jaggumantri et al. (2015); Schjelderup et al. (2021) |
| | All ages | L-Arginine | 400 | 3 | |
| | All ages | L-Glycine | 150 | 3 | |
| | All ages | *S*-Adenosyl methionine | 100 | 2 | |
| | All ages | Betaine | 50–250 | 3 | |
| 15.5 OAT | Adults | Creatine monohydrate | 1.5–2 g per day (1–1.5 g/$m^2$/day) | 2–3 | Heinänen et al. (1999) |
| | Adults | L-Lysine | 10–15 g per day (5 g/$m^2$/ day) | 5[a] | Peltola et al. (2000); Elpeleg and Korman (2001) |
| | Adults | α-Aminoiso butyric acid | 0.1 | 5[a] | Valle et al. (1981) |
| | All ages | L-Proline | 65–488 | 3 | Hayasaka et al. (1985) |

[a]Spread within the diet as evenly as possible through the 24 h

**Beware/Pitfalls**

In CrT deficiency, creatine administration might be efficient in females but less in males.

In OAT deficiency, creatine administration corrects skeletal muscle abnormalities but not progress of ophthalmologic abnormalities.

Studies of the long-term efficacy of these approaches have not been reported or the results are inconclusive.

## References


Almeida LS, Verhoeven NM, Roos B, et al. Creatine and guanidinoacetate: diagnostic markers for inborn errors in creatine biosynthesis and transport. Mol Genet Metab. 2004;82:214–9.

Berends LM, Struys EA, Roos B, et al. Guanidinoacetate methyltransferase activity in lymphocytes, for a fast diagnosis. JIMD Rep. 2017;37:13–7.

Bruun TUJ, Sidky S, Bandeira AO, et al. Treatment outcome of creatine transporter deficiency: international retrospective cohort study. Metab Brain Dis. 2018;33(3):875–84.

Cheillan D, Salomons GS, Acquaviva C, et al. Prenatal diagnosis of guanidinoacetate methyltransferase deficiency: increased guanidinoacetate concentrations in amniotic fluid. Clin Chem. 2006;52:775–7.

Desroches CL, Patel J, Wang P, et al. Carrier frequency of guanidinoacetate methyltransferase deficiency in the general population by functional characterization of missense variants in the GAMT gene. Mol Genet Genomics. 2015;290(6):2163–71.

Dewey KG, Beaton G, Fjeld C, Lönnerdal B, Reeds P. Protein requirements of infants and children. Eur J Clin Nut. 1996;50(Suppl 1):S119–47.

Dunbar M, Jaggumantri S, Sargent M, Stöckler-Ipsiroglu S, van Karnebeek CD. Treatment of X-linked creatine transporter (SLC6A8) deficiency: systematic review of the literature and three new cases. Mol Genet Metab. 2014;112:259–74.

Elpeleg N, Korman SH. Sustained oral lysine supplementation in ornithine delta-aminotransferase deficiency. J Inherit Metab Dis. 2001;24:423–4.

Hanna-El-Daher L, Braissant O. Creatine synthesis and exchanges between brain cells: what can be learned from human creatine deficiencies and various experimental models? Amino Acids. 2016;48:1877–95.

Hayasaka S, Saito T, Nakajima H, et al. Clinical trials of vitamin B6 and proline supplementation for gyrate atrophy of the choroid and retina. Br J Ophthalmol. 1985;69:283–90.

Heinänen K, Näntö-Salonen K, Komu M, et al. Creatine corrects muscle 31P spectrum in gyrate atrophy with hyperornithinaemia. Eur J Clin Invest. 1999;29:1060–5.

Jaggumantri S, Dunbar M, Edgar V, et al. Treatment of creatine transporter (SLC6A8) deficiency with oral s-adenosyl methionine as adjunct to l-arginine, glycine, and creatine supplements. Pediatr Neurol. 2015;53(4):360–3e2.

Joncquel M, Briand G, Valayannopoulos V, et al. Determination of new reference values for GAA and creatine from a large cohort of controls subjects and description of the French patients affected of creatine deficiency disorders (CDS). J Inherit Metab Dis. 2011;34(Suppl 3):S128.

Joncquel-Chevalier Curt M, Bout MA, Fontaine M, et al. Functional assessment of creatine transporter in control and X-linked SLC6A8-deficient fibroblasts. Mol Genet Metab. 2018;123(4):463–71.

Khaikin Y, Sidky S, Abdenur J, et al. Treatment outcome of twenty-two patients with guanidinoacetate methyltransferase deficiency: an international retrospective cohort study. Eur J Paediatr Neurol. 2018;22(3):369–79.

Mercimek-Mahmutoglu S, Salomons GS. Creatine deficiency syndromes. In: Adam MP, Ardinger HH, Pagon RA, Wallace SE, Bean LJH, Stephens K, Amemiya A, editors. GeneReviews® [Internet]. Seattle: University of Washington, Seattle; 1993-2019; 2009. [Updated 2015 Dec 10].

Mercimek-Mahmutoglu S, Connolly MB, Poskitt KJ, et al. Treatment of intractable epilepsy in a female with SLC6A8 deficiency. Mol Genet Metab. 2010;101:409–12.

Mercimek-Mahmutoglu S, Salomons GS, Chan A. Case Study for the evaluation of current treatment recommendations of guanidinoacetate methyltransferase deficiency: ineffectiveness of sodium benzoate. Pediatr Neurol. 2014;51:133–7.

Näntö-Salonen K, Komu M, Lundbom N, et al. Reduced brain creatine in gyrate atrophy of the choroid and retina with hyperornithinemia. Neurology. 1999;53:303–7.

Pasquali M, Schwarz E, Jensen M, et al. Feasibility of newborn screening for guanidinoacetate methyltransferase (GAMT) deficiency. J Inherit Metab Dis. 2014;37(2):231–6.

Peltola K, Heinonen OJ, Näntö-Salonen K, Pulkki K, Simell O. Oral lysine feeding in gyrate atrophy with hyperornithinaemia—a pilot study. J Inherit Metab Dis. 2000;23:305–57.

Reichold M, Klootwijk ED, Reinders J, et al. Glycine amidinotransferase (GATM), renal Fanconi syndrome, and kidney failure. J Am Soc Nephrol. 2018;29(7):1849–58.

Rosenberg EH, Almeida LS, Kleefstra T, et al. High prevalence of SLC6A8 deficiency in X-linked mental retardation. Am J Hum Genet. 2004;75:97–105.

Schjelderup J, Hope S, Vatshelle C, van Karnebeek CDM. Treatment experience in two adults with creatinfe transporter deficiency. Mol Genet Metab Rep. 2021;27:100731.

Schulze A, Ebinger F, Rating D, Mayatepek E. Improving treatment of guanidinoacetate methyltransferase deficiency: reduction of guanidinoacetic acid in body fluids by arginine restriction and ornithine supplementation. Mol Genet Metab. 2001;74:413–9.

Sharer JD, Bodamer O, Longo N, et al. Laboratory diagnosis of creatine deficiency syndromes: a technical standard and guideline of the American College of Medical Genetics and Genomics. Genet Med. 2017;19(2):256–63.

Shih VE. Amino acid analysis. In: Blau N, Duran M, Blaskovics ME, Gibson KM, editors. Physician's guide to the laboratory diagnosis of metabolic diseases. Berlin, Heidelberg, New York: Springer; 2003. p. 11–26.

Sinclair GB, van Karnebeek CD, Ester M, et al. A three-tier algorithm for guanidinoacetate methyltransferase (GAMT) deficiency newborn screening. Mol Genet Metab. 2016;118(3):173–7.

Stöckler-Ipsiroglu S, van Karnebeek CD. Cerebral creatine deficiencies: a group of treatable intellectual developmental disorders. Semin Neurol. 2014;35(3):350–6.

Stöckler-Ipsiroglu S, van Karnebeek C, Longo N, et al. Guanidinoacetate methyltransferase (GAMT) deficiency: outcomes in 48 individuals and recommendations for diagnosis, treatment and monitoring. Mol Genet Metab. 2014;111:16–25.

Stöckler-Ipsiroglu S, Apatean D, Battini R, et al. Arginine:Glycine Amidinotransferase (AGAT) deficiency: clinical features and long term outcomes in 16 patients diagnosed worldwide. Mol Genet Metab. 2015;116(4):252–9.

Struys EA, Verhoeven-Duif N, Jakobs C. Creatine and its metabolites. In: Blau N, Duran M, Gibson MK, editors. Laboratory guide to the methods in biochemical genetics. Berlin, Heidelberg: Springer; 2008. p. 739–49.

Valayannopoulos V, Boddaert N, Chabli A, et al. Treatment by oral creatine, L-arginine and L-glycine in six severely affected patients with creatine transporter defect. J Inherit Metab Dis. 2012; 35:151–7.

Valle D, Simell O. The hyperornithinemias. In: Scriver CR, Beaudet A, Sly WS, Valle D, editors. The metabolic and molecular bases of inherited disease. New York: McGraw Hill; 1995. p. 1147–85.

Valle D, Walser M, Brusilow S, Kaiser-Kupfer MI, Takki K. Gyrate atrophy of the choroid and retina: biochemical considerations and experience with an arginine-restricted diet. Ophthalmology. 1981;88:325–30.

van de Kamp JM, Mancini GM, Pouwels PJ, et al. Clinical features and X-inactivation in females heterozygous for creatine transporter defect. Clin Genet. 2011;79:264–72.

van de Kamp JM, Pouwels PJ, Aarsen FK, et al. Long-term follow-up and treatment in nine boys with X-linked creatine transporter defect. J Inherit Metab Dis. 2012;35(1):141–9.

van de Kamp JM, Betsalel OT, Mercimek-Mahmutoglu S, et al. Phenotype and genotype in 101 males with X-linked creatine transporter deficiency. J Med Genet. 2013;50:463–72.

Verhoeven NM, Schor DS, Roos B, et al. Diagnostic enzyme assay that uses stable-isotope-labeled substrates to detect L-arginine:glycine amidinotransferase deficiency. Clin Chem. 2003;49(5):803–5.

Viau KS, Ernst SL, Pasquali M, et al. Evidence-based treatment of guanidinoacetate methyltransferase (GAMT) deficiency. Mol Genet Metab. 2013;110(3):255–62.

Weleber RG, Kennaway NG. Clinical trial of vitamin B6 for gyrate atrophy of the choroid and retina. Ophthalmology. 1981; 88:316–24.

Young S, Struys E, Wood T (2007) Quantification of creatine and guanidinoacetate using GC-MS and LC-MS/MS for the detection of cerebral creatine deficiency syndromes. Curr Protoc Hum Genet 17.3.1–17.3.18

# Disorder of Glutathione Metabolism

# 16

Verena Peters and Johannes Zschocke

## Contents




**Summary**

Glutathione (GSH), a tripeptide composed of glutamate, cysteine, and glycine, prevents damage caused by reactive oxygen species and is metabolized via the γ-glutamyl cycle. The reduction of glutathione disulfide (GSSG) to the sulfhydryl from glutathione (GSH) is catalyzed by glutathione reductase. Several enzymes involved in the glutathione pathway, such as γ-glutamylcysteine synthetase (GCLC), glutathione synthetase (GSS), glutathione peroxidase 4 (GPX4), and glutathione reductase (GSR), are regulated, at least in part, by Nrf2 through its activation of the Nrf2-antioxidant response element. GPX4 catalyzes the reduction of hydrogen peroxide and lipid hydroperoxides at the expense of GSH.

Defects have been described in all those enzymes, except for the γ-glutamyl cyclotransferase (GGCT). The disorders are inherited in autosomal recessive, Nrf2 superactivity in an autosomal dominant manner. The most frequent disorder in human is the glutathione synthetase (GSS) deficiency, which is often associated with hemolytic anemia, a clinical feature also present in γ-glutamylcysteine (GCLC) deficiency. The severe form of glutathione synthetase (GSS) deficiency is associated with 5-oxoprolinuria, metabolic acidosis, central nervous system damage, and recurrent bacterial infections. 5-Oxoprolinuria can also be



V. Peters (✉)
Centre for Pediatric and Adolescent Medicine, University of Heidelberg, Heidelberg, Germany
e-mail: Verena.Peters@med.uni-heidelberg.de

J. Zschocke
Institute of Human Genetics, Medical University Innsbruck, Innsbruck, Austria
e-mail: johannes.zschocke@i-med.ac.at



N. Blau et al. (eds.), *Physician's Guide to the Diagnosis, Treatment, and Follow-Up of Inherited Metabolic Diseases*,
https://doi.org/10.1007/978-3-030-67727-5_16

caused by mutations in 5-oxoprolinase (OPLAH), a quite rare disease presenting with a high clinical variability. γ-Glutamyl transpeptidase (GCLC) deficiency has been found in patients with CNS involvement and glutathionuria. Dipeptidase (DPEP) deficiency has been described only in one patient with mental retardation, mild motor impairment, and partial deafness. The main clinical features of glutathione reductase (GSR) deficiency are favism and cataract. Diseases associated with glutathione peroxidase 4 (GPX4) are often associated with Sedaghatian-type spondylometaphyseal dysplasia, and Nrf2 superactivity is a multisystem disorder characterized by hypohomocysteinemia, failure to thrive, immunodeficiency, and neurodevelopmental abnormalities.

Diagnosis is made by measuring the concentration of different metabolites in the γ-glutamyl cycle and homocysteine, enzyme activity, and/or mutation analysis. Treatment aims are mainly to prevent hemolytic crises and correction of acidosis.

## Introduction

The tripeptide glutathione (γ-glutamyl-cysteinylglycine, GSH) is the major nonprotein thiol and is present in millimolar concentrations in most mammalian cells. GSH is involved in several fundamental biological functions, including detoxification, scavenging of free radicals, redox reactions, biosynthesis of DNA, proteins, and leukotrienes, neurotransmission, as well as regulation in the cell cycle (Forman et al. 2009). The ratio of reduced (GSH) and oxidized glutathione (GSSG) is used as a measure of cellular oxidative stress. Disorders of glutathione metabolism are associated with a wide range of clinical features reflecting different pathophysiological functions:

- Deficiencies of enzyme involved in the biosynthesis and regeneration of GSH (γ-glutamylcysteine synthetase, glutathione synthetase, and glutathione reductase) are associated with hemolytic anemia due to reduced redox potential in red blood cells, as well as neurological and other symptoms.
- Deficiencies of enzymes involved in the breakdown of GSH (γ-glutamyl transpeptidase, γ-glutamyl cyclotransferase, and 5-oxoprolinase) may show biochemical abnormalities but are associated with no or inconsistent clinical abnormalities or have not been identified as such.
- Other disorders affecting GSH metabolism include superactivity of the Nrf2-antioxidant response element which activates transcription of a range of antioxidant enzymes involved in GSH biosynthesis and glutathione peroxidase 4 deficiency which causes Sedaghatian-type spondylometaphyseal dysplasia presumably due to impaired regeneration of lipid hydroperoxides.

**γ-Glutamylcysteine synthetase (GCLC) deficiency** has been described in very few patients. It is associated with hemolytic anemia and can have a mild non-neurological phenotype or a more severe phenotype with neurological manifestations which is similar to GSS deficiency (Almusafri et al. 2017; Ferguson and Bridge 2016).

**Glutathione synthetase (GSS) deficiency** is the most frequently diagnosed disorder of human glutathione metabolism with more than 70 patients described worldwide (Shi et al. 1996; Signolet et al. 2016; Soylu Ustkoyuncu et al. 2018). Mildly affected patients show hemolytic anemia as their only clinical symptom. Moderately affected patients show additionally metabolic acidosis (without ketosis or hypoglycemia), and severely affected patients also develop progressive neurological symptoms, such as intellectual disability, seizures, or spasticity, and may develop recurrent bacterial infections caused by defective granulocyte function. Several patients died in early life due to acidosis and electrolyte imbalances (Ristoff and Larsson 2007). About 30 different mutations have been described so far. The type of mutation involved can, to some extent, predict a mild versus a more severe phenotype (Njalsson 2005). The diagnosis of GCLC and GSS deficiencies is mainly based on low glutathione levels and low activities of the enzymes in red blood cells or fibroblasts or the presence of mutations in the genes.

Glutathione regeneration is catalyzed by glutathione reductase by reducing GSSG to GSH. **Hereditary glutathione reductase (GSR) deficiency** was first described in 1976 (van Zwieten et al. 2014). GSR is a flavoprotein, and dietary riboflavin deficiency causes a secondary GSR deficiency. In contrast to disorders in the synthesis of glutathione, the clinical outcome of glutathione reductase deficiency seems to be less severe, mainly presenting with hemolytic anemia, favism, and cataract and one patient with severe neonatal jaundice (Kamerbeek et al. 2007).

The initial degradative step of GSH is catalyzed by γ-glutamyl transpeptidase (GGT). There are two known active GGT isoenzymes encoded by different genes, *GGT1* and *GGT5*, which have different expression patterns (Heisterkamp et al. 2008). Both are membrane-bound extracellular enzymes that hydrolyze the γ-glutamyl bond and transfer the γ-glutamyl group to an acceptor, e.g., an amino acid. GSH is resistant to intracellular breakdown as both GGT isoforms are extracellular, and no other enzyme can degrade GSH. Standard GGT biochemical assays measure the GGT1 transpeptidation reaction with an artificial substrate. Only eight patients with **γ-glutamyl transpeptidase (GGT1) deficiency** have been reported in the literature (Darin et al. 2018). The diagnosis is based on the finding of increased levels of GSH in urine and plasma and lowered enzyme activity levels. The exact genetic alteration has only been described for two siblings with glutathionuria (Darin et al. 2018). Most of the described patients have had central nervous system involvement, but causality has not been proven. Abnormalities of leukotriene metabolism have been reported in patients with GGT deficiency (see chapter on leukotriene metabolism).

Two genetic defects in the γ-glutamyl cycle have been described as causes of persistent 5-oxoprolinuria: either GSS deficiency or by **5-oxoprolinase (OPLAH) deficiency**. At least 20 mutations in *OPLAH* have been reported to date (Calpena et al. 2015; Sass et al. 2016). 5-Oxoprolinuria appears not to cause clinical symptoms and has also been observed in patients with defects in other inborn errors of metabolism, homocystinuria, type 2 diabetes, or drug metabolism as well as in other contexts (Ristoff and Larsson 2007). Further, it is considered as a worsening factor of hyperammonemic encephalopathy (Rousseau et al. 2017).

Cysteinylglycine is cleaved into cysteine and glycine by one of possibly several dipeptidases. A tentative **deficiency of cysteinylglycine dipeptidase** has been described in one patient so far, based on increased urinary cysteinylglycine and decreased activity of plasma dipeptidase. The dipeptidase also converts leukotriene D4 to leukotriene E4. Clinically, the patient presented mental retardation, mild motor impairment, and partial deafness (Mayatepek et al. 2004, 2005) (see chapter on leukotriene metabolism). Cysteine is extremely unstable and rapidly auto-oxidizes to cystine extracellularly, which can generate potentially toxic oxygen free radicals.

Glutathione peroxidase 4 (GPX4) catalyzes the reduction of hydrogen peroxide and organic and lipid hydroperoxides and therefore protects cells against oxidative damage. GPX4 is a selenoprotein (Sneddon et al. 2003), and loss of the gene (Gpx4) causes massive lipid peroxidation. **Diseases associated with GPX4** include Sedaghatian-type spondylometaphyseal dysplasia (Smith et al. 2014) and neurodegeneration (Cardoso et al. 2017). Sedaghatian-type spondylometaphyseal dysplasia is characterized by severe metaphyseal chondrodysplasia with mild limb shortening, platyspondyly, cardiac conduction defects, and central nervous system abnormalities.

The regulation of GSH synthesis is under tight control involving key enzymes including γ-glutamylcysteine synthetase, glutathione synthetase, and glutathione reductase. More importantly, these enzymes are all regulated, at least in part, by Nrf2 through its activation of the Nrf2-antioxidant response element (ARE; Abdul-Aziz et al. 2015). **Nrf2 superactivity** has been described in four patients presenting failure to thrive, immunodeficiency, and neurological symptoms (Huppke et al. 2017). Missense mutations were identified in the *NFE2L2* gene, leading to an altered cytosolic redox balance. All four patients described so far display a similar phenotype with several prominent features including developmental delay, failure to thrive, immunodeficiency, leukoencephalopathy, and hypohomocysteinemia. Hypohomocysteinemia together with elevated activity of glucose-6-phosphate dehydrogenase allows early diagnosis (Harvey et al. 2009).

## Nomenclature

| | Disorders of glutathione metabolism | Alternative name | Abbreviation | Gene | Chromosomal localization | Mode of inheritance | Affected protein | Omim |
|---|---|---|---|---|---|---|---|---|
| 16.1 | γ-Glutamyl transpeptidase deficiency | Glutathionuria; γ-glutamyl transferase deficiency | GGT1 | *GGT1* | 22q11.1-q11.2 | AR | Gamma-glutamyl transpeptidase | 612346 |
| 16.2 | 5-Oxoprolinase deficiency | | OPLAHD | *OPLAH* | 8q24.3 | AR, AD | 5-Oxoprolinase | 614243 |
| 16.3 | γ-Glutamylcysteine synthetase deficiency | Glutamate-cysteine ligase deficiency | GGCS | *GCLC* | 6p12 | AR | γ-Glutamylcysteine synthetase | 606857 |
| 16.4 | Glutathione synthetase deficiency, mild | | GSSD | *GSS* | 20q11.2 | AR | Glutathione synthetase | 601002 |
| 16.5 | Glutathione synthetase deficiency, severe | | GSSD | *GSS* | 20q11.2 | AR | Glutathione synthetase | 601002 |
| 16.6 | Dipeptidase deficiency | Membrane-bound dipeptidase deficiency | | *DPEP1* | | AR | Dipeptidase | |
| 16.7 | Glutathione reductase deficiency | Hemolytic anemia due to glutathione reductase deficiency | | *GSR* | 8p12 | AR | Glutathione reductase | 138300 |
| 16.8 | Glutathione peroxidase 4 deficiency | Spondylometaphyseal dysplasia, Sedaghatian type | | *GPX4* | 19p13.3 | AR | Glutathione peroxidase | 138322 |
| 16.9 | Nrf2 superactivity | Immunodeficiency, developmental delay, and hypohomocysteinemia (IEMDHH) | | *NFE2L2* | 2q31.2 | AD | NFE2-related transcription factor 2 (Nrf2) | 600492 |

## Metabolic Pathway

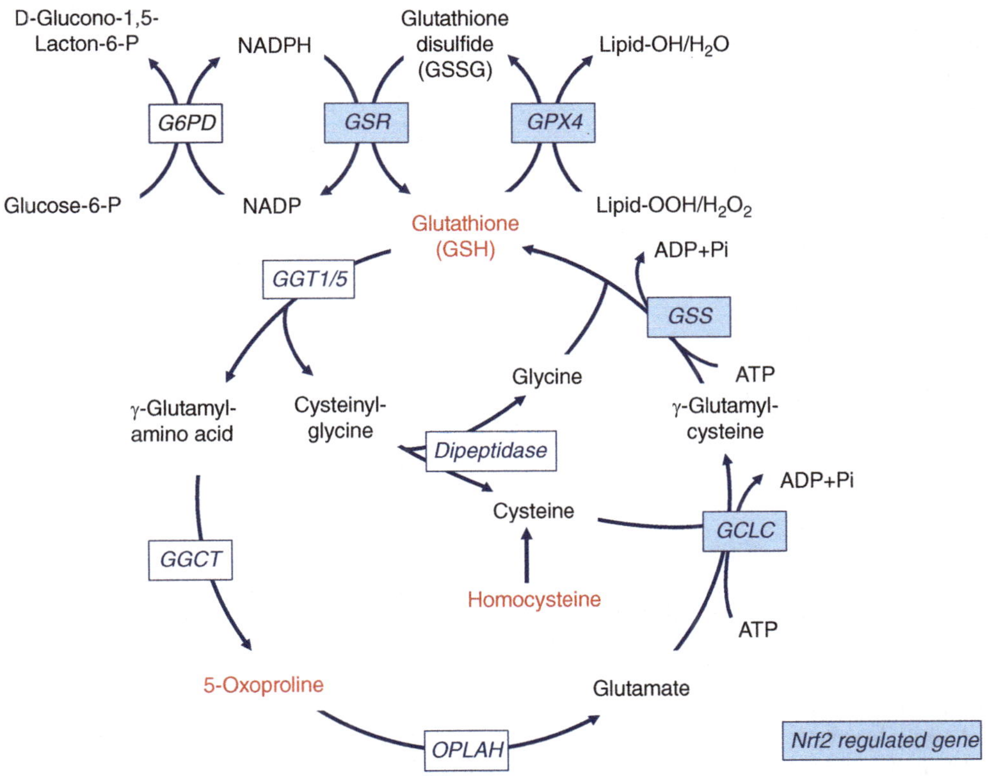


**Fig. 16.1** The γ-glutamyl cycle for the biosynthesis and degradation of glutathione including known metabolic defects: γ-glutamylcysteine synthetase (GCLC), glutathione synthetase (GSS), γ-glutamyl transpeptidase deficiency (GGT1), 5-oxoprolinase (OPLAH), and dipeptidase. The reduction of glutathione disulfide (GSSG) to glutathione (GSH) is catalyzed by glutathione reductase (GSR), and peroxidase 4 (GPX4) catalyzes the reduction of hydrogen peroxide and lipid hydroperoxides at the expense of GSH. γ-Glutamylcysteine synthetase (GCLC), glutathione synthetase (GSS), peroxidase 4 (GPX4), and glutathione reductase (GSR) are regulated, at least in part, by Nrf2 through its activation of the Nrf2-antioxidant response element. No defects have been described or the γ-glutamyl cyclotransferase (GGCT). Glucose-6-phosphate dehydrogenase (G6PD) converts glucose-6-phosphate into 6-phosphoglucono-δ-lactone. Blood glutathione and homocysteine and urinary 5-oxoproline concentrations are important diagnostic markers

## Signs and Symptoms

**Table 16.1** Glutathionuria

| System | Symptoms and biomarkers | Neonatal (birth–1 month) | Infancy (1–18 months) | Childhood (1.5–11 years) | Adolescence (11–16 years) | Adulthood (>16 years) |
|---|---|---|---|---|---|---|
| CNS | Intellectual disability | | | ± | ± | ± |
| | Tremor | | | ± | ± | ± |
| Psychiatric | Psychosis | | | ± | ± | ± |
| Laboratory findings | Gamma-glutamyltranspeptidase (fibroblasts) | ↓ | ↓ | ↓ | ↓ | ↓ |
| | Gamma-glutamyltranspeptidase (white blood cells) | ↓ | ↓ | ↓ | ↓ | ↓ |
| | Glutathione (plasma) | ↑ | ↑ | ↑ | ↑ | ↑ |
| | Glutathione (red blood cells) | n | n | n | n | n |
| | Glutathione (urine) | ↑ | ↑ | ↑ | ↑ | ↑ |
| | Leukotriene LTB4 (plasma) | n | n | n | n | n |
| | Leukotriene LTB4 (urine) | n | n | n | n | n |
| | Leukotriene LTC4 (plasma) | ↑ | ↑ | ↑ | ↑ | ↑ |
| | Leukotriene LTC4 (urine) | ↑ | ↑ | ↑ | ↑ | ↑ |
| | Leukotriene LTD4 (plasma) | ↓ | ↓ | ↓ | ↓ | ↓ |
| | Leukotriene LTD4 (urine) | ↓ | ↓ | ↓ | ↓ | ↓ |
| | Leukotriene LTE4 (plasma) | ↓ | ↓ | ↓ | ↓ | ↓ |
| | Leukotriene LTE4 (urine) | ↓ | ↓ | ↓ | ↓ | ↓ |
| | LTD4-synthesis in nucleated cells (white blood cells) | ↓ | ↓ | ↓ | ↓ | ↓ |

**Table 16.2** Oxoprolinuria

| System | Symptoms and biomarkers | Neonatal (birth–1 month) | Infancy (1–18 months) | Childhood (1.5–11 years) | Adolescence (11–16 years) | Adulthood (>16 years) |
|---|---|---|---|---|---|---|
| CNS | Microcephaly | | ± | ± | | |
| | Retardation, psychomotor | ± | ± | ± | ± | ± |
| Digestive | Colitis | | | | ± | ± |
| | Diarrhea | | | | ± | ± |
| Metabolic | Acidosis | n | n | n | n | n |
| Renal | Urolithiasis | | | ± | ± | ± |
| | Renal colic | | | ± | ± | ± |
| Laboratory findings | 5-Oxoprolinase (fibroblasts) | ↓ | ↓ | ↓ | ↓ | ↓ |
| | 5-Oxoprolinase (white blood cells) | ↓ | ↓ | ↓ | ↓ | ↓ |
| | 5-Oxoproline (urine) | ↑ | ↑ | ↑ | ↑ | ↑ |

**Table 16.3** Gamma-glutamylcysteine synthetase deficiency

| System | Symptoms and biomarkers | Neonatal (birth–1 month) | Infancy (1–18 months) | Childhood (1.5–11 years) | Adolescence (11–16 years) | Adulthood (>16 years) |
|---|---|---|---|---|---|---|
| CNS | Ataxia | ± | ± | ± | ± | ± |
| | Neuropathy | ± | ± | ± | ± | ± |
| Digestive | **Jaundice** | ± | ± | ± | ± | ± |
| Hematological | **Anemia, hemolytic** | + | + | + | + | + |
| Musculoskeletal | Myopathy | ± | ± | ± | ± | ± |
| Psychiatric | Psychosis | ± | ± | ± | ± | ± |
| Laboratory findings | Amino acids, all | n-↑ | n-↑ | n-↑ | n-↑ | n-↑ |
| | Gamma-glutamylcysteine synthetase (fibroblasts) | ↓↓↓ | ↓↓↓ | ↓↓↓ | ↓↓↓ | ↓↓↓ |
| | Gamma-glutamylcysteine synthetase (red blood cells) | ↓↓↓ | ↓↓↓ | ↓↓↓ | ↓↓↓ | ↓↓↓ |
| | Glutathione (red blood cells) | ↓↓↓ | ↓↓↓ | ↓↓↓ | ↓↓↓ | ↓↓↓ |
| | Hemoglobin (blood) | ↓ | ↓ | ↓ | ↓ | ↓ |
| | Reticulocytes (blood) | ↑ | ↑ | ↑ | ↑ | ↑ |

**Table 16.4** Glutathione synthetase deficiency, mild

| System | Symptoms and biomarkers | Neonatal (birth–1 month) | Infancy (1–18 months) | Childhood (1.5–11 years) | Adolescence (11–16 years) | Adulthood (>16 years) |
|---|---|---|---|---|---|---|
| Digestive | Jaundice | ± | ± | ± | ± | ± |
| Hematological | **Anemia, hemolytic** | + | + | + | + | + |
| Laboratory findings | 5-Oxoproline (urine) | n-↑ | n-↑ | n-↑ | n-↑ | n-↑ |
| | Gamma-glutathione synthetase (fibroblasts) | ↓↓↓ | ↓↓↓ | ↓↓↓ | ↓↓↓ | ↓↓↓ |
| | Gamma-glutathione synthetase (red blood cells) | ↓↓↓ | ↓↓↓ | ↓↓↓ | ↓↓↓ | ↓↓↓ |
| | Glutathione (red blood cells) | ↓↓ | ↓↓ | ↓↓ | ↓↓ | ↓↓ |
| | Hemoglobin (blood) | ↓ | ↓ | ↓ | ↓ | ↓ |
| | Reticulocytes (blood) | ↑ | ↑ | ↑ | ↑ | ↑ |

**Table 16.5** Glutathione synthetase deficiency, severe

| System | Symptoms and biomarkers | Neonatal (birth–1 month) | Infancy (1–18 months) | Childhood (1.5–11 years) | Adolescence (11–16 years) | Adulthood (>16 years) |
|---|---|---|---|---|---|---|
| CNS | Ataxia | | ± | ± | ± | ± |
| | Hypertonia | ± | ± | ± | ± | ± |
| | Hypotonia | ± | ± | ± | ± | ± |
| | **Neurological symptoms** | ± | ± | ± | ± | ± |
| | Retardation, psychomotor | ± | ± | ± | ± | ± |
| | Seizures | ± | ± | ± | ± | ± |
| Digestive | Jaundice | ± | ± | ± | ± | ± |
| Eye | Adaptation, dark impaired | | | ± | ± | ± |
| | Corneal clouding | | | ± | ± | ± |
| | Pigmentary retinopathy | | | ± | ± | ± |
| Hematological | **Anemia, hemolytic** | + | + | + | + | + |
| Metabolic | **Acidosis** | + | + | + | + | + |
| | **Lactic acidosis** | + | + | + | + | + |
| Musculoskeletal | Myopathy | ± | ± | ± | ± | ± |
| Other | **Recurrent bacterial infections** | ± | ± | ± | ± | ± |
| | Recurrent bacterial infections | ± | ± | ± | ± | ± |
| Laboratory findings | 5-Oxoproline (urine) | ↑↑↑ | ↑↑↑ | ↑↑↑ | ↑↑↑ | ↑↑↑ |
| | Gamma-glutathione synthetase (fibroblasts) | ↓↓↓ | ↓↓↓ | ↓↓↓ | ↓↓↓ | ↓↓↓ |
| | Gamma-glutathione synthetase (red blood cells) | ↓↓↓ | ↓↓↓ | ↓↓↓ | ↓↓↓ | ↓↓↓ |
| | Glutathione (red blood cells) | ↓↓ | ↓↓ | ↓↓ | ↓↓ | ↓↓ |
| | Hemoglobin (blood) | ↓ | ↓ | ↓ | ↓ | ↓ |
| | Lactate (plasma) | ↑ | ↑ | ↑ | ↑ | ↑ |
| | Reticulocytes (blood) | ↑ | ↑ | ↑ | ↑ | ↑ |

**Table 16.6** Membrane-bound dipeptidase deficiency[a]

| System | Symptoms and biomarkers | Neonatal (birth–1 month) | Infancy (1–18 months) | Childhood (1.5–11 years) | Adolescence (11–16 years) | Adulthood (>16 years) |
|---|---|---|---|---|---|---|
| CNS | EEG, abnormal | | | | + | |
| | Motor impairment | | | | + | |
| | **Neuropathy** | | | | + | |
| | Retardation, psychomotor | | | | + | |
| Ear | Deafness, partial | | | | + | |
| Musculoskeletal | EMG, abnormal | | | | + | |
| | Foot deformity | | | | + | |
| Laboratory findings | Cysteine, bound (urine) | | | | ↑ | |
| | Cystine (urine) | | | | ↑ | |
| | Cysteinylglycine (plasma) | | | | ↑ | |
| | Cysteinylglycine (urine) | | | | ↑ | |
| | Glutathione (red blood cells) | | | | n | |
| | Leukotriene LTD4 (urine) | | | | ↑ | |
| | Leukotriene LTE4 (urine) | | | | ↓ | |

[a]Please check chapter on leukotriene metabolism

**Table 16.7** Glutathione reductase deficiency

| System | Symptoms and biomarkers | Neonatal (birth–1 month) | Infancy (1–18 months) | Childhood (1.5–11 years) | Adolescence (11–16 years) | Adulthood (>16 years) |
|---|---|---|---|---|---|---|
| CNS | Jaundice, severe neonatal | ± | | | | |
| | Migraine | | | | | ± |
| Endocrine | Hypothyroidism | | | | | ± |
| Eye | Cataract, bilateral | | | | | ± |
| Hematological | **Anemia, hemolytic** | | | | | ± |
| | Favism | | | | | ± |
| Laboratory findings | Bilirubin (plasma) | ↑↑ | | | | |
| | Glutathione (plasma) | ↓↓ | | | | ↓↓ |
| | Glutathione reductase activity (red blood cells) | ↓↓↓ | | | | ↓↓↓ |

**Table 16.8** Glutathione peroxidase 4 deficiency

| System | Symptoms and biomarkers | Neonatal (birth–1 month) | Infancy (1–18 months) | Childhood (1.5–11 years) | Adolescence (11–16 years) | Adulthood (>16 years) |
|---|---|---|---|---|---|---|
| Cardiovascular | Cardiorespiratory problems | ± | ± | ± | | |
| CNS | Hypotonia, severe | ± | ± | ± | | |
| | Central nervous system abnormalities | ± | ± | ± | | |
| Musculoskeletal | Metaphyseal chondrodysplasia | ± | ± | ± | | |
| | Platyspondyly | ± | ± | ± | | |
| | Rhizomelic shortening of the upper limbs, mild | ± | ± | ± | | |

**Table 16.9** Nrf2 superactivity

| System | Symptoms and biomarkers | Neonatal (birth–1 month) | Infancy (1–18 months) | Childhood (1.5–11 years) | Adolescence (11–16 years) | Adulthood (>16 years) |
|---|---|---|---|---|---|---|
| Cardiovascular | Heart failure | | | ± | ± | |
| CNS | Absence seizures | | | ± | ± | |
| | **Developmental delay** | | | + | + | |
| Other | **Immunodeficiency** | | | + | + | |
| Laboratory findings | Creatinine (plasma) | | ↓ | ↓ | | |
| | Cysteine (plasma) | | ↓-n | ↓-n | | |
| | Glucose-6-phosphate dehydrogenase activity (erythrocytes) | | n-↑ | n-↑ | | |
| | Glutathione reductase activity (erythrocytes) | | ↓-n | ↓-n | | |
| | Homocysteine (plasma) | | ↓-n | ↓-n | | |

## Reference Values

| Metabolite/activity | |
|---|---|
| 5-Oxoproline (U) | <10 mmol/mol creatinine |
| Glutathione (RBC) | 4.6–10.9 nmol/mg Hb |
| G6PD activity (RBC) | 7.2–10.5 U/g Hb |
| Homocysteine (B) | <2.8 µmol/L (0–12 years) |
| | <4.1 µmol/L (12–18 years) |
| | <10 µmol/L (adults) |

## Pathological Values

| | Glutathione | | | 5-Oxoproline | Acid-base balance | Reticulocytes | Hemolytic anemia | Homocysteine | G6PD activity |
|---|---|---|---|---|---|---|---|---|---|
| | (RBC) (B) | (U) | (P) | (U) | (B) | (B) | (B) | (B) | (B) |
| γ-Glutamyl transpeptidase deficiency | N | ↑ | ↑ | N | N | N | N | | |
| 5-Oxoprolinase deficiency | N | N | N | ↑ | N | N | N | | |
| γ-Glutamylcysteine synthetase deficiency | ↓↓ | N | | N | N | ↑ | ↑ | | |
| Glutathione synthetase deficiency, mild | ↓↓ | N | | N-↑ | N | ↑ | ↑ | | |
| Glutathione synthetase deficiency, severe | ↓↓ | N | | ↑↑↑ | Acidosis | ↑ | ↑ | | |
| Glutathione reductase | N-↓ | | | | | | ↑ | | |
| Nrf2 superactivity | | | | | | | | ↓↓ | ↑↑ |

## Diagnostic Flowchart

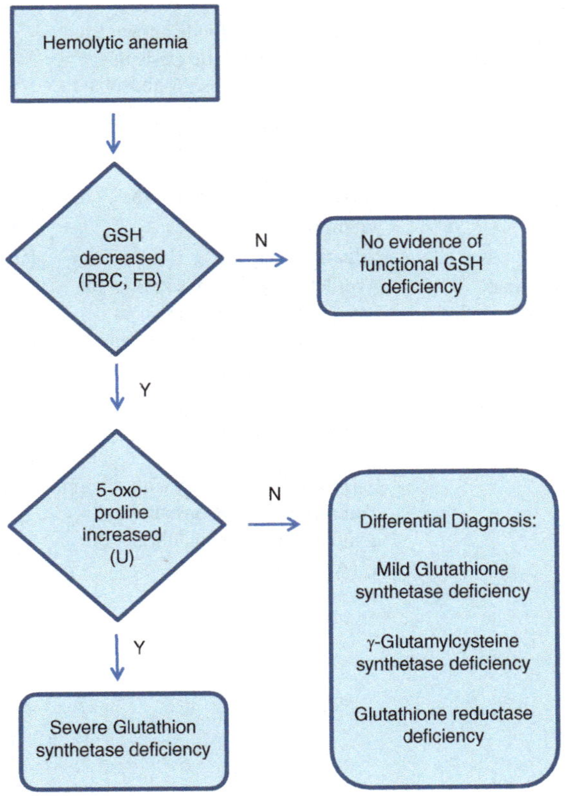


**Fig. 16.2** Biochemical diagnostic flowchart for disorders of the γ-glutamyl cycle presenting with hemolytic anemia

## Specimen Collection

| Test | Material | Handling | Pitfalls |
|---|---|---|---|
| Glutathione | RBC, B, FB | Frozen (−20 °C) | The artificial oxidation of the sulfhydryl (SH) group of GSH, occurring during sample manipulation, may cause inconsistent values |
| γ-Glutamylcysteine synthetase | RBC, LYM, FB | Frozen (−20 °C) | |
| Glutathione synthetase | RBC, LYM, FB | Frozen (−20 °C) | |
| γ-Glutamyl transpeptidase | RBC, FB, P | Frozen (−20 °C) | |
| γ-Glutamyl cyclotransferase | RBC, LYM, FB | Frozen (−20 °C) | |
| 5-Oxoprolinase | WBC, FB | Frozen (−20 °C) | |
| Glutathione reductase | LYM, RBC, tissue extracts | Cells in culture (room temperature) | |
| Glutathione peroxidase 4 | RBC, P, cell extracts | Cells in culture (room temperature) | |
| 5-Oxoproline | U | Frozen (−20 °C) | Excretion of 5-oxoproline has also been observed in patients with defects in other inborn errors of metabolism, homocystinuria, OCT deficiency, cystinosis, or type 2 diabetes or in patients receiving certain drugs (vigabatrin, paracetamol) |
| Homocysteine | P | Frozen (−20 °C) | |
| Glucose-6-phosphate dehydrogenase | RBC | Erythrocytes from EDTA blood | |
| Mutation analysis | FB, WBC, CV, AFC | Cells in culture (room temperature) | Prenatal diagnosis is greatly facilitated if the mutant allele in the specific family is known |

## Treatment Summary

Defects with decreased glutathione levels should avoid drugs that lead to oxidative stress. Also supplementation with antioxidants might be beneficial, but no studies have been made. The clinical goal of management of glutathione synthetase deficiency is the correction acidosis with bicarbonate, THAM, or sodium citrate. Early treatment with vitamin E (10 mg/kg/day) and vitamin C (100 mg/kg/day) has been shown to improve the condition (Ristoff and Larsson 2007; Soylu Ustkoyuncu et al. 2018). *N*-Acetylcysteine used to be recommended since it increases intracellular glutathione levels. However, cysteine has been shown to also accumulate, and since high cysteine levels have neurotoxic effects, treatment with *N*-acetylcysteine is no longer recommended (Ristoff and Larsson 2007). Patients with glutathione synthetase or γ-glutamylcysteine synthetase deficiency should avoid drugs that can induce hemolytic crisis in patients with glucose-6-*P*-dehydrogenase deficiency, e.g., phenobarbital, acetylsalicylic acid, and sulfonamides. Daily oral treatment of Nrf2 superactivity in one patient with 50 mg luteolin and 200 mg ascorbic acid reduced the frequency of infections (Huppke et al. 2017). No specific treatment has been proposed for γ-glutamyl transpeptidase, 5-oxoprolinase, dipeptidase, glutathione peroxidase 4, and glutathione reductase deficiency.

## Standard Treatment

| Disorder | Treatment/diet | Dosage (mg/kg/day) |
|---|---|---|
| γ-Glutamyl transpeptidase deficiency | No treatment has been recommended | |
| 5-Oxoprolinase deficiency | No treatment has been recommended | |
| γ-Glutamylcysteine synthetase deficiency | Avoid drugs and foods known to precipitate hemolytic crisis in patients with glucose-6-phosphate dehydrogenase deficiency, e.g., phenobarbital, acetylsalicylic acid, sulfonamides | |
| | Early supplementation with: | |
| | Vitamin C | 100 |
| | Vitamin E | 10 |
| Glutathione synthetase deficiency | Avoid drugs and foods known to precipitate hemolytic crisis in patients with glucose-6-phosphate dehydrogenase deficiency | |
| | Early supplementation with: | |
| | Vitamin C | 100 |
| | Vitamin E | 10 |
| | Early supplementation with vitamin C and vitamin E. Correction of acidosis (bicarbonate, citrate, or THAM) | |

| Disorder | Treatment/diet | Dosage (mg/kg/day) |
|---|---|---|
| | Avoid drugs and foods known to precipitate hemolytic crisis in patients with glucose-6-phosphate dehydrogenase deficiency. Early supplementation with vitamin C and vitamin E. Correction of acidosis (bicarbonate, citrate, or THAM) | |
| Dipeptidase deficiency | No treatment has been recommended | |
| Glutathione reductase deficiency | No treatment has been recommended | |
| Glutathione peroxidase 4 deficiency | No treatment has been recommended | |

## Experimental Treatment

| Disorder | Treatment/diet | Dosage |
|---|---|---|
| Nrf2 superactivity | Supplementation with luteolin[a] | 50 mg/day |
| | And ascorbic acid [a] | 200 mg/day |

[a]Treatment of one patient with luteolin and ascorbic acid had no side effects but seemed to reduce the frequency of infections and increased muscle strength and endurance and general school performance (Huppke et al. 2017)

## Follow-Up and Monitoring

| Disorder | Clinical investigations | Laboratory investigations |
|---|---|---|
| γ-Glutamyl transpeptidase deficiency | Neurological investigations | |
| 5-Oxoprolinase deficiency | Neurological investigations | Acid-base balance |
| γ-Glutamylcysteine synthetase deficiency | Neurological investigations | Hb, reticulocytes |
| Glutathione synthetase deficiency | Neurological investigations | Acid-base balance |
| | Eye examination (retinal pigmentations, corneal opacities) | Hb, reticulocytes |

## References


Abdul-Aziz A, MacEwan DJ, Bowles KM, Rushworth SA. Oxidative stress responses and NRF2 in human leukaemia. Oxidative Med Cell Longev. 2015;2015:454659.

Almusafri F, Elamin HE, Khalaf TE, Ali A, Ben-Omran T, El-Hattab AW. Clinical and molecular characterization of 6 children with glutamate-cysteine ligase deficiency causing hemolytic anemia. Blood Cells Mol Dis. 2017;65:73–7.

Calpena E, Deshpande AA, Yap S, Kumar A, Manning NJ, Bachhawat AK, Espinos C. New insights into the genetics of 5-oxoprolinase deficiency and further evidence that it is a benign biochemical condition. Eur J Pediatr. 2015;174:407–11.

Cardoso BR, Hare DJ, Bush AI, Roberts BR. Glutathione peroxidase 4: a new player in neurodegeneration? Mol Psychiatry. 2017;22:328–35.

Darin N, Leckstrom K, Sikora P, Lindgren J, Almen G, Asin-Cayuela J. Gamma-glutamyl transpeptidase deficiency caused by a large homozygous intragenic deletion in GGT1. Eur J Hum Genet. 2018;26:808–17.

Ferguson G, Bridge W. Glutamate cysteine ligase and the age-related decline in cellular glutathione: the therapeutic potential of gamma-glutamylcysteine. Arch Biochem Biophys. 2016;593:12–23.

Forman HJ, Zhang H, Rinna A. Glutathione: overview of its protective roles, measurement, and biosynthesis. Mol Asp Med. 2009;30:1–12.

Harvey C, Thimmulappa R, Singh A, Blake D, Ling G, Wakabayashi N, Fujii J, Myers A, Biswal S. Nrf2-regulated glutathione recycling independent of biosynthesis is critical for cell survival during oxidative stress. Free Radic Biol Med. 2009;46:443–53.

Heisterkamp N, Groffen J, Warburton D, Sneddon TP. The human gamma-glutamyltransferase gene family. Hum Genet. 2008;123:321–32.

Huppke P, Weissbach S, Church JA, Schnur R, Krusen M, Dreha-Kulaczewski S, Kuhn-Velten WN, Wolf A, Huppke B, Millan F, et al. Activating de novo mutations in NFE2L2 encoding NRF2 cause a multisystem disorder. Nat Commun. 2017;8:818.

Kamerbeek NM, van Zwieten R, de Boer M, Morren G, Vuil H, Bannink N, Lincke C, Dolman KM, Becker K, Schirmer RH, et al. Molecular basis of glutathione reductase deficiency in human blood cells. Blood. 2007;109:3560–6.

Mayatepek E, Okun JG, Meissner T, Assmann B, Hammond J, Zschocke J, Lehmann WD. Synthesis and metabolism of leukotrienes in gamma-glutamyl transpeptidase deficiency. J Lipid Res. 2004;45:900–4.

Mayatepek E, Badiou S, Bellet H, Lehmann WD. A patient with neurological symptoms and abnormal leukotriene metabolism: a new defect in leukotriene biosynthesis. Ann Neurol. 2005;58:968–70.

Njalsson R. Glutathione synthetase deficiency. Cell Mol Life Sci. 2005;62:1938–45.

Ristoff E, Larsson A. Inborn errors in the metabolism of glutathione. Orphanet J Rare Dis. 2007;2:16.

Rousseau G, Signolet I, Denis MC, Chao de la Barca JM, Mahieu R, Letournel F, Reynier P, Simard G. 5-Oxoprolinuria in hyperammonemic encephalopathy: coincidence or worsening factor? Clin Biochem. 2017;50:1115–7.

Sass JO, Gemperle-Britschgi C, Tarailo-Graovac M, Patel N, Walter M, Jordanova A, Alfadhel M, Baric I, Coker M, Damli-Huber A, et al. Unravelling 5-oxoprolinuria (pyroglutamic aciduria) due to bi-allelic OPLAH mutations: 20 new mutations in 14 families. Mol Genet Metab. 2016;119:44–9.

Shi ZZ, Habib GM, Rhead WJ, Gahl WA, He X, Sazer S, Lieberman MW. Mutations in the glutathione synthetase gene cause 5-oxoprolinuria. Nat Genet. 1996;14:361–5.

Signolet I, Chenouard R, Oca F, Barth M, Reynier P, Denis MC, Simard G. Recurrent isolated neonatal hemolytic anemia: think about glutathione synthetase deficiency. Pediatrics. 2016;138:e20154324.

Smith AC, Mears AJ, Bunker R, Ahmed A, MacKenzie M, Schwartzentruber JA, Beaulieu CL, Ferretti E, Majewski J, Bulman DE, et al. Mutations in the enzyme glutathione peroxidase 4 cause Sedaghatian-type spondylometaphyseal dysplasia. J Med Genet. 2014;51:470–4.

Sneddon AA, Wu HC, Farquharson A, Grant I, Arthur JR, Rotondo D, Choe SN, Wahle KW. Regulation of selenoprotein GPx4 expression and activity in human endothelial cells by fatty acids, cytokines and antioxidants. Atherosclerosis. 2003;171:57–65.

Soylu Ustkoyuncu P, Mutlu FT, Kiraz A, Tag Balkis Z, Yel S. A rare cause of neonatal hemolytic anemia: glutathione synthetase deficiency. J Pediatr Hematol Oncol. 2018;40:e45–9.

van Zwieten R, Verhoeven AJ, Roos D. Inborn defects in the antioxidant systems of human red blood cells. Free Radic Biol Med. 2014;67:377–86.

# Disorders of Ammonia Detoxification

# 17

Johannes Häberle and Vicente Rubio

## Contents



**Summary**

Ammonia, a product of protein catabolism, is detoxified in the liver by the urea cycle in a process that involves mitochondria and cytosol and that is carried out by six enzymes and two mitochondrial amino acid antiporters. Deficiencies in these enzymes and antiporters hamper ammonia detoxification and can cause *primary hyperammonemia*, a life- and cognition-threatening situation that can occur at any age and that can develop within hours from imbalance between ammonia production and detoxification, as in newborns with urea cycle defects following delivery. Hyperammonemia manifestations are generally unspecific and are mainly neurological, gastrointestinal, or psychiatric. Their hallmark is an unexplained change in consciousness and neurological status; indeed, hyperammonemia should be immediately excluded in any unexplained encephalopathy. Acute hyperammonemia is an emergency requiring urgent establishment of anabolism and avoidance of protein catabolism with rapid initiation (except in citrin deficiency, very rare in the West but not in the Orient) of parenteral glucose infusion and protein restriction. Additional urgent measures include dialysis to remove ammonia, and administration of carbamylglutamate and either L-arginine or L-citrulline, to try to enhance residual urea cycle function, and of the nitrogen scavengers sodium benzoate and/or sodium phenylacetate (or its

J. Häberle (✉)
Division of Metabolism and Children's Research Center, University Children's Hospital, Zürich, Switzerland
e-mail: johannes.haeberle@kispi.uzh.ch

V. Rubio
Structural Enzymopathology Unit, Department of Genomics and Proteomics, Instituto de Biomedicina de Valencia of the Spanish National Research Council (CSIC) and Centre for Biomedical Network Research on Rare Diseases (CIBERER-ISCIII), Valencia, Spain
e-mail: rubio@ibv.csic.es


N. Blau et al. (eds.), *Physician's Guide to the Diagnosis, Treatment, and Follow-Up of Inherited Metabolic Diseases*,
https://doi.org/10.1007/978-3-030-67727-5_17

precursor, phenylbutyrate), to excrete nitrogen without use of the urea cycle. Liver transplantation is curative, correcting hepatic urea cycle function. Prognosis of acute hyperammonemia, still poor, is improving with increasing healthcare professionals' awareness.

As urea cycle operation needs substrates (ammonia, aspartate, ATP, bicarbonate, ornithine, glutamate, and acetyl coenzyme A), it can be hampered by substrate depletion or by toxic metabolites, as in *secondary hyperammonemias*. This chapter, in addition to focusing on defects of core urea cycle catalysts, will deal with other genetic conditions that may hamper the supply of ornithine, bicarbonate, glutamate, or ATP and other conditions with an impact on ammonia levels such as glutamine synthetase deficiency and glutamate dehydrogenase superactivity.

## Introduction

Ammonia, the nitrogenous waste product of protein catabolism, crosses biological membranes and reaches the brain, where it is a potent neurotoxin. It causes brain edema possibly because of increased ammonia-dependent glutamine synthesis/accumulation in glial cells, with concomitant osmotically mediated water influx. Oxidative damage may also contribute to ammonia neurotoxicity (Häussinger and Görg 2010). The effects of hyperammonemia are mainly dependent on its duration and severity. Thus, it is essential to control arterial blood ammonia levels within narrow ranges (<100 µmol/L in newborns; <50 µmol/L beyond the neonatal period; Colombo et al. 1984). This is achieved by liver conversion of most of the ammonia to urea for urinary excretion, using for this conversion the urea cycle.

Periportal hepatocytes are the only cells having all the enzymes of the urea cycle (Fig. 17.1) (Grisolia et al. 1976). They extract ammonia from the portal blood (much richer in ammonia than peripheral blood) or produce it from glutamine by glutaminase (Häussinger 1990b) or from glutamate by oxidative deamination catalyzed by glutamate dehydrogenase (Fig. 17.1). In an ATP-consuming process, one molecule of each ammonia and bicarbonate enters the urea cycle inside the mitochondria of periportal hepatocytes, where the first two steps of the urea cycle, catalyzed by carbamoyl phosphate synthetase I (CPS1) and ornithine transcarbamylase (OTC), take place. The remaining three urea cycle steps, catalyzed by argininosuccinate synthetase (ASS), argininosuccinate lyase (ASL), and arginase (ARG1), are cytosolic. ASS incorporates, in an ATP-using reaction, the second ammonia molecule of urea, which is donated by aspartate (Fig. 17.1), with release by ASL of fumarate, which is reconverted to aspartate by incorporation of another ammonia molecule, to be used again by ASS. This involves the shuttling of intermediates in and out of the mitochondria and involving citrin, a liver-specific aspartate-glutamate/$H^+$ mitochondrial antiporter that delivers mitochondrial aspartate to ASS. Overall, urea production from ammonia requires the concerted action of five enzymes and of two mitochondrial transporters (citrin and the ornithine/citrulline mitochondrial antiporter) (Fig. 17.1). Defects in these enzymes and transporters as well as in *N*-acetylglutamate synthase (NAGS), the enzyme that produces the essential activator of CPS1, *N*-acetylglutamate (Tables 17.1, 17.2, 17.3, 17.4, 17.5, 17.6, 17.7 and 17.8), cause *primary hyperammonemia*. Symptoms of hyperammonemia dominate the presentations of CPS1 and OTC deficiencies, while hyperammonemia becomes less prominent more downstream in the cycle, particularly with ARG1 deficiency. Except OTC deficiency, which exhibits X-linked inheritance, all these defects present autosomal recessive inheritance.

This chapter covers, too, inborn errors in which ammonia detoxification can be impaired secondarily, largely by deficiency of urea cycle substrates (ammonia, aspartate, ATP, bicarbonate, ornithine, glutamate, and acetyl coenzyme A) (Häberle 2011). In the deficiency of carbonic anhydrase VA (CAVA; the specific form of carbonic anhydrase expressed in liver mitochondria) (Table 17.9), there is lack of intramitochondrial bicarbonate resulting in functional CPS1 deficiency. In lysinuric protein intolerance (LPI) (Table 17.10), citrulline, arginine, and ornithine are lost in the urine, impairing flux through the urea cycle. In pyrroline-5-carboxylate synthetase (P5CS) deficiency, the endogenous supply of ornithine is compromised (as well as proline synthesis; P5CS catalyzes the first step of both ornithine and proline synthesis). Depending on the mutation, P5CS deficiency presents dominant or recessive inheritance and can manifest (Tables 17.11, 17.12, and 17.13) as an early onset neurocutaneous syndrome or a later onset complicated spastic paraplegia with (recessive) or without (dominant) mental disability (Marco-Marin et al. 2020). Ornithine aminotransferase (OAT) deficiency can lead to neonatal or early infantile hyperammonemia (Table 17.14), reflecting the role of OAT in ornithine synthesis. The autosomal dominant inherited hyperinsulinism-hyperammonemia (HIHA) syndrome (Table 17.15) results from gain-of-function mutations affecting glutamate dehydrogenase (GLUD) that cause nonregulated glutamate deamination. Following conversion of most of the portal blood ammonia to urea by periportal hepatocytes, perivenous hepatocytes further decrease the ammonia level of the liver-exiting blood by making glutamine with glutamine synthetase (GS) (Häussinger 1990a). GS deficiency is an ultra-rare condition included in this chapter because it presents moderate hyperammonemia (Table 17.16) although the urea cycle functions normally. Hyperammonemia due to impaired aspartate availability for ASS function is observed in patients of type B pyruvate carboxylase (PC) deficiency (Table 17.17). Finally, transmembrane protein 70 (TMEM70) deficiency is also included here because hyperammonemia is a manifestation of this complex condition in which oxidative phosphorylation complex V is defective, causing hypertrophic cardiomyopathy (Table 17.18).

When ammonia production exceeds urea synthesis, as in the inborn errors of the urea cycle, blood ammonia levels escalate and can reach in few hours even millimolar concentrations. The *clinical consequences of hyperammonemia* develop in parallel, with rapid escalation towards coma, rendering time crucial in the management of these patients. In about half of the patients, urea cycle disorders present within 2–3 days from birth with somnolence and lethargy accompanied by vomiting, temperature instability, and seizures, with rapid progression to coma (Brusilow and Horwich 2001; Leonard and Morris 2002). The other half of the patients exhibit later presentation (Summar et al. 2008) that can be as severe as in newborns. Indeed, urea cycle disorders can manifest at any age.

*Diagnosis* of the underlying disorder relies on studies of metabolites (Fig. 17.2) followed by molecular genetic (or sometimes enzymatic) confirmation.

*Treatment* of acute hyperammonemia aims at immediate lowering of the ammonia levels by (1) preventing protein catabolism and establishing anabolism by starting parenteral high-dose glucose infusion and stopping protein intake; (2) administering iv. the nitrogen scavengers sodium benzoate and/or sodium phenylacetate to eliminate nitrogen by alternative pathways that circumvent the urea cycle (benzoate conjugates with glycine, yielding hippurate that is excreted in the urine; the same happens for glutamine with phenylacetate, of which phenylbutyrate is a precursor) (Batshaw et al. 2001); (3) stimulating residual urea cycle function by giving, depending on the disorder, L-arginine and/or L-citrulline (these are urea cycle intermediates; Fig. 17.1) and, in NAGS deficiency and in patients with unclear diagnosis, by giving intragastrically *N*-carbamylglutamate (a commercial *N*-acetylglutamate analog that is effective orally (Rubio and Grisolia 1981)) and (4) preparing extracorporeal dialysis to rapidly lower ammonia. Chronic treatment for primary urea cycle disorders includes protein restriction (Leonard 2001; Singh 2007); supplementation of essential amino acids, trace elements, and vitamins; and oral use of nitrogen scavengers and of L-arginine or L-citrulline or, in NAGS deficiency, of *N*-carbamylglutamate. The only definitive cure of most of these conditions is liver transplantation, strongly recommended for patients with neonatal onset (Leonard and McKiernan 2004). Chronic treatment for most conditions that affect the urea cycle indirectly follows the same principles but may require additional action.

*Prognosis* is still bleak, particularly in cases with prolonged, severe, or recurrent episodes of metabolic decompensation (Gropman and Batshaw 2004; Gropman et al. 2007), since the duration and frequency of comatose episodes determine the severity of neurological sequelae (Picca et al. 2001). However, prognosis can be improved by earlier recognition of new patients and earlier specific therapy (Nassogne et al. 2005). Hopefully, enhanced awareness will lead to more widely available diagnosis, earlier start of specific therapy including dialysis, and hence better prognosis, while increased access to liver transplantation should expand the reach of curative therapy. New therapies, some of which still experimental, including gene therapy or editing, chemical chaperoning, nonsense mutation therapeutics, and enzyme substitution will hopefully soon reach clinical practice.

## Nomenclature

| No. | Disorder | Alternative name | Abbreviation | Gene symbol | Chromosomal localization | Affected protein | OMIM no. | Subtype |
|---|---|---|---|---|---|---|---|---|
| 17.1 | *N*-acetylglutamate synthase deficiency | NAGS deficiency | NAGS deficiency | *NAGS* | 17q21.31 | *N*-acetylglutamate synthase | 237310 | All forms |
| 17.2 | Carbamoyl phosphate synthetase I deficiency | CPS1 deficiency | CPS I deficiency | *CPS1* | 2q34 | Carbamoyl phosphate synthetase I | 237300 | All forms |
| 17.3 | Ornithine transcarbamylase deficiency | Ornithine carbamoyltransferase deficiency | OTC deficiency | *OTC* | Xp11.4 | Ornithine transcarbamylase | 311250 | All forms |
| 17.4 | Citrullinemia type I | Argininosuccinate synthetase deficiency | CTLN1 | *ASS1* | 9q34.11 | Argininosuccinate synthetase | 215700 | All forms |
| 17.5 | Argininosuccinic aciduria | Argininosuccinate lyase deficiency | ASL deficiency | *ASL* | 7q11.21 | Argininosuccinate lyase | 207900 | All forms |
| 17.6 | Argininemia | Arginase 1 deficiency | ARG1 deficiency | *ARG1* | 6q23.2 | Arginase 1 | 207800 | All forms |
| 17.7 | HHH syndrome | Hyperammonemia-hyperornithinemia-homocitrullinuria syndrome | HHH syndrome; ORNT1 deficiency | *ORNT1* | 13q14.11 | Mitochondrial ornithine transporter (ORNT1) SLC25A15 | 238970 | All forms |
| 17.8 | Citrin deficiency | Citrin deficiency of the adult neonatal intrahepatic cholestasis caused by citrin deficiency | CTLN2 | *SLC25A13* | 7q21.3 | Aspartate-glutamate carrier (SLC25A13) | 605814, 603471 | All forms |
| 17.9 | Carbonic anhydrase VA deficiency | CAVA deficiency | CAVA deficiency | *CA5A* | 16q24.2 | Carbonic anhydrase VA | 615751 | All forms |
| 17.10 | Lysinuric protein intolerance | Dibasic amino aciduria type 2 | LPI | *SLC7A7* | 14q11.2 | Cationic amino acid transporter, $y^{+}L$ system | 222700 | All forms |
| 17.11 | Pyrroline-5-carboxylate synthetase deficiency | P5CS deficiency, De Barsy syndrome ALDH18A1-associated | P5CS deficiency, ARCL3A, ADCL3 | *ALDH18A1* | 10q24.1 | Pyrroline-5-carboxylate synthetase | 219150, 616603 | Cutis laxa phenotype, dominant and recessive |
| 17.12, 17.13 | Pyrroline-5-carboxylate synthetase deficiency | P5CS deficiency, hereditary spastic paraplegia 9 | P5CS deficiency, SPG9 | *ALDH18A1* | 10q24.1 | Pyrroline-5-carboxylate synthetase | 601162, 616586 | Spastic paraplegia phenotype, dominant and recessive |
| 17.14 | Ornithine aminotransferase deficiency | Gyrate atrophy of choroid and retina | OAT deficiency | *OAT* | 10q26.13 | Ornithine aminotransferase | 258870 | All forms |
| 17.15 | Glutamate dehydrogenase superactivity | Hyperinsulinism-hyperammonemia syndrome; familial hyperinsulinemic hypoglycemia type 6 | HIHA syndrome; HHF6 | *GLUD1* | 10q23.2 | Glutamate dehydrogenase | 606762 | All forms |
| 17.16 | Glutamine synthetase deficiency | GS deficiency | GS deficiency | *GLUL* | 1q25.3 | Glutamine synthetase | 610015 | All forms |
| 17.17 | Pyruvate carboxylase deficiency | Pyruvate carboxylase deficiency of French type | PC deficiency, French type | *PC* | 11q13.2 | Pyruvate carboxylase | 266150 | Type B |
| 17.18 | Transmembrane protein 70 deficiency | Mitochondrial complex V (ATP synthase) deficiency | TMEM70 deficiency, MC5DN2 | *TMEM70* | 8q21.11 | Transmembrane protein 70 | 614052 | All forms |

## Metabolic Pathways

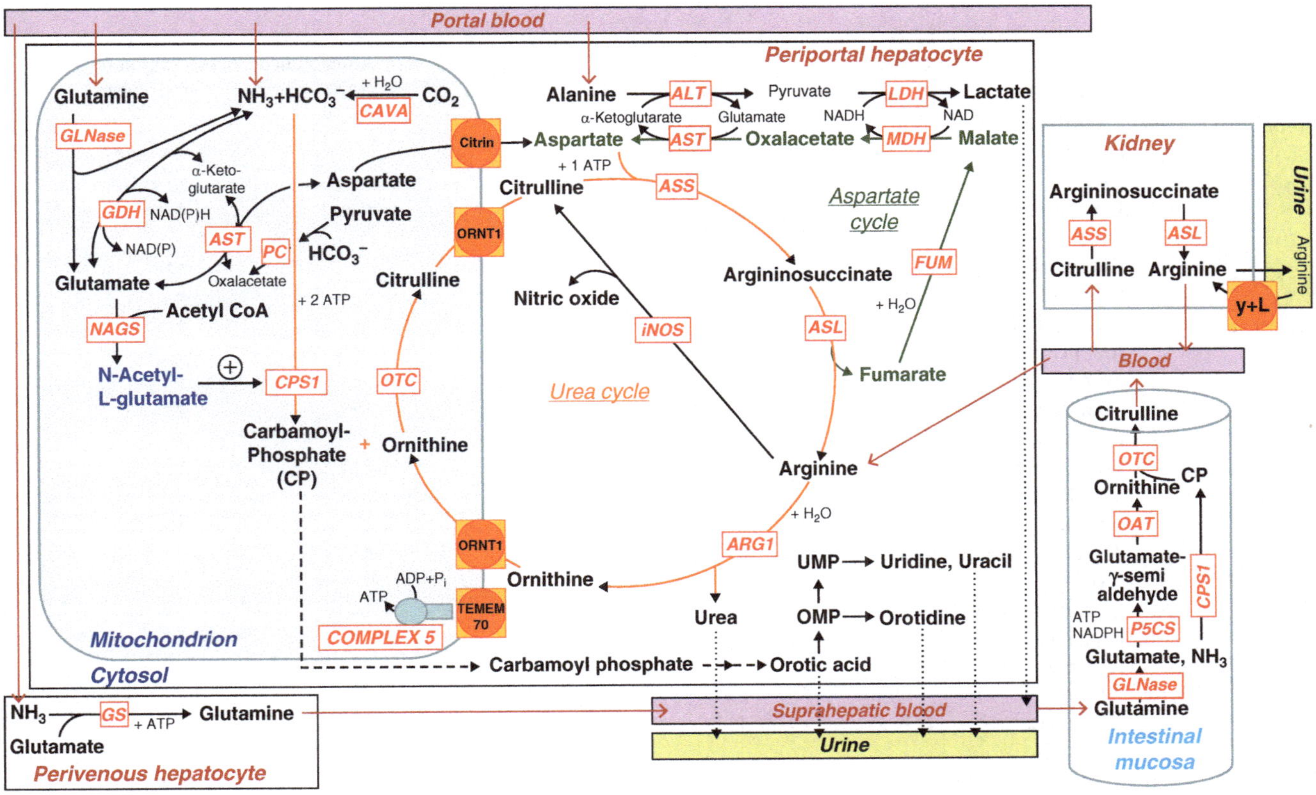


**Fig. 17.1** The urea cycle and associated pathways. The central larger rectangle represents a periportal hepatocyte with the urea cycle and some ancillary reaction within it. For simplicity, not all the substrates and products of each reaction are shown. The main nitrogen-containing compounds taken by urea-synthesizing periportal hepatocytes include ammonia, glutamine, and other amino acids of which alanine is shown as the paradigm. Glutaminase (*GLNase*) and glutamate dehydrogenase (*GDH*) can supply ammonia from glutamine and glutamate, respectively, for entry into the urea cycle at the *CPS1* step. The various transaminases (of which alanine aminotransferase, *ALT*, is shown as the paradigm), coupled to aspartic transaminase (*AST*), provide the other N atom of urea as the aspartate used in the *ASS* reaction. Aspartate can also be provided by exporting it from mitochondria by citrin (in exchange for glutamate and a proton, not shown for simplicity). The fumarate produced in the *ASL* reaction is recycled and reconverted to aspartate in the "aspartate cycle," which combines the actions of fumarase (*FUM*), malate dehydrogenase (*MDH*), and *AST*. This cycle can be carried out in the cytosol if there is an adequate cytosolic supply of NAD as when utilizing alanine (thanks to the conversion of alanine-derived pyruvate to lactate by lactate dehydrogenase, *LDH*). However, if there is little cytosolic NAD supply, the malate produced by fumarase enters the mitochondria (in exchange for α-ketoglutarate), where it is converted to aspartate, which is then exported to the cytosol via citrin (for simplicity, this variant of the aspartate cycle is not shown). For convenience, the mitochondrial ornithine/citrulline antiporter (ORNT1) has been illustrated transporting separately ornithine and citrulline, although it exchanges ornithine for citrulline. A double-lined arrow next to an encircled plus sign indicates allosteric activation of *CPS1* by *N*-acetyl-L-glutamate (in blue). The reactions of pyruvate carboxylase (*PC*) in the context of mitochondrial aspartate production and of carbonic anhydrase type 5 (*CAVA*) supplying bicarbonate to CPS1 are also schematized in the mitochondria. TMEM70 is also shown in the mitochondrial membrane together with the respiratory complex *5* that is built if TMEM70 is functional, schematizing the role of this complex in mitochondrial ATP synthesis. At the bottom of the figure, in a smaller rectangle symbolizing a perivenous hepatocyte, glutamine synthesis by glutamine synthetase (*GS*) is schematized as a "polishing" reaction that converts to glutamine the small amounts of ammonia that have not been used up by periportal hepatocytes to make urea. "De novo" ornithine and citrulline synthesis from glutamate by $\Delta^1$-pyrroline-5-carboxylate synthetase (*P5CS*) and δ-ornithine aminotransferase (*OAT*) is shown on the right, within a cylinder that symbolizes the small intestine, showing also the conversion by the kidney to arginine of the citrulline exported by the intestine to blood, illustrating the fact that this arginine ultimately provides the ornithine used by the liver to make urea. Not shown is the role of the *P5CS* reaction in proline synthesis, since it is also the first step of proline synthesis, where the glutamate semialdehyde cyclizes spontaneously to pyrroline carboxylate, which is then reduced by a reductase to give proline. This reaction occurs in most tissues but not in the intestine. Also shown in the kidney is $y^+L$, the system that reabsorbs dibasic amino acids and that does not work properly in LPI. The figure of the periportal hepatocyte also shows nitric oxide synthase (i*NOS* in the case of hepatocytes) in its position across the cytosolic part of the urea cycle. In macrophages and vascular cells, a reduced cycle involving ASS, ASL, and NOS appears to be operative. NAD(P) and NAD(P)H denote that *GDH* can use both NAD and NADP (and its reduced forms); *OMP* orotidine monophosphate, *UMP* uridine monophosphate. (This figure summarizes information from many sources, all of which cannot be listed because of space constraints. A summary of much knowledge is provided in Grisolia et al. (1976), with more recent data from Häussinger (1990b) and Mori et al. (1998). Data for the citrin transporter is reviewed in Imamura et al. (2003) and Mutoh et al. (2008))

## Signs and Symptoms

**Table 17.1** *N*-acetylglutamate synthase deficiency

| System | Symptoms and biomarkers | Neonatal (birth–1 month) | Infancy (1–18 months) | Childhood (1.5–11 years) | Adolescence (11–16 years) | Adulthood (>16 years) |
|---|---|---|---|---|---|---|
| Autonomic system | Temperature instability[a] | ± | | | | |
| CNS | **Coma** | +++ | +++ | ++ | ++ | ++ |
| | **Developmental delay** | | ±-++ | ±-++ | ±-++ | ±-++ |
| | **Encephalopathy** | +++ | +++ | ++ | ++ | ++ |
| | **Seizures**[a] | +++ | + | + | + | + |
| Digestive | **Feeding difficulties, protein aversion** | ++ | ++ | ++ | ++ | ++ |
| | **Vomiting** | +++ | ++ | ++ | ++ | ++ |
| Other | Failure to thrive | ± | ± | ± | ± | ± |
| Laboratory findings | Ammonia (blood and plasma) | ↑↑↑ | ↑↑↑ | ↑↑↑ | ↑↑↑ | ↑↑↑ |
| | Arginine (plasma) | ↓ | ↓ | ↓ | ↓ | ↓ |
| | Argininosuccinate (urine) | n | n | n | n | n |
| | Citrulline (plasma) | ↓↓↓ | ↓↓ | ↓↓ | ↓↓ | ↓↓ |
| | Glutamine (cerebrospinal fluid) | ↑↑↑ | ↑↑↑ | ↑↑↑ | ↑↑ | ↑↑ |
| | Glutamine (plasma) | ↑↑↑ | ↑↑↑ | ↑↑↑ | ↑↑ | ↑↑ |
| | Orotic acid (urine) | ↓-n | ↓-n | ↓-n | ↓-n | ↓-n |

[a]Mainly in encephalopathic crises

**Table 17.2** Carbamoyl phosphate synthetase I deficiency

| System | Symptoms and biomarkers | Neonatal (birth–1 month) | Infancy (1–18 months) | Childhood (1.5–11 years) | Adolescence (11–16 years) | Adulthood (>16 years) |
|---|---|---|---|---|---|---|
| Autonomic system | Temperature instability[a] | ± | | | | |
| CNS | **Coma** | +++ | +++ | ++ | ++ | ++ |
| | **Developmental delay** | | ±-++ | ±-++ | ±-++ | ±-++ |
| | **Encephalopathy** | +++ | +++ | ++ | ++ | ++ |
| | **Seizures**[a] | +++ | + | + | + | + |
| Digestive | **Feeding difficulties, protein aversion** | ++ | ++ | ++ | ++ | ++ |
| | **Vomiting** | +++ | ++ | ++ | ++ | ++ |
| Other | Failure to thrive | ± | ± | ± | ± | ± |
| Laboratory findings | 3-Methylglutaconic acid (urine) | ↑-n | ↑-n | ↑-n | ↑-n | ↑-n |
| | Ammonia (blood and plasma) | ↑↑↑ | ↑↑↑ | ↑↑↑ | ↑↑↑ | ↑↑↑ |
| | Arginine (plasma) | ↓ | ↓ | ↓ | ↓ | ↓ |
| | Argininosuccinate (urine) | n | n | n | n | n |
| | Citrulline (plasma) | ↓↓↓ | ↓↓ | ↓↓ | ↓↓ | ↓↓ |
| | Glutamine (cerebrospinal fluid) | ↑↑↑ | ↑↑↑ | ↑↑↑ | ↑↑ | ↑↑ |
| | Glutamine (plasma) | ↑↑↑ | ↑↑↑ | ↑↑↑ | ↑↑ | ↑↑ |
| | Orotic acid (urine) | ↓-n | ↓-n | ↓-n | ↓-n | ↓-n |

[a]Mainly in encephalopathic crises

**Table 17.3** Ornithine transcarbamylase deficiency

| System | Symptoms and biomarkers | Neonatal (birth–1 month) | Infancy (1–18 months) | Childhood (1.5–11 years) | Adolescence (11–16 years) | Adulthood (>16 years) |
|---|---|---|---|---|---|---|
| Autonomic system | Temperature instability[a] | ± | | | | |
| CNS | Asterixis | | | | | ± |
| | Ataxia | | | ± | ± | ± |
| | **Coma** | +++ | +++ | ++ | ++ | ++ |
| | Confusion, episodic | | – | ± | ± | ± |
| | **Developmental delay** | | ±-++ | ±-++ | ±-++ | ±-++ |
| | **Encephalopathy** | +++ | +++ | ++ | ++ | ++ |
| | **Seizures**[a] | +++ | ++ | ++ | ++ | ++ |
| | **Stroke-like episodes** | ± | ± | ± | ± | ± |
| Digestive | **Feeding difficulties, protein aversion** | ++ | ++ | ++ | ++ | ++ |
| | Liver failure, acute | | ±-+ | ±-+ | ±-+ | ± |
| | Vomiting | +++ | ++ | ++ | ++ | ++ |
| Eye | Vision, impaired | | | | ± | ± |
| Hematological | Coagulopathy | | ±-+ | ±-+ | ±-+ | ±-+ |
| Other | Failure to thrive | | ±-+ | ±-+ | ±-+ | ±-+ |
| Laboratory findings | Ammonia (blood and plasma) | ↑↑↑ | ↑↑↑ | ↑↑↑ | ↑↑↑ | ↑↑↑ |
| | Arginine (plasma) | ↓ | ↓ | ↓ | ↓ | ↓ |
| | Argininosuccinate (urine) | n | n | n | n | n |
| | ASAT/ALAT (plasma) | n-↑↑ | n-↑↑ | n-↑↑ | n-↑ | n-↑ |
| | Citrulline (plasma) | ↓↓↓ | ↓↓ | ↓↓ | ↓↓ | ↓↓ |
| | Glutamine (cerebrospinal fluid) | ↑↑↑ | ↑↑↑ | ↑↑↑ | ↑↑ | ↑↑ |
| | Glutamine (plasma) | ↑↑↑ | ↑↑↑ | ↑↑↑ | ↑↑ | ↑↑ |
| | Orotic acid (urine) | n-↑↑ | n-↑↑ | n-↑↑ | n-↑↑ | n-↑↑ |
| | Urea (plasma) | ↓-n | ↓-n | ↓-n | ↓-n | ↓-n |

[a]Mainly in encephalopathic crises

**Table 17.4** Argininosuccinate synthetase deficiency

| System | Symptoms and biomarkers | Neonatal (birth–1 month) | Infancy (1–18 months) | Childhood (1.5–11 years) | Adolescence (11–16 years) | Adulthood (>16 years) |
|---|---|---|---|---|---|---|
| Autonomic system | Temperature instability[a] | ± | | | | |
| CNS | Ataxia | | | ± | ± | ± |
| | **Coma** | +++ | +++ | ++ | ++ | ++ |
| | Confusion, episodic | | | ± | ± | ± |
| | **Developmental delay** | | ±-++ | ±-++ | ±-++ | ±-++ |
| | **Encephalopathy** | +++ | +++ | ++ | ++ | ++ |
| | Seizures[a] | +++ | ++ | ++ | ++ | ++ |
| | Stroke-like episodes | ± | ± | ± | ± | ± |
| Digestive | **Feeding difficulties, protein aversion** | ++ | + | + | + | + |
| | Liver failure, acute | | ±-+ | ±-+ | ± | ± |
| | Vomiting | ++ | ++ | + | + | + |
| Other | Failure to thrive | | ±-+ | ±-+ | ±-+ | ±-+ |
| Laboratory findings | Ammonia (blood and plasma) | ↑↑↑ | ↑↑↑ | ↑↑↑ | ↑↑↑ | ↑↑↑ |
| | Arginine (plasma) | ↓ | ↓ | ↓ | ↓ | ↓ |
| | Argininosuccinate (urine) | n | n | n | n | n |
| | ASAT/ALAT (plasma) | n-↑↑ | n-↑↑ | n-↑↑ | n-↑ | n-↑ |
| | Citrulline (plasma) | ↑↑ | ↑↑↑ | ↑↑↑ | ↑↑↑ | ↑↑↑ |
| | Citrulline (urine) | ↑↑ | ↑↑↑ | ↑↑↑ | ↑↑↑ | ↑↑↑ |
| | Glutamine (cerebrospinal fluid) | ↑↑↑ | ↑↑↑ | ↑↑ | ↑↑ | ↑↑ |
| | Glutamine (plasma) | ↑↑↑ | ↑↑↑ | ↑↑ | ↑↑ | ↑↑ |
| | Orotic acid (urine) | n-↑ | n-↑ | n-↑ | n-↑ | n-↑ |
| | Urea (plasma) | ↓-n | ↓-n | ↓-n | ↓-n | ↓-n |

[a]Mainly in encephalopathic crises

**Table 17.5** Argininosuccinate lyase deficiency

| System | Symptoms and biomarkers | Neonatal (birth–1 month) | Infancy (1–18 months) | Childhood (1.5–11 years) | Adolescence (11–16 years) | Adulthood (>16 years) |
|---|---|---|---|---|---|---|
| Autonomic system | Temperature instability[a] | ± | | | | |
| CNS | Ataxia | | | ± | ± | ± |
| | **Coma** | +++ | ++ | + | + | + |
| | Confusion, episodic | | | ± | ± | ± |
| | **Developmental delay** | | ± | + | + | + |
| | **Encephalopathy** | +++ | ++ | + | + | + |
| | Seizures[a] | +++ | ++ | + | + | + |
| | Stroke-like episodes | ± | ± | ± | ± | ± |
| Dermatological | **Brittle hair, trichorrhexis nodosa** | | ± | ±-+ | ±-+ | ±-+ |
| Digestive | Feeding difficulties, protein aversion | ++ | + | + | + | + |
| | Liver disease, chronic | | ± | ± | ±-+ | ±-+ |
| | Vomiting | ++ | ++ | + | + | + |
| Other | Failure to thrive | | ±-+ | ±-+ | ±-+ | ±-+ |
| Laboratory findings | Ammonia (blood and plasma) | ↑↑↑ | ↑↑↑ | ↑↑↑ | ↑↑↑ | ↑↑↑ |
| | Arginine (plasma) | ↓ | ↓ | ↓ | ↓ | ↓ |
| | Argininosuccinate (plasma)[b] | ↑↑ | ↑↑ | ↑↑ | ↑↑ | ↑↑ |
| | Argininosuccinate (urine)[b] | ↑↑↑ | ↑↑↑ | ↑↑↑ | ↑↑↑ | ↑↑↑ |
| | ASAT/ALAT (plasma) | n-↑ | n-↑ | n-↑ | n-↑ | n-↑ |
| | Citrulline (plasma) | ↑ | ↑ | ↑ | ↑ | ↑ |
| | Glutamine (cerebrospinal fluid) | ↑↑↑ | ↑↑↑ | ↑↑ | ↑↑ | ↑↑ |
| | Glutamine (plasma) | ↑↑ | ↑↑ | ↑ | ↑ | ↑ |
| | Orotic acid (urine) | n-↑ | n-↑ | n-↑ | n-↑ | n-↑ |
| | Urea (plasma) | ↓-n | ↓-n | ↓-n | ↓-n | ↓-n |

[a]Mainly in encephalopathic crises
[b]Argininosuccinate is converted spontaneously to its two anhydrides particularly in the urine, depending on the pH and storage conditions of the sample. Modern methods of amino acid analysis identify ASA and its two anhydrides. ASA levels are generally higher in CSF than in plasma

**Table 17.6** Arginase 1 deficiency

| System | Symptoms and biomarkers | Neonatal (birth–1 month) | Infancy (1–18 months) | Childhood (1.5–11 years) | Adolescence (11–16 years) | Adulthood (>16 years) |
|---|---|---|---|---|---|---|
| CNS | Ataxia | | | ± | ± | ± |
| | Confusion, episodic | | | ± | ± | ± |
| | **Developmental delay** | | + | + | + | + |
| | **Seizures** | ± | ± | ± | ±-+ | ±-+ |
| | **Spastic diplegia** | | ± | ±-+ | ++ | ++ |
| Digestive | Feeding, protein aversion | | ± | ± | ± | ± |
| | **Liver diseasea** | ± | ± | ± | ± | ±-+ |
| | Vomiting | ± | ± | ± | ± | ± |
| Hematological | Coagulopathy[a] | | ± | ± | ± | ± |
| Metabolic | **Hyperammonemic episodes** | ± | ± | ± | ± | ± |
| Laboratory findings | Ammonia (blood and plasma) | n-↑ | ↑ | ↑ | ↑ | ↑ |
| | Arginine (plasma)[b] | n-↑ | ↑↑ | ↑↑ | ↑↑ | ↑↑ |
| | ASAT/ALAT (plasma) | n-↑ | n-↑ | n-↑ | n-↑ | n-↑ |
| | Citrulline (plasma) | n-↑ | n-↑ | n-↑ | n-↑ | n-↑ |
| | Glutamine (plasma) | ↑ | ↑ | ↑ | ↑ | ↑ |
| | Orotic acid (urine) | n-↑ | n-↑ | n-↑ | n-↑ | n-↑ |
| | Urea (plasma) | ↓-n | ↓-n | ↓-n | ↓-n | ↓-n |

[a]In the very few neonatal cases reported, intrahepatic cholestasis was found
[b]Typically fourfold to tenfold elevation relative to normal values

**Table 17.7** Mitochondrial ornithine transporter deficiency

| System | Symptoms and biomarkers | Neonatal (birth–1 month) | Infancy (1–18 months) | Childhood (1.5–11 years) | Adolescence (11–16 years) | Adulthood (>16 years) |
|---|---|---|---|---|---|---|
| Autonomic system | Temperature instability | ± | | | | |
| CNS | Asterixis | | | | | ± |
| | Ataxia | | | ± | ± | ± |
| | **Coma** | ± | ± | ± | ± | ± |
| | Confusion, episodic | | | ± | ± | ± |
| | **Developmental delay** | | + | + | + | + |
| | **Encephalopathy** | ± | ± | ± | ± | ± |
| | **Pyramidal signs** | n | n-± | ± | ± | ± |
| | Seizures | ± | ± | ± | ± | ± |
| | **Spastic paresis** | n | n | ± | ± | ± |
| | **Stroke-like episodes** | ± | ± | ± | ± | ± |
| Digestive | Feeding, protein aversion | ± | ± | ± | ± | ± |
| | Liver dysfunction | ± | ± | ± | ± | ± |
| | Liver failure, acute | | ± | ± | ± | ± |
| | Vomiting | ± | ± | ± | ± | ± |
| Eye | Vision, impaired | | | | ± | ± |
| Other | Failure to thrive | n | ± | ± | ± | ± |
| Psychiatric | Behavior, abnormal | | | ± | ± | ± |
| Laboratory findings | $^{14}$C-ornithine incorporation (fibroblasts) | ↓ | ↓ | ↓ | ↓ | ↓ |
| | Ammonia (blood and plasma) | ↑↑ | ↑↑ | ↑↑ | ↑↑ | ↑↑ |
| | Arginine (plasma) | n | n | n | n | n |
| | ASAT/ALAT (plasma) | n-↑ | n-↑ | n-↑ | n-↑ | n-↑ |
| | Citrulline (plasma) | n | n | n | n | n |
| | Creatine (plasma) | n | ↓-n | ↓-n | ↓-n | ↓-n |
| | Factor VII | ↓-n | ↓-n | ↓-n | ↓-n | ↓-n |
| | Factor X | ↓-n | ↓-n | ↓-n | ↓-n | ↓-n |
| | Glutamine (plasma) | n-↑ | n-↑ | n-↑ | n-↑ | n-↑ |
| | Homocitrulline (urine) | ↑↑ | ↑↑ | ↑↑ | ↑↑ | ↑↑ |
| | Ornithine (plasma) | ↑-↑↑ | ↑↑ | ↑↑ | ↑↑ | ↑↑ |
| | Orotic acid (urine) | n-↑ | n-↑ | n-↑ | n-↑ | n-↑ |
| | Urea (plasma) | ↓-n | ↓-n | ↓-n | ↓-n | ↓-n |

**Table 17.8** Citrin deficiency

| System | Symptoms and biomarkers | Neonatal (birth–1 month) | Infancy (1–18 months) | Childhood (1.5–11 years) | Adolescence (11–16 years) | Adulthood (>16 years) |
|---|---|---|---|---|---|---|
| CNS | Ataxia | | | | ± | ± |
| | **Coma** | | | | + | + |
| | Confusion, episodic | | | | ± | ± |
| | Consciousness disturbance | | | | ± | ± |
| | **Developmental delay** | | | | ± | ± |
| | **Encephalopathy** | | | | + | + |
| | Fatigue | | | ± | | |
| Digestive | **Cholestasis, intrahepatic** | ++ | + | | | |
| | Hepatomegaly | + | + | | | |
| | **Jaundice** | ++ | + | | | |
| | Liver dysfunction | ++ | + | | | |
| | Liver steatosis | ± | ± | | ± | ± |
| | **Low carbohydrate, high protein and high fat intake** | | | + | + | + |
| | Pancreatitis, recurrent | | | ± | | ± |
| Hematological | Anemia | ++ | + | | | |
| | Impaired coagulation | + | + | | | |
| Musculoskeletal | Growth retardation | ± | ± | ± | | |
| Other | Failure to thrive | ++ | + | ± | | |
| Psychiatric | **Neuropsychiatric manifestations, sudden onset** | | | | ± | ± |
| Laboratory findings | Albumin (plasma) | ↓↓ | ↓ | n | n | n |
| | Alpha-fetoprotein (serum) | ↑↑ | ↑ | n | n | n |
| | Ammonia (blood and plasma) | n-↑ | n-↑ | n | n-↑↑ | ↑↑ |
| | Arginine (plasma) | n-↑ | n-↑ | n | n | n-↑ |
| | ASAT/ALAT (plasma) | n-↑ | n-↑ | n | n | n |
| | Bilirubin, total/direct (plasma) | ↑↑ | ↑ | n | n | n |
| | Citrulline (plasma) | ↑-↑↑ | ↑-↑↑ | n-↑ | n-↑ | ↑↑ |
| | Erythrocyte count (blood) | ↓↓ | ↓ | n | n | n |
| | Galactose (plasma) | ↑ | ↑ | n | n | n |
| | Galactose (urine) | ↑↑ | ↑ | n | n | n |
| | Gamma-glutamyltransferase (GGT) (plasma) | ↑↑ | ↑-n | n | n | n |
| | Glucose (plasma) | n-↓ | n-↓ | n | n | n |
| | Glutamine (plasma) | n-↑ | n-↑ | n | n | n-↑ |
| | HDL cholesterol (plasma) | n | n | n-↑ | n | n |
| | LDL cholesterol (plasma) | n | n | n-↑ | n | n |
| | Methionine (plasma) | ↑ | ↑ | n | n | ↑ |
| | Phenylalanine (plasma) | ↑ | ↑ | n | n | ↑ |
| | Prothrombin time | n-↑ | n-↑ | n | n | n |
| | Succinylacetone (plasma) | n | n | n | n | n |
| | Threonine (plasma) | ↑ | ↑ | n | n | ↑ |
| | Total protein (plasma) | ↓↓ | ↓ | n | n | n |
| | Tyrosine (plasma) | ↑ | ↑ | n | n | ↑ |

Two forms, neonatal and later form, are distinguished. The neonatal form is dominated by intrahepatic cholestasis and jaundice, generally waning out with carbohydrate-devoid formula. The adult form is dominated by the symptoms and signs of hyperammonemia. Both forms are caused by mutations in the same gene

**Table 17.9** Carbonic anhydrase VA deficiency

| System | Symptoms and biomarkers | Neonatal (birth–1 month) | Infancy (1–18 months) | Childhood (1.5–11 years) | Adolescence (11–16 years) | Adulthood (>16 years) |
|---|---|---|---|---|---|---|
| Autonomic system | **Temperature instability** | + | ± | | | |
| CNS | **Coma** | + | ± | | | |
| | **Encephalopathy** | + | ± | | | |
| Digestive | **Feeding difficulties** | + | ± | | | |
| | **Vomiting** | + | ± | | | |
| Metabolic | **Hypoglycemia** | + | ± | | | |
| Laboratory findings | 2-Oxoglutaric acid (urine) | n-↑ | n-↑ | | | |
| | 3-Hydroxybutyric acid (urine, plasma) | n-↑ | n-↑ | | | |
| | 3-Hydroxyisovaleric acid (urine) | n-↑ | n-↑ | | | |
| | 3-Hydroxypropionic acid (urine) | n-↑ | n-↑ | | | |
| | 3-Methylcrotonylglycine (urine) | n-↑ | n-↑ | | | |
| | Acetoacetate (urine, plasma) | n-↑ | n-↑ | | | |
| | Adipic acid (urine) | n-↑ | n-↑ | | | |
| | Ammonia (blood and plasma) | ↑↑ | ↑ | | | |
| | Arginine (plasma) | ↓-n | ↓-n | | | |
| | Citrulline (plasma) | ↓-n | ↓-n | | | |
| | Fumaric acid (urine) | n-↑ | n-↑ | | | |
| | Glucose (plasma) | ↓ | ↓ | | | |
| | Glutamine (plasma) | n-↑↑↑ | n-↑ | | | |
| | Lactate (plasma) | n-↑↑ | n-↑ | | | |
| | Orotic acid (urine) | n | n | | | |
| | Propionylglycine (urine) | n-↑ | n-↑ | | | |
| | Sebacic acid (urine) | n-↑ | n-↑ | | | |
| | Suberic acid (urine) | n-↑ | n-↑ | | | |

The following combination is unusual and can be seen as typical for this condition: hyperammonemia, decreased plasma citrulline and absence of urinary orotic acid, hypoglycemia, metabolic acidosis, high plasma lactate and urinary ketone bodies, and a urinary profile of organic acids containing carboxylase-related metabolites

**Table 17.10** Lysinuric protein intolerance

| System | Symptoms and biomarkers | Neonatal (birth–1 month) | Infancy (1–18 months) | Childhood (1.5–11 years) | Adolescence (11–16 years) | Adulthood (>16 years) |
|---|---|---|---|---|---|---|
| Autonomic system | Hypertension | | | - | ± | ± |
| CNS | **Coma, hyperammonemic** | | ± | ± | ± | ± |
| | Intellectual disability | | | ± | ± | ± |
| Dermatological | Sparse hair | | | ± | ± | ± |
| Digestive | Diarrhea | | ± | ± | ± | ± |
| | Hepatosplenomegaly | ± | ± | ± | ± | ± |
| | Protein intolerance | | | ± | ± | ± |
| | Vomiting | | ± | ± | ± | ± |
| Hematological | Hemophagocytic lymphohistiocytosis, macrophage activation syndrome | | | ± | ± | ± |
| Musculoskeletal | Bone growth | n | n | ↓-n | ↓-n | ↓-n |
| | Osteoporosis | | | ± | ± | ± |
| Renal | Glomerulonephritis | | | ± | ± | ± |
| | Renal failure, end stage | | | – | ± | ± |
| Respiratory | Chest radiographs, interstitial changes | | | ± | ± | ± |
| | Pulmonary alveolar proteinosis | | | ± | ± | ± |
| | Respiratory insufficiency | | | ± | ± | ± |
| Other | Combined hyperlipidemia | | | ± | ± | ± |
| Laboratory findings | Alanine (plasma) | | | ↑ | ↑ | ↑ |
| | Ammonia (blood) | ↑ | ↑ | ↑ | ↑ | ↑ |
| | Arginine (plasma) | n | n | ↓-n | ↓-n | ↓-n |
| | Arginine (urine) | | | ↑ | ↑ | ↑ |
| | Citrulline (plasma) | | | ↑ | ↑ | ↑ |
| | Ferritin (serum) | n | ↑ | ↑ | ↑ | ↑ |
| | Glutamine (plasma) | | | ↑ | ↑ | ↑ |
| | Glycine (plasma) | | | ↑ | ↑ | ↑ |
| | Lactate dehydrogenase, LDH (plasma) | n | n-↑ | n-↑ | n-↑ | n-↑ |
| | Lysine (plasma) | n | n | ↓-n | ↓-n | ↓-n |
| | Lysine (urine) | | | ↑↑ | ↑↑ | ↑↑ |
| | Ornithine (plasma) | n | n | ↓-n | ↓-n | ↓-n |
| | Ornithine (urine) | | | ↑ | ↑ | ↑ |
| | Orotic acid (urine) | | ↑ | ↑ | ↑ | ↑ |
| | Proline (plasma) | | | ↑ | ↑ | ↑ |

**Table 17.11** Pyrroline-5-carboxylate synthetase deficiency, cutis laxa phenotype 3

| System | Symptoms and biomarkers | Neonatal (birth–1 month) | Infancy (1–18 months) | Childhood (1.5–11 years) | Adolescence (11–16 years) | Adulthood (>16 years) |
|---|---|---|---|---|---|---|
| CNS | Brisk reflexes | | | ± | ± | ± |
| | **Global developmental delay** | | + | + | + | + |
| | Hypoplasia or agenesia of corpus callosum | ± | ± | ± | ± | ± |
| | Hypotonia, truncal | + | + | + | ± | ± |
| | **Intellectual disability** | | + | + | + | + |
| | **Microcephaly** | + | + | + | + | ± |
| | Paucity of white matter | | ± | | | |
| | Pyramidal signs | | | ± | ± | ± |
| | Seizures | ± | ± | - | - | |
| | Speech delayed or absent | | ± | ± | ± | |
| | Tortuous blood vessels | | ± | ± | | |
| Dermatological | **Cutis laxa** | ++ | ++ | ± | ± | |
| | **Wrinkled skin** | ++ | ++ | ± | ± | |
| Digestive | Feeding difficulties | – to ++ | – to ++ | – to ++ | + | |
| | Frequent vomiting | – to ++ | – to ++ | – to ++ | + | |
| | Gastroesophageal reflux | – to ++ | – to ++ | – to ++ | + | |
| Eye | **Cataract** | + | ++ | ++ | | |
| | Corneal clouding | ± | ± | ± | ± | |
| Musculoskeletal | **Facial dysmorphism** | ++ | + | + | + | + |
| | Hernias | ± | ± | ± | ± | |
| | Hip dislocation | ± | ± | ± | ± | |
| | Joint contractures | + | | | | |
| | Joint laxity | ±-++ | ±-++ | ±-+ | | |
| | Osteopenia | | – to ++ | – to ++ | – to ++ | |
| | Osteoporosis | | – to ++ | – to ++ | – to ++ | |
| | **Pes planus** | | ± | ± | ± | ± |
| | **Progeroid appearance** | ++ | + | + | + | + |
| | Short stature | | + | + | + | + |
| Other | **Failure to thrive** | + | ± | + | | |
| | **Intrauterine growth retardation** | ±-++ | | | | |
| | Postnatal growth restriction | | + | + | + | + |
| Laboratory findings | Ammonia (blood) | n-↑ | n-↑ | n-↑ | n-↑ | n-↑ |
| | Arginine (plasma) | ↓-n | ↓-n | ↓-n | ↓-n | ↓-n |
| | Citrulline (plasma) | ↓-n | ↓-n | ↓-n | ↓-n | ↓-n |
| | Creatine (brain MRS) | ↓-n | ↓-n | ↓-n | – | – |
| | Ornithine (plasma) | ↓-n | ↓-n | ↓-n | ↓-n | ↓-n |
| | Proline (plasma) | ↓-n | ↓-n | ↓-n | ↓-n | ↓-n |

This disorder can have recessive inheritance (ARCL3B) or it can be sporadic (ADCL3), associated to monoallelic dominant variants in the *ALDH18A1* gene

**Table 17.12** Pyrroline-5-carboxylate synthetase deficiency, spastic paraplegia type 9B

| System | Symptoms and biomarkers | Neonatal (birth–1 month) | Infancy (1–18 months) | Childhood (1.5–11 years) | Adolescence (11–16 years) | Adulthood (>16 years) |
|---|---|---|---|---|---|---|
| CNS | **Gait disturbance** | | | ±-++ | ++ | ++ |
| | **Global developmental delay** | | + | + | + | + |
| | **Intellectual disability** | | + | + | + | + |
| | Hypoplasia of the corpus callosum | | ± | ± | ± | ± |
| | Microcephaly | ± | ± | ± | ± | ± |
| | Pyramidal signs | | ± | ± | ± | ± |
| | Seizures | | ± | ± | ± | ± |
| | **Spastic paraparesis/ paraplegia/tetraplegia** | | ± | + | ++ | +++ |
| | Speech: abnormal, delayed or absent | | ± | ± | ± | |
| Dermatological | **Cutis laxa** | n | n | n | n | n |
| | **Wrinkled skin** | n | n | n | n | n |
| Eye | Cataract | ± | ± | ± | ± | ± |
| Musculoskeletal | Facial dysmorphism | | | ± | ± | ± |
| | Growth retardation | ± | ± | ± | ± | ± |
| | **Joint laxity** | n | n | n | n | n |
| | Short stature | ± | ± | ± | ± | ± |
| Laboratory findings | Arginine (plasma) | n-↓ | n-↓ | n-↓ | n-↓ | n-↓ |
| | Citrulline (plasma) | n-↓ | n-↓ | n-↓ | n-↓ | n-↓ |
| | Ornithine (plasma) | n-↓ | n-↓ | n-↓ | n-↓ | n-↓ |
| | Proline (plasma) | n-↓ | n-↓ | n-↓ | n-↓ | n-↓ |

This disorder has recessive inheritance

**Table 17.13** Pyrroline-5-carboxylate synthetase deficiency, spastic paraplegia type 9A

| System | Symptoms and biomarkers | Neonatal (birth–1 month) | Infancy (1–18 months) | Childhood (1.5–11 years) | Adolescence (11–16 years) | Adulthood (>16 years) |
|---|---|---|---|---|---|---|
| CNS | Dysarthria | | | – to ± | – to ± | – to ± |
| | Global developmental delay | | – to ± | – to ± | – to ± | – to ± |
| | Intellectual disability | | – to ± | – to ± | – to ± | – to ± |
| | **Increased muscular tone** | | + | + | + | + |
| | Pyramidal signs | | ± | + | + | + |
| | **Spastic paraparesis/ paraplegia** | | ± | ±-+ | ++ | ++ |
| | Spinal cord atrophy | | ± | ± | ± | ± |
| Dermatological | **Cutis laxa** | n | n | n | n | n |
| | **Wrinkled skin** | n | n | n | n | n |
| Digestive | Gastroesophageal reflux | ± | ± | ± | ± | ± |
| | Vomiting | ± | ± | ± | ± | ± |
| Eye | **Cataract** | | ± | ± | + | |
| Musculoskeletal | **Abnormal gait** | | | ±-+ | + | + |
| | Growth retardation | ± | + | + | + | + |
| | Short stature | ± | + | + | + | + |
| | **Joint laxity** | | n | n | n | n |
| | **Muscle weakness** | | + | + | + | + |
| | Muscle wasting | | | ± | ± | ± |
| | Pes cavus | | ± | ± | ± | + |
| Laboratory findings | Arginine (plasma) | n-↓ | n-↓ | n-↓ | n-↓ | n-↓ |
| | Citrulline (plasma) | n-↓ | n-↓ | n-↓ | n-↓ | n-↓ |
| | Ornithine (plasma) | n-↓ | n-↓ | n-↓ | n-↓ | n-↓ |
| | Proline (plasma) | n-↓ | n-↓ | n-↓ | n-↓ | n-↓ |

This disorder is dominantly inherited or has sporadic presentation, in both cases being due to monoallelic mutations in the ALDH18A1 gene

**Table 17.14** Ornithine aminotransferase deficiency

| System | Symptoms and biomarkers | Neonatal (birth–1 month) | Infancy (1–18 months) | Childhood (1.5–11 years) | Adolescence (11–16 years) | Adulthood (>16 years) |
|---|---|---|---|---|---|---|
| CNS | Cortical atrophy (MRI) | | | | ± | ± |
| | Intellectual disability | | | ± | ± | ± |
| | Neuropathy, sensory | | | ± | ± | ± |
| | Seizures | | | | ± | ± |
| | White matter abnormalities (MRI) | | | | ± | ± |
| Digestive | EM, abnormal mitochondria (liver) | | | | ± | ± |
| Eye | **Atrophy, gyrate of choroid and retina** | | | + | ++ | +++ |
| | **Blindness** | | | | | +++[a] |
| | **Cataract, posterior subcapsular** | | | | ± | +++ |
| | **Chorioretinal degeneration** | | | + | ++ | +++ |
| | **Myopia** | | ± | + | ++ | +++ |
| | **Night blindness** | | ± | ++ | 0 | +++ |
| | Retinal detachment | | | ± | ± | ± |
| | **Vision, tunnel** | | | | + | +++ |
| Metabolic | Hyperammonemia (symptomatic) | ± | | | | |
| Musculoskeletal | EM, abnormal mitochondria (muscle) | | | ± | ± | ± |
| | EM, type 2 fiber atrophy (muscle) | | | ± | ± | ± |
| | **EM, type 2 fiber tubular aggregates (muscle)** | | | + | + | ++ |
| | Muscle weakness (mild proximal) | | | ± | ± | ± |
| Laboratory findings | 3-amino-2-piperidone (urine) | n | ↑ | ↑ | ↑ | ↑ |
| | Ammonia (blood and plasma) | n-↑↑ | n | n | n | n |
| | Arginine (urine) | n | ↑ | ↑ | ↑ | ↑ |
| | Creatine (cerebrospinal fluid) | n | ↓↓ | ↓↓ | ↓↓↓ | ↓↓↓ |
| | Creatine (plasma) | n | ↓↓ | ↓↓ | ↓↓↓ | ↓↓↓ |
| | Creatine (urine) | n | ↓↓ | ↓↓ | ↓↓↓ | ↓↓↓ |
| | Creatine/phosphocreatine ratio (brain) (MRS) | n | ↓-n | ↓ | ↓ | ↓ |
| | Creatine/phosphocreatine ratio (muscle) (MRS) | n | ↓-n | ↓ | ↓ | ↓ |
| | Creatinine (plasma) | n | ↓-n | ↓-n | ↓-n | ↓-n |
| | Guanidinoacetate (cerebrospinal fluid) | n | ↓↓ | ↓↓ | ↓↓↓ | ↓↓↓ |
| | Guanidinoacetate (plasma) | n | ↓↓ | ↓↓ | ↓↓↓ | ↓↓↓ |
| | Guanidinoacetate (urine) | n | ↓↓ | ↓↓ | ↓↓↓ | ↓↓↓ |
| | Histology and EM, type 2 fiber atrophy (muscle) | | | + | + | ++-+++ |
| | Lysine (urine) | n | ↑ | ↑ | ↑ | ↑ |
| | Ornithine (plasma) | n | ↑↑↑ | ↑↑↑ | ↑↑↑ | ↑↑↑ |
| | Ornithine (urine) | n | ↑↑↑ | ↑↑↑ | ↑↑↑ | ↑↑↑ |
| | Proline/citrulline ratio | ↑ | n | n | n | n |

[a]>30 years

**Table 17.15** Glutamate dehydrogenase superactivity

| System | Symptoms and biomarkers | Neonatal (birth–1 month) | Infancy (1–18 months) | Childhood (1.5–11 years) | Adolescence (11–16 years) | Adulthood (>16 years) |
|---|---|---|---|---|---|---|
| CNS | Convulsions | ± | ± | ± | ± | ± |
| | EEG, abnormal | + | + | + | ± | ± |
| | **Epilepsy, generalized** | + | ++ | ++ | ± | ± |
| | Intellectual disability | | ± | ± | ± | ± |
| | Seizures | ± | ± | ± | ± | ± |
| Endocrine | **Hyperinsulinism** | + | ++ | ++ | ± | ± |
| Metabolic | **Hypoglycemia** | ++ | ++ | + | + | + |
| | **Hypoglycemia, hypoketotic** | ++ | ++ | + | + | + |
| | **Leucine sensitivity causing hypoglycemia** | ++ | ++ | ++ | ++ | ++ |
| Laboratory findings | Alpha-ketoglutarate (urine) | n-↑ | n-↑ | n-↑ | n-↑ | n-↑ |
| | Ammonia, fasting (blood and plasma) | ↑ | ↑ | ↑ | ↑ | ↑ |
| | Free fatty acids (serum) | ↓ | ↓ | ↓ | ↓ | ↓ |
| | Glucose (plasma) | ↓ | ↓ | ↓ | ↓ | ↓ |
| | Insulin (plasma) | ↑ | ↑ | ↑ | ↑ | ↑ |
| | Ketones (plasma) | ↓ | ↓ | ↓ | ↓ | ↓ |
| | Ketones (urine) | ↓ | ↓ | ↓ | ↓ | ↓ |

**Table 17.16** Glutamine synthetase deficiency

| System | Symptoms and biomarkers | Neonatal (birth–1 month) | Infancy (1–18 months) | Childhood (1.5–11 years) | Adolescence (11–16 years) | Adulthood (>16 years) |
|---|---|---|---|---|---|---|
| CNS | **Absent head control** | + | ++ | ++ | | |
| | Cerebellar hypoplasia | ± | ± | ± | | |
| | **Developmental delay** | + | +++ | +++ | | |
| | EEG, abnormal | + | ++ | ++ | | |
| | **Encephalopathy, epileptic** | ++ | ++ | ++ | | |
| | **Epilepsy, intractable** | ++ | ++ | ++ | | |
| | Myelination, delayed | ± | ± | ± | | |
| Dermatological | Erythema, necrotizing | ± | ± | ± | | |
| Laboratory findings | Ammonia (blood and plasma) | ↑ | ↑ | ↑ | | |
| | Glutamic acid (cerebrospinal fluid) | n | n | n | | |
| | Glutamic acid (plasma) | n | n | n | | |
| | Glutamine (cerebrospinal fluid) | ↓↓ | ↓↓ | ↓↓ | | |
| | Glutamine (plasma) | ↓-↓↓ | ↓↓↓ | ↓↓↓ | | |
| | Glutamine (urine) | ↓ | ↓ | ↓ | | |

**Table 17.17** Pyruvate carboxylase deficiency

| System | Symptoms and biomarkers | Neonatal (birth–1 month) | Infancy (1–18 months) | Childhood (1.5–11 years) | Adolescence (11–16 years) | Adulthood (>16 years) |
|---|---|---|---|---|---|---|
| CNS | Developmental delay | +++ | +++ | +++ | | |
| | Hypokinesia | ++ | + | + | | |
| | **Hypotonia** | +++ | +++ | +++ | | |
| | Parkinsonism, hypokinetic features | ++ | n | n | | |
| | Pyramidal signs | ++ | ++ | ++ | | |
| | **Seizures** | +++ | +++ | +++ | | |
| Digestive | **Vomiting** | +++ | +++ | ++ | | |
| Metabolic | Hypoglycemia | ± | ± | ± | ± | |
| Other | **Failure to thrive** | +++ | +++ | +++ | | |
| Laboratory findings | 3-OH-butyrate/ acetoacetate ratio (plasma) | ↓ | | | | |
| | Alanine (plasma) | ↑ | ↑ | ↑ | | |
| | Ammonia (blood) | n-↑ | n-↑ | n-↑ | | |
| | Citrulline (plasma) | ↑ | ↑ | ↑ | | |
| | Glucose (plasma) | ↓-n | ↓-n | ↓-n | ↓-n | |
| | Ketones (plasma) | ↑ | ↑ | ↑ | | |
| | Ketones (urine) | ↑ | ↑ | ↑ | | |
| | Lactate (plasma) | ↑↑ | ↑ | ↑ | | |
| | Lactate/pyruvate ratio | ↑↑ | n | n | | |
| | Pyruvate (plasma) | ↑↑ | ↑ | ↑ | | |

**Table 17.18** Transmembrane protein 70 deficiency

| System | Symptoms and biomarkers | Neonatal (birth–1 month) | Infancy (1–18 months) | Childhood (1.5–11 years) | Adolescence (11–16 years) | Adulthood (>16 years) |
|---|---|---|---|---|---|---|
| Cardiovascular | **Cardiomyopathy, hypertrophic** | + | + | + | + | + |
| | Wolff-Parkinson-White syndrome | ± | ± | ± | ± | ± |
| CNS | Apnea | ± | ± | ± | ± | ± |
| | Basal ganglia lesions (MRI) | ± | ± | ± | ± | ± |
| | Cerebellar hypoplasia, mild | ± | ± | ± | ± | ± |
| | Cortical atrophy (MRI) | ± | ± | ± | ± | ± |
| | **Encephalopathy** | + | + | + | + | + |
| | **Hypotonia, muscular-axial** | + | + | + | + | + |
| | Microcephaly | ± | ± | ± | ± | ± |
| | **Retardation, psychomotor** | ± | + | + | + | + |
| | Subcortical atrophy (MRI) | ± | ± | ± | ± | ± |
| Digestive | Gastrointestinal dysmotility | ± | ± | ± | ± | ± |
| | Hepatomegaly | + | + | ± | ± | ± |
| | Liver dysfunction | ± | ± | ± | ± | ± |
| Eye | Cataract | ± | ± | ± | ± | ± |
| Genitourinary | Cryptorchidism | ± | ± | ± | ± | ± |
| | Hypospadias | ± | ± | ± | ± | ± |
| Metabolic | **Hyperammonemia, during crisis** | + | + | + | + | ± |
| | **Hyperuricemia, during crisis** | + | + | + | + | ± |
| | **Ketonuria, pronounced during crisis** | + | + | + | + | + |
| | **Lactic acidosis** | + | + | ± | ± | ± |
| | **Metabolic acidosis** | + | + | + | + | ± |
| Musculoskeletal | Contractures | ± | ± | ± | ± | ± |
| | Facial dysmorphism | ± | ± | ± | ± | ± |
| Renal | Renal tubulopathy | ± | ± | ± | ± | ± |
| Respiratory | **Persistent pulmonary hypertension of the newborn** | ± | | | | |
| | Respiratory insufficiency | ± | ± | ± | ± | ± |
| Other | Failure to thrive | + | + | + | + | + |
| | Growth retardation, postnatal | ± | ± | ± | ± | ± |
| | Low birth weight | ± | | | | |
| Laboratory findings | 3-Methylglutaconic acid (urine) | ↑-↑↑ | ↑-↑↑ | ↑-↑↑ | ↑-↑↑ | ↑-↑↑ |
| | Alanine (plasma) | ↑-↑↑ | ↑-↑↑ | ↑-↑↑ | ↑-↑↑ | ↑-↑↑ |
| | Ammonia (blood and plasma) | n-↑↑ | n-↑↑ | n-↑↑ | n-↑↑ | n-↑↑ |
| | Anion gap | ↑ | ↑ | ↑ | ↑ | ↑ |
| | Citrulline (plasma) | n-↑ | n-↑ | n-↑ | n-↑ | n-↑ |
| | Complex V activity (skeletal muscle) | ↓ | ↓ | ↓ | ↓ | ↓ |
| | Creatine kinase (plasma) | n-↑↑ | n-↑↑ | n-↑↑ | n-↑↑ | n-↑↑ |
| | Glutamine (plasma) | n-↑ | n-↑ | n-↑ | n-↑ | n-↑ |
| | Lactate (cerebrospinal fluid) | n-↑↑ | n-↑↑ | n-↑↑ | n-↑↑ | n-↑↑ |
| | Lactate (plasma) | ↑-↑↑↑ | ↑-↑↑↑ | ↑-↑↑↑ | ↑-↑↑↑ | ↑-↑↑↑ |
| | Orotic acid (urine) | n-↑ | n-↑ | n-↑ | n-↑ | n-↑ |
| | Uric acid | n-↑↑ | n-↑↑ | n-↑↑ | n-↑↑ | n-↑↑ |

## Reference Values

| Age | Plasma (μmol/L) | | |
|---|---|---|---|
| | <1 month | 1 month–12 years | >12 years |
| Ammonia, fasting (enzymatic)[a] | <100 | <50 | <50 |
| Arginine[b] | 37–71 | 32–142 | 28–96 |
| Argininosuccinate | <1 | <1 | <1 |
| Citrulline | 8–47 | 8–47 | 19–47 |
| Ornithine[b] | 66–116 | 27–96 | 55–135 |
| Lysine | 154–246 | 85–218 | 135–243 |
| Glutamine[c] | 475–746 | 475–746 | 466–798 |
| Alanine | 274–384 | 148–475 | 146–494 |
| Proline | 150–215 | 40–332 | 100–300 |

| | Urine (mmol/mol creatinine) | | |
|---|---|---|---|
| Age | <1 month | 1–6 months | >6 months |
| Arginine | 0.2–14 | 0.2–14 | 0.2–14 |
| Argininosuccinate | <0.5 | <0.5 | <0.5 |
| Citrulline | 0.2–11 | 0.2–11 | 0.2–11 |
| Ornithine | 0.2–26 | 0.2–26 | 0.2–26 |
| Lysine | 15–199 | 15–199 | 13–80 |
| Glutamine[c] | 52–205 | 52–205 | 45–133 |
| Alanine | 75–244 | 72–206 | 41–130 |
| Proline | 21–213 | 0.2–130 | <14 |
| Orotic acid | <3.4 | <2.35 | <1.44 |
| Orotidine | <5.0 | <1.3 | <0.6 |
| Uracil | 10–50 | 10–50 | 10–50 |

| | Urine (mmol/mol creatinine) | | | | |
|---|---|---|---|---|---|
| Age | <7 days | 8 days–4 months | 5 months–2 years | 3–10 years | >10 years |
| Homocitrulline | <135 | <15 | <4 | <11 | <8 |

| | Cerebrospinal fluid (μmol/L) | |
|---|---|---|
| Age | <1 year | >1 year |
| Glutamine[c] | 390–824 | 352–680 |

Except the values for ammonia, cerebrospinal fluid, and urinary homocitrulline, these reference values are from the Metabolic Diseases Unit of the Vall d'Hebrón Hospital of Barcelona (Drs. J.A. Arranz and E. Riudor)

[a]Preanalytical problems: tourniquet, convulsions, or very heavy resistance. Cooling of the blood and prompt cell removal and ammonia analysis are essential

[b]Cells should be separated soon, since erythrocyte arginase can hydrolyze the arginine and increase the ornithine. Hemolysis must be avoided

[c]Glutamine is unstable on standing unless plasma, CSF, or urine is frozen

## Pathological Values Table

| Disorder | Ammonia (P) | Citrulline[a] (P) | Arginine[b] (P) | Glutamine (P) | Ornithine (P) | Proline (P) | ASA (U) | Orotic acid (U) | Homocitrulline[c] (U) | Lactate (P) | Insulin (P) |
|---|---|---|---|---|---|---|---|---|---|---|---|
| NAGS def. | ↑↑↑ | ↓ | ↓-n | ↑-↑↑ | n | n | nd | n-↓ | n | n-↑ | n |
| CPS1 def. | ↑↑↑ | ↓ | ↓-n | ↑-↑↑ | n | n | nd | n-↓ | n | n-↑ | n |
| OTC def. | ↑↑↑ | ↓ | ↓-n | ↑-↑↑ | n | n | nd | ↑↑-n[d] | n-↑ | n-↑ | n |
| ASS def. | ↑↑ | ↑↑↑ | ↓ | ↑ | n | n | nd | ↑-n | n | n-↑ | n |
| ASL def. | ↑↑ | ↑↑ | ↓ | ↑-n | n | n | ↑↑↑ | ↑-n | n | n-↑ | n |
| ARG1 def. | ↑-↑↑ (not always) | ↑ | n-↑↑ in neonates; ↑↑↑ in infants, children, and adults | ↑-n | n | n | nd | ↑-n | n | n-↑ | n |
| HHH syndrome | ↑↑ | n | n | ↑-↑↑ | ↑↑ but not in neonates | n | nd | ↑-n | ↑↑ | n-↑ | n |
| Citrin def. | ↑↑ (not in neonates) | ↑-↑↑ | (↑)-↑ | n | n | n | nd | n | n | n-↑ | n |
| CAVA deficiency | ↑↑ | n | n | ↑↑ | n | n | n | n | n | n-↑↑ | n |
| LPI | ↑-↑↑ | n | ↓-n | n | ↓-n | n | n | n-↑ | n | n-↑ | n |
| P5CS deficiency(all types)[e] | ↑ (fasting) -n | ↓-n | ↓-n | ↑-n | ↓-n | ↓-n | nd | n | n | n | n |
| OAT deficiency | ↑↑ in neonates | n | n | ↑↑ in neonates | ↑↑ outside neonatal age and early infancy | n | n | n | n | n | n |
| HIHA syndrome | ↑-n | n | n | n | n | n | n | n | n | n | ↑-n |
| GS def. | ↑ | n | n | ↓↓ | n | n | nd | n | n | n | n |
| PC deficiency | ↑↑ | ↑↑ | n | n | n | ↑-n | n | n | n | ↑↑ | n |
| TMEM70 deficiency | ↑-↑↑ | ↑-n | n | ↑-n | n | n | n | n | n | ↑↑ | n |

Ammonia is determined most often enzymatically using glutamate dehydrogenase. Bedside ammonia determination uses a reflectometric method. Amino acids can be determined in different ways, although the classical method is based on ion exchange chromatography with post-column derivatization with ninhydrin and colorimetric detection

*Def.* deficiency, *nd* not detectable, *ASA* argininosuccinate

[a]Watermelon contains citrulline, and its consumption in high amount was reported to increase citrulline levels. Take also into account the possibility that citrulline may have been administered therapeutically to the patient

[b]Exclude arginine load or take into account the possibility that arginine may have been administered therapeutically to the patient

[c]Exclude canned food or milk as a source of the homocitrulline

[d]Normal urinary level of orotic acid has been found in some neonatal onset OTC-deficient patients

[e]Sampling should be done in a fasting state; sampling during fasting is crucial not only for proline but for all the PACO (proline, arginine, citrulline, and ornithine) amino acids

## Diagnostic Flowchart

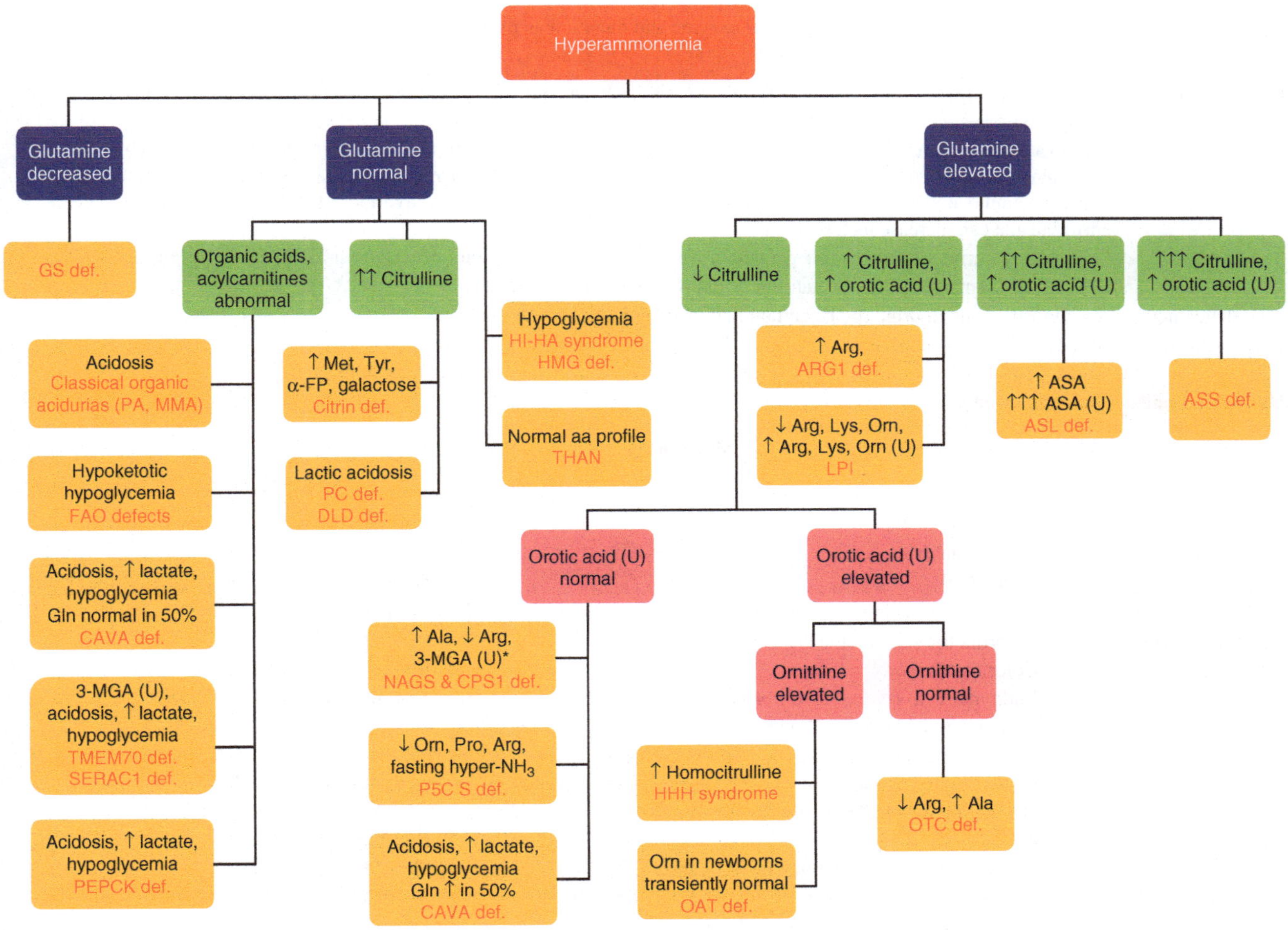


**Fig. 17.2** This diagnostic flowchart describes the typical situation for each disorder; however, some patients will present with different biochemical findings. For this reason, the flowchart should guide diagnosis but must not be taken for absolute exclusion of a disorder. Unless indicated with a (*U*) (urine), the figure refers to plasma levels. Abbreviations not defined in the disease table: *α-FP* α-fetoprotein, *Ala* alanine, *ASA* argininosuccinic acid, *Arg* arginine, *Def.* deficiency, *DLD* dihydrolipoamide dehydrogenase, *FAO* fatty acid oxidation, *Gln* glutamine, *HMG* 3-hydroxy-3-methylglutaryl-CoA lyase, *Met* methionine, *3-MGA* 3-methylglutaconic acid, *MMA* methylmalonic aciduria, *Orn* ornithine, *PA* propionic acidemia, *Pro* proline, *SERAC1* serine active site-containing protein 1, *THAN* transient hyperammonemia of the newborn, *Tyr* tyrosine, *, this asterisk indicates that 3-MGA was only found in few CPS1D patients but not yet in NAGSD. (The figure was adapted from Häberle et al. (2012))

## Specimen Collection

**Table 17.19** Overview on methods and required samples for enzyme and mutation analysis

| | Metabolites |
|---|---|
| For all disorders | Ammonia in plasma (arterial blood preferable; use tourniquets minimally; do not request muscular contractions; refrigerate blood and process at 4 °C; assay within 30 min of blood drawing) |
| | Amino acids in plasma (for routine analysis, draw blood 3–4 h after a meal; use Na heparin; harvest plasma promptly; avoid hemolysis; freeze plasma if analysis is to be delayed, particularly since glutamine is unstable; ASA may not be seen in certain amino acid analyzers; in these cases it can be converted first to its anhydrides by heating; watermelon contains citrulline and can increase its level) |
| | Orotic acid in urine (if urine is refrigerated or frozen, it can precipitate out; heat urine at 37 °C until precipitate dissolved) |
| | Drug levels (benzoate, phenylacetate) in serum if monitoring is required |
| ASL deficiency | Argininosuccinate in urine (make certain that method detects ASA) |
| HHH syndrome | Homocitrulline in the urine |
| LPI | Amino acids in urine: arginine, lysine, ornithine, and cystine (the latter being normal in LPI) |
| HIHA syndrome | Insulin in serum |

| | Mutation analysis |
|---|---|
| For all disorders | DNA |
| | RNA (preferred for CPS1 genetics) |

| | Enzyme analysis | |
|---|---|---|
| Disorder | Method | Sample |
| NAGS deficiency | Stable isotope dilution assay with GC/MS | Liver[a] |
| CPS1 deficiency | Colorimetric[b] or isotopic OTC-coupled assay | **Liver**[a], small intestine |
| OTC deficiency | Colorimetric assay[b] | **Liver**[a,c], small intestine[c] |
| ASS deficiency | Radiometric assay (cultured fibroblasts) | **Skin fibroblasts**, kidney, liver[a] |
| | Isotopically labeled citrulline incorporation[d] (cultured fibroblasts) | |
| | Colorimetric ASL-arginase-coupled assay (liver) | |
| ASL deficiency | Colorimetric, arginase-coupled assay (erythrocytes, liver, kidney) | **Skin fibroblasts**, red blood cells[e], liver[a], kidney |
| | Isotopically labeled citrulline incorporation[d] (cultured fibroblasts) | |
| ARG1 deficiency | Colorimetric assay | **Red blood cells**, liver[a] |
| HHH syndrome | Isotopically labeled ornithine incorporation[d] | **Skin fibroblasts**, liver[a] |
| Citrin deficiency | Transport activity assayed radiometrically in liposomes incorporating the recombinant transporter expressed in *Escherichia coli* | Artificial liposomes |
| P5CS deficiency | Incorporation of isotopically labeled glutamate into protein proline[d] can support the diagnosis[f] | Skin fibroblasts |
| OAT deficiency | Isotopically labeled ornithine incorporation[d] | Skin fibroblasts |
| PC deficiency | Radiometric assay | Skin fibroblasts |

Table adapted from Häberle et al. (2012)

**Bold**: first choice if analysis in more than one tissue is possible

[a]Needle biopsy (>10 mg) sufficient either for NAGS assay or for assay of the other five urea cycle enzymes

Liver tissue should be snap frozen and kept at −80 °C (or below this temperature) until analysis

[b]Treatment with carbamylglutamate might interfere with some colorimetric assays of citrulline, but zero time controls can be used to subtract high blank values

[c]Reliable in males but less so in females due to X-mosaicism in all tissues

[d]Incorporation assays can be considered indirect *in vivo* enzyme assays since the amount of labeled precursor incorporated can be limited by deficiency in one of the enzymatic steps of the route that leads to such incorporation

[e]Caution: conflicting results

[f]Limited experience

## Prenatal Diagnosis Table and Sample Requirements

**Table 17.20** Recommended analyses and sample requirements for prenatal diagnosis

| Disorder | Tests recommended |
|---|---|
| NAGS deficiency | Mutation analysis on DNA from CVS or AFC[a] |
| CPS1 deficiency | **Mutation analysis on DNA from CVS or AFC** |
| | Enzyme analysis, late fetal liver biopsy[b] |
| OTC deficiency | **Mutation analysis on DNA from CVS or AFC**[c] |
| | Enzyme analysis, late fetal liver biopsy[b,d] |
| ASS deficiency | **Mutation analysis on DNA from CVS or AFC** |
| | **Citrulline in amniotic fluid** |
| | Enzyme assays or indirect labeled citrulline incorporation assays using intact or cultured CVS or cultured AFC[e] |
| ASL deficiency | **Mutation analysis on DNA from CVS or AFC** |
| | **Argininosuccinate and its anhydrides in amniotic fluid** |
| | Enzyme assays or indirect labeled citrulline incorporation assays using intact or cultured CVS or cultured AFC[e] |
| ARG1 deficiency | **Mutation analysis on DNA from CVS** |
| | Enzyme assay in fetal blood erythrocytes (mid-gestation sampling) |
| HHH syndrome | **Mutation analysis on DNA from CVS or AFC** |
| | Enzyme assay in CVS or cultured AFC |
| Citrin deficiency | **Mutation analysis on DNA from CVS or AFC** |
| CAVA deficiency | **Mutation analysis on DNA from CVS or AFC** |
| LPI | **Mutation analysis on DNA from CVS or AFC** |
| P5CS deficiency | **Mutation analysis on DNA from CVS or AFC** |
| OAT deficiency | **Mutation analysis on DNA from CVS or AFC** |
| HIHA syndrome | **Mutation analysis on DNA from CVS or AFC** |
| GS deficiency | **Mutation analysis on DNA from CVS or AFC** |
| PC deficiency | **Mutation analysis on DNA from CVS or AFC** |
| | Enzyme assay in CVS or cultured AFC |
| TMEM70 deficiency | **Mutation analysis on DNA from CVS or AFC** |

Table adapted from Häberle et al. (2012)
*CVS* chorionic villous sampling, *AFC* amniotic fluid cells
**Bold**: first choice
[a]In case of a request for prenatal testing, it should be kept in mind that NAGSD is a treatable disorder
[b]Described in single patients but not widely available and very limited experience
[c]In the female fetus, the genotype is only able to exclude *OTC* mutations. Because of the lyonization, it has no predictive value for the resulting phenotype if affected
[d]Interpretation not clear in females due to lyonization, which results in mosaicism for the expression of the X-chromosome
[e]Carried out in few laboratories

## DNA Testing

Mutation analysis is feasible in all disorders described in this chapter. In all disorders, DNA from peripheral blood leukocytes can be used for PCR and direct sequencing; due to the size of the *CPS1* gene and the frequent occurrence of intronic changes, some labs prefer using RNA from stimulated lymphocytes or from cultured fibroblasts for mutation analysis. See also the table in Sect. 17.8.

## Treatment

### Summary

Acute symptomatic hyperammonemia is always an emergency that must be promptly treated (Häberle 2011). Treatment aims at minimizing ammonia production by preventing protein breakdown and at the same time increasing ammonia removal. Dietary protein should be withheld immediately but not for longer than 24–48 h (give thereafter at least essential amino acids). Except in citrin deficiency, in which carbohydrates are contraindicated, high-dose intravenous glucose (with or without insulin) should be given to supply high energy and to prevent endogenous protein catabolism. The nitrogen scavengers sodium benzoate and sodium phenylacetate/phenylbutyrate (or glycerol phenylbutyrate) are given to increase urinary nitrogen excretion bypassing the urea cycle, being excreted as conjugates of glycine and glutamine, respectively (Batshaw et al. 2001; Enns 2010). Administration of L-arginine (oral or intravenous) or L-citrulline (oral) enhances residual urea cycle function and urinary excretion of urea cycle intermediates (Brusilow 1984). Carbamylglutamate administration (oral) restores CPS1 function in NAGS deficiency. Nitrogen scavenger drugs and L-arginine are given at the beginning of treatment of acute hyperammonemia as boluses followed by continuous infusions.

A central venous line is desirable for administration of high glucose concentrations especially if parenteral nutrition is needed for more than 1 or 2 days, also facilitating fluid management and continuous supply of nitrogen scavengers and L-arginine.

If there is severe hyperammonemia with significant associated neurological symptoms, extracorporeal detoxification should be performed to remove ammonia, by either venovenous hemodiafiltration (infants and children) or hemodialysis (adults) (Picca et al. 2001).

Except in citrin deficiency, which is treated with high-protein, low-carbohydrate diet and L-arginine and pyruvate supplementation (Imamura et al. 2003; Mutoh et al. 2008), and in NAGS deficiency, which only requires oral carbamylglutamate, chronic treatment of all other primary urea cycle defects requires lifelong protein restriction, use of scavenger drugs and of L-arginine/L-citrulline, and preparation to cope with catabolic situations. Liver transplantation provides a definitive cure for all urea cycle disorders and for citrin deficiency.

In the case of CAVA deficiency, management of acute hyperammonemia follows the above. LPI is a more complex disorder, with currently mainly symptomatic treatment for its many complications; management of acute hyperammonemia is rarely required. For prevention of hyperammonemia, see below standard management table. In OAT deficiency, hyperammonemia is only described in patients of very young age. Management of acute hyperammonemia in PC and in TMEM70 deficiencies follows the principles of the primary urea cycle disorders.

## Emergency Treatment Table and Medication Requirements

**Table 17.21** Dosages of drugs to be used in acute hyperammonemia and acute decompensations

| Disorder[a] | Sodium benzoate (to be given IV in glucose 10%) | Sodium PBA/sodium phenylacetate (to be given IV in glucose 10%) | L-Arginine hydrochloride (to be given IV in glucose 10%) | *N*-carbamylglutamate (only available as oral/enteral drug) |
|---|---|---|---|---|
| NAGS deficiency | 250 mg/kg as bolus in 90–120 min, then maintenance 250–500 mg/kg/day[b]; >20 kg body weight: 5.5 g/$m^2$/day | 250 mg/kg as bolus in 90–120 min, then maintenance 250–500 mg/kg/day[b]; >20 kg body weight: 5.5 g/$m^2$/day | 250 mg/kg (1.2 mmol/kg) as bolus in 90–120 min, then maintenance 250 mg/kg/day (1.2 mmol/kg/day) | 100 mg/kg bolus per nasogastric tube, then 25–62.5 mg/kg every 6 h |
| CPS1 deficiency and OTC deficiency | Same | Same | Same | – |
| ASS deficiency | Same | Same | Same | – |
| ASL deficiency[c] | Same | Same | 200–400 mg/kg (1–2 mmol/kg) as bolus in 90–120 min, then maintenance 200–400 mg/kg/day (1–2 mmol/kg/day) | – |
| ARG1 deficiency[d] | Same | – | AVOID | – |
| HHH syndrome | Same | Same | – | – |
| Citrin deficiency[e] | Same | Same | 10–15 g/day[f] | – |
| CAVA deficiency | 250 mg/kg as bolus in 90–120 min, then maintenance 250–500 mg/kg/day[b]; >20 kg bw 5.5 g/$m^2$/day | 250 mg/kg as bolus in 90–120 min, then maintenance 250–500 mg/kg/day[b] | 250 mg/kg (1.2 mmol/kg) as bolus in 90–120 min, then maintenance 250 mg/kg/day (1.2 mmol/kg/day) | 100 mg/kg bolus per nasogastric tube, then 25–62.5 mg/kg every 6 h |
| LPI[g] | Same | Same | Same | – |
| P5CS deficiency | Few patients reported with frank hyperammonemia. Arginine or protein feeding should be effective[g] | | | |
| OAT deficiency[h] | 250 mg/kg as bolus in 90–120 min, then maintenance 250–500 mg/kg/day[b]; >20 kg bw 5.5 g/$m^2$/day | 250 mg/kg as bolus in 90–120 min, then maintenance 250–500 mg/kg/day[b] | 250 mg/kg (1.2 mmol/kg) as bolus in 90–120 min, then maintenance 250 mg/kg/day (1.2 mmol/kg/day) | – |
| HIHA syndrome | Not applicable | | | |
| GS deficiency | Not applicable | | | |
| PC deficiency | 250 mg/kg as bolus in 90–120 min, then maintenance 250–500 mg/kg/day[b]; >20 kg bw 5.5 g/$m^2$/day | 250 mg/kg as bolus in 90–120 min, then maintenance 250–500 mg/kg/day[b] | 250 mg/kg (1.2 mmol/kg) as bolus in 90–120 min, then maintenance 250 mg/kg/day (1.2 mmol/kg/day) | – |
| TMEM70 deficiency | Same | Same | Same | – |

Table adapted from Häberle et al. (2012)

Maximal daily drug dosages: sodium benzoate 12 g/day, sodium PBA 12 g/day, L-arginine 12 g/day (15 g/day in citrin deficiency)

*Note*: The doses indicated can be used at the start of treatment but must be adapted depending on plasma ammonia and amino acids

Sodium benzoate and sodium PBA/phenylacetate should be given in parallel in severe acute decompensation. In less severe cases, a stepwise approach with initial sodium benzoate and if hyperammonemia persists or worsens, the addition of sodium PBA/phenylacetate can be chosen

[a]In undiagnosed patients, consider additional use of carnitine 100 mg/kg IV, hydroxycobalamin 1 mg IM/IV, and biotin 10 mg IV/PO

[b]If on hemodialysis/hemodiafiltration, maintenance doses should be increased by 50% without exceeding the top limit given

[c]In ASL deficiency, L-arginine therapy for acute decompensations might be sufficient for some patients

[d]The risk for acute hyperammonemic decompensation is low in ARG1 deficiency

[e]Glucose or other carbohydrates should not be administered (mannitol is allowed) and protein should not be restricted

[f]Limited data in literature; dose of arginine according to Imamura et al. (2003)

[g]Rarely presentation with acute hyperammonemia

[h]Only in neonates and young infants

## Standard Treatment Table and Medication Requirements

**Table 17.22** Dosages of drugs to be used per orally for long-term treatment

| Disorder | Diet | Sodium benzoate[a] (mg/kg/day) | Sodium PBA (g) or glycerol PBA (mL)[a,b] | L-Arginine[a] (hydrochloride and/or free base) (mg/kg/day) | L-Citrulline[a] (mg/kg/day) | Carbamylglutamate[a] (mg/kg/day) |
|---|---|---|---|---|---|---|
| NAGS deficiency | Normal | – | – | – | – | 10–100 |
| CPS1 deficiency | Protein-restricted | Up to 250[c,d] max. 12 g/day | Sodium PBA: <20 kg, up to 0.25 g/kg/day[c,d] >20 kg, 5 g/m²/day max. 12 g/day or glycerol PBA: Dosages in mL equal dosage in g of sodium PBA times 0.85 | <20 kg, 100–200[e] mg/kg/day or 0.5–1 mmol/kg/day >20 kg, 2.5–6 g/m²/day max. 6 g/day | 100–200[e] Max. 6 g/day | – |
| OTC deficiency | Protein-restricted | Same | Same | Same as for CPS1 deficiency | 100–200[e] Max. 6 g/day | – |
| ASS deficiency | Protein-restricted | Same | Same | <20 kg, 100–300[c,d] mg/kg/day or 0.5–1.5 mmol/kg/day >20 kg, 2.5–6 g/m²/day[d] max. 8 g/day | – | – |
| ASL deficiency | Protein-restricted | Same | Same | Same as for ASS deficiency | – | – |
| ARG1 deficiency | Protein-restricted | Same | Same | AVOID | – | – |
| HHH syndrome | Protein-restricted | Same | Same | <20 kg, 100–200[e] mg/kg/day >20 kg, 2.5–6 g/m²/day max. 6 g/day | 100–250[e] Max. 6 g/day | – |
| Citrin deficiency | Low-carbohydrate and protein-rich | For children: fat-soluble vitamins and use of lactose-free formula<br>For adults: L-arginine (5–10 g/day), sodium pyruvate (4–9 g/day), medium chain triglycerides oil (45 mL/day); liver transplantation | | | | |
| CAVA deficiency | Protein-restricted (in neonates during crisis) | No reports on long-term drug treatment available | | | | |
| LPI | Protein-restricted | L-citrulline 100 mg/kg/day in 4 doses<br>Sodium benzoate and/or sodium phenylbutyrate 100–250 mg/kg/day | | | | |
| P5CS deficiency | Normal | Consider ornithine and/or arginine supplementation and perhaps also proline supplementation | | | | |
| OAT deficiency | Protein-restricted, especially low-ornithine | Not applicable | | | | |
| HIHA syndrome | Normal | Diazoxide (for treatment of hyperinsulinism) | | | | |

(continued)

**Table 17.22** (continued)

| Disorder | Diet | Sodium benzoate[a] (mg/kg/day) | Sodium PBA (g) or glycerol PBA (mL)[a,b] | L-Arginine[a] (hydrochloride and/or free base) (mg/kg/day) | L-Citrulline[a] (mg/kg/day) | Carbamylglutamate[a] (mg/kg/day) |
|---|---|---|---|---|---|---|
| GS deficiency | Normal | No treatment available (consider oral/enteral use of glutamine and of nicotinamide) | | | | |
| PC deficiency | Protein-restricted | Not applicable | | | | |
| TMEM70 deficiency | Normal | Not applicable | | | | |

Table adapted from Häberle et al. (2012)

All medications should be divided into three to four doses daily taken with meals and distributed as far as possible throughout the day. Food intake and protein intake are also recommended to be divided in frequent small meals, considering a light evening snack to minimize night fasting catabolism

[a]1 g equal 6.94 mmol sodium benzoate; 5.37 mmol sodium PBA; 4.75 mmol arginine hydrochloride; 5.74 mmol arginine base; 5.71 mmol citrulline; 5.32 mmol carbamylglutamate, respectively. 1 mL glycerol phenylbutyrate delivers 6.22 mmol of phenylbutyrate

[b]PBA is the second-choice drug for long-term treatment and should be given in patients not responsive to benzoate alone (according to Häberle et al. (2019))

[c]Serum/plasma levels of benzoate/PBA and plasma levels of arginine should be monitored

[d]In some patients, higher doses are needed, according to expert advice

[e]If citrulline is given, there is usually no need for concomitant use of L-arginine

## References


Batshaw ML, MacArthur RB, Tuchman M. Alternative pathway therapy for urea cycle disorders: twenty years later. J Pediatr. 2001;138:S46–54; discussion S54–5.

Brusilow SW. Arginine, an indispensable amino acid for patients with inborn errors of urea synthesis. J Clin Invest. 1984;74:2144–8.

Brusilow S, Horwich A. Urea cycle enzymes. In: Scriver C, Beaudet A, Sly W, Valle D, editors. The metabolic & molecular bases of inherited disease. 8th ed. New York: McGraw-Hill; 2001. p. 1909–63.

Colombo JP, Peheim E, Kretschmer R, Dauwalder H, Sidiropoulos D. Plasma ammonia concentrations in newborns and children. Clin Chim Acta. 1984;138:283–91.

Enns GM. Nitrogen sparing therapy revisited 2009. Mol Genet Metab. 2010;100(Suppl 1):S65–71.

Grisolia S, Báguena R, Mayor F, editors. The urea cycle. New York: Wiley; 1976. ISBN 0-471-32791-3.

Gropman AL, Batshaw ML. Cognitive outcome in urea cycle disorders. Mol Genet Metab. 2004;81(Suppl 1):S58–62.

Gropman AL, Summar M, Leonard JV. Neurological implications of urea cycle disorders. J Inherit Metab Dis. 2007;30:865–79.

Häberle J. Clinical practice: the management of hyperammonemia. Eur J Pediatr. 2011;170:21–34.

Häberle J, Burlina A, Chakrapani A, Dixon M, Karall D, Lindner M, Mandel H, Martinelli D, Pintos-Morell G, Santer R, Skouma A, Servais A, Tal G, Rubio V, Huemer M, Dionisi-Vici C. Suggested guidelines for the diagnosis and management of urea cycle disorders: First revision. J Inherit Metab Dis. 2019;42:1192–230.

Häussinger D. Liver glutamine metabolism. J Parenter Enteral Nutr. 1990a;14:56S–62S.

Häussinger D. Nitrogen metabolism in liver: structural and functional organization and physiological relevance. Biochem J. 1990b;267:281–90.

Häussinger D, Görg B. Interaction of oxidative stress, astrocyte swelling and cerebral ammonia toxicity. Curr Opin Clin Nutr Metab Care. 2010;13:87–92.

Imamura Y, Kobayashi K, Shibatou T, Aburada S, Tahara K, Kubozono O, Saheki T. Effectiveness of carbohydrate-restricted diet and arginine granules therapy for adult-onset type II citrullinemia: a case report of siblings showing homozygous SLC25A13 mutation with and without the disease. Hepatol Res. 2003;26:68–72.

Leonard JV. The nutritional management of urea cycle disorders. J Pediatr. 2001;138:S40–44; discussion S44–5.

Leonard JV, McKiernan PJ. The role of liver transplantation in urea cycle disorders. Mol Genet Metab. 2004;81(Suppl 1):S74–8.

Leonard JV, Morris AA. Urea cycle disorders. Semin Neonatol. 2002;7:27–35.

Marco-Marín C, Escamilla-Honrubia JM,Llácer JL, Seri M, Panza E, Rubio V. Δ1-Pyrroline-5-carboxylate synthetase deficiency: An emergent multifaceted urea cycle-related disorder. J Inherit Metab Dis. 2020;43:657–70.

Mori M, Gotoh T, Nagasaki A, Takiguchi M, Sonoki T. Regulation of the urea cycle enzyme genes in nitric oxide synthesis. J Inherit Metab Dis. 1998;21(Suppl 1):59–71.

Mutoh K, Kurokawa K, Kobayashi K, Saheki T. Treatment of a citrin-deficient patient at the early stage of adult-onset type II citrullinaemia with arginine and sodium pyruvate. J Inherit Metab Dis. 2008;31(Suppl 2):S343–7.

Nassogne MC, Heron B, Touati G, Rabier D, Saudubray JM. Urea cycle defects: management and outcome. J Inherit Metab Dis. 2005;28:407–14.

Picca S, Dionisi-Vici C, Abeni D, Pastore A, Rizzo C, Orzalesi M, Sabetta G, Rizzoni G, Bartuli A. Extracorporeal dialysis in neonatal hyperammonemia: modalities and prognostic indicators. Pediatr Nephrol. 2001;16:862–7.

Rubio V, Grisolia S. Treating urea cycle defects. Nature. 1981;292:496.

Singh RH. Nutritional management of patients with urea cycle disorders. J Inherit Metab Dis. 2007;30:880–7.

Summar ML, Dobbelaere D, Brusilow S, Lee B. Diagnosis, symptoms, frequency and mortality of 260 patients with urea cycle disorders from a 21-year, multicentre study of acute hyperammonaemic episodes. Acta Paediatr. 2008;97:1420–5.

# Amino Acid Transport Defects

# 18

Manuel Palacín, Stefan Bröer, and Gaia Novarino

## Contents



M. Palacín (✉)
Institute for Research in Biomedicine (IRB Barcelona), Barcelona Institute of Science and Technology, Barcelona, Spain

Centro de Investigación Biomédica en Red de Enfermedades Raras (CIBERER), Barcelona, Spain

Department of Biochemistry and Molecular Biomedicine, Faculty of Biology, University of Barcelona, Barcelona, Spain
e-mail: manuel.palacin@irbbarcelona.org

S. Bröer
Research School of Biology, The Australian National University, Canberra, ACT, Australia
e-mail: stefan.broeer@anu.edu.au

G. Novarino
Institute of Science and Technology (IST) Austria, Klosterneuburg, Austria
e-mail: gaia.novarino@ist.ac.at

**Summary**

Disorders associated with the malfunction of amino acid transporters mainly affect the function of the intestine, kidney, brain, and liver. Mutations of brain amino acid transporters, for example, alter neuronal excitability (e.g., episodic ataxia due to SLC1A3 (EAAT1) defect and hyperekplexia due to SLC6A5 (GLYT2) deficiency) or brain development (SLC1A1 (EAAT3), SLC3A2/SLC7A5 (CD98hc/LAT1), and SLC1A4 (ASCT1) deficiencies). Mutations of renal and intestinal amino acid transporters SLC3A1/SLC7A9 (rBAT/b$^{0,+}$AT) and SLC1A1 (EAAT3) cause renal problems (cystinuria and dicarboxylic amino-aciduria, respectively) and malabsorption that can affect


N. Blau et al. (eds.), *Physician's Guide to the Diagnosis, Treatment, and Follow-Up of Inherited Metabolic Diseases*,
https://doi.org/10.1007/978-3-030-67727-5_18

whole-body homoeostasis (Hartnup disorder SLC6A19 ($B^0AT1$), lysinuric protein intolerance SLC3A2/SLC7A7 (CD98hc/$y^+LAT1$), and hyperdibasic aminoaciduria type 1). Mutations in the neuronal system A amino acid transporter SLC38A8 (SNAT8) cause eye developmental and visual defects. Inborn errors associated with mitochondrial SLC25 family members such as SLC25A12 (neuronal- and muscle-specific mitochondrial aspartate/glutamate transporter 1; AGC1) (global cerebral hypomyelination), SLC25A13 (aspartate/glutamate transporter 2) (citrin deficiency), SLC25A15 (ornithine-citrulline carrier 2) (homocitrullinuria, hyperornithinemia, and hyperammonemia syndrome), and SLC25A22 (mitochondrial glutamate/H+ symporter 1, GC1) (neonatal myoclonic epilepsy) will be dealt within Chap. 43 (defects of mitochondrial carriers).

## Introduction

Amino acid transporters are essential for the absorption of amino acids from nutrition, mediating the interorgan and intercellular transfer of amino acids and the transport of amino acids between cellular compartments (Bröer and Palacín 2011). To date, 11 SLC families are known to comprise amino acid transporters. Defects due to mutations in amino acid transporters in six of these families affecting renal tubular reabsorption (Fig. 18.1) and intestinal absorption, neurotransmitter reuptake in the synapse (Fig. 18.2), and development of organs are considered in this chapter: (1) Mutations in the members of the glutamate transporter family SLC1A1 (EAAT3) and SLC1A3 (EAAT1) cause the primary inherited aminoaciduria named dicarboxylic aminoaciduria and episodic ataxia type 6, respectively (Bailey et al. 2011; Jen et al. 2005). (2 and 3) Mutations in the heteromeric amino acid transporters (HAT) SLC3A1/SLC7A9 (rBAT/$b^{0,+}AT$) and SLC3A2/SLC7A7 (CD98hc/$y^+LAT1$) cause the primary inherited aminoacidurias cystinuria and lysinuric protein intolerance (LPI), respectively (Borsani et al. 1999; Calonge et al. 1994; Feliubadaló et al. 1999; Torrents et al. 1999). Moreover, mutations in SLC3A1/SLC7A5 (CD98hc/LAT1) cause autism spectrum disorder (ASD) (Tărlungeanu et al. 2016) and in SLC3A1/SLC7A8 (CD98hc/LAT2) contribute to age-related hearing loss (ARHL) (Guarch et al. 2018). In cystinuria, mutations are found in either of the two subunits (SLC3A1 or SLC7A9) (Chillarón et al. 2010), whereas in LPI, ASD, and ARHL, mutations are only present in the light subunit SLC7A7, SLC7A5, or SLC7A8, respectively. (4) Mutations in SLC6A5 (neuronal glycine transporter GLYT2), member of the neurotransmitter branch of the neurotransmitter transporter family, cause hyperekplexia (Rees et al. 2006). Mutations in the members of the metabolic branch of this family SLC6A19 (sodium-dependent neutral amino acid transporter $B^0AT$) and SLC1A4 (sodium-dependent small neutral amino acid exchanger ASCT1) cause the primary inherited aminoaciduria named Hartnup disorder (Kleta et al. 2004; Seow et al. 2004) and brain (Damseh et al. 2015; Heimer et al. 2015; Srour et al. 2015), respectively. (5) Mutations in SLC36A2 (proton-dependent glycine, proline, and hydroxyproline transporter PAT2) cause hyperglycinuria and iminoglycinuria with the modulation of variants in SLC6A20 (system IMINO transporter) (Bröer et al. 2008). (6) Mutations in SLC38A8 (neuronal sodium-dependent system A transporter SNAT8) cause eye and visual defects (Perez et al. 2014; Poulter et al. 2013). Finally, one case with mutations in SLC7A2 (cationic amino acid transporter CAT2) with increased plasma concentration of arginine has been described with not yet associated pathology (Yahyaoui et al. 2019), and for the lysine malabsorption syndrome (Omura et al. 1976), dibasic aminoaciduria type I (Kihara et al. 1973), and the methionine malabsorption syndrome (Hooft et al. 1965; Smith and Strang 1958), only one or two families transmitting each disease have been described and the associated genes are unknown.

The principal biochemical and structural characteristics of these amino acid transporters have been reviewed elsewhere (Bröer and Palacín 2011). SLC1 family members (glutamate/aspartate transporters named EAAT for excitatory amino acid transporters 1–5) mediate high-affinity sodium- and potassium-dependent uptake of glutamate and aspartate in mammalian cells. SLC1A1 (EAAT3) is expressed in the apical membrane of epithelial cells of the kidney proximal convoluted tubule (Fig. 18.1) and the small intestine and in neurons of the brain cortex, particularly in the hippocampus, the basal ganglia, and the olfactory bulb. SLC1A3 (EAAT1) is found in astrocytes throughout the brain (Fig. 18.2). It is the main glutamate transporter in the cerebellum, inner ear, circumventricular organs, and retina. Expression in peripheral organs is limited (Zhou and Danbolt 2013). ASCT1 (SLC1A4) is a sodium-activated exchanger of the L-isomers of alanine, serine, cysteine, and threonine with a chloride channel activity that is thermodynamically uncoupled from amino acid transport (Zerangue and Kavanaugh 1996). ASCT1 also transports the co-agonist of NMDA glutamate receptors D-serine, and being expressed in astrocytes has been suggested to play a key role on the signaling of these receptors (Kaplan et al. 2018) (Fig. 18.2). Structural knowledge on SLC1 transporters is based on crystal structures of bacterial homologues (Reyes et al. 2009) and human EAAT1 (Canul-Tec et al. 2017).

HAT are composed of a heavy subunit (SLC3 family) and a light subunit (LAT branch of the SLC7 family), which are linked by a conserved disulfide bridge (Fig. 18.1). Both subunits are required to form functional transporters at the cell

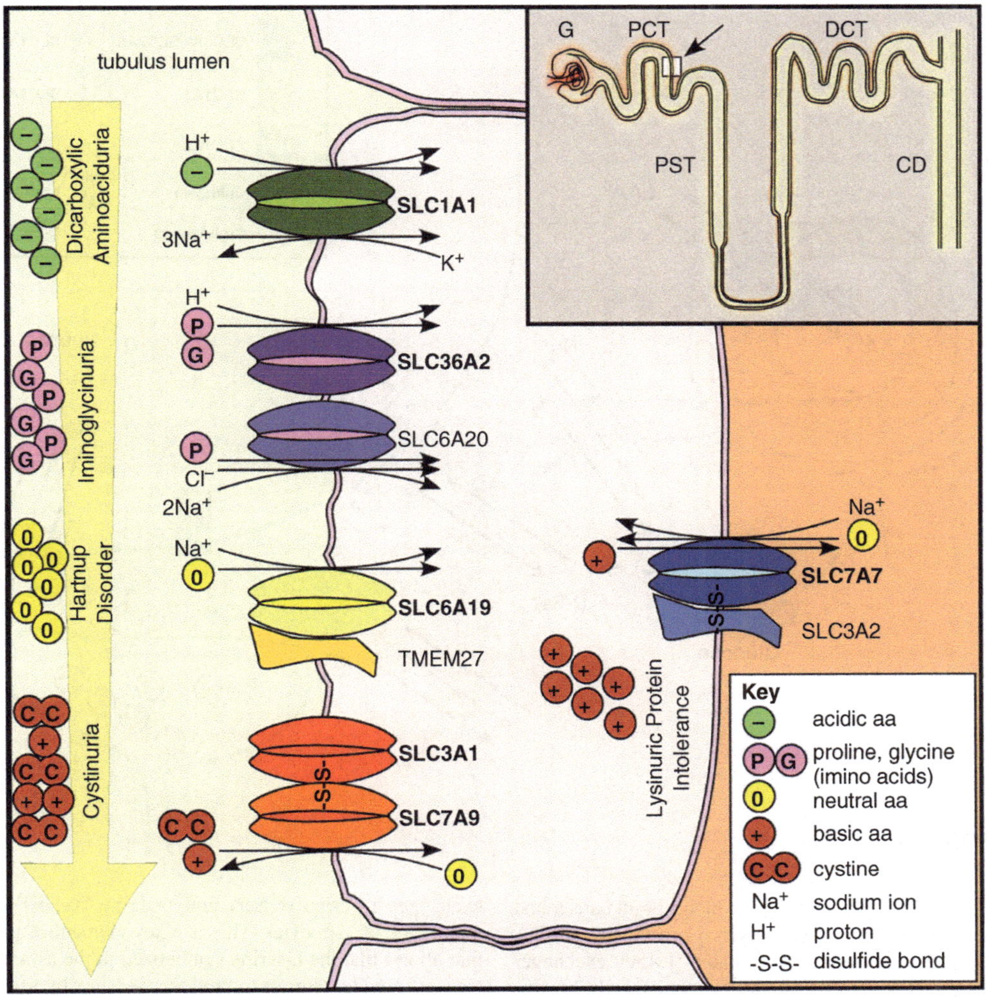


**Fig. 18.1** Principal epithelial transporters involved in amino acid reabsorption, which are mutated in human aminoacidurias. A nephron is depicted (inset), showing the glomerulus (G), proximal convoluted tubule (PCT), proximal straight tubule (PST), distal convoluted tubule (DCT), and collecting duct (CD). A cross section of the proximal convoluted tubule (white square indicated with an arrow) is represented in the main diagram. Four of the aminoacidurias, including dicarboxylic aminoaciduria, iminoglycinuria (and hyperglycinuria), Hartnup disorder, and cystinuria, manifest at the apical surface of the renal tubule, while lysinuric protein intolerance manifests at the basolateral surface (see text for details). The major transporters involved in each aminoaciduria are in bold. Iminoglycinuria results from complete inactivation of SLC36A2, a proline and glycine transporter, or from additional modifying mutations in the high-affinity proline transporter SLC6A20 when SLC36A2 is not completely inactivated (Bröer et al. 2008). Iminoglycinuria is a benign condition with no associated pathology. Mutations in the neutral amino acid transporter, SLC6A19, are responsible for Hartnup disorder (Kleta et al. 2004; Seow et al. 2004). The neutral amino acid transport defect can also be exacerbated by a kidney-specific loss of heterodimerization of mutant SLC6A19 with TMEM27 (Kowalczuk et al. 2008). Finally, no mutations have been identified in SLC3A2, coding for the ancillary protein of y$^+$LAT1 (SLC7A7) in patients with LPI (Bröer and Palacín 2011). Renal amino acid transporters not depicted in the scheme because have not been related to aminoacidurias: (1) SLC3A1/SLC7A13 is expressed in the apical membrane of PST epithelial cells and exchanges cystine and dicarboxylic amino acids (Nagamori et al. 2016), (2) the neutral amino acid exchanger SLC3A2/SLC7A8 and the uniport of aromatic amino acids SLC16A10 are expressed in the basolateral membrane of the PCT epithelial cells where cooperate in the renal reabsorption of neutral amino acids (Vilches et al. 2018). Figure extracted from Bailey et al. (2011)

surface. HAT are amino acid exchangers. Transporter SLC3A1/SLC7A9 (rBAT/b$^{0,+}$AT) is expressed in the apical membrane of epithelial cells of the kidney proximal convoluted tubule and the small intestine (Calonge et al. 1994; Feliubadaló et al. 1999) and transporter SLC3A1/SLC7A13 (rBAT/AGT1) in the kidney proximal straight tubule (Nagamori et al. 2016) (Fig. 18.1). rBAT/b$^{0,+}$AT participates in renal and intestinal (re)absorption of cysteine and cationic amino acids, and rBAT/AGT1 putatively in renal reabsorption of cysteine. Transporter SLC3A2/SLC7A7 (CD98hc/y$^+$LAT1) is mainly expressed in the basolateral plasma membrane of the epithelial cells of the kidney proximal convoluted tubule (Fig. 18.1) and the small intestine, with a role in (re)absorption of cationic amino acids, and in white blood cells (Borsani et al. 1999; Torrents et al. 1999). Transporter SLC3A2/SLC7A5 (CD98hc/LAT1), which exchanges large

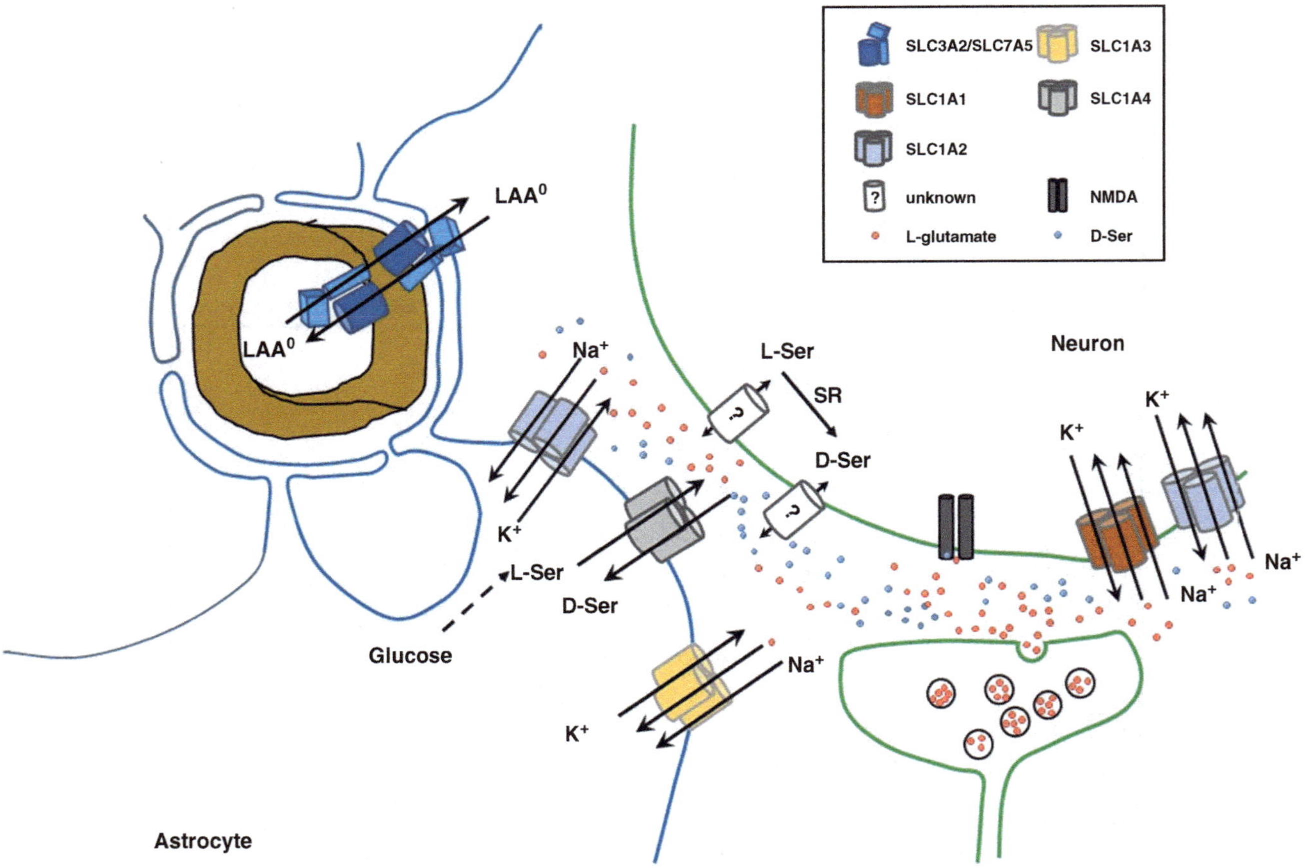


**Fig. 18.2** SLC3A2/SLC7A5 transporter in the blood-brain barrier and principal transporters involved in glutamatergic synapsis with NMDA glutamate receptors. The large neutral amino acid ($LAA^0$) exchanger CD98hc/LAT1 heterodimer is expressed in the endothelial cells (brown) of the blood-brain barrier and mediates access of essential branched chain amino acids to the central nervous system to support proper development. The $Na^+$- and $K^+$-coupled glutamate transporters SLC1A3 (astrocytes), SLC1A1 (neurons), and SLC1A2 (astrocytes and neurons) terminate transmission by active uptake of glutamate from the synaptic cleft in glutamatergic synapses (Zhou and Danbolt 2013). SLC1A4 exchanges L-serine (L-Ser) and D-serine (D-Ser) across the plasma membrane of astrocytes. This is a key element of the "Serine shuttle" that allows that the L-serine synthetized in the astrocytes from glucose is transferred to neurons to produce D-serine, by serine racemase (SR), that acts as a co-agonist of NMDA glutamate receptors (Kaplan et al. 2018). Loss-of-function mutations in SLC7A5 and ASCT1 cause, among other alterations, microcephaly. Loss-of-function mutations in SLC1A1 cause dicarboxylic aminoaciduria with mental retardation and in SLC1A3 cause episodic ataxia. L- and D-serine transporters in neurons and the blood-brain barrier are not depicted here

neutral amino acids, is expressed in the endothelial cells of the blood-brain barrier (Fig. 18.2). Loss-of-function in mouse causes dramatic increase of histidine and depletion of branched chain amino acids in cerebral spinal fluid (Tărlungeanu et al. 2016). Transporter SLC3A2/SLC7A8 (CD98hc/LAT2) has a broad tissue expression, including the basolateral membrane of renal and small intestinal epithelial cells where has a role on renal reabsorption of neutral amino acids (Vilches et al. 2018), and in fibrocytes of the cochlea where supports proper aging of the organ (Guarch et al. 2018). SLC7A2 (CAT2) is a member of the other branch of the SLC7 family, the cationic amino acid transporters (CATs). LATs are exchangers with different amino acid substrate profiles, whereas CATs mediate transport of cationic amino acids in favor of chemical and electrical gradients (see Fotiadis et al. 2013, for a review). The structure of the human heteromeric CD98hc/LAT1 complex has been elucidated (Lee et al. 2019; Yan et al. 2019), as well as that of bacterial homologues of LATs (Errasti-Murugarren et al. 2019) and CATs (Jungnickel et al. 2018) transporters.

The SLC6 family comprises 20 members in humans that can be grouped into four subfamilies, namely, the monoamine transporter branch, the GABA (γ-aminobutyric acid) transporter branch, and the amino acid transporter branches I and II. SLC6A5 (GLYT2) and SLC6A19 ($B^0AT1$) belong to the two latter subfamilies and mediate reuptake of glycine in synapses and the uptake of neutral amino acids in epithelial cells, respectively. GLYT2 is mainly found in the spinal cord where it terminates inhibitory neurotransmission. $B^0AT1$ is found in the apical membrane of kidney proximal tubular epithelial cells (Fig. 18.1) and enterocytes of the small intestine. Structural understanding of this family is derived from the bacterial transporter LeuT, for which structures are available in all conformations (Penmatsa and

Gouaux 2014), the dopamine transporter from *Drosophila* (Penmatsa et al. 2013), and the human serotonin transporter (Coleman et al. 2016).

Finally, transporters of the SLC38 family are found in all cell types of the body. They mediate sodium-dependent net uptake (system A) and sodium- and proton-dependent influx and efflux (system N) of amino acids (see Bröer 2014, for a review). SLC38A8 (SNAT8) is a system A transporter for L-glutamine, L-alanine, L-arginine, L-histidine, and L-aspartate. In mouse, SNAT8 is expressed in adult and fetal brain and in spinal cord and shows weaker expression in other tissues. Protein SNAT8 is present throughout the neuronal retina, with stronger staining in the inner and outer plexiform layers and photoreceptor layer (Perez et al. 2014) and in all neurons, both excitatory and inhibitory, in mouse brain (Hägglund et al. 2015). Structural understanding of this family has been obtained through the crystal structure of the lysosomal member SLC38A9 from zebrafish (Lei et al. 2018).

## Nomenclature

| No. | Disorders of amino acid transport | Alternative name | Abbreviation | Inheritance | Gene symbol | Chromosomal localization | Affected protein | OMIM no. |
|---|---|---|---|---|---|---|---|---|
| 18.1 | Hartnup disorder | | HD | AR | *SLC6A19* | 5p15.33 | Sodium-dependent neutral amino acid transporter ($B^0AT1$) | 234500 |
| 18.2 | Iminoglycinuria | | IG | AR (or digenic) | *SLC36A2* (±*SLC6A20*) | 5q33.1 (3p21.31) | Proton amino acid transporter (PAT2) (system imino transporter SIT) | 242600 |
| 18.3 | Hyperglycinuria | | HG | AD | SLC36A2 | 5q33.1 | Proton amino acid transporter (PAT2) | 138500 |
| 18.4 | Cystinuria type A | | Cystinuria A | AR | *SLC3A1* (1) | 2p16.3 | Amino acid transport system b(0,+) composed by rBAT (SLC3A1) and $b^{0,+}AT$ (SLC7A9) and the cysteine/dicarboxylic amino acid exchanger composed by rBAT (SLC3A) and AGT1 (SLC7A13)[a] | 220100 |
| 18.5 | Cystinuria type B | | Cystinuria B | AD, AR | *SLC7A9* | 19q12 | Amino acid transport system b(0,+) composed by rBAT (SLC3A1) and $b^{0,+}AT$ (SLC7A9) | 220100 |
| 18.6 | Lysinuric protein intolerance | Dibasic aminoaciduria type 2 | LPI | AR | *SLC7A7* | 14q11.2 | Amino acid transport system $y^+L$ (CD98hc/ $y^+LAT1$) (SLC3A2/ SLC7A7)[b] | 222700 |
| 18.7 | Dicarboxylic aminoaciduria | | DA | AR | *SLC1A1* | 9p24 | Neuronal/epithelial high-affinity glutamate transporter, excitatory amino acid transporter 3 (EAAT3) | 222730 |
| 18.8 | Lysine malabsorption syndrome | | | | | | | 247950 |
| 18.9 | Dibasic aminoaciduria type 1 | | | AD | | | | 222690 |
| 18.10 | Methionine malabsorption syndrome | Oasthouse disease; Smith-Strang disease; methioninuria | | | | | | 250900 |

(continued)

| No. | Disorders of amino acid transport | Alternative name | Abbreviation | Inheritance | Gene symbol | Chromosomal localization | Affected protein | OMIM no. |
|---|---|---|---|---|---|---|---|---|
| 18.11 | Cationic amino acid transporter 2 deficiency | | | AR | SLC7A2 | 8p22 | Cationic amino acid transporter 2 (CAT2) | 601872 |
| 18.12 | Large neutral amino acid transporter deficiency | SLC7A5 deficiency | | AR | *SLC7A5* | 16q24.2 | Amino acid exchanger L composed by CD98hc (SLC3A2) and LAT1 (SLC7A5) | 600182 |
| 18.13 | Neuronal system A amino acid transporter deficiency | Foveal hypoplasia type 2 with or without optic nerve misrouting and/or anterior segment dysgenesis | | AR | *SLC38A8* | 16q23.3 | Neuronal sodium-dependent system A amino acid transporter SNAT8 | 609218 |
| 18.14 | Glutamate aspartate transporter deficiency | EAAT1 deficiency; episodic ataxia type 6 | EA6 | AD | *SLC1A3* | 5p13 | Glutamate/aspartate transporter (GLAST); excitatory amino acid transporter 1 (EAAT1) | 612656 |
| 18.15 | ASCT1 transporter deficiency | Spastic tetraplegia, thin corpus callosum, and progressive microcephaly | | AR | *SLC1A4* | 2p14 | Glutamate/neutral amino acid transporter ASCT1 | 616657 |
| 18.16 | Hyperekplexia due to glycine transporter GLYT2 defect | Startle disease, familial | | AR | *SLC6A5* | 11p15.1 | Neuronal glycine transporter GLYT2 | 614618 |

[a]Different recessive contiguous gene deletion syndromes involving PREPL and a variable combination of SLC3A1 (hypotonia-cystinuria syndrome), CAMKMT (atypical hypotonia-cystinuria syndrome), and PPM1B (2p21 deletion syndrome) have been described (Régal et al. 2018)
[b]CD98hc (SLC3A2) is also named 4F2hc

## Signs and Symptoms

**Table 18.1** Hartnup disorder

| System | Symptoms and biomarkers | Neonatal (birth–1 month) | Infancy (1–18 months) | Childhood (1.5–11 years) | Adolescence (11–16 years) | Adulthood (>16 years) |
|---|---|---|---|---|---|---|
| CNS | Ataxia | | ± | ± | ± | |
| Dermatological | **Photosensitivity** | | ± | ± | ± | |
| Psychiatric | Psychosis | | ± | ± | ± | |
| Laboratory findings | Glutamic acid (urine) | n-↑ | n-↑ | n-↑ | n-↑ | n-↑ |
| | Neutral amino acids (urine) | ↑ | ↑ | ↑ | ↑ | ↑ |

**Table 18.2** Iminoglycinuria

| System | Symptoms and biomarkers | Neonatal (birth–1 month) | Infancy (1–18 months) | Childhood (1.5–11 years) | Adolescence (11–16 years) | Adulthood (>16 years) |
|---|---|---|---|---|---|---|
| Other | No clinical significance | + | + | + | + | + |
| Laboratory findings | Glycine (urine) | ↑↑ | ↑↑ | ↑↑ | ↑↑ | ↑↑ |
| | Hydroxyproline (urine) | ↑↑ | ↑↑ | ↑↑ | ↑↑ | ↑↑ |
| | Proline (urine) | ↑↑ | ↑↑ | ↑↑ | ↑↑ | ↑↑ |

**Table 18.3** Hyperglycinuria

| System | Symptoms and biomarkers | Neonatal (birth–1 month) | Infancy (1–18 months) | Childhood (1.5–11 years) | Adolescence (11–16 years) | Adulthood (>16 years) |
|---|---|---|---|---|---|---|
| Other | No clinical significance | + | + | + | + | + |
| Laboratory findings | Glycine (urine) | ↑ | ↑ | ↑ | ↑ | ↑ |

**Table 18.4** Cystinuria type A

| System | Symptoms and biomarkers | Neonatal (birth–1 month) | Infancy (1–18 months) | Childhood (1.5–11 years) | Adolescence (11–16 years) | Adulthood (>16 years) |
|---|---|---|---|---|---|---|
| Metabolic | Hematuria | | ± | ± | ± | ± |
| Renal | Obstructive uropathy | | ± | ± | ± | ± |
| | Renal failure, chronic | | | ± | ± | ± |
| | Urinary infections | | ± | ± | ± | ± |
| | **Urolithiasis, cystine stones** | | ± | ± | ± | ++ |
| Laboratory findings | Arginine (plasma) | | ↓-n | ↓-n | ↓-n | ↓-n |
| | Arginine (urine) | | ↑↑ | ↑↑ | ↑↑ | ↑↑ |
| | Cystine (plasma) | | ↓-n | ↓-n | ↓-n | ↓-n |
| | Cystine (urine) | | ↑↑ | ↑↑ | ↑↑ | ↑↑ |
| | Cystine crystals (urine) | + | + | + | + | + |
| | Lysine (plasma) | | ↓-n | ↓-n | ↓-n | ↓-n |
| | Lysine (urine) | | ↑↑ | ↑↑ | ↑↑ | ↑↑ |
| | Ornithine (plasma) | | ↓-n | ↓-n | ↓-n | ↓-n |
| | Ornithine (urine) | | ↑↑ | ↑↑ | ↑↑ | ↑↑ |

**Table 18.5** Cystinuria type B

| System | Symptoms and biomarkers | Neonatal (birth–1 month) | Infancy (1–18 months) | Childhood (1.5–11 years) | Adolescence (11–16 years) | Adulthood (>16 years) |
|---|---|---|---|---|---|---|
| Metabolic | Hematuria | | ± | ± | ± | ± |
| Renal | Obstructive uropathy | | ± | ± | ± | ± |
| | Renal failure, chronic | | | ± | ± | ± |
| | Urinary infections | | ± | ± | ± | ± |
| | **Urolithiasis** | | ± | ± | ± | + |
| | Urolithiasis, cystine stones | | ± | ± | ± | ++ |
| Laboratory findings | Arginine (plasma) | | ↓-n | ↓-n | ↓-n | ↓-n |
| | Arginine (urine) | | ↑↑ | ↑↑ | ↑↑ | ↑↑ |
| | Cystine (plasma) | | ↓-n | ↓-n | ↓-n | ↓-n |
| | Cystine (urine)[a] | | ↑↑ | ↑↑ | ↑↑ | ↑↑ |
| | Cystine crystals (urine) | + | + | + | + | + |
| | Lysine (plasma) | | ↓-n | ↓-n | ↓-n | ↓-n |
| | Lysine (urine) | | ↑↑ | ↑↑ | ↑↑ | ↑↑ |
| | Ornithine (plasma) | | ↓-n | ↓-n | ↓-n | ↓-n |
| | Ornithine (urine) | | ↑↑ | ↑↑ | ↑↑ | ↑↑ |

[a]Certain mutations in b0,+AT (SLC7A9) (e.g., p.T123M) cause isolated cystinuria (OMIM 238200) in heterozygosis (Eggermann et al. 2007)

**Table 18.6** Lysinuric protein intolerance

| System | Symptoms and biomarkers | Neonatal (birth–1 month) | Infancy (1–18 months) | Childhood (1.5–11 years) | Adolescence (11–16 years) | Adulthood (>16 years) |
|---|---|---|---|---|---|---|
| Autonomic system | Hypertension | | | – | ± | ± |
| CNS | **Coma, hyperammonemic** | | ± | ± | ± | ± |
| | Intellectual disability | | | ± | ± | ± |
| Dermatological | Sparse hair | | | ± | ± | ± |
| Digestive | Diarrhea | | ± | ± | ± | ± |
| | Hepatosplenomegaly | ± | ± | ± | ± | ± |
| | Protein intolerance | | | ± | ± | ± |
| | Vomiting | | ± | ± | ± | ± |
| Hematological | Hemophagocytic lymphohistiocytosis, macrophage activation syndrome | | | ± | ± | ± |
| Musculoskeletal | Bone growth | n | n | ↓-n | ↓-n | ↓-n |
| | Osteoporosis | | | ± | ± | ± |
| Renal | Glomerulonephritis | | | ± | ± | ± |
| | Renal failure, end stage | | | – | ± | ± |
| Respiratory | Chest radiographs, interstitial changes | | | ± | ± | ± |
| | Pulmonary alveolar proteinosis | | | ± | ± | ± |
| | Respiratory insufficiency | | | ± | ± | ± |
| Other | Combined hyperlipidemia | | | ± | ± | ± |
| Laboratory findings | Alanine (plasma) | | | ↑ | ↑ | ↑ |
| | Ammonia (blood) | ↑ | ↑ | ↑ | ↑ | ↑ |
| | Arginine (plasma) | n | n | ↓-n | ↓-n | ↓-n |
| | Arginine (urine) | | | ↑ | ↑ | ↑ |
| | Citrulline (plasma) | | | ↑ | ↑ | ↑ |
| | Ferritin (serum) | n | ↑ | ↑ | ↑ | ↑ |
| | Glutamine (plasma) | | | ↑ | ↑ | ↑ |
| | Glycine (plasma) | | | ↑ | ↑ | ↑ |
| | Lactate dehydrogenase, LDH (plasma) | n | n-↑ | n-↑ | n-↑ | n-↑ |
| | Lysine (plasma) | n | n | ↓-n | ↓-n | ↓-n |
| | Lysine (urine) | | | ↑↑ | ↑↑ | ↑↑ |
| | Ornithine (plasma) | n | n | ↓-n | ↓-n | ↓-n |
| | Ornithine (urine) | | | ↑ | ↑ | ↑ |
| | Orotic acid (urine) | | ↑ | ↑ | ↑ | ↑ |
| | Proline (plasma) | | | ↑ | ↑ | ↑ |

**Table 18.7** Dicarboxylic aminoaciduria

| System | Symptoms and biomarkers | Neonatal (birth–1 month) | Infancy (1–18 months) | Childhood (1.5–11 years) | Adolescence (11–16 years) | Adulthood (>16 years) |
|---|---|---|---|---|---|---|
| CNS | Intellectual disability | | ± | ± | ± | ± |
| Psychiatric | Behavior, psychotic | | | ± | ± | ± |
| Renal | Urolithiasis, glutamate stones | | ± | ± | ± | ± |
| Laboratory findings | Aspartic acid (urine) | ↑ | ↑ | ↑ | ↑ | ↑ |
| | Glutamic acid (urine) | ↑↑ | ↑↑ | ↑↑ | ↑↑ | ↑↑ |

**Table 18.8** Lysine malabsorption syndrome[a]

| System | Symptoms and biomarkers | Neonatal (birth–1 month) | Infancy (1–18 months) | Childhood (1.5–11 years) | Adolescence (11–16 years) | Adulthood (>16 years) |
|---|---|---|---|---|---|---|
| CNS | Ankle clonus | + | + | | | |
| | Convulsions | + | + | | | |
| | Limited deep tendon reflexes | + | + | | | |
| | Mental and physical retardation | + | + | | | |
| Musculoskeletal | Head circumference | + | + | | | |
| | Osteoporosis | + | + | | | |
| Other | Body weight | ↓ | ↓ | | | |
| | Flaccid members | + | + | | | |
| Laboratory findings | Arginine (P, U) | n | n | n | | |
| | Cystine (P, U) | n | n | n | | |
| | Lysine (P) | ↓ | ↓ | ↓ | | |
| | Lysine (U) | ↑ | ↑ | ↑ | | |
| | Ornithine (P, U) | n | n | n | | |

[a]Only a 21-month-old girl has been presented in Omura et al. (1976), which showed increased renal clearance of Lys and malabsorption of Lys after oral load

**Table 18.9** Dibasic aminoaciduria type I

| System | Symptoms and biomarkers | Neonatal (birth–1 month) | Infancy (1–18 months) | Childhood (1.5–11 years) | Adolescence (11–16 years) | Adulthood (>16 years) |
|---|---|---|---|---|---|---|
| CNS | Athetosis | | ± | + | | |
| | Dysarthria | | ± | + | | |
| | **Intellectual disability** | | + | ++ | | |
| Psychiatric | **Hyperactivity** | | + | ++ | | |
| Other | **Adverse reaction to phenothiazines** | | ++ | ++ | | |
| Laboratory findings | Arginine (plasma) | | n | n | n | |
| | Arginine (urine) | | | ↑ | ↑ | |
| | Cystine (plasma) | | n | n | n | |
| | Lysine (plasma) | | n | n | n | |
| | Lysine (urine) | | | ↑ | ↑ | |
| | Lysine, intestinal absorption | | | | ↓ | |
| | Ornithine (plasma) | | n | n | n | |
| | Ornithine (urine) | | | ↑ | ↑ | |

**Table 18.10** Methionine malabsorption syndrome

| System | Symptoms and biomarkers | Neonatal (birth–1 month)[a] | Infancy (1–18 months)[a,b] | Childhood (1.5–11 years) | Adolescence (11–16 years) | Adulthood (>16 years) |
|---|---|---|---|---|---|---|
| CNS | Convulsions | + | + | + | + | |
| | Intellectual disability | + | + | + | + | |
| Digestive | Diarrhea | + | + | + | + | |
| Hair | White hair | + | + | + | ± | |
| Respiratory | Hypernoea (attacks) | + | + | + | + | |
| Other | Oasthouse smell (U) | + | + | + | + | |
| Laboratory findings | 3-Hydroxybutyric acid (U) | ↑ | ↑ | ↑ | | |
| | Branched chain amino acids (U)[c] | ↑ | ↑ | ↑ | | |
| | Methionine (U)[c] | ↑ | ↑ | ↑ | | |
| | Serine (U) | ↑ | ↑ | ↑ | | |

[a]A neonatal girl was first described with the "oasthouse disease" with hyperexcretion in urine of α-hydroxybutyric acid and amino acids (phenylalanine, tyrosine, and methionine) and a suspected phenylketonuria (PKU) mimicked condition (Smith and Strang 1958). A toddler girl presented similar symptoms but without PKU signs (Hooft et al. 1968, 1965). Methionine malabsorption was demonstrated in this patient

[b]Methionine-poor diet introduced at 2 years of age improved all the signs and symptoms with the exception of mental retardation

[c]The indicated aminoaciduria was not detected in the second patient (Hooft et al. 1968, 1965)

**Table 18.11** Cationic amino acid transporter 2 deficiency

| System | Symptoms and biomarkers[a] | Neonatal (birth–1 month) | Infancy (1–18 months) | Childhood (1.5–11 years) | Adolescence (11–16 years) | Adulthood (>16 years) |
|---|---|---|---|---|---|---|
| Other | No clinical symptoms | | | | | |
| Laboratory findings | Arginine (P) | ↑ | ↑ | ↑ | | |
| | Arginine/ornithine ratio (P) | n | | | | |
| | Arginine, lysine, ornithine (U) | ↑ | ↑ | ↑ | | |
| | Asymmetric dimethylarginine (P, U) | n | | n | | |
| | Guanidinoacetate (U) | ↑ | | n | | |
| | Lysine (P) | ↑ | ↑ | ↑ | | |
| | NO (nitrate/nitrite) | n | | n | | |
| | Ornithine (P) | n | n | n | | |
| | Symmetric dimethylarginine (U) | ↑ | | n | | |

[a]Only a 4-year-old boy has been reported (Yahyaoui et al. 2019). After identifying hyperargininemia in newborn screening (dried blood spot) and diagnosis (1 month old), the infant is on protein-restricted diet of 2 g/kg/day with PFD1 formula 30 g/day to control amino acid levels. He has been asymptomatic and presents normal psychomotor development

**Table 18.12** Large neutral amino acid transporter deficiency

| System | Symptoms and biomarkers | Neonatal (birth–1 month) | Infancy (1–18 months) | Childhood (1.5–11 years) | Adolescence (11–16 years) | Adulthood (>16 years) |
|---|---|---|---|---|---|---|
| CNS | **Autism spectrum disorder** | | ++ | ++ | ++ | ++ |
| | **Developmental delay** | ++ | ++ | | | |
| | **Microcephaly** | ++ | ++ | ++ | | |
| | **Motor delay** | – | ++ | ++ | | |
| Laboratory findings | Branched chain amino acid levels (CSF) | + | + | + | + | + |

**Table 18.13** Neuronal system A amino acid transporter deficiency

| System | Symptoms and biomarkers | Neonatal (birth–1 month) | Infancy (1–18 months) | Childhood (1.5–11 years) | Adolescence (11–16 years) | Adulthood (>16 years) | Characteristic |
|---|---|---|---|---|---|---|---|
| Eye | Anterior segment dysgenesis[a] | | | | | ± | |
| | Defective visual acuity | | + | | | + | |
| | Foveal hypoplasia | | + | | | + | |
| | Nystagmus[b] | | + | | | + | |
| | Ocular albinism | | − | | | − | |
| | Optic nerve decussation defects[a] | | | | | + | |
| | Refractive errors[b] | | | | | ± | |
| Other | Albinism | | − | | | − | |

Fifteen patients from seven families of diverse origin and nine patients from three families of Jews Indian (Mumbai region) ancestry have been reported by Perez et al. (2014) and Poulter et al. (2013), respectively

[a]Optic nerve decussation defects (misrouting in the optic chiasm) and dysgenesis of the anterior segment of the eye have only been characterized in Poulter et al. (2013)

[b]Nystagmus and refractive errors have only been characterized in Perez et al. (2014)

**Table 18.14** Glutamate aspartate transporter deficiency

| System | Symptoms and biomarkers | Neonatal (birth–1 month) | Infancy (1–18 months) | Childhood (1.5–11 years) | Adolescence (11–16 years) | Adulthood (>16 years) |
|---|---|---|---|---|---|---|
| CNS | **Ataxia** | | | + | + | + |
| | Epilepsy | | | + | + | + |
| | Hemiplegic migraine | | | + | + | + |
| | Interictal nystagmus | | | + | + | + |
| Digestive | Nausea | | | + | + | + |
| | Vomiting | | | + | + | + |
| Eye | Photophobia | | | + | + | + |

**Table 18.15** ASCT1 transporter deficiency

| System | Symptoms and biomarkers | Neonatal (birth–1 month) | Infancy (1–18 months) | Childhood (1.5–11 years) | Adolescence (11–16 years) | Adulthood (>16 years) |
|---|---|---|---|---|---|---|
| CNS | Brain atrophy (MRI) | ± | ± | ± | ± | |
| | EEG hypsarrhythmia | ± | ± | ± | ± | |
| | EEG epileptic spikes | ± | ± | ± | ± | |
| | Hypomyelination (MRI) | ± | ± | ± | ± | |
| | **Intellectual disability** | +++ | +++ | +++ | +++ | |
| | Microcephaly | ± | ± | ± | ± | |
| | **Motor developmental delay** | ++ | ++ | ++ | ++ | |
| | Musculoskeletal spasticity | ± | ± | ± | ± | |
| | Seizures | ± | ± | ± | ± | |
| | Thin corpus callosum | ± | ± | ± | ± | |

Fifteen patients from ten Ashkenazi and one Ashkenazi-Iraqi Jews families were reported by Damseh et al. (2015), Heimer et al. (2015), and Srour et al. (2015)

**Table 18.16** GLYT2 transporter deficiency

| System | Symptoms and biomarkers | Neonatal (birth–1 month) | Infancy (1–18 months) | Childhood (1.5–11 years) | Adolescence (11–16 years) | Adulthood (>16 years) |
|---|---|---|---|---|---|---|
| CNS | **Head-retraction reflex** | ↑ | ↑ | ↑ | ↑ | ↑ |
| | Intellectual disability, mild | | ± | ± | ± | ± |
| | Periodic limb movements during sleep | ± | ± | ± | ± | ± |
| | Startle reflex | + | + | + | + | + |
| | **Stiffness** | + | + | + | + | ± |
| Musculoskeletal | Hernias | | ± | ± | ± | ± |
| | Hip dislocation | ± | ± | ± | ± | ± |
| Other | Sudden infant death | ± | ± | | | |

## **Metabolic Pathways** (See Figs. 18.1 and 18.2)

## Metabolites Important for Diagnosis

**Hartnup disorder** Metabolites important for diagnosis: neutral amino acids in the urine (glycine is usually normal).

**Iminoglycinuria** Metabolites important for diagnosis: glycine, proline, hydroxyproline in urine.

**Hyperglycinuria** Metabolites important for diagnosis: glycine in urine (proline and hydroxyproline are normal).

**Cystinuria A and Cystinuria B** Due to mutations in SLC3A1 (rBAT) or SLC7A9 (b0,+AT), respectively. Metabolites important for diagnosis: cystine, lysine, arginine, and ornithine in urine.

**Lysinuric protein intolerance** Metabolites important for diagnosis: dibasic amino acids in the plasma (decreased) and urine (increased) and orotic acid in urine (increased).

**Dicarboxylic aminoaciduria** Metabolites important for diagnosis: glutamate and aspartate in the urine.

**Lysine malabsorption syndrome** Metabolites important for diagnosis: Lys, Arg, Orn in urine and plasma.

**Dibasic aminoaciduria type I** Metabolites important for diagnosis: lysine, arginine, and ornithine in urine.

**Methionine malabsorption syndrome** Metabolites important for diagnosis: α-hydroxybutyrate (oasthouse smell), Met, BCAA, and Ser in urine and feces.

**Cationic amino acid transporter 2 deficiency** Metabolites important for diagnosis: Arg, Lys, ornithine, and guanidinoacetic acid.

**Large neutral amino acid transporter LAT1 deficiency** Metabolites important for diagnosis: not identified, but branched chain amino acid levels are expected to be below reference values in patients.

**Neuronal system A SNAT8 transporter deficiency** Metabolites important for diagnosis: not identified.

**Episodic ataxia due to EAAT1 defect** Metabolites important for diagnosis: not identified.

**ASCT1 transporter deficiency** Metabolites important for diagnosis: not identified.

**Hyperekplexia due to GLYT2 deficiency** Metabolites important for diagnosis: not identified.

## Reference Values

Urine amino acid levels (mmol/mol creatinine) (5–95 percentile limits) measured by amino acid analyzer.

| Amino acid | Neonatal | Infancy | Childhood | Adolescence | Adulthood |
|---|---|---|---|---|---|
| | Fasting | Fasting | Fasting | Fasting | Fasting |
| Alanine | 75–244 | 36–206 | 33–130 | 17–92 | 16–68 |
| Arginine | <14 | <11 | <9 | <6 | <5 |
| Asparagine | <84 | <58 | <32 | <24 | <23 |
| Aspartate | 2–12 | 2–16 | 2–10 | 1–10 | 2–7 |
| Citrulline | <10 | <10 | <10 | <10 | <10 |
| Cystine | 24–78 | 12–48 | 8–30 | 7–23 | 6–34 |
| Glutamate | <30 | <29 | <11 | <9 | <12 |
| Glutamine | 52–205 | 63–229 | 45–236 | 20–112 | 20–76 |
| Glycine | 283–1097 | 210–743 | 110–356 | 64–236 | 43–173 |
| Histidine | 80–295 | 72–342 | 61–287 | 43–184 | 26–153 |
| Isoleucine | <6 | <6 | <6 | <6 | <4 |
| Leucine | 3–25 | 4–16 | 3–18 | 3–16 | 2–11 |
| Lysine | 22–171 | 13–199 | 10–69 | 10–56 | 7–58 |
| Methionine | 7–27 | 6–29 | 5–29 | 3–17 | 2–16 |
| Ornithine | <31 | <31 | <14 | <14 | <8 |
| Phenylalanine | 4–32 | 7–28 | 6–31 | 5–20 | 2–19 |
| Proline | 21–213 | <130 | <13 | <9 | <9 |
| Serine | 80–262 | 42–194 | 32–124 | 23–69 | 21–50 |
| Threonine | 20–138 | 14–92 | 9–62 | 8–28 | 7–29 |
| Tyrosine | 6–55 | 11–54 | 9–48 | 6–26 | 2–23 |
| Valine | 3–26 | 4–19 | 3–21 | 3–17 | 3–13 |

Fasting plasma amino acid levels (mM) (range limits) measured by amino acid analyzer (Hospital Sant Joan de Deu, Barcelona, Spain (Rafael Artuch)).

| Amino acid | Neonatal | Infancy | Childhood to adulthood |
|---|---|---|---|
| | Fasting | Fasting | Fasting |
| Alanine | 0.19–0.34 | 0.17–0.44 | 0.23–0.42 |
| Arginine | 0.05–0.08 | 0.05–0.12 | 0.05–0.10 |
| Asparagine | 0.05–0.12 | 0.05–0.12 | 0.03–0.11 |
| Aspartate | <0.02 | <0.02 | <0.02 |
| Citrulline | <0.04 | 0.01–0.05 | 0.01–0.05 |
| Cystine | 0.02–0.06 | 0.02–0.06 | 0.02–0.06 |
| Glutamate | <0.08 | <0.08 | <0.08 |
| Glutamine | 0.42–0.75 | 0.33–0.67 | 0.33–0.63 |
| Glycine | 0.11–0.29 | 0.11–0.29 | 0.11–0.29 |
| Histidine | 0.05–0.10 | 0.05–0.10 | 0.05–0.10 |
| Isoleucine | 0.04–0.09 | 0.04–0.09 | 0.04–0.09 |
| Leucine | 0.08–0.15 | 0.08–0.15 | 0.06–0.16 |
| Lysine | 0.07–0.20 | 0.12–0.24 | 0.11–0.23 |
| Methionine | 0.01–0.04 | 0.01–0.04 | 0.01–0.04 |
| Ornithine | 0.04–0.11 | 0.04–0.11 | 0.04–0.11 |
| Phenylalanine | 0.04–0.07 | 0.04–0.07 | 0.04–0.07 |
| Proline | 0.09–0.27 | 0.09–0.27 | 0.12–0.23 |
| Serine | 0.10–0.20 | 0.10–0.20 | 0.10–0.20 |
| Threonine | 0.06–0.29 | 0.06–0.29 | 0.10–0.20 |
| Tyrosine | 0.04–0.11 | 0.04–0.08 | 0.04–0.09 |
| Valine | 0.13–0.29 | 0.13–0.29 | 0.13–0.29 |

## Pathological Values

**Hartnup disorder** Altered urine amino acid levels (lower and upper values in mmol/mol creatinine) in adults with HD (Potter et al. 2002).

| Amino acid | Patients HD |
|---|---|
| Alanine | 384–1436 |
| Glutamate | 15–29 |
| Glutamine | 515–2010 |
| Glycine | 159–708 |
| Histidine | 325–653 |
| Isoleucine | 14–194 |
| Leucine | 16–200 |
| Lysine | 2–88 |
| Methionine | 5–51 |
| Phenylalanine | 12–122 |
| Serine | 546–842 |
| Threonine | 233–665 |
| Tyrosine | 2–281 |
| Valine | 43–566 |

Urine samples obtained by random collection. Glutamate and lysine are usually slightly elevated, but no in all HD patients

**Iminoglycinuria** Altered urine amino acid levels (lower and upper values in mmol/mol creatinine) in adults with IG (Bröer et al. 2008).

| Amino acid | Patients IG |
|---|---|
| Glycine | 576–1965 |
| Proline | 33–1000 |
| Hydroxyproline | 35–250 |

**Hyperglycinuria** Altered urine amino acid levels (lower and upper values in mmol/mol creatinine) in adults with HG (Bröer et al. 2008).

| Amino acid | Patients HG |
|---|---|
| Glycine | 174–632 |

**Cystinuria A and B** Altered urine amino acid levels (5–95 percentile limits in mmol/mol creatinine) in cystinuria (Font-Llitjós et al. 2005).

| Amino acid | Controls[a] | Cystinuria patients[b] | Type B carriers[c] |
|---|---|---|---|
| Cystine | 3–12 | 73–385 | 15–152 |
| Lysine | 4–56 | 300–1315 | 56–507 |
| Arginine | <5 | 26–946 | 0–38 |
| Ornithine | 1–8 | 66–389 | 2–59 |

Urine samples randomly collected (morning or 24 h) from 83 controls and 34 patients and 127 type B carriers of any age

[a]Controls were relatives of cystinuria patients without mutations in SLC3A1 and SLC7A9

[b]Patients with two mutated SLC3A1 alleles (cystinuria type A); similar ranges of values were obtained from the urine of patients with cystinuria type B (two mutated SLC7A9 alleles)

[c]Values from cystinuria type B carriers ($b^{0,+}$AT heterozygotes) are also shown

**Lysinuric protein intolerance** Altered amino acid plasma concentration (mM) in 20 patients (the range of lower-upper values is shown) (Simell 2001). Altered urine excretion values (mmol/mol creatinine) of amino acids and orotic acid after overnight fasting in one LPI patient (provided by R. Artuch from Gömez et al. 2006). Reference values for urine orotic acid excretion (1.2–6.9 mmol/mol creatinine).

| Amino acid | Plasma | Urine |
|---|---|---|
| Alanine | 0.42–1.02 | 116 |
| Arginine | 0.01–0.06 | 661 |
| Citrulline | 0.14–0.53 | 53 |
| Glutamine | 3.64–7.16 | 149 |
| Glycine | 0.39–0.53 | 240 |
| Lysine | 0.03–0.18 | 1040 |
| Ornithine | <0.08 | 112 |
| Carbamoyl phosphate metabolite | | |
| Orotic acid | – | 30 |

**Dicarboxylic aminoaciduria** Altered urine amino acid levels (lower and upper values in mmol/mol creatinine) in DA (Bailey et al. 2011).

| Amino acid | Reference values | | Patients DA | |
|---|---|---|---|---|
| | Infancy | Adulthood | Infancy | Adulthood |
| Aspartate | <26 | <15 | 50 | 46–51 |
| Glutamate | <63 | <36 | 1225 | 1052–1377 |

Urine samples obtained by random collection

**Lysine malabsorption syndrome** Cationic amino acids and cystine urine levels (mmol/mol creatinine) in the only patient identified (Omura et al. 1976). The normal range reported in this publication is also shown.

| Amino acid | Normal range values | Reported patient |
|---|---|---|
| Lysine | 19–100 | 1414 |
| Arginine | Trace-13 | 13 |
| Ornithine | Trace-21 | 27 |
| Cystine | Trace-14 | 13 |

**Dibasic aminoaciduria type I** Altered urine amino acid levels (range of values in six determinations within 2 years) of the only identified patient with hyperdibasic aminoaciduria type I (mmol/mol creatinine) (Kihara et al. 1973).

| Amino acid | Controls[a] | Patient |
|---|---|---|
| Cystine | 3 | 22–45 |
| Lysine | 12 | 400–803 |
| Arginine | 2 | 11–56 |
| Ornithine | 9 | 21–83 |

[a]Control reference values in the Pacific State Hospital (California, USA) at the time of the study

**Methionine malabsorption syndrome** Metabolite important for diagnosis: α-hydroxybutyrate (oasthouse smell) in urine and feces (Hooft et al. 1968, 1965). To our knowledge, quantitative determination of α-hydroxybutyrate in urine and feces before methionine-poor diet was introduced in the patient has not been reported. Under methionine-poor diet, no α-hydroxybutyrate is detected in urine and feces (Hooft et al. 1968).

**Cationic amino acid transporter 2 deficiency** Metabolites important for diagnosis in plasma and urine in the unique patient described (Yahyaoui et al. 2019).

| | Reference values | Patients DA | |
|---|---|---|---|
| Plasma (μM) | Infancy | Neonate | Infant[a] |
| Lysine | 199–209 | 599 | 392 |
| Arginine | 34–88 | 312 | 261 |
| Ornithine | 1–25 | 177 | 121 |
| Urine (mmol/mol creatinine) | | | |
| Lysine | 25–191 | 1005 | 632 |
| Arginine | 1–19 | 94 | 350 |
| Ornithine | 1–25 | 42 | 108 |
| Guac[b] | 11–168 | 380 | 82 |
| ADMA[b] | 4.7–12 | 50 | 26 |

[a]Analysis performed at 2 years of age. Currently, the child receives a protein-controlled diet of 1.2 g/kg/day with protein- and amino-acid-free infant formula (PFD1), 30 g/day, and is asymptomatic

[b]*Guac* guadinoacetic acid, *ADMA* asymmetric dimethylarginine

**Large neutral amino acid transporter LAT1 deficiency** No pathological values of amino acids in the cerebral spinal fluid of patients are available. According to *Slc7a5* knockout mice amino acid levels in cerebral spinal fluid (Tărlungeanu et al. 2016), branched chain amino acids in cerebral spinal fluid are expected to be below reference values in patients.

## Diagnostic Flowcharts

### Hartnup disorder

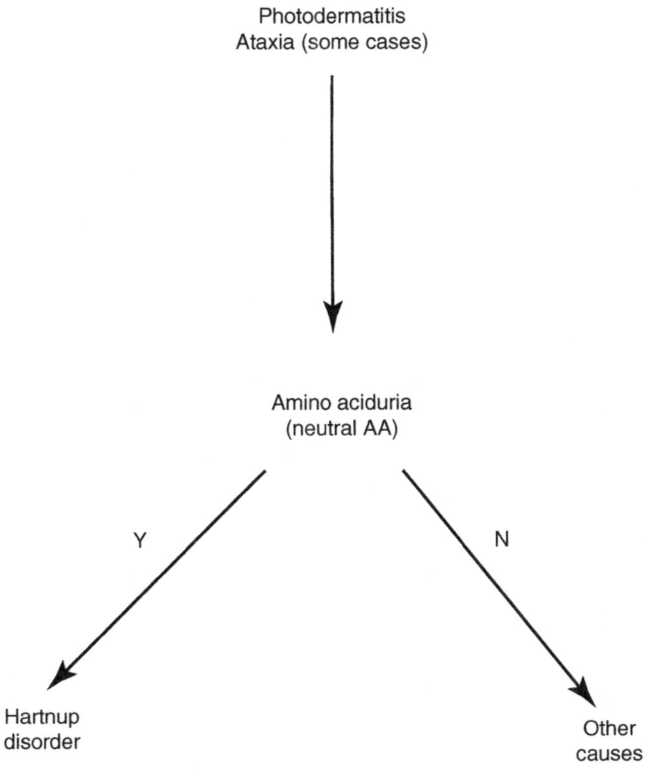


Iminoglycinuria and hyperglycinuria are considered benign and no diagnostic flowchart required. Accidental identification through urine amino acid analysis.

### Cystinuria

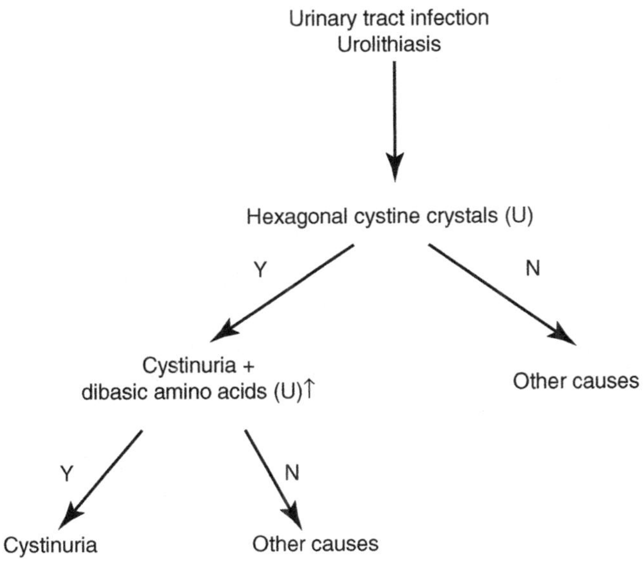


If patients are presented with neonatal seizures, hypotonia, developmental delay, and/or facial dysmorphism, the very rare hypotonia-cystinuria syndrome (OMIM 606407) due to homozygous deletion on chromosome 2p21 should be discarded.

### Lysinuric protein intolerance

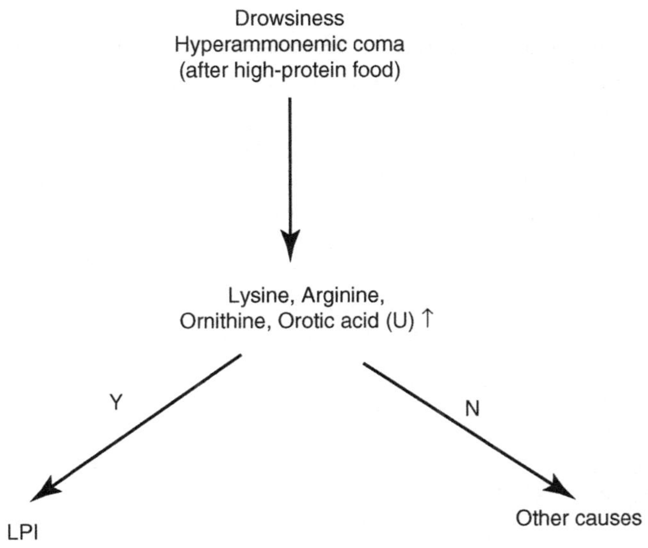


**Dicarboxylic aminoaciduria** Usually detected retrospectively, consider in cases of obsessive-compulsive disorder. Mental retardation most likely diagnosed due to ascertainment bias.

**Lysine malabsorption syndrome** The principal differences between the described patient with lysine malabsorption syndrome and LPI patients are (1) absence of hyperammonemia or protein intolerance and (2) isolate lysninuria (i.e., without argininuria and ornithinuria).

The principal differences between the described patient with lysine malabsorption syndrome and the patient with dibasic aminoaciduria type I are isolate lysninuria without argininuria and ornithinuria.

**Dibasic aminoaciduria type I** The principal differences between the described patient with hyperdibasic aminoaciduria type I and LPI patients are (1) absence of hyperammonemia or protein intolerance and (2) moderate hyperdibasic aminoaciduria in the obligated heterozygotes (e.g., parents) in the former.

**Methionine malabsorption syndrome** The presence of α-hydroxybutyrate in urine and feces with a typical oasthouse smell is a paradigmatic characteristic of this syndrome.

**Cationic amino acid transporter 2 deficiency** The characteristic biochemical profile includes high plasma and urine arginine, ornithine, and lysine levels. Newborn screening centers should know of this disorder since it can be detected in arginase 1 deficiency screening (OMIM 207800).

At present, it is unclear whether this defect is benign or the early establishment of a low-protein diet from the first month of life may have prevented or delayed the onset of symptoms.

**Large neutral amino acid transporter LAT1 deficiency** Diagnostic flowchart for diagnosing large neutral amino acid transporter deficiency. MRI, magnetic resonance imaging; WGS, whole genome sequencing; WES, whole exome sequencing; TGS, targeted genome sequencing; ADOS, Autism Diagnostic Observation Schedule.

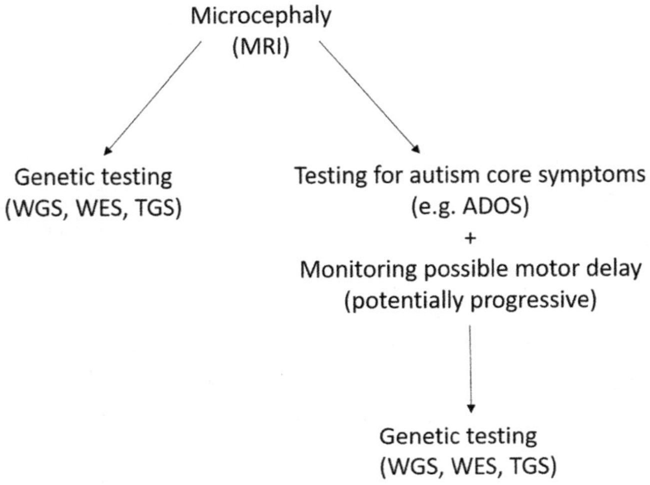


**Neuronal system A amino acid transporter deficiency** Defective SNAT8 (SLC38A8) cause isolated foveal hypoplasia nystagmus and optic nerve misrouting without albinism. Foveal hypoplasia has been identified in association with optic nerve misrouting in cases of ocular (MIM 300500) or oculocutaneous (MIM 203100, OMIM 606952 and 300808) albinism (reviewed) (Perez et al. 2014; Poulter et al. 2013).

**Episodic ataxia due to EAAT1 defect**

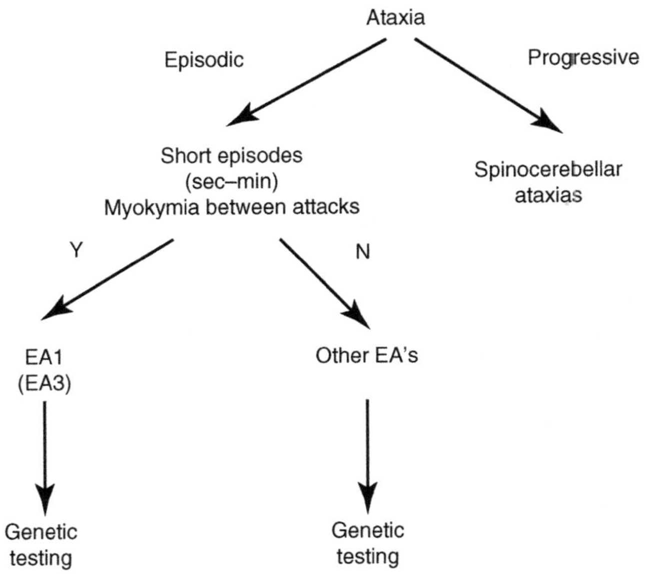


**ASCT1 transporter deficiency** CNS and musculoskeletal symptoms are alike to those of L-serine biosynthesis disorders (developmental delay and intellectual disability, microcephaly, seizures, and dysmyelination) (i.e., OMIM references 601815, 610992, and 614023) (Damseh et al. 2015; Heimer et al. 2015; Srour et al. 2015, for a review).

**Hyperekplexia**

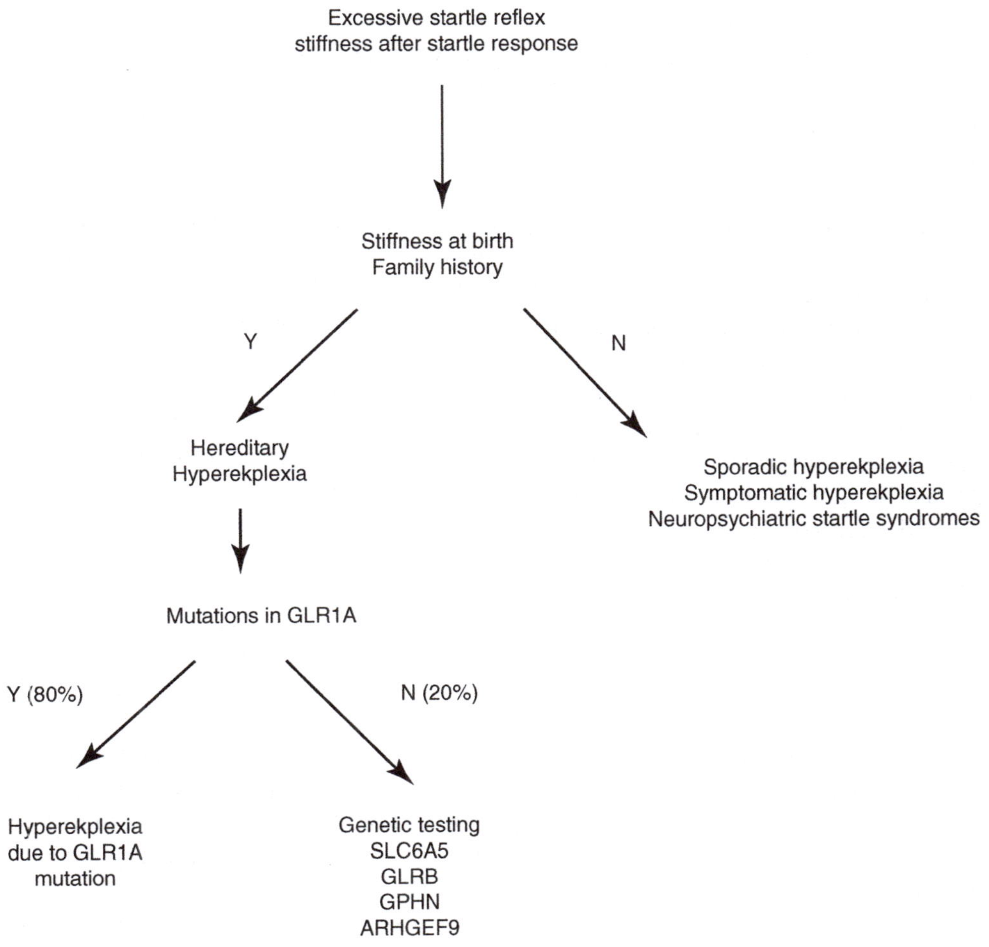


## Specimen Collection

**Aminoacidurias** Standard urine sample collected for 24 h or as single sample where amino acid concentration is referred to creatinine amount.

Large neutral amino acid transporter deficiency, neuronal system A amino acid transporter deficiency, episodic ataxia, ASCT1 and transporter deficiency, and startle disease due to glycine transporter GLYT2 defect, not applicable.

## Prenatal Diagnosis

Prenatal diagnosis is not recommended in cystinuria, dicarboxylic aminoaciduria, Hartnup disorder, and lysinuric protein intolerance. For at-risk pregnancies of episodic ataxia type 6, if mutations have been identified in the family, DNA sequence analysis can be performed by a research laboratory. In Ashkenazi Jewish populations, due to a relatively high carrier rate of ASCT1 (SLC1A4) mutations, mainly c.766G>A, p.(E256K), DNA sequence prenatal diagnosis can be performed for risk pregnancies. If SLC7A5 mutations causing large neutral amino acid transporter deficiency are known in the family, prenatal genetic testing or DNA sequencing of the parents can be used for prenatal diagnosis.

## Neonatal Diagnosis

Expanded newborn screening for amino acid disorders using tandem mass spectrometry includes the possibility to determine arginine levels in dried blood sample specimen to detect possible patients of hyperargininemia in cationic amino acid transporter 2 deficiency, and oasthouse smell might facilitate identification of methionine malabsorption syndrome. Early diagnosis would facilitate protein-deficient diet or methionine-deficient diet in these diseases, respectively.

## DNA Testing

DNA testing can be performed but is not necessary for diagnosis of cystinuria, dicarboxylic aminoaciduria and Hartnup disorder, iminoglycinuria, and hyperglycinuria. In cystinuria, if one mutated allele is already identified in one of the two cystinuria genes (SLC3A1 or SLC7A9), the second mutated allele most probably will be identified in the same gene because digenic inheritance in cystinuria has not been demonstrated. A small proportion (~4%) of carriers of one mutated allele (mainly SLC7A9 heterozygotes) present with cystine lithiasis. LPI: Neonatal DNA screenings for the unique mutation present in Finland (Finnish mutation 1181-2A→T) and a northern part of Iwate (Japan) (mutation R410X) with an incidence in the population of 1:60,000 have been established due to the benefits of an early therapy. DNA testing for common forms of hyperekplexia and episodic ataxia type 6 is available. For the cases associated with SLC6A5 and SLC1A3, respectively, sequencing is only available through research laboratories.

DNA sequencing by specialized laboratories will be necessary for diagnosis in the following cases: (1) SLC7A2 (CAT2) and arginase 1 in cases of hyperargininemia at birth, (2) SLC38A8 (SNAT8) in isolated foveal hypoplasia, (3) SLC1A4 (ASCT1) in the suspicious of central nervous system symptoms due to serine synthesis defects, and (4) large neutral amino acid transporter deficiency if microcephaly is present. In this latter case, skin biopsies for fibroblast primary cultures can be collected to monitor SLC7A5 transporter function via transporter assays.

## Treatment Summary

Methods to reverse the defect in transport that causes the disorders discussed in this chapter have not been developed. Photodermatitis in Hartnup disorder is treated with oral nicotinamide. Treatment and management of cystinuria in children and adults relate to the prevention of stone formation by reducing the absolute amount and increasing the solubility of the poorly soluble cystine that is excreted in the urine by dietary measures and alkalization of urine. If these conservative approaches fail, thiol-chelating drugs that reduce cystine to more soluble cysteine adducts are used. The goal is to maintain cystine urine concentration below 1 mmol/L (~250 mg/L) and excretion below <100 μmol per mmol of creatinine (Chillarón et al. 2010; Knoll et al. 2005). For LPI, they are two main directions of therapy (Sebastio et al. 2011). The first is aimed to reduce the risk of hyperammonemia (low-protein diet and L-citrulline supplementation (to refill urea cycle intermediates) or administration of ammonium scavengers (e.g., sodium benzoate)). The second is aimed at the specific treatment of the severe complications. Treatment is not required for dicarboxylic aminoaciduria, iminoglycinuria, and hyperglycinuria.

Acetazolamide should be tried in any patient with episodic ataxia type 6, but not all are responsive. Clonazepam is used to treat hyperekplexia. Low-protein diet and methionine restricted diet were implemented in the unique cases of cationic amino acid transporter 2 deficiency and methionine malabsorption syndrome, respectively (Hooft et al. 1968; Yahyaoui et al. 2019).

No treatment has been implemented for large neutral amino acid transporter deficiency and neuronal system A transporter deficiency. Serine supplementation could be envisaged as a treatment for ASCT1 transporter deficiency, but this has not been implemented even in mouse models.

## Emergency Treatment

### Cystinuria type A and type B

Urological interventions are often indicated for the management of cystine stones >5 mm in diameter (Chillarón et al. 2010). The almost noninvasive extracorporeal shock wave lithotripsy should be the treatment of choice at least in children (Knoll et al. 2005).

**Pitfalls**: Some cystine stones have crystalline structures (e.g., smooth appearance or low degree of radio-opacity), which make them resistant to extracorporeal shock wave lithotripsy. Ureteroscopy and percutaneous nephrostolithotomy may be preferable in these patients to remove the stones.

### Episodic ataxia due to EAAT1 defect

Antiepileptic drugs: carbamazepine (up 1600 mg/day), sulthiamine (50–200 mg/day), and diphenylhydantoin (150–300 mg/day).

**Dangers/Pitfalls**: Drugs should be used with caution due to significant side effects.

### Hyperekplexia due to GLYT2 defect

Sudden infant death due to apnea (stiffness of respiratory muscles) can occur in cases of hyperekplexia. This can be prevented by the Vigevano maneuver (flexing of head and limbs toward the trunk) (Vigevano et al. 1989).

## Standard Treatment

### Cystinuria type A and type B

| Objective | Strategy | Neonatal | Infancy | Childhood | Adolescence | Adulthood |
|---|---|---|---|---|---|---|
| Decrease in cystine excretion | Dietary sodium intake (upper limit; g/24 h) (Metabolic Nephropathy Work group 2011) | – | – | 2 | 2 | 2 |
| | Animal protein intake (g/kg BW • 24 h) | – | – | – | <1 | <1 |
| Decrease in urine cystine concentration | Fluid intake (L/24 h) | 0.5–1 | 2 | 3–4 | 4 | 4–5 |
| Increase in cystine solubility in urine | Urine alkalization (pH 7.5) Potassium citrate (mmol/24 h) (divided in 2–3 doses/day) | – | 10–20 | 10–60 | 10–60 | 40–90 |
| | Tiopronin[1] (mg/kg BW • 24 h)[2] | – | – | 20–40 | 20–40 | 45–60 |

[a]Alternative treatment with tiopronin (α-mercaptopropionylglycine) produces adducts with cysteine that increase the solubility of cysteine 50-fold. This treatment is recomended to do not exceed 1.2 g/24 h (2021)

**Dangers/Pitfalls**

A high nocturnal fluid intake will delay the achievement of urinary control in childhood. At least two nocturnal fluid intakes are recommended, but good compliance is difficult to achieve in adolescents and adults.

Potassium citrate administration is recommended in three doses (one-quarter of the daily dose in the morning, one-quarter at lunchtime, and half in the evening), which is recommended to monitor urine pH (>7.5) with indicator paper three times per day to adjust treatment.

The incidence of adverse effects is similar for both agents (tiopronin—fever, proteinuria, and hyperlipidemia; D-penicillamine—rash, fever, immune-complex-mediated glomerulonephritis, leucopenia, thrombocytopenia, and taste loss) but is slightly lower with tiopronin. Monitoring of liver enzymes, complete blood cell count, and urinary protein excretion should be performed regularly while patients are on tiopronin or D-penicillamine therapy.

**Hartnup disorder** Oral nicotinamide treatment (50–100 mg/day) may prevent or resolve photodermatitis in Hartnup disorder.

### Lysinuric protein intolerance

| Objective | Strategy | Neonatal | Infancy | Childhood | Adolescence | Adulthood |
|---|---|---|---|---|---|---|
| Prevention of hyperammonemia | Low-protein diet (upper limit; g/kg BW • 24 h) | – | – | 0.8–1.5 | 0.8–1.5 | 0.5–0.8 |
| | Citrulline supplementation (mg/kg BW • 24 h) (in 4 divided doses) | – | – | 100 | 100 | 100 |
| | Sodium benzoate (mg/kg BW • 24 h) (in 4 divided doses) | – | – | 100–250 | 100–250 | 100–250 |
| | L-Carnitine (mg/kg BW • 24 h) (in 2 or more divided doses)[a] | – | – | 25–50 | 25–50 | 25–50 |
| Additional treatments | hGH (for patients with GH deficiency) | – | – | Careful evaluation for patients with severe growth retardation and delayed bone age | | – |
| | L-Lysine (mg/kg BW • 24 h) (in presence of marked hypolysinemia) | – | – | 10–40 | 10–40 | 10–40 |
| | Statins (to treat combined hyperlipidemia) | – | – | Standard protocols | | |
| Severe complications | Pulmonary alveolar proteinosis (PAP) | – | Bronchoalveolar lavage in specialized center. Immunosuppressors | | | |
| | Chronic renal disease | – | – | – | Standard guidelines under the direction of specialist | |
| | Hemophagocytic lymphohistiocytosis | – | – | Standard guidelines under the direction of specialist | | |

[a]Hypocarnitinemia, which strongly correlates with renal insufficiency, low-protein diet, and the use of ammonia scavenger drugs, might present in LPI. Therefore, L-carnitine is supplemented after measurement of plasma carnitine levels (Sebastio et al. 2011)

**Dangers/Pitfalls**

Urinary orotic acid can be used to monitor the protein tolerance and the urea cycle functioning but is not totally reliable.

Nutritional deficiency due to the low-protein diet might require supplementation of calcium, vitamin D, iron, and zinc.

Recurrent fatal pulmonary alveolar proteinosis after heart-lung transplantation in a child highlighted that this complication of LPI is caused by factors external to the lung, most likely macrophages (Santamaria et al. 2004).

Pulmonary alveolar proteinosis (PAP) of different origins is usually treated by whole lung lavage or granulocyte-macrophage colony-stimulating factor (GM-CSF) administration. GM-CSF is a hematopoietic growth factor known to stimulate stem cells to proliferate into granulocytes or monocytes, promote differentiation of monocytes into alveolar macrophages, increase the catabolism within alveolar macrophages, and increase the innate immune potential of neutrophils. Although GM-CSF may have therapeutic advantage in certain types of PAP, it may not be suitable for treating LPI-associated PAP because of the tendency of LPI alveolar macrophages to form granulomas (Douda et al. 2009).

**Episodic ataxia type 6 due to EAAT3 defect** Typical treatment is acetazolamide (125–1000 mg/day) (Pessia 2010). Acetazolamide is a carboanhydrase inhibitor and particularly effective in episodic ataxia type 2 caused by mutations in the calcium channel gene CACNA1A (Jen et al. 2007). Whether bicarbonate homeostasis is deranged in episodic ataxias is unclear.

4-Aminopyridine treatment has been shown to be effective in patients with EA (Jen et al. 2007).

**Dangers/Pitfalls**. Not all cases of EA are responsive to acetazolamide.

**Hyperekplexia** Clonazepam is used to treat hyperekplexia. Initial dose is 0.5 mg twice/day, which can be increased to 2 mg twice a day. Clonazepam modulates the $GABA_A$ receptor, making it more sensitive to GABA. $GABA_A$ receptors and glycine receptors have an overlapping distribution in the brain. Clonazepam is a muscle relaxant counteracting the muscle stiffness observed in hyperekplexia.

**Dangers/Pitfalls**. Hyperekplexia can be misdiagnosed as seizures, but commonly used anticonvulsants are ineffective. The effectiveness of valproic acid, clobazam, and fluoxetine has been reported in a few sporadic cases of unknown genetic etiology (Zhou et al. 2002), but has not been tested in controlled studies.

## Experimental Treatment

**Cystinuria** Real-time atomic force microscopy has been used to identify cystine derivatives (L-cystine dimethyl ester and L-cystine methyl ester) that bind to the surface and reduce the growth of cystine microcrystals in vitro (Rimer et al. 2010). Proof of principle of their antilithiasic activity in vivo is yet lacking.

**Lysinuric protein intolerance** Therapy with bisphosphonates (alendronate 10 mg/kg body weight • 24 h) has been proposed for severe osteoporosis in LPI (Gömez et al. 2006), but a standardized protocol is lacking.

**Episodic ataxia due to EAAT1 defect** See emergency treatment.

**Acknowledgments** The authors thank Dr. Christian Lueck (Canberra Hospital) for clarification of differential diagnosis in cases of episodic ataxia. The authors thank Dr. Rafael Artuch (Hospital San Joan de Deu, Barcelona) for reference values of plasma amino acid concentration. The authors also thank Lisa Kraus (Institute of Science and Technology-Austria) and Dr. Susanna Bodoy (IRB-Barcelona) that helped in preparing tables and bibliography.

## References

Bailey CG, Ryan RM, Thoeng AD, Ng C, King K, Vanslambrouck JM, et al. Loss-of-function mutations in the glutamate transporter SLC1A1 cause human dicarboxylic aminoaciduria. J Clin Invest. 2011. https://doi.org/10.1172/JCI44474.

Borsani G, Bassi MT, Sperandeo MP, De Grandi A, Buoninconti A, Riboni M, et al. SLC7A7, encoding a putative permease-related protein, is mutated in patients with lysinuric protein intolerance. Nat Genet. 1999. https://doi.org/10.1038/6815.

Bröer S. The SLC38 family of sodium-amino acid co-transporters. Pflugers Arch - Eur J Physiol. 2014. https://doi.org/10.1007/s00424-013-1393-y.

Bröer S, Palacín M. The role of amino acid transporters in inherited and acquired diseases. Biochem J. 2011. https://doi.org/10.1042/bj20101912.

Bröer S, Bailey CG, Kowalczuk S, Ng C, Vanslambrouck JM, Rodgers H, et al. Iminoglycinuria and hyperglycinuria are discrete human phenotypes resulting from complex mutations in proline and glycine transporters. J Clin Investig. 2008. https://doi.org/10.1172/JCI36625.

Calonge MJ, Gasparini P, Chillarón J, Chillón M, Gallucci M, Rousaud F, et al. Cystinuria caused by mutations in rBAT, a gene involved in the transport of cystine. Nat Genet. 1994. https://doi.org/10.1038/ng0494-420.

Canul-Tec JC, Assal R, Cirri E, Legrand P, Brier S, Chamot-Rooke J, Reyes N. Structure and allosteric inhibition of excitatory amino acid transporter 1. Nature 2017. https://doi.org/10.1038/nature22064.

Chillarón J, Font-Llitjós M, Fort J, Zorzano A, Goldfarb DS, Nunes V, Palacín M. Pathophysiology and treatment of cystinuria. Nat Rev Nephrol. 2010. https://doi.org/10.1038/nrneph.2010.69.

Coleman JA, Green EM, Gouaux E. X-ray structures and mechanism of the human serotonin transporter. Nature. 2016. https://doi.org/10.1038/nature17629.

Damseh N, Simonin A, Jalas C, Picoraro JA, Shaag A, Cho MT, et al. Mutations in SLC1A4, encoding the brain serine transporter, are associated with developmental delay, microcephaly and hypomyelination. J Med Genet. 2015. https://doi.org/10.1136/jmedgenet-2015-103104.

Douda DN, Farmakovski N, Dell S, Grasemann H, Palaniyar N. SP-D counteracts GM-CSF-mediated increase of granuloma formation by alveolar macrophages in lysinuric protein intolerance. Orphanet J Rare Dis. 2009. https://doi.org/10.1186/1750-1172-4-29.

Eggermann T, Elbracht M, Haverkamp F, Schmidt C, Zerres K. Isolated cystinuria (OMIM 238200) is not a separate entity but is caused by a mutation in the cystinuria gene SLC7 A9 [3]. Clin Genet. 2007. https://doi.org/10.1111/j.1399-0004.2007.00797.x.

Errasti-Murugarren E, Fort J, Bartoccioni P, Díaz L, Pardon E, Carpena X, et al. L amino acid transporter structure and molecular bases for the asymmetry of substrate interaction. Nat Commun. 2019;10(1):1807. https://doi.org/10.1038/s41467-019-09837-z.

Feliubadaló L, Font M, Purroy J, Rousaud F, Estivill X, Nunes V, et al. Non-type I cystinuria caused by mutations in SLC7A9, encoding a subunit (b(o,+)AT) of rBAT. Nat Genet. 1999. https://doi.org/10.1038/12652.

Font-Llitjós M, Jiménez-Vidal M, Bisceglia L, Di Perna M, De Sanctis L, Rousaud F, et al. New insights into cystinuria: 40 New mutations, genotype-phenotype correlation, and digenic inheritance causing partial phenotype. J Med Genet. 2005. https://doi.org/10.1136/jmg.2004.022244.

Fotiadis D, Kanai Y, Palacín M. The SLC3 and SLC7 families of amino acid transporters. Mol Asp Med. 2013. https://doi.org/10.1016/j.mam.2012.10.007.

Gómez L, García-Cazorla A, Gutiérrez A, Artuch R, Varea V, Martín J, et al. Treatment of severe osteoporosis with alendronate in a patient with lysinuric protein intolerance. J Inherit Metab Dis. 2006. https://doi.org/10.1007/s10545-006-0236-9.

Guarch ME, Font-Llitjós M, Murillo-Cuesta S, Errasti-Murugarren E, Celaya AM, Girotto G, et al. Mutations in L-type amino acid transporter-2 support SLC7A8 as a novel gene involved in age-related hearing loss. elife. 2018. https://doi.org/10.7554/eLife.31511.

Hägglund MGA, Hellsten SV, Bagchi S, Philippot G, Löfqvist E, Nilsson VCO, et al. Transport of l-glutamine, l-alanine, l-arginine and l-histidine by the neuron-specific slc38a8 (SNAT8) in cns. J Mol Biol. 2015. https://doi.org/10.1016/j.jmb.2014.10.016.

Heimer G, Marek-Yagel D, Eyal E, Barel O, Oz Levi D, Hoffmann C, et al. SLC1A4 mutations cause a novel disorder of intellectual disability, progressive microcephaly, spasticity and thin corpus callosum. Clin Genet. 2015. https://doi.org/10.1111/cge.12637.

Hooft C, Timmermans J, Snoeck J, Antener I, Oyaert W, Van den Hende C. Methionine malabsorption syndrome. Ann Paediatr Int Rev Pediatr. 1965;205(1):73–104. http://www.ncbi.nlm.nih.gov/pubmed/5897673.

Hooft C, Carton D, Snoeck J, Timmermans J, Antener I, van den HC. Further investigations in the methionine malabsorption syndrome. Helv Paediatr Acta. 1968;23(4):334–49.

Jen JC, Wan J, Palos TP, Howard BD, Baloh RW. Mutation in the glutamate transporter EAAT1 causes episodic ataxia, hemiplegia, and seizures. Neurology. 2005. https://doi.org/10.1212/01.WNL.0000172638.58172.5a.

Jen JC, Graves TD, Hess EJ, Hanna MG, Griggs RC, Baloh RW. Primary episodic ataxias: diagnosis, pathogenesis and treatment. Brain. 2007. https://doi.org/10.1093/brain/awm126.

Jungnickel KEJ, Parker JL, Newstead S. Structural basis for amino acid transport by the CAT family of SLC7 transporters. Nat Commun. 2018. https://doi.org/10.1038/s41467-018-03066-6.

Kaplan E, Zubedat S, Radzishevsky I, Valenta AC, Rechnitz O, Sason H, et al. ASCT1 (Slc1a4) transporter is a physiologic regulator of brain d-serine and neurodevelopment Proc Natl Acad Sci. 2018. https://doi.org/10.1073/pnas.1722677115.

Kihara H, Valente M, Porter MT, Fluharty AL. Hyperdibasicaminoaciduria in a mentally retarded homozygote with a peculiar response to phenothiazines. Pediatrics. 1973.

Kleta R, Romeo E, Ristic Z, Ohura T, Stuart C, Arcos-Burgos M, et al. Mutations in SLC6A19, encoding B0AT1, cause Hartnup disorder. Nat Genet. 2004. https://doi.org/10.1038/ng1405.

Knoll T, Zöllner A, Wendt-Nordahl G, Michel MS, Alken P. Cystinuria in childhood and adolescence: recommendations for diagnosis, treatment, and follow-up. Pediatr Nephrol. 2005. https://doi.org/10.1007/s00467-004-1663-1.

Kowalczuk S, Bröer A, Tietze N, Vanslambrouck JM, Rasko JEJ, Bröer S. A protein complex in the brush-border membrane explains a Hartnup disorder allele. FASEB J. 2008. https://doi.org/10.1096/fj.08-107300.

Lee Y, Wiriyasermkul P, Jin C, Quan L, Ohgaki R, Okuda S, et al. Cryo-EM structure of the human L-type amino acid transporter 1 in complex with glycoprotein CD98hc. BioRxiv. 2019;577551 https://doi.org/10.1101/577551.

Lei HT, Ma J, Sanchez Martinez S, Gonen T. Crystal structure of arginine-bound lysosomal transporter SLC38A9 in the cytosol-open state. Nat Struct Mol Biol. 2018. https://doi.org/10.1038/s41594-018-0072-2.

Metabolic Nephropathy Work group of the European Reference Network for Rare Kidney Diseases (ERKNet) and eUROGEN in Kidney International. 2021;99:48–58; https://doi.org/10.1016/j.kint.2020.06.035/.

Nagamori S, Wiriyasermkul P, Guarch ME, Okuyama H, Nakagomi S, Tadagaki K, et al. Novel cystine transporter in renal proximal tubule identified as a missing partner of cystinuria-related plasma membrane protein rBAT/SLC3A1. Proc Natl Acad Sci. 2016. https://doi.org/10.1073/pnas.1519959113.

Omura K, Yamanaka N, Higami S, Matsuoka O, Fujimoto A. Lysine malabsorption syndrome: a new type of transport defect. Pediatrics. 1976.

Penmatsa A, Gouaux E. How LeuT shapes our understanding of the mechanisms of sodium-coupled neurotransmitter transporters. J Physiol. 2014. https://doi.org/10.1113/jphysiol.2013.259051.

Penmatsa A, Wang KH, Gouaux E. X-ray structure of dopamine transporter elucidates antidepressant mechanism. Nature. 2013. https://doi.org/10.1038/nature12533.

Perez Y, Gradstein L, Flusser H, Markus B, Cohen I, Langer Y, et al. Isolated foveal hypoplasia with secondary nystagmus and low vision is associated with a homozygous SLC38A8 mutation. Eur J Hum Genet. 2014. https://doi.org/10.1038/ejhg.2013.212.

Pessia MHM. Episodic ataxia type 1. In: Pagon RA, Bird TD, editors. Gene reviews. Seattle: University of Washington; 2010.

Potter SJ, Lu A, Wilcken B, Green K, Rasko JEJ. Hartnup disorder: polymorphisms identified in the neutral amino acid transporter SLC1A5. J Inherit Metab Dis. 2002. https://doi.org/10.1023/A:1021286714582.

Poulter JA, Al-Araimi M, Conte I, Van Genderen MM, Sheridan E, Carr IM, et al. Recessive mutations in SLC38a8 cause foveal hypoplasia and optic nerve misrouting without albinism. Am J Hum Genet. 2013. https://doi.org/10.1016/j.ajhg.2013.11.002.

Rees MI, Harvey K, Pearce BR, Chung SK, Duguid IC, Thomas P, et al. Mutations in the gene encoding GlyT2 (SLC6A5) define a presynaptic component of human startle disease. Nat Genet. 2006. https://doi.org/10.1038/ng1814.

Régal L, Mårtensson E, Maystadt I, Voermans N, Lederer D, Burlina A, et al. PREPL deficiency: delineation of the phenotype and development of a functional blood assay. Genet Med. 2018. https://doi.org/10.1038/gim.2017.74.

Reyes N, Ginter C, Boudker O. Transport mechanism of a bacterial homologue of glutamate transporters. Nature. 2009. https://doi.org/10.1038/nature08616.

Rimer JD, An Z, Zhu Z, Lee MH, Goldfarb DS, Wesson JA, Ward MD. Crystal growth inhibitors for the prevention of L-cystine kidney stones through molecular design. Science. 2010. https://doi.org/10.1126/science.1191968.

Santamaria F, Brancaccio G, Parenti G, Francalanci P, Squitieri C, Sebastio G, et al. Recurrent fatal pulmonary alveolar proteinosis after heart-lung transplantation in a child with lysinuric protein intolerance. J Pediatr. 2004. https://doi.org/10.1016/j.jpeds.2004.04.047.

Sebastio G, Sperandeo MP, Andria G. Lysinuric protein intolerance: reviewing concepts on a multisystem disease. Am J Med Genet C: Semin Med Genet. 2011;157(1):54–62. https://doi.org/10.1002/ajmg.c.30287.

Seow HF, Bröer S, Bröer A, Bailey CG, Potter SJ, Cavanaugh JA, Rasko JEJ. Hartnup disorder is caused by mutations in the gene encoding the neutral amino acid transporter SLC6A19. Nat Genet. 2004. https://doi.org/10.1038/ng1406.

Simell O. Lysinuric protein intolerance and another cationic aminoacidurias. In: The metabolic and molecular bases of inherited disease. 8th ed. New York: McGraw-Hill; 2001.

Smith AJ, Strang LB. An inborn error of metabolism with the urinary excretion of α-hydroxy-butyric acid and phenylpyruvic acid. Arch Dis Child. 1958. https://doi.org/10.1136/adc.33.168.109.

Srour M, Hamdan FF, Gan-Or Z, Labuda D, Nassif C, Oskoui M, et al. A homozygous mutation in SLC1A4 in siblings with severe intellectual disability and microcephaly. Clin Genet. 2015. https://doi.org/10.1111/cge.12605.

Tărlungeanu DC, Deliu E, Dotter CP, Kara M, Janiesch PC, Scalise M, et al. Impaired amino acid transport at the blood brain barrier is a cause of autism spectrum disorder. Cell. 2016. https://doi.org/10.1016/j.cell.2016.11.013.

Torrents D, Mykkänen J, Pineda M, Feliubadaló L, Estévez R, De Rafael C, et al. Identification of SLC7A7, encoding y+LAT-1, as the lysinuric protein intolerance gene. Nat Genet. 1999. https://doi.org/10.1038/6809.

Vigevano F, Di Capua M, Bernardina BD. Startle disease: an avoidable cause of sudden infant death. Lancet. 1989. https://doi.org/10.1016/S0140-6736(89)91226-9.

Vilches C, Boiadjieva-Knöpfel E, Bodoy S, Camargo S, López de Heredia M, Prat E, et al. Cooperation of antiporter LAT2/CD98hc with uniporter TAT1 for renal reabsorption of neutral amino acids. J Am Soc Nephrol. 2018. https://doi.org/10.1681/ASN.2017111205.

Yahyaoui R, Blasco-Alonso J, Benito C, Rodríguez-García E, Andrade F, Aldámiz-Echevarría L, et al. A new metabolic disorder in human cationic amino acid transporter-2 that mimics arginase 1 deficiency in newborn screening. J Inherit Metab Dis. 2019. https://doi.org/10.1002/jimd.12063.

Yan R, Zhao X, Lei J, Zhou Q. Structure of the human LAT1-4F2hc heteromeric amino acid transporter complex. Nature. 2019. https://doi.org/10.1038/s41586-019-1011-z.

Zerangue N, Kavanaugh MP. ASCT-1 is a neutral amino acid exchanger with chloride channel activity. J Biol Chem. 1996;271(45):27991–4. http://www.ncbi.nlm.nih.gov/pubmed/8910405.

Zhou Y, Danbolt NC. GABA and glutamate transporters in brain. Front Endocrinol. 2013. https://doi.org/10.3389/fendo.2013.00165.

Zhou L, Chillag KL, Nigro MA. Hyperekplexia: a treatable neurogenetic disease. Brain Dev. 2002. https://doi.org/10.1016/S0387-7604(02)00095-5.

# Disorders of Monoamine Metabolism

# 19

Thomas Opladen and Georg F. Hoffmann

## Contents




## Summary

Neurotransmitters include the catecholamines (dopamine, norepinephrine, and epinephrine) and the indoleamines (serotonin and melatonin). They are chemical messengers, which mediate, amplify, or modulate synaptic transmission between neurons in the brain. Consequently, neurotransmitters are involved in central brain functions including control of movements and behavior, neuronal excitation and inhibition, the regulation of body temperature, pain threshold, memory, and a host of other processes. Inherited deficiencies of monoamine neurotransmitters encompass defects of biosynthesis and catabolism, as well as defects of transporters. They result in a wide variety of clinical signs and symptoms. This chapter will focus on primary disorders of serotonin and dopamine metabolism. Described defects are deficiencies of tyrosine hydroxylase (TH), aromatic L-amino acid decarboxylase (AADC), dopamine $\beta$-hydroxylase (D$\beta$H), monoamine oxidase A, as well as



T. Opladen (✉)
Division of Neuropediatrics and Metabolic Medicine, Department of Pediatrics, University Children's Hospital, Heidelberg, Germany
e-mail: Thomas.opladen@med.uni-heidelberg.de

G. F. Hoffmann (✉)
University Children's Hospital, Heidelberg, Germany
e-mail: georg.hoffmann@med.uni-heidelberg.de





N. Blau et al. (eds.), *Physician's Guide to the Diagnosis, Treatment, and Follow-Up of Inherited Metabolic Diseases*,
https://doi.org/10.1007/978-3-030-67727-5_19

the hereditary dopamine transporter deficiency syndrome (DTDS) and the brain dopamine-serotonin vesicular transport (VMAT2) disease.

Neurotransmitter disorders are important to recognize because early diagnosis and prompt therapeutic intervention seem to improve motor and cognitive outcome. The disease predominantly starts during infancy and early childhood. The specific clinical presentation of neurotransmitter diseases is determined by the type and severity of the underlying disorder. The clinical phenotype is not characteristic but can mimic that of other neurological disorders. Although detailed clinical history and physical examination are essential, the diagnosis is almost exclusively based on the quantitative determination of monoamines or their metabolites in cerebrospinal fluid (CSF). The additional determination of pterin metabolites is needed for the differentiation from deficiencies of $BH_4$ metabolism. Every diagnosis must be confirmed by molecular testing. The aim of treatment is to restore neurotransmitter homeostasis. Bypassing the metabolic block using levodopa/decarboxylase inhibitor together with dopamine agonists has led to remarkable clinical improvement in TH deficiency. In patients with AADC deficiency, treatment options are limited and in many cases not satisfactory. Patients with DβH deficiency benefit from droxidopa administration. While patients with VMAT2 defects benefit from treatment with a dopamine receptor agonist, no specific treatment with sustained effect for MAO-A deficiency or dopamine transporter deficiency syndrome has been described.

## Introduction

The umbrella term "neurotransmitter" subsumes different types of chemical substances involved in synaptic transmission from cell to cell within the central (CNS) and peripheral nervous system (PNS). Neurotransmitters are synthesized in the neuron and stored within vesicles, are essential for intercellular communication, and lay the foundation of basic and complex biological functions, including muscular movement as well as neuropsychological development (Kurian et al. 2011a). Neurotransmitters can be grouped according to their chemical structure into amino acid transmitters (glycine, glutamate, and γ-aminobutyric acid (GABA)), monoamines transmitters (with the subgroup of catecholamines norepinephrine, epinephrine, and dopamine as well as serotonin), and neuropeptides, classified as short proteins or polypeptides (e.g., the hypothalamic hormones oxytocin and vasopressin or orexins) (Brennenstuhl et al. 2019). Inherited defects of neurotransmitter synthesis, breakdown, and transport have become recognized as a cause of early onset, severe, and progressive encephalopathies.

This chapter will focus on primary disorders of serotonin and dopamine (monoamine neurotransmitter) metabolism. Described defects in monoamine metabolism include deficiencies of tyrosine hydroxylase (TH) (EC 1.14.16.2) (Bartholome and Ludecke 1998; Ludecke and Bartholome 1995), aromatic L-amino acid decarboxylase (AADC) (EC 4.1.1.28) (Hyland et al. 1992), dopamine *β*-hydroxylase (D*β*H) (EC 1.14.17.1) (Man in 't Veld et al. 1987; Robertson et al. 1986), monoamine oxidase (MAO) (EC 1.4.3.4) (Brunner et al. 1993a), as well as the recently characterized hereditary dopamine transporter deficiency syndrome (Kurian et al. 2011b) and the brain dopamine-serotonin vesicular transport disease (Rilstone et al. 2013).

The diseases predominantly have their onset during infancy and early childhood. The clinical presentation is determined by the type and severity of the underlying disorder. The phenotype is not characteristic and can be mistaken for other neurological disease entities (Kurian et al. 2011a). Important neurological symptoms are developmental delay, central and peripheral hypotonia, hypo- or hyperkinesia, mixed pyramidal and extrapyramidal motor disorders, epilepsy, and oculogyric crises. Cognitive function is mostly less severely affected (Assmann et al. 2003; Brun et al. 2010; Willemsen et al. 2010).

Identical clinical pictures may result from abnormalities of tetrahydrobiopterin ($BH_4$) metabolism (see Chap. 20). But in contrast to patients with $BH_4$ deficiencies where hyperphenylalaninemia in newborn screening can guide an early way to diagnosis, hyperphenylalaninemia is always missing in neurotransmitter disorders. Recently, an option for newborn screening for AADC deficiency using the determination of 3-*O*-methyldopa (3OMD) was published (Brennenstuhl 2020). However, this investigation is still limited to very few laboratories. Hence, the diagnosis is depending on a diagnostic lumbar puncture, more explicitly the quantitative determination of monoamine metabolites and pterin species in cerebrospinal fluid (CSF) (Hoffmann et al. 1998). Apart from a strictly standardized sampling protocol, neurotransmitter analysis requires special logistics and transport as well as demanding laboratory techniques, adequately established age-related reference values, and finally experienced interpretation in the clinical context (Brautigam et al. 2002; Bräutigam et al. 1998). It is therefore performed in a limited number of specialized laboratories worldwide. As a consequence, only small numbers of patients have been diagnosed, and a substantial number is suspected to remain undiagnosed. A generalized deficiency of dopaminergic transmission can be recognized by raised levels of prolactin in blood. However, this is not a diagnostic test because of insufficient sensitivity as well as specificity. In addition, prolactin levels can change in response to stress. To obtain reliable values, three determinations should be done hourly in a resting relaxed patient. If these are in agreement, the value is to be trusted.

Tyrosine hydroxylase (TH) catalyzes the conversion of L-tyrosine to L-dopa. It is the rate-limiting step in the biosynthesis of dopamine, norepinephrine, and epinephrine. The first committed defect, autosomal recessively inherited TH deficiency (DYT5b, DYT/PARK-TH), is therefore characterized by decreased concentrations of homovanillic acid (HVA) in CSF in combination with normal 5-hydroxyindoleacetic acid (5-HIAA). TH deficiency is associated with a broad phenotypic spectrum. According to the severity of the neurological symptoms and the concentrations of the monoamine in CSF, patients were delineated into two clinical phenotypes: an infantile onset, progressive, hypokinetic-rigid syndrome with dystonia (type A, less severe) and a complex encephalopathy with neonatal onset (type B). However, both phenotypes overlap substantially to a continuum of symptomatology and clinical severity (Willemsen et al. 2010).

Aromatic L-amino acid decarboxylase (AADC) is required for the synthesis of both serotonin and the catecholamines. Therefore, the clinical phenotype of autosomal recessively inherited AADC deficiency is caused by a severe combined deficiency of serotonin and catecholamines and characterized by oculogyric crises, dystonia, and severe neurological dysfunction in addition to vegetative symptoms (Brun et al. 2010; Pons et al. 2004; Swoboda et al. 2003). Biochemically, the deficiency leads to low levels of all neurotransmitters and accumulation of 3-*O*-methyldopa, 5-hydroxytryptophan, and L-dopa in CSF, plasma, and urine.

The aim of treatment in TH and AADC deficiencies is to restore neurotransmitter homeostasis. Bypassing the metabolic block using levodopa/decarboxylase inhibitor (carbidopa or benserazide) together (if required) with dopamine agonists leads to a good to excellent clinical response in most TH-deficient patients. AADC-deficient patients received dopamine receptor agonists, monoamine oxidase inhibitors, anticholinergics, and selective serotonin reuptake inhibitors often in conjunction with vitamin $B_6$ (cofactor for AADC). For the treatment of AADC-D, a consensus guideline was recently published. Nevertheless, the treatment response is often disappointing (Wassenberg et al. 2017), and significant clinical improvement was only observed in attenuated clinical manifestations (Brun et al. 2010). Recently, it has been shown that gene therapy approaches in AADC deficiency improve motor and mental function as well as brain white matter tracts (Kojima et al. 2019; Tseng et al. 2019).

Dopamine $\beta$-hydroxylase (D$\beta$H) catalyzes the conversion of dopamine to norepinephrine presynaptic secretory vesicles. D$\beta$H deficiency represents a very rare disease with 20 cases worldwide (Brennenstuhl et al. 2019). Autosomal recessive D$\beta$H deficiency is characterized by primary autonomic failure with complete absence of norepinephrine and epinephrine in plasma in combination with increased levels of dopamine. Serum D$\beta$H activity is low (Man in 't Veld et al. 1987; Robertson et al. 1986). The initial symptoms can be seen during the perinatal period with hypotension, muscle hypotonia, hypothermia and hypoglycemia, delayed eye opening, and ptosis. Children exhibit a reduced ability to exercise because blood pressure cannot adapt adequately which results in syncopes. Symptoms usually progressively worsen during early adulthood with severe orthostatic hypotension and also eyelid ptosis, nasal stuffiness, and retrograde ejaculation (Senard and Rouet 2006). Treatment is mainly supportive with the aim to relieve orthostatic symptoms. Oral administration of droxidopa (or L-threo-3,4-dihydroxyphenylserine), a synthetic amino acid precursor of norepinephrine which can cross the blood-brain barrier and can be utilized to generate dopamine, has been shown to improve orthostatic hypotension. Very few pathogenic *DBH* mutations have been identified. Variations in the *DBH* gene were further reported in patients with Gilles de la Tourette syndrome, ADHD, and schizophrenia (Haavik et al. 2008).

X chromosome-linked monoamine oxidase (MAO) catalyzes the oxidative deamination of a wide variety of monoamines including dopamine, serotonin, and the catecholamines. Two forms of the enzyme are classified as MAO-A and MAO-B depending on their sensitivity to inhibitors and affinity for substrates. MAO-A prefers serotonin, norepinephrine, and dopamine MAO-B phenylethylamine. While isolated MAO-B deficiency reveals no relevant clinical phenotype, MAO-A deficiency leads conceptually to accumulation of the monoamine neurotransmitters in CSF, while levels of their metabolites in body fluids and compartments are decreased (Brunner et al. 1993a). Male patients presented with mild mental retardation and a tendency toward stereotyped hand movements, as well as behavioral problems with repeated occurrences of aggression (Brunner et al. 1993b). In addition, chronic episodes of flushing, diarrhea, headaches, and psychiatric problems have been reported (Cheung and Earl 2001). Combined deletion of *MAO-A* and *MAO-B* was described in a male patient with severe developmental delay, intermittent hypotonia, and stereotypical hand movements (Whibley et al. 2010). Up to now, no effective treatment for MAO-A deficiency is available. Dietary intervention of avoiding foods rich in amines and cyproheptadine hydrochloride and sertraline hydrochloride have been used with uncertain or with no effect.

In addition to enzyme deficiencies, two transporter defects are known to cause disorders of biogenic amines. The autosomal recessive SLC6A3-related dopamine transporter deficiency syndrome (DTDS) typically presents in infancy and atypically later in childhood, adolescence, or adulthood (Assmann et al. 2004; Kurian et al. 2009; Ng et al. 2014). After initial nonspecific clinical symptoms (including delayed motor development with axial hypotonia), patients with early onset DTDS develop a variable hyperkinetic movement disorder with predominantly choreatic and dystonic features. Over time, hyperkinetic features shift toward parkinsonian symptoms such as tremor, bradykinesia, and hypomimia. In some patients, oculogyric crises occur. Neurodevelopmental milestones are hardly achieved; however, cognitive impairment is usually mild compared with motor deficiencies (Kurian et al. 2011b). The atypical later-onset DTDS can develop during childhood or adulthood after normal psychomotor development in infancy and early childhood (Ng et al. 2014). Symptoms include parkinsonism-dystonia with tremor, progressive bradykinesia, variable tone, and dystonic posturing.

Characteristic biochemical findings are elevated HVA in CSF and raised HVA/5-HIAA ratio in CSF (>4.0; Norm range: 1.0–4.0). All known patients have a homozygous or compound heterozygous mutations in the *SLC6A3* gene. There is no causative treatment available. Treatment attempts include dopamine agonists (e.g., pramipexole) or anticholinergic drugs, such as trihexyphenidyl to control dystonia, benzodiazepines or chloral hydrate to relief chorea, dyskinesia and improve sleep as well as supportive treatment with physiotherapy and/or focal botulinum toxin (Yildiz et al. 2017).

The second transporter defect was identified in eight children from one consanguineous family showing clinical symptoms of deficiencies of dopamine, serotonin, epinephrine, and norepinephrine without detectable deficit of neurotransmitters in CSF. A mutation in *SLC18A2* gene encoding the vesicular monoamine transporter 2 (VMAT2) protein was identified, leading to a defective monoamine loading into synaptic vesicles (Rilstone et al. 2013). While normal CSF monoamine metabolites are not suitable for diagnosis, patients show elevated homovanillic acid and 5-hydroxyindoleacetic acid concentration in urine and present low total serotonin levels in blood (Rath et al. 2017). The use of dopamine receptor agonists resulted in an improvement of movement disorders, while L-dopa/carbidopa worsened the clinical presentation (Ng et al. 2015).

## Nomenclature

| No. | Disease name | Alternative disease name | Disease abbreviation | Gene symbol | Chromosomal localization | Mode of inheritance | Affected protein | OMIM no. |
|---|---|---|---|---|---|---|---|---|
| 19.1 | Tyrosine hydroxylase deficiency | DYT5b, DYT/PARK-TH | TH | *TH* | 11p15.5 | AR | Tyrosine-3-hydroxylase | 191290 |
| 19.2 | Aromatic l-amino acid decarboxylase deficiency | DOPA decarboxylase deficiency | AADC | *DDC* | 7p12.1-12.3 | AR | Aromatic l-amino acid decarboxylase | 107930 |
| 19.3 | Dopamine β-hydroxylase deficiency | | DBH | *DBH* | 9q34 | AR | Dopamine beta-hydroxylase | 609312 |
| 19.4 | Monoamine oxidase A deficiency | Brunner syndrome | MAO-A | *MAOA* | Xp11-21 | XLR | Monoamine oxidase A | 309850 |
| 19.5 | Dopamine transporter deficiency | Infantile Parkinsonism-dystonia | DTDS | *SLC6A3* | 5p15.3 | AR | SLC6A3 transporter | 126455 |
| 19.6 | Vesicular monoamine transporter 2 deficiency | | VMAT2 | *SLC18A2* | | AR | SLC18A2 Vesicular monoamine transporter 2 | 193001 |

## Metabolic Pathways

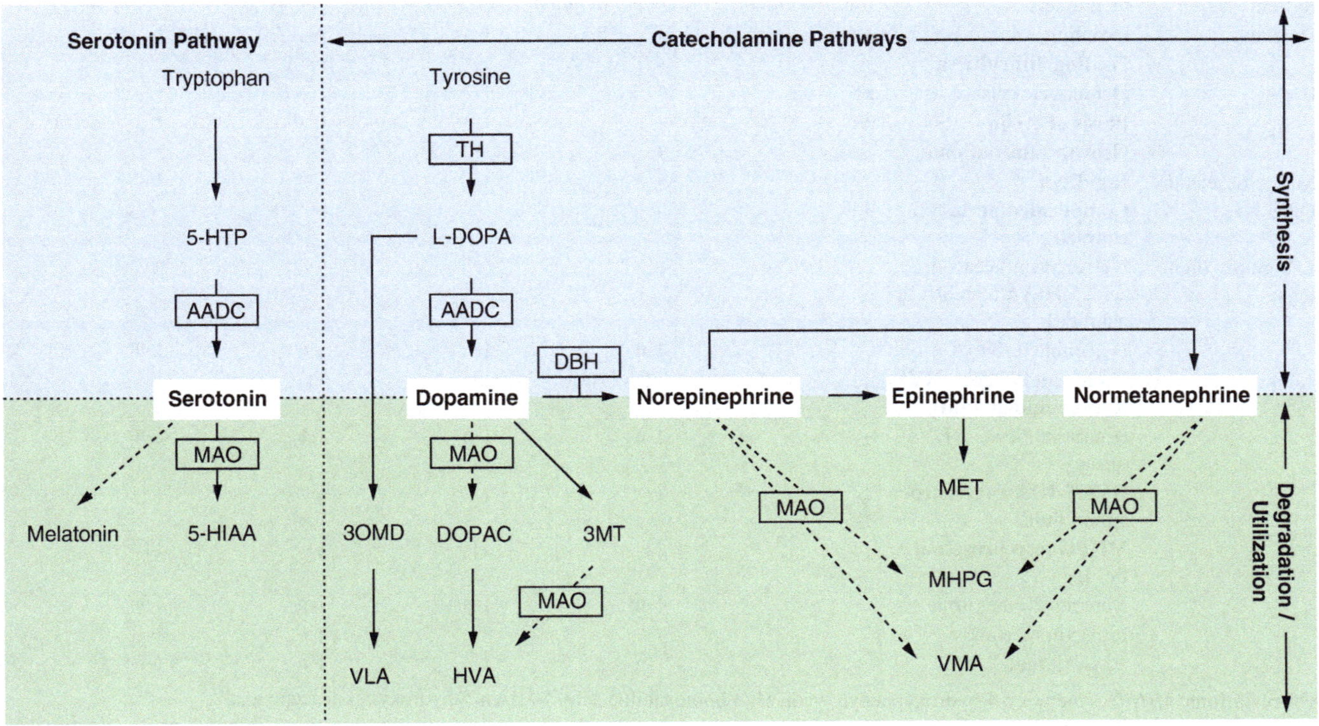


Metabolism of serotonin and the catecholamines: *TH* tyrosine hydroxylase, *AADC* aromatic *l*-amino acid decarboxylase, *DBH* dopamine ß-hydroxylase, *MAO* monoamine oxidase, *VLA* vanillactic acid, *3OMD* 3-*O*-methyldopa, *5-HTP* 5-hydroxytryptophan, *5-HIAA* 5-hydroxyindoleacetic acid, *DOPAC* dihydroxyphenylacetic acid, *HVA* homovanillic acid, *VMA* vanillylmandelic acid, *MHPG* 3-methoxy-4-hydroxyphenylglycol, *MET* metanephrine, *3MT* 3-methoxytyramine. (- - - > represents several steps involved. Pathological metabolites used as markers in the differential diagnosis are shown within boxes)

## Signs and Symptoms

**Table 19.1** Tyrosine hydroxylase deficiency

| System | Symptoms and biomarkers | Neonatal (birth–1 month) | Infancy (1–18 months) | Childhood (1.5–11 years) | Adolescence (11–16 years) | Adulthood (>16 years) |
|---|---|---|---|---|---|---|
| Autonomic system | **Sweating** | ± | + | + | + | + |
| | **Temperature instability** | + | + | + | + | + |
| CNS | **Bradykinesia** | + | + | + | + | + |
| | **Dystonia** | | + | + | + | + |
| | Dystonic crisis[a] | | + | + | + | + |
| | **Epileptic seizures** | | ± | ± | ± | ± |
| | **Hypokinesiaa** | + | + | + | + | + |
| | **Hypotonia** | + | + | + | + | + |
| | **Intellectual disabilitya** | – | + | + | + | + |
| | **Irritability crisis** | ± | + | + | + | + |
| | **Lethargy crisis** | ± | + | + | + | + |
| | **Sleep disturbances** | | + | + | + | + |
| | **Tremor** | | + | + | + | + |

(continued)

**Table 19.1** (continued)

| System | Symptoms and biomarkers | Neonatal (birth–1 month) | Infancy (1–18 months) | Childhood (1.5–11 years) | Adolescence (11–16 years) | Adulthood (>16 years) |
|---|---|---|---|---|---|---|
| Digestive | **Drooling** | ± | + | + | + | + |
| | **Feeding difficulties**[a] | + | + | + | + | + |
| Eye | **Oculogyric crisis** | ± | + | + | + | + |
| | **Ptosis of eyelid** | ± | + | + | + | + |
| | **Growth retardation**[a] | | + | + | + | + |
| Musculoskeletal | **Rigidity**[a] | | + | + | + | + |
| Other | **Complicated perinatal course**[b] | ++ | | | | |
| Laboratory findings | 5-Hydroxyindoleacetic acid, 5-HIAA (cerebrospinal fluid) | n | n | n | n | n |
| | Dopamine (urine) | | ↓-n | ↓-n | ↓-n | ↓-n |
| | **Homovanillic acid, HVA (cerebrospinal fluid)** | ↓↓ | ↓↓ | ↓↓ | ↓↓ | ↓↓ |
| | Homovanillic acid, HVA (urine) | – | ↓-n | ↓-n | ↓-n | ↓-n |
| | **HVA/5-HIAA (cerebrospinal fluid)** | ↓ | ↓ | ↓ | ↓ | ↓ |
| | **MHPG (cerebrospinal fluid)** | ↓↓ | ↓↓ | ↓↓ | ↓↓ | ↓↓ |
| | Norepinephrine (urine) | | ↓-n | ↓-n | ↓-n | ↓-n |
| | Prolactin (plasma) | | ↑ | ↑ | ↑ | ↑ |
| | VMA (urine) | | ↓-n | ↓-n | ↓-n | ↓-n |

**Abbreviations**: *MHPG* 3-methoxy-4-hydroxyphenylglycol, *HVA* homovanillic acid, 5-HIAA 5-hydroxyindoleacetic acid

Based on the presenting neurological features, TH deficiency can be conceptually divided in two phenotypes: an infantile onset, progressive, hypokinetic-rigid syndrome with dystonia (type A, less severe) and a complex encephalopathy with neonatal onset (type B, more severe)

[a]Predominant in type B

[b]Only in type B

**Table 19.2** Aromatic L-amino acid decarboxylase deficiency

| System | Symptoms and biomarkers | Neonatal (birth–1 month) | Infancy (1–18 months) | Childhood (1.5–11 years) | Adolescence (11–16 years) | Adulthood (>16 years) |
|---|---|---|---|---|---|---|
| Autonomic system | **Sweating** | | + | + | + | + |
| | **Temperature instability** | | ± | ± | ± | ± |
| CNS | **Absent head control** | | ± | ± | ± | ± |
| | **Athetosis** | | ± | ± | ± | ± |
| | **Chorea** | | ± | ± | ± | |
| | Dysarthria | | + | + | + | + |
| | Dystonia | | + | + | + | + |
| | **EEG, abnormal** | | **n** | **n** | **n** | **n** |
| | Global developmental delay | | + | + | + | + |
| | Hyperkinesia | | + | + | + | + |
| | **Hypertonia (mainly limbs)** | | + | + | + | + |
| | **Hypokinesia** | | + | + | + | + |
| | **Hypotonia (mainly truncal)** | | ++ | ++ | ++ | ++ |
| | Insomnia | | + | + | + | |
| | **Irritability** | | + | + | + | + |
| | **Poor head control** | | ± | ± | ± | ± |
| | **Swallowing difficulties** | | + | + | | |
| Digestive | **Diarrhea** | | ± | ± | | ± |
| | **Drooling** | | + | + | + | + |
| | **Feeding difficulties** | | + | + | | |
| Eye | **Eye movements, abnormal** | | ++ | ++ | ++ | ++ |
| | **Oculogyric crisis** | | ++ | ++ | ++ | ++ |
| | **Poor visual fixation** | | ± | ± | | |
| | **Ptosis of eyelid** | | + | + | + | − |
| Psychiatric | **Behavioral abnormalities** | | + | + | + | + |
| Respiratory | **Nasal congestion** | | + | + | + | |
| | **3-O-Methyldopa, 3OMD (cerebrospinal fluid)** | | ↑↑ | ↑↑ | ↑↑ | ↑↑ |
| | 3-*O*-Methyldopa, 3OMD (dried blood spot) | ↑↑↑ | ↑↑ | ↑ | ↑/n | ↑/n |
| | **5-Hydroxyindoleacetic acid, 5-HIAA (cerebrospinal fluid)** | | ↓ | ↓ | ↓ | ↓ |
| | **5-Hydroxytryptophan (cerebrospinal fluid)** | | ↑ | ↑ | ↑ | ↑ |
| Laboratory findings | **Homovanillic acid, HVA (cerebrospinal fluid)** | | ↓ | ↓ | ↓ | ↓ |
| | **l-Dopa (cerebrospinal fluid)** | | n-↑ | n-↑ | n-↑ | n-↑ |
| | **MHPG (cerebrospinal fluid)** | | ↓ | ↓ | ↓ | ↓ |
| | Vanillinlactic acid (urine) | | n-↑ | n-↑ | n-↑ | n-↑ |

**Abbreviations**: *3OMD* 3-*O*-methyldopa, *5-HTP* 5-hydroxytryptophan, *HVA* homovanillic acid, *5-HIAA* 5-hydroxyindoleacetic acid

**Table 19.3** Dopamine beta-hydroxylase deficiency

| System | Symptoms and biomarkers | Neonatal (birth–1 month) | Infancy (1–18 months) | Childhood (1.5–11 years) | Adolescence (11–16 years) | Adulthood (>16 years) |
|---|---|---|---|---|---|---|
| Autonomic system | **Hypothermia** | ± | ± | | | |
| Cardiovascular | **Hypotension, orthostatic** | | | ± | ++ | +++ |
| | Syncope | | | ± | ++ | +++ |
| Eye | **Eyes opening, delayed** | ± | | | | |
| | **Ptosis of eyelid** | ± | ± | ± | ± | ± |
| Genitourinary | **Impaired ejaculation** | | | | | ++ |
| Metabolic | **Hypoglycemia** | ± | ± | | | |
| Musculoskeletal | **Exercise intolerance** | | | ± | + | + |
| Psychiatric | Behavioral disorder, mild | | | | ± | ± |
| Laboratory findings | 3-*O*-Methyldopa (plasma) | | | | n-↑ | n-↑ |
| | **Dopamine (plasma)** | | | | ↑↑ | ↑↑ |
| | **Dopamine beta-hydroxylase (plasma)** | | | | ↓↓↓ | ↓↓↓ |
| | **Epinephrine (plasma)** | | | | ↓↓ | ↓↓ |
| | **Glucose (plasma)** | **n-↓** | **n-↓** | | | |
| | **Homovanillic acid, HVA (cerebrospinal fluid)** | | | | ↑ | ↑ |
| | **Homovanillic acid, HVA (urine)** | | | | ↑ | ↑ |
| | **l-Dopa (cerebrospinal fluid)** | | | | ↑ | ↑ |
| | **l-Dopa (plasma)** | | | | ↑ | ↑ |
| | **MHPG (cerebrospinal fluid)** | | | | ↓ | ↓ |
| | **Norepinephrine (plasma)** | | | | ↓↓↓ | ↓↓↓ |
| | Norepinephrine (urine) | | | | ↓↓↓ | ↓↓↓ |
| | **Vanillylmandelic acid, VMA (urine)** | | | | ↓ | ↓ |

**Abbreviations**: *3OMD* 3-*O*-methyldopa, *HVA* homovanillic acid, *MHPG* 3-methoxy-4-hydroxyphenylglycol, *VMA* vanillylmandelic acid
**Please note:** Metabolite values have not been reported in children, but a similar pattern is predicted
Plasma DßH activity can be low to undetectable in normal individuals; therefore, a low value is not diagnostic by itself

**Table 19.4** Monoamine oxidase A deficiency

| System | Symptoms and biomarkers | Neonatal (birth–1 month) | Infancy (1–18 months) | Childhood (1.5–11 years) | Adolescence (11–16 years) | Adulthood (>16 years) |
|---|---|---|---|---|---|---|
| CNS | **Intellectual disability, mild** | | | + | + | + |
| | **Stereotyped hand movements** | | | | ± | ± |
| Dermatological | **Flushing** | | | | ± | ± |
| Psychiatric | **Behavior, aggressive** | | | | + | + |
| Laboratory findings | **3-Methoxytyramine (urine)** | | | | ↑↑ | ↑↑ |
| | **5-Hydroxyindoleacetic acid, 5-HIAA (cerebrospinal fluid)** | | | | ↓ | ↓ |
| | 5-Hydroxyindoleacetic acid, 5-HIAA (urine) | | | | ↓-n | ↓-n |
| | **Homovanillic acid, HVA (cerebrospinal fluid)** | | | | ↓ | ↓ |
| | **Homovanillic acid, HVA (urine)** | | | | ↓ | ↓ |
| | **MAO-A (fibroblasts)** | | | | ↓↓ | ↓↓ |
| | MAO-B (platelets) | | | | n | + |
| | 3-Methoxy-4-hydroxyphenylglycol, MHPG (urine) | | | | ↓-n | ↓-n |
| | MHPG (cerebrospinal fluid) | | | | ↓-n | ↓-n |
| | **Normetanephrine (urine)** | | | | ↑↑ | ↑↑ |
| | **Vanillylmandelic acid, VMA (urine)** | | | | ↓ | ↓ |

**Abbreviations**: *5-HIAA* 5-hydroxyindoleacetic acid, *3OMD* 3-*O*-methyldopa, *HVA* homovanillic acid, *MHPG* 3-methoxy-4-hydroxyphenylglycol, *VMA* vanillylmandelic acid
**Please note**: Metabolite values have not been reported in children, but a similar pattern is predicted

**Table 19.5** Dopamine transporter deficiency syndrome

| System | Symptoms and biomarkers | Neonatal (birth–1 month) | Infancy (1–18 months) | Childhood (1.5–11 years) | Adolescence (11–16 years) | Adulthood (>16 years) |
|---|---|---|---|---|---|---|
| Autonomic system | **Hyperthermia** | | ± | ± | ± | |
| | **Sweating** | | ± | ± | ± | |
| CNS | **Axial hypotonia** | | ± | + | + | |
| | **Bradykinesia** | | ± | + | + | |
| | Bulbar dysfunction | | | ± | + | |
| | **Chorea** | | ± | ± | ± | |
| | **Dysarthria** | | | | ± | ± |
| | Dyskinesia | | ± | + | + | |
| | Dystonia | | ± | + | + | |
| | **Dystonic crisis** | | | ± | ± | |
| | **Hyperkinesia** | | ± | ± | ± | |
| | **Hypokinesia** | | ++ | ++ | ++ | |
| | **Hypomimia** | | ± | + | + | |
| | **Movement disorder** | | ++ | ++ | ++ | |
| | **Neonatal irritability** | ± | | | | |
| | Parkinsonism, hypokinetic features | | ± | + | + | |
| | **Pyramidal signs** | | | ± | ± | |
| | **Tremora** | | ± | ± | ± | |
| Digestive | **Drooling** | | ± | ± | ± | |
| | **Feeding difficulties** | + | | | | |
| Eye | Ocular flutter | | | ± | ± | |
| Psychiatric | **Attention deficit disorder** | | | | ± | ± |
| Laboratory findings | **Homovanillic acid, HVA (urine)** | ↑ | ↑ | ↑ | ↑ | |
| | **HVA/5-HIAA (cerebrospinal fluid)** | ↑↑ | ↑↑ | ↑↑ | ↑↑ | |
| | Prolactin (plasma) | | n-↑ | n-↑ | n-↑ | |
| | **Rigidity** | | ± | + | + | |

**Abbreviations**: *HVA* homovanillic acid, *5-HIAA* 5-hydroxyindoleacetic acid
[a]Predominant in atypical later-onset DTDS

**Table 19.6** Dopamine-serotonin vesicular transport defect

| System | Symptoms and biomarkers | Neonatal (birth–1 month) | Infancy (1–18 months) | Childhood (1.5–11 years) | Adolescence (11–16 years) | Adulthood (>16 years) |
|---|---|---|---|---|---|---|
| Autonomic system | Sweating | | + | + | + | + |
| CNS | Absent head control | n | + | | | |
| | Ataxia | | + | + | + | + |
| | **Cognitive dysfunction** | **n** | **n** | + | ++ | ++ |
| | **Developmental delay** | **n** | + | + | + | + |
| | Dysarthria | | | | ++ | ++ |
| | Dysdiadochokinesis | | | | ++ | ++ |
| | Dystonia | n | + | ++ | ++ | ++ |
| | Hypertonia, extremities | | | + | + | + |
| | Hypomimia | | + | | | |
| | Hypotonia | n | + | ++ | ++ | ++ |
| | **Parkinsonism, hypokinetic features** | | + | + | ++ | ++ |
| | Poor head control | n | + | | | |
| Eye | **Oculogyric crisis** | | ++ | ++ | ++ | ++ |
| | **Ptosis of eyelid** | | | ++ | ++ | ++ |
| Other | Hypernasal speech | | | + | + | + |
| | Profuse nasal secretion | | + | + | + | + |
| Respiratory | Nasal congestion | | ++ | ++ | ++ | ++ |
| Laboratory findings | **5-Hydroxyindoleacetic acid, 5-HIAA (urine)** | | ↑↑ | ↑↑ | ↑↑ | ↑↑ |
| | **Dopamine (urine)** | | ↓ | ↓ | ↓ | ↓ |
| | **Homovanillic acid, HVA (urine)** | | ↑↑ | ↑↑ | ↑↑ | ↑↑ |
| | **Norepinephrine (urine)** | | ↓ | ↓ | ↓ | ↓ |

**Abbreviations**: *HVA* homovanillic acid, *5-HIAA* 5-hydroxyindoleacetic acid

## Reference Values

### Enzyme Analyses

| Age | Plasma L-dopa decarboxylase (pmol/min/mL) | Liver L-Dopa de-carboxylase (pmol/min/mg protein) | Fibroblast MAO-A (pmol/min/mg protein) | Plasma DβH (nmol/min/mL) |
|---|---|---|---|---|
| Fetal | | 720–2590 | – | – |
| <3 years | 36–129 | 125–695 | – | – |
| Adult | 24–43 | | 10–350[a] | 0–100[b] |

[a]After stimulation with dexamethasone (Edelstein et al. 1986) Monoamine oxidases A and B are differentially regulated by glucocorticoids and "aging" in human skin fibroblasts.

[b]Plasma dopamine β-hydroxylase: Approximately 5% of the normal population have undetectable plasma DβH. The diagnosis of DβH deficiency, therefore, cannot be made solely on the basis of undetectable plasma DβH. On the other hand its presence rules out the diagnosis

### Biogenic Amines in CSF

| | HVA [nmol/L] | | 5-HIAA [nmol/L] | | 5-HTP [nmol/L] | | L-Dopa [nmol/L] | | 3OMD [nmol/L] | |
|---|---|---|---|---|---|---|---|---|---|---|
| 0–90 days | 484 | 1146 | 302 | 952 | 0 | 20 | 0 | 15 | 0 | 310 |
| 91–210 days | 427 | 989 | 159 | 528 | 0 | 17 | 0 | 15 | 0 | 128 |
| 211–365 days | 403 | 919 | 170 | 412 | 0 | 17 | 0 | 15 | 0 | 50 |
| 1–2 years | 364 | 870 | 155 | 359 | 0 | 15 | 0 | 15 | 0 | 50 |
| 3–5 years | 313 | 824 | 130 | 362 | 0 | 15 | 0 | 15 | 0 | 50 |
| 6–8 years | 260 | 713 | 110 | 247 | 0 | 15 | 0 | 15 | 0 | 50 |
| 9–12 years | 220 | 560 | 90 | 237 | 0 | 10 | 0 | 15 | 0 | 50 |
| 13–15 years | 190 | 507 | 75 | 203 | 0 | 10 | 0 | 15 | 0 | 50 |
| >16 years | 115 | 455 | 51 | 204 | 0 | 10 | 0 | 15 | 0 | 50 |

These reference ranges were established in the author's laboratory using the second milliliter of CSF (0.5 mL in children <1 year of life). Tubes were placed immediately on ice and kept frozen at −20 °C until shipping

### Blood and Plasma Neurotransmitters and Metabolites (nmol/L) (HPLC, Electrochemical (EC) or Fluorescence (F) Detection)

| Age | 3OMD (F) | L-Dopa (F) | 5-HTP (F) | NE[a] (EC) | DA[a] (EC) | Whole blood serotonin (F) |
|---|---|---|---|---|---|---|
| <3 | <80 | <25 | <20 | – | | 550–1780 |
| Adult | <80 | <25 | <20 | 0.5–3.1 | 0–0.7 | 450–980 |

*3OMD* 3-*O*-methyldopa, *5-HTP* 5-hydroxytryptophan, *NE* norepinephrine, *DA* dopamine

[a]Plasma catecholamines: Age-specific lower limits of plasma norepinephrine and dopamine have not been determined. Plasma norepinephrine varies with posture, activity, volume status and dietary salt, but should be present in plasma even during resting conditions at concentrations of at least 0.3 nmol/L

### Urine Neurotransmitters and Metabolites (nmol/mmol Creatinine) (HPLC, Electrochemical (EC) or Fluorescence (F) Detection)

| Age (years) | 3OMD[a] (F) | L-Dopa[a] (F) | 5-HTP[a] (F) | 5-HIAA[a] (F) | HVA[a] (F) | NE[a] (EC) | E[a] (EC) | DA[a] (EC) | NMN[a] (EC) | 3MT[a] (EC) | VMA[a] (EC) | 5HTa (F) | VLAa (EC) |
|---|---|---|---|---|---|---|---|---|---|---|---|---|---|
| <3 | 152–378 | | | 5500–7300 | 7000–8500 | 22–140 | 2.5–26 | 76–1350 | 5–143 | 45–480 | 500–2500 | 130–170 | <150 |
| Adult | 90–225 | 12–42 | <5 | 300–5100 | 1000–2800 | 10–53 | 2–11 | 60–225 | 55–200 | 60–145 | 800–2200 | 11–68 | <80 |

*3OMD* 3-*O*-methyldopa, *5-HTP* 5-hydroxytryptophan, *NE* norepinephrine, *E* epinephrine, *DA* dopamine, *NMN* nor-metanephrine, *3MT* 3-methoxytyramine, *VMA* vanillylmandelic acid, *5HT* serotonin, *HVA* homovanillic acid, *5-HIAA* 5-hydroxyindoleacetic acid, *VLA* vanillactic acid

[a]Unconjugated

## Pathological Values

| | 5-HIAA (CSF) | HVA (CSF) | HVA/ 5-HIAA | 3OMD (P, U, CSF) | L-Dopa (P, U, CSF) | 5-HTP (P, U, CSF) | MHPG (U, CSF) | DOPAC (P, U) | Pro (P) | NE (P, U) | E (P, U) | DA (P, U) | NMN (U) | 3MT (U) | VMA (U) | VLA (U) | SERO (B) | 5-HIAA (U) | HVA (U) |
|---|---|---|---|---|---|---|---|---|---|---|---|---|---|---|---|---|---|---|---|
| **TH** | n | ↓↓ | ↓↓ | n | | | ↓ | | ↑ | | | ↓-n | | | ↓-n | | | | |
| **AADC** | ↓↓ | ↓↓ | | ↑↑↑ | ↑↑ | ↑↑ | | ↑ (U) | ↑ | ↓↓↓ | ↓ | ↑-n (U) | | ↑ (U) | | ↑ | ↓ | | ↑ |
| **DβH** | n | ↑ (U) | | ↑-n | ↑<br>(P, CSF) | | ↓↓ | ↑↑ (P) | | ↓↓↓ | ↓ | ↑↑↑ | | | ↓ | | | | |
| **MAO-A** | ↓<br>↓-n (U) | ↓<br>↓-n (U) | | n | | | ↓ | | | | | ↑↑ | ↑↑ | ↑↑ | ↓ | | ↑ | | |
| **DTDS** | n | ↑<br>↑-n (U) | ↑↑ | | | | | | n-↑ | | | | | | | | | | |
| **VMAT2** | n | n | | | | | | | | ↓<br>(U) | | ↓<br>(U) | | | | | ↓ | ↑↑ | ↑↑ |

**Abbreviations**: *P* plasma, *U* urine, *CSF* cerebral spinal fluid, *3OMD* 3-*O*-methyldopa, *HVA* homovanillic acid, *MHPG* 3-methoxy-4-hydroxyphenylglycol, *VMA* vanillylmandelic acid, *5-HTP* 5-hydroxytryptophan, *5-HIAA* 5-hydroxyindoleacetic acid, *NE* norepinephrine, *E* epinephrine, *DA* dopamine, *NMN* normetanephrine, *3MT* 3-methoxytyramine, *VMA* vanillylmandelic acid, *VLA* vanillactic acid, *SERO* serotonin, *Pro* prolactin

## Diagnostic Flowchart

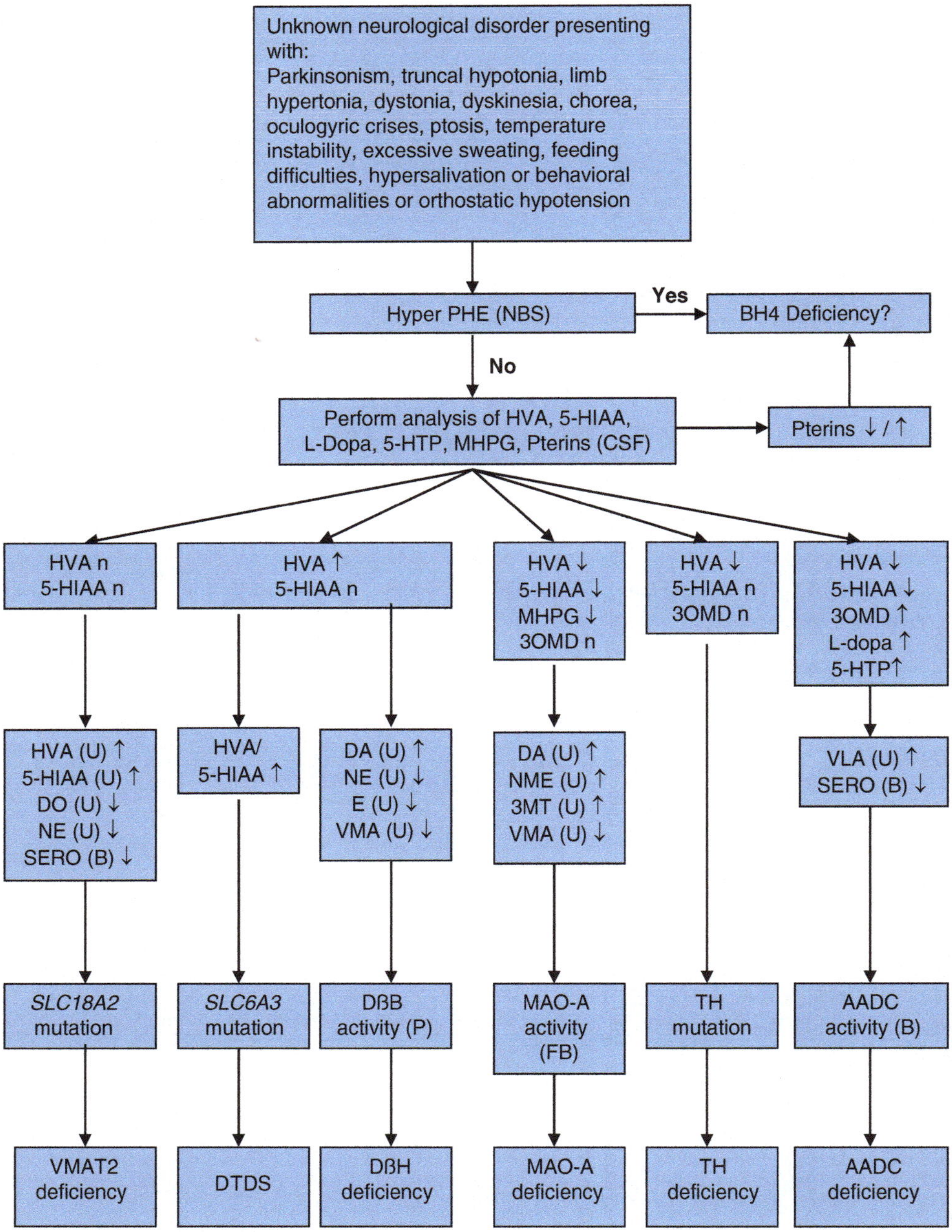


**Abbreviations**: *P* plasma, *B* blood, *U* urine, *CSF* cerebral spinal fluid, *3OMD* 3-*O*-methyldopa, *HVA* homovanillic acid, *MHPG* 3-methoxy-4-hydroxyphenylglycol, *VMA* vanillylmandelic acid, *5-HTP* 5-hydroxytryptophan, *5-HIAA* 5-hydroxyindoleacetic acid, *NE* norepinephrine, *E* epinephrine, *NMN* normetanephrine, *3MT* 3-methoxytyramine, *VMA* vanillylmandelic acid, *VLA* vanillactic acid, *SERO* serotonin

## Specimen Collection

| Test | Material | Preconditions | Handling | Pitfalls |
|---|---|---|---|---|
| 5-HIAA<br>HVA<br>3OMD<br>L-Dopa<br>MHPG<br>$BH_4$<br>$BH_2$<br>Neo | CSF | Before medication | Collect 6 CSF fractions (0.5 mL each for children <1 year; 1 mL for children >1 year)<br>Place tubes immediately on ice and keep frozen at −20 °C<br>Use the 1st fraction for other investigations (CSF cell count, lactate, glucose, etc.)<br>Collect the 4th fraction for pterins ($BH_4$) in tubes containing 1 mg DTE and 1 mg DTPA (diethylene-triaminepentaacetic acid) | Unstable in blood-contaminated samples<br>In the case of blood contamination, centrifuge CSF first |
| AADC enzyme activity | Plasma | | 1 mL, EDTA tube, centrifuge and store immediately at −70 °C | |
| 5HT, 3MT, 3OMD, NMN, 5-HIAA, VMA, HVA, DA, E, MHPG, NE | 24 h urine | Diet free of biogenic amine-containing food-stuffs urine | 24 h urine collected into 6 M HCl, store at −20 °C | Many foods (e.g., bananas, dates) contain biogenic amines and metabolites |
| Serotonin, 5HT | Whole blood | | 2 mL, EDTA tubes containing 6 mg ascorbic acid, store at −20 °C | |
| DßH | Plasma | | 1 mL, heparin tube, store at −70 °C | |
| MAO-A | Fibroblast | | Room temp. | |
| Catecholamines and metabolites | Plasma | | 1 mL, in EDTA tube, store at −70 °C | |
| VLA | Urine | | Urine 10 mL, store at −20 °C organic acid proil | |
| 30MD | DBS | Indicate possible L-Dopa treatment | Guthrie/dried blood spot card, room temperature | In newborn screening can the maternal L-Dopa treatment result in high 3OMD levels in the neonate |

**Abbreviations:** *MHPG* 3-methoxy-4-hydroxyphenylglycol, *HVA* homovanillic acid, *5-HIAA* 5-hydroxyindoleacetic acid, *3OMD* 3-*O*-methyldopa, *VMA* vanillylmandelic acid, *5-HTP* 5-hydroxytryptophan, *NE* norepinephrine, *E* epinephrine, *DA* dopamine, *NMN* normetanephrine, *3MT* 3-methoxytyramine, *VLA* vanillactic acid, *Pro* prolactin, *BH4* tetrahydrobiopterin, *BH2* dihydrobiopterin, *Neo* neopterin, *DA* dopamine, *NMN* normetanephrine, *DβH* dopamineß-hydroxylase

## Prenatal Diagnosis

| | Material | Timing |
|---|---|---|
| TH | **Chorionic villi**<br>**Amniotic fluid cells** (if mutations are known) | I. Trimester |
| AADC | **Chorionic villi**<br>**Amniotic fluid cells** (if mutations are known)<br>Liver biopsy for enzyme analysis (2. trimester) | I. Trimester |
| DßH | – | – |
| MAO-A | – | – |
| DTDS | **Chorionic villi**<br>**Amniotic fluid cells** (if mutations are known) | I. Trimester |
| VMAT2 | **Chorionic villi**<br>**Amniotic fluid cells** (if mutations are known) | I. Trimester |

## DNA Testing

| | Tissue | Methodology |
|---|---|---|
| TH | Genomic DNA (and from **cultures of skin fibroblasts, lymphoblasts, lymphocytes)** | PCR/SSCP sequencing |
| AADC | Genomic DNA (and from **cultures of skin fibroblasts, lymphoblasts, lymphocytes)** | PCR sequencing |
| DßH | Genomic DNA | PCR sequencing |
| MAO-A | Cultured fibroblasts | PCR sequencing |
| DTDS | Genomic DNA (and from **cultures of skin fibroblasts, lymphoblasts, lymphocytes)** | PCR sequencing |
| VMAT2 | Genomic DNA (and from **cultures of skin fibroblasts, lymphoblasts, lymphocytes)** | PCR sequencing |

## Treatment

Treatment in TH deficiency is aimed at correction of the shortage of neurotransmitters. Bypassing the metabolic block using levodopa/carbidopa only or together with dopamine agonists usually leads to a good to excellent clinical response in most TH-deficient patients. In addition to L-dopa, inhibitors of dopamine degradation such as selegiline can be used. Despite appropriate treatment, long-term cognitive development can be subnormal in these patients (Willemsen et al. 2010).

AADC-deficient patients have received dopamine receptor agonists, monoamine oxidase inhibitors, anticholinergics, and selective serotonin reuptake inhibitors in conjunction with vitamin $B_6$ (cofactor for AADC). Therapy is usually initiated with one of the dopamine agonists (bromocriptine or pergolide), sometimes in combination with low-dose pyridoxine. In a second step, a monoamine oxidase inhibitor is added (e.g., selegiline). All other medications are added only if the initial treatment protocol fails to improve neurological symptoms. Treatment should be carefully evaluated for at least 3 months and be discontinued in case of no or questionable positive effects. L-Dopa treatment has been successful in three siblings with mutations affecting the L-dopa binding (Wassenberg et al. 2017). In general, response to treatment in AADC patients is variable, and outcome appears to be better in less severely affected patients and males than females. Gene therapy approaches are promising new treatment options in AADC deficiency leading to improved motor and mental function as well as brain white matter tracts (Kojima et al. 2019; Tseng et al. 2019).

Since orthostatic hypotension is the main symptom in patients with dopamine $\beta$-hydroxylase (D$\beta$H), treatment focuses on this aspect. Droxidopa, a synthetic amino acid precursor of norepinephrine, can cross the blood-brain barrier and can by using the AADC generate dopamine, improving orthostatic hypotension.

Up to now, no effective treatment for MAO-A deficiency is available. Dietary intervention by avoiding foods rich in amines as well as cyproheptadine hydrochloride and sertraline hydrochloride supplementation have been used with uncertain or with no effect.

Various drug treatment strategies and surgical interventions like deep brain stimulators had only little, temporary, or even no effect on the clinical symptoms of DTDS-deficient patients (Kurian et al. 2011b).

In brain dopamine-serotonin vesicular transport disease, treatment was initially started with levodopa leading to a worsening of the movement disorder. In contrast, subsequent treatment with direct dopamine agonists was followed by immediate ambulation, near-complete correction of the movement disorder, and resumption of development (Rilstone et al. 2013).

## Emergency Treatment

**Dangers and Pitfalls**

1. Besides the neurological picture, patients with TH and AADC deficiency developed additional non-neurological symptoms, especially autonomic symptoms including hypoglycemia due to catecholamine deficiency (Manegold et al. 2009).
2. Lack of catecholamines may also render patients susceptible to sudden cardiac arrest, especially when patients are exposed to stressful situations. Therefore, clinical admission and close cardiac monitoring during acute illness and/or for any medical intervention is inevitable (Wassenberg et al. 2017).
3. Use glucose infusion during acute illness and/or during any medical intervention.

## Standard Treatment

| | Medication | Dosage (mg/kg/day) | Dose/day (*n*) |
|---|---|---|---|
| TH | Levodopa (L-dopa) | (0.5) 1–10 | 2–6 |
| | Carbidopa | 10–25% of L-dopa | 2–6 |
| AADC | Pramipexole | 5–10 **µg/kg/day!** | 3 |
| | Bromocriptine | 0.1–0.5 | 3 |
| | Selegiline | 0.1–0.3 | 2–3 |
| | Pyridoxine ($B_6$) | 50–200 **mg/day!** | 2 |
| | Tranylcypromine | 0.1–0.5 | 2 |
| | Trihexyphenidyl | 0.1–0.5 | 3 |
| | Levodopa (L-dopa)[a] | 1–15 | 3 |
| DßH | Droxidopa | 250–500 | 2–3 |
| DTDS | Pramipexole | 5–10 **µg/kg/day!** | 3 |
| | Bromocriptine | 0.1–0.5 | 3 |
| | Selegiline | 0.1–0.3 | 2–3 |
| VMAT2 | Pramipexole | Not known | Not known |

Please note: The dosages given are the range which is usually applied. In individual patients, some adaptations and variations depending on the clinical picture are needed

[a]L-Dopa treatment should be limited to AADC-deficient patients with proven variants at the L-dopa binding site (Wassenberg et al. 2017)

**Dangers/Pitfalls**

1. L-Dopa/carbidopa/5-hydroxytryptophan therapy should be introduced slowly and increased in steps of not more than 1 mg/kg over days or weeks.
2. Changes in dopamine receptor density can cause difficulties with treatment. Receptor hypersensitivity in early diagnosed, severe cases means that treatment with cocareldopa should start at very low doses (0.25–0.5 mg levodopa/kg per day) given frequently up to 6 times a day. Receptor downregulation in late-diagnosed severe forms means that treatment with cocareldopa in the maximally tolerated dose up to 10 mg levodopa/kg per day should be maintained for as much as 6 months before deciding it is unhelpful.
3. L-Dopa/carbidopa/5-hydroxytryptophan therapy may reduce CSF folate (5′-methyltetrohydrofolate in CSF is the major transport species for the brain folate pool and is utilized by the single carbon transfer pathway to methylate L-dopa to 3-*O*-methyl-dopa). Determine 5-methyltetrahydrofolate in CSF. Consider folinic acid (5-formyltetra-hydrofolate) substitution (10–20 mg/day). This may occur "naturally" in AADC deficiency, again requiring folate supplementation (Surtees and Hyland 1990).
4. In AADC deficiency dopamine agonists can produce dyskinesia and increased irritability, and the dose needs to be carefully titrated.
5. The dose of trihexyphenidyl should start at 1 or 2 mg three times a day. The dose is then increased by 1 or 2 mg/day each week until one of three possibilities occur: (1) the child's condition improves; (2) troublesome side-effects occur (dry eyes or mouth, or gastrointestinal disturbance most commonly); or (3) a limit of 10 mg/kg/day is reached.

## Experimental Treatment

To date, there are only very few reports on prenatal treatment in cases with confirmed disorders of monoamine metabolism, and most of them concentrate on disorders in tetrahydrobiopterin metabolism (Bruggemann et al. 2012; Kuseyri et al. 2018). Assuming that adequate catecholamine maintenance is essential for embryonic (synaptic) development, it has been suggested that early administration of L-dopa with a decarboxylase inhibitor can improve long-term outcome of the fetus (Bruggemann et al. 2012).

In addition, the conclusion of a recent study on pregnancy management and outcome in patients with four different tetrahydrobiopterin disorders stating that these patients require an intensive clinical and biochemical supervision by a multidisciplinary team before, during, and after the pregnancy holds also true for patients with disorders of monoamine metabolism (Kuseyri et al. 2018).

| | Medication | Dosage (mg/kg/day) | Dose/day (*n*) |
|---|---|---|---|
| MAO-A | Sertraline hydrochloride | | |
| | Cyproheptadine | | |
| DTDS | Ropinirole? | 2–6 | 2–6 |
| | Levodopa (L-dopa)? | 2–6 | 2–6 |

**Dangers/Pitfalls**

1. Adjunctive treatment with a M AO-B inhibitor such as selegeline, COMT inhibitor such as entacapone, and dopamine agonists such as bromocriptine may be necessary in TH. When introducing a MAO-B inhibitor or a COMT inhibitor, L-dopa should be reduced by approximately 50–30%.
2. Pyridoxine is a natural cofactor of AADC. In most patients, no sustained clinical or biochemical effect is achieved. In one family, in whom kinetic studies showed the mutation to decrease the binding affinity for the substrate, an improvement was achieved by combined therapy of L-dopa, without carbidopa, and pyridoxine.
3. Sertraline hydrochloride should be introduced slowly because of the risk of causing the serotonin syndrome.

## References


Assmann B, Surtees R, Hoffmann GF. Approach to the diagnosis of neurotransmitter diseases exemplified by the differential diagnosis of childhood-onset dystonia. Ann Neurol. 2003;54(Suppl 6):S18–24.

Assmann BE, Robinson RO, Surtees RA, Brautigam C, Heales SJ, Wevers RA, Zschocke J, Hyland K, Sharma R, Hoffmann GF. Infantile Parkinsonism-dystonia and elevated dopamine metabolites in CSF. Neurology. 2004;62(10):1872–4.

Bartholome K, Ludecke B. Mutations in the tyrosine hydroxylase gene cause various forms of L-dopa-responsive dystonia. Adv Pharmacol. 1998;42:48–9.

Bräutigam C, Wevers RA, Jansen RJ, Smeitink JA, de Rijk-van Andel JF, Gabreels FJ, Hoffmann GF. Biochemical hallmarks of tyrosine hydroxylase deficiency. Clin Chem. 1998;44(9):1897–904.

Brautigam C, Hyland K, Wevers R, Sharma R, Wagner L, Stock GJ, Heitmann F, Hoffmann GF. Clinical and laboratory findings in twins with neonatal epileptic encephalopathy mimicking aromatic L-amino acid decarboxylase deficiency. Neuropediatrics. 2002;33(3):113–7.

Brennenstuhl H, Jung-Klawitter S, Assmann B, Opladen T. Inherited disorders of neurotransmitters: classification and practical approaches for diagnosis and treatment. Neuropediatrics. 2019;50(1):2–14.

Brennenstuhl, H. J Inherit Metab Dis. 2020;43(3):602–610.

Bruggemann N, Spiegler J, Hellenbroich Y, Opladen T, Schneider SA, Stephani U, Boor R, Gillessen-Kaesbach G, Sperner J, Klein C. Beneficial prenatal levodopa therapy in autosomal recessive guanosine triphosphate cyclohydrolase 1 deficiency. Arch Neurol. 2012;69(8):1071–5. archneurol.2012.104 [pii].

Brun L, Ngu LH, Keng WT, Ch'ng GS, Choy YS, Hwu WL, Lee WT, et al. Clinical and biochemical features of aromatic L-amino acid decarboxylase deficiency. Neurology. 2010;75(1):64–71.

Brunner HG, Nelen M, Breakefield XO, Ropers HH, van Oost BA. Abnormal behavior associated with a point mutation in the structural gene for monoamine oxidase A. Science. 1993a;262(5133):578–80.

Brunner HG, Nelen MR, van Zandvoort P, Abeling NG, van Gennip AH, Wolters EC, Kuiper MA, Ropers HH, van Oost BA. X-linked borderline mental retardation with prominent behavioral disturbance: phenotype, genetic localization, and evidence for disturbed monoamine metabolism. Am J Hum Genet. 1993b;52(6):1032–9.

Cheung NW, Earl J. Monoamine oxidase deficiency: a cause of flushing and attention-deficit/hyperactivity disorder? Arch Intern Med. 2001;161(20):2503–4. ibr1112-3 [pii].

Edelstein SB, Breakefield XO. Monoamine oxidases A and B are differentially regulated by glucocorticoids and "aging" in human skin fibroblasts. Cell Mol Neurobiol. 1986;6(2):121–50.

Haavik J, Blau N, Thöny B. Mutations in human monoamine-related neurotransmitter pathway genes. Hum Mutat. 2008;29(7):891–902.

Hoffmann GF, Surtees RA, Wevers RA. Cerebrospinal fluid investigations for neurometabolic disorders. Neuropediatrics. 1998;29(2):59–71.

Hyland K, Surtees RA, Rodeck C, Clayton PT. Aromatic L-amino acid decarboxylase deficiency: clinical features, diagnosis, and treatment of a new inborn error of neurotransmitter amine synthesis. Neurology. 1992;42(10):1980–8.

Kojima K, Nakajima T, Taga N, Miyauchi A, Kato M, Matsumoto A, Ikeda T, et al. Gene therapy improves motor and mental function of aromatic l-amino acid decarboxylase deficiency. Brain. 2019;142(2):322–33.

Kurian MA, Zhen J, Cheng SY, Li Y, Mordekar SR, Jardine P, Morgan NV, et al. Homozygous loss-of-function mutations in the gene encoding the dopamine transporter are associated with infantile parkinsonism-dystonia. J Clin Invest. 2009;119(6):1595–603.

Kurian MA, Gissen P, Smith M, Heales SJ, Clayton PT. The monoamine neurotransmitter disorders: an expanding range of neurological syndromes. Lancet Neurol. 2011a;10(8):721–33.

Kurian MA, Li Y, Zhen J, Meyer E, Hai N, Christen H-J, Hoffmann GF, et al. Clinical and molecular characterisation of hereditary dopamine transporter deficiency syndrome: an observational cohort and experimental study. Lancet Neurol. 2011b;10(1):54–62.

Kuseyri O, Weissbach A, Bruggemann N, Klein C, Gizewska M, Karall D, Scholl-Burgi S, et al. Pregnancy management and outcome in patients with four different tetrahydrobiopterin disorders. J Inherit Metab Dis. 2018;41(5):849–63.

Ludecke B, Bartholome K. Frequent sequence variant in the human tyrosine hydroxylase gene. Hum Genet. 1995;95(6):716.

Man in 't Veld AJ, Boomsma F, Moleman P, Schalekamp MA. Congenital dopamine-beta-hydroxylase deficiency. A novel orthostatic syndrome. Lancet. 1987;1(8526):183–8.

Manegold C, Hoffmann GF, Degen I, Ikonomidou H, Knust A, Laass MW, Pritsch M, Wilichowski E, Horster F. Aromatic L-amino acid decarboxylase deficiency: clinical features, drug therapy and follow-up. J Inherit Metab Dis. 2009;32(3):371–80.

Ng J, Zhen J, Meyer E, Erreger K, Li Y, Kakar N, Ahmad J, et al. Dopamine transporter deficiency syndrome: phenotypic spectrum from infancy to adulthood. Brain. 2014;137(Pt 4):1107–19.

Ng J, Papandreou A, Heales SJ, Kurian MA. Monoamine neurotransmitter disorders—clinical advances and future perspectives. Nat Rev Neurol. 2015;11(10):567–84.

Pons R, Ford B, Chiriboga CA, Clayton PT, Hinton V, Hyland K, Sharma R, De Vivo DC. Aromatic L-amino acid decarboxylase deficiency: clinical features, treatment, and prognosis. Neurology. 2004;62(7):1058–65.

Rath M, Korenke GC, Najm J, Hoffmann GF, Hagendorff A, Strom TM, Felbor U. Exome sequencing results in identification and treatment of brain dopamine-serotonin vesicular transport disease. J Neurol Sci. 2017;379:296–7.

Rilstone JJ, Alkhater RA, Minassian BA. Brain dopamine-serotonin vesicular transport disease and its treatment. N Engl J Med. 2013;368(6):543–50.

Robertson D, Goldberg MR, Onrot J, Hollister AS, Wiley R, Thompson JG Jr, Robertson RM. Isolated failure of autonomic noradrenergic neurotransmission. Evidence for impaired beta-hydroxylation of dopamine. N Engl J Med. 1986;314(23):1494–7.

Senard JM, Rouet P. Dopamine beta-hydroxylase deficiency. Orphanet J Rare Dis. 2006;1:7.

Surtees R, Hyland K. L-3,4-dihydroxyphenylalanine (levodopa) lowers central nervous system S-adenosylmethionine concentrations in humans. J Neurol Neurosurg Psychiatry. 1990;53:569–72.

Swoboda KJ, Saul JP, McKenna CE, Speller NB, Hyland K. Aromatic L-amino acid decarboxylase deficiency: overview of clinical features and outcomes. Ann Neurol. 2003;54(Suppl 6):S49–55.

Tseng CH, Chien YH, Lee NC, Hsu YC, Peng SF, Tseng WI, Hwu WL. Gene therapy improves brain white matter in aromatic l-amino acid decarboxylase deficiency. Ann Neurol. 2019;85(5):644–52.

Wassenberg T, Molero-Luis M, Jeltsch K, Hoffmann GF, Assmann B, Blau N, Garcia-Cazorla A, et al. Consensus guideline for the diagnosis and treatment of aromatic l-amino acid decarboxylase (AADC) deficiency. Orphanet J Rare Dis. 2017;12(1):12.

Whibley A, Urquhart J, Dore J, Willatt L, Parkin G, Gaunt L, Black G, Donnai D, Raymond FL. Deletion of MAOA and MAOB in a male patient causes severe developmental delay, intermittent hypotonia and stereotypical hand movements. Eur J Hum Genet. 2010;18(10):1095–9.

Willemsen MA, Verbeek MM, Kamsteeg EJ, de Rijk-van Andel JF, Aeby A, Blau N, Burlina A, et al. Tyrosine hydroxylase deficiency: a treatable disorder of brain catecholamine biosynthesis. Brain. 2010;133(Pt 6):1810–22.

Yildiz Y, Pektas E, Tokatli A, Haliloglu G. Hereditary dopamine transporter deficiency syndrome: challenges in diagnosis and treatment. Neuropediatrics. 2017;48(1):49–52.

# Disorders of Phenylalanine and Tetrahydrobiopterin Metabolism

# 20

Alberto Burlina, Francjan J. van Spronsen, and Nenad Blau

## Contents




A. Burlina (✉)
Division of Inherited Metabolic Diseases, Reference Centre Expanded Newborn Screening, Department of Woman's and Child's Health, University Hospital, Padova, Italy
e-mail: alberto.burlina@unipd.it

F. J. van Spronsen
Division of Metabolic Diseases, University of Groningen, University Medical Center Groningen, Beatrix Children's Hospital, Groningen, The Netherlands
e-mail: f.j.van.spronsen@umcg.nl

N. Blau (✉)
Division of Metabolism, University Children's Hospital, Zürich, Switzerland
e-mail: Nenad.Blau@kispi.uzh.ch





N. Blau et al. (eds.), *Physician's Guide to the Diagnosis, Treatment, and Follow-Up of Inherited Metabolic Diseases*,
https://doi.org/10.1007/978-3-030-67727-5_20

**Summary**

Most countries now identify hyperphenylalaninemia (HPA) immediately after birth through national neonatal screening programs. Rapid identification of HPA allows timely diagnosis of the underlying enzyme defect and application of appropriate therapy: every patient with confirmed HPA who receives appropriate dietary intervention is potentially a child saved from a lifetime of mental retardation. Pharmacological treatment with tetrahydrobiopterin (BH4; sapropterin) and an enzyme substitution therapy with phenylalanine ammonia lyase (PAL; pegvaliase) are recently introduced in some groups of patients with phenylalanine hydroxylase (PAH) deficiency. Approximately 1–2% of cases of HPA detected by screening of neonates will have a disorder of BH4 metabolism (higher in countries with frequent consanguineous marriages). It is important to test for the presence of BH4 deficiency in patients with even mild elevation of blood Phe. Analysis of pterins (neopterin, biopterin, and primapterin) in blood or urine and measurement of dihydropteridine reductase (DHPR) should be carried out on all patients. Some patients with autosomal dominant GTP cyclohydrolase I (GTPCH) deficiency and patients with sepiapterin reductase (SR) deficiency may present with normal blood Phe in the newborn period, however. Measurement of monoamine neurotransmitter metabolites in cerebrospinal fluid adds importantly to the diagnosis of different forms (severe vs. mild) of BH4 deficiencies. Molecular diagnostics for the PAH co-chaperone DNAJC12 variants are mandatory in all patients in which deficiencies of PAH and BH4 are genetically excluded.

## Introduction

Hyperphenylalaninemia (HPA) is a condition caused primarily by genetically based defects in Phe metabolism. HPA is usually caused by a deficiency of the hepatic phenylalanine-4-hydroxylase (PAH), by one of the enzymes involved in its cofactor tetrahydrobiopterin (BH4) biosynthesis (GTP cyclohydrolase I, GTPCH; and 6-pyruvoyl-tetrahydropterin synthase, PTPS) or regeneration (dihydropteridine reductase, DHPR; and pterin carbinolamine-4α-dehydratase, PCD) (Blau et al. 2010), or by the DNAJC12 co-chaperon of the PAH (Anikster et al. 2017). BH4 is known to be the natural cofactor and co-substrate for PAH, tyrosine-3-hydroxylase, and tryptophan-5-hydroxylase as well as all three isoforms of nitric oxide synthase (NOS) (Werner et al. 2011). Tyrosine-3-hydroxylase and tryptophan-5-hydroxylase are the two rate-limiting enzymes in the biosynthesis of the neurotransmitters dopamine and serotonin. Thus, with two exceptions (see below), any cofactor defect will result in a deficiency of biogenic amines accompanied by HPA (Burlina and Blau 2014). Because phenylalanine is a competitive inhibitor of the uptake of tyrosine and tryptophan across the blood-brain barrier and of the hydroxylases of tyrosine and tryptophan in the CNS, depletion of catecholamines and serotonin occurs in untreated patients with PAH deficiency. Both groups of HPA (PAH and BH4 deficiency) are heterogeneous disorders varying from severe, e.g., classical phenylketonuria (PKU), to mild, and benign forms (van Spronsen et al. 2017). Because of the different clinical and biochemical severities in patients with BH4 deficiencies, the terms “severe” or “mild” will be used based upon the type of treatment and involvement of the CNS. For the BH4 defects, symptoms may manifest during the first weeks of life but usually are noted within the first half year of life. Birth is generally uneventful, except for an increased incidence of prematurity and lower birth weights in severe PTPS deficiency (Opladen et al. 2012).

Two disorders of BH4 metabolism may present without HPA. These are autosomal dominant GTPCH deficiency (also addressed as Segawa disease, dopa-responsive dystonia (DRD), DYT5a, DYT/PARK-GCH1) (Segawa 2011) and sepiapterin reductase (SR) (DYT/PARK-SPR) deficiency (Friedman et al. 2012). While DRD is caused by mutations in the *GCH1* gene and is inherited in an autosomal dominant manner, SR deficiency is inherited in an autosomal recessive trait. Both diseases result in severe biogenic amines deficiencies (Brennenstuhl et al. 2019) but appear to decrease PAH activity in a less meaningful way so that it does not result in HPA. DRD usually presents with a dystonic gait and diurnal variation. A wide phenotypic spectrum of *GCH1* variants has been reported ranging from dystonia to “Parkinsonian” symptoms such as tremor, bradykinesia, and impaired fine motor skills. Symptoms can show a circadian fluctuation with worsening during the day and improvement of the symptoms after sleep.

In SR deficiency, the early phenotype includes axial hypotonia, developmental delay of motor functions, and psychiatric symptoms such as increased irritability, behavioral problems, and oculogyric crises (Friedman et al. 2012). Later, the phenotype changes toward dystonia with apparent circadian rhythm. Recently, endocrinological disturbances such as hypoglycemia and growth-hormone deficiency were identified as early symptoms of dopamine depletion in SR deficiency (Zielonka et al. 2015).

Recently, variants in DNAJC12, a co-chaperone of the HSP40/DNAJ family, type III, were described to lead to mild HPA, central biogenic amines deficiency, dystonia, intellectual disability, and parkinsonism, thereby defining a new entity of HPA without PAH or BH4 deficiency (Anikster et al. 2017). DNAJC12 interacts with PAH, TH, and the TPHs, which indicates that DNAJC12 is a specific co-chaperone for the aromatic amino acid hydroxylases that contributes to the maintenance of their intracellular stability (Jung-Kc et al. 2019).

A diagnosis of HPA is usually based upon the confirmation of an elevated blood phenylalanine level obtained on a normal diet, following a positive newborn screening test. Normal breast milk or formula feeding for only 24 h is sufficient to raise the baby's blood phenylalanine sufficiently to trigger a positive test level (>120 μmol/L), while severe illness may also cause HPA even without nutritional intake. In general, an infant will be found to have a positive screening test after 12 h postnatal if the phenylalanine-to-tyrosine ratio rather than the phenylalanine concentration is used. The tandem mass spectrometer (TMS) is today the method of choice for newborn screening. Based on the fact that patients diagnosed early have better outcome, it is logical—although not proven—that detection as early as possible is essential in order to introduce appropriate treatment to not only prevent mental retardation but to guarantee the best optimal mental development.

In PAH and BH4 deficiencies, factors like a relatively high phenylalanine intake in relation to current growth velocity or catabolic situations may be responsible for high phenylalanine concentrations in blood. Once HPA has been detected, a sequence of quantitative tests (see Sect. 20.8) enables the differentiation between variants, i.e., classical PKU (usually the patients with the most severe PAH deficiency), BH4-responsive PKU, BH4 deficiencies, and the DNAJC12 variant. Because the last two forms are actually a group of diseases that may be detected because of HPA, but not simply and routinely identified by neonatal mass screening, selective screening for a BH4 deficiency and DNAJC12 is essential in every newborn with even slightly elevated phenylalanine levels. Differential testing for BH4 deficiencies should be done in all newborns with plasma phenylalanine levels >120 μmol/L (2 mg/dL), as well as in older infants and children with neurological signs and symptoms. DNAJC12 should be genotyped in HPA patients in which deficiencies of PAH and BH4 are excluded (Blau et al. 2018).

Since the two forms of BH4 deficiency presenting *without* HPA (DRD and SR deficiency) cannot be recognized through the newborn screening for PKU, investigation of neurotransmitter metabolites and pterins in CSF is essential in patients with delay in mental development and neurological issues, especially concerning tonus regulation. In patients with DRD, a phenylalanine loading test, a trial with L-dopa, DNA testing, and enzyme activity measurement in cytokine-stimulated fibroblasts are confirmatory for the diagnosis. SR deficiency can be definitely diagnosed by pterins analysis in CSF and urine and by DNA testing, but a phenylalanine-loading test can be indicative as well.

For patients with PAH deficiency, three different treatments are available: diet, chaperone therapy with BH4, and enzyme replacement therapy (Blau and Longo 2015). Future treatment options for lowering the blood phenylalanine in PKU, like gene replacement or repair or manipulation of microbioma are under development (Lichter-Konecki and Vockley 2019) while other strategies such as large neutral amino acids targeting the brain more directly are also under development. In BH4 deficiencies, the goal is to reduce phenylalanine by supplementation with BH4 and to normalize brain neurotransmitters by normalizing blood—and by that brain—phenylalanine but especially by giving the precursors of the neurotransmitters knowing that they will pass the blood-brain barrier oral administration of dopamine and serotonin precursors (L-dopa/carbidopa and 5-hydroxytryptophan, respectively). In instances where the standard treatment approach is not beneficial, drugs like selegiline, entacapone, pramipexole, and rotigotine should be considered (Burlina and Blau 2014; Opladen et al. 2012). In this respect, it should be taken into account that some patients with PAH deficiency, historically only treated by diet, can be treated with BH4 (sapropterin dihydrochloride). At the same time, in patients with DHPR deficiency, in whom historically the HPA was treated with BH4, the diet restricting phenylalanine intake is the treatment of choice, as BH4 administration may result in BH2 accumulation and the BH4/BH2 ratio may then become less optimal. DNAJC12-deficient patients can be treated by oral administration of BH4, dopamine, and serotonin precursors (Straniero et al. 2017), but some patients with a milder phenotype do well on BH4 alone (van Spronsen et al. 2017).

Late introduction of treatment in all the patients called above leads to irreversible brain damage. In contrast to early and continuously treated patients with PAH deficiency, some patients with BH4 deficiencies (DHPR and severe form of PTPS) show progressive neurological deterioration despite treatment. An international working group on neurotransmitter-related disorders (iNTD) focused primarily on epidemiology, diagnosis, and treatment of these disorders is now systematically collecting data for improving the understanding of these disorders (Opladen et al. 2016).

## Nomenclature

| No. | Disorder | Alternative name | Abbreviation | Gene | Chromosomal location | Mode of inheritance | Affected protein | OMIM |
|---|---|---|---|---|---|---|---|---|
| 20.1 | Phenylalanine hydroxylase deficiency | Classic PKU | cPKU | *PAH* | 12q22-24.1 | AR | Phenylalanine hydroxylase | 261600 |
| 20.2 | GTP cyclohydrolase I deficiency | | arGTPCH | *GCH1* | 14q22.1-22.2 | AR | GTP cyclohydrolase I | 233910 |
| 20.3 | 6-Pyruvoyl-tetrahydropterin synthase deficiency | | PTPS | *PTS* | 11q22.3-23.3 | AR | 6-Pyruvoyl-tetrahydropterin synthase | 261640 |
| 20.4 | Dihydropteridine reductase deficiency | | DHPR | *QDPR* | 4p15.3 | AR | Dihydropteridine reductase | 261630 |
| 20.5 | Pterin-4α-carbinolamine dehydratase deficiency | Primapterinuria | PCD | *PCBD1* | 10q22 | AR | Pterin-4α-carbinolamine dehydratase | 264070 |
| 20.6 | Dopa-responsive dystonia | Segawa disease | adGTPCH | *GCH1* | 14q22.1-22.2 | AD | GTP cyclohydrolase I | 600225 |
| 20.7 | Sepiapterin reductase deficiency | | SR | *SPR* | 2p14-p12 | AR | Sepiapterin reductase | 182125 |
| 20.8 | DNAJC12 deficiency | | DNAJC12 | *DNAJC12* | 10q21.3 | AR | DNAJC12 co-chaperon | 617384 |

## Metabolic Pathway

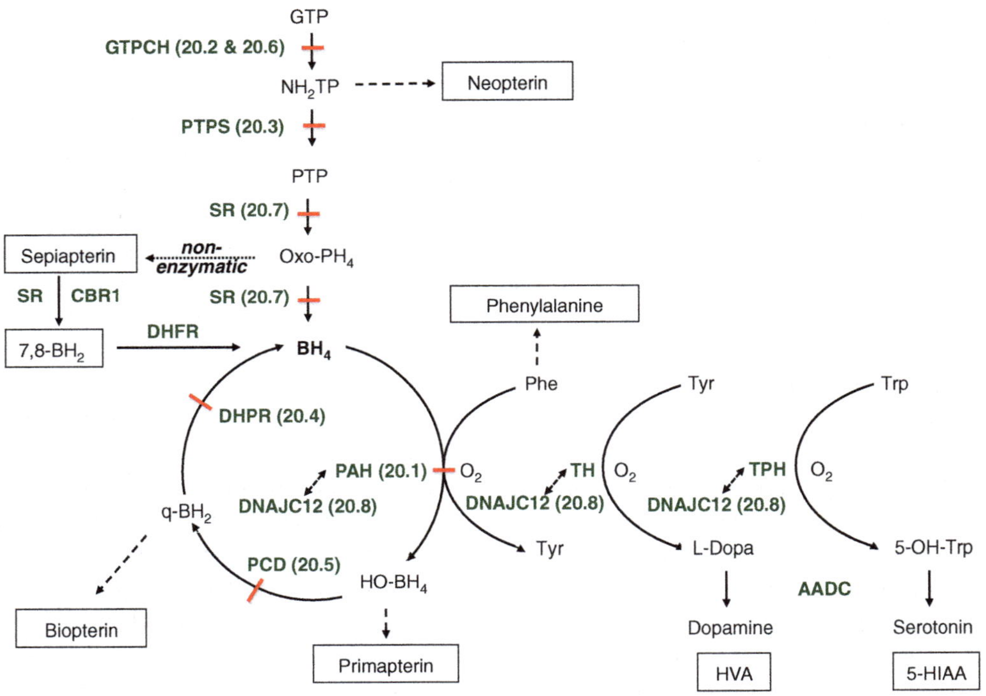


**Fig. 20.1** Biosynthesis and regeneration of tetrahydrobiopterin (BH4) including possible metabolic defects in hyperphenylalaninemia (HPA) and catabolism of phenylalanine. 20.1 = phenylalanine-4-hydroxylase (PAH); 20.2/20.6 = GTP cyclohydrolase I, 20.3 = 6-pyruvoyl-tetrahydropterin synthase (PTPS), 20.4 = dihydropteridine reductase (DHPR), 20.5 = Pterin-4α-carbinolamine dehydratase (PCD), 20.7 = sepiapterin reductase (SR), 20.8 = DNAJC12, carbonyl reductase (CR), aldose reductase (AR), dihydrofolate reductase (DHFR), aromatic amino acid decarboxylase (AADC), tyrosine hydroxylase (TH), tryptophan hydroxylase (TPH). Pathological metabolites used as specific markers in the differential diagnosis are marked in squares

## Signs and Symptoms

**Table 20.1** Phenylalanine hydroxylase deficiency, classic PKU (Phe >1200 μM)

| System | Symptoms and biomarkers | Neonatal (birth–1 month) | Infancy (1–18 months) | Childhood (1.5–11 years) | Adolescence (11–16 years) | Adulthood (>16 years) |
|---|---|---|---|---|---|---|
| CNS | Autism | | | ± | ± | ± |
| | Brain, abnormal (MRI) | | ± | ± | ± | ± |
| | Hypertonia, extremities | | ± | ± | ± | |
| | **Intellectual disability** | ± | + | + | + | + |
| | Irritability | | ± | ± | ± | ± |
| | **Microcephaly** | | + | + | + | + |
| | Seizures | | | ± | ± | ± |
| Dermatological | **Hypopigmentation** | + | + | + | + | + |
| Musculoskeletal | Head circumference | ↓-n | ↓-n | | | |
| | Height | ↓-n | ↓-n | ↓-n | | |
| | Hypotonia, muscular-axial | | ± | ± | ± | |
| Other | Birth weight | ↓-n | | | | |
| | **Odor (U, body)** | ± | + | + | + | + |
| Laboratory findings | 5-Hydroxyindoleacetic acid, 5-HIAA (cerebrospinal fluid) | | ↓-n | ↓-n | ↓ | ↓ |
| | Biopterin (B) | ↑ | ↑ | ↑ | ↑ | ↑ |
| | Homovanillic acid, HVA (cerebrospinal fluid) | ↓-n | ↓-n | ↓-n | ↓ | ↓ |
| | Neopterin (U) | ↑ | ↑ | ↑ | ↑ | ↑ |
| | Phenylalanine (plasma, DBS (dried blood spot), cerebrospinal fluid) | ↑↑↑ | ↑↑↑ | ↑↑↑ | ↑↑↑ | ↑↑↑ |
| | Phenylpyruvic acid (urine) | n-↑ | ↑ | ↑ | ↑ | ↑ |
| | Tetrahydrobiopterin, BH4 (sapropterin dihydrochloride) loading test | n | n | n | n | n |

**Table 20.2** Autosomal recessive GTP cyclohydrolase I deficiency

| System | Symptoms and biomarkers | Neonatal (birth–1 month) | Infancy (1–18 months) | Childhood (1.5–11 years) | Adolescence (11–16 years) | Adulthood (>16 years) |
|---|---|---|---|---|---|---|
| Autonomic system | Temperature instability | + | + | + | | |
| CNS | **Hypertonia, extremities** | + | + | + | + | |
| | Intellectual disability | | + | + | + | |
| | Seizures, myoclonic | | + | + | | |
| | **Swallowing difficulties** | + | + | + | + | + |
| Digestive | Drooling | + | + | + | | |
| | Feeding difficulties | + | + | + | | |
| Eye | Ptosis of eyelid | + | + | + | ± | ± |
| Musculoskeletal | Hypotonia, muscular-axial | ± | + | + | + | |
| | Microcephaly | + | + | + | + | |
| Laboratory findings | 5-Hydroxyindoleacetic acid, 5-HIAA (cerebrospinal fluid) | ↓ | ↓ | ↓ | ↓ | |
| | Biopterin (dried blood spots, urine, cerebrospinal fluid) | ↓↓ | ↓↓ | ↓↓ | ↓↓ | ↓ |
| | GTPCH activity, cytokines-stimulated (fibroblasts) | ↓ | ↓ | ↓ | ↓ | |
| | Homovanillic acid, HVA (cerebrospinal fluid) | ↓↓ | ↓↓ | ↓↓ | ↓↓ | |
| | Neopterin (dried blood spots, urine, cerebrospinal fluid) | ↓↓ | ↓↓ | ↓↓ | ↓↓ | ↓ |
| | Phenylalanine (plasma, DBS, cerebrospinal fluid) | n-↑ | ↑ | ↑ | ↑ | ↑ |
| | Tetrahydrobiopterin loading test, BH4 (sapropterin dihydrochloride) loading test | +++ | +++ | +++ | +++ | |

**Table 20.3** 6-Pyruvoyl-tetrahydropterin synthase deficiency

| System | Symptoms and biomarkers | Neonatal (birth–1 month) | Infancy (1–18 months) | Childhood (1.5–11 years) | Adolescence (11–16 years) | Adulthood (>16 years) |
|---|---|---|---|---|---|---|
| Autonomic system | Temperature instability | + | + | + | | |
| CNS | Choreoathetosis | | + | + | + | |
| | Cortical atrophy (MRI) | + | + | + | + | + |
| | EEG, abnormal | + | + | + | + | + |
| | **Hypertonia, extremities** | ± | ± | + | + | ± |
| | **Intellectual disability** | ± | + | + | + | + |
| | Microcephaly | + | + | + | | |
| | Retardation, psychomotor | | + | + | | |
| | Seizures, myoclonic | | + | + | | |
| | Seizures, tonic-clonic | | + | + | | |
| | Subcortical atrophy (MRI) | + | + | + | + | + |
| | **Swallowing difficulties** | + | + | + | | |
| Dermatological | Hypopigmented hair | | + | + | | |
| | Rash, eczematous | | + | + | + | |
| Digestive | Drooling | + | + | + | + | |
| Eye | **Ptosis of eyelid** | + | + | + | | |
| Musculoskeletal | **Hypotonia, muscular-axial** | ± | + | + | + | + |
| Respiratory | Pneumonia | | + | + | | |
| Other | **Birth weight** | ↓ | | | | |
| | Sudden death | | ± | ± | | |
| Laboratory findings | 5-Hydroxyindoleacetic acid, 5-HIAA (cerebrospinal fluid) | ↓↓ | ↓↓ | ↓↓ | ↓ | ↓ |
| | Biopterin (dried blood spots, urine, cerebrospinal fluid) | ↓↓↓ | ↓↓↓ | ↓↓ | ↓↓ | ↓↓ |
| | Homovanillic acid, HVA (cerebrospinal fluid) | ↓↓ | ↓↓ | ↓↓ | ↓↓ | ↓ |
| | Neopterin (dried blood spots, urine, cerebrospinal fluid) | ↑↑↑ | ↑↑↑ | ↑↑ | ↑↑ | ↑↑ |
| | Phenylalanine (cerebrospinal fluid) | ↑ | ↑ | ↑ | ↑ | ↑ |
| | Phenylalanine (plasma, DBS) | ↑ | ↑ | ↑ | ↑ | ↑ |
| | Prolactin (plasma) | ↑ | ↑ | ↑ | ↑ | ↑ |
| | PTPS activity (red blood cells, fibroblasts) | ↓ | ↓ | ↓ | ↓ | ↓ |
| | Tetrahydrobiopterin loading test, BH4 (sapropterin dihydrochloride) loading test | ++ | ++ | ++ | ++ | ++ |

**Table 20.4** Dihydropteridine reductase deficiency

| System | Symptoms and biomarkers | Neonatal (birth–1 month) | Infancy (1–18 months) | Childhood (1.5–11 years) | Adolescence (11–16 years) | Adulthood (>16 years) |
|---|---|---|---|---|---|---|
| Autonomic system | Temperature instability | + | + | + | | |
| CNS | **Axial hypotonia** | | + | + | + | |
| | **Basal ganglia calcifications (CT)** | | + | + | + | |
| | Choreoathetosis | | + | + | + | |
| | Cortical atrophy (MRI) | ± | + | + | + | + |
| | EEG, abnormal | + | + | + | + | + |
| | Generalized slowing (EEG) | + | + | + | + | + |
| | **Intellectual disability** | ± | + | + | + | + |
| | Microcephaly | + | + | + | | |
| | Retardation, psychomotor | | + | + | | |
| | **Seizures, myoclonic** | | + | + | | |
| | Seizures, tonic-clonic | + | + | + | | |
| | Spike wave discharges (EEG) | + | + | + | + | + |
| | Subcortical atrophy (MRI) | ± | + | + | + | + |
| Dermatological | Hypopigmented hair | | + | + | | |
| | Rash, eczematous | | + | + | + | |
| Digestive | Drooling | + | + | + | + | |
| Musculoskeletal | **Hypotonia, muscular-axial** | ± | + | + | + | + |
| Respiratory | Pneumonia | | + | + | | |
| Other | Sudden death | | + | + | | |
| Laboratory findings | 5-Hydroxyindoleacetic acid, 5-HIAA (cerebrospinal fluid) | ↓↓ | ↓↓ | ↓↓ | ↓ | ↓ |
| | Biopterin (dried blood spots, urine, cerebrospinal fluid) | n-↑ | n-↑ | n-↑ | ↑ | ↑ |
| | Dihydrobiopterin (cerebrospinal fluid) | ↑↑ | ↑↑ | ↑↑ | ↑↑ | ↑↑ |
| | Dihydropteridine reductase, DHPR (dried blood spot) | ↓↓ | ↓↓ | ↓↓ | ↓↓ | ↓↓ |
| | Homovanillic acid, HVA (cerebrospinal fluid) | ↓↓ | ↓↓ | ↓↓ | ↓↓ | ↓ |
| | Neopterin (dried blood spots, urine, cerebrospinal fluid) | n | n | n | n | n |
| | Phenylalanine (plasma, DBS, cerebrospinal fluid) | ↑ | ↑ | ↑ | ↑ | ↑ |
| | Prolactin (plasma) | ↑ | ↑ | ↑ | ↑ | ↑ |
| | Tetrahydrobiopterin loading test, BH4 (sapropterin dihydrochloride) loading test | + | + | + | + | + |

**Table 20.5** Pterin carbinolamine-4α-dehydratase deficiency

| System | Symptoms and biomarkers | Neonatal (birth–1 month) | Infancy (1–18 months) | Childhood (1.5–11 years) | Adolescence (11–16 years) | Adulthood (>16 years) |
|---|---|---|---|---|---|---|
| CNS | Hypotonia, mild | + | | | | |
| | **Transient alteration in tone** | + | | | | |
| Endocrine | **Diabetes MODY3** | | | ± | ± | ± |
| Laboratory findings | Biopterin (dried blood spots, urine) | ↓-n | ↓-n | ↓-n | | |
| | Glucose (plasma) | | | n-↑ | n-↑ | n-↑ |
| | Magnesium (plasma) | | | ↓-n | ↓-n | ↓-n |
| | Neopterin (dried blood spots, urine) | ↑ | ↑ | | | |
| | Phenylalanine (plasma, DBS) | ↑ | n-↑ | n | n | n |
| | Primapterin (dried blood spots, urine) | ↑ | ↑ | ↑ | ↑ | |
| | Tetrahydrobiopterin loading test, BH4 (sapropterin dihydrochloride) loading test | + | + | + | | |

**Table 20.6** Autosomal dominant GTPCH deficiency

| System | Symptoms and biomarkers | Neonatal (birth–1 month) | Infancy (1–18 months) | Childhood (1.5–11 years) | Adolescence (11–16 years) | Adulthood (>16 years) |
|---|---|---|---|---|---|---|
| CNS | Bradykinesia | | ± | ± | ± | ± |
| | **Dystonia** | | + | + | + | + |
| | **Diurnal fluctuation of symptoms** | | ± | + | + | ± |
| | Dyskinesia | | | | ± | ± |
| | Hypertonia | ± | ± | ± | ± | ± |
| | **Hypokinesia** | | + | ++ | ++ | ++ |
| | Hypotonia | | ± | ± | ± | ± |
| | **Parkinsonism** | | | ± | ± | ± |
| | Spasticity | ± | ± | ± | ± | ± |
| | Tendon reflexes, increased | ± | ± | ± | ± | ± |
| | Tremor | | | | + | + |
| Digestive | Dysphagia | | ± | ± | ± | ± |
| Musculoskeletal | Pes equinovarus | | | ± | ± | |
| | **Rigidity** | ± | + | + | + | + |
| | Scoliosis | | | ± | ± | |
| Laboratory findings | 5-Hydroxyindoleacetic acid, 5-HIAA (cerebrospinal fluid) | ↓-n | ↓-n | ↓-n | ↓-n | ↓-n |
| | Biopterin (cerebrospinal fluid) | ↓ | ↓ | ↓ | ↓ | ↓ |
| | Biopterin (urine) | n | n | n | n | n |
| | Homovanillic acid, HVA (cerebrospinal fluid) | ↓ | ↓ | ↓ | ↓ | ↓ |
| | Neopterin (cerebrospinal fluid) | ↓ | ↓ | ↓ | ↓ | ↓ |
| | Neopterin (urine) | n | n | n | n | n |
| | Phe loading test | ± | ± | + | + | + |
| | Phenylalanine (plasma, DBS) | n | n | n | n | n |

**Table 20.7** Sepiapterin reductase deficiency

| System | Symptoms and biomarkers | Neonatal (birth–1 month) | Infancy (1–18 months) | Childhood (1.5–11 years) | Adolescence (11–16 years) | Adulthood (>16 years) |
|---|---|---|---|---|---|---|
| CNS | Axial hypotonia | ++ | ++ | ++ | + | |
| | **Cerebral palsy** | | | ± | ± | ± |
| | **Diurnal fluctuation of symptoms** | | + | + | ± | ± |
| | Dysarthria | ± | ± | ± | ± | |
| | **Hypokinesia** | + | ++ | ± | ± | ± |
| | Language difficulties | | ++ | ++ | + | |
| | Parkinsonism | | ± | ± | ± | |
| | **Retardation, psychomotor** | | ++ | ++ | | |
| | Tendon reflexes, increased | ± | ± | ± | | |
| Digestive | Gastrointestinal dysmotility | ± | ± | ± | | |
| Eye | Eye movements, abnormal | ± | ± | ± | | |
| | Oculogyric crisis | ± | ± | ± | | |
| Musculoskeletal | Muscle weakness | + | ± | ± | ± | |
| Psychiatric | Behavior, psychotic | | ± | ± | ± | ± |
| Laboratory findings | 5-Hydroxyindoleacetic acid, 5-HIAA (cerebrospinal fluid) | ↓↓↓ | ↓↓↓ | ↓↓↓ | ↓↓↓ | ↓↓ |
| | Biopterin (cerebrospinal fluid) | ↑ | ↑ | ↑ | ↑ | ↑ |
| | Biopterin (urine) | n | n | n | n | n |
| | Dihydrobiopterin (cerebrospinal fluid) | ↑↑ | ↑↑ | ↑↑ | ↑↑ | ↑↑ |
| | Homovanillic acid, HVA (cerebrospinal fluid) | ↓↓↓ | ↓↓↓ | ↓↓↓ | ↓↓↓ | ↓↓↓ |
| | Neopterin (dried blood spots, cerebrospinal fluid) | n | n | n | n | n |
| | Neopterin (urine) | n | +/– | n | n | n |
| | Phe loading test | | +/– | +/– | +/– | +/– |
| | Phenylalanine (plasma, DBS) | n | n | n | n | n |
| | Prolactin (plasma) | ↑ | ↑ | ↑ | ↑ | ↑ |
| | Sepiapterin (cerebrospinal fluid) | ↑↑ | ↑↑ | ↑↑ | ↑↑ | ↑↑ |
| | Sepiapterin (urine) | | ↑↑ | ↑↑ | ↑↑ | |

**Table 20.8** DNAJC12-deficient hyperphenylalaninemia

| System | Symptoms and biomarkers | Neonatal (birth–1 month) | Infancy (1–18 months) | Childhood (1.5–11 years) | Adolescence (11–16 years) | Adulthood (>16 years) |
|---|---|---|---|---|---|---|
| CNS | Autism | ± | ± | ± | | |
| | **Developmental delay** | ± | ± | ± | | |
| | Dystonia | ± | ± | ± | | |
| | **Intellectual disability** | ± | ± | ± | | |
| | **Parkinsonism** | | | | | ± |
| Psychiatric | **Attention deficit disorder** | | | ± | ± | |
| Laboratory findings | 5-Hydroxyindoleacetic acid, 5-HIAA (cerebrospinal fluid) | ↓ | ↓ | ↓ | | |
| | Biopterin (cerebrospinal fluid) | n-↑ | n-↑ | n-↑ | | |
| | Biopterin (dried blood spots, urine) | n | n | n | | |
| | Homovanillic acid, HVA (cerebrospinal fluid) | ↓ | ↓ | ↓ | | |
| | Neopterin (dried blood spots, urine, cerebrospinal fluid) | n | n | n | | |
| | Phenylalanine (plasma, DBS) | ↑ | ↑ | ↑ | | |
| | Tetrahydrobiopterin loading test, BH4 (sapropterin dihydrochloride) loading test | + | + | + | + | + |

## Reference Values

Plasma, urine, and dried blood spots[a]

| Age | Phe (P) µmol/L | Neo (P) nmol/L | Bio (P) nmol/L | Neo (U) mmol/mol Creat | Bio (U) mmol/mol Creat | Neo (DBS) nmol/g Hb | Bio (DBS) nmol/g Hb |
|---|---|---|---|---|---|---|---|
| Newborns | <120 | 3–11 | 4–18 | 1.1–4.0 | 0.5–3.0 | 0.19–2.93 | 0.08–1.20 |
| 0–1 year | <80 | 3–11 | 4–18 | 1.1–4.0 | 0.5–3.0 | 0.19–2.93 | 0.08–1.20 |
| 2–4 years | <80 | 3–11 | 4–18 | 1.1–4.0 | 0.5–3.0 | 0.19–2.93 | 0.08–1.20 |
| 5–10 years | <80 | 3–11 | 4–18 | 1.1–4.0 | 0.5–3.0 | 0.19–2.93 | 0.08–1.20 |
| 11–16 years | <70 | 3–11 | 4–18 | 0.2–1.7 | 0.5–2.7 | 0.19–2.93 | 0.08–1.20 |
| >16 years | <70 | 3–11 | 4–18 | 0.2–1.7 | 0.5–2.7 | 0.19–2.93 | 0.08–1.20 |

[a]See also Chap. 19, "Disorders of Monoamine Metabolism"

CSF

| Age | Neo (CSF)[a] nmol/L | BH4 (CSF) nmol/L | BH2 (CSF) nmol/L | Neo (CSF)[a] nmol/L | Bio (CSF)[a] nmol/L | 5-HIAA[b] (CSF) nmol/L | HVA[b] (CSF) nmol/L | 5-MTHF (CSF) nmol/L |
|---|---|---|---|---|---|---|---|---|
| Newborns | 0.5–3.0 | 3–11 | 4–18 | 15–35 | 20–70 | 144–800 | 300–1000 | 64–182 |
| 0–1 year | 0.5–3.0 | 3–11 | 4–18 | 12–30 | 15–40 | 114–336 | 295–932 | 64–182 |
| 2–4 years | 0.5–3.0 | 3–11 | 4–18 | 9–20 | 10–30 | 105–299 | 211–871 | 63–111 |
| 5–10 years | 0.5–3.0 | 3–11 | 4–18 | 9–20 | 10–30 | 88–178 | 144–801 | 41–117 |
| 11–16 years | 0.5–2.7 | 3–11 | 4–18 | 9–20 | 10–30 | 74–163 | 133–551 | 41–117 |
| >16 years | 0.5–2.7 | 3–11 | 4–18 | 9–20 | 10–30 | 66–141 | 115–488 | 41–117 |

[a]Total neopterin or biopterin
[b]See also Chap. 31, "Disorders of Neurotransmitter Metabolism"

Amniotic fluid, amniocytes, and fibroblasts

| | Age | Phe µmol/L | Neo nmol/L | Bio nmol/L | 5-HIAA nmol/L | HVA nmol/L |
|---|---|---|---|---|---|---|
| Amniotic fluid | Fetus | <120 | 16–40 | 6–21 | 32–135 | 50–144 |
| Amniocytes[a] | Fetus | | <14[b] | <115[b] | | |
| Fibroblasts[a] | Infants (0–12 months) | | 11–73[b] | 183–303[b] | | |
| | Children and adults | | 18–98[b] | 154–303[b] | | |

[a]In cytokine-stimulated cells
[b]pmol/mg

Enzymes

| Age | DHPR (RBC) mU/mg Hb | PTPS (RBC) µU/g Hb | SR (RBC) µU/mg protein | GTPCH (FB)[a] µU/mg protein | PTPS (FB) µU/mg protein | DHPR (FB) mU/mg protein | SR (FB) µU/mg protein |
|---|---|---|---|---|---|---|---|
| Fetus | 2.3–3.8 | 35–77 | | 1.5–1.9 | 3.0–3.3 | 5.8–8.8 | |
| Newborns (0–1 month) | 1.8–4.8 | 34–64 | | | | | |
| Infants (0–12 months) | 1.8–4.8 | | 0.33–1.86 | 1.7–4.9 | 0.5–1.7 | 6.3–8.7 | 97–185 |
| Children and adults | 1.8–4.8 | 11–29 | 0.33–1.86 | 1.4–6.5 | 0.4–1.6 | 4.5–8.3 | 99–185 |

[a]In cytokine-stimulated cells

## Pathological Values/Differential Diagnosis

Plasma

| Actual Phe[a] (µmol/L) | Neo (P) nmol/L | Bio (P) nmol/L |
|---|---|---|
| <200 | 3–11 | 4–18 |
| 200–600 | 2–32 | 12–46 |
| 600–1200 | 9–27 | 24–39 |

[a]Plasma neopterin and biopterin values depend strongly upon the actual hyperphenylalaninemia

Plasma, urine, DBS, and CSF

| Variant | Phe (P) | Neo (U) | Bio (U) | %Bio[a] | Neo (DBS) | Bio (DBS) | Neo (CSF) | Bio (CSF) | 5-HIAA (CSF) | HVA (CSF) | 5-MTHF (CSF) |
|---|---|---|---|---|---|---|---|---|---|---|---|
| | µmol/L | mmol/mol Creat | | | nmol/g Hb | | nmol/L | | | | |
| 1.1 PAH def. (classical) | >1200 | 1.1–16.9 | 1.2–8.1 | ~50 | 0.15–4.62 | 0.08–1.68 | 9–118 | 15–143 | 14–471 | 47–1174 | n |
| 1.1 PAH def. (variant) | 600–1200 | 1.1–16.9 | 1.2–8.1 | ~50 | 0.15–4.62 | 0.08–1.68 | 9–118 | 15–143 | n | n | n |
| 1.1 PAH def. (benign) | 120–600 | 1.1–16.9 | 1.2–8.1 | ~50 | 0.15–4.62 | 0.08–1.68 | n | n | n | n | n |
| 1.2. GTPCH def. | 120–1200[b] | <0.2 | <0.2 | ~50 | <0.15 | <0.08 | 0.05–3.0 | 1.5–7.5 | 61–183 | 15–48 | n |
| 1.3. PTPS def. (severe) | 250–2500 | 5.0–51.2 | <0.5 | <5 | 2.2–6.3 | 0 | 47–402 | 1.0–16.0 | 5–113 | 5–223 | n |
| 1.3. PTPS def. (mild) | 240–2200 | 5.0–51.2 | <0.5 | <5 | 2.2–6.3 | 0 | 25–230 | 13–56 | 93–420 | 249–998 | n |
| 1.4. DHPR def. (severe) | 180–2500 | 0.5–23.2 | 3.8–25.6 | >80 | 0.47–2.1 | 0.67–1.5 | 11–70 | 43–117 | 4–75 | 19–204 | ↓ |
| 1.4. DHPR def. (mild) | 280–600 | 0.5–23.2 | 3.8–25.6 | >80 | 0.47–2.1 | 0.67–1.5 | 11–70 | 43–117 | 21–66 | n | ↓-n |
| 1.5. PCD def. (benign) | 180–1200 | 4.1–22.5 | 0.7–1.5[c] | <50 | – | – | 43–117 | 16–96 | n | n | n |
| 1.6 DRD | <120 | n | n | ~50 | n | n | 1.1–6.2 | 3.1–7.6 | 48–97 | 120–239 | n |
| 1.7 SR def. | <120 | n | n | ~50 | n | n | 14–51 | 72–102[d] | 3–15 | 49–111 | n |
| 1.8 DNAJC12 | >120 | n | n | n | n | n | n | n | 20 | 86 | n |

[a]%Bio = 100 * Bio/(Neo + Bio)

[b]Several patients were missed in the newborn screening due to the negative Guthrie test

[c]Primapterin (7-Bio) ↑

[d]7,8-Dihydrobiopterin ↑

## Loading Tests

### Loading Test with BH4 (Sapropterin Dihydrochloride) to Diagnose BH4-Responsive PAH Deficiency

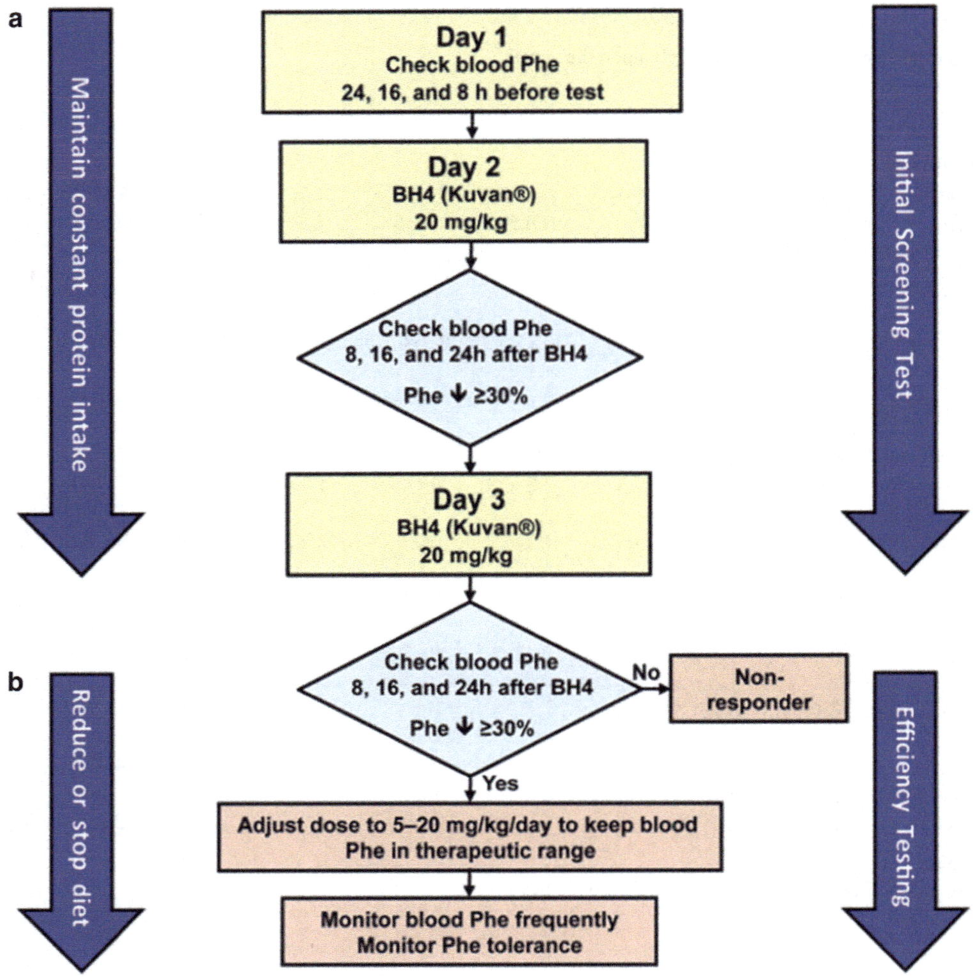


**Fig. 20.2** Suggested European guidelines algorithms for the BH4 (sapropterin dihydrochloride) challenge, screening, and initiating treatment in BH4-responsive PKU patients. (**a**) Initial screening test with blood phenylalanine monitoring on the first day and BH4 (sapropterin dihydrochloride) administration (20 mg/kg) on two following days. (**b**) Efficiency testing in BH4-responsive patients over several weeks with BH4 doses adjusted individually according to phenylalanine tolerance and therapeutic blood phenylalanine levels. Combined phenylalanine (100 mg/kg) and BH4 (20 mg/kg) loading test is sometimes difficult to interpret and is therefore not recommended (Blau et al. 2011). It is of importance to note that this BH4 loading test in neonates must be done over a period of 24 h (blood samples at 4, 6, 8, 12, and 24 h after sapropterin administration) and is useful to differentiate BH4 deficiencies from PAH deficiency (Muntau et al. 2019), rather than proving BH4 responsiveness

## Diagnostic Flowcharts

### Differential Diagnosis of HPAs

Screening for a $BH_4$ deficiency should be done in all newborns and children with even slight HPA (plasma Phe >120 μmol/L) as well as in older children without HPA but with neurological symptoms suggestive of a neurotransmitter deficiency.

The following protocol is suggested:

1. Analysis of pterins in DBS or urine
2. Measurement of DHPR activity in DBS
3. Analysis of phenylalanine and tyrosine in serum or plasma or DBS before and during > not after a $BH_4$ challenge
4. DNA testing

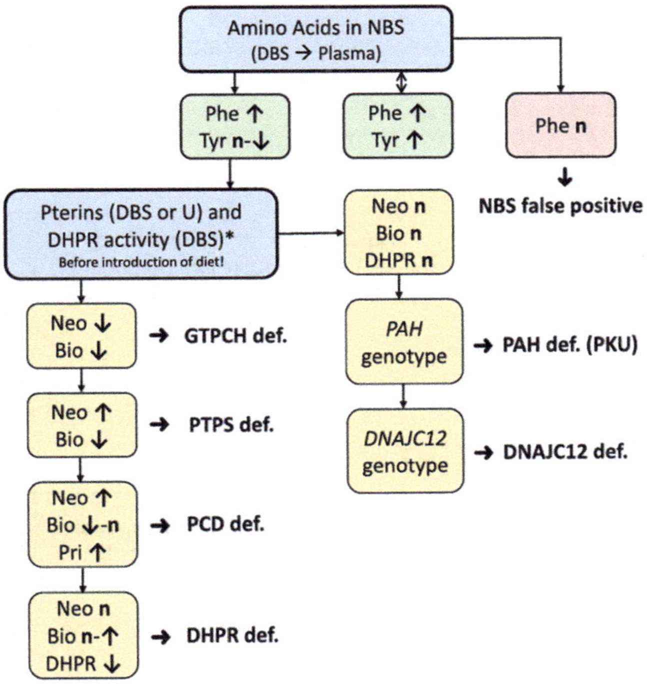


**Fig. 20.3** Diagnostic flowchart for the laboratory diagnosis of PKU, BH4, and DNAJC12 deficiencies. Dried blood spots (DBS) or random urine (U) can be used for the differential diagnosis, and depending on the profile of neopterin (Neo), biopterin (Bio), and primapterin (Pri) and dihydropteridine reductase (DHPR) activity in DBS, diagnosis of following BH4 deficiencies can be established: GTP cyclohydrolase I (GTPCH) deficiency (low or no detectable neopterin and biopterin), 6-pyruvoyl-tetrahydropterin synthase (PTPS) deficiency (high neopterin and low or no detectable biopterin), dihydropteridine reductase (DHPR) deficiency (normal neopterin and normal or elevated biopterin and no DHPR activity), pterin-4α-carbinolamine dehydratase (PCD) deficiency (elevated neopterin, low-normal biopterin, and elevated primapterin), and DNAJC12 (normal pterins and PAH genotype) (modified from Blau et al. (Blau et al. 2018))

The first two tests are essential and will allow the differentiation between all variants with $BH_4$ deficiencies.

With some limitations (DHPR def.), the $BH_4$ loading test (for 24 h) is an additional useful diagnostic tool for the rapid discrimination between classical PKU and biopterin variants (Muntau et al. 2019). This test is particularly useful for identifying the $BH_4$-responsive PAH deficiency. For the interpretation and determination of the various disorders based upon loading tests, see "Pathological Values and Differential Diagnosis."

### Interpretation of the Phenylalanine Loading Test in Patients with DRD

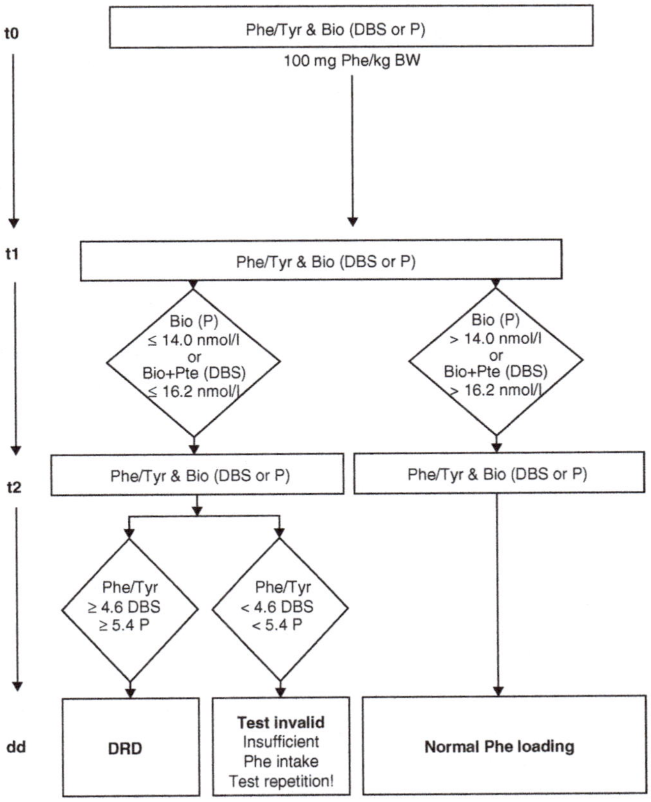


**Fig. 20.4** Phenylalanine (Phe) loading in children: revised shortened test procedure and test interpretation (*Bio* biopterin, *Pte* pterin, Phe/Tyr Phe/tyrosine ratio, *DBS* dried blood spot, *P* plasma, *BW* body weight, *dd* diagnostic decision) (Opladen et al. 2010)

**Diagnostic Flowchart in the Differential Diagnosis of Non-HPA Variants**

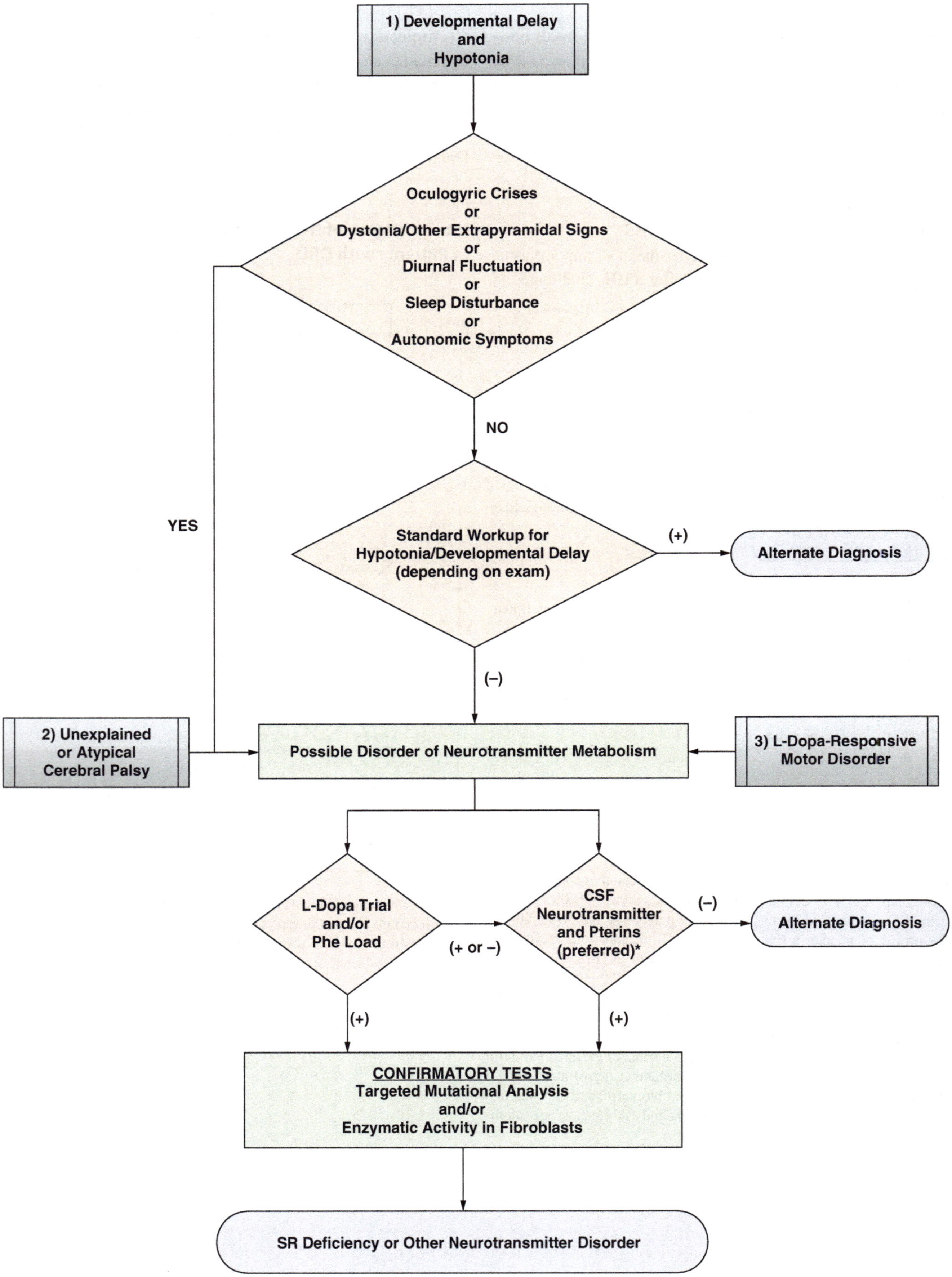

## Specimen Collection

| Test | Preconditions | Material | Handling | Pitfalls |
|---|---|---|---|---|
| Phe | Normal Phe intake | Guthrie card, serum/ plasma, CSF | Keep cool (−20 °C) for serum or plasma Guthrie card at RT | |
| Neo Bio | Normal Phe intake, Phe in plasma high enough | Random urine, Spotted urine | Keep cool, dark (−20 °C) Oxidized sample, dark, RT | Infections (Neo ↑) |
| | | Serum/plasma | Keep cool, dark (−20 °C) | |
| | | CSF | EDTA tube, (−20 °C) | |
| $BH_4$, $BH_2$ | | CSF | DTE/DETAPAC tube, (−80 °C) | |
| HVA 5HIAA 5-MTHF | 1 h before medication, withdraw first 0.5 mL | CSF | EDTA tube, (−80 °C) | |
| DNAJC12 | Normal Phe intake | whole blood | Frozen (−20 °C) | |
| DHPR | | Erythrocytes from heparinized blood | Frozen (−20 °C) | |
| | | Guthrie card | RT | |
| | | Fibroblasts | RT | |
| | Min. 50 mg | Chorionic villi | Frozen (−80 °C) | |
| PTPS | Before medication, no $BH_4$ | Erythrocytes from heparinized blood | Frozen (−20 °C) | |
| | Min. 50 mg | Chorionic villi | Frozen (−80 °C) | |
| GTPCH | | Fibroblasts | RT | |
| SR | | Fibroblasts | RT | |

*RT* room temperature, *DTE/DETAPAC* dithiothreitol and diethylenetriaminepenta-acetic acid

**Fig. 20.5** Diagnostic algorithm for patients with a possible disorder of neurotransmitter metabolism. Sepiapterin reductase (SR) deficiency and other disorders of neurotransmitter metabolism should be considered in patients with (1) developmental delay with hypotonia, (2) suspect but unexplained cerebral palsy (CP) or CP with atypical features, and (3) uncharacterized L-dopa-responsive motor disorders. (1) In a patient with developmental delay and hypotonia, if oculogyric crises, diurnal fluctuation, sleep disturbance, or extrapyramidal or autonomic signs exist, a disorder of neurotransmitter biosynthesis is likely and cerebrospinal fluid (CSF) analysis should be done. If no other signs are present, CSF analysis should be considered if standard workup for hypotonia is unrevealing. If CSF analysis is abnormal, then mutational screening and/or measurement of enzymatic activity can be targeted to confirm the specific disorder suggested by the pattern of CSF abnormalities. If CSF evaluation is impractical, alternative evaluation may include L-dopa trial and/or phenylalanine load. If negative, CSF analysis must still be done to exclude a disorder of neurotransmitter metabolism. If L-dopa trial and/or phenylalanine loading are positive, CSF analysis will allow targeted mutational screening; however, one should keep in mind that phenylalanine load can be positive in heterozygote carriers for PKU. Alternatively, CSF analysis may be skipped, and broad mutational screening undertaken. Mutational and gene dosage screening may be time-consuming and costly, and false negatives may still occur. Therefore, this alternative evaluation route should be reserved for cases in which CSF analysis is not available or is declined, or in which other clinical features lead to suspicion of a specific diagnosis. (2) In a patient with unexplained CP or CP with atypical features, a disorder of neurotransmitter metabolism should be considered and diagnostic algorithm, as outlined above, should be followed. Atypical or unexplained features suggesting need for further metabolic investigation in a child with possible CP include lack of adequate antecedent, nondiagnostic magnetic resonance imaging, progressive symptoms, familial occurrence, episodic encephalopathy, and features not expected in the CPs such as diurnal variation, sleep disturbance, autonomic symptoms, or oculogyric crises. (3) All patients with an L-dopa-responsive motor disorder should be evaluated for a disorder of neurotransmitter metabolism. CSF analysis (after discontinuation of L-dopa therapy for at least 10 days) is the recommended first step. If L-dopa withdrawal is impractical, the results of CSF analyses may still be informative if either pterins or 5-hydroxyindoleacetic acid levels are abnormal. Alternatively, molecular investigations can be done, guided either by results of phenylalanine loading test or clinical symptoms with caveats as noted above. CSF analysis should consist of homovanillic acid, 5-hydroxyindoleacetic acid (5-HIAA), pterins (neopterin, biopterin, and sepiapterin), and 5-methyltetrahydrofolate

## Prenatal Diagnosis

Prenatal diagnosis is only relevant for GTPCH, PTPS, DHPR, and SR deficiencies. Generally, the first choice of method for each of these is mutation analysis in chorionic villous material provided that disease causing mutations and their parental origin has been confirmed. Alternatively, enzyme assay in cultured amniocytes can be performed in some diseases.

## DNA Analysis

All genes (*GCH1*, *PTS*, *QDPR*, *PCBD1*, *SPR*, *DNAJC12*) in this chapter are known, and mutation analysis of genomic DNA isolated from peripheral blood, chorionic villi, amniocytes, or other cells is feasible. Sanger sequencing of individual genes or next generation sequencing of gene panels are used. For mutations suspected to affect splicing, mRNA analysis in appropriate tissues may be necessary.

A locus-specific PNDdb database (http://www.biopku.org/home/pnddb.asp) lists all reported variants.

## Treatment

PKU patients due to a PAH deficiency present with HPA (20.1; see below). In PAH deficiency, European guidelines to optimize PKU care have been released. The main goal of treatment is to reduce or normalize blood phenylalanine levels without causing deficiencies of other amino acids and other nutrients that are usually received by intake of natural intake (Belanger-Quintana et al. 2011). This can be done by introduction of the low-phenylalanine (or low-natural protein) diet. In some patients, administration of the synthetic cofactor BH4 can decrease or even replace the necessity of the diet. In such cases, it is important to be sure that patients use normal amounts of natural protein of high biological value not causing deficiencies of amino acids (van Wegberg et al. 2017).

Untreated blood phenylalanine concentrations determine management of patients with PKU. No intervention is required if the blood phenylalanine concentration is less than 360 μmol/L. Treatment is recommended up to the age of 12 years if the phenylalanine blood concentration is between 360 and 600 μmol/L, and lifelong treatment is recommended if the concentration is more than 600 μmol/L. For women trying to conceive and during pregnancy (maternal PKU), untreated phenylalanine blood concentrations of more than 360 μmol/L need to be reduced. Treatment target concentrations are as follows: 120–360 μmol/L for individuals aged 0–12 years and for maternal PKU, and 120–600 μmol/L for nonpregnant individuals older than 12 years (van Wegberg et al. 2017).

One should be aware that there are individuals with "severe" PKU mutations that have escaped severe mental retardation despite high blood phenylalanine levels and very poor dietary control (van Vliet et al. 2019). One explanation for this phenomenon is that they have near normal brain phenylalanine levels, despite high blood phenylalanine levels. A number of studies have now demonstrated considerably variability in blood vs. brain phenylalanine levels in PKU patients, although this can partly be explained by technical issues with measuring the phenylalanine content in brain. Outcome in PKU appears to be related to both blood and brain phenylalanine levels. This, in all probability, will assume greater importance in making decisions about the strictness and duration of dietary control in the future. It has also been shown that the brain phenylalanine levels of heterozygotes (parents) for PKU are higher than usually seen in PKU patients under very strict dietary control. This would suggest that control levels would probably be higher and safer than are now generally recommended although the neurocognitive functioning of the parents has never been officially studied (Burlina et al. 2019).

In BH4 deficiencies (20.2–20.7; see below), the mode of treatment depends on the type of disease, may differ with the patient's age, and the policies in various countries and centers (Opladen et al. 2012) In addition, patients with HPA due to a cofactor defect need more strict blood phenylalanine control and additional supplementations with the neurotransmitter precursors L-dopa and 5-hydroxytryptophan in combination with the peripheral decarboxylase inhibitor carbidopa. Patients with dihydropteridine reductase deficiency (DHPR, 20.4) need additional folinic acid substitution. In patients revealing levodopa-induced peak-dose dyskinesia, slow-release forms of drugs can be used and reaching the upper therapeutic limits of L-dopa may be an indication for the use of MAO and/or COMT inhibitors.

Patients with dopa-responsive dystonia (DRD, dominant GTPCH cyclohydrolase I deficiency, 20.6) and sepiapterin reductase deficiency (SR, 20.7) respond to low-dosage L-dopa/carbidopa therapy, and patients with SR deficiency need additional supplementation with 5-hydroxytryptophan and probably also BH4 (Friedman et al. 2012).

Prognosis and outcome strongly depend on the age when the diagnosis is made and treatment introduced but also on the type of mutation (Jäggi et al. 2008). Patients with DNAJC12 (20.8) can be treated by oral administration of sapropterin dihydrochloride, dopamine, and serotonin precursors (Straniero et al. 2017).

Recommendations for treatment and monitoring are not completely uniform worldwide. Therefore, where possible and necessary, recommendations have been combined and ranges of values indicating lower and upper limits are reported.

20.1: Phenylalanine hydroxylase deficiency (PKU)

| Age (in years) | Protein requirement g/kg BW/day[a] | Target blood Phe µmol/L | | Minimum frequency of blood Phe measurement (usually home sampling)[b] | Minimum frequency of outpatient visits[b] |
|---|---|---|---|---|---|
| | | Europe[b] | USA[c] | | |
| 0–1 | 1.14–1.77 | 120–360 | 120–360 | Weekly | Every 2 months |
| 1–2 | 0.97–1.14 | 120–360 | 120–360 | Fortnightly | Twice per year |
| 2–4 | 0.90–0.97 | 120–360 | 120–360 | Fortnightly | Twice per year |
| 4–6 | 0.85–0.90 | 120–360 | 120–360 | Fortnightly | Twice per year |
| 6–10 | 0.90–0.92 | 120–360 | 120–360 | Fortnightly | Twice per year |
| 10–12 | 0.89–0.91 | 120–360 | 120–360 | Fortnightly | Twice per year |
| 12–15 | 0.85–0.90 | 120–600 | 120–360 | Monthly | Twice per year |
| >16 | 0.8 | 120–600 | 120–360 | Monthly | Once per year |
| Pregnancy wish | 0.8 | 120–360 | 120–360 | Weekly | Not advised on |
| Pregnancy | 0.8[d] | 120–360 | 120–360 | Twice weekly | Once per trimester |

[a]Based on WHO 2007, in which the European PKU guidelines by van Wegberg et al. (van Wegberg et al. 2017) advise to multiply the "protein" intake from amino acid supplements by 1.4 (40% added) since the bioavailability of amino acids mixtures is not equivalent to natural protein
[b]According to the European guidelines for PKU (van Wegberg et al. 2017)
[c]According to the US consensus for PKU (Vockley et al. 2014)
[d]For trimesters 1, 2, and 3, an additional total protein intake is advised as 1, 10, and 31 g. This is usually achieved by increasing the natural protein as the Phe allowance can be increased

Treatment and monitoring only necessary for pregnant women with blood phenylalanine levels >360 µmol/L (see below).

## Tetrahydrobiopterin (BH4)-Responsive PKU/HPA

The treatment trial starts with at 20 mg/kg BW of BH4 per kg body weight and natural protein intake is increased, the BH4 dose should be adjusted, within blood phenylalanine concentrations maintained in the target (20.1) (van Spronsen et al. 2017

**Beware/Pitfalls**

1. Patients are on an unrestricted (i.e., protein-rich) diet.
2. $BH_4$ may significantly reduce plasma and CSF tyrosine levels. Consider nutrition and tyrosine supplementation.
3. L-Dopa/carbidopa/5-hydroxytryptophan therapy should be introduced slowly but continuously increased according to the clinical picture in steps of 1 mg/kg/day per week. 5-Hydroxytryptophan may not be tolerated due to gastrointestinal side effect. In this case, monotherapy with L-dopa/carbidopa may be sufficient.
4. L-Dopa/carbidopa/5-hydroxytryptophan therapy may reduce CSF folates ($CH_3$-group trapping by L-dopa to 3-*O*-methyldopa). Determine 5-methyltetrahydrofolate in CSF. Consider folinic acid (5-formyltetrahydrofolate, leucovorin) substitution (10–20 mg/day).

20.2: GTP cyclohydrolase I deficiency and 20.3: 6-Pyruvoyl-tetrahydropterin synthase deficiency (severe form)

| No. | Symbol | Age | Medication/diet | Dosage (mg/kg/day) | Dosages per day |
|---|---|---|---|---|---|
| 20.2 | GTPCH | Newborn | L-Dopa | 1–3 | 3–6 |
| 20.3.1 | PTPS | | Carbidopa | 10–25%[a] | 3–6 |
| | (severe) | | 5-Hydroxytryptophan | 1–2 | 3–6 |
| | | | Tetrahydrobiopterin (BH4) | 5–10 | 3 |
| | | <1–2 years | L-Dopa | 4–7 | 3–6 |
| | | | Carbidopa | 10–25%[a] | 3–6 |
| | | | 5-Hydroxytryptophan | 3–5 | 3–6 |
| | | | Tetrahydrobiopterin (BH4) | 5–10 | 2 |
| | | >1–2 years | L-Dopa | 8–15 | 3–6 |
| | | | Carbidopa | 10–25%[a] | 3–6 |
| | | | 5-Hydroxytryptophan | 6–9 | 3–6 |
| | | | Tetrahydrobiopterin (BH4) | 5–10 | 2 |

[a]Percentage compared to L-dopa).

5. Drugs like trimethoprim-sulfamethazole or methotrexate may induce hyperphenylalaninemia by inhibiting DHPR.

20.3: 6-Pyruvoyl-tetrahydropterin synthase deficiency (mild form)

| No. | Symbol | Age | Medication/diet | Dosage (mg/kg/day) | Dosages per day |
|---|---|---|---|---|---|
| 20.3.2 | PTPS (mild) | All ages | Tetrahydrobiopterin (BH4; sapropterin dihydrochloride) | 5–10 | 2 |

**Beware/Pitfalls**

1. Patients are on an unrestricted (i.e., protein-rich) diet.
2. BH4 may significantly reduce plasma and CSF tyrosine levels. Monitor and consider tyrosine supplementation.
3. Drugs like trimethoprim-sulfamethoxazoles or methotrexate may induce hyperphenylalaninemia by inhibiting DHPR.

20.4: Dihydropteridine reductase deficiency

| No. | Symbol | Age | Medication/diet | Dosage (mg/kg/day) | Doses per day |
|---|---|---|---|---|---|
| 20.4 | DHPR | Newborn | l-Dopa | 1–3 | 3–6 |
| | | | Carbidopa | 10–25%[a] | 3–6 |
| | | | 5-Hydroxytryptophan | 1–2 | 3–6 |
| | | | Folinic acid | 15–20 mg/day | 1–2 |
| | | | Diet (see 20.1 PKU) | | |
| | | <1–2 years | l-Dopa | 4–7 | 3–6 |
| | | | Carbidopa | 10–25%[a] | 3–6 |
| | | | 5-Hydroxytryptophan | 3–5 | 3–6 |
| | | | Folinic acid | 15–20 mg/day | 1–2 |
| | | | Diet (see 20.1 PKU) | | |
| | | >1–2 years | l-Dopa | 8–15 | 3–6 |
| | | | Carbidopa | 10–25%[a] | 3–6 |
| | | | 5-Hydroxytryptophan | 6–9 | 3–6 |
| | | | Folinic acid | 15–20 mg/day | 1–2 |
| | | | Diet (see 20.1 PKU) | | |

[a]Percentage compared to l-dopa

**Beware/Pitfalls**

1. Patients are on low-Phe diet (see 20.1); however, blood Phe levels should be close to normal. These patients are more sensitive to high Phe levels than other PKU.
2. L-Dopa/carbidopa/5-hydroxytryptophan therapy should be introduced slowly but continuously increased according to the clinical picture in steps of 1 mg/kg/day per week. 5-Hydroxytryptophan may not be tolerated due to gastrointestinal side effect. In this case, monotherapy with L-dopa/carbidopa may be sufficient.
3. Drugs like trimethoprim-sulfamethoxazoles or methotrexate may induce hyperphenylalaninemia by inhibiting DHPR.

20.5: Pterin-4α-carbinolamine dehydratase deficiency

| No. | Symbol | Age | Medication/diet | Dosage (mg/kg/day) | Doses per day |
|---|---|---|---|---|---|
| 20.5 | PCD | Newborn | Tetrahydrobiopterin (BH4; sapropterin dihydrochloride) | 5–10 | 2 |
| | | >1 year | No treatment | | |

**Beware/Pitfalls**

1. Patients are on an unrestricted (i.e., protein-rich) diet.
2. BH4 may significantly reduce plasma and CSF tyrosine levels. Consider tyrosine supplementation.
3. Drugs like trimethoprim-sulfametazole or methotrexate may induce hyperphenylalaninemia by inhibiting DHPR.

20.6: Dopa-responsive dystonia/autosomal dominant GTPCH deficiency

| No. | Symbol | Age | Medication/diet | Dosage (mg/kg/day) | Doses per day |
|---|---|---|---|---|---|
| 20.6 | DRD | Newborn | l-Dopa<br>Carbidopa | 1–3<br>10–25%[a] | 3–4<br>3–4 |
| | | >1 year | l-Dopa<br>Carbidopa | 4–12<br>10–25%[a] | 3–4<br>3–4 |

[a]Percentage compared to L-dopa

**Beware/Pitfalls**

1. L-Dopa/carbidopa therapy should be introduced slowly but continuously increased according to the clinical picture in steps of 1 mg/kg/day per week.

20.7: Sepiapterin reductase deficiency

| No. | Symbol | Age | Medication/diet | Dosage (mg/kg/day) | Doses per day |
|---|---|---|---|---|---|
| 20.7 | SR | Newborn | l-Dopa<br>Carbidopa<br>5-Hydroxytryptophan | 1–3<br>10–25%[a]<br>1–2 | 3–4<br>3–4<br>3–4 |
| | | >1 year | l-Dopa<br>Carbidopa<br>5-Hydroxytryptophan | 4–10<br>10–25%[a]<br>3–9 | 3–4<br>3–4<br>3–4 |

[a]Percentage compared to l-dopa

20.8: DNAJC12

| No. | Symbol | Age | Medication/diet | Dosage (mg/kg/day) | Doses per day |
|---|---|---|---|---|---|
| 20.8 | DNAJC12 | All ages | Tetrahydrobiopterin (BH4; sapropterin dihydrochloride) | 20 | 2 |
| | | | l-Dopa<br>Carbidopa<br>5-Hydroxytryptophan | 4–10<br>10–25%*<br>3–9 | 3–4<br>3–4<br>3–4 |

**Beware/Pitfalls**

1. L-Dopa/carbidopa/5-hydroxytryptophan therapy should be introduced slowly and increased in steps of not more than 10 mg/day.

## Alternative Therapies/Experimental Trials

| No. | Deficiency symbol | Age | Medication | Dosage (mg/kg/day) | Dosages per day |
|---|---|---|---|---|---|
| 20.1 | BH4-responsive PKU | >4 years | Tetrahydrobiopterin (BH4; sapropterin dihydrochloride)[a] | 10–20 | 1–2 |
| 20.3–20.5 | GTPCH, PTPS, DHPR | All ages | Deprenyl[b]<br>Entacapone[c] | 0.1–0.3<br>~30 | 3–4<br>1–2 |
| 20.7 | SR | All ages | Deprenyl[b]<br>Sertraline[d]<br>Melatonin[e]<br>Bromocriptine | 0.07–0.14<br>0.71–2.14<br>0.01–0.03<br>Not reported | 3–4<br>2–3<br>1–2<br>Not reported |

[a]Tetrahydrobiopterin ($BH_4$; sapropterin dihydrochloride, Kuvan®) treatment has been recently introduced as a standard therapy for children with phenylalanine hydroxylase deficiency that showed a decrease of Phe levels after $BH_4$ loading (see above)
[b]MAO-B inhibitor (selegiline)
[c]COMT inhibitor
[d]Serotonin reuptake inhibitor
[e]Product of serotonin metabolism

### Beware/Pitfalls

1. Administration of MAO-B or COMT inhibitors allows a 30% reduction of the daily dosage of neurotransmitter precursors.

## Follow-Up/Monitoring

### PAH Deficiency

| Age | Biochemical monitoring Phe and Tyr | Clinical monitoring[a] | Intellectual and personality development |
|---|---|---|---|
| 0–3 months | Weekly | 1–3 monthly | |
| 4–12 months | Weekly | 1–3 monthly | X |
| 1–2 years | Weekly | 2–6 monthly | |
| 2–3 years | Weekly | 2–6 monthly | X |
| 4–6 years | Fortnightly | 3–6 monthly | X |
| 7–9 years | Fortnightly | 6 monthly | |
| 10–12 years | Monthly | 6 monthly | X |
| 13–15 years | Monthly | 6 monthly | X |
| Adolescents/adults | Monthly | 6–12 monthly | X |
| Maternal PKU | Weekly[b] | Bimonthly[c] | |

[a]Nutrient intake, body growth, general health, as well as laboratory tests: blood count, calcium, phosphate, magnesium, iron, liver and kidney function tests, alkaline phosphatase, total protein, albumin, prealbumin, cholesterol, triglycerides, vitamins
[b]Plasma AA, albumin, cholesterol, ferritin, folate, vitamin B12
[c]Nutrient intake including micronutrients, body growth, general health

### Standard Protocol for Intercurrent Illness

The best possible intake of fluid, energy, and Phe-free amino acid mixtures (AAM), with special attention for higher need of energy, while taking AAM in these periods may be a real.

### $BH_4$ Deficiencies

Plasma Phe and Tyr are monitored in all forms of HPA, CSF investigations only in disorders affecting $BH_4$ metabolism with and without HPA (20.2–20.7).

| Test | Age | Frequency | Comments |
|---|---|---|---|
| Phe and Tyr (blood) | 1–3 years | Weekly to fortnightly | Phe levels: 40–240 (360) μmol/L[a] |
| | 4–10 years | Fortnightly to monthly | |
| | 11–16 years | Monthly | Phe levels: 40–900 μmol/L[a] |
| | >16 years | Every 2–3 months | Phe levels: 40–1200 μmol/L[a] |
| Neopterin Biopterin 5HIAA HVA Folates (CSF)[b] | <1 months | Fortnightly | Close to normal range |
| | 1 month–1 year | Every 4–8 weeks | Close to normal range |
| | <1 year | Monthly to yearly | Close to normal range |

[a]In DHPR-deficient patients, Phe levels should be close to 240–360 μmol/L at all ages

[b]Lumbar puncture in the morning before medication. Discard first 0.5 mL and collect the next 1–2 mL (−80 °C)

## References


Anikster Y, Haack TB, Vilboux T, Pode-Shakked B, Thony B, Shen N, et al. Biallelic mutations in DNAJC12 cause hyperphenylalaninemia, dystonia, and intellectual disability. Am J Hum Genet. 2017;100(2):257–66.

Belanger-Quintana A, Burlina A, Harding CO, Muntau AC. Up to date knowledge on different treatment strategies for phenylketonuria. Mol Genet Metab. 2011;104(Suppl):S19–25.

Blau N, Hennermann JB, Langenbeck U, Lichter-Konecki U. Diagnosis, classification and genetics of phenylketonuria and tetrahydrobiopterin (BH4) deficiencies. Mol Genet Metab. 2011;104:S2–9.

Blau N, Longo N. Alternative therapies to address the unmet medical needs of patients with phenylketonuria. Expert Opin Pharmacother. 2015;16(6):1–10.

Blau N, Martinez A, Hoffmann GF, Thony B. DNAJC12 deficiency: a new strategy in the diagnosis of hyperphenylalaninemias. Mol Genet Metab. 2018;123:1–5.

Blau N, Van Spronsen FJ, Levy HL. Phenylketonuria. Lancet. 2010;376:1417–27.

Brennenstuhl H, Jung-Klawitter S, Assmann B, Opladen T. Inherited disorders of neurotransmitters: classification and practical approaches for diagnosis and treatment. Neuropediatrics. 2019;50(1):2–14.

Burlina A, Blau N. Tetrahydrobiopterin disorders presenting with hyperphenylalaninemia. In: Hoffmann FG, Blau N, editors. Congenital neurotransmitter disorders: a clinical approach. Huppauge: Nova Publishers Inc; 2014.

Burlina AP, Lachmann RH, Manara R, Cazzorla C, Celato A, van Spronsen FJ, et al. The neurological and psychological phenotype of adult patients with early-treated phenylketonuria: a systematic review. J Inherit Metab Dis. 2019;42(2):209–19.

Friedman J, Roze E, Abdenur JE, Chang R, Gasperini S, Saletti V, et al. Sepiapterin Reductase Deficiency: a treatable mimic of cerebral palsy. Ann Neurol. 2012;71:520–30.

Jäggi L, Zurflüh MR, Schuler A, Ponzone A, Porta F, Fiori L, et al. Outcome and long-term follow-up of 36 patients with tetrahydrobiopterin deficiency. Mol Genet Metab. 2008;93:295–305.

Jung-Kc K, Himmelreich N, Prestegard KS, Shi TS, Scherer T, Ying M, et al. Phenylalanine hydroxylase variants interact with the co-chaperone DNAJC12. Hum Mutat. 2019;40:483–94.

Lichter-Konecki U, Vockley J. Phenylketonuria: current treatments and future developments. Drugs. 2019;79:495–500.

Muntau AC, Adams DJ, Belanger-Quintana A, Bushueva TV, Cerone R, Chien YH, et al. International best practice for the evaluation of responsiveness to sapropterin dihydrochloride in patients with phenylketonuria. Mol Genet Metab. 2019;127:1–11.

Opladen T, Cortes-Saladelafont E, Mastrangelo M, Horvath G, Pons R, Lopez-Laso E, et al. The International Working Group on Neurotransmitter related Disorders (iNTD): a worldwide research project focused on primary and secondary neurotransmitter disorders. Mol Genet Metab Rep. 2016;9:61–6.

Opladen T, Hoffmann FG, Blau N. An international survey of patients with tetrahydrobiopterin deficiencies presenting with hyperphenylalaninaemia. J Inherit Metab Dis. 2012;35(6):963–73.

Opladen T, Okun JG, Burgard P, Blau N, Hoffmann GF. Phenylalanine loading in pediatric patients with dopa-responsive dystonia: revised test protocol and pediatric cut-off values. J Inherit Metab Dis. 2010;33:697–703.

Segawa M. Hereditary progressive dystonia with marked diurnal fluctuation. Brain Dev. 2011;33(3):195–201.

Straniero L, Guella I, Cilia R, Parkkinen L, Rimoldi V, Young A, et al. DNAJC12 and dopa-responsive non-progressive Parkinsonism. Ann Neurol. 2017;82(4):640–6.

van Spronsen FJ, van Wegberg AM, Ahring K, Belanger-Quintana A, Blau N, Bosch AM, et al. Key European guidelines for the diagnosis and management of patients with phenylketonuria. Lancet Diabetes Endocrinol. 2017;5(9):743–56.

van Vliet D, van Wegberg AMJ, Ahring K, Bik-Multanowski M, Casas K, Didycz B, et al. Untreated PKU patients without intellectual disability: what do they teach us? Nutrients. 2019;11(11):2572.

van Wegberg AMJ, MacDonald A, Ahring K, Belanger-Quintana A, Blau N, Bosch AM, et al. The complete European guidelines on phenylketonuria: diagnosis and treatment. Orphanet J Rare Dis. 2017;12(1):162.

Vockley J, Andersson HC, Antshel KM, Braverman NE, Burton BK, Frazier DM, et al. Phenylalanine hydroxylase deficiency: diagnosis and management guideline. Genet Med. 2014;16(2):188–200.

Werner ER, Blau N, Thöny B. Tetrahydrobiopterin: biochemistry and pathophysiology. Biochem J. 2011;438:397–414.

Zielonka M, Makhseed N, Blau N, Bettendorf M, Hoffmann GF, Opladen T. Dopamine-responsive growth-hormone deficiency and central hypothyroidism in sepiapterin reductase deficiency. JIMD Rep. 2015;24:109–13.

# Tyrosine Metabolism

# 21

Francjan J. van Spronsen, Alberto Burlina, and Carlo Dionisi Vici

## Contents



F. J. van Spronsen
Division of Metabolic Diseases, University of Groningen, University Medical Center Groningen, Beatrix Children's Hospital, Groningen, The Netherlands
e-mail: f.j.van.spronsen@umcg.nl

A. Burlina (✉)
Division of Inherited Metabolic Diseases, Reference Centre Expanded Newborn Screening, Department of Woman's and Child's Health, University Hospital, Padova, Italy
e-mail: alberto.burlina@unipd.it

C. Dionisi Vici
Babino Gesù Children's Research Hospital, Rome, Italy
e-mail: carlo.dionisivici@opbg.net

**Summary**

Inherited disorders of tyrosine catabolism have been identified at five of the six enzymatic steps. Under normal conditions tyrosine concentrations are regulated by its synthetic enzyme (phenylalanine hydroxylase) and especially the first catabolic enzyme (tyrosine aminotransferase). Acquired or inherited deficiency of the second catabolic enzyme (4-hydroxyphenylpyruvate dioxygenase) also results in hypertyrosinemia. Tyrosine is mainly degraded in the liver but to a minor extent also in the kidney. In tyrosinemia type I, the primary defect is


N. Blau et al. (eds.), *Physician's Guide to the Diagnosis, Treatment, and Follow-Up of Inherited Metabolic Diseases*,
https://doi.org/10.1007/978-3-030-67727-5_21

in the last enzyme of the pathway, accumulation of toxic metabolites are seen, and the hypertyrosinemia results from secondary deficiency of 4-hydroxyphenylpyruvate dioxygenase, which also is found in severe liver disease in general and in the immature liver. Generally, there is no common phenotype to the different disorders of tyrosine degradation. The occurrence of corneal and skin lesions, as seen in tyrosinemia type II, is a direct effect of high tissue tyrosine. Cognitive impairment is common in tyrosinemia type II, probably common in type III, and increasingly reported in type I. The liver and kidney diseases of tyrosinemia type I are caused by accumulation of toxic metabolites (fumarylacetoacetate and its derivatives) and can be prevented by an inhibitor (nitisinone) of tyrosine degradation at the level of 4-hydroxyphenylpyruvate dioxygenase. Whether maleylacetoacetate hydrolase that essentially gives the same metabolic features as tyrosinemia type I results in clinical features is unclear. In alkaptonuria there is no increase in tyrosine level, and the degradation of tyrosine proceeds at a normal rate to produce homogentisate. Upon oxidation, homogentisate forms reactive intermediates and pigment, which is deposited in various tissues particularly in joints and connective tissue. In hawkinsinuria, a very rare condition, data suggest that an aberrant metabolism of 4-hydroxyphenylpyruvate in some cases may lead to failure to thrive, acidosis, and excretion of a characteristic metabolite pattern.

## Introduction

Hypertyrosinemia in the newborn is usually not due to inborn errors of tyrosine (Tyr) metabolism but rather to immaturity of 4-hydroxyphenylpyruvate dioxygenase (4HPD). This is called transient tyrosinemia of the premature newborn. At any age, liver dysfunction of any cause or postprandial sampling can give mildly increased Tyr levels.

Sustained isolated hypertyrosinemia is strongly suggestive of an inborn error of tyrosine degradation.

The phenotype of tyrosinemia type I (TT1) is variable, and the severity of the disease varies with age at the onset of symptoms (van Spronsen et al. 1994). Newborns detected by neonatal screening by succinylacetone (SA) in blood are clinically asymptomatic, but plasma alpha-fetoprotein (AFP) usually is already increased suggesting prenatal damage to the liver and most children have mild prolongation of coagulation tests. In non-screened patients, the most common presentation is severe liver disease or failure between 2 and 4 months of age, often preceded by a period of nonspecific failure to thrive. Typically, there is a pronounced coagulopathy with highly increased prothrombin time and sometimes thrombocytopenia, with a disproportionately moderate increase in transaminases and normal ammonia and almost normal bilirubin. Plasma AFP can be extremely high. Sepsis is not uncommon. There may be early signs of hypophosphatemic rickets secondary to renal tubulopathy. Plasma Tyr and methionine show moderate to marked increases. In later presenting patients, laboratory signs of tubulopathy and liver disease may be more impressive than the subtle clinical picture, while clinically rickets, porphyria-like neurologic crisis characterized by pain in the limbs and sometimes by paralysis resembling Guillain-Barré, or hepatic noduli that can develop into liver cancer (hepatocellular carcinoma or hepatoblastoma) can be a presenting symptom.

In comparison with the previous edition of this book (Holme and Mithcell 2014), developmental delay in TT1 is increasingly reported and in early diagnosed patients may represent an important clinical feature (van Ginkel et al. 2017a, b), with possible relations to high concentrations of Tyr and to low concentrations of phenylalanine (Phe), showing the importance—as well as the complexity—of adequate dietary management of these patients. If real eye problems (as in tyrosinemia type 2, TT2) are seen, it is believed to be related to higher Tyr concentrations rather than nitisinone itself.

So far, some patients with (mildly) increased SA concentrations appear to have a deficiency of maleylacetoacetate isomerase (MAAI) rather than FAH (Fig. 21.1), also showing that these patients do not have liver or renal failure (Yang et al. 2017).

TT2 is characterized by eye lesions (painful recurrent corneal lesions, frequently with dendritic morphology, that may be diagnosed as herpetic keratitis if the diagnosis is not suspected), skin disease (hyperkeratosis at the pressure points of palms, finger pads, and soles of the feet), and/or developmental delay or intellectual deficiency. The disorder usually presents during infancy but may become manifest at any age. Tyr concentration is grossly elevated in an otherwise normal amino acid profile.

In asymptomatic patients referred for hypertyrosinemia, discovered by neonatal screening or in the course of an investigation for another problem, it is urgent to eliminate type I disease by showing normal liver function and normal SA. After this, the distinction between TT2 and tyrosinemia type 3 (TT3) may be difficult as Tyr level in TT2 tends to be higher, but shows considerably overlap, while organic acids with increased 4HP point at TT3. Since the concentration of blood tyrosine may be normal in some TT1, SA is the recommended biomarker to screen TTI at birth to avoid false-negative results (Stinton et al. 2017). If SA is increased, normal liver functions point at MAAI rather than FAH deficiency.

To obtain a specific diagnosis in chronically hypertyrosinemic patients without skin or eye signs, molecular testing is the approach of choice also because enzyme studies of both TT2 and TT3 require liver tissue. Today, the dietary measures are similar, but knowing the precise diagnosis also in relation to its treatment is important.

TT3 patients have been detected because of high plasma Tyr levels in an otherwise normal amino acid profile, performed in the investigation of neurological symptoms and in mental retardation or neonatal screening programs. Eye or skin lesions have not been reported, while mental retardation and epilepsy as well as vision and language problems have (Blundell et al. 2018).

Hawkinsinuria (HAWK): This rare and incompletely understood disorder is characterized by failure to thrive and acidosis in some, but clearly not all—biochemically affected—infants. No symptoms have been reported after infancy. Autosomal dominant transmission is described. Organic acids (identification of hawkinsin (2-cystenyl-1, 4-dihydroxycyclohexenylacetate)) rather than the just slightly increased Tyr in plasma will result in its diagnosis. After infancy, 4-hydroxycyclohexylacetate appears in urine in addition to hawkinsin. The condition has responded to restriction of dietary protein as well as *N*-acetyl-L-cysteine pointing at glutathione depletion (Gomez-Ospina et al. 2016).

Alkaptonuria (AKU): The earliest physical sign of AKU is abnormal darkening of urine on standing. This sign is frequently overlooked by parents and often not explored by physicians. It should lead to investigation of the excretion of homogentisate. The finding is most likely to be noticed in diapers and is typically not detectable in older patients who live in areas with modern plumbing. Symptoms like patchy grayish pigmentation of the sclera, a blue-gray aspect to the cartilage of the ear, and arthritis, most often in the hip and knee, do not appear until early adulthood, while aortic valve leakage and aorta aneurysm are problems of late adulthood. Periods of acute inflammation may resemble rheumatoid arthritis. The arthritis may be severe and disabling in middle-aged adults. Ankylosis of the lumbosacral region is common. The specific diagnosis may be suggested by radiologists who note reduced intervertebral spacing in the lumbar spine, with calcification of the intervertebral disc and marked degenerative changes in the shoulder and hip joints. Diagnosis is confirmed by identification of homogentisate in urine, often present in millimolar amounts, and DNA mutations found in the gene for 4HPD. Nitisinone has proven to be effective in preventing the formation of homogentisate (Ranganath et al. 2018). Questions to be answered are how early nitisinone needs to be started to prevent these long-term consequences and the strictness of dietary treatment.

## Nomenclature

| No. | Disorder | Alternative name | Abbreviation | Gene symbol | Chromosomal localization | Affected protein | OMIM no. |
|---|---|---|---|---|---|---|---|
| 21.1 | Tyrosinemia type I | Hepatorenal Tyrosinemia Hereditary Tyrosinemia type I Fumarylacetoacetase deficiency | TT1 | *FAH* | 15q25.1 | Fumarylacetoacetase | 276700 |
| 21.2 | Tyrosinemia type II | Tyrosine aminotransferase deficiency | TT2 | *TAT* | 16q22.2 | Tyrosine aminotransferase | 276600 |
| 21.3 | Tyrosinemia type III | 4-hydroxyphenylpyruvate dioxygenase deficiency | TT3 | *HPD* | 12q24.31 | 4-hydroxyphenylpyruvate dioxygenase | 276710 |
| 21.4 | Hawkinsinuria | 4-hydroxyphenylpyruvate dioxygenase change of function | HAWK | *HPD* | 12q24.31 | 4-hydroxyphenylpyruvate hydroxylase | 140350 |
| 21.5 | Alkaptonuria | Homogentisate 1,2-dioxygenase deficiency | AKU | *HGD* | 3q13.33 | Homogentisate 1,2-dioxygenase | 203500 |
| 21.6 | Maleylacetoacetate isomerase deficiency | | MAAI | GSTZ1 | 14q24.3 | Maleylacetoacetate isomerase | 617596 |

## Metabolic Pathway

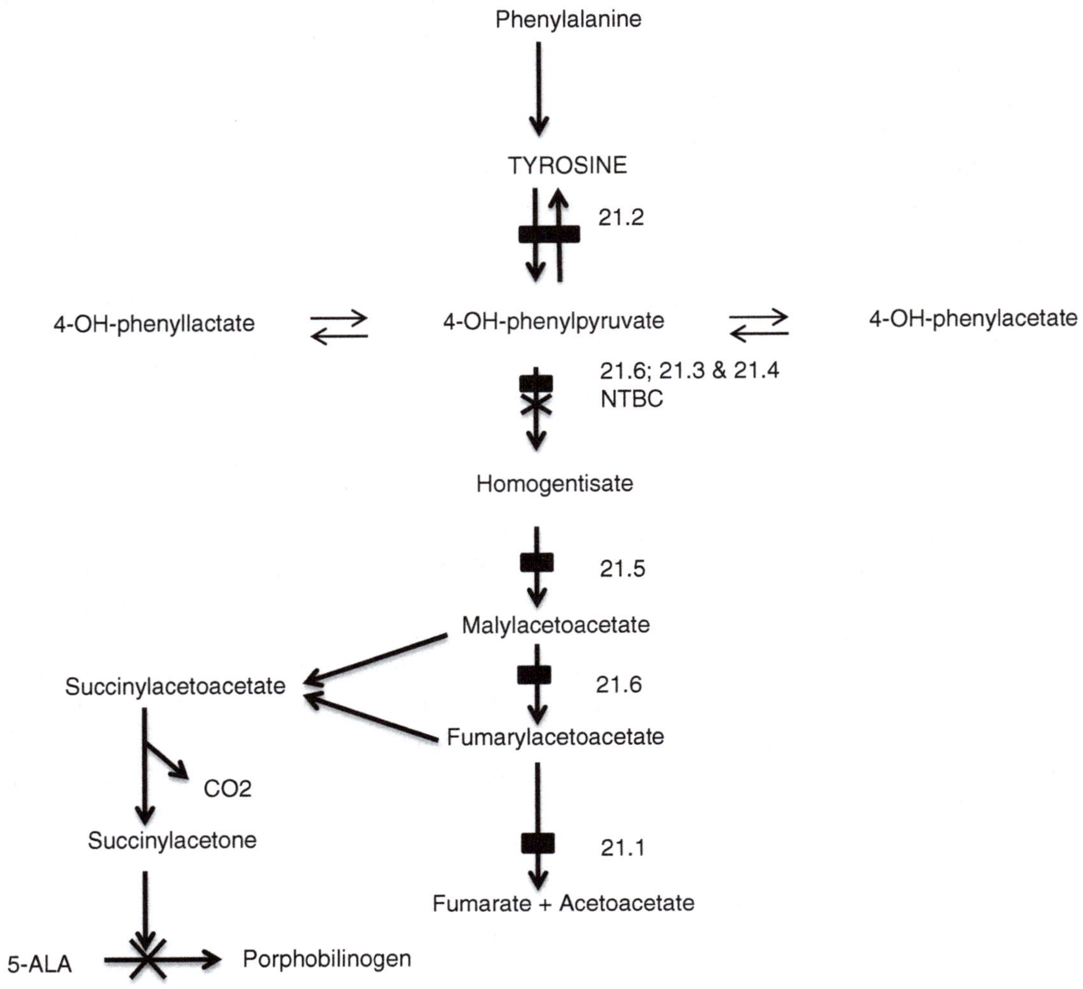


**Fig. 21.1** Tyrosine degradation pathway. Diagnostically important metabolites are framed. The sites of known metabolic disorders are indicated as *filled boxes*. **21.1** fumarylacetoacetase, **21.2** tyrosine aminotransferase, **21.3** & **21.4** 4-hydroxyphenylpyruvate dioxygenase, **21.5** homogentisate dioxygenase, **21.6** maleylacetoacetate isomerase. Inhibition by succinylacetone and nitisinone (NTBC) are indicated by crosses. *5-ALA* 5-aminolevulinate

## Signs and Symptoms

**Table 21.1** Tyrosinemia type I

| System | Symptom | Neonatal screening | Neonatal (birth–1 month) | Infancy (1–18 months) | Childhood (1.5–11 years) | Adolescence (11–16 years) | Adulthood (>16 years) |
|---|---|---|---|---|---|---|---|
| CNS | Neurocognitive and behavioral issues | [a] | [a] | ±[a] | ± | ± | ± |
| | Porphyria-like neurological crisis | | | ± | ± | ± | ± |
| Digestive | Liver carcinoma[b], hepatocellular, hepatoblastoma | | | ± | + | + | + |
| | Liver failure, acute | | ± | ± | | | |
| Eye[c] | Corneal erosion | | | | ± | ± | ± |
| | Lacrimation | | | | ± | ± | ± |
| | Photophobia | | | | ± | ± | ± |
| Musculoskeletal | Rickets | | | | ± | ± | ± |
| Renal | **Hypertension** | | | + | + | + | + |
| | Nephrocalcinosis | | | + | + | ± | ± |
| | Renal enlargement | | ± | + | + | | |
| | Renal failure, chronic | | | | | | ± |
| | **Renal tubulopathy** | | ± | + | + | + | + |

**Table 21.1** (continued)

| System | Symptom | Neonatal screening | Neonatal (birth–1 month) | Infancy (1–18 months) | Childhood (1.5–11 years) | Adolescence (11–16 years) | Adulthood (>16 years) |
|---|---|---|---|---|---|---|---|
| Laboratory findings | 4-Hydroxyphenylacetate (urine) | | ↑ | ↑ | ↑ | ↑ | ↑ |
| | 4-Hydroxyphenyllactate (urine) | | ↑ | ↑ | ↑ | ↑ | ↑ |
| | 4-Hydroxyphenylpyruvate (urine) | | ↑ | ↑ | ↑ | ↑ | ↑ |
| | 5-Aminolevulinic acid (urine) | | ↑ | ↑ | ↑ | ↑ | ↑ |
| | Alpha-fetoprotein (serum) | ↑↑ | ↑↑ | ↑↑ | ↑ | (↑) | (↑) |
| | Methionine (plasma) | | (↑) | (↑) | (↑) | – | – |
| | Porphobilinogen synthase (red blood cells) | | ↓ | | ↓ | ↓ | ↓ |
| | Succinylacetone (urine, DBS, plasma)[d] | ↑/↑↑ | ↑ | ↑ | ↑ | ↑ | ↑ |
| | Tyrosine (DBS, plasma) | (↑) | ↑ | ↑ | ↑ | ↑ | ↑ |
| | Phenylalanine (DBS, plasma) | n | n | | | | |

Succinylacetone is measured rapidly in order to exclude tyrosinemia type I. As measuring succinylacetone is now not that difficult anymore, measuring the decreased activity of porphobilinogen synthase activity in RBC or increased concentrations of delta-aminolevulinic acid strictly speaking is not needed anymore. Of note, increased excretion of phenolic tyrosine metabolites is present in sustained hypertyrosinemia of any cause and is of no differential diagnostic value

[a]Be aware of the risks on mental development as a result of too low Phe concentrations

[b]Lower risk in patients identified at newborn screening and treated early

[c]Higher risk in patients treated with NTBC and noncompliant with dietary treatment

[d]Succinylacetone and/or succinyl acetoacetate and/or 4-oxo-6-hydroxyheptonoate (U).

**Table 21.2** Tyrosinemia type II

| System | Symptom | Neonatal | Infancy | Childhood | Adolescence | Adulthood |
|---|---|---|---|---|---|---|
| CNS | Behavioral disorder | | ± | ± | ± | ± |
| | Mental retardation | | ± | ± | ± | ± |
| Dermatological | Blisters, erosion, hyperkeratosis on palms and soles | | | ± | ± | ± |
| Eye | Corneal erosion | | ± | + | + | + |
| | **Lacrimation** | | + | + | + | + |
| | Photophobia | | ± | + | + | + |
| Laboratory findings | 4-Hydroxyphenylacetate (urine) | ↑↑ | ↑↑ | ↑↑ | ↑↑ | ↑↑ |
| | 4-Hydroxyphenyllactate (urine) | ↑↑ | ↑↑ | ↑↑ | ↑↑ | ↑↑ |
| | 4-Hydroxyphenylpyruvate (urine) | ↑↑ | ↑↑ | ↑↑ | ↑↑ | ↑↑ |
| | Tyrosine (DBS, plasma) | ↑↑↑ | ↑↑↑ | ↑↑↑ | ↑↑↑ | ↑↑↑ |
| | Phenylalanine (DBS, plasma) | n | n | n | n | n |

**Table 21.3** Tyrosinemia type III

| System | Symptom | Neonatal | Infancy | Childhood | Adolescence | Adulthood |
|---|---|---|---|---|---|---|
| CNS | Mental retardation | | ± | ± | ± | ± |
| Laboratory findings | 4-Hydroxyphenylacetic acid (urine) | ↑↑ | ↑↑ | ↑↑ | ↑↑ | ↑↑ |
| | 4-Hydroxyphenyllactate (urine) | ↑↑ | ↑↑ | ↑↑ | ↑↑ | ↑↑ |
| | 4-Hydroxyphenylpyruvate (urine) | ↑↑ | ↑↑ | ↑↑ | ↑↑ | ↑↑ |
| | Tyrosine (DBS, plasma) | ↑↑ | ↑↑ | ↑↑ | ↑↑ | ↓↓ |
| | Phenylalanine (DBS, plasma) | n | n | n | n | n |

**Table 21.4** Hawkinsinuria

| System | Symptom | Neonatal | Infancy | Childhood | Adolescence | Adulthood |
|---|---|---|---|---|---|---|
| Digestive | Unspecified hepatopathy | | + | | | |
| Other | Failure to thrive, acidosis | | + | | | |
| Laboratory findings | 4-Hydroxycyclohexylacetate (urine) | | | ↑ | ↑ | ↑ |
| | 4-Hydroxyphenylacetate (urine) | | ↑ | | | |
| | 4-Hydroxyphenyllactate (urine) | | ↑ | | | |
| | 4-Hydroxyphenylpyruvate (urine) | | ↑ | | | |
| | 5-Oxoproline (urine) | | ↑ | | | |
| | Hawkinsin (urine) | | ↑ | ↑ | ↑ | ↑ |
| | Tyrosine (DBS, plasma) | n | (↑)[a] | n | n | n |
| | Phenylalanine (DBS, plasma) | n | n | n | n | n |

[a]Reported in a single patient

**Table 21.5** Alkaptonuria

| System | Symptom | Neonatal | Infancy | Childhood | Adolescence | Adulthood |
|---|---|---|---|---|---|---|
| Cardiovascular | Mitral and aortic valvulitis | | | | | ± |
| Dermatological | Pigmentation | | | | | ± |
| Eye | Scleral pigmentation | | | | | + |
| Musculoskeletal | Arthritis | | | | | + |
| | Lumbosacral disc degeneration | | | | | + |
| | Ochronosis | | | | | + |
| Other | **Urine darkening on standing** | + | + | + | + | + |
| Special laboratory | Homogentisate (urine) | ↑↑↑ | ↑↑↑ | ↑↑↑ | ↑↑↑ | ↑↑↑ |

**Table 21.6** Maleylacetoacetate isomerase deficiency

| System | Symptom | Neonatal screened patients |
|---|---|---|
| Liver and kidney | Functions proven to be and remain normal | n |
| Special laboratory | Alpha-fetoprotein (serum)<br>Succinylacetone (DBS, urine, plasma) | ↑ |

## Reference Values

| Age | Phe (DBS, P) | Tyr (DBS, P) | Met (P) | SA (P and DBS) | Porphobilinogen synthase (RBC)[a] | SA (U) | 5-Aminolevulinate (U) | Hawkinsin (U) | Homogentisate (U) |
|---|---|---|---|---|---|---|---|---|---|
| Years | | µ mol/L | | | Nkat/g Hgb | Mmol/mol creatinine in random samples | | | |
| Newborn | 30–120 | 50–150 | 10–60 | <0.024 | 0.58–1.25 | <0.1 | <20 | n.d. | <1 |
| 1–12 | 30–80 | 30–130 | 10–50 | <0.024 | 0.58–1.25 | <0.1 | <12 | n.d. | <1 |
| >12 | 30–80 | 30–100 | 10–40 | <0.024 | 0.58–1.25 | <0.1 | <3 | n.d. | <1 |

[a]Enzymatic method. Reference values vary with the methodology

## Pathological Values

| No. | Disorder | Phe (DBS, P) | Tyr (DBS, P) | Met (DBS, P) | SA (P, DBS) | Porphobilinogen synthase activity (RBC) | SA (U) | 5-Aminolevulinate (U) | Hawkinsin (U) | Homogentisate (U) |
|---|---|---|---|---|---|---|---|---|---|---|
| | | µ mol/L | | | | % of normal mean | mmol/mol creatinine in random samples | | | |
| 21.1 | Tyrosinemia I | 20–200 | 150–1300 | 20–1300 | 0.5 to >100 | 1–50 | 0.5 to >1000 | 20 to >100 | ND | <1-trace |
| 21.2 | Tyrosinemia II | Normal | 800 to >2000 | Normal | ND | Normal | ND | Normal | ND | <1 |
| 21.3 | Tyrosinemia III | Normal | 500–1200 | Normal | ND | Normal | ND | Normal | ND | <1 |
| 21.4 | Hawkinsinuria | Normal | Normal to moderate increase | Normal | ND | Normal | ND | Normal | 200–2000 | <1 |
| 21.5 | Alkaptonuria | Normal | Normal | Normal | ND | Normal | ND | Normal | ND | >1000 |
| 21.6 | Maleylacetoacetate isomerase deficiency | Normal | Normal | Normal | 0.2–1.2 | ND | ND | ND | ND | ND |

Increased tyrosine concentration is caused by inborn or acquired deficiency of the first two enzymes of the tyrosine degradation pathway (the increased tyrosine concentration of TT1 is caused by secondary inhibition of 4-hydroxyphenylpyruvate dioxygenase by liver disease in general)

## Diagnostic Flowchart in Hypertyrosinemias
(Fig. 21.2)

**Fig. 21.2** Clinical and biochemical signs suggestive of hereditary tyrosinemias. *Plasma succinylacetone concentrations up to 1282 nmol/L have been reported in maleylacetoacetate isomerase deficiency

| Clinical situation | Symptoms and signs | Diagnosis |
|---|---|---|
| Neonatal screening (Succinylacetone) | Asymptomatic<br>Mild coagulopathy | Tyrosinemia type I if succinylacetone more than mildly increased* |
| | Asymptomatic<br>No coagulopathy or liver abnormalities | Maleylacetoacetate isomerase deficiency if succinylacetone is only mildly increased* |
| Neonatal screening (hypertyrosinaemia) | Transaminases (±)<br>A-Fetoprotein (+)<br>Prothrombine time (±)<br>Porphobilinogen synthase deficiency (+)<br>Succinylacetone (+) | Tyrosinemia type I<br>(tyr(P) 120-1300 µmol/L) |
| ↘ Persistent | No liver disease<br>Succinylcetone (-) | Tyrosinemia type II<br>(tyr(P) 800-2000 µmol/L)<br>Tyrosinemia type III<br>(tyr(P) 500-1300 µmol/L)<br>↓<br>Mutation analysis<br>(Rarely, liver enzyme assay) |
| Failure to thrive | Signs of liver disease (+)<br>Succinylacetone (+) | Tyrosinemia type I |
| | Acidosis (+)<br>Hawkinsin (+)<br>5-oxoproline (+) | Hawkinsinuria |
| Liver disease | Prothrombin time (+)<br>Transaminases (±)<br>α-Fetoprotein (+)<br>Bilirubin (normal-100 µmol/L)<br>Succinylacetone (U)(+) | Tyrosinemia type I |
| Rickets | Hypophosphatemia (+)<br>Alkaline phosphatase (+)<br>General aminoaciduria (+)<br>Complete Fanconi syndrome (+)<br>Signs of liver disease (+)<br>Succinylacetone (U)(+) | Tyrosinemia type I |
| Mental retardation | Eye and/or skin symptoms (+)<br>No other symptoms | Tyrosinemia type II<br>Tyrosinemia type II or III |

*plasma succinylacetone concentrations up to 1282 nmol/l have been reported in Maleylacetoacetate isomerase deficiency.

## Specimen Collection

| Test | Material | Handling | Pitfalls |
|---|---|---|---|
| Phe (Blood) | Plasma | Ambient temp | Liver disease, any cause; false negatives in treated patients |
| | Blood spot | Ambient temp | Variation possible due to various technical issues<br>There are known differences with plasma >20% |
| Tyr (Blood) | Plasma | Ambient temp | Liver disease, any cause; false negatives in dietary treated patients |
| | Blood spot | Ambient temp | Variation possible due to various technical issues<br>Not that many studies on differences with plasma |
| Met (P) | Plasma | Ambient temp | Liver disease, any cause |
| 4-Hydroxyphenylpyruvate, 4-Hydroxyphenyllactate and 4-Hydroxyphenylacetate | Urine | Ambient temp | Nonspecific elevations in liver disease of any cause. Urinary levels highly variable with diet and not generally useful for patient follow-up |
| Succinylacetone (Blood) | Plasma | Ambient temp | Slight increase in severe liver disease; possible false positive on dichloroacetate, treatment |
| | Blood spot | Ambient temp | So far, succinylacetone so far seems not easy to be compared to plasma |
| Porphobilinogen synthase (RBC) | Heparinized blood | Ambient temp | May be close to normal in TT1<br>Primary deficiency of porphobilinogen synthase |
| Succinylacetone (U) | Urine | Ambient temp<br>(Frozen −20 °C) | False negatives possible in dilute urine specimens with some techniques |
| Hawkinsin | Urine | Frozen −20 °C | Failure to recognize hawkinsin and related metabolites if the specific diagnosis is not suggested on requisition |
| Homogentisate | Urine | Frozen −20 °C | – |
| FAH activity | Fibroblasts<br>Lymphocytes<br>Liver | Ambient temp<br>Frozen (−70 °C)<br>Frozen (−70 °C) | False positive: pseudo-deficiency. False negative: back mutation with significant FAH activity in revertant areas (common in liver)<br>Insensitivity: very low normal activity in most available extrahepatic tissues renders enzymatic diagnosis difficult |
| TAT activity | Liver | Frozen (−70 °C) | False positive: highly regulated enzyme with wide normal range of activity depending on physiological state |
| HPD activity | Liver | Frozen (−70 °C) | False positive: secondary deficiency in cirrhotic liver<br>Late maturation prenatally; may be low in premature infants |

In general plasma and urine are stored frozen until assay. Experiences of the laboratory of the late Prof Holme learned that untreated blood and urine samples retain acceptable quality if transported at ambient temperature by same day or overnight courier

## Prenatal Diagnosis

DNA analysis is the preferred method for prenatal diagnosis of all diseases of tyrosine degradation. The pathogenic variation of each biological parent must be known before proposing this technique. Molecular diagnosis can be performed on cells obtained directly or by culture after amniocentesis, from chorionic villus samples or at the preimplantation stage. Measurement of SA in amniotic fluid is an acceptable approach to diagnosis of TT1 for couples in whom the causal DNA variations are not known.

## DNA Testing

DNA analysis is available for all diseases of tyrosine degradation. Standard molecular diagnostic procedures can be applied, using genomic DNA of any source. If the patient comes from a background with a known ethnic founder effect or if the pathogenic variation for which he or she is at risk is known, this can be tested directly. Otherwise, exome sequencing and, if necessary, deletion/duplication analysis are the methods of choice.

## Treatment and Monitoring Summary

### Diet Therapy

In all forms of hypertyrosinemia but MAAI, a mainstay of treatment is dietary restriction of the intake of Tyr and its precursor Phe, plus provision of adequate amounts of other nutrients in a form that is palatable as much as possible. Close supervision is necessary in order to avoid dietary deficiencies. Compliance is an important long-term issue, especially because hypertyrosinemia itself does not directly confer a sense of discomfort. In TT1, expert consensus, without clear data, suggested that plasma Tyr should be maintained below 400 or 500 μmol/L (De Laet et al. 2013; Chinsky et al. 2017). In TT2 and TT3, the ideal levels of plasma Tyr are even less established. Eye and skin lesions have rarely been seen in TT2 patients with plasma Tyr level <800 μmol/L, suggesting that levels should be maintained below this level. However, the repeated observation of developmental delay in many TT2 patients suggests that a lower level, perhaps 400–500 μmol/L, may be more appropriate. The increasing number of studies on intellectual and executive functions as well as social abilities in TT1 has delineated that there might not only be a relation with blood Tyr but also with blood Phe concentrations (van Vliet et al. 2015; van Ginkel et al. 2017a, b) pointing at effects of low Phe and high Tyr concentrations.

### The Place of Liver Transplantation in the Era Without Nitisinone and the Era with Nitisinone

In the era that only dietary treatment was available and nitisinone was not, liver transplantation was the only definitive answer to both the oncological and metabolic problem in TT1 (van Spronsen et al. 1994). This completely changed with nitisinone.

Patients presenting with liver failure usually respond favorably to nitisinone, liver transplantation only being necessary in those patients in which the liver does not respond within some 5 days or when liver failure progresses as can be seen by the increase of ammonia and bilirubin. This implies that nitisinone is an emergency treatment in infants with unexplained liver failure till TT1 has been excluded. Nitisinone is available only for oral administration. In acutely ill patients with suspected and proven TT1, all efforts should be made to administer nitisinone immediately, even not preventing from use when samples for the proof of TT1 have not yet been taken as high SA will remain present for some hours after the first dose.

The other indication for liver transplantation that still may exist is the development of liver cancer. While liver disease, acute porphyria, and renal tubulopathy are not reported anymore on adequate use of nitisinone, liver cancer can be an issue. The older the patient is at start of nitisinone, the higher the risk of pre-malignancy development in the liver till diagnosis resulting in hepatocellular carcinoma (HCC) or hepatoblastoma at presentation or later in life (Mayorandan et al. 2014; van Ginkel et al. 2017b). Patients with an AFP that does not show a normalization of AFP within some 1–2 years of nitisinone are considered to be at risk for later development of liver cancer (Koelink et al. 2006), while patients with an AFP that starts to rise again after its decrease (often not have completely normalized by optimal nitisinone use) and patients with a new nodule seen at ultrasound under nitisinone should be considered to have liver cancer necessitating immediate referral to the liver transplantation team.

Patients who have had a donor liver still show mild increased SA in both blood and urine. It has therefore been advocated to continue nitisinone after liver transplantation. However, to our knowledge, none of the patients without receiving nitisinone after liver transplantation has developed any renal cancer that theoretically could be hypothesized. At the same time, these experiments with nitisinone after liver transplantation revealed that the dose of nitisinone to diminish the SA in blood and urine in a "healthy liver" is only a fraction of the dose needed in the diseased liver in TT1 patients but at the same time may result in still higher blood Tyr concentrations, resembling the situation in AKU (Milan et al. 2017).

### TT1-Nitisinone Treatment

Nitisinone combined with dietary therapy is the medical treatment of choice for patients with TT1 since 1992 (Lindstedt et al. 1992). To date, no instance of liver cancer has occurred in patients detected by neonatal screening and treated with nitisinone rapidly thereafter (Larochelle et al. 2012). Late-treated patients are at greater risk of liver cancer, but no acute episodes of liver failure or neurological crises occurred during nitisinone treatment.

Starting nitisinone in infants with liver failure is an adventure. At the one hand, these patients may still deteriorate the first days before nitisinone start to show its clinical effect (usually within 3 days), and in these patients 2 mg/kg/day might be needed. Nitisinone may increase the already increased Tyr concentrations, but the need for natural protein for anabolism probably is of more importance accepting the higher Tyr concentrations for some days if the liver accepts that amount of nitrogen load without increasing ammonia. In that respect, attention should be paid to give clotting factors rather than fresh frozen plasma in case of too high risk of bleeding.

Starting nitisinone in patients presenting with acute intermittent porphyria caused by TT1 can also show to be very efficacious still necessitating the promotion of anabolism.

Nitisinone has a long half-life in healthy adults of 54 h, permitting once daily administration. However, the healthy situation cannot be transferred to the TT1 patient that easily as can be learned from two issues. First of all, the experiment with nitisinone in patients having or had liver transplantation learned that nitisinone metabolism is different in a healthy compared to a diseased liver. Second, a recent study showed that dividing the total daily dose into two daily doses results in better reduction of SA if compared to taking the total dose in one daily dose (Kienstra et al. 2018). That study also showed that nitisinone levels of >35 µmol/L may suffice to suppress blood SA levels to <0.6 µmol/L. The lack of total depression of SA presumably reflects a state of increased liver cancer risk. It is important to monitor dose and compliance both clinically and by repeated laboratory measurements. Therefore, the use of home sampling methods to frequently monitor not only blood Phe and Tyr but also NTBC and SA is of clinical importance. If that is not provided by the own institutional laboratory, it is advised to collaborate with metabolic institutions that provide this service.

Monitoring TT1 probably can be split into the situation with diagnosis of neonatal screening and clinical presentation, the last group of patients not only having a higher risk of liver cancer when presented after 2–3 months of age (Holme and Lindstedt 1998; Larochelle et al. 2012), but tubular function also needing longer to return to normal than the patients found by newborn screening (Maiorana et al. 2014; Maiorana and Dionisi-Vici 2017).

Therefore, in patients with clinical presentation after 2 months of age, the authors of this chapter would advise a frequency of AFP of four times a year and twice yearly ultrasound and only performing MRI (with contrast) in case of some lesion found with ultrasound if performed by an experienced radiologist, only performing yearly studies on the kidney (tubular and glomerular) when patients show some issues at diagnosis having returned to normal. In case of newborn screening, patients do even need less regular follow-up with AFP and ultrasound (twice yearly and once yearly, respectively), while kidney function measurements are only needed on clinical indication. Both groups of patients will continue to show some very mild abnormalities in prothrombin time, but this seems to be without any clinical relevance.

Instead, increased attention should be given to neurocognitive function and psychosocial development, and both parents and school teams should be aware of the risk of delay in development and behavioral issues, while research is needed in larger series to explore the adequate target concentrations of both Phe and Tyr. This at itself points to the importance of centers of expertise to centralize the experience and learn from that much faster than is being done now.

For all such patients, developmental assessment should be regularly performed, and plasma Phe and Tyr concentrations should be monitored regularly in order that evidence-based conclusions regarding development and metabolic control can be attained in the future. If developmental delay or behavioral issues are present, appropriate educational help is needed.

## TT2 and TT3

These patients are offered dietary treatment as above. Cutaneous and ocular complications are usually rapidly reversed when dietary control of plasma Tyr is achieved. Symptomatic treatment can provide some immediate benefit.

It is reasonable to consider that the development delay seen in some TT2 and TT3 patients may be related to increased levels of plasma Tyr. Controlled trials in large numbers of patients are not available at present because of the rarity of these conditions and the lack of consistent documentation of outcome. This again not only asks for international cooperation in research but also for expert centers that can see as many of these patients as possible to increase and disseminate the expertise. This issue should be discussed with patients and families, and treatment should be offered accordingly. The authors treat patients with these conditions in a similar fashion to the recommendations for nitisinone-treated TT1 patients (De Laet et al. 2013).

## Alkaptonuria (AKU)

Currently most treatment of AKU is still symptomatic, concentrating upon the relief of the symptoms of arthritis and joint pain. Nitisinone results in a marked reduction in homogentisate excretion at small doses of nitisinone (Milan et al. 2017). As these small doses of nitisinone for AKU imply hypertyrosinemia, dietary restriction of Phe and Tyr seems essential again. Results of long-term studies as presently undertaken will be needed to show the effect of adequate reduction of homogentisate in order to prevent the major complications of AKU. However, these studies are performed in adults not knowing whether starting nitisinone (with dietary) treatment already in infancy or childhood is more effective.

### Hawkinsinuria (HAWK)

Reported patients have become asymptomatic after infancy. Patients should be given symptomatic treatment for acidosis. Temporary dietary restriction of Phe and Tyr could be considered in symptomatic patients.

### Maleylacetoacetate Isomerase Deficiency (MAAI)

Reported patients are without symptoms, signs being found with mildly increased SA concentrations at newborn screening for TT1. These patients do not seem to need treatment (Yang et al. 2017).

## Comments

There are six defined inborn errors of tyrosine metabolism: TT1, TT2, TT3, HAWK, AKU, and MAAI. The most common and serious of these disorders is TT1. For this disease efficient drug treatment is available with nitisinone, based on inhibition of Tyr degradation at a level prior to the formation of hepatotoxic metabolites. Early institution of nitisinone therapy is desirable, before complications occur. SA is the most sensitive and specific marker for neonatal screening of TT1, and this is now increasingly practiced in newborn screening programs. The outcome in TT1 patients detected by neonatal screening and treated early with nitisinone is very promising to date (Larochelle et al. 2012; Mayorandan et al. 2014), but attention should be focused on neurocognitive and psychosocial development in addition to liver and kidney function and porphyria-like symptoms. For TT2, dietary control of Tyr levels can prevent skin and ocular complications. Controlled dietary restriction of Phe and Tyr is a reasonable approach to all defects in the catabolism of Tyr except MAAI. Expanded newborn screening with SA efficiently detect TT1 and possibly also MAAI depending on the cut-off at newborn screening, but the other inborn errors of Tyr degradation are generally not detected by newborn screening, and a high index of suspicion by clinicians and diagnostic laboratory personnel is necessary to ensure early diagnosis and treatment.

## References


Blundell J, Frisson S, Chakrapani A, Kearney S, Vijay S, MacDonald A, Gissen P, Hendriksz C, Olson A. Markers of cognitive function in individuals with metabolic disease: Morquio syndrome and tyrosinemia type III. Cogn Neuropsychol. 2018;35(3–4):120–47.

Chinsky JM, Singh R, Ficicioglu C, van Karnebeek CDM, Grompe M, Mitchell G, Waisbren SE, Gucsavas-Calikoglu M, Wasserstein MP, Coakley K, Scott CR. Diagnosis and treatment of tyrosinemia type I: a US and Canadian consensus group review and recommendations. Genet Med. 2017;19(12). https://doi.org/10.1038/gim.2017.101

De Laet C, Dionisi-Vici C, Leonard JV, McKiernan P, Mitchell G, Monti L, de Baulny HO, Pintos-Morell G, Spikerkötter U. Recommendations for the management of tyrosinemia type 1. Orphanet J Rare Dis. 2013;8:8. https://doi.org/10.1186/1750-1172-8-8.

Gomez-Ospina N, Scott AI, Oh GJ, Potter D, Goel VV, Destino L, Baugh N, Enns GM, Niemi AK, Cowan TM. Expanding the phenotype of hawkinsinuria: new insights from response to N-acetyl-L-cysteine. J Inherit Metab Dis. 2016;39(6):821–9.

Holme E, Lindstedt S. Tyrosinaemia type I and NTBC (2-(2-nitro-4-trifluoromethylbenzoyl)-1,3-cyclohexanedione). J Inherit Metab Dis. 1998;21:507–17.

Holme E, Mithcell G. Tyrosine metabolism. In: Blau N, Duran M, Gibson KM, Dinoisi-Vici C, editors. Physician's guide to the diagnosis, treatment, and follow-up of inherited metabolic diseases; 2014. p. 23–31.

Kienstra NS, van Reemst HE, van Ginkel WG, Daly A, van Dam E, MacDonald A, Burgerhof JGM, de Blaauw P, McKiernan PJ, Heiner-Fokkema MR, van Spronsen FJ. Daily variation of NTBC and its relation to succinylacetone in tyrosinemia type 1 patients comparing a single dose to two doses a day. J Inherit Metab Dis. 2018;41(2):181–6.

Koelink CJ, van Hasselt P, van der Ploeg A, van den Heuvel-Eibrink MM, Wijburg FA, Bijleveld CM, van Spronsen FJ. Tyrosinemia type I treated by NTBC: how does AFP predict liver cancer? Mol Genet Metab. 2006;89(4):310–5.

Larochelle J, Alvarez F, Bussières JF, Chevalier I, Dubois J, Faucher F, Fenyves D, Gooyer P, Grenier A, Holme E, Laframboise R, Lambert M, Lindstedt S, Maranda B, Melançon S, Merouani A, Mitchell J, Parizeault G, Pelletier L, Phan V, Rinaldo P, Scott CR, Scriver C, Mitchell GA. Effect of nitisinone (NTBC) treatment on the clinical course of hepatorenal tyrosinemia in Québec. Mol Genet Metab. 2012;107:49–54.

Lindstedt S, Holme E, Lock EA, Hjalmarson O, Strandvik B. Treatment of hereditary tyrosinaemia type I by inhibition of 4-hydroxyphenylpyruvate dioxygenase. Lancet. 1992;340:813–7.

Maiorana A, Dionisi-Vici C. NTBC and correction of renal dysfunction. Adv Exp Med Biol. 2017;959:93–100.

Maiorana A, Malamisura M, Emma F, Boenzi S, Di Ciommo VM, Dionisi-Vici C. Early effect of NTBC on renal tubular dysfunction in hereditary tyrosinemia type I. Mol Genet Metab. 2014;113(3):188–93.

Mayorandan S, Meyer U, Gokcay G, Segarra NG, de Baulny HO, van Spronsen F, Zeman J, de Laet C, Spiekerkoetter U, Thimm E, Maiorana A, Dionisi-Vici C, Moeslinger D, Brunner-Krainz M, Lotz-Havla AS, Cocho de Juan JA, Couce Pico ML, Santer R, Scholl-Bürgi S, Mandel H, Bliksrud YT, Freisinger P, Aldamiz-Echevarria LJ, Hochuli M, Gautschi M, Endig J, Jordan J, McKiernan P, Ernst S, Morlot S, Vogel A, Sander J, Das AM. Cross-sectional study of 168 patients with hepatorenal tyrosinaemia and implications for clinical practice. Orphanet J Rare Dis. 2014;9:107.

Milan AM, Hughes AT, Davison AS, Devine J, Usher J, Curtis S, Khedr M, Gallagher JA, Ranganath LR. The effect of nitisinone on homogentisic acid and tyrosine: a two-year survey of patients attending the National Alkaptonuria Centre, Liverpool. Ann Clin Biochem. 2017;54(3):323–30.

Ranganath LR, Khedr M, Milan AM, Davison AS, Hughes AT, Usher JL, Taylor S, Loftus N, Daroszewska A, West E, Jones A, Briggs M, Fisher M, McCormick M, Judd S, Vinjamuri S, Griffin R, Psarelli EE, Cox TF, Sireau N, Dillon JP, Devine JM, Hughes G, Harrold J, Barton GJ, Jarvis JC, Gallagher JA. Nitisinone arrests ochronosis and decreases rate of progression of Alkaptonuria: evaluation of the effect of nitisinone in the United Kingdom National Alkaptonuria Centre. Mol Genet Metab. 2018;125(1–2):127–34.

Stinton C, Geppert J, Freeman K, Clarke A, Johnson S, Fraser H, Sutcliffe P, Taylor-Phillips S. Newborn screening for Tyrosinemia type 1 using succinylacetone—a systematic review of test accuracy. Orphanet J Rare Dis. 2017;12(1):48.

van Ginkel WG, Jahja R, Huijbregts SCJ, van Spronsen FJ. Neurological and neuropsychological problems in tyrosinemia type I patients. Adv Exp Med Biol. 2017a;959:111–22.

van Ginkel WG, Pennings JP, van Spronsen FJ. Liver cancer in tyrosinemia type 1. Adv Exp Med Biol. 2017b;959:101–9.

van Spronsen FJ, Thomasse Y, Smit GP, Leonard JV, Clayton PT, Fidler V, Berger R, Heymans HS. Hereditary tyrosinemia type I: a new clinical classification with difference in prognosis on dietary treatment. Hepatology. 1994;20:1187–91.

van Vliet D, van Dam E, van Rijn M, Derks TG, Venema-Liefaard G, Hitzert MM, Lunsing RJ, Heiner-Fokkema MR, van Spronsen FJ. Infants with Tyrosinemia Type 1: should phenylalanine be supplemented? JIMD Rep. 2015;18:117–24.

Yang H, Al-Hertani W, Cyr D, Laframboise R, Parizeault G, Wang SP, Rossignol F, Berthier MT, Giguère Y, Waters PJ, Mitchell GA, Québec NTBC Study Group. Hypersuccinylacetonaemia and normal liver function in maleylacetoacetate isomerase deficiency. J Med Genet. 2017;54(4):241–7.

# Disorders of Sulfur Amino Acid and Hydrogen Sulfide Metabolism

# 22

Ivo Barić, Viktor Kožich, and Brian Fowler

## Contents



I. Barić (✉)
Division for Genetics and Metabolic Diseases,
Department of Pediatrics, University Hospital Center Zagreb
and University of Zagreb, School of Medicine, Zagreb, Croatia
e-mail: ibaric@kbc-zagreb.hr

V. Kožich
Department of Pediatrics and Inherited Metabolic Diseases,
Charles University-First Faculty of Medicine and General
University Hospital in Prague, Praha, Czech Republic
e-mail: Viktor.Kozich@vfn.cz

B. Fowler
Labs Pediatrics, University Children's Hospital,
Basel, Switzerland
e-mail: brian.fowler@ukbb.ch


N. Blau et al. (eds.), *Physician's Guide to the Diagnosis, Treatment, and Follow-Up of Inherited Metabolic Diseases*,
https://doi.org/10.1007/978-3-030-67727-5_22

## Summary

The conversion of methionine to inorganic sulfate involves the formation of homocysteine encompassing transmethylation followed by transsulfuration. Several inherited enzyme deficiencies within this pathway have been described. Those causing hypermethioninemia may be confused with the many known secondary causes of increased methionine demanding diagnostic expediency. Most of the disorders have been described in small numbers of patients so that the full clinical spectrum of these is not known. Exceptions are methionine adenosyltransferase (MAT) I/III deficiency and cystathionine ß-synthase deficiency which causes classical homocystinuria, characterized primarily by an increased risk of thrombosis and embolism, lens dislocation, and other connective tissue involvement and cognitive impairment. While methionine adenosyltransferase I/III deficiency is only symptomatic in some patients causing different neurological problems and glycine *N*-methyltransferase deficiency affects liver function, other diseases causing hypermethioninemias may be associated with a multisystem disease of varying severity and progression. MAT II deficiency can be associated with thoracic aortic aneurysms in some heterozygotes for *MAT2* mutations. Methanethiol oxidase deficiency causes cabbage-like breath odor (extraoral halitosis). The association of mercaptopyruvate sulfur transferase deficiency with cognitive impairment, as the only disease characteristic, is questionable. Isolated sulfite oxidase deficiency is characterized by refractory convulsions in early infancy, brain atrophy, severe psychomotor retardation, and lens dislocation. Ethylmalonic encephalopathy is a severe disorder manifesting with seizures, developmental delay and cognitive impairment, orthostatic acrocyanosis and petechia due to vasodilation, failure to thrive, and chronic hemorrhagic diarrhea. Measurement of plasma and urine amino acids and total homocysteine can detect many of the disorders described in this chapter, while other tests are necessary for others. Confirmatory tests are enzyme assays and/or mutation analysis. Treatment combines one or more of dietary restriction of precursors, substitution of essential products, pharmacologic doses of cofactors, and binding and removing of harmful metabolites. Early diagnosis and early treatment favor better outcome.


## Introduction

Sulfur-containing amino acids include methionine, homocysteine, cystathionine, cysteine, and taurine. This chapter deals with inherited deficiencies of enzymes in the transmethylation and transsulfuration pathways that convert sulfur from methionine via homocysteine and cysteine to sulfate, including sulfide metabolism (Fig. 22.1). Since adenosine kinase deficiency also disrupts the methionine cycle, it is included in this chapter.

Most disorders described in this chapter are inherited as autosomal recessive traits. Exceptions are autosomal dominant forms of methionine adenosyltransferase (MAT) II deficiency and a subgroup of MAT I/III deficiency, caused by mutations with dominant negative effect on the wild-type allele (Chamberlin et al. 1997).

**Pathophysiology** of disorders of sulfur-containing amino acids is complex and only partly understood (Kožich et al. 2016). In disorders associated with hypermethioninemia, very high concentrations can be harmful themselves, primarily for the brain. In MAT I/III deficiency, low adenosylmethionine (AdoMet) and subsequent deficient methylation could be contributing factors. There are several hypotheses of how *MAT2A* loss-of-function mutations could lead to aortic disease, and it is possible that they require a second "hit" (Guo et al. 2015). Methionine can be also transaminated yielding methanethiol; deficiency of methanethiol oxidase results in accumulation of malodorous molecules such as methanethiol and dimethylsulfide. In *S*-adenosylhomocysteine (AdoHcy) hydrolase deficiency, high concentrations of AdoHcy inhibit numerous methyltransferases with very variable clinical consequences. Several putative pathogenetic mechanisms of adenosine kinase deficiency are related to increased adenosine and its various toxic effects. Another mechanism could be inhibition of numerous methyltransferases caused by secondary elevation of *S*-adenosylhomocysteine. The latter mechanism could also be important in classical homocystinuria, where a major pathogenetic mechanism seems to be elevation of homocysteine with its adverse effect on coagulation, vessels and secondary to vascular changes in many tissues, and possibly the decreased production of cysteine manifesting in connective tissue including lens zonular fibers. Clinical consequences of sulfite oxidase deficiency are likely due to toxic effects of sulfite, *S*-sulfocysteine, and thiosulfate on the brain and connective tissue. Patients with ethylmalonic encephalopathy accumulate a large amount of hydrogen sulfide, which leads directly to vasodilation and to secondary inhibition of cytochrome c-oxidase with subsequent impairment of short-chain fatty oxidation with typical metabolite changes and of oxidative phosphorylation with lactic acidosis.

**Clinical presentation** can occur at any age and varies widely in its severity.

*MAT I/III deficiency* is asymptomatic in all individuals with the autosomal dominant disease, while about half of the patients with the autosomal recessive form have developed neurological symptoms (Chien et al. 2015). Hypermethioninemia, the biochemical hallmark of this

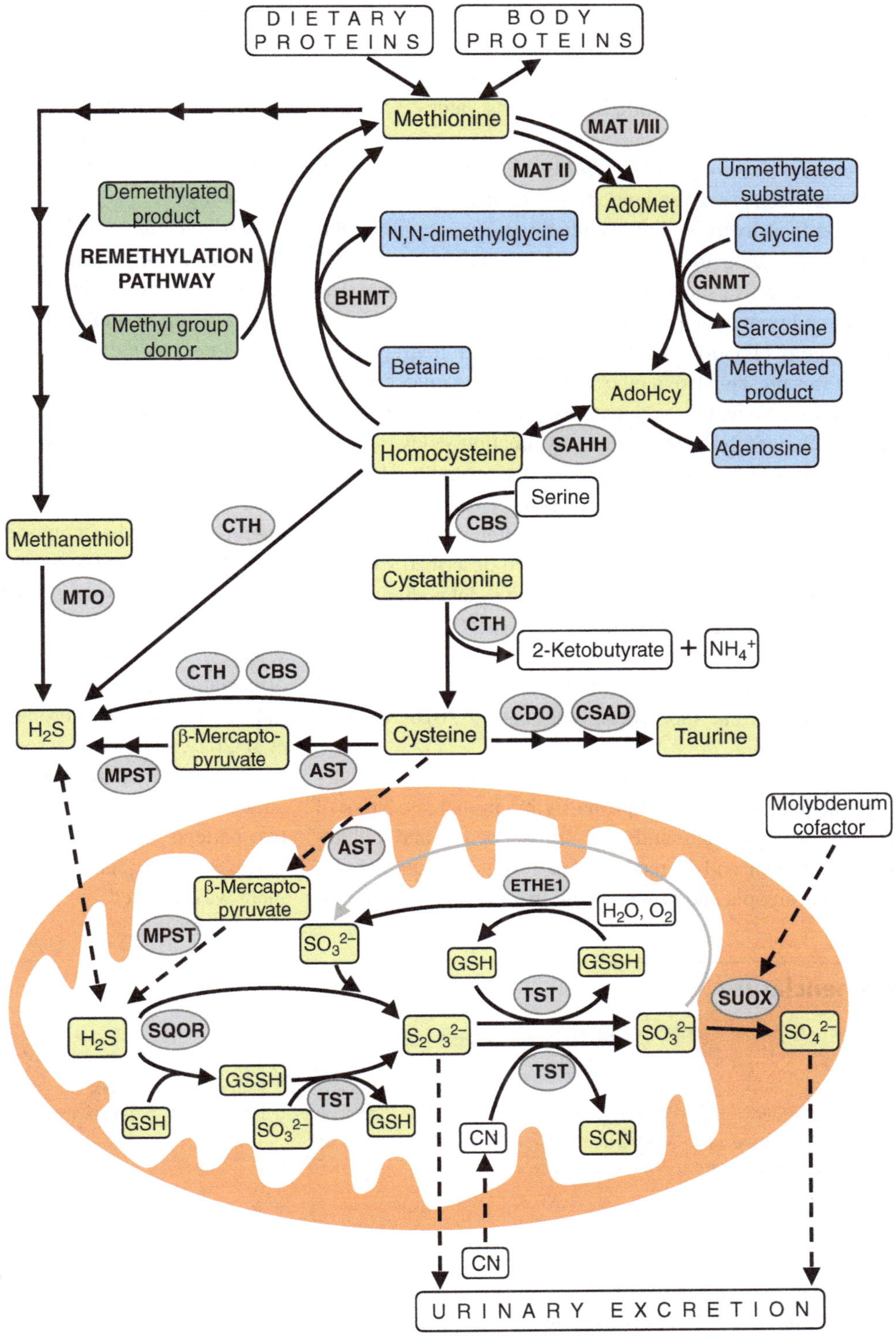


**Fig. 22.1** Metabolism of sulfur amino acids and of hydrogen sulfide. Methionine is converted to cysteine via a series of reactions involving the following enzymes: *MATI/III* methionine adenosyltransferase I/III, *MATII* methionine adenosyltransferase II, *GNMT* glycine *N*-methyltransferase, *SAHH* *S*-adenosylhomocysteine hydrolase, *BHMT* betaine homocysteine methyltransferase, *CBS* cystathionine beta-synthase, *CTH* cystathionine gamma-lyase, *AdoMet* *S*-adenosylmethionine, *AdoHcy* *S*-adenosylhomocysteine. Cysteine serves as the major precursor for synthesis of hydrogen sulfide catalyzed by CBS, CTH, aspartate aminotransferase (AST), and mercaptopyruvate sulfurtransferase (MPST); hydrogen sulfide may be also synthesized by methanethiol oxidase (MTO). Another route of cysteine oxidation to taurine is catalyzed by cysteine dioxygenase (CDO) and cysteine sulfinic acid decarboxylase (CSAD). Mitochondrial oxidation of hydrogen sulfide requires the following enzymes: *SQOR* sulfide:quinone oxidoreductase, *ETHE1* persulfide dioxygenase, *TST* thiosulfate transferase, *SUOX* sulfite oxidase, *GSH* glutathione, *GSSH* glutathione persulfide

disease, if severe, is itself associated with increased risk of various neurological problems (Braverman et al. 2005). The most characteristic brain imaging changes are demyelination with edema of subcortical and deep white matter, more pronounced in dorsal brain stem and resulting in separation of myelin layers—the so-called vacuolating myelinopathy (Braverman et al. 2005). Neurological abnormalities tend to occur in patients with plasma methionine concentrations generally above 800 μmol/L, whereas they have been rare in subjects with lower levels (Chien et al. 2015).

*MAT II deficiency* is only a risk factor for developing thoracic aortic aneurysms in some heterozygotes for *MAT2A* mutations.

*Glycine N-methyltransferase (GNMT) deficiency* (Mudd et al. 2001) has been so far described in only five children. The only clinical sign was mild hepatomegaly present in two siblings. The patients have remained clinically well during follow-up (Barić et al. 2017). Their aminotransferase activities ranged from borderline to fivefold increase. Plasma methionine can reach potentially damaging values (see MAT I/III deficiency).

*S-adenosylhomocysteine hydrolase deficiency* (Barić et al. 2004) has been proven and reported so far in ten patients. Two sibs had fetal hydrops, liver synthetic failure, and muscular hypotonia leading to respiratory failure and death in early infancy. They also showed brain abnormalities including cerebellar and pontine hypoplasia, hypoplastic corpus callosum, and hypomyelination. Muscle disease with high creatine kinase was present also in other patients with a milder phenotype. They also had, in various combinations, developmental delay, behavioral abnormalities, myelination delay, strabismus, coagulopathy, and liver disease. One patient had hepatocellular carcinoma, and there is some evidence that this disease carries increased risk for this malignancy.

*Adenosine kinase deficiency* has been described so far in 19 patients. All had severe developmental delay, hypotonia, and frontal bossing. The majority had hypertelorism, failure to thrive, epilepsy, macrocephaly, neonatal jaundice, and liver disease with elevated aminotransferases. About half of patients had cardiac anomalies (Staufner et al. 2016; Alhusani et al. 2019).

*Cystathionine beta-synthase (CBS) deficiency* is clinically variable and characterized primarily by an increased risk of thrombosis—predominantly in venous beds—and pulmonary embolism and in more severe forms by osteoporosis, lenticular myopia and lens dislocation, developmental delay, and cognitive impairment (Mudd et al. 1985). About half of patients are pyridoxine responsive with a less severe disease (Morris et al. 2017).

*Cystathionase deficiency* is considered a benign condition (Kraus et al. 2009) although it was originally described in patients with psychomotor retardation and other neurological findings.

*Methanethiol oxidase (MTO) deficiency* has been described in only five patients with cabbage-like breath odor (extraoral halitosis) due to accumulation of methanethiol and dimethylsulfide (Pol et al. 2018).

*Isolated sulfite oxidase deficiency* is characterized by refractory convulsions starting in the neonatal or early infantile period, severe psychomotor retardation, brain imaging findings resembling hypoxic-ischemic encephalopathy with development of cysts, and early death. Lens dislocation occurs usually after the neonatal period. Milder and late-onset cases have been reported (Claerhout et al. 2018; Bindu et al. 2017, see Online resources).

*Persulfide dioxygenase (PDO) deficiency* or ethylmalonic encephalopathy (ETHE1) is a severe disorder manifesting in seizures, developmental delay and cognitive impairment, orthostatic acrocyanosis and petechia due to vasodilation, failure to thrive, and chronic hemorrhagic diarrhea (Di Meo et al. 2017, see Online resources).

*Mercaptopyruvate sulfur transferase (MPST) deficiency* and/or excretion of the mercaptolactate has been reported in two patients with mental retardation (Ampola et al. 1969); however, subsequently no association with cognitive impairment was reported.

## Nomenclature

| No. | Disorder | Alternative name | Abbreviation of the disease/ deficiency | Gene symbol | Chromosomal localization | Mode of inheritance | Affected protein | OMIM No. | Subtype |
|---|---|---|---|---|---|---|---|---|---|
| 22.1 | Methionine adenosyltransferase I/III deficiency | MAT deficiency | MAT I/III | *MAT1A* | 10q22 | AR | Methionine adenosyltransferase I/III | 250850 | Potentially symptomatic form |
| 22.1 | Methionine adenosyltransferase I/III deficiency | MAT deficiency | MAT I/III | *MAT1A* | 10q22 | AD | Methionine adenosyltransferase I/III | 250850 | Benign form |
| 22.2 | Methionine adenosyltransferase II deficiency | *S*-adenosylmethionine synthase isoform type 2 deficiency; MATII deficiency | MATII | *MAT2A* | 2p11.2 | AD | Methionine adenosyltransferase II alpha | 601468 | Potentially symptomatic |
| 22.3 | Glycine *N*-methyltransferase deficiency | GNMT deficiency | GNMT | *GNMT* | 6p12 | AR | Glycine *N*-methyltransferase | 606664 | All forms |
| 22.4 | *S*-adenosylhomocysteine hydrolase deficiency | SAHH deficiency | AHCY | *AHCY* | 20q11.22 | AR | Adenosylhomocysteinase, *S*-adenosylhomocysteine hydrolase | 613752 | All forms |

| No. | Disorder | Alternative name | Abbreviation of the disease/ deficiency | Gene symbol | Chromosomal localization | Mode of inheritance | Affected protein | OMIM No. | Subtype |
|---|---|---|---|---|---|---|---|---|---|
| 22.5 | Adenosine kinase deficiency | Hypermethioninemia due to adenosine kinase deficiency | ADK | *ADK* | 10q22.2 | AR | Adenosine kinase | 614300 | All forms |
| 22.6 | Cystathionine beta-synthase deficiency | Classical homocystinuria | CBS | *CBS* | 21q22.3 | AR | Cystathionine beta-synthase | 263200 | All forms |
| 22.7 | Cystathionase deficiency | Cystathionine gamma-lyase deficiency | CTH | *CTH* | 1p31.1 | AR | Cystathionine gamma-lyase | 219500 | All forms (probably benign) |
| 22.8 | Methanethiol oxidase deficiency | Extraoral halitosis, MTO deficiency | MTO | *SELENBP1* | 1q21.3 | AR | Methanethiol oxidase | 604188 | All forms |
| 22.9 | Sulfite oxidase deficiency | Isolated sulfite oxidase deficiency | SUOX | *SUOX* | 12q13.13 | AR | Sulfite oxidase | 272300 | Isolated |
| 22.10 | Mitochondrial sulfur dioxygenase deficiency | Ethylmalonic encephalopathy | ETHE1 | *ETHE1* | 19p13.32 | AR | Mitochondrial persulfide dioxygenase | 602473, 608451 | All forms |
| 22.11 | Mercaptopyruvate sulfur transferase deficiency | β-Mercaptolactate cysteine disulfiduria | MPST | *MPST* | 22q12.3 | AR | Mercaptopyruvate sulfur transferase | 602496 | All forms (probably benign) |

[a]Inheritance of this risk factor with incomplete penetrance is autosomal dominant

## Metabolic Pathway

Metabolism of sulfur amino acids is summarized in Fig. 22.1. Methionine and homocysteine are linked by the remethylation cycle (see Chap. 28 for details) and the transsulfuration pathway. The essential amino acid methionine is derived from the diet or catabolism of proteins. Methionine is first converted to *S*-adenosylmethionine by two methionine *S*-adenosyltransferases, the ubiquitously expressed MATII and liver-expressed MATI/III encoded by *MAT2A* and *MAT1A* genes, respectively. *S*-adenosylmethionine (AdoMet) is the methyl-group donor in a wide range of transmethylation reactions including DNA methylation, creatine, and neurotransmitter synthesis, and surplus amounts are converted to sarcosine by glycine *N*-methyltransferase. The transfer of methyl groups from AdoMet yields *S*-adenosylhomocysteine, which is a strong inhibitor of transmethylation reactions and must be cleaved to adenosine and homocysteine by *S*-adenosylhomocysteine hydrolase. Depending on a number of factors, about half of available homocysteine is recycled into methionine by the folate and cobalamin-dependent remethylation cycle, while the other half is channeled into the transsulfuration pathway. In the latter series of reactions, homocysteine is condensed with serine to form cystathionine via a reaction catalyzed by the pyridoxal phosphate-requiring cystathionine ß-synthase. Cystathionine is cleaved to cysteine, α-ketobutyrate, and ammonia by another pyridoxal phosphate-dependent enzyme, γ-cystathionase. Cysteine is an important precursor for the synthesis of glutathione and taurine and the major source for endogenous production of the signaling molecule hydrogen sulfide. The sulfur atom of cysteine can be fully oxidized to sulfate via two major pathways. Cysteine can be converted to cysteine sulfinic acid by cysteine dioxygenase followed by transamination with α-oxoglutarate yielding pyruvate and sulfite, although cysteine sulfinate can be also decarboxylated and give rise to hypotaurine and finally to taurine. The other pathway utilizes cysteine for the synthesis of the gasotransmitter hydrogen sulfide by catalysis of CBS, CTH, MPST, and cysteinyl-tRNA synthetase; hydrogen sulfide exists in a dynamic equilibrium of dissolved gas, hydrosulfide, and various organic and inorganic polysulfides. Oxidation of hydrogen sulfide occurs in mitochondria and starts with persulfidation of GSH by sulfide:quinone oxidoreductase, followed by release of sulfite under the catalysis of ETHE1. Sulfite is finally oxidized by the molybdenum cofactor-containing sulfite oxidase to the ultimate oxidation product sulfate.

## Signs and Symptoms

**Table 22.1** Methionine adenosyltransferase I/III deficiency (AR and AD[a] forms)

| System | Symptoms and biomarkers | Neonatal (birth–1 month) | Infancy (1–18 months) | Childhood (1.5–11 years) | Adolescence (11–16 years) | Adulthood (>16 years) |
|---|---|---|---|---|---|---|
| CNS | Cognitive dysfunction | | | ± | ± | ± |
| | Demyelination | | | ± | ± | ± |
| | Developmental delay | | | ± | ± | ± |
| | Dysdiadochokinesis | | | ± | ± | ± |
| | Dysmetria | | | ± | ± | ± |
| | Dystonia | | | ± | ± | ± |
| | Headache | | | ± | ± | ± |
| | Language difficulties | | | ± | ± | ± |
| | Tendon reflexes, increased | | | ± | ± | ± |
| | Tremor | | | ± | ± | ± |
| | **Vacuolating myelopathy** | | | ± | ± | ± |
| Eye | Nystagmus | | | ± | ± | ± |
| Other | **Cabbage-like breath odor (dimethylsulfide)** | ± | ± | ± | ± | ± |
| Laboratory findings | Cystathionine (plasma) | n | n | n | n | n |
| | Homocysteine, total (plasma) | n-↑ | n-↑ | n-↑ | n-↑ | n-↑ |
| | Methionine (P, U) | ↑↑↑ | ↑↑↑ | ↑↑↑ | ↑↑↑ | ↑↑↑ |
| | Methionine sulfoxide (urine) | ↑ | ↑ | ↑ | ↑ | ↑ |
| | Methionine-to-cystathionine ratio | ↑↑ | ↑↑ | ↑↑ | ↑↑ | ↑↑ |
| | Methionine-to-total homo-cysteine ratio | ↑↑ | ↑↑ | ↑↑ | ↑↑ | ↑↑ |
| | *S*-Adenosylhomocysteine (plasma) | n | n | n | n | n |
| | *S*-Adenosylmethionine (plasma) | n | n-↓ | n-↓ | n-↓ | n-↓ |

[a]The only reported clinical abnormality in autosomal dominant MATI/III deficiency is the cabbage-like odor

**Table 22.2** Methionine adenosyltransferase II deficiency

| System | Symptoms and biomarkers | Neonatal (birth–1 month) | Infancy (1–18 months) | Childhood (1.5–11 years) | Adolescence (11–16 years) | Adulthood (>16 years) |
|---|---|---|---|---|---|---|
| Cardiovascular | **Thoracic aortic aneurysms** | | | | | ± |

There are no specific biochemical abnormalities in individuals with thoracic aortic aneurysms who are heterozygotes for *MAT2A* mutations

**Table 22.3** Glycine *N*-methyltransferase deficiency

| System | Symptoms and biomarkers | Neonatal (birth–1 month)[a] | Infancy (1–18 months)[a] | Childhood (1.5–11 years) | Adolescence (11–16 years) | Adulthood (>16 years) |
|---|---|---|---|---|---|---|
| Digestive | Hepatomegaly | | ± | ± | | |
| Other | Failure to thrive | | ± | | | |
| Laboratory findings | ALAT (P) | | | ↑ | | |
| | ASAT (P) | | | ↑ | | |
| | Homocysteine, total (P) | | | n-↑ | n-↑ | n-↑ |
| | Methionine (P, U) | | | ↑↑↑ | ↑↑↑ | ↑↑↑ |
| | *S*-Adenosylhomocysteine (P) | | | n | n | n |
| | *S*-Adenosylmethionine (P) | | | ↑↑↑ | ↑↑↑ | ↑↑↑ |
| | Sarcosine (P) | | | n | n | n |

[a]Metabolite levels not yet reported in these age groups, however, expected to be similar to other age groups

**Table 22.4** *S*-adenosylhomocysteine hydrolase deficiency

| System | Symptoms and biomarkers | Neonatal (birth–1 month) | Infancy (1–18 months) | Childhood (1.5–11 years) | Adolescence (11–16 years) | Adulthood (>16 years) |
|---|---|---|---|---|---|---|
| CNS | Cerebellar hypoplasia | ± | ± | | | |
| | Delayed myelination | ± | ± | ± | | |
| | Developmental delay | ±-+++ | +-+++ | + | ± | ± |
| | Hypoplasia of corpus callosum | ± | ± | | | |
| | Hypoplasia of pons | ± | ± | | | |
| Digestive | Hepatocellular carcinoma | | | | | ± |
| | Liver dysfunction | ±-+++ | ±-+++ | ± | ± | ± |
| Eye | Strabismus | ± | ± | ± | ± | − |
| Hematological | Coagulopathy | ±-+++ | ±-+++ | ±-++ | ± | ± |
| Metabolic | Protein synthesis reduced | ±-+++ | ±-+++ | ± | − | − |
| Musculoskeletal | Absent tendon reflexes | + | + | + | + | + |
| | Muscle weakness | +-+++ | +-+++ | +-++ | +-++ | ++ |
| | Myopathy | +-+++ | +-+++ | ++ | ++ | ++ |
| | Weak tendon reflexes | ++-+++ | ++-+++ | ++-+++ | ++-+++ | ++-+++ |
| Psychiatric | Attention deficit disorder | | ± | ±-++ | ±-++ | ±-+++ |
| | Behavior, aggressive | | | ± | ± | ± |
| | Hyperactivity | | | ± | ± | ± |
| Respiratory | Respiratory insufficiency | ±-+++ | ±-+++ | | | |
| Other | Fetal hydrops | ±-++ | | | | |
| Laboratory findings | ALAT (plasma) | n-↑↑ | ↑-↑↑ | ↑-↑↑ | ↑-↑↑ | ↑-↑↑ |
| | Albumin (serum) | ↓↓↓-n | ↓↓↓-n | ↓↓↓-n | ↓↓↓-n | ↓↓↓-n |
| | ASAT (plasma) | n-↑↑ | ↑-↑↑ | ↑-↑↑ | ↑-↑↑ | ↑-↑↑ |
| | Creatine kinase (plasma) | ↑-↑↑ | ↑-↑↑ | ↑↑ | ↑↑ | ↑↑ |
| | Homocysteine, total (plasma) | n-↑ | n-↑ | n-↑ | n-↑ | n-↑ |
| | Methionine (plasma and urine) | n-↑↑ | n-↑↑ | n-↑↑ | n-↑↑ | n-↑↑ |
| | Prothrombin time | n-↑↑ | n-↑↑ | n-↑↑↑ | n-↑↑ | n-↑↑ |
| | *S*-Adenosylhomocysteine (plasma) | ↑↑↑ | ↑↑↑ | ↑↑↑ | ↑↑↑ | ↑↑↑ |
| | *S*-Adenosylmethionine (plasma) | ↑↑↑ | ↑↑↑ | ↑↑↑ | ↑↑↑ | ↑↑↑ |
| | Sarcosine (plasma) | n-↑ | n-↑ | n-↑ | n-↑ | n-↑ |

**Table 22.5** Adenosine kinase deficiency

| System | Symptoms and biomarkers | Neonatal (birth–1 month)[a] | Infancy (1–18 months)[a] | Childhood (1.5–11 years) | Adolescence (11–16 years) | Adulthood (>16 years) |
|---|---|---|---|---|---|---|
| Cardiovascular | Cardiac anomalies, malformations | ± | ± | ± | ± | ± |
| CNS | Epilepsy | | ± | ±-++ | ±-++ | ±-++ |
| | Developmental delay | | ++-+++ | ++-+++ | ++-+++ | ++-+++ |
| | Hypotonia | ±-++ | +-++ | +-++ | +-++ | +-++ |
| | Thin corpus callosum | ± | ± | ± | ± | ± |
| Digestive | Cholestasis | ± | ± | ± | ± | ± |
| | Liver dysfunction | ± | ± | ± | ± | ± |
| | Liver steatosis | ± | + | + | + | + |
| Ear | Hearing loss, sensorineural | − | ±-++ | ±-++ | ±-++ | ±-++ |
| Musculoskeletal | Macrocephaly | | ±-++ | ±-++ | ±-++ | ±-++ |
| | Frontal bossing | | + | + | + | + |
| | Muscle weakness, progressive | | ±-+ | ±-++ | ±-++ | ±-++ |
| | Short stature | ± | ± | ± | ± | ± |
| | Slender hands and feet | ± | ± | ± | ± | ± |
| Other | Failure to thrive | ± | ± | ± | ± | ± |
| Laboratory findings | Adenosine (dried blood spots) | | | n-↑ | n-↑ | n-↑ |
| | Adenosine (urine) | | | n-↑ | n-↑ | n-↑ |
| | ALAT (plasma) | ↑-↑↑ | n-↑↑ | n-↑↑ | n-↑↑ | n-↑↑ |
| | Bilirubin, conjugated (plasma) | ↑ | ↑ | | | |
| | Creatine kinase (plasma) | n-↑ | n-↑ | n-↑ | n-↑ | n-↑ |
| | Glucose (plasma) | n-↓ | n-↓ | n-↓ | n-↓ | |
| | Homocysteine, total (plasma) | n-↑ | n-↑ | n-↑ | n-↑ | n-↑ |
| | Methionine (plasma and urine) | n-↑↑↑ | n-↑↑↑ | n-↑↑↑ | n-↑↑↑ | n-↑↑↑ |
| | Prothrombin time | n-↑ | n-↑ | n-↑ | n-↑ | n-↑ |
| | *S*-Adenosylhomocysteine (plasma) | | | ↑-↑↑ | ↑-↑↑ | ↑-↑↑ |
| | *S*-Adenosylmethionine (plasma) | | | ↑-↑↑ | ↑-↑↑ | ↑-↑↑ |
| | Uric acid (plasma) | | n-↑ | n-↑↑ | n-↑↑ | n-↑ |

[a]Metabolite levels not yet reported in these age groups, however, expected to be similar to other age groups

**Table 22.6** Cystathionine beta-synthase deficiency

| System | Symptoms and biomarkers | Neonatal (birth–1 month) | Infancy (1–18 months) | Childhood (1.5–11 years) | Adolescence (11–16 years) | Adulthood (>16 years) |
|---|---|---|---|---|---|---|
| Cardiovascular | Thromboses, infarcts | | ± | ± | ± | ± |
| CNS | Developmental delay | | n-± | n-+++ | n-+++ | n-+++ |
| | Intellectual disability | | | n-+++ | n-+++ | n-+++ |
| | Psychiatric symptoms | | | ± | ± | ± |
| | Seizures | | ± | ± | ± | ± |
| | Stroke | | ± | ± | ± | ± |
| Dermatological | Malar flush | | | ± | ± | ± |
| Eye | Ectopia lentis | | ± | ± | ± | ± |
| | Iridodonesis | | ± | ± | ± | ± |
| | Myopia | | ± | ± | ± | ± |
| Hematological | Thromboembolism | | ± | ± | ± | ± |
| Musculoskeletal | Arachnodactyly | | | ± | ± | ± |
| | Genu valgum | | | ± | ± | ± |
| | Kyphosis | | | ± | ± | ± |
| | Marfanoid features | | | ± | ± | ± |
| | Osteoporosis | | ± | ± | ± | ± |
| | Pes cavus | | | ± | ± | ± |
| | Scoliosis | | | ± | ± | ± |
| | Sternal deformities | | | ± | ± | ± |
| Laboratory findings | Cystathionine by LC-MS/MS or GC-MS/MS (plasma) | n-↓↓ | n-↓↓ | n-↓↓ | n-↓↓ | n-↓↓ |
| | Cysteine, total (plasma) | ↓↓ | ↓↓ | ↓↓ | ↓↓ | ↓↓ |
| | Cystine (plasma) | ↓↓ | ↓↓ | ↓↓ | ↓↓ | ↓↓ |
| | Homocystine (plasma, urine) | ↑-↑↑ | ↑-↑↑ | ↑-↑↑ | ↑-↑↑ | ↑-↑↑ |
| | Homocysteine, total (DBS) | ↑-↑↑↑ | ↑-↑↑↑ | ↑-↑↑↑ | ↑-↑↑↑ | ↑-↑↑↑ |
| | Homocysteine, total (plasma) | ↑-↑↑↑ | ↑-↑↑↑ | ↑-↑↑↑ | ↑-↑↑↑ | ↑-↑↑↑ |
| | Methionine (DBS) | n-↑↑ | n-↑↑ | n-↑↑ | n-↑↑ | n-↑↑ |
| | Methionine (plasma) | n-↑↑ | n-↑↑ | n-↑↑ | n-↑↑ | n-↑↑ |
| | Methionine-to-cystathionine ratio | ↑-↑↑↑ | ↑-↑↑↑ | ↑-↑↑↑ | ↑-↑↑↑ | ↑-↑↑↑ |
| | Methionine-to-phenylalanine ratio (DBS) | n-↑↑ | n-↑↑ | n-↑↑ | n-↑↑ | n-↑↑ |
| | Methionine-to-total homocysteine ratio | ↓ | ↓ | ↓ | ↓ | ↓ |
| | Nitroprusside test (urine) | | ↑ | ↑ | ↑ | ↑ |
| | *S*-Adenosylhomocysteine (plasma) | ↑-↑↑ | ↑-↑↑ | ↑-↑↑ | ↑-↑↑ | ↑-↑↑ |
| | *S*-Adenosylmethionine (plasma) | ↑↑ | ↑↑ | ↑↑ | ↑↑ | ↑↑ |
| | Sarcosine (plasma) | ↑-↑↑ | ↑-↑↑ | ↑-↑↑ | ↑-↑↑ | ↑-↑↑ |

**Table 22.7** Cystathionase deficiency

| System | Symptoms and biomarkers | Neonatal (birth–1 month) | Infancy (1–18 months) | Childhood (1.5–11 years) | Adolescence (11–16 years) | Adulthood (>16 years) |
|---|---|---|---|---|---|---|
| Other | No clinical significance | + | + | + | + | + |
| Laboratory findings | Cystathionine (plasma) | ↑ | ↑ | ↑ | ↑ | ↑ |
| | Cystathionine (urine) | ↑↑ | ↑↑ | ↑↑ | ↑↑ | ↑↑ |
| | Cystathionine by GC-MS or LC-MS/MS (plasma) | ↑↑↑ | ↑↑↑ | ↑↑↑ | ↑↑↑ | ↑↑↑ |
| | Cystathionine by GC-MS or LC-MS/MS (urine) | ↑↑↑ | ↑↑↑ | ↑↑↑ | ↑↑↑ | ↑↑↑ |
| | Cysteine, total (plasma) | n | n | n | n | n |
| | Homocysteine, total (plasma) | n-↑ | n-↑ | n-↑ | n-↑ | n-↑ |
| | Methionine-to-cystathionine ratio | ↓↓ | ↓↓ | ↓↓ | ↓↓ | ↓↓ |

**Table 22.8** Methanethiol oxidase deficiency

| System | Symptoms and biomarkers | Neonatal (birth–1 month)[a] | Infancy (1–18 months)[a] | Childhood (1.5–11 years) | Adolescence (11–16 years) | Adulthood (>16 years) |
|---|---|---|---|---|---|---|
| Other | Cabbage-like smelling breath | ±-+ | ±-+ | ±-+ | ±-+ | ±-+ |
| Laboratory findings | Dimethylsulfide (breath, blood) | | | ↑↑ | ↑↑ | ↑↑ |
| | Dimethylsulfoxide (blood) | | | ↑↑ | ↑↑ | ↑↑ |
| | Methanethiol (breath) | | | ↑↑ | ↑↑ | ↑↑ |

[a]Metabolite levels not yet reported in these age groups, however, expected to be similar to other age groups

**Table 22.9** Sulfite oxidase deficiency

| System | Symptoms and biomarkers | Neonatal (birth–1 month) | Infancy (1–18 months) | Childhood (1.5–11 years) | Adolescence (11–16 years) | Adulthood (>16 years)[a] |
|---|---|---|---|---|---|---|
| CNS | Acute hemiplegia | | | ± | ± | ± |
| | Axial hypotonia | ± | + | + | ± | ± |
| | Cerebellar atrophy (MRI) | ± | + | + | + | + |
| | Cerebral atrophy (MRI) | ± | + | + | + | + |
| | Cystic white matter changes | ± | + | + | + | + |
| | Microcephaly | ± | + | + | + | + |
| | Movement, abnormal | ± | + | + | + | + |
| | Peripheral hypertonia | ± | + | + | ± | ± |
| | Retardation, psychomotor | ±-+++ | +-+++ | +-+++ | +-+++ | +-+++ |
| | Seizures, pharmacoresistant | ±-+++ | ±-+++ | ±-+++ | ±-+++ | ±-+++ |
| | Ventriculomegaly (brain) | ± | + | + | + | + |
| Digestive | Feeding difficulties | ±-+ | ±-+ | ±-+ | ±-+ | ±-+ |
| Eye | Ectopia lentis | | ± | ± | ± | ± |
| Laboratory findings | Alpha-aminoadipic semi-aldehyde (cerebrospinal fluid) | ↑ | ↑ | ↑ | | |
| | Alpha-aminosemialde-hyde (urine) | ↑ | ↑ | ↑ | | |
| | Homocysteine, total (plasma) | ↓ | ↓ | ↓ | ↓ | ↓ |
| | Methionine (plasma) | n | n | n | n | n |
| | Pipecolic acid (cerebro-spinal fluid) | ↑ | ↑ | ↑ | | |
| | Pyridoxal 5′-phosphate (cerebrospinal fluid) | ↓ | ↓ | ↓ | | |
| | *S*-Sulfocysteine (plasma) | ↑-↑↑ | ↑-↑↑ | ↑-↑↑ | ↑-↑↑ | ↑-↑↑ |
| | *S*-Sulfocysteine (urine) | ↑-↑↑ | ↑-↑↑ | ↑-↑↑ | ↑-↑↑ | ↑-↑↑ |
| | Sulfite (plasma, urine) | ↑-↑↑ | ↑-↑↑ | ↑-↑↑ | ↑-↑↑ | ↑-↑↑ |
| | Taurine (plasma, urine) | ↑-↑↑ | ↑-↑↑ | ↑-↑↑ | ↑-↑↑ | ↑-↑↑ |
| | Thiosulfate (plasma, urine) | ↑↑ | ↑↑ | ↑↑ | ↑↑ | ↑↑ |
| | Uric acid (plasma) | n | n | n | – | – |
| | Uric acid (urine) | n | n | n | – | – |

[a]Data on patients who are alive after age of 16 years are so scarce that the information in that column is only extrapolation from the column of the previous age group

**Table 22.10** Mitochondrial sulfur dioxygenase deficiency

| System | Symptoms and biomarkers | Neonatal (birth–1 month)[a] | Infancy (1–18 months) | Childhood (1.5–11 years) | Adolescence (11–16 years) | Adulthood (>16 years) |
|---|---|---|---|---|---|---|
| Cardiovascular | Orthostatic acrocyanosis | | ±-+++ | ±-+++ | ±-+++ | |
| CNS | Axial hypotonia | ±-++ | +-+++ | +-+++ | +-+++ | |
| | Dystonia | | +-++ | +-++ | +-++ | |
| | Hyperintense lesions in the basal ganglia on MRI (Leigh-like encephalopathy) | | +-+++ | +-+++ | | |
| | Hyperintense patchy T2 changes on MRI in the white matter, brain stem and cerebellum | | ±-+++ | ±-+++ | | |
| | Retardation, psychomotor | | +++ | +++ | +++ | |
| | Seizures | | +-++ | +-++ | +-++ | |
| | Spastic tetraplegia | | +++ | +++ | +++ | |
| Dermatological | Petechiae | | ±-+++ | ±-+++ | ±-+++ | |
| Digestive | Hemorrhagic diarrhea, chronic | | +-+++ | +-+++ | +-+++ | |
| Metabolic | Hematuria | | + | + | + | |
| Other | Failure to thrive | | +-+++ | +-+++ | +-+++ | |
| Laboratory findings | 2-Methylbutyrylglycine (urine) | | ↑↑ | ↑↑ | | |
| | C4 Butyrylcarnitine (plasma, DBS) | ↑↑ | ↑↑ | ↑↑ | | |
| | C4 Isobutyrylcarnitine (plasma, DBS) | | ↑ | ↑ | | |
| | C5 2-Methylbutyrylcarnitine (plasma, DBS) | | ↑ | ↑ | | |
| | C5 Isovalerylcarnitine (plasma, DBS) | | ↑ | ↑ | | |
| | C5-DC Glutarylcarnitine (plasma, DBS) | ↑↑ | ↑↑ | ↑↑ | ↑↑ | ↑↑ |
| | Ethylmalonic acid (urine) | ↑↑ | ↑↑↑ | ↑↑↑ | | |
| | Hydrogen sulfide (plasma) | ↑-↑↑ | ↑-↑↑ | ↑-↑↑ | | |
| | Isovalerylglycine (urine) | | ↑ | ↑ | | |
| | Lactate (plasma) | | ↑↑ | ↑↑ | | |
| | Methylsuccinic acid (urine) | | ↑↑ | ↑↑ | | |
| | *S*-sulfocysteine (urine) | | n-↑ | n-↑ | | |
| | Sulfite (plasma, urine) | ↑↑ | ↑↑ | ↑↑ | | |
| | Taurine (plasma, urine) | | ↑ | ↑ | | |
| | Thiosulfate (plasma, urine) | | ↑↑↑ | ↑↑↑ | | |

Milder course with less expressed neurological signs and symptoms, lack of vascular symptoms, and survival in adulthood is very exceptional. To avoid confusion with much more frequent severe course, this milder form of the disease was not the basis for symbols entered in the table
[a]Metabolite levels not yet reported in these age groups, however, expected to be similar to other age groups

**Table 22.11** Mercaptopyruvate sulfur transferase deficiency

| System | Symptoms and biomarkers | Neonatal (birth–1 month)[a] | Infancy (1–18 months)[a] | Childhood (1.5–11 years) | Adolescence (11–16 years) | Adulthood (>16 years) |
|---|---|---|---|---|---|---|
| CNS | Intellectual disability | | | | ± | ± |
| Laboratory findings | Beta-mercaptolactate cysteine disulfide (urine) | | | | ↑ | |
| | Mercaptopyruvate (urine) | | | | | ↑ |
| | Mercaptolactate (urine) | | | | | ↑ |
| | Nitroprusside test (urine) | | | | ↑ | ↑ |

[a]Metabolite levels not yet reported in these age groups, however, expected to be similar to other age groups

## Reference Values[a]

| Analyte | Infant <1 year | Child 1–12 years | Adolescent 12–18 years | Adult >18 years |
|---|---|---|---|---|
| **Plasma amino acids** (μmol/L) | | | | |
| Methionine | 12–31 | 11–30 | 16–23 | 15–40 |
| Homocystine | Below detection limit (approx. 5 μmol/L) | | | |
| Cystathionine | Below detection limit (approx. 5 μmol/L) | | | |
| Taurine | 15–200 | 19–139 | 10–162 | 6–126 |
| *S*-sulfocysteine | Below detection limit (approx. 5 μmol/L) | | | |
| **Special assays in plasma or blood** (in blood where indicated in brackets) (μmol/L) | | | | |
| Total homocysteine | 3.5–10 | 4–10 | 4–13 | 5–15 |
| Total cysteine | 200–360 (not age stratified) | | | |
| Sarcosine | 0.6–2.5 (not age stratified) | | | |
| *S*-adenosylmethionine | 0.03–0.16 (not age stratified) | | | |
| *S*-adenosylhomocysteine | 0.015–0.06 (not age stratified) | | | |
| Cystathionine (by sensitive GC-MS or LC-MS/MS assays) | 0.08–0.5 (up to 1 in neonates) | | | |
| Methionine-to-cystathionine ratio | 40–200 (not age stratified) | | | |
| Thiosulfate | 0.4–0.7 (not age stratified) | | | |
| Sulfite | 0.2–0.5 (not age stratified) | | | |
| Free sulfide (hydrogen sulfide) | 0.15–0.3 (not age stratified) | | | |
| Dimethylsulfide (blood) | <0.007 (not age stratified) | | | |
| Dimethylsulfoxide (blood) | <1 (not age stratified) | | | |
| Lactate (blood) | Reference ranges for lactate in blood are shown in Chap. 42 of this book | | | |
| **Dried blood spots** (μmol/L blood) | | | | |
| Methionine | 7–40 (not age stratified) | | | |
| Methionine/phenylalanine | 0.15–0.6 | | | |
| Total homocysteine | 2.5–9 | | 5.5–9 | 8–13 |
| Methionine-to-total homocysteine ratio | 2–4 (not age stratified) | | | |
| **Reference ranges for acylcarnitines in dried blood spots are shown in Chap. 5 of this book** | | | | |
| **Urinary amino acids** (mmol/mol creatinine) | | | | |
| Methionine | 7–29 | 5–20 | 3–17 | 2–16 |
| Cystathionine | Usually below detection limit (not age stratified) | | | |
| Homocystine | 0.2–3.7 (not age stratified) | | | |
| **Reference ranges for organic acids in urine are shown in Chap. 4 of this book** | | | | |
| **Urinary special assays** (mmol/mol creatinine) | | | | |
| Total cysteine | 10–50 (not age stratified) | | | |
| Total homocysteine | 1–4 (not age stratified) | | | |
| Thiosulfate | 0.8–2.5 (not age stratified) | | | |
| Sulfite | 0.03–0.15 (not age stratified) | | | |
| *S*-sulfocysteine | 0.3–1 (not age stratified) | | | |
| **Simple tests in urine (qualitative test)** | | | | |
| Nitroprusside test | Negative (not age stratified) | | | |
| **Exhaled air (ppb)** | | | | |
| Dimethylsulfide | 1–19 (not age stratified) | | | |
| Methanethiol | 0.01–0.24 (not age stratified) | | | |

[a]Table shows typical values from literature (Duran et al. 2008, Chap. 2 of this book) and authors' laboratories; due to the lack of harmonization and the use of different analytical platforms for many of the metabolites listed, these reference ranges are not universally applicable. Therefore, it is important to use the reference ranges given by the laboratory which issued the results. Reference ranges can be also found in the Human Metabolome Database (see Sect. 22.17 Online Resources)

## Pathological Values[a,b,c]

| Metabolites | 22.1[b] MAT I/III | 22.3 GNMT | 22.4 SAHH | 22.5 ADK | 22.6 CBS | 22.7 CTH | 22.8 MTO | 22.9 SUOX | 22.10 ETHE1 | 22.11 MPST |
|---|---|---|---|---|---|---|---|---|---|---|
| **Plasma amino acids** | | | | | | | | | | |
| Methionine | ↑↑↑ | ↑↑↑ | n-↑↑ | n-↑↑↑ | n-↑↑↑ | n | n | | | |
| Homocystine | | | | | ↑-↑↑↑ | | | | | |
| Cystathionine | | | | | | ↑ | | | | |
| Taurine | | | | | | | | ↑-↑↑ | ↑ | |
| *S*-sulfocysteine | | | | | | | | ↑-↑↑ | | |
| **Plasma acylcarnitines** | | | | | | | | | | |
| C4 butyrylcarnitine | | | | | | | | | ↑↑ | |
| C4 isobutyrylcarnitine | | | | | | | | | ↑ | |
| C5 2-methylbutyrylcarnitine | | | | | | | | | ↑ | |
| C5 isovalerylcarnitine | | | | | | | | | ↑ | |
| Glutarylcarnitine | | | | | | | | | ↑ | |
| **Special assays in plasma or blood** (in blood where indicated in brackets) | | | | | | | | | | |
| Total homocysteine | n-↑ | n-↑ | n-↑ | n-↑ | ↑-↑↑↑ | n-↑ | | ↓ | n-↓ | |
| Total cysteine | | | | | ↓↓ | n | | ↓ | | |
| Sarcosine | n-↑ | n | n-↑ | | ↑-↑↑ | | | | | |
| *S*-adenosylmethionine | n-↓ | ↑↑↑ | ↑↑↑ | ↑-↑↑ | ↑↑ | | | | | |
| *S*-adenosylhomocysteine | | | ↑↑↑ | ↑-↑↑ | ↑-↑↑ | | | | | |
| Cystathionine (by sensitive GC-MS or LC-MS/MS assays) | | | | | n-↓↓ | ↑↑↑ | | | | |
| Methionine-to-cystathionine ratio | ↑↑ | | | | ↑-↑↑↑ | ↓↓ | | | | |
| Thiosulfate | | | | | | | | ↑↑ | ↑↑ | |
| Sulfite | | | | | | | | ↑↑ | ↑↑ | |
| Free sulfide (hydrogen sulfide) | | | | | | | | ↑ | ↑↑ | |
| Lactate (blood) | | | | | | | | | ↑ | |
| Dimethylsulfoxide (blood) | | | | | | | ↑↑ | | | |
| Dimethylsulfide (blood) | | | | | | | ↑↑ | | | |
| **Dried blood spots** | | | | | | | | | | |
| Methionine | ↑↑-↑↑↑ | | | | n-↑↑ | | | | | |
| Methionine/phenylalanine | ↑↑-↑↑↑ | | | | n-↑↑ | | | | | |
| Total homocysteine | n | | | | ↑-↑↑↑ | | | | | |
| Methionine-to-total homocysteine | ↑↑ | | | | ↓ | | | | | |
| Adenosine | | | | n-↑ | | | | | | |
| C4 butyrylcarnitine | | | | | | | | | ↑↑ | |
| C4 isobutyrylcarnitine | | | | | | | | | ↑ | |
| C5 2-methylbutyrylcarnitine | | | | | | | | | ↑ | |
| C5 isovalerylcarnitine | | | | | | | | | ↑ | |
| Glutarylcarnitine | | | | | | | | | ↑ | |
| **Urinary amino acids** | | | | | | | | | | |
| Methionine | ↑↑↑ | ↑↑↑ | n-↑↑ | ↑↑ | n-↑↑ | | | | | |
| Cystathionine | | | | | n-↓ | ↑↑ | | | | |
| Homocystine | | | | | ↑-↑↑↑ | | | | | |
| **Organic acids in urine** | | | | | | | | | | |
| Ethylmalonic acid | | | | | | | | | ↑↑-↑↑↑ | |
| 2-Methylbutyrylglycine | | | | | | | | | ↑↑ | |
| Methylsuccinic acid | | | | | | | | | ↑↑ | |
| Isovalerylglycine | | | | | | | | | ↑ | |
| **Urinary special assays** | | | | | | | | | | |
| Total homocysteine | | | | | ↑-↑↑↑ | n-↑ | | | | |
| Thiosulfate | | | | | | | | ↑↑↑ | ↑↑ | |
| Sulfite | | | | | | | | ↑↑↑ | ↑↑ | |
| *S*-sulfocysteine | | | | | | | | ↑-↑↑ | n-↑ | |
| Adenosine | | | | n-↑ | | | | | | |

| Metabolites | 22.1[b] MAT I/ III | 22.3 GNMT | 22.4 SAHH | 22.5 ADK | 22.6 CBS | 22.7 CTH | 22.8 MTO | 22.9 SUOX | 22.10 ETHE1 | 22.11 MPST |
|---|---|---|---|---|---|---|---|---|---|---|
| Alpha-aminosemialdehyde | | | | | | | | ↑ | | |
| Mercaptolactate, mercaptopyruvate | | | | | | | | | | ↑↑ |
| Mercaptocysteine disulfide | | | | | | | | | | ↑↑ |
| **Simple tests in urine** | | | | | | | | | | |
| Nitroprusside test[d] | | | | | Positive | | | | | Positive |
| **Exhaled air** | | | | | | | | | | |
| Dimethylsulfide | | | | | | ↑↑ | | | | |
| Methanethiol | | | | | | ↑↑ | | | | |
| **Special assays in cerebrospinal fluid** | | | | | | | | | | |
| Pipecolic acid | | | | | | | | ↑ | | |
| Pyridoxal 5′-phosphate | | | | | | | | ↓ | | |

[a]Pathological values may vary in different age groups and disease forms; for details, see Tables 22.1–22.11

[b]There are no specific biochemical abnormalities in individuals with thoracic aortic aneurysms who are heterozygotes for *MAT2A* mutations. Therefore, related column is not provided

[c]Normal values are denoted by "n" only when particularly important for differential diagnosis. Blank cells indicate that the metabolite is within reference range or that data are not available

[d]Nitroprusside test has limited reliability due to false-negative results

## Diagnostic Flowcharts

Since most of the mentioned diseases are at least partly treatable if diagnosed early and may have rapid course, the *diagnostic work-up* in suspected cases should also be rapid. Suspicion should be raised in all patients having unexplained neurological symptoms, muscle disease, liver disease, lens dislocation and other marfanoid features, orthostatic acrocyanosis, or any other symptom attributable to diseases from this group or unexplained hypermethioninemia and/or hyperhomocysteinemia or hypohomocysteinemia (see Sect. 22.4). Measurement of plasma total homocysteine and amino acids (methionine, taurine, and *S*-sulfocysteine) and special tests for sarcosine, cystathionine, *S*-adenosylmethionine, and *S*-adenosylhomocysteine should be sufficient as the first step to detect all diseases from this group; sulfite and thiosulfate analysis is necessary for diagnosing disorders in the distal part of transsulfuration pathway (for differential diagnosis of hypermethioninemia and hypo- and hyperhomocysteinemia, see Diagnostic flowcharts, Figs. 22.2 and 22.3).

It is useful to keep in mind that in MAT I/III deficiency homocysteine can be sufficiently elevated to mimic CBS deficiency, probably due to less than normal stimulation of CBS by low AdoMet and inhibition of betaine-homocysteine methyltransferase, $N^5$-*methyltetrahydrofolate-homocysteine* methyltransferase and cystathionine gamma-lyase by methionine, in particular in patients with very high methionine values (Stabler et al. 2002). Mild elevations of tHcy, which can be diagnostically misleading, have also been described in other methylation defects and in CTH deficiency.

*Pyridoxine responsiveness test in CBS deficiency.* This test is performed in patients with CBS deficiency to assess pyridoxine responsiveness. Recent guidelines recommended standard tests in patients detected symptomatically using 10 mg/kg/day pyridoxine (maximum of 500 mg/day) for 6 weeks; the plasma tHcy concentration should be measured at least twice before treatment and twice on treatment (by the end of weeks 2 and 6). The test should be done on normal protein intake, folate supplements should be given, and vitamin $B_{12}$ deficiency should be corrected prior to testing. Classification of pyridoxine responsiveness is as follows: full responsiveness, plasma tHcy levels below 50 μmol/L; extreme responsiveness, tHcy below 50 μmol/L on pyridoxine doses <1 mg/kg/day; partial responsiveness, tHcy falls >20% of pre-test average but above 50 μmol/L; and non-responsiveness, tHcy falls by <20% (Morris et al. 2017).

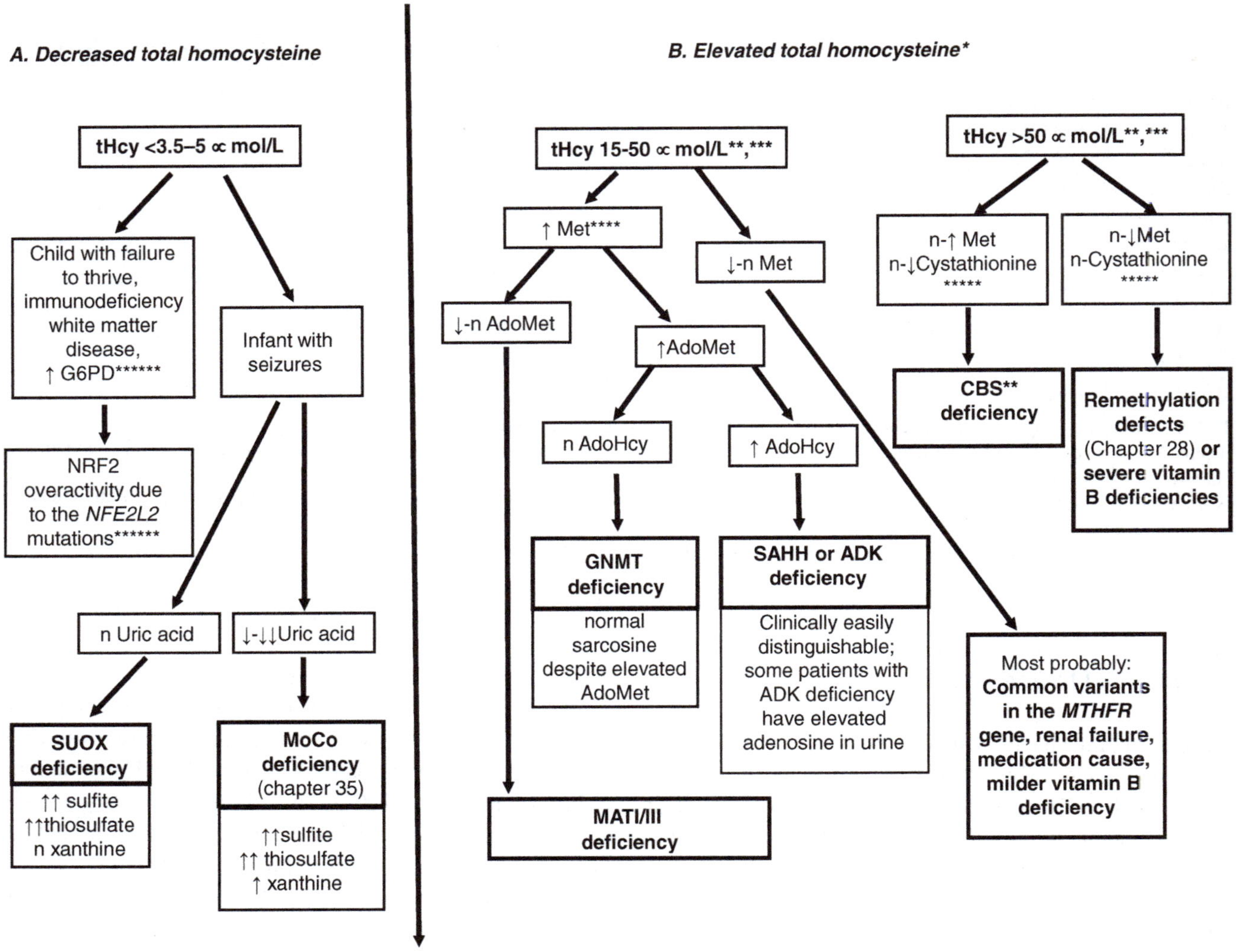


**Fig. 22.2** Diagnostic flowchart for hypo- (**a**) and hyperhomocysteinemia (**b**). * tHcy range of 5–15 μmol/L is used here as reference range for all ages; actually, in children the upper limit of reference range is lower (see Reference Values). ** In non-treated CBS deficiency, tHcy is usually significantly >50 μmol/L but may be lower in mild cases, in particular when on vitamin supplementation (even non-pharmacological doses of pyridoxine). *** In non-CBS hypermethioninemias, tHcy is usually normal or only mildly elevated, and values of about 50 μmol/L are exceptionally seen. **** In ADK and SAHH deficiency, plasma methionine concentrations can occasionally be normal, for instance, in SAHH deficiency in early infancy during lower methionine intake and higher needs for growth. ***** Cystathionine for differential diagnosis of hyperhomocysteinemia cannot be detected by amino acid analyzers and must be determined by sensitive GC-MS or LC-MS/MS assay. ****** This disease has been reported in only few patients (for details, see Chap. 16), and all abnormalities are not necessarily present in all patients. Mild hypohomocysteinemia (below 3.5–5 μmol/L) is sometimes seen without association with a particular disease. *ADK* adenosine kinase, *AdoHcy* *S*-adenosylhomocysteine, *AdoMet* *S*-adenosylmethionine, *CBS* cystathionine beta synthase, *GNMT* glycine *N*-methyltransferase, *G6PD* glucose-6-phosphate dehydrogenase, *MAT I/III* methionine adenosyltransferase I/III, *Met* methionine, *MoCo* molybdenum cofactor, *MTHFR* methylenetetrahydrofolate reductase, *NFE2L2* nuclear factor, erythroid 2 like 2, *NRF2* nuclear factor-erythroid 2-related factor 2, *SAHH* *S*-adenosylhomocysteine hydrolase, *SUOX* sulfite oxidase, *tHcy* plasma total homocysteine

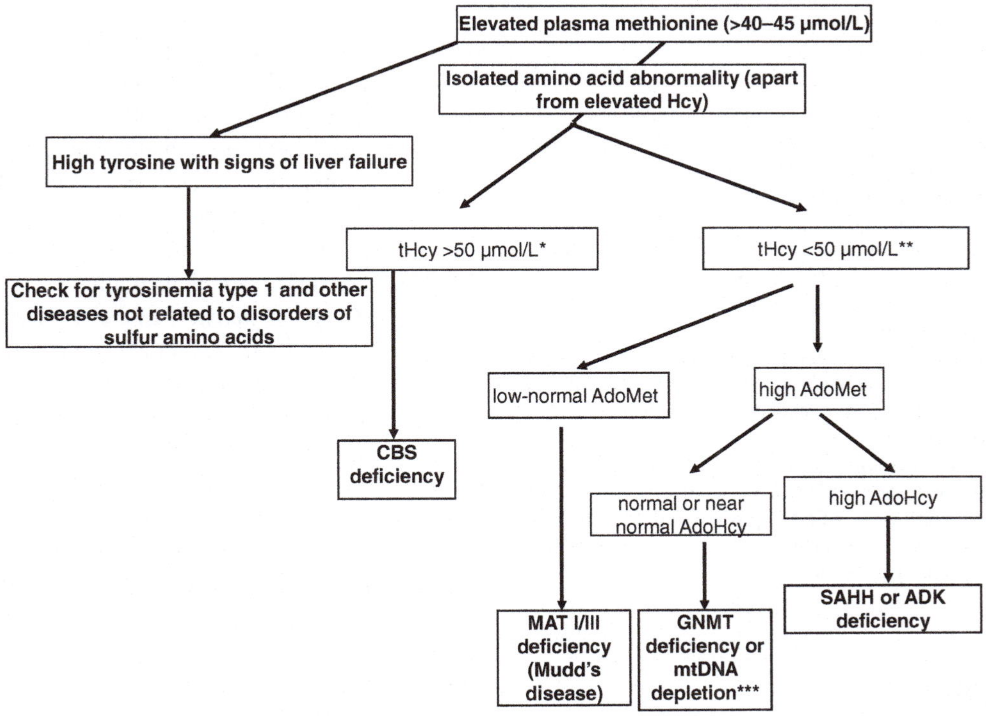


**Fig. 22.3** Diagnostic flowchart in patients with hypermethioninemia. *In untreated CBS deficiency, tHcy is usually >50 µmol/L but may be lower in mild cases, in particular when on vitamin supplementation (non-pharmacological doses). **In non-CBS deficiency hypermethioninemias, tHcy is usually normal or only mildly elevated, and values of about 50 µmol/L are rarely seen. ***Tyrosine can be elevated. *ADK* adenosine kinase, *AdoHcy* S-adenosylhomocysteine, *AdoMet* S-adenosylmethionine, *CBS* cystathionine beta synthase, *GNMT* glycine *N*-methyltransferase, *MAT I/III* methionine adenosyltransferase I/III, *mtDNA* mitochondrial DNA, *SAHH* S-adenosylhomocysteine hydrolase, *tHcy* plasma total homocysteine

## Loading Test

Increase of plasma dimethylsulfone and dimethylsulfoxide in methionine loading test in patients suspected to suffer from extraoral halitosis due to methanethiol oxidase deficiency can point to the cause of the disease. The methionine loading test became obsolete in diagnosis of sulfur-containing amino acids disorders.

## Specimen Collection

Overview on required samples for metabolite, enzyme, and mutation analysis

| Disorder | Metabolite: sample |
|---|---|
| | Amino acids (including taurine): plasma or serum[a] and urine |
| | Organic acids: urine |
| | Acylcarnitines: dried blood spots and plasma/serum |
| | **Special assays** |
| CBS, CTH, SUOX | Total homocysteine and total cysteine: plasma[b] and urine |
| Disorder | Metabolite: sample |
| MATI/III, GNMT, ADK, CBS | *S*-adenosylmethionine: plasma[c], whole blood |
| MATI/III, GNMT, ADK, CBS | *S*-adenosylhomocysteine: plasma[c], whole blood |
| SUOX, ETHE | Thiosulfate: plasma and urine[d,e] |
| SUOX, ETHE | Sulfite: plasma and urine[d,e] |
| SUOX, ETHE | Free sulfide (hydrogen sulfide): plasma[d] |
| MTO | Methanethiol and dimethylsulfide in exhaled air |
| CBS | Methionine, Met/Phe and tHcy in dried blood spots |
| | Other assays: plasma, blood or urine (may require special sampling conditions, consult the laboratory) |
| | **Enzyme assays[f]: specimen** |
| MAT I/III | Liver[g] |
| GNMT | Liver[g] |
| SAHH | Cultured fibroblasts, erythrocytes, liver |
| ADK | Not available |
| CBS | Cultured fibroblasts and plasma[a] |
| CTH | Liver[g] |
| SUOX | Cultured fibroblasts |
| ETHE1 | Not available |
| MPST | Erythrocytes |
| MTO | Erythrocytes |

| Disorder | Metabolite: sample |
|---|---|
| | **Mutation analysis** |
| All disorders | DNA |

[a]Blood for plasma amino acids analysis should be sampled after 3–4 h fasting. For taurine determination only plasma should be used and handled as in [b]. Rapid deproteinization is essential for determination of non-protein bound homocysteine (this analysis is considered obsolete and should be replaced by total homocysteine determination)
[b]Samples should be immediately placed into ice/water slush, separation of plasma within 60 min since collection is essential
[c]EDTA blood on ice, immediate separation of plasma and deproteinization (within 30 min since collection)
[d]Plasma: only lithium heparin plasma should be collected, samples should be immediately placed into ice/water slush, separation of plasma within 15 min since collection, and immediate freezing prior to analysis at −85 °C is essential
[e]Urine: only freshly collected urine should be used for analysis, immediate freezing prior to analysis at −85 °C is essential
[f]In general, enzymatic work-up as a first step is advised. In some cases (common mutation or small gene), mutation analysis as first step
[g]Liver biopsy is not routinely justified

## Prenatal Diagnosis

Prenatal diagnosis is only relevant for SAHH, ADK, CBS, ETHE1, and SUOX deficiencies. Generally the first choice of method for each of these is mutation analysis in chorionic villous material provided that disease-causing mutations and their parental origin have been confirmed. Alternatively, enzyme assay in cultured amniocytes can be performed in some diseases.

## DNA Testing

All genes in this chapter are known, and mutation analysis of genomic DNA isolated from peripheral blood, chorionic villi, amniocytes, or other cells is feasible. Sanger sequencing of individual genes or next-generation sequencing of gene panels are used. For mutations suspected to affect splicing, mRNA analysis in appropriate tissues may be necessary.

## Treatment Summary

The general treatment goal for disorders of sulfur amino acid and hydrogen sulfide metabolism is correcting biochemical abnormalities in order to suppress their adverse effects. This causal treatment primarily consists in various combinations of high doses of cofactors, low-protein or low-methionine or low-cysteine diet, and supplementation of metabolites behind the enzymatic block. Betaine is an additional means to decrease homocysteine concentration.

In *MAT I/III deficiency*, methionine restriction is indicated in symptomatic patients and those with brain imaging changes. It is justified also in asymptomatic patients with severe deficiency and plasma methionine >500–800 µmol/L. AdoMet supplementation may be necessary. It seems that *GNMT deficiency*, *cystathionase deficiency*, and *autosomal dominant MATI/III deficiency* do not require treatment. In *AdoHcy hydrolase deficiency*, low-methionine diet can decrease plasma AdoMet and AdoHcy, with a positive effect on methylation and clinical and biochemical abnormalities (Barić et al. 2005). Phosphatidylcholine, creatine, and cysteine supplementation may be useful. Liver transplantation seemed beneficial in one patient with short follow-up. *CBS-deficient* patients are treated with varying doses of pyridoxine if responsive in the pyridoxine test. Folate and cobalamin should be added to avoid vitamin depletion and stimulate homocysteine remethylation. Betaine and/or a low-methionine diet (sometimes with methionine-free/cystine-enriched amino acid mixture) may also be needed in partial responders but necessary in pyridoxine nonresponsive patients. In *isolated sulfite oxidase deficiency*, partial success with low-protein diet combined with methionine- and cysteine-free amino acid mixture has been reported only in late-onset patients (Touati et al. 2000). Low methionine diet may ameliorate the liver phenotype in *adenosine kinase deficiency*. For *MATII deficiency and mercaptopyruvate sulfurtransferase deficiency*, no successful causal treatment has been reported. In *ethylmalonic encephalopathy*, metronidazole and *N*-acetylcysteine may reduce some symptoms. Early liver transplantation may be an option to reverse otherwise unfavorable outcome. In *MTO deficiency*, metronidazole can reduce methanethiol production by gut bacteria.

## Emergency Treatment

### Methionine Adenosyltransferase I/III Deficiency (AR and ADa forms)

If unexplained neurological signs are present with very high methionine level, discontinuance of methionine intake for 1–3 days followed by low-methionine diet until symptoms disappear, in combination with AdoMet supplementation (for instance, at a dose of 400 mg twice daily, Surtees et al.

1991), seems to be indicated. See also the comment [b] below the standard treatment table.

### *S*-Adenosylhomocysteine Hydrolase Deficiency

Severe cases, such as those presenting with fetal hydrops, insufficiency of liver synthetic function, and severe muscular hypotonia leading to respiratory insufficiency, may potentially benefit from strict methionine restriction and choline and cysteine supplementation in combination with vigorous symptomatic treatment.

### Ethylmalonic Encephalopathy

Continuous renal replacement therapy may help to reestablish metabolic control during acute metabolic decompensations in patients on chronic treatment with *N*-acetylcysteine and metronidazole (Kitzler et al. 2019).

For other disorders from this group, emergency situations amenable to specific disease-related emergency treatment are not likely. A diet low in protein and an amino acid mixture without cystine and methionine may be helpful in mild sulfite oxidase deficiency.

## Standard Treatment

| Disease | Comment | Medication/diet | Dosage[a] | Goals |
|---|---|---|---|---|
| **22.1** MAT I/III deficiency | For the autosomal dominant form of the disease, treatment does not seem to be indicated<br>For the autosomal recessive form, if plasma methionine concentrations are above risky level (clear risk above 800 µmol/L, existing risk above 500–600 µmol/L), a methionine-restricted diet is recommended<br>If the mean plasma methionine is below 500–600 µmol/L, treatment does not seem to be indicated | Low-methionine diet | In infancy ~15–20 mg of methionine/kg/day; later less as expressed in mg/kg/day and according to clinical and biochemical parameters | Disappearance/prevention of clinical symptoms<br>Normalization of brain imaging findings<br>The aim of the diet is to maintain methionine levels around 500–600 µmol/L, even in asymptomatic individuals<br>It should be borne in mind that lowering plasma methionine below 500 µmol/L in patients with some residual MAT I/III activity may further limit the flux through MAT I/III and further decrease the availability of AdoMet (Mudd et al. 2001) |
| | AdoMet supplementation, especially if methionine intake is limited, may be necessary | *S*-adenosylmethionine | 2–3 × 400 mg daily per os[b] | Clinical improvement, normalization of plasma and/or CSF AdoMet; normalization of hyperhomocysteinemia |
| **22.2** Methionine adenosyltransferase II deficiency | No causal treatment; surgery and other measures according to risk assessment of thoracic aorta aneurysm development | | | |
| **22.3** GNMT deficiency | There is no evidence that therapy is necessary; low-methionine diet can correct biochemical abnormalities. It may be indicated when plasma methionine reaches values above 500–600 µmol/L, which may be risky regardless of cause | Low-methionine diet | In infancy ~15–20 mg of methionine/kg/day; later less as expressed in mg/kg/day and according to clinical and biochemical parameters | Correction of biochemical abnormalities and potential neurological problems due to high hypermethioninemia |
| **22.4** AHCY deficiency | Due to small number of patients, these recommendations are based only on pathogenetic hypotheses and limited clinical experience<br>Liver transplantation seemed beneficial in one patient with a short follow-up | Low-methionine diet | In infancy natural protein intake containing ~10–20 mg/kg/day of methionine, depending on the severity of the disease and biochemical findings, in combination with methionine-free amino acid mixture to meet needs for proteins | Clinical improvement and decrease of AdoMet and AdoHcy as close to normal values as possible, while avoiding protein malnutrition |

| Disease | Comment | Medication/diet | Dosage[a] | Goals |
|---|---|---|---|---|
| | | Phosphatidylcholine | 3 × 600–1200 mg/day | Avoidance of possible phosphatidylcholine and choline deficiency |
| | | *N*-acetylcysteine | 3 × 100–200 mg/day | Avoidance of possible glutathione deficiency |
| | | Creatine (may be useful theoretically) | 3–5 g/day | Avoidance of possible creatine deficiency |
| **22.5** ADK deficiency | Low methionine diet should be considered as a therapeutic option, since it ameliorates the liver phenotype clinically and biochemically. Positive effect on the neurological outcome has only been reported in a single case. Diazoxide is recommended for recurrent hypoglycemia when it is due to hyperinsulinism (Barić et al. 2017) | Low methionine diet | Daily intake of 15–20 mg of methionine per kg of body weight in infants and small children; later less as expressed in mg/kg/day and according to clinical and biochemical parameters | Improvement of clinical and biochemical indices of liver disease |
| **22.6** CBS deficiency[c] | *Test of pyridoxine responsiveness* should be done on normal protein intake at the beginning of the treatment (for details, see above)<br>Before test possible folate and cobalamin deficiency should be corrected to assure proper assessment of the test results | A. Pyridoxine responders and partial responders | | **Clinical targets:** For early diagnosed patients, prevention of all the complications of CBS deficiency while maintaining normal growth and nutrition<br>For late-diagnosed patients, prevention of further complications, especially thromboembolic disease<br>**Biochemical targets**: Maintenance of tHcy concentration as close to normal as possible. In fully responsive patients, standard doses can lead to tHcy levels below 50 μmol/L (and sometimes within the normal range in extreme responsive patients). Some patients who are partially responsive to pyridoxine may be able to achieve a tHcy level below 50 μmol/L if they are also on a low-Met diet; for others it is not a realistic goal. Excessive methionine restriction, with plasma methionine concentrations that are sometimes below the normal range, may impair growth and neurodevelopmental progress in children. In pyridoxine unresponsive patients, it is recommended to keep tHcy levels at least below 100 μmol/L, but this may need revision when very long-term data become available (Morris et al. 2017). Plasma methionine levels in patients treated with betaine should be kept below 800 μmol/L (it is probably safer below 500–600 μmol/L) |
| | | Pyridoxine | The pyridoxine dose should be the lowest that achieves the biochemical targets. Recommended doses are up to 10 mg/kg/day divided into 1–3 doses; doses above 500 mg/day should be avoided | |
| | | Folate[d] | Optimal dose is not known; up to 1 mg/day is probably sufficient if folate deficiency is not present | |
| | | Hydroxocobalamin | Vitamin $B_{12}$ should be monitored and supplemented if deficient | |
| | | Low-methionine diet (for partially responsive patients only) | The degree of methionine or natural protein restriction required varies and is determined for each patient according to their plasma tHcy, methionine, and other parameters | |
| | | Betaine (for partially responsive patients only) | Patients' responses to betaine are variable and optimal doses have to be individualized. For children, the initial betaine dose is 50 mg/kg twice daily. For adults, the starting dose is 3 g twice a day. The dose and frequency are adjusted according to response. There is unlikely to be any benefit in exceeding a dose of 150–200 mg/kg/day | |

| Disease | Comment | Medication/diet | Dosage[a] | Goals |
|---|---|---|---|---|
| | Guidelines for protein intake in methionine-restricted diet are very approximate. Diet must be adjusted, in combination with other measures, to achieve therapeutic goal, if possible, but should not jeopardize the patient; therefore strict monitoring of growth and nutritional indices (including aromatic and branched chain amino acids) is necessary | B. Pyridoxine nonresponders | | |
| | | There is no evidence that long-term pyridoxine is beneficial if there is no biochemical response in a properly conducted test (Morris et al. 2017) | | |
| | | Folate[d] | Optimal dose is not known; less than 1 mg/day is probably sufficient if folate deficiency is not present | |
| | In nearly all CBS-deficient patients, high remethylation activity may lead to folate and/or cobalamin depletion; therefore, folate and cobalamin should be added to the therapy | Cobalamin | Vitamin $B_{12}$ should be monitored and supplemented if deficient | |
| | | Low-methionine diet | Patients may require only isolated mild protein/methionine restriction or more severe restriction combined with amino acid mixture administration. The combined intake of low natural protein and methionine-free/cystine-enriched amino acid mixture (total protein equivalent) should follow the WHO/FAO recommendations (Joint FAO/WHO/UNU Expert Consultation on Protein and Amino Acid Requirements in Human Nutrition 2007). Methionine intake in natural protein depends on age and should be adjusted to maintain plasma tHcy levels <100 μmol/L while avoiding protein over-restriction. This can be typically achieved by prescribing 0.4–1.0 g natural protein/kg/day; however, higher or lower intake may be needed. If diet is based on calculation of methionine intake, appropriate amount may be between 4 and 10 mg/kg/day, with higher needs in infancy, particularly early infancy | |
| | | Betaine | See pyridoxine responders | |

| Disease | Comment | Medication/diet | Dosage[a] | Goals |
|---|---|---|---|---|
| **22.7** CTH deficiency | The disorder seems benign and therapy unnecessary | | | |
| **22.8** Methanethiol oxidase deficiency | There is no standard treatment for this recently described disease, and options provided are based on pathogenesis (low methionine diet, metronidazole) and short trial in a single patient (metronidazole), respectively (Pol et al. 2018). Although an effect is expected from metronidazole, it is not recommended as prophylactic treatment | Metronidazole<br>Low-protein/low methionine diet | Metronidazole: children 20–30 mg/kg/day three times daily; adults 400 mg three times daily (doses provided here are those usually used for anaerobic infections and for this indication may depend on the effect, occasion, and duration of the therapy/prophylaxis)<br>Low-protein/low methionine diet can be considered but should not be over-restrictive so that methionine intake carefully adjusted to avoid harmful effects | To minimize the malodor while avoiding side effects |
| **22.9** Isolated SUOX deficiency | The treatment has been useful only in milder forms of the disease. The diet must be carefully monitored to avoid protein malnutrition. Thiamine and pyridoxine can be added to avoid thiamine and pyridoxal-5-phosphate deficiency due to sulfite accumulation | Low-methionine and low-cysteine diet<br>Dextromethorphan (NMDA receptor antagonist) | Dependent on age and biochemical markers of the disease and protein status<br>Dextromethorphan: 12.5 mg/kg daily (dosage reported in patient with molybdenum cofactor deficiency; largely variable dosage has been reported in nonketotic hyperglycinemia) | Clinical improvement, decrease of toxic metabolites (*S*-sulfocysteine, thiosulfate), to limit excitotoxicity (dextromethorphan) |
| **22.10** Ethylmalonic encephalopathy | Metronidazole and *N*-acetylcysteine may improve metabolic abnormalities (decrease $H_2S$ accumulation and the sulfur atom from $H_2S$, respectively), reduce some symptoms, and slow disease progression | Metronidazole<br>*N*-acetylcysteine | Metronidazole 25–50 mg/kg/day three times daily<br>*N*-acetylcysteine 50–100 mg/kg/day in 2–3 doses | Decrease of $H_2S$ accumulation and assimilation of the sulfur atom from $H_2S$, respectively, reducing some symptoms and slowing disease progression |
| **22.11** Mercaptopyruvate sulfurtransferase deficiency | This condition could be benign | Not reported | – | – |

[a]With the exception of CBS deficiency, given doses are arbitrary and frequently not evaluated in a sufficient number of patients for each given indication; therefore, they must be adjusted individually according to the diagnosis, patients' needs, and results of clinical and biochemical monitoring. A common problem is finding a proper balance between the wish to achieve desired therapeutic goals and avoidance of potentially serious side effects of higher doses than recommended/tested

[b]The dosage and route are only for approximate orientation. Information about AdoMet treatment in children is very limited. In adults daily doses from 50 mg to 3 g have been used. Intramuscular and intravenous forms of the drug do exist and should be considered in every patient individually

[c]Besides specific measures listed in table for CBS deficiency, other risk factors for thromboembolism should be checked and, if needed, treated. Dehydration and immobilization should be avoided to reduce the risk of thromboembolic disease. Patients who are poorly controlled or have had a vascular event may need additional treatment with anti-platelet drugs or anticoagulants. Surgery and anesthesia pose an additional risk of thrombosis. Biochemical control should be optimized before elective procedures. Standard anti-thrombotic measures such as elastic stockings, pneumatic leg compression systems, and early mobilization should be followed during and after surgery. Low molecular weight heparin is recommended in cases of prolonged immobilization. Nitrous oxide increases Hcy concentrations and should be avoided. Standard measures for preventing thrombosis are recommended for travel (Morris et al. 2017). Theoretically, phosphatidylcholine and creatine may inhibit transfer of methyl groups and thereby diminish the production of *S*-adenosylhomocysteine and homocysteine

[d]Folinate is probably generally a better option than folate, but folate should be satisfactory in most cases, except in those where parenteral use is necessary (folinate is available for parenteral use and folate is not)

**Warning Boxes/Pitfalls**

1. In patients treated with low-methionine diet, careful clinical and biochemical monitoring is necessary to avoid consequences of protein malnutrition.
2. Long-term folate therapy in high doses may be associated with increased cancer risk.
3. There is a high risk of peripheral neuropathy following long-term treatment with pyridoxine doses above 900 mg/day, but it has not been found in patients treated with less than 500 mg/day. In children, the safe dose is likely to depend on body weight; there are few data but last guidelines suggest using doses up to 10 mg/kg/day, with a maximum of 500 mg/day (Morris et al. 2017).
4. A major potential problem of betaine therapy in CBS deficiency and other disorders with both elevated tHcy and methionine is potential increase of methionine to the concentrations that may be toxic for the brain, leading to cerebral edema and other consequences of excessive hypermethioninemia described above.
5. Accidental inhalation of betaine in powder form can cause pulmonary problems.

## Experimental Treatment

For *CBS deficiency,* molecular chaperones have been investigated in proof of principle studies, while enzyme replacement therapy is in phase I/II of a clinical trial.

For *ethylmalonic encephalopathy*, early liver transplantation may be an option to reverse otherwise poor outcome (Dionisi-Vici et al. 2016). Diet restricted in sulfur-containing amino acids may contribute to better outcome in patients detected by newborn screening, particularly if liver transplantation would be proven as an option. In some patients, improvement in some symptoms has been observed with ubiquinone and/or riboflavin.

## Follow-Up and Monitoring

Recommendations given in the table are only approximate guidelines and should be adjusted individually according to age, severity of the disease, compliance, and other factors.

| Disease | Clinical follow-up and monitoring | Biochemical follow-up and monitoring |
|---|---|---|
| **22.1** MAT I/III deficiency | Both for untreated patients and those on therapy: any neurological sign or symptom should be considered as a possible sign of the disease and reason for further clinical (including brain imaging) and metabolic evaluation. Therefore, neurological and cognitive evaluation should be performed regularly in all patients with the risk of grossly elevated plasma methionine (clear risk above 800 µmol/L and existing risk above 500–600 µmol/L). In these patients neurological testing should take place about once every 2–3 months in infants and every 6–12 months later in life. If indicated, brain MRI should be performed (Chien et al. 2015). For patients on low-methionine diet, additionally, signs of protein malnutrition should be regularly looked for | In untreated patients without symptoms, checking of methionine, AdoMet, and total homocysteine (tHcy) is justified. The frequency depends on the severity of enzyme deficiency and mode of inheritance. The autosomal dominant form of MAT I/III deficiency is considered benign and does not require regular biochemical monitoring. In patients with the autosomal recessive form of the disease with severe enzyme deficiency and previous plasma methionine close to 500 µmol/L or more, or abnormal tHcy values, checking should be more frequent (i.e., in infancy every 3 months, later every 3–12 months and after significant changes in dietary methionine intake). In patients with the autosomal recessive form and mild enzyme deficiency, if highest plasma methionine values, which should be checked after normal and high protein intake, are not close to 500 µmol/L, only sporadic checking of plasma methionine is indicated, i.e., when symptoms attributable to MAT I/III deficiency appear. In patients on low-methionine diet, regular monitoring of protein status and plasma amino acids is indicated (in infancy at least every 3 months, later every 6–12 months and after significant changes in dietary methionine intake). In hyperhomocysteinemic patients in similar intervals, tHcy should be measured and thrombophilia screen should be performed at least once |

| Disease | Clinical follow-up and monitoring | Biochemical follow-up and monitoring |
|---|---|---|
| **22.2** MAT II deficiency | In individuals with *MAT2* mutations, regular cardiac evaluation by ultrasound and if needed other methods to check for possible development of thoracic aorta dilatation are indicated | Not possible due to the lack of biochemical markers |
| **22.3** GNMT deficiency | In GNMT-deficient patients tending to have very high plasma methionine levels which have been related to central nervous system complications (see MAT I/III deficiency above), regular neurological and cognitive testing is justified. [a]Yearly liver ultrasound seems justified | Due to possible hypermethioninemia-related problems, plasma methionine checking in regular intervals is recommended (in infancy every 3 months, if indicated even more frequently, later every 6–12 months or depending on previous values). Liver function tests, alpha-fetoprotein[a] |
| **22.4** AHCY deficiency | Careful evaluation of all body systems, particularly of the nervous system and development, muscles, liver, and coagulation. In infancy every 1–3 months, if indicated even more frequently, later every 3–6 months. This includes imaging studies, particularly regular liver imaging | Careful biochemical monitoring is mandatory to control both disease development and treatment to avoid their complications. The following tests are indicated: protein status, amino acids, AdoMet, AdoHcy, liver function tests, creatine kinase, alpha-fetoprotein, coagulation tests, liver imaging, while others depend on the clinical situation. Follow-up intervals depend on age and clinical course. In infancy this could be every 1–3 months, if indicated even more frequently, later every 3–6 months |
| **22.5** ADK deficiency | Careful clinical evaluation with regular follow-up visits depending on age and severity is recommended (intervals ranging from 1 month to 1 year), including regular monitoring of psychomotor development and neurological examination and regular liver imaging<br>Since epilepsy is often present in ADK deficiency, regular electroencephalography is recommended. In one patient retinal dystrophy was diagnosed; thus ophthalmological examination on a regular basis should be considered. Because of an increased incidence of cardiac defects, echocardiography should be performed in all patients and followed up accordingly. Several patients presented with cholelithiasis; thus abdominal ultrasound should be performed in cases of unexplained pain (colic) | Assays of protein status, plasma amino acids, tHcy, AdoMet, AdoHcy, adenosine in urine and/or dried blood spot, serum aminotransferases, total and direct bilirubin, ammonia, blood glucose, uric acid, coagulation tests, and alpha-fetoprotein are relevant. Regular blood glucose profiles should be performed, depending on the presence and treatment of recurrent hypoglycemia. A full blood count should be included in the regular monitoring to check for megaloblastic anemia |
| **22.6** CBS deficiency | The adequate frequency of monitoring depends on the severity of the disorder, treatment, compliance, age, status of the patient, and previous complications (e.g., thrombosis). Approximate schedule could be the following: Neurological and, depending on age, developmental or mental evaluation in infancy every 3 months, later every 6–12 months. Ophthalmology examination yearly. Bone mineral density once in 1–3 years. Vascular status every 6–12 months, depending on the severity of the disease and clinical course | Plasma amino acids and total homocysteine in infancy every 1–3 months, if indicated even more frequently, later every 3–6 months. If tHcy is monitored in dried blood spots, this test may be done more frequently. In patients on low-methionine diet protein status in the same intervals. Unless on supplementation, serum cobalamin and folate every 3–6 months. Thrombophilia screening should be considered once. Lipids first time at age 2–3 years, afterward, if normal, every 2–3 years, if not every 3 months alongside therapy |
| **22.7** CTH deficiency | Not necessary | |
| **22.8** MTO deficiency | Malodor can be monitored clinically. Possible related psychological burden may need psychologist's evaluation | If metronidazole is used, caution should be taken because of possible side effects. If low-protein/low methionine diet is used, protein status should be checked to avoid methionine deficiency and/or protein malnutrition |
| **22.9** Isolated SUOX deficiency | General and, particularly, neurological (including EEG and imaging) and developmental evaluation in infancy every 1–3 months, later every 3–6 months, if indicated more frequently. Ophthalmology every 6 months, if indicated, more frequently | If on diet, protein status, amino acids, *S*-sulfocysteine, thiosulfate, sulfite in infancy every 1–3 months, if indicated more frequently, later every 3–6 months |

| Disease | Clinical follow-up and monitoring | Biochemical follow-up and monitoring |
|---|---|---|
| **22.10** Ethylmalonic encephalopathy | General and, particularly, neurological (including EEG and imaging) and developmental evaluation in infancy every 1–3 months, later every 3–6 months, if indicated more frequently. Nutritional evaluation | Blood count according to blood losses in stool. Specific markers of the disease activity include lactate, plasma and urinary thiosulfate and sulfite, urinary ethylmalonate, and plasma C4- and C5-acylcarnitines. The frequency of monitoring depends on clinical condition and is more frequent in crises and/or following active treatment attempts, like liver transplantation. Otherwise it can be carried out in parallel with clinical evaluation, every 1–3 months in infancy, later every 3–6 months, if indicated more frequently |
| **22.11** Mercaptopyruvate sulfurtransferase deficiency | If the disease is associated with intellectual disability, regular cognitive assessment seems justified | There is no evidence that intervention in this very rare disorder is needed or effective. Specific markers would be beta-mercaptolactate cysteine disulfide (urine), mercaptopyruvate, and mercaptolactate. It is questionable if this would have practical meaning |

[a]In mice, in the long term significant liver disease may take place, including hepatocellular carcinoma; therefore, liver ultrasound and liver tumor markers checking may be justified

## Online Resources

1. Bindu PS, Nagappa M, Bharath RD, Taly AB (2017) Isolated sulfite oxidase deficiency. GeneReviews® https://www.ncbi.nlm.nih.gov/books/NBK453433/ Sep21, 2017
2. Di Meo I, Lamperti C, Tiranti V (2017) Ethylmalonic encephalopathy. GeneReviews® https://www.ncbi.nlm.nih.gov/books/NBK453432/ Sep21, 2017.
3. Enzyme Commission numbers—http://www.chem.qmul.ac.uk/iubmb/enzyme/
4. Inborn Errors of Metabolism Knowledgebase (IEMbase)—http://www.iembase.org/
5. OMIM catalogue—http://www.ncbi.nlm.nih.gov/omim/
6. The Online Metabolic and Molecular Bases of Inherited Disease—https://ommbid.mhmedical.com/
7. Human Metabolome Database—http://www.hmdb.ca/

**Acknowledgements** The authors would like to acknowledge the help of Ms. Jitka Sokolová, MSc. with the manuscript preparation. Institutional and grant support to V.K. was provided by RVO-VFN 64165 and Progres Q26, and AZV 16-30384A, respectively.

## References

Alhusani A, Obaid A, Blom HJ, Wedell A, Alfadhel M. Adenosine kinase deficiency: report and review. Neuropediatrics. 2019;50:46–50.

Ampola MG, Efron ML, Bixby EM, Meshorer E. Mental deficiency and a new aminoaciduria. Am J Dis Child. 1969;117:66–70.

Barić I, Fumić K, Glenn B, et al. S-adenosylhomocysteine hydrolase deficiency in a human: a genetic disorder of methionine metabolism. Proc Natl Acad Sci U S A. 2004;101:4234–9.

Barić I, Ćuk M, Fumić K, et al. S-Adenosylhomocysteine hydrolase deficiency: a second patient, the younger brother of the index patient, and outcomes during therapy. J Inherit Metab Dis. 2005;28:885–902.

Barić I, Staufner C, Augoustides-Savvopoulou P, et al. Consensus recommendations for the diagnosis, treatment and follow-up of inherited methylation disorders. J Inherit Metab Dis. 2017;40:5–20.

Braverman NE, Mudd SH, Barker PB, Pomper MG. Characteristic MR imaging changes in severe hypermethioninemic states. Am J Neuroradiol. 2005;26:2705–6.

Chamberlin ME, Ubagai T, Mudd SH, Levy H, Chou JY. Dominant inheritance of isolated hypermethioninemia is associated with a mutation in the human methionine adenosyltransferase 1A gene. Am J Hum Genet. 1997;60:540–6.

Chien YH; Abdenur JE, Baronio F, et al. Mudd's disease (MAT I/III deficiency): a survey of data for MAT1A homozygotes and compound heterozygotes. Orphanet J Rare Dis. 2015;10:99.

Claerhout H, Witters P, Régal L, Jansen K, Van Hoestenberghe MR, Breckpot J, Vermeersch P. Isolated sulfite oxidase deficiency. J Inherit Metab Dis. 2018;41:101–8.

Dionisi-Vici C, Diodato D, Torre G, Picca S, Pariante R, Giuseppe Picardo S, Di Meo I, Rizzo C, Tiranti V, Zeviani M, de Ville de Goyet J. Liver transplant in ethylmalonic encephalopathy: a new treatment for an otherwise fatal disease. Brain. 2016;139:1045–51.

Duran M, Blau N, Gibson MK, editors. Laboratory guide to the methods in biochemical genetics. Berlin: Springer; 2008. p. 859.

Guo DC, Gong L, Regalado ES, Santos-Cortez RL, Zhao R, Cai B, et al. MAT2A mutations predispose individuals to thoracic aortic aneurysms. Am J Hum Genet. 2015;96:170–7.

Joint FAO/WHO/UNU Expert Consultation on Protein and Amino Acid Requirements in Human Nutrition (2002: Geneva, Switzerland). Protein and amino acid requirements in human nutrition. Report of a Joint WHO/FAO/UNU Expert Consultation. WHO Technical Report Series 935. Geneva: WHO; 2007.

Kitzler TM, Gupta IR, Osterman B, Poulin C, Trakadis Y, Waters PJ, Buhas DC. Acute and chronic management in an atypical case of ethylmalonic encephalopathy. JIMD Rep. 2019;45:57–63.

Kožich V, Morris AAM, Blom HJ. Disorders of sulfur amino acid metabolism. In: Saudubray JM, Baumgartner MR, Walter J, editors. Inborn metabolic diseases: diagnosis and treatment. 6th ed. Berlin: Springer; 2016. p. 309–20.

Kraus JP, Hasek J, Kozich V, et al. Cystathionine gamma-lyase: clinical, metabolic, genetic, and structural studies. Mol Genet Metab. 2009;97:250–9.

Morris AA, Kožich V, Santra S, et al. Guidelines for the diagnosis and management of cystathionine beta-synthase deficiency. J Inherit Metab Dis. 2017;40:49–74.

Mudd SH, Skovby F, Levy HL, et al. The natural history of homocystinuria due to cystathionine β-synthase deficiency. Am J Hum Genet. 1985;37:1–31.

Mudd SH, Cerone R, Schiaffino MC, et al. Glycine N-methyltransferase deficiency: a novel inborn error causing persistent isolated hypermethioninemia. J Inherit Metab Dis. 2001;24:448–64.

Pol A, Renkema GH, Tangerman A, et al. Mutations in *SELENBP1*, encoding a novel human methanethiol oxidase, cause extraoral halitosis. Nat Genet. 2018;50:120–9.

Stabler SP, Steegborn C, Wahl MC, et al. Elevated plasma total homocysteine in severe methionine adenosyltransferase I/III deficiency. Metabolism. 2002;51:981–8.

Staufner C, Lindner M, Dionisi-Vici C, et al. Adenosine kinase deficiency: expanding the clinical spectrum and evaluating therapeutic options. J Inherit Metab Dis. 2016;39(02):273–83.

Surtees R, Leonard J, Austin S. Association of demyelination with deficiency of cerebrospinal-fluid S-adenosylmethionine in inborn errors of methyl-transfer pathway. Lancet. 1991;338:1550–4.

Touati G, Rusthoven E, Depondt E, et al. Dietary therapy in two patients with a mild form of sulfite oxidase deficiency. Evidence for clinical and biological improvement. J Inherit Metab Dis. 2000;23:45–53.

# Disorders of Branched-Chain Amino Acid Metabolism

# 23

Manuel Schiff, Jean-François Benoist, Anaïs Brassier, and Jerry Vockley

## Contents



M. Schiff (✉) · J.-F. Benoist · A. Brassier
APHP, Reference Center for Inborn Error of Metabolism and Filière G2M, Pediatrics Department, Necker Univ Hospital, Paris, France
e-mail: manuel.schiff@aphp.fr; jean-francois.benoist@aphp.fr; anais.brassier@aphp.fr

J. Vockley
Children's Hospital of Pittsburgh, University of Pittsburgh Medical Center, University of Pittsburgh, Pittsburgh, PA, USA
e-mail: vockleyg@upmc.edu

**Summary**

Disorders in the catabolic pathways of the branched-chain amino acids (BCAA) leucine, isoleucine, and valine encompass diverse organic and amino acidurias. Clinical severity may range from asymptomatic findings in some to life-threatening episodes and multi-organ involvement in others. Several of these defects may reflect a complex pathogenesis related to mitochondrial dysfunction, particularly the 3-methylglutaconic acidurias. As a general rule, treatment includes (1) dietary restriction of the precursor BCAA along with optimal nutritional supply, (2) adjunct therapy (e.g., with L-carnitine, appropriate cofactors, other conjugating compounds), and (3) rapid intervention for acute metabolic decompensation including


N. Blau et al. (eds.), *Physician's Guide to the Diagnosis, Treatment, and Follow-Up of Inherited Metabolic Diseases*,
https://doi.org/10.1007/978-3-030-67727-5_23

home preventative measures strictly following a written sick-day protocol. Late complications of these diseases must be anticipated, such as liver disease, cardiomyopathy, and renal failure. In asymptomatic screened individuals, instructions regarding risks for metabolic stress and fasting avoidance, along with clinical monitoring, represent appropriate prophylactic interventions.

## Introduction

The catabolic pathways of branched-chain amino acids (BCAA), namely, leucine, isoleucine, and valine, consist of multiple steps including transamination, oxidative decarboxylation, and dehydrogenation. Due to irreversible steps early in metabolism, elevated levels of these amino acids do not occur in those disorders that result from blocks in the pathways distal to the site of maple syrup urine disease (MSUD). Rather, they are associated with organic acidemia and aciduria. Severe forms of these disorders usually present as acute, overwhelming neurological deterioration in the neonatal period if not detected through newborn screening. Milder variants may be episodic and not become symptomatic until late childhood or even adult life. Moreover, some patients are asymptomatic and identified only through family studies or newborn screening. Some disorders of BCAA metabolism are exceedingly rare, and the clinical experience in managing these cases is still being defined.

*Branched-Chain Amino Acid (BCAA) Transferase (BCAT1 and BCAT2) Deficiency:* The existence of this disorder in humans remains in question. There is some evidence that transamination of valine and transamination of leucine and isoleucine may be affected differentially. Early reports have described patients with hyperleucine-isoleucinemia and hypervalinemia, attributed to a defect of branched-chain amino acid transamination, who presented with failure to thrive and mental retardation (Reddi et al. 1977).

*Maple syrup urine disease (MSUD)* results from deficient activity of the branched-chain α-ketoacid dehydrogenase complex (BCKDC). During episodes of metabolic decompensation, the BCAA and their corresponding branched-chain α-ketoacids (BCKA) accumulate excessively. The pathophysiology of MSUD is thought to be related primarily to leucine. The enzyme complex BCKDC consists of three catalytic components (E1, E2, and E3) encoded by four different genetic loci. Whereas mutations in all four of the catalytic loci have been associated with clinical disease (MSUD 1a, 1b, 2, 3, respectively), *BCKDHA* and *BCKDHB* are the most frequently involved genes.

Five *clinical forms* of MSUD exist, differentiated by the amount of residual enzymatic activity, age and severity of onset, and responsiveness to thiamine. These include *classic*, *intermediate*, *intermittent*, and *thiamine-responsive* MSUD, in addition to *E3* (lipoamide dehydrogenase) *deficiency*. The latter associates with combined deficiencies of the pyruvate dehydrogenase complex and 2-oxoglutarate dehydrogenase complexes, which share the E3 component with BCKDC. The former is exceedingly rare and doubts exist concerning its reality. The activity of the complex BCKDC is tightly regulated, in particular by phosphorylation under the control of a specific kinase (BCKDHK) and a phosphatase. BCKDC phosphatase deficiency is responsible for a mild form of MSUD, while the kinase deficiency leads to persistently reduced BCAA body fluid levels associated with developmental delay, microcephaly, and autism (Novarino et al. 2012).

*Isovaleric acidemia (IVA)* results from deficient activity of isovaleryl-CoA dehydrogenase, ranging from acute neonatal to an intermittent or chronic presentation. Asymptomatic individuals with only subtle biochemical abnormalities are detected through newborn screening (Ensenauer et al. 2004, 2011; Vockley and Ensenauer 2006). In patients with a severe phenotype, the odor of "sweaty feet" may be detected during metabolic crisis, associated with marked ketoacidosis, bone marrow suppression, and hyperammonemia.

*3-Methylcrotonyl-CoA carboxylase (3MCCC) deficiency (MCCD)* also features a highly variable phenotype, from severe presentation to asymptomatic in patients detected via newborn screening or family association studies (Gibson et al. 1998). Thus far there are no reliable markers to identify the few individuals at risk for clinical symptoms. A more recent study performed whole exome sequencing in individuals exhibiting nonspecific phenotypes attributed to MCCD and showed that such signs were likely not due to mutations in the MCC enzyme but from rare homozygous mutations in other disease genes. These findings suggest that MCCD should be viewed largely as an asymptomatic condition (Shepard et al. 2015). Appropriate testing (urinary organic acids, acylcarnitine profile, and eventually mutation analysis/enzymatic assay) is necessary to differentiate 3MCCC deficiency from the multiple carboxylase deficiencies due to defects in biotin metabolism.

*3-Methylglutaconic aciduria* occurs in multiple forms. Only type I (MGA1), associated with reduced activity of 3-methylglutaconyl-CoA hydratase, is a disorder of the leucine degradation pathway. Barth (MGA2) syndrome is an X-linked multi-system disorder with cardiomyopathy, myopathy, neutropenia, and 3-methylglutaconic aciduria. Costeff syndrome (MGA3) is characterized by optic atrophy and neurological symptoms. MEGDEL syndrome is a recessive disorder featuring sensorineural deafness and encephalopathy with neuroradiological evidence of Leigh disease. Neonatal mitochondrial encephalocardiomyopathy is caused by isolated mitochondrial ATP synthase deficiency, associated with mutation in the TMEM 70 gene. 3-Methylglutaconic aciduria type IV refers to conditions in which the primary etiologies remain to be elucidated. Most of the time and for yet understood reasons, MGA is a biomarker in the setting of mitochondrial respiratory chain disorders (Wortmann et al. 2013). For more details on the mitochondrial etiologies of MGA.

*3-Hydroxy-3-methylglutaric acidemia (HMG-CoA lyase deficiency)* is a dual defect in leucine degradation and ketogenesis that often presents with neonatal hypoketotic hypoglycemia, metabolic acidosis, and hyperammonemia (Gibson et al. 1988). Milder forms of the disorder, including presentation in adulthood, have also been reported. Overwhelming metabolic decompensation and organic aciduria are associated with a characteristic absence of ketone bodies, a hallmark of this disorder.

*2-Methylbutyrylglycinuria or 2-methylbutyryl-CoA dehydrogenase (MBD) deficiency* is a defect in isoleucine degradation caused by mutations in the short/branched-chain acyl-CoA dehydrogenase (*ACADSB*) (Andresen et al. 2000). Diverse clinical symptoms such as hypotonia, mental retardation, autistic features, hypoglycemia, or metabolic acidosis have been reported, but most individuals (especially those identified by newborn screening) have remained asymptomatic (Gibson et al. 2000; Sass et al. 2008). A founder mutation in the Hmong Chinese population has been described (Alfardan et al. 2010).

*2-Methyl-3-hydroxybutyryl-CoA dehydrogenase (MHBD) deficiency (or 17beta-hydroxysteroid dehydrogenase type 10 [HSD10] deficiency)* was first reported in a 2-year-old boy with neurodegenerative symptoms (Zschocke et al. 2000). This defect was also documented in a female patient who was less severely affected, suggesting skewed X-inactivation (Perez-Cerda et al. 2005). Additional patients delineated a clinical spectrum from severe neurological disease to isolated ketoacidosis mimicking beta-ketothiolase deficiency (Fukao et al. 2014). The disease-causing gene, HSD17B10, encodes 17beta-hydroxysteroid dehydrogenase type 10 (HSD10), the latter essential for structural and functional integrity of mitochondria (Rauschenberger et al. 2010; Oerum et al. 2017).

*Beta-ketothiolase deficiency (alpha-methylacetoacetic aciduria, 3-oxothiolase deficiency, methylacetoacetyl-coenzyme A thiolase [MAT] deficiency)* is a defect of ketone body utilization and isoleucine catabolism. It is caused by mutations in the *ACAT1* gene and presents with recurrent episodes of fasting metabolic ketoacidosis with or without hypoglycemia (Grünert et al. 2017). A subset of ACAT1-deficient patients may exhibit chronic movement disorder and basal ganglia abnormalities on neuroimaging independent of ketoacidotic episodes (Paquay et al. 2017).

*Isobutyryl-CoA dehydrogenase deficiency (IBD deficiency)* is a disorder of valine degradation. The original patient presented with anemia and dilated cardiomyopathy, probably related to secondary carnitine deficiency (Roe et al. 1998). Thus far, more individuals have been described who are mostly asymptomatic, largely identified via newborn screening (Koeberl et al. 2003; Sass et al. 2004; Oglesbee et al. 2007).

*Short-chain enoyl-CoA hydratase or crotonase deficiency (SCEH/ECHS1 deficiency)* is a disorder of both valine degradation and short-chain fatty acid oxidation (Peters et al. 2014). Pathogenesis is thought to be ascribed mainly to the former. Clinical presentation includes infantile-onset severe developmental delay with regression and seizures, with elevated plasma lactate and brain MRI abnormalities consistent with Leigh-like disease. In urine, 2,3-dihydroxy-2-methylbutyric acid and *N*-acetyl-*S*-(2-carboxypropyl)cysteine, the metabolites of acrylyl-CoA and methacrylyl-CoA, are the most specific markers of the disease (Fitzsimons et al. 2018; Sharpe and McKenzie 2018); other unspecific markers such as 3-methylglutaconic can be found. Molecular studies revealed variants in the *ECHS1* gene.

*3-Hydroxyisobutyryl-CoA deacylase deficiency (or methacrylic aciduria)* has been confirmed in a few patients with variants in the *HIBCH* gene (Tan et al. 2018). They presented with failure to thrive, developmental delay, and neurological symptoms in infancy with neuroradiological findings compatible with Leigh-like disease. Unusual cysteine and cysteamine conjugates of methacrylic acid were detected in urine. With the exception of 3-hydroxyisobutyryl carnitine, the metabolite abnormalities are essentially the same as those observed in ECHS1 patients. In fibroblasts from the initial patients, 3-hydroxyisobutyryl-CoA hydrolase activity was deficient (Loupatty et al. 2007).

*3-Hydroxyisobutyric aciduria* may be caused by a primary defect of 3-hydroxyisobutyrate dehydrogenase, active in valine metabolism, or via secondary inhibition of 3-hydroxyisobutyrate dehydrogenase in selected respiratory chain defects (Loupatty et al. 2006). The clinical phenotype is variable, but the majority of patients reported in the literature presented with dysmorphic features, neurodevelopmental symptoms, ketoacidotic episodes, and lactic acidemia.

*Methylmalonate semialdehyde dehydrogenase (MMSDH) deficiency* is a rare disorder of the valine catabolic pathway associated with variable clinical and biochemical phenotype from vomiting and dehydration (Chambliss et al. 2000) to neurodevelopmental disease with delayed myelination (Marcadier et al. 2013). To date four patients were reported with mutations in *ALDH6A1* encoding for MMSDH.

Isoleucine and valine share the propionate pathway for their terminal steps of catabolism, and *propionic acidemia* (PA, propionyl-CoA carboxylase deficiency) and *methylmalonic acidemia* (MMA, methylmalonyl-CoA mutase deficiency) are disorders of propionate degradation derived in part from the catabolism of isoleucine and valine, as well as other propionate precursors (threonine, methionine, odd-chain fatty acids, and cholesterol). MMA and PA usually present with life-threatening episodes of ketoacidosis, hyperammonemia, encephalopathy, and hematological manifestations. Late complications of these disorders include renal failure (particularly in MMA), pancreatitis, liver disease, cardiomyopathy (particularly in PA), long QT syndrome (particularly in PA), basal ganglion infarction, optic neuropathy, or impaired hearing ability (Grünert et al. 2013; Tuncel et al. 2018). Secondary mitochondrial respiratory chain deficiencies have been demonstrated in both disorders (De Keyzer et al. 2009). In addition to the primary deficiencies of propionyl-CoA carboxylase (PCCA and PCCB) and methylmalonyl-CoA mutase (MMUT), secondary defects of these enzymes can be associated with genetic disorders in the metabolism of their respective cofactors, i.e., biotin and cobalamin.

*Methylmalonic aciduria due to methylmalonyl-CoA epimerase deficiency* is a rare recessive disorder identified through moderate methylmalonic accumulation in urine. The clinical significance and biochemical characteristics of this rare condition have been incompletely defined. Some patients may present with an acute decompensation and other with progressive neurological symptoms (Waters et al. 2016). At least two patients were also affected by a second inherited disorder, a sepiapterin reductase deficiency (Mazzuca et al. 2015); the link between the two disorders is not understood.

*Malonic aciduria* (MA) is caused by malonyl-CoA decarboxylase deficiency leading to a block in fatty acid metabolism. Patients present with cardiomyopathy, developmental delay, short stature, seizures, hypoglycemia, and metabolic acidosis (Salomons et al. 2007).

*Combined malonic and methylmalonic aciduria* (CMAMMA) is a rare recessive disorder caused by a defect in the *ACSF3* gene, which encodes an acyl-CoA synthetase. Initial CMAMMA patients were reported with developmental delay, seizures, cognitive decline, cardiomyopathy, and metabolic acidosis (Sloan et al. 2011). More recently, a significant number of asymptomatic CMAMMA patients from Quebec identified through urine newborn screening have been reported (Levtova et al. 2019).

## Nomenclature

| No. | Disorder | Alternative name | Abbreviation | Gene Symbol | Chromosomal Localization | Affected protein | OMIM No. |
|---|---|---|---|---|---|---|---|
| 23.1 | BCAA aminotransferase deficiency | Hypervalinemia and hyperleucine-isoleucinemia | | | | BCAA aminotransferase | 238340 |
| | | | | *BCAT1* | 12p12.1 | BCAA transferase 1 | 113520 |
| | | | | *BCAT2* | 19q13.33 | BCAA transferase 2 | 113530 |
| 23.2 | Maple syrup urine disease | Branched-chain alpha-ketoacid dehydrogenase complex deficiency | MSUD | | | Branched-chain alpha-ketoacid dehydrogenase complex | 248600 |
| | | Maple syrup urine disease 1a | MSUD1A | *BCKDHA* | 19q132 | E1 α-subunit | 608348 |
| | | Maple syrup urine disease 1b | MSUD1B | *BCKDHB* | 6q14.1 | E1 β-subunit | 248611 |
| | | Maple syrup urine disease type 2 | MSUD2 | *DBT* | 1p31 | Dihydrolipoamide branched-chain transacylase (DBT, E2) | 248610 |
| 23.3 | | E3 deficiency | MSUD3 | *DLD* | 7q31-q32 | Dihydrolipoamide dehydrogenase (E3) | 238331 |
| 23.4 | Branched-chain ketoacid dehydrogenase phosphatase deficiency | | | *PPM1K* | 4q22.1 | Protein phosphatase 2C | 611065 |
| 23.5 | Branched-chain ketoacid dehydrogenase kinase deficiency | | | *BCKDK* | 16p11.2 | Branched-chain ketoacid dehydrogenase kinase | 614923 |
| 23.6 | Isovaleric acidemia | Isovaleryl-CoA dehydrogenase deficiency | IVA | *IVD* | 15q15.1 | Isovaleryl-CoA dehydrogenase | 243500 |
| 23.7 | Isobutyryl-CoA dehydrogenase deficiency | Isobutyrylglycinuria | IBD | *ACAD8* | 11q25 | Isobutyryl-CoA dehydrogenase | 611283 |
| 23.8 | 2-Methylbutyryl-CoA dehydrogenase deficiency | Short/branched-chain acyl-CoA dehydrogenase deficiency; 2-methylbutyrylglycinuria | MBD | *ACADSB* | 10q26.13 | 2-Methylbutyryl-CoA dehydrogenase | 610006 |
| 23.9 | Methylcrotonyl-CoA carboxylase deficiency | Methylcrotonylglycinuria | MCC | | | Methylcrotonyl-CoA carboxylase | |
| | | Methylcrotonyl-CoA carboxylase 1 deficiency; Methylcrotonylglycinuria type 1 | | *MCCC1* | 3q27.1 | | 210200 |
| | | Methylcrotonyl-CoA carboxylase 2 deficiency; Methylcrotonylglycinuria type 2 | | *MCCC2* | 5q12-13.2 | | 210210 |
| 23.10 | 3-Methylglutaconyl-CoA hydratase deficiency | 3-methylglutaconic aciduria type 1 | | *AUH* | 9q22.31 | 3-Methylglutaconyl-CoA hydratase | 250950 |
| 23.11 | Mitochondrial Short-chain enoyl-CoA hydratase 1 deficiency | Crotonase deficiency | SCEH | *ECHS1* | 10q26.3 | Short-chain enoyl-CoA hydratase | 602292 |
| 23.12 | 3-hydroxyisobutyryl-CoA hydrolase deficiency | β-Hydroxyisobutyryl-CoA deacylase deficiency | HIBCH | *HIBCH* | 2q32.2 | 3-Hydroxyisobutyryl-CoA deacylase | 610690 |

(continued)

| No. | Disorder | Alternative name | Abbreviation | Gene Symbol | Chromosomal Localization | Affected protein | OMIM No. |
|---|---|---|---|---|---|---|---|
| 23.13 | 3-Hydroxyisobutyrate dehydrogenase deficiency | 3-Hydroxyisobutyric aciduria | HIBDH | *HIBADH* | 7p15.2 | 3-Hydroxyisobutyrate dehydrogenase | 608475 |
| 23.14 | HSD10 mitochondrial deficiency | 2-Methyl-3-hydroxybutyryl-CoA dehydrogenase deficiency | MHBD | *HSD17B10* | Xp11.22 | 17-beta-hydroxysteroid dehydrogenase type 10 | 300438 |
| 23.15 | 3-Hydroxy-3-methylglutaryl-CoA lyase deficiency | 3-Hydroxy-3-methyl glutaric aciduria | HGMCLD | *HMGCL* | 1p35-36 | 3-Hydroxy-3-methylglutaryl-CoA lyase | 246450 |
| 23.16 | Methylmalonate semialdehyde dehydrogenase deficiency | Combined semialdehyde dehydrogenase deficiency | MMSDH | *ALDH6A1* | 14q24.3 | Methylmalonate semialdehyde dehydrogenase | 603178 |
| 23.17 | Propionyl-CoA carboxylase deficiency | Propionic acidemia | PA | | | Propionyl-CoA carboxylase | 606054 |
| | | Propionyl-CoA carboxylase α subunit deficiency | | *PCCA* | 13q32.3 | Propionyl-CoA carboxylase α subunit | 232000 |
| | | Propionyl-CoA carboxylase β subunit deficiency | | *PCCB* | 3q23.3 | Propionyl-CoA carboxylase β subunit | 232050 |
| 23.18 | Methylmalonyl-CoA epimerase deficiency | | | *MCEE* | 2p13.3 | Methylmalonyl-CoA epimerase | 251120 |
| 23.19 | Methylmalonic aciduria due to methylmalonyl-CoA mutase deficiency | Methylmalonyl-CoA mutase deficiency | MMA | *MMUT* | 6p12.3 | Methylmalonyl-CoA mutase | 251000 |
| 23.20 | Acyl-CoA synthetase family member 3 deficiency | Combined malonic and methylmalonic aciduria | CMAMMA | *ACSF3* | 16q24.3 | Acyl-CoA synthetase 3 | 614265 |
| 23.21 | Malonyl-CoA decarboxylase deficiency | Malonic aciduria | | *MLYCD* | 16q23.3 | Malonyl-CoA decarboxylase | 248360 |
| 23.22 | Mitochondrial acetoacetyl-CoA thiolase deficiency | Beta-ketothiolase deficiency; β-methylacetoacetic aciduria | MAT | *ACAT1* | 11q22.3 | 3-Oxothiolase | 203750 |
| 23.23 | Large neutral amino acid transporter deficiency | | | *SLC7A5* | 16q24.2 | LAT1 | |

## Metabolic Pathway

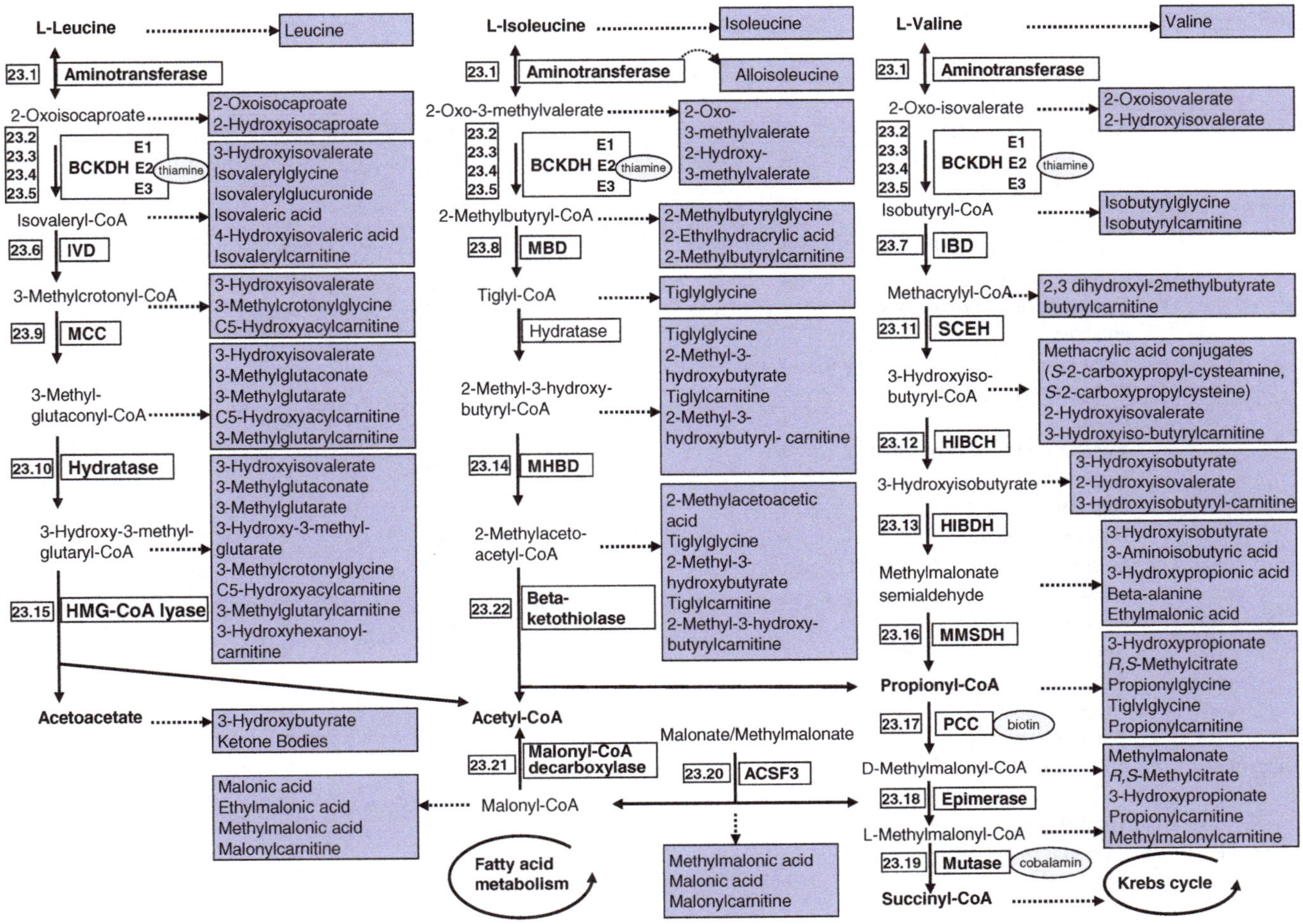


**Fig. 23.1** Metabolic pathways

## Signs and Symptoms

**Table 23.1** Branched-chain aminotransferase deficiency (BCAT1/2)

| System | Symptoms and biomarkers | Neonatal (birth–1 month) | Infancy (1–18 months) | Childhood (1.5–11 years) | Adolescence (11–16 years) | Adulthood (>16 years) |
|---|---|---|---|---|---|---|
| CNS | Developmental delay | | | ± | ± | ± |
| Laboratory findings | Isoleucine (plasma) | | ↑ | ↑ | ↑ | ↑ |
| | Leucine (plasma) | | ↑ | ↑ | ↑ | ↑ |
| | Valine (plasma) | | ↑↑ | ↑↑ | ↑↑ | ↑↑ |

**Table 23.2** Maple syrup urine disease, all types (*BCKDHA, BCKDHB, DBT*)

| System | Symptoms and biomarkers | Neonatal (birth–1 month) | Infancy (1–18 months) | Childhood (1.5–11 years) | Adolescence (11–16 years) | Adulthood (>16 years) |
|---|---|---|---|---|---|---|
| CNS | Apnea | ± | ± | ± | ± | ± |
| | **Ataxia** | ± | ± | ± | ± | ± |
| | Axonal sensory motor polyneuropathy, chronic | ± | ± | ± | ± | ± |
| | **Brain edema (MRI)** | ± | ± | ± | ± | ± |
| | Brain edema (MRI) | ± | ± | ± | ± | ± |
| | Brain edema, cytotoxic | ± | ± | ± | ± | ± |
| | Brainstem edema (MRI) | ± | ± | ± | ± | ± |
| | Cerebellar edema (MRI) | ± | ± | ± | ± | ± |
| | Cerebral atrophy (MRI) | ± | ± | ± | ± | ± |
| | **Coma, during ketoacidotic episodes** | + | + | + | + | + |
| | Deep gray matter structural lesions | ± | ± | ± | ± | ± |
| | Delayed myelination | ± | ± | ± | ± | ± |
| | Dystonia | ± | ± | ± | ± | ± |
| | **Encephalopathic crisis, acute** | ± | ± | ± | ± | ± |
| | Hypertonia | ± | ± | ± | ± | ± |
| | Hypotonia | ± | ± | ± | ± | ± |
| | **Irritability, episodic** | ± | ± | ± | ± | ± |
| | **Lethargy, during ketoacidotic episodes** | + | + | + | + | + |
| | Opisthotonus | ± | ± | ± | ± | ± |
| | **Retardation, psychomotor** | ± | ± | ± | ± | ± |
| | Seizures | ± | ± | ± | ± | ± |
| | Vacuolating myelinopathy | ± | ± | ± | ± | ± |
| | White matter changes (MRI) | ± | ± | ± | ± | ± |
| Digestive | **Feeding difficulties** | + | + | + | ± | ± |
| | Pancreatitis | ± | ± | ± | ± | ± |
| | **Vomiting, episodic** | + | + | + | ± | ± |
| Metabolic | Hypoglycemia | ± | ± | ± | ± | ± |
| | Ketoacidosis | + | + | + | + | + |
| | **Metabolic acidosis** | + | + | + | + | + |
| Musculoskeletal | Hypotonia, muscular-axial | ± | ± | ± | ± | ± |
| Other | Failure to thrive | ± | ± | ± | ± | ± |
| | Hypothermia during crisis | ± | ± | ± | | |
| | **Odor of maple syrup** | ± | ± | ± | ± | ± |
| Laboratory findings | 2,4-Dinitrophenylhydrazine test (urine) | ± | ± | ± | ± | ± |
| | Alloisoleucine (plasma) | ↑-↑↑↑ | ↑-↑↑↑ | ↑-↑↑↑ | ↑-↑↑↑ | ↑-↑↑↑ |
| | Ammonia (blood) | n-↑ | n-↑ | n-↑ | n-↑ | n-↑ |
| | Anion gap | + | + | + | + | + |
| | BCKDC activity (fibroblasts) | ↓ | ↓ | ↓ | ↓ | ↓ |
| | Branched-chain oxoacids (plasma) | ↑-↑↑↑ | ↑-↑↑↑ | ↑-↑↑↑ | ↑-↑↑↑ | ↑-↑↑↑ |
| | Branched-chain oxoacids (urine) | ↑-↑↑↑ | ↑-↑↑↑ | ↑-↑↑↑ | ↑-↑↑↑ | ↑-↑↑↑ |
| | Ferric chloride test (urine) | ± | ± | ± | ± | ± |
| | Glucose (plasma) | ↓-n | ↓-n | ↓-n | ↓-n | ↓-n |
| | Isoleucine (plasma) | ↑-↑↑↑ | ↑-↑↑↑ | ↑-↑↑↑ | ↑-↑↑↑ | ↑-↑↑↑ |
| | Leucine (plasma) | ↑-↑↑↑ | ↑-↑↑↑ | ↑-↑↑↑ | ↑-↑↑↑ | ↑-↑↑↑ |
| | *N*-acetylaspartic acid (NAA) peak during crisis (MRS) | ↓ | ↓ | ↓ | ↓ | ↓ |
| | Osmolality (serum) | ↓-n | ↓-n | ↓-n | ↓-n | ↓-n |
| | Sodium (plasma) | ↓-n | ↓-n | ↓-n | ↓-n | ↓-n |
| | Valine (plasma) | ↑-↑↑↑ | ↑-↑↑↑ | ↑-↑↑↑ | ↑-↑↑↑ | ↑-↑↑↑ |

**Table 23.3** Pyruvate dehydrogenase complex deficiency E3 (DLD)

| System | Symptoms and biomarkers | Neonatal (birth–1 month) | Infancy (1–18 months) | Childhood (1.5–11 years) | Adolescence (11–16 years) | Adulthood (>16 years) |
|---|---|---|---|---|---|---|
| CNS | Agenesis, corpus callosum (MRI) | + | + | + | | |
| | Developmental delay | ++ | ++ | ++ | | |
| | Hypogenesis, corpus callosum | + | + | + | | |
| | **Hypotonia, progressive generalized** | ++ | ++ | ++ | | |
| | Leigh syndrome | ± | ++ | ++ | | |
| | **Microcephaly** | + | ++ | ++ | | |
| | Spasticity | ± | ++ | ++ | | |
| Digestive | **Liver failure, acute recurrent** | + | + | + | + | + |
| Musculoskeletal | Myoglobinuria | | | | + | + |
| | **Myopathy** | n | | | + | + |
| Laboratory findings | 2-Oxoadipate (urine) | ↑ | ↑ | ↑ | ↑ | ↑ |
| | 2-Oxoglutaric acid (urine) | ↑ | ↑ | ↑ | ↑ | ↑ |
| | Isoleucine (plasma) | ↑ | ↑ | ↑ | ↑ | ↑ |
| | Lactate (urine) | ↑ | ↑ | ↑ | ↑ | ↑ |
| | Lactate/pyruvate ratio | n | n | n | n | n |
| | Leucine (plasma) | ↑ | ↑ | ↑ | ↑ | ↑ |
| | Valine (plasma) | ↑ | ↑ | ↑ | ↑ | ↑ |

**Table 23.4** Branched-chain ketoacid dehydrogenase phosphatase deficiency (PPM1K)

| System | Symptoms and biomarkers | Neonatal (birth–1 month) | Infancy (1–18 months) | Childhood (1.5–11 years) | Adolescence (11–16 years) | Adulthood (> 16 years) |
|---|---|---|---|---|---|---|
| Other | No clinical significance | | | | | |
| Laboratory findings | Isoleucine (plasma) | ↑ | | | | ↑ |
| | Leucine (plasma) | ↑ | | | | ↑ |
| | Valine (plasma) | ↑ | | | | ↑ |

**Table 23.5** Branched-chain ketoacid dehydrogenase kinase deficiency (BCKDK)

| System | Symptoms and biomarkers | Neonatal (birth–1 month) | Infancy (1–18 months) | Childhood (1.5–11 years) | Adolescence (11–16 years) | Adulthood (>16 years) |
|---|---|---|---|---|---|---|
| CNS | **Autism** | | | + | + | |
| | **Intellectual disability** | | | + | + | |
| | Seizures | | ± | ± | ± | |
| | Speech delay | | + | + | + | |
| | Stereotyped hand movements | | | ± | ± | |
| Laboratory findings | Isoleucine (plasma) | | ↓ | ↓ | ↓ | |
| | Leucine (plasma) | | ↓ | ↓ | ↓ | |
| | Valine (plasma) | | ↓ | ↓ | ↓ | |

**Table 23.6** Isovaleric acidemia (IVD)

| System | Symptoms and biomarkers | Neonatal (birth–1 month) | Infancy (1–18 months) | Childhood (1.5–11 years) | Adolescence (11–16 years) | Adulthood (>16 years) |
|---|---|---|---|---|---|---|
| Cardiovascular | Cardiac arrhythmia | ± | ± | ± | ± | ± |
| CNS | Abnormalities in the globus pallidus (MRI) | ± | ± | ± | ± | ± |
| | Altered consciousness | ± | ± | ± | ± | ± |
| | Ataxia | | ± | ± | ± | ± |
| | Coma, during ketoacidotic episodes | + | + | + | + | + |
| | Developmental delay | ± | ± | ± | ± | ± |
| | Encephalopathic crisis, acute | ± | ± | ± | ± | ± |
| | Hypertonia | ± | ± | ± | ± | ± |
| | Hypotonia | ± | ± | ± | ± | ± |
| | Lethargy, during ketoacidotic episodes | + | + | + | + | + |
| | Retardation, psychomotor | ± | ± | ± | ± | ± |
| | Seizures | ± | ± | ± | ± | ± |
| | White matter changes (MRI) | ± | ± | ± | ± | ± |
| Dermatological | Alopecia | | ± | ± | | |
| Digestive | Feeding difficulties | + | + | + | ± | ± |
| | Hepatomegaly | ± | ± | ± | ± | ± |
| | Pancreatitis | ± | ± | ± | ± | ± |
| | Vomiting, episodic | + | + | + | ± | ± |
| Hematological | Leukopenia | ± | ± | ± | ± | ± |
| | Neutropenia | ± | ± | ± | ± | ± |
| | Pancytopenia | ± | ± | ± | ± | ± |
| | Thrombocytopenia | ± | ± | ± | ± | ± |
| Metabolic | Hypoglycemia | ± | ± | ± | ± | ± |
| | Ketoacidosis | + | + | + | + | + |
| | Metabolic acidosis | + | + | + | + | + |
| Musculoskeletal | Hypotonia, muscular-axial | ± | ± | ± | ± | ± |
| Other | Failure to thrive | ± | ± | ± | ± | ± |
| | Hypothermia during crisis | ± | ± | ± | | |
| | Odor of sweaty feet | ± | ± | ± | ± | ± |
| Laboratory findings | 3-Hydroxyisovaleric acid (urine) | ↑-↑↑↑ | ↑-↑↑↑ | ↑-↑↑↑ | ↑-↑↑↑ | ↑-↑↑↑ |
| | Ammonia (blood) | n-↑ | n-↑ | n-↑ | n-↑ | n-↑ |
| | Anion gap | + | + | + | + | + |
| | C5 Acylcarnitine (blood) | ↑-↑↑↑ | ↑-↑↑↑ | ↑-↑↑↑ | ↑-↑↑↑ | ↑-↑↑↑ |
| | C5 Acylcarnitine (plasma) | ↑-↑↑↑ | ↑-↑↑↑ | ↑-↑↑↑ | ↑-↑↑↑ | ↑-↑↑↑ |
| | C5 Isovaleryl carnitine (blood) | ↑-↑↑↑ | ↑-↑↑↑ | ↑-↑↑↑ | ↑-↑↑↑ | ↑-↑↑↑ |
| | C5/C2 Acylcarnitines ratio | ↑ | ↑ | ↑ | ↑ | ↑ |
| | Calcium (plasma) | ↓-n | ↓-n | ↓-n | ↓-n | ↓-n |
| | Carnitine, esterified (plasma) | ↑ | ↑ | ↑ | ↑ | ↑ |
| | Carnitine, free (dried blood spot) | ↓ | ↓ | ↓ | ↓ | ↓ |
| | Carnitine, free (plasma) | ↓ | ↓ | ↓ | ↓ | ↓ |
| | Glucose (plasma) | ↓-n | ↓-n | ↓-n | ↓-n | ↓-n |
| | Glycine (plasma) | n-↑ | n-↑ | n-↑ | n-↑ | n-↑ |
| | Homocysteine (plasma) | n | n | n | n | n |
| | Isovaleric acid (plasma) | ↑-↑↑ | ↑-↑↑ | ↑-↑↑ | ↑-↑↑ | ↑-↑↑ |
| | Isovaleryl glycine (urine) | ↑-↑↑↑ | ↑-↑↑↑ | ↑-↑↑↑ | ↑-↑↑↑ | ↑-↑↑↑ |
| | Isovaleryl-CoA dehydrogenase (fibroblasts) | ↓ | ↓ | ↓ | ↓ | ↓ |
| | Lactate (plasma) | n-↑ | n-↑ | n-↑ | n-↑ | n-↑ |
| | Lactate/*N*-acetylaspartic acid (NAA) ratio (MRS) | n-↑ | n-↑ | n-↑ | n-↑ | n-↑ |
| | Uric acid (plasma) | n-↑ | n-↑ | n-↑ | n-↑ | n-↑ |

**Table 23.7** Isobutyryl-CoA dehydrogenase deficiency (ACAD8)

| System | Symptoms and biomarkers | Neonatal (birth–1 month) | Infancy (1–18 months) | Childhood (1.5–11 years) | Adolescence (11–16 years) | Adulthood (>16 years) |
|---|---|---|---|---|---|---|
| Cardiovascular | Cardiomyopathy, dilated | ± | ± | ± | ± | ± |
| Digestive | Vomiting, episodic | ± | ± | ± | ± | ± |
| Hematological | Anemia | ± | ± | ± | ± | ± |
| Other | Most patients appear to be asymptomatic | ± | ± | ± | ± | ± |
| Laboratory findings | C4 Acylcarnitine | ↑ | ↑ | ↑ | ↑ | ↑ |
| | Carnitine, esterified (plasma) | ↑ | ↑ | ↑ | ↑ | ↑ |
| | Carnitine, free (dried blood spot) | ↓ | ↓ | ↓ | ↓ | ↓ |
| | Carnitine, free (plasma) | ↓ | ↓ | ↓ | ↓ | ↓ |
| | Isobutyryl-CoA dehydrogenase (fibroblasts) | ↓ | ↓ | ↓ | ↓ | ↓ |
| | Isobutyrylglycine (urine) | ↑ | ↑ | ↑ | ↑ | ↑ |

**Table 23.8** 2-Methylbutyrylglycinuria (ACADSB)

| System | Symptoms and biomarkers | Neonatal (birth–1 month) | Infancy (1–18 months) | Childhood (1.5–11 years) | Adolescence (11–16 years) | Adulthood (>16 years) |
|---|---|---|---|---|---|---|
| CNS | Autistic spectrum disorder | ± | ± | ± | ± | ± |
| | Decreased cortical sulci | ± | ± | | | |
| | Retardation, psychomotor | ± | ± | ± | ± | ± |
| Metabolic | Hypoglycemia | ± | ± | ± | | |
| Musculoskeletal | Hypotonia, muscular-axial | ± | ± | ± | ± | ± |
| Other | Patients may remain asymptomatic | ± | ± | ± | ± | ± |
| Laboratory findings | 2-Ethylhydracrylic acid (blood) | n-↑ | n-↑ | n-↑ | n-↑ | n-↑ |
| | 2-Ethylhydracrylic acid (plasma) | n-↑ | n-↑ | n-↑ | n-↑ | n-↑ |
| | 2-Methylbutyric acid (urine) | ↑↑ | ↑↑ | ↑↑ | ↑↑ | ↑↑ |
| | 2-Methylbutyryl-CoA dehydrogenase (fibroblasts) | ↓ | ↓ | ↓ | ↓ | ↓ |
| | 2-Methylbutyrylglycine (urine) | ↑↑ | ↑↑ | ↑↑ | ↑↑ | ↑↑ |
| | Anion gap | ± | ± | ± | ± | ± |
| | C5 2-Methylbutyrylcarnitine (blood) | ↑-↑↑ | ↑-↑↑ | ↑-↑↑ | ↑-↑↑ | ↑-↑↑ |
| | C5 2-Methylbutyrylcarnitine (plasma) | ↑-↑↑ | ↑-↑↑ | ↑-↑↑ | ↑-↑↑ | ↑-↑↑ |
| | C5/C2 Acylcarnitines ratio | ↑ | ↑ | ↑ | ↑ | ↑ |
| | Glucose (plasma) | ↓-n | ↓-n | ↓-n | | |
| | Isobutyrylglycine (urine) | n-↑ | n-↑ | n-↑ | n-↑ | n-↑ |

**Table 23.9** Methylcrotonylglycinuria A and B (MCCC1/2)

| System | Symptoms and biomarkers | Neonatal (birth–1 month) | Infancy (1–18 months) | Childhood (1.5–11 years) | Adolescence (11–16 years) | Adulthood (>16 years) |
|---|---|---|---|---|---|---|
| Cardiovascular | Cardiomyopathy | ± | ± | ± | ± | ± |
| | Cerebral atrophy (MRI) | ± | ± | ± | ± | ± |
| | Encephalopathy acute, precipitated by infection | ± | ± | ± | ± | ± |
| | Hypertonia | ± | ± | ± | ± | ± |
| | Hypotonia | ± | ± | ± | ± | ± |
| | Metabolic stroke | ± | ± | ± | ± | ± |
| CNS | Retardation, psychomotor | ± | ± | ± | ± | ± |
| | White matter changes (MRI) | ± | ± | ± | ± | ± |

(continued)

**Table 23.9** (continued)

| System | Symptoms and biomarkers | Neonatal (birth–1 month) | Infancy (1–18 months) | Childhood (1.5–11 years) | Adolescence (11–16 years) | Adulthood (>16 years) |
|---|---|---|---|---|---|---|
| Hematological | Neutropenia | ± | ± | ± | ± | ± |
| | Thrombocytopenia | ± | ± | ± | ± | ± |
| Metabolic | Hypoglycemia | ± | ± | ± | ± | ± |
| | Ketoacidosis | ± | ± | ± | ± | ± |
| | Metabolic acidosis | ± | ± | ± | ± | ± |
| Musculoskeletal | Muscle pain | ± | ± | ± | ± | ± |
| | Muscle weakness | ± | ± | ± | ± | ± |
| Other | Failure to thrive | ± | ± | ± | ± | ± |
| | Highly variable phenotype incl. asymptomatic individuals | ± | ± | ± | ± | ± |
| | Odor, acrid (urine) | ± | ± | ± | ± | ± |
| Laboratory findings | 3-Hydroxyisovaleric acid (urine) | ↑-↑↑↑ | ↑-↑↑↑ | ↑-↑↑↑ | ↑-↑↑↑ | ↑-↑↑↑ |
| | 3-Methylcrotonylcarnitine | n-↑↑ | n-↑↑ | n-↑↑ | n-↑↑ | n-↑↑ |
| | 3-Methylcrotonylglycine (urine) | ↑-↑↑↑ | ↑-↑↑↑ | ↑-↑↑↑ | ↑-↑↑↑ | ↑-↑↑↑ |
| | Ammonia (blood) | n-↑ | n-↑ | n-↑ | n-↑ | n-↑ |
| | Anion gap | ± | ± | ± | ± | ± |
| | ASAT/ALAT (plasma) | n-↑ | n-↑ | n-↑ | n-↑ | n-↑ |
| | Base excess | ± | ± | ± | ± | ± |
| | C5-OH Acylcarnitine (dried blood spot) | ↑-↑↑↑ | ↑-↑↑↑ | ↑-↑↑↑ | ↑-↑↑↑ | ↑-↑↑↑ |
| | C5-OH Acylcarnitine (plasma) | ↑-↑↑↑ | ↑-↑↑↑ | ↑-↑↑↑ | ↑-↑↑↑ | ↑-↑↑↑ |
| | Carnitine, esterified (plasma) | n-↑ | n-↑ | n-↑ | n-↑ | n-↑ |
| | Carnitine, free (dried blood spot) | ↓-n | ↓-n | ↓-n | ↓-n | ↓-n |
| | Carnitine, free (plasma) | ↓-n | ↓-n | ↓-n | ↓-n | ↓-n |
| | Glucose (plasma) | ↓-n | ↓-n | ↓-n | ↓-n | ↓-n |
| | Methylcrotonyl-CoA carboxylase (fibroblasts) | ↓ | ↓ | ↓ | ↓ | ↓ |
| | Uric acid (plasma) | n-↑ | n-↑ | n-↑ | n-↑ | n-↑ |

**Table 23.10** Methylglutaconic aciduria type I (AUH)

| System | Symptoms and biomarkers | Neonatal (birth–1 month) | Infancy (1–18 months) | Childhood (1.5–11 years) | Adolescence (11–16 years) | Adulthood (>16 years) |
|---|---|---|---|---|---|---|
| CNS | Ataxia | ± | ± | ± | + | + |
| | Athetosis | ± | ± | ± | ± | ± |
| | Basal ganglia lesions (MRI) | ± | ± | ± | ± | ± |
| | Cerebellar abnormalities | ± | ± | ± | ± | ± |
| | Cerebellar abnormalities | ± | ± | ± | ± | ± |
| | Cerebral atrophy (MRI) | ± | ± | ± | ± | ± |
| | Dementia | ± | ± | ± | ± | ± |
| | Fits | ± | ± | ± | | |
| | Leukoencephalopathy | ± | ± | + | + | + |
| | Regression | + | + | + | + | + |
| | Retardation | + | + | + | + | + |
| | Retardation, psychomotor | ± | + | + | ± | ± |
| | Seizures, febrile | ± | ± | ± | | |
| | Spasticity, limbs | ± | ± | ± | ± | + |
| | White matter changes (MRI) | ± | ± | ± | ± | ± |
| Digestive | Hepatomegaly | ± | ± | ± | ± | ± |
| | Liver dysfunction | ± | ± | ± | ± | ± |
| Eye | Nystagmus | ± | ± | ± | ± | ± |
| | Optic atrophy | ± | ± | ± | ± | ± |
| Hematological | Thrombocytopenia | ± | ± | ± | | |

**Table 23.10** (continued)

| System | Symptoms and biomarkers | Neonatal (birth–1 month) | Infancy (1–18 months) | Childhood (1.5–11 years) | Adolescence (11–16 years) | Adulthood (>16 years) |
|---|---|---|---|---|---|---|
| Metabolic | Hypoglycemia | ± | ± | ± | | |
| | Metabolic acidosis | ± | ± | ± | | |
| Laboratory findings | 3-Hydroxyisovaleric acid (MRS) | n-↑ | n-↑ | n-↑ | n-↑ | n-↑ |
| | 3-Hydroxyisovaleric acid (urine) | ↑-↑↑↑ | ↑-↑↑↑ | ↑-↑↑↑ | ↑-↑↑↑ | ↑-↑↑↑ |
| | 3-Methylglutaconic acid (urine) | ↑-↑↑↑ | ↑-↑↑↑ | ↑-↑↑↑ | ↑-↑↑↑ | ↑-↑↑↑ |
| | 3-Methylglutaconyl-CoA hydratase (fibroblasts) | ↓ | ↓ | ↓ | ↓ | ↓ |
| | 3-Methylglutaric acid (urine) | ↑-↑↑ | ↑-↑↑ | ↑-↑↑ | ↑-↑↑ | ↑-↑↑ |
| | Ammonia (blood) | n-↑ | n-↑ | n-↑ | n-↑ | n-↑ |
| | ASAT/ALAT (plasma) | n-↑ | n-↑ | n-↑ | n-↑ | n-↑ |
| | C5-OH Acylcarnitine (dried blood spot) | ↑-↑↑↑ | ↑-↑↑↑ | ↑-↑↑↑ | ↑-↑↑↑ | ↑-↑↑↑ |
| | C5-OH Acylcarnitine (plasma) | ↑-↑↑↑ | ↑-↑↑↑ | ↑-↑↑↑ | ↑-↑↑↑ | ↑-↑↑↑ |
| | C6-Unsaturated acylcarnitine (blood) | ↑-↑↑ | ↑-↑↑ | ↑-↑↑ | ↑-↑↑ | ↑-↑↑ |
| | C6-Unsaturated acylcarnitine (plasma) | ↑-↑↑ | ↑-↑↑ | ↑-↑↑ | ↑-↑↑ | ↑-↑↑ |
| | Carnitine, esterified (plasma) | n-↑ | n-↑ | n-↑ | n-↑ | n-↑ |
| | Carnitine, free (dried blood spot) | ↓-n | ↓-n | ↓-n | ↓-n | ↓-n |
| | Carnitine, free (plasma) | ↓-n | ↓-n | ↓-n | ↓-n | ↓-n |
| | Creatine kinase (plasma) | n-↑ | n-↑ | n-↑ | | |
| | Glucose (plasma) | ↓-n | ↓-n | ↓-n | | |
| | N-acetylaspartate (MRS) | ↓-n | ↓-n | ↓-n | ↓-n | ↓-n |

**Table 23.11** Mitochondrial short-chain enoyl-CoA hydratase 1 deficiency (ECHS1)

| System | Symptoms and biomarkers | Neonatal (birth–1 month) | Infancy (1–18 months) | Childhood (1.5–11 years) | Adolescence (11–16 years) | Adulthood (>16 years) |
|---|---|---|---|---|---|---|
| Cardiovascular | Cardiomyopathy, hypertrophic | + | | | | |
| CNS | Apnea | + | | | | |
| | Basal ganglia lesions (MRI) | + | | | | |
| | Brain, abnormal (MRI) | + | | | | |
| | Dystonia | + | | | | |
| | Hypotonia | + | | | | |
| | Optic atrophy | ± | | | | |
| | Regression, psychomotor | + | | | | |
| | Seizures | + | | | | |
| Ear | Hearing loss | ± | | | | |
| Laboratory findings | 2-Methyl-2,3-dihydroxybutyrate (urine) | ↑ | | | | |
| | C4 acylcarnitine | ↑ | | | | |
| | Lactate (plasma) | ↑ | | | | |
| | Lactate/pyruvate ratio | n | | | | |
| | Pyruvate (plasma) | ↑ | | | | |
| | S-(2-carboxypropyl)-cysteine (urine) | ↑ | | | | |

**Table 23.12** 3-Hydroxyisobutyryl-CoA deacylase deficiency (HIBCH)

| System | Symptoms and biomarkers | Neonatal (birth–1 month) | Infancy (1–18 months) | Childhood (1.5–11 years) | Adolescence (11–16 years) | Adulthood (>16 years) |
|---|---|---|---|---|---|---|
| CNS | Abnormalities in the globus pallidus (MRI) | ± | ± | ± | ± | ± |
| | Abnormalities in the midbrain | ± | ± | ± | ± | ± |
| | Agenesis of the cingulate gyrus | ± | ± | ± | ± | ± |
| | Agenesis, corpus callosum (MRI) | ± | ± | ± | ± | ± |
| | Developmental delay | + | ± | + | + | + |
| | Dystonia | ± | ± | ± | ± | ± |
| | Encephalopathy acute, precipitated by infection | ± | ± | ± | ± | ± |
| | Regression | ± | ± | ± | ± | ± |
| | Retardation | ± | ± | ± | ± | ± |
| | Truncal ataxia | ± | ± | ± | ± | ± |
| Digestive | Feeding difficulties | + | + | + | + | + |
| Metabolic | Metabolic acidosis | ± | ± | ± | ± | ± |
| Musculoskeletal | Hypotonia, muscular-axial | ± | ± | ± | ± | ± |
| Other | Dysmorphism | ± | ± | ± | ± | ± |
| Laboratory findings | 2-Hydroxyisovaleric acid (urine) | ↑ | ↑ | ↑ | ↑ | ↑ |
| | 3-Hydroxyisobutyryl-CoA deacylase (fibroblasts) | ↓ | ↓ | ↓ | ↓ | ↓ |
| | Anion gap | ± | ± | ± | ± | ± |
| | C4-OH 3-Hydroxyisobutyryl-carnitine (dried blood spot) | ↑ | ↑ | ↑ | ↑ | ↑ |
| | C4-OH 3-Hydroxyisobutyryl-carnitine (plasma) | ↑ | ↑ | ↑ | ↑ | ↑ |
| | Methacrylic acid conjugates (urine) | ↑ | ↑ | ↑ | ↑ | ↑ |
| | S-2-carboxypropyl-cysteamine (urine) | ↑ | ↑ | ↑ | ↑ | ↑ |
| | S-2-carboxypropyl-cysteine (urine) | ↑ | ↑ | ↑ | ↑ | ↑ |

**Table 23.13** 3-Hydroxyisobutyrate dehydrogenase deficiency (HIBADH)

| System | Symptoms and biomarkers | Neonatal (birth–1 month) | Infancy (1–18 months) | Childhood (1.5–11 years) | Adolescence (11–16 years) | Adulthood (>16 years) |
|---|---|---|---|---|---|---|
| CNS | Developmental delay | ± | ± | ± | ± | ± |
| | Focal white matter lesions | ± | ± | ± | ± | ± |
| | Intracerebral calcification (CT) | ± | ± | ± | ± | ± |
| | Microcephaly | ± | ± | ± | ± | ± |
| | White matter changes (MRI) | ± | ± | ± | ± | ± |
| Metabolic | Ketoacidosis | + | + | + | + | ± |
| | Metabolic acidosis | + | + | + | + | ± |
| Musculoskeletal | Dysmorphic features | ± | ± | ± | ± | ± |
| Other | Failure to thrive | ± | + | + | ± | ± |
| Laboratory findings | 2-Hydroxyisovaleric acid (urine) | ↑-↑↑ | ↑-↑↑ | ↑-↑↑ | ↑-↑↑ | ↑-↑↑ |
| | 3-Hydroxyisobutyrate dehydrogenase (fibroblasts) | ↓ | ↓ | ↓ | ↓ | ↓ |
| | 3-Hydroxyisobutyric acid (urine) | ↑-↑↑ | ↑-↑↑ | ↑-↑↑ | ↑-↑↑ | ↑-↑↑ |
| | C4-OH 3-Hydroxyisobutyryl-carnitine (dried blood spot) | n-↑ | n-↑ | n-↑ | n-↑ | n-↑ |
| | C4-OH 3-Hydroxyisobutyryl-carnitine (plasma) | n-↑ | n-↑ | n-↑ | n-↑ | n-↑ |
| | Carnitine, esterified (plasma) | n-↑ | n-↑ | n-↑ | n-↑ | n-↑ |
| | Carnitine, free (dried blood spot) | ↓-n | ↓-n | ↓-n | ↓-n | ↓-n |
| | Carnitine, free (plasma) | ↓-n | ↓-n | ↓-n | ↓-n | ↓-n |
| | Lactate (plasma) | n-↑ | n-↑ | n-↑ | n-↑ | n-↑ |

**Table 23.14** 2-Methyl-3-hydroxybutyryl-CoA dehydrogenase deficiency (HSD17B10)

| System | Symptoms and biomarkers | Neonatal (birth–1 month) | Infancy (1–18 months) | Childhood (1.5–11 years) | Adolescence (11–16 years) | Adulthood (>16 years) |
|---|---|---|---|---|---|---|
| Cardiovascular | Cardiomyopathy | ± | + | + | ± | ± |
| CNS | Basal ganglia lesions (MRI) | ± | ± | ± | ± | ± |
| | Brain atrophy (MRI) | ± | ± | ± | ± | ± |
| | Choreoathetosis | ± | ± | ± | ± | ± |
| | Dysarthria | ± | ± | + | + | + |
| | Dystonia | ± | + | + | + | + |
| | Frontotemporal atrophy (MRI) | ± | ± | ± | ± | ± |
| | Frontotemporal atrophy (MRI) | ± | ± | + | + | + |
| | Movement disorder | ± | ± | ± | ± | ± |
| | Periventricular white matter changes | ± | ± | ± | ± | ± |
| | Regression, psychomotor | ± | + | + | + | + |
| | Retardation, psychomotor | ± | + | + | + | + |
| | Seizures | ± | + | + | ± | ± |
| | Spasticity | ± | ± | ± | ± | ± |
| Ear | Hearing loss, sensorineural | ± | ± | ± | ± | ± |
| Eye | Vision, decreased | ± | ± | ± | ± | ± |
| Metabolic | Hypoglycemia | ± | ± | ± | ± | ± |
| | Ketoacidosis | ± | ± | ± | ± | ± |
| | Lactic acidosis | ± | + | + | ± | ± |
| | Metabolic acidosis | ± | ± | ± | ± | ± |
| Musculoskeletal | Rigidity | | | ± | ± | ± |
| Other | Most patients are male | + | + | + | + | + |
| Laboratory findings | 17-Beta-hydroxysteroid dehydrogenase type 10 (fibroblasts) | ↓ | ↓ | ↓ | ↓ | ↓ |
| | 2-Methyl-3-hydroxybutyric acid (urine) | ↑ | ↑ | ↑ | ↑ | ↑ |
| | C5:1 Tiglylcarnitine (blood) | n-↑ | n-↑ | n-↑ | n-↑ | n-↑ |
| | C5:1 Tiglylcarnitine (plasma) | n-↑ | n-↑ | n-↑ | n-↑ | n-↑ |
| | C5-OH 2-Methyl-3-hydroxy-butyrylcarnitine (blood) | n-↑ | n-↑ | n-↑ | n-↑ | n-↑ |
| | C5-OH 2-Methyl-3-hydroxy-butyrylcarnitine (plasma) | n-↑ | n-↑ | n-↑ | n-↑ | n-↑ |
| | Glucose (plasma) | ↓-n | ↓-n | ↓-n | ↓-n | ↓-n |
| | Lactate (cerebrospinal fluid) | n-↑ | n-↑ | n-↑ | n-↑ | n-↑ |
| | Lactate (plasma) | n-↑ | n-↑ | n-↑ | n-↑ | n-↑ |
| | Lactate (plasma) | n-↑ | ↑ | ↑ | n-↑ | n-↑ |
| | Tiglylglycine (urine) | ↑ | ↑ | ↑ | ↑ | ↑ |

**Table 23.15** 3-Hydroxy-3-methyl glutaric aciduria (HMGCL)

| System | Symptoms and biomarkers | Neonatal (birth–1 month) | Infancy (1–18 months) | Childhood (1.5–11 years) | Adolescence (11–16 years) | Adulthood (>16 years) |
|---|---|---|---|---|---|---|
| Cardiovascular | Cardiomyopathy, dilated | | ± | ± | ± | ± |
| CNS | Basal ganglia lesions (MRI) | ± | ± | ± | ± | ± |
| | Cerebral atrophy (MRI) | ± | ± | ± | ± | ± |
| | Cerebral infarction | ± | ± | ± | ± | ± |
| | Coma, during crisis | + | + | + | + | + |
| | Convulsions | + | + | | | |
| | Lethargy, during crisis | + | + | + | + | + |
| | Occipital lesions | ± | ± | ± | ± | ± |
| | Retardation, psychomotor | ± | ± | ± | ± | ± |
| | Seizures | ± | ± | ± | ± | ± |
| | Stroke-like encephalopathy | ± | ± | ± | ± | ± |
| | White matter abnormalities (MRI) | ± | ± | ± | ± | ± |

(continued)

**Table 23.15** (continued)

| System | Symptoms and biomarkers | Neonatal (birth–1 month) | Infancy (1–18 months) | Childhood (1.5–11 years) | Adolescence (11–16 years) | Adulthood (>16 years) |
|---|---|---|---|---|---|---|
| Digestive | Hepatomegaly | + | + | ± | ± | ± |
| | Liver dysfunction | + | + | + | + | + |
| | Pancreatitis | ± | ± | ± | ± | ± |
| | Vomiting, episodic | + | + | ± | ± | ± |
| Metabolic | Hypoglycemia, hypoketotic | + | + | + | + | + |
| | Lactic acidosis | + | + | + | + | + |
| | Metabolic acidosis | + | + | + | + | + |
| Musculoskeletal | Hypotonia, muscular-axial | ± | ± | ± | ± | ± |
| Respiratory | Respiratory distress | ± | ± | ± | ± | ± |
| Laboratory findings | 3-Hydroxy-3-methylglutaric acid (urine) | ↑-↑↑↑ | ↑-↑↑↑ | ↑-↑↑↑ | ↑-↑↑↑ | ↑-↑↑↑ |
| | 3-Hydroxy-3-methylglutaryl-CoA lyase (fibroblasts, immortalized lymphocytes) | ↓ | ↓ | ↓ | ↓ | ↓ |
| | 3-Hydroxyisovaleric acid (urine) | ↑-↑↑↑ | ↑-↑↑↑ | ↑-↑↑↑ | ↑-↑↑↑ | ↑-↑↑↑ |
| | 3-Methylcrotonylglycine (urine) | n-↑ | n-↑ | n-↑ | n-↑ | n-↑ |
| | 3-Methylglutaconic acid (urine) | ↑-↑↑↑ | ↑-↑↑↑ | ↑-↑↑↑ | ↑-↑↑↑ | ↑-↑↑↑ |
| | 3-Methylglutaric acid (urine) | ↑-↑↑↑ | ↑-↑↑↑ | ↑-↑↑↑ | ↑-↑↑↑ | ↑-↑↑↑ |
| | Adipic acid (urine) | n-↑ | n-↑ | n-↑ | n-↑ | n-↑ |
| | Ammonia (blood) | n-↑ | n-↑ | n-↑ | n-↑ | n-↑ |
| | ASAT/ALAT (plasma) | n-↑ | n-↑ | n-↑ | n-↑ | n-↑ |
| | C5-OH Acylcarnitine (dried blood spot) | ↑-↑↑↑ | ↑-↑↑↑ | ↑-↑↑↑ | ↑-↑↑↑ | ↑-↑↑↑ |
| | C5-OH Acylcarnitine (plasma) | ↑-↑↑↑ | ↑-↑↑↑ | ↑-↑↑↑ | ↑-↑↑↑ | ↑-↑↑↑ |
| | C6:1 Acylcarnitine (blood) | ↑-↑↑↑ | ↑-↑↑↑ | ↑-↑↑↑ | ↑-↑↑↑ | ↑-↑↑↑ |
| | C6:1 Acylcarnitine (plasma) | ↑-↑↑↑ | ↑-↑↑↑ | ↑-↑↑↑ | ↑-↑↑↑ | ↑-↑↑↑ |
| | C6DC Acylcarnitine (blood) | ↑-↑↑↑ | ↑-↑↑↑ | ↑-↑↑↑ | ↑-↑↑↑ | ↑-↑↑↑ |
| | C6DC Acylcarnitine (plasma) | ↑-↑↑↑ | ↑-↑↑↑ | ↑-↑↑↑ | ↑-↑↑↑ | ↑-↑↑↑ |
| | Carnitine, free | ↓-n | ↓-n | ↓-n | ↓-n | ↓-n |
| | Free fatty acids (serum) | n-↑ | n-↑ | n-↑ | n-↑ | n-↑ |
| | Glucose (plasma) | ↓-n | ↓-n | ↓-n | ↓-n | ↓-n |
| | Glutaric acid (urine) | n-↑ | n-↑ | n-↑ | n-↑ | n-↑ |
| | Ketones (plasma) | ↓ | ↓ | ↓ | ↓ | ↓ |
| | Lactate (plasma) | n-↑↑ | n-↑↑ | n-↑↑ | n-↑↑ | n-↑↑ |
| | Sebacic acid (urine) | n-↑ | n-↑ | n-↑ | n-↑ | n-↑ |
| | Suberic acid (urine) | n-↑ | n-↑ | n-↑ | n-↑ | n-↑ |

**Table 23.16** Methylmalonate semialdehyde dehydrogenase deficiency (ALDH6A1)

| System | Symptoms and biomarkers | Neonatal (birth–1 month) | Infancy (1–18 months) | Childhood (1.5–11 years) | Adolescence (11–16 years) | Adulthood (>16 years) |
|---|---|---|---|---|---|---|
| CNS | Developmental delay | ± | ± | ± | ± | ± |
| Digestive | Hepatomegaly | ± | ± | ± | ± | ± |
| | Vomiting, episodic | ± | ± | ± | ± | ± |
| Other | Failure to thrive | ± | ± | ± | ± | ± |
| Laboratory findings | 2-Aminoisobutyrate | n-↑ | n-↑ | n-↑ | n-↑ | n-↑ |
| | 3-Aminoisobutyric acid (urine) | n-↑ | n-↑ | n-↑ | n-↑ | n-↑ |
| | 3-Hydroxyisobutyric acid (urine) | n-↑ | n-↑ | n-↑ | n-↑ | n-↑ |
| | 3-Hydroxypropionic acid (urine) | n-↑ | n-↑ | n-↑ | n-↑ | n-↑ |
| | Beta-alanine (urine) | n-↑ | n-↑ | n-↑ | n-↑ | n-↑ |
| | Ethylmalonic acid (urine) | n-↑ | n-↑ | n-↑ | n-↑ | n-↑ |
| | Lactate (plasma) | n-↑ | n-↑ | n-↑ | n-↑ | n-↑ |
| | Methionine (plasma) | n-↑ | n-↑ | n-↑ | n-↑ | n-↑ |
| | Methylmalonic semialdehyde dehydrogenase (fibroblasts) | ↓ | ↓ | ↓ | ↓ | ↓ |

**Table 23.17** Propionic acidemia (PCCA/B)

| System | Symptoms and biomarkers | Neonatal (birth–1 month) | Infancy (1–18 months) | Childhood (1.5–11 years) | Adolescence (11–16 years) | Adulthood (>16 years) |
|---|---|---|---|---|---|---|
| Cardiovascular | Arrhythmia | ± | ± | ± | ± | ± |
| | Cardiomyopathy | ± | ± | ± | ± | ± |
| | Cardiomyopathy, dilated | | | ± | ± | ± |
| | QT interval prolongation | ± | ± | ± | ± | ± |
| CNS | Ataxia | ± | ± | ± | ± | ± |
| | Basal ganglia abnormalities (MRI) | ± | ± | ± | ± | ± |
| | Basal ganglia lesions (MRI) | ± | ± | ± | ± | ± |
| | Brain edema (MRI) | ± | ± | ± | ± | ± |
| | Cerebral atrophy (MRI) | ± | ± | ± | ± | ± |
| | Choreoathetosis | ± | ± | ± | ± | ± |
| | Coma, during ketoacidotic episodes | + | + | + | + | + |
| | Delayed myelination | ± | ± | ± | ± | ± |
| | Dystonia | ± | ± | ± | ± | ± |
| | Encephalopathy acute, precipitated by infection | + | + | + | + | + |
| | Extrapyramidal signs | ± | ± | ± | ± | ± |
| | Hypertonia | + | + | + | + | + |
| | Hypotonia | + | + | + | + | + |
| | Lethargy, during ketoacidotic episodes | + | + | + | + | + |
| | Metabolic stroke | ± | ± | ± | ± | ± |
| | Retardation, psychomotor | + | + | + | + | + |
| | Seizures | ± | ± | ± | ± | ± |
| | White matter changes (MRI) | ± | ± | ± | ± | ± |
| Digestive | Feeding difficulties | + | + | + | + | + |
| | Hepatomegaly | + | + | ± | ± | ± |
| | Liver dysfunction | ± | ± | ± | ± | ± |
| | Pancreatitis | ± | ± | ± | ± | ± |
| | Vomiting | ± | ± | ± | ± | ± |
| Ear | Hearing loss, sensorineural | ± | ± | ± | ± | ± |
| Endocrine | Decreased body height | ± | ± | ± | ± | ± |
| | Hypergonadotropic hypogonadism, female | | | | ± | ± |
| Eye | Optic atrophy | ± | ± | ± | ± | ± |
| Hematological | Anemia | + | + | + | + | + |
| | Myelodysplasia | ± | ± | ± | ± | ± |
| | Neutropenia | + | + | + | + | + |
| | Thrombocytopenia | + | + | + | + | + |
| Metabolic | Hypoglycemia | ± | ± | ± | ± | ± |
| | Ketoacidosis | + | + | + | + | + |
| | Metabolic acidosis | + | + | + | + | + |
| Musculoskeletal | Hypotonia, muscular-axial | + | + | + | ± | ± |
| | Osteopenia | | ± | ± | ± | ± |
| Renal | Renal failure, chronic | | | | | ± |
| | Temporary impairment of renal function | ± | ± | ± | ± | ± |
| Respiratory | Respiratory insufficiency | ± | ± | ± | ± | ± |
| Other | Failure to thrive | ± | ± | ± | ± | ± |
| | Low body temperature during crisis | ± | ± | ± | | |

(continued)

**Table 23.17** (continued)

| System | Symptoms and biomarkers | Neonatal (birth–1 month) | Infancy (1–18 months) | Childhood (1.5–11 years) | Adolescence (11–16 years) | Adulthood (>16 years) |
|---|---|---|---|---|---|---|
| Laboratory findings | 2-Methylbutyrylglycine (urine) | n-↑ | n-↑ | n-↑ | n-↑ | n-↑ |
| | 3-Hydroxypropionic acid (urine) | ↑ | ↑ | ↑ | ↑ | ↑ |
| | 3-Methylcrotonylglycine (urine) | n-↑ | n-↑ | n-↑ | n-↑ | n-↑ |
| | Ammonia (blood) | n-↑↑ | n-↑↑ | n-↑↑ | n-↑↑ | n-↑↑ |
| | Anion gap | + | + | + | + | + |
| | Butyrylglycine (urine) | n-↑ | n-↑ | n-↑ | n-↑ | n-↑ |
| | C3 Propionylcarnitine (blood) | ↑ | ↑ | ↑ | ↑ | ↑ |
| | C3 Propionylcarnitine (blood) | ↑ | ↑ | ↑ | ↑ | ↑ |
| | C3 Propionylcarnitine (plasma) | ↑ | ↑ | ↑ | ↑ | ↑ |
| | C3 Propionylcarnitine (plasma) | ↑ | ↑ | ↑ | ↑ | ↑ |
| | C3/C0 Acylcarnitines ratio | ↑ | ↑ | ↑ | ↑ | ↑ |
| | C3/C2 Acylcarnitines ratio | ↑ | ↑ | ↑ | ↑ | ↑ |
| | C3/C4DC Acylcarnitines ratio | ↑ | ↑ | ↑ | ↑ | ↑ |
| | Carnitine, esterified (plasma) | ↑ | ↑ | ↑ | ↑ | ↑ |
| | Carnitine, free (dried blood spot) | ↓-n | ↓-n | ↓-n | ↓-n | ↓-n |
| | Carnitine, free (plasma) | ↓-n | ↓-n | ↓-n | ↓-n | ↓-n |
| | Glucose (plasma) | ↓-n | ↓-n | ↓-n | ↓-n | ↓-n |
| | Glutamine (cerebrospinal fluid) | n-↑ | n-↑ | n-↑ | n-↑ | n-↑ |
| | Glutamine (plasma) | ↓-n | ↓-n | ↓-n | ↓-n | ↓-n |
| | Glutamine/glutamate ratio (MRS) | n-↑ | n-↑ | n-↑ | n-↑ | n-↑ |
| | Glycine (cerebrospinal fluid) | ↑ | ↑ | ↑ | ↑ | ↑ |
| | Glycine (plasma) | ↑ | ↑ | ↑ | ↑ | ↑ |
| | Glycine (urine) | ↑ | ↑ | ↑ | ↑ | ↑ |
| | Isobutyrylglycine (urine) | n-↑ | n-↑ | n-↑ | n-↑ | n-↑ |
| | Ketones (plasma) | n-↑↑ | n-↑↑ | n-↑↑ | n-↑↑ | n-↑↑ |
| | Ketones (urine) | n-↑↑ | n-↑↑ | n-↑↑ | n-↑↑ | n-↑↑ |
| | Lactate (MRS) | n-↑ | n-↑ | n-↑ | n-↑ | n-↑ |
| | Lactate (plasma) | n-↑ | n-↑ | n-↑ | n-↑ | n-↑ |
| | Lactate (urine) | ↑ | ↑ | ↑ | ↑ | ↑ |
| | Methylcitric acid (urine) | ↑ | ↑ | ↑ | ↑ | ↑ |
| | *N*-acetylaspartate (MRS) | ↓-n | ↓-n | ↓-n | ↓-n | ↓-n |
| | Propionyl-CoA-carboxylase activity (fibroblasts) | ↓ | ↓ | ↓ | ↓ | ↓ |
| | Propionyl-CoA-carboxylase activity (white blood cells) | ↓ | ↓ | ↓ | ↓ | ↓ |
| | Propionylglycine (urine) | ↑↑↑ | ↑↑↑ | ↑↑↑ | ↑↑↑ | ↑↑↑ |
| | Tiglylglycine (urine) | ↑↑ | ↑↑ | ↑↑ | ↑↑ | ↑↑ |
| | Uric acid (plasma) | n-↑ | n-↑ | n-↑ | n-↑ | n-↑ |

**Table 23.18** Methylmalonyl-CoA epimerase deficiency (MCEE)

| System | Symptoms and biomarkers | Neonatal (birth–1 month) | Infancy (1–18 months) | Childhood (1.5–11 years) | Adolescence (11–16 years) | Adulthood (>16 years) |
|---|---|---|---|---|---|---|
| Other | No clinical significance | + | + | + | + | + |
| Laboratory findings | Methylmalonic acid (urine) | ↑ | ↑ | ↑ | ↑ | |

**Table 23.19** Methylmalonic aciduria due to methylmalonyl-CoA mutase deficiency (MMUT)

| System | Symptoms and biomarkers | Neonatal (birth–1 month) | Infancy (1–18 months) | Childhood (1.5–11 years) | Adolescence (11–16 years) | Adulthood (>16 years) |
|---|---|---|---|---|---|---|
| Cardiovascular | Cardiomyopathy | ± | ± | ± | ± | ± |
| CNS | Ataxia | ± | ± | ± | ± | ± |
| | Basal ganglia abnormalities (MRI) | ± | ± | ± | ± | ± |
| | Basal ganglia lesions (MRI) | ± | ± | ± | ± | ± |
| | Brain edema (MRI) | ± | ± | ± | ± | ± |
| | Cerebral atrophy (MRI) | ± | ± | ± | ± | ± |
| | Choreoathetosis | ± | ± | ± | ± | ± |
| | Coma, during ketoacidotic episodes | + | + | + | + | + |
| | Delayed myelination | ± | ± | ± | ± | ± |
| | Dystonia | ± | ± | ± | ± | ± |
| | Encephalopathy acute, precipitated by infection | + | + | + | + | + |
| | Extrapyramidal signs | ± | ± | ± | ± | ± |
| | Hypertonia | ± | ± | ± | ± | ± |
| | Hypotonia | ± | ± | ± | ± | ± |
| | Lethargy, during ketoacidotic episodes | + | + | + | + | + |
| | Metabolic stroke | ± | ± | ± | ± | ± |
| | Retardation, psychomotor | + | + | + | + | + |
| | Seizures | ± | ± | ± | ± | ± |
| | White matter changes (MRI) | ± | ± | ± | ± | ± |
| Digestive | Feeding difficulties | + | + | + | + | + |
| | Hepatomegaly | + | + | ± | ± | ± |
| | Liver dysfunction | ± | ± | ± | ± | ± |
| | Pancreatitis | ± | ± | ± | ± | ± |
| | Vomiting | ± | ± | ± | ± | ± |
| Endocrine | Decreased body height | ± | ± | ± | ± | ± |
| | Hyperglycemia | ± | ± | | | |
| Eye | Optic neuropathy | ± | ± | ± | ± | ± |
| Hematological | Anemia | + | + | + | + | + |
| | Neutropenia | + | + | + | + | + |
| | Thrombocytopenia | + | + | + | + | + |
| Metabolic | Ketoacidosis | + | + | + | + | + |
| | Metabolic acidosis | + | + | + | + | + |
| Musculoskeletal | Hypotonia, muscular-axial | + | + | + | ± | ± |
| | Osteopenia | | ± | ± | ± | ± |
| Renal | Progressive renal impairment | ± | + | + | + | + |
| | Reduced glomerular filtration rate | | ± | + | + | + |
| | Renal tubulopathy | ± | ± | ± | ± | ± |
| | Tubulointerstitial nephritis | ± | ± | ± | ± | ± |
| Respiratory | Respiratory insufficiency | ± | ± | ± | ± | ± |
| Other | Failure to thrive | ± | ± | ± | ± | ± |
| | Hypothermia during crisis | ± | ± | ± | | |
| Laboratory findings | 14C-Propionate incorporation assay (fibroblasts) | ↓ | ↓ | ↓ | ↓ | ↓ |
| | 3-Hydroxypropionic acid (urine) | ↑ | ↑ | ↑ | ↑ | ↑ |
| | Ammonia (blood) | n-↑↑ | n-↑↑ | n-↑↑ | n-↑↑ | n-↑↑ |
| | Anion gap | + | + | + | + | + |
| | C3 Propionylcarnitine (blood) | ↑ | ↑ | ↑ | ↑ | ↑ |
| | C3 Propionylcarnitine (plasma) | ↑ | ↑ | ↑ | ↑ | ↑ |
| | C3-DC Methylmalonylcarnitine (dried blood spot) | ↑ | ↑ | ↑ | ↑ | ↑ |

(continued)

**Table 23.19** (continued)

| System | Symptoms and biomarkers | Neonatal (birth–1 month) | Infancy (1–18 months) | Childhood (1.5–11 years) | Adolescence (11–16 years) | Adulthood (>16 years) |
|---|---|---|---|---|---|---|
| | C3-DC Methylmalonylcarnitine (plasma) | ↑ | ↑ | ↑ | ↑ | ↑ |
| | Carnitine, esterified (plasma) | ↑ | ↑ | ↑ | ↑ | ↑ |
| | Carnitine, free (dried blood spot) | ↓-n | ↓-n | ↓-n | ↓-n | ↓-n |
| | Carnitine, free (plasma) | ↓-n | ↓-n | ↓-n | ↓-n | ↓-n |
| | Glucose (plasma) | ↓-n | ↓-n | ↓-n | ↓-n | ↓-n |
| | Glutamine (plasma) | ↓-n | ↓-n | ↓-n | ↓-n | ↓-n |
| | Glycine (plasma) | ↑ | ↑ | ↑ | ↑ | ↑ |
| | Glycine (urine) | ↑ | ↑ | ↑ | ↑ | ↑ |
| | Ketones (plasma) | n-↑↑ | n-↑↑ | n-↑↑ | n-↑↑ | n-↑↑ |
| | Ketones (urine) | n-↑↑ | n-↑↑ | n-↑↑ | n-↑↑ | n-↑↑ |
| | Lactate (MRS) | n-↑ | n-↑ | n-↑ | n-↑ | n-↑ |
| | Lactate (plasma) | n-↑ | n-↑ | n-↑ | n-↑ | n-↑ |
| | Lactate (urine) | ↑ | ↑ | ↑ | ↑ | ↑ |
| | Methylcitric acid (urine) | ↑ | ↑ | ↑ | ↑ | ↑ |
| | Methylmalonic acid (plasma) | ↑-↑↑↑ | ↑-↑↑↑ | ↑-↑↑↑ | ↑-↑↑↑ | ↑-↑↑↑ |
| | Methylmalonic acid (urine) | ↑-↑↑↑ | ↑-↑↑↑ | ↑-↑↑↑ | ↑-↑↑↑ | ↑-↑↑↑ |
| | Methylmalonyl-CoA mutase activity (fibroblasts) | ↓ | ↓ | ↓ | ↓ | ↓ |
| | *N*-acetylaspartate (MRS) | ↓-n | ↓-n | ↓-n | ↓-n | ↓-n |
| | Uric acid (plasma) | n-↑ | n-↑ | n-↑ | n-↑ | n-↑ |

**Table 23.20** Combined MA and MMA (ACSF3)

| System | Symptoms and biomarkers | Neonatal (birth–1 month) | Infancy (1–18 months) | Childhood (1.5–11 years) | Adolescence (11–16 years) | Adulthood (>16 years) |
|---|---|---|---|---|---|---|
| Cardiovascular | Cardiomyopathy | ± | ± | ± | ± | ± |
| CNS | Autistic spectrum disorder | ± | ± | ± | ± | ± |
| | Coma | ± | ± | ± | ± | ± |
| | Developmental delay | ± | ± | ± | ± | ± |
| | Dystonia | ± | ± | ± | ± | ± |
| | Hyperintensities, T2 (MRI) | ± | ± | ± | ± | ± |
| | Lethargy | ± | ± | ± | ± | ± |
| | Loss of speech | | ± | ± | ± | ± |
| | Memory problems | | ± | ± | ± | ± |
| | Microcephaly | ± | ± | ± | | |
| | Migraine, ocular | | | ± | ± | ± |
| | Seizures | ± | ± | ± | ± | ± |
| Digestive | Feeding difficulties | ± | ± | ± | ± | ± |
| | Liver dysfunction | ± | ± | ± | ± | ± |
| | Vomiting | ± | ± | ± | ± | ± |
| Metabolic | Hypoglycemia | ± | ± | ± | ± | ± |
| | Ketoacidosis | ± | ± | ± | ± | ± |
| | Metabolic acidosis | ± | ± | ± | ± | ± |
| Musculoskeletal | Hypotonia, muscular-axial | ± | ± | ± | ± | ± |
| Other | Failure to thrive | ± | ± | ± | ± | ± |
| | Mild dysmorphic features | ± | ± | ± | ± | ± |

**Table 23.20** (continued)

| System | Symptoms and biomarkers | Neonatal (birth–1 month) | Infancy (1–18 months) | Childhood (1.5–11 years) | Adolescence (11–16 years) | Adulthood (>16 years) |
|---|---|---|---|---|---|---|
| Laboratory findings | Base excess | ± | ± | ± | ± | ± |
| | C3 Propionylcarnitine (blood) | n | n | n | n | n |
| | C3 Propionylcarnitine (plasma) | n | n | n | n | n |
| | C3-DC Malonylcarnitine | ↑ | ↑ | ↑ | ↑ | ↑ |
| | Carnitine, free (dried blood spot) | ↓-n | ↓-n | ↓-n | ↓-n | ↓-n |
| | Carnitine, free (plasma) | ↓-n | ↓-n | ↓-n | ↓-n | ↓-n |
| | Cholesterol (serum) | ↓-n | ↓-n | ↓-n | ↓-n | ↓-n |
| | Glucose (plasma) | ↓-n | ↓-n | ↓-n | ↓-n | ↓-n |
| | Lactate (plasma) | n-↑↑ | n-↑↑ | n-↑↑ | n-↑↑ | n-↑↑ |
| | Malonic acid (urine) | n-↑↑ | n-↑↑ | n-↑↑ | n-↑↑ | n-↑↑ |
| | Methylmalonic acid (plasma) | ↑-↑↑↑ | ↑-↑↑↑ | ↑-↑↑↑ | ↑-↑↑↑ | ↑-↑↑↑ |
| | Methylmalonic acid (urine) | ↑-↑↑↑ | ↑-↑↑↑ | ↑-↑↑↑ | ↑-↑↑↑ | ↑-↑↑↑ |
| | Urine MMA/MA ratio | ↑ | ↑ | ↑ | ↑ | ↑ |

**Table 23.21** Malonic aciduria (MLYCD)

| System | Symptoms and biomarkers | Neonatal (birth–1 month) | Infancy (1–18 months) | Childhood (1.5–11 years) | Adolescence (11–16 years) | Adulthood (>16 years) |
|---|---|---|---|---|---|---|
| Cardiovascular | Cardiomyopathy | ± | + | + | + | + |
| CNS | Basal ganglia lesions (MRI) | ± | ± | ± | ± | ± |
| | Developmental delay | ± | + | + | ± | ± |
| | Dystonia | ± | ± | ± | ± | ± |
| | Encephalopathy acute, precipitated by infection | ± | ± | ± | ± | ± |
| | Epilepsy | ± | ± | ± | ± | ± |
| | Frontotemporal atrophy (MRI) | ± | ± | ± | ± | ± |
| | White matter abnormalities (MRI) | ± | ± | ± | ± | ± |
| Digestive | Hepatomegaly | + | + | ± | ± | ± |
| | Vomiting | + | + | + | ± | ± |
| Metabolic | Hypoglycemia | ± | ± | ± | ± | ± |
| | Metabolic acidosis | ± | ± | ± | ± | ± |
| Musculoskeletal | Hypotonia, muscular-axial | ± | ± | ± | ± | ± |
| Laboratory findings | 3-Hydroxybutyric acid (urine) | n-↑↑ | n-↑↑ | n-↑↑ | n-↑↑ | n-↑↑ |
| | Adipic acid (urine) | n-↑↑ | n-↑↑ | n-↑↑ | n-↑↑ | n-↑↑ |
| | Ammonia (blood) | n-↑ | n-↑ | n-↑ | n-↑ | n-↑ |
| | Base excess | ± | ± | ± | ± | ± |
| | C3-DC Malonylcarnitine | ↑ | ↑ | ↑ | ↑ | ↑ |
| | C4-DC Methylmalonylcarnitine (urine) | ↑ | ↑ | ↑ | ↑ | ↑ |
| | Carnitine, free (dried blood spot) | ↓-n | ↓-n | ↓-n | ↓-n | ↓-n |
| | Carnitine, free (plasma) | ↓-n | ↓-n | ↓-n | ↓-n | ↓-n |
| | Cholesterol (serum) | ↓-n | ↓-n | ↓-n | ↓-n | ↓-n |
| | Ethylmalonic acid (urine) | n-↑↑ | n-↑↑ | n-↑↑ | n-↑↑ | n-↑↑ |
| | Fumaric acid (urine) | n-↑↑ | n-↑↑ | n-↑↑ | n-↑↑ | n-↑↑ |
| | Glucose (plasma) | ↓-n | ↓-n | ↓-n | ↓-n | ↓-n |
| | Glutaric acid (urine) | n-↑ | n-↑ | n-↑ | n-↑ | n-↑ |
| | Ketones (plasma) | n-↑↑ | n-↑↑ | n-↑↑ | n-↑↑ | n-↑↑ |
| | Ketones (urine) | n-↑↑ | n-↑↑ | n-↑↑ | n-↑↑ | n-↑↑ |

(continued)

**Table 23.21** (continued)

| System | Symptoms and biomarkers | Neonatal (birth–1 month) | Infancy (1–18 months) | Childhood (1.5–11 years) | Adolescence (11–16 years) | Adulthood (>16 years) |
|---|---|---|---|---|---|---|
| | Lactate (plasma) | n-↑↑ | n-↑↑ | n-↑↑ | n-↑↑ | n-↑↑ |
| | Malic acid (urine) | n-↑↑ | n-↑↑ | n-↑↑ | n-↑↑ | n-↑↑ |
| | Malonic acid (urine) | ↑-↑↑↑ | ↑-↑↑↑ | ↑-↑↑↑ | ↑-↑↑↑ | ↑-↑↑↑ |
| | Malonyl-CoA decarboxylase activity | ↓ | ↓ | ↓ | ↓ | ↓ |
| | Methylmalonic acid (urine) | n-↑ | n-↑ | n-↑ | n-↑ | n-↑ |
| | Sebacic acid (urine) | n-↑↑ | n-↑↑ | n-↑↑ | n-↑↑ | n-↑↑ |
| | Suberic acid (urine) | n-↑↑ | n-↑↑ | n-↑↑ | n-↑↑ | n-↑↑ |
| | Succinic acid (urine) | n-↑↑ | n-↑↑ | n-↑↑ | n-↑↑ | n-↑↑ |
| | Urine MMA/MA ratio | ↓ | ↓ | ↓ | ↓ | ↓ |

**Table 23.22** Monocarboxylate transporter-1 deficiency (ACAT1)

| System | Symptoms and biomarkers | Neonatal (birth–1 month) | Infancy (1–18 months) | Childhood (1.5–11 years) | Adolescence (11–16 years) | Adulthood (>16 years) |
|---|---|---|---|---|---|---|
| Cardiovascular | Cardiomyopathy | ± | ± | ± | ± | ± |
| CNS | Abnormalities in the putamen | ± | ± | ± | ± | ± |
| | Ataxia | ± | ± | ± | ± | ± |
| | Basal ganglia abnormalities (MRI) | ± | ± | ± | ± | ± |
| | Basal ganglia lesions (MRI) | ± | ± | ± | ± | ± |
| | Brain edema (MRI) | ± | ± | ± | ± | ± |
| | Coma, during ketoacidotic episodes | ± | ± | ± | ± | ± |
| | Dentate nucleus lesions (MRI) | ± | ± | ± | ± | ± |
| | Hyperintensities (T2) of the globus pallidus (MRI) | ± | ± | ± | ± | ± |
| | Hypertonia | ± | ± | ± | ± | ± |
| | Hypotonia | ± | ± | ± | ± | ± |
| | Lethargy, during ketoacidotic episodes | ± | ± | ± | ± | ± |
| | Movement disorder | ± | ± | ± | ± | ± |
| | Pyramidal signs | ± | ± | ± | ± | ± |
| | Retardation, psychomotor | ± | ± | ± | ± | ± |
| | Seizures | ± | ± | ± | ± | ± |
| Digestive | Hepatomegaly | + | + | + | ± | ± |
| | Liver dysfunction | ± | + | + | ± | ± |
| | Vomiting, episodic | + | + | + | + | + |
| Hematological | Neutropenia | ± | ± | ± | ± | ± |
| | Thrombocytopenia | ± | ± | ± | ± | ± |
| Metabolic | Ketoacidosis | + | + | + | + | + |
| | Metabolic acidosis | + | + | + | + | + |
| Musculoskeletal | Hypotonia, muscular-axial | ± | ± | ± | ± | ± |
| Respiratory | Respiratory distress | ± | ± | ± | ± | ± |
| Other | Acetone-like odor to the breath | ± | ± | | | |
| | Failure to thrive | ± | ± | ± | ± | ± |
| Laboratory findings | 2-Ethylhydracrylic acid (urine) | ↑ | ↑ | ↑ | ↑ | ↑ |
| | 2-Methyl-3-hydroxybutyric acid (urine) | ↑ | ↑ | ↑ | ↑ | ↑ |
| | 2-Methylacetoacetic acid (urine) | ↑ | ↑ | ↑ | ↑ | ↑ |
| | 3-Hydroxy-*n*-butyric acid (blood) | ↑ | ↑ | ↑ | | |
| | 3-Hydroxy-*n*-butyric acid (urine) | ↑ | ↑ | ↑ | | |

**Table 23.22** (continued)

| System | Symptoms and biomarkers | Neonatal (birth–1 month) | Infancy (1–18 months) | Childhood (1.5–11 years) | Adolescence (11–16 years) | Adulthood (>16 years) |
|---|---|---|---|---|---|---|
| | 3-Oxothiolase activity (fibroblasts) | ↓ | ↓ | ↓ | ↓ | ↓ |
| | Acetoacetate (blood) | ↑ | ↑ | ↑ | | |
| | Acetoacetate (urine) | ↑ | ↑ | ↑ | | |
| | Ammonia (blood) | n-↑ | n-↑ | n-↑ | n-↑ | n-↑ |
| | Anion gap | + | + | + | + | + |
| | C5:1 Tiglylcarnitine (blood) | ↑ | ↑ | ↑ | ↑ | ↑ |
| | C5:1 Tiglylcarnitine (plasma) | ↑ | ↑ | ↑ | ↑ | ↑ |
| | C5-OH 2-Methyl-3-hydroxy-butyrylcarnitine (blood) | ↑ | ↑ | ↑ | ↑ | ↑ |
| | C5-OH 2-Methyl-3-hydroxy-butyrylcarnitine (plasma) | ↑ | ↑ | ↑ | ↑ | ↑ |
| | Carnitine, esterified (plasma) | ↑ | ↑ | ↑ | ↑ | ↑ |
| | Carnitine, free (dried blood spot) | ↓ | ↓ | ↓ | ↓ | ↓ |
| | Carnitine, free (plasma) | ↓ | ↓ | ↓ | ↓ | ↓ |
| | Choline (MRS) | n-↑ | n-↑ | n-↑ | n-↑ | n-↑ |
| | Dicarboxylic acids (urine) | n | n | n | n | n |
| | Free fatty acids (serum) | n | n | n | | |
| | Glucose (plasma) | ↓-↑ | ↓-↑ | ↓-↑ | ↓-↑ | ↓-↑ |
| | Glycine (plasma) | n-↑ | n-↑ | n-↑ | n-↑ | n-↑ |
| | Ketones (plasma) | ↑ | ↑ | ↑ | ↑ | ↑ |
| | Ketones (urine) | ↑ | ↑ | ↑ | ↑ | ↑ |
| | Lactate (MRS) | n-↑ | n-↑ | n-↑ | n-↑ | n-↑ |
| | Tiglylglycine (urine) | ↑-↑↑↑ | ↑-↑↑↑ | ↑-↑↑↑ | ↑-↑↑↑ | ↑-↑↑↑ |
| | Uric acid (plasma) | n-↑ | n-↑ | n-↑ | n-↑ | n-↑ |

## Diagnostic Flowchart

A positive newborn screening test for elevated leucine should be confirmed by quantitative plasma amino acid analysis and usually is seen only in MSUD. High-risk newborns require an early newborn screening, e.g., at day 1 of life, along with preventative dietary intervention. Abnormal blood acylcarnitine species may be seen in the other disorders in this pathway, and making the correct diagnosis depends on analysis of urinary organic acids by combined gas chromatography/mass spectrometry (GCMS). Further diagnostic information is obtained through analysis of urinary acylglycines. Essentially, the detection of unusual body odor (maple syrup, sweaty feet), acidosis, ketosis, elevated ammonia, hypoglycemia, or carnitine deficiency suggests that urine organic acid analysis should be performed. Patients with many of these disorders may be asymptomatic at birth and are identified only on the basis of an abnormal newborn screening using tandem mass spectrometry. In patients not screened as newborns, non-specific symptoms such as failure to thrive or developmental delay should trigger a metabolic evaluation that may identify a diagnostic metabolite. Blood acylcarnitines and urinary organic acid profiling are again essential for the correct differential diagnosis followed by confirmatory analysis. The disorders of isoleucine and valine metabolism are also detected in a sequential process that begins with the evaluation of the symptoms and signs displayed by the patient (selective metabolic screening) or in some countries on newborn screening. Clinical chemistry is helpful in the assessment of ketogenesis by urinary tests for ketone bodies or quantification of 3-hydroxybutyrate and acetoacetate in the blood. Electrolytes, blood gases, and pH provide evidence of acidosis, and it is important to test for hyperammonemia. Analysis of plasma amino acids and blood acylcarnitines is helpful. In virtually all instances, the definitive diagnosis will come from organic acid analysis of the urine, followed by further molecular testing. Enzymatic testing is not a first-line analysis and should be reserved to unsolved cases.

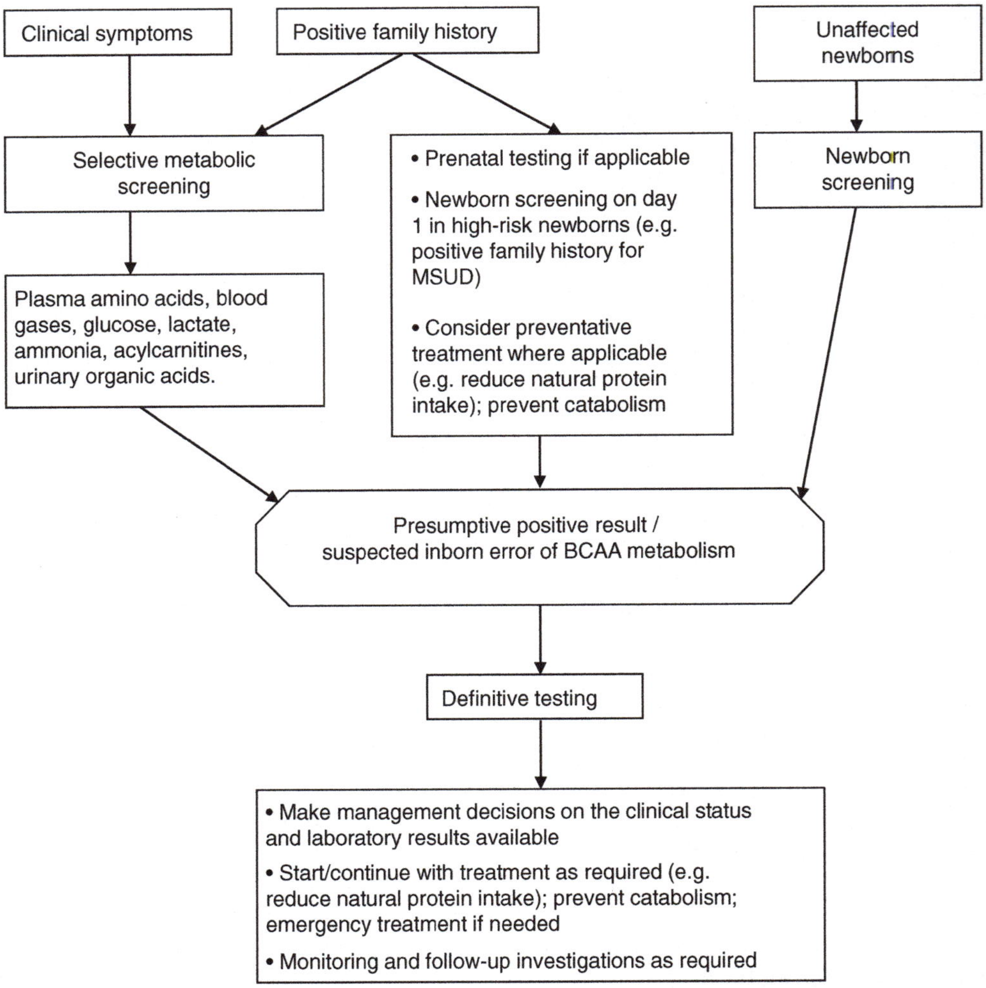


**Fig. 23.2** Diagnostic flowchart

## Reference Values

- Urine/spot tests

| | 2,4-Dinitrophenylhydrazine (DNPH) test | Ferric chloride test |
|---|---|---|
| Normal | No precipitate | No color change |

- Plasma quantitative amino acids (μmol/L)
  (Ion exchange column chromatography or high-performance liquid chromatography, HPLC)

| Age | Valine | Isoleucine | Leucine | Alloisoleucine |
|---|---|---|---|---|
| Newborn[a] | 86–220 | 23–95 | 48–180 | 0 |
| Child | 64–320 | 30–105 | 59–180 | 0 |
| Adult | 99–286 | 30–108 | 61–162 | 0 |

| Age | Glycine | Methionine | Threonine |
|---|---|---|---|
| Newborn[a] | 220–500 | 6–40 | 60–200 |
| Child | 130–400 | 9–45 | 60–200 |
| Adult | 120–550 | 9–59 | 43–130 |

[a]The national standards and local reference ranges for newborn screening or selective screening tests should be used

- Organic acids in urine (mmol/mol creatinine), blood plasma or serum (μmol/L), or dried blood spots (DBS, μmol/L)
  (Gas chromatography (GC)/mass spectrometry, GC/MS)

| Age | Urine 2-oxoiso-caproic acid | Urine 2-oxo-3-methyl-valeric acid | Urine 2-oxoiso-valeric acid | Urine 2-hydroxy-isovaleric acid | Urine 2-hydroxy-isocaproic acid | Urine 2-hydroxy-3-methyl-valeric acid | Urine lactate | Venous blood lactate (mmol/L) |
|---|---|---|---|---|---|---|---|---|
| All | <2 | <2 | <2 | <2 | <2 | <2 | <197 | <2.2 |

| Age | Plasma/serum isovaleric acid | DBS isovaleryl-glycine | Urine isovalery-glycine | Urine 3-hydroxy-isovaleric acid | Urine 4-hydroxy-isovaleric acid | Urine isovaleryl-glucuronide | Urine 3-methyl-crotonyl-glycine | Urine 3-methyl-glutaconic acid | Urine 3-methyl-glutaric acid | Urine 3-hydroxy-3-methyl glutaric acid |
|---|---|---|---|---|---|---|---|---|---|---|
| All | <10 | <0.5 | <10 | <16 | <2 | ND | <2 | <6 | <7 | <36 |

| Age | Urine 3-hydroxy-propionate | DBS 3-hydroxy-propionate | Urine methyl-citrate | Urine propionyl-glycine | Urine 2-methyl-butyryl-glycine | Urine methyl-malonate | DBS methyl-malonate | Urine 2-methyl-3-hydroxy butyrate | Urine 3-hydroxy-isobutyrate | Urine 2-methyl-acetoacetate |
|---|---|---|---|---|---|---|---|---|---|---|
| All | <2 | ND | <2 | <2 | <2 | <2 | <0.4 | <12 | <24 | <2 |

| Age | Urine 2-methyl-butyryl-glycine | Urine 2-ethyl-hydra-crylic acid | Urine 2-methyl-3-hydroxy butyrate | Urine tiglyl-glycine | Urine isobutyryl-glycine | Urine *S*-2-carboxy-propyl-cysteamine and *S*-2-carboxy-propylcysteine | Urine 3-hydroxy-isobutyrate |
|---|---|---|---|---|---|---|---|
| All | <2 | <2 | <11 | <2 | <3.8 | ND | <33 |

| Age | Urine 3-hydroxy-propionate | DBS 3-hydroxy-propionate | Urine methyl-citrate | Urine tiglyl-glycine | Urine propionyl-glycine | Urine methyl-malonate | DBS methyl-malonate | Plasma/serum methyl-malonate | Urine malonic acid |
|---|---|---|---|---|---|---|---|---|---|
| All | <10 | ND | <8 | <2 | <2 | <2 | <0.4 | <0.2 | <5 |

- Acylcarnitines in dried blood spots (DBS, µmol/L) (Tandem mass spectrometry)[a]

| Age | Free carnitine (C0) | C3-/ propionyl-carnitine | C3-DC/ malonyl-carnitine | C4-/ butyryl-carnitine + isobutyryl-carnitine | C4-DC-/ methyl-malonyl-carnitine | C4-OH-/3-OH-isobutyryl-carnitine | C5-/isovaleryl-/2-methyl-butyryl-carnitine | C5:1-/pentanoyl-/ tiglyl-carnitine | C5-OH-/3-hydroxy-isovaleryl-/2-methyl-3-OH-butyryl-carnitine |
|---|---|---|---|---|---|---|---|---|---|
| All[b] | 10–60 | <3.60 | <0.20 | <0.50 | <0.54 | <0.39 | <0.20 | <0.03 | <0.36 |

[a]The national standards and local reference ranges for newborn screening or selective screening tests should be used
[b]Of note, acylcarnitine reference values are age-dependent (see special literature)

## Pathological Values

- Urine/spot tests

| Disorder | 2,4-Dinitrophenylhydrazine (DNPH) test[a] | Ferric chloride test[a] |
|---|---|---|
| 23.2 Maple syrup disease (MSUD) | Yellow precipitate | Greenish-gray color |

[a]This test has historical importance but has since been replaced (e.g., through newborn screening or selective metabolic screening using tandem mass spectrometry)

- Plasma quantitative amino acids (μmol/L)
  (Ion exchange column chromatography or high-performance liquid chromatography, HPLC)

| Disorder | Valine | Isoleucine | Leucine | Alloisoleucine | % Normal activity of BCKD[a] complex |
|---|---|---|---|---|---|
| 23.1 BCAT deficiency | 220–1500 | Increased | Increased | – | Normal |
| 23.2–23.4 MSUD | | | | | |
| Clinical forms: | | | | | |
| Classic | To 7550 | To 4800 | To 10,800 | ≥5–970 | 0–2 |
| Intermediate[a] | To 1000 | To 1000 | To 2000 | 2–220 | 3–30 |
| Intermittent[a] | To 1000 | To 1000 | To 4000 | 2–220 | 3–30 |
| Thiamin-responsive | To 1000 | To 1000 | To 5000 | Present | 2–40 |

[a]Levels may only be abnormal during acute episodes of ketoacidosis in the intermittent/intermediate form

- Comments/Additions
  1. Leucine, isoleucine, and valine are usually not elevated in metabolic defects distal from the BCKD complex as this complex catalyzes an irreversible enzymic reaction.
  2. Secondary findings, such as elevated plasma glycine and alanine concentrations, are not listed separately.

- Organic acids in urine (mmol/mol creatinine), blood plasma or serum (μmol/L) or dried blood spots (DBS, μmol/L)
  (Gas chromatography (GC)/mass spectrometry, GC/MS)[a]

| Disorder abbreviation | Urine 2-oxoiso-caproic acid | Urine 2-oxo-3-methyl-valeric acid | Urine 2-oxoiso-valeric acid | Urine 2-hydroxy-isovaleric acid | Urine 2-hydroxy-isocaproic acid | Urine 2-hydroxy-3-methyl-valeric acid | Urine lactate[b] | Venous blood lactate (mmol/L)[b] |
|---|---|---|---|---|---|---|---|---|
| 23.1 BCAA transferase deficiency | – | – | – | – | – | – | | |
| 23.2–23.4 MSUD | To 4400 | To 2500 | To 800 | To 3600 | To 80 | To 400 | n-↑ | n-↑ |

| Disorder abbreviation | Plasma/serum isovaleric acid | DBS isovaleryl-glycine | Urine isovalery-glycine | Urine 3-hydroxy-isovaleric acid | Urine 4-hydroxy-isovaleric acid | Urine isovaleryl-glucuronide | Urine 3-methyl-crotonyl-glycine |
|---|---|---|---|---|---|---|---|
| 23.6 IVA | 600–5000 (with episodes); 10–50 (between episodes) | 1.3–80.0 | To 4980 | To 2000 | 20–300 | Detectable[c] | – |
| 23.9 methylcrotonylglycinuria | – | – | – | 96–8850 | – | – | 40–4042 |

| Disorder abbreviation | Urine 3-hydroxy-isovaleric acid | Urine 3-methyl-crotonyl-glycine | Urine 3-methyl-glutaconic acid | Urine 3-methyl-glutaric acid | Urine 3-hydroxy-3-methyl-glutaric acid |
|---|---|---|---|---|---|
| 23.10 3-methylglutaconic aciduria type 1 | 47–3840 | – | 168–2900 | 4.5–9.0 | – |
| 23.15 hydroxymethylglutaric aciduria | 60–9600 | 0–400 | 140–24,200 | 14–3000 | 200–11,000 |

| Disorder abbreviation | Urine 2-methyl-butyryl-glycine | Urine 2-ethyl-hydra-crylic acid | Urine 2-methyl-3-hydroxy butyrate | Urine tiglyl-glycine | Urine 2-methyl-acetoacetate | Urine isobutyryl-glycine | Urine *S*-2-carboxy-propyl-cysteamine + *S*-2-carboxy-propylcysteine | 2,3-dihydroxy-2-methylbutyrate | Urine 3-hydroxy-isobutyrate |
|---|---|---|---|---|---|---|---|---|---|
| 23.7 Isobutyryl-CoA dehydrogenase deficiency | – | – | – | – | | ↑ | – | | |
| 23.8 methylbutyrylglycinuria | 3–37 | ↑ | – | | | – | – | | |
| 23.11 Crotonase deficiency | | | | | | | | ↑ | |
| 23.12 HIBCH deficiency | – | – | | | | | ↑ | | |
| 23.13 HIBADH Deficiency | – | – | | | | | | | |
| 23.14 2-methyl-3-hydroxybutyryl-COA deficiency | – | n-↑ | 11–30 | ↑ | | – | – | | |
| 23.22 β-ketothiolase deficiency | – | | 11–4400 | 2–1000 | 2–650 | – | – | | |

| Disorder abbreviation | Urine 3-hydroxy-propionate | DBS 3-hydroxy-propionate | Urine methyl-citrate | Urine tiglyl-glycine | Urine propionyl-glycine | Urine methyl-malonate | Plasma/(DBS) methyl-malonate | Urine malonic acid |
|---|---|---|---|---|---|---|---|---|
| 23.16 MMSDH deficiency[d] | n-↑ | n-↑ | | | | n (-↑) | n (-↑) | |
| 23.17 PA | 20–2000 | 69–107 | 150–2800 | 13–497 | 2–450 | – | – | |
| 23.19 MMA | 4–1000 | 11–32 | To 2800 | (↑) | (↑) | 20–16,543 | 24–6129 (2–2920) | – |
| 23.20 CMAMMA | | | | | | 21–1830 | 0.4–48 | 3–600 |
| 23.21 MA | | | | | | 17–210 | n-↑ | 100–5440 |

[a]Levels may only be abnormal in variant forms during metabolic decompensation. Range of (but not all) metabolites are given

[b]As an elevated concentration of lactate is a frequent finding, lactate is therefore not listed repeatedly

[c]Isovalerylglucuronide is more likely to be excreted when the concentration of 3-hydroxyisovaleric acid is high

[d]3-hydroxy-/3-aminoisobutyric acids, 2-aminoisobutyrate, 3-hydroxypropionic acids, and ethylmalonate may also be increased in methylmalonate semialdehyde dehydrogenase deficiency

- Acylcarnitines in dried blood spots (DBS, μmol/L) (Tandem mass spectrometry)[a,b]

| Disorder abbreviation | Free carnitine (C0) | C3-/ propionyl-carnitine | C4-/ butyryl-carnitine + isobutyryl-carnitine | C3-DC/ malonylcarnitine | C4-DC-/ methyl-malonyl-carnitine | C4-OH-/3-OH-isobutyryl-carnitine | C5-/ isovaleryl-/2-methyl-butyryl-carnitine | C5:1-/ pentanoyl-/ tiglyl-carnitine | C5-OH-/3-hydroxy-isovaleryl-/2-methyl-3-OH-butyryl-carnitine |
|---|---|---|---|---|---|---|---|---|---|
| 23.1 BCAA aminotransferase deficiency | n | | | | | | | | |
| 23.2–23.4 MSUD | n | | | | | | | | |
| 23.6 IVA | ↓-n | | | | | | ↑ | | |
| 23.7 isobutyryl-CoA dehydrogenase deficiency | ↓-n | | ↑ | | | | | | ↑ |
| 23.8 methylbutyrylglycinuria | ↓-n | | | | | | ↑ | | |
| 23.9 3-methylcrotonylglycinuria type 1 | ↓-n | | | | | | | | ↑ |
| 23.10 3-methylglutaconic aciduria MGA1 | ↓-n | | | | | | | | ↑ |
| 23.11 crotonase deficiency | | | n-(↑) | | | | | | |
| 23.12 β-hydroxyisobutyryl-CoA deacylase deficiency | ↓-n | | | | | ↑ | | | |
| 23.13 3-hydroxyisobutyrate dehydrogenase deficiency | ↓-n | | | | | ↑ | | | |
| 23.14 2-methyl-3-hydroxybutyryl-CoA dehydrogenase deficiency | ↓-n | | | | | | | ↑ | ↑ |
| 23.15 Hydroxymethylglutaric aciduria | ↓-n | | | | | | | | ↑ |
| 23.16 MMSDH deficiency | (n) | | | | | | | | |
| 23.17 PA[c] | ↓-n | ↑ | | | | | | | |
| 23.18–23.19 MMA[c] | ↓-n | ↑ | | | ↑ | | | | |
| 23.20 CMAMMA | ↓-n | n | | ↑ | | | | | |
| 23.21 MA | ↓-n | | | ↑ | | | | | |

[a]Levels may only be abnormal in patients with variant forms during metabolic decompensation
[b]Acylcarnitine concentration may increase following L-carnitine supplementation
[c]Molar ratios should be applied for diagnostic purposes, e.g., C3/acetylcarnitine (C2) and C3/C0

## Specimen Collection

| Tests | Sample requirements |
|---|---|
| Urine | 5–10 mL, random, fresh or frozen without preservatives and shipped frozen (packed in dry-ice) or lyophilized and shipped at room temperature with original volume specified or shipped as fresh sample with 1–2 drops of chloroform for preservation. |
| Amino acids | Test urinary amino acids, e.g., in patients with hyperammonemia or kidney dysfunction, otherwise plasma sample preferred |
| Organic acids | |
| Carnitine (free/total) | |
| Acylglycines | |
| 2,4-Dinitrophenylhydrazine (DNPH) test | Fresh or frozen random<br>This test has historical importance but has since been replaced<br>May give false-negative results<br>Usually positive if blood leucine is greater than 800 μmol/L<br>May be positive in other conditions with oxoacids<br>False positives with methenamine and radio-opaque contrast material |
| Ferric chloride test | Fresh or frozen random<br>This test has historical importance but has since been replaced<br>Turned colors to various abnormal urinary metabolites |
| Plasma | Plasma, 0.5–1.0 mL for each determination from heparinized or EDTA blood (or serum) supernatant from clinical centrifugation (within 20 min), fresh or promptly frozen and shipped frozen (packed with dry-ice) or lyophilized and shipped at room temperature with original volume specified. For quantitative amino acids: random or semi-fasting conditions (i.e., 4 hrs) |
| Amino acids | Plasma ketone body concentration changes with fasting over time, check glucose simultaneously |
| Organic acids | |
| Carnitine (free/total) | |
| Acylcarnitine profile | |
| Organic acids (such as methylmalonic acid) ketone bodies | |
| Dried blood spots | Drops of whole blood correctly collected on filter paper.<br>It is important neither to overload nor to dilute the sample.<br>Blood spots should dry completely before storage or transportation (at room temperature) |
| Acylcarnitine profile | |
| Amino acids | |
| Organic acids (such as methylmalonic acid) | |
| Cerebrospinal fluid | 0.5–1 mL for each investigation (standard plastic lumbar puncture tube), fresh or frozen and shipped frozen (packed with dry-ice). Check plasma amino acids simultaneously |
| Amino acids | |

## Prenatal Diagnosis[a]

| Disorder | | Type of analysis[a] | Timing, trimester |
|---|---|---|---|
| 23.1 | BCAA aminotransferase deficiency | | |
| 23.2 | Maple syrup disease | Molecular analysis | I, II |
| 23.2 | | | |
| 23.2 | | | |
| 23.3 | E3 deficiency | Molecular analysis | I, II |
| 23.4 | Branched-chain ketoacid dehydrogenase phosphatase deficiency | | |
| 23.5 | Branched-chain ketoacid dehydrogenase kinase deficiency | Molecular analysis | I, II |
| 23.6 | Isovaleric acidemia | Molecular analysis | I, II |
| 23.7 | Isobutyryl-CoA dehydrogenase deficiency | Molecular analysis | I, II |
| 23.8 | 2-Methylbutyrylglycinuria | Molecular analysis | I, II |
| 23.9 | 3-Methylcrotonylglycinuria type 1 | Molecular analysis | I, II |
| 23.9 | 3-Methylcrotonylglycinuria type 2 | Molecular analysis | I, II |
| 23.10 | 3-Methylglutaconic aciduria type 1 | Molecular analysis | I, II |
| 23.11 | Crotonase deficiency | Molecular analysis | I, II |
| 23.12 | β-Hydroxyisobutyryl-CoA deacylase deficiency | Molecular analysis | I, II |

| Disorder | | Type of analysis[a] | Timing, trimester |
|---|---|---|---|
| 23.13 | 3-Hydroxyisobutyrate dehydrogenase deficiency | Molecular analysis | I, II |
| 23.14 | 2-Methyl-3-hydroxybutyryl-CoA dehydrogenase deficiency | Molecular analysis | I, II |
| 23.15 | Hydroxymethylglutaric aciduria | Molecular analysis | I, II |
| 23.16 | Methylmalonate semialdehyde dehydrogenase deficiency[a] | Molecular analysis | I, II |
| 23.17 | Propionic acidemia (propionyl-CoA carboxylase α subunit deficiency) | Molecular analysis | I, II |
| 23.17 | Propionic acidemia (propionyl-CoA carboxylase β-subunit deficiency) | Molecular analysis | I, II |
| 23.18 | Methylmalonyl-CoA epimerase deficiency[a] | Molecular analysis | I, II |
| 23.19 | Methylmalonic aciduria (methylmalonyl-CoA mutase deficiency) | Molecular analysis | I, II |
| 23.20 | Combined methylmalonic and malonic aciduria[a] | Molecular analysis | I, II |
| 23.21 | Malonic aciduria | Molecular analysis | I, II |
| 23.22 | β-ketothiolase deficiency | Molecular analysis | I, II |
| 23.23 | Large neutral amino acid transporter deficiency | | |

[a]Thus far, studies have been limited

## DNA Analysis

| Disorder | | Material | Methodology |
|---|---|---|---|
| 23.1 | Branched-chain aminotransferase 2 deficiency[a] | *For all entities*: WBC, FB, or other suitable cells or tissue samples may be used | *For all entities*: Direct genomic DNA sequencing or RT-PCR (reverse transcription-polymerase chain reaction)/ genomic amplification and sequencing<br>In some cases allele-specific oligonucleotide hybridization or single-stranded conformational polymorphism analysis may be used |
| 23.2 | Maple syrup urine disease type 1a | | |
| 23.2 | Maple syrup urine disease type 1b | | |
| 23.2 | Maple syrup urine disease type 2 | | |
| 23.3 | E3 deficiency | | |
| 23.4 | Branched-chain ketoacid dehydrogenase phosphatase deficiency | | |
| 23.5 | Branched-chain ketoacid dehydrogenase kinase deficiency | | |
| 23.6 | Isovaleric acidemia | | |
| 23.7 | Isobutyryl-CoA dehydrogenase deficiency | | |
| 23.8 | 2-Methylbutyrylglycinuria | | |
| 23.9 | 3-Methylcrotonylglycinuria type 1 | | |
| 23.9 | 3-Methylcrotonylglycinuria type 2 | | |
| 23.10 | 3-Methylglutaconic aciduria type 1 | | |
| 23.11 | Crotonase deficiency | | |
| 23.12 | β-Hydroxyisobutyryl-CoA deacylase deficiency[a] | | |
| 23.13 | 3-Hydroxyisobutyrate dehydrogenase deficiency | | |
| 23.14 | 2-Methyl-3-hydroxybutyryl-CoA dehydrogenase deficiency | | |
| 23.15 | Hydroxymethylglutaric aciduria | | |
| 23.16 | Methylmalonate semialdehyde dehydrogenase deficiency[a] | | |
| 23.17 | Propionic acidemia (propionyl-CoA carboxylase α subunit deficiency) | | |
| 23.17 | Propionic acidemia (propionyl-CoA carboxylase β subunit deficiency) | | |
| 23.18 | Methylmalonyl-CoA epimerase deficiency | | |
| 23.19 | Methylmalonic aciduria due to methylmalonyl-CoA mutase deficiency | | |
| 23.20 | Combined malonic and methylmalonic aciduria[a] | | |
| 23.21 | Malonic aciduria | | |
| 23.22 | Mitochondrial acetoacetyl-CoA thiolase deficiency | | |
| 23.23 | Large neutral amino acid transporter deficiency[a] | | |

[a]Very limited evidence

## Treatment Summary

The mainstay of treatment for all of the disorders is to limit intake of the affected amino acid(s) while preventing catabolism. With severe forms of the disorders, special medical foods (devoid of all or some BCAA, as required for the different conditions) are needed to allow for adequate caloric, protein, and other nutrient intake. In MSUD and IVA, the medical food is Leu-free. This Leu-free medical food should always be used for all of the MSUD patients. Milder IVA forms may only require a moderately reduced natural protein intake without medical food. Further, in PA and MMA, the use of the amino acid medical food devoid of Met, Thr, Val, and Ile is controversial (Manoli et al. 2016). The amount of natural protein tolerated is determined by monitoring parameters such as growth, control of acidosis, excretion of abnormal metabolites, and blood amino acid levels. The least restrictive dietary approach should be taken in order to avoid over-treatment and nutritional deficiencies. Emergency treatment includes promotion of anabolism using a special high-calorie diet, transient stop of natural protein intake or of the precursor amino acids, carefully adjusted IV treatment including adequate amounts of IV dextrose, correction of acidosis, detoxification, prevention of brain edema, and emergency hemodialysis in case of coma/encephalopathy with severe hyperammonemia or profound metabolic acidosis in classic forms of the disorders. Carnitine is used in a quantity of conditions to support excretion of organic acids as carnitine adducts, thus sparing coenzyme A and preserving the function of the Krebs cycle. Hyperammonemia may occur, particularly in PA and MMA, but conjugating agents are typically not indicated for therapy as ammonia normalizes with reversal of the primary metabolic derangement. *N*-carbamylglutamate may be useful in the setting of acute hyperammonemia in PA and MMA. If severe, hemodialysis may be indicated. The chronic treatment of severe forms of the disorders, particularly of PA and MMA, is also challenging. Late complications must be anticipated, including neurologic complications, renal failure (particularly in MMA), or cardiomyopathy (particularly in PA). Liver transplantation (PA and MMA) and combined liver/kidney transplantation (MMA) have been applied in a number of cases, and there is substantial evidence of benefits. Novel therapies such as mRNA (An et al. 2017) are currently under evaluation in MMA and PA patients.

## Emergency Treatment

- **Branched-chain aminotransferase 2 deficiency**
  - The existence of this disorder in humans is not established.
- **Branched-chain ketoacid dehydrogenase E1α deficiency**
- **Branched-chain ketoacid dehydrogenase E1β deficiency**
- **Dihydrolipoyl transacylase deficiency**
- **Branched-chain ketoacid dehydrogenase phosphatase deficiency**
  - Emergency treatment table (includes management of ill neonates)

| Objective | Treatment |
|---|---|
| 1. Correct dehydration | Normal saline bolus as clinically indicated. Start IV dextrose 10–12.5% at 1–1.5 times maintenance; add NaCl and KCl depending on renal output and serum electrolyte levels. Plan rehydration over a 48 h period to prevent cerebral edema. Do not use hypoosmolar solutions |
| 2. Maintain normal plasma sodium and osmolality levels. High risk for SIADH | (a) Check plasma sodium (aim for 140–145 mEq/L with minimal fluctuation) and plasma osmolality (290–300 mosm/L) regularly; monitor intake and output, body weight; urine osmolality (≤300–400 mosm/L), urine electrolytes and output (2–4 mL/kg/h)<br>(b) Give 3% NaCl, dosage carefully calculated to replace deficit if hyponatremic. May also need furosemide 0.50 (0.25–1) mg/kg per dose every 6–8 h if plasma osmolality falls<br>(c) Limit free water intake, observe for fluid overload due to excessive vasopressin production<br>(d) Monitor for signs of increased intracranial pressure |
| 3. Correct hyperglycemia (blood glucose >200 mg/dL) induced by IV fluids | Regular insulin drip, e.g., 0.05–0.1 units/kg per hour until blood glucose is controlled |
| 4. Re-establish anabolism | (a) BCAA-free formula and/or IV fluids to provide total caloric intake of 120–150% of maintenance or give step 1 sick-day diet by PO or NG/G-tube (see table Protocol for intercurrent illness)[a]<br>(b) Add intralipid i.v. 1.5–2 g/kg/day<br>(c) Add back natural protein beginning with, e.g., 100 mg of leucine per day after 24 h; total protein including BCAA-free supplements 2.5–3.5 g/kg per day |
| 5. Reduce persistently elevated leucine levels or encephalopathy | (a) Hemodialysis (HD) or hemofiltration (HF) in encephalopathic patients if intensified treatment (measure 1–4) is insufficient over a period of 2–4 h<br>(b) Expect rate of decrease in plasma leucine levels >750 µmol/L per 24 h |

[a]Isoleucine and valine levels should be high during crisis, at over 400–600 µM, to suppress entry of leucine into the brain. Isoleucine and valine usually need to be added early (after 24 h) into treatment (e.g., 40–100 mg/kg per day each). Leucine is reintroduced when its plasma level falls close to the normal range (e.g., total daily dose of 100 mg of leucine per day when plasma level below 400 µmol/L, 200 mg per day when level below 300 µmol/L; provide in total 2.0–2.5 g/kg per day of protein equivalent). Aim at target ratios of approximately 1:2:2 for plasma leucine, isoleucine, and valine, respectively

- **Comments/Additions**
  1. Stop all natural protein sources initially but add back leucine restricted source after 24 h to re-establish protein anabolism.
  2. Monitor laboratory studies including blood glucose, electrolytes, lactate, osmolality, plasma amino acids, urinary organic acids, and dipstick for ketones as indicated by the clinical history and examination.
  3. Patients with the E3 subunit deficiency may experience severe lactic acidosis and abnormal blood glucose.
  4. Thiamine 10 mg/kg per day (50–500 mg per day) may be given until genotype is known but is usually of low/no benefit.

- **Protocol for intercurrent illness**

| Treatment | Branched-chain amino acid-free special medical food | Natural food leucine intake |
|---|---|---|
| First 24 h | 1.2–1.5 times usual daily amount with additional isoleucine and valine[a] | None |
| 24–48 h | 1.2–1.5 times usual daily amount with additional isoleucine and valine[a] | None to half usual dietary intake |
| >48 h or when well | Usual daily amount | Gradual increase to usual full dietary intake |

[a]Additions of isoleucine and valine should be increased during sick days. Goal is to keep levels of isoleucine and valine between 150–350 and 200–400 μM, respectively, when the patient is well and at over 400–600 μM when ill

- **Comments/Additions**
  1. Families/individuals should start sick-day formula (to decrease leucine intake, increase isoleucine and valine intake, and suppress catabolism) with the onset of intercurrent illness or symptoms related to loss of metabolic control. Fluids without calories or electrolytes should be avoided or intake minimized.
  2. If the patient is unable to take in oral fluids and has persistent vomiting, or the clinical condition deteriorates, they should proceed urgently to an experienced emergency care facility.

- **Dihydrolipoamide dehydrogenase deficiency**

  – Management may be adapted according to the three mitochondrial enzyme complex deficiencies that can be observed. See table for disorder 23.2, (MSUD) for the branched-chain ketoacid dehydrogenase deficiency and for the PDH complex: ketogenic diet, trial of dichloroacetate (DCA), and thiamine supplementation. Management of the primarily liver presentation (recurrent Reye-like liver failure) typically involves supportive therapy during times of acute liver injury or failure, including nutritional support, IV glucose for hypoglycemia, correction of metabolic acidosis, correction of coagulopathy, and avoidance of liver-toxic medications. Riboflavin should be used in the myopathic form of the disease.

- **Branched-chain ketoacid dehydrogenase kinase deficiency**
  – BCAA supplementation could be proposed in an attempt to prevent irreversible brain damage.
- **Isovaleric acidemia**
- **3-Methylcrotonylglycinuria type 1**[a]
- **3-Methylcrotonylglycinuria type 2**[a]
- **3-Methylglutaconic aciduria type 1**[b]
- **Hydroxymethylglutaric aciduria**[c]
- Emergency treatment table (includes management of ill neonates)

| Objective | Treatment |
|---|---|
| 1. Treat dehydration | Normal saline bolus as clinically indicated. Start IV dextrose 10–12.5% at 1–1.5 times maintenance; add NaCl and KCl depending on renal output and serum electrolyte levels |
| 2. Correct acidosis | Usually corrects with re-establishment of anabolic state. In extremis, give 1–2 mEq/kg of Na bicarbonate |
| 3. Correct hyperglycemia (blood glucose >200 mg/dL) induced by IV fluids | Regular insulin drip, e.g., 0.05 units/kg per hour until blood glucose is controlled |
| 4. Re-establish anabolism | (a) Leucine-free formula or IV fluids (plus low-fat in HMGCL deficiency/disorder 23.9) with caloric intake 120–150% of maintenance<br>(b) Can add intralipids for additional calories except for HMGCL deficiency (disorder 23.9) |
| 6. Metabolite conjugation | Carnitine: 100 mg/kg per day in 3 divided doses IV or PO<br>Glycine (IVA only): usual daily dose (e.g., 250 mg/kg per day) in sick-day enteral formula or TPN |

[a]Most patients do not become acutely ill
[b]Treatment is mainly symptomatic
[c]Patients with HMGCL (disorder 23.9) usually present with acute hypoketotic or nonketotic hypoglycemia and dehydration may be underestimated. Give IV glucose bolus (e.g., 2 mL/kg of dextrose 10%) in a hypoglycemic patient

- **Comments/Additions**
  1. Stop all natural protein sources initially. Begin to add back leucine restricted protein after 24 h and complete protein after 48 h.
  2. Monitor laboratory studies including blood glucose, electrolytes, pH, blood gases, ammonia, lactate, plasma amino acids, urinary organic acids, acylcarni-

tine profile, liver function tests, CK, and any other laboratory tests indicated by the clinical history and examination.

- **Protocol for intercurrent illness: initial measures**

| Treatment | Leucine-free special medical food[a] | Natural food leucine intake | L-carnitine (mg/kg/day) |
|---|---|---|---|
| First 24 h | 1.2–1.5 times usual daily amount | None | 100 |
| 24–48 h | 1.2–1.5 times usual daily amount | None to half usual dietary intake | 100 |
| >48 h or when well | Usual daily amount | Gradual increase to usual full dietary intake | 100 |

[a]Leucine-free and low fat for HMGCL (disorder 23.15)

- **Comments/Additions**
  1. Families/individuals should start sick-day formula (to decrease leucine intake and suppress catabolism). Start carnitine if not used routinely. Fluids without calories or electrolytes should be avoided or intake minimized.
  2. In patients with HMGCL deficiency (disorder 23.15), prompt administration of carbohydrates/IV dextrose is mandatory. IV lipids are contraindicated. Monitor urine ketones, which will become positive with loss of metabolic control or inadequate caloric intake except in patients who are unable to produce ketones.
  3. If the patient is unable to take in oral fluids and has persistent vomiting, or the clinical condition deteriorates, they should proceed urgently to an experienced emergency care facility.

- **Isoleucine catabolic pathway:**
  - **2-Methylbutyrylglycinuria**[1a]
  - **2-Methyl-3-hydroxybutyryl-CoA dehydrogenase deficiency**
  - **β-ketothiolase deficiency**
- **Valine catabolic pathway:**
  - **Isobutyryl-CoA dehydrogenase deficiency**[1]
  - **Crotonase deficiency**
  - **3-Hydroxyisobutyryl-CoA deacylase deficiency**
  - **3-Hydroxyisobutyrate dehydrogenase deficiency**
  - **Methylmalonate semialdehyde dehydrogenase deficiency**

Treatment is similar to the leucine pathway disorders except that isoleucine or valine reduced concentration formulae are required. Check carnitine status and add L-carnitine as required (e.g., 50–100 mg/kg per day). In patients with beta-ketothiolase deficiency (disorder 23.22), oral or IV carbohydrate administration is most effective in suppressing ketogenesis; metabolic acidosis should be treated cautiously to prevent hypernatremia and paradoxical CNS acidosis. Treatment mostly relies on preventative measures: avoidance of fasting. Risk of acute metabolic decompensation in SBCAD and IBD deficiencies appears to be small and chronic dietary therapy is likely not necessary.

[1]Patients not usually acutely ill

- **Propionic academia (α-subunit)**
- **Propionic acidemia (β-subunit)**
- **Methylmalonic aciduria due to methylmalonyl-CoA epimerase deficiency**[a]
- **Methylmalonic aciduria due to methylmalonyl-CoA mutase deficiency**

- Emergency treatment table (includes management of ill neonates):

| Objective | Treatment |
|---|---|
| 1. Treat dehydration | Normal saline bolus as clinically indicated. Start IV dextrose 10–12.5% at 1–1.5 times maintenance; add NaCl and KCl depending on renal output and serum electrolyte levels. Plan rehydration over a 48 h period to prevent cerebral edema. |
| 2. Correct acidosis | Usually corrects with re-establishment of anabolic state. In extremis, give 1–2 mEq/kg of Na bicarbonate. |
| 3. Correct hyperglycemia (blood glucose >200 mg/dL) | If lactate <3 mM: regular insulin drip, e.g., 0.05–0.1 units/kg per hour until blood glucose is controlled. But if lactate >3 mM, consider to reduce glucose intake first |
| 4. Re-establish anabolism | (b) If able to feed enterally, use Ile-/Met-/Thr-/Val-free formula to provide total caloric intake of 120–150% of maintenance<br>(c) Adjust IV treatment as required (peripheral/central line)<br>(d) 20% fat emulsion, rate 1–3 g/kg/day IV<br>(e) If NPO use lowered Ile/Met/Thr/Val-free TPN |
| 6. Metabolite conjugation and reduction | (b) L-carnitine 100 mg/kg per day IV or PO/NG[a]<br>(c) Add metronidazole PO or NG for intermittent treatment (10 mg/kg per day for 1 week)<br>(d) Urgently consider HD/HF in encephalopathic patients or if blood ammonia is ≥300–400 μM or in case of persistent severe acidosis, particularly if intensified treatment is insufficient over a period of 2–4 h |
| 7. Enhance residual enzyme activity | Cobalamin-responsive MMA: 1 mg hydroxocobalamin/dose IM daily[b,c] |

| Objective | Treatment |
|---|---|
| 10. Other | (b) Treat infections effectively. Note that neutropenia and thrombocytopenia are frequent findings during metabolic crisis<br>(c) Monitor for further complications (e.g., cerebral edema, acute pancreatitis) |

[a]Most patients do not become acutely ill
[b]Higher doses of L-carnitine have also been used (200–400 mg/kg per day). It is reasonable to increase the IV dose, e.g., when the patient undergoes HD/HF
[c]Each patient with MMA should be tested for B12 responsiveness by a trial of parenteral hydroxocobalamin in a dose of 1 mg/day. In those who respond, therapy is continued but the oral route may be used. Cyanocobalamin may be used if hydroxocobalamin is not available
[d]In PA, biotin responsiveness is doubtful. Biotin supplementation (10 mg daily) is therefore rarely beneficial
[e]*N*-carbamylglutamate may be started as a bridge, e.g., while waiting for HD/HF. In undiagnosed patients presenting with hyperammonemia, sodium benzoate/phenylacetate may be given but should be stopped once PA or MMA has been diagnosed

- **Comments/Additions**
  1. Stop all natural protein sources initially, and then reintroduce restricted natural protein by 24 h (0.2–0.5 g/kg/day), and begin addition of complete protein by 48 h with escalation to normal intake thereafter. Use additional Ile-/Met-/Thr-/Val-free formula for adequate amino acid supply.
  2. Laboratory studies including blood gases, pH, ammonia, blood glucose, lactate, electrolytes, osmolality, plasma amino acids, acylcarnitines, ALT, AST, coagulation screen, CK, full blood count, urinary ketones, and urinary organic acids and any other laboratory tests indicated by the clinical history and examination.
  3. A few patients with methylmalonic aciduria due to methylmalonyl-CoA epimerase deficiency have been described with an associated sepiapterin reductase deficiency without knowing the mechanism that links the two disorders. Sepiapterin reductase deficiency should be treated as specified in Chapter.

- **Protocol for intercurrent illness: initial measures**

| Treatment | Ile-/Met-/Thr-/Val-free special medical food | Natural food protein intake |
|---|---|---|
| First 24 h | 1.2–1.5 times usual daily amount | None |
| 24–48 h | 1.2–1.5 times usual daily amount | None to half usual dietary intake |
| >48 h or when well | Usual daily amount | Gradual increase to usual full dietary intake |

- **Combined malonic aciduria and methylmalonic aciduria**
- **Malonic aciduria**
- **Emergency treatment table (includes management of ill neonates)**[a]

| Objective | Treatment |
|---|---|
| 1. Treat hypoglycemia | Give IV glucose bolus (e.g., 2 mL/kg of dextrose 10%); start IV dextrose 10–12.5% at maintenance and add NaCl and KCl depending on serum electrolyte levels |
| 2. Metabolite conjugation | Carnitine: 100 mg/kg per day in 3 divided doses IV or PO |
| 3. Correct acidosis | Usually corrects with re-establishment of anabolic state. In extremis, give 1–2 mEq/kg of Na bicarbonate |
| 4. Other | (a) Monitor cardiac function<br>(b) Monitor for further complications (e.g., lactic acidemia, seizures) |

[a]There is limited experience in managing this condition

- **Comments/Additions**
  1. If the patient is feeding orally, increase the amount of calories from carbohydrate relative to fat, introduce MCT fat, and prevent fasting.
  2. Laboratory studies including blood gases, pH, blood glucose, lactate, electrolytes, full blood count, osmolality, CK, ALT, AST, acylcarnitines, cholesterol, ketones, and urinary organic acids and any other laboratory tests indicated by the clinical history and examination.

## Chronic Treatment

- **Branched-chain aminotransferase 2 deficiency**
  – The existence of this disorder in humans remains in question.
- **Branched-chain ketoacid dehydrogenase E1α deficiency**
- **Branched-chain ketoacid dehydrogenase E1β deficiency**
- **Dihydrolipoyl transacylase deficiency**
- **E3 deficiency**
- **Branched-chain ketoacid dehydrogenase phosphatase deficiency**

- Standard treatment table

| No. | Disease/symbol | Age | Medication/diet | Dosage | Target plasma levels |
|---|---|---|---|---|---|
| 23.2<br>23.2<br>23.2 | MSUD—Severe forms (MSUD 1a, 1b, 2) | All ages | Lowered BCAA diet[a]<br>Isoleucine and valine supplements[b] | See table below<br>Adjusted to blood levels | Leucine 100–300 μM<br>Isoleucine 150–350 μM<br>Valine 200–400 μM[c] |
| | | | NaCl[d]<br>Thiamine[e] | 3–5 mEq/kg/day<br>50–300 mg/day | Within normal limits |
| 23.2<br>23.2<br>23.4 | MSUD—Milder forms (1a, 2, BCKDH phosphatase) | All ages | Reduced natural protein diet[f]<br>Multivitamin with minerals<br>Thiamine[e] | See table below<br>As required<br>50–300 mg/day | See above (severe forms) |
| 23.2 | MSUD—Thiamine-responsive forms (2) | All ages | Reduced natural protein diet[f]<br>Multivitamin with minerals<br>Thiamine | See table below<br>As required<br>10 mg/kg/day (50–500 mg/day) | See above (severe forms) |
| 23.3 | MSUD 3 (combined dehydrogenase deficiency; E3 deficiency) | All ages | See above (severe forms)[g] | | See above (severe forms) |

[a]Special medical food devoid of the branched-chain amino acids and enriched with micronutrients (see table Nutritional treatment for patients with maple syrup urine disease)
[b]Typically as 10 mg/mL solutions
[c]Target ratios of approximately 1:2:2 for leucine, isoleucine, and valine, respectively
[d]Calculate the amount present in the diet and add supplements to meet the recommended intake
[e]Thiamine given until molecular genotype known. Not given in patients with the Mennonite mutation Y393N
[f]Protein intake of approximately 1.5–2.0 g/kg/day in young infants and 0.6–1.5 g/kg/day in older children and adults
[g]Attempts at treatment with diet and co-factors have been unsuccessful in some patients in preventing CNS deterioration; usually not thiamine-responsive

- **Comments/Additions**
  1. Intake of whole protein and supplements of individual amino acids is adjusted based on plasma quantitative amino acids levels and individual needs to meet the target levels.
  2. All patients with MSUD 1a, MSUD 1b, and MSUD 2 should be given a trial of thiamine therapy for at least 3 weeks or until the molecular genotype is known. Patients homozygous for the Y393N Mennonite mutation are not thiamine-responsive.

- Standard nutritional treatment for patients with maple syrup urine disease[a]

| Age | Total protein requirement[b] (g/kg/day) | Leucine tolerance[c] (mg/kg/day) | Isoleucine intake (mg/kg/day) | Valine intake (mg/kg/day) | Energy requirement[d] (kcal/kg/day) |
|---|---|---|---|---|---|
| Neonates | 2.7–3.5 | 40–100 | 30–90 | 40–95 | 100–145 |
| Infants | 2.5–3.2 | 35–75 | 20–70 | 30–80 | 80–135 |
| Young children | 1.8–2.6 | 20–65 | 10–30 | 20–50 | 60–130 |
| Older children and adults | 1.4–1.8 | 5–50 | 5–30 | 15–30 | 35–70 |

[a]Modified from Strauss et al. (2010), Acosta and Yannicelli (2001), and Marriage (2010). These recommendations are only a guide and must be individualized for each patient, based on the severity of their disorder, actual needs, and blood quantitative amino acid levels
[b]Includes protein intake from special medical foods devoid of BCAA plus that from natural whole protein sources
[c]Leucine (mg/kcal ratio of 0.5–0.8 for neonates, 0.4–0.6 for infants; ratio of 0.25:0.30 in children and older)
[d]Lipids should comprise 40–50% of total calories. Formula concentrations over 24 kcal/oz. may result in loose stools, diarrhea, and dehydration

- **Isovaleric acidemia**
- Standard treatment table

| No. | Symbol | Age | Medication/diet | Dosage | Target plasma levels |
|---|---|---|---|---|---|
| 23.6 | IVA—Severe forms | All ages | Lowered leucine diet[a] | See tables below | Leucine 50–180 μM, or normal range for laboratory |
| | | | L-Carnitine | 100 mg/kg/day in 3 doses[b] | Normal to high normal range for free carnitine |
| | | | Glycine | 250 (150–300) mg/kg/day in 3 doses[c] | Glycine 200–400 μM |

| No. | Symbol | Age | Medication/diet | Dosage | Target plasma levels |
|---|---|---|---|---|---|
| 23.6 | IVA-Mild forms | All ages | Reduced natural protein diet[d]<br>Multivitamin with minerals<br>L-Carnitine | See tables below<br>As required<br>30–100 mg/kg/day in 3 doses[b] | Normal free carnitine |
| | | | Glycine | 150–250 mg/kg/day in 3 doses[d,e] | Glycine 200–400 μM |

[a]Special medical food devoid of leucine and enriched with micronutrients may be needed for severe forms of the disorder. Patients with milder forms of the disorder will only require a reduced natural protein intake. The least restrictive diet sufficient to maintain metabolic control should be used

[b]Calculate the amount present in the special medical food or protein-free product and add supplements to meet the recommended intake

[c]Glycine is often omitted from chronic therapy. If used, it is added to the daily special formula as weighed dry powder or 100 mg/mL solution

[d]Natural protein intake of approximately 1.5–2.0 g/kg per day in young infants and 0.6–1.5 g/kg per day in older children and adults. Patients with a mild IVA form and the missense mutation 932C>T (A282V) usually do not require protein restriction

[e]Patients with a mild IVA form may not require glycine supplements

- Standard nutritional treatment for patients with isovaleric acidemia[a]

| Age | Protein requirement[a] (g/kg/day) | Leucine intake[b] from whole natural protein (mg/kg/day) | Energy requirement[c] (kcal/kg/day) |
|---|---|---|---|
| Neonates | 2.5–3.5 | 65–150 | 95–145 |
| Infants | 2.0–3.0 | 50–140 | 80–135 |
| Young children | 1.5–2.0 | 40–90 | 60–130 |
| Older children and adults | 1.1–1.8 | 30–60 | 35–70 |

[a]Includes protein intake from special medical food devoid of leucine plus that from natural whole protein sources

[b]These figures reflect leucine intake if special medical foods devoid of leucine are used and may be too low for some actively growing infants and children

[c]Formula concentrations over 24 Kcal/oz. may result in loose stools, diarrhea, and dehydration

[d]Modified from Acosta and Yannicelli (2001) and Marriage (2010). These recommendations are only a guide and must be individualized for each patient, based on the severity of their disorder. Patients with milder forms of the disorder will tolerate a higher leucine intake and may only require a reduced natural protein diet

- **Comments/Additions**
  1. Although leucine is the precursor amino acid for the disorder, it is the organic acids that are toxic to the patients and not the leucine per se as with MSUD. Monitoring leucine levels gives an indication as to whether there is sufficient intake of natural protein to support growth, losses, and tissue repair, but it does not rise in catabolism. The plasma leucine range of 50–150 μM, however, may be too low for some growing infants and children. Many affected patients are able to tolerate a near-normal leucine intake and may be treated with a lowered natural protein diet, without selective leucine restriction. The least restrictive dietary approach allowing metabolic control should be used in order to avoid over-treatment and leucine deficiency.

- **3-Methylcrotonylglycinuria type 1**
- **3-Methylcrotonylglycinuria type 2**
- Standard Treatment Table

| No. | Symbol | Age | Medication/diet | Dosage | Target plasma levels |
|---|---|---|---|---|---|
| 23.9 | 3MCCC1<br>3MCCC2 | All ages | Lowered leucine diet[a] | See tables for IVA/disorder 23.2 | Leucine 50–180 μM, or normal range for laboratory |
| | | | L-Carnitine | 50–100 mg/kg per day in 2–3 doses[b] | Normal free carnitine |

[a]Special medical food devoid of leucine may be needed for severe forms of the disorder. Patients with milder forms of the disorder will only require a reduced natural protein intake. The least restrictive diet should be used. Glycine is usually not given, though it might be considered in severe cases (175–250 mg/kg per day) as it increases 3-methylcrotonylglycine excretion

[b]Calculate the amount present in the special medical food if used and add supplements to meet the recommended intake

- **Comments/Additions**
  1. Special medical food devoid of leucine and enriched with micronutrients may be needed for severe forms of the disorder. Patients with milder forms of the disorder will only require a reduced natural protein intake. The least restrictive diet allowing metabolic control should be used.
  2. Patients are not responsive to biotin therapy.
  3. Asymptomatic individuals may not need dietary restrictions or L-carnitine but may occasionally need blood and urine monitoring.

- **3-Methylglutaconic aciduria, type 1**
- Standard treatment table

| No. | Symbol | Age | Medication/diet | Dosage | Target plasma levels |
|---|---|---|---|---|---|
| 23.10 | 3MG1 | All ages | L-Carnitine | 100 mg/kg per day in 3 doses[a] | Normal free carnitine |
| | | | Lowered leucine diet[b] | See tables for IVA/disorder 23.6 | Leucine 50–180 μM, or normal range for laboratory |

[a]Calculate the amount present in the special medical food if used and add supplements to this to meet the recommended intake
[b]No dietary regimen has been therapeutically proven. Special medical food devoid of leucine may be used for severe forms of the disorder. Patients with milder forms of the disorder might require a reduced natural protein intake. The least restrictive diet allowing metabolic control should be used

- **Comments/Additions**
  1. See comment 1 for Isovaleric acidemia.

- **Hydroxymethylglutaric aciduria**
- Standard treatment table

| No. | Symbol | Age | Medication/diet | Dosage | Target plasma levels |
|---|---|---|---|---|---|
| 23.15 | HMGCL | All ages | Lowered leucine and fat, high carbohydrate diet[a] | See tables for IVA/disorder 7.3<br>Of note, fat is limited to 20–25% of total daily caloric intake | Leucine 50–180 μM, or normal range for laboratory |
| | | | L-Carnitine | 100 mg/kg/day in 3 doses | Normal free carnitine |

[a]Special medical food devoid of leucine may be needed for severe forms of the disorder. Patients with milder forms of the disorder will only require a reduced natural protein intake and low-fat diet. Avoid fasting. The least restrictive diet that allows metabolic control should be used

- Comments/**Additions**
  1. See comment 1 for Isovaleric acidemia.
  2. In addition to leucine restriction, daily caloric intake of fat is limited to 20–25% of total caloric intake per day. Use a leucine-free product that contains carbohydrates and other nutrients, but no or very low fat.
  3. Avoid fasting. Overnight drip nasogastric or gastrostomy feedings may be needed.
  4. Uncooked cornstarch added to the special metabolic formula may be used to prevent hypoglycemia.

- **2-Methylbutyrylglycinuria**
- **2-Methyl-3-hydroxybutyryl-CoA dehydrogenase deficiency**
- **α-Methylacetoacetic aciduria**
- **Isobutyryl-CoA dehydrogenase deficiency**
- **Crotonase deficiency**
- **3-Hydroxyisobutyryl-CoA deacylase deficiency**
- **3-Hydroxyisobutyrate dehydrogenase deficiency**
- **Methylmalonate semialdehyde dehydrogenase deficiency**
- Standard nutritional treatment for patients with disorders limited to isoleucine or valine[a]

| Age | Isoleucine intake[b] | Valine intake | Natural protein requirement[d] (g/kg/day) | Total protein requirement (g/kg/day) | Energy requirement (kcal/kg/day) |
|---|---|---|---|---|---|
| Neonates | 90–150 mg/kg/day | 65–110 mg/kg/day | 1.5–2.5 | 2.8–3.5 | 95–145 |
| Infants | 50–115 mg/kg/day | 40–90 mg/kg/day | 1.2–2.0 | 2.5–3.2 | 80–135 |
| Young children | 630–1250 mg per day | 600–1100 mg per day | 0.8–1.5 | 1.8–2.6 | 60–130 |
| Older children and adults | 965–1900 mg per day | 900–2015 mg per day | 0.5–1.4 | 1.4–1.8 | 35–70 |

[a]Modified from Yanicelli (2010). These recommendations are only a guide and must be individualized for each patient, based on the severity of their disorder, actual needs, and blood quantitative amino acid levels
[b]The targets relating to isoleucine curtailment would apply to MBD deficiency (disorder 23.8), to MHBD deficiency (disorder 23.14), and in principle to beta-ketothiolase deficiency (disorder 23.22)
[c]The targets relating to valine curtailment would apply to MMSDH deficiency (disorder 23.16), to HIBDH deficiency (disorder 23.13), to IBD deficiency (disorder 23.7), and in principle to HIBCH deficiency (disorder 23.12)
[d]In addition to the natural protein intake, special medical food (devoid of Ile or Val as appropriate) provides adequate total protein intake. The least restrictive diet should be used. These are approximate therapeutic strategies, and individual patient's requirements may vary substantially. Also, for a given patient, variations must be anticipated in relationship to growth rate, physical activity, intercurrent illness, etc.
[e]Monitor carnitine status and add L-carnitine as required (e.g., 50–100 mg/kg per day)
[f]In beta-ketothiolase deficiency (disorder 23.22): avoid fasting and high-fat intake; carbohydrate-rich meals and frequent feeding have been effective to avoid ketonuria

- **Propionic academia (α-subunit)**
- **Propionic acidemia (β-subunit)**
- **Methylmalonic aciduria due to methylmalonyl-CoA epimerase deficiency (the need for dietary treatment of this condition remains questionable)**
- **Methylmalonic aciduria due to methylmalonyl-CoA mutase deficiency**

- Standard treatment table

| No. | Symbol | Age | Medication/diet | Dosage | Target plasma levels |
|---|---|---|---|---|---|
| 23.17 | PA | All ages | Lowered Ile/Val/Met/Thr diet[a] | See table below | Low normal to normal range of age for laboratory for Ile/Val/Met/Thr[b]; normal ammonia; normal acid-base status |
| | | | l-Carnitine | 100 mg/kg/day in 3 doses | Normal to high normal range for free carnitine |
| | | | Metronidazole | 10 mg/kg per day for intermittent treatment PO[c,d] | |
| 23.19 | MMA | All ages | Lowered Ile/Val/Met/Thr diet[a] | See table below | Low normal to normal range of age for laboratory for Ile/Val/Met/Thr[b]; normal plasma ammonia; normal acid-base status |
| | | | l-Carnitine | 100 mg/kg/day in 3 doses | Normal to high normal range for free carnitine |
| | | | In cobalamin-responsive MMA: hydroxocobalamin | 1 mg per day IM[e] | |
| | | | Metronidazole | 10 mg/kg per day for intermittent treatment PO[c] | |
| | | | In renal failure: symptomatic therapy | As required | |

This plan must be individualized for each patient, based on the severity and type of their disorder

[a]Individualize depending upon tolerance to protein, growth, and nutritional adequacy, guided by parameters in table Standard nutritional treatment for propionic acidemia and methylmalonic acidemia. Benefits from lowered Ile/Val/Met/Thr medical food is controversial (Manoli et al. 2016)

[b]Provide an adequate intake; prevent deficiencies

[c]Short-course or intermittent treatment (e.g., 1 week per month; >6 months)

[d]In PA, biotin responsiveness is doubtful and supplementation rarely beneficial

[e]Each patient with MMA should be tested for B12 responsiveness by a trial of parenteral hydroxocobalamin in a dose of 1 mg/day IM. In those that respond (decrease in urinary MMA excretion by ≥50%), therapy is continued, but the oral route may be used and the dose may be adjusted. Cyanocobalamin may be used if hydroxocobalamin is not available

- Standard nutritional treatment for propionic acidemia and methylmalonic acidemia[a]

| Age | Isoleucine intake | Methionine intake | Threonine intake | Valine intake | Natural protein requirement[b] | Total protein requirement[c] | Energy requirement[d] |
|---|---|---|---|---|---|---|---|
| Neonates | 60–110 mg/kg/day | 20–50 mg/kg/day | 50–125 mg/kg/day | 60–105 mg/kg/day | 1.2–1.8 g/kg/day | 2.7–3.5 g/kg/day | 125–145 kcal/kg/day |
| Infants | 40–90 mg/kg/day | 15–40 mg/kg/day | 20–75 mg/kg/day | 40–80 mg/kg/day | 0.8–1.5 g/kg/day | 2.5–3.2 g/kg/day | 115–140 kcal/kg/day |
| Young children | 485–735 mg per day | 275–390 mg per day | 415–600 mg per day | 550–830 mg per day | 0.7–1.2 g/kg/day | 1.8–2.6 g/kg/day | 900–1800 kcal per day |
| Older children and adults | 630–1470 mg per day | 360–950 mg per day | 540–1455 mg per day | 720–2000 mg per day | 0.5–0.8 g/kg/day | 1.4–1.7 g/kg/day | 1500–3200 kcal per day |

[a]Modified from Yanicelli (2010). These recommendations are only a guide and must be individualized for each patient, based on the severity of their disorder, actual needs, and blood quantitative amino acid levels

[b]In addition to the whole protein, specialized formulas (devoid of Ile/Met/Thr/Val) are needed. Of note, individual patient's requirements may vary substantially

[c]Includes protein intake from special medical foods devoid of Ile/Met/Thr/Val plus that from natural whole protein sources. Total protein recommendation is higher when the majority of protein is supplied by free amino acids (Ile–/Met-/Thr-/Val-free formula). However, patients with hyperammonemia or MMA patients with renal impairment require carefully adjusted protein amounts

[d]Energy requirement is usually lower during well state compared with unwell state in patients

- **Combined malonic aciduria and methylmalonic aciduria**
- **Malonic aciduria**
- Standard treatment table[a]

| No. | Symbol | Age | Medication/diet | Dosage[a] | Target plasma levels |
|---|---|---|---|---|---|
| 23.19 | MMA | All ages | High carbohydrate and low long-chain triglycerides (LCT) fat diet; medium chain triglycerides (MCT) fat supplements | Dietary fat may comprise 30–50% LCT and 50–70% MCT | Normal blood glucose, normal essential fatty acids, normal cholesterol |
| | | | l-Carnitine | 100 mg/kg/day in 3 doses | Normal free carnitine |
| 23.20 | CMAMMA | All ages | High carbohydrate and low long-chain triglycerides (LCT) fat diet; medium chain triglycerides (MCT) fat supplements; moderate restriction of natural protein | Dietary fat may comprise 30–50% LCT and 50–70% MCT | Normal blood glucose, normal essential fatty acids, normal cholesterol |
| | | | l-Carnitine | 100 mg/kg/day in 2–3 doses | Normal free carnitine |

[a]There are no established treatment recommendations and dosage may vary considerably
[b]Little information published and effectiveness of treatment has yet to be determined
[c]Check whether metabolite levels are responsive to (moderate) protein restriction in patients with combined malonic aciduria and methylmalonic aciduria (disorder 23.20)

- **Comments/Additions**
  1. Avoid fasting to prevent hypoglycemia.
  2. The management of a patient with cardiomyopathy should be done in consultation with a cardiologist; a beta blocker or angiotensin-converting enzyme inhibitor or other medications might be given depending on individual needs.
  3. Cholesterol supplementation should be given in patients with reduced cholesterol levels.

## Experimental Treatment

| Disorder no. | Symbol | Substance |
|---|---|---|
| 23.2 | MSUD 1a<br>MSUD 1b<br>MSUD 2<br>MSUD 1a | Coenzyme Q10 (5 mg/kg/day; electron carrier of the respiratory chain with antioxidant properties; in addition to standard therapy during crisis)[a]<br>Phenylbutyrate (500 mg/kg/day; to activate E1α/BCKDC enzyme activity; in addition to standard therapy) |
| 23.17 | PA | Citric acid (as K-Na-hydrogen citrate, 80–120 mg/kg/day PO; might improve TCA cycle flux; in addition to standard therapy during crisis with lactic acidosis)[c] |

[a]Knerr et al. (2011)
[b]Brunetti-Pierri et al. (2011)
[c]Siekmeyer et al. (2013)

## Flowcharts: Standard Therapy and Emergency Therapy

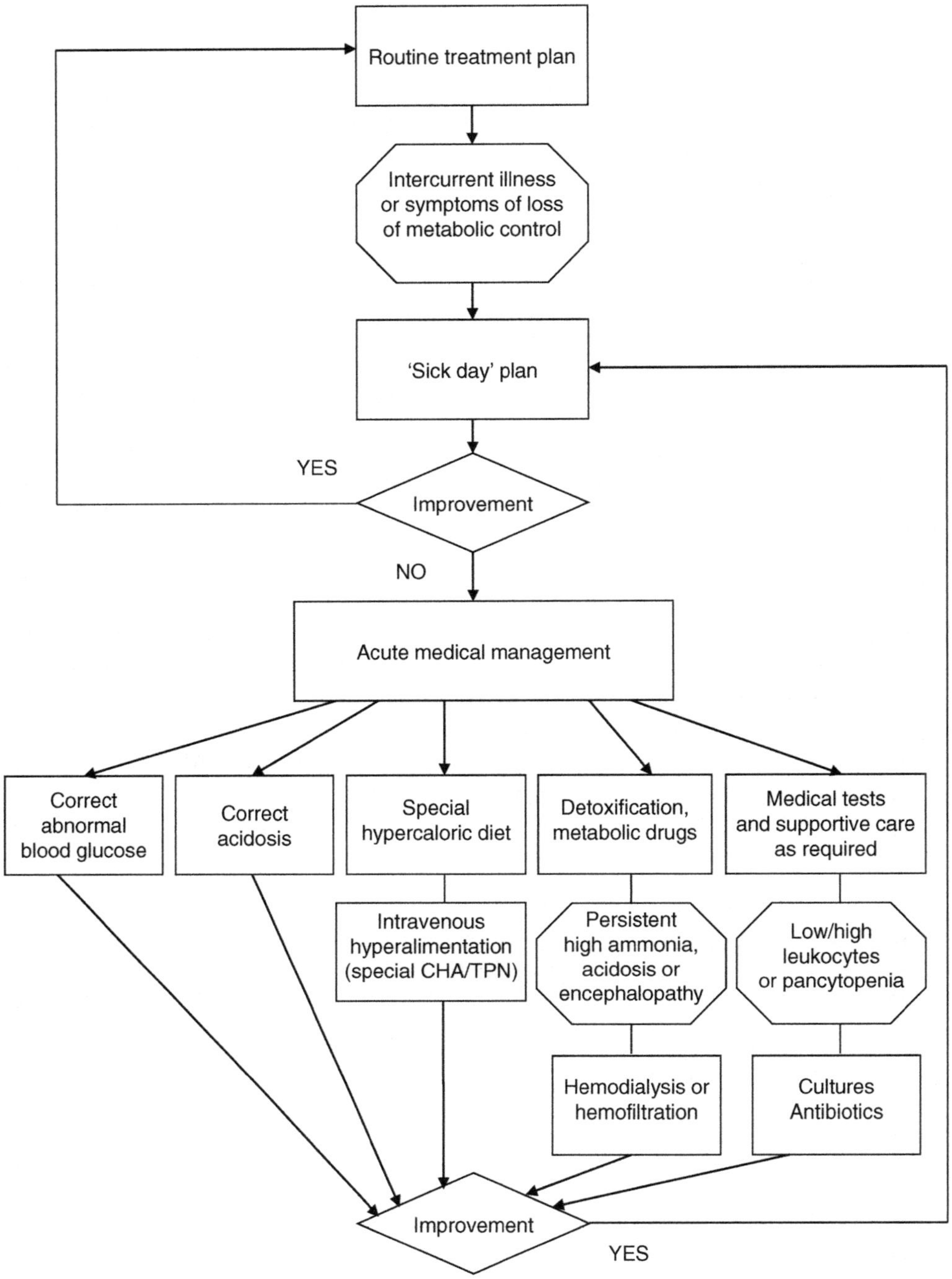


Disorders 23.2–23.6: management of patients with disorders of BCAA metabolism[a]. [a]These are approximate guidelines, and individual patient's requirements may vary substantially

## References


Acosta PB, Yannicelli. The Ross metabolic formula system, nutrition support protocols, 4th edn. Columbus: Ross Products Division, Abbott Laboratories; 2001.

Alfardan J, Mohsen AW, Copeland S, Ellison J, Keppen-Davis L, Rohrbach M, Powell BR, Gillis J, Matern D, Kant J, Vockley J. Characterization of new ACADSB gene sequence mutations and clinical implications in patients with 2-methylbutyrylglycinuria identified by newborn screening. Mol Genet Metab. 2010;100:333–8.

An D, Schneller JL, Frassetto A, Liang S, Zhu X, Park JS, Theisen M, Hong SJ, Zhou J, Rajendran R, Levy B, Howell R, Besin G, Presnyak V, Sabnis S, Murphy-Benenato KE, Kumarasinghe ES, Salerno T, Mihai C, Lukacs CM, Chandler RJ, Guey LT, Venditti CP, Martini PGV. Systemic messenger RNA therapy as a treatment for methylmalonic acidemia. Cell Rep. 2017;21:3548–58.

Andresen BS, Christensen E, Corydon TJ, Bross P, Pilgaard B, Wanders RJ, Ruiter JP, Simonsen H, Winter V, Knudsen I, Schroeder LD, Gregersen N, Skovby F. Isolated 2-methylbutyrylglycinuria caused by short/branched-chain acyl-CoA dehydrogenase deficiency: identification of a new enzyme defect, resolution of its molecular basis, and evidence for distinct acyl-CoA dehydrogenases in isoleucine and valine metabolism. Am J Hum Genet. 2000;67:1095–103.

Brunetti-Pierri N, Lanpher B, Erez A, Ananieva EA, Islam M, Marini JC, Sun Q, Yu C, Hegde M, Li J, Wynn RM, Chuang DT, Hutson S, Lee B. Phenylbutyrate therapy for maple syrup urine disease. Hum Mol Genet. 2011;20:631–40.

Chambliss KL, Gray RG, Rylance G, Pollitt RJ, Gibson KM. Molecular characterization of methylmalonate semialdehyde dehydrogenase deficiency. J Inherit Metab Dis. 2000;23:497–504.

De Keyzer Y, Valayannopoulos V, Benoist JF, Batteux F, Lacaille F, Hubert L, Chrétien D, Chadefeaux-Vekemans B, Niaudet P, Touati G, Munnich A, de Lonlay P. Multiple OXPHOS deficiency in the liver, kidney, heart, and skeletal muscle of patients with methylmalonic aciduria and propionic aciduria. Pediatr Res. 2009;66:91–5.

Ensenauer R, Vockley J, Willard JM, Huey JC, Sass JO, Edland SD, Burton BK, Berry SA, Santer R, Grünert S, Koch HG, Marquardt I, Rinaldo P, Hahn S, Matern D. A common mutation is associated with a mild, potentially asymptomatic phenotype in patients with isovaleric acidemia diagnosed by newborn screening. Am J Hum Genet. 2004;75:1136–42.

Ensenauer R, Fingerhut R, Maier EM, Polanetz R, Olgemöller B, Röschinger W, Muntau AC. Newborn screening for isovaleric acidemia using tandem mass spectrometry: data from 1.6 million newborns. Clin Chem. 2011;57:623–6.

Fitzsimons PE, Alston CL, Bonnen PE, Hughes J, Crushell E, Geraghty MT, Tetreault M, O'Reilly P, Twomey E, Sheikh Y, Walsh R, Waterham HR, Ferdinandusse S, Wanders RJA, Taylor RW, Pitt JJ, Mayne PD. Clinical, biochemical, and genetic features of four patients with short-chain enoyl-CoA hydratase (ECHS1) deficiency. Am J Med Genet A. 2018;176:1115–27.

Fukao T, Akiba K, Goto M, Kuwayama N, Morita M, Hori T, Aoyama Y, Venkatesan R, Wierenga R, Moriyama Y, Hashimoto T, Usuda N, Murayama K, Ohtake A, Hasegawa Y, Shigematsu Y, Hasegawa Y. The first case in Asia of 2-methyl-3-hydroxybutyryl-CoA dehydrogenase deficiency (HSD10 disease) with atypical presentation. J Hum Genet. 2014;59:609–14.

Gibson KM, Breuer J, Nyhan WL. 3-Hydroxy-3-methylglutaryl-coenzyme A lyase deficiency. Review of 18 reported patients. Eur J Pediatr. 1988;148:180–6.

Gibson KM, Bennett MJ, Naylor EW, Morton DH. 3-Methylcrotonyl-coenzyme A carboxylase deficiency in Amish/Mennonite adults identified by detection of increased acylcarnitines in blood spots of their children. J Pediatr. 1998;132:519–23.

Gibson KM, Burlingame TG, Hogema B, Jakobs C, Schutgens RB, Millington D, Roe CR, Roe DS, Sweetman L, Steiner RD, Linck L, Pohowalla P, Sacks M, Kiss D, Rinaldo P, Vockley J. 2-Methylbutyryl-coenzyme A dehydrogenase deficiency: a new inborn error of L-isoleucine metabolism. Pediatr Res. 2000;47:830–3.

Grünert SC, Müllerleile S, De Silva L, Barth M, Walter M, Walter K, Meissner T, Lindner M, Ensenauer R, Santer R, Bodamer OA, Baumgartner MR, Brunner-Krainz M, Karall D, Haase C, Knerr I, Marquardt T, et al. Propionic acidemia: clinical course and outcome in 55 pediatric and adolescent patients. Orphanet J Rare Dis. 2013;8:6.

Grünert SC, Schmitt RN, Schlatter SM, Gemperle-Britschgi C, Balcı MC, Berg V, Çoker M, Das AM, Demirkol M, Derks TGJ, Gökçay G, Uçar SK, Konstantopoulou V, Christoph Korenke G, Lotz-Havla AS, Schlune A, Staufner C, Tran C, Visser G, Schwab KO, Fukao T, Sass JO. Clinical presentation and outcome in a series of 32 patients with 2-methylacetoacetyl-coenzyme A thiolase (MAT) deficiency. Mol Genet Metab. 2017;122:67–75.

Knerr I, Crushell E, Mayne P, Deverell D, Monovari AA, Treacy E. Assessment of biochemical profiles during metabolic decompensation in 14 patients with maple syrup urine disease (MSUD). J Inher Metab Dis. 2011;34(Suppl 3):S80.

Koeberl DD, Young SP, Gregersen NS, Vockley J, Smith WE, Benjamin DK Jr, An Y, Weavil SD, Chaing SH, Bali D, McDonald MT, Kishnani PS, Chen YT, Millington DS. Rare disorders of metabolism with elevated butyryl- and isobutyryl-carnitine detected by tandem mass spectrometry newborn screening. Pediatr Res. 2003;54:219–23.

Levtova A, Waters PJ, Buhas D, Lévesque S, Auray-Blais C, Clarke JTR, Laframboise R, Maranda B, Mitchell GA, Brunel-Guitton C, Braverman NE. Combined malonic and methylmalonic aciduria due to ACSF3 mutations: benign clinical course in an unselected cohort. J Inherit Metab Dis. 2019;42:107–16.

Loupatty FJ, van der Steen A, Ijlst L, Ruiter JP, Ofman R, Baumgartner MR, Ballhausen D, Yamaguchi S, Duran M, Wanders RJ. Clinical, biochemical, and molecular findings in three patients with 3-hydroxyisobutyric aciduria. Mol Genet Metab. 2006;87:243–8.

Loupatty FJ, Clayton PT, Ruiter JP, Ofman R, Ijlst L, Brown GK, Thorburn DR, Harris RA, Duran M, Desousa C, Krywawych S, Heales SJ, Wanders RJ. Mutations in the gene encoding 3-hydroxyisobutyryl-CoA hydrolase results in progressive infantile neurodegeneration. Am J Hum Genet. 2007;80:195–9.

Manoli I, Myles JG, Sloan JL, Shchelochkov OA, Venditti CP. A critical reappraisal of dietary practices in methylmalonic acidemia raises concerns about the safety of medical foods. Part 1: isolated methylmalonic acidemias. Genet Med. 2016;18:386–95.

Marcadier JL, Smith AM, Pohl D, Schwartzentruber J, Al-Dirbashi OY, FORGE Canada Consortium, Majewski J, Ferdinandusse S, Wanders RJ, Bulman DE, Boycott KM, Chakraborty P, Geraghty MT. Mutations in ALDH6A1 encoding methylmalonate semialdehyde dehydrogenase are associated with dysmyelination and transient methylmalonic aciduria. Orphanet J Rare Dis. 2013;8:98.

Marriage. Nutritional management of patients with inherited disorders of branched-chain amino acid metabolism. In: Acosta PB, editor. Nutritional management of patients with inherited metabolic disorders. 1st ed. Sudbury: Jones and Bartlett Publishers; 2010. p. 175–236.

Mazzuca M, Maubert MA, Damaj L, Clot F, Cadoudal M, Dubourg C, Odent S, Benoit JF, Bahi-Buisson N, Christa L, de Lonlay P. Combined sepiapterin reductase and methylmalonyl-CoA epimerase deficiency in a second patient: cerebrospinal fluid polyunsaturated fatty acid level and follow-up under L-DOPA, 5-HTP and BH4 trials. JIMD Rep. 2015;22:47–55.

Novarino G, El-Fishawy P, Kayserili H, Meguid NA, Scott EM, Schroth J, Silhavy JL, Kara M, Khalil RO, Ben-Omran T, Ercan-Sencicek

AG, Hashish AF, Sanders SJ, Gupta AR, Hashem HS, Matern D, Gabriel S, Sweetman L, Rahimi Y, Harris RA, State MW, Gleeson JG. Mutations in BCKD-kinase lead to a potentially treatable form of autism with epilepsy. Science. 2012;338:394–7.

Oerum S, Roovers M, Leichsenring M, Acquaviva-Bourdain C, Beermann F, Gemperle-Britschgi C, Fouilhoux A, Korwitz-Reichelt A, Bailey HJ, Droogmans L, Oppermann U, Sass JO, Yue WW. Novel patient missense mutations in the HSD17B10 gene affect dehydrogenase and mitochondrial tRNA modification functions of the encoded protein. Biochim Biophys Acta Mol basis Dis. 2017;1863:3294–302.

Oglesbee D, He M, Majumder N, Vockley J, Ahmad A, Angle B, Burton B, Charrow J, Ensenauer R, Ficicioglu CH, Keppen LD, Marsden D, Tortorelli S, Hahn SH, Matern D. Development of a newborn screening follow-up algorithm for the diagnosis of isobutyryl-CoA dehydrogenase deficiency. Genet Med. 2007;9:108–16.

Paquay S, Bourillon A, Pichard S, Benoist JF, de Lonlay P, Dobbelaere D, Fouilhoux A, Guffon N, Rouvet I, Labarthe F, Mention K, Touati G, Valayannopoulos V, Ogier de Baulny H, Elmaleh-Bergès M, Acquaviva-Bourdain C, Vianey-Saban C, Schiff M. Mitochondrial acetoacetyl-CoA thiolase deficiency: basal ganglia impairment may occur independently of ketoacidosis. J Inherit Metab Dis. 2017;40:415–22.

Perez-Cerda C, García-Villoria J, Ofman R, Sala PR, Merinero B, Ramos J, García-Silva MT, Beseler B, Dalmau J, Wanders RJ, Ugarte M, Ribes A. 2-Methyl-3-hydroxybutyryl-CoA dehydrogenase (MHBD) deficiency: an X-linked inborn error of isoleucine metabolism that may mimic a mitochondrial disease. Pediatr Res. 2005;58:488–91.

Peters H, Buck N, Wanders R, Ruiter J, Waterham H, Koster J, Yaplito-Lee J, Ferdinandusse S, Pitt J. ECHS1 mutations in Leigh disease: a new inborn error of metabolism affecting valine metabolism. Brain. 2014;137:2903–8.

Rauschenberger K, Schöler K, Sass JO, Sauer S, Djuric Z, Rumig C, Wolf NI, Okun JG, Kölker S, Schwarz H, Fischer C, Grziwa B, Runz H, Nümann A, Shafqat N, Kavanagh KL, Hämmerling G, Wanders RJ, Shield JP, Wendel U, Stern D, Nawroth P, Hoffmann GF, Bartram CR, Arnold B, Bierhaus A, Oppermann U, Steinbeisser H, Zschocke J. A non-enzymatic function of 17beta-hydroxysteroid dehydrogenase type 10 is required for mitochondrial integrity and cell survival. EMBO Mol Med. 2010;2:51–62.

Reddi OS, Reddy SV, Reddy KR. A sibship with hypervalinemia. Hum Genet. 1977;39:139–42.

Roe CR, Cederbaum SD, Roe DS, Mardach R, Galindo A, Sweetman L. Isolated isobutyryl-CoA dehydrogenase deficiency: an unrecognized defect in human valine metabolism. Mol Genet Metab. 1998;65:264–71.

Salomons GS, Jakobs C, Pope LL, Errami A, Potter M, Nowaczyk M, Olpin S, Manning N, Raiman JA, Slade T, Champion MP, Peck D, Gavrilov D, Hillman R, Hoganson GE, Donaldson K, Shield JP, Ketteridge D, Wasserstein M, Gibson KM. Clinical, enzymatic and molecular characterization of nine new patients with malonyl-coenzyme A decarboxylase deficiency. J Inherit Metab Dis. 2007;30:23–8.

Sass JO, Sander S, Zschocke J. Isobutyryl-CoA dehydrogenase deficiency: isobutyrylglycinuria and ACAD8 gene mutations in two infants. J Inherit Metab Dis. 2004;27:741–5.

Sass JO, Ensenauer R, Röschinger W, Reich H, Steuerwald U, Schirrmacher O, Engel K, Häberle J, Andresen BS, Mégarbané A, Lehnert W, Zschocke J. 2-Methylbutyryl-coenzyme A dehydrogenase deficiency: functional and molecular studies on a defect in isoleucine catabolism. Mol Genet Metab. 2008;93:30–5.

Sharpe AJ, McKenzie M. Mitochondrial fatty acid oxidation disorders associated with short-chain enoyl-CoA hydratase (ECHS1) deficiency. Cells. 2018;23. pii: E46.

Shepard PJ, Barshop BA, Baumgartner MR, Hansen JB, Jepsen K, Smith EN, Frazer KA. Consanguinity and rare mutations outside of MCCC genes underlie nonspecific phenotypes of MCCD. Genet Med. 2015;17:660–7.

Siekmeyer M, Petzold-Quinque S, Terpe F, Beblo S, Gebhardt R, Schlensog-Schuster F, Kiess W, Siekmeyer W. Citric acid as the last therapeutic approach in an acute life-threatening metabolic decompensation of propionic acidaemia. J Pediatr Endocrinol Metab. 2013;26:569–74.

Sloan JL, Johnston JJ, Manoli I, Chandler RJ, Krause C, Carrillo-Carrasco N, Chandrasekaran SD, Sysol JR, O'Brien K, Hauser NS, Sapp JC, Dorward HM, Huizing M, NIH Intramural Sequencing Center Group, Barshop BA, Berry SA, James PM, Champaigne NL, de Lonlay P, Valayannopoulos V, Geschwind MD, Gavrilov DK, Nyhan WL, Biesecker LG, Venditti CP. Exome sequencing identifies ACSF3 as a cause of combined malonic and methylmalonic aciduria. Nat Genet. 2011;43:883–6.

Strauss KA, Wardley B, Robinson D, Hendrickson C, Rider NL, Puffenberger EG, Shelmer D, Moser AB, Morton DH. Classical maple syrup urine disease and brain development: principles of management and formula design. Mol Genet Metab. 2010;99: 333–45.

Tan H, Chen X, Lv W, Linpeng S, Liang D, Wu L. Truncating mutations of HIBCH tend to cause severe phenotypes in cases with HIBCH deficiency: a case report and brief literature review. J Hum Genet. 2018;63:851–5.

Tuncel AT, Boy N, Morath MA, Hörster F, Mütze U, Kölker S. Organic acidurias in adults: late complications and management. J Inherit Metab Dis. 2018;41:765–76.

Vockley J, Ensenauer R. Isovaleric acidemia: new aspects of genetic and phenotypic heterogeneity. Am J Med Genet C Semin Med Genet. 2006;142C:95–103.

Waters PJ, Thuriot F, Clarke JT, Gravel S, Watkins D, Rosenblatt DS, Lévesque S. Methylmalonyl-coA epimerase deficiency: a new case, with an acute metabolic presentation and an intronic splicing mutation in the MCEE gene. Mol Genet Metab Rep. 2016;9: 19–24.

Wortmann SB, Kluijtmans LA, Rodenburg RJ, Sass JO, Nouws J, van Kaauwen EP, Kleefstra T, Tranebjaerg L, de Vries MC, Isohanni P, Walter K, Alkuraya FS, Smuts I, Reinecke CJ, van der Westhuizen FH, Thorburn D, Smeitink JA, Morava E, Wevers RA. 3-Methylglutaconic aciduria-lessons from 50 genes and 977 patients. J Inherit Metab Dis. 2013;36:913–21.

Yanicelli S. Nutritional management of patients with inherited disorders of organic acid metabolism. In: Acosta PB, editor. Nutritional management of patients with inherited metabolic disorders. 1st ed. Sudbury: Jones and Bartlett Publishers; 2010. p. 283–341.

Zschocke J, Ruiter JP, Brand J, Lindner M, Hoffmann GF, Wanders RJ, Mayatepek E. Progressive infantile neurodegeneration caused by 2-methyl-3-hydroxybutyryl-CoA dehydrogenase deficiency: a novel inborn error of branched-chain fatty acid and isoleucine metabolism. Pediatr Res. 2000;48:852–5.

# Disorders of Beta and Gamma Amino Acids

24

Phillip L. Pearl and Lance Rodan

## Contents



**Summary**

Disorders of beta amino acid synthesis, specifically dihydropyrimidine dehydrogenase, dihydropyrimidinase, and beta-ureidopropionase deficiency, manifest with neurodevelopmental impairment including epilepsy, sensitivity to fluropyrimidine chemotherapeutics, and abnormal urine pyrimidines on diagnostic testing. Of the disorders of beta amino acid degradation, hyper-beta-alaninemia and methylmalonate semialdehyde dehydrogenase deficiency have neurological phenotypes. In contrast, beta-aminoisobutyric aciduria is asymptomatic. Carnosinase deficiency leads to homocarnosinosis, with elevated urinary carnosine and CSF homocarnosine, although a phenotype has not been confirmed. The disorders of gamma amino acid metabolism are manifest by impaired GABA degradation in GABA transaminase deficiency and the more common succinic semialdehyde dehydrogenase (SSADH) deficiency. GABA transaminase deficiency leads to an early-onset epileptic encephalopathy associated with choreoathetosis, hypersomnolence, and sometimes growth acceleration, the latter attributed to GABA-mediated enhancing effects on growth hormone production. SSADH typically has the phenotype of a nonprogressive neurodevelopmental disorder with profound effects on expressive language, mild hypotonia and ataxia, and later development of epilepsy. There are other cases with prominent choreoathetosis and sometimes regression associated with systemic illnesses in infancy. GABA transporter deficiency may manifest as myoclonic-atonic epilepsy. There are a variety of GABA receptor subunit deficiencies, each with a handful of affected patients identified, and mostly manifest as early infantile or childhood *epileptic* encephalopathy.

P. L. Pearl (✉) · L. Rodan
Department of Neurology, Boston Children's Hospital, Harvard Medical School, Boston, MA, USA
e-mail: Phillip.Pearl@childrens.harvard.edu; Lance.Rodan@childrens.harvard.edu


N. Blau et al. (eds.), *Physician's Guide to the Diagnosis, Treatment, and Follow-Up of Inherited Metabolic Diseases*,
https://doi.org/10.1007/978-3-030-67727-5_24

## Introduction

Beta and gamma amino acids are non-essential, non-proteinogenic amino acids containing an amine group attached to a beta or gamma carbon atom, respectively. The beta and gamma amino acids serve diverse cellular functions in humans, including an important role in the nervous system. They are present in both free and dipeptide forms. The free-form beta amino acids include beta-alanine, beta-aminoisobutyrate, and beta-leucine, and dipeptides include carnosine and anserine. The only gamma amino acid in humans is gamma aminobutyric acid (GABA), which exists in both free form and as the dipeptide homocarnosine (Pearl et al. 2019).

### Beta-Alanine

β-alanine is produced through the degradation of the pyrimidine base uracil. Free-form beta-alanine acts as a neurotransmitter/neuromodulator in the central nervous system and as a precursor for pantothenic acid, which is required for synthesis of Coenzyme A. Beta-alanine is catabolized to acetyl-CoA, which can be used for anaplerosis and for synthesis of ketone bodies, fatty acids, and other compounds.

### Beta-Aminoisobutyrate

Beta-aminoisobutyrate exists in two enantiomers in humans: an R-enantiomer derived from catabolism of the pyrimidine base thymine and an S-enantiomer derived from valine catabolism. In plasma, the S-enantiomer is the predominant form due to active renal reabsorption, whereas in urine the R-enantiomer is the predominant form, eliminated by renal filtration and tubular secretion. It has been suggested that there may be non-enzymatic interconversion between these enantiomers. The functions of beta-aminoisobutyrate have not been fully elucidated. It may play a role as a myokine involved in the browning of white fat through a PPARalpha-mediated mechanism. In addition, beta-aminoisobutyrate is a structural analogue of gamma aminobutyric acid (GABA) and glycine and may play a role in neurotransmission. Beta-aminoisobutyrate is catabolized to the anaplerotic metabolite propionyl-CoA.

### Beta-Leucine

Beta-leucine is converted to alpha-leucine in a reversible reaction catalyzed by the B12-dependent enzyme leucine 2,3-aminomutase. The biological role of beta-leucine has not been established. Beta-leucine accounts for a very small percentage of the total leucine pool in tissues, other than in the testes where it accounts for approximately one-third. Elevated beta-leucine is a biomarker of vitamin B12 deficiency.

### Gamma-Aminobutyric Acid (GABA)

GABA is synthesized through decarboxylation of the amino acid glutamate via the enzyme glutamic acid decarboxylase (GAD) and to a lesser degree through metabolism of the polyamine putrescine. GABA is the principal inhibitory neurotransmitter in the human central nervous system. It facilitates neuronal inhibition by binding to specific transmembrane GABA receptors. There are two classes of receptors: GABA-A and GABA-B receptors. GABA-A receptors are ligand-activated chloride channels, and GABA-B receptors are metabotropic, G protein-coupled receptors that activate potassium channels. GABA is catabolized to the Krebs cycle intermediate succinate.

### Beta and Gamma Amino Acid Dipeptides

β-alanine and GABA both occur as imidazole dipeptides. The β-alanine dipeptides include carnosine (β-alanyl-L-histidine) and anserine (β-alanyl-1-methyl-L-histidine). Carnosine is synthesized endogenously through the enzyme carnosine synthetase. Most carnosine obtained from the diet is excreted intact in urine. Carnosine contains the largest pool of beta-alanine in humans. Carnosine is primarily stored within skeletal muscle and central nervous system. In skeletal muscle, it acts as an intracellular buffer and antioxidant during glycolysis. In the central nervous system, it may play a role as a neurotransmitter. Carnosine is hydrolyzed to its constituent amino acids, beta-alanine and histidine, by carnosine dipeptidase. Anserine is not a constituent of human tissue and is obtained solely from dietary sources. It is hydrolyzed to beta-alanine and 1-methylhistidine by carnosine dipeptidase (Pearl et al. 2019).

GABA exists as the dipeptide homocarnosine (β-aminobutyryl-L-histidine). It is synthesized through the enzyme carnosine synthetase. Homocarnosine is found only in the brain. The function of homocarnosine has not been established. It is hydrolyzed to its constituent amino acids by the enzyme carnosine dipeptidase.

## Nomenclature

| No. | Disorder | Alternate disease name | Disease abbreviation | Gene symbol | Chromosome localization | Mode of inheritance | Altered protein | OMIM # |
|---|---|---|---|---|---|---|---|---|
| 24.1 | Dihydropyrimidine dehydrogenase deficiency | Thymine-uraciluria | | DPYD | 1p21.3 | AR | Dihydropyrimidine dehydrogenase | 274270; 612779 |
| 24.2 | Dihydropyrimidinase deficiency | Dihydropyrimidinuria | | DPYS | 8q22.3 | AR | Dihydropyrimidinase | 222748; 613326 |
| 24.3 | Beta-ureidopropionase deficiency | β-alanine synthase deficiency | | UPB1 | 22q11.23 | AR | Beta-ureidopropionase | 613161 |
| 24.4 | Hyper-β-aminoisobutyric aciduria | Beta-aminoisobutyric aciduria | AGXT2 | AGXT2 | 5p13.2 | AR | d-beta-aminoisobutyrate:pyruvate aminotransferase | 210100 |
| 24.5 | Hyper-β-alaninemia | | | Gene unknown | Locus unknown | AR | ? beta-alanyl-alpha-ketoglutarate transaminase | 237400 |
| 24.6 | GABA transaminase deficiency | GABA-T | GABA-T | ABAT | 16p13.2 | AR | GABA transaminase | 613163; 137150 |
| 24.7 | Succinic semialdehyde dehydrogenase deficiency | 4-Hydroxybutyric aciduria, SSADH deficiency | SSADH | ALDH5A1 | 6p22.3 | AR | Succinic semialdehyde dehydrogenase | 271980; 610045 |
| 24.8 | GABA transporter deficiency | Myoclonic-atonic epilepsy | MAE | SLC6A1 | 3p25.3 | AD | GABA transporter | 137165 |
| 24.9 | GABA type A receptor α1 subunit deficiency | EIEE type 19 | EIEE19 | GABRA1 | 5q34 | AD | GABA-A receptor, alpha 1 | 137160 |
| 24.10 | GABA type A receptor α6 subunit deficiency | | | GABRA6 | 5q34 | AD | GABA-A receptor, alpha 6 | 137143 |
| 24.11 | GABA type A receptor β1 subunit deficiency | EIEE type 45 | EIEE45 | GABRB1 | 4p12 | AD | GABA-A receptor, beta 1 | 137190 |
| 24.12 | GABA type A receptor β2 subunit deficiency | Infantile or early childhood epileptic encephalopathy type 2 | IECEE2 | GABRB2 | 5q34 | AD | GABA-A receptor, beta 2 | 600232; 617829 |
| 24.13 | GABA type A receptor β3 subunit deficiency | EIEE type 43 | EIEE43 | GABRB3 | 15q12 | AD | GABA-A receptor, beta 3 | 137192 |
| 24.14 | GABA type A receptor γ2 subunit deficiency | EIEE type 74, GEFS+ type 3 | GEFSP3 | GABRG2 | 5q34 | AD | GABA-A receptor, gamma 2 | 137164; 611277 |
| 24.15 | GABA type A receptor δ subunit deficiency | GEFS+, type 5 | | GABRD | 1p36.33 | AD | GABA-A receptor, delta | 137163 |
| 24.16 | GABA type B receptor subunit 2 deficiency | EIEE, type 59; Rett like phenotype | EIEE59 | GABBR2 | 9q22.23 | AD | GABA-B receptor, R2 | 607340; 617904 |
| 24.17 | Serum carnosinase deficiency/ homocarnosinosis | Carnosinemia; homocarnosinosis | CARN | CNDP1 | 18q22.3 | AR | Carnosinase | 212200; 236130 |
| 24.18 | Methylmalonate semialdehyde dehydrogenase deficiency | Combined semialdehyde dehydrogenase deficiency | MMSDH | ALDH6A1 | 14q24.3 | AR | Methylmalonate semialdehyde dehydrogenase | 614105; 603178 |

*EIEE* early infantile epileptic encephalopathy, *GEFS+* genetic epilepsy with febrile seizures plus (other seizure types)

## Metabolic Pathways and Disorders

### Disorders of Beta Amino Acid Synthesis

Beta-alanine and beta-aminoisobutyrate are synthesized in the liver and kidney through the degradation of the pyrimidine bases, uracil and thymine, respectively, in three sequential steps utilizing enzymes shared by both pathways.

#### Dihydropyrimidine Dehydrogenase Deficiency

Dihydropyrimidine dehydrogenase is the first and rate-limiting enzyme of the pyrimidine degradation pathway. It catalyzes the reduction of uracil to 5,6-dihydrouracil and thymine to 5,6-dihydrothymine. Dihydropyrimidine dehydrogenase is ubiquitously expressed. It is encoded by the DPYD gene.

Dihydropyrimidine dehydrogenase deficiency is an autosomal recessive disorder resulting from mutations in the DPYD gene. More than 75 patients have been reported to date (Fang et al. 2019). It has incomplete penetrance and variable expressivity. Affected individuals variably present with developmental delays, hypotonia, autism, epilepsy, growth restriction, microcephaly, dysmorphic features, and ophthalmological abnormalities. There may be nonspecific MRI abnormalities including cerebral volume loss, white matter abnormalities, and abnormalities of corpus callosum (Chen et al. 2014). In contrast, some individuals with DPYD gene mutations and classic biochemical abnormalities may remain entirely asymptomatic, suggesting a role of modifier genes or environmental factors. Individuals with dihydropyrimidine dehydrogenase deficiency are unable to normally metabolize fluoropyrimidine chemotherapy medications, 5-fluorouracil and capecitabine, resulting in drug toxicity if they are unknowingly treated. Clinical manifestations include myelosuppression, diarrhea, mucositis, stomatitis, neurotoxicity, and potentially death. Heterozygous carriers for dihydropyrimidine dehydrogenase deficiency may also have adverse reactions to these medications. Biochemical diagnosis is established through measurement of urine pyrimidines, demonstrating accumulation of uracil and thymine. These abnormalities may also be detected in blood and CSF. Treatment of dihydropyrimidine dehydrogenase deficiency is supportive, aimed at managing neurological manifestations and avoiding medications in the fluoropyrimidine category.

#### Dihydropyrimidinase Deficiency

In the second step of pyrimidine degradation, dihydropyrimidinase catalyzes the hydrolytic ring opening of the dihydropyrimidines, 5,6-dihydrouracil and 5,6-dihydrothymine, to *N*-carbamyl-beta-alanine and *N*-carbamyl-beta-aminoisobutyric acid, respectively. The enzyme is primarily expressed in the liver and kidneys. It is encoded by the DPYS gene.

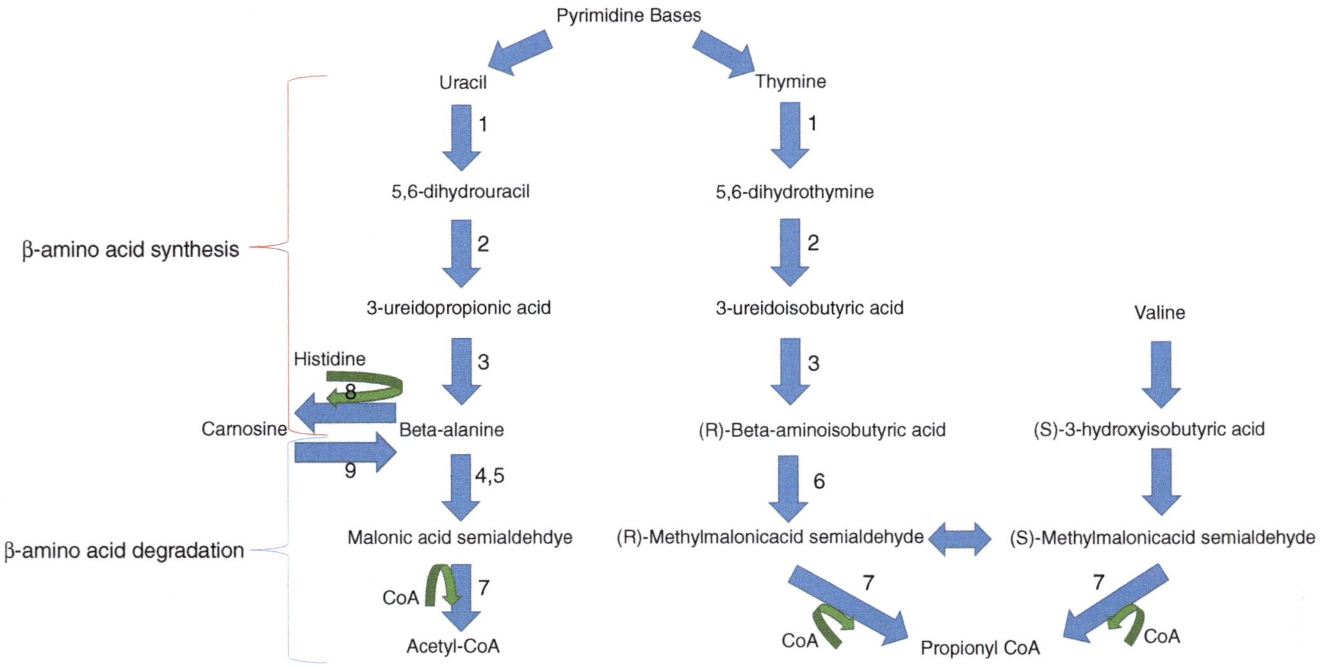


**Fig. 24.1** Beta amino acid metabolism. (1) Dihydropyrimidine dehydrogenase. (2) Dihydropyrimidinase. (3) Beta-ureidopropionase. (4) β-alanine-α-ketoglutarate transaminase. (5) β-alanine-pyruvate transaminase. (6) β-aminoisobutyrate-pyruvate transaminase. (7) Methylmalonate semialdehyde dehydrogenase. (8) Carnosine synthetase. (9) Carnosinase

Dihydropyrimidinase deficiency is an autosomal recessive disorder resulting from mutations in the DPYS gene. Approximately 30 patients with confirmed dihydropyrimidinase deficiency have been reported to date (Nakahima et al. 2017). Similar to dihydropyrimidine dehydrogenase deficiency, dihydropyrimidinase deficiency has incomplete penetrance and variable expressivity. Affected individuals variably present with developmental delay, epilepsy, growth restriction, and dysmorphic features. Autism has been rarely reported. Some affected individuals may be asymptomatic (Nakahima et al. 2017). Similar to dihydropyrimidine dehydrogenase deficiency, this disorder may be associated with adverse reactions to the fluropyrimidine chemotherapies. Neuroimaging may variably demonstrate cerebral atrophy and white matter abnormalities (Nakahima et al. 2017). Biochemical diagnosis is established through measurement of urine pyrimidines, demonstrating accumulation of 5,6-dihydrouracil and 5,6-dihydrothymine. A similar profile may be detected in plasma and cerebrospinal fluid. Enzyme activity can be measured in liver biopsy. Treatment of dihydropyrimidinase deficiency is supportive.

#### Beta-Ureidopropionase Deficiency

In the third step of pyrimidine degradation, beta-ureidopropionase catalyzes the conversion of *N*-carbamyl-beta-alanine and *N*-carbamyl-beta-aminoisobutyric acid to beta-alanine and beta-aminoisobutyric acid, respectively. The enzyme is primarily expressed in the liver and kidneys. It is encoded by the UPB1 gene.

Beta-ureidopropionase deficiency is an autosomal recessive disorder resulting from biallelic variants in the UPB1 gene. Approximately 40 patients have been reported to date (Fang et al. 2019). Similar to other defects in pyrimidine degradation, the clinical presentation is variable, ranging from asymptomatic individuals to individuals affected with a severe neurodevelopmental disorder associated with developmental delay, hypotonia, dystonia, epilepsy, autism, microcephaly, growth restriction, dysmorphic features, optic atrophy, retinal pigmentary abnormalities, and gastrointestinal dysmotility. Individuals with beta-ureidopropionase deficiency and carriers also appear to be at increased risk of fluoropyrimidine-related toxicity. Neuroimaging is inconsistent, and various abnormalities have been described, including cortical malformations, atrophy, cerebellar and brainstem dysplasia, and white matter abnormalities. Biochemical diagnosis is established through measurement of urine pyrimidines, demonstrating highly elevated levels of *N*-carbamyl-beta-alanine and *N*-carbamyl-beta-aminoisobutyric acid and moderately elevated levels of 5,6-dihydrouracil and 5,6-dihydrothymine. A similar profile may be detected in plasma and cerebrospinal fluid. Enzyme activity can be measured in liver biopsy. Treatment of beta-ureidopropionase deficiency remains supportive. Treatment with ß-alanine is not effective.

### Disorders of Beta Amino Acid Degradation

#### Hyper-Beta-Alaninemia

Beta-alanine is catabolized in two sequential steps. Beta-alanine is first transaminated in the liver by either beta-alanine-alpha-ketoglutarate transaminase (AKT) or beta-alanine-pyruvate transaminase to malonate semialdehyde (beta-ketopropionate). In the second step, malonate semialdehyde is oxidized by methylmalonate semialdehyde dehydrogenase to acetyl-CoA.

Hyper-beta-alaninemia was first described in 1966. It has been reported in two individuals to date, one of which also carried a clinical diagnosis of Cohen syndrome (Higgins et al. 1994). Reported clinical features include epilepsy, encephalopathy, lethargy, and hypotonia. The molecular basis has not yet been established. It is hypothesized to result from deficiency of beta-alanine transaminase activity, either beta-alanine pyruvate aminotransferase or beta-alanine alpha ketoglutarate aminotransferase. The biochemical features of hyper-beta-alaninemia have been induced experimentally in vitro by administration of aminooxyacetate, an inhibitor of aminotransferases. In addition, one of the reported individuals with hyper-beta-alaninemia was found to have reduced beta-alanyl-alpha-ketoglutarate transaminase (AKT) activity in cultured skin fibroblasts. Biochemical evaluation in this disorder demonstrates elevations of plasma and urine beta-alanine, as well as elevated urine levels of GABA and beta-aminoisobutyrate. The mechanism of neurotoxicity has not yet been elucidated, although it has been suggested that it may result from increased oxidative stress, depletion of taurine, and mitochondrial damage. In the index case, pyridoxine supplementation resulted in biochemical but not clinical improvement. Dietary modifications, pantothenic acid supplementation, and antibiotic therapy were also not found to be beneficial (Scriver et al. 1966). In the second case, pyridoxine supplementation resulted in both biochemical correction and clinical improvement. Pyridoxine is a precursor of the transaminase cofactor.

#### Beta-Aminoisobutyric Aciduria

Similar to beta-alanine, beta-aminoisobutyric acid is catabolized into two sequential steps. It is first deaminated by beta-aminoisobutyrate aminotransferases to methylmalonate semialdehyde and then oxidized by methylmalonate semialdehyde dehydrogenase to propionyl-CoA.

Beta-aminoisobutyric aciduria is considered a benign biochemical variant and occurs at a high frequency in certain populations: 5–10% in Caucasians and 40–95% in Asian populations. The disorder results from deficiency of hepatic D-beta-aminoisobutyrate:pyruvate aminotransferase, encoded by the AGXT2 gene. Inheritance is autosomal recessive, with incomplete penetrance. Individuals with beta-aminoisobutyric aciduria excrete large amounts of (R) beta-aminoisobutyric acid in their urine but have no clinical symptoms (Pearl et al. 2019).

#### Methylmalonate Semialdehyde Dehydrogenase Deficiency

Methylmalonate semialdehyde dehydrogenase is involved in the second step of both beta-alanine and beta-aminoisobutyrate degradation. It is also involved in the valine catabolic pathway. It is a member of the aldehyde dehydrogenase superfamily but uniquely requires CoA as a substrate. It is located in the mitochondrial matrix.

Methylmalonate semialdehyde dehydrogenase deficiency is an autosomal recessive disorder resulting from mutations in the ALDH6A1 gene. Four patients have been reported to date. This disorder presents with variable developmental delays, microcephaly, dysmorphic features, epilepsy, ophthalmological abnormalities, hypotonia, and dystonia. Imaging may demonstrate delayed myelination and thinning of the corpus callosum. Metabolic evaluation variably demonstrates metabolic acidosis and increased urinary excretion of 3-hydroxyisobutyric acid, beta-aminoisobutyric acid, beta-alanine, 3-hydroxypropionate, lactate, and methylmalonic acid. Management is supportive (Marcadier et al. 2013).

### Disorders of Beta and Gamma Amino Acid Dipeptide Metabolism

#### Serum Carnosinase Deficiency and Homocarnosinosis

Both carnosine and homocarnosine are hydrolyzed to their constituent amino acids by the enzyme carnosine dipeptidase (also known as carnosinase). There are separate serum and tissue forms, encoded by different genes. The serum form is encoded by the CNDP1 gene. Deficiency of serum carnosine dipeptidase was initially reported in association with two distinct disorders, serum carnosinase deficiency and homocarnosinosis. It is now appreciated that these likely represent the same biochemical defect. Biochemical features include increased urinary excretion of carnosine and elevated levels of CSF homocarnosine. While about half of the patients with this biochemical finding have been reported to present with neurological disease (spasticity, retinal degeneration, epilepsy), the association between this biochemical finding and clinical disease has not been firmly established. Multiple cases of asymptomatic family members with serum carnosinase deficiency have been ascertained after diagnosis of symptomatic probands (Pearl et al. 2019). Further, the index family with homocarnosinosis was determined to have had SPG11 gene-related hereditary spastic paraplegia as the likely cause of their symptoms (Sjaastad et al. 2018).

### Disorders of Gamma Amino Acids

#### GABA Transaminase Deficiency

Gamma transaminase (GABA-T), or ABAT (4-aminobutyrate aminotransferase), converts GABA to succinic semialdehyde, leading to the oxidative metabolism of GABA through the Krebs cycle. If GABA-T is absent, there is a resultant accumulation of GABA and beta-alanine, homocarnosine, and the GABA ketone, 2-pyrrolidinone. GABA-T deficiency is caused by biallelic pathogenic variants in the ABAT gene (OMIM 613163). While initially characterized as an early-onset epileptic encephalopathy with mortality within the first 2 years of life, an expanded phenotypic spectrum has been identified with further case series, including survival into adulthood (Hegde et al. 2019).

The typical presentation is neonatal or early infantile-onset encephalopathy along with hypotonia, hypersomnolence, epilepsy, choreoathetosis, and in some cases, accelerated linear growth. EEG recordings manifest burst-suppression, modified hypsarrhythmia, multifocal spikes, or generalized spike-wave. MRI demonstrates cerebral atrophy, thalamic lesions, and increased diffusion-weighted signal intensity involving the internal and external capsules and cerebral white matter (Ichikawa et al. 2019). MR spectroscopy may be helpful in demonstrating elevated GABA levels (Ichikawa et al. 2019). There is no specific treatment. Flumazenil, a GABA-A benzodiazepine receptor antagonist, has been utilized with variable effects (Koenig et al. 2017).

#### Succinic Semialdehyde Dehydrogenase (SSADH) Deficiency

GABA is normally deaminated to succinic semialdehyde, itself an unstable intermediate, by GABA-T and then converted to succinic acid via SSADH. Deficiency of SSADH

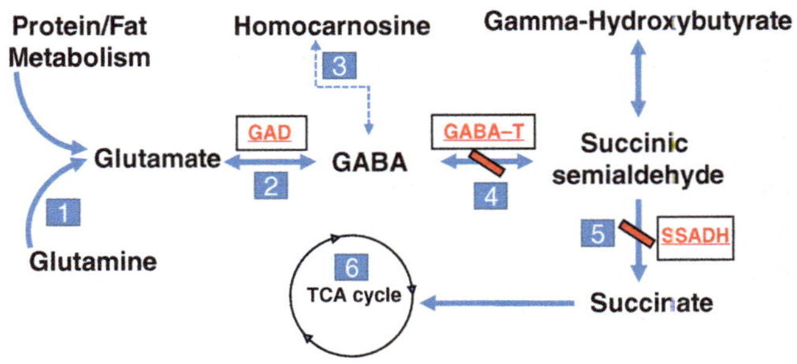


Fig. 24.2 GABA metabolism. (1) Glutaminase. (2) Glutamic acid decarboxylase. (3) Homocarnosinase/carnosinase. (4) GABA transaminase. (5) Succinic semialdehyde dehydrogenase. (6) Tricarboxylic acid cycle

leads to the pathological accumulation of gamma-hydroxybutyrate (GHB) as well as D-2-hydroxyglutaric acid and 4,5-dihydroxyhexanoic acid (DHHA). SSADH deficiency is caused by inactivating variants of the ALDH5A1 gene and is an autosomal recessively inherited disorder (OMIM 271980). The true prevalence is unknown, although at least 350 patients have been estimated to have been diagnosed based on laboratory experience, and 182 confirmed cases from 40 countries had been published as of 2016 based on a literature review along with our database (Attri et al. 2017). The true prevalence is likely underestimated, given the nonspecific neurologic phenotype, absence of systemic abnormalities or neurodegenerative course in most cases, potential for misdiagnosis, and increasing number of cases diagnosed with more widespread use of next-generation sequencing. The typical presentation is that of a relatively static encephalopathy with hypotonia and developmental delay having onset in the first 2 years, with subsequent manifestations being intellectual deficiency, severe expressive language impairment, mild ataxia, and a neuropsychiatric profile characterized by ADHD and sometimes aggression and autistic behavior in childhood with increasingly incapacitating anxiety and obsessive-compulsive disorder in adulthood (DiBacco et al. 2018). About half of patients develop epilepsy, and there appears to be a risk for SUDEP (sudden unexplained death in epilepsy patients) in as high as 10–15% of the adult cohort with otherwise normal or nearly normal life expectancy (Lapalme-Remis et al. 2015).

The diagnosis is made by elevation of 4-hydroxybutyric acid (GHB) which is detected on urine organic acids as the most common metabolic pathway to clinical suspicion, although more clinicians are recently using targeted gene sequencing panels with nonspecific neurologic phenotypes or whole exome sequencing and arriving at the diagnosis. GHB is elevated in all physiologic body fluids, owing to impaired GABA degradation by SSADH. SSADH deficiency was first described in two patients with high levels of GHB found in blood, urine, and cerebrospinal fluid in 1983 (Gibson et al. 1983), followed by purification of mammalian SSADH, molecular cloning of ALDH5A1 gene and identification of mutations (Chambliss et al. 1998), and elaboration of the phenotype (Pearl et al. 2007).

A murine genetic degradation model has led to extensive therapeutic insight, leading to translational trials demonstrating downregulation of GABA(A) and (B) receptor activity in both clinical studies and animal models (Reis et al. 2012; Pearl et al. 2009a). Additional clinical studies have indicated sleep disturbances and polysomnographic abnormalities consistent with decreased stage REM, consistent with a hyper-GABA'ergic effect, as well as clinical trials that have either shown no definite benefit or are in progress (Pearl et al. 2009b, 2014). A natural history study is currently underway, along with the international working group on neurotransmitter related diseases (iNTD) and sponsored by the National Institute of Child Health and Development (NICHD) of the National Institutes of Health (NIH) (www.clinicaltrials.gov).

#### GABA Transporter Deficiency

The GABA transporter that removes GABA from the synaptic cleft is coded by the solute carrier gene SLC6A1, which maps to chromosomal locus 3p25-p24. Mutations in the transporter were reported to cause epilepsy of the myoclonic-atonic type in seven individuals, with six mutations characterized by two truncations and four missense alterations (Carvill et al. 2015). Interestingly, Slc6a1-knockout mice develop spike-wave discharges characteristic of absence seizures. A large cohort of 24 patients with pathogenic SLC6A1 variants were reported to have the phenotype of myoclonic atonic epilepsy (MAE) along with language delay plus mild or moderate intellectual deficiency before epilepsy onset (Johannesen et al. 2018). Excellent clinical response to the ketogenic diet has been reported, which is well known to occur in a subset of patients with the syndrome of MAE, or myoclonic atonic epilepsy of Doose (Palmer et al. 2016).

#### GABA Receptor Subunit Deficiencies

GABA type A receptors are composed of five homologous, variable subunits that form a central channel that functions as a chloride ion pore. Each subunit has a long, variable extracellular region, four transmembrane domains, and a variable cytoplasmic region. Zinc ions play a critical role in regulating GABA-A receptors via an allosteric mechanism dependent on the subunit receptor composition. There are distinct binding sites for benzodiazepines and neurosteroids. A number of GABA type A receptor subunit deficiencies have been described, each in a handful or less of patients. The associated nomenclature and clinical disorders are shown in Nomenclature Table.

In contrast to the ionotropic GABA-A receptors, metabotropic GABA type B receptors' inhibitory properties are mediated through G protein-coupled second messenger systems which regulate potassium conductance. The GABA-B receptor R2 subunit is encoded by the gene GABBR2, with cytogenetic location 9q22.33. Pathogenic variants have been associated with an early infantile epileptic encephalopathy as well as a neurodevelopmental disorder with speech impairment and loss of purposeful hand skills (Hamdan et al. 2017; Lopes et al. 2016).

## Signs and Symptoms

**Table 24.1** Dihydropyrimidine dehydrogenase deficiency

| System | Symptoms and biomarkers | Neonatal (birth–1 month) | Infancy (1–18 months) | Childhood (1.5–11 years) | Adolescence (11–16 years) | Adulthood (>16 years) |
|---|---|---|---|---|---|---|
| CNS | **Autism** | | ± | ± | ± | ± |
| | Cerebral atrophy (MRI) | ± | ± | ± | ± | ± |
| | Epilepsy | ± | ± | ± | ± | ± |
| | Hypertonia | ± | ± | ± | ± | ± |
| | Hypotonia | ± | ± | ± | ± | ± |
| | **Intellectual disability** | | ± | ± | ± | ± |
| | Microcephaly | | ± | ± | ± | ± |
| | Retardation, motor | | ± | ± | ± | ± |
| | Seizures | ± | ± | ± | ± | ± |
| | White matter abnormalities (MRI) | | ± | ± | ± | ± |
| Digestive | Feeding difficulties | ± | | | | |
| Eye | Coloboma | | ± | ± | ± | ± |
| | Eye movements, abnormal | ± | ± | ± | ± | ± |
| | **Nystagmus** | | ± | ± | ± | ± |
| | Optic atrophy | | ± | ± | ± | ± |
| Psychiatric | Hyperactivity | ± | ± | ± | ± | ± |
| Other | Severe 5-Fluorouracil toxicity, heterogotes | | | | | +++ |
| | Severe 5-Fluorouracil toxicity, homozygotes | | | | | +++ |
| Laboratory findings | 5-OH-Methyluracil | ↑↑ | ↑↑ | ↑↑ | ↑↑ | ↑↑ |
| | Dihydropyrimidine dehydrogenase (white blood cells) | ↓ | ↓ | ↓ | ↓ | ↓ |
| | Thymine (plasma) | ↑↑ | ↑↑ | ↑↑ | ↑↑ | ↑↑ |
| | Thymine (urine) | ↑↑↑ | ↑↑↑ | ↑↑↑ | ↑↑↑ | ↑↑↑ |
| | Uracil (plasma) | ↑↑ | ↑↑ | ↑↑ | ↑↑ | ↑↑ |
| | Uracil (urine) | ↑↑↑ | ↑↑↑ | ↑↑↑ | ↑↑↑ | ↑↑↑ |

**Table 24.2** Dihydropyrimidinase deficiency

| System | Symptoms and biomarkers | Neonatal (birth–1 month) | Infancy (1–18 months) | Childhood (1.5–11 years) | Adolescence (11–16 years) | Adulthood (>16 years) |
|---|---|---|---|---|---|---|
| CNS | **Intellectual disability** | | ± | ± | ± | ± |
| | **Seizures** | ± | ± | ± | ± | ± |
| Musculoskeletal | **Dysmorphic features** | ± | ± | ± | ± | ± |
| Laboratory findings | Dihydrothymine (plasma) | ↑↑ | ↑↑ | ↑↑ | ↑↑ | ↑↑ |
| | Dihydrothymine (urine) | ↑↑↑ | ↑↑↑ | ↑↑↑ | ↑↑↑ | ↑↑↑ |
| | Dihydrouracil (plasma) | ↑↑ | ↑↑ | ↑↑ | ↑↑ | ↑↑ |
| | Dihydrouracil (urine) | ↑↑↑ | ↑↑↑ | ↑↑↑ | ↑↑↑ | ↑↑↑ |

**Table 24.3** Beta-ureidopropionase deficiency

| System | Symptoms and biomarkers | Neonatal (birth–1 month) | Infancy (1–18 months) | Childhood (1.5–11 years) | Adolescence (11–16 years) | Adulthood (>16 years) |
|---|---|---|---|---|---|---|
| CNS | Dystonia | ± | ± | ± | ± | ± |
| | **Hypotonia** | + | + | | | |
| | Retardation, psychomotor | ± | ± | ± | ± | ± |
| | Seizures | ± | ± | ± | ± | ± |
| | **Speech disturbances** | | | ± | ± | ± |
| Musculoskeletal | Dysmorphic features | ± | ± | ± | ± | ± |
| Laboratory findings | Dihydrothymine (plasma) | ↑ | ↑ | ↑ | ↑ | ↑ |
| | Dihydrothymine (urine) | ↑ | ↑ | ↑ | ↑ | ↑ |
| | Dihydrouracil (plasma) | ↑ | ↑ | ↑ | ↑ | ↑ |
| | Dihydrouracil (urine) | ↑ | ↑ | ↑ | ↑ | ↑ |
| | *N*-Carbamyl-β-alanine (plasma) | ↑↑ | ↑↑ | ↑↑ | ↑↑ | ↑↑ |
| | *N*-Carbamyl-β-alanine (urine) | ↑↑↑ | ↑↑↑ | ↑↑↑ | ↑↑↑ | ↑↑↑ |
| | *N*-Carbamyl-β-aminoisobutyric acid (plasma) | ↑↑ | ↑↑ | ↑↑ | ↑↑ | ↑↑ |

**Table 24.4** Hyper-β-aminoisobutyric aciduria

| System | **Symptoms and biomarkers** | Neonatal (birth–1 month) | Infancy (1–18 months) | Childhood (1.5–11 years) | Adolescence (11–16 years) | Adulthood (>16 years) |
|---|---|---|---|---|---|---|
| Other | No clinical significance | + | + | + | + | + |
| Laboratory findings | Beta-aminoisobutyric acid (urine) | ↑ | ↑ | ↑ | | |

**Table 24.5** Hyper-β-alaninemia

| System | **Symptoms and biomarkers** | Neonatal (birth–1 month) | Infancy (1–18 months) | Childhood (1.5–11 years) | Adolescence (11–16 years) | Adulthood (>16 years) |
|---|---|---|---|---|---|---|
| CNS | Encephalopathy | + | + | + | | |
| | Hypotonia | + | + | + | | |
| | Lethargy | + | + | + | | |
| | Movement disorder | + | + | + | | |
| | Seizures | + | + | + | | |
| Laboratory findings | Beta-aminoisobutyric acid (urine) | ↑ | ↑ | ↑ | | |

**Table 24.6** GABA transaminase deficiency

| System | **Symptoms and biomarkers** | Neonatal (birth–1 month) | Infancy (1–18 months) | Childhood (1.5–11 years) | Adolescence (11–16 years) | Adulthood (>16 years) |
|---|---|---|---|---|---|---|
| CNS | Diffusion restriction in the external capsule (MRI) | + | + | + | + | + |
| | Diffusion restriction in the internal capsule (MRI) | + | + | + | + | + |
| | Diffusion restriction in the subcortical white matter (MRI) | + | + | + | + | + |
| | Hypotonia | ++ | ++ | + | | |
| | Lethargy | ++ | + | + | | |
| | Pitched cry, high | ++ | ++ | + | | |
| | **Retardation, psychomotor** | + | +++ | +++ | +++ | +++ |
| | **Seizures** | +++ | +++ | +++ | + | + |
| | Spasticity | ± | + | ++ | ++ | ++ |
| | Tendon reflexes, increased | ++ | ++ | ++ | ++ | ++ |
| Digestive | Feeding difficulties | ++ | ++ | ++ | ++ | ++ |
| Endocrine | Growth hormone | | ↑ | ↑ | | |
| Other | Accelerated growth | + | + | + | | |
| Laboratory findings | Beta-alanine (cerebrospinal fluid) | ↑ | ↑ | ↑ | ↑ | ↑ |
| | GABA (MRS) | ↑ | ↑ | ↑ | ↑ | ↑ |
| | GABA free (cerebrospinal fluid) | ↑ | ↑ | ↑ | ↑ | ↑ |
| | Homocarnosine (cerebrospinal fluid) | ↑ | ↑ | ↑ | ↑ | ↑ |

**Table 24.7** Succinic semialdehyde dehydrogenase deficiency

| System | Symptoms and biomarkers | Neonatal (birth–1 month) | Infancy (1–18 months) | Childhood (1.5–11 years) | Adolescence (11–16 years) | Adulthood (>16 years) |
|---|---|---|---|---|---|---|
| CNS | **Ataxia** | | + | ++ | + | + |
| | Cerebellar atrophy (MRI) | + | + | + | + | + |
| | Cerebral atrophy (MRI) | + | + | + | + | + |
| | **EEG, abnormal** | + | + | + | ++ | ++ |
| | **Generalized slowing (EEG)** | + | + | + | + | + |
| | **Hyperintensities (T2) of the globus pallidus (MRI)** | + | + | + | + | + |
| | **Hypotonia** | ++ | ++ | ++ | + | |
| | Increased T2 signal in the brain stem (MRI) | + | + | + | + | + |
| | Increased T2 signal in the cerebellar dentate nucleus (MRI) | + | + | + | + | + |
| | Increased T2 signal in the subcortical white matter (MRI) | + | + | + | + | + |
| | **Language difficulties** | | ++ | ++ | ++ | ++ |
| | Oculomotor dyspraxia | | + | ++ | ++ | ++ |
| | **Retardation, psychomotor** | + | ++ | ++ | ++ | ++ |
| | **Seizures** | | + | + | ++ | ++ |
| | Sleep disturbances | + | ++ | ++ | ++ | |
| | **Spike wave discharges (EEG)** | | | + | ++ | ++ |
| | Tendon reflexes, decreased | + | ++ | ++ | + | + |
| Digestive | Feeding difficulties | + | + | + | | |
| Eye | Strabismus | | + | + | + | + |
| Psychiatric | Anxiety | | + | ++ | +++ | +++ |
| | Attention disorder | | + | ++ | + | + |
| | Behavior, aggressive | | + | ++ | ++ | + |
| | Hyperactivity | | | ++ | + | |
| Laboratory findings | 4-Hydroxybutyric acid (urine) | ↑↑ | ↑↑ | ↑↑ | ↑↑ | ↑ |

**Table 24.8** GABA transporter deficiency

| System | Symptoms and biomarkers | Neonatal (birth–1 month) | Infancy (1–18 months) | Childhood (1.5–11 years) | Adolescence (11–16 years) | Adulthood (>16 years) |
|---|---|---|---|---|---|---|
| CNS | Developmental delay | + | + | + | | |
| | Intellectual disability | | | + | + | + |
| | Language delay | | + | + | | |
| | **Seizures, myoclonic-atonic** | | | + | + | + |

**Table 24.9** GABA type A receptor α1 subunit deficiency

| System | Symptoms and biomarkers | Neonatal (birth–1 month) | Infancy (1–18 months) | Childhood (1.5–11 years) | Adolescence (11–16 years) | Adulthood (>16 years) |
|---|---|---|---|---|---|---|
| CNS | Seizures (multiple types described) | + | + | + | | |

Table 24.10 GABA type A receptor α6 subunit deficiency

| System | Symptoms and biomarkers | Neonatal (birth–1 month) | Infancy (1–18 months) | Childhood (1.5–11 years) | Adolescence (11–16 years) | Adulthood (>16 years) |
|---|---|---|---|---|---|---|
| | No clinical significance | + | + | + | + | + |

Table 24.11 GABA type A receptor β1 subunit deficiency

| System | Symptoms and biomarkers | Neonatal (birth–1 month) | Infancy (1–18 months) | Childhood (1.5–11 years) | Adolescence (11–16 years) | Adulthood (>16 years) |
|---|---|---|---|---|---|---|
| CNS | Developmental Delay | + | + | | | |
| | Hypotonia | + | + | | | |
| | Seizures | + | + | + | | |

Table 24.12 GABA type A receptor β2 subunit deficiency

| System | Symptoms and biomarkers | Neonatal (birth–1 month) | Infancy (1–18 months) | Childhood (1.5–11 years) | Adolescence (11–16 years) | Adulthood (>16 years) |
|---|---|---|---|---|---|---|
| CNS | Developmental Delay | + | + | | | |
| | Intellectual disability | + | + | + | + | |
| | Seizures (type varies) | + | + | + | + | |

Table 24.13 GABA type A receptor β3 subunit deficiency

| System | Symptoms and biomarkers | Neonatal (birth–1 month) | Infancy (1–18 months) | Childhood (1.5–11 years) | Adolescence (11–16 years) | Adulthood (>16 years) |
|---|---|---|---|---|---|---|
| CNS | Seizures (absence) | | + | + | | |

Table 24.14 GABA type A receptor γ2 subunit deficiency

| System | Symptoms and biomarkers | Neonatal (birth–1 month) | Infancy (1–18 months) | Childhood (1.5–11 years) | Adolescence (11–16 years) | Adulthood (>16 years) |
|---|---|---|---|---|---|---|
| CNS | Seizures (absence, myoclonic) | + | + | + | | |

Table 24.15 GABA type A receptor δ subunit deficiency

| System | Symptoms and biomarkers | Neonatal (birth–1 month) | Infancy (1–18 months) | Childhood (1.5–11 years) | Adolescence (11–16 years) | Adulthood (>16 years) |
|---|---|---|---|---|---|---|
| CNS | Seizures (multiple types: myoclonic) | + | + | | | |

**Table 24.16** GABA type B receptor subunit 2 deficiency

| System | Symptoms and biomarkers | Neonatal (birth–1 month) | Infancy (1–18 months) | Childhood (1.5–11 years) | Adolescence (11–16 years) | Adulthood (>16 years) |
|---|---|---|---|---|---|---|
| CNS | Developmental delay | + | + | + | | |
| | Early Infantile Encephalopathy | + | + | | | |
| | Hypotonia | + | + | + | + | + |
| | Intellectual disability | | | + | + | + |
| | Loss of purposeful hand movements | | | + | | |
| | Rett Like Phenotype | | | + | | |
| | Seizures | + | + | ± | | |
| | Speech disturbances | | + | + | + | + |

**Table 24.17** Serum carnosinase deficiency/ homocarnosinosis

| System | Symptoms and biomarkers | Neonatal (birth–1 month) | Infancy (1–18 months) | Childhood (1.5–11 years) | Adolescence (11–16 years) | Adulthood (>16 years) |
|---|---|---|---|---|---|---|
| Other | No clinical significance | + | + | + | + | + |
| Laboratory findings | Anserine (urine) | ↑ | ↑ | ↑ | ↑ | ↑ |
| | Carnosine (plasma) | ↑ | ↑ | ↑ | ↑ | ↑ |
| | Carnosine (urine) | ↑ | ↑ | ↑ | ↑ | ↑ |
| | Homocarnosine (cerebrospinal fluid) | ↑ | ↑ | ↑ | ↑ | ↑ |

**Table 24.18** Methylmalonate semialdehyde dehydrogenase deficiency

| System | Symptoms and biomarkers | Neonatal (birth–1 month) | Infancy (1–18 months) | Childhood (1.5–11 years) | Adolescence (11–16 years) | Adulthood (>16 years) |
|---|---|---|---|---|---|---|
| CNS | Developmental delay | ± | ± | ± | ± | ± |
| Digestive | Hepatomegaly | ± | ± | ± | ± | ± |
| | Vomiting, episodic | ± | ± | ± | ± | ± |
| Other | **Failure to thrive** | ± | ± | ± | ± | ± |
| Laboratory findings | 2-Aminoisobutyrate | n-↑ | n-↑ | n-↑ | n-↑ | n-↑ |
| | 3-Aminoisobutyric acid (urine) | n-↑ | n-↑ | n-↑ | n-↑ | n-↑ |
| | 3-Hydroxyisobutyric acid (urine) | n-↑ | n-↑ | n-↑ | n-↑ | n-↑ |
| | 3-Hydroxypropionic acid (urine) | n-↑ | n-↑ | n-↑ | n-↑ | n-↑ |
| | Beta-alanine (urine) | n-↑ | n-↑ | n-↑ | n-↑ | n-↑ |
| | Ethylmalonic acid (urine) | n-↑ | n-↑ | n-↑ | n-↑ | n-↑ |
| | Lactate (plasma) | n-↑ | n-↑ | n-↑ | n-↑ | n-↑ |
| | Methionine (plasma) | n-↑ | n-↑ | n-↑ | n-↑ | n-↑ |
| | Methylmalonic semialdehyde dehydrogenase (fibroblasts) | ↓ | ↓ | ↓ | ↓ | ↓ |

## Reference Values and Pathological Values

**Table 24.19** Normal and pathological values

| Beta amino acid disorders | Normal | Dihydropyrimidine dehydrogenase deficiency | Dihydropyrimidinase deficiency | Beta-ureidopropionase deficiency | Hyper-β-aminoisobutyric aciduria | Hyper-β-alaninemia | Methylmalonic semialdehyde dehydrogenase deficiency |
|---|---|---|---|---|---|---|---|
| Thymine (urine) mmol/mol creatinine | 0–3 years: 0–3<br>4–6 years: 0–3<br>7–12 years: 0–3<br>13–18 years: 0–3<br>>18 years: 0–3 | ↑ | | | | | |
| Thymine (plasma) nmol/mL | 0–1 year: 0–2<br>1–4 years: 0–2<br>5–18 years: 0–2<br>>18 years: 0–2 | ↑ | | | | | |
| Dihydrothymine (urine) mmol/mol creatinine | 0–3 years: 0–11<br>4–6 years: 0–3<br>7–12 years: 0–3<br>13–18 years: 0–3<br>>18 years: 0–3 | | ↑ | ↑ | | | |
| Dihydrothymine (plasma) nmol/mL | 0–1 year: 0–2<br>1–4 years: 0–2<br>5–18 years: 0–2<br>>18 years: 0–2 | | ↑ | ↑ | | | |
| Uracil (urine) mmol/mol creatinine | 0–3 years: 0–50<br>4–6 years: 0–30<br>7–12 years: 0–25<br>13–18 years: 0–20<br>>18 years: 0–20 | ↑ | | | | | |
| Uracil (plasma) nmol/mL | 0–1 year: 0–2<br>1–4 years: 0–2<br>5–18 years: 0–2<br>>18 years: 0–2 | ↑ | | | | | |
| Dihydrouracil (urine mmol/mol creatinine) | 0–3 years: 0–15<br>4–6 years: 0–6<br>7–12 years: 0–3<br>13–18 years: 0–6<br>>18 years: 0–6 | | ↑ | ↑ | | | |
| Dihydrouracil (plasma) nmol/mL | 0–1 year: 0–3<br>1–4 years: 0–3<br>5–18 years: 0–3<br>>18 years: 0–3 | | ↑ | ↑ | | | |

**Table 24.19** (continued)

| Beta amino acid disorders | | | | | | | |
|---|---|---|---|---|---|---|---|
| | Normal | Dihydropyrimidine dehydrogenase deficiency | Dihydropyrimidinase deficiency | Beta-ureidopropionase deficiency | Hyper-β-aminoisobutyric aciduria | Hyper-β-alaninemia | Methylmalonic semialdehyde dehydrogenase deficiency |
| 5-OH-methyluracil (urine) mmol/mol creatinine | 0–1 year: 0–4.9<br>1–5 years: 0–10.1<br>5–16 years: 0–2.0<br>>16 years: 0–3.6 | Elevated | | | | | |
| *N*-Carbamyl-β-alanine (urine) mmol/mol creatinine | 0–3 years: 0–30<br>4–6 years: 0–10<br>7–12 years: 0–10<br>13–18 years: 0–10<br>>18 years: 0–10 | | | ↑ | | | |
| *N*-Carbamyl-β-alanine (plasma) nmol/mL | 0–1 year: 0–2<br>1–4 years: 0–2<br>5–18 years: 0–2<br>>18 years: 0–2 | | | ↑ | | | |
| *N*-Carbamyl-β-aminoisobutyric acid (urine) mmol/mol creatinine | 0–3 years: 0–20<br>4–6 years: 0–3<br>7–12 years: 0–3<br>13–18 years: 0–3<br>>18 year: 0–3 | | | ↑ | | | |
| *N*-Carbamyl-β-aminoisobutyric acid (plasma) nmol/mL | 0–1 year: 0–2<br>1–4 years: 0–2<br>5–18 years: 0–2<br>>18 years: 0–2 | | | ↑ | | | |
| Beta-aminoisobutyric acid (urine) mmol/mol creatinine | 0–30 days: 0–269<br>1–23 months: 0–309<br>2–17 years: 0–133<br>>18 years: 0–88 | | | ↑ | ↑ | ↑ | |
| Methylmalonate (plasma) | 0–0.4 μmol/L | | | | | | ↑ |
| Methylmalonate (urine) | 0–3.6 mmol/mol creatinine | | | | | | (↑) |
| 3-hydroxyisobutyric acid (urine) | 0–3 mmol/mol creatinine | | | | | | ↑ |

| GABA disorders | | | | |
|---|---|---|---|---|
| | Normal | SSADH | GABA-T | Serum carnosinase deficiency/homocarnosinosis |
| 4-Hydroxybutyric acid (urine) | 0–7 mmol/mol creatinine | 100–1200 | | |
| 4-Hydroxybutyric acid (plasma) | 0–3 µmol/L | 35–600 | | |
| 4-Hydroxybutyric acid (CSF) | 0–2 µmol/L | 100–850 | | |
| Free GABA (serum) | 0.12–0.50 µmol/L | | 2.1 | |
| Free GABA (CSF) | <2 years 0.017–0.067 µmol/L<br>>2 years 0.032–0.167 µmol/L | | 1.26 | |
| Total GABA (CSF)<br>µmol/L | <3 months: <1<br>3–23 months: <1<br>2–10 years: 0–2<br>>10 years: 0–3 | | 38 | |
| Beta-alanine (plasma)<br>µmol/L | 0–30 days: 0–8<br>1–23 months: 0–8<br>2–17 years: 0–5<br>>18 years: 0–5 | | 23 | |
| Beta-alanine (CSF) | <0.1 µmol/L | | 0.48 | |
| Homocarnosine (CSF) | <0.02–10 µmol/L | | | 50–75 |
| Anserine (urine)<br>nmol/mg Cr | 0–30 days: 0–3<br>1–23 months: 0–5<br>2–17 years: 0<br>>18 years: 0 | | | ↑ |
| Carnosine (urine)<br>nmol/mg Cr | 0–30 days: 97–665<br>1–23 months: 203–635<br>2–17 years: 72–402<br>>18 years: 10–90 | | | ↑ |
| Carnosine (plasma)<br>µmol/L | 0–30 days: 0–19<br>1–23 months: 0<br>2–17 years: 0<br>>18 years: 0 | | | 0.005–0.03 |

(continued)

## Diagnostic Flowcharts

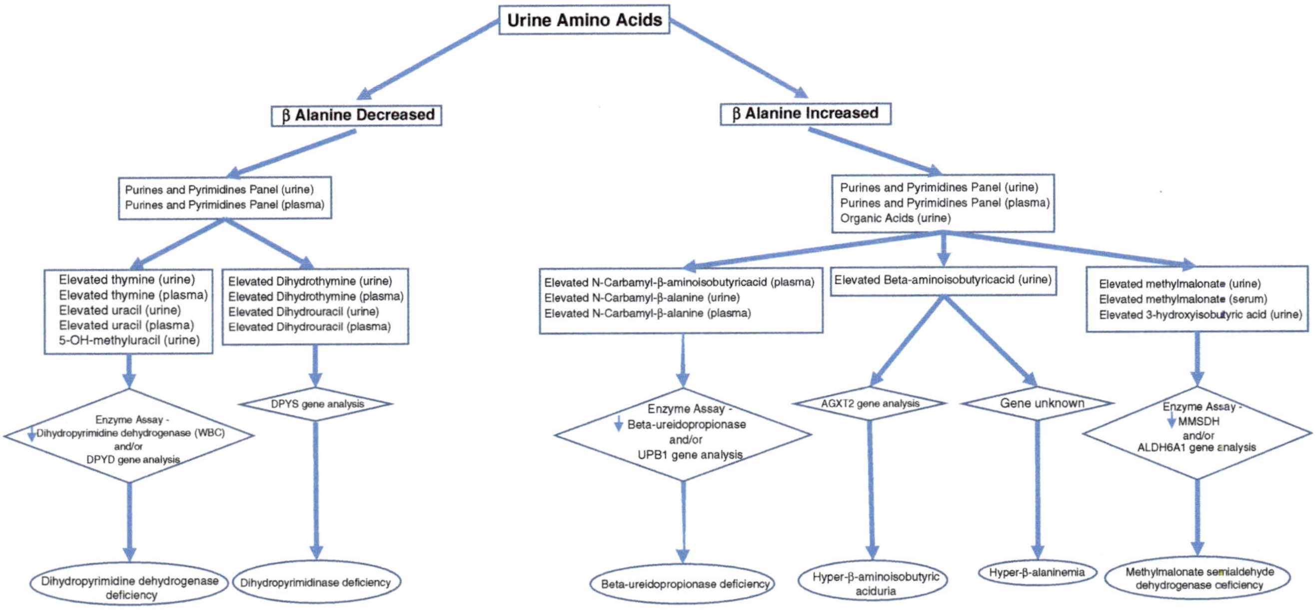


**Fig. 24.3** Diagnostic flowchart beta amino acid disorders

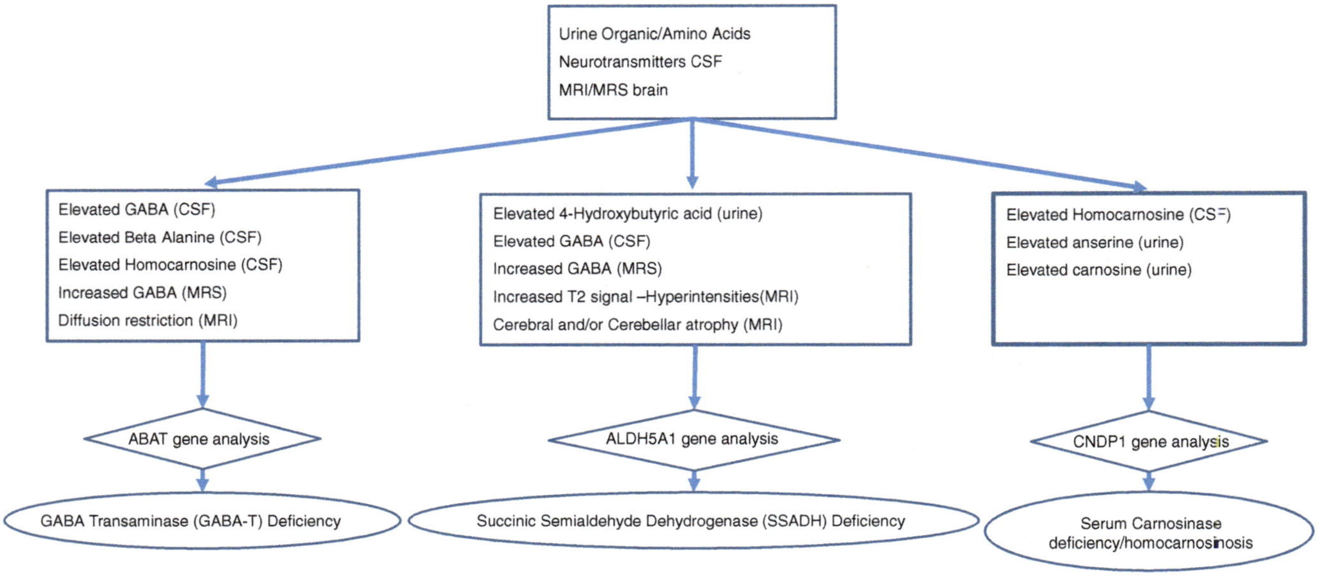


**Fig. 24.4** Diagnostic flowchart GABA disorders

## Specimen Collection

**Table 24.20** Specimen collection and interpretation pitfalls

| Metabolite | Material | Handling | Pitfalls |
|---|---|---|---|
| Amino acids | Urine | First morning urine preferred. Keep refrigerated in short term (24 h). Freeze at −20 °C for up to 1 month | |
| Neurotransmitters | CSF | Freeze immediately; store at −80 °C | |
| Organic acids | Urine | Freeze at −20 °C | |
| Organic acids | Plasma | Obtained from blood anticoagulated with heparin<br>Plasma samples should be stored at −20 °C or at −80 °C | |
| Purines and pyrimidines panel | Urine | 24 h collection is preferred, but random urine specimen can be used. During the collection period, the urine aliquots are kept refrigerated (4 °C), and after completion stored frozen at −20 °C for 1 week to 2 months. If storing longer than 2 months, storage at −80 °C is recommended | Need aged matched reference range |
| Purines and pyrimidines panel | Plasma | Obtained from blood anticoagulated with heparin, as well as EDTA. Plasma samples should be stored at −20 °C or at −80 °C | Need aged matched reference range |
| GABA | Serum | Freeze immediately; store at −80 °C | Vigabatrin ↑ |
| GABA | CSF | Freeze immediately; store at −80 °C | Vigabatrin ↑<br>Hyperprolinemia<br>Immaturity of transporter or polymorphism in transporter |
| 4-Hydroxybutyric acid | Urine | First morning urine preferred. Keep refrigerated in short term (24 h). Freeze at −20 °C for up to 1 month | Treatment with 4-hydroxybutyric acid ↑<br>Vigabatrin ↓ |
| 4-Hydroxybutyric acid | CSF | Freeze at −20 °C | Treatment with 4-hydroxybutyric acid ↑<br>Vigabatrin ↓ |

## Diagnosis

Diagnosis of the disorders of beta and gamma amino acids may follow clinical suspicion, although the phenotypes are nonspecific and generally involve early infantile onset epileptic encephalopathies, although can also manifest as autism spectrum, neurodevelopmental disability with profound language impairment, and extrapyramidal syndromes, e.g., choreoathetosis or dystonia. Urine organic acids are often useful as a laboratory screening tool. More specific metabolic analytes are identified in Table 24.21 (Diagnosis) and include urine purines and pyrimidines and potentially CSF GABA. Enzyme assays are available for some conditions. Generally, mutation analysis, whether through targeted screening or whole exome sequencing, is used to establish the diagnosis.

**Table 24.21** Diagnosis

| No. | Disorder | Prenatal diagnosis | Diagnosis |
|---|---|---|---|
| 24.1 | Dihydropyrimidine dehydrogenase deficiency | Mutation analysis | Urine purines and pyrimidines panel: elevated uracil and thymine<br>Mutation analysis |
| 24.2 | Dihydropyrimidinase deficiency | Mutation analysis | Urine purines and pyrimidines panel: elevated dihydrouracil and dihydrothymine<br>Enzyme assay of liver biopsy<br>Mutation analysis |
| 24.3 | Beta-ureidopropionase deficiency | Mutation analysis | Urine purines and pyrimidines panel: elevated *N*-Carbamyl-β-alanine and *N*-carbamyl-β-aminoisobutyric acid<br>Enzyme assay of liver biopsy<br>Mutation analysis |
| 24.4 | Hyper-β-aminoisobutyric aciduria | Mutation analysis | Beta-aminoisobutyric acid (urine)<br>Mutation analysis |
| 24.5 | Hyper-β-alaninemia | | Beta-aminoisobutyric acid (urine) |
| 24.6 | GABA transaminase deficiency | Mutation analysis | Neurotransmitters CSF: elevated GABA<br>Mutation analysis |
| 24.7 | Succinic semialdehyde dehydrogenase deficiency | Metabolite: 4-hydroxybutyric acid in amniotic fluid<br>Enzyme assay in CVS or cultured amniocytes<br>Mutation analysis | Urine organic acids: elevated 4-hydroxybutyric acid<br>Mutation analysis |
| 24.8 | GABA transporter deficiency | Mutation analysis | Mutation analysis |
| 24.9 | GABA type A receptor α1 subunit deficiency | Mutation analysis | Mutation analysis |
| 24.10 | GABA type A receptor α6 subunit deficiency | Mutation analysis | Mutation analysis |
| 24.11 | GABA type A receptor β1 subunit deficiency | Mutation analysis | Mutation analysis |
| 24.12 | GABA type A receptor β2 subunit deficiency | Mutation analysis | Mutation analysis |
| 24.13 | GABA type A receptor β3 subunit deficiency | Mutation analysis | Mutation analysis |
| 24.14 | GABA type A receptor γ2 subunit deficiency | Mutation analysis | Mutation analysis |
| 24.15 | GABA type A receptor δ subunit deficiency | Mutation analysis | Mutation analysis |
| 24.16 | GABA type B receptor subunit 2 deficiency | Mutation analysis | Mutation analysis |
| 24.17 | Serum carnosinase deficiency/ homocarnosinosis | Enzyme assay | Neurotransmitters CSF: elevated GABA, elevated homocarnosinase<br>Mutation analysis |
| 24.18 | Methylmalonate semialdehyde dehydrogenase deficiency | Molecular analysis<br>WBC, FB or other suitable cells or tissue samples may be used | Mutation analysis<br>Molecular analysis<br>WBC, FB, or other suitable cells or tissue samples may be used |

## Treatment Summary

The treatment of the disorders of beta and gamma amino acids is supportive and largely consists of antiseizure medications and, when indicated, anxiolytics and psychoactive medications. The chemotherapeutic 5-fluorouracil and related compounds should be avoided in the beta amino acid synthesis deficiencies of dihydropyrimidine dehydrogenase, dihydropyrimidinase, and beta-ureidopropionase. Valproate is generally contraindicated in SSADH deficiency because it can inhibit any residual enzymatic activity. Targeted therapy is not currently available, including enzyme replacement or gene therapy. Attempts have been made for more specific therapies such as flumazenil as a benzodiazepine receptor antagonist of the GABA(A) receptor in GABA transaminase deficiency, and there may be a role for the cofactor pyridoxine in hyper-beta-alaninemia (cf Table 24.22).

**Table 24.22** Treatment

| No. | Disorder | Emergency treatment | Long-term treatment | Experimental treatment |
|---|---|---|---|---|
| 24.1 | Dihydropyrimidine dehydrogenase deficiency | Supportive | No specific treatment<br>The use of 5-halogenated pyrimidines (5-fluorouracil) should be avoided at any time | None |
| 24.2 | Dihydropyrimidinase deficiency | Supportive | No specific treatment<br>The use of 5-halogenated pyrimidines (5-fluorouracil) should be avoided at any time | None |
| 24.3 | Beta-ureidopropionase deficiency | Supportive | No specific treatment<br>The use of 5-halogenated pyrimidines (5-fluorouracil) should be avoided at any time | None |
| 24.4 | Hyper-β-aminoisobutyric aciduria | No treatment needed | No treatment needed | None |
| 24.5 | Hyper-β-alaninemia | Supportive | 10–100 mg/day of pyridoxine may be beneficial | None |
| 24.6 | GABA transaminase deficiency | Supportive | No specific treatment<br>Supportive | Flumazenil |
| 24.7 | Succinic semialdehyde dehydrogenase deficiency | Supportive | No specific treatment<br>Supportive | SGS-742 Phase 2 Clinical Trial (GABA B receptor antagonist) |
| 24.8 | GABA transporter deficiency | Supportive | Ketogenic diet has been beneficial | None |
| 24.9 | GABA type A receptor α1 subunit deficiency | Supportive | No specific treatment<br>Supportive | None |
| 24.10 | GABA type A receptor α6 subunit deficiency | Supportive | No specific treatment<br>Supportive | None |
| 24.11 | GABA type A receptor β1 subunit deficiency | Supportive | No specific treatment<br>Supportive | None |
| 24.12 | GABA type A receptor β2 subunit deficiency | Supportive | No specific treatment<br>Supportive | None |
| 24.13 | GABA type A receptor β3 subunit deficiency | Supportive | No specific treatment<br>Supportive | None |
| 24.14 | GABA type A receptor γ2 subunit deficiency | Supportive | No specific treatment<br>Supportive | None |
| 24.15 | GABA type A receptor δ subunit deficiency | Supportive | No specific treatment<br>Supportive | None |
| 24.16 | GABA type B receptor subunit 2 deficiency | Supportive | No specific treatment<br>Supportive | None |
| 24.17 | Serum carnosinase deficiency/ homocarnosinosis | Supportive | Vegetarian diet<br>Supportive | None |
| 24.18 | Methylmalonate semialdehyde dehydrogenase deficiency | Supportive | Supportive | None |

## Follow-Up and Monitoring

Clinical follow-up at regular intervals is indicated in these chronic disorders, including electroencephalography with associated seizure disorders and neuroimaging for baseline and then later studies depending upon the clinical course. Serial testing of metabolic analytes has an unknown role in these disorders.

## References


Attri SV, Singhi P, Wiwattanadittakul N, et al. Incidence and geographic distribution of SSADH deficiency. JIMD Rep. 2017;34:111–5.

Carvill GL, McMahon JM, Schneider A, et al. Mutations in the GABA transporter SLC6A1 cause epilepsy with myoclonic-atonic seizures. Am J Hum Genet. 2015;96:808–15.

Chambliss KL, Hinson DD, Trettel F, et al. Two exon-skipping mutations as the molecular basis of succinic semialdehyde dehydrogenase deficiency (4-hydroxybutyric aciduria). Am J Hum Genet. 1998;63:399–408.

Chen BC, Mohd Rawi R, Meinsma R, et al. Dihydropyrimidine dehydrogenase deficiency in two Malaysian siblings with abnormal MRI findings. Mol Syndromol. 2014;5(6):299–303.

DiBacco ML, Roullet JB, Kapur K, et al. Age-related phenotype and biomarker changes in SSADH deficiency. Ann Clin Transl Neurol. 2018;6:114–20.

Fang Y, Cai C, Wang C. Clinical and genetic analysis of 7 Chinese patients with β-ureidopropionase deficiency. Medicine (Baltimore). 2019;98(1):e14021.

Gibson KM, Sweetman L, Nyhan WL, et al. Succinic semialdehyde dehydrogenase deficiency: an inborn error of gamma-aminobutyric acid metabolism. Clin Chim Acta. 1983;133:33–42.

Hamdan FF, Myers CT, Cossette P, et al. High rate of recurrent de novo mutations in developmental and epileptic encephalopathies. Am J Hum Genet. 2017;101:664–85.

Hegde AU, Karnavat PK, Vyas R, DiBacco ML, Grant PE, Pearl PL. GABA transaminase deficiency with survival into adulthood. J Child Neurol. 2019;34:216–20.

Higgins JJ, Kaneski CR, Bernardini I, et al. Pyridoxine-responsive hyper-beta-alaninemia associated with Cohen's syndrome. Neurology. 1994;44(9):1728–32.

Ichikawa K, Tsuji M, Tsuyusaki Y, Tomiyasu M, Aida N, Goto T. Serial magnetic resonance imaging and $^{1}$H-magnetic resonance spectroscopy in GABA transaminase deficiency: a case report. JIMD Rep. 2019;43:7–12.

Johannesen KM, Gardella E, Linnankivi T, et al. Defining the phenotypic spectrum of SLC6A1 mutations. Epilepsia. 2018;59: 389–402.

Koenig MD, Hodgeman R, Riviello JJ, Chung W, Bain J, Chiriboga CA, Ichikawa K, Osaka H, Tsuji M, Gibson GM, Bonnen PE, Pearl PL. Phenotype of GABA-transaminase deficiency. Neurology. 2017;88:1–6.

Lapalme-Remis S, Lewis EC, De Meulemeester C, et al. Natural history of SSADH deficiency through adulthood. Neurology. 2015;85:861–5.

Lopes F, Barbosa M, Ameur A, et al. Identification of novel genetic causes of Rett syndrome-like phenotypes. J Med Genet. 2016;53:190–9.

Marcadier JL, Smith AM, Pohl D, et al. Mutations in ALDH6A1 encoding methylmalonate semialdehyde dehydrogenase are associated with dysmyelination and transient methylmalonic aciduria. Orphanet J Rare Dis. 2013;8:98.

Nakahima Y, Meijer J, Dobritzsch D, et al. Dihydropyrimidinase deficiency in four East Asian patients due to novel and rare DPYS mutations affecting protein structural integrity and catalytic activity. Mol Genet Metab. 2017;122(4):216–22.

Palmer S, Towne MC, Pearl PL, et al. SLC6A1 mutation and ketogenic diet in epilepsy with myoclonic-atonic seizures. Pediatr Neurol. 2016;64:77–9.

Pearl PL, Jakobs C, Gibson M. Online metabolic and molecular bases of inherited disease. Chapter 91: Disorders of β- and γ-amino acids in free and peptide-linked forms. 2007. Accessed April 2019.

Pearl PL, Gibson KM, Cortez MA, et al. Succinic semialdehyde dehydrogenase deficiency: lessons from mice and men. J Inherit Metab Dis. 2009a;32:343–52.

Pearl PL, Gibson KM, Quezado Z, et al. Decreased GABA-A binding on FMZ-PET in succinic semialdehyde dehydrogenase deficiency. Neurology. 2009b;73:423–9.

Pearl PL, Schreiber J, Theodore WH, et al. Taurine trial in SSADH deficiency and elevated CNS GABA. Neurology. 2014;82:940–4.

Reis J, Cohen LG, Pearl PL, et al. GABA(B)-ergic motor cortex dysfunction in SSADH deficiency. Neurology. 2012;79:47–54.

Scriver CR, Pueschel S, Davies E. Hyper-beta-alaninemia associated with beta-aminoaciduria and gamma-aminobutyricaciduaia, somnolence and seizures. N Engl J Med. 1966;274(12):635–43.

Sjaastad O, Blau N, Rydning SL, et al. Homocarnosinosis: a historical update and findings in the SPG11 gene. Acta Neurol Scand. 2018;138(3):245–50.

# Amino Acid Synthesis Deficiencies

# 25

Tom J. de Koning and Gajja Salomons

## Contents



**Summary**

In recent years the list of disorders affecting amino acid synthesis has grown rapidly. Not only the number of defects has increased, but also the associated clinical phenotypes have expanded spectacular, the latter mainly due to the advances of next-generation sequencing diagnostics.

An important reason for the contribution of NGS in the diagnosis of amino acid synthesis disorders is the fact that the biochemical diagnosis of some of these synthesis disorders can be quite challenging, synthesis defects may present with low values of amino acids, or their concentrations can even be completely normal. Defects in the synthesis pathways of serine metabolism, glutamine, glutamate, proline, and asparagine have been reported, and all pose specific challenges to a biochemical diagnosis. An exception to this are the disorders of pyrroline-5-carboxylate (P5C) synthesis where ornithine or proline is strongly elevated and easily detected by plasma amino acid analysis. Finally, Snyder-Robinson, a defect in the synthesis of the polyamine spermine, is discussed here as well, and molecular testing is advised for this disorder as well.

Although the amino acid synthesis defects in this chapter are not all in related metabolic pathways, they do share some clinical features. In children the central nervous system is primarily affected, giving rise to (congenital) microcephaly, early-onset seizures, and mental retardation to a variable degree. The brain abnormalities can be accompanied by skin disorders such as cutis laxa in proline defects, collodion-like skin and ichthyosis in serine deficiency, necrolytic erythema in glutamine deficiency, and difficult to classify skin abnormalities in glutaminase hyperactivity. In adults with serine or proline disorders, several forms of polyneuropathy with or without intellectual disability appear to be the major presenting symptom. An exception to this is ornithine aminotransferase deficiency which primarily affects the choroid and retina and Snyder-Robinson syndrome in which mental retardation is accompanied by seizures, dysmorphic features, and severe osteoporosis.

T. J. de Koning (✉)
Department of Clinical Sciences, Lund University, Lund, Sweden

Departments of Genetics and Neurology, University Medical Center Groningen, Groningen, The Netherlands
e-mail: tom.j_de_koning@med.lu.se; t.j.de.koning@umcg.nl

G. Salomons
Department of Genetic Metabolic Diseases, Amsterdam University Medical Centers, Amsterdam, The Netherlands
e-mail: g.salomons@amsterdamumc.nl


N. Blau et al. (eds.), *Physician's Guide to the Diagnosis, Treatment, and Follow-Up of Inherited Metabolic Diseases*,
https://doi.org/10.1007/978-3-030-67727-5_25

## Introduction

By tradition the biochemical analysis of elevated levels of amino acids or their degradation products in body fluids has been the cornerstone in diagnosing inborn errors of metabolism. In 1996 (Jaeken et al. 1996), for the first time, defects in the pathway of serine synthesis were reported and identified through low concentrations of amino acids. Since then defects in the synthesis pathways of serine, proline, glutamine, glutamate, and asparagine have all been reported. In this chapter the defects in the synthesis of pyrroline-5-carboxylate (P5C) are discussed as well, namely, ornithine aminotransferase (OAT) deficiency and hyperprolinemia type I and II as well as Snyder-Robinson syndrome, a defect in the synthesis of the polyamine spermine (Fig. 25.1).

Some of these disorders present with low values of amino acids, for instance, serine and glutamine deficiency, whereas in others amino acid concentrations are variable or completely normal (proline and asparagine synthesis defects) or highly elevated as in OAT deficiency, hyperprolinemia type I and II, and glutaminase deficiency. Only the latter disorders are easily diagnosed through elevated concentrations of an amino acid, namely, ornithine, glutamine, or proline (Fig. 25.2).

With the discovery of these amino disorders, it became evident that they can give rise to a whole spectrum of clinical symptoms ranging from lethal developmental defects to late-onset adult neurologic disease. The disorders do have some clinical features in common as well. In children the brain is primarily affected, giving rise to (congenital) microcephaly, early-onset seizures, and mental retardation to a variable degree. These neurological symptoms can be accompanied by skin disorders such as cutis laxa in proline defects, collodion-like skin and ichthyosis in serine deficiency, necrolytic erythema in glutamine deficiency, and difficult to classify skin abnormalities in glutaminase hyperactivity. On brain MRI hypomyelination can be seen in serine, proline, mild glutamine, glutaminase hyperactivity, and asparagine deficiency, whereas structural abnormalities are present in severe serine, glutamine, and glutaminase deficiency as well as in proline deficiency. The adulthood-onset phenotypes of serine and proline synthesis defects have a different presentation with several forms of polyneuropathy with or without intellectual disability.

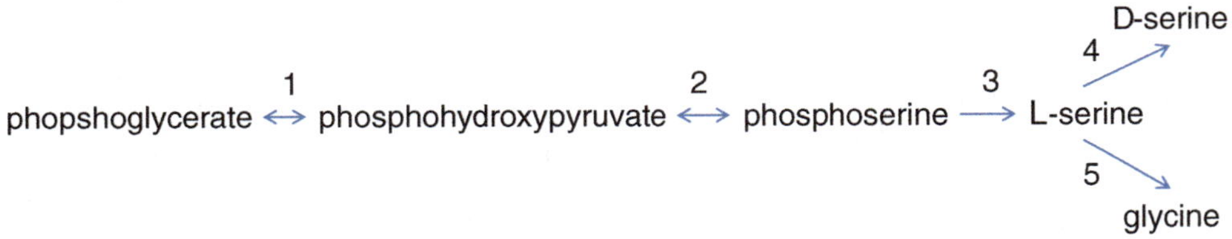


**Fig. 25.1** Serine synthesis. (1) Phosphoglycerate dehydrogenase, (2) phosphohydroxyamino transferase, (3) phosphoserine phosphatase, (4) serine racemase, (5) serine hydroxymethyltransferases

**Fig. 25.2** Glutamine, glutamate and asparagine synthesis. (1) Glutamine synthetase, (2) glutaminase, (3) ornthine aminotransferase, (4) asparagine synthetase

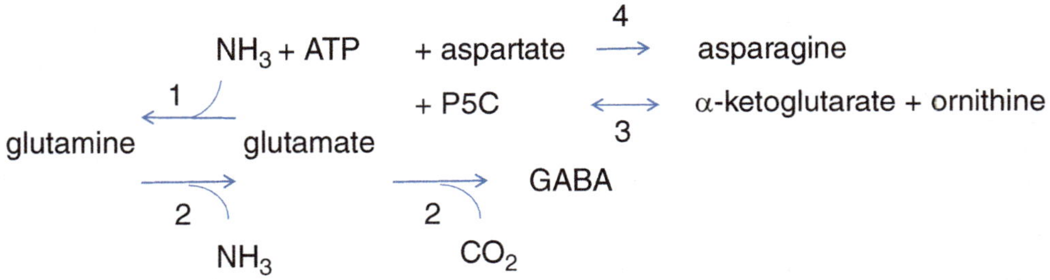

## Serine Deficiency

L-serine is synthesized in three steps from the glycolytic intermediate phosphoglycerate, and defects in any of these three enzymes give rise to identical clinical phenotypes. Serine deficiency is associated with a wide spectrum of clinical presentations ranging from Neu-Laxova syndrome, a lethal fetal developmental defect, to adult-onset neuropathy (Acuna-Hidalgo et al. 2014; van der Crabben et al. 2013). The majority of patients present as infants with congenital microcephaly, severe psychomotor retardation, spastic paraplegia, and intractable seizures. On MRI extensive developmental defects are seen in Neu-Laxova syndrome with lissencephaly, absence of corpus callosum, and hypoplasia of pons and cerebellum, whereas in infantile cases hypomyelination is the major finding on MRI. In juvenile and adulthood presentations, normal MRIs are found.

## Glutamine Deficiency

Glutamine deficiency appears to be an ultra-rare disorder among the synthesis defects and is caused by a deficiency of glutamine synthetase. Only four patients have been reported so far. The first two patients reported were severely affected and presented as newborns with respiratory failure, hypotonia, absence of spontaneous movement, and generalized seizures and died soon after birth (Häberle et al. 2005). The children also suffered from necrolytic skin abnormalities. The two other patients reported had a somewhat milder phenotype with psychomotor retardation and intractable seizures. In only one of them episodic necrolytic skin abnormalities were also present. MRI showed structural abnormalities in severe cases and hypomyelination in a milder case (Häberle et al. 2012).

## Glutaminase Deficiency and Hyperactivity

Very recently both a deficiency and hyperactivity of glutaminase were reported, an enzyme that regulates the synthesis of glutamate from glutamine and plays an important role in brain homeostasis of glutamate, ammonia, and GABA.

Although very little patients were reported so far, glutaminase deficiency apparently also causes a spectrum of symptoms ranging from severe hypotonia, respiratory insufficiency, and early-onset intractable seizures to infantile presentation with motor and speech delay evolving into progressive ataxia (Rumping et al. 2019a; van Kuilenburg et al. 2019). On MRI simplified gyration and white matter abnormalities were present in early-onset presentation, and cerebellar atrophy may be seen during follow-up of the infantile presentation.

The case with glutaminase hyperactivity presented with congenital cataracts and developed hypotonia, significant developmental delay, behavioral abnormalities, and specific skin abnormalities (Tessadori et al. 2019b). Low glutamate and high glutamine were present on MRS, but CSF and plasma analyses were unremarkable. High glutamine and low glutamate excretion was observed in urine, but with some samples being close to the levels of reference samples.

## Disorders of Proline and P5C Synthesis

In contrast to most metabolic disorders are the proline synthesis defects mostly known by their gene symbols and usually not classified according to the corresponding enzymes. The proline defects are pyrroline-5-carboxylate synthase (P5CS or *ALDH18A1*) deficiency, pyrroline-5-carboxylate reductase 1 (*PYCR1*) deficiency, and pyrroline-5-carboxylate reductase 2 (*PYCR2*) deficiency.

The phenotypes of P5CS deficiency and PYCR1 deficiency are overlapping, and most patients have prominent cutis laxa and therefore classified as autosomal recessive cutis laxa syndromes. The cutis laxa can be associated with microcephaly, progeroid features, mental retardation, hypotonia, seizures, joint laxity (intrauterine), growth retardation, cataract, and corneal abnormalities (Baumgartner et al. 2000; Reversade et al. 2009; Skidmore et al. 2011; Zampatti et al. 2012). In some patients movement disorders such as tremor and dystonia were reported as well. On MRI, hypomyelination with a thin corpus callosum can be seen as well as cerebellar abnormalities. Adults with P5CS deficiency present with late-onset spastic paraparesis, a phenotype very different from that in children (Coutelier et al. 2015).

PYCR2 deficiency was first classified as hypomyelinating leukodystrophy-10 reported with secondary microcephaly and hypomyelination (Nakayama et al. 2015). In subsequent reports the phenotype (Zaki et al. 2016) expanded to that of a lethal neurodegenerative disorder with microcephaly, severe failure to thrive, profound psychomotor retardation, dysmorphism, ataxia and hyperkinetic movement disorders, seizures, and spastic tetraplegia. The MRI findings can be more variable with regard to the white matter abnormalities, and many patients had extensive cortical atrophy and thin corpus callosum.

The two forms of hyperprolinemia can be regarded as a synthesis disorder of P5C, the intermediate metabolite in proline and ornithine metabolism. The clinical significance of a deficiency of proline dehydrogenase causing hyperprolinemia type I is still unclear; at present it is considered a risk factor for schizophrenia, but associations with autism and neurological symptoms such as seizures have been suggested. In hyperprolinemia type I, elevated proline is often an incidental finding, but it is important to realize this can be caused by a deletion of 22q11 (DiGeorge syndrome), the region that contains proline dehydrogenase. In contrast, in hyperprolinemia type II, drug-resistant seizures typically starting in the first year of life are the major clinical symptoms. The seizures are pyridoxine responsive, and when the disorder is not treated in time developmental delay can occur.

Ornithine aminotransferase (OAT) deficiency or gyrate atrophy of the retina and choroidea is also a disorder of P5C synthesis; OAT is a pyridoxal phosphate-dependent enzyme and converts ornithine into P5C. A deficiency of OAT causes a progressive disorder of the retina and choroid resulting in myopia in childhood, impaired night vision in adolescence and young adulthood, and progressive retinopathy in adulthood ultimately leading to blindness. In rare cases newborns can present with hyperammonemia identical to a urea cycle defect (Cleary et al. 2005). Developmental outcomes are not systematically investigated in this disorder, but developmental delay and learning these disabilities were observed in OAT deficiency patients, in combination with a significant reduced creatine peak on MR spectroscopy (Valayannopoulos et al. 2009) (Fig. 25.3).

## Asparagine Synthetase Deficiency

Asparagine synthetase catalyzes the transfer of ammonia from glutamine to aspartic acid to form asparagine. A deficiency causes an epileptic encephalopathy with intractable seizures, progressive (congenital) microcephaly, severe developmental disabilities, axial hypotonia, and spastic tetraplegia (Ruzzo et al. 2013). In many patients abnormal gyration patterns are seen on MRI with decreased cerebral volume, thin corpus callosum, and ventriculomegaly. In patients for whom follow-up was reported, it showed that, similar to PYCR2 deficiency, it is a slowly progressive disorder with progressive microcephaly and MRI abnormalities.

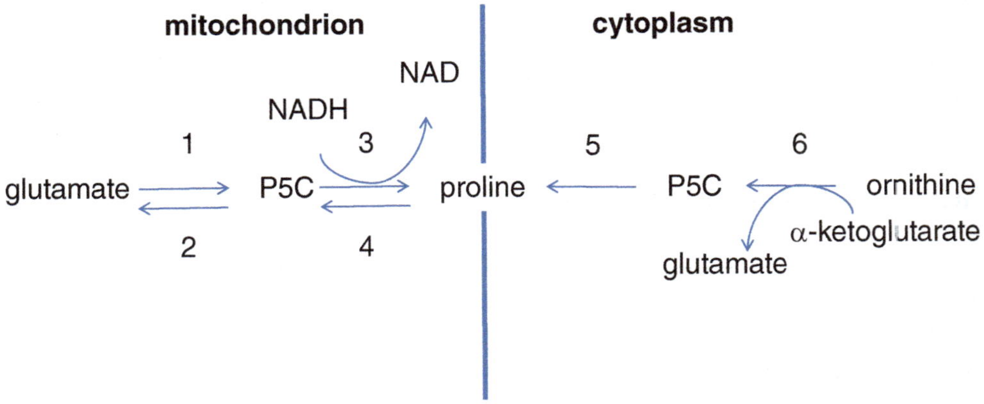


**Fig. 25.3** Proline and P5C synthesis. (1) P5C synthase, (2) P5C dehydrogenase, (3) PYCR1 and PYCR2, (4) proline dehydrogenase, (5) PYCRL, (6) ornthine aminotransferase. *P5C* $\Delta^1$-pyrroline-5-carboxylate, pyrroline-5-carboxylate reductase (PYCR, three isoforms 1, 2 and L)

### Snyder-Robinson Syndrome (SRS)

This X-linked disorder is caused by a deficiency of spermine synthase, which converts spermidine into spermine, a primary synthesis route for polyamines that starts with L-ornithine (Li et al. 2017). Affected males present with profound mental retardation, hypotonia, asthenic body built, dysmorphic features, and seizures. In addition they have early onset osteoporosis starting in the first decade of life, leading to fractures in the absence of trauma. In rare cases the phenotype can be present in females as well.

## Nomenclature

| No. | Disorder | Alternative name | Abbreviation | Gene symbol | Chromosomal localization | Affected protein | OMIM |
|---|---|---|---|---|---|---|---|
| 25.1 | 3-Phosphoglycerate dehydrogenase deficiency | Serine deficiency | 3-PGDH | *PHGDH* | 1p12 | Phosphoglycerate dehydrogenase | 606879, 256520 |
| 25.2 | 3-Phosphoserine aminotransferase deficiency | Serine deficiency | PSAT | *PSAT1* | 9q21.2 | Phosphoserine aminotransferase | 172480, 616038 |
| 25.3 | Phosphoserine phosphatase deficiency | Serine deficiency | PSP | *PSPH* | 7p11.2 | Phosphoserine phosphatase | 614023 |
| 25.4 | Glutamine synthetase deficiency | Glutamine deficiency | GS | *GLUL* | 1q25.3 | Glutamine synthetase | 610015 |
| 25.5 | Glutaminase deficiency | Glutamate deficiency | GLS | *GLS* | 2q32.2 | Glutaminase | 618328, 618412 |
| 25.6 | Glutaminase hyperactivity | Glutamate hyperactivity | GLS | *GLS* | 2q32.2 | Glutaminase | 618339 |
| 25.7 | Pyrroline-5-carboxylate synthase (P5CS) deficiency | Proline deficiency<br>ALDH18A1 deficiency | P5CS | *ALDH18A1* | 10q24.1 | Pyrroline-5-carboxylate synthase | 616603, 219150<br>601162, 616586 |
| 25.8 | Pyrroline-5-carboxylate reductase 1 (PYCR1) deficiency | Proline deficiency | PYCR1 | *PYCR1* | 17q25.3 | Pyrroline-5-carboxylate reductase 1 | 612940, 614438 |
| 25.9 | Pyrroline-5-carboxylate reductase 2 (PYCR2) deficiency | | PYCR2 | *PYCR2* | 1q42.12 | Pyrroline-5-carboxylate reductase 2 | 616420 |
| 25.10 | Proline dehydrogenase | Hyperprolinemia type I<br>Proline oxidase deficiency | PRODH | *PRODH* | 22q11.21 | Proline dehydrogenase | 606810 |
| 25.11 | Pyrroline-5-carboxylate dehydrogenase | Hyperprolinemia type II | P5CDH | *ALDH4A1* | 1p36.13 | Pyrroline-5-carboxylate dehydrogenase | 606811 |
| 25.12 | Asparagine synthetase deficiency | Asparagine deficiency | ASNS | *ASNS* | 7q21.3 | Asparagine synthetase | 615574 |
| 25.13 | Ornithine aminotransferase deficiency | Gyrate atrophy of retina and choroidea<br>OAT deficiency | OAT | *OAT* | 10q26.13 | Ornithine aminotransferase | 613349 |

## Signs and Symptoms

**Table 25.1** Phosphoglycerate dehydrogenase deficiency

| System | Symptoms and biomarkers | Neonatal (birth–1 month) | Infancy (1–18 months) | Childhood (1.5–11 years) | Adolescence (11–16 years) | Adulthood (>16 years) |
|---|---|---|---|---|---|---|
| CNS | **Absent myelination** | +++ | +++ | +++ | +++ | |
| | Ataxia | ± | ± | ± | + | + |
| | Axonal sensory motor polyneuropathy, chronic | ± | ± | ± | + | ++ |
| | **Cortical atrophy (MRI)** | ++ | +++ | +++ | +++ | |
| | **Delayed myelination** | +++ | +++ | +++ | +++ | |
| | Hyperexcitability | + | ++ | ++ | ++ | |
| | **Hypsarrhythmia (EEG)** | | +++ | ++ | | |
| | **Lennox-Gastaut syndrome** | | ++ | ++ | + | |
| | **Multifocal epilepsy (EEG)** | +++ | +++ | +++ | +++ | |
| | Retardation, psychomotor | ++ | +++ | +++ | ++ | + |
| | **Seizures** | +++ | +++ | ++ | ++ | + |
| | Spastic tetraplegia | + | +++ | +++ | +++ | |
| | **Subcortical atrophy (MRI)** | ++ | +++ | +++ | +++ | |
| Endocrine | Hypogonadism | + | + | + | + | |
| Eye | **Cataract** | + | + | + | + | + |
| | Nystagmus | ++ | ++ | ++ | + | |
| Hematological | Anemia, megaloblastic | + | + | + | + | |
| Musculoskeletal | Adducted thumbs | + | ++ | ++ | ++ | |
| | **Microcephaly** | +++ | +++ | +++ | +++ | |
| Laboratory findings | 5-Methyl-THF (cerebrospinal fluid) | ↓ | ↓ | ↓ | ↓ | ↓ |
| | Choline/creatine ratio (MRS) | ↑ | ↑ | ↑ | ↑ | |
| | Glycine (cerebrospinal fluid) | ↓ | ↓ | ↓ | ↓ | ↓ |
| | Glycine, fasting (plasma) | ↓ | ↓ | ↓ | ↓ | ↓ |
| | *N*-Acetylaspartate/creatine ratio (MRS) | ↓ | ↓ | ↓ | ↓ | |
| | Serine (cerebrospinal fluid) | ↓↓↓ | ↓↓↓ | ↓↓↓ | ↓↓↓ | ↓↓↓ |
| | Serine, fasting (plasma) | ↓ | ↓ | ↓ | ↓ | ↓ |
| Fetal (Neu-Laxova syndrome) | Cataract + | | | | | |
| | Cerebellar hypoplasia +++ | | | | | |
| | Cleft lip and or palate + | | | | | |
| | Collodion-like skin defect + | | | | | |
| | Congenital heart defects + | | | | | |
| | Contractures +++ | | | | | |
| | Corpus callosum agenesis + | | | | | |
| | Dandy-Walker abnormality + | | | | | |
| | Dysmorphism + | | | | | |
| | Limb defects + | | | | | |
| | Lissencephaly + | | | | | |
| | Lung hypoplasia ++ | | | | | |
| | Microcephaly +++ | | | | | |
| | Neural tube defects + | | | | | |
| | Protruding eyes + | | | | | |
| | Pterygia + | | | | | |
| | Severe intrauterine growth retardation (IUGR) +++ | | | | | |
| | Small mouth + | | | | | |
| | Syndactyly ++ | | | | | |

**Table 25.2** Phosphoserine aminotransferase deficiency

| System | Symptoms and biomarkers | Neonatal (birth–1 month) | Infancy (1–18 months) | Childhood (1.5–11 years) | Adolescence (11–16 years) | Adulthood (>16 years) |
|---|---|---|---|---|---|---|
| CNS | Cerebellar vermis hypoplasia (MRI) | + | ++ | ++ | | |
| | Generalized atrophy (MRI) | + | ++ | ++ | | |
| | Hypertonia | + | ++ | ++ | | |
| | **Seizures, intractable** | ++ | ++ | ++ | | |
| Musculoskeletal | Microcephaly | | ++ | ++ | | |
| Laboratory findings | Glycine (cerebrospinal fluid) | ↓ | ↓ | ↓ | | |
| | Glycine (plasma) | ↓ | ↓ | ↓ | | |
| | Serine (cerebrospinal fluid) | ↓↓ | ↓↓ | ↓↓ | | |
| | Serine (plasma) | ↓ | ↓ | ↓ | | |
| Fetal (Neu-Laxova syndrome) | Cataract + | | | | | |
| | Cleft lip and or palate + | | | | | |
| | Collodion-like skin defect + | | | | | |
| | Congenital heart defects + | | | | | |
| | Contractures +++ | | | | | |
| | Dysmorphism + | | | | | |
| | Limb defects + | | | | | |
| | Lung hypoplasia ++ | | | | | |
| | Microcephaly +++ | | | | | |
| | Neural tube defects + | | | | | |
| | Protruding eyes + | | | | | |
| | Severe intrauterine growth retardation (IUGR) +++ | | | | | |
| | Small mouth + | | | | | |

**Table 25.3** Phosphoserine phosphatase deficiency

| System | Symptoms and biomarkers | Neonatal (birth–1 month) | Infancy (1–18 months) | Childhood (1.5–11 years) | Adolescence (11–16 years) | Adulthood (>16 years) |
|---|---|---|---|---|---|---|
| CNS | **Retardation, psychomotor** | | ++ | ++ | ++ | |
| Musculoskeletal | Growth retardation | | ++ | ++ | ++ | |
| Laboratory findings | Serine (cerebrospinal fluid) | | ↓↓ | ↓↓ | ↓↓ | |
| | Serine (plasma) | | ↓-n | ↓-n | ↓-n | |
| Fetal (Neu-Laxova syndrome) | Cataract + | | | | | |
| | Cerebellar hypoplasia +++ | | | | | |
| | Cleft lip and or palate + | | | | | |
| | Congenital heart defects + | | | | | |
| | Contractures +++ | | | | | |
| | Collodion-like skin defect + | | | | | |
| | Corpus callosum agenesis + | | | | | |
| | Dandy-Walker abnormality + | | | | | |
| | Dysmorphism + | | | | | |
| | Lissencephaly + | | | | | |
| | Limb defects + | | | | | |
| | Lung hypoplasia ++ | | | | | |
| | Microcephaly +++ | | | | | |
| | Neural tube defects + | | | | | |
| | Protruding eyes + | | | | | |
| | Pterygia + | | | | | |
| | Severe intrauterine growth retardation (IUGR) +++ | | | | | |
| | Small mouth + | | | | | |
| | Syndactyly ++ | | | | | |

**Table 25.4** Glutamine synthetase deficiency

| System | Symptoms and biomarkers | Neonatal (birth–1 month) | Infancy (1–18 months) | Childhood (1.5–11 years) | Adolescence (11–16 yreas) | Adulthood (>16 years) |
|---|---|---|---|---|---|---|
| CNS | **Absent head control** | + | ++ | ++ | | |
| | Cerebellar hypoplasia | ± | | | | |
| | **Developmental delay** | + | +++ | +++ | | |
| | EEG, abnormal | + | ++ | ++ | | |
| | **Encephalopathy, epileptic** | ++ | ++ | ++ | | |
| | **Epilepsy, intractable** | ++ | ++ | ++ | | |
| Dermatological | Erythema, necrotizing | + | ± | ± | | |
| Laboratory findings | Ammonia (blood) | n↑ | n↑ | n↑ | | |
| | Glutamic acid (cerebrospinal fluid) | n | n | n | | |
| | Glutamic acid (plasma) | n | n | n | | |
| | Glutamine (cerebrospinal fluid) | ↓↓ | ↓↓ | ↓↓ | | |
| | Glutamine (plasma) | ↓↓ | ↓↓↓ | ↓↓↓ | | |
| | Glutamine (urine) | ↓ | ↓ | ↓ | | |

**Table 25.5** Glutaminase deficiency

| System | Symptoms and biomarkers | Neonatal (birth–1 month) | Infancy (1–18 months) | Childhood (1.5–11 years) | Adolescence (11–16 years) | Adulthood (>16 years) |
|---|---|---|---|---|---|---|
| CNS | Burst-suppression pattern EEG | + | | | | |
| | Developmental delay | | + | + | + | |
| | Febrile seizures | | | + | | |
| | Hypotonia | + | | | | |
| | Intractable seizures | + | | | | |
| | MRI cerebellar atrophy | | | | ± | |
| | MRI simplified gyration pattern | | + | | | |
| | Progressive ataxia | | | | + | |
| Respiratory | Respiratory insufficiency | + | | | | |
| Laboratory findings | Glutamine (plasma) | ↑↑ | ↑↑ | ↑↑↑ | ↑↑↑ | |
| | Orotic acid (urine) | n | n | n | n | |

**Table 25.6** Glutaminase hyperactivity

| System | Symptoms and biomarkers | Neonatal (birth–1 month) | Infancy (1–18 months) | Childhood (1.5–11 years) | Adolescence (11–16 years) | Adulthood (>16 years) |
|---|---|---|---|---|---|---|
| CNS | Absent myelination | | | + | + | |
| | Delayed myelination | | | + | + | |
| | **Developmental delay** | | + | + | | |
| | Hypotonia | | + | + | + | |
| | Loss of speech | | | + | + | |
| Dermatological | **Skin abnormalities** | | | + | + | |
| Eye | **Cataract** | | + | | | |
| Musculoskeletal | Kyphoscoliosis | | | + | + | |
| | **Microcephaly** | | + | + | | |
| Laboratory findings | Glutamine on MRS | | | ↓-n | ↓-n | |
| | Glutamate on MRS | | | ↑↑ | ↑↑ | |
| | Ratio glutamate/glutamine in urine | | | ↑ | ↑ | |

**Table 25.7** Pyrroline-5-carboxylate synthetase deficiency, cutis laxa phenotype 3

| System | Symptoms and biomarkers | Neonatal (birth–1 month) | Infancy (1–18 months) | Childhood (1.5–11 years) | Adolescence (11–16 years) | Adulthood (>16 years) |
|---|---|---|---|---|---|---|
| Cardiovascular | Congenital heart abnormalities | + | | | | |
| | **Valvulitis, mitral** | + | + | + | | |
| CNS | Absent corpus callosum | + | | | | |
| | **Developmental delay** | | ± | ± | | |
| | Dystonia | | + | + | | |
| | Hypotonia | + | + | + | | |
| | Paucity of white matter | | ± | | | |
| | Pyramidal signs | | | ± | ± | |
| | Seizures | + | | | | |
| | Thin corpus callosum | | ± | | | |
| | Tortuous blood vessels | + | ± | | | |
| Dermatological | **Cutis laxa** | ++ | ++ | ++ | ++ | |
| | **Wrinkly skin** | ++ | ++ | + | | |
| Digestive | Feeding difficulties | ++ | ++ | ++ | + | |
| Eye | **Cataract** | + | ++ | ++ | | |
| | Corneal clouding | | + | + | + | |
| Hair | Sparse hair | | + | + | + | |
| Musculoskeletal | Hernias | | + | + | + | |
| | Hip dislocation | + | + | + | + | |
| | Joint contractures | + | | | | |
| | Joint laxity | + | + | + | | |
| | **Microcephaly** | + | + | + | | |
| | Osteopenia | | ± | ± | | |
| | Osteoporosis | | + | ++ | ++ | |
| | Pes planus | | + | + | + | |
| | Rhizomelia | | + | + | | |
| | Short stature | | + | + | + | |
| | Wormian bones | | + | + | | |
| Other | Failure to thrive | | ± | + | | |
| | Intrauterine growth retardation | + | | | | |
| | **Progeroid appearance** | ++ | + | + | | |
| Psychiatric | Behavior difficulties | | + | + | + | |
| Laboratory findings | Ammonia (blood) | n-↑ | n-↑ | n-↑ | | |
| | Arginine (plasma) | ↓-n | ↓-n | ↓-n | | ↓-n |
| | Citrulline (plasma) | ↓-n | ↓-n | ↓-n | | ↓-n |
| | Creatine (MRS) | ↓-n | ↓-n | ↓-n | | |
| | Ornithine (plasma) | ↓-n | ↓-n | ↓-n | | ↓-n |
| | Proline (plasma) | ↓-n | ↓-n | ↓-n | | ↓-n |

Table 25.8 Pyrroline-5-carboxylate reductase 1 deficiency

| System | Symptoms and biomarkers | Neonatal (birth–1 month) | Infancy (1–18 months) | Childhood (1.5–11 years) | Adolescence (11—16 years) | Adulthcod (>16 years) |
|---|---|---|---|---|---|---|
| CNS | Agenesis, corpus callosum (MRI) | | ± | ± | | |
| | **Developmental delay** | | + | + | | |
| | Hydrocephalus | | ± | ± | | |
| Dermatological | **Cutis laxa** | | + | + | | |
| | **Wrinkly skin** | | + | | | |
| Digestive | Gastroesophageal reflux | | + | + | | |
| Ear | **Prominent ears** | + | + | + | | |
| Eye | **Blue sclerae** | + | + | + | | |
| | Deeply set eyes | | ± | ± | | |
| | Hypotelorism | | ± | ± | | |
| Musculoskeletal | Bulbous nose | | ± | ± | | |
| | Clasped thumb | | ± | ± | | |
| | Fontanel enlarged | + | | | | |
| | Hip dislocation | | + | + | | |
| | Joint hyperextensibility | + | + | + | ± | ± |
| | Long digits | | ± | ± | | |
| | **Microcephaly** | + | + | + | | |
| | Midface hypoplasia | + | + | + | | |
| | **Osteopenia** | | + | + | | |
| | **Sagging cheeks** | + | + | + | + | ± |
| | Scoliosis | | ± | ± | | |
| | **Triangular face** | + | + | + | ± | ± |
| | **Wide forehead** | + | + | + | | |
| Other | Failure to thrive | + | | | | |
| | Intrauterine growth retardation | + | | | | |

Table 25.9 Pyrroline-5-carboxylate reductase 2 deficiency

| System | Symptoms and biomarkers | Neonatal (birth–1 month) | Infancy (1–18 months) | Childhood (1.5–11 years) | Adolescence (11–16 years) | Adulthood (>16 years) |
|---|---|---|---|---|---|---|
| CNS | **Cerebral atrophy (MRI)** | + | + | | | |
| | **Cortical atrophy (MRI)** | + | + | | | |
| | **Hyperkinesia** | + | + | + | | |
| | **Hyperreflexia** | + | + | + | | |
| | **Hypomyelination (MRI)** | + | + | + | | |
| | Loss of speech | | + | + | | |
| | Retardation, psychomotor | | + | + | | |
| | Seizures | ± | ± | ± | | |
| | **Spasticity** | + | + | + | | |
| | Thin corpus callosum | + | + | + | | |
| | Truncal hypotonia | + | + | + | | |
| Ear | **Hearing loss** | | + | + | | |
| | **Large malformed ears** | + | + | + | | |
| | **Low-set ears** | + | + | + | | |
| Eye | Downslanting palpebral fissures | | + | + | | |
| | Nystagmus | | ± | ± | | |
| | **Upslanting palpebral fissures** | + | + | + | | |

(continued)

**Table 25.9** (continued)

| System | Symptoms and biomarkers | Neonatal (birth–1 month) | Infancy (1–18 months) | Childhood (1.5–11 years) | Adolescence (11–16 years) | Adulthood (>16 years) |
|---|---|---|---|---|---|---|
| Musculoskeletal | **Arachnodactyly** | | + | + | | |
| | **Bitemporal narrowing** | + | + | + | | |
| | **Bulbous nose** | + | + | + | | |
| | **Facial dysmorphism** | + | + | + | | |
| | **Growth retardation** | + | + | + | | |
| | Inability to walk | | + | + | | |
| | Joint hyperextensibility | | + | + | | |
| | **Long philtrum** | + | + | + | | |
| | **Malar hypoplasia** | + | + | + | | |
| | **Microcephaly** | + | + | + | | |
| | Short nose | + | + | + | | |
| | **Triangular face** | + | + | + | | |
| | Upturned nose | + | + | + | | |
| Other | Death | | | + | | |
| | **Failure to thrive** | + | + | | | |

**Table 25.10** Proline dehydrogenase deficiency

| System | Symptoms and biomarkers | Neonatal (birth–1 month) | Infancy (1–18 months) | Childhood (1.5–11 years) | Adolescence (11–16 years) | Adulthood (>16 years) |
|---|---|---|---|---|---|---|
| Other | **No clinical significance** | ± | ± | ± | ± | ± |
| CNS | Developmental delay | | | | ± | ± |
| | Epilepsy | | | | ± | ± |
| Psychiatric | Autism | | | ± | ± | ± |
| | **Schizophrenia susceptibility** | | | | ± | + |
| Laboratory findings | Glycine (urine) | n-↑ | n-↑ | n-↑ | n-↑ | n-↑ |
| | Hydroxyproline (urine) | n-↑ | n-↑ | n-↑ | n-↑ | n-↑ |
| | Proline (plasma) | ↑↑ | ↑↑ | ↑↑ | ↑↑ | ↑↑ |
| | Proline (urine) | n-↑ | n-↑ | n-↑ | n-↑ | n-↑ |

**Table 25.11** Pyrroline-5-carboxylate dehydrogenase deficiency

| System | Symptoms and biomarkers | Neonatal (birth–1 month) | Infancy (1–18 months) | Childhood (1.5–11 years) | Adolescence (11–16 years) | Adulthood (>16 years) |
|---|---|---|---|---|---|---|
| CNS | Intellectual disability | | ± | ± | ± | ± |
| | **Seizures, febrile** | | ± | ± | n | n |
| | **Seizures, pharmacoresistant** | | ± | ± | ± | ± |
| Laboratory findings | Hydroxyproline (plasma) | n | n | n | n | n |
| | Hydroxyproline (urine) | n-↑↑↑ | n-↑↑↑ | n-↑↑↑ | n-↑↑↑ | n-↑↑↑ |
| | Proline (plasma) | ↑-↑↑↑ | ↑-↑↑↑ | ↑-↑↑↑ | ↑-↑↑↑ | ↑-↑↑↑ |
| | Proline (urine) | ↑↑↑ | ↑↑↑ | ↑↑↑ | ↑↑↑ | ↑↑↑ |
| | Pyrroline-5-carboxylate, P5C (urine) | ↑ | ↑ | ↑ | ↑ | ↑ |

**Table 25.12** Asparagine synthetase deficiency

| System | Symptoms and biomarkers | Neonatal (birth–1 month) | Infancy (1–18 months) | Childhood (1.5–11 years) | Adolescence (11–16 years) | Adulthood (>16 years) |
|---|---|---|---|---|---|---|
| CNS | **Burst-suppression (EEG)** | + | + | | | |
| | **Cerebellar hypoplasia** | + | + | | | |
| | **Cortical atrophy (MRI)** | + | + | | | |
| | **Delayed myelination** | + | + | | | |
| | **Encephalopathy, progressive** | + | + | | | |
| | **Hyperekplexia** | + | + | + | | |
| | Hyperreflexia | + | + | + | | |
| | **Hypsarrhythmia (EEG)** | + | + | | | |
| | **Seizures** | + | + | + | | |
| | **Spastic tetraplegia** | + | + | | | |
| | Thin corpus callosum | + | + | | | |
| | Truncal hypotonia | + | + | + | | |
| | **Ventriculomegaly** | + | + | | | |
| Digestive | Feeding difficulties | ± | ± | | | |
| Ear | **Large malformed ears** | + | + | + | | |
| Eye | **Blindness, cortical** | + | + | + | | |
| Musculoskeletal | **Large feet** | + | + | + | | |
| | **Large hands** | + | + | + | | |
| | Microcephaly | + | + | + | | |
| | **Micrognathia** | + | + | + | | |
| Other | **Failure to thrive** | + | + | | | |
| Respiratory | **Respiratory insufficiency** | + | + | | | |
| Laboratory findings | Asparagine (CSF) | | | ↓-n | | |
| | Asparagine (plasma) | ↓-n | ↓-n | | | |

**Table 25.13** Ornithine aminotransferase deficiency

| System | Symptoms and biomarkers | Neonatal (birth–1 month) | Infancy (1–18 months) | Childhood (1.5–11 years) | Adolescence (11–16 years) | Adulthood (>16 years) |
|---|---|---|---|---|---|---|
| CNS | Cortical atrophy (MRI) | | | | ± | ± |
| | EEG, abnormal | | | | ± | ± |
| | Intellectual disability | | | ± | ± | ± |
| | Neuropathy, sensory | | | ± | ± | ± |
| | Seizures | | | | ± | ± |
| | White matter abnormalities (MRI) | | | | ± | ± |
| Digestive | EM, abnormal mitochondria (liver) | | | | ± | ± |
| Eye | **Adaptation, dark impaired/night blindness** | | ± | ++ | +++ | +++ |
| | **Atrophy, gyrate of choroid and retina** | | | + | ++ | +++ |
| | **Cataract, posterior subcapsular** | | | | ± | +++ |
| | **Chorioretinal degeneration** | | | + | ++ | +++ |
| | **Myopia** | | ± | + | ++ | +++ |
| | **Night blindness** | | | | | +++ |
| | Retinal detachment | | | ± | ± | ± |
| | **Vision, tunnel** | | | | + | +++ |

(continued)

**Table 25.13** (continued)

| System | Symptoms and biomarkers | Neonatal (birth–1 month) | Infancy (1–18 months) | Childhood (1.5–11 years) | Adolescence (11–16 years) | Adulthood (>16 years) |
|---|---|---|---|---|---|---|
| Musculoskeletal | EM, abnormal mitochondria (muscle) | | | ± | ± | ± |
| | EM, type 2 fiber atrophy (muscle) | | | ± | ± | ± |
| | EM, type 2 fiber tubular aggregates (muscle) | | | ± | ± | ± |
| | Muscle weakness | | | ± | ± | ± |
| Laboratory findings | 3-Amino-2-piperidone (urine) | ± | ↑ | ↑ | ↑ | ↑ |
| | Ammonia (blood) | n-↑↑ | n | n | n | n |
| | Arginine (urine) | n-↑ | ↑ | ↑ | ↑ | ↑ |
| | Creatine (cerebrospinal fluid) | | ↓↓ | ↓↓ | ↓↓↓ | ↓↓↓ |
| | Creatine (plasma) | | ↓↓ | ↓↓ | ↓↓↓ | ↓↓↓ |
| | Creatine (urine) | | ↓↓ | ↓↓ | ↓↓↓ | ↓↓↓ |
| | Creatine/phosphocreatine ratio (brain) (MRS) | | | ↓ | ↓ | ↓ |
| | Creatine/phosphocreatine ratio (muscle) (MRS) | | | ↓ | ↓ | ↓ |
| | Creatinine (plasma) | | ↓-n | ↓-n | ↓-n | ↓-n |
| | Guanidinoacetate (cerebrospinal fluid) | | ↓↓ | ↓↓ | ↓↓↓ | ↓↓↓ |
| | Guanidinoacetate (plasma) | | ↓↓ | ↓↓ | ↓↓↓ | ↓↓↓ |
| | Guanidinoacetate (urine) | | ↓↓ | ↓↓ | ↓↓↓ | ↓↓↓ |
| | Histology and EM, type 2 fiber atrophy (muscle) | | | + | + | ++-+++ |
| | Lysine (urine) | n-↑ | ↑ | ↑ | ↑ | ↑ |
| | Ornithine (plasma) | ± | ↑↑↑ | ↑↑↑ | ↑↑↑ | ↑↑↑ |
| | Ornithine (urine) | ± | ↑↑↑ | ↑↑↑ | ↑↑↑ | ↑↑↑ |
| | Proline/citrulline ratio | ↑ | n | n | n | n |

## Diagnosis of Amino Acid Synthesis Disorders

In most of the amino acid synthesis disorders discussed here, molecular diagnostic techniques are preferred over biochemical testing. An exception to this are OAT deficiency, glutaminase deficiency, and hyperprolinemia type I and II where elevated concentrations of ornithine, glutamine, and proline are easily detected in plasma. In the other disorders, pitfalls in biochemical testing hamper the use of it, either because of preanalytical confounders (non-fasted plasma samples in serine deficiency or near-normal glutamine in milder glutamine synthetase deficiency), inconsistent findings in patients (P5CS deficiency and asparagine synthase), or the fact that no abnormalities can be detected at all in body fluids (PYCR1, PYCR2, and SRS). One must be aware of the fact that heterozygous mutations can cause a phenotype in these disorders either because of dominant negative effects on dimerization of protein complexes (*ALDH18A1*) or gain of function (*GLS*). Unfortunately the lack of easily available functional assays may cause difficulties in interpreting variants of unknown significance (VUS) in the genes involved.

## Treatment

Of all the synthesis defects, serine deficiency appears most amendable for therapy (van der Crabben et al. 2013). Except for Neu-Laxova syndrome, therapy with L-serine has been successfully applied, and even in the severe infantile form seizures can be treated. However, to prevent psychomotor retardation, patients must be treated during pregnancy on within the first month of life (de Koning et al. 2004). In the other disorders, reports of treatment are anecdotal, but it is very likely that, for instance, in glutamine deficiency similar to serine deficiency, treatment with L-glutamine and nicotinamide must start early to treat seizures and prevent psychomotor retardation. In OAT deficiency treatment consists of protein restriction, pyridoxine, and creatine monohydrate, the latter because there is evidence of low creatine on MRS (Valayannopoulos et al. 2009).

Of course in all disorders discussed, symptomatic treatment of associated findings is warranted, for instance, treatment of seizures or osteoporosis.

## Follow-Up and Monitoring

Monitoring L-serine therapy in serine deficiency would require repeated lumbar punctures, but normalization of CSF serine occurs with the dosages recommended. Therefore, we would advise follow-up based on clinical response, for instance, on improvement of well-being and drop in seizure frequency, albeit that improvement in EEG patterns can take months. For glutamine deficiency clinical follow-up is recommended as well; in the case treated with high dosages of L-glutamine, therapy resulted in partial correction of CSF glutamine, but in a significant improvement of EEG abnormalities. Follow-up on clinical findings may be more important than monitoring correction of CSF deficiency of the amino acid (Häberle et al. 2012).

In OAT deficiency lowering ornithine concentrations delays the progression of the retinal abnormalities in most patients, and this can be done by arginine/protein restriction, but the diet is difficult to adhere to. Plasma values should be at least below 400–500 μmol/L (Kaiser-Kupfer et al. 2004). In a minority of patients, this can be achieved by pyridoxine therapy alone. Beware of the fact that long-term treatment with high-dose pyridoxine can cause polyneuropathy, and this should be monitored as well. It is unsure whether creatine therapy in this disorder does result in reduced risk for retinopathy but likely results in better brain and muscular function.

In all disorders discussed here, potential complications of the defects should be monitored at regular intervals during clinical follow-up.

## References

Acuna-Hidalgo R, Schanze D, Kariminejad A, Nordgren A, Kariminejad MH, Conner P, Grigelioniene G, Nilsson D, Nordenskjöld M, Wedell A, Freyer C, Wredenberg A, Wieczorek D, Gillessen-Kaesbach G, Kayserili H, Elcioglu N, Ghaderi-Sohi S, Goodarzi P, Setayesh H, van deVorst M, Steehouwer M, Pfundt R, Krabichler B, Curry C, MacKenzie MG, Boycott KM, Gilissen C, Janecke AR, Hoischen A, Zenker M. Neu-Laxova syndrome is a heterogeneous metabolic disorder caused by defects in enzymes of the L-serine biosynthesis pathway. Am J Hum Genet. 2014;95:285–93.

Baumgartner MR, Hu CA, Almashanu S, Steel G, Obie C, Aral B, Rabier D, Kamoun P, Saudubray JM, Valle D. Hyperammonemia with reduced ornithine, citrulline, arginine and proline: a new inborn error caused by a mutation in the gene encoding delta(1)-pyrroline-5-carboxylate synthase. Hum Mol Genet. 2000;9:2853–8.

Cleary MA, Dorland L, de Koning TJ, Poll-The BT, Duran M, Mandell R, Shih VE, Berger R, Olpin SE, Besley GT. Ornithine aminotransferase deficiency: diagnostic difficulties in neonatal presentation. J Inherit Metab Dis. 2005;28:673–9.

Coutelier M, Goizet C, Durr A, Habarou F, Morais S, Dionne-Laporte A, Tao F, Konop J, Stoll M, Charles P, Jacoupy M, Matusiak R, Alonso I, Tallaksen C, Mairey M, Kennerson M, Gaussen M, Schule R, Janin M, Morice-Picard F, Durand CM, Depienne C, Calvas P, Coutinho P, Saudubray JM, Rouleau G, Brice A, Nicholson G, Darios F, Loureiro JL, Zuchner S, Ottolenghi C, Mochel F, Stevanin G. Alteration of ornithine metabolism leads to dominant and recessive hereditary spastic paraplegia. Brain. 2015;38:2191–205.

de Koning TJ, Klomp LW, van Oppen AC, et al. Prenatal and early postnatal treatment in 3-phosphoglycerate-dehydrogenase deficiency. Lancet. 2004;364:2221–2.

Häberle J, Gorg B, Rutch F, Schimdt E, Toutain A, Benoist JF, Gelot A, Suc AL, Höhne W, Schliess F, Häussinger D, Koch HG. Congenital glutamine deficiency with glutamine synthetase deficiency. N Engl J Med. 2005;353:1926–33.

Häberle J, Shahbeck N, Ibrahim K, Schmitt B, Scheer I, O'Gorman R, Chaudhry FA, Ben-Omran T. Glutamine supplementation in a child with inherited GS deficiency improves the clinical status and partially corrects the peripheral and central amino acid imbalance. Orphanet J Rare Dis. 2012;7:48.

Jaeken J, Detheux M, Van Maldergem L, Frijns JP, Alliet P, Foulon M, Carchon H, Van Schaftingen E. 3-Phosphoglycerate dehydrogenase deficiency and 3-phosphoserine phosphatase deficiency: inborn errors of serine biosynthesis. J Inherit Metab Dis. 1996;19:223–6.

Kaiser-Kupfer MI, Caruso RC, Valle D, Reed GF. Use of an arginine-restricted diet to slow progression of visual loss in patients with gyrate atrophy. Arch Ophthalmol. 2004;122:982–4.

Li C, Brazill JM, Liu S, Bello C, Zhu Y, Morimoto M, Cascio L, Pauly R, Diaz-Perez Z, Malicdan MCV, Wang H, Boccuto L, Schwartz CE, Gahl WA, Boerkoel CF, Zhai RG. Spermine synthase deficiency causes lysosomal dysfunction and oxidative stress in models of Snyder-Robinson syndrome. Nat Commun. 2017;8:1257.

Nakayama T, Al-Maawali A, El-Quessny M, Rajab A, Khalil S, Stoler JM, Tan WH, Nasir R, Schmitz-Abe K, Hill RS, Partlow JN, Al-Saffar M, Servattalab S, LaCoursiere CM, Tambunan DE, Coulter ME, Elhosary PC, Gorski G, Barkovich AJ, Markianos K, Poduri A, Mochida GH. Mutations in PYCR2, encoding Pyrroline-5-carboxylate Reductase 2, cause microcephaly and Hypomyelination. Am J Hum Genet. 2015;96:709–19.

Reversade B, Escande-Beillard N, Dimopoulou A, Fischer B, Chng SC, Li Y, Shboul M, Tham PY, Kayserili H, Al-Gazali L, Shahwan M, Brancati F, Lee H, O'Connor BD, Schmidt-von Kegler M, Merriman B, Nelson SF, Masri A, Alkazaleh F, Guerra D, Ferrari P, Nanda A, Rajab A, Markie D, Gray M, Nelson J, Grix A, Sommer A, Savarirayan R, Janecke AR, Steichen E, Sillence D, Hausser I, Budde B, Nürnberg G, Nürnberg P, Seemann P, Kunkel D, Zambruno G, Dallapiccola B, Schuelke M, Robertson S, Hamamy H, Wollnik B, Van Maldergem L, Mundlos S, Kornak U. Mutations in PYCR1 cause cutis laxa with progeroid features. Nat Genet. 2009;41:1016–21.

Rumping L, Büttner B, Maier O, Rehmann H, Lequin M, Schlump JU, Schmitt B, Schiebergen-Bronkhorst B, Prinsen HCMT, Losa M, Fingerhut R, Lemke JR, Zwartkruis FJT, Houwen RHJ, Jans JJM, Verhoeven-Duif NM, van Hasselt PM, Jamra R. Identification of a loss-of-function mutation in the context of glutaminase deficiency and neonatal epileptic encephalopathy. JAMA Neurol. 2019a;76:342–50.

Rumping L, Tessadori F, Pouwels PJW, Vringer E, Wijnen JP, Bhogal AA, Savelberg SMC, Duran KJ, Bakkers MJG, Ramos RJJ, Schellekens PAW, Kroes HY, Klomp DWJ, Black GCM, Taylor RL, Bakkers JPW, Prinsen HCMT, van der Knaap MS, Dansen TB, Rehmann H, Zwartkruis FJT, Houwen RHJ, van Haaften G,

Verhoeven-Duif NM, Jans JJM, van Hasselt PM. GLS hyperactivity causes glutamate excess, infantile cataract and profound developmental delay. Hum Mol Genet. 2019b;28:96–104.

Ruzzo EK, Capo-Chichi JM, Ben-Zeev B, Chitayat D, Mao H, Pappas AL, Hitomi Y, Lu YF, Yao X, Hamdan FF, Pelak K, Reznik-Wolf H, Bar-Joseph I, Oz-Levi D, Lev D, Lerman-Sagie T, Leshinsky-Silver E, Anikster Y, Ben-Asher E, Olender T, Colleaux L, Décarie JC, Blaser S, Banwell B, Joshi RB, He XP, Patry L, Silver RJ, Dobrzeniecka S, Islam MS, Hasnat A, Samuels ME, Aryal DK, Rodriguiz RM, Jiang YH, Wetsel WC, McNamara JO, Rouleau GA, Silver DL, Lancet D, Pras E, Mitchell GA, Michaud JL, Goldstein DB. Deficiency of asparagine synthetase causes congenital microcephaly and a progressive form of encephalopathy. Neuron. 2013;80:429–41.

Skidmore DL, Chitayat D, Morgan T, Hinek A, Fischer B, Dimopoulou A, Somers G, Halliday W, Blaser S, Diambomba Y, Lemire EG, Kornak U, Robertson SP. Further expansion of the phenotypic spectrum associated with mutations in ALDH18A1, encoding Δ1-pyrroline-5-carboxylate synthase (P5CS). Am J Med Genet A. 2011;155A:1848–56.

Valayannopoulos V, Boddaert N, Mention K, Touati G, Barbier V, Chabli A, Sedel F, Kaplan J, Dufier JL, Seidenwurm D, Rabier D, Saudubray JM, de Lonlay P. Secondary creatine deficiency in ornithine delta-aminotransferase deficiency. Mol Genet Metab. 2009;97:109–13.

van der Crabben SN, Verhoeven-Duif NM, Brilstra EH, Van Maldergem L, Coskun T, Rubio-Gozalbo E, Berger R, de Koning TJ. An update on serine deficiency disorders. J Inherit Metab Dis. 2013;36(4):613–9.

van Kuilenburg ABP, Tarailo-Graovac M, Richmond PA, Drögemöller BI, Pouladi MA, Leen R, Brand-Arzamendi K, Dobritzsch D, Dolzhenko E, Eberle MA, Hayward B, Jones MJ, Karbassi F, Kobor MS, Koster J, Kumari D, Li M, MacIsaac J, McDonald C, Meijer J, Nguyen C, Rajan-Babu IS, Scherer SW, Sim B, Trost B, Tseng LA, Turkenburg M, van Vugt JJFA, Veldink JH, Walia JS, Wang Y, van Weeghel M, Wright GEB, Xu X, Yuen RKC, Zhang J, Ross CJ, Wasserman WW, Geraghty MT, Santra S, Wanders RJA, Wen XY, Waterham HR, Usdin K, van Karnebeek CDM. Glutaminase deficiency caused by short tandem repeat expansion in *GLS*. N Engl J Med. 2019;380:1433–41.

Zaki MS, Bhat G, Sultan T, Issa M, Jung HJ, Dikoglu E, Selim L, Mahmoud GI, Abdel-Hamid MS, Abdel-Salam G, Marin-Valencia I, Gleeson JG. PYCR2 mutations cause a lethal syndrome of microcephaly and failure to thrive. Ann Neurol. 2016;80:59–70.

Zampatti S, Castori M, Fischer B, Ferrari P, Garavelli L, Dionisi-Vici C, Agolini E, Wischmeijer A, Morava E, Novelli G, Häberle J, Kornak U, Brancati F. De Barsy syndrome: a genetically heterogeneous autosomal recessive cutis laxa syndrome related to P5CS and PYCR1 dysfunction. Am J Med Genet A. 2012;158A:927–31.

# Disorders of Glycine Metabolism

# 26

Johan L. K. Van Hove, Curtis R. Coughlin II, and Michael A. Swanson

## Contents



**Summary**

Glycine is broken down by the glycine cleavage enzyme, which is composed of the P-protein, T-protein, H-protein, and L-protein. Its deficient activity causes accumulation of glycine in all tissues, including the brain, which defines nonketotic hyperglycinemia (NKH). It is caused by mutations in the genes *GLDC* encoding the P-protein and *AMT* encoding the T-protein. Children with the severe phenotype have two mutations without residual activity and present in the first days to weeks of life with transient apnea, coma, hypotonia, hiccups, burst-suppression pattern, and myoclonic epilepsy. Patients have very limited or no developmental progress and develop intractable multifocal epilepsy, axial hypotonia and peripheral spasticity, cortical blindness, and poor feeding. In childhood they can develop scoliosis, hip dysplasia, and poor airway maintenance resulting in pneumonia. Children with the attenuated form have at least one mutation with residual

J. L. K. Van Hove (✉) · C. R. Coughlin II · M. A. Swanson
Section of Clinical Genetics and Metabolism, Department of Pediatrics, University of Colorado, Children's Hospital Colorado, Aurora, CO, USA
e-mail: Johan.Vanhove@childrenscolorado.org; Curtis.Coughlin@childrenscolorado.org; Mike.Swanson@cuanschutz.edu


N. Blau et al. (eds.), *Physician's Guide to the Diagnosis, Treatment, and Follow-Up of Inherited Metabolic Diseases*,
https://doi.org/10.1007/978-3-030-67727-5_26

enzyme activity. Many children also present in the neonatal period, but some present in infancy or later. Patients make variable developmental progress, have little or no spasticity, chorea, and pronounced hyperactivity, episodic lethargy, or ataxia. Patients have no seizures or seizures that are controlled with treatment. Infants with NKH have a diagnostic pattern of diffusion restriction in the posterior limb of the internal capsule, anterior brain stem tracts, posterior tegmental tracts, and cerebellar white matter. Hypoplastic corpus callosum is frequent. Specific treatment of NKH includes reduction of glycine with sodium benzoate and use of dextromethorphan to reduce neurotransmission at the NMDA receptor. This treatment improves developmental outcome when initiated early in attenuated NKH patients. In severe NKH, treatment can improve alertness and seizure control in patients without changing the lack of development.

The glycine transporter GLYT1 encoded by the gene *SLC6A9* provides uptake of glycine at the cell membrane in astrocytes. Patients with mutations in this gene present with prolonged apnea requiring ventilation or hypotonia developing into spasticity with axial hypotonia. Reported congenital anomalies include hydrops, polyhydramnios, and arthrogryposis. Patients also develop excessive startles and hyperekplexia. They have mildly elevated glycine in cerebrospinal fluid (CSF) but not in blood. There is no specific treatment.

Primary differential diagnosis for the disorders with elevated glycine in the CSF includes disorders of the cofactors pyridoxal-phosphate and lipoate, medication interference by valproate, and loss of the integrity of the blood brain barrier such as in hypoxic-ischemic injury.

## Introduction

The primary enzyme in the catabolism of glycine is the glycine cleavage enzyme (GCE). The GCE is located in hepatocytes and in astrocytes and consists of four proteins (P, T, H, and L) and has two cofactors lipoate and pyridoxal phosphate.

### Nonketotic Hyperglycinemia

Disorders caused by pathogenic mutations in the genes encoding for P-protein (*GLDC* gene) and for T-protein (*AMT* gene) cause nonketotic hyperglycinemia (NKH). This condition is phenotypically distinguished into the severe form and an attenuated form based on severity of outcome (Swanson et al. 2015; Hennermann et al. 2012). Patients with the severe form have two mutations without residual activity, whereas patients with the attenuated form have at least one mutation with some residual activity (Swanson et al. 2015).

Patients with the severe form present in the first month of life with neonatal epileptic encephalopathy. Patients can have hiccups in utero, and at birth, rare patients have club feet or cleft palate (Hennermann et al. 2012). In the first days of life, neonates develop a comatose episode with myoclonia, hiccups, and often a burst-suppression pattern on EEG. Up to 85% of severe patients have apnea requiring ventilation which spontaneously resolves by the end of the first month (Hennermann et al. 2012; Hoover-Fong et al. 2004). Over the next year, they lack any developmental progress and develop treatment-resistant epilepsy, progressive peripheral spasticity with axial hypotonia, cortical blindness, and poor swallowing requiring gastric tube feeding. Long-term complications include the development of scoliosis, hip dysplasia, and poor airway maintenance (Ramirez et al. 2012).

Most patients with the attenuated form present in the neonatal period essentially similar to the severe form at that age, but some patients may present later in life with developmental delays or epilepsy (Swanson et al. 2015; Hennermann et al. 2012; Hoover-Fong et al. 2004). Patients with the attenuated form are divided based on severity into poor, intermediate, and good outcome categories (Swanson et al. 2015). Patients with attenuated poor outcome still develop epilepsy which is usually treatable with antiepileptics, have moderate spasticity, and make some limited developmental progress. They usually only use sign language. Patients with the attenuated intermediate phenotype have a developmental quotient (DQ) of 20–50, often are very hyperactive, and can have choreatic movements, intermittent ataxia, and intermittent episodes of lethargy. If they have epilepsy, it is readily treatable. Receptive language is fair but expressive language is poor. Patients with the attenuated good outcome category make substantial developmental progress (DQ > 50). They tend to have pronounced hyperactivity, clumsy walk and movements, and some developmental delays but do not have epilepsy. They too can have intermittent episodes of lethargy.

On brain MRI, all NKH patients in the neonatal period and early infancy have a recognizable pattern of diffusion restriction of the posterior limb of the internal capsule, the corticospinal tract into the brain stem, the posterior tegmental tracts, and the cerebellar white matter (Stence et al. 2019) (Fig. 26.1). This evolves over time and is less recognizable in late infancy. The corpus callosum is thin and shortened and, in severe NKH, does not grow over time. In severe NKH, there is gradual development of atrophy. A few patients with severe NKH develop hydrocephalus often with a large retrocerebellar cystic area (Hoover-Fong et al. 2004; Van Hove et al. 2000).

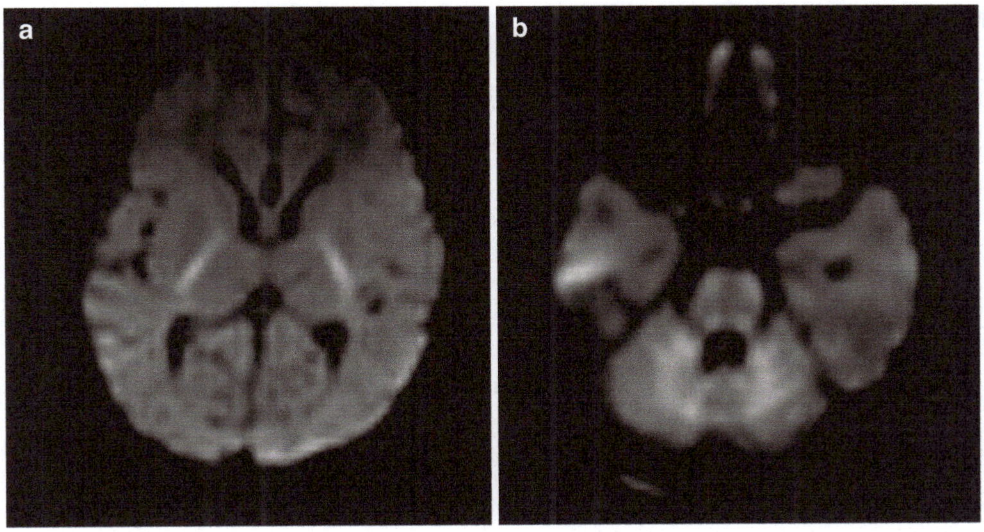


**Fig. 26.1** Brain MRI of a neonate with nonketotic hyperglycinemia
Legend: Diffusion weighted images of a neonate with NKH showing diffusion restriction (**a**) at the level of the posterior limb of the internal capsule and (**b**) in the anterior part of the brain stem, the posterior tegmental tracts, and the white matter of the cerebellum. Reproduced with permission from GeneReviews®, University of Washington, Seattle (Van Hove et al. 2002)

Plasma glycine is often but not always elevated. CSF glycine is always elevated with the elevation related to outcome, as a high CSF glycine is predictive of severe NKH (Swanson et al. 2015). The ratio of CSF-plasma glycine is elevated, and a low ratio is predictive of attenuated NKH (Swanson et al. 2015). Mutations are identified either in the *GLDC* gene in 80% of cases or in the *AMT* gene in 20% of cases (Coughlin II et al. 2017). It is unclear if any rare cases of *GCSH* mutations exist. Exonic copy number variants are common in *GLDC*. The primary differential diagnosis involves the disorders of the synthesis and metabolism of the co-factors pyridoxal-phosphate (PLP) and lipoate (Coughlin II et al. 2017; Van Hove et al. 2002; Wilson et al. 2019). Particularly, some patients with lipoate deficiency have presented biochemically similarly to patients with nonketotic hyperglycinemia (Baker et al. 2014). Some patients with PLP disorders have presented symptomatically similar to nonketotic hyperglycinemia and can have elevated CSF glycine (Wilson et al. 2019). Some patients with perinatal hypoxic ischemic injury can present with a transient comatose episode with elevated CSF glycine likely due to blood-brain barrier dysfunction (Aburahma et al. 2011). This resolves over time resulting in normalization of the biochemistry and often symptoms, and was historically called transient nonketotic hyperglycinemia (Aburahma et al. 2011; Aliefendioğlu et al. 2003). None of these differential diagnostic conditions has the full typical pattern of diffusion restriction on brain MRI, which can rapidly guide to the correct diagnosis (Stence et al. 2019). A peak of increased glycine, more in severe than in attenuated NKH patients, is noticeable on brain magnetic resonance spectroscopy (MRS) best recognizable in intermediate or long echo times (Stence et al. 2019).

## Glycine Transporter Defect (GLYT1, SLC6A9)

The glycine transporter GLYT1 is responsible for the transport of glycine into the astrocyte where it becomes accessible to the glycine cleavage enzyme. Its absence results in increased brain glycine (Kurolap et al. 2016).

Patients with the glycine transporter defect presented in the neonatal period (Kurolap et al. 2016; Alfadhel et al. 2016; Kurolap et al. 2017). Prenatal findings may include hydrops, polyhydramnios, and arthrogryposis (Kurolap et al. 2016; Alfadhel et al. 2016). In the neonatal period, they have severe hypotonia and poor breathing requiring prolonged ventilation, which they can only be weaned off after months. They can be encephalopathic and unresponsive. They have profound hypotonia and lack of almost all developmental progress. They have joint laxity or arthrogryposis, particularly club feet. They develop severe global developmental delays, axial hypotonia with peripheral spasticity, and contractures, some present since birth. They have sudden startle-like movements to any stimuli, but no seizures and are not accompanied by epileptic elements on EEG, and may represent hyperekplexia movements, which tends to resolve in late infancy.

They have normal levels of plasma glycine but mildly elevated levels of CSF glycine with an elevated CSF-plasma glycine ratio. Brain imaging can show ventriculomegaly, optic atrophy, thin or normal corpus callosum, and white matter abnormalities. Some have abnormal signal in the basal ganglia. A polyneuropathy and abnormal visual and auditory evoked potentials were reported. Many children have died in infancy (Kurolap et al. 2017).

## Nomenclature

| No. | Disorder | Alternative name | Abbreviation | Gene | Chromosomal location | Mode of inheritance | Affected protein | Disease OMIM# |
|---|---|---|---|---|---|---|---|---|
| 26.1 | Nonketotic hyperglycinemia | Severe nonketotic hyperglycinemia | NKH | *GLDC*<br>*AMT*<br>*GCSH* | 9p24.1<br>3p21.31<br>16q23.2 | AR | P-protein<br>T-protein<br>H-protein | 605899 |
| 26.2 | Nonketotic hyperglycinemia | Attenuated nonketotic hyperglycinemia | NKH | *GLDC*<br>*AMT*<br>*GCSH* | 9p24.1<br>3p21.31<br>16q23.2 | AR | P-protein<br>T-protein<br>H-protein | 605899 |
| 26.3 | Glycine transporter GLYT1 encephalopathy | Glycine encephalopathy with normal serum glycine | – | *SLC6A9* | 1p34.1 | AR | GLYT1-protein | 617301 |

Subtypes

- Severe nonketotic hyperglycinemia
- Attenuated nonketotic hyperglycinemia
  - Attenuated poor nonketotic hyperglycinemia
  - Attenuated intermediate nonketotic hyperglycinemia
  - Attenuated good nonketotic hyperglycinemia

## Metabolic Pathways

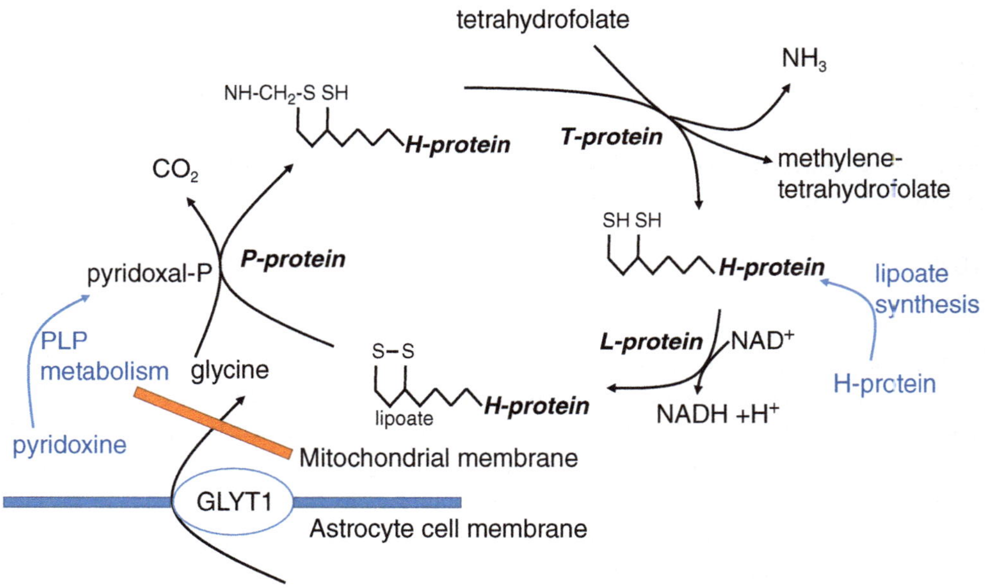


**Fig. 26.2** Metabolic pathways of glycine metabolism
Legend: Glycine is metabolized by the P-protein with pyridoxal-phosphate as cofactor. The T-protein transfers the methyl group to tetrahydrofolate synthesizing methylene-tetrahydrofolate. The L-protein reoxidizes the lipoate group, which is carried by the H-protein. The lipoate cofactor is synthesized on the H-protein in a multistep process

## Signs and Symptoms

**Table 26.1** Nonketotic hyperglycinemia, severe phenotype

| System | Symptoms and biomarkers | Neonatal (birth–1 month) | Infancy (1–18 months) | Childhood (1.5–11 years) | Adolescence (11–16 years) | Adulthood (>16 years) |
|---|---|---|---|---|---|---|
| CNS | Apnea | ++ | + | | | |
| | **Burst-suppression (EEG)** | +++ | ++ | | | |
| | Hiccups | ++ | ± | | | |
| | Hydrocephalus | + | + | + | + | |
| | **Hypoplasia, corpus callosum** | ++ | +++ | +++ | +++ | |
| | **Hypotonia** | +++ | ++ | ++ | ++ | |
| | **Hypsarrhythmia (EEG)** | **n** | ++ | | | |
| | Lethargy | +++ | +++ | ++ | + | |
| | **Multifocal epilepsy (EEG)** | + | ++ | +++ | +++ | |
| | Myoclonic epilepsy | ++ | ++ | + | + | |
| | Posterior fossa anormalies (MRI) | + | + | + | + | |
| | Retardation, psychomotor | +++ | +++ | +++ | +++ | |
| | **Seizures** | + | +++ | +++ | +++ | |
| | **Spasticity** | ± | ++ | +++ | +++ | |
| Digestive | Feeding difficulties | ++ | +++ | +++ | +++ | |
| Eye | Cortical blindness | + | ++ | ++ | ++ | |
| Musculoskeletal | Hip dysplasia | | | + | ++ | |
| | Scoliosis | | | ++ | ++ | |
| Respiratory | Difficulties airway management | + | + | ++ | +++ | |
| Other | Age at presentation | +++ | + | | | |
| Laboratory findings | Glycine (cerebrospinal fluid) | ↑↑ | ↑↑ | ↑↑ | ↑↑ | |
| | Glycine (CSF)/ Glycine (P) ratio | ↑↑ | ↑↑ | ↑↑ | ↑↑ | |
| | Glycine (plasma) | ↑↑ | ↑↑ | ↑↑ | ↑↑ | |

**Table 26.2** Nonketotic hyperglycinemia, attenuated phenotype

| System | Symptoms and biomarkers | Neonatal (birth–1 month) | Infancy (1–18 months) | Childhood (1.5–11 years) | Adolescence (11–16 years) | Adulthood (>16 years) |
|---|---|---|---|---|---|---|
| CNS | Apnea | ++ | ± | | | |
| | Ataxia | | ± | ± | ± | |
| | **Burst-suppression (EEG)** | ± | ± | | | |
| | Chorea | n | + | ++ | ++ | |
| | Episodic lethargy | + | + | ++ | ++ | |
| | Hiccups | ± | | | | |
| | Hydrocephalus | | | | | |
| | **Hypoplasia, corpus callosum** | ± | + | + | + | |
| | **Hypotonia** | ++ | ++ | ++ | + | |
| | Hypsarrhythmia (EEG) | | ± | | | |
| | Lethargy | + | + | + | + | |
| | Multifocal epilepsy (EEG) | + | + | + | + | |
| | Neurologic deterioration | ± | ± | ± | ± | |
| | Retardation, psychomotor | + | ++ | +++ | +++ | |
| | **Seizures** | ± | + | + | + | |
| | Spasticity | ± | ± | ± | ± | |
| | Hyperactivity | | + | +++ | +++ | |
| Psychiatric | Age at symptom onset | ++ | ++ | ± | | |
| Other | Glycine (cerebrospinal fluid) | ↑↑ | ↑↑ | ↑↑ | ↑↑ | |
| Laboratory findings | Glycine (CSF)-glycine (P) ratio | ↑↑ | ↑↑ | ↑↑ | ↑↑ | |
| | Glycine (plasma) | ↑ | ↑ | ↑ | ↑ | |

**Table 26.3** Glycine transporter 1 deficiency

| System | Symptoms and biomarkers | Neonatal (birth–1 month) | Infancy (1–18 months) | Childhood (1.5–11 years) | Adolescence (11–16 years) | Adulthood (>16 years) |
|---|---|---|---|---|---|---|
| CNS | **Apnea** | +++ | ++ | | | |
| | Coma | ++ | ++ | ++ | | |
| | **Developmental delay** | +++ | +++ | +++ | | |
| | **Hyperekplexia** | + | +++ | + | | |
| | Hypotonia | +++ | ++ | + | | |
| | **Increased startle** | + | +++ | + | | |
| | No seizures | + | + | + | | |
| | Polyneuropathy | ± | + | + | | |
| | **Spasticity** | +++ | +++ | +++ | | |
| | Thin corpus callosum | ± | ± | ± | | |
| | Ventriculomegaly | ± | ± | ± | | |
| Coma | Lethargy | ++ | ++ | ++ | | |
| Digestive | **Feeding difficulties** | +++ | +++ | +++ | | |
| Musculoskeletal | Contractures | +++ | ++ | ++ | | |
| Other | Age of symptom onset | +++ | + | | | |
| | Hydrops | ± | | | | |
| | Polyhydramnios | ± | | | | |
| Laboratory findings | Glycine (cerebrospinal fluid) | ↑ | ↑ | | | |
| | Glycine (CSF)-glycine (P) ratio | ↑ | ↑ | | | |
| | Glycine (plasma) | n | n | | | |

## Diagnostic Flowchart

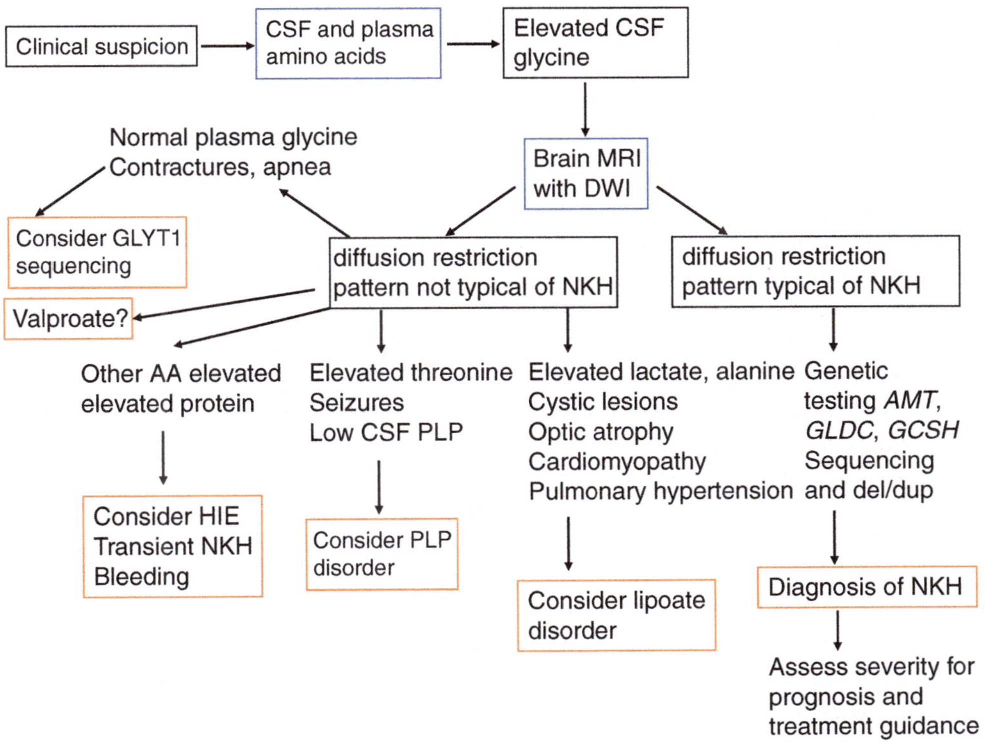


**Fig. 26.3** Diagnostic flowchart for children <3 months of age Legend: Upon clinical suspicion, CSF amino acids are obtained. A brain magnetic resonance imaging (MRI) with diffusion weighted images (DWI) is obtained when elevated CSF glycine is found. If a pattern of diffusion restriction typical of nonketotic hyperglycinemia (NKH) is identified, then molecular testing for genes of NKH can provide a confirmed diagnosis. If the pattern is not present or is different, then alternative diagnoses should be considered, such as GLYT1 disorder, valproate use, hypoxic ischemic injury (HIE) with blood-brain barrier damage, a disorder of pyridoxal-phosphate (PLP), or a disorder or lipoate synthesis and metabolism

## Reference Values

| Parameter | Control values <6 months | >6 months |
|---|---|---|
| Plasma glycine in µM | 125–450 | 125–350 |
| CSF glycine in µM | 3–20 | 3–12 |
| CSF-plasma glycine ratio | <0.02 | <0.02 |

## Pathological Values

| Parameter | Severe NKH | Attenuated NKH | GLYT1 |
|---|---|---|---|
| Plasma glycine in µM | 1133 (342–2363) | 822 (342–1590) | 228; 275 |
| CSF glycine in µM | 228 (40–510) | 99 (41–230) | 25 (21–31) |
| CSF-plasma glycine ratio | 0.22 (0.09–0.45) | 0.13 (0.04–0.22) | 0.07; 0.08 |

Values from: Swanson et al. (2015), Kurolap et al. (2016), and Alfadhel et al. (2016)

## Loading Tests

A glycine loading test shows higher glycine levels and lack of an expected rise in serine (von Wendt et al. 1978). A glycine breath test using $^{13}$C-glycine shows lack of increase in $^{13}CO_2$ exhalation (Kure et al. 2006).

## Specimen Collection

Plasma glycine: Obtain plasma glycine at least 3–4 h after a meal. It is elevated with the following: (1) valproate; (2) diet low in essential amino acids and increase in non-essential amino acids or kwashiorkor; (3) disorders of vitamin B6 pyridoxal phosphate including pyridoxine-dependent epilepsy due to mutations in *ALDH7A1*, pyridox(am)ine oxidase deficiency (*PNPO*), and pyridoxal binding protein PLPBP (*PROSC*); (4) severe liver failure, in particular with disseminated neonatal herpes infection; (5) exogenous loading with large amounts of glycine (e.g., certain immunoglobulins in a glycine buffer); (6) disorders of lipoate synthesis; and (7) newborns identified on newborn screening with very elevated glycine levels who remain asymptomatic; the cause is currently unknown.

CSF glycine: CSF glycine must be obtained on a clean tap (Korman and Gutman 2002). We recommend measuring all amino acids. The CSF glycine is increased in the following: (1) blood contamination or serum contamination (including at the level of the puncture or from intracranial bleeding)—look for elevated CSF protein and for elevation of CSF branched chain amino acids as an indicator; (2) use of valproate and to a small extent certain other anticonvulsants such as vigabatrin; (3) breakthrough of the blood-brain barrier, e.g., after hypoxic-ischemic injury (look for elevated branched chain amino acids); (4) mild elevation in certain neurological conditions such as vanishing white matter disease; mild elevations in disorders affecting the formation of pyridoxal-phosphate (pyridoxine-dependent epilepsy ALDH7A1, pyridox(am)ine oxidase deficiency (*PNPO*), and pyridoxal binding protein PLPBP (*PROSC*)); and (5) disorders affecting lipoate synthesis.

CSF-plasma glycine ratio: This ratio is calculated from a simultaneously obtained plasma and CSF glycine value. The ratio is increased in the same circumstances where CSF glycine is elevated.

## Prenatal Diagnosis

Prenatal diagnosis is almost always done by molecular analysis. This is possible in chorionic villus biopsy or amniocentesis. Preimplantation genetic diagnosis has also been successfully accomplished. For molecular diagnosis, the pathogenic variants in the family should be known, which is best performed prior to pregnancy. When only a single pathogenic variant is known, then intragenic linkage using intragenic single nucleotide polymorphisms can be done.

If the mutation is not known, then enzyme assays on chorionic villus biopsy are possible. A false-negative rate of at least 1% can occur, more commonly so in attenuated NKH or in NKH due to defects in the T-protein (Hennermann et al. 2012; Applegarth et al. 2000).

## DNA Testing Table and Sample Requirements

DNA testing can be done on blood or on any tissue.

Testing in *GLDC* requires sequencing, which can be either Sanger sequencing or next-generation sequencing. Copy number alternations occur in 20% of the alleles. These can be identified by gene-targeted microarray, by multiplex ligation-dependent probe amplification (MLPA), by quantitative PCR, or in some cases by next-generation sequencing at sufficient read depth. Rare, very long deletions have been identified by fluorescent in situ hybridization (FISH) or genome-wide microarray.

Testing in *AMT* requires sequencing, which can be either Sanger sequencing or next-generation sequencing. Care must be taken to include the 5′ UTR region as pathogenic mutations in this region have been reported (Coughlin II et al. 2017). Thus far, intragenic copy number alterations in this gene have not yet been reported, but labs often test for them using gene-targeted microarray or in some cases next-generation sequencing at sufficient read depth.

Testing in *GCSH* requires sequencing, which can be either Sanger sequencing or next-generation sequencing. No proven pathogenic mutation in *GCSH* has been reported. Large deletions encompassing the entire GCSH gene have been identified by fluorescent in situ hybridization (FISH) or genome-wide microarray.

Testing in *SLC6A9* requires sequencing, which can be either Sanger sequencing or next-generation sequencing. Limited information about the span of mutations in this condition has been reported thus far.

## Treatment Summary

Current treatment of nonketotic hyperglycinemia is based on decreasing glycine levels and by blocking the effect of the stimulation of glycine on the NMDA receptor (Van Hove et al. 2002).

Benzoate treatment is used to decrease plasma glycine levels. Benzoate is activated to benzoyl-Coenzyme A, which then conjugates with glycine to hippurate using glycine-N-acyltransferase, an enzyme only present in the liver and kidney, and hippurate is then excreted in urine. The dose of benzoate is increased and individually tailored to such an extent that glycine levels remain in a targeted treatment range of 120 to 300 μmol/L when obtained 1–2 h after a dose of benzoate. In infancy, very regular monitoring of plasma glycine levels is necessary for a safe and effective treatment. Patients with severe NKH require a higher dose (500–750 mg/kg/day) than patients with attenuated NKH (250–550 mg/kg/day) (Van Hove et al. 2005). Medication dosing should be divided in no less than three samples per day, more in infants, starting with six doses in neonates. Gastric irritation is common, and antacids, preferably proton pump inhibitors, are indicated (Hennermann et al. 2012). Some infants can have low carnitine levels which may require substitution (Van Hove et al. 1995). Overdosing of benzoate begins with nausea, vomiting, and hypocalcemia, but if severe can be very toxic and lethal. The contribution of dietary glycine to the overall metabolism of glycine is limited (Van Hove et al. 2005). Some reduction in glycine levels can be achieved through a glycine-restricted diet, but this is usually reserved for severe NKH already treated with high doses of benzoate. Dietary glycine restriction alone has no effect. A ketogenic diet, often initiated for anticonvulsant properties, strongly reduces glycine levels, and benzoate dosing should be appropriately reduced to avoid toxicity (Cusmaiu et al. 2012).

Blocking overstimulation of the NMDA receptor has been done with partial antagonists dextromethorphan or ketamine. High doses of dextromethorphan are used starting at 10 mg/kg/day in an infant, 5 mg/kg/day in a child, and 3 mg/kg/day in an adolescent or adult. Dosing is divided in three or four doses, but for the slow release version, twice daily dosing is possible. Pharmacogenomic differences in the metabolism of dextromethorphan at CYP2D6 and CYP3A4 should be taken into account, as for poor metabolizers the dose should be sharply reduced.

The clinical effect of the combination treatment of lowering plasma glycine levels with benzoate and of dextromethorphan has resulted in improvement in attenuated NKH in cognitive outcome and epilepsy when initiated in very early infancy (Bjoraker et al. 2016). In severe NKH, it results in improvements in alertness, breathing, and seizure control but does not prevent lack of development, therapy-resistant epilepsy, or spasticity (Hennermann et al. 2012). The role of dextromethorphan is very limited in severe NKH, whereas in some children with attenuated NKH, it can improve chorea and attentiveness (Van Hove et al. 2002). Benzoate treatment in attenuated NKH prevents episodic neurological depression. Up to 80% of neonatal presenting NKH patients have transient apnea, and the utility of intensive care treatment should be reviewed. Some families have elected to withdraw intensive care support during this time (Boneh et al. 2008). After resumption of breathing, some untreated infants may die in the next 2 years, but many survive long term (Hoover-Fong et al. 2004).

Seizure control is difficult in severe NKH. First-line treatment for neonates with myoclonic epilepsy treatment are benzodiazepine class medications in particular clobazam, with phenobarbital second. Later seizures respond variably to medications. Valproate, which inhibits the glycine cleavage enzyme, and vigabatrin should be avoided as severe neurological regressions have been reported. Ketogenic diet has variable success on infantile spasms but rarely controls the hypsarrhythmic background (Cusmaiu et al. 2012). Older patients with difficult to control seizures have responded to vagal nerve stimulator.

Symptomatic treatment in severe NKH includes placement of a gastric tube to enable feeding, monitoring, and as needed surgical treatment for scoliosis and hip dislocation (Hennermann et al. 2012; Hoover-Fong et al. 2004; Ramirez et al. 2012). Maintaining good airway management is essential for older children with severe NKH.

Treatment of GLYT1 deficiency is symptomatic. Treatment with sodium benzoate and dextromethorphan has no effect. Ventilatory support may need to be continued for several months, but most infants can eventually be weaned. Hyperekplexia responds to benzodiazepines. Tone management is important and physical therapy is usually indicated, and most children require gastrostomy feeding (Kurolap et al. 2017; Alfallaj and Alfadhel 2019).

## Experimental Treatment

Treatment with increased co-factors can sometimes improve activity. Treatment of patients with missense mutations in GLDC have occasionally responded to treatment with pyridoxal phosphate with increased cognitive abilities. However, in most no effect is seen, and occasional worsening of chorea and behavior is known. Treatment of patients with missense mutations in AMT has occasionally appeared to improve to treatment with folinic acid.

## Follow-Up and Monitoring

It is essential that patients treated with benzoate have regular plasma glycine levels monitored, and medication dosage should be adjusted frequently in infancy. Glycine levels should be obtained 1–2 h after a dose of benzoate. Occasional monitoring of carnitine levels is appropriate in benzoate-treated infants. The changing epileptic propensity in infancy requires frequent neurological and, as indicated, EEG monitoring. Older children with severe NKH should be monitored for orthopedic problems and for airway management.

## Online Resources

GLYT1 Encephalopathy: GeneReviews: accessible at: https://www.ncbi.nlm.nih.gov/books/NBK465013/

Nonketotic hyperglycinemia: GeneReviews: accessible at: https://www.ncbi.nlm.nih.gov/books/NBK1357/

NKH Crusaders, accessible at: https://www.nkhcrusaders.com/

Joseph's goal, accessible at: http://www.josephsgoal.org/

## References


Aburahma S, Khassawneh M, Griebel M, Sharp G, Gibson J. Pitfalls in measuring cerebrospinal fluid glycine levels in infants with encephalopathy. J Child Neurol. 2011;26:703–6.

Alfadhel M, Nashabat M, Qahtani HA, Alfares A, Mutairi FA, Shaalan HA, Douglas GV, Wieringa K, Juusola J, Alrifai MT, Arold ST, Alkuraya F, Ali QA. Mutation in SLC6A9 encoding a glycine transporter causes a novel form of non-ketotic hyperglycinemia in humans. Hum Genet. 2016;135:1263–8.

Alfallaj R, Alfadhel M. Glycine transporter 1 encephalopathy from biochemical Pathway to clinical disease: review. Child Neurol Open. 2019;6:2329048X19831486.

Aliefendioğlu D, Aslan AT, Coşkun T, Dursun A, Çakmak FN, Keismer M. Transient nonketotic hyperglycinemia: two case reports and literature review. Pediatr Neurol. 2003;28:151–5.

Applegarth DA, Toone JR, Rolland MO, Black SH, Yim DK, Bemis G. Non-concordance of CVS and liver glycine cleavage enzyme in three families with non-ketotic hyperglycinemia (NKH) leading to false negative prenatal diagnoses. Prenat Diagn. 2000;20:367–70.

Baker PR, Friederich MW, Swanson MA, Shaikh T, Battacharya K, Scharer GH, Aicher J, Creadon-Swindell G, Geiger E, MacLean KN, Lee W-T, Deshpande C, Freckmann M-L, Shih L-Y, Wasserstein M, Rasmussen MB, Lund AM, Procopis P, Cameron JM, Robinson BH, Brown GK, Brown RM, Compton AG, Dieckmann CL, Collard R, Coughlin CR II, Spector E, Wempe MF, Van Hove JLK. Variant nonketotic hyperglycinaemia is caused by mutations in *LIAS*, *BOLA3*, and the novel gene *GLRX5*. Brain. 2014;173(Pt 2): 366–79.

Bjoraker KJ, Swanson MA, Coughlin CR II, Christodoulou J, Tan ES, Fergeson M, Dyack S, Ahmad A, Friederich MW, Spector E, Creadon-Swindell G, Hodge MA, Gaughan S, Burns C, Van Hove JLK. Neurodevelopmental outcome and treatment efficacy of benzoate and dextromethorphan in siblings with attenuated Nonketotic hyperglycinemia. J Pediatr. 2016;170:234–9.

Boneh A, Allen S, Mendelson D, Spriggs M, Gillam LH, Korman SH. Clinical, ethical and legal considerations in the treatment of newborns with non-ketotic hyperglycinaemia. Mol Genet Metab. 2008;94:143–7.

Coughlin CR II, Swanson MA, Kronquist K, Acquaviva C, Hutchin T, Rodriguez-Pombo P, Vaisänen M-L, Spector E, Creadon-Swindell G, Brás-Goldberg A, Rahikkala E, Moilanen JS, Mahieu V, Matthijs G, Bravo-Alonso I, Pérez-Cerdá C, Ugarte M, Vianey-Saban C, Scharer GH, Van Hove JLK. The genetic basis of classic nonketotic hyperglycinemia due to mutations in GLDC and AMT. Genet Med. 2017;19:104–11.

Cusmaiu R, Martinelli D, Moavero R, Dionisi Vici C, Vigevano F, Castaa C, Elia M, Bernabei S, Bevivino E. Ketogenic diet in early myoclonic encephalopathy due to non ketotic hyperglycinemia. Eur J Paediatr Neurol. 2012;16:509–13.

Hennermann JB, Berger J-M, Grieben U, Scharer G, Van Hove JLK. Prediction of long-term outcome in glycine encephalopathy: a clinical survey. J Inherit Metab Dis. 2012;35:253–61.

Hoover-Fong JE, Shah S, Van Hove JLK, Applegarth D, Toone J, Hamosh A. Natural history of nonketotic hyperglycinemia in 65 patients. Neurology. 2004;63:1847–53.

Korman SH, Gutman A. Pitfalls in the diagnosis of glycine encephalopathy (non-ketotic hyperglycinemia). Dev Med Child Neurol. 2002;44:712–20.

Kure S, Korman SH, Kanno J, Narisawa A, Kubota M, Takayanagi T, Takayanagi M, Saito T, Matsui A, Kamada F, Aoki Y, Ohura T, Matsubara Y. Rapid diagnosis of glycine encephalopathy by 13C-glycine breath test. Ann Neurol. 2006;59:862–7.

Kurolap A, Ambruster A, Hershkovitz T, Hauf K, Mory A, Paperna T, Hannapel E, Tal G, Nijem Y, Sella E, Mahajnah M, Ilivitzki A, Harshkovitz D, Ekhilevitch N, Mandel H, Eulenburg V, Baris HN. Loss of glycine transporter 1 causes a subtype of glycine encephalopathy with arthrogryposis and mildly elevated cerebrospinal fluid glycine. Am J Hum Genet. 2016;99:1172–80.

Kurolap A, Hershkovitz T, Baris HN. GLYT1 encephalopathy. In: Adam MP, Ardinger HH, Pagon RA, Wallace SE, Bean LJH, Stephens K, Amemiya A, editors. GeneReviews® [internet]. Seattle, WA: University of Washington, Seattle; 2017. p. 1993–2020.

Ramirez N, Flynn JM, Csalduc F, Rodriguez S, Cornier AS, Calro S. Musculoskeletal manifestations of neonatal nonketotic hyperglycinemia. J Child Orthop. 2012;6:199–203.

Stence NV, Fenton LZ, Levek C, Tong S, Coughlin CR II, Hennermann JB, Wortmann SB, Van Hove JLK. Brain imaging in classic nonketotic hyperglycinemia: quantitative analysis and relation to phenotype. J Inherit Metab Dis. 2019;42:438–50.

Swanson MA, Coughlin CR II, Scharer GH, Szerlong HJ, Bjoraker KJ, Spector EB, Creadon-Swindell G, Mahieu V, Matthijs G, Hennermann JB, Applegarth DA, Toone JR, Tong S, Williams K, Van Hove JLK, Swanson MA, et al. Biochemical and molecular predictors for prognosis in nonketotic hyperglycinemia. Ann Neurol. 2015;78:606–18.

Van Hove JL, Coughlin C, Swanson M, Hennermann JB. Nonketotic hyperglycinemia. In: Adam MP, Ardinger HH, Pagon RA, Wallace SE, Bean LJH, Stephens K, Amemiya A, editors. GeneReviews® [internet]. Seattle, WA: University of Washington, Seattle; 2002. p. 1993–2019, [Updated 2019 May 23].

Van Hove JLK, Kishnani PS, Demaerel P, Kahler SG, Miller C, Jaeken J, Rutledge SL. Acute hydrocephalus in nonketotic hyperglycinemia. Neurology. 2000;54:754–6.

Van Hove JLK, Kishnani P, Muenzer J, Wenstrup RJ, Summar ML, Brummond MR, Lachiewicz AM, Millington DS, Kahler SG. Benzoate therapy and carnitine deficiency in non-ketotic hyperglycinemia. Am J Med Genet. 1995;59:444–53.

Van Hove JLK, Vande Kerckhove K, Hennermann JB, Mahieu V, Declercq P, Mertens S, De Becker M, Kishnani PS, Jaeken J. Benzoate treatment and the glycine index in nonketotic hyperglycinaemia. J Inherit Metab Dis. 2005;28:651–63.

von Wendt L, Similä S, Hirvasniemi A, Suvanto E. Nonketotic hyperglycinemia. A clinical analysis of 19 Finnish patients. Monogr Hum Genet. 1978;9:58–64.

Wilson MP, Plecko B, Mills PB, Clayton PT. Disorders affecting vitamin $B_6$ metabolism. J Inherit Metab Dis. 2019;42(4):629–46.

# Disorders of Lipoic Acid and Iron-Sulfur Protein Metabolism

# 27

Antonia Ribes and Frederic Tort

## Contents



**Summary**

Iron-sulfur (Fe-S) clusters are one of the most ancient, ubiquitous, and versatile classes of metal cofactors found in nature. In contrast to its simple structure, the biogenesis of Fe-S clusters is an extremely complex process. It involves a large number of proteins necessary for assembly, maturation, and delivery of Fe-S to their target proteins, including subunits of the mitochondrial respiratory chain complexes I, II, and III, aconitase, heme biosynthesis, and lipoic acid synthase (LIAS). Lipoic acid (LA) is an essential cofactor required for the activity of five multienzyme complexes (the 2-oxoacid dehydrogenase complexes and the glycine cleavage system) that play a central role in the mitochondrial energy metabolism. Four well-defined clinical entities, Friedreich ataxia, myopathy with lactic acidosis and exercise intolerance (ISCU), X-linked sideroblastic anemia with ataxia (ABCB7), and sideroblastic anemia associated with particular mutations in GLRX5, were the first-described diseases related to Fe-S cluster biosynthesis or transport defects. However, the progress in the knowledge of these diseases started when two parallel and independent studies identified mutations in the genes encoding for the Fe-S cluster proteins NFU1 and BOLA3, in patients with a fatal mitochondrial encephalopathy, lactic acidemia, hyperglycinemia, and deficiencies in the activity of LA-dependent enzymes. Later on, new diseases with similar clinical and biochemical characteristics were described. LA supplementation has been speculated as a potential treatment for patients with lipoic acid deficiency, but eukaryotic cells cannot use exogenously supplied LA. Therefore, for the moment, no specific treatment is available. This chapter focuses on the diagnosis and clinical description of 17 diseases due to lipoic acid and iron sulfur cluster biogenesis defects.

A. Ribes (✉) · F. Tort
Section of Inborn Errors of Metabolism-IBC, Department of Biochemistry and Molecular Genetics, Hospital Clínic de Barcelona, CIBERER, Barcelona, Spain
e-mail: aribes@clinic.cat; ftort@ciberer.es


N. Blau et al. (eds.), *Physician's Guide to the Diagnosis, Treatment, and Follow-Up of Inherited Metabolic Diseases*,
https://doi.org/10.1007/978-3-030-67727-5_27

## Introduction

Iron-sulfur (Fe-S) clusters are one of the most ancient, ubiquitous, and versatile classes of metal cofactors found in nature. Proteins that contain Fe-S clusters constitute one of the largest protein families that are localized within mitochondria, cytosol, and nucleus (Stehling et al. 2014). The biogenesis of Fe-S clusters is performed by two main protein machineries, the mitochondrial iron-sulfur cluster (ISC) assembly system and the cytosolic iron-sulfur protein assembly (CIA) machinery. The most common stoichiometric species of Fe-S include [2Fe-2S], [3Fe-4S], and [4Fe-4S] (Lill et al. 2012). The biogenesis is Fe-S is a complex process and involves a large number of proteins necessary for assembly, maturation, and delivery of Fe-S clusters to their target proteins, including subunits of the mitochondrial respiratory chain; complexes I,II, and III; aconitase; heme biosynthesis; and lipoic acid synthase (Stehling et al. 2014). As indicated in Fig. 27.1, de novo synthesis of [2Fe-2S] cluster is accomplished on the scaffold protein, ISCU. Ferrous iron is imported into the mitochondria through the MFRN1 transporter and with the participation of FXN is delivered to ISCU. The sulfur required for Fe-S synthesis is provided by the conversion of a cysteine to alanine, a reaction catalyzed by the NFS1-ISD11 desulfurase complex. Then, the coordinated action of FDX1, FDX2, and FDXR allows the final assembly of the [2Fe-2S] cluster on the ISCU scaffold protein. After that, the [2Fe-2S] cluster is released from the scaffold protein by the action of a chaperone system (HSCB, GRPEL1, HSPA9) and GLXR5 protein. On the other hand, the [2Fe-2S] cluster can be directly used for the assembly of [2Fe–2S] proteins (such as complex III subunits), or exported to the cytosol through the ABCB7 transporter to take part in the CIA machinery, or delivered to the IBA57-ISCA1-ISCA2 complex for maturation to [4Fe–4S] clusters. The mature [4Fe–4S] clusters are specifically delivered to target proteins by the action of late-acting factors, such as NFU1 and BOLA3. These proteins are required for the proper assembly of mitochondrial respiratory chain complexes I and II as well as for lipoic acid synthase (LIAS) activity, the enzyme responsible of lipoic acid (LA) synthesis. LA is an essential cofactor required for the activity of five multienzymatic complexes that play a central role in the mitochondrial energy metabolism: the 2-oxoacid dehydrogenase complexes (pyruvate dehydrogenase, 2-ketoglutarate dehydrogenase, 2-oxoadipate dehydrogenase, and branched-chain ketoacid dehydrogenase) and the glycine cleavage system (GCS). The activity of these enzymes depends exclusively on de novo intramitochondrial LA synthesis, which requires the appropriate function of LIAS, LIPT1, and LIPT2. In addition, the mitochondrial fatty acid synthesis (mtFASII) and the biogenesis of iron-sulfur (Fe-S) clusters are also essential for LA synthesis (Tort et al. 2016). Therefore, it is not surprising that mutations in genes involved in LA biosynthesis could potentially lead to multiple and severe defects of the mitochondrial energy metabolism.

## Nomenclature

| No. | Disease name | Alternative disease name | Disease abbreviation | Gene symbol | Chromosomal localization | Mode of inheritance | Affected protein | Disease OMIM |
|---|---|---|---|---|---|---|---|---|
| 27.1 | Lipoyltransferase 2 deficiency | Neonatal severe encephalopathy with lactic acidosis and brain abnormalities | NELABA | *LIPT2* | 11q13.4 | AR | Lipoyl(octanoyl)transferase 2 (LIPT2) | 617668 |
| 27.2 | Lipoic acid synthase deficiency | Hyperglycinemia, lactic acidosis, and seizures | HGCLAS | *LIAS* | 4p14 | AR | Lipoic acid synthase (LIAS) | 614462 |
| 27.3 | Lipoyltransferase 1 deficiency | – | LIPT1D | *LIPT1* | 2q11.2 | AR | Lipoyltransferase 1 (LIPT1) | 616299 |
| 27.4 | NFU1 deficiency | Multiple mitochondrial dysfunction syndrome type 1 | MMDS1 | *NFU1* | 2p13.3 | AR | NFU1 Iron-sulfur cluster scaffold (NFU1) | 605711 |
| 27.5 | BOLA3 deficiency | Multiple mitochondrial dysfunction syndrome type 2 | MMDS2 | *BOLA3* | 2p13.1 | AR | BolA family member 3 (BOLA3) | 614299 |
| 27.6 | Glutaredoxin 5 deficiency | Spasticity, childhood-onset, with hyperglycinemia | SPAHGC | *GLRX5* | 14q32.13 | AR | Glutaredoxin 5 (GLRX5) | 616859 |
| 27.6 | Glutaredoxin 5 deficiency | Pyridoxine-refractory sideroblastic anemia type 3 | SIDBA3 | *GLRX5* | 14q32.13 | AR | Glutaredoxin 5 (GLRX5) | 616860 |
| 27.7 | IBA57 deficiency | Multiple mitochondrial dysfunction syndrome type 3 | MMDS3 | *IBA57* | 1q42.13 | AR | Iron-sulfur cluster assembly factor IBA57 (IBA57) | 615330 |
| 27.7 | IBA57 deficiency | Spastic paraplegia 74, autosomal recessive | SPG74 | *IBA57* | 1q42.13 | AR | Iron-sulfur cluster assembly factor IBA57 (IBA57) | 616451 |
| 27.8 | ISCA1 deficiency | Multiple mitochondrial dysfunctions syndrome type 5 | MMDS5 | *ISCA1* | 9q21.33 | AR | Iron-sulfur cluster assembly 1 (ISCA1) | 617613 |
| 27.9 | ISCA2 deficiency | Multiple mitochondrial dysfunctions syndrome type 4 | MMDS4 | *ISCA2* | 14q24.3 | AR | Iron-sulfur cluster assembly 2 (ISCA2) | 616370 |
| 27.10 | ISCU deficiency | Hereditary myopathy with lactic acidosis, Swedish type myopathy with exercise intolerance | HML | *ISCU* | 12q23.3 | AD, AR | Iron-sulfur cluster assembly enzyme ISCU | 255125 |
| 27.11 | ABCB7 deficiency | Sideroblastic anemia and spinocerebellar ataxia | ASAT | *ABCB7* | Xq13.3 | XLR | ATP binding cassette subfamily B member 7 (ABCB7) | 301310 |
| 27.12 | Ferredoxin 2 deficiency | Mitochondrial myopathy, episodic, with optic atrophy and reversible leukoencephalopathy | MEOAL | *FDX1L* | 19p13.2 | AR | Ferredoxin 2 (FDX2) | 251900 |
| 27.13 | Ferredoxin reductase deficiency | Auditory neuropathy and optic atrophy | ANOA | *FDXR* | 17q25.1 | AR | Ferredoxin reductase (FDXR) | 617717 |
| 27.14 | ISD11 deficiency | Combined oxidative phosphorylation deficiency 19 | COXPD19 | *LYRM4* | 6p25.1 | AR | ISD11 | 615595 |
| 27.15 | NFS1 deficiency | Infantile mitochondrial complex II/III deficiency | IMC23D | *NFS1* | 20q11.22 | AR | NFS1 cysteine Desulfurase (NFS1) | 603485 |
| 27.16 | Frataxin deficiency | Friedreich ataxia | FRDA | *FXN* | 9q21.11 | AR | Frataxin (FXN) | 229300 |
| 27.17 | HSPA9 deficiency | Sideroblastic anemia type 4; | SIDBA4 | *HSPA9* | 5q31.2 | AR | Heat shock 70 kDa protein 9 (Mortalin) (HSPA9) | 182170 |
| 27.17 | HSPA9 deficiency | Epiphyseal, vertebral, ear, nose, plus associated malformations (EVEN-plus) syndrome | EVPLS | *HSPA9* | 5q31.2 | AR | Heat shock 70 kDa protein 9 (Mortalin) (HSPA9) | 616854 |

## Metabolic Pathway

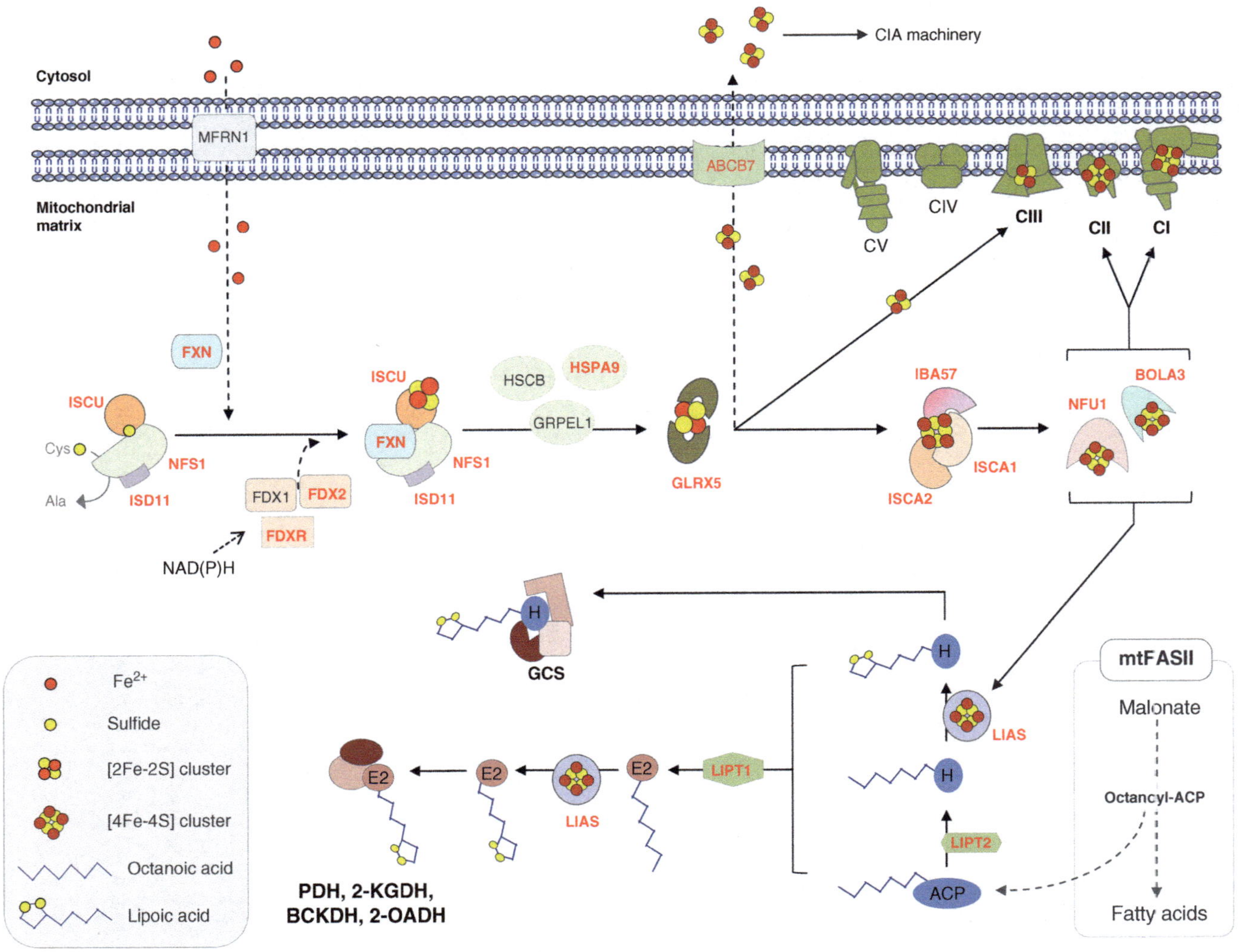


**Fig. 27.1** Fe-S Clusters and Lipoic Acid Synthesis Pathways
The synthesis of Fe-S is orchestrated by a complex molecular machinery and consists of three main steps: (1) iron import into the mitochondria and assembly of the [2Fe–2S] clusters on the ISCU scaffold protein, (2) maturation of the [2Fe–2S] clusters, and (3) delivery of the [2Fe–2S] and [4Fe–4S] clusters to their target proteins, by the action of late-acting factors. During this process Fe-S clusters can also be specifically exported to the cytosol to be incorporated to the cytosolic and nuclear proteins, through CIA machinery. Fe-S clusters are essential for the activity of a wide variety of enzymes, including several subunits of the mitochondrial respiratory chain complexes I, II, and III and also for other processes such as LA synthesis, a reaction catalyzed by LIAS. LA is synthetized in a multistep process that, in addition to Fe-S cluster biogenesis, requires the proper function of the mtFASII, a complex biochemical pathway that synthesizes saturated fatty acids from mevalonate. Octanoic acid bound to ACP is transferred to the H protein of the GCS by the action LIPT2. The octanoylated H protein is the substrate for the insertion of two sulfur atoms at C-6 and C-8 positions by LIAS. LIPT1 is responsible for the octanoylation and the subsequent lipoylation of the E2 subunits of the 2-oxoacid dehydrogenase complexes (PDH, 2-KGDH, BCKDH, and 2-OADH)
Fe-S cluster and lipoic acid metabolism enzymes associated with human disease are highlighted in red color
CIA, cytosolic iron-sulfur cluster assembly; CI-V, mitochondrial respiratory chain complexes I–V; mtFASII, mitochondrial fatty acid synthesis pathway; ACP, acyl-carrier protein; LIAS, lipoic acid synthase; LIPT1, lipoyltransferase 1; LIPT2, lipoyl(octanoyl) transferase 2; PDH, pyruvate dehydrogenase; BCKDH, branched-chain ketoacid dehydrogenase; 2-KGDH, 2-ketoglutarate dehydrogenase; 2-OADH, 2-oxoadipate dehydrogenase; GCS, glycine cleavage system

## Signs and Symptoms

**Table 27.1** Lipoyltransferase 2 deficiency

| System | Symptoms and biomarkers | Neonatal (birth–1 month) | Infancy (1–18 months) | Childhood (1.5–11 years) | Adolescence (11–16 years) | Adulthood (>16 years) |
|---|---|---|---|---|---|---|
| Cardiovascular | **Ventricular dilatation** | +++ | | | | |
| CNS | Abnormal EEG | ± | | | | |
| | **Cortical atrophy with white matter abnormalities and cysts** | +++ | | | | |
| | Dystonia | ± | | | | |
| | **Encephalopathy** | +++ | | | | |
| | Epilepsy | ± | | | | |
| | Hypotonia | ++ | | | | |
| | Microcephaly | ± | | | | |
| | Tetraparesis | ± | | | | |
| Respiratory | Respiratory distress | ± | | | | |
| Laboratory findings | 2-Ketoglutarate dehydrogenase (fibroblasts) | ↓↓↓ | | | | |
| | Complexes I–IV (fibroblasts) | n | | | | |
| | Glycine (plasma) | ↑ | | | | |
| | Lactate (cerebrospinal fluid) | ↑ | | | | |
| | Lactate (plasma) | ↑↑ | | | | |
| | Lactate (urine) | ↑↑ | | | | |
| | Protein-bound lipoic acid (fibroblasts) | ↓↓↓ | | | | |
| | Pyruvate dehydrogenase (fibroblasts) | ↓↓↓ | | | | |

**Table 27.2** Lipoic acid synthase deficiency

| System | Symptoms and biomarkers | Neonatal (birth–1 month) | Infancy (1–18 months) | Childhood (1.5–11 years) | Adolescence (11–16 years) | Adulthood (>16 years) |
|---|---|---|---|---|---|---|
| CNS | **Brain atrophy of the white matter** | ++ | | ++ | | ++ |
| | Delayed motor and mental development | | | + | | +++ |
| | **Hypotonia** | ++ | | ++ | | |
| | Involuntary movements | | | ± | | |
| | Microcephaly | | | + | | |
| | **Seizures** | +++ | | +++ | | +++ |
| Digestive | Feeding difficulties | + | | ++ | | +++ |
| Laboratory findings | Complexes I–IV (muscle, fibroblasts) | n | | | | |
| | Glycine (cerebrospinal fluid) | ↑↑ | | ↑↑ | | |
| | Glycine (plasma) | ↑↑ | | ↑↑ | | |
| | Glycine (urine) | ↑↑ | | | | |
| | Lactate (plasma) | ↑↑ | | n-↑ | | |
| | Protein-bound lipoic acid (fibroblasts) | ↓↓↓ | | | | |
| | Pyruvate dehydrogenase (fibroblasts) | ↓↓↓ | | | | |

**Table 27.3** Lipoyltransferase 1 deficiency

| System | Symptoms and biomarkers | Neonatal (birth–1 month) | Infancy (1–18 months) | Childhood (1.5–11 years) | Adolescence (11–16 years) | Adulthood (>16 years) |
|---|---|---|---|---|---|---|
| Cardiovascular | Bradycardia | ± | ± | | | |
| CNS | Cortical atrophy (MRI) | | ± | + + + | | |
| | **Delayed myelination** | | + | + + + | | |
| | Dystonia | ± | ± | | | |
| | Hypertonia | ± | | | | |
| | Hypotonia | | ± | + | | |
| | Irritability | | ± | | | |
| | Leigh syndrome | | + + + | | | |
| | **Psychomotor delay** | | + + + | + | | |
| | **Seizures** | | + + + | ± | | |
| | **Spastic tetraparesis** | | + + + | ± | | |
| Digestive | Vomiting | | + + + | | | |
| Pulmonary | Pulmonary hypertension | ± | | | | |
| Respiratory | Respiratory distress | ± | | | | |
| Others | Dehydration | ± | ± | | | |
| Laboratory findings | 2-Ketoglutarate (urine) | ↑↑↑ | ↑↑ | ↑↑ | | |
| | 2-Ketoglutarate dehydrogenase (fibroblasts) | | ↓↓ | ↓-n | | |
| | Alanine (cerebrospinal fluid) | | n-↑ | | | |
| | Alanine (plasma) | ↑↑ | ↑↑ | ↑↑ | | |
| | Alanine (urine) | | ↑↑ | | | |
| | ASAT/ALAT (plasma) | ↑↑ | ↑↑ | | | |
| | Glutamic acid (plasma) | | ↑↑ | n-↑ | | |
| | Glycine (cerebrospinal fluid) | n | n | | | |
| | Glycine (plasma) | n | n | n | | |
| | Glycine (urine) | n | n | | | |
| | Lactate (plasma) | ↑↑ | ↑↑ | ↑↑ | | |
| | Lactate (urine) | ↑↑↑ | ↑↑↑ | ↑↑ | | |
| | Proline (plasma) | ↑↑ | ↑↑ | n-↑ | | |
| | Protein-bound lipoic acid (fibroblasts) | ↓↓↓ | ↓↓↓ | ↓↓↓ | | |
| | Pyruvate dehydrogenase (fibroblasts) | ↓↓ | ↓↓ | ↓↓ | | |

**Table 27.4** NFU1 deficiency

| System | Symptoms and biomarkers | Neonatal (birth–1 month) | Infancy (1–18 months) | Childhood (1.5–11 years) | Adolescence (11–16 years) | Adulthood (>16 years)[a] |
|---|---|---|---|---|---|---|
| CNS | Cerebral atrophy (MRI) | | + + | | | |
| | **Cystic leukoencephalopathy** | | + + | | | |
| | Dystonia | | ± | | | |
| | Epileptic seizures | | ± | | | |
| | Hypotonia | | ± | | | |
| | Intellectual disability | | + + | | | |
| | Lethargy | + ++ | | | | |
| | **Leukodystrophy** | | + + | | | |
| | **Neurological regression** | | + + + | | | |
| | Spastic paraparesis | | | | | + |
| | Spasticity | | + | | | + |
| | Subacute demyelinating mixed motor sensory neuropathy | | | | | + |
| Digestive | Feeding difficulties | + ++ | | | | |
| Musculoskeletal | Scoliosis | | | | | + |
| | Weakness | + ++ | | | | |
| Pulmonary | **Pulmonary hypertension** | | + + | | | n |

**Table 27.4** (continued)

| System | Symptoms and biomarkers | Neonatal (birth–1 month) | Infancy (1–18 months) | Childhood (1.5–11 years) | Adolescence (11–16 years) | Adulthood (>16 years)[a] |
|---|---|---|---|---|---|---|
| Other | Failure to thrive | | + + | | | |
| | Stress-induced deterioration followed by partial recovery | | | | | + |
| | Unable to walk | | | | | + |
| Laboratory findings | 2-Hydroxyadipate (urine) | | n-↑ | | | |
| | 2-Hydroxyglutarate (urine) | | n-↑ | | | |
| | 2-Ketoadipate (urine) | | ↑ | | | |
| | 2-Ketoglutarate (urine) | | ↑↑ | | | |
| | 2-Ketoglutarate dehydrogenase (fibroblasts) | ↓↓↓ | ↓↓ | | | ↓↓↓ |
| | Complexes I–II (muscle, fibroblasts) | ↓↓ | ↓↓ | | | ↓-n |
| | Glutamic acid (plasma) | | ↑ | | | |
| | Glycine (cerebrospinal fluid) | | ↑↑↑ | | | ↑↑ |
| | Glycine (plasma) | ↑↑↑ | ↑↑↑ | | | ↑↑ |
| | Glycine (urine) | | ↑↑↑ | | | ↑↑ |
| | Lactate (cerebrospinal fluid) | | ↑ | | | |
| | Lactate (plasma) | ↑↑ | ↑ | | | n-↑ |
| | Lactate (urine) | ↑↑ | n-↑ | | | |
| | Protein-bound lipoic acid (fibroblasts) | ↓↓↓ | ↓↓↓ | | | |
| | Pyruvate dehydrogenase (fibroblasts) | ↓↓↓ | ↓↓ | | | ↓↓↓ |

[a]Only one adulthood patient

**Table 27.5** BOLA3 deficiency

| System | Symptoms and biomarkers | Neonatal (birth–1 month) | Infancy (1–18 months) | Childhood (1.5–11 years) | Adolescence (11–16 years) | Adulthood (>16 years) |
|---|---|---|---|---|---|---|
| Cardiovascular | **Cardiomyopathy** | + + + | + + + | | | |
| CNS | Developmental delay | | + + | | | |
| | Dystonia | | + | | | |
| | Hypotonia | | + + | | | |
| | Irritability | | ± | | | |
| | Lethargy | | ± | | | |
| | **Leukodystrophy** | | + + + | | | |
| | **Leukoencephalopathy** | + + | + + + | | | |
| | **Neurological regression** | | + + | | | |
| | **Seizures, myoclonic** | | + + + | | | |
| | Spasticity | | ± | | | |
| Digestive | Feeding difficulties | + + + | ± | | | |
| | Hepatomegaly | | ± | | | |
| Eye | Optic atrophy | | + + | | | |
| Respiratory | Respiratory distress | | ± | | | |
| Others | Failure to thrive | + + | + | | | |
| Laboratory findings | 2-ketoglutarate dehydrogenase (fibroblasts) | | ↓ | | | |
| | Complexes I–III (muscle, fibroblasts) | ↓ | ↓ | | | |
| | Glycine (cerebrospinal fluid) | | ↑↑↑ | | | |
| | Glycine (plasma) | ↑ | ↑↑ | | | |
| | Lactate (cerebrospinal fluid) | ↑↑↑ | ↑↑↑ | | | |
| | Lactate (plasma) | ↑↑↑ | ↑↑↑ | | | |
| | Lactate (urine) | ↑↑↑ | | | | |
| | Protein-bound lipoic acid (fibroblasts) | | ↓-n | | | |
| | Pyruvate dehydrogenase (fibroblasts) | ↓ | ↓↓ | | | |

**Table 27.6** Glutaredoxin 5 deficiency

| System | Symptoms and biomarkers | Neonatal (birth–1 month) | Infancy (1–18 months) | Childhood (1.5–11 years) | Adolescence (11–16 years) | Adulthood (>16 years) |
|---|---|---|---|---|---|---|
| CNS | Cervical spinal cord lesions | | | + | | |
| | Spasticity | | | + ++ | | |
| Eye | Nystagmus | | | ± | | |
| | Optic atrophy | | | ± | | |
| Hematological | **Anemia, sideroblastic** | | | | | + ++ |
| Laboratory findings | Complexes I–III (muscle, fibroblasts) | | | ↓-n | | |
| | Ferritin (serum) | | | | | ↑ |
| | Glycine (cerebrospinal fluid) | | | ↑ | | |
| | Glycine (plasma) | | | ↑ | | |
| | Lactate (cerebrospinal fluid) | | | n-↑ | | |
| | Lactate (plasma) | | | n-↑ | | |
| | Protein-bound lipoic acid (fibroblasts) | | | ↓ | | |
| | Pyruvate dehydrogenase (fibroblasts) | | | ↓ | | |
| | Transferrin (serum) | | | | | ↑ |

**Table 27.7** IBA57 deficiency

| System | Symptoms and biomarkers | Neonatal (birth–1 month)[a] | Infancy (1–18 months) | Childhood (1.5–11 years)[b] | Adolescence (11–16 years) | Adulthood (>16 years) |
|---|---|---|---|---|---|---|
| CNS | Cerebral atrophy (MRI) | + ++ | + + | | | |
| | Epileptic seizures | | ± | | | |
| | Hypotonia | + ++ | + + | | | |
| | **Intellectual disability** | | + + | | | |
| | **Leukodystrophy** | | + + + | | | |
| | Neuropathy, peripheral | | | + ++ | | |
| | Spastic paraplegia | | | + ++ | | |
| | Spastic tetraparesis | | + | | | |
| Digestive | **Feeding difficulties** | | + ++ | | | |
| Eye | Optic atrophy | | | + ++ | | |
| Respiratory | Respiratory insufficiency | + ++ | | | | |
| Others | Intrauterine growth retardation | + ++ | | | | |
| | Perinatal death | + ++ | | | | |
| | Polyhydramnios | + ++ | | | | |
| Laboratory findings | 2-Ketoglutarate dehydrogenase (fibroblasts) | | ↓↓ | | | |
| | Branched-chain ketoacid dehydrogenase (fibroblasts) | | ↓↓ | | | |
| | Complexes I–IV (muscle, fibroblasts) | ↓↓ | ↓↓ | | | |
| | Glycine (cerebrospinal fluid) | ↑↑↑ | n-↑↑ | | | |
| | Glycine (plasma) | ↑↑↑ | n-↑↑ | | | |
| | Lactate (cerebrospinal fluid) | ↑↑ | ↑↑ | | | |
| | Lactate (plasma) | ↑↑ | ↑ | | | |
| | Lactate (urine) | ↑↑ | | | | |
| | Protein-bound lipoic acid (fibroblasts) | ↓↓↓ | ↓↓↓ | | | |
| | Pyruvate dehydrogenase (fibroblasts) | | ↓↓↓ | | | |

[a]Two members of a single family
[b]Ten members of a single family

**Table 27.8** ISCA1 deficiency

| System | Symptoms and biomarkers | Neonatal (birth–1 month) | Infancy (1–18 months) | Childhood (1.5–11 years) | Adolescence (11–16 years) | Adulthood (>16 years) |
|---|---|---|---|---|---|---|
| CNS | Deep tendon reflexes | | ++ | | | |
| | Developmental delay | | ++ | | | |
| | **Leukodystrophy** | | +++ | | | |
| | Neurologic deterioration | | ++ | | | |
| | Poor head control | | + | | | |
| | Seizures | | ++ | | | |
| | Spasticity | | ++ | | | |
| | Ventriculomegaly | | ++ | | | |
| Digestive | **Feeding difficulties** | | +++ | | | |
| Eye | Nystagmus | | ± | | | |
| | Strabismus | | ± | | | |
| Laboratory findings | Complexes I–IV (muscle) | | ↓↓ | | | |
| | Creatine kinase (plasma) | | n-↑ | | | |
| | Glycine (plasma) | | n | | | |
| | Glycine (urine) | | n | | | |
| | Lactate (plasma) | | ↑ | | | |
| | Lactate (urine) | | n | | | |
| | Protein-bound lipoic acid (fibroblasts) | | ↓↓↓ | | | |
| | Pyruvate dehydrogenase (fibroblasts) | | ↓↓ | | | |

**Table 27.9** ISCA2 deficiency

| System | Symptoms and biomarkers | Neonatal (birth–1 month) | Infancy (1–18 months) | Childhood (1.5–11 years) | Adolescence (11–16 years) | Adulthood (>16 years) |
|---|---|---|---|---|---|---|
| CNS | **Axial hypotonia** | | +++ | | | |
| | **Cerebellar white matter abnormalities (MRI)** | | +++ | | | |
| | **Diffuse bilateral cerebral white matter abnormalities (MRI)** | | +++ | | | |
| | **Neurodevelopmental regression** | | +++ | | | |
| | Seizures | | ± | | | |
| | **Spasticity, limbs** | | +++ | | | |
| | Spinal cord abnormalities (MRI) | | + | | | |
| Digestive | Gastroesophageal reflux | | ± | | | |
| Eye | **Nystagmus** | | +++ | | | |
| | **Optic atrophy** | | +++ | | | |
| Laboratory findings | 2-Ketoglutarate dehydrogenase (fibroblasts) | | ↓↓ | | | |
| | Complexes I–IV (fibroblasts) | | ↓-n | | | |
| | Glycine (cerebrospinal fluid) | | ↑ | | | |
| | Glycine (plasma) | | n-↑ | | | |
| | Glycine (urine) | | n-↑ | | | |
| | Lactate (cerebrospinal fluid) | | ↑ | | | |
| | Lactate (plasma) | | n-↑ | | | |
| | mtDNA content (fibroblasts) | | ↓-n | | | |
| | Protein-bound lipoic acid (fibroblasts) | | ↓↓ | | | |
| | Pyruvate dehydrogenase (fibroblasts) | | ↓↓ | | | |

**Table 27.10** ISCU deficiency

| System | Symptoms and biomarkers | Neonatal (birth–1 month) | Infancy (1–18 months) | Childhood (1.5–11 years) | Adolescence (11–16 years) | Adulthood (>16 years) |
|---|---|---|---|---|---|---|
| Cardiovascular | Cardiomyopathy | | | ± | ± | ± |
| Musculoskeletal | **Exercise intolerance** | | | + | +++ | +++ |
| | **Muscle weakness** | | | + | +++ | +++ |
| | Myoglobinuria | | | ± | ± | +++ |
| | **Myopathy** | | | +++ | +++ | +++ |
| | Rhabdomyolysis | | | ± | ± | +++ |
| Laboratory findings | Aconitase (muscle) | | | ↓ | ↓ | ↓ |
| | Complexes I–III (muscle) | | | ↓ | ↓ | ↓ |
| | Creatine kinase (plasma) | | | n-↑ | n-↑ | ↑ |
| | Lactate (plasma) | | | ↑↑ | ↑↑ | ↑↑ |
| | Myoglobin (urine) | | | n-↑ | n-↑ | ↑↑↑ |
| | SDH histochemistry (muscle) | | | ↓ | ↓ | ↓ |

**Table 27.11** ABCB7 deficiency

| System | Symptoms and biomarkers | Neonatal (birth–1 month) | Infancy (1–18 months) | Childhood (1.5–11 years) | Adolescence (11–16 years) | Adulthood (>16 years) |
|---|---|---|---|---|---|---|
| CNS | **Cerebellar ataxia, nonprogressive** | | | +++ | +++ | +++ |
| | **Dysarthria** | | | +++ | +++ | +++ |
| Other | **Ringed sideroblasts on bone marrow** | | | +++ | +++ | +++ |
| Laboratory findings | Protoporphyrin (red blood cells) | | | ↑ | ↑ | ↑ |

**Table 27.12** Ferredoxin 2 deficiency

| System | Symptoms and biomarkers | Neonatal (birth–1 month) | Infancy (1–18 months) | Childhood (1.5–11 years) | Adolescence (11–16 years) | Adulthood (>16 years) |
|---|---|---|---|---|---|---|
| CNS | Axonal sensorimotor neuropathy | | ± | | ++ | |
| | Delayed motor development | | ++ | | | |
| | Learning disability | | ± | | | |
| | **Reversible leukoencephalopathy** | | ++ | ++ | | |
| Eye | Nystagmus | | +++ | +++ | ++ | |
| | Optic atrophy | | +++ | +++ | ++ | |
| Hematological | Anemia, microcytic | | ++ | | | |
| | Neutropenia | | ++ | | | |
| Musculoskeletal | **Exercise intolerance** | | | ++ | +++ | |
| | Muscle cramps | | | ++ | +++ | |
| | **Muscle weakness** | | | ++ | +++ | |
| | Myoglobinuria | | | | +++ | |
| Laboratory findings | 3-Methylglutaconic acid (urine) | | | | ↑ | |
| | Complexes I–IV (muscle, fibroblasts)) | | | | ↓ | |
| | Creatine kinase (plasma) | | | | ↑↑↑ | |
| | Lactate (plasma) | | | | ↑↑ | |
| | Lactate (urine) | | | | ↑↑ | |
| | Myoglobin (urine) | | | | ↑↑↑ | |
| | Pyruvate dehydrogenase (fibroblasts) | | | | ↓ | |

**Table 27.13** Ferredoxin reductase deficiency

| System | Symptoms and biomarkers | Neonatal (birth–1 month) | Infancy (1–18 months) | Childhood (1.5–11 years) | Adolescence (11–16 years) | Adulthood (>16 years) |
|---|---|---|---|---|---|---|
| CNS | **Ataxia** | | | ++ | ++ | |
| | Cerebral atrophy (MRI) | | + | + | | |
| | **Developmental delay** | | +++ | ++ | | |
| | **Dysarthria** | | | +++ | +++ | +++ |
| | Encephalopathy, progressive | | ± | ± | | |
| | **Hypotonia** | | ++ | ++ | | |
| | Irritability | | | ± | | |
| | Microcephaly | | ± | + | | + |
| | Motor developmental delay | | + | ++ | ± | |
| | **Neuropathy, sensory axonal** | | | + | ++ | +++ |
| | Seizures | | ± | ± | | |
| | Sleep disturbances | | ± | | | |
| | Spasticity | | | ++ | ++ | |
| | Swallowing difficulties | | + | + | | |
| Dermatological | Café au lait spot | | ± | | ± | |
| Digestive | Feeding difficulties | | + | + | | |
| Ear | Hearing loss, sensorineural | | + | + | +++ | +++ |
| Eye | Nystagmus | | | + | | ± |
| | **Optic atrophy** | | + | +++ | ++ | +++ |
| | Retinitis pigmentosa | | ± | ++ | ± | |
| | Strabismus | | + | | | |
| | Unable to track visually | | ++ | | | |
| | **Visual impairment** | | +++ | +++ | | |
| Musculoskeletal | Muscle weakness | | | + | | |
| Other | Failure to thrive | | ++ | + | | |
| | Wheelchair bound | | | ++ | ++ | ++ |
| Laboratory findings | Complexes I–IV (muscle) | | ↓-n | ↓-n | | |

**Table 27.14** ISD11 deficiency

| System | Symptoms and biomarkers | Neonatal (birth–1 month)[a] | Infancy (1–18 months) | Childhood (1.5–11 years) | Adolescence (11–16 years) | Adulthood (>16 years) |
|---|---|---|---|---|---|---|
| CNS | Epilepsy | ± | | | | |
| | Hypotonia | + | | | | |
| | Lethargy | ± | | | | |
| Digestive | Feeding difficulties | + | | | | |
| | Gastroesophageal reflux | + | | | | |
| | Hepatomegaly | ± | | | | |
| Respiratory | **Respiratory distress** | ++ | | | | |
| | **Stridor, inspiratory** | ++ | | | | |
| Others | Low weight gain | + | | | | |
| Laboratory findings | ASAT/ALAT (plasma) | ↑ | | | | |
| | Complexes I–IV (muscle, fibroblasts, leucocytes) | n-↓ | | | | |
| | Gamma-glutamyl transpeptidase, GGT (plasma) | ↑ | | | | |
| | Lactate (cerebrospinal fluid) | ↑↑ | | | | |
| | Lactate (plasma) | ↑↑ | | | | |
| | Lactate (urine) | ↑↑ | | | | |

[a]Two patients of the same family: one patient died during infancy and the other was alive and asymptomatic at 20 years of age

**Table 27.15** NFS1 deficiency

| System | Symptoms and biomarkers | Neonatal (birth–1 month) | Infancy (1–18 months)[a] | Childhood (1.5–11 years) | Adolescence (11–16 years) | Adulthood (>16 years) |
|---|---|---|---|---|---|---|
| Cardiovascular | Cardiac failure | | + + | | | |
| CNS | Cerebral infarction | | ± | | | |
| | Developmental and gross motor delay | | ± | | | |
| | **Hypotonia** | | +++ | | | |
| | **Lethargy** | | +++ | | | |
| | Seizures | | + + | | | |
| Digestive | **Anorexia** | | +++ | | | |
| | Hemorrhagic pancreatitis | | ± | | | |
| | Vomiting | | ± | | | |
| Metabolic | Hypoglycemia | | ++ | | | |
| Renal | Renal failure | | ++ | | | |
| Respiratory | Respiratory failure | | ++ | | | |
| Laboratory findings | ASAT/ALAT (plasma) | | ↑ | | | |
| | Complexes I–IV (muscle) | | ↓↓ | | | |
| | Creatine kinase (plasma) | | ↑ | | | |
| | Disseminated intravascular coagulation | | + | | | |
| | Glucose (plasma) | | ↓ | | | |
| | Lactate (plasma) | | ↑↑ | | | |

[a]Only one family with three siblings

**Table 27.16** Frataxin deficiency

| System | Symptoms and biomarkers | Neonatal (birth–1 month) | Infancy (1–18 months) | Childhood (1.5–11 years) | Adolescence (11–16 years) | Adulthood (>16 years) |
|---|---|---|---|---|---|---|
| Cardiovascular | Cardiomyopathy | | | | ++ | ++ |
| CNS | **Absent lower limb reflexes** | | | | +++ | +++ |
| | **Ataxia** | | | | +++ | +++ |
| | **Dysarthria** | | | | +++ | +++ |
| | Hearing, impaired | | | | ± | ± |
| | Sphincter control problems | | | | ± | ± |
| | Spinal cord atrophy | | | | ++ | ++ |
| | Swallowing difficulties | | | | ± | ± |
| Endocrine | Abnormal glucose tolerance | | | | ± | ± |
| | Diabetes | | | | ± | ± |
| Eye | Vision, decreased | | | | ± | ± |
| Musculoskeletal | Pes cavus | | | | ++ | ++ |
| | Scoliosis | | | | ++ | ++ |

Four well-defined clinical entities, Friedreich ataxia (FXN) (Table 27.16), myopathy with lactic acidosis and exercise intolerance (ISCU) (Table 27.10), X-linked sideroblastic anemia with ataxia (ABCB7) (Table 27.11), and sideroblastic anemia associated with particular mutations in GLRX5 (Table 27.6), were the first-described diseases related to Fe-S cluster biosynthesis or transport defects. In addition, patients with mutations in HSPA9 also presenting two well-defined phenotypes consisting in sideroblastic anemia (Schmitz-Abe et al. 2015) or EVEN-plus syndrome (Royer-Bertrand et al. 2015) (Table 27.17) were described later on. In these cases diagnosis goes directly from the clinical suspicion to molecular studies.

The progress in the knowledge of these diseases started in 2011 when two parallel and independent studies identified mutations in the genes encoding for the Fe-S cluster proteins NFU1 and BOLA3 (Tables 27.4 and 27.5) in patients with a fatal mitochondrial encephalopathy with lactic acidosis, hyperglycinemia, and deficient activities of LA-dependent enzymes (Navarro-Sastre et al. 2011; Cameron et al. 2011).

**Table 27.17** HSPA9 deficiency

| System | Symptoms and biomarkers | Neonatal (birth–1 month) | Infancy (1–18 months) | Childhood (1.5–11 years) | Adolescence (11–16 years) | Adulthood (>16 years) |
|---|---|---|---|---|---|---|
| Cardiovascular | Heart abnormalities | | ± | + | | |
| CNS | Abnormal gait | | | ± | | |
| | Agenesis of the corpus callosum | | ± | ± | | |
| | Agenesis of the septum pellucidum | | ± | | | |
| | Developmental delay | | ± | ± | | |
| | Hypotonia | | | ± | | |
| Hematological | Anemia, sideroblastic | | | | | +++ |
| Musculoskeletal | Anal atresia | + | | | | |
| | Aplasia cutis congenita on skull vertex | ++ | | | | |
| | **Hypoplastic nose** | + | ± | +++ | | |
| | **Microtia** | + | | +++ | | |
| | **Short stature** | +++ | | +++ | | |
| | Shortened limbs | ++ | | | | |
| | **Skeletal abnormalities** | + | + | +++ | | |
| | **Synophrys** | + | | +++ | | |
| Renal | Hypoplastic kidney | | | ± | | |
| | Vesicouretral reflux | | | ± | | |
| Others | **Low weight** | +++ | | +++ | | |
| | Teeth abnormalities | | | ± | | |
| Laboratory findings | Microcytic or macrocytic red blood cells | | | | | +++ |
| | Ringed sideroblasts in bone marrow | | | | | +++ |

Later on, six new diseases, LIPT2, LIAS (Tables 27.1 and 27.2), GLRX5, IBA57, ISCA1, and ISCA2 (Tables 27.6, 27.7, 27.8, and 27.9), with very close clinical and biochemical phenotype to NFU1 and BOLA3 were described. It is important to remark that patients with mutations in GLRX5 can present two different phenotypes: the abovementioned sideroblastic anemia into adulthood or progressive spasticity and MRI abnormalities consistent with leukodystrophy in childhood (Table 27.6). These two phenotypes are mutation dependent. In fact, it has been demonstrated that GLRX5 protein is multifunctional and defects of the different amino acids of the protein will lead to distinct effects downstream Fe-S biosynthesis (Baker et al. 2014; Lui et al. 2016).

Neonatal encephalopathy with lactic acidosis and normal glycine was observed in a patient with mutation in *LIPT1* (Table 27.3) (Tort et al. 2014). This could be explained by the fact that LIPT1 is required for lipoylation, and subsequent activation, of the 2-oxoacid dehydrogenases but is not involved in the regulation of the GCS. On the other hand, other diseases, ISCU (Table 27.10) FDX2 (Table 27.12), ISD11, and NFS1 (Tables 27.14 and 27.15), presenting also with lactic acidosis but normal glycine completed the spectrum of mitochondrial encephalopathies associated with LA and Fe-S cluster disorders.

It is interesting that patients carrying mutations in *ISCU* and *FDX2* had a similar clinical phenotype showing late-onset presentation, even into adulthood, with myopathy, rhabdomyolysis, and myoglobinuria. In addition, the recent report of patients with normal lactate, hearing loss, and visual impairment in childhood, associated with *FDXR* mutations (Table 27.13) highlight the wide clinical and biochemical heterogeneity of mitochondrial disorders related to Fe-S metabolism (Peng et al., 2017; Paul et al. 2017; Slone et al. 2018).

To summarize, the clinical suspicion is always the first step for the diagnosis. As mentioned above, in the well-defined clinical syndromes, the diagnosis goes from the clinical suspicion to molecular studies, but for other diseases the analysis of both LA- and Fe-S cluster-dependent pathways is very useful to direct the defect. With few exceptions, high lactate is a common finding of these diseases (Figs. 27.2 and 27.3). Glycine elevation, due to the defective lipoylation of the H-protein of GCS, is observed in all patients with defects in LA synthesis (LIAS, LIPT2, NFU1, BOLA3, IBA57, GLRX5, and ISCA2). In contrast, glycine levels remained unaltered in individuals with mutations in *LIPT1*, *FDX1L*, *LYRM4* (ISD11 protein), *FDXR*, and *NFS1*. On the other hand, analysis of LA levels is also a useful parameter. This analysis is performed using a specific antibody that recognizes the lipoylated forms of the E2 subunits of 2-oxoacid dehydrogenase complexes as well as the lipoylated H-protein of the GCS. This approach is mainly used as a research resource. Nevertheless, the fact that this antibody does not react against non-lipoylated proteins provides an efficient and cost-effective tool to identify lipoylation defects. Another useful parameter is the measurement of the respiratory chain activities, which are frequently altered in the patients with defects in biosynthesis, maturation, and delivery of Fe-S clusters but are unaltered in other defects (Figs. 27.2 and 27.3) (Tort et al. 2016; Mayr et al. 2014).

The *inheritance* of these diseases is autosomal recessive, except for ABCB7 that is X-linked and ISCU that can be autosomal recessive or dominant (Olsson et al. 2008; Mochel et al. 2008; Legati et al. 2017).

Concerning *frequency*, apart from the high number of reported patients with Friedreich ataxia, the first-described Fe-S cluster disorder (Campuzano et al. 1996), the most frequently described disease is NFU1, with more than 70 reported patients. It is remarkable that 27 patients with the recently described FDXR deficiency have already been reported (Peng et al., 2017; Paul et al. 2017; Slone et al. 2018).

## Reference Values

| Metabolites | | | | |
|---|---|---|---|---|
| | Plasma (μmol/L) | CSF (μmol/L) | Urine (mmol/mol creatinine) | CSF/plasma |
| **Lactate** | 0.5–2 | 0.8–2.8 | | |
| **Glycine** | 81–436 | 3.7–8 | 110–356 | <0.04 |
| *Enzyme activities*[a] | | | | |
| **MRC** | **Muscle** | **Fibroblasts** | | |
| Complex I | 25–54 | | | |
| Complexes I + III | 18–37 | 15–42 | | |
| Complex II | 37–82 | 22–35 | | |
| Complexes II + III | 27–48 | 11–20 | | |
| Complex III | 103–207 | 25–48 | | |
| Complex IV | 78–186 | 33–57 | | |
| Citrate synthase | 127–222 | 41–62 | | |
| **PDH** | | | | |
| PDH (total) | 0.8–3.4 | 0.34–2.6 | | |

[a]nmol $min^{-1}$ $mg^{-1}$ protein; *MRC* Mitochondrial respiratory chain, *PDH* Pyruvate dehydrogenase

## Diagnostic Flowchart

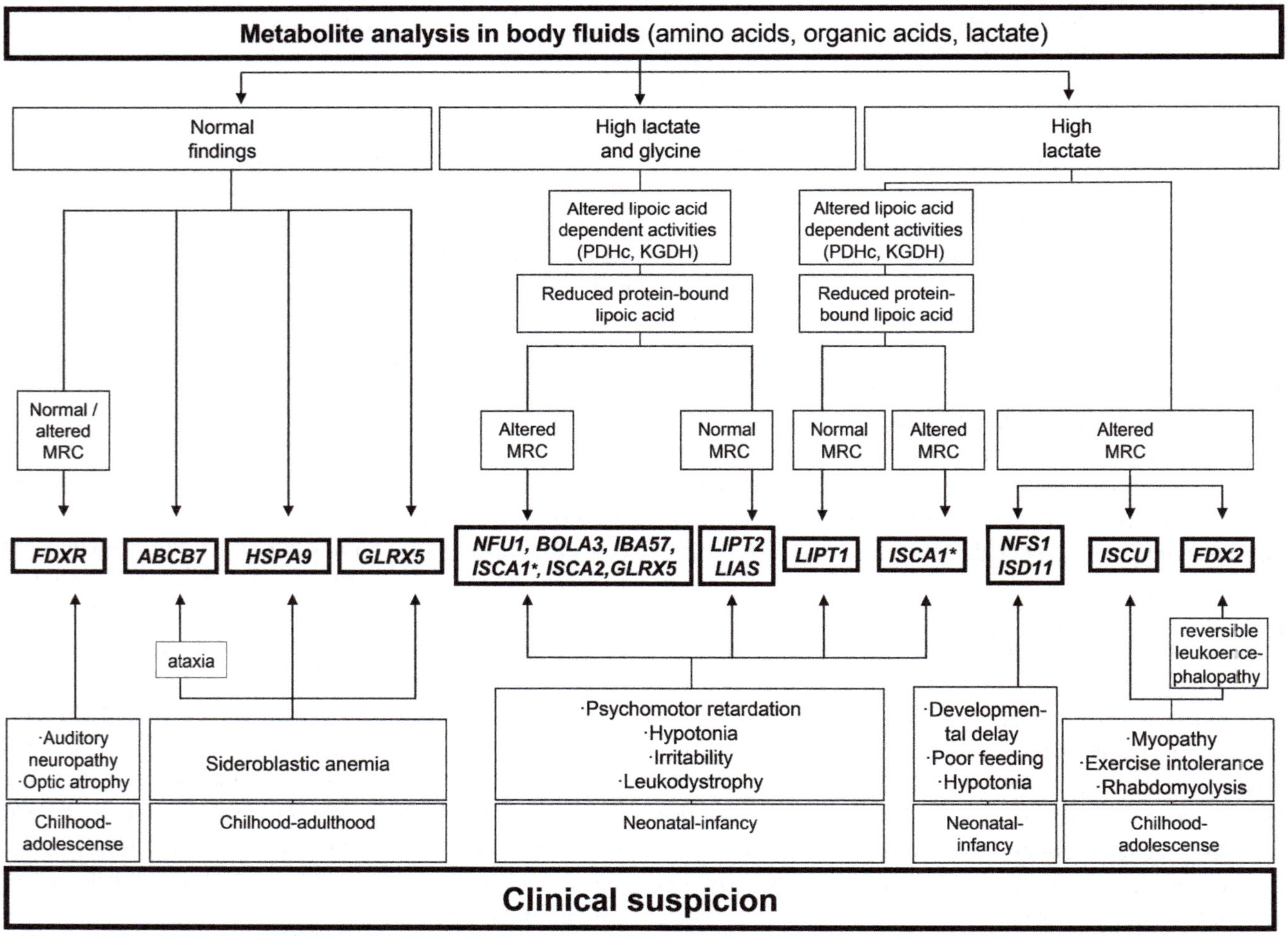


* Glycine elevation has not been documented in ISCA1 patients. ISCA1 is involved in a protein complex together with IBA57 and ISCA2, both deficiencies presenting with hyperglycinemia. Therefore, hyperglycinemia can not be excluded in this disease.

**Fig. 27.2** Diagnostic flowchart

| | Iron-sulfur clusters (Fe-S) | | Lipoic acid | |
|---|---|---|---|---|
| | biosynthesis | maturation-delivery | biosynthesis | transport |
| | ISCU · FDX2 · ISD11 NFS1 · FDXR · FDXR | NFU1 · BOLA3 · IBA57 ISCA1 · ISCA2 · GLRX5 | LIAS LIPT2 | LIPT1 |
| **Lactate** | n-↑ | ↑ | ↑ | ↑ |
| **Glycine*** | n | ↑↑ | ↑↑ | n |
| **MRC activities** | n-↓ | ↓ | n | n |
| **Lipoic acid (LA)** | n / nr | ↓↓ | ↓↓ | ↓↓ |
| **LA-dependent activities ** ** | n-↓ | ↓ | ↓ | ↓ |

*Hyperglycinemia in body fluids but normal CSF/plasma ratio; **PDH, 2-KGDH; MRC, mitochondrial respiratory chain; n, normal; nr, not reported

**Fig. 27.3** Biochemical characteristics of lipoic acid and Fe-S protein disorders

## Genetic Diagnosis

To reach the genetic diagnosis, the use of whole exome or targeted exome sequencing is strongly recommended. In this context, accurate clinical and biochemical characterization of patients will be determinant for the interpretation of genetic data and to narrow down the potential disease-causing mutations identified in each case. Therefore, this combined strategy is a good approach to reach a final diagnosis.

## Treatment

LA supplementation has been speculated as a potential treatment for patients with LA deficiency, but eukaryotic cells cannot use exogenously supplied LA. In fact it has been demonstrated that endogenous production of LA was essential for mouse development as LIAS knock-out mice died during early embryonic development and supplementation with LA to the heterozygous mothers during pregnancy did not revert the prenatal death of LIAS knock-out mice (Yi and Maeda 2005). Therefore, at present, no specific treatment for these patients is available.

## Specimen Collection

| Enzymatic activities | | |
|---|---|---|
| | Method | Sample |
| **PDH** | $^{14}CO2$ production from [1-$^{14}$C]-labeled pyruvate after activation with $Ca^{++}$ and $Mg^{++}$ and addition of carnitine and cytochrome C | Skin fibroblasts, muscle biopsy |
| **MRC** | Spectrophotometric determinations or BN-PAGE (in gel activity) | Skin fibroblasts, muscle biopsy |
| **Protein-bound lipoic acid**[a] | Western blot (SDS-PAGE) | Skin fibroblasts, muscle biopsy, liver necropsy |
| | Immunofluorescence | Skin fibroblasts |
| Genetic analysis | | |
| | **Method** | **Sample** |
| **Identification of disease-causing mutations** | Whole exome sequencing/ targeted exome sequencing | Genomic DNA |

*PDH* Pyruvate dehydrogenase, *MRC* Mitochondrial respiratory chain
[a]Using commercially available anti protein-bound lipoic acid antibodies

## References


Baker PR, Friederich MW, Swanson MA, Shaikh T, Bhattacharya K, Scharer GH, Aicher J, Creadon-Swindell G, Geiger E, MacLean KN, Lee WT, Deshpande C, Freckmann ML, Shih LY, Wasserstein M, Rasmussen MB, Lund AM, Procopis P, Cameron JM, Robinson BH, Brown GK, Brown RM, Compton AG, Dieckmann CL, Collard R, Coughlin CR 2nd, Spector E, Wempe MF, Van Hove JL. Variant non ketotic hyperglycinemia is caused by mutations in LIAS, BOLA3 and the novel gene GLRX5. Brain. 2014;137:366–79.

Cameron JM, Janer A, Levandovskiy V, Mackay N, Rouault TA, Tong WH, Ogilvie I, Shoubridge EA, Robinson BH. Mutations in iron-sulfur cluster scaffold genes NFU1 and BOLA3 cause a fatal deficiency of multiple respiratory chain and 2-oxoacid dehydrogenase enzymes. Am J Hum Genet. 2011;89:486–95.

Campuzano V, Montermini L, Moltò MD, Pianese L, Cossée M, Cavalcanti F, Monros E, Rodius F, Duclos F, Monticelli A, Zara F, Cañizares J, Koutnikova H, Bidichandani SI, Gellera C, Brice A, Trouillas P, De Michele G, Filla A, De Frutos R, Palau F, Patel PI, Di Donato S, Mandel JL, Cocozza S, Koenig M, Pandolfo M. Friedreich's ataxia: autosomal recessive disease caused by an intronic GAA triplet repeat expansion. Science. 1996;271:1423–7.

Legati A, Reyes A, Ceccatelli Berti C, Stehling O, Marchet S, Lamperti C, Ferrari A, Robinson AJ, Mühlenhoff U, Lill R, Zeviani M, Goffrini P, Ghezzi D. A novel de novo dominant mutation in ISCU associated with mitochondrial myopathy. J Med Genet. 2017;54:815–24.

Lill R, Hoffmann B, Molik S, Pierik AJ, Rietzschel N, Stehling O, Uzarska MA, Webert H, Wilbrecht C, Mühlenhoff U. The role of mitochondria in cellular iron-sulfur protein biogenesis and iron metabolism. Biochim Biophys Acta. 2012;1823:1491–508.

Liu G, Wang Y, Anderson GJ, Camaschella C, Chang Y, Nie G. Functional analysis of GLRX5 mutants reveals distinct functionalities of GLRX5 protein. J Cell Biochem. 2016;117:207–17.

Mayr JA, Feichtinger RG, Tort F, Ribes A, Sperl W. Lipoic acid biosynthesis defects. J Inherit Metab Dis. 2014;37:553–63.

Mochel F, Knight MA, Tong WH, Hernandez D, Ayyad K, Taivassalo T, Andersen PM, Singleton A, Rouault TA, Fischbeck KH, Haller RG. Splice mutation in the iron-sulfur cluster scaffold protein ISCU causes myopathy with exercise intolerance. Am J Hum Genet. 2008;82:652–60.

Navarro-Sastre A, Tort F, Stehling O, Uzarska MA, Arranz JA, Del Toro M, Labayru MT, Landa J, Font A, Garcia-Villoria J, Merinero B, Ugarte M, Gutierrez-Solana LG, Campistol J, Garcia-Cazorla A, Vaquerizo J, Riudor E, Briones P, Elpeleg O, Ribes A, Lill R. A fatal mitochondrial disease is associated with defective NFU1 function in the maturation of a subset of mitochondrial Fe-S proteins. Am J Hum Genet. 2011;89:656–67.

Olsson A, Lind L, Thornell LE, Holmberg M. Myopathy with lactic acidosis is linked to chromosome 12q23.3-24.11 and caused by an intron mutation in the ISCU gene resulting in a splicing defect. Hum Mol Genet. 2008;17:1666–72.

Paul A, Drecourt A, Petit F, Deguine DD, Vasnier C, Oufadem M, Masson C, Bonnet C, Masmoudi S, Mosnier I, Mahieu L, Bouccara D, Kaplan J, Challe G, Domange C, Mochel F, Sterkers O, Gerber S, Nitschke P, Bole-Feysot C, Jonard L, Gherbi S, Mercati O, Ben Aissa I, Lyonnet S, Rötig A, Delahodde A, Marlin S. FDXR mutations cause sensorial neuropathies and expand the spectrum of mitochondrial Fe-S-synthesis diseases. Am J Hum Genet. 2017;101:630–7.

Peng Y, Shinde DN, Valencia CA, Mo JS, Rosenfeld J, Truitt Cho M, Chamberlin A, Li Z, Liu J, Gui B, Brockhage R, Basinger A, Alvarez-Leon B, Heydemann P, Magoulas PL, Lewis AM, Scaglia F, Gril S, Chong SC, Bower M, Monaghan KG, Willaert R, Plona MR, Dineen R, Milan F, Hoganson G, Powis Z, Helbig KL, Keller-Ramey J, Harris B, Anderson LC, Green T, Sukoff Rizzo SJ, Kaylor J, Chen J, Guan MX, Sellars E, Sparagana SP, Gibson JB, Reinholdt LG, Tang S, Huang T. Biallelic mutations in the ferredoxin reductase gene cause novel mitochondriopathy with optic atrophy. Hum Mol Genet. 2017;26:4937–50.

Royer-Bertrand B, Castillo-Taucher S, Moreno-Salinas R, Cho TJ, Chae JH, Choi M, Kim OH, Dikoglu E, Campos-Xavier B, Girardi E, Superti-Furga G, Bonafé L, Rivolta C, Unger S, Superti-Furga A. Mutations in the heat-shock protein A9 (HSPA9) gene cause the EVEN-PLUS syndrome of congenital malformations and skeletal dysplasia. Sci Rep. 2015;5:17154.

Schmitz-Abe K, Ciesielski SJ, Schmidt PJ, Campagna DR, Rahimov F, Schilke BA, Cuijpers M, Rieneck K, Lausen B, Linenberger ML, Sendamarai AK, Guo C, Hofmann I, Newburger PE, Matthews D, Shimamura A, Snijders PJ, Towne MC, Niemeyer CM, Watson HG, Dziegiel MH, Heeney MM, May A, Bottomley SS, Swinkels DW, Markianos K, Craig EA, Fleming MD. Congenital sideroblastic anemia due to mutations in the mitochondrial HSP70 homologue HSPA9. Blood. 2015;126:2734–8.

Slone J, Peng Y, Chamberlin A, Harris B, Kaylor J, McDonald MT, Lemmon M, El-Dairi MA, Tchapyjnikov D, Gonzalez-Krellwitz LA, Sellars EA, McConkie-Rosell A, Reinholdt LG, Huang T. Biallelic mutations in FDXR cause neurodegeneration associated with inflammation. J Hum Genet. 2018;63:1211–22.

Stehling O, Wilbrecht C, Lill R. Mitochondrial iron-sulfur protein biogenesis and human disease. Biochimie. 2014;100:61–77.

Tort F, Ferrer-Cortes X, Ribes A. Differential diagnosis of lipoic acid synthesis defects. J Inherit Metab Dis. 2016;39:781–93.

Tort F, Ferrer-Cortès X, Thió M, Navarro-Sastre A, Matalonga L, Quintana E, Bujan N, Arias A, García-Villoria J, Acquaviva C, Vianey-Saban C, Artuch R, García-Cazorla À, Briones P, Ribes A. Mutations in the lipoyltransferase LIPT1 gene cause a fatal disease associated with a specific lipoylation defect of the 2-ketoacid dehydrogenase complexes. Hum Mol Genet. 2014;23:1907–15.

Yi X, Maeda N. Endogenous production of lipoic acid is essential for mouse development. Mol Cell Biol. 2005;25:8387–92.

# Part III

# Disorders of Vitamins, Cofactors, Metals and Minerals

# Disorders of Cobalamin Metabolism

# 28

Matthias R. Baumgartner and D. Sean Froese

## Contents




**Summary**

Vitamin $B_{12}$ (Cbl) is needed for just two metabolic reactions in man, the methylation of homocysteine to methionine (cofactor methyl-Cbl) and the conversion of methylmalonyl-CoA to succinyl-CoA (cofactor adenosyl-Cbl). A complex sequence of processes is required to convert dietary Cbl to its cofactors and to correctly deliver them to the target enzymes. A wide range of acquired or hereditary disorders of absorption, transport and intracellular processing of Cbl are known, resulting in combined methylmalonic aciduria and homocystinuria or each in isolation. Seventeen distinct genetic disorders have been identified involving transcription factors, carrier proteins, receptors, membrane proteins, molecular chaperones and enzymes, and the genes have been characterised for each of these, although the exact function of some of the proteins remains to be elucidated. Main clinical hallmarks of these disorders are haematological and neurological disease of varying severity. Diagnosis centres on measurement of the two precursors of the Cbl enzymes, methylmalonic acid and homocysteine, together with



M. R. Baumgartner (✉) · D. S. Froese
Division of Metabolism and Children's Research Center, University Children's Hospital Zürich, University of Zürich, Zürich, Switzerland
e-mail: matthias.baumgartner@kispi.uzh.ch; sean.froese@kispi.uzh.ch




N. Blau et al. (eds.), *Physician's Guide to the Diagnosis, Treatment, and Follow-Up of Inherited Metabolic Diseases*,
https://doi.org/10.1007/978-3-030-67727-5_28

measurements of other parameters such as total vitamin $B_{12}$, holotranscobalamin, 3-hydroxypropionic acid and methylcitric acid, C3-acylcarnitine and methionine. Absorption and transport defects respond well to treatment with Cbl. Intracellular processing defects also respond to Cbl, but biochemical and clinical abnormalities may not fully resolve, and long-term outcome can be poor. Prenatal diagnosis can be reliably performed in those disorders where this is indicated.

## Introduction

Vitamin $B_{12}$ (cobalamin, Cbl) is a complex molecule with a cobalt-containing corrin ring. It is derived almost exclusively from animal sources, secondary to production by microorganisms. Cbl is needed for just two metabolic reactions in man, methylation of homocysteine to methionine and conversion of methylmalonyl-CoA to succinyl-CoA (Fig. 28.1). Deficiency of Cbl, inability to absorb Cbl normally or inability to process Cbl to its two active cofactors can result in elevated circulating and urinary levels of the precursors methylmalonic acid (MMA) and homocysteine which are useful diagnostic markers for Cbl disorders.

In children, causes of Cbl deficiency fall into three categories: (1) dietary deficiency, (2) abnormal absorption and transport and inborn errors of cellular uptake and (3) inborn errors of intracellular processing. While the first category is an acquired form of Cbl deficiency, the two latter categories represent mostly inherited disorders (Watkins and Rosenblatt 2017).

Abnormal Cbl absorption and transport may result from hereditary causes such as absent or abnormal intrinsic factor (IF), defective ileal receptors or deficient transport into cells or from a wide range of nonhereditary absorption disorders such as surgery involving the stomach or terminal ileum, decreased Cbl release from food protein, competi-

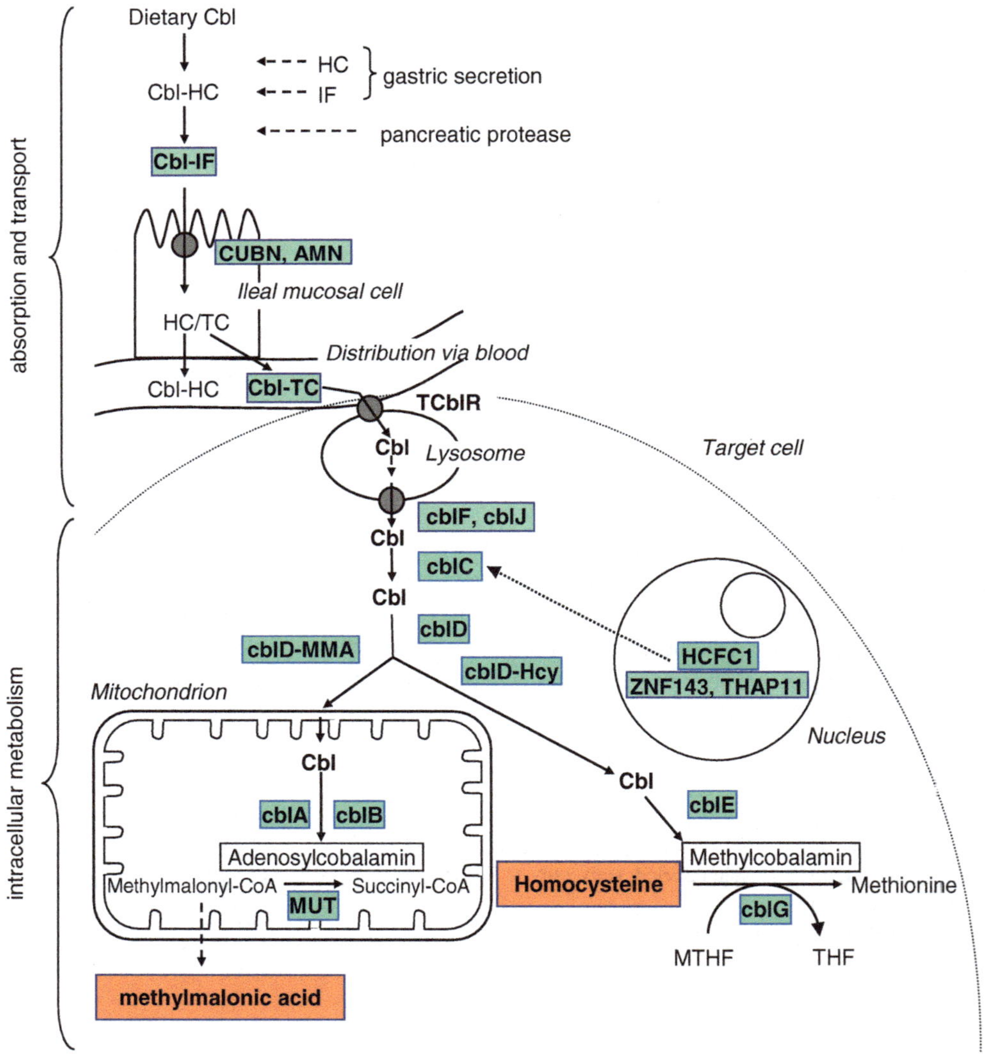


**Fig. 28.1** Cobalamin and its metabolism. For details see text. *Cbl* Cobalamin, *HC* Haptocorrin, *IF* Intrinsic factor, *CUBN* Cubilin, *AMN* Amnionless, *TC* Transcobalamin, *Cbl-TC* Holotranscobalamin, *MMA* Methylmalonic acid, *Hcy* Homocysteine, *THF* Tetrahydrofolate, *MTHF* Methyltetrahydrofolate

tion for Cbl in the ileum or loss of the ileal absorptive surface. Cbl malabsorption (or juvenile Cbl deficiency, JCD) is a potentially fatal condition that is mostly hereditary in nature in children since the classic adult form of autoimmune pernicious anaemia is rare in early life. Two main forms of inherited JCD exist: intrinsic factor deficiency (IFD) and Imerslund-Najman-Gräsbeck syndrome (IGS), also known as juvenile/hereditary megaloblastic anaemia, MGA1 or juvenile pernicious anaemia with proteinuria. IFD is caused by mutations in the gastric IF gene (*GIF*, (Tanner et al. 2005)). In IGS, deleterious mutations in the genes encoding the ileal Cbl receptor cubilin (*CUBN*, (Aminoff et al. 1999)) or its facilitator amnionless (*AMN*, (Tanner et al. 2003)) cause malabsorption of Cbl. Both proteins are involved in intestinal absorption and renal tubular reabsorption and form the heterodimer named CUBAM that accomplishes the internalisation of the IF-Cbl complex (Fyfe et al. 2004).

Conversion of Cbl to its active cofactors, methylcobalamin (MeCbl) and adenosylcobalamin (AdoCbl), requires a series of biochemical modifications that have been classified as Cbl complementation groups A–J, each of which represents a distinct autosomal recessive genetic disease (Fig. 28.1).

Patients belonging to the complementation groups *cblF*, *cblJ*, *cblC* and one form of *cblD* have combined deficiencies of AdoCbl and MeCbl synthesis and are thus characterised by both methylmalonic aciduria (MMAuria) and elevated total homocysteine (tHcy) which is often associated with low plasma methionine and *S*-adenosylmethionine (SAM). The *cblF* defect is a rare disorder described in less than 20 unrelated families. The gene responsible for the defect (*LMBRD1*) encodes a lysosomal membrane protein that is thought to act as an accessory protein for lysosomal export of Cbl (Rutsch et al. 2009; Fettelschoss et al. 2017). The *cblJ* defect has been described in only six unrelated patients with a biochemical phenotype similar to *cblF*. The gene responsible for the defect, *ABCD4*, encodes a presumed ABC transporter that interacts with and is targeted to the lysosome by the cblF protein (Fettelschoss et al. 2017; Coelho et al. 2012). *cblC* disease is the most frequent inborn error of Cbl metabolism with over 500 patients known in the Western world, a number that may be doubled when accounting for recent publications from mainland China (Liu et al. 2018; Hu et al. 2018). The gene responsible for *cblC*, designated *MMACHC* for MMAuria *cblC* type with homocystinuria, is thought to be a porter that carries out targeted delivery of Cbl from the lysosome to other Cbl-related proteins but also functions as a decyanase and dealkylase (Lerner-Ellis et al. 2006; Hannibal et al. 2009; Kim et al. 2008). Loss of expression of *MMACHC* due to mutation of the gene *PRDX1*, which results in epigenetic silencing of *MMACHC*, has recently been described in the heterozygous state combined with genetic *MMACHC* mutation in three patients with *cblC* disease (Gueant et al. 2018). Alternatively, loss of *MMACHC* expression due to mutation of the transcriptional co-regulator *HCFC1* (sometimes termed *cblX* disease) (Yu et al. 2013) or its interacting transcription factors *THAP11* (also called Ronin) (Quintana et al. 2017) and *ZNF143* (Pupavac et al. 2016) has been described in 19, 1 and 1 patient, respectively. The *cblD* defect has only recently been elucidated, over 30 years after the first description of the complementation group in two siblings. Approximately 20 patients are known worldwide (Coelho et al. 2008; Parini et al. 2013; Stucki et al. 2012). The *cblD* defect is remarkable in that mutations in the same gene (*MMADHC* for MMAuria, *cblD* type, with homocystinuria) cause three distinct biochemical phenotypes: (1) deficient synthesis of both Cbl coenzymes causing combined MMAuria and homocystinuria (*cblD*-MMA/HC) associated with truncating mutations in the middle part of the gene, (2) deficiency of MeCbl synthesis causing isolated homocystinuria (*cblD*-HC) associated with missense mutations in the C-terminal part and (3) deficient synthesis of AdoCbl causing isolated MMAuria (*cblD*-MMA), associated with truncating mutations in the N-terminal region (Fig. 28.1).

The *cblD-HC*, *cblE* and *cblG* defects are associated with deficient methionine synthesis associated with elevated tHcy, low methionine and SAM in plasma with normal MMA. The *cblE* defect is caused by deficiency of methionine synthase reductase (*MTRR*), which is required for the activation of the methionine synthase apoenzyme by reductive methylation (Fig. 28.1). The *cblG* defect is caused by deficient activity of the methionine synthase apoenzyme (*MTR*) itself. The genes for both defects have been described (Watkins and Rosenblatt 2017).

MMAurias are a heterogeneous group of inborn errors of metabolism biochemically characterised by the accumulation of MMA in body fluids and tissues. They result from deficiency of the mitochondrial enzyme methylmalonyl-CoA mutase (*MMUT*) or by a defect in the synthesis of its cofactor AdoCbl (*cblA*, *cblB* and *cblD-MMA*) (Fig. 28.1). MMUT deficiencies are further subdivided into defects without ($mut^0$) and with residual activity ($mut^-$). The conversion of L-methylmalonyl-CoA to succinyl-CoA, catalysed by MMUT, links the final catabolic pathways of branched-chain amino acids, odd-chain fatty acids and cholesterol to the Krebs cycle (Fowler et al. 2008). In the final step of AdoCbl synthesis in the mitochondrion, adenosyltransferase encoded by the *cblB* locus (*MMAB*) converts cob(II)alamin to AdoCbl and transfers the product directly to MMUT, in a process gated by the protein encoded by the *cblA* locus (*MMAA*) (Banerjee et al. 2009; Plessl et al. 2017).

## Nomenclature

| No. | Disorder | Alternative name | Abbreviation | Gene symbol | Chromosomal localisation | Affected protein | OMIM No. |
|---|---|---|---|---|---|---|---|
| 28.1 | Hereditary intrinsic factor deficiency | Congenital pernicious anaemia | IFD | *GIF* | 11q13 | Transcobalamin III | 261000 |
| 28.2 | Cubilin deficiency | Imerslund-Najman-Gräsbeck syndrome (IGS) due to CUBN | IGS | *CUBN* | 10p12.1 | Cubilin | 261100 |
| 28.3 | Amnionless deficiency | Imerslund-Najman-Gräsbeck syndrome due to AMN | IGS | *AMN* | 14q32.32 | Amnionless | 261100 |
| 28.4 | Haptocorrin deficiency | TC I (TCN1) deficiency | HCD | *TCN1* | 11q12.1 | $B_{12}$-binding alpha-globulin | 193090 |
| 28.5 | Transcobalamin deficiency | TC II deficiency | TCD | *TCN2* | 22q12.2 | Vitamin $B_{12}$-binding protein 2? | 275350 |
| 28.6 | Transcobalamin receptor deficiency | TCR/CD320 defect | TCR | *CD320* | 19p13.2 | CD320 receptor | 613646 |
| 28.7 | Adenosylcobalamin and methylcobalamin synthesis defect – cblF | Methylmalonic aciduria and homocystinuria, cblF type | cblF | *LMBRD1* | 6q13 | Lysosomal export of cobalamin? | 277380 |
| 28.8 | Adenosylcobalamin and methylcobalamin synthesis defect—cblJ | Methylmalonic aciduria and homocystinuria, cblJ type | cblJ | *ABCD4* | 14q24 | Lysosomal export of cobalamin? | 614857 |
| 28.9 | Adenosylcobalamin and methylcobalamin synthesis defect—cblC | Methylmalonic aciduria and homocystinuria, cblC type | cblC | *MMACHC* | 1p34.1 | Intracellular cobalamin chaperone and upper axial ligand cleavage? | 277400 |
| 28.10 | Adenosylcobalamin and methylcobalamin synthesis defect—cblC | Methylmalonic aciduria and homocystinuria, cblC type, digenic | epi-cblC | *PRDX1* | 1p34.1 | | 176763 |
| 28.11 | Adenosylcobalamin and methylcobalamin synthesis defect—cblD-MMA/HC | Methylmalonic aciduria and homocystinuria, cblD- type | cblD-MMA/HC | *MMADHC* | 2q32.2 | Intracellular cobalamin targeting? | 277410 |
| 28.15 | Methylcobalamin synthesis defect—cblD-HC | Homocystinuria, cblD-HC type | cblD-HC | *MMADHC* | 2q32.2 | | 277410 |
| 28.18 | Adenosylcobalamin synthesis defect—cblD-MMA | Methylmalonic aciduria, cblD-MMA type | cblD-MMA | *MMADHC* | 2q32.2 | | 277410 |
| 28.12 | Methylmalonic aciduria and homocystinuria, cblX type | | cblX | *HCFC1* | Xq28 | Host cell factor C1 | 309541 |
| 28.13 | Methylmalonic aciduria and homocystinuria due to ZNF143 deficiency | | | *ZNF143* | 11p15.4 | SPH-binding factor | |
| 28.14 | Methylmalonic aciduria and homocystinuria due to Ronin deficiency | | | *THAP11* | 16q22.1 | Ronin | |

| No. | Disorder | Alternative name | Abbreviation | Gene symbol | Chromosomal localisation | Affected protein | OMIM No. |
|---|---|---|---|---|---|---|---|
| 28.16 | Methionine synthase reductase deficiency—cblE | Methylcobalamin deficiency, cblE type | cblE | *MTRR* | 5p15.31 | Methionine synthase reductase, 5-methyltetrahydrofolate-homocysteine methyltransferase reductase | 236270 |
| 28.17 | Methionine synthase deficiency—cblG | Methylcobalamin deficiency, cblG type | cblG | *MTR* | 1q43 | Methionine synthase, 5-methyltetrahydrofolate-homocysteine methyltransferase | 250940 |
| 28.19 | Adenosylcobalamin synthesis defect—cblA | Methylmalonic aciduria, cblA type | cblA | *MMAA* | 4q31.21 | Gating and ejection of misincorporated cobalamin on MMUT? | 251100 |
| 28.20 | Adenosylcobalamin synthesis defect—cblB | Methylmalonic aciduria, cblB type | cblB | *MMAB* | 12q24.11 | Adenosyltransferase | 251110 |

## Metabolic Pathway

Cobalamin and its metabolism are shown in Fig. 28.1. Cbl is released from food proteins in the acidity of the stomach and binds to haptocorrin (HC), produced in saliva and in the stomach. In the duodenum, pancreatic enzymes degrade the Cbl-HC complexes releasing free Cbl which forms a complex with intrinsic factor (IF) from gastric parietal cells. The Cbl-IF factor complex is taken up by epithelial cells in the terminal ileum via specific receptor-mediated endocytosis. Free Cbl then enters the portal circulation bound to transcobalamin (TC) and is transported to tissues where the Cbl-TC complex binds to the TC receptor and is internalised (Nielsen et al. 2012). In the cell, conversion of Cbl to its active cofactors, methylcobalamin (MeCbl) and adenosylcobalamin (AdoCbl), requires a series of biochemical modifications that have been classified as Cbl complementation groups A–J (Fig. 28.1).

## Signs and Symptoms

The characteristic hallmark of Cbl disorders is haematologic abnormalities with megaloblastic anaemia, hypersegmentation of neutrophils and (pan)cytopenia. However, these symptoms may only manifest late or not at all. In most disorders, the phenotypes encompass a spectrum ranging from early-onset to late-onset clinical forms. The clinical presentation and characteristic laboratory findings of each disease are summarised in Tables 28.1, 28.2 and 28.3, 28.4, 28.5, 28.6, 28.7, 28.8, 28.9, 28.10, and 28.11; 28.12, 28.13 and 28.14; 28.15, 28.16, and 28.17; and 28.18, 28.19 and 28.20.

### Absorption and Transport Disorders

In disorders of Cbl absorption and transport, the symptoms are usually indistinguishable from those caused by dietary deficiency of vitamin $B_{12}$. Unspecific clinical signs and symptoms may already arise in the first months of life including failure to thrive (weight and head circumference), developmental regression, irritability, apathy, anorexia and refusal of solid foods (Whitehead 2006). Clinically, Imerslund-Najman-Gräsbeck syndrome (IGS) and intrinsic factor deficiency (IFD) overlap considerably; mild, Cbl-resistant proteinuria (not obligatory) in IGS may help to distinguish the two disorders. While patients with IGS and IFD usually present between age 1 and 10 (Tables 28.1, 28.2 and 28.3), those with transcobalamin (TC) deficiency present much earlier, mainly in the first weeks to months of life (Table 28.5). Although haptocorrin deficiency has been associated with low serum Cbl levels, there is no evidence that these low levels result in clinical manifestation of Cbl deficiency (Table 28.4) (Watkins and Rosenblatt 2017). Nine patients with defects in the TC receptor have come to medical attention, mostly as the result of positive newborn screening results for MMAuria (Hannah-Shmouni et al. 2018). Homocysteine was also elevated in most patients (Table 28.6). Eight of the nine patients have remained asymptomatic, with the ninth suffering from bilateral central retinal artery occlusions (Karth et al. 2012). The long-term effects of this condition are yet to be unravelled.

**Tables 28.1–28.3** Hereditary Intrinsic factor deficiency (28.1), and Imerslund-Najman-Gräsbeck syndrome including Cubilin deficiency (28.2), and Amnionless deficiency (28.3)

| System | Symptoms and biomarkers | Neonatal (birth–1 month)[a] | Infancy (1–18 months) | Childhood (1.5–11 years) | Adolescence (11–16 years) | Adulthood (>16 years)[b] |
|---|---|---|---|---|---|---|
| CNS | **Apathy** | | ± | ± | ± | |
| | Deep tendon reflexes | | ↓-n | ↓-n | ↓-n | |
| | Dementia | | | ± | ± | |
| | Developmental regression | | ± | ± | ± | |
| | Hypotonia | | ± | ± | ± | |
| | Intellectual disability | | ± | ± | ± | |
| | **Irritability** | | ± | ± | | |
| | Movement disorder | | ± | ± | ± | |
| | Seizures | | ± | ± | ± | |
| Digestive | **Anorexia** | | ± | ± | ± | |
| Haematological | (pan)cytopenia | | ± | ± | ± | |
| | **Anaemia, megaloblastic** | | ± | + | ± | |
| | Neutrophils, hypersegmented | | ± | + | ± | |
| | Pancytopenia | | ± | ± | ± | |
| Psychiatric | Psychosis | | | ± | ± | |
| Other | **Failure to thrive** | | ± | ± | ± | |
| Laboratory findings | Holotranscobalamin (plasma)[c] | | ↓ | ↓ | ↓ | |
| | Homocysteine (urine) | | ↑ | ↑ | ↑ | |
| | Homocysteine, total (plasma) | | ↑ | ↑ | ↑ | |
| | Methylmalonic acid (plasma) | | ↑ | ↑ | ↑ | |
| | Methylmalonic acid (urine) | | ↑ | ↑ | ↑ | |
| | Proteins, total (urine)[d] | n-↑ | n-↑ | n-↑ | n-↑ | n-↑ |
| | Vitamin B12 (serum) | | ↓ | ↓↓ | ↓ | |

[a]Neonatal presentation extremely rare

[b]Solid data on adult patients not available

[c]Following oral vitamin $B_{12}$ load (Bor et al. 2005)

[d]Mild Cbl-resistant proteinuria may be present in IGS (not obligatory) and help to distinguish from IFD

**Table 28.4** Haptocorrin deficiency

| System | Symptoms and biomarkers | Neonatal (birth–1 month) | Infancy (1–18 months) | Childhood (1.5–11 years) | Adolescence (11–16 years) | Adulthood (>16 years) |
|---|---|---|---|---|---|---|
| Others | **No consistent clinical picture** | | | + | + | |
| Laboratory findings | Holotranscobalamin (plasma) | | | n | n | |
| | Homocysteine, total (plasma) | | | n | n | |
| | Vitamin B12 (serum) | | | ↓ | ↓ | |

## Intracellular Disorders

Although disorders of intracellular Cbl metabolism share many clinical features with the forms of Cbl deficiency due to abnormal absorption and transport, some clinical manifestations are unique. Symptoms are generally more severe, and in most cases there is only a partial or no response to parenteral hydroxo-Cbl treatment (Watkins et al. 2016).

Patients with combined deficiency of MeCbl and AdoCbl synthesis (*cblC*, *cblD*, *cblF*, *cblJ*) usually present within the first year of life with poor feeding, failure to thrive, developmental delay, megaloblastic anaemia and (pan)cytopenia (Tables 28.7, 28.8, 28.9, 28.10 and 28.11). In *cblF* and *cblJ*, low birth weight, minor facial abnormalities and congenital heart defects have been reported as well, while most *cblJ* patients have been reported to have skin hyperpigmentation and grey hair. In *cblC* patients, at least two distinct pheno-

**Table 28.5** Transcobalamin deficiency

| System | Symptoms and biomarkers | Neonatal (birth–1 month) | Infancy (1–18 months) | Childhood (1.5–11 years) | Adolescence (11–16 years) | Adulthood[a] (>16 years) |
|---|---|---|---|---|---|---|
| CNS | **Apathy** | ± | + | + | | |
| | Deep tendon reflexes | | ↓-n | ↓-n | | |
| | Developmental delay | | ± | ± | ± | |
| | Hypotonia | | ± | ± | ± | |
| | Neurologic dysfunction | | ± | ± | ± | |
| Digestive | **Diarrhoea, chronic** | ± | ++ | + | | |
| Haematological | (pan)cytopenia | ± | + | + | | |
| | **Anaemia, megaloblastic** | ± | ++ | + | + | ± |
| | Neutrophils, hypersegmented | ± | ± | ± | ± | |
| | Pancytopenia | ± | + | + | | |
| Others | **Failure to thrive** | ± | ++ | + | | |
| Laboratory findings | Holotranscobalamin (plasma) | | ↓ | ↓ | ↓ | |
| | Homocysteine (urine) | | ↑ | ↑ | | |
| | Homocysteine, total (plasma) | | ↑ | ↑ | | |
| | Methylmalonic acid (plasma) | ↑ | ↑ | ↑ | | |
| | Methylmalonic acid (urine) | ↑ | ↑ | ↑ | | |
| | Vitamin B12 (serum) | | ↓-n | ↓-n | ↓-n | |

[a]Solid data on adult patients not available

**Table 28.6** Transcobalamin receptor defect

| System | Symptoms and biomarkers | Neonatal (birth–1 month) | Infancy (1–18 months) | Childhood[a] (1.5–11 years) | Adolescence[a] (11–16 years) | Adulthood[a] (>16 years) |
|---|---|---|---|---|---|---|
| Others | **No consistent clinical picture** | + | + | | | |
| Laboratory findings | Homocysteine, total (plasma) | (↑) | (↑) | | | |
| | Methylmalonic acid (urine) | ↑ | ↑ | | | |

[a]Few patients described, none beyond infancy

types differentiated by age of onset have been delineated and are related to specific mutations in *MMACHC* (Lerner-Ellis et al. 2009). Early-onset patients present in the first year of life with feeding problems, failure to thrive, neurological symptoms including muscular hypotonia, developmental delay and seizures (Fischer et al. 2014; Huemer et al. 2018) and more rarely with atypical haemolytic uremic syndrome and pulmonary hypertension (Beck et al. 2017). These patients may develop multisystem pathology, which mainly presents as persistent failure to thrive, cognitive dysfunction and eye disease, which is resistant to therapy (Fischer et al. 2014; Huemer et al. 2018). In contrast, a few *cblC* patients have come to clinical attention after the first year of life and have presented as late as in the fourth decade (Thauvin-Robinet et al. 2008). Clinical findings in this group are mainly neurologic and include gait abnormalities, confusion, disorientation, psychosis and dementia (Fischer et al. 2014; Huemer et al. 2018). Macrocytic anaemia is found in less than half of these patients. Only three patients with epimutation of *MMACHC* due to genetic mutation of *PRDX1* have so far been described, and these were consistent with early onset *cblC* disease (Gueant et al. 2018). Alternatively, 19 patients with mutation of *HCFC1* (Yu et al. 2013; Gerard et al. 2015; Koufaris et al. 2016) and one patient each with mutation of *ZNF143* (Pupavac et al. 2016) and *THAP11* (Quintana et al. 2017) have presented in the first months of life with a somewhat similar clinical presentation to early-onset *cblC* patients (Tables 28.12, 28.13 and 28.14). However, in these patients the metabolic abnormalities were milder, while the neurological presentation more severe and often included intractable seizures and severe intellectual disability.

**Tables 28.7–28.11** Adenosylcobalamin and methylcobalamin synthesis defect—cblF (28.7), cblJ (28.8), cblC (28.9), epi-cblC (28.10) and cblD-MMA-HC (28.11)

| System | Symptoms and biomarkers | Neonatal (birth–1 month) | Infancy (1–18 months) | Childhood (1.5–11 years) | Adolescence (11–16 years) | Adulthood (>16 years)[a] |
|---|---|---|---|---|---|---|
| Cardiovascular | Cardiac, anomalies, malformations | ± | ± | | | |
| | Cardiomyopathy | ± | ± | | | |
| CNS | Cerebral atrophy (MRI) | | ± | ± | ± | ± |
| | Dementia | | | | ± | ± |
| | Developmental delay | | ± | ± | ± | |
| | Extrapyramidal signs | | ± | ± | ± | ± |
| | Hypotonia | + | ++ | + | + | + |
| | Myelopathy | n | n | ± | ± | ± |
| | **Neurologic dysfunction** | + | ++ | ++ | ++ | ++ |
| | **Psychiatric symptoms** | | | | ± | ± |
| | Seizures | ± | ± | ± | ± | ± |
| | White mater changes (MRI) | | ± | ± | ± | ± |
| Digestive | Feeding difficulties | + | + | + | ± | ± |
| | Liver dysfunction | | ± | ± | ± | ± |
| Eye | Maculopathy | | ± | ± | ± | ± |
| | Nystagmus | | ± | ± | ± | ± |
| | Retinopathy | | ± | ± | ± | ± |
| | **Vision, impaired** | | ± | ± | ± | ± |
| Haematological | **Anaemia, megaloblastic** | ± | + | + | + | ± |
| | Neutrophils, hypersegmented | ± | ± | ± | ± | ± |
| Musculoskeletal | Dysmorphic features | ± | ± | | | |
| Renal | Haemolytic uraemic syndrome | | ± | ± | ± | |
| Others | **Failure to thrive** | ± | ++ | + | | |
| | Life-threatening illness | + | + | ± | ± | ± |
| | Low birth weight | ± | | | | |
| Laboratory findings | 3-Hydroxypropionic acid (urine) | ↑ | ↑ | ↑ | ↑ | ↑ |
| | C3 propionylcarnitine (blood) | ↑ | ↑ | ↑ | ↑ | ↑ |
| | C3 propionylcarnitine (plasma) | ↑ | ↑ | ↑ | ↑ | ↑ |
| | Homocysteine (urine) | ↑ | ↑ | ↑ | ↑ | ↑ |
| | Homocysteine, total (plasma) | ↑ | ↑ | ↑ | ↑ | ↑ |
| | Methionine (plasma) | ↓-n | ↓-n | ↓-n | ↓-n | ↓-n |
| | Methylcitric acid (urine) | ↑ | ↑ | ↑ | ↑ | ↑ |
| | Methylmalonic acid (plasma) | ↑ | ↑ | ↑ | ↑ | ↑ |
| | Methylmalonic acid (urine) | ↑ | ↑ | ↑ | ↑ | ↑ |
| | S-Adenosylmethionine (cerebrospinal fluid) | | ↓ | ↓ | ↓ | ↓ |
| | S-Adenosylmethionine (plasma) | | ↓ | ↓ | ↓ | ↓ |

[a]Combined deficiencies in adulthood only reported in cblC deficiency to date

**Tables 28.12–28.14** cblC-like adensoylcobalamin and methylcobalamin defect—HCFC1(28.12), ZNF143 (28.13) and THAP11 (28.14)

| System | Symptoms and biomarkers | Neonatal (birth–1 month) | Infancy (1–18 months) | Childhood (1.5–11 years) | Adolescence (11–16 years) | Adulthood (>16 years) |
|---|---|---|---|---|---|---|
| CNS | Choreoathetosis | + | + | | | |
| | Cortical malformations | ± | ± | | | |
| | **Developmental delay** | ± | +++ | | | |
| | Hypotonia | + | + | | | |
| | Infantile spasms with hypsarrhythmia | + | + | | | |
| | Movement disorder | ± | ± | | | |
| | **Neurologic dysfunction** | ++ | ++ | | | |
| | **Seizures, intractable** | + | +++ | | | |
| Eye | Vision, impaired | | ± | | | |
| Haematological | Macrocytosis | ± | ± | | | |
| Musculoskeletal | Dysmorphic features | ± | ± | | | |
| | Microcephaly | + | + | | | |
| Others | **Failure to thrive** | ± | ++ | | | |
| | Life-threatening illness | + | + | | | |
| Laboratory findings | C3 propionylcarnitine (blood) | n-↑ | n-↑ | n-↑ | | |
| | Glycine (cerebrospinal fluid) | ↑ | ↑ | ↑ | | |
| | Glycine (plasma) | n-↑ | n-↑ | n-↑ | | |
| | Homocysteine, total (plasma) | n-↑ | n-↑ | | | |
| | Methylmalonic acid (plasma) | ↑ | ↑ | ↑ | | |
| | Methylmalonic acid (urine) | ↑ | ↑ | ↑ | | |

The clinical features of the isolated homocystinuria defects (*cblE*, *cblG*, *cblD*-HC) include poor feeding and vomiting with failure to thrive, megaloblastic anaemia, and neurological disease including developmental delay, cerebral atrophy, hypotonia or hypertonia, ataxia, neonatal seizures, nystagmus and visual disturbances (Huemer et al. 2015; Huemer et al. 2017) (Tables 28.15, 28.16 and 28.17). Most patients are symptomatic in the first year of life, but isolated cases with later onset and minimal findings have also been reported (Vilaseca et al. 2003).

The majority of patients with isolated MMAuria (*cblA*, *cblB*, *cblD*-MMA and *mut*) present during the newborn period or infancy with metabolic crises, often precipitated by catabolic stress, e.g. induced by febrile illness. Symptoms include vomiting, dehydration, tachypnea, lethargy, failure to thrive, developmental delay, hypotonia and encephalopathy (Tables 28.18, 28.19 and 28.20). Long-term complications include chronic renal failure, developmental delay, metabolic stroke, extrapyramidal movement disorder and optic neuropathy (Baumgartner et al. 2014; Kolker et al. 2015). Patients with $mut^0$ and *cblB* defects tend to have earlier onset of symptoms and a higher frequency of complications and deaths than those with $mut^-$ and *cblA* defects (Horster et al. 2007).

**Tables 28.15–28.17** Methylcobalamin synthesis defect—cblD-HC (28.15), cblE (28.16) and cblG (28.17)

| System | Symptoms and biomarkers | Neonatal (birth–1 month) | Infancy (1–18 months) | Childhood (1.5–11 years) | Adolescence (11–16 years) | Adulthood (>16 years) |
|---|---|---|---|---|---|---|
| CNS | Ataxia | | ± | ± | ± | ± |
| | Cerebral atrophy (MRI) | | ± | ± | ± | ± |
| | Developmental delay | ± | + | + | ± | |
| | Hypertonia | ± | ± | ± | ± | ± |
| | Hypotonia | ± | ± | ± | ± | ± |
| | Lethargy | ± | ± | ± | ± | ± |
| | Myelopathy | n | n | n | ± | ± |
| | **Neurological symptoms** | ± | ++ | + | + | + |
| | **Psychiatric symptoms** | **n** | **n** | **n** | ± | ± |
| | Seizures | ± | ± | ± | ± | ± |
| Digestive | Vomiting | ± | ± | ± | ± | ± |
| Eye | Nystagmus | | ± | ± | ± | ± |
| | Vision, impaired | | ± | ± | ± | ± |
| Haematological | **Anaemia, megaloblastic** | ± | ++ | + | + | ± |
| Others | **Failure to thrive** | ± | + | + | ± | |
| Laboratory findings | Homocysteine (urine) | ↑ | ↑ | ↑ | ↑ | ↑ |
| | Homocysteine, total (plasma) | ↑ | ↑↑ | ↑↑ | ↑↑ | ↑↑ |
| | Methionine (plasma) | ↓-n | ↓-n | ↓-n | ↓-n | ↓-n |
| | Methylmalonic acid (plasma)[a] | n | n | n | n | n |
| | Methylmalonic acid (urine)[a] | n | n | n | n | n |
| | S-Adenosylmethionine (cerebrospinal fluid) | | ↓ | ↓ | ↓ | ↓ |
| | S-Adenosylmethionine (plasma) | | ↓ | ↓ | ↓ | ↓ |

[a]Elevated MMA in isolated cases with cblE

**Tables 28.18–28.20** Adenosylcobalamin synthesis defect—cblD-MMA (28.18), cblA (28.19) and cblB (28.20)

| System | Symptoms and biomarkers | Neonatal (birth–1 month) | Infancy (1–18 months) | Childhood (1.5–11 years) | Adolescence (11–16 years) | Adulthood (>16 years) |
|---|---|---|---|---|---|---|
| Cardiovascular | Cardiomyopathy | | | ± | ? | ? |
| CNS | Basal ganglia lesions (MRI) | | ± | ± | ± | ± |
| | **Encephalopathic crisis, acute** | ± | ± | ± | ± | ± |
| | Extrapyramidal movement disorder | | ± | ± | ± | ± |
| | Hypotonia | ± | ± | ± | ± | ± |
| | Intellectual disability | | ± | ± | ± | ± |
| | Metabolic stroke | ± | ± | ± | ± | ± |
| | Seizures | ± | ± | ± | ± | ± |
| Digestive | Pancreatitis | | ± | ± | ± | ± |
| | **Vomiting** | ++ | + | ± | ± | ± |
| Eye | Optic neuropathy | | | | + | + |
| Haematological | (pan)cytopenia | ± | ± | ± | ± | ± |
| | Pancytopenia | ± | ± | ± | ± | ± |
| Metabolic | **Acidosis** | ++ | + | + | ± | ± |
| | **Ketosis** | ++ | + | + | ± | ± |
| | Metabolic acidosis | +++ | ++ | ± | ± | ± |
| Renal | Renal failure, chronic | | ± | ± | + | ++ |
| Others | **Dehydration** | ++ | + | ± | ± | ± |
| | **Failure to thrive** | | ± | ± | ± | |
| | **Life-threatening illness** | ++ | + | + | ± | ± |

**Tables 28.18–28.20** (continued)

| System | Symptoms and biomarkers | Neonatal (birth–1 month) | Infancy (1–18 months) | Childhood (1.5–11 years) | Adolescence (11–16 years) | Adulthood (>16 years) |
|---|---|---|---|---|---|---|
| Laboratory findings | 3-Hydroxypropionic acid (urine) | ↑ | ↑ | ↑ | ↑ | ↑ |
| | Ammonia (blood) | ↑↑ | n-↑ | n-↑ | n-↑ | n-↑ |
| | Anion gap | + | + | + | ± | ± |
| | C3 propionylcarnitine (blood) | ↑↑ | ↑↑ | ↑↑ | ↑↑ | ↑↑ |
| | C3 propionylcarnitine (plasma) | ↑↑ | ↑↑ | ↑↑ | ↑↑ | ↑↑ |
| | C3/C0 acylcarnitines ratio | ↑ | ↑ | ↑ | ↑ | ↑ |
| | C3/C2 acylcarnitines ratio | ↑ | ↑ | ↑ | ↑ | ↑ |
| | C3/C4DC Acylcarnitines ratio | ↑ | ↑ | ↑ | ↑ | ↑ |
| | Carnitine, free (dried blood spot) | ↓↓ | ↓↓ | ↓↓ | ↓↓ | ↓↓ |
| | Carnitine, free (plasma) | ↓↓ | ↓↓ | ↓↓ | ↓↓ | ↓↓ |
| | Homocysteine, total (plasma) | n | n | n | n | n |
| | Lactate (plasma) | n-↑ | n-↑ | n-↑ | n-↑ | n-↑ |
| | Methylcitric acid (urine) | ↑↑ | ↑↑ | ↑↑ | ↑↑ | ↑↑ |
| | Methylmalonic acid (plasma) | ↑↑↑ | ↑↑↑ | ↑↑↑ | ↑↑↑ | ↑↑↑ |
| | Methylmalonic acid (urine) | ↑↑↑ | ↑↑↑ | ↑↑↑ | ↑↑↑ | ↑↑↑ |

## Diagnosis

Haematologic investigations and measurement of serum Cbl can be helpful. Cbl levels below 125 pmol/L are almost always indicative of Cbl deficiency. However, symptomatic patients with low-normal Cbl that are responsive to Cbl treatment have been reported. Accumulating evidence indicates that plasma measurements of the biologically active Cbl holotranscobalamin may be superior to serum Cbl, and these are being introduced increasingly into the clinical setting (Nexo and Hoffmann-Lucke 2011). However, both markers may be normal in patients with TC deficiency and inborn errors of intracellular Cbl metabolism. In these disorders, measurement of the two metabolic markers MMA and tHcy, which are sensitive indicators of Cbl deficiency, is indicated. Limitations are the specificity of tHcy which is also increased in folate deficiency and the complexity and cost of the assay for MMA. Further studies are usually required to determine the cause of Cbl deficiency, e.g. mutation analysis and/or tests for investigating Cbl absorption or enzymatic and genetic complementation studies in defects of Cbl metabolism. These tests should be performed in laboratories with specific expertise.

## Reference Values

| Analyte | Infant | Child | Adolescent | Adult |
|---|---|---|---|---|
| | <1 year | 1–12 years | 12–18 years | >18 years |
| Serum holotranscobalamin (pmol/L) | >50 | | | |
| Plasma propionylcarnitine (C3) (μmol/L) | <0.54 | | | |
| Blood propionylcarnitine (C3) (μmol/L) | <3.2 | | | |
| Plasma quantitative amino acids (μmol/L) | | | | |
| Total homocysteine[a] | 2.9–10 | 2.8–8.5 | 4.1–13.4 | <10 |
| Methionine | 9–53 | 9–29 | 16–36 | 12–32 |
| S-Adenosylmethionine (nmol/L) | 27–159 | | | 30–118 |
| Urinary quantitative amino acids (mmol/mol creatinine) | | | | |
| Homocyst(e)ine | <8 | | <3 | |
| Plasma (P: μmol/L) and urinary (U: mmol/mol creatinine) quantitative organic acids | | | | |
| Methylmalonic acid (P) | 0.073–0.27 | | | |
| Methylmalonic acid (U) | <3.6 | | | |
| Methylcitric acid (U) | <25 | <18.8 | <8.6 | |
| 3-Hydroxypropionic acid (U) | <21 | <23 | <9 | |
| Amino acids in CSF (μmol/L) | | | | |
| Methionine | 2–7 | <5 | | <9 |
| S-Adenosylmethionine (nmol/L) | 189–243 | 61–201 | | |

[a]Caveat: preanalytics

## Pathological Values

| Disorder | Megaloblastic anaemia | Vitamin $B_{12}$ (S) | Holotranscobalamin (S) | MMA (P) | C3 propionylcarnitine (B) | MMA (U) | Methylcitric acid (U) | 3-Hydroxypropionic acid (U) | Homocysteine (P) | Homocyst(e)ine (U) | Methionine (P) |
|---|---|---|---|---|---|---|---|---|---|---|---|
| 28.1 IFD | + | ↓↓ | | ↑-↑↑ | n-↑ | ↑-↑↑ | n-↑ | n-↑ | ↑↑ | ↑↑ | n-↓ |
| 28.2 CUB | + | ↓↓ | | ↑-↑↑ | n-↑ | ↑-↑↑ | n-↑ | n-↑ | ↑↑ | ↑↑ | n-↓ |
| 28.3 AMN | + | ↓↓ | | ↑-↑↑ | n-↑ | ↑-↑↑ | n-↑ | n-↑ | ↑↑ | ↑↑ | n-↓ |
| 28.4 HCD | n | ↓ | n | | | | | | n | | |
| 28.5 TCD | + | n-↓ | | ↑-↑↑ | n-↑ | ↑-↑↑ | n-↑ | n-↑ | ↑↑ | ↑↑ | n-↓ |
| 28.6 TCR | | ↓↓ | | | | ↑ | | | n-↑ | | |
| 28.7 cblF | + | n | n | ↑-↑↑ | ↑ | ↑-↑↑ | ↑ | ↑ | ↑↑ | ↑↑ | ↓ |
| 28.8 cblJ | (+) | n | n | ↑-↑↑ | ↑ | ↑-↑↑ | ↑ | ↑ | ↑↑ | ↑↑ | ↓ |
| 28.9 cblC | + | n | n | ↑-↑↑ | ↑ | ↑-↑↑ | ↑ | ↑ | ↑↑↑ | ↑↑↑ | ↓↓ |
| 28.10 epi-cblC | + | n | n | ↑-↑↑ | ↑ | ↑-↑↑ | ↑ | ↑ | ↑↑↑ | ↑↑↑ | ↓↓ |
| 28.11 cblD-MMA/HC | + | n | n | ↑-↑↑ | ↑ | ↑-↑↑ | ↑ | ↑ | ↑↑ | ↑↑ | ↓ |
| 28.15 cblD-HC | + | n | n | n | n | n | n | n | ↑↑ | ↑↑ | ↓ |
| 28.18 cblD-MMA | n | n | n | ↑-↑↑ | ↑ | ↑-↑↑ | ↑ | ↑ | n | n | n |
| 28.12 HCFC1 | | n | n | ↑ | n-↑ | ↑ | | | n-↑ | | |
| 28.13 ZNF143 | | n | n | ↑ | n-↑ | ↑ | | | n-↑ | | |
| 28.14 THAP11 | | n | n | ↑ | n-↑ | ↑ | | | n-↑ | | |
| 28.16 cblE | + | n | n | n | n | n | n | n | ↑↑ | ↑↑ | ↓ |
| 28.17 cblG | + | n | n | n | n | n | n | n | ↑↑ | ↑↑ | ↓ |
| 28.19 cblA | n | n | n | ↑↑ | ↑-↑↑ | ↑↑ | ↑-↑↑ | ↑-↑↑ | n | n | n |
| 28.20 cblB | n | n | n | ↑↑↑ | ↑↑ | ↑↑↑ | ↑↑ | ↑↑ | n | n | n |

## Diagnostic Flowchart

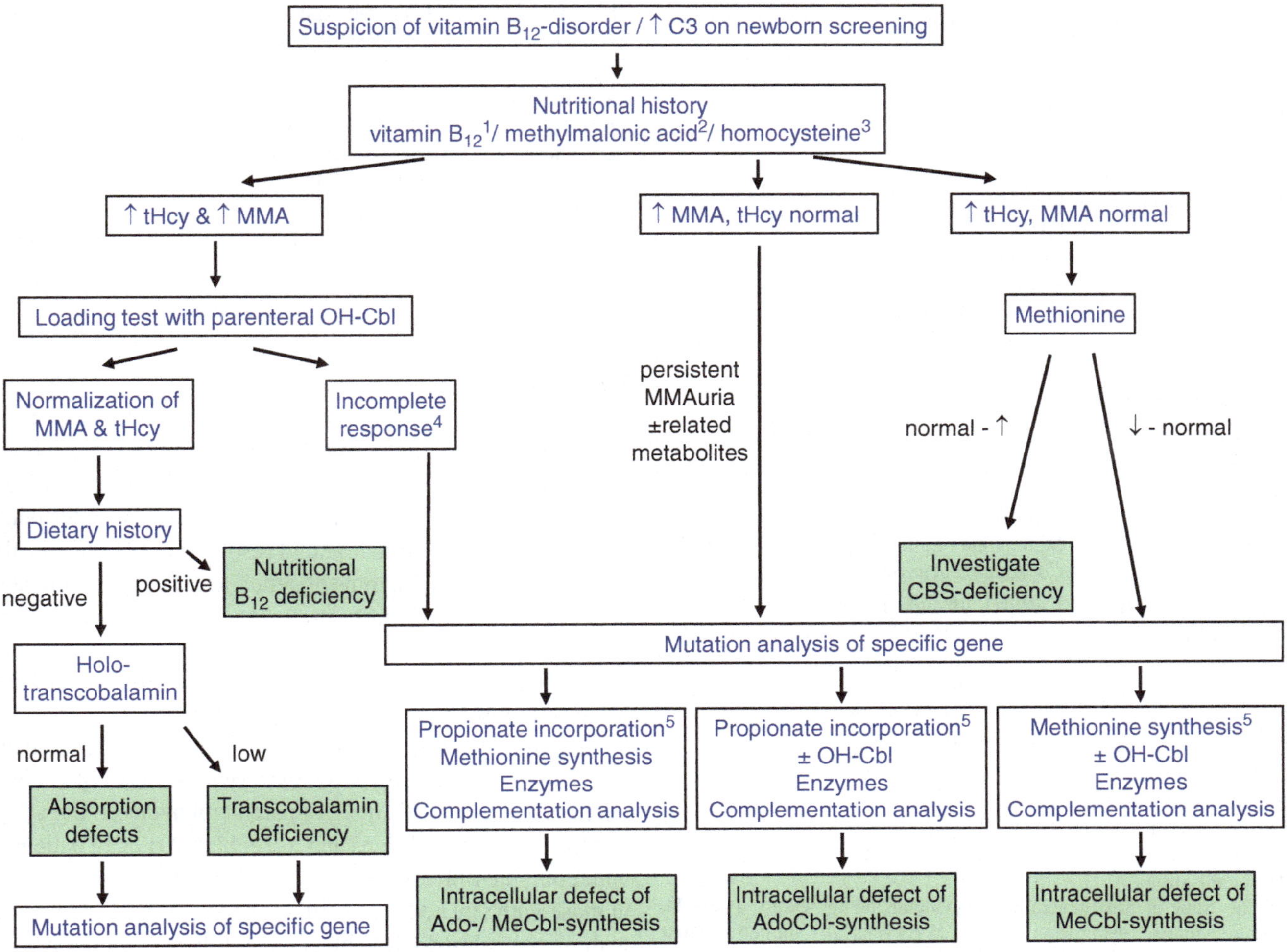


[1]serum vitamin $B_{12}$; [2]plasma or urinary methylmalonic acid (MMA); [3]plasma total homocysteine (tHcy); [4]cblF may show complete response
[5]functional/enzymatic studies in cultured fibroblasts

## Specimen Collection

Overview on methods and required samples for enzyme and mutation analysis

| Metabolite | Sample |
|---|---|
| Methylmalonic acid | Plasma |
| Total homocysteine | Plasma[a] |
| Holo-transcobalamin[b] | Plasma or serum |
| *S*-Adenosylmethionine | Plasma[c]<br>CSF |
| **Disorder** | **Enzyme assays[d]: Method** |
| **28.7 cblF**<br>**28.8 cblJ**<br>**28.9 cblC**<br>**28.10 epi-cblC**<br>**28.11 cblD-MMA/HC**<br>**28.12 HCFC1**<br>**28.13 ZNF143**<br>**28.14 THAP11** | **Cultured fibroblasts:**<br>Propionate fixation<br>Methionine synthesis from formate/MeTHF<br>Cobalamin coenzyme synthesis |
| **28.15 cblD-HC**<br>**28.16 cblE**<br>**28.17 cblG** | **Cultured fibroblasts:**<br>Methionine synthesis from formate/MeTHF<br>Cobalamin coenzyme synthesis |
| **28.18 cblD-MMA**<br>**28.19 cblA**<br>**28.20 cblB** | **Cultured fibroblasts:**<br>Propionate fixation, methylmalonyl-CoA mutase<br>**Lymphocytes:**<br>Methylmalonyl-CoA mutase |
| | **Mutation analysis** |
| All disorders | DNA analysis possible |

[a]Immediate separation of plasma essential
[b]Stable parameter (Nexo and Hoffmann-Lucke 2011)
[c]EDTA blood on ice, immediate separation of plasma and deproteinisation
[d]In the light of next-generation sequencing being widely available, mutation analysis using gene panels or WES is usually applied as a first step; enzymatic workup is advised in all unclear cases. In some cases (common mutation or small gene), single gene/exon analysis is advised as first step

## Prenatal Diagnosis

| Disorder | Tests recommended and sample requirements |
|---|---|
| **28.7 cblF**<br>**28.8 cblJ**<br>**28.9 cblC**<br>**28.10 epi-cblC**<br>**28.11 cblD-MMA/HC** | **CVS DNA[a]**<br>**Cultured amniocytes—Enzymatic assays**<br>**Cell-free amniotic fluid—tHcy, MMA, methylcitrate** |
| **28.12 HCFC1**<br>**28.13 ZNF143**<br>**28.14 THAP11** | **CVS DNA[a]** |
| **28.15 cblD-HC**<br>**28.16 cblE**<br>**28.17 cblG** | **CVS DNA[a]**<br>**Cultured amniocytes—Enzymatic assays**<br>**Cell-free amniotic fluid—tHcy** |
| **28.18 cblD-MMA**<br>**28.19 cblA**<br>**28.20 cblB** | **CVS DNA[a]**<br>**Cultured amniocytes—Enzymatic assays**<br>**Cell-free amniotic fluid—MMA, methylcitrate** |

*CVS* Chorionic villous sampling
[a]First choice if disease causing mutations and their parental origin confirmed

## Treatment

In patients with defects of Cbl absorption and transport, treatment with relatively small amounts of Cbl, administered by injection to circumvent the barrier of the intestinal mucosa, generally results in rapid resolution of biochemical abnormalities and symptoms of deficiency. The conventional therapy is 1000 μg of parenteral cyano-Cbl or hydroxo-Cbl daily for 1 week, followed by 100–1000 μg cyano-Cbl weekly for 1 month and monthly thereafter. This therapy is believed to replete and sustain body Cbl stores.

Treatment of diseases caused by defects of intracellular processing of Cbl usually requires very large doses of cofactor, i.e. 1000 μg or even more of parenteral hydroxo-Cbl several times weekly (Watkins and Rosenblatt 2017). In patients with combined MMA and Hcy (cblC, cblD, cblF, cblJ) and in those with isolated Hcy (cblE, cblG, cblD-HC), treatment with parenteral hydroxo-Cbl, betaine, folinic acid/methylfolinic acid and theoretically methionine usually corrects the haematologic abnormalities and improves but usually does not completely correct the biochemical abnormalities. Moreover, neurological symptoms respond only partially, and severe neurological deficits, including eye disease, often persist. Treatment of isolated MMAurias consists of dietary restriction of protein, carnitine supplementation and, in Cbl-responsive patients, parenteral hydroxo-Cbl. While most patients with *cblA* will respond even to oral hydroxo-Cbl, only about one third of *cblB* patients and even fewer patients with *mut* will do so (Matsui et al. 1983). Thus, it is important to reliably classify these patients and identify those who genuinely benefit from hydroxo-Cbl treatment using a standardised test (Fowler et al. 2008).

## Drugs and Dosages to be Used in Acute Presentation of Suspected Disorders of Vitamin $B_{12}$ Metabolism

Emergency and standard treatment tables and medication requirements. Acute presentation

| Disorder | Hydroxo-Cbl (CN-Cbl less effective) | Folic or folinic acid (never give without Cbl) | L-Carnitine | L-Arginine hydrochloride (to be given IV in glucose 10%) | Sodium benzoate (to be given IV in glucose 10%) |
|---|---|---|---|---|---|
| All disorders | 1–5 mg/day i.m., i.v. or s.c. | Folic acid: 15 mg/kg/day (i.v. in three doses)<br>Folinic acid (preferred, if available): 3 mg/kg/day (i.v. in one dose) | 50–100 mg/kg/day[a] | – | – |
| Disorders with MMA only (cblA, cblB, cblD-MMA)[b] | Same | Optional | 50–200 mg/kg/day i.v. | 250 mg/kg (1.2 mmol/kg) as bolus in 90–120 min, then maintenance 250 mg/kg/day (1.2 mmol/kg/day) | 250 mg/kg as bolus in 90–120 min, then maintenance 250–500 mg/kg/day[c]<br>>20 kg bw: 5.5 g/m²/day |

[a]Optional
[b]For more details see methylmalonyl-CoA mutase deficiency in Chap. 23 (disorder **23.23**)
[c]If on haemodialysis/haemodiafiltration, doses should be increased to 350 mg/kg/day (maintenance dose)

Dosages of drugs to be used for long-term treatment

| Disorder | Hydroxo-Cbl (Cyano-Cbl generally less effective) | Folinic/folic acid (never give without Cbl) | L-Carnitine | Diet | Betaine |
|---|---|---|---|---|---|
| 28.1 IFD | 1 mg i.m. or s.c. every 1–3 months | Folic acid up to 10 mg 4× daily | – | – | – |
| 28.2 and 28.3 IGS | | | | | |
| 28.4 HCD | – | – | – | – | – |
| 28.5 TCD | 0.5–1 mg p.o. 2× weekly or 1 mg i.m. 1× weekly | Folic acid up to 10 mg 4× daily | – | – | – |
| 28.6 TCR | – | – | – | – | – |
| 28.7 cblF | 1 mg i.m. or s.c. daily[a] | Folinic acid 15 mg/day[b] | 50 mg/kg/day[b] | Moderate protein restriction[b] | Up to 250 mg/kg/day |
| 28.8 cblJ | | | | | |
| 28.9 cblC | | | | | |
| 28.10 epi-cblC | | | | | |
| 28.11 cblD-MMA/HC | | | | | |
| 28.12 HCFC1 | | | | | |
| 28.13 ZNF143 | | | | | |
| 28.14 THAP11 | | | | | |
| 28.15 cblD-HC | 1 mg i.m. or s.c. daily | Folinic acid 15 mg/day[b] | – | – | Up to 250 mg/kg/day |
| 28.16 cblE | | | | | |
| 28.17 cblG | | | | | |
| 28.18 cblD-MMA[c] | 1 mg i.m. or s.c. 1–7× weekly[d] | – | 50–100 mg/kg/day | Protein restriction and supplementation of precursor-free amino acid mixture[b] | – |
| 28.19 cblA | | | | | |
| 28.20 cblB | | | | | |

[a]In cblC OHCbl should be titrated individually based on metabolic response; up to 20 mg OHCbl daily have been used; even with such doses tHcy mostly cannot be normalised; levels between 40 and 60 µmol/L are typicaslly reached in infantile-onset cblC. In some late-onset patients, tHcy has been normalised
[b]Optional
[c]See also methylmalonyl-CoA mutase deficiency in Chap. 23 (disorder **23.23**)
[d]Cbl responsiveness should be carefully tested starting with 1–2 mg OHCbl i.m. or s.c. for several days followed by titrating cobalamin dosage against methylmalonate excretion and clinical status in cobalamin-responsive patients

## Experimental Treatment

In the cblC defect, prenatal diagnosis and treatment of the affected foetus by administration of hydroxo-Cbl i.m. in the mother have been reported (Huemer et al. 2005; Trefz et al. 2016). Furthermore, attempts to treat this disorder with antioxidants and creatine have been made. In the cblA and cblB defects, transplantation of the kidney and/or the liver has been reported. It must be borne in mind that such treatment does not prevent neurological damage such as metabolic stroke.

## References


Aminoff M, Carter JE, Chadwick RB, Johnson C, Grasbeck R, Abdelaal MA, et al. Mutations in CUBN, encoding the intrinsic factor-vitamin B-12 receptor, cubilin, cause hereditary megaloblastic anaemia 1. Nat Genet. 1999;21(3):309–13.

Banerjee R, Gherasim C, Padovani D. The tinker, tailor, soldier in intracellular B12 trafficking. Curr Opin Chem Biol. 2009;13(4):484–91.

Baumgartner MR, Horster F, Dionisi-Vici C, Haliloglu G, Karall D, Chapman KA, et al. Proposed guidelines for the diagnosis and management of methylmalonic and propionic acidemia. Orphanet J Rare Dis. 2014;9:130.

Beck BB, van Spronsen F, Diepstra A, Berger RM, Komhoff M. Renal thrombotic microangiopathy in patients with cblC defect: review of an under-recognized entity. Pediatr Nephrol. 2017;32(5):733–41.

Bor MV, Cetin M, Aytac S, Altay C, Nexo E. Nonradioactive vitamin B12 absorption test evaluated in controls and in patients with inherited malabsorption of vitamin B12. Clin Chem. 2005;51(11):2151–5.

Coelho D, Suormala T, Stucki M, Lerner-Ellis JP, Rosenblatt DS, Newbold RF, et al. Gene identification for the cblD defect of vitamin B12 metabolism. N Engl J Med. 2008;358(14):1454–64.

Coelho D, Kim JC, Miousse IR, Fung S, du Moulin M, Buers I, et al. Mutations in ABCD4 cause a new inborn error of vitamin B12 metabolism. Nat Genet. 2012;44(10):1152–5.

Fettelschoss V, Burda P, Sagne C, Coelho D, De Laet C, Lutz S, et al. Clinical or ATPase domain mutations in ABCD4 disrupt the interaction between the vitamin B12-trafficking proteins ABCD4 and LMBD1. J Biol Chem. 2017;292(28):11980–91.

Fischer S, Huemer M, Baumgartner M, Deodato F, Ballhausen D, Boneh A, et al. Clinical presentation and outcome in a series of 88 patients with the cblC defect. J Inherit Metab Dis. 2014;

Fowler B, Leonard JV, Baumgartner MR. Causes of and diagnostic approach to methylmalonic acidurias. J Inherit Metab Dis. 2008;31(3):350–60.

Fyfe JC, Madsen M, Hojrup P, Christensen EI, Tanner SM, de la Chapelle A, et al. The functional cobalamin (vitamin B-12)-intrinsic factor receptor is a novel complex of cubilin and amnionless. Blood. 2004;103(5):1573–9.

Gerard M, Morin G, Bourillon A, Colson C, Mathieu S, Rabier D, et al. Multiple congenital anomalies in two boys with mutation in HCFC1 and cobalamin disorder. Eur J Med Genet. 2015;58(3):148–53.

Gueant JL, Chery C, Oussalah A, Nadaf J, Coelho D, Josse T, et al. Publisher correction: a PRDX1 mutant allele causes a MMACHC secondary epimutation in cblC patients. Nat Commun. 2018;9(1):554.

Hannah-Shmouni F, Cruz V, Schulze A, Mercimek-Andrews S. Transcobalamin receptor defect: identification of two new cases through positive newborn screening for propionic/methylmalonic aciduria and long-term outcome. Am J Med Genet A. 2018;176(6):1411–5.

Hannibal L, Kim J, Brasch NE, Wang S, Rosenblatt DS, Banerjee R, et al. Processing of alkylcobalamins in mammalian cells: a role for the MMACHC (cblC) gene product. Mol Genet Metab. 2009;97(4):260–6.

Horster F, Baumgartner MR, Viardot C, Suormala T, Burgard P, Fowler B, et al. Long-term outcome in methylmalonic acidurias is influenced by the underlying defect (mut0, mut-, cblA, cblB). Pediatr Res. 2007;62(2):225–30.

Hu S, Mei S, Liu N, Kong X. Molecular genetic characterization of cblC defects in 126 pedigrees and prenatal genetic diagnosis of pedigrees with combined methylmalonic aciduria and homocystinuria. BMC Med Genet. 2018;19(1):154.

Huemer M, Simma B, Fowler B, Suormala T, Bodamer OA, Sass JO. Prenatal and postnatal treatment in cobalamin C defect. J Pediatr. 2005;147(4):469–72.

Huemer M, Burer C, Jesina P, Kozich V, Landolt MA, Suormala T, et al. Clinical onset and course, response to treatment and outcome in 24 patients with the cblE or cblG remethylation defect complemented by genetic and in vitro enzyme study data. J Inherit Metab Dis. 2015;38(5):957–67.

Huemer M, Diodato D, Schwahn B, Schiff M, Bandeira A, Benoist JF, et al. Guidelines for diagnosis and management of the cobalamin-related remethylation disorders cblC, cblD, cblE, cblF, cblG, cblJ and MTHFR deficiency. J Inherit Metab Dis. 2017;40(1):21–48.

Huemer M, Diodato D, Martinelli D, Olivieri G, Blom H, Gleich F, et al. Phenotype, treatment practice and outcome in the cobalamin-dependent remethylation disorders and MTHFR deficiency: data from the E-HOD registry. J Inherit Metab Dis. 2018;

Karth P, Singh R, Kim J, Costakos D. Bilateral central retinal artery occlusions in an infant with hyperhomocysteinemia. J AAPOS. 2012;16(4):398–400.

Kim J, Gherasim C, Banerjee R. Decyanation of vitamin B12 by a trafficking chaperone. Proc Natl Acad Sci U S A. 2008;105(38):14551–4.

Kolker S, Valayannopoulos V, Burlina AB, Sykut-Cegielska J, Wijburg FA, Teles EL, et al. The phenotypic spectrum of organic acidurias and urea cycle disorders. Part 2: the evolving clinical phenotype. J Inherit Metab Dis. 2015;38(6):1059–74.

Koufaris C, Alexandrou A, Tanteles GA, Anastasiadou V, Sismani C. A novel HCFC1 variant in male siblings with intellectual disability and microcephaly in the absence of cobalamin disorder. Biomed Rep. 2016;4(2):215–8.

Lerner-Ellis JP, Tirone JC, Pawelek PD, Dore C, Atkinson JL, Watkins D, et al. Identification of the gene responsible for methylmalonic aciduria and homocystinuria, cblC type. Nat Genet. 2006;38(1):93–100.

Lerner-Ellis JP, Anastasio N, Liu J, Coelho D, Suormala T, Stucki M, et al. Spectrum of mutations in MMACHC, allelic expression, and evidence for genotype-phenotype correlations. Hum Mutat. 2009;30(7):1072–81.

Liu Y, Liu YP, Zhang Y, Song JQ, Zheng H, Dong H, et al. Heterogeneous phenotypes, genotypes, treatment and prevention of 1 003 patients with methylmalonic acidemia in the mainland of China. Zhonghua Er Ke Za Zhi. 2018;56(6):414–20.

Matsui SM, Mahoney MJ, Rosenberg LE. The natural-history of the inherited methylmalonic acidemias. N Engl J Med. 1983;308(15):857–61.

Nexo E, Hoffmann-Lucke E. Holotranscobalamin, a marker of vitamin B-12 status: analytical aspects and clinical utility. Am J Clin Nutr. 2011;94(1):359S–65S.

Nielsen MJ, Rasmussen MR, Andersen CBF, Nexo E, Moestrup SK. Vitamin B-12 transport from food to the body's cells-a sophisticated, multistep pathway. Nat Rev Gastro Hepat. 2012;9(6):345–54.

Parini R, Furlan F, Brambilla A, Codazzi D, Vedovati S, Corbetta C, et al. Severe neonatal metabolic decompensation in methylmalonic acidemia caused by CblD defect. JIMD Rep. 2013;11:133–7.

Plessl T, Burer C, Lutz S, Yue WW, Baumgartner MR, Froese DS. Protein destabilization and loss of protein-protein interaction are fundamental mechanisms in cblA-type methylmalonic aciduria. Hum Mutat. 2017;38(8):988–1001.

Pupavac M, Watkins D, Petrella F, Fahiminiya S, Janer A, Cheung W, et al. Inborn error of cobalamin metabolism associated with the intracellular accumulation of transcobalamin-bound cobalamin and mutations in ZNF143, which codes for a transcriptional activator. Hum Mutat. 2016;37(9):976–82.

Quintana AM, Yu HC, Brebner A, Pupavac M, Geiger EA, Watson A, et al. Mutations in THAP11 cause an inborn error of cobalamin metabolism and developmental abnormalities. Hum Mol Genet. 2017;

Rutsch F, Gailus S, Miousse IR, Suormala T, Sagne C, Toliat MR, et al. Identification of a putative lysosomal cobalamin exporter altered in the cblF defect of vitamin B12 metabolism. Nat Genet. 2009;41(2):234–9.

Stucki M, Coelho D, Suormala T, Burda P, Fowler B, Baumgartner MR. Molecular mechanisms leading to three different phenotypes in the cblD defect of intracellular cobalamin metabolism. Hum Mol Genet. 2012;21(6):1410–8.

Tanner SM, Aminoff M, Wright FA, Liyanarachchi S, Kuronen M, Saarinen A, et al. Amnionless, essential for mouse gastrulation, is mutated in recessive hereditary megaloblastic anemia. Nat Genet. 2003;33(3):426–9.

Tanner SM, Li Z, Perko JD, Oner C, Cetin M, Altay C, et al. Hereditary juvenile cobalamin deficiency caused by mutations in the intrinsic factor gene. Proc Natl Acad Sci U S A. 2005;102(11):4130–3.

Thauvin-Robinet C, Roze E, Couvreur G, Horellou MH, Sedel F, Grabli D, et al. The adolescent and adult form of cobalamin C disease: clinical and molecular spectrum. J Neurol Neurosurg Psychiatry. 2008;79(6):725–8.

Trefz FK, Scheible D, Frauendienst-Egger G, Huemer M, Suomala T, Fowler B, et al. Successful intrauterine treatment of a patient with cobalamin C defect. Mol Genet Metab Rep. 2016;6:55–9.

Vilaseca MA, Vilarinho L, Zavadakova P, Vela E, Cleto E, Pineda M, et al. CblE type of homocystinuria: mild clinical phenotype in two patients homozygous for a novel mutation in the MTRR gene. J Inherit Metab Dis. 2003;26(4):361–9.

Watkins D, Rosenblatt DS. Inherited disorders of folate and cobalamin transport and metabolism. In: Valle D, Beaudet AL, Vogelstein B, Kinzler KW, Antonarakis SE, Ballabio A, et al., editors. The online metabolic and molecular bases of inherited disease. New York: McGraw-Hill Medical; 2017.

Watkins D, Rosenblatt DS, Fowler B. Disorders of cobalamin and folate transport and metabolism. In: Saudubray JM, Baumgartner MR, Walter J, editors. Inborn metabolic diseases. Diagnosis and treatment. 6th ed. Berlin, Heidelberg: Springer; 2016. p. 385–400.

Whitehead VM. Acquired and inherited disorders of cobalamin and folate in children. Br J Haematol. 2006;134(2):125–36.

Yu HC, Sloan JL, Scharer G, Brebner A, Quintana AM, Achilly NP, et al. An X-linked cobalamin disorder caused by mutations in transcriptional coregulator HCFC1. Am J Hum Genet. 2013;93(3):506–14.

# Disorders of Folate Metabolism and Transport

# 29

Robert Steinfeld and Nenad Blau

## Contents




**Summary**

Folates play an essential role in one-carbon methyl transfer reactions, mediating several biological processes including DNA synthesis, regulation of gene expression through methylation and formylation reactions, embryonic central nervous system development, synthesis and breakdown of amino acids, and synthesis of thymidines, purines, and neurotransmitters (Blount et al. 1997; Linhart et al. 2009; Ghoshal et al. 2006; Pogribny et al. 2008; Fournier et al. 2002). In mammals, folates are mostly derived from exogenous sources as folate is stored in the liver for few months. The biologically active folate derivative is 5,6,7,8-tetrahydrofolate (THF). Dietary folate is absorbed in the intestine via the proton-coupled folate transporter (PCFT). In the cytoplasm, interconversion of 5,10-methylene-THF and 5,10-methenyl-THF, interconversion of 5,10-methenyl-THF and 10-formyl-THF, and reaction of THF with formate to synthesize 10-formyl-THF are mediated by the MTHFD1 gene that encodes a trifunctional protein. Metabolism of 5,10-methylene-THF to 5-methyl-THF in the liver is catalyzed by methylene-THF reductase (MTHFR). 5-Methyl-THF is then widely distributed in the bloodstream. The transport of 5-methyl-THF inside the cells is mediated by different transport systems that include the proton-coupled folate transporter (PCFT), the reduced folate carrier 1 (RFC1), and the two GPI-anchored receptors, folate receptor alpha (FRα) and beta (FRβ) (Matherly and Goldman 2003). The physiological form of folate, 5-methyl-THF, is actively transported to the central nervous system by FRα-mediated endocytosis in choroid epithelial cells, reaching a higher concentration in the cerebrospinal



R. Steinfeld (✉)
Division of Pediatric Neurology, University Children's Hospital Zürich, Zürich, Switzerland
e-mail: robert.steinfeld@kispi.uzh.ch

N. Blau
Division of Metabolism, University Children's Hospital, Zürich, Switzerland
e-mail: nenad.blau@kispi.uzh.ch




N. Blau et al. (eds.), *Physician's Guide to the Diagnosis, Treatment, and Follow-Up of Inherited Metabolic Diseases*,
https://doi.org/10.1007/978-3-030-67727-5_29

fluid when compared to the serum. FRα is a high-affinity low-capacity receptor that functions at a nanomolar range of extracellular folate concentrations (Weitman et al. 1992). Glutamate formiminotransferase-cyclodeaminase (FTCD) is a bifunctional enzyme that catalyzes the folate-dependent degradation of N-formimino-L-glutamic acid (FIGLU) to form 5,10-methenyltetrahydrofolate, glutamate, and ammonia, the final two reactions of the pathway responsible for the degradation of L-histidine. Thus far, seven different inherited disorders of folate metabolism are known which lead to folate deficiency including hereditary folate malabsorption, folate receptor alpha deficiency, 5,10-methylenete-THF reductase deficiency, 5,10-methenyl-THF synthetase deficiency, dihydrofolate reductase deficiency, and 5,10-methylenete-THF dehydrogenase deficiency (Watkins et al. 2011; Watkins and Rosenblatt 2012). Reduced folate carrier deficiency presenting with recurrent megaloblastic anemia has been reported very recently in a single patient carrying a homozygous deletion of the Phe212 residue (Svaton et al. 2020). Glutamate formimino transferase deficiency is considered as a non-disease, despite being former characterized by megaloblastic anemia, mental retardation and elevated urine FIGLU following a histidine load (Hilton et al. 2003). Mitochondrial 10-formyltetrahydrofolate dehydrogenase, encoded by *ALDH1L2*, affects mitochondrial pool of metabolites relevant to beta-oxidation of fatty acids and presents with neuro-ichthyotic syndrome (Sarret et al. 2019). For more details on FIGLU-uria, see Chap. 71.

## Introduction

Hereditary folate malabsorption is an autosomal recessive condition where infants present at 2–6 months of age with clinical features suggestive of megaloblastic anemia, failure to thrive, diarrhea, frequent infections, mucositis, immune deficiency, and neurological features including epilepsy, developmental delay, and intellectual disability due to a defect in the uptake of folates from the intestine and the blood-brain barrier of the choroid plexus. Folate levels on both serum and cerebrospinal fluid are low (see Table 29.1). This condition is caused by variants in the *SLC46A1* gene that maps to 17q11.2 and encodes the PCFT (Qiu et al. 2006). Several variants have been reported including missense, nonsense, and splice site variants, and it has been demonstrated that they affect folate transport in an in vitro system (Qiu et al. 2006). The therapy of this condition has involved the parenteral administration of folate. However, oral therapy has been successfully implemented in some cases (Watkins et al. 2011). Folate receptor alpha deficiency is an autosomal recessive condition caused by loss of function variants in the *FOLR1* gene encoding the folate receptor alpha that leads to impaired transport of folate to the CNS (see Table 29.2). The patients initially described exhibit null variants causing severe cerebral folate deficiency (CFD) (Steinfeld et al. 2009). These patients have an initial period of normal development until the age of 2 years, and they eventually exhibit psychomotor decline, progressive movement disturbance, white matter disease, and epilepsy (Steinfeld et al. 2009; Cario et al. 2009). Myoclonic-astatic seizures have been described in the most affected patients, and the epilepsy in these patients seems to be drug refractory (Steinfeld et al. 2009; Cario et al. 2009) although a case associated with progressive myoclonic epilepsy has responded to high dose of folinic acid supplementation (Perez-Duenas et al. 2011). These patients have almost undetectable levels of cerebrospinal fluid (CSF) 5-methyl-THF. MR-based in vivo metabolite analysis indicates depletion of white matter choline and inositol. Folinic acid therapy restores glial choline and inositol contents, CSF 5-methyl-THF and ameliorates symptoms in these patients. Folate receptor alpha deficiency caused by a homozygous p.(Arg204*) variant in the *FOLR1* gene has been described in a patient with congenital deafness, labyrinthine aplasia, microtia, and microdontia (LAMM) syndrome (Dill et al. 2011). Folinic acid treatment helped to regain consciousness, but the epilepsy was controlled with pyridoxal 5′-phosphate.

Methylenete-THF reductase (MTHFR) deficiency is an autosomal recessive condition caused by variants in the *MTHFR* gene that maps to 1p36.22 (Goyette et al. 1994). This condition represents the most common of the known inborn errors of folate metabolism with more than 160 subjects identified (Huemer et al. 2019). Methylene-THF reductase mediates the conversion of 5,10-methylene-THF to 5-methyl-THF. Biochemically, patients with this condition have hyperhomocysteinemia with low or low-normal methionine levels, reflecting decreased activity of methionine synthase. Clinical features of this disorder include developmental delay, intellectual disability, neurological and psychiatric features, thrombotic events, and serious disease leading to death (Strauss et al. 2007) (see Table 29.3). Severe MTHFR deficiency should be a diagnostic consideration in infantile epileptic encephalopathy and infantile communicating hydrocephalus (Prasad et al.

2011; Baethmann et al. 2000). Microcephaly and developmental regression become noticeable following the onset of seizures. Patients with this condition do not exhibit megaloblastic anemia. Other subjects may present later in childhood with developmental delay and other neurological manifestations. The striking changes of demyelination do not necessarily reflect an effect from the vascular lesions, suggesting the participation of other factors such as inadequate methionine synthesis, a deficiency of *S*-adenosylmethionine or accumulation of toxic intermediates from the elevated levels of homocysteine (Prasad et al. 2011). Among different therapeutic strategies, the best outcome has been seen with betaine-homocysteine methyltransferase that converts homocysteine to methionine without requiring folate when started prenatally or soon after birth (Strauss et al. 2007). MTHFR deficiency can be pre-clinically diagnosed through the newborn screening for total homocysteine (Huemer et al. 2019).

Dihydrofolate reductase (DHFR) deficiency is a rare inborn error of folate metabolism (Cario et al. 2011; Banka et al. 2011) (see Table 29.4). DHFR is a key enzyme in folate metabolism and an important target of several pharmacological compounds. Three individuals from two families were described, who presented with megaloblastic anemia and/or pancytopenia, severe CFD, and cerebral tetrahydrobiopterin deficiency due to a germline missense variant in *DHFR*, leading to profound enzymatic deficiency. Cerebral folate levels, anemia, and pancytopenia were corrected by treatment with folinic acid. These individuals presented in the first weeks of life with epilepsy, developmental delay, and cerebral and cerebellar atrophy (Banka et al. 2011). Individuals from a third family presented at 2–11 years, and two exhibited atypical childhood absence epilepsy (Cario et al. 2011). All of these subjects were homozygous for variants in the *DHFR* gene that maps to 5q14.1. Therapy with folinic acid has corrected the biochemical abnormalities. However, in some cases, the epilepsy became persistent when the treatment with folinic acid was not given in a consistent basis (Cario et al. 2011).

Variants in the *MTHFD1* gene mapping to 14q23.3 have been identified by exome sequencing in an infant who presented at 2 months of age with megaloblastic anemia, atypical hemolytic uremic syndrome, and severe combined immunodeficiency (see Table 29.5). The *MTHFD1* gene encodes the trifunctional enzyme that mediates the 5,10-methylene-THF dehydrogenase, 5,10-methenyl-THF cyclohydrolase, and 10-formyl-THF synthetase reactions (Watkins and Rosenblatt 2012). Homocysteine and methylmalonic acid were increased. In vitro studies demonstrated decreased synthesis of methylcobalamin, required for the activity of methionine synthase. Serum folate was normal (Keller et al. 2013; Bidla et al. 2020).

Several patients with *MTHFS* variants and with frequent seizures and cerebral hypomyelination, unresponsive to folinic acid administration, were reported with very low CSF 5MTHF (see Table 29.6). All other biochemical parameters were normal, and there were no signs of anemia. MTHFS converts 5-formyl-THF to 5,10-methenyl-THF, thus making folinic acid not a therapeutic option. CFD may be associated with autistic features in a subset of children with developmental regression, intellectual disability, epilepsy, dyskinesia, and autism (Moretti et al. 2008; Rodan et al. 2018) (see Table 29.7).

A single patient presenting with a folate-dependent megaloblastic anemia, hyperhomocysteinemia, low total vitamin B12 levels, and normal serum folates due to a homozygous Phe212 deletion in the *SLC19A1* gene responded well to treatment with cyanocobalamin and folate (Svaton et al. 2020).

Two phenotypes of the glutamate formimino transferase deficiency, a severe and a mild form, have been described with their genetic basis not yet fully elucidated (Hilton et al. 2003).

## Nomenclature

| No. | Disorder | Alternative name | Abbreviation | Gene symbol | Chromosomal localization | Affected protein | OMIM No. |
|---|---|---|---|---|---|---|---|
| 29.1 | Hereditary folate malabsorption | Proton-coupled folate transporter (PCFT) deficiency | HFM | *SLC46A1* | 17q11.2 | SLC46A1 transporter | 229050 |
| 29.2 | Folate receptor alpha deficiency | Cerebral folate deficiency | CFD | *FOLR1* | 11q13.4 | FOLR1 transporter | 613068 |
| 29.3 | 5,10-methylene-tetrahydrofolate reductase deficiency | Homocystinuria due to deficiency of MTHFR activity | MTHFR | *MTHFR* | 1p36.22 | 5,10-methylenetetrahydrofolate reductase | 236250 |
| 29.4 | 5,10-methylene-tetrahydrofolate dehydrogenase deficiency | Trifunctional dehydrogenase/ cyclohydrolase/synthetase | MTHFD1 | *MTHFD1* | 14q23.3 | 5,10-methylene-tetrahydrofolate dehydrogenase/5,10-Methenyl-tetrahydrofolate cyclohydrolase/Formyl-tetrahydrofolate synthase | 172460 |
| 29.5 | Dihydrofolate reductase deficiency | Megaloblastic anemia due to DHFR deficiency | DHFRD | *DHFR* | 5q14.1 | Dihydrofolate reductase | 126060 |
| 29.6 | Glutamate formimino transferase deficiency | Formiminoglutamic aciduria | FIGLU | *FTCD* | 21q22.3 | Formimino transferase | 229100 |
| 29.7 | 5,10-Methenylte-trahydrofolate synthetase deficiency | 5-Formyltetrahydrofolate cycloligase | MTHFS | *MTHFS* | 15q24.3 | 5,10-Methenyltetrahydrofolate synthetase | 604197 |
| 29.8 | Reduced folate carrier deficiency | Folate-dependent recurrent megaloblastic anemia | RFCD | *SLC19A1* | 21q22.3 | Reduced folate carrier | 600424 |
| 29.9 | Mitochondrial 10-formyltetrahydrofolate dehydrogenase deficiency | | FTHFDH | *ALDH1L2* | 12q23.3 | Mitochondrial 10-formyltetrahydrofolate dehydrogenase | 613584 |

## Metabolic Pathway

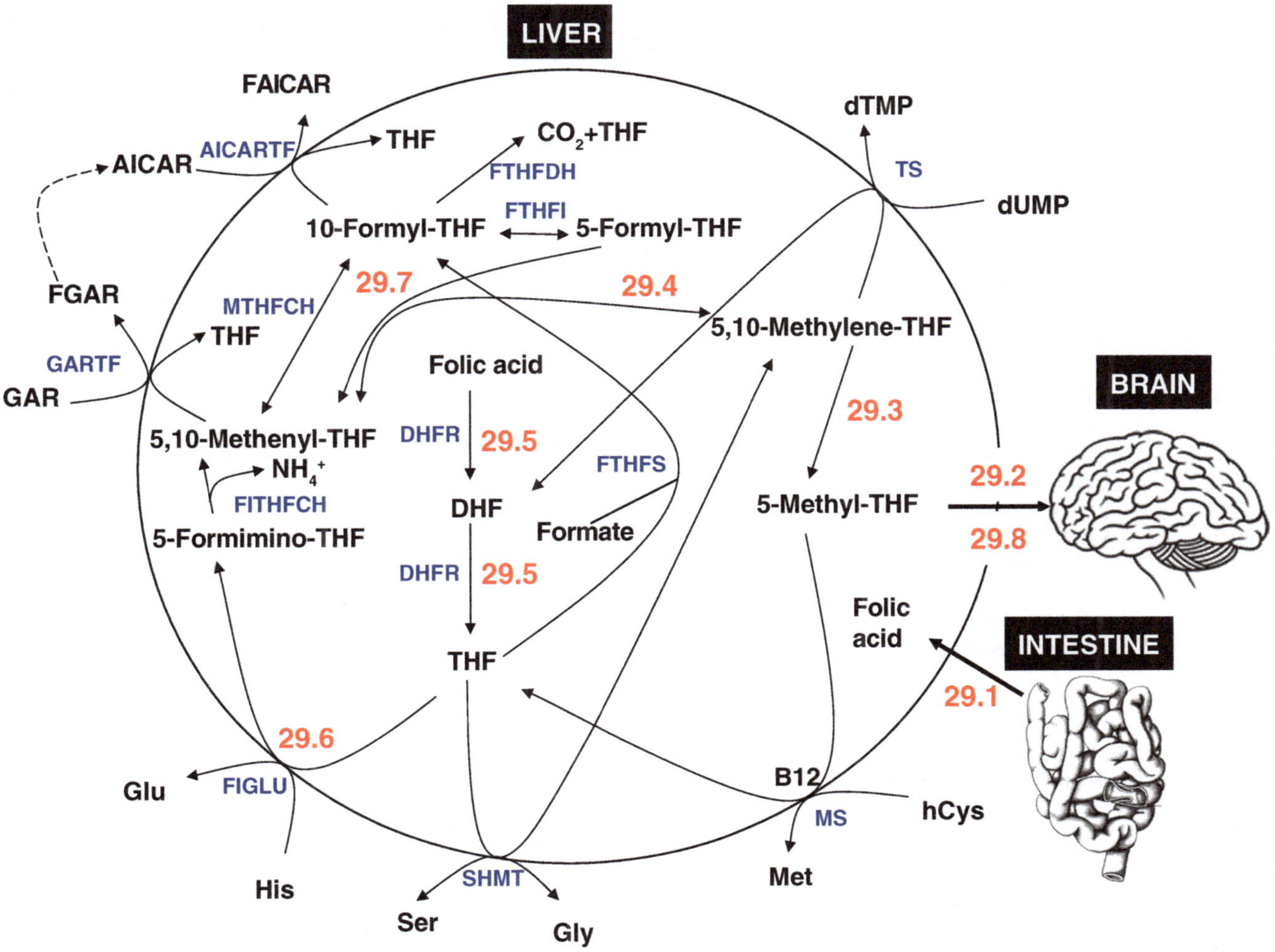


**Fig. 29.1** Metabolic pathway; functions in purines, pyrimidines, and amino acid metabolism and transport of folates in human body; and inherited metabolic disorders (in *red*) resulting in cerebral folate deficiency. Metabolites: *AICAR* 5′-Phosphoribosyl-5-aminoimidazole-4-carboxamide, *DHF* Dihydrofolate, *dTMP* Deoxythymidine monophosphate, *dUMP* Deoxyuridine monophosphate, *FAICAR* Formyl-5′-phosphoribosyl-5- aminoimidazole-4-carboxamide, *FGAR* Formyl-5′-phosphoribosylglycinamide, *GAR* 5′-Phosphoribosylglycinamide, *hCys* Homocysteine, *THF* Tetrahydrofolate. Enzymes: *AICART* 5′-Phosphoribosyl-5-aminoimidazole-4-carboxamide transformylase, *FITHFCH* Formimino-THF cyclodeaminase, *FTHFDH* Formyl-THF dehydrogenase, *FTHFI* Formyl-THF isomerase, *FTHFS* 10-Formyl-THF synthase, *GARTF* 5′-Phosphoribosylglycinamide transformylase, *MTHFCH* Methenyl-THF cyclohydrolase

## Signs and Symptoms

**Table 29.1** Hereditary folate malabsorption (*SLC46A1*)

| System | Symptoms and biomarkers | Neonatal (birth–1 month) | Infancy (1–18 months) | Childhood (1.5–11 years) | Adolescence (11–16 years) | Adulthood (>16 years) |
|---|---|---|---|---|---|---|
| Cardiovascular | Heart failure | | | ± | | |
| CNS | Intellectual disability | | | ± | | |
| | Movement disorder | | | ± | | |
| | **Neurologic deterioration** | | + | + | | |
| | Neuropathy, peripheral | | | ± | | |
| | Seizures | | ± | ± | | |
| Digestive | Diarrhea | | ± | ± | | |
| | Stomatitis | | ± | ± | | |
| Hematological | **Anemia, megaloblastic** | | + | + | | |
| | Pancytopenia | | ± | ± | | |
| Others | Failure to thrive | | ± | ± | | |
| | **Frequent infections** | | + | + | | |
| Laboratory findings | 5-Methyl-THF (cerebrospinal fluid) | | ↓ | ↓ | | |
| | Cobalamins (plasma) | | | n | | |
| | Folate (serum) | | ↓ | ↓ | | |
| | Formiminoglutamic acid, FIGLU (urine) | | | n-↑ | | |
| | Homocysteine (plasma) | | n-↑ | n-↑ | | |
| | Immunoglobulins | | ↓-n | ↓-n | | |

**Table 29.2** Folate receptor alpha deficiency (*FOLR1*)

| System | Symptoms and biomarkers | Neonatal (birth–1 month) | Infancy (1–18 months) | Childhood (1.5–11 years) | Adolescence (11–16 years) | Adulthood (>16 years) |
|---|---|---|---|---|---|---|
| CNS | **Ataxia** | | + | ++ | + | |
| | Cerebellar atrophy (MRI) | | ± | ± | ± | |
| | **Cerebral atrophy (MRI)** | | ± | ± | ± | |
| | Developmental regression | | + | + | ++ | |
| | EEG, abnormal | | + | + | + | |
| | Gait disturbance | | ± | ± | ± | |
| | **Hypertonia** | | + | ++ | + | |
| | **Hypomyelination (MRI)** | | + | + | + | |
| | Movement disorder | | | ± | | |
| | **Seizures** | | + | ++ | ++ | |
| | **Seizures, myoclonic-astatic** | | + | ++ | ++ | |
| | Seizures, tonic-clonic | | ± | ± | ± | |
| | Tendon reflexes, increased | | ± | ± | ± | |
| | Tremor | | ± | ± | ± | |
| Musculoskeletal | Microcephaly | | | ± | | |
| Psychiatric | Autistic spectrum disorder | | ± | ± | ± | |
| | Behavior, aggressive | | ± | ± | ± | |
| Laboratory findings | 5-Methyl-THF (cerebrospinal fluid) | | ↓↓↓ | ↓↓↓ | ↓-n | |
| | Choline (MRS) | | ↓ | ↓ | ↓ | |
| | Folate (serum) | n | n | n | n | n |
| | Inositol (MRS) | | ↓ | ↓ | ↓ | |

Infantile symptoms only in patients with additional genetic defects?

**Table 29.3** Methylenetetrahydrofolate reductase deficiency (*MTHFR*)

| System | Symptoms and biomarkers | Neonatal (birth–1 month) | Infancy (1–18 months) | Childhood (1.5–11 years) | Adolescence (11–16 years) | Adulthood (>16 years) |
|---|---|---|---|---|---|---|
| CNS | **Developmental regression** | | + | + | + | + |
| | Gait disturbance | | | ± | ± | ± |
| | Hydrocephalus | | | + | | |
| | Infantile spasms | | + | ± | ± | ± |
| | **Intellectual disability** | | | ± | ± | ± |
| | Neuropathy, peripheral | | | | | + |
| | Psychiatric symptoms | | | | | ± |
| | Seizures, myoclonic | | + | ± | ± | ± |
| | Seizures, tonic-clonic | | + | ± | ± | ± |
| Digestive | Feeding difficulties | | + | | | |
| Hematological | Thromboembolic episodes | | | ± | | |
| Musculoskeletal | Microcephaly | | | ± | ± | ± |
| | Muscle weakness | | | ± | ± | ± |
| Respiratory | Apnea | | ± | ± | ± | ± |
| | 5-Hydroxyindoleacetic acid, 5HIAA (cerebrospinal fluid) | | | ↓-n | ↓-n | ↓-n |
| Laboratory findings | 5-Methyl-THF (cerebrospinal fluid) | | | ↓ | ↓ | ↓ |
| | Homocysteine (plasma) | | | ↑ | ↑ | ↑ |
| | Homovanillic acid, HVA (cerebrospinal fluid) | | | ↓-n | ↓-n | ↓-n |
| | Methionine (plasma) | | | ↓-n | ↓-n | ↓-n |

**Table 29.4** 5,10-Methylene-tetrahydrofolate dehydrogenase deficiency (*MTHFD1*)

| System | Symptoms and biomarkers | Neonatal (birth–1 month) | Infancy (1–18 months) | Childhood (1.5–11 years) | Adolescence (11–16 years) | Adulthood (>16 years) |
|---|---|---|---|---|---|---|
| Cardiovascular | Microangiopathy | | ± | | | |
| Hematological | **Anemia, megaloblastic** | | + | | | |
| | **Anisocytosis** | | + | + | | |
| | **Hemolytic uremic syndrome (atypical)** | | + | | | |
| | **Immunodeficiency, severe combined (SCID)** | | + | + | | |
| | **Thrombocytopenia** | | + | + | | |
| Eye | Retinopathy | | ± | | | |
| Laboratory findings | 5-methyl-THF (cerebrospinal fluid) | | ↓ | ↓ | | |
| | Cobalamins (plasma) | | n | n | | |
| | Folate (serum) | | n | n | | |
| | Homocysteine, total (plasma) | | ↑ | | | |
| | Methylcobalamin synthesis (fibroblasts) | | ↓ | | | |
| | Methylmalonic acid (plasma) | | ↑ | | | |

**Table 29.5** Dihydrofolate reductase deficiency (*DHFR*)

| System | Symptoms and biomarkers | Neonatal (birth–1 month) | Infancy (1–18 months) | Childhood (1.5–11 years) | Adolescence (11–16 years) | Adulthood (>16 years) |
|---|---|---|---|---|---|---|
| CNS | Cerebral atrophy (MRI) | | + | | | |
| | **Delayed myelination** | | + | | | |
| | Epilepsy | | + | + | + | |
| Eye | Eye movements, abnormal | | | ± | ± | |
| | Oculogyric crisis | | | ± | ± | |
| Hematological | **Anemia, megaloblastic** | | + | ++ | ++ | |
| | Pancytopenia | | | + | + | |
| Musculoskeletal | Microcephaly | | + | | | |
| Others | Failure to thrive | | + | | | |
| Laboratory findings | 5-Hydroxyindoleacetic acid, 5HIAA (cerebrospinal fluid) | | | ↓-n | ↓-n | |
| | 5-methyl-THF (cerebrospinal fluid) | | | ↓↓↓ | ↓↓↓ | |
| | Folic acid (blood) | | | ↓↓ | ↓↓ | |
| | Formiminoglutamic acid, FIGLU (urine) | | | n-↑ | n-↑ | |
| | Hemoglobin (blood) | | | ↓ | ↓ | |
| | Homocysteine (plasma) | | n | | | |
| | Homovanillic acid, HVA (cerebrospinal fluid) | | | ↓-n | ↓-n | |
| | Lactate dehydrogenase, LDH (plasma) | | | ↑ | ↑ | |
| | Methylmalonic acid (urine) | | | n-↑ | n-↑ | |
| | Orotic acid (urine) | | | n-↑ | n-↑ | |
| | Tetrahydrobiopterin, BH4 (cerebrospinal fluid) | | | ↓-n | ↓-n | |

**Table 29.6** Glutamate formimino transferase deficiency (*FTCD*)

| System | Symptoms and biomarkers | Neonatal (birth–1 month) | Infancy (1–18 months) | Childhood (1.5–11 years) | Adolescence (11–16 years) | Adulthood (>16 years) |
|---|---|---|---|---|---|---|
| Others | No clinical significance | + | + | + | + | + |
| Laboratory findings | Formiminoglutamic acid, FIGLU (urine) | ↑ | ↑ | ↑ | ↑ | ↑ |
| | Hydantoin-5-propionic acid (urine) | ↑ | ↑ | ↑ | ↑ | ↑ |

**Table 29.7** 5,10-Methenyltetrahydrofolate synthetase deficiency (*MTHFS*)

| System | Symptoms and biomarkers | Neonatal (birth–1 month) | Infancy (1–18 months) | Childhood (1.5–11 years) | Adolescence (11–16 years) | Adulthood (>16 years) |
|---|---|---|---|---|---|---|
| Autonomic system | Hyperthermia | | | ± | | |
| CNS | **Delayed myelination** | | + | + | | |
| | Intellectual disability | | | ± | ± | |
| | **Seizures** | | + | + | + | |
| | **Speech delay** | | + | + | + | |
| Digestive | Feeding difficulties | | ± | | | |
| Hematological | Macrocytic anemia | | ± | | | |
| Musculoskeletal | **Microcephaly** | | + | + | | |
| | Short stature | | + | + | | |
| Others | Recurrent infections | | | + | + | |
| Laboratory findings | 5-methyl-THF (cerebrospinal fluid) | | | ↓↓ | | |

**Table 29.8** Reduced folate carrier deficiency

| System | Symptoms and biomarkers | Neonatal (birth–1 month) | Infancy (1–18 months) | Childhood (1.5–11 years) | Adolescence (11–16 years) | Adulthood (>16 years) |
|---|---|---|---|---|---|---|
| Hematological | **Anemia, megaloblastic** | | | | + | |
| Laboratory findings | Folate (serum) | | | | n | |
| | Hemoglobin (blood) | | | | ↓ | |
| | Homocysteine (plasma) | | | | ↑ | |
| | Vitamin B12 (serum) | | | | ↓-n | |

**Table 29.9** Mitochondrial 10-formyltetrahydrofolate dehydrogenase deficiency (ALDH1L2)

| System | Symptoms and biomarkers | Neonatal (birth–1 month) | Infancy (1–18 months) | Childhood (1.5–11 years) | Adolescence (11–16 years) | Adulthood (>16 years) |
|---|---|---|---|---|---|---|
| CNS | Hypomyelination (MRI) | | | | + | |
| | Hypotonia | + | | | | |
| | Regression, motor | | + | + | + | |
| Dermatological | **Ichthyosis** | + | + | + | + | |
| Musculoskeletal | **Facial dysmorphism** | | + | + | + | |
| Psdychiatric | Attention disorder | | | | + | |
| | Hyperactivity | | | | + | |

## Reference Values

| Age (yrs) | 5MTHF (CSF) | 5HIAA (CSF) | HVA (CSF) | H-Cys (P) | Met (P) | FIGLU (U) | Folates (B) |
|---|---|---|---|---|---|---|---|
| | nmol/L | nmol/L | nmol/L | µmol/L | µmol/L | µmol/L | nmol/L |
| <0.5 | 64–182 | 280 (150–800) | 720 (310–1100) | 3.3–8.3 | 11–31 | <11 | 4–20 |
| 0.6–1.9 | 64–182 | 224 (114–336) | 660 (295–932) | 3.3–8.3 | 11–30 | <11 | 4–20 |
| 2.0–4.9 | 63–111 | 202 (105–299) | 603 (211–871) | 3.3–8.3 | 11–30 | <11 | 4–20 |
| 5.0–10.9 | 41–117 | 133 (88–178) | 523 (144–801) | 3.3–8.3 | 11–30 | <11 | 4–20 |
| 11.0–15.9 | 41–117 | 118 (74–163) | 399 (133–551) | 4.7–10.3 | 16–23 | <11 | 4–20 |
| >16 | 64–182 | 103 (66–141) | 261 (115–488) | <15 | 14–34 | <11 | 4–20 |

nd: not detectable

## Pathological Values

| | 5MTHF (CSF) | 5MTHF (S) | hCys (P) | FIGLU (U) | Clb (P) | Inositol (MRS) | Choline (MRS) | 5HIAA, HVA (CSF) |
|---|---|---|---|---|---|---|---|---|
| 29.1 | ↓ | ↓ | n-↑ | n-↑ | n | | | |
| 29.2 | ↓↓↓ | n | n-↑ | | | ↓ | ↓ | |
| 29.3 | ↓↓ | | ↑ | | | | | ↓-n |
| 29.4 | ↓ | n | ↑ | | n | | | |
| 29.5 | ↓↓↓ | ↓↓ | n | n-↑ | | | | ↓-n |
| 29.6 | | | ↑ | | | | | |
| 29.7 | ↓ | n | | | | | | n |
| 29.8 | | n | ↑ | | ↓-n | | | |

*5MTHF* 5-Methyl-tetrahydrofolate, *hCys* Homocysteine, *FIGLU* N-Formimino-L-glutamic acid, *5HIAA* 5-Hydroxyindoleacetic acid, *HVA* Homovanillic acid

## Specimen Collection

| Test | Material | Handling | Pitfalls |
|---|---|---|---|
| Cobalamins | Plasma or serum | Frozen (−20 °C) | |
| Homocysteine<br>Methionine | Plasma | Frozen (−20 °C) | Immediate separation from plasma essential |
| FIGLU | Urine | Frozen (−20 °C) | |
| Folates | Serum | Frozen (−20 °C) | |
| 5-Methyl-THF | CSF | Frozen (−80 °C) | |
| HVA, 5HIAA | CSF | Frozen (−80 °C) | |
| BH4 | CSF | Frozen (−80 °C)<br>Add DTE + | |

## Prenatal Diagnosis and DNA Testing

No data available for prenatal diagnosis. DNA testing possible for disorders 29.1–29.8.

## Treatment

Drugs and dosages to be used in acute/chronic presentations of suspected disorders of folate transport and metabolism

| Disorder | Folinic acid/folic acid | Betaine | Hydroxocobalamin/ cyanocobalamin | Methionine | Vitamin B6 |
|---|---|---|---|---|---|
| 29.1<br>Hereditary folate malabsorption | Folinic acid parenterally (intravenous in acute presentation and intramuscular for chronic treatment) 4 mg/day | | | | |
| 29.2<br>Folate receptor alpha deficiency | Folinic acid orally 2–5 mg/kg/day.<br>100 mg intravenously or once a week have been used concomitantly with 5 mg per kilo per day of oral folinic acid.<br>Preliminary results indicate that intrathecal administration may be more efficient than oral administration. However, no doses have been reported (Grapp et al. 2012) | | | | |
| 29.3<br>5,10-methylene-THF reductase deficiency | Folinic acid orally 15 mg/day | Betaine orally 100–250 mg/kg/day in neonates and infants. In children and adults, 6–9 g/day in three divided doses with a maximum daily dose of up to 20 g/day | Hydroxocobalamin 0.5–1 mg orally or 1 mg IM monthly | Methionine orally 40–50 mg/kg/day | Vitamin B6 orally 100–250 mg/day |
| 29.4<br>5,10-methylene-THF dehydrogenase deficiency | L-methyl-THF 3 mg compounded with 35 mg of pyridoxal 5′-phosphate and 2 mg of methylcobalamin given orally once a day | | | | |

| Disorder | Folinic acid/folic acid | Betaine | | Hydroxocobalamin/ cyanocobalamin | Methionine | Vitamin B6 |
|---|---|---|---|---|---|---|
| 29.5 Dihydrofolate reductase deficiency | Folinic acid orally 1 mg/kg/ day | | | | | |
| 29.6 | No treatment needed | | | | | |
| 29.7 5,10-Methenyl-THF synthetase deficiency | L-methyl-THF 3 mg compounded with 35 mg of pyridoxal 5′-phosphate and 2 mg of methylcobalamin given orally once a day | | | | | |
| 29.8 Reduced folate carrier deficiency | Folic acid 10 mg/day | | | Cyanocobalamin i.m. 1000 µg twice a week | | |

Folic acid *should not* be used to treat these disorders since it is not a physiologic form of folate and binds in an irreversible way to folate receptor alpha, inhibiting the binding of 5-methylTHF and blocking the transport of folate across the choroid plexus. In addition, folate has to be converted by a series of enzymatic reactions to the biological active 5MTHF

## Hereditary Folate Malabsorption

Folic acid should not be used to treat hereditary folate malabsorption. Folic acid is the most common pharmacologic form of folate and very stable. However, it is not a physiologic form of folate. It binds in an irreversibly way to folate receptors and may block these receptors from transporting folate across the choroid plexus (Kamen and Smith 2004). 5-Formyl-tetrahydrofolate (5-formyl-THF), also known as folinic acid (Ca-Folinate), is a racemic and stable form of folate that is found in human tissues and can be used in oral and parenteral formulations. The active L-isomer may also be used for parenteral administration. The active isomer, L-5-methyltetrahydrofolate (L-5MTHF), is the principal folate in the diet, the form that is absorbed in the intestine and circulating in the blood. It is available commercially but only for oral and not parenteral supplementation. No controlled studies have been conducted in order to provide guidelines for optimal treatment. The required dose of reduced folate seems to vary among patients. The dose of reduced folate needed to improve the neurological features is much higher than that needed to improve the hematological problems. Dosing should be done and guided by its effect on reaching normal age ranges for trough CSF 5MTHF concentrations. Oral doses of 150–200 mg of 5-formyl-THF have been associated with good clinical outcomes (Geller et al. 2002). An appropriate starting dose of a reduced folate in an infant could be 50 mg or 10–15 mg/kg given daily as a single dose. Appropriate dosing of a reduced folate should be tailored to achieve a normal CSF 5MTHF concentration for age. The parenteral dose used to achieve adequate blood folate levels is lower than the oral dose. The hematological abnormalities have corrected with intramuscular injections of 1.0 mg/day of 5-formyl-THF. Nevertheless, the normalization of CSF 5MTHF levels requires higher reduced folate doses. Dosing should be adjusted in each individual to achieve a CSF 5MTHF level normal for age (Grapp et al. 2012).

## Folate Receptor Alpha Deficiency

Since this is a rare autosomal recessive disorder, no controlled studies have been conducted in order to provide guidelines for optimal treatment. It has been presumed that alternative or residual transport pathways into the central nervous system can be used by increasing the plasma 5MTHF concentrations. Thus, most patients have been treated with folinic acid at oral doses of 2–5 mg per kg/body weight daily. Folic acid should not be used to treat folate receptor alpha deficiency since it is not a physiologic form of folate (Kamen and Smith 2004). In addition, folate has to be converted by a series of enzymatic reactions to the biological active 5MTHF. 5-formyl-THF is a racemic and stable form of folate found in human tissues. It can be used in oral formulation. The active L-isomer (Isovorin) may also be used for oral administration. Most patients benefit from this treatment and respond within 2–6 months of therapy with reduced frequency of seizures, almost complete normalization of neurological status, improved motor skills, and increase of the CSF 5MTHF concentration in the CSF (Steinfeld et al. 2009; Cario et al. 2009; Grapp et al. 2012). In addition, after 6 months of treatment, the white matter choline and inositol signals normalized, and signs of remyelination were observed on brain MRI (Steinfeld et al. 2009). In one additional case of folate receptor alpha deficiency, a trial with 30 mg/day of folinic acid at the age of 26 months controlled the seizures completely in 1 month and ameliorated the myoclonic jerks and choreic movements presented by the patient (Perez-Duenas et al. 2010). In few patients, alternative routes of folinic acid supplementation (intravenous and/or intrathecal) have been tried, and the results indicate better treatment efficacy (Grapp et al. 2012).

## Methylenetetrahydrofolate Reductase Deficiency

The aim of the treatment is the decrease of homocysteine levels by using the compound betaine (Huemer et al. 2019). Betaine is a substrate of the enzyme betaine-homocysteine S-methyltransferase (BHMT) that catalyzes remethylation of homocysteine to methionine in kidney and liver causing hypermethioninemia in these patients. Betaine is administered orally, and treatment is begun with 100 mg/kg/day. Doses may range from 100 to 250 mg/kg/day in neonates and infants. In children and adults, doses can range to 6–9 g/day in two to six divided doses, and the total daily dose can be increased up to 20 g/day (Prasad et al. 2011). Since the expression of BHMT is low in the central nervous system, it is not surprising to find out that the best therapeutic outcome with betaine has been observed when started prenatally or soon after birth with restoration of plasma SAM levels and attainment of normal brain growth and development (Strauss et al. 2007). Frequent dosing of orally administered betaine (six divided doses) normalized total plasma homocysteine levels in one infant with MTHFR deficiency (Ucar et al. 2010). Supplementation with methionine (40–50 mg/kg/day), folinic acid (5–30 mg/day), vitamin B6 (100–250 mg/day), and vitamin B12 (0.5–1 mg/day orally) may be contemplated based on the fact that they play a role as cofactors in different enzymatic reactions of the folate utilization pathway that ultimately leads to the synthesis of 5MTHF (Schiff et al. 2011).

## Methylene-THF Dehydrogenase Deficiency

No treatment was initially reported in the only patient identified with this particular inborn error of metabolism (Watkins and Rosenblatt 2012). However, the treatment was subsequently reported as consisting of 3 mg of L-methyl-THF compounded with 35 mg of pyridoxal 5′-phosphate and 2 mg of methyl-cobalamin given orally once a day. This treatment provided partial immune reconstitution (Keller et al. 2013).

## Dihydrofolate Reductase Deficiency

Therapy with 1 mg/kg per day of folinic acid corrects the biochemical abnormalities including cerebral 5MTHF levels, total red blood cell folate levels, anemia, and pancytopenia (Cario et al. 2011). The treatment can also improve school performance and control the epilepsy; however, irregular treatment with folinic acid is associated with recurrence of epilepsy of enzymatic (Cario et al. 2011). In another report, treatment with 10–30 mg of daily folinic acid corrected the cerebral 5MTHF level and improved the anemia and the seizure control (Banka et al. 2011).

## Glutamate Formimino Transferase Deficiency

No treatment required.

## Methenyl-THF Synthetase Deficiency

No treatment has been reported so far.

## Reduced Folate Carrier Deficiency

A combined therapy with cyanocobalamin (1000 mg, i.m.) and folic acid (10 mg/day) seems to be beneficial in a single patient.

## Mitochondrial 10-formyltetrahydrofolate Dehydrogenase Deficiency

No treatment has been reported so far.

## References


Baethmann M, Wendel U, Hoffmann GF, Gohlich-Ratmann G, Kleinlein B, Seiffert P, et al. Hydrocephalus internus in two patients with 5,10-methylenetetrahydrofolate reductase deficiency. Neuropediatrics. 2000;31(6):314–7.

Banka S, Blom HJ, Walter J, Aziz M, Urquhart J, Clouthier CM, et al. Identification and characterization of an inborn error of metabolism caused by dihydrofolate reductase deficiency. Am J Hum Genet. 2011;88(2):216–25.

Bidla G, Watkins D, Chery C, Froese DS, Ells C, Kerachian M, et al. Biochemical analysis of patients with mutations in MTHFD1 and a diagnosis of methylenetetrahydrofolate dehydrogenase 1 deficiency. Mol Genet Metab. 2020;130:179–82.

Blount BC, Mack MM, Wehr CM, MacGregor JT, Hiatt RA, Wang G, et al. Folate deficiency causes uracil misincorporation into human DNA and chromosome breakage: implications for cancer and neuronal damage. Proc Natl Acad Sci U S A. 1997;94(7):3290–5.

Cario H, Bode H, Debatin KM, Opladen T, Schwarz K. Congenital null mutations of the FOLR1 gene: a progressive neurologic disease and its treatment. Neurology. 2009;73(24):2127–9.

Cario H, Smith DEC, Bloom HJ, Blau N, Bode H, Holzmann K, et al. Dihydrofolate reductase deficiency caused by a homozygous DHFR mutation, leads to congenital megaloblastic anemia and severe neurologic disease due to cerebral folate deficiency. Am J Hum Genet. 2011;88:226–31.

Dill P, Schneider J, Weber P, Trachsel D, Tekin M, Jakobs C, et al. Pyridoxal phosphate-responsive seizures in a patient with cerebral folate deficiency (CFD) and congenital deafness with labyrinthine aplasia, microtia and microdontia (LAMM). Mol Genet Metab. 2011;104:362–8.

Fournier I, Ploye F, Cottet-Emard JM, Brun J, Claustrat B. Folate deficiency alters melatonin secretion in rats. J Nutr. 2002;132(9):2781–4.

Geller J, Kronn D, Jayabose S, Sandoval C. Hereditary folate malabsorption: family report and review of the literature. Medicine (Baltimore). 2002;81(1):51–68.

Ghoshal K, Li X, Datta J, Bai S, Pogribny I, Pogribny M, et al. A folate- and methyl-deficient diet alters the expression of DNA methyltransferases and methyl CpG binding proteins involved in epigenetic gene silencing in livers of F344 rats. J Nutr. 2006;136(6):1522–7.

Goyette P, Sumner JS, Milos R, Duncan AM, Rosenblatt DS, Matthews RG, et al. Human methylenetetrahydrofolate reductase: isolation of cDNA, mapping and mutation identification. Nat Genet. 1994;7(2):195–200.

Grapp M, Just IA, Linnankivi T, Wolf P, Lucke T, Hausler M, et al. Molecular characterization of folate receptor 1 mutations delineates cerebral folate transport deficiency. Brain. 2012;135:2022.

Hilton JF, Christensen KE, Watkins D, Raby BA, Renaud Y, de la Luna S, et al. The molecular basis of glutamate formiminotransferase deficiency. Hum Mutat. 2003;22(1):67–73.

Huemer M, Diodato D, Martinelli D, Olivieri G, Blom H, Gleich F, et al. Phenotype, treatment practice and outcome in the cobalamin-dependent remethylation disorders and MTHFR deficiency: data from the E-HOD registry. J Inherit Metab Dis. 2019;42(2):333–52.

Kamen BA, Smith AK. A review of folate receptor alpha cycling and 5-methyltetrahydrofolate accumulation with an emphasis on cell models in vitro. Adv Drug Deliv Rev. 2004;56(8):1085–97.

Keller MD, Ganesh J, Heltzer M, Paessler M, Bergqvist AG, Baluarte HJ, et al. Severe combined immunodeficiency resulting from mutations in MTHFD1. Pediatrics. 2013;131(2):e629–34.

Linhart HG, Troen A, Bell GW, Cantu E, Chao WH, Moran E, et al. Folate deficiency induces genomic uracil misincorporation and hypomethylation but does not increase DNA point mutations. Gastroenterology. 2009;136(1):227–35.e3.

Matherly LH, Goldman DI. Membrane transport of folates. Vitam Horm. 2003;66:403–56.

Moretti P, Peters SU, Del Gaudio D, Sahoo T, Hyland K, Bottiglieri T, et al. Brief report: autistic symptoms, developmental regression, mental retardation, epilepsy, and dyskinesias in CNS folate deficiency. J Autism Dev Disord. 2008;38(6):1170–7.

Perez-Duenas B, Toma C, Ormazabal A, Muchart J, Sanmarti F, Bombau G, et al. Progressive ataxia and myoclonic epilepsy in a patient with a homozygous mutation in the FOLR1 gene. J Inherit Metab Dis. 2010;33(6):795–802.

Perez-Duenas B, Ormazabal A, Toma C, Torrico B, Cormand B, Serrano M, et al. Cerebral folate deficiency syndromes in childhood: clinical, analytical, and etiologic aspects. Arch Neurol. 2011;68(5):615–21.

Pogribny IP, Karpf AR, James SR, Melnyk S, Han T, Tryndyak VP. Epigenetic alterations in the brains of fisher 344 rats induced by long-term administration of folate/methyl-deficient diet. Brain Res. 2008;1237:25–34.

Prasad AN, Rupar CA, Prasad C. Methylenetetrahydrofolate reductase (MTHFR) deficiency and infantile epilepsy. Brain and Development. 2011;33(9):758–69.

Qiu A, Jansen M, Sakaris A, Min SH, Chattopadhyay S, Tsai E, et al. Identification of an intestinal folate transporter and the molecular basis for hereditary folate malabsorption. Cell. 2006;127(5):917–28.

Rodan LH, Qi W, Ducker GS, Demirbas D, Laine R, Yang E, et al. 5,10-methenyltetrahydrofolate synthetase deficiency causes a neurometabolic disorder associated with microcephaly, epilepsy, and cerebral hypomyelination. Mol Genet Metab. 2018;125(1–2):118–26.

Sarret C, Ashkavand Z, Paules E, Dorboz I, Pediaditakis P, Sumner S, et al. Deleterious mutations in ALDH1L2 suggest a novel cause for neuro-ichthyotic syndrome. NPJ Genom Med. 2019;4(1).

Schiff M, Benoist JF, Tilea B, Royer N, Giraudier S. Ogier de Baulny H. isolated remethylation disorders: do our treatments benefit patients? J Inherit Metab Dis. 2011;34(1):137–45.

Steinfeld R, Grapp M, Kraetzner R, Dreha-Kulaczewski S, Helms G, Dechent P, et al. Folate receptor alpha defect causes cerebral folate transport deficiency: a treatable neurodegenerative disorder associated with disturbed myelin metabolism. Am J Hum Genet. 2009;85(3):354–63.

Strauss KA, Morton DH, Puffenberger EG, Hendrickson C, Robinson DL, Wagner C, et al. Prevention of brain disease from severe 5,10-methylenetetrahydrofolate reductase deficiency. Mol Genet Metab. 2007;91(2):165–75.

Svaton M, Skvarova Kramarzova K, Kanderova V, Mancikova A, Smisek P, Jesina P, et al. A homozygous deletion in the SLC19A1 gene as a cause of folate-dependent recurrent megaloblastic anemia. Blood. 2020;135(26):2427–31.

Ucar SK, Koroglu OA, Berk O, Yalaz M, Kultursay N, Blom HJ, et al. Titration of betaine therapy to optimize therapy in an infant with 5,10-methylenetetrahydrofolate reductase deficiency. Eur J Pediatr. 2010;169(2):241–3.

Watkins D, Rosenblatt DS. Update and new concepts in vitamin responsive disorders of folate transport and metabolism. J Inherit Metab Dis. 2012;35:665–70.

Watkins D, Schwartzentruber JA, Ganesh J, Orange JS, Kaplan BS, Nunez LD, et al. Novel inborn error of folate metabolism: identification by exome capture and sequencing of mutations in the MTHFD1 gene in a single proband. J Med Genet. 2011;48(9):590–2.

Weitman SD, Weinberg AG, Coney LR, Zurawski VR, Jennings DS, Kamen BA. Cellular localization of the folate receptor: potential role in drug toxicity and folate homeostasis. Cancer Res. 1992;52(23):6708–11.

# Disorders of Biotin Metabolism

# 30

Bruce A. Barshop

## Contents



**Summary**

Disorders in the processing of biotin present with deficiencies of the biotin-dependent carboxylases, i.e., multiple carboxylase deficiency. The biochemical and clinical abnormalities reflect those observed in individual, isolated defects of three mitochondrial carboxylases: methylcrotonyl-CoA carboxylase, propionyl-CoA carboxylase, and pyruvate carboxylase. Dietary deficiency of biotin is very rare in general, but may occur with prolonged insufficiency or with a defect of absorption and transport. Multiple carboxylase deficiency is caused by defects in holocarboxylase synthetase or in biotinidase. Treatment of biotinidase deficiency with biotin supplementation is highly effective in reversing the abnormalities, and that is usually also the case for the treatment of holocarboxylase deficiency, though there may be some variability of response.

B. A. Barshop (✉)
Department of Pediatrics, University of California San Diego, La Jolla, CA, USA
e-mail: bbarshop@ucsd.edu

## Introduction

Biotin is a vitamin cofactor used in carboxylation reactions which fix $CO_2$ from bicarbonate to substrates, to generate carboxylic acid moieties; in fact each biotin-dependent reaction in human metabolism converts a carboxylic acid (or CoA ester) to a dicarboxylic acid (or CoA ester).


N. Blau et al. (eds.), *Physician's Guide to the Diagnosis, Treatment, and Follow-Up of Inherited Metabolic Diseases*,
https://doi.org/10.1007/978-3-030-67727-5_30

In its active form, biotin is covalently bound to lysine in the active site of a carboxylase holoenzyme. Utilization of biotin requires its transfer to the correct lysine residue of the carboxylase apoenzyme to generate the active holoenzyme, a reaction carried out by holocarboxylase synthetase (HCS). Ingested biotin may be free, or as most often ingested, protein-bound, in the form of the lysine conjugate (biocytin). Absorption and cellular uptake of free biotin involves the transporter SLC5A6 (also known as the sodium-dependent multivitamin transporter, SMVT) which mediates biotin, pantothenic acid, and lipoate uptake in a variety of cellular systems (Prasad and Ganapathy 2000). Recovery of protein-bound biotin from dietary sources, and retention of biotin from endogenous carboxylase proteins as they are proteolyzed, requires cleavage of biocytin, a reaction catalyzed by the enzyme biotinidase. Biotinidase deficiency or HCS deficiency (HCSD) causes a functional defect in all the carboxylases, termed multiple carboxylase deficiency (MCD).

HCS is a complex enzyme which activates biotin to form D-biotinyl-5′-adenylate and then catalyzes the covalent attachment of the biotin to an active site ε-amino group of a lysine residue of a newly synthesized apocarboxylase protein, converting it into an active holocarboxylase enzyme.

There are four biotin-dependent enzymes in human metabolism (Fig. 30.1). Acetyl-CoA carboxylase (ACC) is used to generate malonyl-CoA which is important in initiation of the synthesis of fatty acids and regulation of their oxidation. ACC is present in two isomers, one of which (ACC1) is cytoplasmic and the other of which (ACC2) is associated with the endomembrane system (including primarily the cytosolic side of the outer mitochondrial membrane). There are as yet no known disorders due to defects in ACC, but the other three carboxylases, which are all localized to the mitochondrial matrix, each have a disease state associated with its deficiency. These include methylcrotonyl-CoA carboxylase (two subunits, MCCC1 and MCCC2), propionyl-CoA carboxylase (two subunits, PCCA and PCCB), and pyruvate carboxylase (PC).

The first patient ascertained with MCD had HCSD and was described in 1971 by Gompertz et al. as having an abnormality of leucine metabolism due to identification of 3-methylcrotonylglycine and 3-hydroxyisovaleric acid in the urine. A defect in 3-methylcrotonyl-CoA carboxylase was documented by Gompertz et al. in 1973. When methylcitric and hydroxypropionic acids were also found to be increased in the same patient in 1977 by Sweetman et al., enzymatic analysis revealed defective activity of propionyl-CoA carboxylase in addition. The third mitochondrial carboxylase, pyruvate carboxylase, was also shown to be defective in 1979, and the disorder was then renamed multiple carboxylase deficiency (Saunders et al. 1979).

## Nomenclature

| # | Disorder | Alternative name | Abbr | Gene symbol | Chromosomal location | Affected protein | Mode of inheritance | OMIM |
|---|---|---|---|---|---|---|---|---|
| 30.1 | Biotinidase deficiency | Late-onset multiple carboxylase deficiency | BTDD | *BTD* | 3p25.1 | Biotinidase | AR | 253260 |
| 30.2 | Holocarboxylase synthetase deficiency | Infantile-onset multiple carboxylase deficiency | HCSD | *HLCS* | 21q22.13 | Holocarboxylase synthetase | AR | 253270 |
| 30.3 | Sodium-dependent multivitamin transporter deficiency | Biotin transporter defect | | *SLC5A6* | 2p23.3 | Sodium-dependent vitamin transporter | AR | 604024 |

## Metabolic Pathway

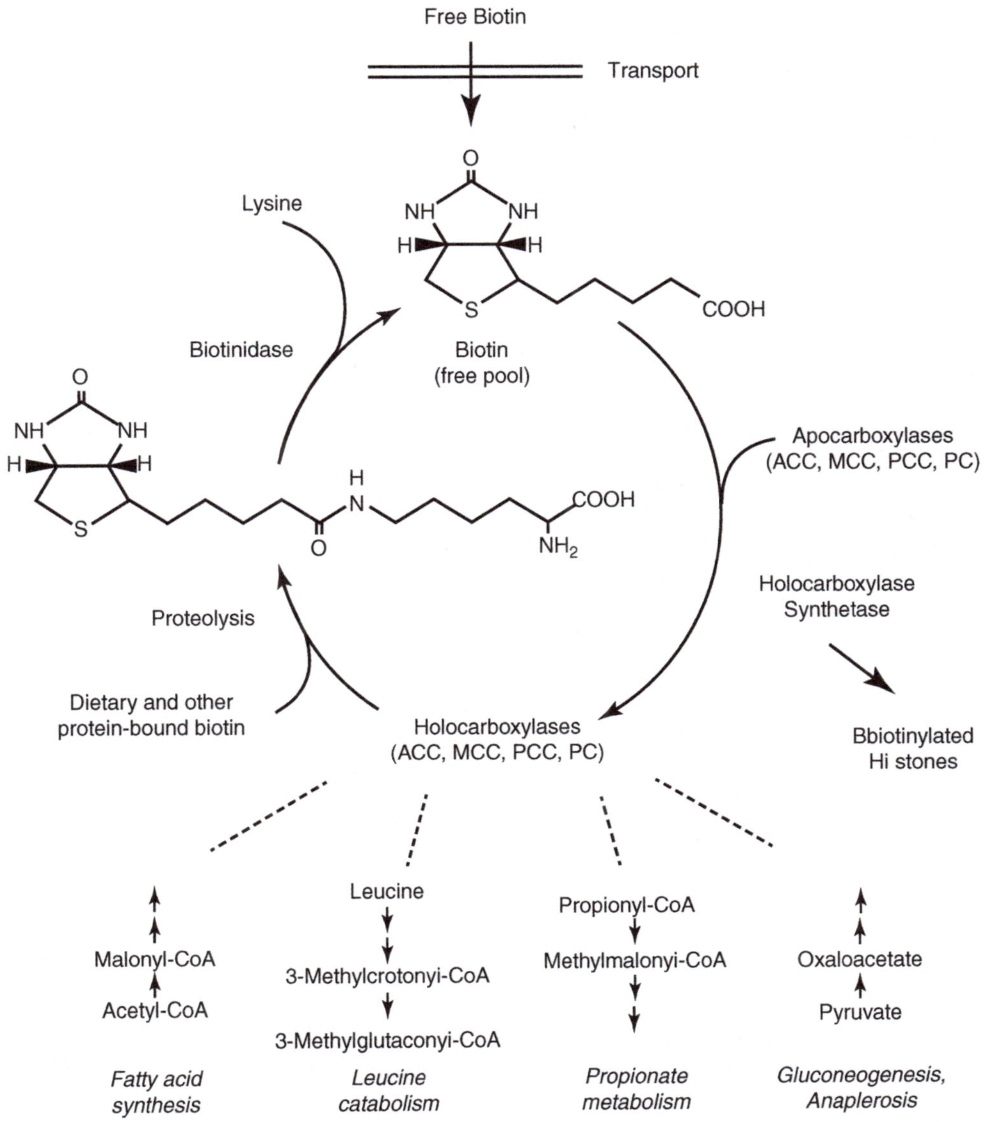


**Fig. 30.1** Pathways of biotin metabolism

## Signs and Symptoms

**Table 30.1** Biotinidase deficiency

| System | Symptoms and biomarkers | Neonatal (birth–1 month) | Infancy (1–18 months) | Childhood (1.5–11 years) | Adolescence (11–16 years) | Adulthood (>16 years) |
|---|---|---|---|---|---|---|
| Digestive | **Glossitis** | ± | ++ | + | | |
| Cardiovascular | **Valvulitis, mitral** | ± | ++ | ++ | | |
| CNS | Ataxia | ± | + | ++ | | |
| | Bulbar dysfunction | ± | ± | + | | |
| | Developmental delay | ± | + | ++ | | |
| | Seizures | ± | + | ++ | | |
| Dermatological | Alopecia | ± | + | ++ | | |
| | Skin rash | ± | + | ++ | | |
| Digestive | **Stomatitis** | ± | ++ | + | | |
| Ear | Hearing loss | − | + | ++ | | |
| Eye | Corneal erosion | − | + | ++ | | |
| | Optic atrophy | − | ± | + | | |
| Respiratory | Stridor, inspiratory | ± | ± | ± | | |
| Laboratory findings | 3-Hydroxyisovaleric acid (urine) | n-↑ | ↑↑ | ↑↑↑ | | |
| | 3-Hydroxypropionic acid (urine) | n-↑ | ↑↑ | ↑↑↑ | | |
| | 3-Methylcrotonylglycine (urine) | n-↑ | ↑↑ | ↑↑↑ | | |
| | Biotinidase (plasma) | ↓ | ↓ | ↓ | ↓ | ↓ |
| | C5-OH acylcarnitine (dried blood spot) | n-↑ | ↑↑ | ↑↑↑ | | |
| | C5-OH acylcarnitine (plasma) | n-↑ | ↑↑ | ↑↑↑ | | |
| | Lactate (plasma) | n-↑ | ↑ | ↑↑ | | |
| | Methylcitric acid (urine) | n-↑ | ↑↑ | ↑↑↑ | | |

**Table 30.2** Holocarboxylase synthetase deficiency

| System | Symptoms and biomarkers | Neonatal (birth–1 month) | Infancy (1–18 months) | Childhood (1.5–11 years) | Adolescence (11–16 years) | Adulthood (>16 years) |
|---|---|---|---|---|---|---|
| CNS | **Ataxia** | ± | ++ | ++ | | |
| | Bulbar dysfunction | ± | ± | + | | |
| | Developmental delay | + | ++ | +++ | | |
| | Seizures | + | ++ | +++ | | |
| Dermatological | **Alopecia** | ++ | +++ | +++ | | |
| | **Skin rash** | ++ | +++ | +++ | | |
| Laboratory findings | 3-Hydroxypropionic acid (urine) | ↑ | ↑↑ | ↑↑↑ | | |
| | 3-Methylcrotonylglycine (urine) | ↑ | ↑↑ | ↑↑↑ | | |
| | C5-OH acylcarnitine (dried blood spot) | ↑ | ↑↑ | ↑↑↑ | | |
| | C5-OH acylcarnitine (plasma) | ↑ | ↑↑ | ↑↑↑ | | |
| | Lactate (plasma) | ↑ | ↑↑↑ | ↑↑↑ | | |
| | Methylcitric acid (urine) | ↑ | ↑↑ | ↑↑↑ | | |

**Table 30.3** Sodium-dependent multivitamin transporter deficiency

| System | Symptoms and biomarkers | Neonatal (birth–1 month) | Infancy (1–18 months) | Childhood (1.5–11 years) | Adolescence (11–16 years) | Adulthood (>16 years) |
|---|---|---|---|---|---|---|
| CNS | Brain changes on MRI – Atrophy | ± | ++ | | | |
| | Brain changes on MRI – Polymicrogyria | ± | | | | |
| | Developmental delay | ++ | ++ | ++ | | |
| | Hypoplasia of pons | | | ++ | | |
| | Thin corpus callosum | | | ++ | | |
| Digestive | Severe gastroesophageal reflux | ++ | ++ | ++ | | |
| Musculoskeletal | Microcephaly | ± | ++ | | | |
| | Osteoporosis | | | ++ | | |
| Others | Failure to thrive | ++ | ++ | ++ | | |
| | Variable immunodeficiency | + | + | + | | |

## Biotinidase Deficiency

Biotinidase deficiency presents with a median age of 3 months (Wolf et al. 1983), but it may present in the second decade of life (Wolf et al. 1998). In earlier literature biotinidase deficiency was referred to as the later infantile form of multiple carboxylase deficiency (Wolf et al. 1983) to distinguish it from the usual neonatal presentation of holocarboxylase synthetase deficiency. It is also possible for adults with profound biotinidase deficiency to remain asymptomatic, although those individuals would be predicted to be at ongoing risk for symptoms to arise at times of intercurrent infection or other stress. Such individuals have been ascertained because of abnormal results on newborn screening of their babies (Wolf et al. 1997).

The cutaneous lesions tend to be patchy, in contrast to the total body eruption seen in holocarboxylase synthetase deficiency, or there may be severe generalized involvement of the skin with redness and desquamation. Concomitant mucocutaneous candidiasis is common. The alopecia may be progressive to alopecia totalis but is usually less than total.

Neurological manifestations of biotinidase deficiency (Wolf 2011) tend to be indolent and significant. Ataxia is a prominent feature and may interfere with walking. Seizures are common and may be the only obvious symptom; they may be general or myoclonic or may present as infantile spasms. There may be developmental delay and neurodevelopmental regression. Stridorous breathing and apnea have been reported in some patients, may be a presenting sign, and may be expected to resolve with biotin treatment. The untreated disease may be fatal.

Visual and auditory neurosensory abnormalities have been reported in a considerable number of patients, often as late complications. Loss of visual function is associated with optic atrophy and appears to be encountered only in patients for whom diagnosis and treatment is delayed (Wolf 2011). Neurosensory hearing loss seems to follow the same pattern (Wolf 2011). Many of the neurological features of disease disappear in response to treatment with biotin, as do the cutaneous and metabolic features; but sensorineural abnormalities involving the optic and auditory nerves are among those which are not reversible once they have appeared and neurologic signs may persist if there is a long delay instituting treatment (Ferreira et al. 2017).

## Holocarboxylase Synthetase Deficiency

Patients with HCS deficiency generally present in the first days or months of life with overwhelming illness identical to those of propionic acidemia or other classic organic acidemia. The age of onset of clinical symptoms generally has generally been before 6 weeks of life, but it is clear that patients with an abnormal holocarboxylase synthetase can present at any age from 1 day to 6 years of age (Suormala et al. 1997).

In the acute episode of illness, the infant has massive ketosis and metabolic acidosis with an anion gap. There may be tachypnea or Kussmaul breathing, and blood ammonia may be elevated. The episode may progress to dehydration and deep coma, and a number of patients have died of this disease; the initial episode may be lethal within hours of birth (Sweetman et al. 1982). Cutaneous features are an integral part of the untreated disease, though some patients have died before the development of skin lesions, and now patients are being treated before the development of cutaneous lesions. An erythematous eruption may involve the entire body, with bright red, scaly, or desquamative lesions. Complicating monilial infection is common. Varying degrees of alopecia are seen, including alopecia totalis, with absence of eyelashes, eyebrows, and lanugo, as well as the hair of the head. There may be persistent vomiting and failure to thrive. Neurological abnormalities appear to be related to the effects of the initial or subsequent episodes of illness, which might include decreased brain perfusion and hyperammonemia; with treatment and while compensated, the neurological function is otherwise expected to be normal, and the neurological examination may be normal despite a hyperammonemic episode (Dabbagh et al. 1994). Muscular hypotonia and hypertonia have been described, as have more severe forms of dystonia and movement disorders, including athetosis and opisthotonus. There may be electroencephalographic abnormalities and abnormal findings on cranial computed tomography or magnetic resonance imaging, particularly involving the white matter. Subependymal cysts were observed in one infant and reported to disappear following 6 months of treatment (Squires et al. 1997), and subependymal cysts were also observed in seven Samoan infants who had severe disease, incomplete responsiveness to biotin, and early life-threatening metabolic events (Wilson et al. 2005), as well as a Samoan infant in an earlier series, who had a poor dermatological response to biotin (Sweetman et al. 1982).

The biochemical hallmark of this disease is the excretion of 3-hydroxyisovaleric acid and 3-methylcrotonylglycine, plus elevated quantities of lactic acid in blood and urine. The first clinical chemical clue to the disease may be the discovery of lactic acidemia. Organic acid analysis during an acute acidosis also reveals methylcitric and 3-hydroxypropionic acids and may also include tiglylglycine (Sweetman et al. 1982). The excretion of 3-hydroxyisovaleric acid is almost always greater than that of 3-methylcrotonylglycine and may be as high as 200 times normal (Sweetman et al. 1977).

### Biotin Transporter Defect

Using whole genome-scanning, a child was found to have mutations in the SLC5A6 gene (Subramanian et al. 2017). The proband, identified at 15 months of age, presented with failure to thrive, developmental delay, microcephaly, generalized atrophy and thin corpus callosum on MRI, variable immunodeficiency, gastroesophageal reflux, and osteoporosis and pathologic bone fractures. The patient responded clinically to supplemental administration of biotin, pantothenic acid, and lipoate (Subramanian et al. 2017), but interestingly was said to have normal organic acids and other metabolic testing. It may be that another patient reported earlier (Mardach et al. 2002) had this or a similar defect, although the phenotype was slightly different (encephalopathy during episode of viral gastroenteritis at 18 months, findings of biotin-dependent MCD with normal activities of BTD and HCS, but moderately reduced rate of biotin uptake in vitro), and no mutations were found in SLC5A6.

This entity is distinct from the so-called biotin-thiamine-dependent basal ganglion, first described as a biotin-responsive entity, but subsequently proven to be caused by a defect in a thiamine transporter SLC19A3 (Zeng et al. 2005). The reported effect of biotin is presumed to be due to increased expression of the SLC19A3 gene in response to biotin (Leon-Del-Rio 2019). This entity is discussed in Chap. 31 (Disorders of Thiamine).

## Diagnosis

Biotinidase deficiency is diagnosed by enzyme assay. It is generally conducted as a fluorometric assay and routinely performed on bloodspots in newborn screening programs worldwide (Heard et al. 1986); serum or plasma samples may be assayed also, and that is usually done for confirmation. The enzyme defect can be demonstrated whether the patient takes biotin or not, and the objective is to make the diagnosis prior to other biochemical changes. In the event of delayed treatment, the first biochemical changes generally include elevation of blood lactate and urine 3-hydroxyisovalerate and 3-methylcrotonylglycine. The diagnostic findings of holocarboxylase synthetase deficiency are similar in terms of organic acid changes, but enzymatic confirmation is more complicated. The assay may involve formation of acid-precipitable radiolabel from $H^{14}CO_2$ in the presence of apocarboxylases prepared from biotin-deficient rats (Burri et al. 1981), but that is a difficult assay to validate to clinical standards. Presumptive diagnosis may be made in fibroblast cultures which are grown in biotin-depleted media to check the activities of carboxylases. A practical solution may be to use p67, a peptide comprising the 67 C-terminal amino acids of propionyl-CoA carboxylase, as the substrate (Rios-Avila et al. 2011). Molecular methodology to document DNA mutations is possible as a primary diagnostic step, but in the present era of newborn screening, molecular studies are more often recommended to confirm an enzymatic diagnosis. Similarly, for diagnosis of SLC5A6 defects, it might in principle be possible to perform assay of biotin uptake in biopsies as in experimental cell culture systems (Subramanian et al. 2017), but that is not practical in general, and it is disconcerting that urine organic acids were reportedly normal in the sole reported case (Subramanian et al. 2017).

## Reference Values

| Compound | Fluid | Method | Age/gender | Reference range |
|---|---|---|---|---|
| **3-Hydroxyisovaleric acid** | Urine | GC-MS | All | 0–58 mmol/mol creatinine |
| **3-Methylcrotonylglycine** | Urine | GC-MS | All | 0–2 mmol/mol creatinine |
| **Lactic acid** | Blood, CSF | Enzymatic | All | 0.5–1.5 mmol/L |
| **Lactic acid** | Urine | GC-MS or enzymatic | All | 10–200 mmol/mol creatinine |
| Methylcitric acid | Urine | GC-MS | All | 0–5 mmol/mol creatinine |
| 3-Hydroxypropionic acid | Urine | GC-MS | All | 0–24 mmol/mol creatinine |
| Tiglylglycine | Urine | GC-MS | All | 0–2 mmol/mol creatinine |

## Specimen Collection

| Test | Material | Handling | Pitfalls |
|---|---|---|---|
| Organic acids | Urine | Preservative-free, frozen | Results may be uninformative if responsive patient being treated. Sample thawing, bacterial contamination |
| Lactic acid | Serum | Prompt separation, freezing | Tourniquet/agitation effects. Delayed processing, thawing |
| Carboxylase assays | Whole blood | Yellow-top tube, room temp | Results may be uninformative if responsive patient being treated. Freezing, temp extremes or delays in shipping. |
| | Fibroblasts | Skin biopsy, plates to reference lab | Temperature extremes or delays in shipping. Bacterial or mycoplasma contamination. |

## Prenatal Diagnosis

Though feasibility of prenatal diagnosis of biotinidase deficiency by enzymatic assay activity in amniocytes was demonstrated as early as 1984, prenatal diagnosis is rarely undertaken, probably because outcome is expected to be favorable with treatment. Prenatal testing of amniocytes and chorionic villi has yielded evidence of normal fetuses and heterozygotes. If disease-causing mutations have been identified in the family, it is recommended to use DNA-based methods if prenatal diagnosis is desired. In holocarboxylase synthetase deficiency, amniotic fluid at 16 weeks of gestation showed methylcitrate and 3-hydroxyisovalerate to be only slightly elevated, but enzyme assay was diagnostic in amniocytes and may also be applied to chorionic villi. Given the complexity of the enzyme assay for HCS, molecular analysis affords advantages. Prenatal diagnosis of SLC5A6 dysfunction has never been performed, but there are special concerns, since unlike other forms of MCD, systemic biotin deficiency may be present prenatally in a biotin transporter defect and features such as structural brain abnormalities may reflect early effects on fetal development and organogenesis.

## Treatment

Supplementation with pharmacologic doses of biotin is the cornerstone of therapy. Doses of 5–20 mg daily are generally used. In most cases, patients respond quickly, and most symptoms are reversible; when dosage is inadequate or is stopped due to error or noncompliance, symptoms may reappear. Currently, dosage of biotin in the range of 5–10 mg per day appears to be adequate and effective during childhood (Wolf 2010). Usually the dose is not changed, so with growth, the body mass-normalized dosage tends to decrease. To assure that the dosage is adequate and that the patient is in compliance, some have monitored urinary organic acids (3-hydroxyisovleric and 3-methylcrotonylglycine) and/or plasma acylcarnitines (C5OH-carnitine) (Wolf 2010). There is some concern arising from anecdotal reports of several females with biotinidase deficiency who have begun to lose hair when entering puberty, with reversal when the dose is increased to 15–20 mg from 10 mg.

Supplementation must be in the form of free biotin in biotinidase deficiency (as opposed to some formulations marketed in the health food industry which are derived from yeast extracts and are composed of biocytin). The dosage is determined only by the body's requirements for biotin, since the supplemented biotin does not interact directly with the biotinidase enzyme. In HCSD, however, there is a direct interaction at the biotin binding site of the enzyme, so the effectiveness may be determined by the concentration of biotin. A few cases have been encountered which have been incompletely responsive or unresponsive to biotin (Wilson et al. 2005; Santer et al. 2003), and those have proven to correspond to mutations outside of the biotin binding domain (exons 4–8), resulting in decreased Vmax. However, most cases of HCSD have been found to alterations in Km and relatively normal levels for Vmax, so those are all responsive to high doses of biotin (Bartlett et al. 1980).

Individuals with partial biotinidase deficiency (10%–30% of mean normal serum biotinidase activity) may not exhibit symptoms, but they are at risk of developing symptoms when stressed, such as during infection. Although it is uncommon for individuals with partial deficiency to develop symptoms, given the safety of biotin, it is recommended that they be treated with 1–10 mg oral biotin daily. Patients who are homozygous for the p.D444H biotinidase variant are expected to have approximately 45%–50% of mean normal serum biotinidase enzyme activity (similar to heterozygotes for profound biotinidase deficiency mutations) and do not require biotin therapy (Wolf 2016).

As opposed to biotinidase and HCS deficiency, the rationale is not clear for using biotin to treat isolated deficiencies of the individual carboxylases (primary forms of propionic acidemia, 3-methylcrotonyl-CoA carboxylase deficiency, and pyruvate carboxylase deficiency). Since biotin is covalently bound to the apocarboxylases through the action of HCS, it is not easy to imagine a mutation in the apocarboxylase itself which would affect that process but which would also be remediated with higher biotin concentrations, since the reversible binding of biotin is supposed to be limited to its interaction with HCS. It is a common practice to conduct a trial of biotin in newly diagnosed cases of isolated carboxylase deficiency, and there is one mutation in methylcrotonyl-CoA carboxylase (R385S) which is reported to be biotin-responsive (Baumgartner et al. 2004), but a response to biotin supplementation is virtually never observed in isolated individual carboxylase deficiencies.

If there is an incomplete response to biotin in an individual case of HCSD, alteration of the diet may be indicated, to limit protein and provide supplements of carnitine (and possibly glycine) as appropriate, in the same manner that isolated carboxylase deficiencies are managed. In general, a complete response is expected with adequate amounts of biotin in most cases of HCSD and all cases of biotinidase deficiency; in such cases, dietary modification is not necessary.

## Follow-Up and Monitoring

Ongoing monitoring is recommended, including annual ophthalmologic examination and auditory testing for profound biotinidase deficiency and every 2 years for partial biotinidase deficiency. The interval for follow-up in HCS deficiency should be individualized depending upon responsiveness to therapy.

Adequacy of treatment may be confirmed with periodic monitoring of urine organic acids, to look for an increase in 3-hydroxyisovalerate, 3-methylcrotonylglycine, and related metabolites. Even in cases where a complete response is documented, it is a common practice to monitor organic acids annually.

Raw eggs should be avoided because the undenatured egg white protein avidin tightly binds biotin and decreases its bioavailability. It has also been noted that there needs to be awareness that results of biotin-binding diagnostic bioassays can be compromised when patients are taking pharmacologic doses of biotin.

## References


Bartlett K, Ng H, Leonard JV. A combined defect of three mitochondrial carboxylases presenting as biotin-responsive 3-methylcrotonyl glycinuria and 3-hydroxyisovaleric aciduria. Clin Chim Acta. 1980;100:183–6.

Baumgartner MR, Dantas MF, Suormala T, et al. Isolated 3-methylcrotonyl-CoA carboxylase deficiency: evidence for an allele-specific dominant negative effect and responsiveness to biotin therapy. Am J Hum Genet. 2004;75:790–800.

Burri BJ, Sweetman L, Nyhan WL. Mutant holocarboxylase synthetase: evidence for the enzyme defect in early infantile biotin-responsive multiple carboxylase deficiency. J Clin Invest. 1981;68:1491–5.

Dabbagh O, Brismar J, Gascon GG, Ozand PT. The clinical spectrum of biotin-treatable encephalopathies in Saudi Arabia. Brain Dev. 1994;16(Suppl):72–80.

Ferreira P, Chan A, Wolf B. Irreversibility of symptoms with biotin therapy in an adult with profound Biotinidase deficiency. JIMD Reports. 2017;36:117–20.

Heard GS, Wolf B, Jefferson LG, et al. Neonatal screening for biotinidase deficiency: results of a 1-year pilot study. J Pediatr. 1986;108:40–6.

Leon-Del-Rio A. Biotin in metabolism, gene expression, and human disease. J Inherit Metab Dis. 2019;42:647–54.

Mardach R, Zempleni J, Wolf B, et al. Biotin dependency due to a defect in biotin transport. J Clin Invest. 2002;109:1617–23.

Prasad PD, Ganapathy V. Structure and function of mammalian sodium-dependent multivitamin transporter. Curr Opin Clin Nutr Metab Care. 2000;3:263–6.

Rios-Avila L, Prince SA, Wijeratne SS, Zempleni J. A 96-well plate assay for high-throughput analysis of holocarboxylase synthetase activity. Clin Chim Acta. 2011;412:735–9.

Santer R, Muhle H, Suormala T, et al. Partial response to biotin therapy in a patient with holocarboxylase synthetase deficiency: clinical, biochemical, and molecular genetic aspects. Mol Genet Metab. 2003;79:160–6.

Saunders M, Sweetman L, Robinson B, Roth K, Cohn R, Gravel RA. Biotin-response organicaciduria. Multiple carboxylase defects and complementation studies with propionic acidemia in cultured fibroblasts. J Clin Invest. 1979;64:1695–702.

Squires L, Betz B, Umfleet J, Kelley R. Resolution of subependymal cysts in neonatal holocarboxylase synthetase deficiency. Dev Med Child Neurol. 1997;39:267–9.

Subramanian VS, Constantinescu AR, Benke PJ, Said HM. Mutations in SLC5A6 associated with brain, immune, bone, and intestinal dysfunction in a young child. Hum Genet. 2017;136:253–61.

Suormala T, Fowler B, Duran M, et al. Five patients with a biotin-responsive defect in holocarboxylase formation: evaluation of responsiveness to biotin therapy in vivo and comparative biochemical studies in vitro. Pediatr Res. 1997;41:666–73.

Sweetman L, Bates SP, Hull D, Nyhan WL. Propionyl-CoA carboxylase deficiency in a patient with biotin-responsive 3-methylcrotonylglycinuria. Pediatr Res. 1977;11:1144–7.

Sweetman L, Nyhan WL, Sakati NA, et al. Organic aciduria in neonatal multiple carboxylase deficiency. J Inherit Metab Dis. 1982;5:49–53.

Wilson CJ, Myer M, Darlow BA, et al. Severe holocarboxylase synthetase deficiency with incomplete biotin responsiveness resulting in antenatal insult in samoan neonates. J Pediatr. 2005;147:115–8.

Wolf B. Clinical issues and frequent questions about biotinidase deficiency. Mol Genet Metab. 2010;100:6–13.

Wolf B. The neurology of biotinidase deficiency. Mol Genet Metab. 2011;104:27–34.

Wolf B. Biotinidase deficiency. In: Pagon RA, Adam MP, Bird TD, editors. GeneReviews. Seattle: University of Washington, Seattle; 2016.

Wolf B, Grier RE, Allen RJ, et al. Phenotypic variation in biotinidase deficiency. J Pediatr. 1983;103:233–7.

Wolf B, Norrgard K, Pomponio RJ, et al. Profound biotinidase deficiency in two asymptomatic adults. Am J Med Genet. 1997;73:5–9.

Wolf B, Pomponio RJ, Norrgard KJ, et al. Delayed-onset profound biotinidase deficiency. J Pediatr. 1998;132:362–5.

Zeng WQ, Al-Yamani E, Acierno JS Jr, et al. Biotin-responsive basal ganglia disease maps to 2q36.3 and is due to mutations in SLC19A3. Am J Hum Genet. 2005;77:16–26.

# Thiamine Disorders

# 31

Majid Alfadhel and Marwan Nashabat

## Contents



**Summary**

Thiamine or vitamin B1 is an essential water-soluble vitamin for which human body relies solely on external dietary intake. Once absorbed by two thiamine transporters, hTHTR1 and hTHTR2, the free thiamine is phosphorylated to the active form, thiamine pyrophosphate (TPP), by thiamine phosphokinase (TPK1). TPP acts as a cofactor for multiple enzymes in the cytosol, mitochondria, and peroxisomes. Thiamine-related diseases in humans are either primary or secondary. Four diseases were described so far related to primary thiamine metabolism dysfunction. Thiamine-responsive megaloblastic anemia syndrome or Rogers syndrome is caused by mutations in *SLC19A2*, encoding the first thiamine transporter and characterized by a triad of megaloblastic anemia, non-type 1 diabetes mellitus, and sensory neural hearing loss. Biotin-thiamine-responsive basal ganglia disease (BTBGD) is caused by mutations in the gene encoding for the second thiamine transporter (*SLC19A3*). The disease is classified into three phenotypes: classical childhood BTBGD, early infantile (< 3 months) Leigh-like/atypical infantile spasms, and adult Wernicke's-like encephalopathy. The subacute encephalopathy is usually provoked by a stressor. Thiamine pyrophosphokinase deficiency is caused by mutations in *TPK1* gene resulting in episodic encephalopathy with psychomotor developmental delay, ataxia, seizures, and dystonia. Mutations in *SLC25A19* are responsible for mitochondrial thiamine pyrophosphate carrier deficiency with two distinct phenotypes: Amish microcephaly and neuropathy and bilateral striatal necrosis. Thiamine metabolism disorders are considered generally among the treatable metabolic conditions. Clinicians should have a low threshold to start thiamine supplementation upon suspicion due to the huge difference in the outcome based on the time of treatment initiation.

M. Alfadhel (✉)
King Abdullah International Medical Research Centre,
King Saud bin Abdulaziz University for Health Sciences,
Riyadh, Saudi Arabia
e-mail: dralfadhelma@gmail.com

M. Nashabat
King Abdulaziz Medical City, Riyadh, Saudi Arabia


N. Blau et al. (eds.), *Physician's Guide to the Diagnosis, Treatment, and Follow-Up of Inherited Metabolic Diseases*,
https://doi.org/10.1007/978-3-030-67727-5_31

## Introduction

Thiamine or vitamin B1 is an essential water-soluble vitamin for which human body relies solely on external dietary intake. The main sources of dietary thiamin are meats, whole grains, nuts, and legumes. The limited stores and short half-life of thiamine necessitate a regular supply of the vitamin. The recommended daily intake of thiamine differs according to age, sex, pregnancy and lactation status, and carbohydrate intake. For females and males, it is recommended to take 1.1 mg/day and 1.2 mg/day, respectively (WHO and FAO 2005). As a hydrophilic micronutrient, thiamin is absorbed in the upper part of the small intestine in exchange with hydrogen at physiological concentrations. However, at high concentrations, it can be absorbed by passive diffusion (Brown 2014). The intestinal phosphatases convert the ingested phosphate attached thiamine to the free form, which is absorbed by two thiamine transporters, hTHTR1 and hTHTR2, encoded by *SLC19A2* and *SLC19A3* genes, respectively (Ganapathy et al. 2004). Once absorbed, the free thiamine is phosphorylated to the active form, thiamine pyrophosphate (TPP), by thiamine phosphokinase (TPK1). TPP acts as a cofactor for multiple enzymes in the cytosol, mitochondria, and peroxisomes. In the cytosol, TPP is required for the transketolase enzyme in the pentose phosphate pathway, to produce NADPH in addition to the ribose sugar needed for the DNA and RNA synthesis. Additionally, TPP is transported to the mitochondria through SLC25A19 (Kang and Samuels 2008), where it is utilized by pyruvate dehydrogenase complex to produce acetyl-CoA, which takes place in the citric acid cycle to produce energy. Furthermore, within the citric acid cycle, 2-oxoglutarate dehydrogenase complex converts alpha-ketoglutarate to succinate only in the presence of TPP as a cofactor. Branched-chain alpha-ketoacid dehydrogenase complex located in the inner membrane of the mitochondria catalyzes the branched chain amino acids, valine, leucine, and isoleucine, catabolism in the presence of TPP (Lonsdale 2006). The alpha oxidation of fatty acids takes place only in peroxisomes by the enzyme 2-hydroxy acyl-CoA lyase (HACL1), which requires TPP as a cofactor (Fraccascia et al. 2011).

Thiamine-related diseases in humans are either primary or secondary. Four diseases were described so far related to primary thiamine metabolism dysfunction, thiamine-responsive megaloblastic anemia syndrome or Rogers syndrome (SLC19A2), biotin-thiamine-responsive basal ganglia disease or thiamine metabolism dysfunction syndrome 2 (SLC19A3), thiamine pyrophosphokinase deficiency or thiamine metabolism dysfunction syndrome 5 (TPK1), and mitochondrial thiamine pyrophosphate carrier deficiency or bilateral striatal necrosis or Amish microcephaly (SLD25A19). Secondary causes of thiamine disorders are related to the nutritional deficiency of thiamine like beriberi and Wernicke's encephalopathy.

Thiamine-responsive megaloblastic anemia (TRMA) syndrome or Rogers syndrome is caused by homozygous or compound heterozygous mutations in *SLC19A2*, encoding the first thiamine transporter. The classic triad of the disease since its first description (Porter et al. 1969) includes megaloblastic anemia, non-type 1 diabetes mellitus, and sensory neural hearing loss. The hTHTR1 is the sole thiamine transporter in the marrow, beta cells of the pancreas, and the cochlear inner hair cells, which might explain the cardinal features of the disease (Bergmann et al. 2009). The age of onset of the symptoms ranges from infancy to adulthood, noting that deafness usually starts at a later age. Other reported associated symptoms include cardiac abnormalities like arrhythmia, atrial and ventricular septal defects, visual impairments particularly optic nerve atrophy and retinal dystrophy, neurological symptoms like seizures, and stroke-like symptoms. Short stature was also reported in multiple cases (Bergmann et al. 2009; Ricketts et al. 2006). The thiamine level can be normal or slightly reduced. Additionally, patients do not manifest lactic acidosis or organic aciduria (Ortigoza Escobar and Duenas 2016).

The dysfunction of the second thiamine transporter (hTHTR2) encoded by *SLC19A3* causes biotin-thiamine-responsive basal ganglia disease (BTBGD) or thiamine metabolism dysfunction syndrome type 2. The disease was first described by Ozand et al. in 1998, (Ozand et al. 1998) who reported ten cases mostly from Saudi Arabia presented with subacute encephalopathy and improved on biotin supplementation. Thereafter, more cases were reported, and the disease phenotypes were further delineated and classified into three main subtypes; classical childhood BTBGD, early infantile (<3 months) Leigh-like/atypical infantile spasms, and adult Wernicke's-like encephalopathy (Alfadhel and Tabarki 2018). The patients with classical phenotype present with subacute encephalopathy, usually triggered by a stressor like fever, vaccine, or trauma, with confusion, dysarthria and dysphagia, supranuclear facial nerve palsy, seizures, and external ophthalmoplegia, progressing to severe cogwheel rigidity, dystonia, and quadriparesis or even death if not treated. The second phenotype presents in early infantile life either in the form of Leigh-like syndrome with poor feeding, encephalopathy, and severe lactic acidosis (Perez-Duenas et al. 2013) or as atypical infantile spasm with poor outcome (Yamada et al. 2010). The third adult Wernicke's-like encephalopathy phenotype manifests with status epilepticus, diplopia, nystagmus, ptosis, ophthalmoplegia, and ataxia (Kono et al. 2009). The genotype-phenotype correlation is still not clear (Alfadhel and Tabarki 2018). Biochemically, patients may have lactic acidosis, elevated serum alanine, leucine, and isoleucine, in addition to the increase in the excretion of α-Ketoglutarate in urine. Brain MRI findings vary according to the phenotype; bilateral symmetrical lesions in the basal ganglia in addition to the involvement of the thalami, cerebellum, and brain stem are characteristic in the classical phenotype (Kassem et al. 2014). In the early infantile phenotype, brain MRI may mimic the classical phenotype, but with restricted diffusion in various regions of the cortex and white matter (Yamada et al. 2010).

Thiamine pyrophosphokinase deficiency is caused by mutations in *TPK1* gene. This disease was the most recent thiamine metabolism disorder reported. Most of the patients present with episodic encephalopathy with psychomotor developmental delay, ataxia, seizures, and dystonia. So far, only nine patients were reported in the literature, only one of them presented with progressive (non-episodic) Leigh-like encephalopathy. The symptoms for most of the patients were provoked by a febrile illness. Investigations may show lactic acidosis and elevated α-Ketoglutarate in urine. The reported radiological findings in brain MRI include the involvement of the basal ganglia, thalamus in addition to white matter involvement in some patients (Banka et al. 2014; Fraser et al. 2014; Mayr et al. 2011).

Mutations in *SLC25A19* are responsible for mitochondrial thiamine pyrophosphate carrier deficiency with two distinct phenotypes: Amish microcephaly and neuropathy and bilateral striatal necrosis. Amish microcephaly was reported in Amish population with microcephaly evident as early as the 20th week of gestation. The patients showed severe frontal sloping and absent fontanels. Hepatomegaly, seizures, exaggerated startle reflex, and irritability were also reported. Most of the patients died in the first year of life. Biochemically, patients had lactic acidosis and marked elevation in α-Ketoglutarate in urine. Brain MRI might show an immature brain with absent gyri (lissencephaly) and cerebellar vermis hypoplasia. Viral infections were reported to provoke metabolic acidosis crises and worsening of the patients' conditions (Kelley et al. 2002). Sui, VM. et al. reported another case with similar genotype but with a more favorable outcome. They expanded the phenotype to include partial agenesis of the corpus callosum and neural tube defect (Siu et al. 2010). The second phenotype was reported in Arab patients by Spiegel et al. presented with episodic flaccid paralysis attacks starting at ages from 3 to 6 years. The attacks are usually preceded by a viral infection with near-complete recovery. However, patients suffered from slowly progressive polyneuropathy. The cognitive abilities of the patients were maintained. Brain MRI findings included bilateral caudate and putamen hyperintensity (Spiegel et al. 2009).

## Nomenclature

| No. | Disorder | Alternative name | Disease abbreviation | Gene symbol | Chromosomal location | Mode of inheritance | Affected protein | Disease OMIM# |
|---|---|---|---|---|---|---|---|---|
| 31.1 | Thiamine-responsive megaloblastic anemia | Rogers syndrome; thiamine metabolism dysfunction syndrome type 1 | TRMA | *SLC19A2* | 1q23.3 | AR | THTR1 transporter | 249270 |
| 31.2 | Biotin-thiamine-responsive basal ganglia disease | Thiamine metabolism dysfunction syndrome type 2 | BTBGD, THMD2, BBGD | *SLC19A3* | 2q36.3 | AR | THTR2 transporter | 607483 |
| 31.3 | Thiamine pyrophosphokinase deficiency | Thiamine metabolism dysfunction syndrome type 5 | THMD5 | *TPK1* | 7q35 | AR | Thiamine pyrophosphokinase | 614458 |
| 31.4 | Mitochondrial thiamine pyrophosphate carrier deficiency | Amish lethal microcephaly, thiamine metabolism dysfunction syndrome type 3 (severe) | MCPHA, THMD3 | *SLC25A19* | 17q25.1 | AR | Mitochondrial thiamine pyrophosphate carrier | 607196 |
| | | Bilateral striatal necrosis and progressive polyneuropathy, thiamine metabolism dysfunction syndrome type 4 (milder) | THMD4 | *SLC25A19* | 17q25.1 | AR | Mitochondrial thiamine pyrophosphate carrier | 613710 |

## Metabolic Pathways

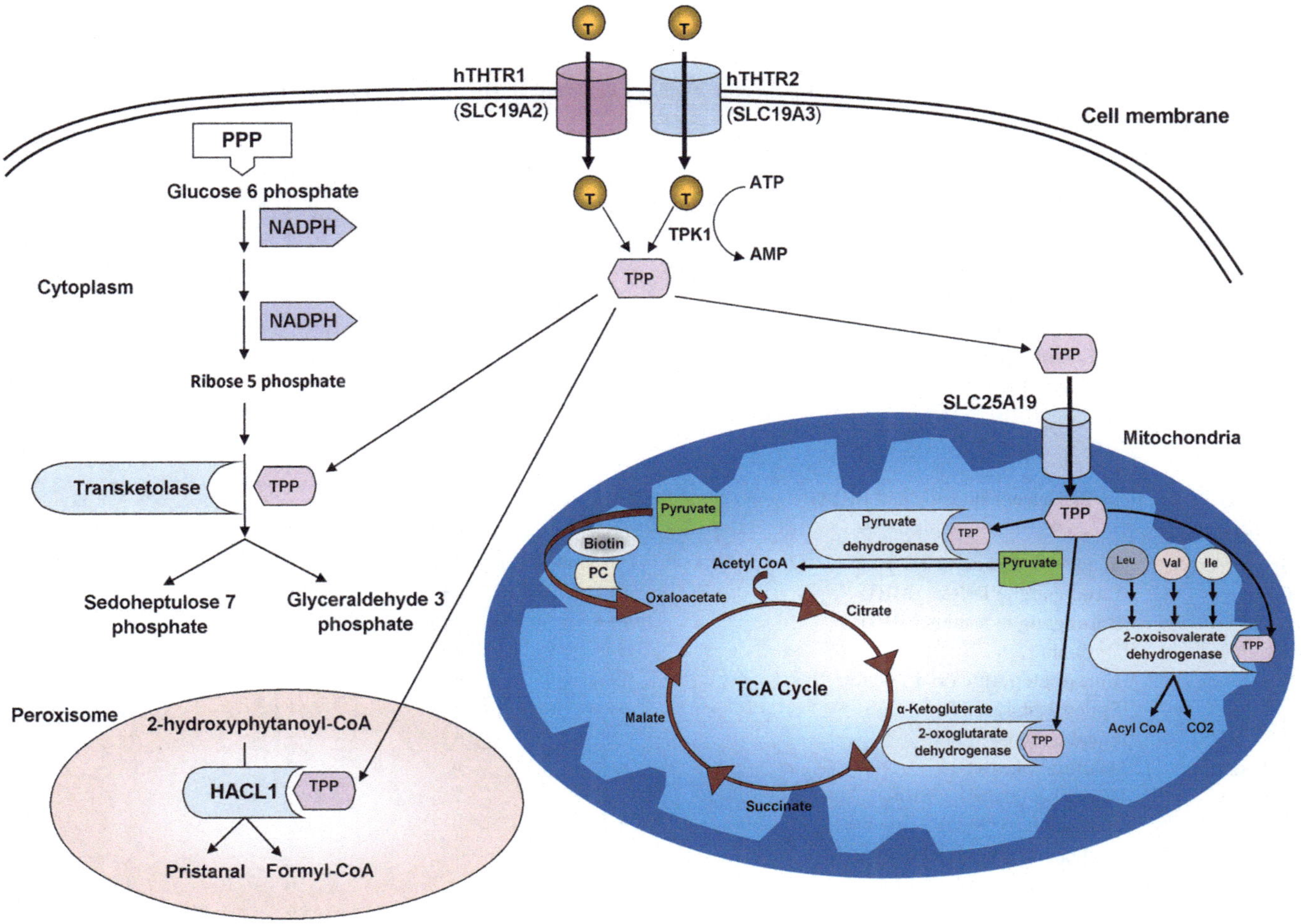


**Fig. 31.1** Thiamine enters the cells through two transporters (hTHTR1 and hTHTR2). In the cytoplasm, thiamine undergoes phosphorylation to produce the active form (thiamine pyrophosphate (TPP)) by thiamine pyrophosphate kinase (TPK1). TPP is transported to the mitochondria by thiamine pyrophosphate carrier encoded by *SLC25A19*, where it acts as a cofactor for three main enzymes; pyruvate dehydrogenase, 2-oxoglutarate dehydrogenase (α ketoglutarate dehydrogenase), and 2-oxoisovalerate dehydrogenase (α-ketoacid dehydrogenase). In the cytoplasm, TPP acts as a cofactor for transketolase in the pentose phosphate pathway (PPP). In the peroxisomes, TPP acts as a cofactor with 2-hydroxy acyl-CoA lyase (HACL1) in the α-oxidation of fatty acids like phytanic acid
*AMP* Adenosine monophosphate, *ATP* Adenosine triphosphate, *hTHTR1* Human thiamine transporter 1, *hTHTR2* Human thiamine transporter 2, *NADPH* Reduced form of nicotinamide adenine dinucleotide phosphate, *PC* Pyruvate carboxylase, *SLC19A3* Solute Carrier Family 19, Member 3, *T* Thiamine, *SLC25A19* Solute Carrier Family 25, Member 19, *TCA* Tricarboxylic acid

## Signs and Symptoms

**Table 31.1** Thiamine-responsive megaloblastic anemia syndrome

| System | Symptoms and biomarkers | Neonatal (birth–1 month) | Infancy (1–18 months) | Childhood (1.5–11 years) | Adolescence (11–16 years) | Adulthood (>16 years) |
|---|---|---|---|---|---|---|
| Cardiovascular | Cardiomyopathy | | ± | ± | ± | ± |
| CNS | Epilepsy | | + | + | + | + |
| Ear | **Deafness** | | ± | +++ | +++ | ++ |
| Endocrine | **Diabetes mellitus** | | ++ | ++ | +++ | +++ |
| Eye | Optic neuropathy | | ± | + | + | + |
| Hematological | **Anemia, sideroblastic** | | ++ | ++ | ++ | ++ |
| | **Thrombocytopenia** | | ± | ++ | ++ | ++ |
| Laboratory findings | **Glucose (plasma)** | | ↑ | ↑ | ↑ | ↑ |
| | **Lactate (plasma)** | **n** | **n** | **n** | **n** | **n** |
| | **Thiamine (plasma)** | **n** | **n** | **n** | **n** | **n** |

**Table 31.2** Wernicke-like encephalopathy and BRBG

| System | Symptoms and biomarkers | Neonatal (birth–1 month) | Infancy (1–18 months) | Childhood (1.5–11 years) | Adolescence (11–16 years) | Adulthood (>15 years) |
|---|---|---|---|---|---|---|
| CNS | **Basal ganglia lesions (MRI)** | | +++ | +++ | +++ | +++ |
| | **Basal ganglia lesions (MRI)** | | +++ | +++ | +++ | +++ |
| | Dystonia | ± | ± | ++ | ++ | ++ |
| | **Encephalopathic crisis, acute** | | +++ | +++ | +++ | +++ |
| | Epilepsy, intractable | | ++ | ± | ± | ± |
| | **Focal epilepsy** | | | ++ | ++ | ++ |
| Laboratory findings | **Alanine (plasma)** | **n** | **n-↑** | **n** | **n** | **n** |
| | Alpha-ketoglutarate (urine) | | ↑ | ↑ | | |
| | Hemoglobin (blood) | | n | n | n | n |
| | Lactate (cerebrospinal fluid) | | ↑ | ↑ | | |
| | **Lactate (plasma)** | | **n-↑** | **n-↑** | **n** | **n** |
| | Pyruvate (plasma) | n | n | n | n | n |
| | Thiamine (plasma) | | | ↓-n | n | n |

**Table 31.3** Thiamine metabolism dysfunction syndrome 5

| System | Symptoms and biomarkers | Neonatal (birth–1 month) | Infancy (1–18 months) | Childhood (1.5–11 years) | Adolescence (11–16 years) | Adulthood (>16 years) |
|---|---|---|---|---|---|---|
| CNS | Ataxia | | | + | + | |
| | Dystonia | | | + | + | |
| | **Encephalopathy, episodic** | | | + | + | |
| | Hyperintensities (T2) of the globus pallidus (MRI) | | | + | + | |
| Laboratory findings | **Alpha-ketoglutarate (urine)** | | | ↑ | ↑ | |
| | **Lactate (cerebrospinal fluid)** | | | ↑ | ↑ | |
| | **Lactate (plasma)** | | | ↑ | ↑ | |

**Table 31.4** Mitochondrial thiamine pyrophosphate carrier deficiency

| System | Symptoms and biomarkers | Neonatal (birth–1 month) | Infancy (1–18 months) | Childhood (1.5–11 years) | Adolescence (11–16 years) | Adulthood (>16 years) |
|---|---|---|---|---|---|---|
| CNS | **Basal ganglia lesions (MRI)** | | | +++ | +++ | +++ |
| | **Dystonia** | | | ++ | ++ | ++ |
| | **Encephalopathy acute, precipitated by infection** | | | +++ | +++ | +++ |
| | **Polyneuropathy** | | | +++ | +++ | +++ |
| Laboratory findings | Alpha-ketoglutarate (urine) | | | ↑ | ↑ | ↑ |
| | **Lactate (cerebrospinal fluid)** | | | **n-↑** | **n-↑** | **n-↑** |

## Reference Values Table

Plasma

| Compound | Infants | Childhood | Adolescence | Adult |
|---|---|---|---|---|
| Lactic acid (mmol/L) | <2.1 | 0.45–2.2 | 1–1.55 | 1–1.55 |
| Thiamine (ng/mL) | | 30–90 | | 20–50 |
| Alanine (umol/L) | 134–416 | 148–475 | 193–545 | 259–407 |

Urine

| Compound | Infants | Childhood | Adolescence | Adult |
|---|---|---|---|---|
| Lactic acid (umol/mmol creatinine) | 50.73 ± 53.54 | <52 | 3.6–29.3 | 3.6–29.3 |
| Oxoglutaric acid (α-ketoglutarate) (umol/mmol creatinine) | <110 | <95 | <80 | <75 |

CSF

| Compound | Infants | Childhood | Adolescence | Adult |
|---|---|---|---|---|
| Lactic acid (mmol/L) | 0.5–2.2 | <2 | 0.45–2.1 | 0.45–2.1 |
| Alanine (umol/L) | 28.5–38 | 6–47 | | 19–73 |

## Pathological Values Table

Thiamine-responsive megaloblastic anemia syndrome

| Compound | Neonatal (birth–1 month) | Infancy (1–18 months) | Childhood (1.5–11 years) | Adolescence (11–16 years) | Adulthood (>16 years) |
|---|---|---|---|---|---|
| Lactate (plasma) | n | n | n | n | n |
| Thiamine (plasma) | n | n | n | n | n |
| Glucose (plasma) | | ↑ | ↑ | ↑ | ↑ |

Biotin-thiamine-responsive basal ganglia disease

| Symptom name | Neonatal (birth–1 month) | Infancy (1–18 months) | Childhood (1.5–11 years) | Adolescence (11–16 years) | Adulthood (>16 years) |
|---|---|---|---|---|---|
| Lactate (plasma) | | n-↑ | n-↑ | n | n |
| Pyruvate (plasma) | n | n | n | n | n |
| Thiamine (plasma) | | | ↓-n | n | n |
| Hemoglobin (blood) | | n | n | n | n |
| Alanine (plasma) | n | n-↑ | n | n | n |
| Lactate (cerebrospinal fluid) | | ↑ | ↑ | | |
| Alpha-ketoglutarate (urine) | | ↑ | ↑ | | |

Thiamine pyrophosphokinase deficiency

| Symptom name | Neonatal (birth–1 month) | Infancy (1–18 months) | Childhood (1.5–11 years) | Adolescence (11–16 years) |
|---|---|---|---|---|
| Lactate (cerebrospinal fluid) | | | ↑ | ↑ |
| Alpha-ketoglutarate (urine) | | | ↑ | ↑ |
| Lactate (plasma) | | | ↑ | ↑ |

Mitochondrial thiamine pyrophosphate carrier deficiency

| Symptom name | Neonatal (birth–1 month) | Infancy (1–18 months) | Childhood (1.5–11 years) | Adolescence (11–16 years) | Adulthood (>16 years) |
|---|---|---|---|---|---|
| Lactate (cerebrospinal fluid) | | | n-↑ | n-↑ | n-↑ |
| Alpha-ketoglutarate (urine) | | | ↑ | ↑ | ↑ |

## Diagnostic Flowchart

Molecular investigations are the mainstay in diagnosing thiamine metabolism disorders as the signs and symptoms are general and may not give a clue for the diagnosis. TRMA could be an exception, where the presentation with the classic triad of the syndrome might ease reaching the diagnosis. Although the phenotypes of BTBGD were described thoroughly in the literature, the unspecific presenting symptoms, which might mimic other diseases including mitochondrial diseases, and the lack of specific biomarkers, make the molecular test as the best initial diagnostic tool. The lactic acidosis and the elevation of the urine alpha ketoglutarate are not specific nor consistent in all patients with TPK1 deficiency and mitochondrial thiamine pyrophosphate carrier deficiency. However, the presence of marked microcephaly in addition to the biochemical findings should raise the suspicion of SLC25A19 gene mutation. Combining the clinical presentations, biochemical findings and the brain MRI could narrow the differential diagnosis.

## Prenatal Diagnosis Table

In families with diagnosed patients, it is highly recommended to go for prenatal genetic testing in each pregnancy. No other prenatal tests or biomarkers could confirm the diagnosis of any thiamine metabolism disorder.

## Treatment Summary

Given the fact that thiamine metabolism disorders are considered generally among the treatable metabolic conditions, clinicians should have a low threshold to start thiamine supplementation upon suspicion due to the huge difference in the outcome based on the time of treatment initiation, in addition to the safety of the medication (thiamine) in all age groups, as there were no significant adverse effects reported so far (Ortigoza-Escobar et al. 2016).

Thiamine supplementation was proven to improve the clinical features of TRMA patients. A prompt hematological response was observed after thiamine supplementation mainly in thrombocytes and neutropenia; however, the sideroblasts and macrocytic anemia may persist. The need for insulin is reduced after thiamine treatment, and some patients were successfully off insulin. However, in the adolescence, they may develop insulin-dependent diabetes. On the other hand, thiamine did not improve the hearing loss, and the patients may benefit from cochlear implant. The thiamine dose for TRMA ranges from 1 to 4 mg/kg/day (Porter et al. 1969; Bergmann et al. 2009; Ricketts et al. 2006; Ortigoza-Escobar et al. 2016).

BTBGD patients usually recover immediately after thiamine and biotin supplementation; however, the level of neurological sequelae depends on the time of treatment initiation. It is recommended to give biotin and thiamine supplements for life as the discontinuation of the treatment might result in the recurrence of the encephalopathy and neurological deficit. The exact role of biotin in the management is still not fully understood; however, it might improve the expression of hTHTR2 and may bypass the oxaloacetate supply for the citric acid cycle through the pyruvate carboxylase (Alfadhel and Tabarki 2018; Ortigoza-Escobar et al. 2016). It is recommended to use biotin as an adjunct treatment with thiamine, which is considered the main treatment for this disease. The recommended doses of biotin range from 5 to 10 mg/kg/day and thiamine 10 to 40 mg/kg/day (Tabarki et al. 2015).

Most of the patients with TPK1 deficiency were treated using either thiamine alone or with other treatment modalities like mitochondrial cocktail and ketogenic diet. The thiamine doses used ranged from 100 up to 500 mg per day. Significant improvements were observed on the treated patients particularly the early diagnosed and treated patients. However, there was a limited benefit for late diagnosed patients (Banka et al. 2014; Fraser et al. 2014; Mayr et al. 2011). Banka et al. used the ketogenic diet for one of their patients before adding the thiamine, which resulted in severe metabolic acidosis and serious consequences on the patient. Hence they recommended not to use the ketogenic diet alone for TPK1 deficiency patients (Banka et al. 2014).

The first reported cases of Amish microcephaly did not receive any management and died early (Kelley et al. 2002). On the other hand, the case reported by Sui et al. was managed with low-protein, high-fat diet in addition to a vitamin cocktail including thiamin 50 mg per day, which resulted in resolving the lactic acidosis and improvement of the patient's condition (Siu et al. 2010). The polyneuropathy phenotype was managed by Spiegel et al. using high thiamine doses, which were not expected to improve the neurological impairment of the patients; however, it hopefully might prevent future deterioration (Spiegel et al. 2009).

## Follow-Up and Monitoring

TRMA patients need annual monitoring for the complete blood count with differential and reticulocytes count. In addition to serum glucose and the glycosylated hemoglobin, hearing assessment, ophthalmology evaluation, and cardiac evaluation are also recommended.

A regular follow-up for BTBGD patients to monitor the compliance of treatment and to monitor any progression of the neurological symptoms. The prognosis depends on the age of onset and the age of establishing the diagnosis, the age of initiating the treatment, and the nature of the mutation.

The literature lacks long-term follow-up data for patients with TPK1 deficiency and mitochondrial thiamine pyrophosphate carrier deficiency (SLC25A19). However, it is recommended to keep all the patients on thiamine supplementation and to monitor the patients closely for any neurological deterioration. Additionally, serum lactic acid level and urine alpha ketoglutarate level urine should be monitored.

## References


Alfadhel M, Tabarki B. SLC19A3 gene defects sorting the phenotype and acronyms: review. Neuropediatrics. 2018;49(2):83–92.

Banka S, et al. Expanding the clinical and molecular spectrum of thiamine pyrophosphokinase deficiency: a treatable neurological disorder caused by TPK1 mutations. Mol Genet Metab. 2014;113(4):301–6.

Bergmann AK, et al. Thiamine-responsive megaloblastic anemia: identification of novel compound heterozygotes and mutation update. J Pediatr. 2009;155(6):888–892.e1.

Brown G. Defects of thiamine transport and metabolism. J Inherit Metab Dis. 2014;37(4):577–85.

Fraccascia P, et al. Role of thiamine pyrophosphate in oligomerisation, functioning and import of peroxisomal 2-hydroxyacyl-CoA lyase. Biochim Biophys Acta. 2011;1814(10):1226–33.

Fraser JL, et al. Thiamine pyrophosphokinase deficiency causes a Leigh disease like phenotype in a sibling pair: identification through whole exome sequencing and management strategies. Mol Genet Metab Rep. 2014;1:66–70.

Ganapathy V, Smith SB, Prasad PD. SLC19: the folate/thiamine transporter family. Pflugers Arch. 2004;447(5):641–6.

Kang J, Samuels DC. The evidence that the DNC (SLC25A19) is not the mitochondrial deoxyribonucleotide carrier. Mitochondrion. 2008;8(2):103–8.

Kassem H, et al. Biotin-responsive basal ganglia disease: neuroimaging features before and after treatment. AJNR Am J Neuroradiol. 2014;35(10):1990–5.

Kelley RI, et al. Amish lethal microcephaly: a new metabolic disorder with severe congenital microcephaly and 2-ketoglutaric aciduria. Am J Med Genet. 2002;112(4):318–26.

Kono S, et al. Mutations in a thiamine-transporter gene and Wernicke's-like encephalopathy. N Engl J Med. 2009;360(17):1792–4.

Lonsdale D. A review of the biochemistry, metabolism and clinical benefits of thiamin(e) and its derivatives. Evid Based Complement Alternat Med. 2006;3(1):49–59.

Mayr JA, et al. Thiamine pyrophosphokinase deficiency in encephalopathic children with defects in the pyruvate oxidation pathway. Am J Hum Genet. 2011;89(6):806–12.

Ortigoza Escobar JD, Duenas BP. Treatable inborn errors of metabolism due to membrane vitamin transporters deficiency. Semin Pediatr Neurol. 2016;23(4):341–50.

Ortigoza-Escobar JD, et al. Treatment of genetic defects of thiamine transport and metabolism. Expert Rev Neurother. 2016;16(7):755–63.

Ozand PT, et al. Biotin-responsive basal ganglia disease: a novel entity. Brain. 1998;121(Pt 7):1267–79.

Perez-Duenas B, et al. Reversible lactic acidosis in a newborn with thiamine transporter-2 deficiency. Pediatrics. 2013;131(5):e1670–5.

Porter FS, Rogers LE, Sidbury JB Jr. Thiamine-responsive megaloblastic anemia. J Pediatr. 1969;74(4):494–504.

Ricketts CJ, et al. Thiamine-responsive megaloblastic anaemia syndrome: long-term follow-up and mutation analysis of seven families. Acta Paediatr. 2006;95(1):99–104.

Siu VM, et al. Amish microcephaly: long-term survival and biochemical characterization. Am J Med Genet A. 2010;152A(7):1747–51.

Spiegel R, et al. SLC25A19 mutation as a cause of neuropathy and bilateral striatal necrosis. Ann Neurol. 2009;66(3):419–24.

Tabarki B, et al. Treatment of biotin-responsive basal ganglia disease: open comparative study between the combination of biotin plus thiamine versus thiamine alone. Eur J Paediatr Neurol. 2015;19(5):547–52.

WHO and FAO. Vitamin and mineral requirements in human nutrition. Geneva: World Health Organization; 2005.

Yamada K, et al. A wide spectrum of clinical and brain MRI findings in patients with SLC19A3 mutations. BMC Med Genet. 2010;11:171.

# Disorders of Riboflavin Metabolism

# 32

Christine Vianey-Saban, Cécile Acquaviva, and Annet M. Bosch

## Contents



**Summary**

Riboflavin or vitamin B2, a water-soluble vitamin supplied by dairy products, is the precursor of flavin mononucleotide (FMN) and flavin adenine dinucleotide (FAD). FAD is the essential cofactor for the two electron transporters Electron Transfer Flavoprotein (ETF) and ETF-ubiQuinone Oxidoreductase (ETF-QO) involved in multiple acyl-CoA dehydrogenase deficiency (MADD). A genetic defect in ETF or in ETF-QO results in an impairment of mitochondrial fatty acid oxidation, branched-chain amino acids, lysine, and choline metabolisms. The clinical phenotype of MADD patients is highly variable, ranging from severe neonatal non-ketotic hypoglycaemia, cardiomyopathy, metabolic acidosis, sometimes associated with congenital abnormalities and a poor prognosis despite dietary and 3-hydroxybutyrate treatment, to muscle weakness or exercise intolerance in adulthood, which responds well to riboflavin.

C. Vianey-Saban (✉) · C. Acquaviva
CHU de Lyon, Department of Biochemistry & Molecular Biology, Division of Inborn Errors of Metabolism, Lyon University Hospital Centre, Bron, France
e-mail: christine.vianeysaban@gmail.com; cecile.acquaviva-bourdain@chu-lyon.fr

A. M. Bosch
Department of Pediatrics, Emma Children's Hospital, Amsterdam University Medical Centers, Amsterdam, The Netherlands
e-mail: A.M.Bosch@amsterdamumc.nl


N. Blau et al. (eds.), *Physician's Guide to the Diagnosis, Treatment, and Follow-Up of Inherited Metabolic Diseases*,
https://doi.org/10.1007/978-3-030-67727-5_32

FAD and FMN are the cofactors for at least 80 enzymes. Dietary depletion of riboflavin is rare in developed countries. The intestinal absorption and the uptake of riboflavin by the different organs are mediated by three riboflavin transporters: RFVT1 (*SLC52A1* gene), RFVT2 (*SLC52A2* gene), and RFVT3 (*SLC52A3* gene). In the cytoplasmic compartment, the conversion of riboflavin into FMN and FAD is catalysed by riboflavin kinase and FAD synthase (*FLAD1* gene). The uptake of FAD in mitochondria is mediated by the mitochondrial FAD transporter (MFT, *SLC25A32* gene). Genetic defects of RFVT2 or RFVT3 cause Riboflavin Transporter Deficiencies (RTD) type 2 and 3, which were formerly known as Brown-Vialetto-van Laere or Fazio-Londe syndrome. RTD patients may present from infancy into adulthood with progressive cranial neuropathy, muscle weakness, (sensory) ataxia, and respiratory insufficiency. FAD synthase deficiency is associated either with an early-onset severe hypotonia of poor prognosis or with a mild phenotype with muscle weakness and exercise intolerance. MFT-deficient patients present with exercise intolerance, muscle weakness, and vomiting during exercise, starting in infancy or adolescence, leading to a more severe neuromuscular phenotype without treatment. High-dose oral riboflavin supplementation (minimum 20 mg/kg/day) is life-saving in RTD patients and has to be tried in patients with the severe form of FAD synthase deficiency. Patients with late-onset FAD synthase and MTF deficiency respond dramatically to lower riboflavin doses (3 mg/kg/day).

## Introduction

Riboflavin or vitamin B2 is a water-soluble vitamin. Milk and dairy products make the greatest contribution of its intake in Western diets. Meat, fish, and green vegetables are also good sources. Unknown amounts are generated by intestinal bacteria. Recommended intakes range from 0.4 mg/day in infancy to 1.8 mg/day in adult females during lactation. Riboflavin is degraded by light but is relatively heat-stable. Biochemical signs of depletion arise within only a few days of dietary deprivation. Poor riboflavin status interferes with iron handling and contributes to anaemia when iron intakes are low. Riboflavin depletion has been described as a risk factor for cancer, cardiovascular disease, and neurodegeneration.

Riboflavin is the precursor of flavin mononucleotide (FMN) and flavin adenine dinucleotide (FAD). FAD is the essential cofactor for the two electron transporters Electron Transfer Flavoprotein (ETF) and Electron Transfer Flavoprotein-ubiQuinone Oxidoreductase (ETF-QO), involved in multiple acyl-CoA dehydrogenase deficiency (MADD). Eleven ETF-dependent dehydrogenases have been identified, and this concerns five different metabolisms: (1) fatty acid oxidation (very long-chain acyl-CoA dehydrogenase, VLCAD; long-chain acyl-CoA dehydrogenase, LCAD; medium-chain acyl-CoA dehydrogenase, MCAD; and short-chain acyl-CoA dehydrogenase, SCAD), (2) branched-chain amino acid metabolism (isovaleryl-CoA dehydrogenase, 2-methylbutyryl-CoA dehydrogenase, and isobutyryl-CoA dehydrogenase), (3) lysine and tryptophan metabolism (glutaryl-CoA dehydrogenase), (4) choline metabolism (sarcosine dehydrogenase and dimethylglycine dehydrogenase), and (5) D-2-hydroxyglutarate dehydrogenase.

FAD and FMN are the cofactors for at least 80 other enzymes called flavoproteins. The majority of human flavoproteins are mitochondrial oxidoreductases. A number of them are involved in the biosynthesis of other cofactors such as coenzyme-A, coenzyme-Q (ubiquinone), heme, and pyridoxal 5′-phosphate, highlighting the involvement of riboflavin in the metabolism of folate, cobalamins, and other vitamins. In the nucleus, FAD-dependent oxidases play some role in epigenic events, controlling the expression of genes involved in energy metabolism.

A small amount of riboflavin is present in food as free riboflavin: most is present as FAD, and a smaller amount occurs as FMN, both non-covalently bound to enzymes. To be absorbed FMN and FAD have to be hydrolysed to riboflavin by non-specific phosphatases in the brush border membranes of enterocytes. Absorption takes place mainly in the proximal small intestine and partly in colon via carrier-mediated processes. Three riboflavin transporters have been identified almost 10 years ago, belonging to the SLC52 family of solute carriers: riboflavin transporter 1 (RFVT1, *SLC52A1* gene, Yonezawa et al. 2008), riboflavin transporter 2 (RFVT2, *SLC52A2* gene, Yao et al. 2010), and riboflavin transporter 3 (RFVT3, *SLC52A3* gene, Yamamoto et al. 2009). RFVT1 is a high-affinity transporter, located in the plasma membrane, mainly expressed in the small intestine, placenta, and kidney, but ubiquitous. It could play an important role in the homeostasis of riboflavin. *SLC52A1* gene is highly conserved among species, so likely an important gene for survival. RFVT2 is ubiquitously expressed, especially in the brain and salivary glands, but also in the intestine and kidney. RFVT3 plays a major role in intestinal absorption of riboflavin. Located at the apical membrane domain, it is highly expressed in ileum and jejunum, stomach, testis, pancreas, and prostate. It is efficient in acidic conditions and saturable but inhibited by FMN and FAD. Following intestinal absorption, riboflavin may enter blood circulation as the free form or as FMN. Free riboflavin is transported in the plasma bound to albumin and some immunoglobulins, but most endogenous blood flavins are located in erythrocytes, mainly as enzyme-bound FAD (or FMN). That is why measurement of blood flavins has to be performed in whole blood. In tissues, most riboflavin is enzyme bound, such as FAD bound to succinate dehydrogenase.

The intracellular metabolism of riboflavin is not fully elucidated. The uptake of riboflavin by the different organs and tissues is mediated by all RFVTs, but not the uptake of FMN and FAD (Jin et al. 2017). In the cytoplasmic compartment, the conversion of riboflavin into its active cofactors FMN and FAD is catalysed by riboflavin kinase and FAD synthase. Riboflavin kinase also called flavokinase (EC 2.7.1.26, *RFK* gene) is a cytosolic enzyme which catalyses the phosphorylation of riboflavin to form flavin mononucleotide (FMN) in the presence of ATP and Mg(2+). FAD synthase FADS (EC 2.7.7.2, *FLAD1* gene) converts FMN to FAD in an ATP-dependent reaction. Two different isoforms have been identified: hFADS1, localised in mitochondria, and hFADS2, a soluble cytosolic isoform. FAD synthase is organised in two domains: the phosphoadenosine-5′-phosphosulfate (PAPS) reductase domain, also called FADS domain, which catalyses the synthesis of FAD and acts as a FAD chaperone for the delivery of FAD for the synthesis of flavoproteins, and the molybdenum-pterin-binding (MPTb) domain, which has a $Co^{++}$ dependent FAD hydrolytic activity (Gianscapero et al. 2015). The uptake of FAD in mitochondria is mediated by the mitochondrial FAD transporter (MFT) (Spaan et al. 2005), previously identified as the human mitochondrial folate transporter: it facilitates the transport of FAD from the cytosol to the mitochondria or vice versa, therefore controlling the flavin homeostasis in the mitochondria. Little is known about the assembly of FAD (and FMN) to apoenzymes, the FAD cleavage and the flavoprotein turnover.

There is little or no storage of riboflavin in the body. Renal reabsorption, by possibly RFVT1 and RFVT2, is saturable. Any surplus is eliminated in urine, and this possibly explains why there is no toxicity to administrate high doses of riboflavin.

Multiple acyl-CoA dehydrogenase deficiency (MADD) has been identified more than 30 years ago (Frerman and Goodman 1985). It is sometimes called glutaric aciduria type 2, but this denomination is misleading, since glutaric acid excretion can be normal and therefore has to be abandoned. MADD is caused by a deficiency of either ETF (*ETFA* or *ETFB* genes) or of ETF-QO (*ETFDH* gene). Conversely, the inborn errors of riboflavin transport and intracellular metabolism have been identified much more recently. The association of Brown-Vialetto-Van Laere syndrome and Fazio Londe syndrome with RFVT2 and RFVT3 deficiency has been reported in 2010 (Green et al. 2010; Bosch et al. 2011), while deficiency of FAD synthase and of the mitochondrial FAD transporter (MFT) have been reported in 2016 (Olsen et al. 2016; Schiff et al. 2016). Regarding RFVT1 deficiency, two case reports were published of transient riboflavin deficiency in infants of mothers who harboured only one heterozygous mutation, in one case in combination with a maternal dietary riboflavin deficiency (Ho et al. 2011; Mosegaard et al. 2017) that can cause a transient MADD.

## Multiple Acyl-CoA Dehydrogenase Deficiency

More than 500 patients have been reported with heterogeneous clinical presentation and have been classified into three groups: (1) severe neonatal form, associated with congenital abnormalities (polycystic kidneys, midface hypoplasia), (2) severe neonatal form without congenital abnormalities, both with a poor prognosis, and (3) late-onset milder phenotype. Neonates usually present with severe metabolic acidosis, hypoketotic hypoglycaemia, hyperammonaemia, hypotonia, and frequently cardiomyopathy. They usually have an unpleasant odour of sweaty feet, similar to that of isovaleric acidaemia. The prognosis is poor, leading to early death. Neonatal form can be due to mutations in *ETFA*, *ETFB*, or *ETFDH* genes. Milder phenotypes can present at any age. In infancy, symptoms are mainly acute decompensation with hypoglycaemia and acidosis triggered by fast or infections, and possibly cardiomyopathy, while in adolescence and adulthood, symptoms are chronic, dominated by exercise intolerance and muscle weakness (Grünert 2014; Béhin et al. 2016). The majority of late-onset MADD patients responds well to riboflavin and harbour mutations in the *ETFDH* gene. All patients present with an abnormal plasma/DBS acylcarnitine profile, with an increase in all chain-length acylcarnitines (C4 to C18) with or without glutarylcarnitine (C5DC), and an abnormal urinary organic acid profile, characterised by an increase of ethylmalonic acid (EMA), 2-hydroxyglutaric acid, glutaric acid, and acylglycine conjugates. In late-onset MADD, the biochemical abnormalities can be less obvious and normalise with riboflavin supplementation. When performed, most patients present a massive lipid storage myopathy.

## Riboflavin Transporter Deficiency

The phenotype was previously known as the "Brown-Vialetto-van Laere syndrome" or "Fazio-Londe syndrome" which may have been a more heterogeneous group of patients before the possibility of a molecular diagnosis (Bosch et al. 2012). Patients may present at all ages. The youngest patients present within the first year of life, usually with a rapidly progressive life-threatening hypotonia, muscular weakness, bulbar palsy, and respiratory insufficiency resulting from muscle weakness and diaphragmatic paralysis. At older ages, symptoms of sensorimotor axial neuropathy and hearing loss are more prominent. Approximately 50% of patients demonstrate an abnormal plasma/DBS acylcarnitine profile when untreated, with an increase in short-, medium-, and long-chain acylcarnitines. Urinary organic acid profile may demonstrate increased ethylmalonic acid (EMA). Flavins in blood may be normal or low. Untreated patients all rapidly deteriorate with a limited life expectancy. Oral supplementation of riboflavin is life-saving, and most patients demonstrate striking improvement, while a minority only shows stabilisation of symptoms. Patients with riboflavin transporter deficiency type 2 (RFVT2) and type 3 (RFVT3) are reported to have similar phenotypes (Jaeger and Bosch 2016; O'Callaghan et al. 2019).

## Disorders of Intracellular Riboflavin Metabolism

### FAD Synthase Deficiency

Patients with FAD synthase deficiency present either an early-onset form with severe progressive generalised hypotonia in the neonatal period or early infancy, sometimes associated with cardiomyopathy, leading to respiratory failure or cardiac arrest and early death, or a late-onset form with exercise intolerance and muscle weakness in childhood or adolescence (Olsen et al. 2016; Auranen et al. 2017; Yıldız et al. 2018; García-Villoria et al. 2018; Muru et al. 2019). Conversely to transporter defects, no cranial and no peripheral neuropathy are present.

Although it was inconstant in one patient, all patients presented with abnormal plasma or dried blood spot (DBS) acylcarnitine profile, exhibiting an increase in short-, medium-, and long-chain acylcarnitines, like in MADD, even if this profile can be incomplete. Urinary organic acid profile was dominated by an increase in ethylmalonic acid (EMA), lactic acid, and, less constantly, glutaric acid, 2-hydroxyglutaric acid, and acylglycine derivatives. Increase of lactataemia and mild increase of CK, allowing differential diagnosis with congenital myopathies, were also reported. Blood flavin levels were decreased or normal. Interestingly, one patient with a severe phenotype was misdiagnosed as MCAD deficiency at newborn screening. Mutation analysis of the *FLAD1* gene (exome, gene panels, or Sanger sequencing) revealed that mutations in the FADS domain (FAD synthesis) are associated with the late-onset phenotype, while mutations in the MPTb domain (FAD cleavage) are associated with the severe early phenotype. When performed, a massive lipid storage myopathy, with faint SDH and/or COX staining, has been observed.

No clinical improvement was reported with riboflavin treatment in the early-onset form of the disease, although one patient presented a slight clinical improvement with high doses. This patient died of aspiration pneumonia (Yıldız et al. 2018). The prognosis is severe with death occurring before the first year of life. Conversely, the late-onset form is associated with a clear clinical improvement with low doses of riboflavin.

### Mitochondrial FAD Transporter (MFT) Deficiency

The two published patients with MFT deficiency (Schiff et al. 2016; Hellebrekers et al. 2017) presented with exercise intolerance, muscle weakness, and vomiting during exercise, starting in infancy or adolescence, leading to a more severe neuromuscular phenotype with progressive dysarthria, swallowing difficulties, myoclonic jerks, and need of wheelchair around 50 years in one of them (Hellebrekers et al. 2017).

The acylcarnitine and organic acid profiles were "MADD-like", with additionally an increase of urinary dimethylglycine and sarcosine levels in one of them. Hyperlactataemia was also reported, but nothing is known about CK or flavin levels. The diagnosis has to be confirmed by mutation analysis of the *SLC25A32* gene. Both patients presented a massive lipid storage myopathy with ragged-red fibres, faint SDH, and/or COX staining and complex II deficiency (suggestive of mitochondrial myopathy) at muscle histology.

Treatment with low doses of riboflavin (30 mg/day and 3 mg/kg/day) resulted in a dramatic improvement of symptoms and a normalisation of biochemical biomarkers. Symptoms reappeared when B2 was stopped in one patient (Schiff et al. 2016).

## Nomenclature

| No. | Disorder | Alternative name | Abbreviation | Inheritance | Gene symbol | Chromosomal localisation | Affected protein | OMIM N° |
|---|---|---|---|---|---|---|---|---|
| 32.1 | Riboflavin transporter 2 deficiency | Brown-Vialetto-van Laere syndrome type 1 | RFVT2 deficiency | AR | *SLC52A3* | 20p13 | Riboflavin transporter 2 | 613350 |
| 32.2 | Riboflavin transporter 3 deficiency | Brown-Vialetto-van Laere syndrome type 2 | RFVT3 deficiency | AR | *SLC52A2* | 8q24.3 | Riboflavin transporter 3 | 607882 |
| 32.3 | Flavin adenine dinucleotide synthase deficiency (early-onset form) | FAD synthase deficiency (early-onset form) | FADS deficiency | AR | *FLAD1* | 1q21.3 | FAD synthase | 610595 |
| 32.4 | Flavin adenine dinucleotide synthase deficiency (late-onset form) | FAD synthase deficiency (late-onset form) | FADS deficiency | AR | *FLAD1* | 1q21.3 | FAD synthase | 610595 |
| 32.5 | Mitochondrial flavin adenine dinucleotide transporter deficiency | Riboflavin-responsive exercise intolerance | MFT deficiency | AR | *SLC25A32* | 8q22.3 | Mitochondrial FAD transporter | 610815 |
| 32.6 | Electron transfer flavoprotein deficiency | Multiple acyl-CoA dehydrogenase deficiency (ETF) | MADD (ETF) | AR | *ETFA*, *ETFB* | *ETFA* 15q24.2-q24.3 *ETFB* 19q13.41 | Electron transfer flavoprotein (ETF) | ETFA 608053 ETFB 130410 |
| 32.7 | Electron transfer flavoprotein dehydrogenase deficiency | Multiple acyl-CoA dehydrogenase deficiency (ETFDH) | MADD (ETFDH) | AR | *ETFDH* | 4q32-qter | ETF-ubiquinone oxidoreductase (ETF-QO) | 231675 |
| 32.8 | Riboflavin-responsive electron transfer flavoprotein dehydrogenase deficiency | Riboflavin-responsive multiple acyl-CoA dehydrogenase deficiency (ETFDH) | RR-MADD (ETFDH) | AR | *ETFDH* | 4q32-qter | ETF-ubiquinone oxidoreductase (ETF-QO) | 231675 |
| 32.9 | Riboflavin transporter 1 deficiency | Transient riboflavin deficiency | RFVT1 deficiency | | *SLC52A1* | 17p13.2 | Riboflavin transporter 1 | 607883 |

## Metabolic Pathways

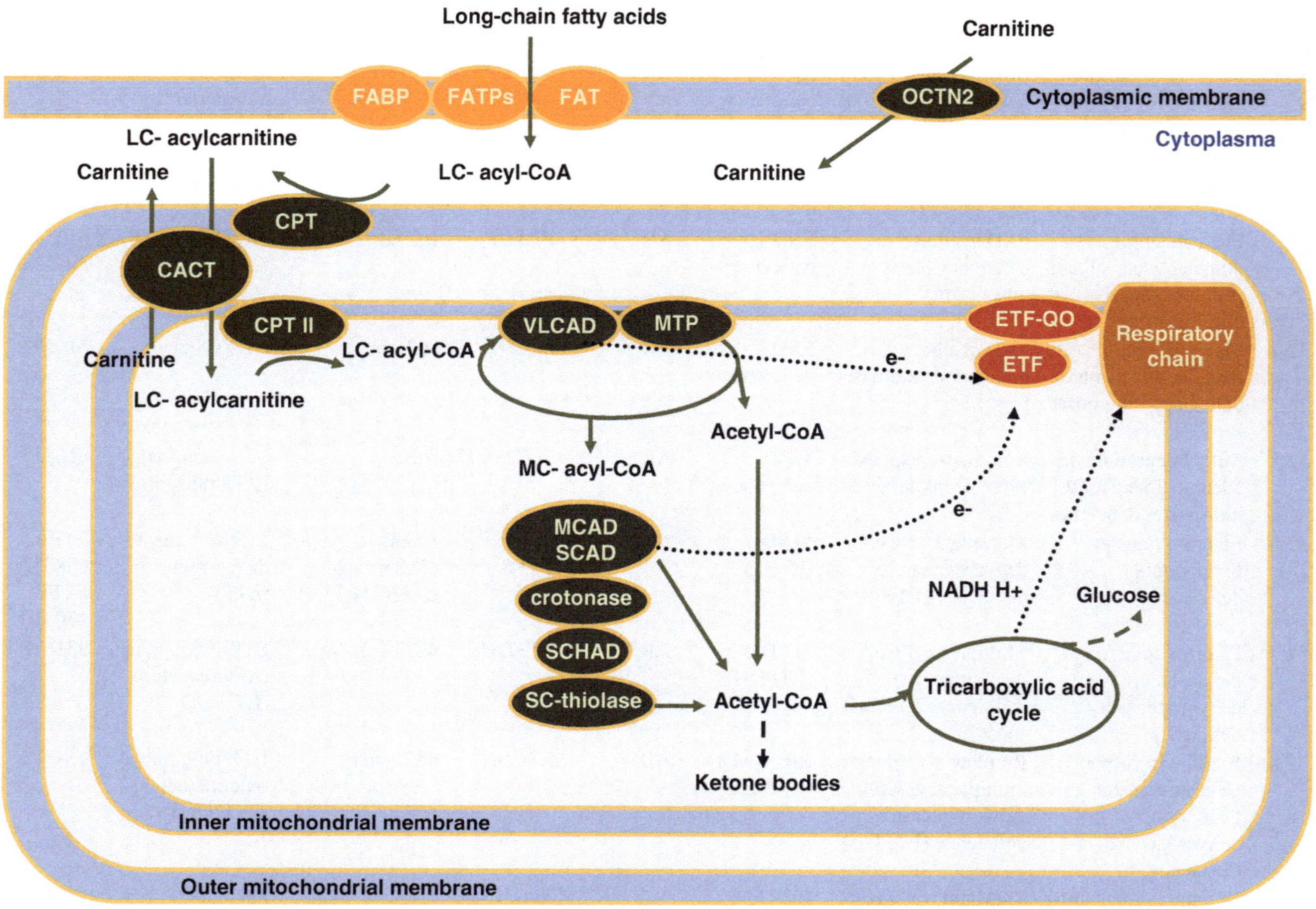


**Fig. 32.1** Simplified scheme of mitochondrial fatty acid oxidation. ETF (Electron Transfer Flavoprotein) and ETF-QO (ETF-ubiQuinone Oxidoreductase) are the two electron transporters which transfer electrons from VLCAD (very long-chain acyl-CoA dehydrogenase), MCAD (medium-chain acyl-CoA dehydrogenase), and SCAD (short-chain acyl-CoA dehydrogenase) to coenzyme $Q_{10}$ and then to complex II of the respiratory chain. ETF is a matrix soluble protein, while ETF-QO is linked to inner mitochondrial membrane

**Fig. 32.2** Simplified scheme of electron transfer from acyl-CoA dehydrogenases to coenzyme $Q_{10}$. *$CoQ_{10}$* Coenzyme $Q_{10}$, *ETF* Electron transfer flavoprotein, *ETF-QO* ETF-ubiQuinone Oxidoreductase, *red*, Reduced

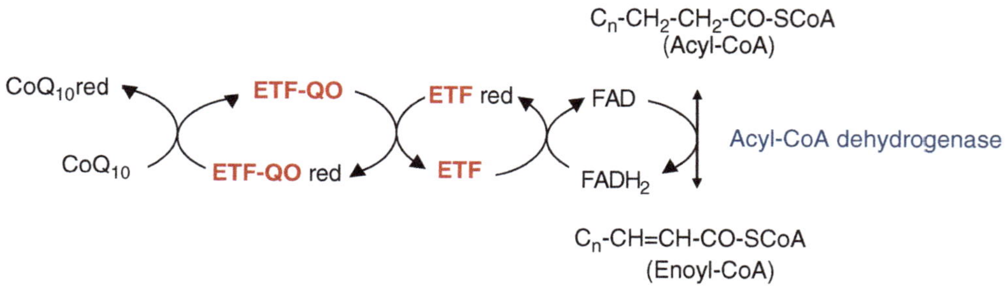

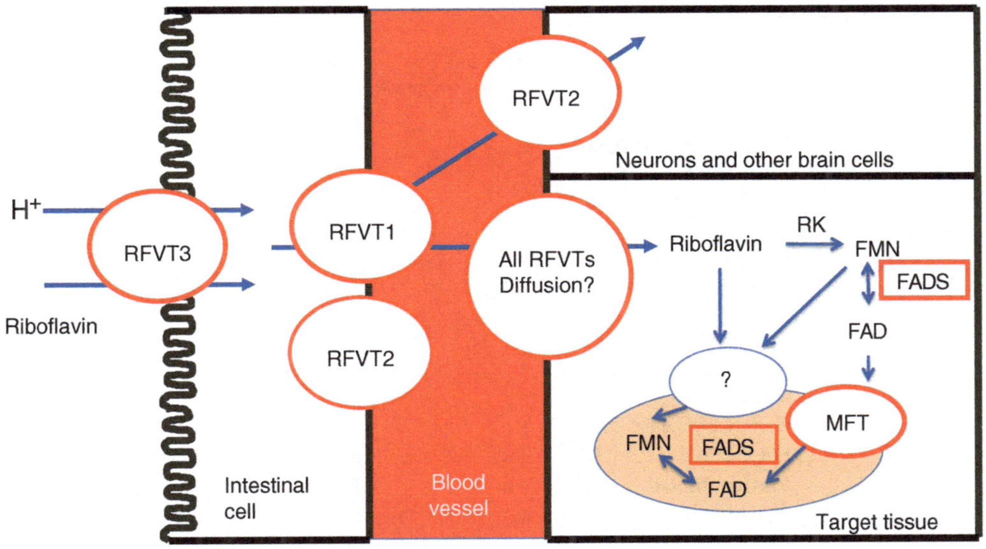


**Fig. 32.3** Simplified scheme of riboflavin metabolism. *FAD* Flavin adenine dinucleotide, *FADS* FAD synthase, *FMN* Flavin mononucleotide, *MFT* Mitochondrial FAD transporter, *RFVT* Riboflavin transporter, *RK* Riboflavin kinase

## Signs and Symptoms

**Table 32.1** Riboflavin transporter 2 deficiency—RTD2-RFVT2 deficiency (Brown-Vialetto-van Laere syndrome or Fazio-Londe syndrome)

| System | Symptoms and biomarkers | Neonatal (birth–1 month) | Infancy (1–18 months) | Childhood (1.5–11 years) | Adolescence (11–16 years) | Adulthood (>16 years) |
|---|---|---|---|---|---|---|
| CNS | **Ataxia** | | ± | ± | ± | ± |
| | **Pontobulbar palsy** | ± | ± | ± | ± | ± |
| Ear | **Deafness, sensorineural** | | ± | + | + | ++ |
| Eye | **Vision loss/optic atrophy** | | ± | ± | ± | ± |
| Musculoskeletal | **Muscle weakness** | ± | ± | + | + | + |
| | **Respiratory insufficiency (muscle weakness, diaphragm paralysis)** | ± | ± | ± | ± | ± |
| Others | **Riboflavin responsiveness** | + | + | + | + | + |
| Laboratory findings | C4-C18 Acylcarnitine (P, DBS) | n-↑ | n-↑ | n-↑ | n-↑ | n-↑ |
| | C6-C10 dicarboxylic acids—adipic, suberic, sebacic acids (U) | n-↑ | n-↑ | n-↑ | n-↑ | n-↑ |
| | Carnitine, free (P, DBS) | ↓-n | ↓-n | ↓-n | ↓-n | ↓-n |
| | Ethylmalonic acid (U) | n-↑ | n-↑ | n-↑ | n-↑ | n-↑ |
| | **Flavins (blood)** | ↓-n | ↓-n | ↓-n | ↓-n | ↓-n |
| | Glutaric acid (U) | n-↑ | n-↑ | n-↑ | n-↑ | n-↑ |

**Table 32.2** Riboflavin transporter 3 deficiency—RTD3-RFVT3 deficiency (Brown-Vialetto-Van Laere syndrome or Fazio-Londe syndrome)

| System | Symptoms and biomarkers | Neonatal (birth–1 month) | Infancy (1–18 months) | Childhood (1.5–11 years) | Adolescence (11–16 years) | Adulthood (>16 years) |
|---|---|---|---|---|---|---|
| CNS | **Ataxia** | | ± | ± | ± | ± |
| | **Pontobulbar palsy** | ± | ± | ± | ± | ± |
| Ear | **Deafness, sensorineural** | | ± | + | + | ++ |
| Eye | **Vision loss/optic atrophy** | | ± | ± | ± | ± |

(continued)

**Table 32.2** (continued)

| System | Symptoms and biomarkers | Neonatal (birth–1 month) | Infancy (1–18 months) | Childhood (1.5–11 years) | Adolescence (11–16 years) | Adulthood (>16 years) |
|---|---|---|---|---|---|---|
| Musculoskeletal | **Muscle weakness** | ± | ± | + | + | + |
| | **Respiratory insufficiency (muscle weakness, diaphragm paralysis)** | ± | ± | ± | ± | ± |
| Others | **Riboflavin responsiveness** | + | + | + | + | + |
| Laboratory findings | C4-C18 acylcarnitine (P, DBS) | n-↑ | n-↑ | n-↑ | n-↑ | n-↑ |
| | C6-C10 dicarboxylic acids—adipic, suberic, sebacic acids (U) | n-↑ | n-↑ | n-↑ | n-↑ | n-↑ |
| | Carnitine, free (P, DBS) | ↓-n | ↓-n | ↓-n | ↓-n | ↓-n |
| | Ethylmalonic acid (U) | n-↑ | n-↑ | n-↑ | n-↑ | n-↑ |
| | **Flavins (blood)** | ↓-n | ↓-n | ↓-n | ↓-n | ↓-n |
| | Glutaric acid (U) | n-↑ | n-↑ | n-↑ | n-↑ | n-↑ |

**Table 32.3** Flavin adenine dinucleotide (FAD) synthase deficiency (early-onset form)

| System | Symptoms and biomarkers | Neonatal (birth–1 month) | Infancy (1–18 months) | Childhood (1.5–11 years) | Adolescence (11–16 years) | Adulthood (>16 years) |
|---|---|---|---|---|---|---|
| Cardiovascular | Cardiomyopathy | + | + | | | |
| CNS | **Hypotonia** | +++ | +++ | | | |
| Eye | Cataract | | | ± | | |
| | Ptosis | | | ± | | |
| Musculoskeletal | **Muscle weakness** | ++ | ++ | | | |
| | Myopathy | | | ± | | |
| Others | Riboflavin responsiveness | ± | ± | + | | |
| Laboratory findings | 2-Hydroxyglutaric acid (U) | n-↑ | n-↑ | n-↑ | | |
| | **C4-C18 acylcarnitines (P, DBS): Not all acylcarnitines** | ↑↑ | ↑↑ | ↑↑ | | |
| | **CK** | ↑ | ↑ | | | |
| | **Ethylmalonic acid (U)** | ↑↑ | ↑↑ | ↑↑ | | |
| | Flavins (blood) | ↓-n | ↓-n | ↓-n | | |
| | Glutarylcarnitine (P, DBS) | n-↑ | n-↑ | n-↑ | | |
| | Hexanoylglycine (U) | n-↑ | n-↑ | n-↑ | | |
| | Isovalerylgycine (U) | n-↑ | n-↑ | n-↑ | | |
| | **Massive lipid storage myopathy** | +++ | +++ | ++ | | |

**Table 32.4** Flavin adenine dinucleotide (FAD) synthase deficiency (late-onset form)

| System | Symptoms and biomarkers | Neonatal (birth–1 month) | Infancy (1–18 months) | Childhood (1.5–11 years) | Adolescence (11–16 years) | Adulthood (>16 years) |
|---|---|---|---|---|---|---|
| Musculoskeletal | Acute rhabdomyolysis episodes | | | | + | + |
| | **Exercise intolerance** | | | ± | + | ++ |
| | **Muscle weakness** | | | | | ++ |
| | Scoliosis | | | | ± | |
| Others | Riboflavin responsiveness | | | ± | ± | ++ |
| Laboratory findings | **2-Hydroxyglutaric acid (U)** | | | ↑ | ↑ | ↑ |
| | Acylglycines (U) | | | n | n | n |
| | **C4-C18 acylcarnitines (P, DBS): Not all acylcarnitines** | | | ↑ | ↑ | ↑ |
| | **Ethylmalonic acid (U)** | | | ↑ | ↑ | ↑ |
| | Flavins (blood) | | | ↓-n | ↓-n | ↓-n |
| | Glutaric acid (U) | | | n-↑ | n-↑ | n-↑ |
| | Glutarylcarnitine (P, DBS) | | | n | n | n |
| | **Massive lipid storage myopathy** | | | +++ | +++ | +++ |

**Table 32.5** Mitochondrial flavin adenine dinucleotide transporter (MFT) deficiency (two patients)

| System | Symptoms and biomarkers | Neonatal (birth–1 month) | Infancy (1–18 months) | Childhood (1.5–11 years) | Adolescence (11–16 years) | Adulthood (>16 years) |
|---|---|---|---|---|---|---|
| CNS | Dysarthria | | | | | ± |
| | Swallowing difficulties | | | | | ± |
| Musculoskeletal | **Exercise intolerance** with nausea or vomiting during exercise | | | | + | + |
| | Muscle weakness | | | ± | ± | ± |
| Others | **Riboflavin responsiveness** | | | ++ | ++ | ++ |
| Laboratory findings | 2-Hydroxyglutaric acid (U) | | | | n to ↑ | n-↑ |
| | **2-Methylbutyrylglycine (U)** | | | | ↑ | ↑ |
| | **C4-C10 acylcarnitines (P, DBS)** | | | | ↑↑ | ↑↑ |
| | **Ethylmalonic acid (U)** | | | | ↑↑ | ↑↑ |
| | Glutaric acid (U) | | | | n to ↑↑ | n-↑ |
| | Glutarylcarnitine (P, DBS) | | | | ↑ | ↑ |
| | Hexanoylglycine (U) | | | | n | n |
| | **Isobutyrylglycine (U)** | | | | ↑ | ↑ |
| | **Isovalerylglycine (U)** | | | | ↑ | ↑ |
| | Lactate (B) | | | | ↑ | ↑ |
| | **Lipid storage myopathy with ragged-red fibres** | | | | + | + |
| | Suberylglycine (U) | | | | n | n |

**Table 32.6** Multiple acyl-CoA dehydrogenase deficiency (MADD)—Electron transfer flavoprotein (ETF) deficiency (*ETFA* or *ETFB* gene)

| System | Symptoms and biomarkers | Neonatal (birth–1 month) | Infancy (1–18 months) | Childhood (1.5–11 years) | Adolescence (11–16 years) | Adulthood (>16 years) |
|---|---|---|---|---|---|---|
| Cardiovascular | Cardiomyopathy | ± | ± | ± | n | n |
| CNS | Coma | ± | ± | ± | n | n |
| | Hypotonia, muscular-axial | ± | ± | ± | ± | ± |
| | Lethargy | ± | ± | ± | n | n |
| Digestive | Liver dysfunction | ± | ± | ± | ± | ± |
| Musculoskeletal | Rhabdomyolysis, exercise induced | n | ± | ++ | ++ | ++ |
| | Skeletal myopathy | ± | ± | ± | ± | ± |
| Others | Congenital anomalies (brain, kidney) | + | + | | | |
| | Riboflavin responsiveness | – | – | – | – | – |
| Laboratory findings | **2-Methylbutyrylglycine (U)** | ↑ | ↑ | ↑ | ↑ | ↑ |
| | Ammonia (P) | ↑ | ↑ | n-↑ | n-↑ | n-↑ |
| | **C4-C18 acylcarnitine (P, DBS)** | ↑ | ↑ | ↑ | ↑ | ↑ |
| | C6-C10 dicarboxylic acids: adipic, suberic, sebacic acids (U) | n-↑ | n-↑ | n-↑ | n-↑ | n-↑ |
| | Carnitine, free (P, DBS) | ↓-n | ↓-n | ↓-n | ↓-n | ↓-n |
| | Creatine kinase (P) | n-↑ | n-↑ | n-↑↑ | n-↑↑ | n-↑↑ |
| | **D-2-Hydroxyglutaric acid (U)** | ↑ | ↑ | ↑ | ↑ | ↑ |
| | Dimethylglycine (P, U) | ↑ | ↑ | ↑ | ↑ | ↑ |
| | **Ethylmalonic acid (U)** | ↑ | ↑ | ↑ | ↑ | ↑ |
| | Glucose (P) | ↓-n | ↓-n | ↓-n | | |
| | Glutaric acid (U) | ↑ | ↑ | ↑ | n-↑ | n-↑ |
| | Glutarylcarnitine—C5DC (P, DBS) | ↑ | ↑ | ↑ | n-↑ | n-↑ |
| | **Hexanoylglycine (U)** | ↑ | ↑ | ↑ | ↑ | ↑ |
| | **Isobutyrylglycine (U)** | ↑ | ↑ | ↑ | ↑ | ↑ |
| | **Isovalerylglycine (U)** | ↑ | ↑ | ↑ | ↑ | ↑ |
| | Ketones, during hypoglycaemia (P, U) | ↓ | ↓ | ↓-n | | |
| | **Lipid storage myopathy** | | | ++ | ++ | ++ |
| | Metabolic acidosis (P) | + | + | ± | ± | ± |
| | Sarcosine (P, U) | ↑ | ↑ | ↑ | ↑ | ↑ |
| | Transaminase (P) | n-↑ | n-↑ | n-↑ | n-↑ | n-↑ |

**Table 32.7** Multiple acyl-CoA dehydrogenase deficiency (MADD)—Electron transfer flavoprotein ubiquinone oxidoreductase (ETF-QO) deficiency (*ETFDH* gene)

| System | Symptoms and biomarkers | Neonatal (birth–1 month) | Infancy (1–18 months) | Childhood (1.5–11 years) | Adolescence (11–16 years) | Adulthood (>16 years) |
|---|---|---|---|---|---|---|
| Cardiovascular | Cardiomyopathy | ± | ± | ± | ± | ± |
| CNS | Coma | ± | ± | ± | n | n |
| | Hypotonia, muscular-axial | ± | ± | ± | ± | ± |
| | Lethargy | ± | ± | ± | n | n |
| Digestive | Liver dysfunction | ± | ± | ± | ± | ± |
| Musculoskeletal | Rhabdomyolysis, exercise induced | n | ± | ++ | ++ | ++ |
| | Skeletal myopathy | ± | ± | ± | n | n |
| Others | Congenital anomalies (brain, kidney) | + | + | | | |
| | Riboflavin responsiveness | − | − | − | − | − |
| Laboratory findings | **2-Methylbutyrylglycine (U)** | ↑ | ↑ | ↑ | ↑ | ↑ |
| | Ammonia (P) | ↑ | ↑ | n-↑ | n-↑ | n-↑ |
| | **C4-C18 acylcarnitine (P, DBS)** | ↑ | ↑ | ↑ | ↑ | ↑ |
| | C6-C10 dicarboxylic acids: adipic, suberic, sebacic acids (U) | n-↑ | n-↑ | n-↑ | n-↑ | n-↑ |
| | Carnitine, free (P, DBS) | ↓-n | ↓-n | ↓-n | ↓-n | ↓-n |
| | Creatine kinase (P) | n-↑ | n-↑ | n-↑↑ | n-↑↑ | n-↑↑ |
| | **D-2-Hydroxyglutaric acid (U)** | ↑ | ↑ | ↑ | ↑ | ↑ |
| | Dimethylglycine (P, U) | ↑ | ↑ | ↑ | ↑ | ↑ |
| | **Ethylmalonic acid (U)** | ↑ | ↑ | ↑ | ↑ | ↑ |
| | Glucose (P) | ↓-n | ↓-n | ↓-n | | |
| | Glutaric acid (U) | ↑ | ↑ | ↑ | n-↑ | n-↑ |
| | Glutarylcarnitine—C5DC (P, DBS) | ↑ | ↑ | ↑ | n-↑ | n-↑ |
| | **Hexanoylglycine (U)** | ↑ | ↑ | ↑ | ↑ | ↑ |
| | **Isobutyrylglycine (U)** | ↑ | ↑ | ↑ | ↑ | ↑ |
| | **Isovalerylglycine (U)** | ↑ | ↑ | ↑ | ↑ | ↑ |
| | Ketones, during hypoglycaemia (P, U) | ↓ | ↓ | ↓-n | | |
| | **Lipid storage myopathy** | | | + + | + + | + + |
| | Metabolic acidosis (P) | + | + | ± | ± | ± |
| | Sarcosine (P, U) | ↑ | ↑ | ↑ | ↑ | ↑ |
| | Transaminase (P) | n-↑ | n-↑ | n-↑ | n-↑ | n-↑ |

**Table 32.8** Riboflavin-responsive multiple acyl-CoA dehydrogenase deficiency (RR-MADD)—Electron transfer flavoprotein ubiquinone oxidoreductase (ETF-QO) deficiency (*ETFDH* gene)

| System | Symptoms and biomarkers | Neonatal (birth–1 month) | Infancy (1–18 months) | Childhood (1.5–11 years) | Adolescence (11–16 years) | Adulthood (>16 years) |
|---|---|---|---|---|---|---|
| CNS | Encephalopathy, episodic | | | ± | ± | ± |
| Digestive | Liver dysfunction | | | ± | ± | ± |
| | Vomiting | | | ± | ± | ± |
| Musculoskeletal | Exercise intolerance, muscle pain | ± | + | ++ | +++ | +++ |
| | Muscle weakness | ± | + | ++ | +++ | +++ |
| Others | **Riboflavin responsiveness** | | + | + | + | + |

Table 32.8 (continued)

| System | Symptoms and biomarkers | Neonatal (birth–1 month) | Infancy (1–18 months) | Childhood (1.5–11 years) | Adolescence (11–16 years) | Adulthood (>16 years) |
|---|---|---|---|---|---|---|
| Laboratory findings | **2-Methylbutyrylglycine (U)** | | n-↑ | n-↑ | n-↑ | n-↑ |
| | **C4-C18 acylcarnitine (P, DBS)** | n-↑ | n-↑ | n-↑ | n-↑ | n-↑ |
| | C6-C10 dicarboxylic acids: adipic, suberic, sebacic acids (U) | | n-↑ | n-↑ | n-↑ | n-↑ |
| | Carnitine, free (P, DBS) | ↓-n | ↓-n | ↓-n | ↓-n | ↓-n |
| | Creatine kinase (P) | n-↑ | n-↑ | n-↑ | n-↑ | n-↑ |
| | **D-2-Hydroxyglutaric acid (U)** | | ↑ | ↑ | ↑ | ↑ |
| | Dimethylglycine (P, U) | | n-↑ | n-↑ | n-↑ | n-↑ |
| | **Ethylmalonic acid (U)** | | ↑ | ↑ | ↑ | ↑ |
| | Glutaric acid (U) | | n-↑ | n-↑ | n-↑ | n-↑ |
| | Glutarylcarnitine—C5DC (P, DBS) | n | n | n | n | n |
| | **Hexanoylglycine (U)** | | n-↑ | n-↑ | n-↑ | n-↑ |
| | **Isobutyrylglycine (U)** | | n-↑ | n-↑ | n-↑ | n-↑ |
| | **Isovalerylglycine (U)** | | n-↑ | n-↑ | n-↑ | n-↑ |
| | **Lipid storage myopathy** | | | + + | + + | + + |
| | Sarcosine (P, U) | | n-↑ | n-↑ | n-↑ | n-↑ |

No signs and symptoms table has been issued for RFVT1 deficiency since the two described affected heterozygous mothers were asymptomatic and biochemical investigation was normal away from delivery.

## Reference Values

Reference values for free carnitine and acylcarnitine species in plasma and dried blood spots are given in Chap. 5. Reference values for urinary organic acids are given in Chap. 4

| Compound | Plasma | Whole blood |
|---|---|---|
| Riboflavin | 5–38 nmol/L | |
| FAD | 57–170 nmol/L | 174–471 nmol/L |
| FMN | 4–14 nmol/L | |
| CK | ♂ 46–171 U/L<br>♀ 34–145 U/L | |

## Pathological Values

Patients with MADD, FAD synthase, and MFT deficiency usually present with an abnormal plasma/DBS acylcarnitine profile, exhibiting an increase of all chain-length acylcarnitines (C4, C5, C6, C8, C10:1, C10, C12:1, C12, C14:1, C14, C16:1, C16, C18:1, C18) and, in the severe form of these diseases, glutarylcarnitine (C5DC), associated with a decrease in free carnitine levels. The concentrations of these acylcarnitines are highly variable and depend of the patient's status and of the severity of the disease. Their urinary organic acid profile is characterised by an increase of ethylmalonic acid, 2-hydroxyglutaric acid, and, most of the time but non constantly, glutaric acid, dicarboxylic acids, and acylglycine conjugates (isovalerylglycine, 2-methylbutyrylglycine, isobutyrylglycine, hexanoylglycine, suberylglycine). Plasma/DBS acylcarnitine and urinary organic acid profiles usually normalise after riboflavin supplementation, except for the severe form of MADD and FAD synthase. An increase of CK is often reported in acute episodes, as well as an increase of transaminases.

In RTD, the acylcarnitine profile and the urinary organic acid profile can be "MADD-like" or normal, and flavin levels can be decreased or normal. That is why the diagnosis relies on genetic studies.

## Diagnostic Flowchart

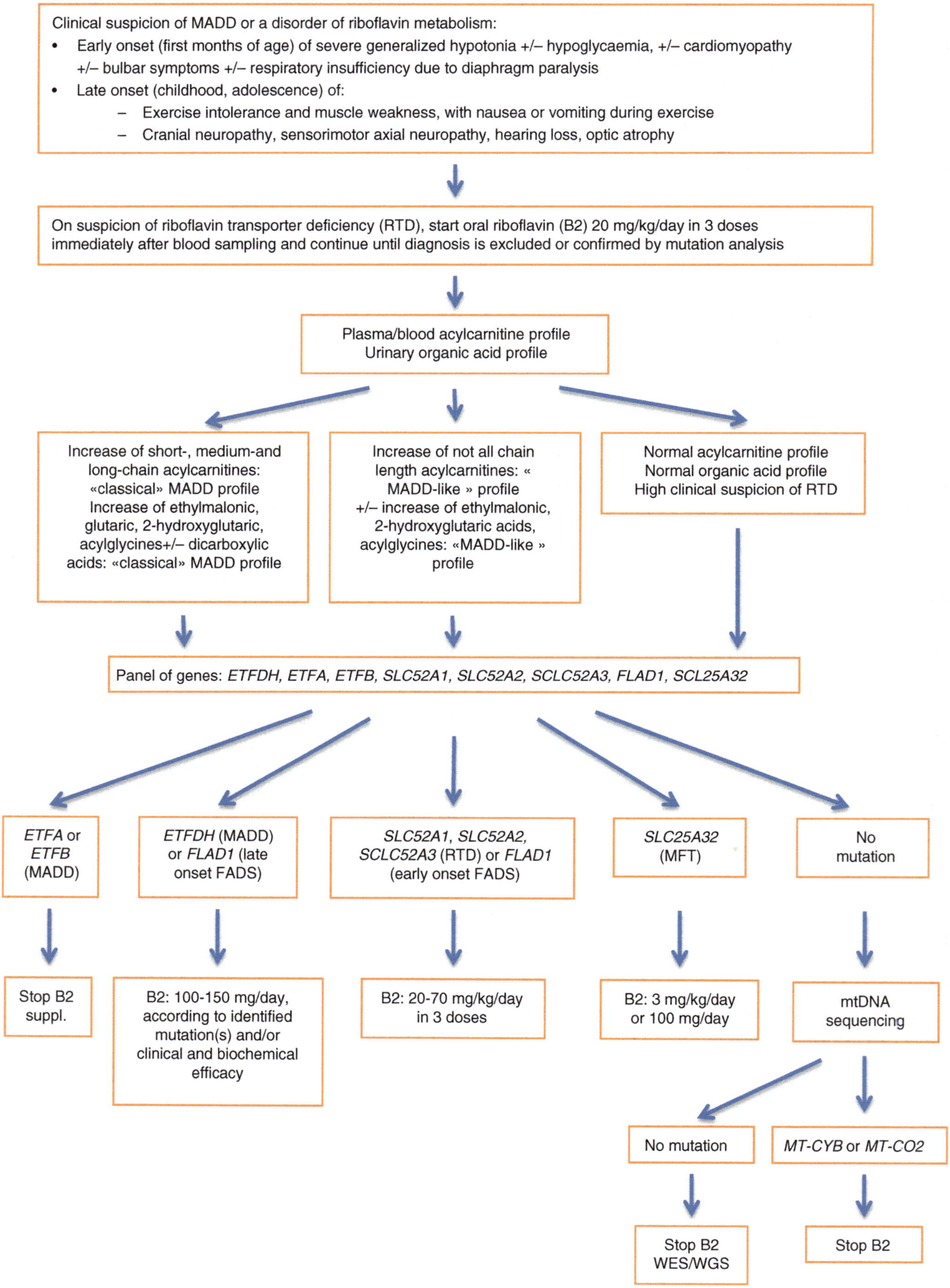

This diagnosis flowchart shows how to reach a diagnosis. However, if the clinical picture is highly suggestive of MADD or of an inborn error of riboflavin metabolism, an **immediate treatment** with riboflavin has to be tried, directly after taking the first biological samples: minimum dose is 20 mg/kg/day in three doses in patients with neurological symptoms, while it can be lower (3 mg/kg/day) in patients with only muscular symptoms.

*B2* Riboflavin, *FADS* FAD synthase, *MADD* Multiple acyl-CoA dehydrogenase deficiency, *MFT* Mitochondrial FAD transporter, *mtDNA* Mitochondrial DNA, *RTD* Riboflavin transporter defects, *WES* Whole exome sequencing, *WGS* Whole genome sequencing.

## Specimen Collection

| Test | Precondition | Material | Handling | Pitfalls |
|---|---|---|---|---|
| **Acylcarnitines** | During an acute episode (if any)<br>Fasting state<br>Before B2 supplementation | Plasma<br>Dried blood spot (DBS) | Frozen (−20 °C): Plasma<br>Room temperature: DBS | False negative: Possible normal profile in RTD, lack of diagnostic acylcarnitines when severe secondary carnitine deficiency<br>False positive: Anoxia can induce a "MADD-like" profile |
| **Carnitine** | During an acute episode (if any)<br>Fasting state<br>Before B2 supplementation | Plasma<br>Dried blood spot (DBS) | Frozen (−20 °C): Plasma<br>Room temperature: DBS | False negative: Frequently normal in RTD |
| **Organic acids** | During an acute episode (if any)<br>First morning urine sample, preferably<br>Before B2 supplementation | Spot urine (no addition of preservatives) | Frozen (−20 °C) | False negative: Possible normal profile in RTD.<br>Late-onset MADD and FAD synthase deficiency: Increase of only ethylmalonic and 2-hydroxyglutaric acids |
| **Flavins (riboflavin, FAD, FMN)** | Before B2 supplementation | EDTA plasma<br>EDTA whole blood | Frozen (−20 °C) and protected from light: Plasma and whole blood | False negative: Can be normal in all disorders<br>False positive: Decrease due to light degradation |
| **Functional tests in lymphocytes** | Before B2 supplementation | EDTA blood | Don't centrifuge<br>Room temperature<br>Has to reach the lab within 48 h | False negative: Can be normal in all disorders |
| **Functional tests in cultured fibroblasts** | – | Skin biopsy | Room temperature in culture medium | Cell culture medium depleted in riboflavin is necessary for RR-MADD and IEM of riboflavin metabolism |
| **Molecular analysis** | – | EDTA blood | Room temperature | Identification of only one heterozygous mutation does not rule out a diagnosis |

## Prenatal Diagnosis

Prenatal diagnosis is available for MADD and disorders of riboflavin metabolism. Mutation analysis in DNA extracted from chorionic villi or from amniocytes is the more reliable technique, provided that the index case's genotype has been determined. RTD deficiency can be diagnosed by mutation analysis only. Quantification of acylcarnitines and acylglycines in the supernatant of amniotic fluid can be used when an abnormal plasma acylcarnitine profile and an abnormal urinary organic acid profile have been observed in the index case, but only abnormal levels of short- and medium-chain acylcarnitines can be detected, since long-chain acylcarnitines are not excreted in urine and therefore are absent from amniotic fluid. Functional tests, such acylcarnitine profiling or fatty acid flux in cultured chorionic villi cells or amniocytes, can only be used in severe form of MADD.

| Disorder | Prenatal diagnosis suggested | Reliability of mutation analysis | Reliability of acylcarnitines/acylglycines quantification in AF | Reliability of functional tests | Remarks |
|---|---|---|---|---|---|
| RFVT1 | – | + | – | – | No patients with two mutations of *SLC52A1* gene have been identified. Heterozygous patients are asymptomatic |
| RFVT2 | + | + | – | – | |
| RFVT3 | + | + | – | – | |
| FADS early-onset form | + | + | ± | – | Severe outcome |
| FADS late-onset form | – | + | – | – | Favourable outcome with riboflavin supplementation |
| MFT | – | + | ± | – | Favourable outcome with riboflavin supplementation |
| MADD (ETF or ETF-QO) early-onset form | + | + | + | + | Severe outcome |
| MADD (ETF or ETF-QO) late onset form | ± | + | ± | ± | Depend of the severity of the clinical phenotype |
| RR-MADD | – | + | – | – | Favourable outcome with riboflavin supplementation |

## DNA Testing

Multiple acyl-CoA dehydrogenase deficiency and all disorders in the transport or metabolism of riboflavin are inherited in an autosomal recessive pattern. Molecular genetic testing of all genes involved in these disorders can be performed in genomic DNA (from blood or any tissue) by Sanger methods or by MPS (massive parallel sequencing). No prevalent mutations have been identified, except three common riboflavin-responsive mutations in the *ETFDH* gene mainly found in the Chinese and Taiwanese population: c.250G>A; c.770G>A; and c.1227A>C (Xi et al. 2014).

## Treatment

### Summary

Early-onset forms of MADD are treated with an emergency regime, avoidance of fasting, and a diet restricted in fat. Late-onset forms of MADD may respond to riboflavin supplementation (3 mg/kg/day or 100–150 mg/day) (Grünert 2014).

On suspicion of RTD, supplementation of high-dose oral riboflavin (20–70 mg/kg/day in three doses) must be started immediately without awaiting a final diagnosis. Clinical improvement is observed in the majority of RTD patients, but sometimes it is not observed for months following the beginning of riboflavin supplementation. Supplementation with oral riboflavin has to be considered in all other disorders of riboflavin metabolism.

### Emergency Treatment

Emergency treatment for early-onset forms of MADD is high-dose glucose infusion, in association with insulin when high doses of glucose are required, and carnitine supplementation in case of carnitine depletion. Late-onset MADD may demonstrate clinical improvement with riboflavin supplementation (Grünert 2014).

Immediate start of oral riboflavin supplementation on suspicion of RTD is life-saving, and supplementation needs to be continued until the diagnosis is confirmed or excluded by genetic analysis (O'Callaghan et al. 2019).

In FAD synthase deficiency, especially late onset, patients demonstrate riboflavin responsivity; however riboflavin supplementation should initially be started in all patients (Olsen et al. 2016).

In mitochondrial FAD transporter deficiency, riboflavin supplementation was highly effective in the two described patients (Schiff et al. 2016; Hellebrekers et al. 2017).

### Standard Treatment

Early-onset forms of MADD are treated with an emergency regime, avoidance of fasting, and a diet restricted in fat. Due to the accumulation of carnitine conjugates, MADD patients are prone to carnitine deficiency, which may require oral carnitine supplementation (Grünert 2014).

Recommended doses of riboflavin supplementation depend of the disease. There is no literature report on effective dosing of riboflavin in MADD. Morris and Spiekekotter (2011) propose 100 mg/day, while Zschocke and Hoffmann

(2011) recommend 150 mg/day in the Vademecum Metabolicum. RTD patients have demonstrated strong clinical improvements on doses of 10–70 mg/kg/day in three doses (Jaeger and Bosch 2016). There is no evidence for riboflavin dosing in FAD synthase deficiency, but a high dose seems advisable. In two patients with mitochondrial FAD transporter deficiency, a striking effect of riboflavin supplementation has been reported with doses of 30 mg/day and 3 mg/kg/day, respectively.

### Experimental Treatment

Long-term treatment of severe MADD patients with 3-hydroxybutyrate has been proposed, with clinical improvement in 70% of patients (reviewed by van Rijt et al. 2020). Prescribed doses ranged between 100 and 2600 mg/kg/day, divided in one to six daily doses. Cornelius et al. (2014) reported that $CoQ_{10}$ treatment can decrease ROS production in fibroblasts from RR-MADD patients and may relieve oxidative stress. This suggests that late-onset MADD patients could benefit from a combined treatment of riboflavin and $CoQ_{10}$.

For RTD esterified derivatives of riboflavin may increase bioavailability (Manole et al. 2017). The effects of $CoQ_{10}$ in RTD are presently unclear.

## Follow-Up and Monitoring

The biological monitoring of patients with MADD, FAD synthase, and MFT deficiency usually associates CK, transaminases, plasma/blood acylcarnitine profile including free and total carnitine levels, and eventually urinary organic acids. Normalisation of these parameters after riboflavin supplementation is an indication of the efficacy of this treatment. General indices of nutrition in patients on a restricted diet (severe MADD), echocardiogram, liver ultrasound, and eventually nerve conduction studies should also be monitored. In adults, the monitoring is usually on an annual basis, whereas it has to be more frequent in younger patients.

In RTD patients with abnormal plasma/blood acylcarnitine profiles, or urinary organic acid profiles, or abnormal flavins, a rapid normalisation is seen after supplementation of riboflavin, and these parameters may be used for monitoring. Clinical follow-up by a neurologist, ophthalmologist, and ENT specialist is warranted. In case of hearing loss, cochlear implantates are reported to be effective (Anderson et al. 2019).

## References


Anderson P, Schaefer S, Henderson L, Bruce IA. Cochlear implantation in children with auditory neuropathy: Lessons from Brown-Vialetto-Van Laere syndrome. Cochlear Implants Int. 2019;20(1):31–8.

Auranen M, Paetau A, Piirilä P, Pohju A, Salmi T, Lamminen A, Löfberg M, Mosegaard S, Olsen RK, Tyni T. Patient with multiple acyl-CoA dehydrogenation deficiency disease and FLAD1 mutations benefits from riboflavin therapy. Neuromuscul Disord. 2017;27(6):581–4.

Béhin A, Acquaviva-Bourdain C, Souvannanorath S, Streichenberger N, Attarian S, Bassez G, Brivet M, Fouilhoux A, Labarre-Villa A, Laquerrière A, Pérard L, Kaminsky P, Pouget J, Rigal O, Vanhulle C, Eymard B, Vianey-Saban C, Laforêt P. Multiple acyl-CoA dehydrogenase deficiency (MADD) as a cause of late-onset treatable metabolic disease. Rev Neurol (Paris). 2016;172:231–41.

Bosch AM, Abeling NG, Ijlst L, Knoester H, van der Pol WL, Stroomer AE, Wanders RJ, Visser G, Wijburg FA, Duran M, Waterham HR. Brown-Vialetto-Van Laere and Fazio Londe syndrome is associated with a riboflavin transporter defect mimicking mild MADD: a new inborn error of metabolism with potential treatment. J Inherit Metab Dis. 2011;34:159–64.

Bosch AM, Stroek K, Abeling NG, Waterham HR, Ijlst L, Wanders RJ. The Brown-Vialetto-Van Laere and Fazio Londe syndrome revisited: natural history, genetics, treatment and future perspectives. Orphanet J Rare Dis. 2012;7:83.

Cornelius N, Corydon TJ, Gregersen N, Olsen RK. Cellular consequences of oxidative stress in riboflavin responsive multiple acyl-CoA dehydrogenation deficiency patient fibroblasts. Hum Mol Genet. 2014;23(16):4285–301.

Frerman FE, Goodman SI. Deficiency of electron transfer flavoprotein or electron transfer flavoprotein:ubiquinone oxidoreductase in glutaric acidemia type II fibroblasts. Proc Natl Acad Sci U S A. 1985;82(13):4517–20.

García-Villoria J, De Azua B, Tort F, Mosegaard S, Ugarteburu O, Texidó L, Morales-Romero B, Olsen RKJ, Ribes A. *FLAD1*, encoding FAD synthase, is mutated in a patient with myopathy, scoliosis and cataracts. Clin Genet. 2018;94(6):592–3.

Gianscapero TA, Galluccio M, Miccolis A, Leone P, Eberini I, Iametti S, Indiveri C, Barile M. Human FAD synthase is a bi-functional enzyme with a FAD hydrolase activity in the molybdopterin binding domain. Biochem Biophys Res Commun. 2015;465(3):443–9.

Green P, Wiseman M, Crow YJ, Houlden H, Riphagen S, Lin JP, Raymond FL, Childs AM, Sheridan E, Edwards S, Josifova DJ. Brown-Vialetto-Van Laere syndrome, a ponto-bulbar palsy with deafness, is caused by mutations in *c20orf54*. Am J Hum Genet. 2010;86:485–9.

Grünert SC. Clinical and genetical heterogeneity of late-onset multiple acyl-coenzyme A dehydrogenase deficiency. Orphanet J Rare Dis. 2014;9:117–25.

Hellebrekers DMEI, Sallevelt SCEH, Theunissen TEJ, Hendrickx ATM, Gottschalk RW, Hoeijmakers JGJ, Habets DD, Bierau J, Schoonderwoerd KG, Smeets HJM. Novel *SLC25A32* mutation in a patient with a severe neuromuscular phenotype. Eur J Hum Genet. 2017;25(7):886–8.

Ho G, Yonezawa A, Masuda S, Inui K, Sim KG, Carpenter K, Olsen RK, Mitchell JJ, Rhead WJ, Peters G, Christodoulou J. Maternal riboflavin deficiency, resulting in transient neonatalonset glutaric aciduria type 2, is caused by a microdeletion in the riboflavin transporter gene *GPR172B*. Hum Mutat. 2011;32(1):E1976–84.

Jaeger B, Bosch AM. Clinical presentation and outcome of riboflavin transporter deficiency: mini review after five years of experience. J Inherit Metab Dis. 2016;39(4):559–64.

Jin C, Yao Y, Yonezawa A, Imai S, Yoshimatsu H, Otani Y, Omura T, Nakagawa S, Nakagawa T, Matsubara K. Riboflavin transporters RFVT/SLC52A mediate translocation of riboflavin, rather than FMN or FAD, across plasma membrane. Biol Pharm Bull. 2017;40(11):1990–5.

Manole A, Jaunmuktane Z, Hargreaves I, Ludtmann MHR, Salpietro V, Bello OD, Pope S, Pandraud A, Horga A, Scalco RS, Li A, Ashokkumar B, Lourenço CM, Heales S, Horvath R, Chinnery PF, Toro C, Singleton AB, Jacques TS, Abramov AY, Muntoni F, Hanna MG, Reilly MM, Revesz T, Kullmann DM, Jepson JEC, Houlden H. Clinical, pathological and functional characterization of riboflavin-responsive neuropathy. Brain. 2017;140(11):2820–37.

Morris A, Spiekekotter U. Disorders of mitochondrial fatty acid oxidation and riboflavin metabolism. In: Saudubray JM, Baumgartner MR, Walter J, editors. Inborn metabolic diseases, diagnosis and treatment. Berlin Heidelberg New York: Springer Verlag; 2011. p. 201–14.

Mosegaard S, Bruun GH, Flyvbjerg KF, Bliksrud YT, Gregersen N, Dembic M, Annexstad E, Tangeraas T, Olsen RKJ, Andresen BS. An intronic variation in *SLC52A1* causes exon skipping and transient riboflavin responsive multiple acyl CoA dehydrogenase deficiency. Mol Genet Metab. 2017;122:182–8.

Muru K, Reinson K, Künnapas K, Lilleväli H, Nochi Z, Mosegaard S, Pajusalu S, Olsen RKJ, Õunap K. *FLAD1*-associated multiple acyl-CoA dehydrogenase deficiency identified by newborn screening. Mol Genet Genomic Med. 2019;7(9):e915.

O'Callaghan B, Bosch AM, Houlden H. An update on the genetics, clinical presentation, and pathomechanisms of human riboflavin transporter deficiency. J Inherit Metab Dis. 2019;42(4):598–607.

Olsen RKJ, Koňaříková E, Giancaspero TA, Mosegaard S, Boczonadi V, Mataković L, Veauville-Merllié A, Terrile C, Schwarzmayr T, Haack TB, Auranen M, Leone P, Galluccio M, Imbard A, Gutierrez-Rios P, Palmfeldt J, Graf E, Vianey-Saban C, Oppenheim M, Schiff M, Pichard S, Rigal O, Pyle A, Chinnery PF, Konstantopoulou V, Möslinger D, Feichtinger RG, Talim B, Topaloglu H, Coskun T, Gucer S, Botta A, Pegoraro E, Malena A, Vergani L, Mazzà D, Zollino M, Ghezzi D, Acquaviva C, Tyni T, Boneh A, Meitinger T, Strom TM, Gregersen N, Mayr JA, Horvath R, Barile M, Prokisch H. Riboflavin-responsive and -non-responsive mutations in FAD synthase cause multiple acyl-CoA dehydrogenase and combined respiratory-chain deficiency. Am J Hum Genet. 2016;98(6):1130–45.

Schiff M, Veauville-Merllié A, Su CH, Tzagoloff A, Rak M, Ogier de Baulny H, Boutron A, Smedts-Walters H, Romero NB, Rigal O, Rustin P, Vianey-Saban C, Acquaviva-Bourdain C. *SLC25A32* mutations and riboflavin-responsive exercise intolerance. N Engl J Med. 2016;374:795–7.

Spaan AN, Ijlst L, van Roermund CW, Wijburg FA, Wijburg FA, Wanders RJ, Waterham HR. Identification of the human mitochondrial FAD transporter and its potential role in multiple acyl-CoA dehydrogenase deficiency. Mol Genet Metab. 2005;86(4):441–7.

van Rijt WJ, Jager EA, Allersma DP, Aktuğlu Zeybek AÇ, Bhattacharya K, Debray FG, Ellaway CJ, Gautschi M, Geraghty MT, Gil-Ortega D, Larson AA, Moore F, Morava E, Morris AA, Oishi K, Schiff M, Scholl-Bürgi S, Tchan MC, Vockley J, Witters P, Wortmann SB, van Spronsen F, Van Hove JLK, Derks TGJ. Efficacy and safety of D,L-3-hydroxybutyrate (D,L-3-HB) treatment in multiple acyl-CoA dehydrogenase deficiency. Genet Med. 2020;22(5):908–16.

Xi J, Wen B, Lin J, Zhu W, Luo S, Zhao C, Li D, Lin P, Lu J, Yan C. Clinical features and *ETFDH* mutation spectrum in a cohort of 90 Chinese patients with late-onset multiple acyl-CoA dehydrogenase deficiency. J Inherit Metab Dis. 2014;37(3):399–404.

Yamamoto S, Inoue K, Ohta KY, Fukatsu R, Maeda JY, Yoshida Y, Yuasa H. Identification and functional characterization of rat riboflavin transporter 2. J Biochem. 2009;145(4):437–43.

Yao Y, Yonezawa A, Yoshimatsu H, Masuda S, Katsura T, Inui K. Identification and comparative functional characterization of a new human riboflavin transporter hRFT3 expressed in the brain. J Nutr. 2010;140(7):1220–6.

Yıldız Y, Jentoft Olsen RK, Serap Sivri A, Sivri HS, Akçören Z, Nygaard HH, Tokatlı A. Post-mortem detection of *FLAD1* mutations in 2 Turkish siblings with hypotonia in early infancy. Neuromuscul Disord. 2018;28(9):787–90.

Yonezawa A, Masuda S, Katsura T, Inui K. Identification and functional characterization of a novel human and rat riboflavin transporter, RFT1. Am J Physiol Cell Physiol. 2008;295(3):C632–41.

Zschocke J, Hoffmann G. Vademecum metabolicum. Friedrichsdorf, Germany: Milupa Metabolics GmbH; 2011.

# Disorders of Niacin, NAD, and Pantothenate Metabolism

# 33

Anna Ardissone, Daria Diodato, Ivano Di Meo, and Valeria Tiranti

## Contents



**Summary**

Niacin or vitamin B3 and pantothenate or vitamin B5 are water-soluble vitamins acting as precursors of nicotinamide adenine dinucleotide (NAD) and Coenzyme A (CoA), respectively, two fundamental elements for every cell.

The niacin-derived coenzymes NAD and NADP carry out similar oxidation and reduction reactions: NADP is mainly involved in biosynthetic pathways, while NAD, in its reduced form NADH, supplies the mitochondrial electron transport chain with reducing equivalent and, in doing so, propels the oxidative phosphorylation.

Pantothenate-derived CoA is a crucial molecule for hundred of metabolic reactions, including, among others, the Krebs cycle and the oxidation and synthesis of fatty acids. Both coenzymes play crucial roles not only in metabolism and in maintaining mitochondrial functionality but also in complex mechanisms of signalling. Moreover, by modulating deacetylation (NAD) and acetylation (CoA) of histones and transcription factors, these coenzymes also regulate gene expression.

NAD biosynthetic pathways originate from four major molecules: (i) the amino acid tryptophan (Trp), (ii) nicotinic acid (NA), (iii) nicotinamide (NAM), and (iv) nicotinamide riboside (NR). Nicotinamide mononucleotide (NMN) generated from NAM and NR can also be a source of NAD.

CoA is instead synthesized through the sequential activity of five enzymatic reactions belonging to the same

A. Ardissone
Unit of Child Neurology, Fondazione IRCCS Istituto Neurologico Carlo Besta, Milan, Italy
e-mail: anna.ardissone@istituto-besta.it

D. Diodato
Neuromuscular and Neurodegenerative Disease Unit, Children Hospital Bambino Gesù, Rome, Italy
e-mail: daria.diodato@opbg.net

I. Di Meo · V. Tiranti (✉)
Unit of Medical Genetics and Neurogenetics, Fondazione IRCCS Istituto Neurologico Carlo Besta, Milan, Italy
e-mail: ivano.dimeo@istituto-besta.it; valeria.tiranti@istituto-besta.it


N. Blau et al. (eds.), *Physician's Guide to the Diagnosis, Treatment, and Follow-Up of Inherited Metabolic Diseases*,
https://doi.org/10.1007/978-3-030-67727-5_33

metabolic pathway, in which pantothenate is the starting molecule.

Considering the vital roles of NAD and CoA, their deficiency either due to shortage of vitamins in the diet or to genetic causes impinging on the biochemical pathways responsible for their production and proper maintenance could give rise to human diseases.

We will discuss disorders of niacin and NAD separately from disorders of pantothenate for the sake of clarity even if it is clear that NAD and CoA play convergent roles in energetic metabolism and regulate common pathways.

## Introduction

### Disorders of Niacin and NAD Metabolism

Niacin is the term that defines both NAM and NA and is necessary to synthesize the two coenzymes NAD and NADP.

Tryptophan, NA, NAM, and NR are used to generate NAD through different metabolic pathways (Fig. 33.1): NAD synthesized from NA is known as Preiss-Handler pathway; tryptophan is the starting amino acid in the de novo synthesis (kynurenine pathway); the salvage pathway converts NR and NAM through two enzymatic steps into nicotinamide mononucleotide (NMN).

The best-known disorder due to niacin deficiency is pellagra that was endemic a century ago in rural areas and nowadays is present, in developed countries, as secondary effect to other disorders such as tuberculosis, malabsorption, and alcoholism. Distinctive features of pellagra include diarrhoea, peculiar pigmented skin rash, and dementia, which can be reversed by NAM and NA administration.

Disorders of niacin and NAD metabolism are also due to genetic causes affecting different genes coding for enzymes designed to synthesize NAD, synthesize and modify NADP, remove toxic metabolites, and transport tryptophan.

These disorders mainly impair brain functions and, in some instances, give rise to pellagra-like clinical manifestations.

Deficiency of nicotinamide mononucleotide adenylyl transferase 1 (*NMNAT1*), a central enzyme in the Preiss-Handler NAD biosynthetic pathway, catalysing the condensation of nicotinic acid mononucleotide (NaMN) with AMP (Zhang et al., 2003), leads to Leber congenital amaurosis (LCA), an early-onset neurodegenerative condition of the human retina causing congenital blindness (Koenekoop et al., 2012).

The mitochondrial kinase coded by the *NADK2* gene synthesizes NADP+ (Ohashi et al., 2012). Exome sequence investigation revealed the presence of a nonsense mutation in this gene in one subject with deficiency of 2,4-dienoyl-CoA reductase (DECR; OMIM#616034) (Houten et al., 2014) and early-onset encephalopathy, developmental delay, movement disorder, lactic acidosis, and premature death. Mitochondria derived from patient fibroblasts displayed reduction of NADP(H) level, and real-time measurement of oxygen consumption demonstrated a reduction of the respiratory rate with a parallel increase in extracellular acidification. In addition to decreased activity of DECR, laboratory tests also showed hyperlysinaemia due to impaired activity of alpha-aminoadipic semialdehyde synthase coded by the *AASS* gene (OMIM#605113).

The very severe phenotype observed in this patient could be ascribed not only to the combined deficiency of DECR and AASS, two NADP-dependent mitochondrial enzymes, but also to a global deficiency of additional NADP-dependent processes inside the mitochondria.

Recently and thanks to exome sequencing in subjects with complex clinical neurological presentations, new genes coding for proteins responsible for elimination of damaged metabolites have been identified.

Two genes belonging to the metabolite repair system denominated *NAXE* (Kremer et al., 2016) and *NAXD* (van Bergen et al., 2019) were found mutated in a childhood-onset lethal metabolic disorder with neurological involvement and in an early-onset encephalopathy with brain oedema and leucoencephalopathy, respectively.

The *NAXE* gene encodes an epimerase involved in the repair of NADHX and NADPHX, toxic compounds inhibiting several dehydrogenase activities. The epimerase catalyses the conversion of R-NAD(P)HX to S-NAD(P)HX so that S-NAD(P)HX can be reconverted to S-NAD(P)H by the dehydratase *NAXD*. In patient-derived fibroblasts, elevated concentrations of toxic compounds S-NADHX, R-NADHX, and cyclic NADHX were identified (Kremer et al., 2016; van Bergen et al., 2019).

Homozygous or compound heterozygous mutations in the gene *NNT*, coding for a pyridine nucleotide transhydrogenase protein located in the inner mitochondrial membrane, cause glucocorticoid deficiency type 4 with or without mineralocorticoid deficiency (Meimaridou et al., 2012; Yamaguchi et al., 2013; Hershkovitz et al., 2015; Weinberg-Shukron et al., 2015; Roucher-Boulez et al., 2016). This protein transfers a hydride ion between NAD, NAD(H), and NADP(H) (Zieger and Ware, 1997), and it contributes to functioning of the mitochondrial respiratory chain system playing a role in removing excess of reactive oxygen species in adrenal glands (Meimaridou et al., 2012).

Hartnup disorder is an autosomal recessive disorder due to defective transport of neutral amino acids across epithelial cells in renal proximal tubules and intestinal mucosa causing increased level of amino acids in urine. It is characterized by symptoms like pellagra, cerebellar ataxia, and neurological manifestation. The genetic cause of this disorder was identified in 2004 (Kleta et al. 2004) as due to mutation in the *SLC6A19* gene coding for a neutral amino acid transporter. One particular amino acid transported includes tryptophan, which is required to generate NAD, and this would be the reason for the clinical manifestations resembling pellagra.

Kynureninase and 3-hydroxyanthranilate 3,4-dioxygenase deficiencies are caused by mutations in the *KYNU* and *HAAO* genes, respectively, which code for enzymes involved in the kynurenine pathway leading to NAD cofactor production from tryptophan. A first missense mutation in *KYNU* gene was identified in 2007 (Christensen et al. 2007) in two brothers with no pathological phenotype except for increased level of xanthurenic acid, kynurenine, and 3-hydroxykynurenine in urine. In 2017 additional patients with a complicated multisystem syndrome were proved to carry out truncating mutations in *KYNU* and *HAAO* (Shi et al., 2017). In one affected patient analysis of plasma revealed the presence of high level of 3-hydroxykynurenine and low level of NAD, which was hypothesized to be responsible for the complicated clinical presentation characterized by vertebral, cardiac, renal, and limb defects (VCRL) observed in these patients.

## Disorders of Pantothenate Metabolism

Coenzyme A is synthesized from pantothenate in a pathway composed of five enzymatic reactions (Fig. 33.1). CoA has a relevant role not only in bioenergetic metabolism but contributes to the synthesis of cholesterol, amino acids, phospholipids, fatty acids, and neurotransmitters. This multiplicity of activities impacts massively, even if not exclusively, on the structure and function of the brain.

While there are almost no reports describing deficiency of pantothenic acid due to nutritional deficits, mutations in genes coding for the first (PANK2) and last (COASY) enzymes of the CoA biosynthetic pathway are associated with neurodegenerative disorders hallmarked by iron accumulation in specific regions of the brain (NBIA). The pathogenic mechanisms linking iron accumulation to impaired CoA biosynthesis is still under investigation, but defective mitochondrial functionality seems to be one of the triggering causes of the disease as demonstrated in cellular and animal models (Orellana et al., 2016; Brunetti et al., 2012; Berti et al., 2015). Recently, mutations in *PPCS* gene coding for the second enzyme in the CoA synthetic pathway have been identified in a completely different clinical phenotype characterized by dilated cardiomyopathy and altered acylcarnitine profile (Iuso et al., 2018). It remains to be clarified why malfunctioning of enzymes belonging to the same metabolic pathway results in great clinical heterogeneity.

Mutations in *SLC25A42* coding for a mitochondrial CoA transporter were found in a patient with mitochondrial myopathy and delayed motor development (Shamseldin et al. 2016) and in additional cases presenting with encephalopathy and metabolic crisis (Almannai et al., 2018; Iuso et al., 2019). Instrumental investigations demonstrated increased serum lactate and basal ganglia lesions on MRI, in one case associated with iron deposition; muscle biopsy was performed in few cases and showed ragged-red-like fibers.

## Nomenclature

| No. | Disease name | Alternative disease name | Disease Abbreviation | Gene Symbol | Chromosomal localization | Mode of inheritance | Affected protein | Disease OMIM |
|---|---|---|---|---|---|---|---|---|
| 33.1 | Leber congenital amaurosis 9 | Nicotinamide mononucleotide adenylyl transferase 1 deficiency | LCA9 | *NMNAT1* | 1p36.22 | AR | Nicotinamide nucleotide adenylyltransferase 1 | 608553 |
| 33.2 | Mitochondrial NAD kinase 2 deficiency | 2,4-dienoyl-CoA reductase deficiency with hyperlysinemia | DECRD | *NADK2* | 5p13.2 | AR | 2,4-dienoyl-CoA reductase | 616034 |
| 33.3 | NAD(P)HX epimerase deficiency | Apolipoprotein A-I binding protein deficiency | PEBEL | *NAXE* | 1q22 | AR | Apolipoprotein A-I binding protein | 617186 |
| 33.4 | NAD(P)HX dehydratase deficiency | CARKD deficiency | PEBEL2 | *NAXD* | 13q34 | AR | Carbohydrate kinase domain-containing protein | 618321 |
| 33.5 | Nicotinamide nucleotide transhydrogenase deficiency | Glucocorticoid deficiency type 4 | GCCD4 | *NNT* | 5p12 | AR | Nicotinamide nucleotide transhydrogenase | 614736 |
| 33.6 | Hartnup disorder | | HND | *SLC6A19* | 5p15.33 | AR | B(0)AT1 | 234500 |
| 33.7 | Kynureninase deficiency | Xanthurenic aciduria; vertebral, cardiac, renal, and limb defects syndrome type 2 | VCRL2 | *KYNU* | 2q22.2 | AR | L-kynurenine hydrolase | 617661 |
| 33.8 | 3-hydroxyanthranilic acid 3,4-dioxygenase deficiency | Vertebral, cardiac, renal, and limb defects syndrome type 1 | VCRL1 | *HAAO* | 2p21 | AR | 3-Hydroxyanthranilate 3,4-dioxygenase | 617660 |
| 33.9 | Pantothenate kinase 2 deficiency | Pantothenate kinase-associated neurodegeneration (PKAN); neurodegeneration with brain iron accumulation type 1 | PKAN | *PANK2* | 20p13 | AR | Pantothenate kinase type | 2234200 |
| 33.10 | Phosphopantothenoylcysteine synthetase deficiency | Autosomal recessive dilated cardiomyopathy | CMD2C | *PPCS* | 1p34.2 | AR | Phosphopantothenoylcysteine synthetase | 618189 |
| 33.11 | Coenzyme A synthase deficiency | CoA synthase protein-associated neurodegeneration (CoPAN); neurodegeneration with brain iron accumulation type 6 | COPAN | *COASY* | 17q21.2 | AR | Phosphopantetheine adenylytransferase/ dephosphocoenzyme A | 615643 |
| 33.12 | Mitochondrial coenzyme A transporter deficiency | | | *SLC25A42* | 19p13.11 | AR | Mitochondrial coenzyme A transporter | 610823 |

## Metabolic Pathway

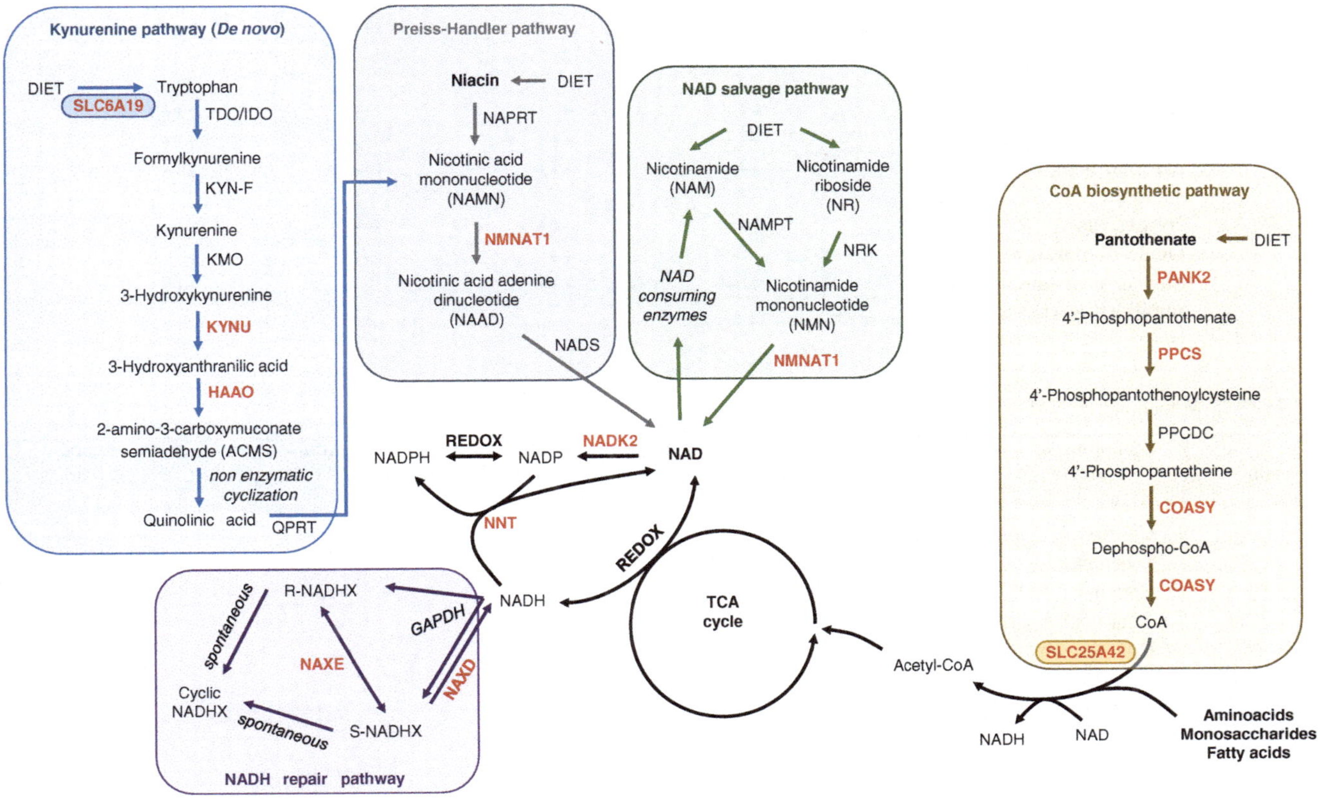


**Fig. 33.1** Schematic representation of niacin, NAD, and pantothenate pathways and their interconnections

For simplicity, different pathways are grouped by different colors. Proteins mutated in human diseases are in red. NAD is synthesized through two main ways: it is produced either in a de novo pathway from amino acids or in salvage pathways by recycling preformed components such as nicotinamide (NAM) back to NAD. In the kynurenine (de novo) pathway (blue), a series of enzymatic and non-enzymatic reactions converts the amino acid tryptophan to nicotinic acid mononucleotide (NAMN), which is also produced in the Preiss-Handler pathway (grey) starting from niacin. NAMN is then converted to NAD by two further enzymatic reactions. NAD and its phosphorylated derivative NADP are reduced to NADH and NADPH by catabolic and anabolic redox reactions. In the NAD salvage pathway (green), NAM molecule, which is produced by NAD consuming enzymes such as sirtuins, Poly (ADP-ribose) polymerases (PARPs), CD38, and CD157, is recycled into nicotinamide mononucleotide (NMN), which in turn is re-converted to NAD. Hydrated forms of NADH and NADPH, called NADHX and NADPHX, respectively, can be formed spontaneously under acidic conditions or enzymatically by glyceraldehyde-3-phosphate dehydrogenase (GAPDH). NADHX and NADPHX, which are inhibitors of several dehydrogenases, are both converted back to NADH and NADPH by a series of enzymatic reactions in the repair pathway (purple) In the CoA biosynthetic pathway (yellow), pantothenate is sequentially converted to CoA by a series of five enzymatic reactions. CoA is then used as an acyl group carrier and carbonyl-activating group in a multitude of biochemical transformations, including tricarboxylic acid (TCA) cycle and fatty acid metabolism. Enzymes: TDO tryptophan 2,3-dioxygenase, IDO indoleamine 2,3-dioxygenase, KYN-F kynurenine formamidase, KMO kynurenine 3-monoxygenase, KYNU kynunerinase, HAAO 3-hydroxyanthranilate 3,4-dioxygenase, QPRT nicotinate-nucleotide pyrophosphorylase, NAPRT nicotinate phosphoribosyltransferase, NMNAT1 nicotinamide mononucleotide adenyltransferase 1, NADS glutamine-dependent NAD(+) synthetase, NAMPT nicotinamide phosphoribosyltransferase, NRK nicotinamide riboside kinase, NADK2 NAD kinase 2, NNT nicotinamide nucleotide transhydrogenase, GAPDH glyceraldehyde-3-phosphate dehydrogenase, NAXE NAD(P)HX epimerase, NAXD NAD(P)HX dehydratase, PANK2 pantothenate kinase 2, PPCS phosphopantothenoylcysteine synthetase, PPCDC phosphopantothenoylcysteine decarboxylase, COASY coenzyme A synthetase. Transporters: SLC6A19 sodium-dependent neutral amino acid transporter B(0)AT1, SLC25A42 mitochondrial coenzyme A transporter

## Signs and Symptoms

**Table 33.1** Nicotinamide mononucleotide adenylyl transferase 1 deficiency

| System | Symptoms and biomarkers | Neonatal (birth–1 month) | Infancy (1–18 months) | Childhood (1.5–11 years) | Adolescence (11–16 years) | Adulthood (>16 years) |
|---|---|---|---|---|---|---|
| Eye | **Attenuated retinal vessels/pigmentary retinal changes** | ++ | +++ | +++ | +++ | +++ |
| | **Blindness** | ++ | +++ | +++ | +++ | +++ |
| | **Hyperopia** | ++ | +++ | +++ | +++ | +++ |
| | **Macular atrophy/ coloboma** | ++ | +++ | +++ | +++ | +++ |
| | **Nystagmus** | ++ | +++ | +++ | +++ | +++ |
| | **Oculo-digital sign** | ++ | ++ | ++ | ++ | ++ |
| | **Slow or near-absent pupillary reactions** | ++ | +++ | +++ | +++ | +++ |

**Table 33.2** Mitochondrial NAD kinase 2 deficiency

| System | Symptoms and biomarkers | Neonatal (birth–1 month) | Infancy (1–18 months) | Childhood (1.5–11 years) | Adolescence (11–16 years) | Adulthood (>16 years) |
|---|---|---|---|---|---|---|
| CNS | Ataxia | ± | ± | + | + | |
| | Chorea | ± | ± | ± | | |
| | Dystonia | ± | ± | ± | | |
| | Epilepsy | + | + | + | | |
| | Neuropathy, peripheral | | | + | + | |
| Eye | Optic atrophy | | | + | + | |
| Metabolic | Lactic acidosis | + | + | + | | |
| Laboratory findings | **C10:2 acylcarnitine (plasma)** | ↑ | ↑ | ↑ | n-↑ | |
| | **Lysine (plasma)** | ↑↑↑ | ↑↑↑ | ↑↑↑ | ↑↑↑ | |
| | Proline (plasma) | | | | ↑↑↑ | |

**Table 33.3** NAD(P)HX epimerase deficiency

| System | Symptoms and biomarkers | Neonatal (birth–1 month) | Infancy (1–18 months) | Childhood (1.5–11 years) | Adolescence (11–16 years) | Adulthood (>16 years) |
|---|---|---|---|---|---|---|
| CNS | Ataxia | | + + + | + + + | | |
| | Hypotonia | | + + + | + + + | | |
| Dermatological | **Skin lesions** | | + + + | + + + | | |
| Respiratory | Respiratory failure | | + + + | + + + | | |
| Laboratory findings | Lactate (cerebrospinal fluid) | | ↑↑ | ↑↑ | | |

**Table 33.4** NAD(P)HX dehydratase deficiency

| System | Symptoms and biomarkers | Neonatal (birth–1 month) | Infancy (1–18 months) | Childhood (1.5–11 years) | Adolescence (11–16 years) | Adulthood (>16 years) |
|---|---|---|---|---|---|---|
| CNS | **Ataxia** | | | ++ | ++ | |
| | Dystonia | | | ++ | ++ | |
| | Psychiatric disturbances | | | ± | ± | |
| | **Psychomotor regression** | | | +++ | +++ | |
| Skin | **Lesions** | | | +++ | +++ | |
| Blood | Pancytopenia | | | ± | ± | |
| Heart | Cardiomyopathy | | | ± | ± | |

**Table 33.5** Nicotinamide nucleotide transhydrogenase deficiency

| System | Symptoms and biomarkers | Neonatal (birth–1 month) | Infancy (1–18 months) | Childhood (1.5–11 years) | Adolescence (11–16 years) | Adulthood (>16 years) |
|---|---|---|---|---|---|---|
| CNS | **Addison crisis** | ± | ± | ± | ± | ± |
| Dermatological | **Hyperpigmentation** | | +++ | +++ | +++ | +++ |
| Endocrine | Precocious puberty | | ± | ± | ± | ± |
| Genitourinary | Azoospermia | | | ± | | |
| | Cryptorchidism | | | ± | | |
| | Testicular nodules | | ± | ± | ± | ± |
| | Testicular tumour | | ± | ± | ± | ± |
| Metabolic | **Hypoglycaemia** | | +++ | +++ | +++ | +++ |
| Laboratory findings | ACTH (plasma) | ↑↑↑ | ↑↑↑ | ↑↑↑ | ↑↑↑ | ↑↑↑ |
| | Aldosterone (plasma) | ↓↓↓ | ↓↓↓ | ↓↓↓ | ↓↓↓ | ↓↓↓ |
| | Cortisol (plasma) | ↓↓↓ | ↓↓↓ | ↓↓↓ | ↓↓↓ | ↓↓↓ |
| | Glucose (plasma | | ↓↓↓ | ↓↓↓ | ↓↓↓ | ↓↓↓ |
| | Renin (plasma) | ↑↑↑ | ↑↑↑ | ↑↑↑ | ↑↑↑ | ↑↑↑ |
| | Testosterone (plasma) | | | | ↓-n | ↓-n |

**Table 33.6** Hartnup disorder

| System | Symptoms and biomarkers | Neonatal (birth–1 month) | Infancy (1–18 months) | Childhood (1.5–11 years) | Adolescence (11–16 years) | Adulthood (>16 years) |
|---|---|---|---|---|---|---|
| CNS | **Ataxia** | | ± | ± | ± | |
| | Seizures | | | ± | | |
| Dermatological | **Photosensitivity** | | ± | ± | ± | |
| Psychiatric | Psychosis | | ± | ± | ± | |
| Laboratory findings | Glutamic acid (urine) | n-↑ | n-↑ | n-↑ | n-↑ | n-↑ |
| | Neutral amino acids (urine) | ↑ | ↑ | ↑ | ↑ | ↑ |

**Table 33.7** 3-Hydroxykynureninase deficiency

| System | Symptoms and biomarkers | Neonatal (birth–1 month) | Infancy (1–18 months) | Childhood (1.5–11 years) | Adolescence (11–16 years) | Adulthood (>16 yreas) |
|---|---|---|---|---|---|---|
| Autonomic system | **Talipes** | ± | ± | | | |
| Cardiovascular | Hypoplastic left heart | ± | ± | | | |
| | Patent ductus arteriosus | ± | ± | | | |
| CNS | Speech delay | ± | ± | | | |
| Digestive | Anteriorly placed anus | ± | | | | |
| Musculoskeletal | Rhizomelia | ± | ± | | | |
| | **Short stature** | + | + | | | |
| | Syndactyly | ± | ± | | | |
| Renal | **Renal hypoplasia** | + | + | | | |
| Laboratory findings | 3-Hydroxykynurenine (urine) | | ↑ | ↑ | ↑ | |
| | 3-Hydroxykynurenine; 3HK (plasma) | ↑ | ↑ | | | |
| | Kynurenine (urine) | | ↑ | ↑ | ↑ | |
| | NAD+ (plasma) | ↓ | ↓ | | | |
| | Xanthurenic acid (urine) | | ↑ | ↑ | ↑ | |

**Table 33.8** 3-Hydroxyanthranilate 3,4-dioxygenase deficiency

| System | Symptoms and biomarkers | Neonatal (birth–1 month) | Infancy (1–18 months) | Childhood (1.5–11 years) | Adolescence (11–16 years) | Adulthood (>16 years) |
|---|---|---|---|---|---|---|
| Autonomic system | Talipes | ± | ± | ± | | |
| Cardiovascular | Atrial septal defect | ± | ± | ± | | |
| | Hypoplastic left heart | ± | ± | ± | | |
| CNS | Intellectual disability | | ± | ± | | |
| Ear | **Hearing loss, sensorineural** | + | + | ± | | |
| Musculoskeletal | **Short stature** | + | + | ± | | |
| Renal | **Renal hypoplasia** | + | + | ± | | |
| Laboratory findings | 3-Hydroxyanthranilic acid; 3HAA (plasma) | ↑ | ↑ | ↓ | | |
| | NAD+ (plasma) | ↓ | ↓ | ↓ | | |

**Table 33.9** Neurodegeneration with brain iron accumulation 1

| System | Symptoms and biomarkers | Neonatal (birth–1 month) | Infancy (1–18 months) | Childhood (1.5–11 years) | Adolescence (11–16 years) | Adulthood (>16 years) |
|---|---|---|---|---|---|---|
| CNS | **Dystonia** | ± | ± | + + | + + + | + + + |
| | **Extrapyramidal signs** | | ± | ++ | ++ | ++ |
| | Intellectual disability | | ± | + | + | + |
| | Parkinsonism | | | + | + | + |
| | **Rigidity** | | ± | ++ | ++ | ++ |
| | Seizures | | | ± | ± | ± |
| | **Spasticity** | | ± | + + | + + | + + |
| Eye | Abnormal eye movement | | | + | + | + |
| | Optic atrophy | | | + | + | + |
| | Retinopathy | ± | ± | ++ | ++ | ++ |
| Musculoskeletal | **Eye-of-the-tiger-sign** | | ± | + + + | + + + | + + |
| Psychiatric | **Depression, other psychiatric symptoms** | | | ± | ± | + |
| Laboratory findings | Iron (brain) | | | ↑ | ↑ | ↑ |

**Table 33.10** Phosphopantothenoylcysteine synthetase deficiency

| System | Symptoms and biomarkers | Neonatal (birth–1 month) | Infancy (1–18 months) | Childhood (1.5–11 years) | Adolescence (11–16 years) | Adulthood (>16 yreas) |
|---|---|---|---|---|---|---|
| Cardiovascular | **Cardiomyopathy, dilated** | + | + + + | + + + | + + + | |
| CNS | Hypotonia, muscular | ± | ± | ± | ± | |
| Musculoskeletal | Dysmorphic features | ± | ± | ± | ± | |
| Laboratory findings | Lactate (plasma) | n-↑ | n-↑ | n-↑ | n-↑ | |

**Table 33.11** Neurodegeneration with brain iron accumulation 6

| System | Symptoms and biomarkers | Neonatal (birth–1 month) | Infancy (1–18 months) | Childhood (1.5–11 years) | Adolescence (11–16 years) | Adulthood (>16 years) |
|---|---|---|---|---|---|---|
| CNS | Areflexia | | | + | + | + |
| | Ataxia | | | Infancy (1–18 months) | + | + |
| | **Axonal neuropathy** | | | ++ | ++ | ++ |
| | **Basal ganglia abnormalities (MRI)** | | ± | ++ | ++ | ++ |
| | Bradykinesia | | | - | + | + |
| | Development delay | | + | + | ++ | ++ |
| | **Dystonia** | | | + | ++ | ++ |
| | Gait disturbance | | ± | + | + | + |
| | Intellectual disability | | + | + | ++ | ++ |
| | **Parkinsonism** | | | + | + | + |
| | **Spastic paraplegia** | | ± | + | ++ | ++ |
| | Thin corpus callosum | | | ± | ± | ± |
| Psychiatric | **Behavioural abnormalities** | | | + | ++ | ++ |
| Laboratory findings | C0/C16 + C18 acylcarnitines ratio (dried blood spot) | ↑ | ↓ | ↓ | | |
| | C16:0 acylcarnitine (dried blood spot) | ↓ | ↓ | ↓ | | |
| | C18:0 acylcarnitine (dried blood spot) | ↓ | ↓ | ↓ | | |
| | Carnitine, free | ↑ | ↑ | ↑ | | |
| | Iron (brain) | | | ↑ | ↑ | |

**Table 33.12** Mitochondrial coenzyme A transporter deficiency

| System | Symptoms and biomarkers | Neonatal (birth–1 month) | Infancy (1–18 months) | Childhood (1.5–11 years) | Adolescence (11–16 years) | Adulthood (>16 years) |
|---|---|---|---|---|---|---|
| Cardiovascular | Cardiomyopathy | ± | ± | ± | ± | ± |
| CNS | Basal ganglia abnormalities (MRI)[a] | ± | ± | ± | + | + |
| | Developmental delay | + | + | + | ± | ± |
| | Intellectual disability | + | + | + | ± | ± |
| | Movement disorder | ± | ± | ± | ± | ± |
| | Seizures | ± | ± | ± | ± | ± |
| Metabolic | Metabolic crisis | + | + | + | ± | ± |
| Musculoskeletal | Myopathy | + | + | + | + | + |
| Laboratory findings | Acylcarnitines (medium and long chain) | n-↑ | n-↑ | n-↑ | n-↑ | |
| | Ammonia (plasma) | n-↑ | n-↑ | n-↑ | n-↑ | |
| | Carnitine, free | ↓-n | ↓-n | ↓-n | ↓-n | |
| | Creatine kinase (plasma) | n-↑ | n-↑ | n-↑ | n-↑ | |
| | Lactate (plasma) | ↑ | ↑ | ↑ | ↑ | |

[a] *signal alteration or iron deposition or atrophy*

## Diagnostic Flowcharts

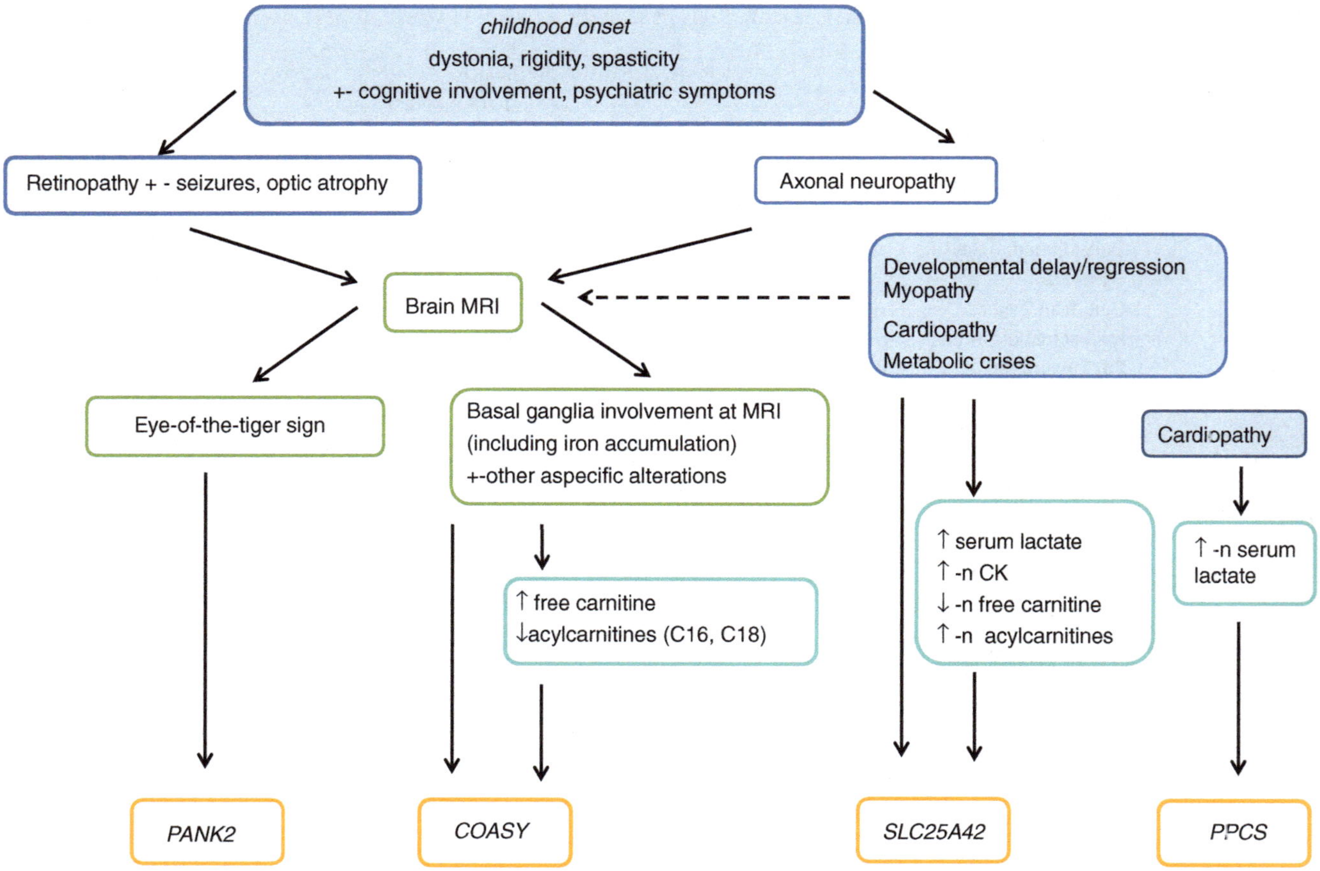


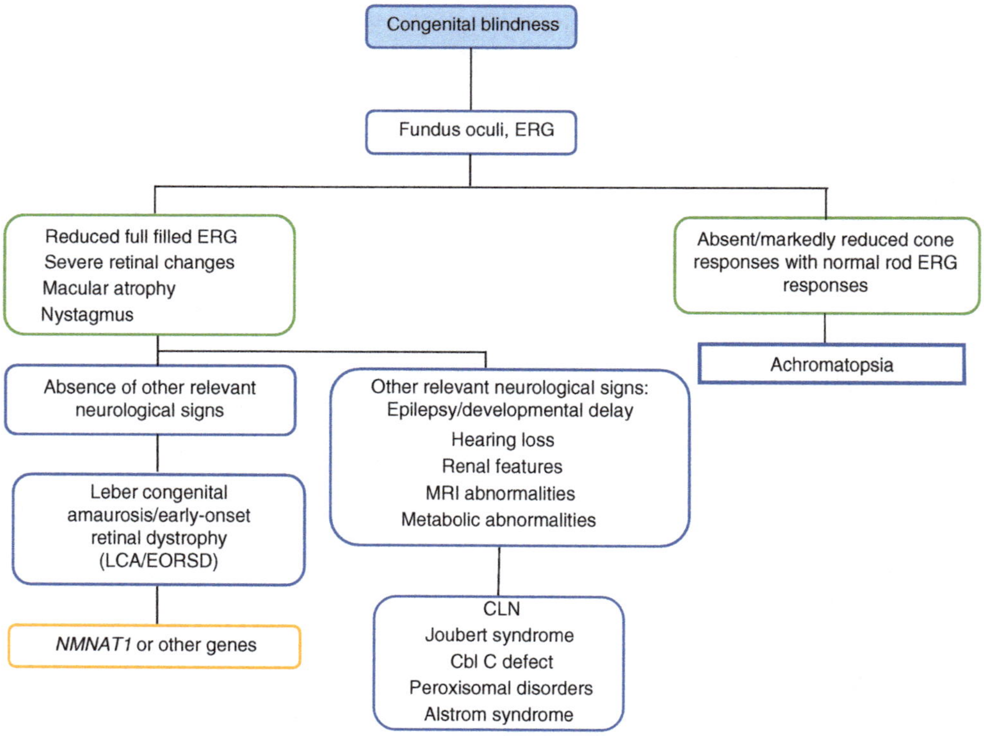

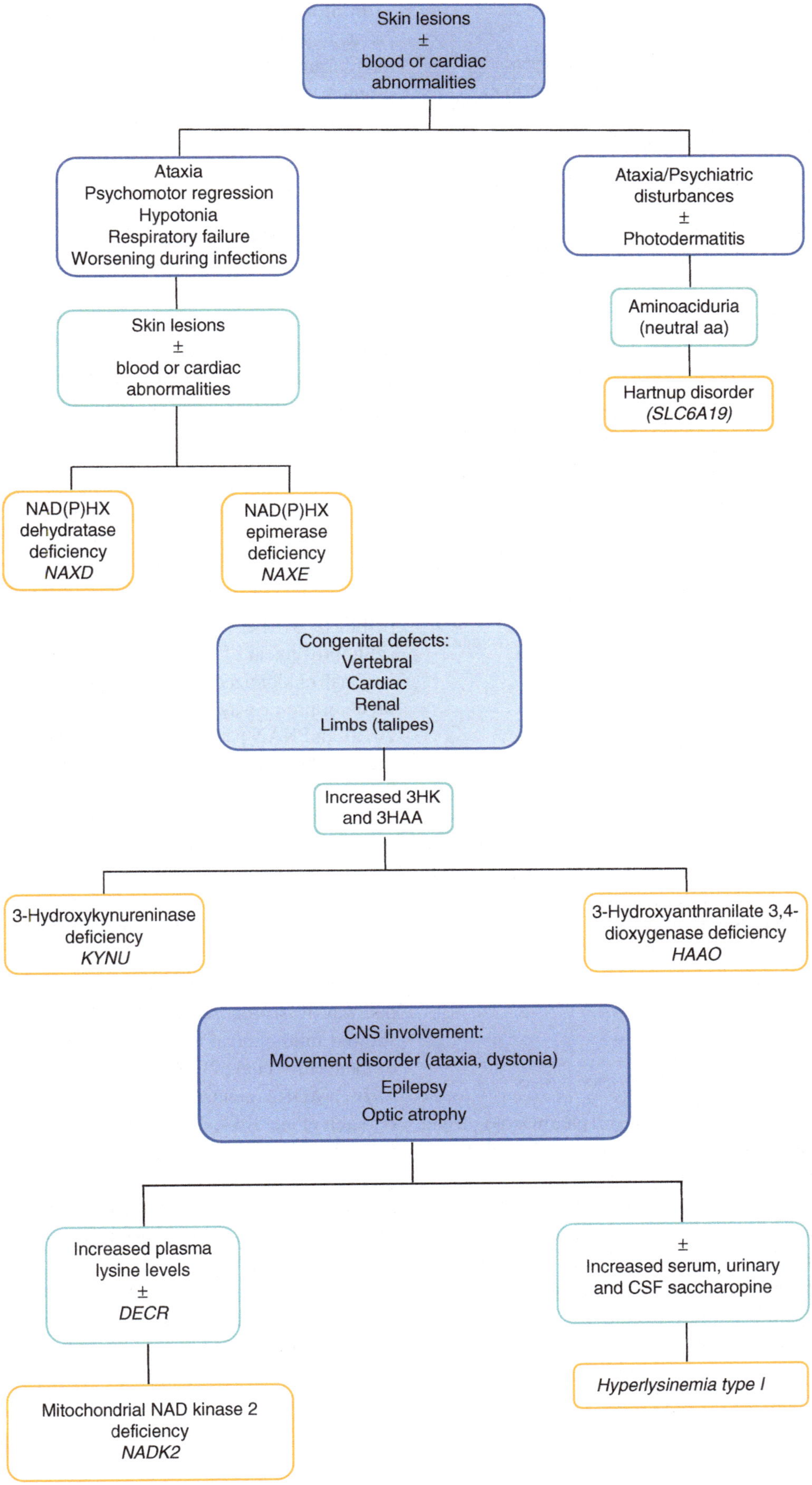
Skin lesions
±
blood or cardiac abnormalities
Ataxia
Psychomotor regression
Hypotonia
Respiratory failure
Worsening during infections
Skin lesions
±
blood or cardiac abnormalities
NAD(P)HX dehydratase deficiency
*NAXD*
NAD(P)HX epimerase deficiency
*NAXE*
Ataxia/Psychiatric disturbances
±
Photodermatitis
Aminoaciduria (neutral aa)
Hartnup disorder *(SLC6A19)*
Congenital defects:
Vertebral
Cardiac
Renal
Limbs (talipes)
Increased 3HK and 3HAA
3-Hydroxykynureninase deficiency
*KYNU*
3-Hydroxyanthranilate 3,4-dioxygenase deficiency
*HAAO*
CNS involvement:
Movement disorder (ataxia, dystonia)
Epilepsy
Optic atrophy
Increased plasma lysine levels
±
*DECR*
Mitochondrial NAD kinase 2 deficiency
*NADK2*
±
Increased serum, urinary and CSF saccharopine
*Hyperlysinemia type I*

## Prenatal Diagnosis

| Disorder | Tests recommended |
|---|---|
| Nicotinamide mononucleotide adenylyl transferase 1 deficiency | Mutation analysis on DNA from CVS or AFC |
| Mitochondrial NAD kinase 2 deficiency | Mutation analysis on DNA from CVS or AFC |
| NAD(P)HX epimerase deficiency | Mutation analysis on DNA from CVS or AFC |
| NAD(P)HX dehydratase deficiency | Mutation analysis on DNA from CVS or AFC |
| Nicotinamide nucleotide transhydrogenase deficiency | Mutation analysis on DNA from CVS or AFC |
| Hartnup disorder | Mutation analysis on DNA from CVS or AFC |
| Kynureninase deficiency | Mutation analysis on DNA from CVS or AFC |
| 3-Hydroxyanthranilic acid 3,4-dioxygenase deficiency | Mutation analysis on DNA from CVS or AFC |
| Pantothenate kinase 2 deficiency | Mutation analysis on DNA from CVS or AFC |
| Phosphopantothenoylcysteine synthetase deficiency | Mutation analysis on DNA from CVS or AFC |
| Coenzyme A synthase deficiency | Mutation analysis on DNA from CVS or AFC |
| Mitochondrial coenzyme A transporter deficiency | Mutation analysis on DNA from CVS or AFC |

*CVS Chorionic villous sampling, AFC Amniotic fluid cells*

## DNA Testing

Genetic investigation is performed for all the diseases described in this chapter, on DNA extracted from peripheral blood mononuclear cells (PBMC). PCR amplification and direct sequencing are carried out for mutation detection. In some laboratories, usage of genes panel followed by next-generation sequencing (NGS) is available.

## Treatment

### Summary

In disorders of pantothenate metabolism, pharmacologic and surgical interventions have focused on palliation of symptoms according to consensus clinical management guideline available for PKAN (Hogarth et al., 2017). Symptomatic treatment is aimed primarily at the dystonia, which can be profoundly debilitating to the affected individual and caregivers. Different treatments have been commonly used including oral baclofen, trihexyphenidyl, and clonazepam, intrathecal and intraventricular baclofen, and deep brain stimulation.

In SLC25A42-related disorders, affected individuals are prone to metabolic decompensations with relatively mild intercurrent illnesses and therefore should be managed to promote anabolism; in acute metabolic crisis management with intravenous fluids and bicarbonate infusion will prevent permanent neurological sequela (Almannai et al., 2018).

### Experimental Treatment

Clinical and experimental studies are currently underway in disorders of pantothenate metabolism, and treatments will mainly target pathogenic mechanisms. The potential for iron chelation using deferiprone (an iron chelator that is able to cross the blood–brain barrier) to modify disease and improve clinical symptoms is highly topical at present. To date, good tolerability of deferiprone, with reduction of radiologically discernible brain iron, and clinical improvement in some PKAN patients was reported (Abbruzzese et al., 2011). Another pilot phase II trial showed that deferiprone was well tolerated in the nine PKAN patients who completed the study, with statistically significant reduction of iron in the pallida by MRI evaluation but disappointingly without clinical improvement of symptoms (Zorzi et al., 2011). An international randomized, double-blind, placebo-controlled trial of deferiprone was recently completed (Klopstock et al., 2019). In PKAN patients who have residual PANK2 activity, the possibility of using high-dose pantothenate therapy has been considered. Pantothenate is well tolerated with no known toxicity. The effect of pantothenate supplementation in PKAN is currently unknown although patients with atypical PKAN have anecdotally reported improvement in motor symptoms, speech, cognition, and general wellbeing while on treatment (Kurian and Hayflick 2013).

Oral pantethine supplementation as targeted treatmente aimed to bypass the deficient enzyme in the CoA synthesis pathway was proposed in two PPCS mutated patients and showed mild clinical and instrumental improvement in one of them (Iuso et al., 2018).

In NADK2 deficiency, low-lysine diet has been tried (Houten et al., 2014; Tort et al., 2016) with reported beneficial effect in one case in association with other cofactors (ubidecarenone, idebenone, vitamin E, creatine) (Tort et al., 2016). NADPH supplementation has been tried in a recently reported case with a milder phenotype with initial beneficial effect (Pomerantz et al., 2018). Treatment with nicotinic acid has been speculated for individuals with NAXE defect (Kremer et al., 2016). Oral nicotinamide treatment (50–100 mg/day) may prevent or resolve photodermatitis in Hartnup disorder.

## References


Abbruzzese G, Cossu G, Balocco M, Marchese R, Murgia D, Melis M, et al. A pilot trial of deferiprone for neurodegeneration with brain iron accumulation. Haematologica. 2011;96:1708–171.

Almannai M, Alasmari A, Alqasmi A, Faqeih E, Al Mutairi F, Alotaibi M, Samman MM, Eyaid W, Aljadhai YI, Shamseldin HE, Craigen W, Alkuraya FS. Expanding the phenotype of SLC25A42-associated mitochondrial encephalomyopathy. Clin Genet. 2018 May;93(5):1097–102.

Berti CC, Dallabona C, Lazzaretti M, Dusi S, Tosi E, Tiranti V, Goffrini P. Modeling human Coenzyme A synthase mutation in yeast reveals altered mitochondrial function, lipid content and iron metabolism. Microb Cell. 2015;2(4):126–35.

Brunetti D, Dusi S, Morbin M, Uggetti A, Moda F, D'Amato I, Giordano C, d'Amati G, Cozzi A, Levi S, Hayflick S, Tiranti V. Pantothenate kinase-associated neurodegeneration: altered mitochondria membrane potential and defective respiration in Pank2 knock-out mouse model. Hum Mol Genet. 2012;21(24):5294–305.

Christensen M, Duno M, Lund AM, Skovby F, Christensen E. Xanthurenic aciduria due to a mutation in KYNU encoding kynureninase. J Inherit Metab Dis. 2007;30:248–55.

Hershkovitz E, Arafat M, Loewenthal N, Haim A, Parvari R. Combined adrenal failure and testicular adrenal rest tumor in a patient with nicotinamide nucleotide transhydrogenase deficiency. J Pediat Endocr Metab. 2015;28:1187–90.

Hogarth P, Kurian MA, Gregory A, Csányi B, Zagustin T, Kmiec T, Wood P, Klucken A, Scalise N, Sofia F, Klopstock T, Zorzi G, Nardocci N, Hayflick SJ. Consensus clinical management guideline for pantothenate kinase-associated neurodegeneration (PKAN). Mol Genet Metab. 2017;120:278–87.

Houten SM, Denis S, Te Brinke H, Jongejan A, van Kampen AH, Bradley EJ, Baas F, Hennekam RC, Millington DS, Young SP, Frazier DM, Gucsavas-Calikoglu M, Wanders RJ. Mitochondrial NADP(H) deficiency due to a mutation in NADK2 causes dienoyl-CoA reductase deficiency with hyperlysinemia. Hum Mol Genet. 2014;23(18):5009–16.

Iuso A, Alhaddad B, Weigel C, Kotzaeridou U, Mastantuono E, Schwarzmayr T, Graf E, Terrile C, Prokisch H, Strom TM, Hoffmann GF, Meitinger T, Haack TB. A homozygous splice site mutation in SLC25A42, encoding the mitochondrial transporter of Coenzyme A, causes metabolic crises and epileptic encephalopathy. JIMD Rep. 2019;44:1–7.

Iuso A, Wiersma M, Schüller HJ, Pode-Shakked B, Marek-Yagel D, Grigat M, Schwarzmayr T, Berutti R, Alhaddad B, Kanon B, Grzeschik NA, Okun JG, Perles Z, Salem Y, Barel O, Vardi A, Rubinshtein M, Tirosh T, Dubnov-Raz G, Messias AC, Terrile C, Barshack I, Volkov A, Avivi C, Eyal E, Mastantuono E, Kumbar M, Abudi S, Braunisch M, Strom TM, Meitinger T, Hoffmann GF, Prokisch H, Haack TB, BJJM B, Haas D, OCM S, Anikster Y. Mutations in PPCS, encoding phosphopantothenoylcysteine synthetase, cause autosomal-recessive dilated cardiomyopathy. Am J Hum Genet. 2018;102(6):1018–30.

Kleta R, Romeo E, Ristic Z, Ohura T, Stuart C, Arcos-Burgos M, Dave MH, Wagner CA, Camargo SR, Inoue S, Matsuura N, Helip-Wooley A, Bockenhauer D, Warth R, Bernardini I, Visser G, Eggermann T, Lee P, Chairoungdua A, Jutabha P, Babu E, Nilwarangkoon S, Anzai N, Kanai Y, Verrey F, Gahl WA, Koizumi A. Mutations in SLC6A19, encoding B0AT1, cause Hartnup disorder. Nat Genet. 2004;36(9):999–1002.

Klopstock T, Tricta F, Neumayr L, Karin I, Zorzi G, Fradette C, Kmieć T, Büchner B, Steele HE, Horvath R, Chinnery PF, Basu A, Küpper C, Neuhofer C, Kálmán B, Dušek P, Yapici Z, Wilson I, Zhao F, Zibordi F, Nardocci N, Aguilar C, Hayflick SJ, Spino M, Blamire AM, Hogarth P, Vichinsky E. Safety and efficacy of deferiprone for pantothenate kinase-associated neurodegeneration: a randomised, double-blind, controlled trial and an open-label extension study. Lancet Neurol. 2019;18(7):631–42.

Koenekoop RK, Wang H, Majewski J, Wang X, Lopez I, Ren H, Chen Y, Li Y, Fishman GA, Genead M, Schwartzentruber J, Solanki N, Traboulsi EI, Cheng J, Logan CV, McKibbin M, Hayward BE, Parry DA, Johnson CA, Nageeb M, Finding of Rare Disease Genes (FORGE) Canada Consortium, Poulter JA, Mohamed MD, Jafri H, Rashid Y, Taylor GR, Keser V, Mardon G, Xu H, Inglehearn CF, Fu Q, Toomes C, Chen R. Mutations in NMNAT1 cause Leber congenital amaurosis and identify a new disease pathway for retinal degeneration. Nat Genet. 2012;44(9):1035–9.

Kremer LS, Danhauser K, Herebian D, Petkovic Ramadža D, Piekutowska-Abramczuk D, Seibt A, Müller-Felber W, Haack TB, Płoski R, Lohmeier K, Schneider D, Klee D, Rokicki D, Mayatepek E, Strom TM, Meitinger T, Klopstock T, Pronicka E, Mayr JA, Baric I, Distelmaier F, Prokisch H. NAXE mutations disrupt the cellular NAD(P)HX repair system and cause a lethal neurometabolic disorder of early childhood. Am J Hum Genet. 2016;99(4):894–902.

Kurian MA, Hayflick SJ. Pantothenate kinase-associated neurodegeneration (PKAN) and PLA2G6-associated neurodegeneration (PLAN): review of two major neurodegeneration with brain iron accumulation (NBIA) phenotypes. Int Rev Neurobiol. 2013;110:49–71.

Meimaridou E, Kowalczyk J, Guasti L, Hughes CR, Wagner F, Frommolt P, Nurnberg P, Mann NP, Banerjee R, Saka HN, Chapple JP, King PJ, Clark AJL, Metherell LA. Mutations in NNT encoding nicotinamide nucleotide transhydrogenase cause familial glucocorticoid deficiency. Nature Genet. 2012;44:740–2.

Ohashi K, Kawai S, Murata K. Identification and characterization of a human mitochondrial NAD kinase. Nat Commun. 2012;3:1248.

Orellana DI, Santambrogio P, Rubio A, Yekhlef L, Cancellieri C, Dusi S, Giannelli SG, Venco P, Mazzara PG, Cozzi A, Ferrari M, Garavaglia B, Taverna S, Tiranti V, Broccoli V, Levi S. Coenzyme a corrects pathological defects in human neurons of PANK2-associated neurodegeneration. EMBO Mol Med. 2016;8(10):1197–211.

Pomerantz DJ, Ferdinandusse S, Cogan J, Cooper DN, Reimschisel T, Robertson A, Bican A, McGregor T, Gauthier J, Millington DS, Andrae JLW, Tschannen MR, Helbling DC, Demos WM, Denis S, Wanders RJA, Newman JN, Hamid R, Phillips JA 3rd, Collaborators of UDN. Clinical heterogeneity of mitochondrial NAD kinase deficiency caused by a NADK2 start loss variant. Am J Med Genet A. 2018;176(3):692–8.

Roucher-Boulez F, Mallet-Motak D, Samara-Boustani D, Jilani H, Ladjouze A, Souchon P-F, Simon D, Nivot S, Heinrichs C, Ronze M, Bertagna X, Groisne L, Leheup B, Naud-Saudreau C, Blondin G, Lefevre C, Lemarchand L, Morel Y. NNT mutations: a cause of primary adrenal insufficiency, oxidative stress and extra-adrenal defects. Europ J Endocr. 2016;175:73–84.

Shamseldin HE, Smith LL, Kentab A, Alkhalidi H, Summers B, Alsedairy H, Xiong Y, Gupta VA, Alkuraya FS. Mutation of the mitochondrial carrier SLC25A42 causes a novel form of mitochondrial myopathy in humans. Hum Genet. 2016;135(1):21–30.

Shi H, Enriquez A, Rapadas M, Martin EMMA, Wang R, Moreau J, Lim CK, Szot JO, Ip E, Hughes JN, Sugimoto K, Humphreys DT, et al. NAD deficiency, congenital malformations, and niacin supplementation. N Engl J Med. 2017;377:544–52.

Tort F, Ugarteburu O, Torres MA, García-Villoria J, Girós M, Ruiz A, Ribes A. Lysine restriction and pyridoxal phosphate administration in a NADK2 patient. Pediatrics. 2016;138(5):e20154534.

Van Bergen NJ, Guo Y, Rankin J, Paczia N, Becker-Kettern J, Kremer LS, Pyle A, Conrotte JF, Ellaway C, Procopis P, Prelog K, Homfray T, Baptista J, Baple E, Wakeling M, Massey S, Kay DP, Shukla A, Girisha KM, LES L, Santra S, Power R, Daubeney P, Montoya J,

Ruiz-Pesini E, Kovacs-Nagy R, Pritsch M, Ahting U, Thorburn DR, Prokisch H, Taylor RW, Christodoulou J, Linster CL, Ellard S, Hakonarson H. NAD(P)HX dehydratase (NAXD) deficiency: a novel neurodegenerative disorder exacerbated by febrile illnesses. Brain. 2019;142(1):50–8.

Weinberg-Shukron A, Abu-Libdeh A, Zhadeh F, Carmel L, Kogot-Levin A, Kamal L, Kanaan M, Zeligson S, Renbaum P, Levy-Lahad E, Zangen D. Combined mineralocorticoid and glucocorticoid deficiency is caused by a novel founder nicotinamide nucleotide transhydrogenase mutation that alters mitochondrial morphology and increases oxidative stress. J Med Genet. 2015;52:636–41.

Yamaguchi R, Kato F, Hasegawa T, Katsumata N, Fukami M, Matsui T, Nagasaki K, Ogata T. A novel homozygous mutation of the nicotinamide nucleotide transhydrogenase gene in a Japanese patient with familial glucocorticoid deficiency. Endocr J. 2013;60:855–9.

Zhang X, Kurnasov OV, Karthikeyan S, Grishin NV, Osterman AL, Zhang H. Structural characterization of a human cytosolic NMN/NaMN adenylyltransferase and implication in human NAD biosynthesis. J Biol Chem. 2003;278(15):13503–11.

Zieger B, Ware J. Cloning and deduced amino acid sequence of human nicotinamide nucleotide transhydrogenase. DNA Seq. 1997;7(6):369–73.

Zorzi G, Zibordi F, Chiapparini L, Bertini E, Russo L, Piga A, Longo F, Garavaglia B, Aquino D, Savoiardo M, Solari A, Nardocci N. Iron-related MRI images in patients with pantothenate kinase-associated neurodegeneration (PKAN) treated with deferiprone: results of a phase II pilot trial. Mov Disord. 2011;26:1756–9.

# Vitamin $B_6$-Dependent and Vitamin $B_6$-Responsive Disorders

34

Barbara Plecko and Eduard A. Struys

## Contents



**Summary**

The importance of vitamin $B_6$ is evident by its role as the most abundant cofactor in human metabolism. A total of six different $B_6$ vitamers follow a complex pathway of absorption and transformation into the final active cofactor, pyridoxal 5′-phosphate (PLP), which catalyses over 100 reactions, mainly in amino acid and neurotransmitter metabolism. Over recent years, a number of genetic defects have been identified as the underlying cause of vitamin $B_6$-dependent epilepsies that need to be considered particularly in therapy-resistant seizures of unclear aetiology in the neonatal period, but also later in life. With diagnostic delay, these disorders can be fatal or may lead to irreversible brain damage. A standardised vitamin $B_6$ trial should be part of a protocol for neonatal seizures in every institution caring for the critically ill newborn. The underlying mechanisms of vitamin $B_6$-dependent epilepsies can be assigned to either reduced synthesis and recycling of PLP (pyridox(am)ine 5′-phosphate oxidase (PNPO) deficiency), reduced cellular uptake (congenital hypophosphatasia, HPP), inactivation of PLP by accumulating compounds (antiquitin deficiency and hyperprolinaemia type II) or disturbed intracellular PLP homeostasis (PLP-binding protein (formerly PROSC) deficiency). The disorders can be distinguished by specific biomarkers in urine, plasma or CSF and confirmed by molecular testing. Affected patients need a lifelong oral treatment with pyridoxine or pyridoxal 5′-phosphate,

B. Plecko (✉)
Department of Pediatrics and Adolescent Medicine, Division of General Pediatrics, Medical University of Graz, Graz, Austria
e-mail: barbara.plecko@medunigraz.at

E. A. Struys
Metabolic Unit, Clinical Chemistry, VUmc Medical Center, Amsterdam, The Netherlands
e-mail: e.struys@vumc.nl


N. Blau et al. (eds.), *Physician's Guide to the Diagnosis, Treatment, and Follow-Up of Inherited Metabolic Diseases*,
https://doi.org/10.1007/978-3-030-67727-5_34

and withdrawal will inevitably lead to seizure recurrence. Pyridoxine has less severe potential side effects compared to PLP and should be the preferred vitamer wherever possible. Add-on of folinic acid may be considered in case of partial response to pyridoxine or PLP. Lysine-restricted diet and high-dose arginine supplementation are being evaluated as add-on therapy in patients with ATQ deficiency. Due to autosomal recessive inheritance, recurrence risk for all disorders discussed here is 25% and intrauterine treatment with vitamin $B_6$ from early pregnancy may be considered in forthcoming pregnancies. Prenatal testing is available by molecular analysis.

## Introduction

Vitamin $B_6$ is a water-soluble vitamin derived from various animal and plant food sources as well as intestinal bacterial flora in six different vitamers: pyridoxal, pyridoxine-glucoside, pyridoxamine and their 5′-phosphorylated esters. Pyridoxal 5′-phosphate is the only active cofactor and catalyses over 140 enzymatic reactions, mainly in amino acid metabolism (e.g. the glycine cleavage system, serine dehydratase, threonine dehydratase) as well as in neurotransmitter metabolism (e.g. GABA formation by glutamate decarboxylase; aromatic acid decarboxylase/AADC). The demand of vitamin $B_6$ is 0.1–0.3 mg/day during infancy and around 1.2–1.4 mg/day in adulthood. As cellular uptake and transport across the blood-brain barrier is only possible for free bases of vitamin $B_6$, phosphorylated vitamers undergo hydrolysation by intestinal phosphatases and tissue non-specific alkaline phosphatase (TNSALP), respectively (Fig. 34.1). The latter is attached to the cellular membrane by a PIGV anchor system. Within cells pyridoxine, pyridoxamine and pyridoxal undergo rephosphorylation by pyridoxal kinase with consecutive oxidation of pyridoxine 5′-phosphate and pyridoxamine 5′-phosphate into pyridoxal 5′-phosphate (PLP) by flavin mononucleotide-dependent pyridox(am)ine 5′-phosphate oxidase (PNPO), which can also recycle pyridoxamine monophosphate back to PLP (salvage pathway). Though the liver seems to play an important role in the formation of PLP, expression of PNPO has also been shown in human intestinal and muscle cells, as well as in neurons. Enzymes involved in PLP synthesis are regulated by a feedback mechanism to avoid toxic PLP concentrations. Recently the PLP-binding protein (PLPBP, formerly named PROSC) has been shown to be crucial for intracellular PLP homeostasis (Fig. 34.1).

The role of vitamin $B_6$ in epileptogenesis has been well recognised by the occurrence of seizures in nutritional deficiency as well as in genetic disorders. Nutritional vitamin $B_6$ deficiency is rare nowadays, eventually seen in children with severe chronic disease or on high dosages of the tuberculostatic isoniazid and cured by adequate vitamin supply.

In contrast, genetically determined vitamin $B_6$-dependent epilepsies are caused by inborn errors of metabolism that lead to reduced PLP availability (Wilson et al. 2019, Clayton 2006). To date, five different disorders are known that can be assigned to four different mechanisms:

- Reduced synthesis and recycling of PLP (pyridox(am)ine 5′-phosphate oxidase (PNPO) deficiency), MIM#610090
- Reduced cellular uptake of PLP (congenital hypophosphatasia, HPP, MIM#241500)
- Inactivation of PLP by accumulating compounds (antiquitin deficiency, MIM#266100 and hyperprolinaemia type II, MIM#239500)
- Disturbed intracellular PLP homeostasis (PLP-binding protein (PLPBP, formerly PROSC) deficiency, MIM#617290)

Seizures with resistance to common anticonvulsants occur as a consequence of imbalance in PLP-dependent neurotransmitter—as well as in cerebral amino acid metabolism. Prematurity, poor adaptation, abdominal distension, lactic acidosis and hypoglycaemia have been described as confounding factors in severe manifestations of PNPO, ATQ as well as PLPBP deficiency (Wilson et al. 2019). A standardised vitamin $B_6$ trial with the administration of 100 mg of pyridoxine i.v. followed by a 3-day trial with pyridoxine, 30 mg/kg/day in two single dosages is recommended for every neonate with therapy-resistant seizures of unclear aetiology. Specific biomarkers serve in the differentiation of these disorders and complement the diagnostic value of a vitamin $B_6$ trial. A variety of secondary biochemical findings has been described in patients with vitamin $B_6$-dependent epilepsies. These include lactic acidosis, elevated threonine and glycine in plasma or CSF and abnormal metabolites of biogenic amines in CSF, as low homovanillic acid, low hydroxyindoleacetic acid, increased 3-methoxytyrosine and high vanillactate in urine. These secondary findings are all explained by impaired function of PLP-dependent enzymes in amino acid or neurotransmitter metabolism. They are nevertheless inconsistent and non-specific and may be found in all circumstances of (cerebral) PLP depletion. While administration of PLP would serve all five disorders, pyridoxine is ineffective in most cases of classical PNPO deficiency as well as in severe PLPBP deficiency. In case of a positive treatment effect, pyridoxine or PLP therapy should be continued until results of biochemical and molecular testing are available.

Due to recent reports on attenuated phenotypes, administration of vitamin $B_6$ should also be considered in older patients with therapy-resistant epilepsy.

## Antiquitin (ATQ) Deficiency

ATQ deficiency is the most prevalent form of pyridoxine-dependent epilepsy (PDE) and has an estimated incidence of 1:64.000 (Coughlin II et al. 2019). Patients with ATQ deficiency usually present with seizures soon after birth (Gospe 2017, Stockler et al. 2011). Seizures are myoclonic, tonic or clonic with variable EEG patterns (Schmitt et al. 2010). Cranial imaging may be normal or may show some grey and white matter atrophy, hydrocephalus, thin corpus callosum mega cisterna magna and also cortical dysplasia (Toldo et al. 2018). Seizures are typically refractory to common anticonvulsants with a high tendency towards status epilepticus (SE). Partial response to phenobarbitone is possible. About 30% of PDE patients suffer from birth asphyxia or may have signs of encephalopathy. Abdominal distension with bile-stained vomiting, elevated lactate or hypoglycaemia may be confusing confounders. Atypical presentations with onset of seizures beyond infancy, initial response to common anticonvulsants or response to extremely low dose of pyridoxine have been observed (van Karnebeek et al. 2016, Srinivasaraghavan et al. 2018).

The *antiquitin* gene is located on 5q31 and encodes alpha-aminoadipic semialdehyde dehydrogenase, an enzyme involved in the L-lysine degradation pathway (Figs. 34.2, 34.3, 34.4 and 34.5). The accumulating compound alpha-aminoadipic semialdehyde (AASA) is in equilibrium with L-$\Delta^1$-piperideine-6-carboxylate (P6C). The latter inactivates pyridoxal 5′-phosphate by a so-called Knoevenagel condensation, leading to profound cerebral PLP deficiency (Mills et al. 2006, Footitt et al. 2011). Elevated AASA in urine serves as a specific biomarker for ATQ deficiency (Table 34.1), though it may also be elevated in molybdenum cofactor—or sulfite oxidase deficiency due to secondary inhibition of antiquitin by accumulating sulfite (Struys et al. 2012a, b). Pipecolic acid (PA) is an unspecific biomarker for ATQ deficiency and is found elevated in urine, plasma and CSF prior to pyridoxine treatment (Plecko et al. 2000, 2007), while urinary levels always normalise, and also plasma levels may normalise on pyridoxine therapy. 6-Oxo-pipecolate (6-oxo-PIP) was described as a potential novel biomarker in plasma, urine and CSF of four patients with ATQ deficiency, with stability at room temperature and measured by LC-MS/MS, but warrants confirmation in larger cohorts (Wempe et al. 2019). Recent labelled isotope studies in cultured human brain cells (Crowther et al. 2019) support data from studies in human fibroblast (Struys et al. 2014) and mice (Pena et al. 2017a, b) that PA is built via the saccharopine pathway by conversion of P6C. Diagnosis is confirmed by molecular analysis of the *ALDH7A1* gene also known as antiquitin, and to date a total of 165 different mutations have been described (Coughlin II et al. 2019).

In 2009, folinic acid-responsive seizures were found to be allelic to antiquitin deficiency (Gallagher et al. 2009). The effect may rely on overlapping cofactor functions of folinic acid and PLP. Add-on of folinic acid, 3–5 mg/kg/day, may be considered, if the initial response to pyridoxine is limited. Inheritance of ATQ deficiency is autosomal recessive with a 25% recurrence risk in forthcoming pregnancies. Patients, who never received pyridoxine experience high mortality, as shown by a considerable rate of deceased siblings diagnosed retrospectively as well as some patients who had been on folinic acid monotherapy. Outcome of patients with ATQ deficiency treated with pyridoxine is variable, and about 70% have some degree of cognitive impairment (Plecko et al. 2007; Mills et al. 2010; Bok et al. 2012). Normal IQ has been described in single patients despite prolonged status epilepticus (Kluger et al. 2008).

## Hyperprolinaemia Type II (HP II)

This inborn error has first been described in Irish travellers, with primary generalised seizures in late infancy or childhood in 50% of affected individuals. Mental retardation may be present, but several individuals were reported with normal school performance (Flynn et al. 1989). A recent series reported on additional anxiety problems and hallucinations (van de Ven et al. 2014). In many patients, seizures are triggered by fever, are relatively benign and can be controlled by common anticonvulsants. Thus, several patients with this autosomal recessive disorder may remain undiagnosed.

HP II is caused by defective $\Delta^1$-pyrroline 5-carboxylate dehydrogenase, leading to increased utilisation of PLP. In analogy to the pathophysiologic mechanism in ATQ deficiency, L-D1-pyrroline-5-carboxylate (P5C) inactivates PLP by a Knoevenagel condensation (Farrant et al. 2001). Patients show high proline on plasma amino acid analysis as well as elevated P5C in urine, plasma and CSF (Fig. 34.6).

## Pyridoxal 5′- Phosphate (PLP)-Dependent Epilepsy (PNPO) Deficiency

Pyridoxal 5′-phosphate-dependent seizures were first described in 2002 (Kuo and Wang 2002). The clinical presentation is indistinguishable from ATQ deficiency except for a higher rate of prematurity seen in about 60% of cases

(Mills et al. 2005; Levtova et al. 2015). Again, about a third of patients have perinatal distress with low APGAR scores, requiring primary intubation in some. Patients typically present with neonatal myoclonic seizures up to 2 weeks of age, sometimes accompanied by roving eye movements and most often severely abnormal EEG (Mills et al. 2005; Hoffmann et al. 2007). One patient has been reported with infantile spasms, presenting at age 5 months (Mills et al. 2014). Recently, a patient with PNPO deficiency was reported with seizures that could initially be controlled by common anticonvulsants over a period of 3 years (Xue et al. 2017). Cranial imaging may be normal or show marked white matter changes. Patients with PNPO deficiency may suffer from anaemia, coagulopathy, renal dysfunction as well as failure to thrive. This broader range of symptoms and very high mortality rate in untreated patients is explained by systemic PLP deficiency. Many patients have deceased siblings with a history of neonatal epileptic encephalopathy and burst suppression EEG, falsely assigned to Ohtahara syndrome. Prognosis of patients with PNPO deficiency relies on early initiation of specific treatment and may result in normal outcome (Porri et al. 2014; Hatch et al. 2016). Seizures and EEG changes respond to pyridoxal 5′-phosphate (PLP) within hours or days. While first patients identified with classical PNPO deficiency had seizures that were resistant to pyridoxine, it became apparent that a subgroup of patients with PNPO mutations allowing residual enzyme activity may respond to pyridoxine and paradoxically have worsening of seizures upon PLP administration (Plecko et al. 2014; Mills et al. 2014).

Pyridoxal 5′-phosphate-dependent epilepsy is caused by autosomal recessive mutations in the *PNPO* gene (Mills et al. 2005). *PNPO* encodes pyridox(am)ine 5′-phosphate oxidase, an enzyme needed for the oxidation of pyridoxine and pyridoxamine into the only active vitamin $B_6$ cofactor, which is pyridoxal 5′-phosphate (PLP). This enzyme is expressed in all human cell types and, aside from PLP synthesis, is involved in the recycling of pyridoxamine monophosphate back to PLP (salvage pathway) as well as PLP trafficking within the cell.

Elevated pyridoxamine (Footitt et al. 2013; Ware et al. 2014) and, even more specific, an elevated pyridoxamine to pyridoxic acid ratio in plasma (and CSF) serve as reliable biomarkers for PNPO deficiency and can be determined while on treatment (Mathis et al. 2016). Elevated plasma glycine, threonine, elevated urinary vanillactate as well as abnormal biogenic amines are inconsistent secondary findings. Glycine elevation can be marked and may mislead clinicians to consider non-ketotic hypoglycaemia instead of going for a vitamin $B_6$ trial. Recently an LC-MS/MS-based assay for the measurement of PNPO activity in dried blood spots has been developed (Wilson et al. 2019).

Diagnosis has to be confirmed by molecular analysis of the *PNPO* gene; prenatal diagnosis is possible. Twenty seven different mutations have been identified to date (Wilson et al. 2019).

## Congenital Hypophosphatasia

The main impact of congenital hypophosphatasia is poor bone mineralisation and early death due to respiratory insufficiency. Only patients with the severe, congenital, autosomal recessive form of this disease may present with therapy-resistant seizures from birth, even before skeletal signs become more prominent (Balasubramaniam et al. 2010, Baumgartner-Sigl et al. 2007). EEG is usually severely abnormal and may show a burst suppression pattern. While seizures are resistant to common anticonvulsants, a favourable response to oral or i.v. administration of pyridoxine has been reported in single cases (Nunes et al. 2002, Baumgartner-Sigl et al. 2007) while in other seizures were resistant to pyridoxine and the encephalopathy was fatal (de Roo et al. 2014). The recently licensed enzyme replacement therapy (ERT) is considered unlikely to alter CNS involvement, as ERT does not cross the blood-brain barrier.

The diagnostic hallmark of congenital hypophosphatasia is a markedly decreased concentration of alkaline phosphatase in plasma, while decreased phosphate and elevated calcium concentrations can be inconsistent. Tissue non-specific alkaline phosphatase (TNSALP) is a multifunctional enzyme that processes three substrates, namely, inorganic pyrophosphate, phosphoethanolamine and PLP for cellular uptake.

With respect to seizure aetiology, impaired TNSALP function leads to reduced intracellular availability of PLP, while plasma levels of PLP are (extremely) high. To date it is not well understood why patients do not show signs of systemic PLP deficiency, if there is toxicity of high extracellular PLP concentrations or if other mechanisms as morphologic changes in neurons as observed in a knock-out mouse model (Sebastián-Serrano et al. 2016) may contribute to human disease. Diagnosis is confirmed by molecular analysis of the *ALPL* gene.

## Pyridoxal-Binding Protein (PLPBP) Formerly PROSC Deficiency

With the application of a standardised vitamin trial and new techniques in genetic testing, another genetic defect causing vitamin $B_6$-dependent epilepsy has been unravelled by Darin et al. in 2016 in seven patients of four families. To date a total of 15 patients with PLPBP deficiency have been described (Darin et al. 2016, Plecko et al. 2017, Shiraku et al. 2018), all presenting with seizures from birth to 3 months of age. There is overlap with ATQ and PNPO deficiency according to seizure type as well as accompanying signs of prematurity or foetal distress, but within the cohort of PLPBP deficiency, four patients had microcephaly at birth and another four developed acquired microcephaly during the course of disease. Seven patients had a burst suppression pattern on EEG, while the remainder had diffuse slowing or (multi)focal discharges. Cranial MRI was normal in eight cases and in all other cases showed broad gyri, shallow sulcy, abnormal white matter and eventually also periventricular cysts. Ten patients were treated with pyridoxine, while five were receiving PLP at dosages ranging from a total of 100 mg to 450 mg/day. Nine were seizure-free aside from febrile breakthrough seizures, but only five patients were on vitamin $B_6$ monotherapy. Thirteen patients have intellectual impairment of variable degree, some of them with considerable delay of first vitamin $B_6$ administration.

In contrast to the aforementioned entities, PLPBP deficiency does not have a specific biomarker. Low PLP concentrations were found in CSF as unspecific clues to vitamin $B_6$-dependent epilepsies, but alterations of amino acids and biogenic amines were inconsistent.

*PLPBP* encodes for a protein with non-enzymatic function. It is most likely a key regulator of intracellular PLP homeostasis and important in protecting PLP from intracellular inactivation by phosphatases.

Diagnosis of PLPBP deficiency relies on genetic testing, either by gene panels for epileptic encephalopathies or by next-generation sequencing. A positive vitamin $B_6$ response to either pyridoxine or PLP but normal biomarkers for ATQ-PNPO as well as TNSALP deficiency may suggest PLPBP deficiency. So far a total of 14 pathogenic variants in PLPBP have been identified.

## Nomenclature

| No. | Disorder | Alternative name | Abbreviation | Gene symbol | Chromosomal localisation | Mode of inheritance | Affected protein | OMIM no. |
|---|---|---|---|---|---|---|---|---|
| 34.1 | Pyridoxine-dependent epilepsy (PDE) | Alpha-amino adipic semialdehyde (AASA) dehydrogenase deficiency | AASADHD | *ALDH7A1* | 5q31 | AR | Alpha-amino adipic semialdehyde dehydrogenase | 266100 |
| 34.2 | Pyridox(am)ine 5′-phosphate oxidase deficiency | Pyridoxal 5′-phosphate (PLP)-dependent seizures | PNPOD | *PNPO* | 17q21.32 | AR | Pyridox(am)ine 5′-phosphate oxidase | 610090 |
| 34.3 | Hyperprolinaemia type II | Pyrroline-5-carboxylate dehydrogenase deficiency | P5CDH | *ALDH4A1* | 1p36.13 | AR | Pyrroline-5-carboxylate dehydrogenase | 239510 |
| 34.4 | Congenital hypophosphatasia | Phosphoethanolaminuria | HOPS | *ALPL* | 1p36.12 | AR | Alkaline phosphatase | 241500 |
| 34.5 | PLP-binding protein deficiency | (Formerly PROSC deficiency) | PLPBP | *PLPBP* | 8p11.23 | AR | PLPBP | 604430 |

## Metabolic Pathways

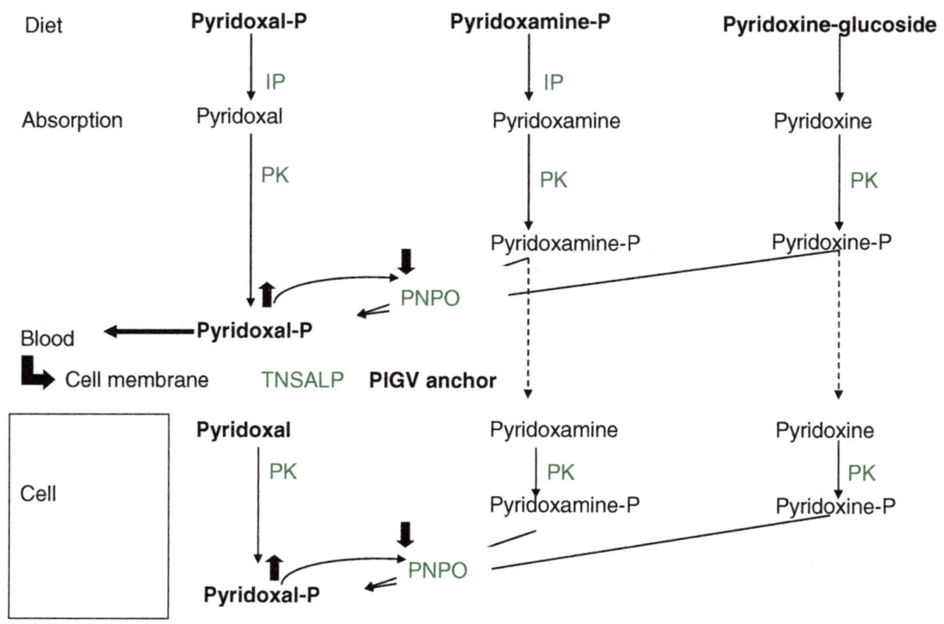


**Fig. 34.1** Vitamin $B_6$ is absorbed in different vitamers that are dephosphorylated by intestinal alkaline phosphatases (IP). In the liver they are then rephosphorylated to their 5′-phosphate esters by phosphate kinase (PK), and pyridox(am)ine is consequently converted into pyridoxal 5′-phosphate (PLP) by pyridoxamine 5′-phosphate oxidase (PNPO) and partly released into circulation. For cellular uptake or transport across the blood-brain barrier, phosphorylated vitamers (mainly PLP) are hydrolysed by tissue non-specific alkaline phosphatase (TNSALP). Within the (brain) cell, rephosphorylation of PL as the major source and oxidation of pyridox(am)ine by PNPO provides PLP as the only active cofactor for intracellular enzyme reactions. Pyridoxal 5′-phosphate exhibits feedback inhibition upon PNPO activity. PLP-binding protein (PLPBP) has a non-enzymatic function and is considered a key regulator of intracellular PLP homeostasis

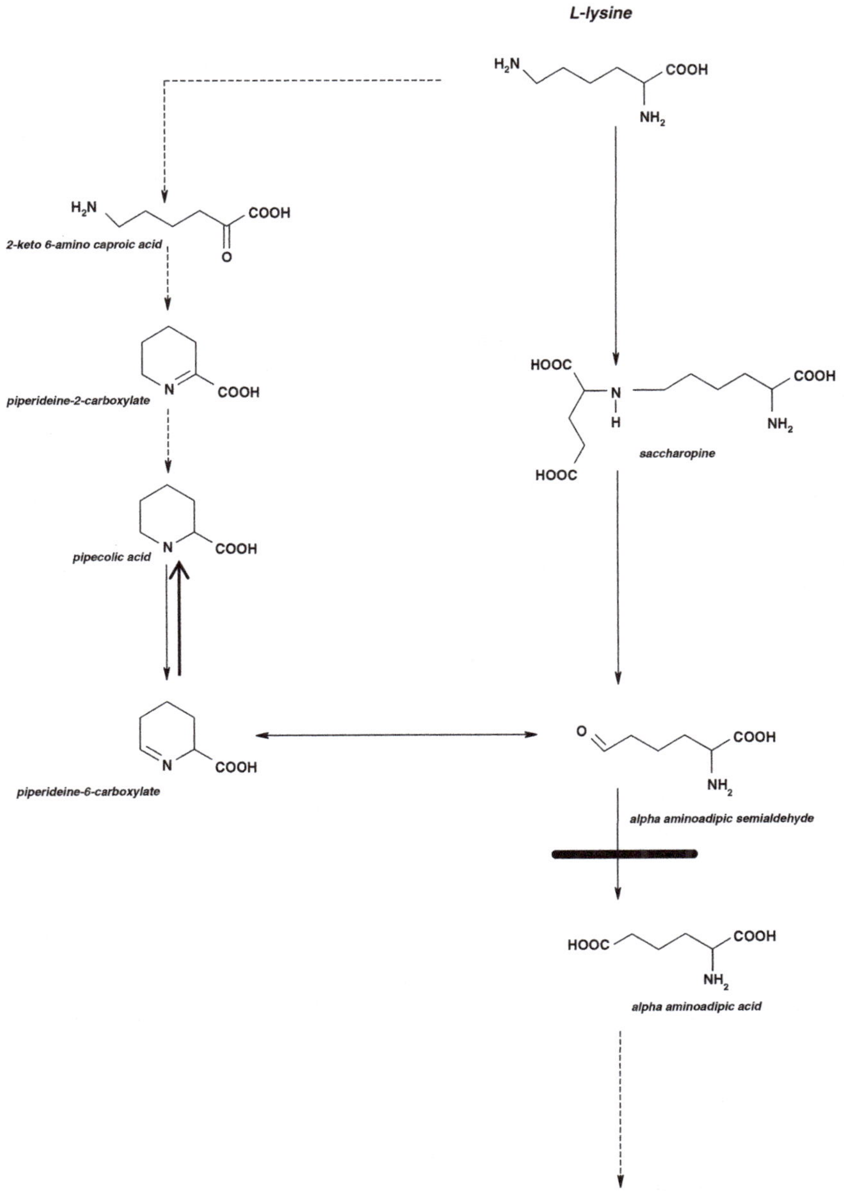


**Fig. 34.2** Lysine degradation pathway. Antiquitin deficiency leads to accumulation of alpha-aminoadipic semialdehyde and piperideine-6-carboxylate and is accompanied by elevated pipecolic acid. It is now assumed that pipecolic acid is formed via the saccharopine pathway by conversion of piperideine-6-carboxylate. Piperideine-6-carboxylate inactivates PLP by a Knoevenagel condensation, leading to cerebral PLP deficiency

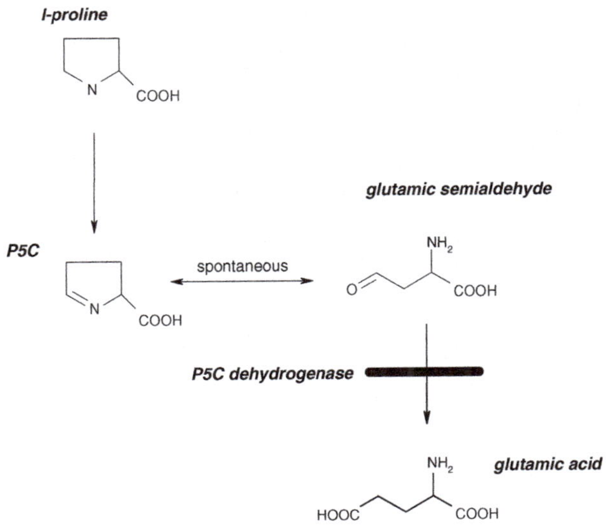


**Fig. 34.3** Catabolism of L-proline. In hyperprolinaemia type II, deficiency of $\Delta^1$-pyrroline-5-carboxylate (*P5C*) dehydrogenase leads to accumulation of glutamic acid γ semialdehyde and P5C. P5C inactivates PLP by a Knoevenagel condensation

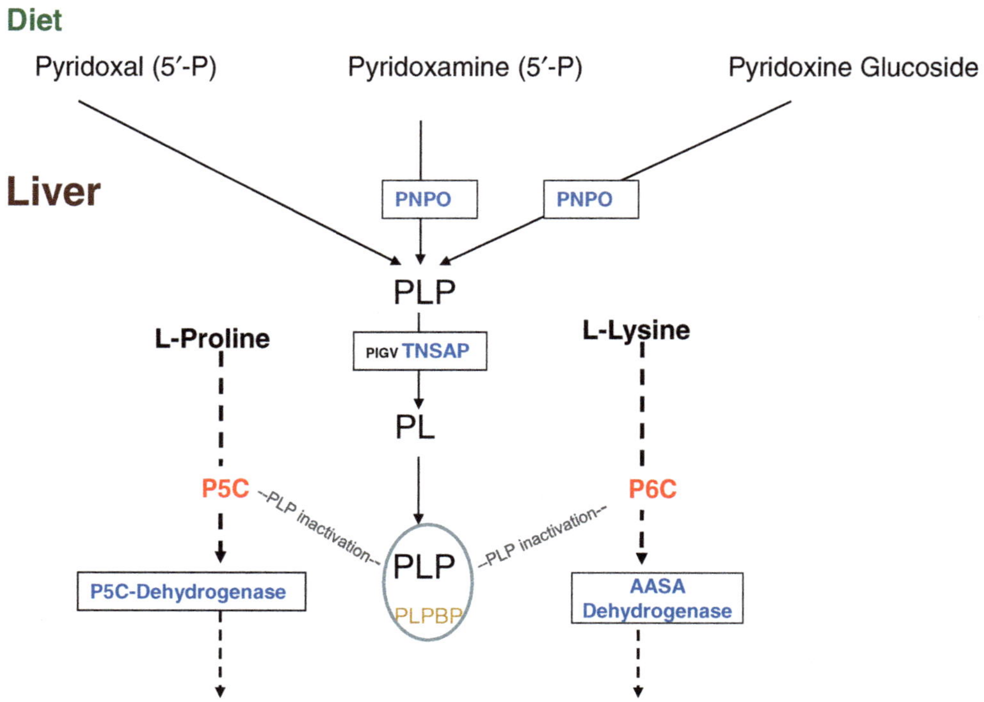


**Fig. 34.4** Scheme illustrating all five inborn errors leading to vitamin $B_6$-dependent epilepsy. Two inborn errors within vitamin $B_6$ metabolism leading to reduced synthesis of pyridoxal 5′-phosphate (*PLP*): pyridox(am)ine 5′-phosphate oxidase (*PNPO*) deficiency and tissue non-specific alkaline phosphatase (*TNSALP*) deficiency in congenital hypophosphatasia, two inborn errors leading to inactivation of PLP by a Knoevenagel condensation, hyperprolinaemia type II (P5C dehydrogenase deficiency) and antiquitin (alpha-AASA dehydrogenase) deficiency and one inborn error with impaired intracellular PLP homeostasis, PLPBP deficiency

## Signs and Symptoms

**Table 34.1** Antiquitin deficiency

| System | Symptoms and biomarkers | Neonatal (birth–1 month) | Infancy (1–18 months) | Childhood (1.5–11 years) | Adolescence (11–16 years) | Adulthood (>16 years) |
|---|---|---|---|---|---|---|
| CNS | Agenesis/hypogenesis, corpus callosum | ± | ± | ± | ± | ± |
| | Developmental delay | | ± | ± | ± | ± |
| | Hypotonia | ± | ± | ± | ± | ± |
| | Mega cisterna magna | ± | ± | ± | ± | ± |
| | **Seizures, pharmacoresistant** | +++ | ++ | ++ | | |
| Digestive | Intestinal pseudo obstruction | ± | | | | |
| | Vomiting | ± | ± | | | |
| Others | Alpha-aminosemialdehyde pre-treatment (U, P, CSF) | ↑↑↑ | ↑↑↑ | ↑↑↑ | | |
| | Alpha-aminosemialdehyde under B6 treatment (U, P, CSF) | ↑↑ | ↑(↑↑) | ↑ | ↑ | ↑ |
| | Low APGAR scores | ± | | | | |
| Laboratory findings | Glucose (P) | ↓-n | n | n | n | n |
| | Lactate (P) | n-↑ | n | n | n | n |
| | PA pretreatment (U, P, CSF) | ↑↑↑ | ↑↑↑ | ↑↑↑ | | |
| | PA under B6 treatment (CSF) | ↑↑↑ | ↑↑ | ↑ | ↑ | |
| | PA under B6 treatment (P) | ↑↑ | ↑ | ↑ | n-↑ | n-↑ |
| | PA under B6 treatment (U) | ↑↑↑ | n-↑ | n | n | n |
| | PLP (CSF) | ↓↓↓ | ↓↓↓ | | | |

**Table 34.2** Pyridox(am)ine 5′-phosphate oxidase deficiency

| System | Symptoms and biomarkers | Neonatal (birth–1 month) | Infancy (1–18 months) | Childhood (1.5–11 years) | Adolescence (11–16 years) | Adulthood (>16 years) |
|---|---|---|---|---|---|---|
| CNS | Developmental delay | ++ | +-+++ | +-+++ | | |
| | Hypotonia | ++ | ++ | ± | | |
| | **Seizures, pharmacoresistant** | +++ | ++ | ++ | | |
| Digestive | Vomiting | ± | ± | | | |
| Others | Low APGAR scores | ± | | | | |
| | Prematurity | +++ | | | | |
| Laboratory findings | 3-Methoxytyrosine (CSF) | ↑↑ | ↑↑ | | | |
| | 5-Hydroxyindoleacetic acid, 5-HIAA (CSF) | ↓ | ↓ | | | |
| | Glucose (P) | ↓-n | n | n | n | n |
| | Glycine (P) | n-↑ | n-↑ | | | |
| | Homovanillic acid, HVA (CSF) | ↓-n | ↓-n | | | |
| | Lactate (P) | n-↑ | n | n | n | n |
| | PLP (CSF) | n-↓↓ | n-↓↓ | | | |
| | Pyridoxamine /pyridoxic acid ratio | ↑↑ | ↑↑ | ↑↑ | | |
| | Threonine (CSF) | n-↑ | n-↑ | | | |
| | Threonine (P) | n-↑ | n-↑ | | | |
| | Vanillactic acid (U) | n-↑ | n-↑ | | | |

**Table 34.3** Hyperprolinaemia type II

| System | Symptoms and biomarkers | Neonatal (birth–1 month) | Infancy (1–18 months) | Childhood (1.5–11 years) | Adolescence (11–16 years) | Adulthood (>16 years) |
|---|---|---|---|---|---|---|
| CNS | Mental retardation | | ± | ± | ± | ± |
| | Seizures, febrile | | ± | ± | | |
| | Seizures, pharmacoresistant | | ± | ± | ± | ± |
| Laboratory findings | Hydroxyproline (P) | n | n | n | n | n |
| | Hydroxyproline (U) | n-↑↑↑ | n-↑↑↑ | n-↑↑↑ | n-↑↑↑ | n-↑↑↑ |
| | P5C (U) | ↑ | ↑ | ↑ | ↑ | ↑ |
| | Proline (P) | ↑-↑↑↑ | ↑-↑↑↑ | ↑-↑↑↑ | ↑-↑↑↑ | ↑-↑↑↑ |
| | Proline (U) | ↑↑↑ | ↑↑↑ | ↑↑↑ | ↑↑↑ | ↑↑↑ |

**Table 34.4** Congenital hypophosphatasia

| System | Symptoms and biomarkers | Neonatal (birth–1 month) | Infancy (1–18 months) | Childhood (1.5–11 years) | Adolescence (11–16 years) | Adulthood (>16 years) |
|---|---|---|---|---|---|---|
| CNS | Seizures | n-+++ | n-+++ | | | |
| Respiratory | Respiratory failure | ++ | ++ | + | | |
| Others | Skeletal hypomineralisation | +++ | +++ | ++ | ++ | ++ |
| Laboratory findings | Alkaline phosphatase (P) | ↓↓↓ | ↓↓↓ | ↓↓ | ↓↓ | ↓↓ |
| | Ca++ (P) | n-↑↑ | n-↑↑ | ↑↑ | ↑-↑↑ | ↑-↑↑ |
| | Phosphate (P) | n-↓↓ | n-↓↓ | ↓ | ↓ | ↓ |
| | PLP (P) | ↑↑↑ | ↑↑↑ | ↑↑ | ↑↑ | ↑↑ |

**Table 34.5** PLP-binding protein (PLPBP) – formerly PROSC deficiency

| System | Symptoms and biomarkers | Neonatal (birth–1 month) | Infancy (1–18 months) | Childhood (1.5–11 years) | Adolescence (11–16 years) | Adulthood (>16 years) |
|---|---|---|---|---|---|---|
| CNS | Seizures | +++ | n-+++ | | | |
| Skeletal | Microcephaly | n-+++ | n-+++ | n-+++ | n-+++ | n-+++ |
| Laboratory findings | Alanine (CSF) | ↑↑ | | | | |
| | Glycine (CSF) | ↑↑ | | | | |
| | Proline (CSF) | n-↑↑ | | | | |
| | Threonine (CSF) | n-↑↑ | | | | |
| | Valine (CSF) | n-↑↑ | | | | |

## Reference and Pathologic Values

Pyridoxine-dependent epilepsy reference values

| Age | Alpha-AASA (U) mmol/mol creatinine | Alpha-AASA (P, CSF) µmol/L | Pipecolic acid (P) µmol/L | Pipecolic acid (CSF) µmol/L |
|---|---|---|---|---|
| <0.5 year | <2 | <0.1 | <1 week 0.55–10.8 | All ages: 0.009–0.12 |
| >0.5 < 1 year | <1 | <0.1 | >1 week 0.54–2.46 | |
| >1 year | <0.5 | <0.1 | | |

Pathological values

| Age | Alpha-AASA (U) mmol/mol creatinine | Alpha-AASA (P, CSF) µmol/L | Pipecolic acid (P) µmol/L | Pipecolic acid (CSF) µmol/L |
|---|---|---|---|---|
| <0.5 year | >3–90 | All ages: | All ages: | All ages: |
| >0.5 < 1 year | >2–40 | 0.5–25 (P) | 2.7–18 | 1.4–14 |
| >1 year | >2–20 | 1–15 (CSF) | | |

Hyperprolinaemia type II reference values

| Proline | | Hydroxyproline | | P5C-glycine conjugate (U) |
|---|---|---|---|---|
| All ages | 50–400 (P) (µM) | All ages | Trace-90 (P) (µM) | Not detectable |
| Age | | Age | | |
| 0–6 months | Trace-190 (U) | 0–6 months | Trace-400 (U) | |
| >6 months | Trace-18 (U) | >6 months | Trace-50 (U) | |
| | | >1 year | Trace-10 (U) | |

Plasma values in µM; urinary values in mmol/mol creatinine

Pathological values

| Proline | | Hydroxyproline | | P5C-glycine conjugate (U) |
|---|---|---|---|---|
| All ages | 500–3700 (P) | All ages | 1–46 (P) | Present |
| | 2100–40,125 (U) | | 84–3769 (U) | |

Plasma values in µM; urinary values in mmol/mol creatinine

Pyridoxal 5′-phosphate (PLP)-dependent epilepsy reference values

| PLP (CSF) nM | HVA (CSF) nM | 5-HIAA (CSF) nM | 3-Methoxytyrosine (3-OMD) nM | Threonine (CSF) µM | Threonine (P) µM | VLA (U) |
|---|---|---|---|---|---|---|
| 49–89 | 300–1100 | 200–600 | <300 | 10–45 | 70–220 | Nd |

Please note that the reference values are age dependent and those depicted here of informative nature

Pathological values

| PLP (CSF) nM | HVA (CSF) nM | 5-HIAA (CSF) nM | 3-Methoxytyrosine (3-OMD) nM | Threonine (CSF) µM | Threonine (P) µM | VLA (U) |
|---|---|---|---|---|---|---|
| <20 | 150–500 | 117–193 | 885–5600 | 34–242 | 53–484 | Present |

Congenital hypophosphatasia reference values

| Serum alkaline phosphatase (I.U.) | PLP (P) nM |
|---|---|
| 80–340 | 10–100 |

Pathological values

| Serum alkaline phosphatase (I.U.) | PLP (P) nM |
|---|---|
| <30 | 200–20,000 |

## Diagnostic Flowchart

neonatal seizures of unknown etiology

↓

"resistance" to first line drug (eg. phb, benzodiazepins)

↓

save serum, urine, evt. CSF (freeze at -80°)

↓

pyridoxine, 100 mg iv. followed by 30 mg/kg/day in 2–3 SD over 1–3 days

↓

if ineffective add on of folinic acid 3–5 mg/kg/day in 1–2 SD

Switch to PLP 30 to 60 mg/kg/day in 3–4 SD over 3 days
(may need adjustment for break through seizures)

↓

if seizures stop, continue pyridoxine or PLP until results are available

**Fig. 34.5** Diagnostic algorithm for neonatal seizures

## Specimen Collection

All specific biomarkers of inborn errors leading to vitamin B$_6$-dependent epilepsy can be determined on or off pyridoxine or PLP supplementation. Urine is the best material to test for AASA. As AASA and P6C are quite unstable, samples should be frozen immediately and kept at −20 °C until analysis (Struys et al. 2012a, b). AASA and P6C may be secondarily elevated in patients with molybdenum cofactor deficiency; therefore simultaneous determination of sulfocysteine prevents diagnostic error. Cerebrospinal fluid specimens should be free of blood contamination. In those with blood contamination, a centrifugal step at low speed can be performed to pellet the erythrocytes. For measurement of pyridoxamine and pyridoxic acid, blood samples should be centrifuged immediately and plasma as well as CSF samples be protected from light and stored at −80° until analysis (Albersen et al. 2012).

## Prenatal Diagnosis

For all entities discussed in this chapter, prenatal diagnosis is feasible by molecular analysis of the respective gene in chorionic villi or amniotic fluid and should be accompanied by genetic counselling.

## DNA Testing

DNA testing for all entities discussed in this chapter is available in specialised laboratories and some commercial institutions. In antiquitin deficiency, patients may harbour deletions and may need MLPA analysis in the presence of normal sequencing of the ALDH7A1 gene.

BIOMARKERS VITAMIN B$_6$ DEPENDENT SEIZURES

| | URINE | PLASMA | CSF | Gene |
|---|---|---|---|---|
| PNPO def | (vanillactate) | pyridoxamine | | *PNPO* |
| Cong. HP | | Alk Phosph, Ca, Ph, PLP | | *ALPL* |
| ALDH7A1 | AASA, P6C (PA) | AASA, (PA) | AASA, PA | *ALDH7A1* |
| HP II | AA, P5C | AA, P5C | AA, P5C | *ALDH4A1* |

**Fig. 34.6** Selective screening for vitamin B$_6$-dependent seizures. *Plp dep. E* Pyridoxalphosphate-dependent epilepsy, *AA* Amino acids, *HP* Hypophosphatasia, *AASA* Alpha aminoadipic semialdehyde, *PA* Pipecolic acid, *L-Δ 1* Piperideine-6-carboxylate HP II hyperprolinaemia type II, *P5C Δ 1* Pyrolline-5-carboxylate. *Red ovals* mark the best biomarker/specimen for the respective entity

## Treatment

### Established Treatment Options

Figure 34.5 illustrates a standardised diagnostic and treatment algorithm that should be performed in every neonate with therapy-resistant seizures of unclear aetiology. Though the scheme suggests time lines, the duration of each individual step is at the discretion of the treating physician and should be adapted to individual scenarios. As severe apnoea may occur in responders along a first vitamin $B_6$ trial, resuscitation equipment should be at hand. In any case, determination of respective biomarkers should be performed in parallel and will help to differentiate among the different disorders. In the presence of diagnostic biomarkers, a diagnostic vitamin $B_6$ withdrawal is contraindicated. Patients with confirmed diagnoses will need a lifelong substitution with pharmacological doses of pyridoxine or PLP. While PLP is effective in all five inborn errors discussed in this chapter, pyridoxine may fail in most cases of PNPO deficiency as well as in severe PLPBP deficiency. The usual pyridoxine dose in a neonate is 100 mg i.v., followed by 30 mg/kg/day in two single i.v. or oral dosages over three consecutive days in order to also identify patients with ambiguous or delayed response. Simultaneous EEG recording with first administration is of no clear benefit (Bok et al. 2010a, b), but an EEG control should be performed at least at the end of the trial in order to verify any improvement regarding epileptic discharges or background activity. 90% of patients with ATQ deficiency will stay seizure-free on pyridoxine monotherapy, which is adapted to weight until a total daily dose of 200–300 mg of pyridoxine is reached. In case of febrile break-through seizures, the pyridoxine dose may be doubled for the first 3–5 days of future febrile illnesses. Long-term doses of pyridoxine above 200–300 mg/day should be avoided as they may lead to sensory (and at dosages above 1000 mg/day also to motor) neuropathy. Pyridoxine monotherapy should be tempted, once a clear pyridoxine effect has been observed. In case patients respond to pyridoxine, but are later identified to harbour pyridoxine-responsive PNPO mutations by molecular analysis, a switch to PLP therapy should only be performed if patients are not seizure-free and should be done at very low pace over several days, as PLP in some of these patients may aggravate seizures or even cause SE (Plecko et al. 2014).

In case pyridoxine fails, folinic acid may be added at 3–5 mg/kg/day given in two single dosages i.v. or orally, and neonates should be switched to PLP starting from 30 to 60 mg/kg/day in three to four single oral dosages. PLP is unlicensed outside of Asia and in most countries is only available as a chemical compound for oral administration. PNPO deficiency is more difficult to treat, as patients need shorter intervals with four (to six) single daily administrations and PLP dosages of 30 up to 60 mg/kg/day. Recently severe side effects of hepatopathy and liver cirrhosis were reported in single patients with PNPO deficiency under high-dose PLP treatment (Sudarsanam et al. 2014, Coman et al. 2016) so that the lowest effective dose of PLP should be used. PLP should be light protected and dissolved immediately before administration to avoid oxidation and build-up of potentially toxic compounds (Mohamed-Ahmed et al. 2017).

Recently a new subgroup of patients harbouring pyridoxine-responsive PNPO mutations has been described (Plecko et al. 2014, Mills et al. 2014). Interestingly these patients may have seizure aggravation upon PLP administration. The comparably higher incidence of antiquitin deficiency, the availability of pyridoxine as a licensed drug and the less severe side effects are in favour of pyridoxine as the first-line drug in standardised vitamin $B_6$ trials. As long-term administration of PLP has led to liver fibrosis in single patients with PNPO deficiency, pyridoxine may be the preferred vitamer wherever possible.

### Experimental Therapies

Since 2012 dietary lysine restriction and high-dose arginine supplementation have emerged as additional treatment modalities for ATQ deficiency (van Karnebeek et al. 2012, 2014; Mercimek-Mahmutoglu et al. 2014; Coughlin 2nd et al. 2015, Yuzyuk et al. 2016) and were shown to decrease concentrations of potentially neurotoxic AASA in plasma, urine and CFS in a so far limited number of patients. While dietary lysine restriction is based on reduction of precursors, arginine supplementation is acting by competitive inhibition of lysine uptake in the gut and also at the blood-brain barrier. Early initiation of lysine restriction and arginine supplementation were associated with better outcomes. Robust long-term data on cognitive outcome are pending.

Intrauterine treatment with pyridoxine, 100 mg/day given from early pregnancy, may benefit offsprings of forthcoming pregnancies that are at risk for antiquitin deficiency (Bok et al. 2010a, b). In these offsprings, molecular and biochemical confirmation should be sought immediately after birth to prevent potential neuronal pyridoxine toxicity in unaffected newborns (Hartmann et al. 2011).

The rational would also argue for administration of low-dose PLP in pregnancies at risk for PNPO deficiency, but no data have been published so far.

As PNPO is a riboflavin-dependent enzyme, mutations with residual activity may benefit from the administration of riboflavin in addition to PLP, but so far no clinical experience on this hypothesis has been reported. For congenital hypophosphatasia, recombinant enzyme replacement therapy is available but may not be effective in preventing fatal encephalopathy observed in single cases.

Very recently animal models have been established for ATQ deficiency in zebrafish (Zabinyakov et al. 2017, Pena et al. 2017a, b), PNPO deficiency in drosophila (Chi et al. 2019) as well as PLPBP deficiency in zebrafish (Johnstone et al. 2019) and will give further insight into disease mechanisms and provide opportunities for new drug discovery .

## References


Albersen M, Groenendaal F, van der Ham M, de Koning TJ, Bosma M, Visser WF, Visser G, de Sain-van der Velden MG, Verhoeven-Duif NM. Vitamin B $_6$ vitamer concentrations in cerebrospinal fluid differ between preterm and term newborn infants. Pediatrics. 2012;130(1):e191–8.

Balasubramaniam S, Bowling F, Carpenter K, Earl J, Chaitow J, Pitt J, Mornet E, Sillence D, Ellaway C. Perinatal hypophosphatasia presenting as neonatal epileptic encephalopathy with abnormal neurotransmitter metabolism secondary to reduced co-factor pyridoxal-5′-phosphate availability. J Inherit Metab Dis. 2010;33(Suppl 3):25–33.

Baumgartner-Sigl S, Haberlandt E, Mumm S, Scholl-Bürgi S, Sergi C, Ryan L, Ericson KL, Whyte MP, Högler W. Pyridoxine-responsive seizures as the first symptom of infantile hypophosphatasia caused by two novel missense mutations (c.677T>C, p.M226T; c.1112C>T, p.T371I) of the tissue-nonspecific alkaline phosphatase gene. Bone. 2007;40:1655–61.

Bok LA, Maurits NM, Willemsen MA, Jakobs C, Teune LK, Poll-The BT, de Coo IF, Toet MC, Hagebeuk EE, Brouwer OF, van der Hoeven JH, Sival DA. The EEG response to pyridoxine-IV neither identifies nor excludes pyridoxine-dependent epilepsy. Epilepsia. 2010a;51:2406–11.

Bok LA, Been JV, Struys EA, Jakobs C, Rijper EA, Willemsen MA. Antenatal treatment in two Dutch families with pyridoxine-dependent seizures. Eur J Pediatr. 2010b;169(3):297–303.

Bok LA, Halbertsma FJ, Houterman S, Wevers RA, Vreeswijk C, Jakobs C, Struys EA, Van Der Hoeven JH, Sival DA, Willemsen MA. Long-term outcome in pyridoxine-dependent epilepsy. Dev Med Child Neurol. 2012;54:849–54.

Chi W, Iyengar ASR, Albersen M, Bosma M, Verhoeven-Duif NM, Wu CF, Zhuang X. Pyridox(am)ine 5′-phosphate oxidase deficiency induces seizures in Drosophila melanogaster. Hum Mol Genet. 2019; https://doi.org/10.1093/hmg/ddz143.

Clayton PT. B6-responsive disorders: a model of vitamin dependency. J Inherit Metab Dis. 2006;29:317–26. Review

Coman D, Lewindon P, Clayton P, Riney K. PNPO deficiency and cirrhosis: expanding the clinical phenotype? JIMD Rep. 2016;25:71–5.

Coughlin CR 2nd, van Karnebeek CD, Al-Hertani W, Shuen AY, Jaggumantri S, Jack RM, Gaughan S, Burns C, Mirsky DM, Gallagher RC, Van Hove JL. Triple therapy with pyridoxine, arginine supplementation and dietary lysine restriction in pyridoxine-dependent epilepsy: neurodevelopmental outcome. Mol Genet Metab. 2015;116:35–43.

Coughlin CR II, Swanson MA, Spector E, Meeks NJL, Kronquist KE, Aslamy M, Wempe MF, van Karnebeek CDM, Gospe SM Jr, Aziz V, Tsai BP, Gao H, Nagy PL, Hyland K, van Dooren SJM, Salomons GS, Van Hove JLK. The genotypic spectrum of ALDH7A1 mutations resulting in pyridoxine dependent epilepsy: a common epileptic encephalopathy. J Inherit Metab Dis. 2019;42:353–61.

Crowther LM, Mathis D, Poms M, Plecko B. New insights into human lysine degradation pathways with relevance to pyridoxine-dependent epilepsy due to antiquitin deficiency. J Inherit Metab Dis. 2019;42:620–8.

Darin N, Reid E, Prunetti L, Samuelsson L, Husain RA, Wilson M, Prunty H, Pope S, Heales S, Lascelles K, Champion M, Wassmer E, Veggiotti P, de Crécy-Lagard V, Mills PB, Clayton PT. Mutations in PROSC disrupt cellular pyridoxal phosphate homeostasis and cause vitamin B6 dependent epilepsy. Am J Hum Genet. 2016;99:1325–37.

Farrant RD, Walker V, Mills G, Mellor JM, Langley GJ. Pyridoxal phosphate de-activation by pyrroline-5-carboxylic acid. J Biol Chem. 2001;276:15107–16.

Flynn MP, Martin MC, Moore PT, Stafford JA, Fleming GA, Phang JM. Type II hyperprolinaemia in a pedigree of Irish travellers (nomads). Arch Dis Child. 1989;64:1699–707.

Footitt EJ, Heales SJ, Mills PB, Allen GF, Oppenheim M, Clayton PT. Pyridoxal 5′-phosphate in cerebrospinal fluid; factors affecting concentration. J Inherit Metab Dis. 2011;34:529–38.

Footitt EJ, Clayton PT, Mills K, Heales SJ, Neergheen V, Oppenheim M, Mills PB. Measurement of plasma B(6) vitamer profiles in children with inborn errors of vitamin B6 metabolism using an LC-MS/MS method. J Inherit Metab Dis. 2013;36(1):139–45.

Gallagher RC, Van Hove JL, Scharer G, Hyland K, Plecko B, Waters PJ, Mercimek-Mahmutoglu S, Stockler-Ipsiroglu S, Salomons GS, Rosenberg EH, Struys EA, Jakobs C. Folinic acid-responsive seizures are caused by α-amino adipic semialdehyde dehydrogenase deficiency and are genetically identical to pyridoxine-dependent epilepsy. Ann Neurol. 2009;65:550–6.

Gospe SM. Pyridoxine-dependent epilepsy. Gene Rev. 2017. http://www.genereviews.org/.

Hartmann H, Fingerhut M, Jakobs C, Plecko B. Status epilepticus in a neonate treated with pyridoxine because of a familial recurrence risk for antiquitin deficiency: pyridoxine toxicity? Dev Med Child Neurol. 2011;53:1150–3.

Hatch J, Coman D, Clayton P, Mills P, Calvert S, Webster RI, Riney K. Normal neurodevelopmental outcomes in PNPO deficiency: a case series and literature review. JIMD Rep. 2016;26:91–7.

Hoffmann GF, Schmitt B, Windfuhr M, Wagner N, Strehl H, Bagci S, Franz AR, Mills PB, Clayton PT, Baumgartner MR, Steinmann B, Bast T, Wolf NI, Zschocke J. Pyridoxal 5′-phosphate may be curative in early-onset epileptic encephalopathy. J Inherit Metab Dis. 2007;30:96–9.

Johnstone DL, Al-Shekaili HH, Tarailo-Graovac M, Wolf NI, Ivy AS, Demarest S, Roussel Y, Ciapaite J, van Roermund CWT, Kernohan KD, Kosuta C, Ban K, Ito Y, McBride S, Al-Thihli K, Abdelrahim RA, Koul R, Al Futaisi A, Haaxma CA, Olson H, Sigurdardottir LY, Arnold GL, Gerkes EH, Boon M, Heiner-Fokkema MR, Noble S, Bosma M, Jans J, Koolen DA, Kamsteeg EJ, Drögemöller B, Ross CJ, Majewski J, Cho MT, Begtrup A, Wasserman WW, Bui T, Brimble E, Violante S, Houten SM, Wevers RA, van Faassen M, Kema IP, Lepage N, Care4Rare Canada Consortium, Lines MA, Dyment DA, Wanders RJA, Verhoeven-Duif N, Ekker M, Boycott KM, Friedman JM, Pena IA, van Karnebeek CDM. PLPHP deficiency: clinical, genetic, biochemical, and mechanistic insights. Brain. 2019;142:542–59.

Kluger G, Blank R, Paul K, Paschke E, Jansen E, Jakobs C, Wörle H, Plecko B. Pyridoxine-dependent epilepsy: normal outcome in a patient with late diagnosis after prolonged status epilepticus causing cortical blindness. Neuropediatrics. 2008;39:276–9.

Kuo MF, Wang HS. Pyridoxal phosphate-responsive epilepsy with resistance to pyridoxine. Pediatr Neurol. 2002;26:146–7.

Levtova A, Camuzeaux S, Laberge AM, Allard P, Brunel-Guitton C, Diadori P, Rossignol E, Hyland K, Clayton PT, Mills PB, Mitchell GA. Normal cerebrospinal fluid pyridoxal 5′-phosphate level in a PNPO-deficient patient with neonatal-onset epileptic encephalopathy. JIMD Rep. 2015;22:67–75.

Mathis D, Abela L, Albersen M, Bürer C, Crowther L, Beese K, Hartmann H, Bok LA, Struys E, Papuc SM, Rauch A, Hersberger M, Verhoeven-Duif NM, Plecko B. The value of plasma vitamin B6 profiles in early onset epileptic encephalopathies. J Inherit Metab Dis. 2016;39:733–41.

Mercimek-Mahmutoglu S, Cordeiro D, Cruz V, Hyland K, Struys EA, Kyriakopoulou L, Mamak E. Novel therapy for pyridoxine dependent epilepsy due to ALDH7A1 genetic defect: L-arginine supplementation alternative to lysine-restricted diet. Eur J Paediatr Neurol. 2014;18:741–6.
Mills PB, Surtees RA, Champion MP, Beesley CE, Dalton N, Scambler PJ, Heales SJ, Briddon A, Scheimberg I, Hoffmann GF, Zschocke J, Clayton PT. Neonatal epileptic encephalopathy caused by mutations in the PNPO gene encoding pyridox(am)ine 5′-phosphate oxidase. Hum Mol Genet. 2005;14:1077–86.
Mills PB, Struys EA, Jakobs C, Plecko B, Baxter P, Baumgartner M, Willemsen MA, Omran H, Tacke U, Uhlenberg B, Weschke B, Clayton PT. Mutations in the antiquitin (ALDH7A1) gene in patients with pyridoxine-dependent seizures. Nat Med. 2006;12:307–9.
Mills PB, Footitt EJ, Mills KA, Tuschl K, Aylett S, Varadkar S, Hemingway C, Marlow N, Rennie J, Baxter P, Dulac O, Nabbout R, Craigen WJ, Schmitt B, Feillet F, Christensen E, De Lonlay P, Pike MG, Hughes MI, Struys EA, Jakobs C, Zuberi SM, Clayton PT. Genotypic and phenotypic spectrum of pyridoxine-dependent epilepsy (ALDH7A1 deficiency). Brain. 2010;133:2148–59.
Mills PB, Camuzeaux SS, Footitt EJ, Mills KA, Gissen P, Fisher L, Das KB, Varadkar SM, Zuberi S, McWilliam R, Stödberg T, Plecko B, Baumgartner MR, Maier O, Calvert S, Riney K, Wolf NI, Livingston JH, Bala P, Morel CF, Feillet F, Raimondi F, Del Giudice E, Chong WK, Pitt M, Clayton PT. Epilepsy due to PNPO mutations: genotype, environment and treatment affect presentation and outcome. Brain. 2014;137:1350–60.
Mohamed-Ahmed AH, Wilson MP, Albuera M, Chen T, Mills PB, Footitt EJ, Clayton PT, Tuleu C. Quality and stability of extemporaneous pyridoxal phosphate preparations used in the treatment of paediatric epilepsy. Pharm Pharmacol. 2017;69:480–8.
Nunes ML, Mugnol F, Bica I, Fiori RM. Pyridoxine-dependent seizures associated with hypophosphatasia in a newborn. J Child Neurol. 2002;17:222–4.
Pena IA, Marques LA, Laranjeira ÂB, Yunes JA, Eberlin MN, MacKenzie A, Arruda P. Mouse lysine catabolism to aminoadipate occurs primarily through the saccharopine pathway; implications for pyridoxine dependent epilepsy (PDE). Biochim Biophys Acta Mol Basis Dis. 2017a:121–8.
Pena IA, Roussel Y, Daniel K, Mongeon K, Johnstone D, Weinschutz Mendes H, Bosma M, Saxena V, Lepage N, Chakraborty P, Dyment DA, van Karnebeek CDM, Verhoeven-Duif N, Bui TV, Boycott KM, Ekker M, MacKenzie A. Pyridoxine-dependent epilepsy in zebrafish caused by Aldh7a1 deficiency. Genetics. 2017b;207:1501–18.
Plecko B, Stöckler-Ipsiroglu S, Paschke E, Erwa W, Struys EA, Jakobs C. Pipecolic acid elevation in plasma and cerebrospinal fluid of two patients with pyridoxine-dependent epilepsy. Ann Neurol. 2000;48:121–5.
Plecko B, Paul K, Paschke E, Stoeckler-Ipsiroglu S, Struys EA, Jakobs C, Hartmann H, Luecke T, di Capua M, Korenke C, Hikel C, Reutershahn E, Freilinger M, Baumeister F, Bosch F, Erwa W. Biochemical and molecular characterization of 18 patients with pyridoxine-dependent epilepsy. Hum Mutat. 2007;28:19–26.
Plecko B, Karl P, Mills P, Clayton P, Paschke E, Maier O, Hasselmann O, Schmiedl G, Kanz S, Connolly M, Wolf N, Struys E, Stockler S, Abela L, Hofer D. Pyridoxine responsiveness in novel PNPO mutations. Neurology. 2014;82:1425–33.
Plecko B, Zweier M, Begemann A, Mathis D, Schmitt B, Striano P, Vari MS, Beccaria F, Zara F, Crowther LM, Joset P, Sticht H, Papuc SM, Rauch A. Confirmation of mutations in PROSC as a novel cause of vitamin $B_6$-dependent epilepsy. J Med Genetics. 2017;54:809–14.
Porri S, Fluss J, Plecko B, Paschke E, Korff CM, Kern I. Positive outcome following early diagnosis and treatment of pyridoxal-5′-phosphate oxidase deficiency: a case report. Neuropediatrics. 2014;45:64–8.
de Roo MGA, Abeling NGGM, Majoie CB, Bosch AM, Koelman JHTM, Cobben JM, Duran M, Poll-The BT. Infantile hypophosphatasia without bone deformities presenting with severe pyridoxine-resistant seizures. Mol Genet Metab. 2014;111:404–7.
Schmitt B, Baumgartner M, Mills PB, Clayton PT, Jakobs C, Keller E, Wohlrab G. Seizures and paroxysmal events: symptoms pointing to the diagnosis of pyridoxine-dependent epilepsy and pyridoxine phosphate oxidase deficiency. Dev Med Child Neurol. 2010;52:133–42.
Sebastián-Serrano Á, Engel T, de Diego-García L, Olivos-Oré LA, Arribas-Blázquez M, Martínez-Frailes C, Pérez-Díaz C, Millán JL, Artalejo AR, Miras-Portugal MT, Henshall DC, Díaz-Hernández M. Neurodevelopmental alterations and seizures developed by mouse model of infantile hypophosphatasia are associated with purinergic signalling deregulation. Hum Mol Genet. 2016;25:4143–56.
Shiraku H, Nakashima K, Nakajima K, Ohta M, Okanishi T, Kanai S, Fujimoto A, Saitsu H, Matsumoto N, Kato M. PLPBP mutations cause variable phenotypes of developmental and epileptic encephalopathy. Epilepsia Open. 2018;3(4):495–502.
Srinivasaraghavan R, Parameswaran N, Mathis D, Bürer C, Plecko B. Antiquitin deficiency with adolescent onset epilepsy: molecular diagnosis in a mother of affected offsprings. Neuropediatrics. 2018;49:154–7.
Stockler S, Plecko B, Gospe SM, Coulter-Mackie M, Connolly M, van Karnebeek C, Mercimek-Mahmutoglu S, Hartmann H, Scharer G, Struys E, Tein I, Jakobs C, Clayton P, Van Hove JL. Pyridoxine dependent epilepsy and antiquitin deficiency: clinical and molecular characteristics and recommendations for diagnosis, treatment and follow-up. Mol Genet Metab. 2011;104(1–2):48–60.
Struys EA, Bok LA, Emal D, Houterman S, Willemsen MA, Jakobs C. The measurement of urinary $\Delta(1)$-piperideine-6-carboxylate, the alter ego of $\alpha$-aminoadipic semialdehyde, in Antiquitin deficiency. J Inherit Metab Dis. 2012a;5:909–16.
Struys EA, Nota B, Bakkali A, Al Shahwan S, Salomons GS, Tabarki B. Pyridoxine-dependent epilepsy with elevated urinary $\alpha$-amino adipic semialdehyde in molybdenum cofactor deficiency. Pediatrics. 2012b;130:1716–9.
Struys EA, Jansen EE, Salomons GS. Human pyrroline-5-carboxylate reductase (PYCR1) acts on $\Delta(1)$-piperideine-6-carboxylate generating L-pipecolic acid. J Inherit Metab Dis. 2014;37:327–32.
Sudarsanam A, Singh H, Wilcken B, Stormon M, Arbuckle S, Schmitt B, Clayton P, Earl J, Webster R. Cirrhosis associated with pyridoxal 5′-phosphate treatment of pyridoxamine 5′-phosphate oxidase deficiency. JIMD Rep. 2014;17:67–70.
Toldo I, Bonardi CM, Bettella E, Polli R, Talenti G, Burlina A, Sartori S, Murgia A. Brain malformations associated to Aldh7a1 gene mutations: Report of a novel homozygous mutation and literature review. Eur J Paediatr Neurol. 2018;6:1042–53.
van de Ven S, Gardeitchik T, Kouwenberg D, Kluijtmans L, Wevers R, Morava E. Long-term clinical outcome, therapy and mild mitochondrial dysfunction in hyperprolinemia. J Inherit Metab Dis. 2014;37:383–90.
van Karnebeek CD, Hartmann H, Jaggumantri S, Bok LA, Cheng B, Connolly M, Coughlin CR 2nd, Das AM, Gospe SM Jr, Jakobs C, van der Lee JH, Mercimek-Mahmutoglu S, Meyer U, Struys E, Sinclair G, Van Hove J, Collet JP, Plecko BR, Stockler S. Lysine restricted diet for pyridoxine-dependent epilepsy: first evidence and future trials. Mol Genet Metab. 2012;107:335–44.
van Karnebeek CD, Stockler-Ipsiroglu S, Jaggumantri S, Assmann B, Baxter P, Buhas D, Bok LA, Cheng B, Coughlin CR 2nd, Das AM,

Giezen A, Al-Hertani W, Ho G, Meyer U, Mills P, Plecko B, Struys E, Ueda K, Albersen M, Verhoeven N, Gospe SM Jr, Gallagher RC, Van Hove JK, Hartmann H. Lysine-restricted diet as adjunct therapy for pyridoxine-dependent epilepsy: the pde consortium consensus recommendations. JIMD Rep. 2014;15:1–11.

van Karnebeek CD, Tiebout SA, Niermeijer J, Poll-The BT, Ghani A, Coughlin CR 2nd, Van Hove JL, Richter JW, Christen HJ, Gallagher R, Hartmann H, Stockler-Ipsiroglu S. Pyridoxine-dependent epilepsy: an expanding clinical spectrum. Pediatr Neurol. 2016;59:6–12.

Ware TL, Earl J, Salomons GS, Struys EA, Peters HL, Howell KB, Pitt JJ, Freeman JL. Typical and atypical phenotypes of PNPO deficiency with elevated CSF and plasma pyridoxamine on treatment. Dev Med Child Neurol. 2014;56:498–502.

Wempe MF, Kumar A, Kumar V, Choi YJ, Swanson MA, Friederich MW, Hyland K, Yue WW, Van Hove JLK, Coughlin CR 2nd. Identification of a novel biomarker for pyridoxine-dependent epilepsy: Implications for newborn screening. J Inherit Metab Dis. 2019;42:565–74.

Wilson MP, Plecko B, Mills PB, Clayton P. Disorders affecting vitamin $B_6$ metabolism. J Inherit Metab Dis. 2019;42:1–18.

Xue J, Chang X, Zhang Y, Yang Z. Novel phenotypes of pyridox(am)ine-5′-phosphate oxidase deficiency and high prevalence of c.445_448del mutation in Chinese patients. Metab Brain Dis. 2017;32:1081–7.

Yuzyuk T, Thomas A, Viau K, Liu A, De Biase I, Botto LD, Pasquali M, Longo N. Effect of dietary lysine restriction and arginine supplementation in two patients with pyridoxine-dependent epilepsy. Mol Genet Metab. 2016;118:167–72.

Zabinyakov N, Bullivant G, Cao F, Fernandez Ojeda M, Jia ZP, Wen XY, Dowling JJ, Salomons GS, Mercimek-Andrews S. Characterization of the first knock-out aldh7a1 zebrafish model for pyridoxine-dependent epilepsy using CRISPR-Cas9 technology. PLoS One. 2017;12(10):e0186645.

# Molybdenum Cofactor Disorders

# 35

Guenter Schwarz and Bernd C. Schwahn

## Contents



**Summary**

Molybdenum (Mo) cofactor deficiency (MoCD) is characterized by neonatal-onset myoclonic epileptic encephalopathy and dystonia with cerebral MRI changes similar to hypoxic-ischemic lesions. The initial presentation is unspecific, and diagnosis is often delayed owing to the absence of easily accessible specific tests. Surviving children suffer from severe static cerebral palsy characterized by myoclonus, generalized seizures, dystonic movements, spasticity, and lack of developmental progress. After the neonatal period, the diagnosis can be ascertained by recognising a typical combination of facial dysmorphism, lens dislocation, and severe atrophy and cystic transformation of the brain or by untargeted genetic testing. Attenuated and atypical cases have been described.

The molecular cause of the disease is the loss of sulfite oxidase activity, one out of four molybdenum cofactor (Moco)-dependent enzymes. The resulting accumulation of toxic sulfite causes a secondary increase of metabolites

G. Schwarz (✉)
Department of Chemistry, Center for Molecular Medicine, Institute of Biochemistry, University of Cologne, Koeln, Germany
e-mail: gschwarz@uni-koeln.de

B. C. Schwahn
Willink Metabolic Unit, Manchester Centre for Genomic Medicine, Manchester University Hospitals NHS Foundation Trust, Saint Mary's Hospital, Manchester, UK
e-mail: bernd.schwahn@mft.nhs.uk



N. Blau et al. (eds.), *Physician's Guide to the Diagnosis, Treatment, and Follow-Up of Inherited Metabolic Diseases*,
https://doi.org/10.1007/978-3-030-67727-5_35

such as S-sulfocysteine and thiosulfate as well as a decrease in L-cystine. A second important Mo-dependent enzyme is xanthine oxidoreductase which catalyzes the conversion of hypoxanthine to xanthine and further to uric acid representing the final steps in purine catabolism. Moco is synthesized by a three-step biosynthetic pathway, which involves gene products of *MOCS1*, *MOCS2*, *MOCS3*, and *GPHN*. Depending on which synthetic step is compromised, MoCD is biochemically classified as type A, B, or C. This distinction is clinically relevant for patient management because the metabolic block in MoCD type A can be circumvented by administering the product of the impaired reaction, cyclic pyranopterin monophosphate (cPMP). A substitution therapy with cPMP is highly effective in reducing sulfite toxicity and restoring the biochemical homeostasis, but the clinical outcome critically depends on the degree of brain injury prior to the start of treatment. There is currently no specific treatment for MoCD type B or MoCD type C.

## Introduction

Four molybdenum (Mo)-enzymes are known in humans, each catalyzing either catabolic or detoxifying reactions (Schwarz et al. 2009). Sulfite oxidase (SO) is localized in the intermembrane space of mitochondria and couples sulfite oxidation to the reduction of cytochrome c. The two cytosolic Mo-enzymes, xanthine oxidoreductase (XO) and aldehyde oxidase, are closely related Mo-iron-flavin enzymes catalyzing hydroxylation reactions of purines and other heterocyclic substrates, respectively (Schwarz et al. 2009). In these enzymes, Moco requires the addition of a terminal sulfido ligand, which is dependent on the Moco sulfurylase MOCOS (Ichida et al. 2001). The mitochondrial amidoxime-reducing component has been identified as a fourth vertebrate Mo-enzyme (Havemeyer et al. 2006) and reduces N-hydroxylated prodrugs as well as metabolites such as N-hydroxy-L-arginine.

Patients with isolated deficiencies in SO or xanthine oxidase (xanthinuria type I) are well-known in the field, while isolated deficiencies in aldehyde oxidase and the amidoxime-reducing component have not been reported yet. Mutations in *MOCOS* cause a deficiency of xanthine oxidase and aldehyde oxidase, named xanthinuria type II (see Sect. 35.4, Table 35.4).

### Moco Biosynthesis

Moco biosynthesis is divided into three major steps based on the two intermediates cyclic pyranopterin monophosphate (cPMP) (Santamaria-Araujo et al. 2004) and molybdopterin (MPT) (Johnson et al. 1984) (Fig. 35.1). The first step in Moco biosynthesis, the conversion of GTP into cPMP, is catalyzed by two proteins encoded by the *MOCS1* gene. *MOCS1* expression undergoes alternative splicing with two different transcripts, one bicistronic and one monocistronic mRNA (Gray and Nicholls 2000). The bicistronic transcript encodes for two open reading frames, MOCS1A and MOCS1B (Reiss et al. 1998), of which only the first is translated yielding a functional MOCS1A protein. MOCS1A catalyzes the S-adenosyl-methionine and [4Fe-4S] cluster-dependent radical conversion of GTP to 3′ 8-cyclo-7,8 dihydro GTP. The second, monocistronic transcript, produces a MOCS1AB fusion protein that is targeted (independent of MOCS1A) to mitochondria and proteolytically cleaved to release a MOCS1B protein, which converts 3′ 8-cyclo-7,8 dihydro GTP to cPMP (Mayr et al. 2020).

The second step in Moco biosynthesis is catalyzed by MPT synthase, which converts cPMP into molybdopterin (MPT) and is encoded by the bicistronic *MOCS2* gene producing both subunits (MOCS2A and MOCS2B) by a ribosomal leaky scanning mechanism (Stallmeyer et al. 1999). *MOCS3* encodes for the Moco sulfurase (Matthies et al. 2004), which is required for the ATP-dependent thiolation of MOCS2A.

The third and final step in Moco synthesis involves the synthesis of MPT-AMP and subsequent molybdate-dependent hydrolysis of MPT-AMP releasing Moco. Both reactions are dependent on the *GPHN* gene, which encodes for a multi-domain cytosolic protein composed of an N-terminal G-domain (GPHN-G), a central domain, and a C-terminal E-domain (GPHN-E, Fig. 35.1). Besides Moco biosynthesis, gephyrin functions as cytosolic membrane-associated receptor clustering protein, being essential for the formation of inhibitory synapses (Fritschy et al. 2008).

### Genetics of MoCD

MoCD is characterized by the simultaneous loss of all Mo-enzyme activities due to biallelic pathogenic variants in either *MOCS1*, *MOCS2*, *MOCS3*, or *GPHN* (Huijmans et al. 2017; Reiss and Hahnewald 2011), and prenatal diagnosis in carrier families has been established. In nearly all cases, disease-causing mutations result in a complete loss of enzyme function due to frame shifts, splice site and nonsense mutations, or missense mutations affecting highly conserved or invariant residues. Approximately 60% of all MoCD patients carry mutations in the *MOCS*1 gene (Reiss and Hahnewald 2011). Most of the remaining MoCD patients are affected in the *MOCS2* gene. Recently, the first patient with a *MOCS3* mutation has been reported (Huijmans et al. 2017) presenting residual SO activity and attenuated disease symptoms. Due to an additional function of MOCS3 in tRNA thiolation (Chowdhury et al. 2012), it is likely that a total loss of MOCS3 function is embryonic lethal. Only two cases with homozygous *GPHN* mutations have been described in the last two decades both representing severe disease manifestation and neonatal death due to a loss of both gephyrin functions, Moco synthesis, and synaptic inhibition (Reiss et al. 2001; Reiss et al. 2011). Homozygosity for private mutations is common, reflecting a low rate of spontaneous mutations and founder effects in consanguineous communities. In addition, heterozygous gephyrin mutations and deletions have been reported in various cases presenting with different forms of epilepsy (Dejanovic et al. 2015; Dejanovic et al. 2014).

## Clinical Presentation

The three biochemically distinct forms of MoCD cannot clinically be reliably distinguished from each other or from isolated SO deficiency (ISOD; see 22.10), and all are childhood onset disorders. ISOD has been reported in more than 50 cases (Claerhout et al. 2018), whereas over 200 cases of MoCD have been described (Misko et al. 2020, Spiegel et al. submitted), and many more are known to metabolic clinicians. Children with MoCD present with a spectrum of clinical severity, with a clear majority being severely affected from the neonatal age. Affected newborns are usually born at term. They may initially appear healthy and have normal proportions including head circumference, although they can display typical minor dysmorphic facial features and may have solitary cerebral parenchymal cysts and a hypoplastic pons and cerebellum. The most common presentation of severe MoCD as first described in 1978 (Duran et al. 1978) is of early myoclonic encephalopathy, often starting within hours to days after birth with poor feeding, irritability, and a distressed facial expression and quickly progressing to myoclonic seizures, decreased consciousness, and apnea. The EEG can initially be normal, advancing to a generalized burst suppression pattern. After a period of 1–2 weeks, children may regain alertness but show persistent hyperexcitability, frequent myoclonus, tonic spasms, and focal seizures with eye deviation and facial flushing. Seizures are often refractive to anticonvulsants. Infants can display dystonic episodes with prominent limb hypertonia, spasticity and opisthotonus. Cerebral visual impairment and bulbar dysfunction and a lack of speech and motor development are common. A proportion of children develop lens dislocation after infancy. Nephrolithiasis has been reported. Mortality is high due to intercurrent lower respiratory tract infections and seizures, with a reported median survival between 2.4 (Spiegel et al., submitted) and 3.0 years (Mechler et al., 2015).

Neuroimaging usually demonstrates severe abnormalities. An early stage of generalized edema is quickly followed by features mimicking severe generalized hypoxic-ischemic encephalopathy (Vijayakumar et al. 2011), which evolves within a few weeks to a characteristic appearance including in decreasing frequency cortical atrophy and loss of white matter with cyst formation, hypoplastic corpus callosum, abnormal basal ganglia, hydrocephalus ex vacuo, dilated ventricles, cerebellar and brainstem hypoplasia, and mega cisterna magna (Arslanoglu et al. 2001; Bayram et al. 2013; Vijayakumar et al. 2011).

Increasingly, cases with symptom onset later in childhood and attenuated severity are being described. Occasionally, children present merely with dystonia and speech delay (Mayr et al., 2018, Scelsa et al. 2019), and the cranial imaging may only show changes to the basal ganglia or even appear normal (Del Rizzo et al. 2013, Spiegel et al., submitted). Attenuated disease probably reflects a slightly higher residual activity of SO, and the diagnosis is easily missed if specific diagnostic investigations are not undertaken. Secondary deterioration can occur with intercurrent illness.

## Disease Mechanism

MoCD is clinically very similar to isolated SOX deficiency, implicating sulfite toxicity as a major underlying cause for neurotoxicity in MoCD patients. Sulfite is a strong reducing agent that attacks disulfide bonds in proteins and small molecules. As a highly abundant disulfide, cystine reacts with accumulating sulfite leading to the formation of S-sulfocysteine (SSC, Fig. 35.2) (Rupar et al. 1996). SSC accumulates in MoCD patients, and its excretion in urine is detectable shortly after birth and increases over the first few days of life (Veldman et al. 2010) supporting the view that sulfite is removed via placental clearance during pregnancy (Belaidi et al. 2012; Reiss et al. 2005). SSC is structurally similar to glutamate and able to bind to NMDA receptors (Olney et al. 1975). We have recently shown that SSC mediated excitotoxicity is NMDA-receptor dependent and causes $Ca^{2+}$ influx, calpain activation, and inhibitory synapse depletion. Treatment with the NMDA receptor antagonist memantine was able to rescue neurodevelopmental deficits in a pharmacological model of MoCD in mice (Kumar et al. 2017). SSC formation results in L-cystine depletion in plasma (Barbot et al. 1995; Johnson and Duran 2001). Deficiency of L-cysteine, the precursor of GSH, might contribute to ferroptosis, a novel form of non-apoptotic cell death that involves glutathione-dependent clearance of lipid peroxidation (Stockwell et al. 2017). MoCD patients have lowered plasma total homocysteine concentrations (Graf et al. 1998; Sass et al. 2003). The molecular cause has not been explored further, but probably reflects, similar to SSC formation, a sulfite-dependent liberation of protein-bound homocysteine as S-sulfohomocysteine. Additional pro-excitatory effects of sulfite might also contribute to the disease pathology given that a sulfite-dependent reduction of pyridoxal 5′-phosphate (PLP) in cerebrospinal fluid of MoCD patients has been reported (Footitt et al. 2011).

The primary route of cysteine catabolism proceeds via the oxidative catabolism (Bagley and Stipanuk 1994) that involves cysteine dioxygenase and aspartate aminotransferase. In addition, there is growing evidence for a significant role of the hydrogen sulfide ($H_2S$)-dependent degradation of cysteine. Formation of $H_2S$ involves at least four enzymes (cystathionine γ-lyase, CSE, cystathionine β-synthase, CBS, and aspartate amino transferase together with 3-mercaptopyruvate sulfurtransferase, MSPT, Fig. 35.2) in three distinct pathways. As a signaling molecule (Abe and Kimura 1996), the half-life of $H_2S$ is rather short, and one mode of action is the $H_2S$-dependent formation of cysteine persulfides, which have been shown to protect protein-bound cysteines from irreversible oxidation (Zivanovic et al. 2019). $H_2S$ is further oxidized to sulfite and thiosulfate in mitochondria by three enzymatic reactions (Fig. 35.2) (Hildebrandt and Grieshaber 2008). First, the mitochondrial membrane flavoprotein sulfur quinone oxidoreductase (SQR) converts $H_2S$ to a GSH-bound persulfide and transfers two electrons to the ubiquinone pool (Kabil and Banerjee 2010). Next, the glutathione persulfide is handed over either to a persulfide dioxygenase releasing sulfite. Alternatively, thiosulfate sulfur transferase transfers the glutathione persulfide to sulfite yielding thiosulfate (Hildebrandt and Grieshaber 2008).

MoCD and SOX deficiency are characterized by high levels of thiosulfate excretion, suggesting an increased sulfur flux via the $H_2S$ pathway. A similar imbalance is seen in cysteine dioxygenase deficiency observed in the *CDO*$^{-/-}$ mice (Ueki et al. 2011). Finally, ethylmalonic encephalopathy (ETHE1 deficiency) is caused by genetic variants in persulfide dioxygenase leading to $H_2S$ accumulation, respiratory chain deficiency, and massively increased thiosulfate excretion (Tiranti et al. 2009). Based on the collective accumulation of thiosulfate in MoCD, SOXD, and ETHE1 deficiency, a recent study identified similar principles of mitochondrial dysfunction in these disorders (Grings et al. 2019).

## Nomenclature

| No. | Disorder | Alt Name | Abbreviation | Gene symbol | Chromosomal localization | Affected protein | OMIM No. |
|---|---|---|---|---|---|---|---|
| 35.1 | Molybdenum cofactor deficiency A | MoCo deficiency, complementation group A | MoCD-A | *MOCS1* | 6p21.3 | MOCS1A, MOCS1AB | 603707 |
| 35.2 | Molybdenum cofactor deficiency B | MoCo deficiency, complementation group B | MoCD-B | *MOCS2* | 5q11 | MOCS2A MOCS2B | 603708 |
| 35.3 | Molybdenum cofactor deficiency C | MoCo deficiency, complementation group C | MoCD-C | *GPHN* | 14q23.3 | Gephyrin | 603930 |
| 35.4 | Molybdenum cofactor sulfurase deficiency | Xanthinuria type II | MCSD | *MOCOS* | 18q12.2 | MOCOS | 613274 |

## Metabolic Pathways

**Fig. 35.1** *Moco biosynthesis, Mo enzymes, and deficiencies.* Intermediates of Moco synthesis are 3′ 8-cyclo 7,8-dihydro-GTP, cyclic pyranopterin monophosphate (cPMP), metal binding pterin (MPT), and adenylated MPT (MPT-AMP). Moco undergoes an additional sulfuration prior to its incorporation into xanthine oxidase and aldehyde oxidase. A deficiency in the latter step leads to xanthinuria type II (35.04). Proteins and domains (GPHN) involved in Moco synthesis are shown. Deficiencies in *MOCS1*, *MOCS2/3*, and *GPHN* cause MoCD type A (35.01), type B (35.02), and type C (35.03), respectively. Isolated deficiencies in SOX and XO cause ISOD 22.10 and XOD 13.19

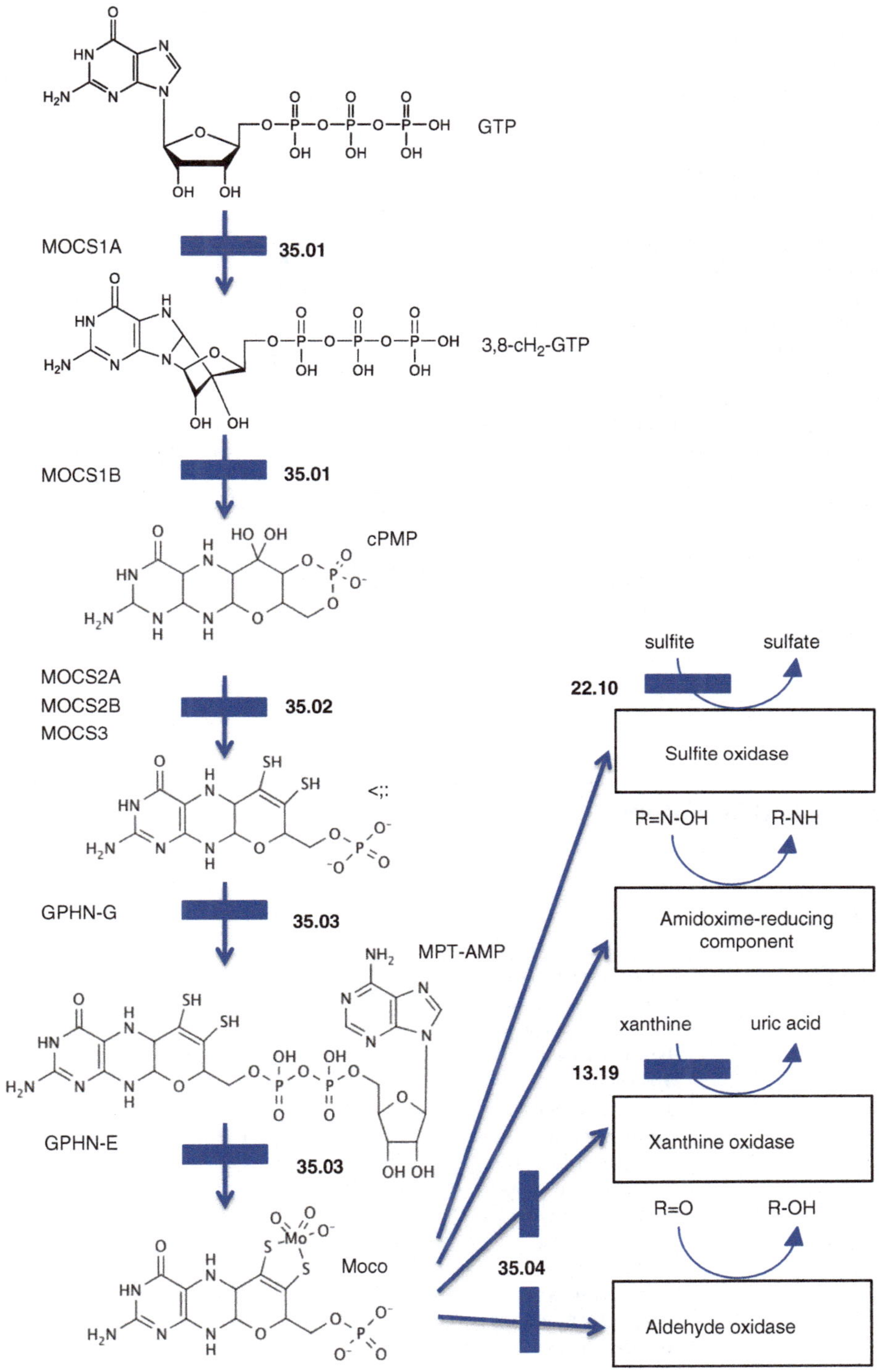

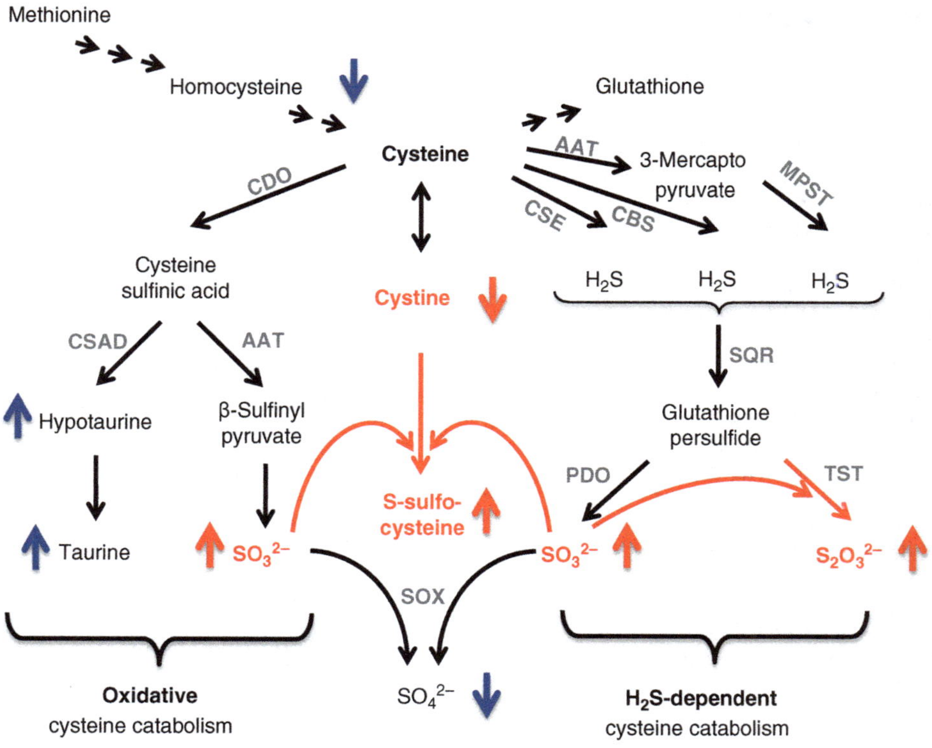


**Fig. 35.2** *Cysteine catabolism and S-containing metabolites that are altered in MoCD and SOX deficiency.* Oxidative and $H_2S$-dependent cysteine catabolism are summarized with the involved enzymes and metabolites. Changes in metabolite concentrations in MoCD and ISOD are highlighted in blue/red with corresponding arrows indicating an increase or decrease in concentration in comparison to controls. Strongly increased sulfur fluxes/metabolite changes in response to MoCD/ISOD are indicated by red arrows. Enzyme abbreviations are *CBS* Cystathionine β-synthase, *CSE* Cystathionine γ-lyase, *CDO* Cysteine dioxygenase, *CSD* Cysteine sulfinate decarboxylase, *AAT* Aspartate aminotransferase, *SO* sulfite oxidase, *MPST* 3-Mercaptopyruvate sulfurtransferase, *SQR* Quinone oxidoreductase, *PSD* Persulfide dioxygenase, *TST* Thiosulfate sulfur transferase

## Signs and Symptoms

**Table 35.1** Molybdenum cofactor deficiency A

| System | Symptoms and biomarkers | Neonatal (birth–1 month) | Infancy (1–18 months) | Childhood (1.5–11 years) | Adolescence (11–16 years) | Adulthood (>16 years) |
|---|---|---|---|---|---|---|
| CNS | **Dystonic cerebral palsy** | | + | ++ | +++ | +++ |
| | **Exaggerated startle response** | +++ | +++ | ++ | | |
| | **Hypertonia, limbs** | + | ++ | ++ | ++ | ++ |
| | **Myoclonus** | ++ | ++ | ++ | ++ | ++ |
| | **Orobulbar dysfunction** | ++ | +++ | +++ | +++ | +++ |
| | **Profound global developmental delay** | | ++ | +++ | +++ | +++ |
| | Reduced consciousness | ++ | | | | |
| | **Seizures, tonic clonic** | +++ | +++ | +++ | ++ | ++ |
| Digestive | **Feeding difficulties** | +++ | +++ | +++ | +++ | +++ |
| Eye | **Cerebral visual impairment** | + | ++ | ++ | ++ | ++ |
| | **Lens dislocation** | | ± | ± | ± | ± |
| Musculoskeletal | **Dysmorphic features** | ++ | + | + | | |
| | **Hypotonia, muscular-axial** | +++ | ++ | ± | | |
| | **Microcephaly** | | ++ | ++ | ++ | ++ |
| Renal | Nephrolithiasis | | ± | ± | ± | ± |
| Respiratory | Apnea | ± | | | | |

**Table 35.1** (continued)

| System | Symptoms and biomarkers | Neonatal (birth–1 month) | Infancy (1–18 months) | Childhood (1.5–11 years) | Adolescence (11–16 years) | Adulthood (>16 years) |
|---|---|---|---|---|---|---|
| Laboratory findings | Alpha-aminosemialdehyde (cerebrospinal fluid) | ↑ | ↑ | ↑ | | |
| | Alpha-aminosemialdehyde (urine) | ↑ | ↑ | ↑ | | |
| | Cyclic pyranopterin monophosphate, cPMP (urine) | n | n | n | n | |
| | Cystine (plasma) | ↓↓ | ↓↓↓ | ↓↓↓ | ↓↓↓ | ↓↓↓ |
| | Homocysteine (plasma) | ↓↓ | ↓↓ | ↓↓ | ↓↓ | ↓↓ |
| | Pipecolic acid (cerebrospinal fluid) | ↑ | ↑ | ↑ | | |
| | Pyridoxal phosphate, PLP (cerebrospinal fluid) | ↓ | ↓ | ↓ | | |
| | Pyridoxal phosphate, PLP (plasma) | ↓ | ↓ | ↓ | ↓ | ↓ |
| | Sulfite (urine) | ↑↑↑ | ↑↑↑ | ↑↑↑ | ↑↑↑ | |
| | Sulfocysteine (plasma) | ↑↑↑ | ↑↑↑ | ↑↑↑ | ↑↑↑ | |
| | Sulfocysteine (urine) | ↑↑↑ | ↑↑↑ | ↑↑↑ | ↑↑↑ | |
| | Taurine (plasma) | ↑ | ↑↑ | ↑↑ | ↑↑ | ↑↑ |
| | Taurine (urine) | ↑ | ↑↑ | ↑↑ | ↑↑ | ↑↑ |
| | Uric acid (plasma) | ↓↓ | ↓↓↓ | ↓↓↓ | ↓↓↓ | |
| | Urothione (urine) | ↓↓↓ | ↓↓↓ | ↓↓↓ | ↓↓↓ | ↓↓↓ |
| | Xanthine (plasma) | ↑↑↑ | ↑↑↑ | ↑↑↑ | ↑↑↑ | |
| | Xanthine (urine) | ↑↑↑ | ↑↑↑ | ↑↑↑ | ↑↑↑ | |

**Table 35.2** Molybdenum cofactor deficiency B

| System | Symptoms and biomarkers | Neonatal (birth–1 month) | Infancy (1–18 months) | Childhood (1.5–11 years) | Adolescence (11–16 years) | Adulthood (>16 years) |
|---|---|---|---|---|---|---|
| CNS | **Dystonic cerebral palsy** | | + | ++ | +++ | +++ |
| | **Exaggerated startle response** | +++ | +++ | ++ | | |
| | **Hypertonia, limbs** | + | ++ | ++ | ++ | ++ |
| | **Myoclonus** | ++ | ++ | ++ | ++ | ++ |
| | **Orobulbar dysfunction** | ++ | +++ | +++ | +++ | +++ |
| | **Profound global developmental delay** | | ++ | +++ | +++ | +++ |
| | Reduced consciousness | ++ | | | | |
| | **Seizures, tonic clonic** | +++ | +++ | +++ | ++ | ++ |
| Digestive | **Feeding difficulties** | +++ | +++ | +++ | +++ | +++ |
| Eye | **Cerebral visual impairment** | + | ++ | ++ | ++ | ++ |
| | **Lens dislocation** | | ± | ± | ± | ± |
| Musculoskeletal | **Dysmorphic features** | ++ | + | + | | |
| | **Hypotonia, muscular-axial** | +++ | ++ | ± | | |
| | **Microcephaly** | | ++ | ++ | ++ | ++ |
| Renal | Nephrolithiasis | | ± | ± | ± | ± |
| Respiratory | Apnea | ± | | | | |
| Laboratory findings | Alpha-aminosemialdehyde (cerebrospinal fluid) | ↑ | ↑ | ↑ | | |
| | Alpha-aminosemialdehyde (urine) | ↑ | ↑ | ↑ | | |
| | Cyclic pyranopterin monophosphate, cPMP (urine) | ↑↑ | ↑↑ | ↑↑ | ↑↑ | |
| | Cystine (plasma) | ↓↓ | ↓↓↓ | ↓↓↓ | ↓↓↓ | ↓↓↓ |
| | Homocysteine (plasma) | ↓↓ | ↓↓ | ↓↓ | ↓↓ | ↓↓ |
| | Pipecolic acid (cerebrospinal fluid) | ↑ | ↑ | ↑ | | |
| | Pyridoxal phosphate, PLP (cerebrospinal fluid) | ↓ | ↓ | ↓ | | |
| | Pyridoxal phosphate, PLP (plasma) | ↓ | ↓ | ↓ | ↓ | ↓ |
| | Sulfite (urine) | ↑↑↑ | ↑↑↑ | ↑↑↑ | ↑↑↑ | |
| | Sulfocysteine (plasma) | ↑↑↑ | ↑↑↑ | ↑↑↑ | ↑↑↑ | |
| | Sulfocysteine (urine) | ↑↑↑ | ↑↑↑ | ↑↑↑ | ↑↑↑ | |
| | Taurine (plasma) | ↑↑ | ↑↑ | ↑↑ | ↑↑ | ↑↑ |
| | Taurine (urine) | ↑↑ | ↑↑ | ↑↑ | ↑↑ | ↑↑ |
| | Trimethylamine (urine) | ↑↑↑ | ↑↑↑ | ↑↑↑ | ↑↑↑ | |
| | Uric acid (plasma) | ↓↓ | ↓↓↓ | ↓↓↓ | ↓↓↓ | |
| | Urothione (urine) | ↓↓ | ↓↓ | ↓↓↓ | ↓↓↓ | ↓↓↓ |
| | Xanthine (urine) | ↑↑↑ | ↑↑↑ | ↑↑↑ | ↑↑↑ | |

**Table 35.3** Molybdenum cofactor deficiency C

| System | Symptoms and biomarkers | Neonatal (birth–1 month) | Infancy (1–18 months) | Childhood (1.5–11 years) | Adolescence (11–16 years) | Adulthood (>16 years) |
|---|---|---|---|---|---|---|
| CNS | Dystonic cerebral palsy | | + | ++ | +++ | |
| | **Exaggerated startle response** | ++ | + | | | |
| | **Hypertonia, limbs** | + | ++ | +++ | +++ | |
| | **Myoclonus** | ++ | ++ | + | | |
| | **Orobulbar dysfunction** | +++ | +++ | +++ | +++ | |
| | **Profound global developmental delay** | | ++ | +++ | +++ | |
| | Reduced consciousness | ++ | + | | | |
| | **Seizures, tonic clonic** | +++ | +++ | +++ | ++ | |
| Digestive | **Feeding difficulties** | +++ | +++ | +++ | | |
| Eye | **Cerebral visual impairment** | | + | + | + | |
| | **Lens dislocation** | | + | + | + | |
| Musculoskeletal | Dysmorphic features | ± | + | + | ++ | |
| | Hypotonia, muscular-axial | +++ | + | + | + | + |
| | **Microcephaly** | ± | ++ | ++ | ++ | |
| Renal | Nephrolithiasis | | ± | ± | ± | |
| Respiratory | Apnea | ± | ± | | | |
| Laboratory findings | Alpha-aminosemialdehyde (cerebrospinal fluid) | ↑ | ↑ | | | |
| | Alpha-aminosemialdehyde (urine) | ↑ | ↑ | | | |
| | Cyclic pyranopterin monophosphate, cPMP (urine) | n–↑ | n–↑ | n–↑ | n–↑ | |
| | Cystine (plasma) | ↓↓ | ↓↓↓ | ↓↓↓ | ↓↓↓ | ↓↓↓ |
| | Homocysteine (plasma) | ↓-↑ | ↓↓ | ↓↓ | ↓↓ | ↓↓ |
| | Pipecolic acid (cerebrospinal fluid) | ↑ | ↑ | | | |
| | Pyridoxal phosphate, PLP (cerebrospinal fluid) | ↓ | ↓ | | | |
| | Pyridoxal phosphate, PLP (plasma) | ↓ | ↓ | ↓ | ↓ | ↓ |
| | Sulfite (urine) | ↑↑↑ | ↑↑↑ | ↑↑↑ | ↑↑↑ | |
| | Sulfocysteine (plasma) | ↑↑↑ | ↑↑↑ | ↑↑↑ | ↑↑↑ | |
| | Sulfocysteine (urine) | ↑↑↑ | ↑↑↑ | ↑↑↑ | ↑↑↑ | |
| | Taurine (plasma) | ↑↑ | ↑↑ | ↑↑ | ↑↑ | ↑↑ |
| | Taurine (urine) | ↑↑ | ↑↑ | ↑↑ | ↑↑ | ↑↑ |
| | Uric acid (plasma) | ↓↓ | ↓↓↓ | ↓↓↓ | ↓↓↓ | |
| | Urothione (urine) | n–↑ | n–↑ | n–↑ | n–↑ | n–↑ |
| | Xanthine (plasma) | ↑↑↑ | ↑↑↑ | ↑↑↑ | ↑↑↑ | |
| | Xanthine (urine) | ↑↑↑ | ↑↑↑ | ↑↑↑ | ↑↑↑ | |

**Table 35.4** Molybdenum cofactor sulfurase deficiency

| System | Symptoms and biomarkers | Neonatal (birth–1 month) | Infancy (1–18 months) | Childhood (1.5–11 years) | Adolescence (11–16 years) | Adulthood (>16 years) |
|---|---|---|---|---|---|---|
| Metabolic | Allopurinol to oxipurinol conversion | ↓ | ↓ | ↓ | ↓ | ↓ |
| Musculoskeletal | Myopathy | | | | ± | ± |
| Renal | **Renal failure, acute** | ± | ± | ± | ± | ± |
| | **Urolithiasis** | ± | ± | ± | ± | ± |
| | **Urolithiasis, xanthine stones** | ± | ± | ± | ± | ± |
| Laboratory findings | Hypoxanthine (plasma) | ↑ | ↑ | ↑ | ↑ | ↑ |
| | Hypoxanthine (urine) | ↑↑ | ↑↑ | ↑↑ | ↑↑ | ↑↑ |
| | Uric acid (plasma) | ↓↓ | ↓↓ | ↓↓ | ↓↓↓ | ↓↓ |
| | Uric acid (urine) | ↓↓ | ↓↓ | ↓↓ | ↓↓↓ | ↓↓ |
| | Xanthine (plasma) | ↑ | ↑ | ↑ | ↑ | ↑ |
| | Xanthine (urine) | ↑↑ | ↑↑ | ↑↑ | ↑↑ | ↑↑ |

## Reference and Pathological Values

Purines in urine and plasma (HPLC-UV and LC-MS/MS)

| | Urine | | | | | Plasma |
|---|---|---|---|---|---|---|
| Compound range[a] | 0–1 year (*n* = 16) | 1–5 years (*n* = 47) | 5–16 years (*n* = 27) | > 16 years (*n* = 26) | Pathological values[b] | 0–100 years (*n* = 100) |
| Uric acid[c] | 820–1026 | 527–790 | 326–436 | 222–287 | < 100 | 120–340 |
| Hypoxanthine | 1–71.9 | 1–88.1 | 1–14.1 | 1–14.0 | >100 | 0–10.0 |
| Xanthine | 0–63.4 | 0–54.7 | 0–21.7 | 0.3–10.7 | > 70 | 0–7.0 |

See also 13.19
[a]µmol/mmol creatinine
[b]In MoCD, xanthinuria type I and II
[c]95% Cl

Sulfite-related metabolites in urine and plasma

| | Urine | | | | | Plasma |
|---|---|---|---|---|---|---|
| Compound range[a] | 0–1 year (*n* = 16) | 1–5 years (*n* = 47) | 5–16 years (*n* = 27) | >16 years (*n* = 26) | Pathological values[b] | 0–100 years (*n* = 100) |
| Total homocysteine[c] | 3.3–8.3 | 4.7–10.3 | <15 | <15 | 0 | 5–15 |
| S-sulfocysteine[d] | 0–18 | | | 0-25 | >50 | 0–3 |
| Thiosulfate[e] | 0–55 | | | | <100 | <9 |
| Cystine[f] | 57–200 µmol/g | | | | <10 | 23–58 |
| Taurine[g] | 30–100 | | | | 400–2000 | 35–245 |
| PLP[h] | 26–69 | 8–136 | 8–41 | | 0–5 | |

[a]µmol/mmol creatinine
[b]In MoCD and SO deficiency
[c]See also Chap. 22
[d]Belaidi et al. (2012)
[e]Reynolds and Harkness (1991)
[f]Plasma: (Bamforth et al. 1990), Urine (van Gennip et al. 1991)
[g]Plasma: (Arslanoglu et al. 2001) Urine: (Belaidi and Schwarz 2013)
[h]CSF: (Footitt et al. 2011)

## Diagnostic Flowchart

**Fig. 35.3** Flowchart to establish the differential diagnosis of ISOD or MoCD subtypes. Sample matrices, urine (U), plasma (P), cerebrospinal fluid (C)

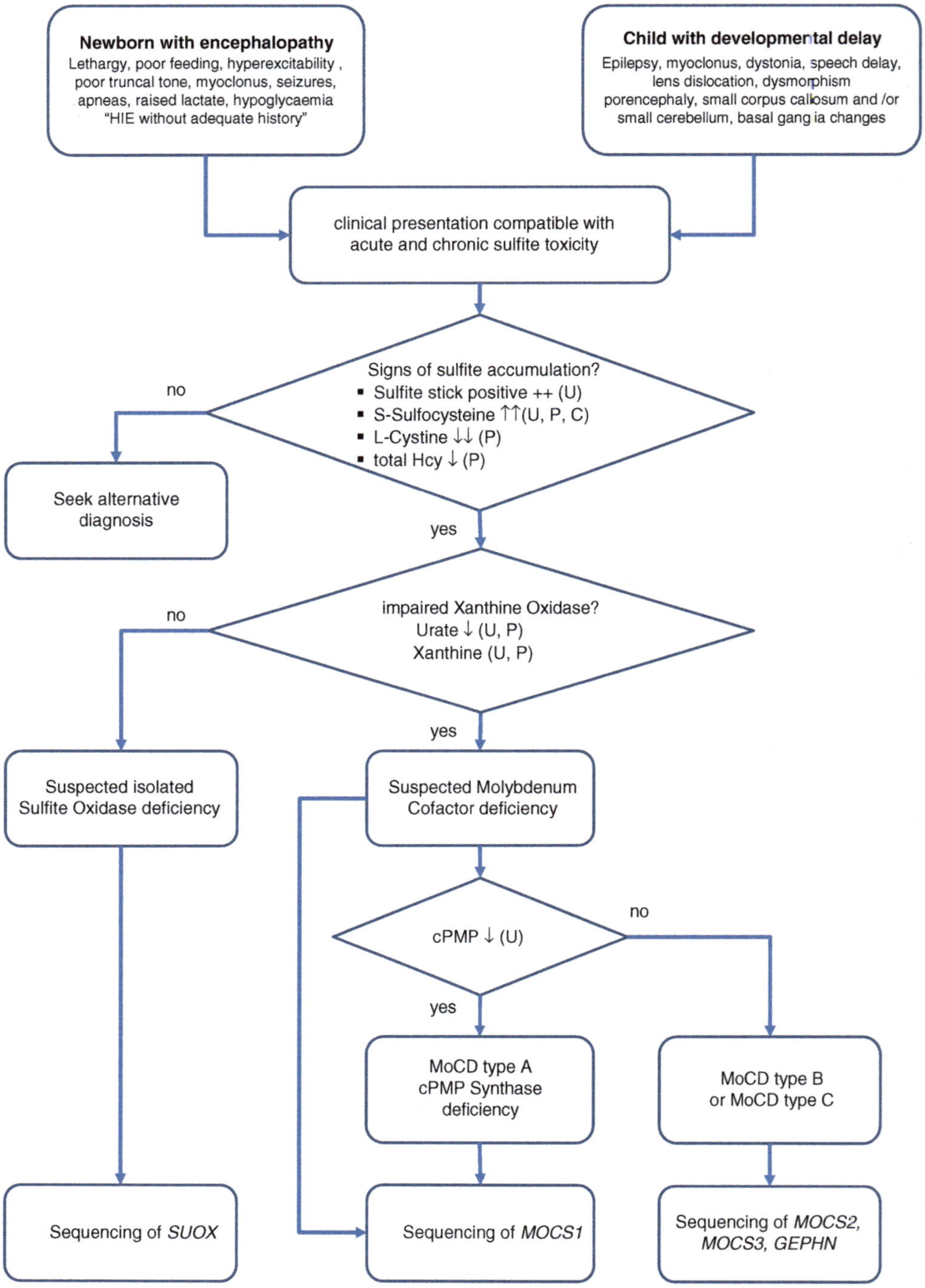

## Specimen Collection

Specimen collection as early as possible, in those cases in which a treatment attempt with cPMP is undertaken; specimen to be collected prior to the first dose of cPMP.

Specimen collection

| Test | Sample requirement |
|---|---|
| Sulfite dipstick | Fresh urine, bedside dipstick test |
| S-Sulfocysteine in urine | Urine, frozen 1 mL |
| S-Sulfocysteine in plasma | Plasma, 0.5 mL |
| Uric acid in urine | Urine |
| Uric acid in plasma | Plasma, 0.5 mL |
| Xanthine in urine | Urine |
| Xanthine in plasma | Plasma, 0.5 mL |

## Prenatal Diagnosis

When pathogenic variants have been identified in the index case, prenatal diagnosis is possible by mutation analysis of DNA extracted from chorionic villi or amniocytes.

Prenatal diagnosis sample requirement

| Disorder | Material | Timing/ trimester |
|---|---|---|
| All MoCD types | Chorionic villus cells | I |
| | Cultured amniocytes | II |
| | Amniotic fluid (might be positive for SSC, unclear diagnostic accuracy) | III |

## DNA Testing

In MoCD patients pathogenic variants have been found in *MOCS1*, *MOCS2, MOCS3*, and *GEPH*. Given the higher prevalence of *MOCS1* mutations, analysis of this gene is suggested before testing for the *MOCS2* gene. Only if no variant has been found in either *MOCS1 or MOCS2*, sequence analysis of *GEPH* or *MOCS3* is suggested. Primers and protocols for Sanger sequencing have been published previously (Reiss et al. 1998; Reiss et al. 1999; Reiss et al. 2001).

## Treatment

Early manifesting neonates often require medical intensive care to survive the initial acute encephalopathic period. Symptomatic treatment afterward focuses on improving quality of life and medication to manage cerebral palsy, myoclonus, dystonia, and treatment-resistant seizures. Most children are immobile and require tube feeding owing to orobulbar dysfunction. Diets restricted in L-methionine and L-cystine have been tried to reduce the accumulation of sulfite. A reduction of about one third of the usual daily intake can be achieved in infants without compromising growth, and while such diets lead to a modest biochemical improvement, the clinical effects in severely affected children have been disappointing. A low-sulfur diet and pyridoxine supplementation have been found to improve seizure control in some patients with attenuated MoCD although those would also be expected to respond to conventional anticonvulsive treatment (Boles et al. 1993; Del Rizzo et al. 2013; Touati et al. 2000).

After the proof of concept of treating MoCD type A with cyclic pyranopterin monophosphate (cPMP) was established in a mouse model (Schwarz et al. 2004), daily intravenous replacement therapy has been used since 2008 to treat amenable patients (Veldman et al. 2010) for as long as 12 years. Results of treatment of the first cohort of 11 patients for up to 5 years within a prospective cohort study suggests that cPMP substitution is generally safe and biochemically effective, leading to rapid and sustained normalization of biomarkers without adverse drug reactions or tachyphylaxis (Schwahn et al. 2015). The clinical outcome of treated patients critically depends on the timing of treatment in relation to the cascade of neurotoxic events triggered by sulfite accumulation after birth and in particular on whether it is started before excitotoxic neuronal cell death occurs (Kumar et al. 2017, Plate et al. 2019). Timely cPMP treatment of neonates with severe MoCD type A can prevent severe neurocognitive sequelae. However, the requirement for daily IV administration causes a significant burden of care and requires permanent venous access. While the treatment with cPMP must be started urgently, the decision whether to continue the treatment long-term needs to be well reflected, with the best interest of the child and family in mind.

In practical terms, cPMP has recently been granted a license for medical use and is available from the manufacturer Origin BioSciences Inc. A single daily dose of cPMP is administered as slow intravenous injection or short infusion. Doses from 0.24 to 1.2 mg per kg body weight per day have been successfully used.

Treatment with cPMP should include close monitoring of biomarkers to establish a biochemical response, which can also help to differentiate MoCD subtypes if genetic test results are not immediately available. A fall in urinary sulfite and SSC concentrations is seen within the first 24 h after administration, and a rise in plasma urate and L-cystine concentrations can be expected within a few days.

### Emergency Treatment

Anticonvulsant treatment, airway protection, and neuromonitoring according to standard algorithms of pediatric emergency medicine and intensive care.

Given the risk-benefit ratio, it appears appropriate to commence cPMP replacement therapy in suspected cases prior to diagnostic confirmation and consider discontinuation after more information has become available.

## Standard Treatment

Supportive treatment and anticonvulsive therapy according to local standards.

cPMP replacement is likely to become established as standard of care for pre-symptomatic infants with MoCD type A.

## Experimental Treatment

Hemofiltration has been proposed as emergency treatment option to protect the neonatal brain against sulfite toxicity. During hemofiltration, careful monitoring of anticonvulsant plasma levels is required. Premature delivery of affected fetuses has been suggested to minimize exposure of the fetal brain to rising sulfite levels during late pregnancy. There is currently no evidence to support the efficacy of either proposition.

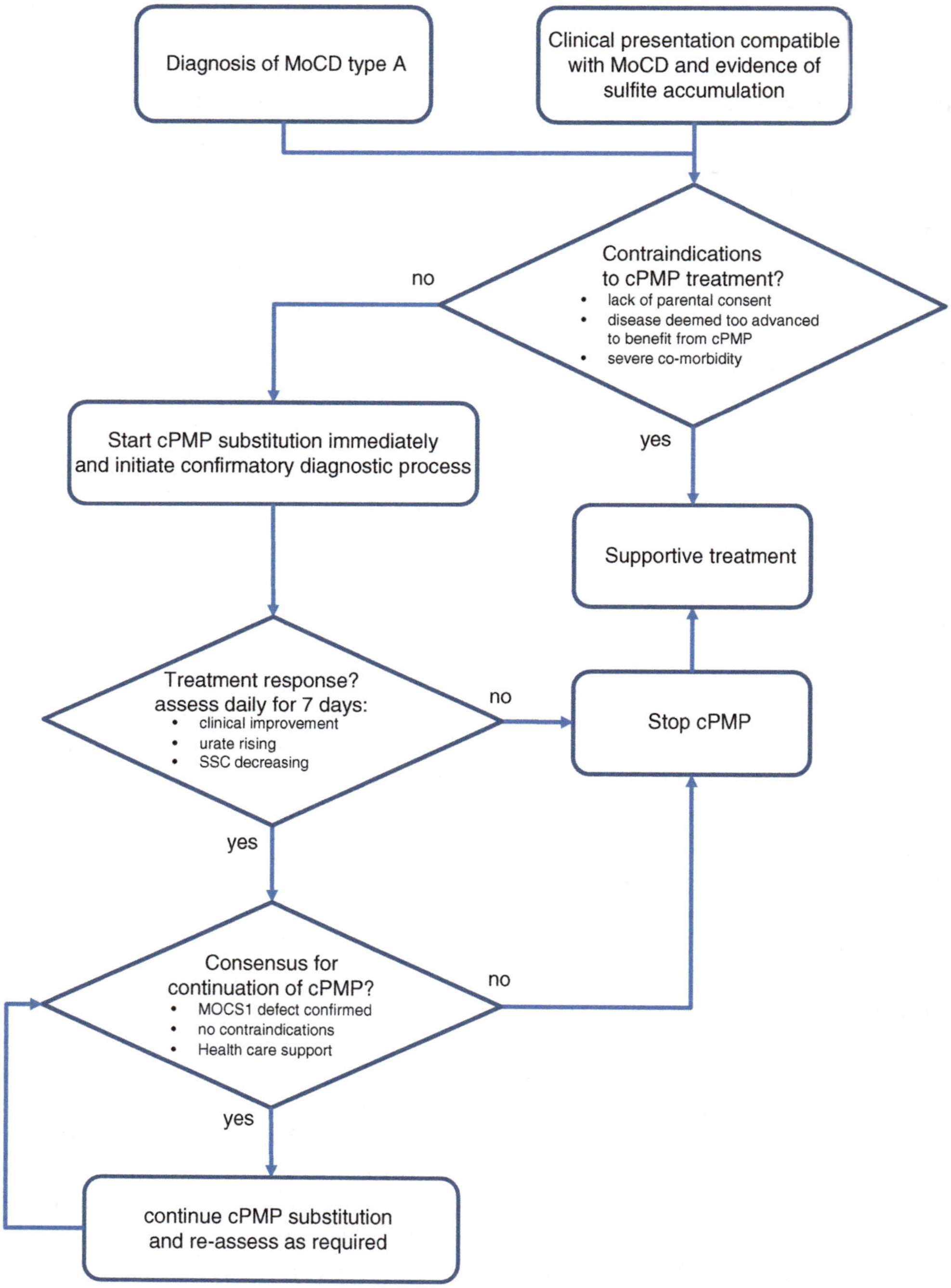


**Fig. 35.4** Suggested decision-making process for the use of cPMP

### Follow-Up and Monitoring

Plasma urate as well as urinary SSC and xanthine are suitable markers of biochemical efficacy, and the latter are stable compounds. This allows urine samples to be collected every few weeks at home and be sent to centralized laboratories for analysis. The ongoing evaluation of biochemical and clinical efficacy will establish justification for continuation of this novel treatment. Clinical monitoring includes regular assessments of nutritional status, motor and bulbar function, as well as cognitive developmental progress, to establish support needs.

## References


Abe K, Kimura H. The possible role of hydrogen sulfide as an endogenous neuromodulator. J Neurosci. 1996;16:1066–71.

Arslanoglu S, Yalaz M, Goksen D, Coker M, Tutuncuoglu S, Akisu M, Darcan S, Kultursay N, Ciris M, Demirtas E. Molybdenum cofactor deficiency associated with Dandy-Walker complex. Brain and Development. 2001;23:815–8.

Bagley PJ, Stipanuk MH. The activities of rat hepatic cysteine dioxygenase and cysteinesulfinate decarboxylase are regulated in a reciprocal manner in response to dietary casein level. J Nutr. 1994;124:2410–21.

Bamforth FJ, Johnson JL, Davidson AGF, Wong LTK, Lockitsch G, Applegrath DA. Biochemical investigation of a child with molybdenum deficiency. Clin Biochem. 1990;23:537–42.

Barbot C, Martins E, Vilarinho L, Dorche C, Cardoso ML. A mild form of infantile isolated sulphite oxidase deficiency. Neuropediatrics. 1995;26:322–4.

Bayram E, Topcu Y, Karakaya P, Yis U, Cakmakci H, Ichida K, Kurul SH. Molybdenum cofactor deficiency: review of 12 cases (MoCD and review). Eur J Paediatr Neurol. 2013;17:1–6.

Belaidi AA, Arjune S, Santamaria-Araujo JA, Sass JO, Schwarz G. Molybdenum cofactor deficiency: a new HPLC method for fast quantification of s-sulfocysteine in urine and serum. JIMD Rep. 2012;5:35–43.

Belaidi AA, Schwarz G. Molybdenum cofactor deficiency: metabolic link between taurine and S-sulfocysteine. Adv Exp Med Biol. 2013;776:13–9.

Boles RG, Ment LR, Meyn MS, Horwich AL, Kratz LE, Rinaldo P. Short-term response to dietary therapy in molybdenum cofactor deficiency. Ann Neurol. 1993;34:742–4.

Chowdhury MM, Dosche C, Lohmannsroben HG, Leimkuhler S. Dual role of the molybdenum cofactor biosynthesis protein MOCS3 in tRNA thiolation and molybdenum cofactor biosynthesis in humans. J Biol Chem. 2012;287:17297–307.

Claerhout H, Witters P, Régal L, Jansen K, Van Hoestenberghe MR, Breckpot J, Vermeersch P. Isolated sulfite oxidase deficiency. J Inherit Metab Dis. 2018;41(1):101–8.

Dejanovic B, Djemie T, Grunewald N, Suls A, Kress V, Hetsch F, Craiu D, Zemel M, Gormley P, Lal D, et al. Simultaneous impairment of neuronal and metabolic function of mutated gephyrin in a patient with epileptic encephalopathy. EMBO Mol Med. 2015;7:1580–94.

Dejanovic B, Lal D, Catarino CB, Arjune S, Belaidi AA, Trucks H, Vollmar C, Surges R, Kunz WS, Motameny S, et al. Exonic microdeletions of the gephyrin gene impair GABAergic synaptic inhibition in patients with idiopathic generalized epilepsy. Neurobiol Dis. 2014;67:88–96.

Del Rizzo M, Burlina AP, Sass JO, Beermann F, Zanco C, Cazzorla C, Bordugo A, Giordano L, Manara R, Burlina AB. Metabolic stroke in a late-onset form of isolated sulfite oxidase deficiency. Mol Genet Metab. 2013;108:263–6.

Duran M, Beemer FA, van de Heiden C, Korteland J, de Bree PK, Brink M, Wadman SK, Lombeck I. Combined deficiency of xanthine oxidase and sulphite oxidase: a defect of molybdenum metabolism or transport? J Inherit Metab Dis. 1978;1:175–8.

Footitt EJ, Heales SJ, Mills PB, Allen GF, Oppenheim M, Clayton PT. Pyridoxal 5′-phosphate in cerebrospinal fluid; factors affecting concentration. J Inherit Metab Dis. 2011;34:529–38.

Fritschy JM, Harvey RJ, Schwarz G. Gephyrin: where do we stand, where do we go? Trends Neurosci. 2008;31:257–64.

Graf WD, Oleinik OE, Jack RM, Weiss AH, Johnson JL. Ahomocysteinemia in molybdenum cofactor deficiency. Neurology. 1998;51:860–2.

Gray TA, Nicholls RD. Diverse splicing mechanisms fuse the evolutionarily conserved bicistronic MOCS1A and MOCS1B open reading frames. RNA. 2000;6:928–36.

Grings M, Seminotti B, Karunanidhi A, Ghaloul-Gonzalez L, Mohsen AW, Wipf P, Palmfeldt J, Vockley J, Leipnitz G. ETHE1 and MOCS1 deficiencies: disruption of mitochondrial bioenergetics, dynamics, redox homeostasis and endoplasmic reticulum-mitochondria crosstalk in patient fibroblasts. Sci Rep. 2019;9:12651.

Havemeyer A, Bittner F, Wollers S, Mendel R, Kunze T, Clement B. Identification of the missing component in the mitochondrial benzamidoxime prodrug-converting system as a novel molybdenum enzyme. J Biol Chem. 2006;281:34796–802.

Hildebrandt TM, Grieshaber MK. Three enzymatic activities catalyze the oxidation of sulfide to thiosulfate in mammalian and invertebrate mitochondria. FEBS J. 2008;275:3352–61.

Huijmans JGM, Schot R, de Klerk JBC, Williams M, de Coo RFM, Duran M, Verheijen FW, van Slegtenhorst M, Mancini GMS. Molybdenum cofactor deficiency: identification of a patient with homozygote mutation in the MOCS3 gene. Am J Med Genet A. 2017;173:1601–6.

Ichida K, Matsumura T, Sakuma R, Hosoya T, Nishino T. Mutation of human molybdenum cofactor sulfurase gene is responsible for classical xanthinuria type II. Biochem Biophys Res Commun. 2001;282:1194–200.

Johnson JL, Duran M. Molybdenum cofactor deficiency and isolated sulfite oxidase deficiency. In: Scriver C, Beaudet A, Sly W, Valle D, editors. The metabolic and molecular bases of inherited disease. McGraw-Hill: New York; 2001. p. 3163–77.

Johnson JL, Hainline BE, Rajagopalan KV, Arison BH. The pterin component of the molybdenum cofactor. Structural characterization of two fluorescent derivatives. J Biol Chem. 1984;259:5414–22.

Kabil O, Banerjee R. Redox biochemistry of hydrogen sulfide. J Biol Chem. 2010;285:21,903–7.

Kumar A, Dejanovic B, Hetsch F, Semtner M, Fusca D, Arjune S, Santamaria-Araujo JA, Winkelmann A, Ayton S, Bush AI, et al. S-sulfocysteine/NMDA receptor-dependent signaling underlies neurodegeneration in molybdenum cofactor deficiency. J Clin Invest. 2017;127:4365–78.

Matthies A, Rajagopalan KV, Mendel RR, Leimkuhler S. Evidence for the physiological role of a rhodanese-like protein for the biosynthesis of the molybdenum cofactor in humans. Proc Natl Acad Sci U S A. 2004;101:5946–51.

Mayr SJ, Sass JO, Vry J, et al. A mild case of molybdenum cofactor deficiency defines an alternative route of MOCS1 protein maturation. J Inherit Metab Dis. 2018;41(2):187–96.

Mayr SJ, Mendel RR, Schwarz G. Molybdenum cofactor biology, evolution and deficiency. Biochim Biophys Acta Mol Cell Res. 2021;1868(1):118883. https://doi.org/:10.1016/j.bbamcr.2020.118883. Epub 2020 Oct 2.

Mechler K, Mountford WK, Hoffmann GF, Ries M. Ultra-orphan diseases: a quantitative analysis of the natural history of molybdenum cofactor deficiency. Genet Med. 2015;17(12):965–70.

Misko AL, Liang Y, Kohl JB, Eichler F. Delineating the phenotypic spectrum of sulfite oxidase and molybdenum cofactor deficiency. Neurol Genet. 2020;6(4):e486.

Olney JW, Misra CH, de Gubareff T. Cysteine-S-sulfate: brain damaging metabolite in sulfite oxidase deficiency. J Neuropathol Exp Neurol. 1975;34:167–77.

Plate J, Sassen WA, Hassan AH, Lehne F, Köster RW, Kruse T. S-Sulfocysteine Induces Seizure-Like Behaviors in Zebrafish. Front Pharmacol. 2019;10:122.

Reiss J, Bonin M, Schwegler H, Sass JO, Garattini E, Wagner S, Lee HJ, Engel W, Riess O, Schwarz G. The pathogenesis of molybdenum cofactor deficiency, its delay by maternal clearance, and its expression pattern in microarray analysis. Mol Genet Metab. 2005;85:12–20.

Reiss J, Cohen N, Dorche C, Mandel H, Mendel RR, Stallmeyer B, Zabot MT, Dierks T. Mutations in a polycistronic nuclear gene associated with molybdenum cofactor deficiency. Nat Genet. 1998;20:51–3.

Reiss J, Dorche C, Stallmeyer B, Mendel RR, Cohen N, Zabot MT. Human molybdopterin synthase gene: genomic structure and mutations in molybdenum cofactor deficiency type B. Am J Hum Genet. 1999;64:706–11.

Reiss J, Gross-Hardt S, Christensen E, Schmidt P, Mendel RR, Schwarz G. A mutation in the gene for the neurotransmitter receptor-clustering protein gephyrin causes a novel form of molybdenum cofactor deficiency. Am J Hum Genet. 2001;68:208–13.

Reiss J, Hahnewald R. Molybdenum cofactor deficiency: mutations in GPHN, MOCS1, and MOCS2. Hum Mutat. 2011;32:10–8.

Reiss J, Lenz U, Aquaviva-Bourdain C, Joriot-Chekaf S, Mention-Mulliez K, Holder-Espinasse M. A GPHN point mutation leading to molybdenum cofactor deficiency. Clin Genet. 2011;80:598–9.

Reynolds AP, Harkness RA. Urinary thiosulphate/creatinine concentration ratio in hospitalized children. J Inherit Metab Dis. 1991;14:938–9.

Rupar CA, Gillett J, Gordon BA, Ramsay DA, Johnson JL, Garrett RM, Rajagopalan KV, Jung JH, Bacheyie GS, Sellers AR. Isolated sulfite oxidase deficiency. Neuropediatrics. 1996;27:299–304.

Santamaria-Araujo JA, Fischer B, Otte T, Nimtz M, Mendel RR, Wray V, Schwarz G. The tetrahydropyranopterin structure of the sulfur-free and metal-free molybdenum cofactor precursor. J Biol Chem. 2004;279:15994–9.

Sass JO, Kishikawa M, Puttinger R, Reiss J, Erwa W, Shimizu A, Sperl W. Hypohomocysteinaemia and highly increased proportion of S-sulfonated plasma transthyretin in molybdenum cofactor deficiency. J Inherit Metab Dis. 2003;26:80–2.

Scelsa B, Gasperini S, Righini A, Iascone M, Brazzoduro VG, Veggiotti P. Mild phenotype in molybdenum cofactor deficiency: a new patient and review of the literature. Mol Genet Genomic Med. 2019;7(6):e657.

Schwahn BC, Van Spronsen FJ, Belaidi AA, et al. Efficacy and safety of cyclic pyranopterin monophosphate substitution in severe molybdenum cofactor deficiency type A: a prospective cohort study. Lancet. 2015;386(10007):1955–63.

Schwarz G, Santamaria-Araujo JA, Wolf S, Lee HJ, Adham IM, Grone HJ, Schwegler H, Sass JO, Otte T, Hanzelmann P, et al. Rescue of lethal molybdenum cofactor deficiency by a biosynthetic precursor from Escherichia coli. Hum Mol Gen. 2004;13:1249–55.

Schwarz G, Mendel RR, Ribbe MW. Molybdenum cofactors, enzymes and pathways. Nature. 2009;460:839–47.

Spiegel R, Schwahn BC, Squires L, Confer N. Molybdenum cofactor deficiencies: a natural history study (submitted).

Stallmeyer B, Drugeon G, Reiss J, Haenni AL, Mendel RR. Human molybdopterin synthase gene: identification of a bicistronic transcript with overlapping reading frames. Am J Hum Genet. 1999;64:698–705.

Stockwell BR, Friedmann Angeli JP, Bayir H, Bush AI, Conrad M, Dixon SJ, Fulda S, Gascon S, Hatzios SK, Kagan VE, et al. Ferroptosis: a regulated cell death Nexus linking metabolism, redox biology, and disease. Cell. 2017;171:273–85.

Tiranti V, Viscomi C, Hildebrandt T, Di Meo I, Mineri R, Tiveron C, Levitt MD, Prelle A, Fagiolari G, Rimoldi M, et al. Loss of ETHE1, a mitochondrial dioxygenase, causes fatal sulfide toxicity in ethylmalonic encephalopathy. Nat Med. 2009;15:200–5.

Touati G, Rusthoven E, Depondt E, Dorche C, Duran M, Heron B, Rabier D, Russo M, Saudubray JM. Dietary therapy in two patients with a mild form of sulphite oxidase deficiency. Evidence for clinical and biological improvement. J Inherit Metab Dis. 2000;23:45–53.

Ueki I, Roman HB, Valli A, Fieselmann K, Lam J, Peters R, Hirschberger LL, Stipanuk MH. Knockout of the cysteine dioxygenase gene results in severe impairment in taurine synthesis and increased catabolism of cysteine to hydrogen sulfide. Am J Physiol Endocrinol Metab. 2011;310:E668.

van Gennip AH, Stroomer A, Plandsoen WG, Abeling NG. The effect of molybdenum cofactor deficiency on the purine pattern of cerebrospinal fluid. J Inherit Metab Dis. 1991;14:364–6.

Veldman A, Santamaria-Araujo JA, Sollazzo S, Pitt J, Gianello R, Yaplito-Lee J, Wong F, Ramsden CA, Reiss J, Cook I, et al. Successful treatment of molybdenum cofactor deficiency type a with cPMP. Pediatrics. 2010;125:e1249–54.

Vijayakumar K, Gunny R, Grunewald S, Carr L, Chong KW, DeVile C, Robinson R, McSweeney N, Prabhakar P. Clinical neuroimaging features and outcome in molybdenum cofactor deficiency. Pediatr Neurol. 2011;45:246–52.

Zivanovic J, Kouroussis E, Kohl JB, Adhikari B, Bursac B, Schott-Roux S, Petrovic D, Miljkovic JL, Thomas-Lopez D, Jung Y, et al. Selective persulfide detection reveals evolutionarily conserved anti-aging effects of S-sulfhydration. Cell Metab. 2019;30:1152–1170.e1113.

# Disorders of Copper, Zinc, and Selenium Metabolism

# 36

Diego Martinelli

## Contents



## Summary

Copper, zinc, and selenium are essential trace elements serving as cofactors of many important metalloenzymes. Copper and zinc uptake requires specific carriers in the intestine. Selenium absorption occurs in the duodenum via an active transport sodium pump. Copper excretion takes place only in the liver. Copper metabolism is regulated by two closely related ATPases that differ in tissue expression: ATP7A, present in most non-hepatic tissues; and ATP7B, predominantly expressed in liver.

Wilson's disease, associated to ATP7B defect, shows neuropsychiatric, ocular, and hepatic symptoms, caused by tissue copper overload due to impaired export into the bile.

Menkes disease, a devastating neurocutaneous disorder, and its milder variant occipital horn syndrome (OHS), due to ATP7A defect, cause systemic copper deficiency, impairing copper-dependent enzymes such as lysyl oxidase, tyrosinase, superoxide dismutase, dopamine beta-monooxygenase, and cytocrome oxidase.

Recently, five additional copper metabolism disorders have been described: (1) ATP7A-related distal hereditary

D. Martinelli (✉)
Division of Metabolic Diseases, Bambino Gesù Children's Hospital, IRCCS, Rome, Italy
e-mail: diego.martinelli@opbg.net


N. Blau et al. (eds.), *Physician's Guide to the Diagnosis, Treatment, and Follow-Up of Inherited Metabolic Diseases*,
https://doi.org/10.1007/978-3-030-67727-5_36

neuropathy, due to specific mutations affecting ATP7A trafficking; (2) Huppke-Brendel syndrome, caused by mutations in an acetyl-CoA transporter involved in copper proteins acetylation; (3) CCS deficiency, caused by defect of copper chaperone to SOD; (4) MEDNIK; and (5) MEDNIK-like syndrome, associated with defects in subunits of adaptor protein complex 1, which regulates copper pump trafficking. Aceruloplasminemia, due to mutations in *CP*, encoding the copper-containing enzyme ceruloplasmin, is discussed in the chapter on iron metabolism.

Zinc is involved in all major metabolic pathways, so its deficiency is highly detrimental. Conversely, high serum zinc is rarely toxic, probably because it binds to albumin and $\alpha_2$-macroglobulin. Acrodermatitis enteropathica, the main inborn error of zinc metabolism, causes a cutaneous disorder associated with diarrhea, infections, and growth retardation. Rarer zinc metabolism disorders are Spondylocheirodysplastic Ehlers-Danlos syndrome, Birk-Landau-Perez syndrome, and Hyperzincemia with Hypercalprotectinemia.

Selenium is involved in antioxidant defenses, immune response, and thyroid function. Two genetic disorders have been associated so far with selenium metabolism.

## Introduction

*Wilson disease* is an autosomal recessive disorder of copper metabolism due to mutations in *ATP7B*, encoding the copper transporting ATP-ase ATP7B (de Bie et al. 2007; Ala et al. 2007) (see Fig. 36.1). In Wilson disease, tissue copper overload, mainly in brain and liver, causes neurological, ocular (Kayser-Fleisher ring), and psychiatric symptoms, along with hepatic cirrhosis and liver failure due to impaired copper export into the bile (Ala et al. 2007). Younger patients generally present with hepatic symptoms, and even with fulminant liver failure, while at an adult age, a neurological presentation is more prevalent. However, even older patients (5th–6th decade of life) can manifest hepatic symptoms at onset (Ferenci et al. 2007), while in the pediatric age group, a neurological presentation is not unusual. The most common neurological syndrome is a movement disorder, particularly dysarthria and dysgraphia, tremor, dystonic rigidity, and drooling. In some patients, psychiatric symptoms (from impulsivity and irritability to psychosis) are predominant. Brain MRI usually shows striatal hyperintensity at T2-weighted images (Table 36.1).

As ATP7B is required for copper incorporation into ceruloplasmin, a defect in this copper pump causes the excretion of shorter half-life ceruloplasmin into the circulation without copper (apo-ceruloplasmin), explaining the characteristic low serum ceruloplasmin levels observed in Wilson disease. As 95% of serum copper is bound to ceruloplasmin, a low level of this protein also causes low serum copper. In Wilson disease, however, serum copper could be in the normal range, due to high release of copper from liver in severely affected patients. Most of this copper is unbound (so-called free serum copper), is toxic to erythrocytes, and can induce hemolysis. However, also subjects heterozygous for an *ATP7B* mutation, as well as patients with aceruloplasminemia, can show low serum ceruloplasmin, making this parameter alone insufficient for the diagnosis. Patients with neurological Wilson disease almost invariably present with Kayser-Fleischer rings, a greenish-brown deposit of copper molecules at the limbus of the cornea (Descemet membrane), which is absent in up to 50% of patients presenting with hepatic symptoms. This ocular sign is not specific, as it can be present also in other cholestatic liver diseases. Most characteristically, 24-h urinary copper excretion is elevated in Wilson disease, but also this parameter can be falsely elevated, for example, in other severe liver diseases. At the same time, 24-h urinary copper excretion can be normal in Wilson disease patients with a low copper load, such as in younger asymptomatic siblings of a known patient (Nicastro et al. 2010). Liver copper is usually elevated in Wilson disease, but it can also be abnormal in patients with cholestatic liver diseases. Therefore, none of the available laboratory tests is perfect or specific for Wilson disease, so the diagnosis is generally made through the combination of several parameters. A numerical value is given to the absence or presence of clinical signs (Kayser-Fleischer rings, neurologic symptoms) and laboratory features (copper in serum, urine, liver; serum ceruloplasmin; genetic testing), scoring from 0 (absent) to 2 (present), and the so-called Leipzig score is calculated (Ferenci et al. 2003). If the score is $\geq 4$, the diagnosis of Wilson disease is very likely (see also the diagnostic flowchart in Fig. 36.2). Wilson disease has been associated with more than 500 possible pathogenic variants in *ATP7B*, mostly rare mutations. Recent improvements in next-generation sequencing techniques have made the genetic diagnosis easier, so it is now reasonable to perform molecular analysis of *ATP7B* gene in any patient who has a provisional diagnosis of Wilson disease, both for confirmation purposes and to facilitate the subsequent screening of family members.

*Menkes disease* is an X-linked recessive disorder due to mutations in *ATP7A*, encoding ATP7A, a copper-transporting ATPase, present in all tissues except the liver. As a consequence, cellular uptake of copper is normal, but it cannot be exported (Kaler 1998). Copper efflux from enterocytes is severely reduced, and insufficient copper reaches the circulation, affecting the metallation of copper-dependent enzymes. Relevant cuproenzymes in the brain include dopamine-β-hydroxylase (DBH), crucial in catecholamine biosynthesis, and peptidyl glycine mono-oxygenase, required for the processing of neuropeptide precursors. Defect of these enzymes, and others like cytochrome c oxidase, which is essential for mitochondrial respiration, are probably responsible for the progressive neurological deterioration in Menkes disease, which generally starts at the age of 2–3 months. Other enzymes influenced by copper deficiency are sulfhydryl oxidase, involved in keratin crosslinking, causing sparse, fragile, greyish, and discolored hair ("pili torti"), and lysyl oxidase, essential for collagen crosslinking. Skin and joint laxity, as well as vascular tortuosity and bladder diverticula, are therefore characteristic features of this disease. Typical biochemical abnormalities in Menkes disease are low serum levels of copper and ceruloplasmin. However, at birth, serum copper and ceruloplasmin may be just below the usual range, making the diagnosis less straightforward. Abnormal levels of cathecholamines and their metabolites are instead quite specific for Menkes disease, especially the ratio between dopamine and norepinephrine as well as the ratio of dihydroxyphenylacetic acid to dihydroxyphenylglycol in plasma (Kaler et al. 2008) (Table 36.2). In cultured fibroblasts, it is possible to demonstrate an increase of copper content and retention rate, whereas egression rate is usually reduced, but these analyses are not available in most laboratories (Kim et al. 2003). Molecular testing of *ATP7A* gene allows the final diagnosis.

*Occipital horn syndrome* is a mild allelic variant of Menkes disease, caused by *ATP7A* mutations retaining a certain degree of protein function (Moeller et al. 2000). The clinical presentation is that of a connective tissue disorder, with skin and joint laxity, bone demineralization, and exostoses, predominantly at the occipital insertion of the paraspinal muscles, hence the origin of its name (Tsukahara et al. 1994). In addition, these patients have urinary tract diverticula and vascular tortuosity. Survival into adult life is usual (Tsukahara et al. 1994). A variable degree of intellectual disability may be present. Additionally, some patients have signs of autonomic dysfunction that point to DBH deficiency (Kaler et al. 2008). Serum copper and ceruloplasmin levels are in the low-normal range, whereas copper retention and egress rate in cultured fibroblasts are similar to those in Menkes disease (Table 36.3). A mutation analysis of *ATP7A* gene clarifies the diagnosis.

*X-linked distal hereditary neuropathy* is the third allelic variant associated with ATP7A defect and is caused by three unique missense mutations (p.A991D, p.T994I and p.P1386S) impairing the intracellular trafficking of this protein. The clinical phenotype is that of a late distal motor neuropathy with normal or slight low serum copper and ceruloplasmin levels and normal neurochemical ratios (Gualandi et al. 2019; Kennerson et al. 2010) (Table 36.4).

*CCS deficiency* has been reported in a patient with *SLC33A1* defect and a homozygous mutation (c.487C->T; p.Arg163Trp) in the *CCS* gene, encoding the intracellular chaperone involved in copper delivery to Cu/Zn superoxide dismutase (SOD1) (Huppke et al. 2012b). This patient, along with the clinical and biochemical features of Huppke-Brendel syndrome, presented additional symptoms not reported in that disease, namely severe muscular hypotonia, hypoglycemia, pericardial effusion, epilepsy, and persistent bilateral thalamic lesions at brain MRI. Although functional studies confirmed a pathogenic role of the *CCS* mutation and reduced SOD1 activity, it is not clear if this particular phenotype was a consequence of CCS defect with concomitant reduced metallation of SOD1.

*MEDNIK* (acronym for Mental retardation, Enteropathy, Deafness, Neuropathy, Ichthyosis, and Keratoderma) syndrome is a rare neurocutaneous disorder, originally described in consanguineous families from the Kamouraska region of Quebec (Martinelli et al. 2013). Aside from those clinical features, patients also presented a mild increase in plasma very long-chain fatty acid levels (VLCFA). Other relevant features reported by Martinelli and colleagues included bilateral T2-weighted hyperintensities of the basal ganglia and hepatopathy with elevated transaminases and cholestasis, reduced serum ceruloplasmin and copper although with increased non-ceruloplasmin bound copper, increased urine copper excretion, and increased liver copper concentration (Table 36.5). Liver biopsies showed intrahepatic cholestasis in one patient, and fibrosis and/or cirrhosis in the other two (Martinelli et al. 2013). The complete phenotype of the disease should therefore better be described as MEDNIK syndrome plus hepatopathy and copper abnormalities (MEDNIK-HC or Martinelli syndrome). MEDNIK syndrome has been associated with truncating mutations (c.364dupG and c.301-2A>G), in the *AP1S1* gene, which encodes for the σ1A subunit of adaptor protein complex 1 (AP-1). Adaptor protein complexes regulate clathrin-coated vesicle assembly, protein cargo sorting, and vesicular trafficking between organelles in eukaryotic cells (Martinelli et al. 2013). In basal conditions, the copper ATPases are localized at the level of the trans-Golgi network, where they transport copper to cuproenzymes synthesized within the secretory compartments. When the intracellular copper level rises, they translocate to the plasma membrane to traffic copper to the plasma membrane (ATP7A) or relocate it to cytoplasmic vesicles associated with bile ducts canalicular membrane (ATP7B). The trafficking of both copper pumps is clathrin-dependent and is mediated by the adaptor protein complex, thus explaining the clinical and biochemical findings of the disease, which combines some aspects of both

Menkes disease and Wilson disease, as well as other symptoms.

Interestingly, two novel missense *AP1S1* mutations, c.269T>C (p.Leu90Pro) and c.346G>A (p.Glu116Lys), have been recently associated with a non-syndromic form of congenital diarrhea in three patients who died within the first 3 months of life due to intractable diarrhea, without showing other symptoms of MEDNIK syndrome, such as sensorineural deafness and ichthyosis (Klee et al. 2020). It is not known, however, if these missense mutations may represent hypomorphs allowing for residual AP-1 complex function in the inner ear or skin, or if the patients have died before manifesting the characteristic features of MEDNIK disease.

*MEDNIK-like syndrome* is a recently described disease associated with two homozygous null variants in *AP1B1*, encoding the large β subunit of the AP-1 complex (Alsaif et al. 2019). Affected individuals showed the same neurocutaneous phenotype as MEDNIK patients, and abnormal copper metabolism highlighted by low plasma copper and ceruloplasmin, but lacked evidence of copper overload in the liver. Plasma VLCFA were also increased.

*Acetyl-CoA transporter deficiency (Huppke-Brendel syndrome)* is a rare disorder caused by mutations in the *SLC33A1* gene, encoding for a transporter (AT-1) that translocates acetyl-CoA into the ER lumen (Huppke et al. 2012a). Disease phenotypes include developmental delay, congenital cataracts, nystagmus, hearing loss, white matter hypomyelination, cerebral and cerebellar atrophy, early death, and low serum copper and ceruloplasmin levels, with normal urine copper. The pathogenesis has not been completely elucidated so far, but an abnormal acetylation of ceruloplasmin could lead to decreased secretion, with secondarily reduced serum copper (Table 36.6).

*Acrodermatitis enteropathica* is an autosomal recessive disorder of zinc transport caused by mutations in the *SLC39A4* gene encoding ZIP4, a zinc transporter expressed at the apical membrane of the enterocytes (Wang et al. 2002), affecting zinc absorption from the gut. Clinical symptoms develop after breastfeeding is stopped, whereas babies fed with infant formula develop the disorder as early as the first 2–4 weeks of life. Patients usually show severe erythematous dermatitis, initially localized at the acral and peri-orificial sites (Neldner and Hambidge 1975). Later on, these lesions become more pustular and hyperkeratotic. Mucosal lesions include gingivitis, stomatitis, and glossitis. Total alopecia is frequent, as well as nail deformities and ophthalmologic problems (blepharitis, conjunctivitis, photophobia, and impaired dark adaption). In addition, some patients present with watery diarrhea and failure to thrive. Behavioral disturbances such as irritability, apathy, and depression are common (Table 36.7). Patients are prone to frequent infections, as zinc deficiency affects cellular and humoral immunity. If untreated, the disease worsens and can even be fatal.

When the diagnosis is suspected on a clinical basis, serum zinc levels should be measured, as they are often severely reduced. Up to 15% of patients, however, show normal values because of zinc release from catabolized tissues (Van Wouwe 1989). Measurement of zinc in other tissues, such as hair or blood cells, does not improve diagnostic accuracy. In addition, several conditions, such as chronic diarrhea or infections, can be associated with secondary reduced serum zinc levels. Low urinary zinc excretion or low alkaline phosphatase (a zinc-dependent enzyme) activity can support the diagnosis. The recent improvement in genetic testing owing to NGS methodologies has made other approaches, such as intestinal zinc transport studies with radiolabeled zinc, archaic.

While waiting for the molecular results, zinc therapy should be started, and a positive response should be obtained within a week. The relapse of skin abnormalities after zinc withdrawal is conclusive.

Additional biochemical abnormalities that can be observed are increased blood ammonia (due to the defect of ornithine transcarbamylase deficiency), hypobetalipoproteinemia, and an altered fatty acid pattern. Biochemical evidence of depressed humoral and cell-mediated immunity may coexist.

#### *Transient Neonatal Zinc Deficiency*

Transient neonatal zinc deficiency is due to maternal heterozygous mutations in *SLC30A2*, which encodes ZnT2, a zinc transporter in mammary epithelial cells. This disorder causes low maternal milk zinc concentrations. Therefore, during breastfeeding, infants show signs of zinc deficiency, resembling acrodermatitis enteropathica, but they resolve after weaning (Chowanadisai et al. 2006) (Table 36.8).

#### *Spondylocheirodysplastic Ehlers-Danlos Syndrome (SCD-EDS)*

The zinc transporter protein ZIP13, encoded by *SLC39A13*, plays a crucial role in bone, tooth, and connective tissue development. Biallelic mutations in this gene cause the spondylocheirodysplastic form of Ehlers-Danlos syndrome (SCD-EDS). Affected patients exhibit both the common features of EDS, like articular hypermobility and skin hyperelasticity, and distinct physical signs such as short stature, tapering fingers, wrinkled palms, and downslanted palpebral fissures with a lack of periorbital tissue.

Skeletal radiographs show platyspondyly, osteopenia, irregular endplates of the vertebral bodies, metaphyseal widening, and epiphyseal flattening (Giunta et al. 2008). A useful biomarker of the disease is a fivefold increase of urinary deoxypyridinoline-to-pyridinoline ratio compared to normal (Table 36.9). Serum zinc levels are normal, but the intracellular distribution of zinc is abnormal, affecting proper nuclear translocation of transcription factor SMADs, which respond to BMP and TGF-β, and are critical for connective tissue development. Electron microscopy studies on skin biopsies documented normal elastic fibers and collagen fibrils (Giunta et al. 2008).

*Birk-Landau-Perez Syndrome* is an autosomal recessive disorder caused by mutations in *SLC30A9*, encoding ZnT9 (Ferreira and Gahl 2017). The ZnT9 defect causes a cerebro-renal syndrome with early-onset intellectual disability and tubulointerstitial nephropathy. After a normal psychomotor development, patients show progressive neurodegeneration, starting at 1–2 years of life. Brain MRI is normal (Table 36.10). ZnT9 is located in the endoplasmic reticulum, and its deficiency affects zinc homeostasis, leading to decreased cytosolic zinc concentrations (Ferreira and Gahl 2017).

*Asymptomatic Familial Hyperzincemia* occurs as a consequence of a variant form of albumin (the major transport protein in blood for zinc) with higher affinity to this metal. Therefore, serum zinc excess is caused by increased binding to albumin (Table 36.11). The condition has no clinical effects, and it is also called Familial Dysalbuminemic Hyperzincemia.

*Hyperzincemia and Hypercalprotectinemia* is an autoinflammatory disorder characterized by pustular and ulcerative inflammatory cutaneous lesions, recurrent arthritis, hepatosplenomegaly, pancytopenia, and growth failure caused by a mutation in the proline-serine-threonine phosphatase-interacting protein 1 (*PSTPIP1*) gene, leading to dysregulation of the metabolism of calprotectin (Holzinger et al. 2015). This protein has zinc-binding capacity, as well as antimicrobial and proinflammatory activity. Laboratory tests show extremely high serum levels of zinc and mostly calprotectin (500–12,000 times the normal levels) (Table 36.12).

*SBP2 Deficiency* is due to biallelic mutations in *SECISBP2*, encoding SBP2. In all reported patients, the deficiency of deiodinases causes abnormal thyroid metabolism, with elevated T4 and rT3, high/normal TSH, and low T3 levels.

Additional clinical symptoms, variably present, include psychomotor or speech delay, sensorineural hearing loss, oligospermia, and progressive congenital myopathy (Ferreira and Gahl 2017). Serum selenium concentration is low, indicating a global selenoprotein synthesis deficiency (Table 36.13). Organic or inorganic selenium supplementation is not able to revert thyroid function abnormalities (Ferreira and Gahl 2017).

*Progressive Cerebellocerebral Atrophy* is caused by biallelic mutations in the *SEPSECS* (Sep (O-phosphoserine) tRNA:Sec (selenocysteine tRNA synthetase) gene, responsible for a severe neurodegenerative disease with intellectual disability, postnatal microcephaly and spasticity, progressive atrophy of the cerebrum and cerebellum, and variable myoclonic or generalized tonic-clonic seizures (Agamy et al. 2010). Serum selenium is normal, and thyroid function has not been investigated in detail (Table 36.14).

## Nomenclature

| No. | Disorder | Alternative name | Abbreviation | Gene symbol | Chromosomal localization | Affected protein | OMIM No. |
|---|---|---|---|---|---|---|---|
| 36.1 | Wilson disease | Hepatolenticular degeneration | WND (WD) | *ATP7B* | 13q14.3 | ATP7B | 277900 |
| 36.2 | Menkes disease | Kinky (steely) hair disease | MNK (MK) | *ATP7A* | Xq21.1 | ATP7A | 309400 |
| 36.3 | Occipital horn syndrome | X-linked cutis laxa | OHS | *ATP7A* | Xq21.1 | ATP7A | 304150 |
| 36.4 | X-linked distal spinal muscular atrophy | | SMAX3 | *ATP7A* | Xq21.1 | ATP7A | 300489 |
| 36.5 | MEDNIK syndrome | Martinelli syndrome | AP1S1 | *AP1S1* | 7q22.1 | Adaptor-related complex protein 1 | 609313 |
| 36.6 | Acetyl-CoA transporter deficiency | Congenital cataracts, hearing loss, and low serum copper and ceruloplasmin | CCHLND | *SLC33A1* | 3q25.31 | SLC33A1 | 614482 |
| 36.7 | Acrodermatitis enteropathica | Zinc-deficiency type (AEZ) | AEZ (AE) | *SLC39A4* | 8q24.3 | ZIP4 | 201100 |
| 36.8 | Zinc transporter 2 deficiency | Transient neonatal zinc deficiency | TNZD | *SLC30A2* | 1p36.11 | ZnT2 | 608118 |
| 36.9 | Spondylocheirodysplastic Ehlers-Danlos syndrome | SCD-EDS | EDSSPD3 | *SLC39A13* | 11p11.2 | ZIP13 | 612350 |
| 36.10 | Birk-Landau-Perez syndrome | | BILAPES | *SLC30A9* | 4p13 | ZnT9 | 617595 |

(continued)

| No. | Disorder | Alternative name | Abbreviation | Gene symbol | Chromosomal localization | Affected protein | OMIM No. |
|---|---|---|---|---|---|---|---|
| 36.11 | Asymptomatic familial hyperzincemia | | | | | | |
| 36.12 | Hyperzincemia and hypercalprotectinemia | | | *PSTPIP1* | 15q24.3 | Proline-serine-threonine phosphatase-interacting protein 1 | |
| 36.13 | Selenocysteine insertion sequence-binding protein 2 deficiency | | | *SECISBP2* | 9q22.2 | SECIS-binding protein 2;SBP2 | 609698 |
| 36.14 | O-phosphoseryl-tRNA(sec) selenium transferase deficiency | Selenocysteinyl-tRNA(sec) synthase deficiency, progressive cerebellocerebral atrophy; Pontocerebellar hypoplasia type 2D | PCH2D | *SEPSECS* | 4p15.2 | O-phosphoseryl-tRNA(sec) selenium transferase | 613811 |

## Metabolic Pathways

### Metabolic Pathway for Copper (see Fig. 36.1)

### Metabolic Pathway for Zinc

Zinc is involved in a variety of biological processes, as a structural, catalytic, and intracellular and intercellular signaling component. Zinc is a cofactor for several enzymes, including ornithine transcarbamylase, alkaline phosphatase, carbonic anhydrase, superoxide dismutase, DNA and RNA polymerases, lactate dehydrogenase, and alcohol dehydrogenase. Two groups of proteins involved in zinc transport are involved in cellular zinc homeostasis: the Zip family that mediates zinc transport from outside the cell into the cytoplasm and the ZnT family that mediates export of zinc, either into the extracellular space or into intracellular organelles. The exact role of each of these zinc transport proteins in the various cell types has not been completely elucidated. In humans, there are nine known ZnT transporters and 15 Zip transporters. The ZIP4 defect has been associated with a zinc absorption defect in the enterocytes, leading to Acrodermatitis Enteropathica. ZIP13 is relevant for bone and connective tissue development, and its loss of function is causative for the spondylocheirodysplastic form of Ehlers-Danlos syndrome. For the zinc export proteins identified in humans, the ZnT2 defect has been associated with low breast milk concentration, whereas the ZnT9 defect causes a cerebro-renal disease, Birk-Landau-Perez syndrome.

### Metabolic Pathway for Selenium

Selenium salts are toxic in large amounts, but trace amounts are crucial for cellular function in humans. Selenium is mainly found in foods in its organic form—selenomethionine in plant sources, selenocysteine in animal sources—while the inorganic forms of selenium—selenate and selenite—are mainly found in dietary supplements.

More than 80% of the ingested selenium is absorbed through the small intestines.

Most biological effects of Se are mediated by selenoproteins, proteins containing the 21st proteinogenic amino acid, selenocysteine (Sec), a cysteine analogue with a selenium-containing selenol group in place of the sulfur-containing thiol group. There are 25 human selenoproteins, including five forms of glutathione peroxidase, three forms of thioredoxin reductase, and three deiodinases, those three participating in thyroid hormone metabolism

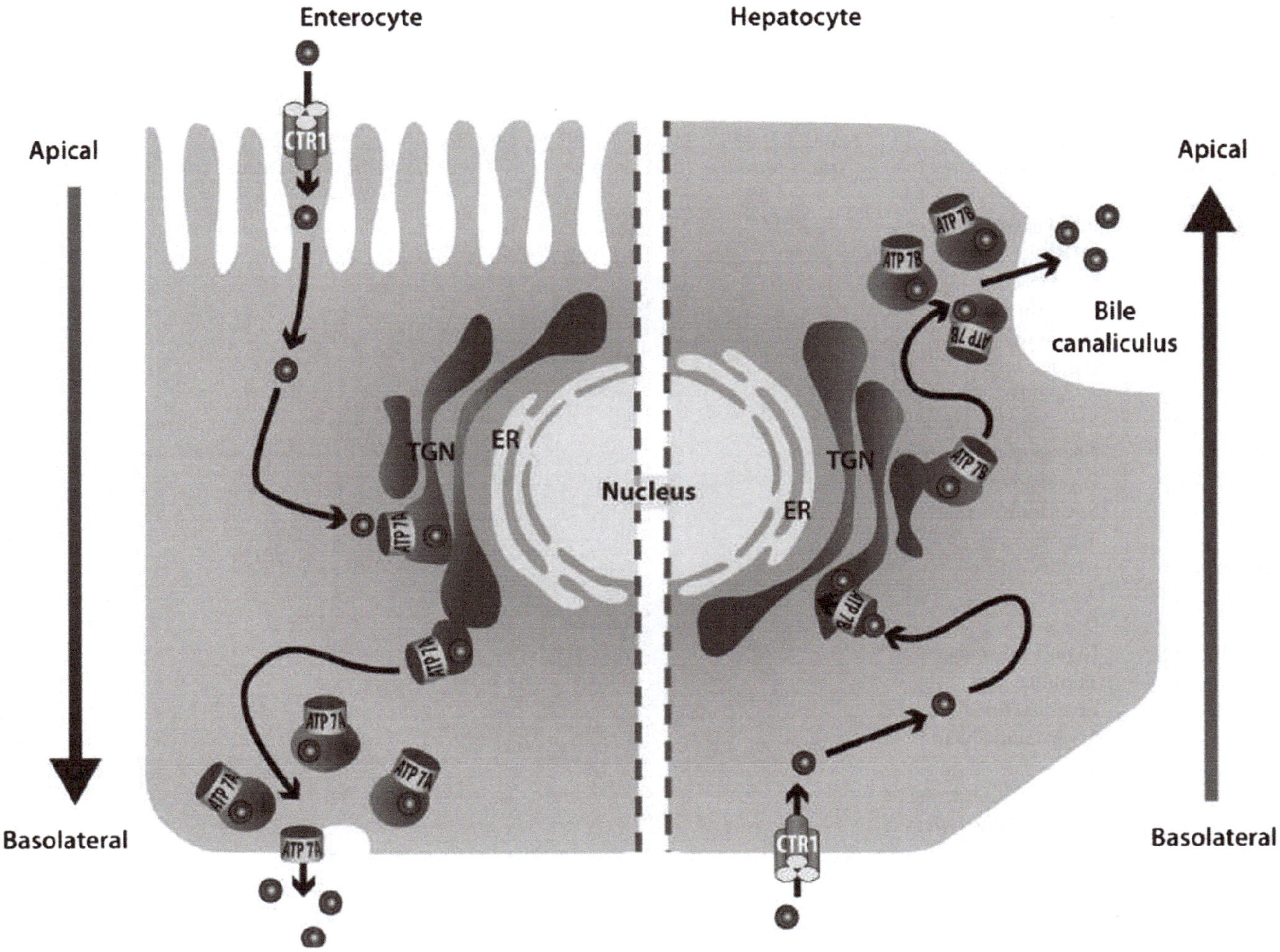


**Fig. 36.1** Schematic representation of the key elements of copper homeostasis (adapted from Agamy et al. (2010)). Left panel: Copper is required for numerous processes, including mitochondrial respiration, antioxidant defense, neurotransmitter synthesis, connective tissue formation, and skin pigmentation. Dietary copper from the intestine is taken up by the enterocytes through CTR1 and transported intracellularly to ATP7A, localized in the trans-Golgi network (TGN). This protein will export copper to the portal circulation. When ATP7A is defective, as in Menkes disease, no copper can leave the enterocyte, resulting in a systemic shortage of copper. Right panel: copper from the portal circulation is taken up through CTR1, transported to ATP7B in the trans-Golgi network (TGN). This protein will export copper to the bile canaliculus. When this pathway is defective, as in Wilson disease, the hepatocytes will gradually accumulate copper, which above a threshold level will induce cellular damage

(Ferreira and Gahl 2017). There is no specific codon for Sec; instead, the UGA codon, usually a stop codon, is made to encode selenocysteine by the presence of a selenocysteine insertion sequence (SECIS), a stem–loop structure present in the 3′-untranslated region of mRNA. Selenocysteine synthesis occurs on a specialized tRNA, called tRNA[Ser]Sec, but there are no tRNA synthetases specific for Sec, so serine is charged onto tRNA[Ser]Sec by Seryl-tRNA synthetase first. Ser-tRNA[Ser]Sec is then converted into Sec-tRNA[Ser]Sec by selenocysteine synthase (SEPSECS). A specific elongation factor, EF-Sec, directs Sec-tRNA[Ser]Sec to the ribosome, which translates UGA as selenocysteine (Sec) instead of termination. SECIS-binding protein 2 (SECISBP2) is crucial for the interaction with the SECIS element (Agamy et al. 2010).

## Signs and Symptoms

**Table 36.1** Wilson disease

| System | Symptoms and biomarkers | Neonatal (birth–1 month) | Infancy (1–18 months) | Childhood (1.5–11 years) | Adolescence (11–16 years) | Adulthood (>16 years) |
|---|---|---|---|---|---|---|
| CNS | Ataxia | | | ± | + | ++ |
| | **Basal ganglia lesions (MRI)** | | | ± | + | ++ |
| | Clumsiness | | | ± | + | + |
| | **Dysarthria** | | | n | + | ++ |
| | **Dystonia** | | | ± | + | ++ |
| | Handwriting | | | ± | + | + |
| | Irritability | | | ± | + | + |
| | **Movement, abnormal** | | | ± | + | ++ |
| | **Neurological symptoms** | | | ± | + | ++ |
| | Psychiatric symptoms | | | n | ± | ± |
| | **Speech disturbances** | | | n | + | ++ |
| | Tremor | | | ± | + | + |
| Digestive | Abdominal pain | | | ± | ± | ± |
| | Ascites | | | ++ | ++ | + |
| | Drooling | | | ± | + | + |
| | **Hepatosplenomegaly** | | | ++ | ++ | ++ |
| | **Jaundice** | | | ++ | ++ | + |
| | **Liver dysfunction** | | | ++ | ++ | ++ |
| | **Liver failure, acute** | | | ++ | ++ | + |
| Eye | Cataract | | | ± | ± | ± |
| | Kayser-Fleischer ring | | | + | + | + |
| Hematological | **Anemia, hemolytic** | | | + | ++ | + |
| | Coagulopathy | | | + | ++ | ++ |
| | Hemolysis | | | + | ++ | + |
| | Leukopenia | | | + | ++ | ++ |
| | Thrombocytopenia | | | + | ++ | ++ |
| Renal | Renal tubular acidosis | | | + | + | + |
| Laboratory findings | Albumin (serum) | n | n | ↓–n | ↓–n | ↓–n |
| | ASAT/ALAT (plasma) | n | n | ↑ | ↑ | ↑ |
| | Bilirubin (plasma) | n | n | n–↑ | n–↑ | n–↑ |
| | Ceruloplasmin (serum) | ↓–n | ↓–n | ↓–n | ↓–n | ↓–n |
| | Copper (liver) | n | n-↑ | ↑ | ↑ | ↑ |
| | Copper (serum) | ↓–n | ↓–n | ↓–n | ↓–n | ↓–n |
| | Copper (urine) | n | n–↑ | n–↑ | ↑ | ↑↑ |
| | Prothrombin ratio | n | n | n–↑ | ↑ | ↑ |

**Table 36.2** Menkes disease

| System | Symptoms and biomarkers | Neonatal (birth–1 month) | Infancy (1–18 months) | Childhood (1.5–11 years) | Adolescence (11–16 years) | Adulthood (>16 years) |
|---|---|---|---|---|---|---|
| Autonomic system | **Hypothermia** | + | + | + | | |
| Cardiovascular | Arterial ruptures | | ± | ± | | |
| | Tortuous arteries | | ± | ± | | |
| CNS | **Convulsions** | | + | + | | |
| | Encephalopathy, progressive | ± | ± | + | | |
| | Intellectual disability | ± | + | + | | |
| | **Retardation, psychomotor** | | + | + | | |
| | Spasticity | ± | ± | + | | |
| Dermatological | **Cutis laxa** | ± | + | + | | |
| Digestive | **Feeding difficulties** | ± | + | + | | |
| Genitourinary | Bladder diverticula | | ± | ± | | |
| Hair | **Hair abnormality** | ± | + | + | | |
| | **Kinky hair** | ± | + | ++ | | |
| Hematological | **Anemia** | ± | ± | ± | | |
| | Neutropenia | ± | ± | ± | | |
| Musculoskeletal | **Connective tissue abnormalities** | ± | + | + | | |
| | Hernias | | ± | ± | | |
| | **Peculiar facies** | + | + | + | | |
| Laboratory findings | Ceruloplasmin (serum) | ↓ | ↓ | ↓ | | |
| | Copper (cerebrospinal fluid) | ↓ | ↓ | ↓ | | |
| | Copper (duodenal) | ↑ | ↑ | ↑ | | |
| | Copper (liver) | ↓ | ↓ | ↓ | | |
| | Copper (serum) | ↓ | ↓ | ↓ | | |

**Table 36.3** Occipital horn syndrome

| System | Symptoms and biomarkers | Neonatal (birth–1 month) | Infancy (1–18 months) | Childhood (1.5–11 years) | Adolescence (11–16 years) | Adulthood (>16 years) |
|---|---|---|---|---|---|---|
| Cardiovascular | **Hypotension, orthostatic** | | | + | + | + |
| Dermatological | **Cutis laxa** | ± | ± | + | + | + |
| Digestive | **Diarrhea** | ± | ± | + | + | + |
| Genitourinary | Bladder diverticula | | ± | + | + | + |
| Musculoskeletal | **Exostosis, occipital horn** | ± | ± | + | + | + |
| Renal | Urinary infections | n | ± | + | + | + |
| Laboratory findings | Ceruloplasmin (serum) | ↓–n | ↓–n | ↓–n | ↓–n | ↓–n |
| | Copper (serum) | ↓–n | ↓–n | ↓–n | ↓–n | ↓–n |

**Table 36.4** X-linked distal spinal muscular atrophy

| System | Symptoms and biomarkers | Neonatal (birth–1 month) | Infancy (1–18 months) | Childhood (1.5–11 years) | Adolescence (11–16 years) | Adulthood (>16 years) |
|---|---|---|---|---|---|---|
| Musculoskeletal | Absent tendon reflexes | | | | | ± |
| | **Muscle weakness, distal** | | | | | + |
| | Weak tendon reflexes | | | | | ± |
| Laboratory findings | Copper (serum) | n | n | n | n | n |

**Table 36.5** MEDNIK syndrome

| System | Symptoms and biomarkers | Neonatal (birth–1 month) | Infancy (1–18 months) | Childhood (1.5–11 years) | Adolescence (11–16 years) | Adulthood (>16 years) |
|---|---|---|---|---|---|---|
| CNS | Cerebral atrophy (MRI) | | + | + | + | + |
| | **Neuropathy, peripheral** | | | + | + | + |
| | **Retardation, psychomotor** | | + | + | + | + |
| Dermatological | **Erythroderma** | | | + | + | + |
| | Hyperkeratosis | | | + | + | + |
| | **Ichthyosis** | | + | + | + | + |
| Digestive | Intestinal pseudo obstruction | ± | + | + | + | + |
| | **Liver dysfunction** | | + | + | + | + |
| Ear | **Deafness** | | | + | + | + |
| Laboratory findings | ASAT/ALAT (plasma) | ↑ | ↑ | ↑ | ↑ | ↑ |
| | Bile acids (enzyme assay) (plasma) | | | ↑ | ↑ | ↑ |
| | Ceruloplasmin (serum) | | ↓ | ↓ | ↓ | ↓ |
| | Copper (serum) | | ↓ | ↓ | ↓ | ↓ |
| | Very-long-chain fatty acids (plasma) | | ↑ | ↑ | ↑ | ↑ |

**Table 36.6** Acetyl-CoA transporter deficiency

| System | Symptoms and biomarkers | Neonatal (birth–1 month) | Infancy (1–18 months) | Childhood (1.5–11 years) | Adolescence (11–16 years) | Adulthood (>16 years) |
|---|---|---|---|---|---|---|
| CNS | Cerebellar atrophy (MRI) | + | ++ | ++ | | |
| | Cerebral atrophy (MRI) | + | ++ | ++ | | |
| | **Hypomyelination (MRI)** | + | ++ | ++ | | |
| Ear | **Hearing loss** | + | ++ | ++ | | |
| Eye | **Cataract** | + | + | + | | |
| Musculoskeletal | **Hypotonia, muscular-axial** | + | ++ | ++ | | |
| Laboratory findings | Ceruloplasmin (serum) | ↓ | ↓ | ↓ | | |
| | Copper (serum) | ↓ | ↓ | ↓ | | |

**Table 36.7** Acrodermatitis enteropathica

| System | Symptoms and biomarkers | Neonatal (birth–1 month) | Infancy (1–18 months) | Childhood (1.5–11 years) | Adolescence (11–16 years) | Adulthood (>16 years) |
|---|---|---|---|---|---|---|
| CNS | **Irritability** | ± | ++ | ++ | + | + |
| Dermatological | **Alopecia** | | + | ++ | ++ | ++ |
| | **Dermatitis** | ± | ++ | +++ | ++ | ++ |
| Digestive | **Anorexia** | | ++ | ++ | + | + |
| | **Diarrhea** | ± | ++ | ++ | + | + |
| Other | **Failure to thrive** | | + | ++ | ++ | ++ |
| | Frequent infections | | + | + | ± | ± |
| Psychiatric | Apathy | ± | + | + | ± | ± |
| | Depression | | | ± | ± | ± |
| Laboratory findings | Alkaline phosphatase (plasma) | ↓–n | ↓ | ↓ | ↓ | ↓ |
| | Zinc (serum) | ↓–n | ↓–n | ↓–n | ↓–n | ↓–n |
| | Zinc uptake (duodenal) | ↓ | ↓ | ↓ | ↓ | ↓ |

**Table 36.8** Zinc transporter 2 deficiency

| System | Symptoms and biomarkers | Neonatal (birth–1 month) | Infancy (1–18 months) | Childhood (1.5–11 years) | Adolescence (11–16 years) | Adulthood (>16 years) |
|---|---|---|---|---|---|---|
| Dermatological | Acrodermatitis enteropathica | + | + | + | | |
| | Alopecia | | + | + | | |
| | Dermatitis | + | + | + | | |
| Laboratory findings | Zinc (serum) | ↓ | n | **n** | | |

**Table 36.9** Spondylocheirodysplastic Ehlers-Danlos syndrome

| System | Symptoms and biomarkers | Neonatal (birth–1 month) | Infancy (1–18 months) | Childhood (1.5–11 years) | Adolescence (11–16 years) | Adulthood (>16 years) |
|---|---|---|---|---|---|---|
| Cardiovascular | Skin veins, prominent | + | + | + | + | |
| Dermatological | **Hyperelastic, loose skin** | + | + | + | + | |
| | **Thin skin** | + | + | + | + | |
| | **Velvety, smooth skin** | + | + | + | + | |
| Digestive | **Bifid uvula** | + | + | + | + | |
| Eye | Blue sclerae | + | + | + | + | |
| | **Downslanting palpebral fissures** | + | + | + | + | |
| | Protuberant eyes | + | + | + | + | |
| Musculoskeletal | **Delayed tooth eruption** | | + | + | | |
| | Flexion contractures of fingers | + | + | + | + | |
| | **Growth retardation** | + | + | + | + | |
| | High palate | + | + | + | + | |
| | Hypodontia | | + | + | + | |
| | Joint laxity | + | + | + | + | |
| | Malocclusion | | + | + | + | |
| | Muscle atrophy | | + | + | + | |
| | **Osteopenia** | + | + | + | + | |
| | **Pes planus** | + | + | + | + | |
| | Platyspondyly | + | + | + | + | |
| | **Short metacarpals** | + | + | + | + | |
| | **Short phalanges** | + | + | + | + | |
| | **Short stature** | | + | + | + | + |
| | Short, wide femoral neck | + | + | + | + | |
| | Slender, tapered fingers | | + | + | + | |
| | **Small ilia with snail-like appearance** | + | + | + | + | |
| | Widened metaphyses (elbows and knees) | + | + | + | + | |
| Other | Low birth weight | + | | | | |
| Laboratory findings | Lysyl hydroxylase activity | | n | n | n | |
| | Lysyl pyridinoline/hydroxylysyl pyridinoline (LP/HP) ratio (urine) | | ↑ | ↑ | ↑ | |
| | Prolyl 4-hydroxylase activity | | n | n | n | |

**Table 36.10** Birk-Landau-Perez syndrome

| System | Symptoms and biomarkers | Neonatal (birth–1 month) | Infancy (1–18 months) | Childhood (1.5–11 years) | Adolescence (11–16 years) | Adulthood (>16 years) |
|---|---|---|---|---|---|---|
| Autonomic system | Hypertension | | | + | + | |
| CNS | **Ataxia** | | | + | + | |
| | **Choreoathetosis** | | | + | + | |
| | **Dystonia** | | | + | + | |
| | Intellectual disability | | | + | + | |
| | **Loss of speech** | | | + | + | |
| Eye | Ptosis of eyelid | | | + | + | |
| | **Strabismus** | | | + | + | |
| Renal | Tubulointerstitial nephritis | | | + | + | |
| Laboratory findings | Potassium (plasma) | | | ↑ | ↑ | |

**Table 36.11** Asymptomatic familial hyperzincemia

| System | Symptoms and biomarkers | Neonatal (birth–1 month) | Infancy (1–18 months) | Childhood (1.5–11 years) | Adolescence (11–16 years) | Adulthood (>16 years) |
|---|---|---|---|---|---|---|
| Other | No clinical symptoms | + | + | + | + | + |
| Laboratory findings | Albumin (serum) | | | n | n | n |
| | Zinc (serum) | | | ↑ | ↑ | ↑ |

**Table 36.12** Hyperzincemia with hypercalprotectinemia

| System | Symptoms and biomarkers | Neonatal (birth–1 month) | Infancy (1–18 months) | Childhood (1.5–11 years) | Adolescence (11–16 years) | Adulthood (>16 years) |
|---|---|---|---|---|---|---|
| Digestive | **Hepatosplenomegaly** | | | | + | + |
| Hematological | **Anemia** | | | | + | + |
| | **Autoinflammation** | | | | + | + |
| Other | Failure to thrive | | ± | ± | | |
| | **Frequent infections** | | | | + | + |
| Laboratory findings | Calprotectin (serum) | | | | ↑ | ↑ |
| | Zinc (serum) | | | | ↑ | ↑ |

**Table 36.13** Selenocysteine insertion sequence-binding protein 2 deficiency

| System | Symptoms and biomarkers | Neonatal (birth–1 month) | Infancy (1–18 months) | Childhood (1.5–11 years) | Adolescence (11–16 years) | Adulthood (>16 years) |
|---|---|---|---|---|---|---|
| Musculoskeletal | **Fatty infiltration of muscles** | | + | + | + | |
| | **Short stature** | | + | + | + | |
| Laboratory findings | Selenium (serum) | | ↓ | ↓ | ↓ | |
| | Thyrotropin | | ↑ | ↑ | ↑ | |
| | Thyroxine T4 (serum) | | ↑ | ↑ | ↑ | |
| | Triiodothyronin T3 (serum) | | ↓ | ↓ | ↓ | |
| | Triiodothyronine, reverse rT3 (serum) | | ↑ | ↑ | ↑ | |

**Table 36.14** O-phosphoseryl-tRNA(Sec) selenium transferase deficiency

| System | Symptoms and biomarkers | Neonatal (birth–1 month) | Infancy (1–18 months) | Childhood (1.5–11 years) | Adolescence (11–16 years) | Adulthood (>16 years) |
|---|---|---|---|---|---|---|
| CNS | **Ataxia** | | | + | + | |
| | Intellectual disability | | + | + | + | |
| | Microcephaly | | + | + | + | |
| | Seizures | | + | + | | |

## Reference Values

| Copper, ceruloplasmin, zinc, and selenium | | | | | |
|---|---|---|---|---|---|
| Serum copper | 11–22 μmol/L[a] | Serum zinc | 11.9–19.4 μmol/L[a] | Serum selenium | 70–150 ng/mL[a] |
| Serum ceruloplasmin | 1.5–3.7 μmol/L | | | | |
| Urinary copper | <0.6 μmol/24 h[a] | Urinary zinc | 4.6 ± 2.6 μmol/24 h[a] | | |
| Liver copper | <55 μg/g dry weight[a] | | | | |

[a]Atomic absorption. Ala et al. (2007) and Van Wouwe (1989)

## Pathological Values

| | Cu (S) μmol/L | Cu (U) μmol/24 h | Cpl (S) μmol/L | Liver copper μg/g dry weight | Zn (S) μmol/L | Zn (U) μmol/24 h | Se (S) ng/mL[a] |
|---|---|---|---|---|---|---|---|
| Wilson disease | | | | | | | |
| – presymptomatic | | >0.6 | <1.5 | 250 | | | |
| – symptomatic | | >1.6 | <1.5 | 250 | | | |
| Menkes disease | <11 | | <1.5 | | | | |
| Occipital Horn syndrome | n–↓ | | n–↓ | | | | |
| X-linked distal spinal muscular atrophy | n | | | | | | |
| Huppke-Brendel syndrome | <11 | n | <0.07 | n[a] | | | |
| CCS deficiency | 0.5[a] | | 0.15[a] | | | | |
| MEDNIK syndrome | 2.4–8.3 | >0.6[a] | 0.1–0.7 | ↑[a] | n[a] | | |
| MEDNIK-like syndrome | <10 | | <0.9 | n[a] | n–↓ | | |
| Acrodermatitis Enteropathica | | | | | 7.1 ± 5.0 | 1.5 ± 0.9 | |
| Asymptomatic Familial Hyperzincemia | | | | | ↑ | | |
| Hyperzincemia and Hypercalprotectinemia | | | | | ↑ | | |
| SCD-EDS | | | | | n | | |
| Birk-Landau-Perez syndrome | | | | | n | | |
| SBP2 deficiency | | | | | | | ↓ |
| Progressive cerebello – cerebral atrophy | | | | | | | n |

Ala et al. (2007), Nicastro et al. (2010), Kaler (1998), Tsukahara et al. (1994), Kennerson et al. 2010, Martinelli et al. (2013), Alsaif et al. (2019), Van Wouwe (1989), Holzinger et al. (2015), Ferreira and Gahl (2017)

[a]One patient

## Diagnostic Flowchart

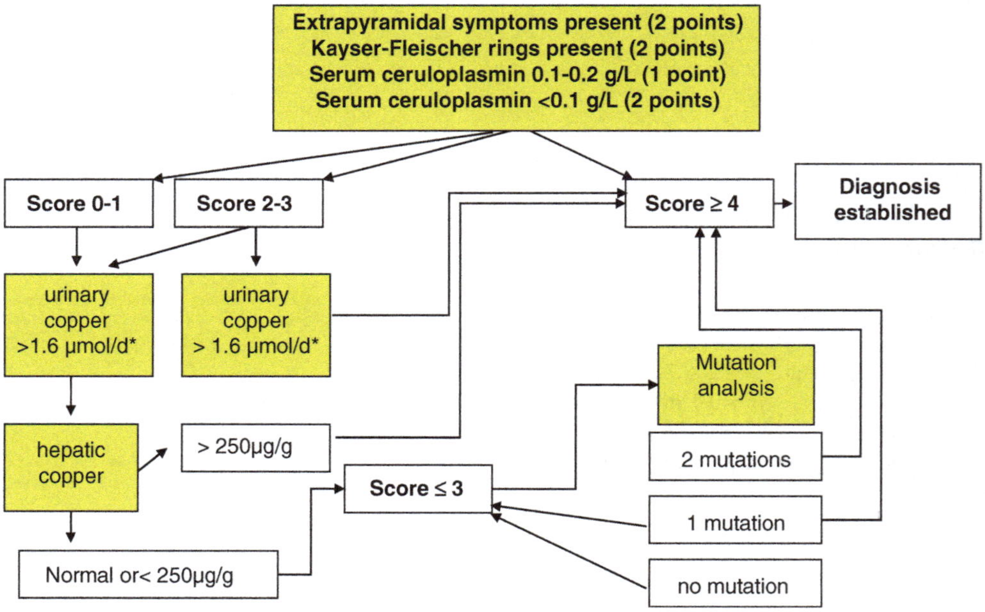


**Fig. 36.2** Diagnostic flowchart for Wilson disease (Modified from Ferenci et al. (2003) and European Association for the study of the Liver (2012). *In asymptomatic children the cut-off can be lowered to 0.6 µmol/day (Ala et al. 2007)

### Menkes Disease

Diagnosis should be suspected in any child with symptoms suggestive of Menkes disease or a positive family history. A quick confirmation is essential, as an early diagnosis is a prerequisite for effective treatment. This can be obtained by determining the ratio of plasma dopamine to norepinephrine (N: 0.04 ± 0.03; Menkes: 0.83 ± 0.71), as well as the ratio of plasma dihydroxyphenylacetic acid to dihydroxyphenylglycol (N: 1.5 ± 0.4; Menkes: 13.0 ± 6.6) (Kaler et al. 2008). Serum copper and ceruloplasmin are generally low, but this may not be discriminatory as levels tend to be low in infancy. An analysis of *ATP7A* for mutations confirms a biochemical diagnosis.

### Occipital Horn Syndrome

In a patient with symptoms suggestive of occipital horn syndrome, serum copper and serum ceruloplasmin are generally low, but can be normal too. Therefore, a genetic analysis of *ATP7A* is mandatory for establishing a diagnosis.

### Acetyl-CoA Transporter Deficiency

The presence of the characteristic constellation of clinical signs, as well as low serum copper and ceruloplasmin, should prompt to sequence the *SLC33A1* gene.

### CCS Deficiency

As this disorder was described only in one patient, who also carried pathogenic mutations in *SLC33A1*, there is not at the moment a definite flowchart to direct the diagnosis.

### MEDNIK and MEDNIK-Like Syndrome

These two disorders should be suspected in presence of the characteristic clinical phenotype associated with low serum copper and ceruloplasmin, and a slight increase in VLCFA. Some symptoms (such as peripheral neuropathy) may not be present in the first phases of the disease. A genetic analysis of *AP1S1* and *AP1B1* gene is required to differentiate between the two disorders.

### Acrodermatitis Enteropathica

Patients who develop the characteristic erythematous dermatitis at the acral and periorificial areas when breastfeeding is stopped should be investigated for *acrodermatitis enteropathica*.

Serum zinc levels are usually low, but 15% of the patients have levels in the normal range (Van Wouwe 1989). The diagnosis is confirmed by disease-causing mutations in *SLC39A4*. All suspected patients should receive zinc therapy waiting for genetic results. A response should be obtained within a week.

**SCD-EDS and Birk-Landau-Perez Syndrome** may be suspected only on the basis of the phenotype, due to the absence of overt serum zinc abnormalities, except for a mild increase in the urinary deoxypyridinoline-to-pyridinoline ratio in SCD-EDS.

**Familial Asymptomatic Hyperzincemia** may be suspected in subjects with persistent evidence of increases in serum zinc, without clinical signs of disease. Conversely, an autoinflammatory disorder with ulcerative cutaneous lesions and systemic involvement may suggest to measure calprotectin. In the presence of a dramatic increase in this protein, serum zinc should be measured, to aid in the diagnosis of *hyperzincemia and hypercalprotectinemia.*

In **SBP2 deficiency**, abnormal thyroid function and low selenium are diagnostic handles whereas in **progressive cerebello-cerebral atrophy** there are no reliable biomarkers.

## Specimen Collection

Tubes for routine blood collection in fasting subjects should be copper, zinc, selenium, and other trace metals free. Copper measurement on dry liver tissue should be performed by collecting the fresh samples in metal-free specimen vials and immediately freezing them in liquid nitrogen. The sample should be store at −80 °C until analysis.

For copper measurement in urine over 24 hr, it is crucial to use copper-free urine collection containers to exclude false positives due to contamination of the collection vessels.

For 24-hr urine collection, it is recommended to keep the urine aliquots refrigerated (at 4 °C), and after completion to send the samples to the laboratory in a well-isolated package. Urine can be stored in the refrigerator at 4 °C for a maximum of 1 week until analysis, or stored frozen at −20 °C (1 week–2 months).

## Prenatal Diagnosis

Prenatal diagnosis in each condition discussed is possible by gene sequencing when the defect in the family is known.

## DNA Testing

For each of the disorders discussed, the gene is known. Molecular analyses could be performed on DNA extracted from blood collected in EDTA tubes. Available options include sequencing of all coding exons and intron–exon boundaries of the gene of interest by Sanger, or as part of a targeted gene panel for Mendelian syndromes, or by exome or whole-genome sequencing. Exon or whole-gene deletions/duplications may be identified by diverse methods including quantitative PCR, long-range PCR, multiplex ligation-dependent probe amplification, and chromosomal microarray that include that gene/chromosome segment.

## Treatment Summary

*Wilson disease* treatment is based on reducing the amount of copper in the body. Several copper chelators are available, that is, penicillamine and trientine, as well as zinc. Penicillamine is the drug of choice in patients with hepatic problems, while in patients with neurologic problems, zinc should be considered (European association for the study of the liver 2012). Zinc treatment is also advisable in patients still without clinical symptoms, for example, those identified through family screening. Many patients, both those with mainly neurological symptoms and those with hepatic disease, especially in the phase of end-stage cirrhosis or liver failure, do not respond to the therapy. For those patients, liver transplantation is an option.

Earlier, *Menkes disease* patients died mostly before the age of 3, but with current supportive care, a longer survival is possible. Treatment with subcutaneous injections of copper histidine or copper chloride before age 10 days is able to normalize the developmental outcome in some patients and improves the neurologic outcome in others (Kaler et al. 2008). However, it is evident that some infants show poor or no significant response at all, also after starting copper histidine treatment very early in life, depending on the residual functional activity of ATP7A protein (Kaler et al. 2008).

In *Occipital horn syndrome*, there is no evidence so far that copper replacement therapy can be clinically beneficial, although it seems reasonable to expect better neurodevelopmental and neurocognitive outcomes in these individuals if they are treated with copper during their first 3 years of age.

*Acetyl-CoA transporter deficiency.* Four patients were treated with copper replacement therapy without reasonable evidence of improvement (Huppke et al. 2012a).

*MEDNIK syndrome* might respond to zinc acetate therapy. In the only patient tested with this treatment, oral zinc acetate therapy at a dose of 50 mg/day was associated with a relevant improvement of both clinical and laboratory abnormalities.

*Acrodermatitis Enteropathica.* Zinc supplementation results in the disappearance of skin lesions within a week and normalization of plasma and urinary excretion of zinc, as well as serum alkaline phosphatase values. The usual therapeutic dose ranges between 30 and 50 mg Zn/day (10–30 μmol elemental zinc/kg/day, 0.5–2 mg/kg elemental zinc/day) and most patients are kept at the same total dose per day during their entire childhood. Zinc is usually provided as zinc salts (gluconate, acetate, and, more often, sulfate), administered in three divided doses daily if gastric problems occur. As zinc competes with copper for absorption at the intestinal level, plasma copper should be monitored to avoid hypocupremia.

Long-term prognosis is excellent and the good response to zinc therapy suggests that other, low-affinity transporters, may be involved in importing this cation at higher luminal concentrations (Neldner and Hambidge 1975; Van Wouwe 1989).

**Standard Treatment**

| | Therapy | Application | Dose | Duration |
|---|---|---|---|---|
| 36.1 Wilson disease | Chelating agents (D-penicillamine, trientine) | Orally | Children: 25 mg/kg/day<br>Adults: 1–2 g in 4 doses | Lifelong |
| | Zinc salts (zinc acetate) | Orally | 1–5 years: 2 × 25 mg/day<br>6–16 years: 3 × 25 mg/day<br>>16 years: 3 × 50 mg/day | Lifelong |
| 36.2 Menkes disease | Cu-histidinate | SC | 250 μg twice daily<br>250 μg daily after 1 year | Lifelong |
| 36.3 Acrodermatitis enteropathica | Zinc sulphate<br>Zinc acetate | Orally | 50–90 mg $Zn^{2+}$/day | Lifelong |
| 36.4 MEDNIK syndrome | Zinc acetate | Orally | 50 mg/day | Lifelong? |

## Follow-Up

*Wilson disease:* Each follow-up visit should include a clinical evaluation, both neurological and hepatological, and laboratory tests of copper metabolism (mainly 24-h urinary copper excretion) and liver function (synthesis, bilirubin, transaminases). These parameters should all improve. On stable, long-term chelator therapy, urinary copper excretion should be 3–8 μmol/24 h, while a urinary copper excretion in excess of 1.6 μmol/24 h after 2 days cessation of chelators may indicate insufficient decoppering or non-adherence to therapy [European association for the study of the Liver]. Similarly, on stable, long-term zinc treatment, urinary copper excretion should be below 1.6 μmol/24 h.

*Menkes disease* patients on copper histidine treatment must be regularly monitored with special emphasis on neurodevelopmental outcome and renal side effects. Serum copper and ceruloplasmin values should normalize under therapy and need to be checked to avoid supranormal levels (Kaler et al. 2008). Serum copper levels, however, are poor predictors of long-term neurodevelopmental outcome.

*Acrodermatitis enteropathica* patients will be monitored clinically to follow the effect of zinc supplementation on symptomatology. Therapy will rapidly improve dermatological signs. Biochemical parameters (serum zinc level, serum alkaline phosphatase, and urinary zinc excretion) will also normalize.

For MEDNIK syndrome, it is not possible at the moment to give recommendations. As for all the other disorders reported in this chapter, for which a therapy is not available, long-term management is mainly directed at preventing disease complications.

## References

Agamy O, Ben Zeev B, Lev D, et al. Mutations disrupting selenocysteine formation cause progressive cerebello-cerebral atrophy. Am J Hum Genet. 2010;87:538–44.

Ala A, Walker AP, Ashkan K, Dooley JS, Schilsky ML. Wilson's disease. Lancet. 2007;369:397–408.

Alsaif HS, Al-Owain M, Barrios-Llerena ME, et al. Homozygous loss-of-function mutations in AP1B1, encoding beta-1 subunit of adaptor-related protein complex 1, cause MEDNIK-like syndrome. Am J Hum Genet. 2019;105:1016–22.

de Bie P, Muller P, Wijmenga C, Klomp LWJ. Molecular pathogenesis of Wilson and Menkes disease: correlation of mutations with molecular defects and disease phenotypes. J Med Genet. 2007;44:673–88.

Chowanadisai W, Lonnerdal B, Kelleher SL. Identification of a mutation in SLC30A2 (ZnT-2) in women with low milk zinc concentration that results in transient neonatal zinc deficiency. J Biol Chem. 2006;28:39,699–707.

European Association for the study of the Liver. EASL clinical practice guidelines: Wilson's disease. J Hepatol. 2012;56:671–85.

Ferenci P, Caca K, Loudianos G, et al. Diagnosis and phenotypic classification of Wilson disease. Liver Int. 2003;23:139–42.

Ferenci P, Czlonkowska A, Merle U, et al. Late-onset Wilson's disease. Gastroenterology. 2007;132:1294–8.

Ferreira CR, Gahl WA. Disorders of metal metabolism. Transl Sci Rare Dis. 2017;2:101–39.

Giunta C, Elçioglu NH, Albrecht B, et al. Spondylocheirodysplastic form of the Ehlers-Danlos syndrome–an autosomal-recessive entity caused by mutations in the zinc transporter gene SLC39A13. Am J Hum Genet. 2008;82:1290–305.

Gualandi F, Sette E, Fortunato F, et al. Report of a novel ATP7A mutation causing distal motor neuropathy. Neuromuscul Disord. 2019;29:776–85.

Holzinger D, Fassl SK, de Jager W, et al. Single amino acid charge switch defines clinically distinct proline-serine-threonine phosphatase-interacting protein 1 (PSTPIP1)-associated inflammatory diseases. J Allergy Clin Immunol. 2015;136:1337–45.

Huppke P, Brendel C, Kalscheuer V, et al. Mutations in *SLC33A1* cause a lethal autosomal-recessive disorder with congenital cataracts, hearing loss, and low serum copper and ceruloplasmin. Am J Hum Genet. 2012a;90:61–8.

Huppke P, Brendel C, Korenke GC, et al. Molecular and biochemical characterization of a unique mutation in CCS, the human copper chaperone to superoxide dismutase. Hum Mutat. 2012b;33:1207–15.

Kaler SG. Diagnosis and therapy of Menkes syndrome, a genetic form of copper deficiency. Am J Clin Nutr. 1998;67S:1029S–34S.

Kaler SG, Holmes CS, Goldstein DS, et al. Neonatal diagnosis and treatment of Menkes disease. New Engl J Med. 2008;358:605–14.

Kennerson ML, Nicholson GA, Kaler SG, et al. Missense mutations in the copper transporter gene *ATP7A* cause X-linked distal hereditary motor neuropathy. Am J Hum Genet. 2010;86:343–52.

Kim BE, Smith K, Petris MJ. A copper treatable Menkes disease mutation associated with defective trafficking of a functional Menkes copper ATPase. J Med Genet. 2003;40:290–5.

Klee KMC, Janecke AR, Civan HA, et al. AP1S1 missense mutations cause a congenital enteropathy via an epithelial barrier defect. Hum Genet. 2020; https://doi.org/10.1007/s00439-020-02168-w. Online ahead of print.

Martinelli D, Travaglini L, Drouin CA, et al. MEDNIK syndrome: a novel defect of copper metabolism treatable by zinc acetate therapy. Brain. 2013;136:872–81.

Moeller LB, Tuemer Z, Lund C, et al. Similar splice site mutations of the *ATP7A* gene lead to different phenotypes: classical Menkes disease or occipital horn syndrome. Am J Hum Genet. 2000;66:1211–20.

Neldner KH, Hambidge KM. Zinc therapy of acrodermatitis enteropathica. N Engl J Med. 1975;292:879–82.

Nicastro E, Ranucci G, Vajro P, Vegnente A, Iorio R. Re-evaluation of the diagnostic criteria for Wilson disease in children with mild liver disease. Hepatology. 2010;52:1948–56.

Tsukahara M, Imaizumi K, Kawai S, Kajii T. Occipital horn syndrome: report of a patient and review of the literature. Clin Genet. 1994;45:32–5.

Van Wouwe JP. Clinical and laboratory diagnosis of acrodermatitis enteropathica. Eur J Pediatr. 1989;149:2–8.

Wang K, Zhou B, Kuo YM, et al. A novel member of a zinc transporter family is defective in acrodermatitis enteropathica. Am J Hum Genet. 2002;71:66–73.

# Disorders of Iron Metabolism

# 37

Maria Domenica Cappellini

## Contents



**Summary**

Iron (Fe) is an essential element for almost every living organism. In humans and other mammals, iron homeostasis evolved to prevent iron excess, which leads to reactive and toxic oxygen species causing cell damage. This situation is attained by mechanisms for efficient regulation and internal iron recycling; however, this sophisticated control limiting iron absorption may easily promote the development of iron deficiency. Other than secondary iron overload conditions (i.e., transfusional iron overload or iron-loading anemias) and secondary iron deficiency, there are several genetically determined iron disorders. The first type of inherited iron-related disorder is "Hereditary Hemochromatosis (HH)," caused by mutations in genes maintaining Fe homeostasis. Different types of HH have been discovered; however, regardless of the mutated gene, the final outcome is an inappropriate hepcidin expression. The most common type of HH (type I) is caused by a mutation in *HFE*, with adult onset, and it accounts for >80% of all hemochromatosis patients, mostly Caucasian. The prevalent p.Cys282Tyr substitution leads to the inability of HFE to sense increased levels of Fe and interact with TfR1, which causes decreased hepcidin expression. Type II or juvenile HH, due to hemojuvelin (HJV) or hepcidin mutations, is a more severe disorder that affects younger individuals and causes a fast and heavy Fe overload in the liver and parenchyma. Type III HH is rare; it is similar to type 1, but is caused by mutations in the *TFR2* gene. Type IV HH differs from the other ones for having an autosomal dominant transmission and for not directly affecting hepcidin expression. It is caused by mutations in the *SLC40A1* gene, which encodes the Fe exporter ferroportin (Fpn), namely the hepcidin target. HH in general is not associated with anemia, whereas the conditions with iron overload associated with anemia suggest congenital atransferrinemia, hereditary aceruloplasminemia, and divalent cation transporter 1 (DMT1)-related iron overload. Finally, there are genetic defects that cause iron deficiency such as mutations occurring in *TMPRSS6* (matriptase 2) responsible for an iron-refractory iron deficiency anemia (IRIDA).

M. D. Cappellini (✉)
Fondazione Ca Granda Policlinico IRCCS, Università di Milano, Milan, Spain
e-mail: Maria.cappellini@unimi.it


N. Blau et al. (eds.), *Physician's Guide to the Diagnosis, Treatment, and Follow-Up of Inherited Metabolic Diseases*,
https://doi.org/10.1007/978-3-030-67727-5_37

## Introduction

Iron (Fe) is an essential element that is involved in a variety of vital functions, including oxygen transport, DNA synthesis, metabolic energy, and cellular respiration. However, excess iron can lead to the generation of reactive oxygen species (ROS), which cause oxidative stress, lipid peroxidation, and DNA damage, compromising cell viability and promoting cell death (Coffey and Ganz 2017). Under physiologic conditions these deleterious effects are prevented by sophisticated regulatory mechanisms, which maintain systemic and cellular Fe homeostasis (Anderson and Frazer 2017). Iron homeostasis is the result of balanced cooperation between functional compartments (erythroid and proliferating cells), uptake and recycling systems (enterocytes and splenic macrophages), storage elements (hepatocytes), and mobilization processes. The intracellular iron homeostasis is maintained by a posttranscriptional mechanism based on iron responsive elements (IREs) and iron regulatory proteins (IRPs) that bind to the IREs (Muckenthaler et al. 2008). In humans, there is no regulated excretion of iron, thus the iron balance is primarily controlled at the level of intestinal absorption, which takes place in the proximal portion of the duodenum. $Fe^{2+}$ iron enters enterocytes through DMT1 localized to the apical membrane and to subapical endosomes. DMT1 remains the primary transmembrane iron transporter and its expression is highly induced in iron deficiency. Once inside the intestinal epithelial cells, a portion of iron remains in the cell for use or storage and it is sloughed into the gut lumen when enterocytes become senescent; the rest is exported across the basolateral membrane of the enterocytes through the iron exporter ferroportin. Iron entry into the bloodstream is critical for systemic iron homeostasis and is negatively regulated by hepcidin, the iron regulatory hormone (Papanikolaou and Pantopoulos 2017; Ganz 2013). Hepcidin, a peptide hormone produced in the liver, is responsible for modulating iron availability to meet iron needs. Hepcidin operates by binding to ferroportin in tissue macrophages, duodenal enterocytes, and other target cells, triggering its tyrosine phosphorylation, internalization, and ubiquitin-mediated degradation in lysosomes. By removing ferroportin from the plasma membrane, hepcidin shuts off cellular iron export. The final consequence is the decrease in serum iron. Iron and inflammation are the major hepcidin inducers. Following iron intake or an increase in body iron stores, hepcidin is mainly upregulated through the activation of the Bone Morphogenetic Proteins, BMP/SMAD signaling, to prevent further dietary iron absorption. Under inflammatory conditions, hepcidin induction serves to promote hypoferremia and iron sequestration in macrophages (Nemeth et al. 2004; Ganz and Nemeth 2015). On the other hand, hepcidin expression is suppressed in iron deficiency, hypoxia, and erythropoietic expansion (stress erythropoiesis). Hepcidin inhibitors are the liver protease matriptase 2, encoded by the transmembrane serine protease 6 (*TMPRSS6*) gene and the erythroid-released hormone erythroferrone (*ERFE*). In iron deficiency, matriptase 2 inhibits hepcidin by cleaving the BMP coreceptor hemojuvelin (HJV) on the hepatocyte membrane (Silvestri et al. 2008). *ERFE* is an EPO target gene activated by Janus Kinase 2-Signal transducer and activator of transcription. It is widely expressed, and it is increased by EPO only in the erythropoietic (bone marrow and spleen) tissues. There are many observations that strengthen the role of *ERFE* in stress erythropoiesis, although *TMPRSS6* has a dominant effect over *ERFE* (Arezes et al. 2018).

The human iron disorders are invariably disorders of iron balance or iron distribution, either in terms of iron overload or iron deficiency. Hence, understanding iron homeostasis is critical for understanding these disorders, as well as understanding genetic iron disorders (Table 1). The first type of inherited iron-related disorder is hemochromatosis (HH). This term must be reserved for iron overload of genetic origin related to hepcidin deficiency. According to the most recent classification updated in 2018 (Brissot et al. 2018, 2019), hemochromatosis encompasses the following entities:

1. hemochromatosis type 1, related to mutations of the *HFE* gene (the *C282Y* mutation in the homozygous state is prevalent), which is by far the most common form, affecting mainly Caucasian populations (Allen et al. 2008)
2. hemochromatosis type 2 (the so-called juvenile hemochromatosis) corresponding to mutations in the hemojuvelin (*HJV*) gene (type 2A hemochromatosis) or to mutations in the hepcidin gene (*HAMP*) (type 2B hemochromatosis) (Kong et al. 2019)
3. hemochromatosis type 3 due to mutations in the transferrin receptor 2 (*TFR2*) gene (Kawabata 2019)
4. hemochromatosis type 4 due to mutations in the ferroportin gene (*SLC40A1*) in rare cases where these mutations lead to a refractory state to hepcidin ("gain-of-function"). There are different mutations in the ferroportin gene that affect the subcellular localization or transporter function of ferroportin ("loss-of-function"); this condition is characterized by macrophage iron loading and preferentially should be called "ferroportin disease." Both are autosomal dominant disorders (Pietrangelo 2017)

Thus, based on the current understanding, the molecular pathogenesis of "hemochromatosis" can be divided into three classes: first, mutations in the hepcidin gene itself (*HAMP*) that cause hemochromatosis by preventing the production of functional hepcidin protein; second, mutations in the genes encoding HFE (*HFE*), TFR2 (*TFR2*), and hemojuvelin (*HFE2*) inactivating signaling pathways that normally upregulate hepcidin expression; and finally, mutations in the gene encoding ferroportin (*SLC40A1*) that can cause hemochromatosis by rendering the transporter insensitive to hepcidin regulation. These different types of hemochromatosis are characterized by common signs including increased plasma iron, increased transferrin saturation, and parenchymal iron accumulation primarily into hepatocytes. The clinical expression may differ in severity among the different forms (Andrews 2008). Anemia is not a manifestation of hemochromatosis; however, there are interesting genetic conditions presenting with microcytic iron deficiency anemia associated with tissue iron overload; it is the case of atransferrinemia (Beaumont-Epinette et al. 2015), DMT1 deficiency (Iolascon et al. 2008), and aceruloplasminemia (Piperno and Alessio 2018). Congenital atransferrinemia is a rare, early onset autosomal recessive disorder caused by transferrin deficiency (<20 mg/dL) due to mutations in the transferrin-encoding *TF* gene on chromosome 3q22.1. The disease is also referred to as hypotransferrinemia, as the complete absence of functional transferrin is lethal. Patients exhibit very low to undetectable levels of plasma transferrin. This leads to impaired erythropoiesis, microcytic hypochromic anemia, growth retardation, and iron overload in parenchymal cells of the liver, heart, and pancreas (Beaumont-Epinette et al. 2015). Mutations in the genes encoding DMT1 (*SLC11A2*) are associated with autosomal recessive hypochromic, microcytic anemia (given the role of DMT1 in the uptake of iron at the apex of duodenal cells), but also have hepatic iron overload. Aceruloplasminemia is a rare autosomal recessive disorder caused by loss of ceruloplasmin function caused by mutations in the *CP* gene on chromosome 3q23-q24 (Kono 2013). The phenotype is quite heterogeneous but is always characterized by iron-restricted erythropoiesis leading to microcytic anemia, diabetes, and in some cases late in life to progressive retinal and neurological degeneration. An impaired iron absorption due to mutations in *TMPRSS6*, leading to an inability to cleave the BMP coreceptor HJV and inhibiting hepcidin, is observed in a recessive condition named IRIDA (congenital, iron-refractory, iron deficiency anemia). IRIDA patients are refractory to oral iron supplementation (Camaschella 2019).

Hyperferritinemia-cataract syndrome is a dominant condition due to IRE-IRP deregulation in which mutations in the IRE of L-ferritin mRNA make L-ferritin refractory to IRP binding; as a result, the protein synthesis becomes iron-independent. Ferritin is high but total body iron is normal. L-ferritin may accumulate in the lens, leading to early onset of cataract (Tsantoula et al. 2014). A dominant rare disease named neuroferritinopathy may be due to nucleotide insertions in the C-terminus of L-ferritin leading to neurodegeneration because of increased oxidation and cell death (Kuwata et al. 2019).

## Nomenclature

| No. | Disorder | Alternative name | Abbreviation | Gene symbol | Chromosomal localization | Affected protein | OMIM No. |
|---|---|---|---|---|---|---|---|
| 37.1 | Hereditary Hemochromasis type 1 | | HH | *HFE* | 6p21.3 | Homeostatic iron regulator | 613609 |
| 37.2 | Hemojuvelin deficiency | Hereditary hemochromatosis Type 2A | HJV | *HFE2* | 1q21 | Hemojuvelin | 608374 |
| 37.3 | Hepcidin deficiency | Hereditary hemochromatosis Type 2B | HH | *HAMP* | 19q13 | Hepcidin | 606464 |
| 37.4 | Transferrin Receptor 2 deficiency | Hereditary hemochromatosis Type 3 | Tfr2 HH | *TFR2* | 7q22 | Transferrin receptor 2 | 604720 |
| 37.5 | Ferroportin deficiency | Hemochromatosis type 4 | FPN HH | *SLC40A1* | 2q32 | Ferroportin | 604653 |
| 37.6 | Ferritin Heavy chain dysregulation | Hereditary hemochromatosis type 5 | HH | *FTH1* | 11q12 | Subunit of ferritin | 134770 |
| 37.7 | Ferritin light chain deficiency | Hereditary L-ferritin deficiency | | *FTL* | 19 | Subunit of ferritin | 134790 |
| 37.8 | Ferritin light chain superactivity | Neuroferritinopathy; neurodegeneration with brain iron accumulation 3 | | *FTL* | 19 | Subunit of ferritin | 134790 |
| 37.7 | Ferritin light chain dysregulation | Hyperferritinemia-cataract syndrome | | *FTL* | 19 | Subunit of ferritin | 134790 |
| 37.8 | Hereditary ceruloplasmin deficiency | Aceruloplasminemia | | *CP* | 3q23-q24 | Ceruloplasmin | 117700 |

(continued)

| No. | Disorder | Alternative name | Abbreviation | Gene symbol | Chromosomal localization | Affected protein | OMIM No. |
|---|---|---|---|---|---|---|---|
| 37.9 | Matriptrase 2 deficiency | Iron-refractory iron deficiency anemia | IRIDA | *TMPRSS6* | 22 | Matriptase 2 | 609862 |
| 37.10 | Hereditary transferrin deficiency | Atransferrinemia | | *TF* | 3q22.1 | Transferrin | 190000 |
| 37.11 | Transferrin receptor deficiency | Immunodeficiency type 46 | | *TFRC* | 3q29 | Transferrin receptor | 190010 |
| 37.12 | Divalent metal transporter 1 deficiency | Hypochromic microcytic anemia with iron overload type 1 | DMT1 | *SLC11A2* | 12q13 | DMT1 | 600523 |

## Metabolic Pathway

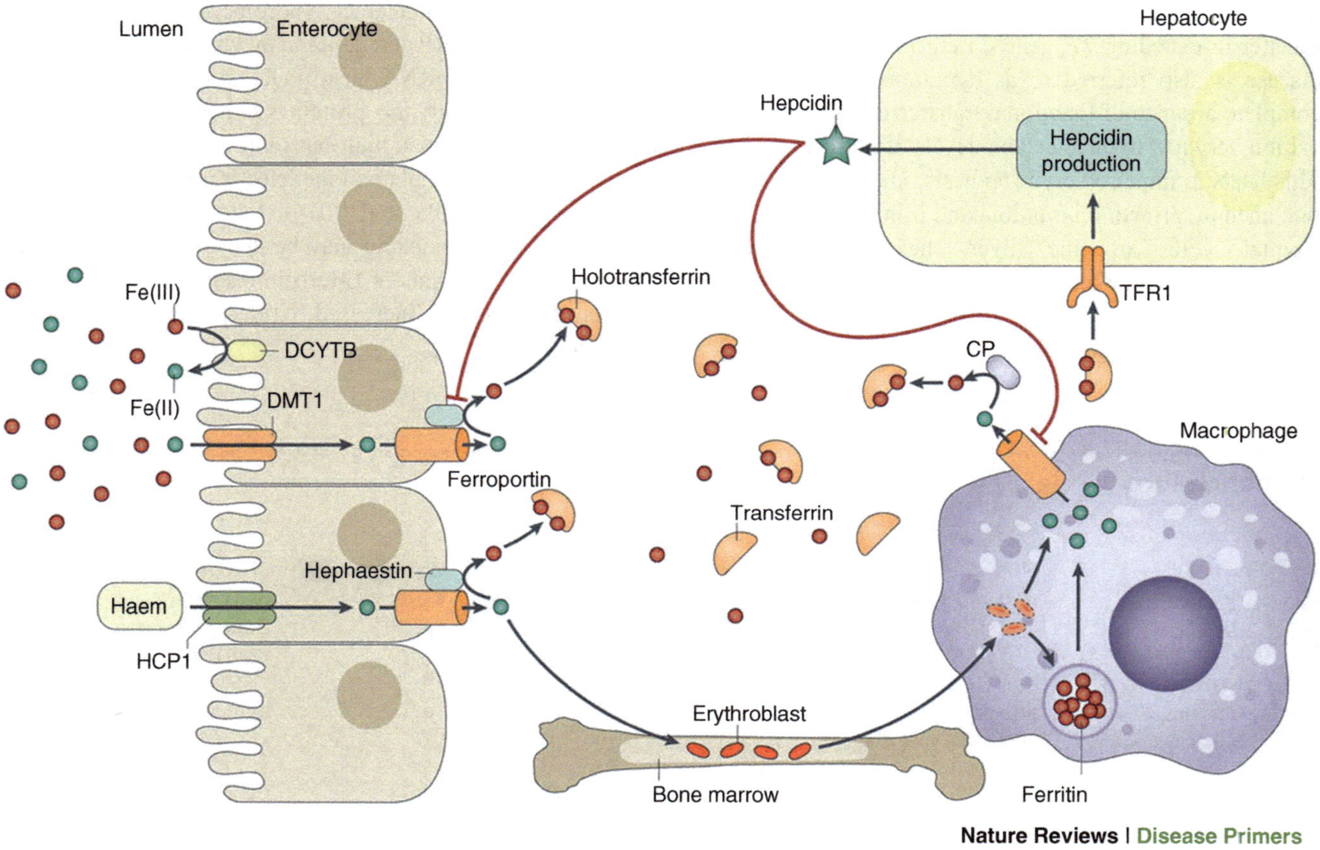


Brissot, P. et al. (2018) Haemochromatosis (Brissot et al. 2018) *Nat. Rev. Dis. Primers*. doi: https://doi.org/10.1038/nrdp.2018.16

## Signs and Symptoms

Hemochromatosis overview

| Symptom | Neonatal[a] | Infancy | Childhood[b] | Adolescence[b] | Adulthood[c] |
|---|---|---|---|---|---|
| Chronic fatigue | | | | + | ++ |
| Hepatomegaly | +++ | | + | ++ | ++ |
| Cirrhosis | +++ | | | ++ | ++ |
| Hepatocellular carcinoma | | | | | + |
| Join pain | | | + | ++ | ++ |
| Osteoporosis | | | | + | + |
| Diabetes mellitus | | | | ++ | + |
| Melanoderma | | | +/– | ++ | + |
| Skin dryness | | | +/– | ++ | + |
| Hypopituitarism | | | + | ++ | +/– |
| Cardiac rhythm disorder | | | | + | + |
| Heart failure | | | | ++ | |

[a]Neonatal hemochromatosis: very rare
[b]Hemochromatosis type 2 and 2B
[c]Hemochromatosis type 1, 3 and 4

Despite the high prevalence of C282Y homozygosity, only a minority of individuals will accumulate enough iron to cause organ damage. Given the autosomal recessive inheritance of C282Y, the frequency of C282Y homozygosity is similar in men and women, but the prevalence of clinical manifestations is much higher in men.

Overview of hematological signs of iron deficiency anemia with tissue iron overload and IRIDA

| | Atransferrinemia | DMT1 deficiency | Aceruloplasminemia | IRIDA |
|---|---|---|---|---|
| Hb | ↓ | ↓ | ↓ | ↓ |
| MCV | ↓ | ↓ | Normal | ↓ |
| Fe | ↑ | ↑ | ↓ | ↓ |
| Transferrin | ↓ Undetectable | ↓ | ↑ | ↑ |
| Transferrin saturation | ↑ | ↑ | ↓ | ↓ |
| S. Ferritin | ↑ | ↑ | ↑ | Normal |
| S. Hepcidin | ↓ | ↓ Normal | ↓ | ↑ |

**Table 37.1** Hereditary hemochromatosis (type 1)

| System | Symptoms and biomarkers | Neonatal (birth–1 month) | Infancy (1–18 months) | Childhood (1.5–11 years) | Adolescence (11–16 years) | Adulthood (>16 years) |
|---|---|---|---|---|---|---|
| Cardiovascular | **Cardiomyopathy** | | | | | ± |
| Dermatological | Hyperpigmentation | | | | | ± |
| Digestive | Abdominal pain | | ± | ± | ± | ± |
| | **Liver fibrosis** | | | | ± | + |
| Endocrine | **Hypogonadism** | | | | ± | + |
| Musculoskeletal | Arthralgia | | | ± | ± | + |
| Laboratory findings | ASAT/ALAT (plasma) | n | n | n | n–↑ | ↑ |
| | Bilirubin (plasma) | n | n | n | n–↑ | n–↑ |
| | Ferritin (serum) | n | ↑ | ↑ | ↑ | ↑ |
| | Glucose (plasma) | n | n | n | n | n–↑ |
| | Iron (liver) | n | n | n–↑ | ↑ | ↑ |
| | Iron (urine) | n | n | n | Possible/borderline increase | ↑ |
| | Transferrin saturation | n | ↑ | ↑ | ↑ | ↑ |

**Table 37.2** Herediatry hemochromatosis (type 2a)

| System | Symptoms and biomarkers | Neonatal (birth–1 month) | Infancy (1–18 months) | Childhood (1.5–11 years) | Adolescence (11–16 years) | Adulthood (>16 years) |
|---|---|---|---|---|---|---|
| Cardiovascular | **Cardiomyopathy** | | | ± | ± | ++ |
| CNS | **Fatigue** | | | | ± | + |
| Digestive | **Hapatopathy** | ± | ± | ± | + | + |
| | **Liver cirrhosis** | | | ± | ± | + |
| Endocrine | **Hypogonadism** | | | ± | + | ++ |
| Musculoskeletal | **Arthralgia** | | | | ± | + |
| Laboratory findings | Ferritin (serum) | n–↑ | n–↑ | n–↑ | ↑ | ↑ |
| | Glucose (plasma) | n | n | n | n–↑ | n–↑ |
| | Iron (liver) | n | n–↑ | n–↑ | n–↑ | ↑ |
| | Transferrin saturation | n–↑ | n–↑ | n–↑ | ↑ | ↑ |

**Table 37.3** Hereditary hemochromatosis (typ 2b)

| System | Symptoms and biomarkers | Neonatal (birth–1 month) | Infancy (1–18 months) | Childhood (1.5–11 years) | Adolescence (11–16 years) | Adulthood (>16 years) |
|---|---|---|---|---|---|---|
| Cardiovascular | **Cardiomyopathy** | | | | | + |
| Endocrine | **Hypogonadism** | | | | | + |
| Laboratory findings | Ferritin (serum) | | | | | ↑ |
| | Glucose (plasma) | | | | | ↑ |
| | Iron (liver) | | | | | ↑ |
| | Transferrin saturation | | | | | ↑ |

**Table 37.4** Hereditary hemochromatosis (type 3)

| System | Symptoms and biomarkers | Neonatal (birth–1 month) | Infancy (1–18 months) | Childhood (1.5–11 years) | Adolescence (11–16 years) | Adulthood (>16 years) |
|---|---|---|---|---|---|---|
| Cardiovascular | **Cardiomyopathy** | | | | ± | + |
| Dermatological | Hyperpigmentation | | | | | + |
| Digestive | Abdominal pain | | ± | ± | ± | ± |
| | **Liver fibrosis** | | | | ± | + |
| Endocrine | **Hypogonadism** | | | | ± | + |
| Musculoskeletal | **Arthralgia** | | | ± | ± | + |
| Laboratory findings | Ferritin (serum) | n | ↑ | ↑ | ↑ | ↑ |
| | Glucose (plasma) | n | n | n | n | n–↑ |
| | Iron (liver) | n | | ↑ | ↑ | ↑ |
| | Transferrin saturation | n | ↑ | ↑ | ↑ | ↑ |

**Table 37.5** Ferroportin 1 deficiency

| System | Symptoms and biomarkers | Neonatal (birth–1 month) | Infancy (1–18 months) | Childhood (1.5–11 years) | Adolescence (11–16 years) | Adulthood (>16 years) |
|---|---|---|---|---|---|---|
| Cardiovascular | Cardiopathy | | | | | ± |
| Digestive | Liver fibrosis/ cirrhosis | | | | | + |
| Endocrine | Diabetes | | | | | ± |
| | Hypogonadism | | | | ± | ± |
| Musculoskeletal | Arthrophaty | | | | | ± |
| Laboratory findings | Ferritin (serum) | n | n | n | n | ↑ |
| | Transferrin saturation | n | n | n | n | n–↑ |

**Table 37.6** Ferritin heavy chain dysregulation

| System | Symptoms and biomarkers | Neonatal (birth–1 month) | Infancy (1–18 months) | Childhood (1.5–11 years) | Adolescence (11–16 years) | Adulthood (>16 years) |
|---|---|---|---|---|---|---|
| Other | Frequently asymptomatic. No clear link with liver damage. | ± | ± | ± | ± | ± |
| Laboratory findings | Ferritin (serum) | n–↑ | n–↑ | n–↑ | n–↑ | n–↑ |

**Table 37.7** Ferritin light chain dysregulation

| System | Symptoms and biomarkers | Neonatal (birth–1 month) | Infancy (1–18 months) | Childhood (1.5–11 years) | Adolescence (11–16 years) | Adulthood (>16 years) |
|---|---|---|---|---|---|---|
| Eye | Cataract | | | ± | + | + |
| Laboratory findings | Ferritin (serum) | n | n | n–↑ | ↑ | ↑ |

**Table 37.8** Hereditary ceruloplasmin deficiency

| System | Symptoms and biomarkers | Neonatal (birth–1 month) | Infancy (1–18 months) | Childhood (1.5–11 years) | Adolescence (11–16 years) | Adulthood (>16 years) |
|---|---|---|---|---|---|---|
| Endocrine | Diabetes | | | | ± | + |
| Eye | Retinal degeneration | | | | ± | + |
| Hematological | Anemia, microcytic | | | | ± | + |
| Psychiatric | Neuropsychiatric symptoms | | | | ± | ± |
| Laboratory findings | Ceruloplasmin (serum) | ↓ | ↓ | ↓ | ↓ | ↓ |
| | Ferritin (serum) | n–↑ | n–↑ | n–↑ | ↑ | ↑ |
| | Transferrin saturation | ↓–n | ↓–n | ↓–n | ↓–n | ↓–n |

**Table 37.9** Matriptrase 2 deficiency

| System | Symptoms and biomarkers | Neonatal (birth–1 month) | Infancy (1–18 months) | Childhood (1.5–11 years) | Adolescence (11–16 years) | Adulthood (>16 years) |
|---|---|---|---|---|---|---|
| Hematological | Anemia, microcytic | ± | + | + | + | + |
| Laboratory findings | Ferritin (serum) | ↓ | ↓ | ↓ | ↓ | ↓ |
| | Hepcidin (plasma) | ↑ | ↑ | ↑ | ↑ | ↑ |
| | Transferrin saturation | ↓ | ↓ | ↓ | ↓ | ↓ |

**Table 37.10** Atransferrinemia

| System | Symptoms and biomarkers | Neonatal (birth–1 month) | Infancy (1–18 months) | Childhood (1.5–11 years) | Adolescence (11–16 years) | Adulthood (>16 years) |
|---|---|---|---|---|---|---|
| Digestive | **Hemosiderosis** | | | + | + | |
| Hematological | **Anemia, hypochromic** | | | + | + | |
| Musculoskeletal | **Growth retardation** | | | + | + | |
| Other | **Recurrent infections** | | | + | + | |
| Laboratory findings | Iron (liver) | | | | ↑ | |
| | Transferrin (serum) | | | ↓ | ↓ | |

**Table 37.11** Transferrin receptor 1 deficiency

| System | Symptoms and biomarkers | Neonatal (birth–1 month) | Infancy (1–18 months) | Childhood (1.5–11 years) | Adolescence (11–16 years) | Adulthood (>16 years) |
|---|---|---|---|---|---|---|
| Cardiovascular | Cardiomyopathy | | | | | ± |
| Digestive | Liver cirrhosis | | | | ± | + |
| Endocrine | Diabetes | | | | | + |
| | Hypogonadism | | | | ± | + |
| Laboratory findings | ASAT/ALAT (plasma) | | | ↑ | ↑ | ↑ |
| | Ferritin (serum) | n-↑ | n-↑ | ↑ | ↑ | ↑ |

**Table 37.12** Divalent metal transporter 1 deficiency

| System | Symptoms and biomarkers | Neonatal (birth–1 month) | Infancy (1–18 months) | Childhood (1.5–11 years) | Adolescence (11–16 years) | Adulthood (>16 years) |
|---|---|---|---|---|---|---|
| Hematological | Anemia, microcytic | + | + | + | + | + |
| Musculoskeletal | Growth retardation | ± | + | + | + | ± |
| Laboratory findings | Ferritin (serum) | n–↑ | n–↑ | n–↑ | n–↑ | n–↑ |
| | Iron (liver) | ↑ | ↑ | ↑ | ↑ | ↑ |
| | Iron (serum) | ↑ | ↑ | ↑ | ↑ | ↑ |
| | Transferrin saturation | ↑ | ↑ | ↑ | ↑ | ↑ |

## Reference and Pathological Values

| Serum | Hb (g/L) ± 2SD | Iron (μmol/L) | Ferritin (μg/L) | Transferrin (g/L; range) |
|---|---|---|---|---|
| Newborn | 185 ± 30 | 6.4–33.0 | 110–503 | 1.8 (1.42.29) |
| 3–6 months | 115 ± 20 | 6.4–33.0 | 4–405 | 2.03 (1.58–2.57) |
| 6–12 months | 120 ± 15 | 6.4–33.0 | 4–405 | – |
| 2–6 years | 125 ± 10 | 6.4–33.0 | 4–405 | 2.39 (1.86–3.03) |
| 6–12 years | 135 ± 20 | 6.4–33.0 | 4–405 | 2.17 (1.97–3.19) |
| 12–18 years (w) | 140 ± 20 | 6.4–33.0 | 9–79 | 2.17 (1.97–3.19) |
| 12–18 years (m) | 145 ± 15 | 6.4–33.0 | 9–59 | 2.17 (1.97–3.19) |
| >18 years (w) | 140 ± 20 | 6.6–26.0 | 6–81 | 2.0–3.4 |
| >18 years (m) | 155 ± 20 | 10.6–28.0 | 30–233 | – |
| CSF | – | 0.4 (0.2–0.6) | – | 14.4 mg/L |
| **HFE** | | >30 | >300 (up to 5000) | >70 |

## Diagnostic Flowchart

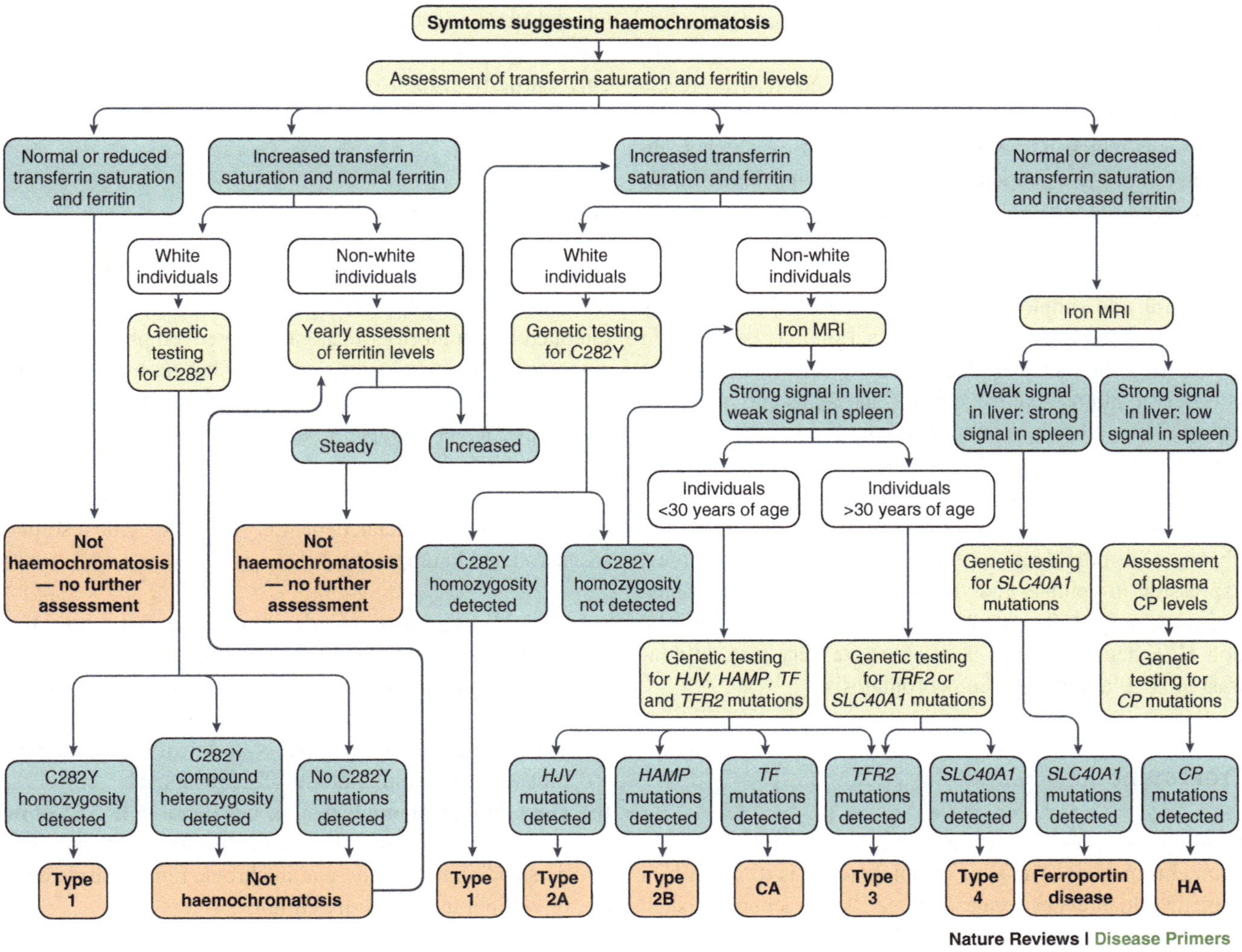


Brissot, P. et al. (2018) Haemochromatosis (Brissot et al. 2018) *Nat. Rev. Dis. Primers*. doi: https://doi.org/10.1038/nrdp.2018.16

In genetic conditions characterized by iron overload, transferrin saturation and ferritin levels are the key parameters to be assessed. However, increased ferritin levels (>300 mcg/L for men and >200 mcg/L for women) need rigorous interpretation before they are assigned to iron overload. Several conditions can be associated with increased ferritin levels independent of substantial iron overload such as metabolic syndrome (which is the most frequent cause), alcoholism, inflammation, and marked cytolysis. Despite these limitations, increased ferritin levels are critical for the diagnosis of hemochromatosis. Any acquired iron overload situation must be excluded (i.e., blood transfusions, dyserythropoiesis, or parenteral iron supplementation) by clinical history; family history could be helpful in some cases. Ethnicity is important considering the fact that *HFE*-associated hemochromatosis is observed almost exclusively in Caucasians and more frequently in men because the phenotypic expression of hemochromatosis is usually less pronounced in women. Age of onset is also important as *HFE*-associated (type 1) and *TFR2*-associated (type 3) hemochromatosis are generally observed in individuals >30 years of age, whereas clinical expression in younger individuals is typical of *HJV*-related (type 2A) or *HAMP*-related (type 2B) hemochromatosis. The non-*HFE* hemochromatosis diseases are very rare, in contrast to *HFE*-associated hemochromatosis.

## Treatment

Phlebotomy (weekly) remains the key of treatment for hemochromatosis. The goal of phlebotomy is to reach iron depletion to prevent tissue damage. After achieving such iron balance, maintenance phlebotomy (1–4 yearly) is advisable lifelong. In the most severe cases with decompensated cirrhosis or heart failure (for example, individuals with severe juvenile hemochromatosis) that badly tolerate phlebotomy, adjunctive oral chelation can be used. Phlebotomies are also efficient for treatment of patients with loss-of-function ferroportin disease but should be carried out on a less intensive schedule given the risk of anemia (Kowdley et al. 2019).

Although randomized clinical trials are missing, a sufficient body of data has suggested that phlebotomy therapy can improve chronic fatigue and cardiac function, stabilize liver disease, reverse hepatic fibrosis, and reduce skin pigmentation in patients with hemochromatosis (Adams and Barton 2010). The effectiveness of phlebotomy is much better if it starts before the development of severe organ damage such as cirrhosis. An alternative to phlebotomy could be erythrocytapheresis; this procedure could be useful in patients suffering from hypoproteinemia or thrombocytopenia (Rombout-Sestrienkova et al. 2016). A phase I/II clinical trial with Deferasirox in non-cirrhotic HFE hemochromatosis patients has been conducted, showing a dose-dependent ferritin reduction.

IRIDA, differently than classical iron deficiency anemia where hepcidin levels are low or even undetectable, has normal or high hepcidin levels, and is resistant to oral iron and only partially responsive to intravenous iron, which still remains the advisable treatment.

## Future Treatments

Although phlebotomy is inexpensive, safe, and effective in reversing many complications of iron overload, it is not well tolerated by a minority of patients. Moreover, phlebotomy is not feasible in iron-loading anemias because the patients become even more anemic. For these reasons, there is a consensus that novel therapeutic approaches are needed for all iron overload diseases. As hepcidin represents the iron homeostasis controller, the use of hepcidin agonists or antagonists could be beneficial, depending on the specific disorder (Katsarou and Pantopoulos 2018).

(a) **Hepcidin agonists** include compounds that mimic the activity of hepcidin and agents that increase the production of hepcidin by targeting hepcidin-regulatory molecules. The potential of these future drugs includes the improvement in erythropoiesis as shown in thalassemia mouse models and in phase I/II clinical trial.
(b) **Hepcidin antagonists** may be beneficial in IRIDA or in anemias associated with a variety of inflammatory disorders and malignancies, and in chronic renal disease with or without inflammatory etiology.

## References


Adams PC, Barton JC. How I treat hemochromatosis. Blood. 2010;116:317–25.

Allen KJ, Gurrin LC, Constantine CC, Osborne NJ, et al. Iron-overload-related disease in HFE hereditary hemochromatosis. N Engl J Med. 2008;358(3):221–30.

Anderson GJ, Frazer DM. Current understanding of iron homeostasis. Am J Clin Nutr. 2017;106:1559S–66S.

Andrews NC. Forging a field: the golden age of iron biology. Blood. 2008;112:219–30.

Arezes J, Foy N, McHugh K, et al. Erythroferrone inhibits the induction of hepcidin by BMP6. Blood. 2018;132:1473–7.

Beaumont-Epinette MP, Delobel JB, Ropert M, et al. Hereditary hypotransferrinemia can lead to elevated transferrin saturation and when associated to HFE or HAMP mutations to iron overload. Blood Cells Mol Dis. 2015;54:151–4.

Brissot P, Pietrangelo A, Adams PC. Hemochromatosis. Nat Rev Dis Primers. 2018; article 18016.

Brissot P, Troadec MB, Loréal O, Brissot E. Pathophysiology and classification of iron overload diseases; update 2018. Transfus Clin Biol. 2019;26:80–8.

Camaschella C. Iron deficiency. Blood. 2019;133:30–9.

Coffey R, Ganz T. Iron Homestasis: an anthropocentric perspective. J Biol Chem. 2017;292(31):12727–34.

Ganz T. Systemic iron homeostasis. Physiol Rev. 2013;93:1721–41.

Ganz T, Nemeth E. Iron homeostasis in host defence and inflammation. Nat Rev Immunol. 2015;15:500–10.

Iolascon A, Camaschella C, Pospisilova D, et al. Natural history of recessive inheritance of DMT1 mutations. J Pediatr. 2008;152:136–9.

Katsarou A, Pantopoulos K. Hepcidin therapeutics. Pharmaceuticals. 2018;11:E127.

Kawabata H. Transferrin and transferrin receptors update. Free Radic Biol Med. 2019;133:46–54.

Kong X, Xie L, Zhu H, et al. Genotypic and phenotypic spectra of hemojuvelin mutations in primary hemochromatosis patients: a systematic review. Orphanet J Rare Dis. 2019;14:171.

Kono S. Aceruloplasminemia: an update. Int Rev Neurobiol. 2013;110:125–51.

Kowdley KV, Brown KE, Ahn J, Sundaram V. ACG clinical guideline: hereditary hemochromatosis. Am J Gastroenterol. 2019;114:1202–18.

Kuwata T, Okada Y, Yamamoto T, et al. Structure, function, folding and aggregation of a Neuroferritinopathy-related ferritin variant. Biochemistry. 2019;58:2318–25.

Muckenthaler MU, Galy B, Hentze MW. Systemic iron homeostasis and the iron-responsive element/iron-regulatory protein (IRE/IRP) regulatory network. Annu Rev Nutr. 2008;28:197–213.

Nemeth E, Tuttle MS, Powelson J, et al. Hepcidin regulates cellular iron efflux by binding to ferroportin and inducing its internalization. Science. 2004;306:2090–3.

Papanikolaou G, Pantopoulos K. Systemic iron homeostasis and erythropoiesis. IUBMB Life. 2017;69:399–413.

Pietrangelo A. Ferroportin disease: pathogenesis, diagnosis and treatment. Haematologica. 2017;102(12):1972–84.

Piperno A, Alessio M. Aceruloplasminemia: waiting for an efficient therapy. Front Neurosci. 2018;12:903.

Rombout-Sestrienkova E, van Kraij MG, Koek GH. How we manage patients with hereditary hemochromatosis. Br J Haematol. 2016;175:759–70.

Silvestri L, Pagani A, Nai A, et al. The serine pro- tease matriptase-2 (TMPRSS6) inhibits hepcidin activation by cleaving membrane hemojuvelin. Cell Metab. 2008;8(6):502–11.

Tsantoula F, Kioumi A, Germenis AE, Speletas M. Hereditary hyperferritinemia cataract syndrome as a cause of childhood hyperferritinemia. J Pediatr Hematol Oncol. 2014;36:304.

# Disorders of Manganese Metabolism

# 38

Karin Tuschl, Philippa B. Mills, and Peter T. Clayton

## Contents



## Summary

Manganese is an essential trace metal that is a constituent of metalloenzymes and is required as an enzyme activator. Blood manganese levels are under tight homeostatic control by the liver as both manganese overload and deficiency impair neuronal function and integrity.

To date, three inherited manganese transporter defects have been identified that lead to abnormal blood manganese levels: mutations in *SLC30A10* (hypermanganesaemia with dystonia 1, HMNDYT1) and *SLC39A14* (hypermanganesaemia with dystonia 2, HMNDYT2) cause manganese overload, while mutations in *SLC39A8* (Congenital Disorder of Glycosylation, Type IIn; CDG2N) cause manganese deficiency. SLC39A14 and SLC30A10 are required for hepatic uptake and adequate biliary excretion of manganese, respec-

K. Tuschl (✉)
Department of Developmental Neurobiology, Kings College, London, UK

Department of Cell and Developmental Biology, University College, London, UK

UCL GOS Institute of Child Health, University College, London, UK
e-mail: k.tuschl@ucl.ac.uk

P. B. Mills · P. T. Clayton
UCL GOS Institute of Child Health, University College, London, UK
e-mail: p.mills@ucl.ac.uk; peter.clayton@ucl.ac.uk


N. Blau et al. (eds.), *Physician's Guide to the Diagnosis, Treatment, and Follow-Up of Inherited Metabolic Diseases*,
https://doi.org/10.1007/978-3-030-67727-5_38

tively. Both these transporter defects are characterised by childhood-onset, progressive Parkinsonism-dystonia due to the accumulation of manganese in the basal ganglia, particularly the globus pallidus, with pathognomonic MRI brain appearances of hyperintensity on T1-weighted images. Whole blood manganese levels are highly raised. In addition to the movement disorder, SLC30A10 loss-of-function causes liver disease, polycythaemia and depletion of iron stores. Intravenous chelation with disodium calcium edetate and iron supplementation effectively lowers the manganese load and can lead to significant improvement in neurological symptoms and halt the progress of liver disease.

SLC39A8 is required for manganese uptake into the organism. Loss-of-function leads to a manganese deficiency syndrome characterised by neurodevelopmental delay, seizures, dystonia and short stature. Biochemically, SLC39A8 deficiency causes hypomanganesaemia and a characteristic dysglycosylation pattern corresponding to a type II congenital disorder of glycosylation because manganese acts as a cofactor for the β-1,4-galactosyltransferase. In addition, manganese deficiency leads to respiratory chain abnormalities and Leigh-like mitochondrial disease. Manganese supplementation can improve clinical symptoms and normalise biochemical findings.

Manganese dyshomeostasis has also been observed in a juvenile type of Parkinson's disease associated with supranuclear gaze palsy, spasticity and dementia due to mutations in *ATP13A2* (PARK9), also known as Kufor-Rakeb Syndrome. ATP13A2 has been shown to transport manganese from the cytosol to the lysosome. In addition, the phenotype can vary from neuronal ceroid lipofuscinosis type 12 (CLN12) to complicated hereditary spastic paraplegia (HSP).

## Introduction

Manganese is one of the six transition metals essential for human metabolism. It is required as a cofactor for numerous enzymatic reactions including glycosylation and phosphorylation, and is involved in amino acid, lipid and carbohydrate metabolism, immune function, bone and connective tissue growth and blood clotting. As a constituent of metalloenzymes such as the manganese superoxide dismutase, it acts as a scavenger of reactive oxygen species (Chen et al. 2015).

Manganese levels are under precise homeostatic control because both excess and deficiency of manganese are deleterious for neuronal function and integrity. Excess manganese accumulates in the basal ganglia and causes a clinical syndrome known as manganism—an extrapyramidal movement disorder characterised by dystonia, bradykinesia and rigidity, accompanied by psychiatric and cognitive defects (Chen et al. 2015). Manganese overload can occur in inherited manganese transporter defects (HMNDYT1 and HMNDYT2 caused by mutations in *SLC30A10* and *SLC39A14*, respectively) or as a result of environmental overexposure, excess manganese in parenteral nutrition or impaired hepatic excretion in patients with liver cirrhosis (Tuschl et al. 2012, 2016; Quadri et al. 2012). Manganese deficiency, on the other hand, leads to dysglycosylation and impaired mitochondrial function. Due to its ubiquitous presence in the diet, acquired manganese deficiency rarely occurs and, hence, deficiency of manganese is only observed in an inherited manganese transporter defect caused by *SLC39A8* mutations (congenital disorder of glycosylation type IIn) (Park et al. 2015a; Boycott et al. 2015; Riley et al. 2017).

Tight homeostatic control of intestinal absorption and biliary excretion of manganese maintains stable tissue concentrations of the metal. This requires a group of solute carrier (SLC) transporters localised at the cell membrane. SLC39A8 and SLC39A14 facilitate uptake of manganese into the cell, while SLC30A10 mediates manganese efflux (Leyva-Illades et al. 2014; Clayton 2017). SLC39A14 appears to be the main transporter allowing for the uptake of manganese into the liver, the primary regulator of manganese homeostasis. Manganese transport also occurs at iron transporters including DMT1, transferrin/transferrin receptor complex and ferroportin, as well as the dopamine (DAT) and citrate transporters (Peres et al. 2016). Because iron competes with manganese for transport, iron supplementation can reduce manganese levels in disorders associated with excess manganese (Clayton 2017). Within the cell, manganese is transported via a number of transporters including ATP13A1 at the endoplasmic reticulum, SPCA1 at the Golgi, ATP13A2 at the lysosome and Mfrn-1 and DMT1 at the mitochondria (Chen et al. 2015; Sorensen et al. 2018; Christenson et al. 2018).

Hypermanganesaemia with dystonia 1 (HMNDYT1) caused by biallelic mutations in *SLC30A10* was the first inherited manganese transporter defect described. Impaired biliary excretion leads to accumulation of manganese in the liver and brain, resulting in liver disease and generalised dystonia. Manganese deposition in the brain causes characteristic neurodegenerative features including severe neuronal loss in the globus pallidus and a vacuolated myelinopathy. MRI brain appearances are pathognomonic with hyperintensity on T1-weighted images of the globus pallidus and striatum, and the white matter of the cerebrum and cerebellum, midbrain, dorsal pons and medulla, while the ventral pons is typically spared (Fig. 38.1a, b). T2-weighted images show corresponding hypointensity of the globus pallidus and striatum (Fig. 38.1c). Activation of erythropoietin

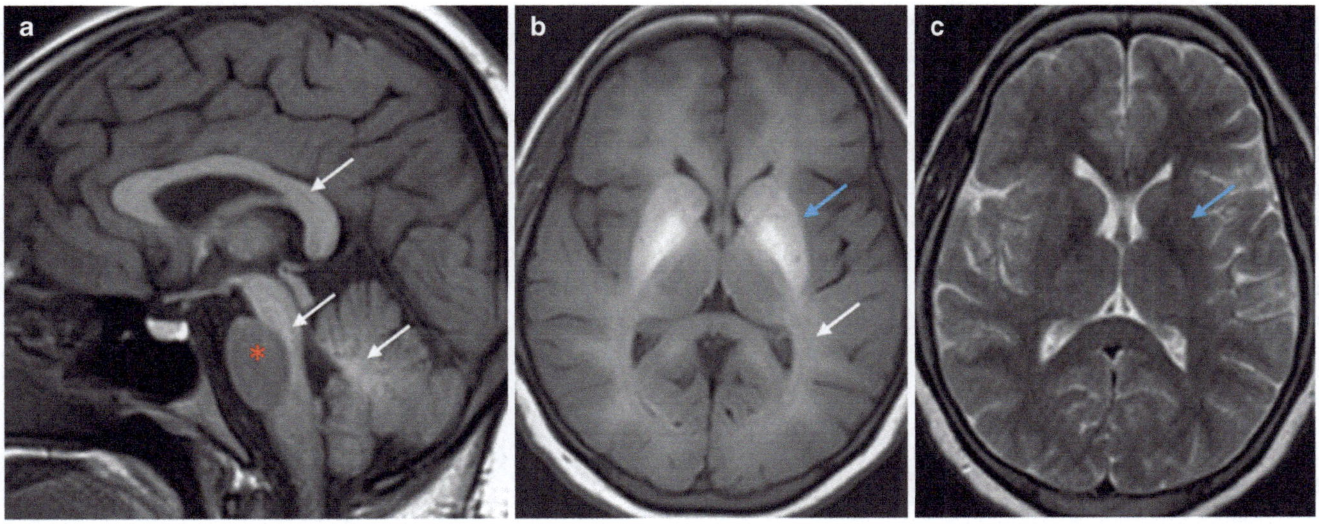


**Fig. 38.1** Characteristic MRI brain appearances due to manganese overload in SLC30A10 (HMNDYT1) and SLC39A14 (HMNDYT2) transporter defects (Tuschl et al. 2016). (**a**, **b**) T1-weighted MR imaging shows hyperintensity of the globus pallidus and striatum (blue arrow), and the white matter in the cerebrum, cerebellum, midbrain, dorsal pons (white arrows) with a pathognomonic sparing of the ventral pons (red star). (**c**) T2-weighted MR imaging shows corresponding hypointensity of the globus pallidus and striatum (blue arrow)

gene expression due to excess manganese leads to polycythaemia, which often precedes clinical symptoms. Whole blood manganese levels are significantly raised and usually exceed 1000 nmol/L. Another characteristic is a depletion of iron stores with increased total iron-binding capacity and low ferritin values. Some patients develop hypothyroidism, which is consistent with findings in SLC30A10 knockout mice (Hutchens et al. 2017). Disease onset is usually within the first few years of life with progressive, generalised dystonia; however, cases of adult-onset atypical Parkinson's disease have been described. Some patients have also presented with primary hypotonia or spastic paraplegia (Gospe Jr. et al. 2000; Gulab et al. 2018; Zaki et al. 2018). Manganese chelation with intravenous disodium calcium edetate, in combination with iron supplementation to reduce the uptake of manganese, reduces manganese blood and tissue levels, improves neurological symptoms and halts liver disease progression (Tuschl et al. 2012, 1993; Quadri et al. 2012, 2015).

Biallelic mutations in *SLC39A14* cause hypermanganesaemia with dystonia 2 (HMNDYT2) due to impaired uptake of manganese into the liver for subsequent biliary excretion. Manganese accumulates in extrahepatic tissues, causing an isolated neurological phenotype of rapidly progressive Parkinsonism-dystonia with onset in infancy or childhood. Whole blood manganese levels are highly raised and MRI brain appearances are identical to that of HMNDYT1 (Fig. 38.1). Hypointensity of the globus pallidus and striatum on T2-weighted images is often pronounced and may be mistaken as the eye of the tiger sign observed in neurodegeneration with brain iron accumulation (NBIA) disorder. Chelation therapy with disodium calcium edetate has been used with some success; however, clinical response is poor in most patients, most likely due to advanced disease progression and significant degree of neurodegeneration (Tuschl et al. 2016, 1993; Zeglam et al. 2018).

Inherited manganese deficiency with low blood manganese levels is caused by biallelic mutations in *SLC39A8* and leads to a type II congenital disorder of glycosylation (Type IIn; CDG2N). Dysglycosylation occurs because manganese is a cofactor for the β-1,4-galactosyltransferase, essential for galactosylation of glycan chains. Affected individuals present as early as infancy with neurodevelopmental delay, hypotonia, seizures, dystonia, ataxia, vision and hearing impairment, dysmorphism and short stature/dwarfism (Park et al. 2015a; Boycott et al. 2015). This disorder may also manifest with Leigh-like mitochondrial disease including features such as raised CSF lactate, respiratory chain abnormalities, bilateral basal ganglia hyperintensities on T2-weighted imaging and cerebellar atrophy (Riley et al. 2017). Treatment has been attempted with oral manganese sulphate with remarkable clinical and biochemical improvement. Upon manganese supplementation, the glycosylation pattern and blood manganese levels normalised. Clinically, this was associated with cessation of seizures and improvement in hearing, vision and motor abilities (Park et al. 2017).

There is evidence that manganese dyshomeostasis also plays a role in individuals with mutations in *ATP13A2*. ATP13A2 facilitates manganese transport into the lysosome and thereby protects cells from manganese toxicity. Biallelic mutations in *ATP13A2* have been reported in three neurodegenerative disorders with parkinsonism as a shared clinical feature: (1) Juvenile-onset Parkinson's disease (PARK9), also known as Kufor-Rakeb-Syndrome, which is accompanied by supranuclear gaze palsy, dementia and generalised brain atrophy (Racette et al. 2012). (2) Neuronal ceroid lipofuscinosis (CLN12) with typical accumulation of autofluorescent lipopigment, which presents with learning difficulties, parkinsonism, spinocerebellar ataxia, bulbar syndrome and pyramidal involvement (Bras et al. 2012). (3) Complex hereditary spastic paraplegia (SPG78), which is accompanied by ataxia and neuropathy, parkinsonism and cognitive decline (Estrada-Cuzcano et al. 2017). The parkinsonian features tend to respond well to treatment with levodopa; however, dyskinesias develop early. In addition, heterozygous mutations in *ATP13A2* pose a genetic risk factor for early-onset Parkinson's disease (Park et al. 2015b). Despite the fact that ATP13A2 is involved in manganese transport, blood manganese levels are normal in affected individuals. T2-weighted MR images show iron accumulation in the basal ganglia, and, hence, *ATP13A2* mutations are also classified as an NBIA disorder (Schneider et al. 2010) (Fig. 38.2).

## Nomenclature

| No. | Disorder | Alternative name | Abbreviation | Gene symbol | Chromosomal location | Mode of Inheritance | Affected protein | OMIM |
|---|---|---|---|---|---|---|---|---|
| 38.1 | Hypermanganesemia with Dystonia 1 | SLC30A10 deficiency; Syndrome of Hepatic Cirrhosis, Dystonia, Polycythemia, and Hypermanganesemia | HMNDYT1 | *SLC30A10* | 1q41 | AR | SLC30A10 (ZNT10) | 613280 |
| 38.2 | Hypermanganesemia with Dystonia 2 | SLC39A14 deficiency | HMNDYT2 | *SLC39A14* | 8p21.3 | AR | SLC39A14 (ZIP14) | 617013 |
| 38.3 | Congenital Disorder of Glycosylation, Type IIn | SLC39A8 deficiency | CDG2N | *SLC39A8* | 4q24 | AR | SLC39A8 (ZIP8) | 616721 |
| 38.4 | Parkinson disease 9 | Kufor-Rakeb Syndrome; Neuronal ceroid lipofuscinosis 12; Complex hereditary spastic paraplegia 78 | PARK9, NCL12, SPG78 | *ATP13A2* | 1p36 | AR | ATP13A2 | 606693 |

## Metabolic Pathways

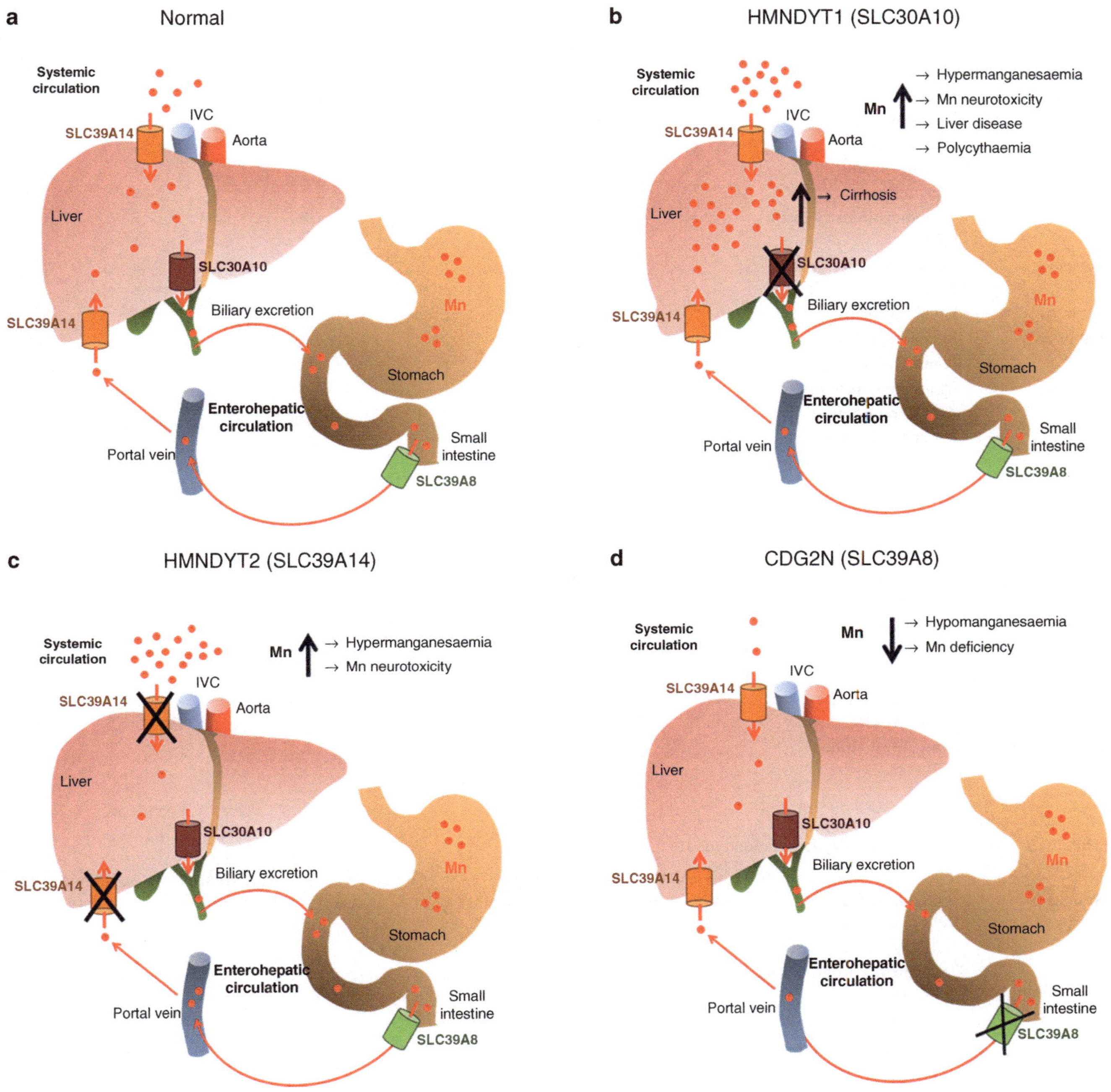


**Fig. 38.2** Our current understanding of how manganese homeostasis (**a**) is maintained under physiological conditions and (**b–d**) is impaired in manganese transporter defects (Tuschl et al. 2016). (**a**) In healthy individuals, manganese from the diet is taken up in the small intestine via SLC39A8 and enters the liver via SLC39A14. The liver regulates blood manganese levels via biliary excretion through SLC30A10. (**b**) In SLC30A10 deficiency (HMNDYT1), biliary excretion of manganese is impaired leading to accumulation of manganese in the liver (causing liver cirrhosis and polycythaemia), the blood (hypermanganesaemia) and the brain where it causes neurotoxicity within the globus pallidus resulting in dystonia. (**c**) In SLC39A14 deficiency (HMNDYT2), manganese uptake into the liver is reduced and manganese accumulates in extrahepatic tissues. (**d**) In SLC39A8 deficiency (CDG2N), uptake of manganese is impaired resulting in systemic manganese deficiency

## Signs and Symptoms

**Table 38.1** Hypermanganesemia with dystonia type 1

| System | Symptoms and biomarkers | Neonatal (birth–1 month) | Infancy (1–18 months) | Childhood (1.5–11 years) | Adolescence (11–16 years) | Adulthood (>16 years) |
|---|---|---|---|---|---|---|
| CNS | **Dysarthria** | | ± | + | + | + |
| | **Dystonia** | | ± | + | + | + |
| | **Hypotonia** | | ± | ± | ± | ± |
| | **Parkinsonism** | | ± | + | + | + |
| | **Spasticity** | | ± | ± | ± | ± |
| | **T1 hyperintensity brain (MRI)** | | ± | + | + | + |
| Digestive | **Hepatomegaly** | | ± | ± | ± | ± |
| | **Jaundice** | | ± | ± | ± | ± |
| | **Liver cirrhosis** | | ± | ± | ± | ± |
| Laboratory findings | **Ferritin (serum)** | | ↓ | ↓ | ↓ | ↓ |
| | **Hemoglobin (blood)** | | ↑ | ↑ | ↑ | ↑ |
| | **Manganese (blood)** | | ↑ | ↑ | ↑ | ↑ |
| | **Total iron binding capacity (TIBC)** | | ↑ | ↑ | ↑ | ↑ |

**Table 38.2** Hypermanganesemia with dystonia type 2

| System | Symptoms and biomarkers | Neonatal (birth–1 month) | Infancy (1–18 months) | Childhood (1.5–11 years) | Adolescence (11–16 years) | Adulthood (>16 years) |
|---|---|---|---|---|---|---|
| CNS | **Dysarthria** | | ± | + | + | + |
| | **Dystonia** | | ± | + | + | + |
| | **Parkinsonism** | | ± | + | + | + |
| | **T1 hyperintensity brain (MRI)** | | ± | + | + | + |
| Laboratory findings | **Manganese (blood)** | | ↑ | ↑ | ↑ | ↑ |

**Table 38.3** Congenital disorder of glycosylation type IIn

| System | Symptoms and biomarkers | Neonatal (birth–1 month) | Infancy (1–18 months) | Childhood (1.5–11 years) | Adolescence (11–16 years) | Adulthood (>16 years) |
|---|---|---|---|---|---|---|
| CNS | **Cerebellar atrophy (MRI)** | | ± | ± | ± | ± |
| | **Cerebral atrophy (MRI)** | | ± | ± | ± | ± |
| | Hyperreflexia | | | ± | ± | |
| | Hypotonia | + | + | + | + | + |
| | Intellectual disability | | ++ | ++ | ++ | ++ |
| | Seizures | | ± | ± | ± | ± |
| Eye | **Strabismus** | | + | + | + | + |
| Musculoskeletal | Osteopenia | | | ± | ± | ± |
| | **Scoliosis** | | ± | ± | ± | ± |
| | **Short stature** | | ± | ± | ± | ± |
| Other | Recurrent infections | | | ± | ± | |
| Laboratory findings | Manganese (blood) | | ↓↓ | ↓↓ | ↓↓ | |
| | Manganese (urine) | | n–↑ | n–↑ | n–↑ | |
| | Sialotransferrins, type 2 pattern (serum) | + | + | + | + | |
| | Zinc (serum) | | ↓ | ↓ | ↓ | |
| | Zinc (urine) | | n | n | n | |

**Table 38.4** Parkinson disease type 9

| System | Symptoms and biomarkers | Neonatal (birth–1 month) | Infancy (1–18 months) | Childhood (1.5–11 years) | Adolescence (11–16 years) | Adulthood (>16 years) |
|---|---|---|---|---|---|---|
| CNS | **Akinesia** | **n** | **n** | **n** | ++ | +++ |
| | Cognitive dysfunction | n | n | + | ++ | +++ |
| | Dysarthria | n | n | n | + | ++ |
| | Extrapyramidal movement disorder | n | n | n | + | ++ |
| | Gait disturbance | n | n | n | ++ | +++ |
| | **Movement disorder** | **n** | **n** | **n** | + | ++ |
| | **Myoclonus** | **n** | **n** | **n** | + | +++ |
| | Neurodegenerative disease | n | n | n | + | ++ |
| Metabolic | EM, storage material | | | | +++ | +++ |
| Musculoskeletal | **Rigidity** | **n** | **n** | **n** | ++ | +++ |
| Psychiatric | **Behavioral abnormalities** | **n** | **n** | **n** | + | ++ |

## Reference Values

| | | Reference value |
|---|---|---|
| Mn (B) | | 73–325 nmol/L |
| Zn (S) | | 8–20 µmol/L |
| Hb (B) | Prepubertal | |
| | 0–6 days | 145–220 g/L |
| | 7 days | 140–186 g/L |
| | 8 days–3 months | 95–125 g/L |
| | 3 months–4 years | 110–140 g/L |
| | 5–12 years | 115–140 g/L |
| | Postpubertal | |
| | Female | 131–175 g/L |
| | Male | 130–175 g/L |
| TIBC (S) | | 50–90 µmol/L |
| Ferritin (S) | | 7–150 µg/L |

## Pathological Values

| | Mn (B) | Zn (S) | Hb (B) | TIBC (S) | Ferritin (S) |
|---|---|---|---|---|---|
| HMNDYT1 (SLC30A10 deficiency) | ↑ | N | ↑ | ↑ | ↓ |
| HMNDYT2 (SLC39A14 deficiency) | ↑ | N | N | N | N |
| CDG2N (SLC39A8 deficiency) | ↓ | ↓/N | N | N | N |

N = normal, ↑ = increased relative to reference range, ↓ = decreased relative to reference range

## Diagnostic Flowchart

### HMNDYT1 and HMNDYT2

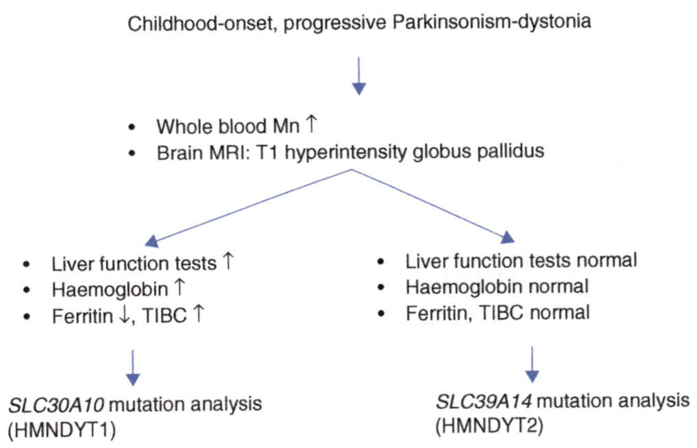


In any individuals with childhood-onset, progressive Parkinsonism-dystonia, whole blood manganese levels should be determined as well as brain MR imaging obtained. If features of manganese accumulation are identified, the above diagnostic algorithm should be followed.

## Specimen Collection

| Test | Precondition | Material | Handling | Pitfalls |
|---|---|---|---|---|
| Mn (B) | – | Blood | Ambient | False elevation due to contamination. Secondary causes of hypermanganesaemia due to liver disease, environmental manganese exposure, parenteral nutrition. |

Ideally, blood for metal determination should be collected in trace-metal-free EDTA blood containers. Alternatively, if such containers are unavailable, common EDTA blood containers can be used and an empty blood container analysed in parallel to rule out background contamination of the container.

## Prenatal Diagnosis

Prenatal diagnosis can be performed by molecular analysis of all four disorders of manganese transport provided the mutation of each biological parent is known. DNA can be isolated from cells directly or by culture after amniocentesis, from chorionic villous samples, from maternal blood, or at the preimplantation stage.

## DNA Testing

Genetic diagnosis can be made by standard molecular diagnostic procedures including gene sequencing of *SLC30A10*, *SLC39A14*, *SLC39A8* and *ATP13A2*, whole exome sequencing, and deletion/duplication analysis using genomic DNA of any source.

## Treatment Summary

### HMNDYT1 and HMNDYT2

The recommended treatment for disorders of manganese overload including HMNDYT1 and HMNDYT2 is the regular chelation of manganese with intravenous disodium calcium edetate in combination with iron supplementation to maintain iron parameters (TIBC, ferritin) within the high normal range. Individuals with HMNDYT1 deficiency seem to respond well with improvement of Parkinsonism-dystonia and liver disease, normalization of haemoglobin, reduction in blood manganese levels and manganese accumulation on brain MRI. However, individuals with HMNDYT2 have a less favourable response, probably due to advanced disease progression and different disease pathogenesis. Chelation treatment can lead to a deficiency of calcium, zinc, copper and selenium, which need frequent monitoring and supplementation as required (Tuschl et al. 2016, 1993).

### CDG2N

High-dose manganese supplementation in individuals with CDG2N can improve neurological symptoms and normalise glycosylation and blood manganese levels. Therapy requires close monitoring of glycosylation assays and blood manganese to prevent manganese toxicity (Park et al. 2017). In addition, galactose and uridine supplementation can normalise glycosylation patterns (Park et al. 2015a; Riley et al. 2017).

### PARK9

Initially, the parkinsonian features in individuals with *ATP13A2* mutations tend to respond well to the standard treatment of Parkinson's disease with levodopa. However, early development of dyskinesias and visual hallucinations complicates treatment (Schneider et al. 2010; Di Fonzo et al. 2007).

## Standard Treatment

| | Therapy | Application | Dose | Duration |
|---|---|---|---|---|
| HMNDYT1 | Disodium calcium edetate | iv | 20 mg/kg/dose (max 1 g) twice daily for 5–8 days every 4 weeks | Lifelong |
| | Ferrous sulphate/fumarate | po | To keep iron parameters within the normal range (TIBC low normal, ferritin high normal) | Lifelong |
| HMNDYT2 | Disodium calcium edetate | iv | 20 mg/kg/dose (max 1 g) twice daily for 5–8 days every 4 weeks | Lifelong |
| | Ferrous sulphate/fumarate | po | To keep iron parameters within the normal range (TIBC low normal, ferritin high normal) | Lifelong |
| CDG2N | Manganese sulphate | po | 15–20 mg/kg to keep blood manganese within the normal range | Lifelong |
| PARK9 | Carbidopa/levodopa (and standard Parkinson's disease treatment) | po | 150–1000 mg daily in 3–4 divided doses | Lifelong |

iv = intravenous, po = peroral

## References

Boycott KM, Beaulieu CL, Kernohan KD, Gebril OH, Mhanni A, Chudley AE, et al. Autosomal-recessive intellectual disability with cerebellar atrophy syndrome caused by mutation of the manganese and zinc transporter gene SLC39A8. Am J Hum Genet. 2015;97(6):886–93.

Bras J, Verloes A, Schneider SA, Mole SE, Guerreiro RJ. Mutation of the parkinsonism gene ATP13A2 causes neuronal ceroid-lipofuscinosis. Hum Mol Genet. 2012;21(12):2646–50.

Chen P, Chakraborty S, Mukhopadhyay S, Lee E, Paoliello MM, Bowman AB, et al. Manganese homeostasis in the nervous system. J Neurochem. 2015;134(4):601–10.

Christenson ET, Gallegos AS, Banerjee A. In vitro reconstitution, functional dissection, and mutational analysis of metal ion transport by mitoferrin-1. J Biol Chem. 2018;293(10):3819–28.

Clayton PT. Inherited disorders of transition metal metabolism: an update. J Inherit Metab Dis. 2017;40(4):519–29.

Di Fonzo A, Chien HF, Socal M, Giraudo S, Tassorelli C, Iliceto G, et al. ATP13A2 missense mutations in juvenile parkinsonism and young onset Parkinson disease. Neurology. 2007;68(19):1557–62.

Estrada-Cuzcano A, Martin S, Chamova T, Synofzik M, Timmann D, Holemans T, et al. Loss-of-function mutations in the ATP13A2/PARK9 gene cause complicated hereditary spastic paraplegia (SPG78). Brain. 2017;140(2):287–305.

Gospe SM Jr, Caruso RD, Clegg MS, Keen CL, Pimstone NR, Ducore JM, et al. Paraparesis, hypermanganesaemia, and polycythaemia: a novel presentation of cirrhosis. Arch Dis Child. 2000;83(5):439–42.

Gulab S, Kayyali HR, Al-Said Y. Atypical neurologic phenotype and novel SLC30A10 mutation in two brothers with hereditary hypermanganesemia. Neuropediatrics. 2018;49(1):72–5.

Hutchens S, Liu C, Jursa T, Shawlot W, Chaffee BK, Yin W, et al. Deficiency in the manganese efflux transporter SLC30A10 induces severe hypothyroidism in mice. J Biol Chem. 2017;292(23):9760–73.

Leyva-Illades D, Chen P, Zogzas CE, Hutchens S, Mercado JM, Swaim CD, et al. SLC30A10 is a cell surface-localized manganese efflux transporter, and Parkinsonism-causing mutations block its intracellular trafficking and efflux activity. J Neurosci. 2014;34(42):14079–95.

Park JH, Hogrebe M, Gruneberg M, DuChesne I, von der Heiden AL, Reunert J, et al. SLC39A8 deficiency: a disorder of manganese transport and glycosylation. Am J Hum Genet. 2015a;97(6):894–903.

Park JS, Blair NF, Sue CM. The role of ATP13A2 in Parkinson's disease: Clinical phenotypes and molecular mechanisms. Mov Disord. 2015b;30(6):770–9.

Park JH, Hogrebe M, Fobker M, Brackmann R, Fiedler B, Reunert J, et al. SLC39A8 deficiency: biochemical correction and major clinical improvement by manganese therapy. Genet Med. 2017;20(2):259–68.

Peres TV, Schettinger MR, Chen P, Carvalho F, Avila DS, Bowman AB, et al. Manganese-induced neurotoxicity: a review of its behavioral consequences and neuroprotective strategies. BMC Pharmacol Toxicol. 2016;17(1):57.

Quadri M, Federico A, Zhao T, Breedveld GJ, Battisti C, Delnooz C, et al. Mutations in SLC30A10 cause parkinsonism and dystonia with hypermanganesemia, polycythemia, and chronic liver disease. Am J Hum Genet. 2012;90(3):467–77.

Quadri M, Kamate M, Sharma S, Olgiati S, Graafland J, Breedveld GJ, et al. Manganese transport disorder: Novel SLC30A10 mutations and early phenotypes. Mov Disord. 2015;30(7):996–1001.

Racette BA, Aschner M, Guilarte TR, Dydak U, Criswell SR, Zheng W. Pathophysiology of manganese-associated neurotoxicity. Neurotoxicology. 2012;33(4):881–6.

Riley LG, Cowley MJ, Gayevskiy V, Roscioli T, Thorburn DR, Prelog K, et al. A SLC39A8 variant causes manganese deficiency, and glycosylation and mitochondrial disorders. J Inherit Metab Dis. 2017;40(2):261–9.

Schneider SA, Paisan-Ruiz C, Quinn NP, Lees AJ, Houlden H, Hardy J, et al. ATP13A2 mutations (PARK9) cause neurodegeneration with brain iron accumulation. Mov Disord. 2010;25(8):979–84.

Sorensen DM, Holemans T, van Veen S, Martin S, Arslan T, Haagendahl IW, et al. Parkinson disease related ATP13A2 evolved early in animal evolution. uPLoS One. 2018;13(3):e0193228.

Tuschl K, Clayton PT, Gospe SM, Mills PB. Dystonia/parkinsonism, hypermanganesemia, polycythemia, and chronic liver disease. In: Adam MP, Ardinger HH, Pagon RA, Wallace SE, LJH B, Stephens K, Amemiya A, editors. SourceGeneReviews®. Seattle, WA: University of Washington, Seattle; 1993–2019.

Tuschl K, Gregory A, Meyer E, Clayton PT, Hayflick SJ, Mills PB, et al. SLC39A14 deficiency. In: Adam MP, Ardinger HH, Pagon RA, Wallace SE, Bean LJH, Stephens K, Amemiya A, editors. SourceGeneReviews®. Seattle, WA: University of Washington, Seattle; 1993–2019.

Tuschl K, Clayton PT, Gospe SM Jr, Gulab S, Ibrahim S, Singhi P, et al. Syndrome of hepatic cirrhosis, dystonia, polycythemia, and hypermanganesemia caused by mutations in SLC30A10, a manganese transporter in man. Am J Hum Genet. 2012;90(3):457–66.

Tuschl K, Meyer E, Valdivia LE, Zhao N, Dadswell C, Abdul-Sada A, et al. Mutations in SLC39A14 disrupt manganese homeostasis and cause childhood-onset parkinsonism-dystonia. Nat Commun. 2016;7:11601.

Zaki MS, Issa MY, Elbendary HM, El-Karaksy H, Hosny H, Ghobrial C, et al. Hypermanganesemia with dystonia, polycythemia and cirrhosis in 10 patients: Six novel SLC30A10 mutations and further phenotype delineation. Clin Genet. 2018;93(4):905–12.

Zeglam A, Abugrara A, Kabuka M. Autosomal-recessive iron deficiency anemia, dystonia and hypermanganesemia caused by new variant mutation of the manganese transporter gene SLC39A14. Acta Neurol Belg. 2018; https://doi.org/10.1007/s13760-018-1024-7.

# Part IV

# Disorders of Carbohydrates

# Disorders of Carbohydrate Absorption, Transmembrane Transport and Metabolism

# 39

Terry G. J. Derks, Charlotte M. A. Lubout, Mathias Woidy, and René Santer

## Contents




**Summary**

Carbohydrates are an important source of energy in the human organism. Within the body, glucose is the most abundant monosaccharide that can be stored as glycogen, a branched polymer with a protein core (glycogenin), mainly in liver and muscle. Inborn errors of metabolism may affect the uptake, distribution and reabsorption of monosaccharides in different organs, a process that is meticulously regulated by a system of transporter proteins. Congenital disorders may impair the intestinal digestion of disaccharides and the conversion of monosaccharides (fructose, galactose) into glucose. They can further affect glycogen synthesis, glycogen breakdown (glycogenolysis), glucose metabolism to acetyl-CoA (glycolysis) and de novo synthesis of glucose (gluconeogenesis).

Glucose absorption and transport disorders present with a very variable clinical picture depending on which of the organ- and substrate-specific transporters is affected. Likewise, disorders of galactose and fructose metabolism affect different organs due to the accumulation of toxic intermediates. After the introduction of these monosaccharides with the diet, impaired liver function is frequently among the first signs.



T. G. J. Derks · C. M. A. Lubout
Section of Metabolic Diseases, Beatrix Children's Hospital, University Medical Center Groningen, Groningen, The Netherlands
e-mail: t.g.j.derks@umcg.nl; c.m.a.lubout@umcg.nl

M. Woidy · R. Santer (✉)
Department of Paediatrics, University Medical Center Eppendorf, Hamburg, Germany
e-mail: m.woidy@uke.de; r.santer@uke.de





N. Blau et al. (eds.), *Physician's Guide to the Diagnosis, Treatment, and Follow-Up of Inherited Metabolic Diseases*, https://doi.org/10.1007/978-3-030-67727-5_39

Glycogen storage diseases can be divided into those mainly presenting with hepatic manifestations (hepatomegaly, fasting intolerance, hypoglycaemia) and those with muscular presentations (exertion intolerance, rhabdomyolysis). Some show a combination of these symptoms, cardiomyopathy may be an additional feature and further accompanying signs, *for example,* haemolytic anaemia, may be observed depending on tissue distribution of the affected protein.

Management of most carbohydrate disorders requires symptomatic measures, supportive care and a multidisciplinary approach. In some conditions, dietetic treatment is possible which may have its basis in an exclusion of certain di- or monosaccharides. Outcome, however, is highly variable and mainly depends on the underlying type of disorder. Causal treatment is not available for most diseases and for some patients, organ transplantation (liver, kidney, heart) is an option. Experimental treatments may include enzyme replacement therapy (available, *e.g.,* for lysosomal α-glucosidase deficiency, GSD-IIa) and gene therapy.

## Introduction

The disorders in this chapter can be divided into disorders of carbohydrate absorption and transmembrane transport, galactose and fructose metabolism, glycolysis, glycogen synthesis, glycogenolysis and gluconeogenesis (Nomenclature Table). Most are inherited according to an autosomal recessive trait. The clinical presentations can be acute or chronic, mild or severe, in some even life threatening. The clinical features are highly variable and can be understood when considering age- and organ-specific pathophysiology. Other groups of metabolic disorders of carbohydrate metabolism are mentioned in Chaps. 40 (pentose phosphate pathway and polyol metabolism), 41 (insulin secretion and signalling) and 61 (oligosaccharidoses and sialic acid disorders).

### Disorders of Carbohydrate Absorption and Transmembrane Transport

Dietary carbohydrates (disaccharides, oligo- and polysaccharides, starch) have to be digested to monosaccharides before entering the human organism. Congenital defects at this step include congenital lactase, sucrose-isomaltase and trehalase deficiencies.

The cellular uptake and release of glucose and other monosaccharides is a protein-mediated process. Such proteins are embedded into the cell membrane and can be regarded as hydrophilic pores within the hydrophobic lipid bilayer. Monosaccharide transporters are substrate- and stereospecific. Their action is saturable and, like for an enzymatic reaction, kinetic characteristics can be described by affinity constants. The number of transporter protein molecules determines maximal transport velocity ($v_{max}$).

Three classes of monosaccharide transporters have been associated with human diseases. The SGLT (*s*odium-dependent *gl*ucose *t*ransporter) family is characterised by the fact that glucose transport is coupled with sodium transport. Since the driving force for this type of transport is the electrochemical gradient for sodium (produced by the cellular $Na^+/K^+$-ATPase system), glucose can be (actively) transported against its own gradient. A second family, the GLUT (*glu*cose *t*ransporter) proteins, mediates so-called facilitative diffusion along an existing glucose gradient and, in the past, members of this family have been regarded to function as 'passive' transporters. However, GLUT proteins are hormonally and substrate regulated; thus, they play a pivotal role in the regulation of carbohydrate metabolism. As an example, one of the key functions of insulin is the translocation of GLUT4-bearing vesicles to the cell membrane of muscle cells and adipocytes, allowing glucose influx.

The genes of the growing number of members of both the SGLT and GLUT families have been identified during recent years. This was a key step in the study of the function of these proteins, of their tissue-specific expression and in the identification of genetic defects. Knowledge of the tissue-specific expression of monosaccharide transporter proteins helps define the clinical picture of the different disease entities. Many tissues carry more than one type of transporter and many members of the monosaccharide transporter families are expressed in more than one tissue. Therefore, congenital disorders of different isoforms of monosaccharide transporters may present with a complex clinical picture and may involve different organ systems. Well-characterised disease entities are congenital intestinal glucose-galactose malabsorption (GGM, *SGLT1* defect), the glucose transporter-1 deficiency syndrome (GLUT1-D) and the Fanconi-Bickel syndrome (FBS, *GLUT2* defect). In contrast, due to the high solubility of glucose, renal glucosuria due to SGLT2 deficiency (SGLT2-D) or due to the rare defect of an SGLT2-associated protein in the renal tubular cell membrane (MAP17), is rarely accompanied by specific clinical symptoms and, like some of the amino acid transporter defects, it can be classified as a '*non*-disease'. The diagnosis has, however, a clinical significance as it prevents repeated investigation for diabetes mellitus in these patients.

Only recently, an inborn error affecting a member of a third monosaccharide transporter family, the glucose/proton cotransporters (encoded by the *SLC45* gene family), has been described. In this condition, glucose supply to neuronal cells is impaired with symptoms of developmental delay, psychiatric features, and epilepsy (Srour et al. 2017).

## Disorders of Galactose and Fructose Metabolism

There are four known disorders of galactose metabolism affecting the enzymes of the Leloir pathway: galactose mutarotase deficiency (GALM-D), galactokinase deficiency (GALK-D), galactose-1-phosphate uridyltransferase deficiency (galactosaemia, GALT-D), and uridine diphosphate galactose-4-epimerase deficiency (GALE-D). Among these disorders, galactosaemia is the most common and can be the most severe. Several partial defects of transferase deficiency have been reported, of which the best known is the Duarte-2 variant (Berry et al. 2016).

Unlike most disorders in this chapter that highly depend on clinical ascertainment/clinical and biochemical pattern recognition, all four disorders of galactose metabolism can be identified by newborn screening programs. These programs are based on enzymatic investigations and detection of increased amounts of galactose and galactose-1-phosphate in dried blood spots. The clinical manifestations of classic galactosaemia occur after galactose is introduced with the diet and the accumulation of metabolic intermediates is responsible for organ damage. Galactitol causes cataract formation, while galactose-1-phosphate (together with phosphate depletion) is a key factor for hepatic, renal tubular and central nervous manifestations.

Four disorders affecting fructose metabolism are known: fructokinase deficiency (FK-D), fructose-1-phosphate aldolase deficiency (hereditary fructose intolerance, HFI), fructose-1,6-bisphosphatase deficiency (FBP-D) and glycerate kinase deficiency (GLYCTK-D). While FK-D is a *non*-disease, severe symptoms in HFI occur after the ingestion of fructose and are the consequence of accumulation of fructose-1-phosphate, with secondary effects mainly on liver cell metabolism, phosphate depletion and protein glycosylation. FBP-D is a disorder of gluconeogenesis; symptoms may occur in the fasted state and without fructose ingestion, although fructose may enhance these effects. For GLYCTK-D, which is related to fructose metabolism but also impairs several other metabolic pathways, *see* Chap. 71.

## Disorders of Glycolysis

Defects in the glycolysis pathway may present as muscle glycogen storage disorders, while others result in haemolysis as they affect erythrocyte metabolism (Bianchi et al. 2019, Tarnopolsky 2018). Some present with both muscle symptoms and haemolysis or give rise to mostly neurological symptoms (Fermo et al. 2019). Genetic variants in *HK1*, the gene coding for hexokinase 1, can present as four distinct clinical pictures: haemolytic anaemia due to loss of hexokinase enzymatic activity on one side, and hereditary motor and sensory neuropathy (Russe type, HMSNR), retinitis pigmentosa type 79 (RP79), and a recently described neurodevelopmental disorder with visual defects and brain anomalies (NEDVIBA) on the other (Jamwal et al. 2019, Okur et al. 2019).

## Disorders of Glycogen Synthesis and Glycogenolysis

Glycogen storage disorders (GSDs) result from enzymatic blocks or impaired transporter function in the pathway of glycogen degradation (glycogenolysis) but defects of glycogen synthesis in liver and muscle have also been termed 'glycogenoses' (GSD-0, GSD-IV). Simply speaking, glycogen storage disorders with cytosolic glycogen accumulation may present as a disease of liver only (GSD-I, GSD-III, GSD-VI and GSD-IX), of liver and kidney (FBS, GSD-I), with liver involvement and (cardio)myopathy (GSD-III, GSD-IX) and myopathy without liver involvement (GSD-V, GSD-VII, rare muscular types (Tarnopolsky 2018)). Lysosomal storage of glycogen results in a multisystem disorder generally presenting with cardiac and/or muscular problems (GSD-II).

GSD-I, GSD-III, GSD-VI and GSD-IX are similar in physical appearance and are usually detected during infancy or childhood because of fasting intolerance, failure to thrive and marked hepatomegaly (and, generally, without splenomegaly or cholestasis) (Fig. 39.1). Hypoglycaemia is another leading sign in hepatic GSDs, which is most severe in GSD-I where both glycogenolysis and gluconeogenesis are affected.

Muscle is unable to produce glucose for systemic use, because glucose-6-phosphatase activity is absent. Classical muscle GSDs involve skeletal muscle and present with muscle weakness, exertion intolerance and/or myoglobinuria, but are usually not diagnosed before late childhood and adolescence. Rare muscle GSDs with defects in the glycolysis pathway of muscle may, however, present with a more complex clinical picture.

Disorders in which detection of polyglucosan bodies is a hallmark are related to GSDs. Examples are muscle glycogenin-1 deficiency, Laforin deficiency and Malin deficiency. Polyglucosan bodies can be found in many tissues but are typically found in muscle or brain. The presence of such insoluble aggregates of abnormally branched glycogen with increased phosphorylation and (in brain) ubiquitination is associated with impaired autophagy. Since such cases with unstable glycogen are rare, the clinical and biochemical phenotypes of the disorders are incompletely defined (Sullivan et al. 2017).

Finally, glycogenolysis is impaired in a congenital disorder of glycosylation, phosphoglucomutase-1 deficiency, which is discussed in more detail elsewhere in this book (*see* Chaps. 58 and 66).

## Disorders of Gluconeogenesis

Glucose can be formed from *non*-hexose precursors such as lactate, pyruvate, glycerol and amino acids, a metabolic pathway called gluconeogenesis. Three *non*-reversible reactions of glycolysis characterise the disorders of gluconeogenesis, which are featured by fasting intolerance with associated recurrent hypoglycaemia and lactic acidosis, with or without ketosis. The mitochondrial matrix enzyme pyruvate carboxylase converts pyruvate to oxaloacetate, a central metabolite involved in gluconeogenesis, the urea cycle, the citric acid cycle, the glyoxylate cycle, amino acid synthesis and fatty acid synthesis. Hence, central nervous system signs and symptoms are part of the clinical phenotype and hyperammonaemia and severe metabolic acidosis may occur. In phosphoenolpyruvate carboxykinase deficiency, an extremely rare condition which may result from deficiency of a mitochondrial or a cytosolic enzyme, the conversion of oxaloacetate into phosphoenolpyruvate is deficient. Fructose-1,6-bisphosphatase deficiency causes relatively mild fasting intolerance, severe lactic acidosis and moderate hepatomegaly during metabolic crises. The disorders involved in the conversion of glucose-6-phosphate into glucose affect both glycogenolysis and gluconeogenesis. Defects of the hepatic proteins result in severe fasting intolerance; in patients with glucose-6-phosphatase catalytic subunit-3 deficiency, the neutrophil enzyme, severe congenital neutropenia is found.

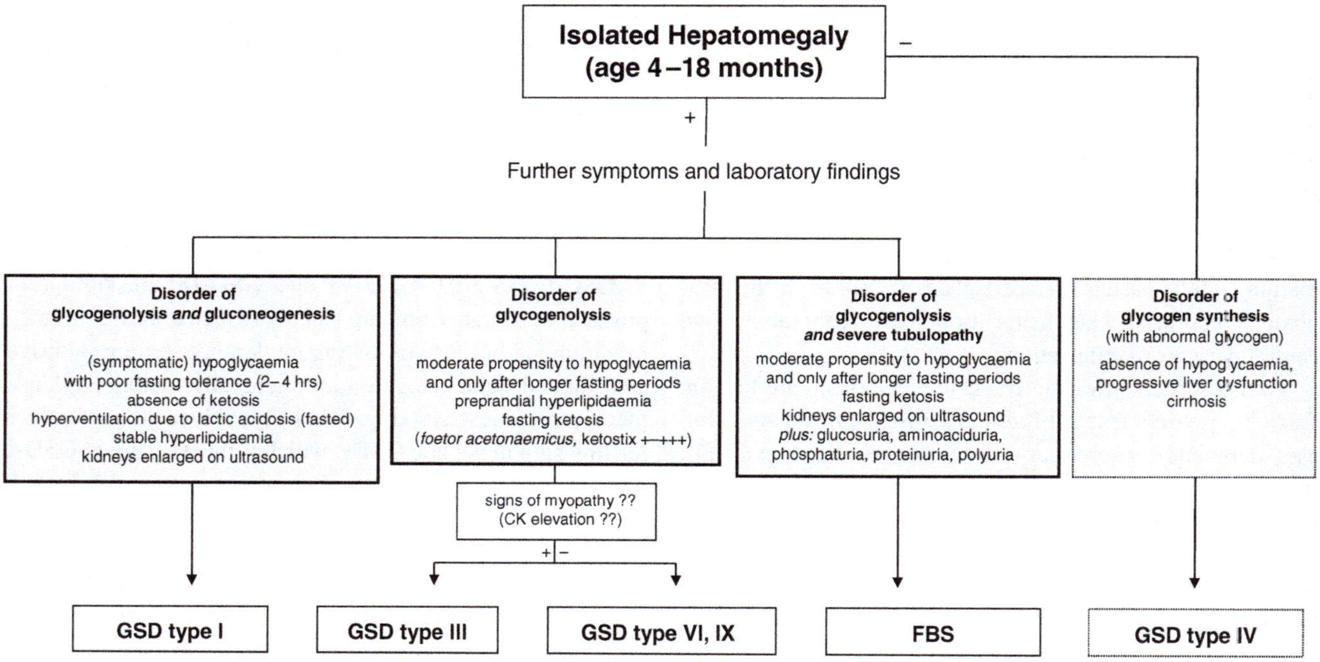


**Fig. 39.1** Flowchart for clinical differentiation of hepatic glycogen storage disorders

## Nomenclature

| No | Disease Name | Alternative Disease Name 1 | Alternative Disease Name 2 | Disease Abbreviation | Gene Symbol | Chromosomal Localisation | Mode of Inheritance | Affected Protein | Disease OMIM |
|---|---|---|---|---|---|---|---|---|---|
| | **Disorders of carbohydrate absorption and transmembrane transport** | | | | | | | | |
| 39.1 | Congenital lactase deficiency | Congenital alactasia | | CL-D | *LCT* | 2q21.3 | AR | Lactase | 223000 |
| 39.2 | Congenital sucrase-isomaltase deficiency | | | CSI-D | *SI* | 3q26.1 | AR | Sucrase-isomaltase | 222900 |
| 39.3 | Trehalase deficiency | Trehalose intolerance | | TREH-D | *TREH* | 11q23.3 | AR | Trehalase | 612119 |
| 39.4 | Intestinal sodium-glucose cotransporter 1 deficiency | Glucose-galactose malabsorption | SGLT1 deficiency | GGM | *SLC5A1* | 22q12.3 | AR | Sodium-glucose cotransporter-1 | 606824 |
| 39.5 | Renal sodium-glucose cotransporter 2 deficiency | Familial renal glucosuria type 1 | SGLT2 deficiency | SGLT2-D | *SLC5A2* | 16p11.2 | AD, AR | Sodium-glucose cotransporter-2 | 233100 |
| 39.6 | MAP17 deficiency | Familial renal glucosuria type 2 | | MAP17-D | *PDZK1IP1* | 1p33 | AR | Membrane-associated protein (MAP17) | 607178 |
| 39.7 | Blood-brain barrier glucose transporter 1 deficiency | Glucose transporter-1 deficiency | | GLUT1-D | *SLC2A1* | 1p34.2 | AD, AR | Glucose transporter 1 | 601042; 606777; 612126; 614847; 608885 |
| 39.8 | Neuronal glucose transporter deficiency | Intellectual developmental disorder with neuropsychiatric features | Brain glucose transporter SLC45A1 deficiency | IDDNPF | *SLC45A1* | 1p36.23 | AR | Solute carrier family 45, member 1 | 617532 |
| 39.9 | Glucose transporter 2 deficiency | Fanconi-Bickel syndrome | | FBS | *SLC2A2* | 3q26.2 | AR | Glucose transporter-2 | 227810 |
| | **Disorders of galactose and fructose metabolism** | | | | | | | | |
| 39.10 | Galactose mutarotase deficiency | Galactosaemia type 4 | | GALM-D | *GALM* | 2p22.1 | AR | Galactose mutarotase | 618881 |
| 39.11 | Galactokinase deficiency | Galactosaemia type 2 | | GALK-D | *GALK1* | 17q25.1 | AR | Galactokinase | 230200 |
| 39.12 | Galactose-1-phosphate uridyltransferase deficiency | Galactosaemia type 1 | | GALT-D | *GALT* | 9p13.3 | AR | Galactose-1-phosphate uridyltransferase | 230400 |
| 39.13 | Galactose epimerase deficiency | Galactosaemia type 3 | | GALE-D | *GALE* | 1p36.11 | AR | Galactose epimerase | 230350 |
| 39.14 | Essential fructosuria | Fructokinase deficiency | Ketohexokinase deficiency | FK-D | *KHK* | 2p23.3 | AR | Fructokinase | 229800 |

(continued)

| No | Disease Name | Alternative Disease Name 1 | Alternative Disease Name 2 | Disease Abbreviation | Gene Symbol | Chromosomal Localisation | Mode of Inheritance | Affected Protein | Disease OMIM |
|---|---|---|---|---|---|---|---|---|---|
| 39.15 | Hereditary fructose intolerance | Fructose-1-phosphate aldolase deficiency | Aldolase B deficiency | HFI | *ALDOB* | 9q31.1 | AR | Fructose-1-phosphate aldolase | 229600 |
| | **Disorders of glycolysis** | | | | | | | | |
| 39.16 | Haemolytic anaemia due to hexokinase deficiency | | | HK1-D | *HK1* | 10q22.1 | AR | Hexokinase 1 | 235700 |
| 39.17 | Neurodevelopmental disorder with visual defects and brain anomalies | | | NEDVIBA | *HK1* | 10q22.1 | AD | Hexokinase 1 | 618547 |
| 39.18 | Hereditary motor and sensory neuropathy, Russe type | Charcot-Marie-Tooth disease type 4G | | HMSNR | *HK1* | 10q22.1 | AR | Hexokinase 1 | 605285 |
| 39.19 | Retinitis pigmentosa type 79 | | | RP79 | *HK1* | 10q22.1 | AD | Hexokinase 1 | 617460 |
| 39.20 | Glucokinase deficiency | Permanent neonatal diabetes mellitus; MODY type 2 | | MODY2 | *GCK* | 7p13 | AD | Glucokinase | 606176; 125851 |
| 39.21 | Glucokinase superactivity | Familial hyperinsulinaemic hypoglycaemia type 3 | | HHF3 | *GCK* | 7p13 | AD | Glucokinase | 602485 |
| 39.22 | Glucose-6-phosphate isomerase deficiency | Haemolytic anaemia, nonspheric, due to GPI deficency | | G6PI-D | *GPI* | 19q13.11 | AR | Glucose phosphate isomerase | 613470 |
| 39.23 | Muscle phosphofructokinase deficiency | Glycogen storage disease type VII | Tarui disease | GSD-VII | *PFKM* | 12q13.11 | AR | Muscle phosphofructokinase | 232800 |
| 39.24 | Aldolase A deficiency | Glycogen storage disease type XII | | ALDOA-D | *ALDOA* | 16p11.2 | AR | Aldolase A | 611881 |
| 39.25 | Triose phosphate isomerase deficiency | Haemolytic anaemia due to triosephosphate isomerase deficiency | | TPI-D | *TPI1* | 12p13.31 | AR | Triosephosphate isomerase | 615512 |
| 39.26 | Phosphoglycerate kinase deficiency | | | PGK-D | *PGK1* | Xq21.1 | XLR | Phosphoglycerate kinase | 300653 |
| 39.27 | Muscle phosphoglycerate mutase deficiency | Glycogen storage disease type X | DiMauro disease | GSD-X | *PGAM2* | 7p13 | AR | Muscle phosphoglycerate mutase | 261670 |
| 39.28 | Enolase β deficiency | Glycogen storage disease type XIII | | GSD-XIII | *ENO3* | 17p13.2 | AR | Enolase β | 612932 |
| 39.29 | Pyruvate kinase deficiency | | | PK-D | *PKLR* | 1q22 | AR | Pyruvate kinase | 266200 |
| 39.30 | Lactate dehydrogenase A deficiency | Glycogen storage disease type XI | | LDHA-D | *LDHA* | 11p15.1 | AR | Lactate dehydrogenase subunit M | 612933 |
| 39.31 | Lactate dehydrogenase B deficiency | | | LDHB-D | *LDHB* | 12p12.1 | AD, AR | Lactate dehydrogenase subunit H | 614128 |

| No | Disease Name | Alternative Disease Name 1 | Alternative Disease Name 2 | Disease Abbreviation | Gene Symbol | Chromosomal Localisation | Mode of Inheritance | Affected Protein | Disease OMIM |
|---|---|---|---|---|---|---|---|---|---|
| 39.32 | D-Lactate dehydrogenase deficiency | Hereditary D-lactic aciduria | | D-LDH-D | *LDHD* | 16q23.1 | AR | D-lactate dehydrogenase | 245450 |
| | **Disorders of glycogen synthesis** | | | | | | | | |
| 39.33 | Muscle glycogenin 1 deficiency | Glycogen storage disease type XV | Polyglucosan body myopathy type 2 | GSD-XV | *GYG1* | 3q24 | AR | Glycogenin 1 | 613507; 616199 |
| 39.34 | Muscle glycogen synthase deficiency | Glycogen storage disease type 0b | | GSD-0b | *GYS1* | 19q13.33 | AR | Glycogen synthase 1 | 611556 |
| 39.35 | Hepatic glycogen synthase deficiency | Glycogen storage disease type 0a | | GSD-0a | *GYS2* | 12p12.1 | AR | Glycogen synthase 2 | 240600 |
| 39.36 | Glycogen branching enzyme deficiency | Glycogen storage disease type IV | Andersen disease | GSD-IV | *GBE1* | 3p12.2 | AR | Glycogen branching enzyme | 232500; 263570 |
| | **Disorders of glycogenolysis** | | | | | | | | |
| 39.37 | Muscle phosphorylase kinase α1 subunit deficiency | Glycogen storage disease type IXd | | GSD-IXd | *PHKA1* | Xq13.1 | XLR | Muscle phosphorylase kinase α1 subunit | 300559 |
| 39.38 | Hepatic phosphorylase kinase α2 subunit deficiency | Glycogen storage disease type IXa | | GSD-IXa | *PHKA2* | Xp22.13 | XLR | Hepatic phosphorylase kinase α2 subunit | 306000 |
| 39.39 | Phosphorylase kinase β subunit deficiency | Glycogen storage disease type IXb | | GSD-IXb | *PHKB* | 16q12.1 | AR | Hepatic and muscle phosphorylase kinase β subunit | 261750 |
| 39.40 | Hepatic phosphorylase kinase γ2 subunit deficiency | Glycogen storage disease type IXc | | GSD-IXc | *PHKG2* | 16p11.2 | AR | Hepatic phosphorylase kinase γ2 subunit | 613027 |
| 39.41 | Constitutional AMP-activated protein kinase activation | | | AMPK-A | *PRKAG2* | 7q36.1 | AD | AMP-activated protein kinase γ2 subunit | 261740; 600858; 194200 |
| 39.42 | Muscle glycogen phosphorylase deficiency | Glycogen storage disease type V | McArdle disease | GSD-V | *PYGM* | 11q13.1 | AR | Muscle glycogen phosphorylase | 232600 |
| 39.43 | Hepatic glycogen phosphorylase deficiency | Glycogen storage disease type VI | Hers disease | GSD-VI | *PYGL* | 14q22.1 | AR | Liver glycogen phosphorylase | 232700 |
| 39.44 | Glycogen debranching enzyme deficiency | Glycogen storage disease type III | Cori disease | GSD-III | *AGL* | 1p21.2 | AR | Amylo-1,6-glucosidase | 232400 |
| 39.45 | Glucose-6-phosphatase deficiency | Glycogen storage disease type Ia | von Gierke disease | GSD-Ia | *G6PC* | 17q21.31 | AR | Glucose-6-phosphatase | 232200 |
| 39.46 | Glucose-6-phosphatase catalytic subunit 3 deficiency | Neutropenia, severe, congenital, type 4 | Dursun syndrome | G6PC3-D | *G6PC3* | 17q21.31 | AR | Glucose-6-phosphatase catalytic subunit 3 | 612541 |

(continued)

| No | Disease Name | Alternative Disease Name 1 | Alternative Disease Name 2 | Disease Abbreviation | Gene Symbol | Chromosomal Localisation | Mode of Inheritance | Affected Protein | Disease OMIM |
|---|---|---|---|---|---|---|---|---|---|
| 39.47 | Glucose-6-phosphate translocase deficiency | Glycogen storage disease type Ib | Glycogen storage disease type I *non*-a | GSD-Ib | *SLC37A4* | 11q23.3 | AR | Glucose-6-phosphate translocase | 232220 |
| 39.48 | HOIL1 deficiency | Polyglucosan body myopathy type 1 | | HOIL1-D | *RBCK1* | 20p13 | AR | Linear ubiquitin chain assembly complex | 615895 |
| 39.49 | HOIL1 interacting protein deficiency | | | HOIL1-IP-D | *RNF31* | 14q12 | AR | Ring finger protein 31 | 612487 |
| 39.50 | Laforin deficiency | Progressive myoclonic epilepsy type 2A | | EPM2A-D | *EPM2A* | 6q24.3 | AR | Laforin glucan phosphatase | 254780 |
| 39.51 | Malin deficiency | Progressive myoclonic epilepsy type 2B | | EPM2B-D | *NHLRC1* | 6p22.3 | AR | Malin | 254780 |
| 39.52 | Lysosomal α-1,4-glucosidase deficiency | Glycogen storage disease type IIa | Pompe disease | GSD-IIa | *GAA* | 17q25.3 | AR | Alpha-1,4-glucosidase | 232300 |
| 39.53 | Lysosome-associated membrane protein 2 deficiency | Glycogen storage disease type IIb | Danon disease | GSD-IIb | *LAMP2* | Xq24 | XLD | Lysosome-associated membrane protein 2 | 300257 |
| | **Disorders of gluconeogenesis** | | | | | | | | |
| 39.54 | Pyruvate carboxylase deficiency | | | PC-D | *PC* | 11q13.2 | AR | Pyruvate carboxylase | 266150 |
| 39.55 | Mitochondrial phosphoenolpyruvate carboxykinase deficiency | PEPCK deficiency, mitochondrial | | mtPCK-D | *PCK2* | 14q11-q12 | AR | Mitochondrial phosphoenolpyruvate carboxykinase | 261650 |
| 39.56 | Cytosolic phosphoenolpyruvate carboxykinase deficiency | PEPCK deficiency, cytosolic | | cPCK-D | *PCK1* | 20q13.31 | AR | Cytosolic phosphoenolpyruvate carboxykinase | 261680 |
| 39.57 | Fructose-1,6-bisphosphatase deficiency | | | FBP-D | *FBP1* | 9q22.32 | AR | Fructose-1,6-bisphosphatase | 229700 |

## Metabolic Pathways

Metabolic pathways of carbohydrate metabolism discussed in this chapter are divided into (i) carbohydrate absorption and transmembrane transport in different organs, (ii) the intracellular pathways linking the metabolism of other monosaccharides to glucose metabolism, (iii) glycolysis, glycogen synthesis and glycogenolysis and (iv) gluconeogenesis.

Accordingly, disorders of organ-specific glucose transport are systematically depicted in Fig. 39.2, galactose and fructose metabolism are presented in Figs. 39.3 and 39.4, respectively. The major steps in disorders affecting glycogen synthesis and breakdown and defects of glycolysis and gluconeogenesis are presented in Fig. 39.5. The steps of glycogenolysis impaired in the different types of glycogen storage diseases are shown in detail in Fig. 39.6.

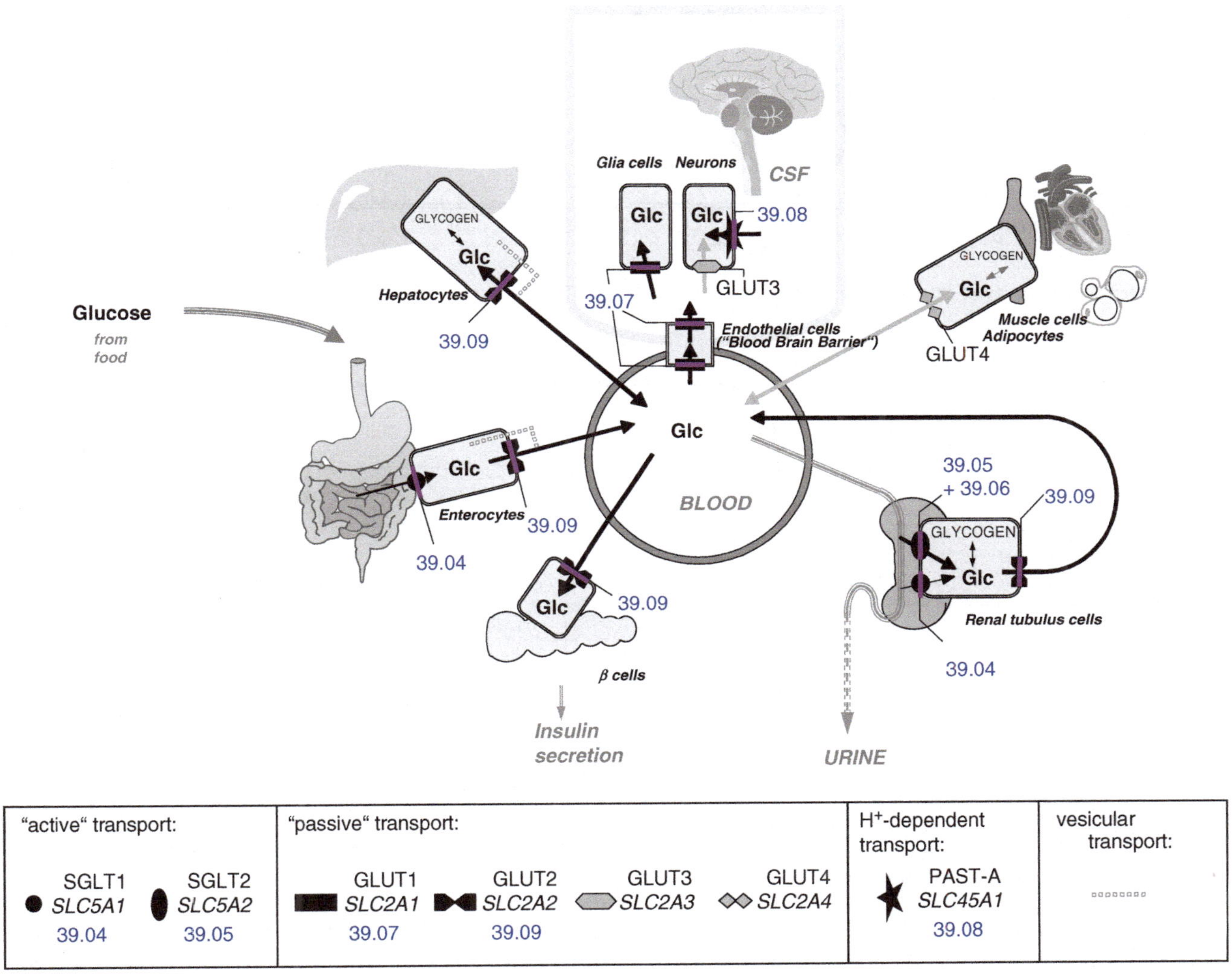


**Fig. 39.2** Cellular uptake and release of glucose and transcellular transport mediated by specific transporter proteins. Transport across cell membranes is indicated by arrows. Transporter proteins are depicted by different symbols. Round symbols represent sodium-dependent '*active*' transporters (encoded by genes of the *SLC5* family), rectangular symbols stand for facilitative, so-called '*passive*' transporters (encoded by genes of the *SLC2* family), and the star-shaped symbol represents a member of the novel glucose/proton cotransporters (encoded by genes of the *SLC45* family). Known defects are shown by pink bars and the respective number. *GLUT3* Glucose transporter-3, *GLUT4* Glucose transporter-4, *CSF* Cerebrospinal fluid

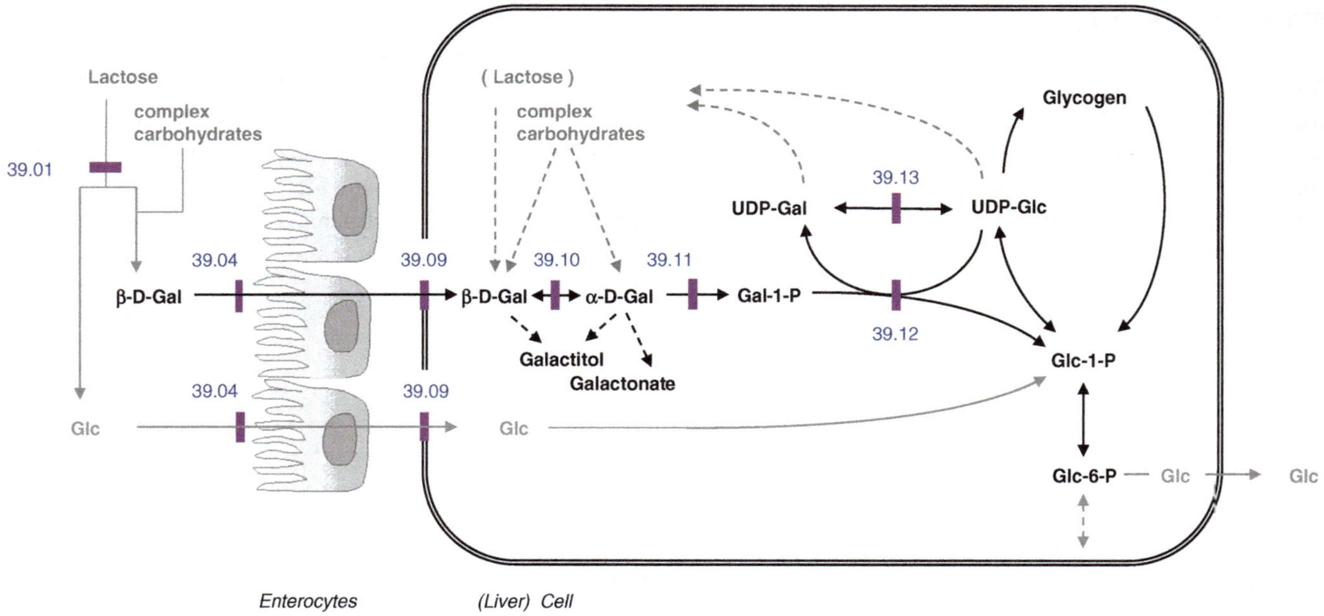


**Fig. 39.3** Metabolic pathway of galactose metabolism

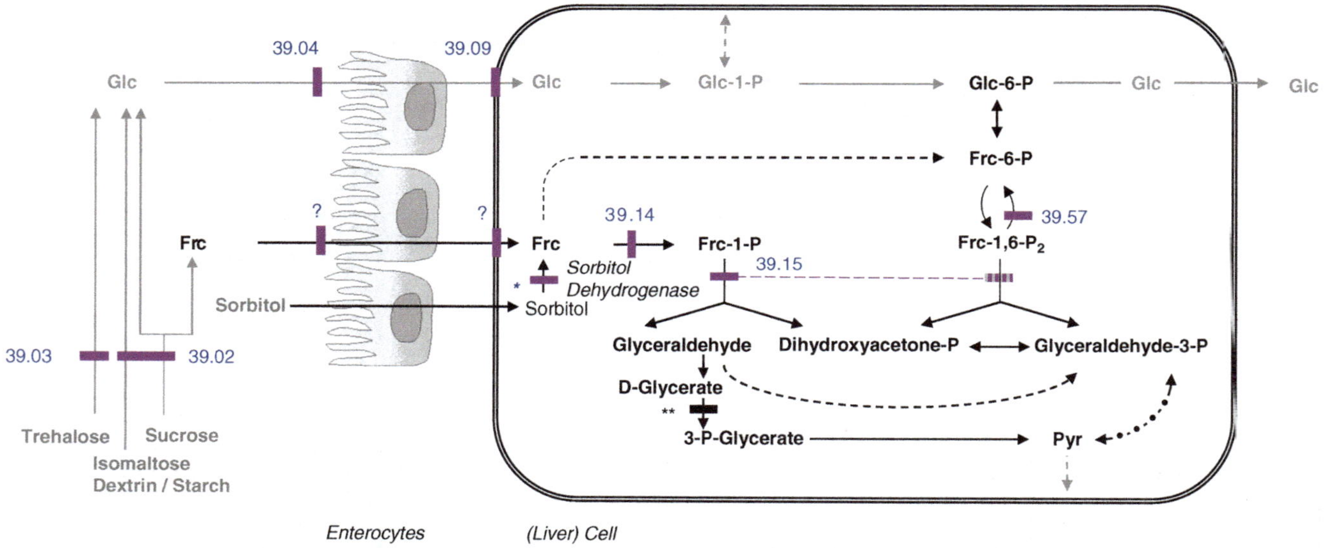


**Fig. 39.4** Metabolic pathway of fructose metabolism
(* *Note added in proof:* Biallelic variants in the gene of sorbitol dehydrogenase (*asterisk*) have only recently been reported as a cause of a common and potentially treatable hereditary neuropathy; *see* Cortese et al. 2020), ** for glycerate kinase deficiency (D-glyceric acidemia, GLYCTK-D) *see* Chap. 71

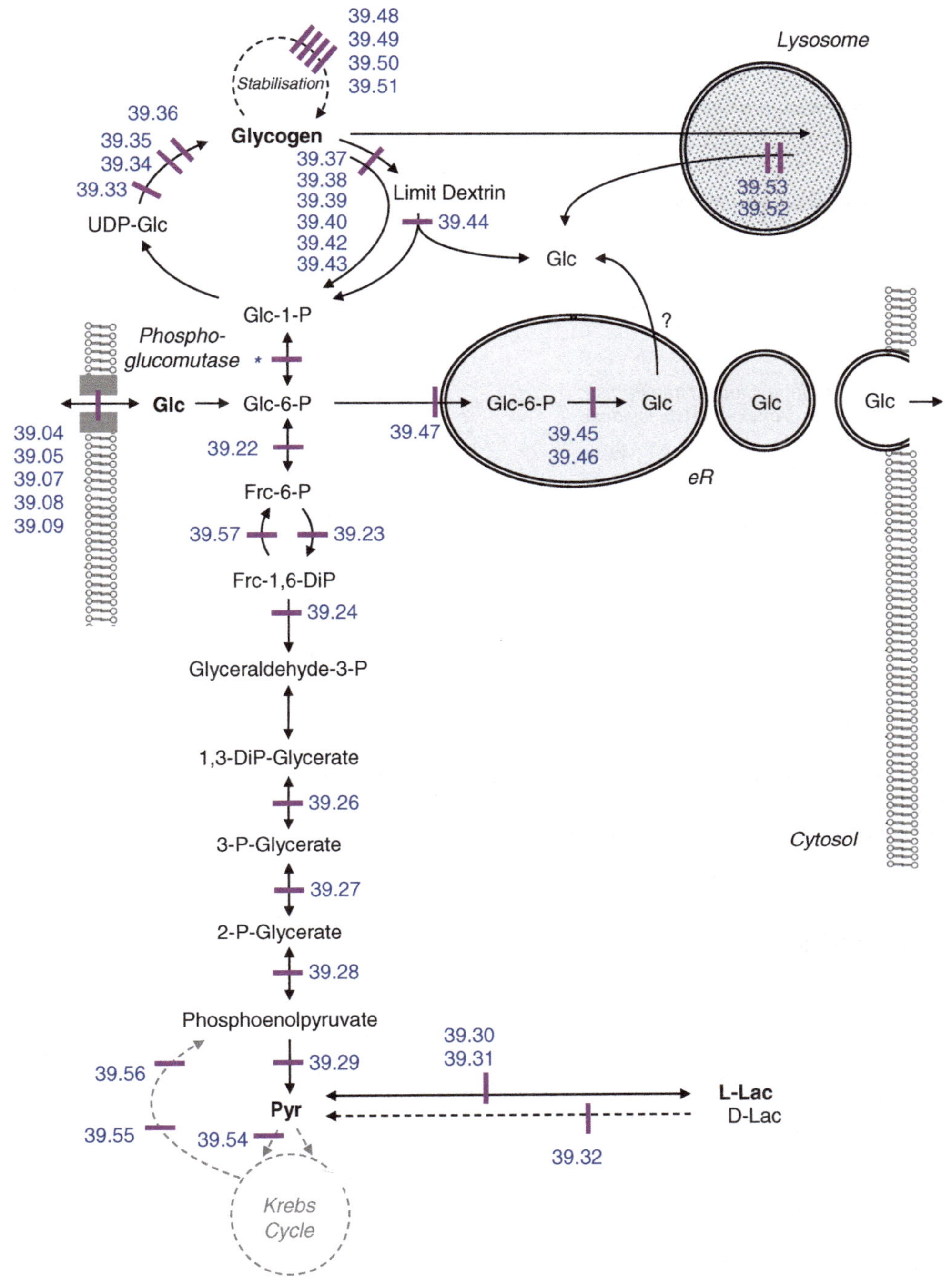


**Fig. 39.5** Principal steps in glycogen synthesis and degradation. *Note* that the scheme is a summary of pathways in different tissues. Tissue-specific isoforms of enzymes (*e.g.*, in liver and muscle) may result in different disease entities with tissue-related signs and symptoms. *eR* endoplasmic reticulum, * *see* Chaps. 58 and 66

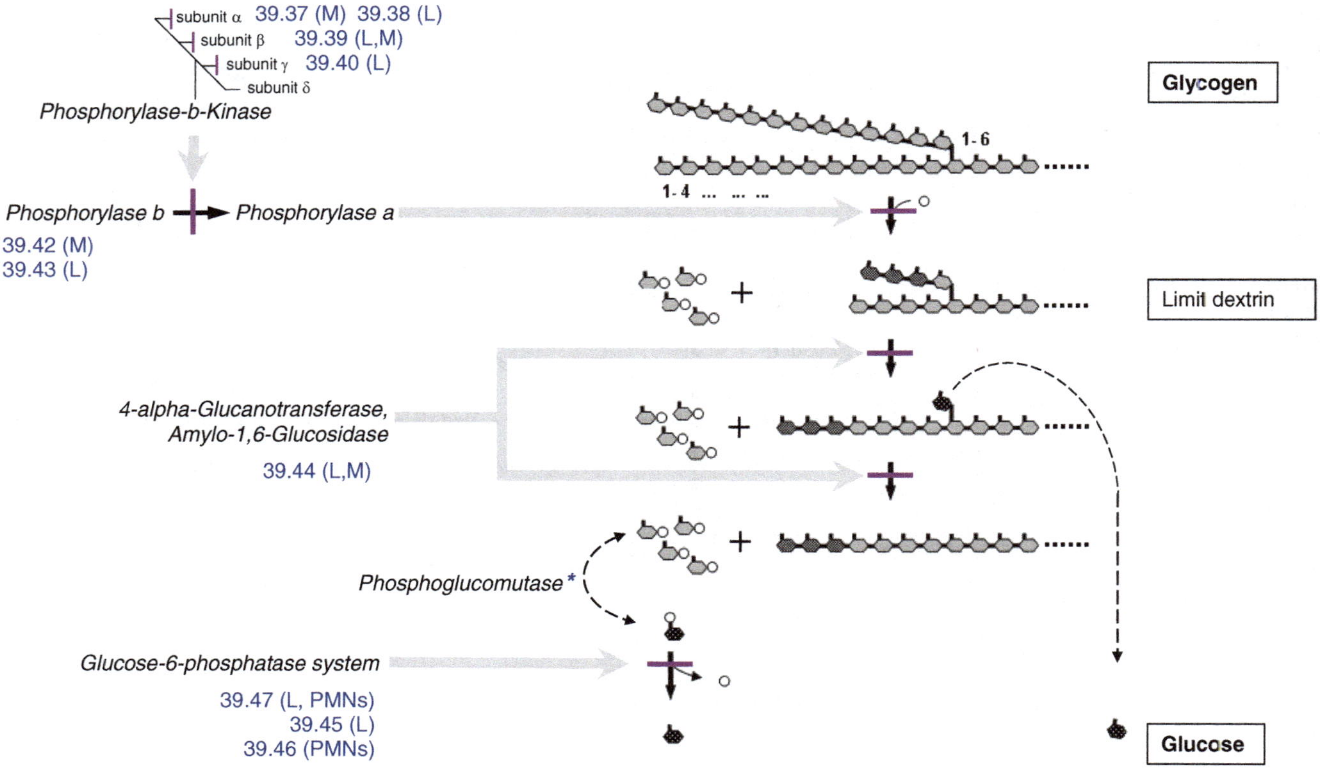


**Fig. 39.6** Metabolic pathway of glycogen degradation. *Note* that the scheme is a summary of pathways in different tissues. Impairment of tissue-specific isoforms of enzymes (L, liver; M, muscle, PMNs, polymorph nuclear cells) results in different disease entities with tissue-related signs and symptoms. **see* Chaps. 58 and 66

## Signs and Symptoms

**Table 39.1** Congenital lactase deficiency (*see also* Wanes et al. 2019)

| System | Symptoms and biomarkers | Neonatal (birth–1 month) | Infancy (1–18 months) | Childhood (1.5–11 years) | Adolescence (11–16 years) | Adulthood (>16 years) |
|---|---|---|---|---|---|---|
| Digestive | **Diarrhea, profuse, osmotic**[a] | +++ | +++ | ++ | ++ | ++ |
| Other | **Dehydration**[a] | +++ | +++ | ++ | ++ | ++ |
| | Failure to thrive[a] | ± | ± | ± | ± | ± |
| | Hypovolaemic shock[a] | ± | ± | ± | ± | ± |
| Renal | Urolithiasis[a] | ± | ± | ± | ± | ± |
| Laboratory findings | Isomaltase activity (intestinal mucosa) | n | n | n | | |
| | Lactase activity in intestinal biopsy | ↓ - ↓↓↓ | ↓ - ↓↓↓ | ↓ - ↓↓↓ | ↓ - ↓↓↓ | ↓ - ↓↓↓ |
| | Maltase activity (intestinal mucosa) | n | n | n | | |
| | pH[a] | n - ↓↓↓ | n - ↓↓↓ | n - ↓ | n - ↓ | n - ↓ |
| | Reducing sugars (stool)[a] | ↑ | ↑ | ↑ | ↑ | ↑ |
| | **Sodium (plasma)**[a] | n - ↑↑↑ | n - ↑↑↑ | n - ↑↑↑ | n - ↑↑↑ | n - ↑↑↑ |
| | Sucrase activity (intestinal mucosa) | n | n | n | | |

[a]Disease features occur on a lactose-containing diet

**Table 39.2** Congenital sucrase-isomaltase deficiency

| System | Symptoms and biomarkers | Neonatal (birth–1 month) | Infancy (1–18 months) | Childhood (1.5–11 years) | Adolescence (11–16 years) | Adulthood (>16 years) |
|---|---|---|---|---|---|---|
| Digestive | Dehydration[a] | n | ± | ± | ± | ± |
| | Diarrhea, profuse, osmotic[a] | n | ± | ± | ± | ± |
| | Diarrhea[a,b] | n | ± | ± | ± | ± |
| Other | Failure to thrive[a,b] | n | ± | ± | ± | ± |
| | Malabsorption[a,b] | n | ± | ± | ± | ± |
| Renal | Urolithiasis[a] | n | ± | ± | ± | ± |
| Laboratory findings | pH[a,b] | n | n - ↓ | n - ↓ | n - ↓ | n - ↓ |
| | Reducing sugars (stool) | n | n | n | n | n |
| | Sodium (plasma)[a,b] | n | n - ↓ | n - ↓ | n - ↓ | n - ↓ |
| | Sucrase-Isomaltase activity in intestinal biopsy | ↓ - ↓↓↓ | ↓ - ↓↓↓ | ↓ - ↓↓↓ | ↓ - ↓↓↓ | ↓ - ↓↓↓ |

[a]Disease features occur on a sucrose-containing diet
[b]Disease features occur on a oligosaccharide/starch-containing diet

**Table 39.3** Trehalase deficiency

| System | Symptoms and biomarkers | Neonatal (birth–1 month) | Infancy (1–18 months) | Childhood (1.5–11 years) | Adolescence (11–16 years) | Adulthood (>16 years) |
|---|---|---|---|---|---|---|
| Digestive | Abdominal pain[a] | | | | + | + |
| | Diarrhea[a] | | | | + | + |
| | Rectal flatulence[a] | | | | + | + |
| Laboratory findings | Reducing sugars (stool)[a] | | | | n | n |
| | Treahalase activity in intestinal biopsy | ↓ - ↓↓↓ | ↓ - ↓↓↓ | ↓ - ↓↓↓ | ↓ - ↓↓↓ | ↓ - ↓↓↓ |

[a]Disease features occur on a trehalose-containing diet

**Table 39.4** Intestinal glucose-galactose malabsorption

| System | Symptoms and biomarkers | Neonatal (birth–1 month) | Infancy (1–18 months) | Childhood (1.5–11 years) | Adolescence (11–16 years) | Adulthood (>16 years) |
|---|---|---|---|---|---|---|
| Digestive | **Diarrhea, profuse, osmotic**[a] | +++ | +++ | ++ | ++ | ++ |
| Other | **Dehydration**[a] | +++ | +++ | ++ | ++ | ++ |
| | Failure to thrive[a] | n | ± | ± | ± | ± |
| | Hypovolaemic shock[a] | ± | ± | ± | ± | ± |
| Renal | Urolithiasis[a] | n | ± | ± | ± | ± |
| Laboratory findings | Fructose loading test, p.o. | n | n | n | n | n |
| | Galactose loading test, p.o. | + | + | + | + | + |
| | Galactose uptake by enterocytes | ↓ | ↓ | ↓ | ↓ | ↓ |
| | Glucose (urine) | n-↑ | n-↑ | n-↑ | n-↑ | n-↑ |
| | Glucose loading test, p.o. | + | + | + | + | + |
| | Glucose uptake by enterocytes | ↓ | ↓ | ↓ | ↓ | ↓ |
| | pH[a] | n-↓↓↓ | n-↓↓↓ | n-↓ | n-↓ | n-↓ |
| | Reducing sugars (stool)[a] | ↑ | ↑ | ↑ | ↑ | ↑ |
| | **Sodium (plasma)**[a] | n-↑↑↑ | n-↑↑↑ | n-↑↑↑ | n-↑↑↑ | n-↑↑↑ |

[a]Disease features occur on a glucose- nd/or galactose-containing diet

**Table 39.5** Renal glucosuria (*see also* Santer and Calado 2010; Ghezzi et al. 2018)

| System | Symptoms and biomarkers | Neonatal (birth–1 month) | Infancy (1–18 months) | Childhood (1.5–11 years) | Adolescence (11–16 years) | Adulthood (>16 years) |
|---|---|---|---|---|---|---|
| Laboratory findings | Amino acids (urine) | n-↑ | n-↑ | n-↑ | n-↑ | n-↑ |
| | Glucose (plasma) | n | n | n | n | n |
| | **Glucose (urine)** | ↑ - ↑↑↑ | ↑ - ↑↑↑ | ↑ - ↑↑↑ | ↑ - ↑↑↑ | ↑ - ↑↑↑ |

**Table 39.6** MAP17 deficiency (*see also* Coady et al. 2016)

| System | Symptoms and biomarkers | Neonatal (birth–1 month) | Infancy (1–18 months) | Childhood (1.5–11 years) | Adolescence (11–16 years) | Adulthood (>16 years) |
|---|---|---|---|---|---|---|
| Laboratory findings | Glucose (plasma) | n | n | n | n | n |
| | **Glucose (urine)** | | | ↑ - ↑↑ | | |

**Table 39.7** Glucose transporter-1 deficiency

| System | Symptoms and biomarkers | Neonatal (birth–1 month) | Infancy (1–18 months) | Childhood (1.5–11 years) | Adolescence (11–16 years) | Adulthood (>16 years) |
|---|---|---|---|---|---|---|
| CNS | **Aquired microcephaly** | | ± | ± | ± | ± |
| | Ataxia | | ± | ± | ± | ± |
| | **Developmental delay** | | ± | ± | ± | ± |
| | Dystonia | | ± | ± | ± | ± |
| | Hypotonia, muscular-axial | | ± | ± | ± | ± |
| | **Intellectual disability** | | ± | ± | ± | ± |
| | **Movement disorder, complex, paroxysmal** | | ± | ± | ± | ± |
| | **Seizures**[a] | | ± | ± | ± | ± |
| Haematological | Anaemia, haemolytic, induced by cold exposure | | ± | ± | ± | ± |
| Laboratory findings | Glucose (cerebrospinal fluid) / Glucose (plasma) ratio[c] | ↓ | ↓ | ↓ | ↓ | ↓ |
| | Glucose (cerebrospinal fluid)[b] | ↓ | ↓ | ↓ | ↓ | ↓ |
| | Glucose uptake (red blood cells) | ↓ | ↓ | ↓ | ↓ | ↓ |
| | GLUT1 in RBC (Western blot) | ↓ | ↓ | ↓ | ↓ | ↓ |
| | Lactate (cerebrospinal fluid) | ↓-n | ↓-n | ↓-n | ↓-n | ↓-n |

[a]In classical GLUT1-D seizures often start before age 2 years
[b]Do not misinterpret the results of random postictal lumbar punctures that can give false-high blood glucose concentrations and an abnormal ratio
[c]In case of a clinical suspicion perform determination of CSF/plasma glucose ratio in samples drawn after at least 4 h of fasting with sample for blood glucose drawn first. The ratio is less reliable than the absolute glucose in CSF

**Table 39.8** Neuronal glucose transporter deficiency (SLC45A1 deficiency)

| System | Symptoms and biomarkers | Neonatal (birth–1 month) | Infancy (1–18 months) | Childhood (1.5–11 years) | Adolescence (11–16 years) | Adulthood (>16 years) |
|---|---|---|---|---|---|---|
| CNS | **Intellectual disability** | | | + | + | + |
| | Seizures | | | ± | + | + |
| | Stereotyped hand movements | | | | | ± |
| Musculoskeletal | **Dysmorphic features** | | | + | | + |
| Psychiatric | Anxiety | | | | | + |
| | Autism | | | + | | ± |
| | Behavioral abnormalities | | | | | + |
| Laboratory findings | Glucose (cerebrospinal fluid) | | | n | | n |
| | Glucose (plasma) | | | n | | n |

**Table 39.9** Glucose transporter 2 deficiency (Fanconi-Bickel syndrome)

| System | Symptoms and biomarkers | Neonatal (birth–1 month) | Infancy (1–18 months) | Childhood (1.5–11 years) | Adolescence (11–16 years) | Adulthood (>16 years) |
|---|---|---|---|---|---|---|
| Digestive | **Hepatomegaly** | n | n - ↑↑↑ | n - ↑↑↑ | n - ↑↑ | n - ↑↑ |
| | Loose stools | ± | ± | | | |
| | Malabsorption | ± | ± | | | |
| Eye | Cataract | | ± | | | |
| Musculoskeletal | **Rickets** | | ± | ± | ± | |
| | **Short stature** | n | ++ | +++ | +++ | +++ |
| Renal | Hyperfiltration | | | | ± | ± |
| | Nephromegaly | n | ± | ± | ± | ± |
| | Renal failure | | | | ± | ± |
| | **Renal tubulopathy, generalised** | ± | ± | ± | ± | ± |

**Table 39.9** (continued)

| System | Symptoms and biomarkers | Neonatal (birth–1 month) | Infancy (1–18 months) | Childhood (1.5–11 years) | Adolescence (11–16 years) | Adulthood (>16 years) |
|---|---|---|---|---|---|---|
| Laboratory findings | Alkaline Phosphatase (plasma) | n-↑ | n-↑ | n-↑ | n-↑ | |
| | Amino acids (urine) | n-↑ | n-↑ | n-↑ | n-↑ | n-↑ |
| | ASAT/ALAT (plasma) | n-↑ | n-↑ | n-↑ | n-↑ | n-↑ |
| | Calcium (urine) | n-↑ | n-↑ | n-↑ | n-↑ | n-↑ |
| | Cholesterol (serum) | n-↑ | n-↑ | n-↑ | n-↑ | n-↑ |
| | Enzymes of galactose metabolism | n | n | n | n | n |
| | Galactitol (urine)[a] | n-↑ | n-↑ | n-↑ | n-↑ | n-↑ |
| | **Galactose (blood spot)** | ± | | | | |
| | **Galactose (plasma)**[a] | ± | ± | ± | ± | ± |
| | Galactose (urine)[a] | n-↑ | n-↑ | n-↑ | n-↑ | n-↑ |
| | **Glucose (urine)** | ↑-↑↑↑ | ↑-↑↑↑ | ↑-↑↑↑ | ↑-↑↑↑ | ↑-↑↑↑ |
| | **Glucose, fasted (plasma)** | ↓-n | ↓-n | ↓-n | ↓-n | ↓-n |
| | **Glucose, fed (plasma)** | n - ↑ | n - ↑↑ | n - ↑↑ | n - ↑↑ | n - ↑↑ |
| | **Glycogen (liver)** | n-↑ | ↑-↑↑↑ | ↑-↑↑↑ | ↑-↑↑ | ↑-↑↑ |
| | Glycogenolytic enzymes (all tissues) | n | n | n | n | n |
| | Phosphate (plasma) | n -↓ | n -↓ | n -↓ | n -↓ | n -↓ |
| | Phosphate (urine) | n-↑ | n-↑ | n-↑ | n-↑ | n-↑ |
| | Rrenal tubular acidosis | ± | ± | ± | ± | ± |
| | Triglycerides (serum) | n-↑ | n-↑ | n-↑ | n-↑ | n-↑ |
| | Uric acid (plasma) | ↑ | ↑ | ↑ | ↑ | ↑ |

[a]On a galactose-containing diet

**Table 39.10** Galactose mutarotase deficiency (*see also* Wada et al. 2019)

| System | Symptoms and biomarkers | Neonatal (birth–1 month) | Infancy (1–18 months) | Childhood (1.5–11 years) | Adolescence (11–16 years) | Adulthood (>16 years) |
|---|---|---|---|---|---|---|
| Eye | **Cataract**[a] | + | + | | | |
| Laboratory findings | Galactose (plasma)[a] | ↑ | ↑ | | | |
| | Galactose (urine)[a] | ↑ | ↑ | | | |
| | Galactose mutarotase activity (lymphocytes) | ↓ | ↓ | | | |
| | Galactose-1-phosphate (red blood cells)[a] | ↑ | n-↑ | | | |

[a]On a galactose-containing diet

**Table 39.11** Galactokinase deficiency

| System | Symptoms and biomarkers | Neonatal (birth–1 month) | Infancy (1–18 months) | Childhood (1.5–11 years) | Adolescence (11–16 years) | Adulthood (>16 years) |
|---|---|---|---|---|---|---|
| Eye | **Cataract**[a] | + | + | + | + | + |
| Other | Pseudotumor cerebri[a] | + | + | | | |
| Laboratory findings | Galactitol (urine)[a] | ↑ | ↑ | ↑ | ↑ | ↑ |
| | Galactokinase (fibroblasts) | ↓ | ↓ | ↓ | ↓ | ↓ |
| | Galactokinase (red blood cells)[a] | ↓ | ↓ | ↓ | ↓ | ↓ |
| | Galactose (plasma)[a] | ↑ | ↑ | ↑ | ↑ | ↑ |
| | Galactose (urine)[a] | ↑ | ↑ | ↑ | ↑ | ↑ |
| | Galactose-1-phosphate (red blood cells)[a] | n | n | n | n | n |
| | Galactose-1-phosphate uridyltransferase (red blood cells) | n | n | n | n | n |
| | Reducing substances (urine)[a] | + | + | + | + | + |

[a]On a galactose-containing diet

**Table 39.12** Galactose-1-phosphate uridyltransferase (deficiency Galactosaemia)

| System | Symptoms and biomarkers | Neonatal (birth–1 month) | Infancy (1–18 months) | Childhood (1.5–11 years) | Adolescence (11–16 years) | Adulthood (>16 years) |
|---|---|---|---|---|---|---|
| CNS | Brain edema (MRI)[a] | + | | | | |
| | Intellectual disability | | | ± | ± | ± |
| Digestive | **Anorexia[a]** | + | + | | | |
| | **Hepatomegaly[a]** | + | + | | | |
| | **Liver cirrhosis[a]** | | + | + | | |
| | **Liver failure[a]** | + | + | | | |
| | **Vomiting[a]** | + | + | | | |
| Endocrine | Hypergonadotropic hypogonadism, female | | | | + | + |
| Eye | **Cataract[a]** | + | + | ± | ± | ± |
| Genitourinary | Ovarian failure | | | | + | + |
| Haematological | Anaemia, hemolytic[a] | + | + | | | |
| Other | *E. coli* sepsis[a] | + | | | | |
| | **Early death[a]** | + | + | | | |
| Laboratory findings | Amino acids (urine)[a] | ↑ | ↑ | n-↑ | n-↑ | n-↑ |
| | ASAT/ALAT (plasma)[a] | ↑ | ↑ | n-↑ | n-↑ | n-↑ |
| | Bilirubin (plasma)[a] | ↑ | ↑ | n-↑ | n-↑ | n-↑ |
| | Calcium (urine)[a] | ↑ | ↑ | n-↑ | n-↑ | n-↑ |
| | Coagulation factors (plasma) a | ↓ | ↓ | ↓-n | ↓-n | ↓-n |
| | Galactitol (urine)[a] | ↑ | ↑ | ↑ | ↑ | ↑ |
| | Galactose (blood spot) | | | | | |
| | Galactose (plasma)[a] | ↑ | ↑ | ↑ | ↑ | ↑ |
| | Galactose (urine)[a] | ↑ | ↑ | ↑ | ↑ | ↑ |
| | Galactose-1-phosphate (red blood cells) | ↑ | ↑ | ↑ | ↑ | ↑ |
| | Galactose-1-phosphate uridyltransferase (red blood cells) | ↓ | ↓ | ↓ | ↓ | ↓ |
| | Glucose (urine)[a] | ↑ | ↑ | n-↑ | n-↑ | n-↑ |
| | Phosphate (urine)[a] | ↑ | ↑ | n-↑ | n-↑ | n-↑ |
| | Proteins, total (urine)[a] | ↑ | ↑ | n-↑ | n-↑ | n-↑ |
| | Reducing substances (urine)[a] | + | + | + | + | + |
| | Sialotransferrins, type 1 pattern (serum)[a] | | n-↑ | n-↑ | n-↑ | n-↑ |

[a]On a galactose-containing diet

**Table 39.13** Uridine diphosphate galactose-4-epimerase deficiency

| System | Symptoms and biomarkers | Neonatal (birth–1 month) | Infancy (1–18 months) | Childhood (1.5–11 years) | Adolescence (11–16 years) | Adulthood (>16 years) |
|---|---|---|---|---|---|---|
| Digestive | **Anorexia[a]** | ± | ± | | | |
| | **Hepatomegaly[a]** | ± | ± | | | |
| | **Liver cirrhosis[a]** | | ± | ± | | |
| | **Liver failure[a]** | ± | ± | | | |
| | **Vomiting[a]** | ± | ± | | | |
| Eye | **Cataract[a]** | ± | ± | | | |
| Other | **Early death[a]** | ± | ± | | | |
| Laboratory findings | Amino acids (urine)[a] | n-↑ | n-↑ | n-↑ | n-↑ | n-↑ |
| | ASAT/ALAT (plasma)[a] | n-↑ | n-↑ | n-↑ | n-↑ | n-↑ |
| | Bilirubin (plasma)[a] | n-↑ | n-↑ | n-↑ | n-↑ | n-↑ |
| | Calcium (urine)[a] | n-↑ | n-↑ | n-↑ | n-↑ | n-↑ |
| | Coagulation factors (plasma)[a] | ↓-n | ↓-n | ↓-n | ↓-n | ↓-n |
| | Galactose (plasma)[a] | n-↑ | n-↑ | n-↑ | n-↑ | n-↑ |
| | Galactose (urine)[a] | n-↑ | n-↑ | n-↑ | n-↑ | n-↑ |
| | Galactose-1-phosphate (red blood cells)[a] | n-↑ | n-↑ | n-↑ | n-↑ | n-↑ |
| | Glucose (urine)[a] | n-↑ | n-↑ | n-↑ | n-↑ | n-↑ |
| | Phosphate (urine)[a] | n-↑ | n-↑ | n-↑ | n-↑ | n-↑ |
| | Proteins, total (urine)[a] | n-↑ | n-↑ | n-↑ | n-↑ | n-↑ |
| | Reducing substances (urine)[a] | ± | ± | ± | ± | ± |
| | UPD-Gal epimerase (liver) | n-↓ | n-↓ | n-↓ | n-↓ | n-↓ |
| | UPD-Gal epimerase (red blood cells) | ↓ | ↓ | ↓ | ↓ | ↓ |

[a]On a galactose-containing diet

**Table 39.14** Essential fructosuria

| System | Symptoms and biomarkers | Neonatal (birth–1 month) | Infancy (1–18 months) | Childhood (1.5–11 years) | Adolescence (11–16 years) | Adulthood (>16 years) |
|---|---|---|---|---|---|---|
| Other | No clinical significance | + | + | + | + | + |
| Laboratory findings | Glucose (urine) | n | n | n | n | n |
| | Ketohexokinase (liver) | ↓ | ↓ | ↓ | ↓ | ↓ |
| | Reducing substances (urine)[a] | + | + | + | + | + |

[a]On a fructose-containing diet

**Table 39.15** Hereditary fructose intolerance

| System | Symptoms and biomarkers | Neonatal (birth–1 month) | Infancy (1–18 months) | Childhood (1.5–11 years) | Adolescence (11–16 years) | Adulthood (>16 years) |
|---|---|---|---|---|---|---|
| Digestive | Abdominal pain[a] | | + | + | ± | ± |
| | Feeding habits, abnormal[a] | | + | + | | |
| | **Hepatomegaly**[a] | | + | + | ± | ± |
| | Liver cirrhosis[a] | | | ± | ± | ± |
| | **Liver failure**[a] | | + | + | ± | ± |
| | Steatorrhea[a] | | ± | ± | ± | ± |
| | Vomiting[a] | | + | + | ± | ± |
| Other | **Failure to thrive**[a] | | + | + | ± | ± |
| | No dental caries[b] | | | + | + | + |
| Renal | **Renal tubulopathy**[a] | | + | + | ± | ± |
| Laboratory findings | ASAT/ALAT (plasma)[a] | | ↑ | ↑ | n-↑ | n-↑ |
| | Bilirubin, conjugated (plasma)[a] | | ↑ | ↑ | n-↑ | n-↑ |
| | **Coagulation factors (plasma)**[a] | | ↓ | ↓ | ↓ | ↓-n |
| | **Fructose-1-phosphate aldolase (liver)** | ↓ | ↓ | ↓ | ↓ | ↓ |
| | **Glucose (plasma)** | | ↓-n | ↓-n | ↓-n | ↓-n |
| | Glycerol (urine)[a] | | ↑ | ↑ | ↑ | ↑ |
| | Magnesium (plasma)[a] | | ↓-n | ↓-n | ↓-n | ↓-n |
| | Phosphate (plasma)[a] | | ↓-n | ↓-n | ↓-n | ↓-n |
| | Sialotransferrins, type 1 pattern (serum)[a] | | n-↑ | n-↑ | n-↑ | n-↑ |
| | Triglycerides (serum)[a,c] | | n-↑ | n-↑ | n-↑ | n-↑ |
| | Uric acid (plasma)[a] | | ↑ | ↑ | n-↑ | n-↑ |

[a]On a fructose-containing diet
[b]On fructose/sucrose restriction
[c]Pseudo(!)-hypertriglyceridaemia due to glycerol accumulation

**Table 39.16** Haemolytic anaemia due to hexokinase 1 deficiency

| System | Symptoms and biomarkers | Neonatal (birth–1 month) | Infancy (1–18 months) | Childhood (1.5–11 years) | Adolescence (11–16 years) | Adulthood (>16 years) |
|---|---|---|---|---|---|---|
| Digestive | **Jaundice** | + | + | + | + | + |
| | **Splenomegaly** | ± | ± | ± | ± | ± |
| Haematological | **Anaemia, hemolytic** | + | + | + | + | + |
| Other | Chronic transfusion dependency | ± | ± | ± | ± | ± |
| | Hydrops fetalis | ± | | | | |
| Laboratory findings | Bilirubin (plasma) | ↑ | ↑ | ↑ | ↑ | ↑ |
| | Fetal haemoglobin (blood) | ↑ | ↑ | ↑ | | |
| | Haemoglobin (blood) | ↓ to ↓↓↓ | ↓ to ↓↓↓ | ↓ to ↓↓↓ | ↓ to ↓↓↓ | ↓ to ↓↓↓ |
| | Hexokinase activity (red blood cells)[a] | ↓-n | ↓-n | ↓-n | ↓-n | ↓-n |
| | Reticulocytes (blood) | ↑ to ↑↑↑ | ↑ to ↑↑↑ | ↑ to ↑↑↑ | ↑ to ↑↑↑ | ↑ to ↑↑↑ |

[a]Enzyme testing might not be reliable after erythrocyte transfusion or when there is reticulocytosis (*see also* Jamwal et al. 2019)

**Table 39.17** Neurodevelopmental disorder wih visual defects and brain anomalies, NEDVIBA (*see also* Okur et al. 2019)

| System | Symptoms and biomarkers | Neonatal (birth–1 month) | Infancy (1–18 months) | Childhood (1.5–11 years) | Adolescence (11–16 years) | Adulthood (>16 years) |
|---|---|---|---|---|---|---|
| CNS | Anomalies of corpus callosum | + | + | | | |
| | Ataxia | + | + | | | |
| | **Brain anomalies** | + | + | | | |
| | **Global developmental delay** | + | + | | | |
| | Hypotonia, axial | + | + | | | |
| | Movement Disorder | + | + | | | |
| Digestive | Feeding difficulties | + | + | | | |
| Eye | **Optic atrophy** | + | + | | | |
| | **Retinitis pigmentosa** | + | + | | | |
| | Visual impairment | + | + | | | |
| Musculoskeletal | Dysmorphic features | + | + | | | |
| Laboratory findings | Hexokinase activity (red blood cells) | n | n | n | | |
| | No biochemical markers | + | + | + | | |

**Table 39.18** Hereditary motor and sensory neuropathy, Russe type

| System | Symptoms and biomarkers | Neonatal (birth–1 month) | Infancy (1–18 months) | Childhood (1.5–11 years) | Adolescence (11–16 years) | Adulthood (>16 years) |
|---|---|---|---|---|---|---|
| CNS | Abnormal motor and sensory nerve conduction studies | | | + | + | + |
| | Cranial nerve involvement | | | ± | ± | ± |
| | Distal sensory loss with areflexia | | ± | + | ++ | +++ |
| Musculoskeletal | Foot deformity (pes cavus), hand deformity (clawing), scoliosis | | | + | + | + |
| | Progressive weakness with onset in the distal lower limbs | | ± | + | ++ | +++ |
| Laboratory findings | Hexokinase activity (red blood cells) | | n | n | n | n |
| | No biochemical markers | | + | + | + | + |

**Table 39.19** Retinitis pigmentosa type 79

| System | Symptoms and biomarkers | Neonatal (birth–1 month) | Infancy (1–18 months) | Childhood (1.5–11 years) | Adolescence (11–16 years) | Adulthood (>16 years) |
|---|---|---|---|---|---|---|
| Eye | Changes electroretinogram | | | ±[a] | + | + |
| | Macular atrophy | | | ±[a] | + | + |
| | Nyctalopia | | | ±[a] | + | + |
| | Optic disc pallor | | | ±[a] | + | + |
| | Pigmentary deposits of the retina | | | ±[a] | + | + |
| | Progressive (peripheral) vision loss | | | ±[a] | + | + |
| | Retinal vascular attenuation | | | ±[a] | + | + |
| Laboratory findings | Hexokinase activity (red blood cells) | | | n | n | n |
| | No biochemical markers | | | + | + | + |

[a]A severe presentation in the first decade has been described in a patient with homozygosity for a *HK1* variant

**Table 39.20** Glucokinase deficiency

| System | Symptoms and biomarkers | Neonatal (birth–1 month) | Infancy (1–18 months) | Childhood (1.5–11 years) | Adolescence (11–16 years) | Adulthood (>16 years) |
|---|---|---|---|---|---|---|
| Endocrine | Diabetes mellitus | | | | | + |
| Laboratory findings | Glucose (plasma) | | ↑ | ↑ | ↑ | ↑ |
| | Glucose (urine) | | ↑ | ↑ | ↑ | ↑ |
| | Insulin (serum) | | ↓ | ↓ | ↓ | ↓ |
| | Ketones (urine) | | n | n | n | n |

**Table 39.21** Glucokinase superactivity

| System | Symptoms and biomarkers | Neonatal (birth–1 month) | Infancy (1–18 months) | Childhood (1.5–11 years) | Adolescence (11–16 years) | Adulthood (>16 years) |
|---|---|---|---|---|---|---|
| CNS | Epilepsy | ± | ± | ± | ± | ± |
| | Intellectual disability | | ± | ± | ± | ± |
| Endocrine | Diabetes mellitus, type 2 | | | + | + | ++ |
| | **Hyperinsulinism** | ++ | ++ | ++ | ++ | ++ |
| Metabolic | Hypoglycaemia | ++ | ++ | ++ | ++ | ± |
| | **Hypoglycaemia, hypoketotic** | ++ | ++ | ++ | ++ | ± |
| Laboratory findings | Free fatty acids (serum)[a] | ↓ | ↓ | ↓ | ↓ | ↓ - ↑ |
| | **Glucose (plasma)** | ↓ - ↓↓↓ | ↓ - ↓↓↓ | ↓ - ↓↓↓ | ↓ - ↓↓↓ | ↓↓↓ - ↑↑↑ |
| | Insulin (plasma)[a] | ↑ - ↑↑↑ | ↑ - ↑↑↑ | ↑ - ↑↑↑ | ↑ - ↑↑↑ | ↑ - ↑↑↑ |
| | Ketones (plasma, urine)[a] | ↓ | ↓ | ↓ | ↓ | ↓ - ↑ |

[a]During hypoglycaemia

**Table 39.22** Glucose-6-phosphate isomerase deficiency (*see also* Fermo et al. 2019)

| System | Symptoms and biomarkers | Neonatal (birth–1 month) | Infancy (1–18 months) | Childhood (1.5–11 years) | Adolescence (11–16 years) | Adulthood (>16 years) |
|---|---|---|---|---|---|---|
| CNS | Intelectual disability/ neurologic symptoms | | | ± | ± | ± |
| Digestive | Pigment gallstones | ± | ± | ± | ± | ± |
| | Splenomegaly | ± | + | + | + | + |
| Haematological | **Chronic haemolytic anaemia improving with age** | ± | + | + | + | + |
| | Haemolytic crisis | ± | ± | ± | ± | ± |
| | Transfusion dependency | ± | ± | ± | ± | ± |
| Musculoskeletal | Muscle weakness | | | ± | ± | ± |
| Other | Hydrops fetalis | ± | | | | |
| | **Stillbirth** | ± | | | | |
| Laboratory findings | Glucosephosphate isomerase activity (red blood cells, leukocytes) | ↓ | ↓ | ↓ | ↓ | ↓ |
| | Haemoglobin (blood) | ↓-n | ↓ to ↓↓↓ | ↓ to ↓↓↓ | ↓ to ↓↓↓ | ↓ to ↓↓↓ |
| | Mean corpuscular volume (MCV) | n-↑ | ↑ | ↑ | ↑ | ↑ |
| | Osmotic fragility (red blood cells) | n | n | n | n | n |
| | Oxidative burst (leukocytes) | ↓ | ↓ | ↓ | ↓ | ↓ |
| | Reticulocytes | n-↑ | ↑ | ↑ | ↑ | ↑ |
| | Unconjugated bilirubin | n-↑ | ↑ | ↑ | ↑ | ↑ |

**Table 39.23** Glycogen storage disease type VII (Muscle phosphofructokinase deficiency)

| System | Symptoms and biomarkers | Neonatal (birth–1 month) | Infancy (1–18 months) | Childhood (1.5–11 years) | Adolescence (11–16 years) | Adulthood (>16 years) |
|---|---|---|---|---|---|---|
| Digestive | Gallstones | | | ± | + | + |
| | Jaundice | | | + | + | + |
| Haematological | **Anaemia, haemolytic** | | | + | + | + |
| | Low RBC life span | | + | + | + | + |
| Musculoskeletal | **Exertion intolerance** | | ++ | + | + | + |
| | **Muscle cramps** | | ++ | + | + | + |
| | **Muscle pain** | | ++ | + | + | + |
| | **Muscle weakness** | | ++ | + | + | + |
| | Second wind phenomenon | | – | – | – | – |
| Laboratory findings | 2,3-Diphosphoglycerate (red blood cells) | | ↓ | ↓ | ↓ | ↓ |
| | Ammonia rise in forearm exercise test (blood) | | | n | n | n |
| | Bilirubin (plasma) | | n | ↑ | ↑ | ↑ |
| | Creatine kinase (plasma) | | ↑ | ↑ | ↑ | ↑ |
| | Glycogen (muscle) | ↑ | ↑ | ↑ | ↑ | ↑ |
| | Lactate rise in forearm exercise test (plasma) | | | ↓ | ↓ | ↓ |
| | Myoglobin (urine) | | ± | ± | ± | ± |
| | Phosphofructokinase (blood cells) | ↓ | ↓ | ↓ | ↓ | ↓ |
| | Phosphofructokinase (fibroblasts) | ↓ | ↓ | ↓ | ↓ | ↓ |
| | Phosphofructokinase (muscle) | ↓ | ↓ | ↓ | ↓ | ↓ |
| | Reticulocytes (blood) | | n | ↑ | ↑ | ↑ |
| | Uric acid (plasma) | | ↑ | ↑ | ↑ | ↑ |

**Table 39.24** Glycogen storage disease type XII (Aldolase A deficiency)

| System | Symptoms and biomarkers | Neonatal (birth–1 month) | Infancy (1–18 months) | Childhood (1.5–11 years) | Adolescence (11–16 years) | Adulthood (>16 years) |
|---|---|---|---|---|---|---|
| CNS | **Intellectual disability** | | ± | ± | ± | ± |
| Haematological | **Anaemia, haemolytic** | | + | + | + | + |
| Musculoskeletal | **Dysmorphic features** | | ± | ± | ± | ± |
| | **Muscle weakness** | | ± | ± | ± | ± |
| | **Rhabdomyolysis** | | ± | ± | ± | ± |
| | **Short stature** | | ± | ± | ± | ± |
| Laboratory findings | Aldolase A (red blood cells) | | ↓ | ↓ | ↓ | ↓ |
| | Bilirubin (plasma) | | ↑ | ↑ | ↑ | ↑ |
| | Creatine kinase (plasma) | | n-↑ | n-↑ | n-↑ | n-↑ |
| | Glycogen (liver) | | n-↑ | n-↑ | n-↑ | n-↑ |
| | Glycogen (muscle) | | n-↑ | n-↑ | n-↑ | n-↑ |
| | Reticulocytes (blood) | | ↑ | ↑ | ↑ | ↑ |

**Table 39.25** Triosephosphate isomerase deficiency

| System | Symptoms and biomarkers | Neonatal (birth–1 month) | Infancy (1–18 months) | Childhood (1.5–11 years) | Adolescence (11–16 years) | Adulthood (>16 years) |
|---|---|---|---|---|---|---|
| Cardiovascular | Cardiomyopathy | | ± | ± | ± | |
| CNS | Dystonia | | ± | ± | ± | |
| | **Intellectual disability** | | ± | ± | ± | |
| | Seizures | | ± | ± | ± | |
| | Stroke | | ± | ± | ± | |
| | Tremor | | ± | ± | ± | |
| Haematological | **Anaemia, haemolytic** | | + | + | + | |
| Musculoskeletal | Progressive muscle weakness | | ± | ± | ± | |
| Other | **Recurrent infections** | | + | + | + | |
| Laboratory findings | Dihydroxyacetone phosphate (red blood cells) | | ↑ | ↑ | ↑ | |
| | Triosephosphate isomerase (red blood cells) | ↓ | ↓ | ↓ | ↓ | |

**Table 39.26** Muscle phosphoglycerate kinase deficiency

| System | Symptoms and biomarkers | Neonatal (birth–1 month) | Infancy (1–18 months) | Childhood (1.5–11 years) | Adolescence (11–16 years) | Adulthood (>16 years) |
|---|---|---|---|---|---|---|
| CNS | Retardation, motor | | ± | ± | ± | ± |
| | Seizures | | ± | ± | ± | ± |
| Eye | Retinal dystrophy | | ± | ± | ± | ± |
| Haematological | **Anaemia, haemolytic** | | ± | ± | ± | ± |
| | RBC life span | | ↓-n | ↓-n | ↓-n | ↓-n |
| Musculoskeletal | **Exertion intolerance** | | ± | ± | ± | ± |
| | **Muscle cramps** | | ± | ± | ± | ± |
| | **Muscle pain** | | ± | ± | ± | ± |
| | **Muscle weakness** | | ± | ± | ± | ± |
| Laboratory findings | Bilirubin (plasma) | | n-↑ | n-↑ | n-↑ | n-↑ |
| | Creatine kinase (plasma) | | n-↑ | n-↑ | n-↑ | n-↑ |
| | Myoglobin (urine) | | n-↑ | n-↑ | n-↑ | n-↑ |
| | Phosphoglycerate kinase (blood cells) | | ↓ | ↓ | ↓ | ↓ |
| | Phosphoglycerate kinase (muscle) | | ↓ | ↓ | ↓ | ↓ |
| | Reticulocytes (blood) | | n-↑ | n-↑ | n-↑ | n-↑ |

**Table 39.27** Glycogen storage disease type X (Muscle phosphoglycerate mutase deficiency)

| System | Symptoms and biomarkers | Neonatal (birth–1 month) | Infancy (1–18 months) | Childhood (1.5–11 years) | Adolescence (11–16 years) | Adulthood (>16 years) |
|---|---|---|---|---|---|---|
| Musculoskeletal | **Exertion intolerance** | | | | + | + |
| | **Muscle cramps** | | | | + | + |
| | **Muscle pain** | | | | + | + |
| | **Muscle weakness** | | | | + | + |
| Laboratory findings | Creatine kinase (plasma) | | | | ↑ | ↑ |
| | Glycogen (muscle) | | | | n-↑ | n-↑ |
| | Myoglobin (urine) | | | | ↑ | ↑ |
| | Phosphoglycerate mutase (muscle) | | | | ↓ | ↓ |

**Table 39.28** Enolase β deficiency (GSD XIII)

| System | Symptoms and biomarkers | Neonatal (birth–1 month) | Infancy (1–18 months) | Childhood (1.5–11 years) | Adolescence (11–16 years) | Adulthood (>16 years) |
|---|---|---|---|---|---|---|
| Musculoskeletal | **Exertion intolerance** | | | | | + |
| | **Muscle cramps** | | | | | + |
| | **Muscle pain** | | | | | + |
| | **Muscle weakness** | | | | | + |
| Laboratory findings | Creatine kinase (plasma) | | | | | ↑ |
| | Enolase beta (muscle) | | | | | ↓ |
| | Glycogen (muscle) | | | | | ↑ |

**Table 39.29** Pyruvate kinase deficiency

| System | Symptoms and biomarkers | Neonatal (birth–1 month) | Infancy (1–18 months) | Childhood (1.5–11 years) | Adolescence (11–16 years) | Adulthood (>16 years) |
|---|---|---|---|---|---|---|
| Cardiovascular | Pulmonary hypertension | ± | ± | ± | ± | ± |
| Digestive | Cholecystitis | | | ± | ± | ± |
| | Cholelithiasis | | | ± | ± | ± |
| | Liver cirrhosis | | | | | + |
| | Neonatal jaundice (severe) | ± | | | | |
| | Neonatal liver failure | ± | | | | |
| | Splenomegaly | ± | ± | ± | ± | ± |
| Haematological | Anaemia, haemolytic | + to +++ | + to +++ | + to +++ | + to +++ | + to +++ |
| | **Haemolytic crisis** | ± | ± | ± | ± | ± |
| | Post-splenectomy thrombosis | | | ± | ± | ± |
| | **Transfusion dependency** | ± | ± | ± | ± | ± |

(continued)

**Table 39.29** (continued)

| System | Symptoms and biomarkers | Neonatal (birth–1 month) | Infancy (1–18 months) | Childhood (1.5–11 years) | Adolescence (11–16 years) | Adulthood (>16 years) |
|---|---|---|---|---|---|---|
| Other | Hydrops fetalis | ± | | | | |
| | Intrauterine growth retardation | ± | | | | |
| Laboratory findings | Bilirubin, unconjugated (plasma) | ↑ | ↑ | ↑ | ↑ | ↑ |
| | Ferritin | | ↑ - ↑↑↑ | ↑ - ↑↑↑ | ↑ - ↑↑↑ | ↑ - ↑↑↑ |
| | Haemoglobin (blood) | ↓ - ↓↓↓ | ↓ - ↓↓↓ | ↓ - ↓↓↓ | ↓ - ↓↓↓ | ↓ - ↓↓↓ |
| | Mean corpuscular volume (MCV) | n - ↑ | n - ↑ | n - ↑ | n - ↑ | n - ↑ |
| | Osmotic fragility | n - ↑ | n - ↑ | n - ↑ | n - ↑ | n - ↑ |
| | Pyruvate kinase activity (spectrophotometric assay, red blood cell)[a] | + | + | + | + | + |
| | Reticulocytes (blood) | ↑ | ↑ | ↑ | ↑ | ↑ |

[a]False normal values can be due to reticulocytosis or recent transfusion (Bianchi et al. 2019)

**Table 39.30** Glycogen storage disease type XI (Lactate dehydrogenase A deficiency)

| System | Symptoms and biomarkers | Neonatal (birth–1 month) | Infancy (1–18 months) | Childhood (1.5–11 years) | Adolescence (11–16 years) | Adulthood (>16 years) |
|---|---|---|---|---|---|---|
| Dermatological | Skin rash[a] | | | | ± | ± |
| Genitourinary | Uterine muscle stiffness, in pregnancy | | | | | + |
| Musculoskeletal | **Exertion intolerance** | | | | + | + |
| | **Muscle cramps** | | | | + | + |
| | **Muscle pain** | | | | + | + |
| | **Muscle weakness** | | | | + | + |
| Laboratory findings | Ammonia rise in forearm exercise test (blood) | | | | n | n |
| | Creatine kinase (plasma) | | | | ↑ | ↑ |
| | Glycogen (muscle) | | | | n-↑ | n-↑ |
| | Lactate (plasma) | | | | ↑ | ↑ |
| | Lactate dehydrogenase (muscle) | | | | ↓ | ↓ |
| | Lactate dehydrogenase (red blood cells) | | | | ↓ | ↓ |
| | Lactate rise in forearm exercise test (plasma) | | | | ↑ | ↑ |
| | Myoglobin (urine) | | | | ↑ | ↑ |

[a]Psoriasis-like lesions

**Table 39.31** Lactate dehydrogenase B deficiency

| System | Symptoms and biomarkers | Neonatal (birth–1 month) | Infancy (1–18 months) | Childhood (1.5–11 years) | Adolescence (11–16 years) | Adulthood (>16 years) |
|---|---|---|---|---|---|---|
| Musculoskeletal | Myoglobinuria | | | | | ± |
| Other | No clinical significance | | | | | + |
| Laboratory findings | Lactate dehydrogenase, LDH (plasma) | | | | | ↓ |
| | Myoglobine (urine) | | | | | ↑ |

**Table 39.32** D-Lactate dehydrogenase deficiency (*see also* Monroe et al. 2019)

| System | Symptoms and biomarkers | Neonatal (birth–1 month) | Infancy (1–18 months) | Childhood (1.5–11 years) | Adolescence (11–16 years) | Adulthood (>16 years) |
|---|---|---|---|---|---|---|
| Other | Gout | | ± | ± | ± | ± |
| | No clinical significance[a] | + | + | + | + | + |
| Metabolic | Acidosis | ± | ± | ± | ± | ± |
| Laboratory findings | Anion gap (plasma) | ± | ± | ± | ± | ± |
| | d-2-Hydroxyisocaproic acid (urine) | n-↑ | n-↑ | n-↑ | n-↑ | n-↑ |
| | d-2-Hydroxyisovaleric acid (urine) | n-↑ | n-↑ | n-↑ | n-↑ | n-↑ |
| | d-Lactate (plasma) | n-↑ | n-↑ | n-↑ | n-↑ | n-↑ |
| | d-Lactate (urine)[c] | n-↑ | n-↑ | n-↑ | n-↑ | n-↑ |
| | Lactate dehydrogenase, LDH (plasma) | n | n | n | n | n |
| | l-Lactate (plasma)[b] | n | n | n | n | n |
| | Uric Acid (P) | | n-↑ | n-↑ | n-↑ | |
| | Uric Acid (U) | | n-↑ | n-↑ | n-↑ | |

[a]But may be relevant in bacterial overgrowth in short bowel patients
[b]Routine lactate (plasma) determinations are specific for l-lactate
[c]Routine lactate (urine) determinations (by GC-MS) detect both l- and d-lactate

**Table 39.33** Glycogen storage disease type XV (Muscle glycogenin 1 deficiency)

| System | Symptoms and biomarkers | Neonatal (birth–1 month) | Infancy (1–18 months) | Childhood (1.5–11 years) | Adolescence (11–16 years) | Adulthood (>16 years) |
|---|---|---|---|---|---|---|
| Cardiovascular | **Cardiomyopathy, hypertrophic** | | | | + | + |
| | **Ventricular arrhythmia** | | | | + | + |
| Musculoskeletal | **Exertion intolerance** | | ± | ± | + | + |
| | **Muscle weakness** | | ± | ± | + | + |
| Laboratory findings | Glycogen (muscle) | ↓↓ | ↓↓ | ↓↓ | ↓↓ | ↓↓ |

**Table 39.34** Glycogen storage disease type 0b (Muscle glycogen synthase deficiency)

| System | Symptoms and biomarkers | Neonatal (birth–1 month) | Infancy (1–18 months) | Childhood (1.5–11 years) | Adolescence (11–16 years) | Adulthood (>16 years) |
|---|---|---|---|---|---|---|
| Cardiovascular | Cardiac arrest, sudden | | | ± | ± | ± |
| | **Cardiomyopathy, hypertrophic** | | | + | + | + |
| | Syncope | | | ± | ± | ± |
| CNS | Seizures | | | ± | ± | ± |
| Musculoskeletal | **Exertion intolerance** | | | + | + | + |
| | **Muscle weakness** | | | + | + | + |
| Laboratory findings | Glycogen (muscle) | ↓↓↓ | ↓↓↓ | ↓↓↓ | ↓↓↓ | ↓↓↓ |
| | Glycogen synthase (muscle) | ↓ | ↓ | ↓ | ↓ | ↓ |

**Table 39.35** Glycogen storage disease type 0a (Hepatic glycogen synthase deficiency)

| System | Symptoms and biomarkers | Neonatal (birth–1 month) | Infancy (1–18 months) | Childhood (1.5–11 years) | Adolescence (11–16 years) | Adulthood (>16 years) |
|---|---|---|---|---|---|---|
| CNS | Seizures | ± | ± | ± | | |
| Digestive | Hepatomegaly | n | n | n | n | n |
| Metabolic | **Hypoglycaemia (fasting)** | ± | ± | ± | | |
| Laboratory findings | Glucose, fasted (plasma) | ↓ | ↓ | ↓ | ↓-n | ↓-n |
| | Glucose, fed (plasma) | n-↑ | n-↑ | n-↑ | n-↑ | n-↑ |
| | Glycogen (liver) | ↓-n | ↓-n | ↓-n | ↓-n | ↓-n |
| | Glycogen synthase (liver) | ↓ | ↓ | ↓ | ↓ | ↓ |
| | Ketones, fasted (plasma) | ↑ | ↑ | ↑ | n-↑ | n-↑ |
| | Ketones, fasted (urine) | ↑ | ↑ | ↑ | n-↑ | n-↑ |
| | Lactate, fed (plasma) | ↑ | ↑ | ↑ | n-↑ | n-↑ |

**Table 39.36** Glycogen storage disease type IV (Glycogen branching enzyme deficiency)

| System | Symptoms and biomarkers | Neonatal (birth–1 month) | Infancy (1–18 months) | Childhood (1.5–11 years) | Adolescence (11–16 years) | Adulthood (>16 years) |
|---|---|---|---|---|---|---|
| Cardiovascular | Cardiomyopathy | | ± | ± | | |
| Digestive | **Hepatopathy** | ± | + | + | | |
| | **Liver cirrhosis** | | + | + | | |
| | **Splenomegaly** | | + | + | | |
| Metabolic | Fasting intolerance | | + | + | | |
| Musculoskeletal | Arthrogryposis multiplex[a] | ± | ± | | | |
| | Hypotonia, muscular-axial | | + | + | | |
| | Muscle weakness | | + | + | | |
| | Muscular atrophy | | + | + | | |
| Other | Adult polyglucosan body disease[a] | | | | | + |
| | **Early death** | | + | + | | |
| | Failure to thrive | | + | + | | |
| Laboratory findings | ASAT/ALAT (plasma) | n-↑ | ↑ | ↑ | | |
| | Bilirubin (plasma) | n-↑ | ↑ | ↑ | | |
| | Branching enzyme (fibroblasts) | ↓ | ↓ | ↓ | | |
| | Branching enzyme (liver) | ↓ | ↓ | ↓ | | |
| | Branching enzyme (muscle) | ↓ | ↓ | ↓ | | |
| | Branching enzyme (red blood cells) | ↓ | ↓ | ↓ | | |
| | Branching enzyme (white blood cells) | ↓ | ↓ | ↓ | | |
| | Coagulation factors (plasma) | ↓-n | ↓ | ↓ | | |
| | Glycogen (liver) | ↑ | ↑ | ↑ | | |
| | Prothrombin time | n | ↑ | ↑ | ↑ | |

[a]Allelic presentations to GSD-IV but rarely found with identical genetic variants

**Table 39.37** Glycogen storage disease type IXd (Muscle phosphorylase kinase α1 subunit deficiency) (*see also* Kishnani et al. 2019)

| System | Symptoms and biomarkers | Neonatal (birth–1 month) | Infancy (1–18 months) | Childhood (1.5–11 years) | Adolescence (11–16 years) | Adulthood (>16 years) |
|---|---|---|---|---|---|---|
| Musculoskeletal | **Exertion intolerance** | | | ± | ± | + |
| | **Muscle cramps** | | | ± | ± | + |
| | **Muscle pain** | | | ± | ± | + |
| | **Muscle weakness** | | | ± | ± | + |
| | Second wind phenomenon | | | ± | ± | + |
| Laboratory findings | Ammonia rise in forearm exercise test (blood) | | | | n | n |
| | Creatine kinase (plasma) | | | | ↑ | ↑ |
| | Glycogen (muscle) | ↑ | ↑ | ↑ | ↑ | ↑ |
| | Lactate rise in forearm exercise test (plasma) | | | | ↓ | ↓ |
| | Myoglobin (urine) | | | | n-↑ | n-↑ |
| | Phosphorylase kinase (muscle) | ↓ | ↓ | ↓ | ↓ | ↓ |
| | Uric acid (plasma) | | | | ↑ | ↑ |

**Table 39.38** Glycogen storage disease type IXa (Hepatic phosphorylase kinase α2 subunit deficiency) (*see also* Kishnani et al. 2019)

| System | Symptoms and biomarkers | Neonatal (birth–1 month) | Infancy (1–18 months) | Childhood (1.5–11 years) | Adolescence (11–16 years) | Adulthood (>16 years) |
|---|---|---|---|---|---|---|
| Digestive | **Hepatomegaly** | ± | ± | ± | | |
| Metabolic | **Hypoglycaemia** | ± | ± | ± | ± | ± |
| Musculoskeletal | Short stature | | ± | + | + | |
| Other | Adiposity (doll-like facies) | | ± | + | + | |
| Laboratory findings | ASAT/ALAT (plasma) | n-↑ | n-↑ | n-↑ | n-↑ | n-↑ |
| | Biotinidase (plasma) | n-↑ | n-↑ | n-↑ | n-↑ | n-↑ |
| | Cholesterol (serum) | n-↑ | n-↑ | n-↑ | n-↑ | n-↑ |
| | Glucose, fasted (plasma) | ↓-n | ↓-n | ↓-n | ↓-n | ↓-n |
| | Glycogen (liver) | n-↑↑ | ↑↑ | ↑↑ | n-↑ | n-↑ |
| | Ketones, fasted (plasma) | ↑ | ↑ | ↑ | n-↑ | n-↑ |
| | Ketones, fasted (urine) | ↑ | ↑ | ↑ | n-↑ | n-↑ |
| | Lactate, fasted (plasma) | n | n | n | n | n |
| | Lactate, fasted (urine) | n | n | n | n | n |
| | Phosphorylase kinase (blood cells) | n-↓ | n-↓ | n-↓ | n-↓ | n-↓ |
| | Phosphorylase kinase (liver) | ↓ | ↓ | ↓ | ↓ | ↓ |
| | Triglyceride (serum) | n-↑ | n-↑ | n-↑ | n-↑ | n-↑ |
| | Uric acid (plasma) | n | n | n | n | n |
| | Uric acid (urine) | n | n | n | n | n |

**Table 39.39** Glycogen storage disease type IXb (Phosphorylase kinase β subunit deficiency) (*see also* Kishnani et al. 2019)

| System | Symptoms and biomarkers | Neonatal (birth–1 month) | Infancy (1–18 months) | Childhood (1.5–11 years) | Adolescence (11–16 years) | Adulthood (>16 years) |
|---|---|---|---|---|---|---|
| Digestive | **Hepatomegaly** | ± | ± | ± | | |
| Metabolic | **Hypoglycaemia** | ± | ± | ± | ± | ± |
| Musculoskeletal | Short stature | | ± | + | + | |
| Other | Adiposity (doll-like facies) | | ± | + | + | |
| Laboratory findings | ASAT/ALAT (plasma) | n-↑ | n-↑ | n-↑ | n-↑ | n-↑ |
| | Biotinidase (plasma) | n-↑ | n-↑ | n-↑ | n-↑ | n-↑ |
| | Cholesterol (serum) | n-↑ | n-↑ | n-↑ | n-↑ | n-↑ |
| | Glucose, fasted (plasma) | ↓-n | ↓-n | ↓-n | ↓-n | ↓-n |
| | Glycogen (liver) | n-↑↑ | ↑↑ | ↑↑ | n-↑ | n-↑ |
| | Ketones, fasted (plasma) | ↑ | ↑ | ↑ | n-↑ | n-↑ |
| | Ketones, fasted (urine) | ↑ | ↑ | ↑ | n-↑ | n-↑ |
| | Lactate, fasted (plasma) | n | n | n | n | n |
| | Lactate, fasted (urine) | n | n | n | n | n |
| | Phosphorylase kinase (blood cells) | ↓ | ↓ | ↓ | ↓ | ↓ |
| | Phosphorylase kinase (liver) | ↓ | ↓ | ↓ | ↓ | ↓ |
| | Triglyceride (serum) | n-↑ | n-↑ | n-↑ | n-↑ | n-↑ |
| | Uric acid (plasma) | n | n | n | n | n |
| | Uric acid (urine) | n | n | n | n | n |

**Table 39.40** Glycogen storage disease type IXc (Hepatic phosphorylase kinase γ2 subunit deficiency) (*see also* Kishnani et al. 2019)

| System | Symptoms and biomarkers | Neonatal (birth–1 month) | Infancy (1–18 months) | Childhood (1.5–11 years) | Adolescence (11–16 years) | Adulthood (>16 years) |
|---|---|---|---|---|---|---|
| Digestive | **Hepatomegaly** | ± | ± | ± | | |
| | Liver cirrhosis | | | ± | ± | ± |
| | Liver fibrosis | | | ± | ± | ± |
| | Splenomegaly | | | ± | ± | ± |
| Metabolic | **Hypoglycaemia** | ± | ± | ± | ± | ± |
| Musculoskeletal | Short stature | | ± | + | + | |
| Other | Adiposity (doll-like facies) | | ± | + | + | |

Table 39.40 (continued)

| System | Symptoms and biomarkers | Neonatal (birth–1 month) | Infancy (1–18 months) | Childhood (1.5–11 years) | Adolescence (11–16 years) | Adulthood (>16 years) |
|---|---|---|---|---|---|---|
| Laboratory findings | ASAT/ALAT (plasma) | n-↑ | n-↑ | n-↑ | n-↑ | n-↑ |
| | Biotinidase (plasma) | n-↑ | n-↑ | n-↑ | n-↑ | n-↑ |
| | Cholesterol (serum) | n-↑ | n-↑ | n-↑ | n-↑ | n-↑ |
| | Glucose, fasted (plasma) | ↓-n | ↓-n | ↓-n | ↓-n | ↓-n |
| | Glycogen (liver) | n-↑↑ | ↑↑ | ↑↑ | n-↑ | n-↑ |
| | Ketones, fasted (plasma) | ↑ | ↑ | ↑ | n-↑ | n-↑ |
| | Ketones, fasted (urine) | ↑ | ↑ | ↑ | n-↑ | n-↑ |
| | Lactate, fasted (plasma) | n | n | n | n | n |
| | Lactate, fasted (urine) | n | n | n | n | n |
| | Phosphorylase kinase (blood cells) | ↓ | ↓ | ↓ | ↓ | ↓ |
| | Phosphorylase kinase (liver) | ↓ | ↓ | ↓ | ↓ | ↓ |
| | Triglyceride (serum) | n-↑ | n-↑ | n-↑ | n-↑ | n-↑ |
| | Uric acid (plasma) | n | n | n | n | n |
| | Uric acid (urine) | n | n | n | n | n |

Table 39.41 Constitutional AMP-activated protein kinase activation

| System | Symptoms and biomarkers | Neonatal (birth–1 month) | Infancy (1–18 months) | Childhood (1.5–11 years) | Adolescence (11–16 years) | Adulthood (>16 years) |
|---|---|---|---|---|---|---|
| Cardiovascular | **Cardiac preexcitation syndrome** | + | + | + | + | + |
| | **Cardiomyopathy, hypertrophic** | + | + | + | + | + |
| | **Heart block (variable types)** | + | + | + | + | + |
| Metabolic | **Hypoglycaemia** | + | + | | | |
| Other | **Early death** | +[a] | +[a] | | | |
| Laboratory findings | Creatine kinase (plasma) | n-↑ | n-↑ | n-↑ | n-↑ | n-↑ |
| | Glucose (plasma) | ↓ | ↓ | | | |
| | Glycogen (heart) | ↑↑[a] | ↑↑[a] | ↑ | ↑ | ↑ |
| | Glycogen (muscle) | n-↑ | n-↑ | n-↑ | n-↑ | n-↑ |
| | Phosphorylase kinase (heart) | ↓[a] | ↓[a] | | | |
| | Protein kinase, AMP-activated (heart) | ↑↑[a] | ↑↑[a] | ↑ | ↑ | ↑ |
| | Protein kinase, AMP-activated (muscle) | ↑↑[a] | ↑↑[a] | ↑ | ↑ | ↑ |

[a]Severe neonatal type ('fatal congenital heart glycogenosis')

Table 39.42 Glycogen storage disease type V (Muscle glycogen phosphorylase deficiency)

| System | Symptoms and biomarkers | Neonatal (birth–1 month) | Infancy (1–18 months) | Childhood (1.5–11 years) | Adolescence (11–16 years) | Adulthood (>16 years) |
|---|---|---|---|---|---|---|
| Musculoskeletal | **Exertion intolerance** | | | | ± | + |
| | **Muscle cramps** | | | | ± | + |
| | **Muscle pain** | | | | ± | + |
| | **Muscle weakness** | | | | ± | + |
| | Second wind phenomenon | | | | ± | + |
| Laboratory findings | Ammonia rise in forearm exercise test (blood) | | | | n | n |
| | Creatine kinase (plasma) | | | | ↑ | ↑ |
| | Glycogen (muscle) | | ↑ | ↑ | ↑ | ↑ |
| | Lactate rise in forearm exercise test (plasma) | | | | ↓ | ↓ |
| | Myoglobin (urine) | | | | n-↑ | n-↑ |
| | Phosphorylase (muscle) | ↓ | ↓ | ↓ | ↓ | ↓ |
| | Uric acid (plasma) | | | | ↑ | ↑ |

**Table 39.43** Glycogen storage disease type VI (Hepatic glycogen phosphorylase deficiency) (*see also* Kishnani et al. 2019)

| System | Symptoms and biomarkers | Neonatal (birth–1 month) | Infancy (1–18 months) | Childhood (1.5–11 years) | Adolescence (11–16 years) | Adulthood (>16 years) |
|---|---|---|---|---|---|---|
| Digestive | **Hepatomegaly** | ± | ± | ± | | |
| Metabolic | **Hypoglycaemia** | ± | ± | ± | ± | ± |
| Musculoskeletal | Short stature | | ± | + | + | |
| Other | Adiposity (doll-like facies) | | ± | + | + | |
| Laboratory findings | ASAT/ALAT (plasma) | n-↑ | n-↑ | n-↑ | n-↑ | n-↑ |
| | Biotinidase (plasma) | n-↑ | n-↑ | n-↑ | n-↑ | n-↑ |
| | Cholesterol (serum) | n-↑ | n-↑ | n-↑ | n-↑ | n-↑ |
| | Glucose, fasted (plasma) | ↓-n | ↓-n | ↓-n | ↓-n | ↓-n |
| | Glycogen (liver) | n-↑↑ | ↑↑ | ↑↑ | n-↑ | n-↑ |
| | Glycogen phosphorylase (liver) | ↓ | ↓ | ↓ | ↓ | ↓ |
| | Ketones, fasted (plasma) | ↑ | ↑ | ↑ | n-↑ | n-↑ |
| | Ketones, fasted (urine) | ↑ | ↑ | ↑ | n-↑ | n-↑ |
| | Lactate, fasted (plasma) | n | n | n | n | n |
| | Lactate, fasted (urine) | n | n | n | n | n |
| | Triglyceride (serum) | ↑ | ↑ | ↑ | ↑ | ↑ |
| | Uric acid (plasma) | n | n | n | n | n |
| | Uric acid (urine) | n | n | n | n | n |

**Table 39.44** Glycogen storage disease type III (Glycogen debranching enzyme deficiency>) (*see also* Kishnani et al. 2010; Sentner et al. 2016)

| System | Symptoms and biomarkers | Neonatal (birth–1 month) | Infancy (1–18 months) | Childhood (1.5–11 years) | Adolescence (11–16 years) | Adulthood (>16 years) |
|---|---|---|---|---|---|---|
| Cardiovascular | Cardiomyopathy | | + | + | + | + |
| Digestive | Biliary cirrhosis | | | ± | ± | ± |
| | **Hepatomegaly** | | ± | ++ | + | + |
| | Liver adenoma | | | | | ± |
| | Liver carcinoma | | | | | ± |
| | Liver fibrosis | | | ± | ± | ± |
| Metabolic | **Hypoglycaemia** | + | + | + | ± | ± |
| Musculoskeletal | Exertion intolerance | | | ± | ± | + |
| | Muscle weakness | | | + | + | ++ |
| | Osteopenia | | | | | + |
| | Short stature | | ± | + | + | + |
| Other | Adiposity (doll-like facies) | | ± | + | + | + |
| Laboratory findings | Amylo-1,6-glucosidase (liver) | ↓ | ↓ | ↓ | ↓ | ↓ |
| | Amylo-1,6-glucosidase (white blood cells) | ↓ | ↓ | ↓ | ↓ | ↓ |
| | ASAT/ALAT (plasma) | ↑↑ | ↑↑ | ↑↑ | ↑↑ | ↑↑ |
| | Biotinidase (plasma) | n-↑ | ↑-↑↑↑ | ↑-↑↑↑ | ↑-↑↑ | n-↑ |
| | Cholesterol (serum) | ↑ | ↑ | ↑ | ↑ | ↑ |
| | Creatine kinase (plasma) | n-↑ | n-↑ | n-↑ | n-↑ | n-↑ |
| | Glucose, fasted (plasma) | ↓ | ↓ | ↓ | ↓-n | ↓-n |
| | Glycogen (liver) | n-↑↑↑ | ↑↑↑ | ↑↑↑ | ↑↑↑ | ↑↑↑ |
| | Ketones, fasted (plasma) | ↑↑ | ↑↑ | ↑↑ | ↑↑ | ↑↑ |
| | Ketones, fasted (urine) | ↑↑ | ↑↑ | ↑↑ | ↑↑ | ↑↑ |
| | Lactate, fasted (plasma) | n | n | n | n | n |
| | Lactate, fasted (urine) | n | n | n | n | n |
| | Triglyceride (serum) | ↑ | ↑ | ↑ | ↑ | ↑ |
| | Uric acid (plasma) | n | n | n | n | n |
| | Uric acid (urine) | n | n | n | n | n |

**Table 39.45** Glycogen storage disease type Ia (Glucose-6-phosphatase deficiency) (*see also* Chen 2001; Rake et al. 2002; Kishnani et al. 2014)

| System | Symptoms and biomarkers | Neonatal (birth–1 month) | Infancy (1–18 months) | Childhood (1.5–11 years) | Adolescence (11–16 years) | Adulthood (>16 years) |
|---|---|---|---|---|---|---|
| Digestive | Diarrhea | ± | ± | ± | ± | ± |
| | **Hepatomegaly** | | ± | ++ | + | + |
| | Liver adenoma | | | | | ± |
| | Liver carcinoma | | | | | ± |
| | Pancreatitis | | | ± | ± | ± |
| Haematological | Bleeding tendency | ± | ± | ± | ± | ± |
| Metabolic | **Hypoglycaemia** | + | + | + | + | + |
| Musculoskeletal | Osteopenia | ± | ± | ± | + | + |
| | Short stature | | ± | + | + | + |
| Other | Adiposity (doll-like facies) | | ± | + | + | + |
| Renal | Glomerulosclerosis | | | | ± | + |
| | Hyperfiltration | | | | ± | + |
| | Renal enlargement | + | + | + | + | + |
| Respiratory | Tachypnea | + | + | + | | |
| Laboratory findings | ASAT/ALAT (plasma) | n-↑ | n-↑ | n-↑ | n-↑ | n-↑ |
| | Biotinidase (plasma) | n-↑ | ↑-↑↑↑ | ↑-↑↑↑ | ↑-↑↑ | n-↑ |
| | Cholesterol (serum) | ↑ | ↑ | ↑ | ↑ | ↑ |
| | Glucose, fasted (plasma) | ↓ | ↓ | ↓ | ↓ | ↓ |
| | Glucose-6-phosphatase (liver) | ↓ | ↓ | ↓ | ↓ | ↓ |
| | Glycogen (liver) | n-↑↑↑ | ↑↑↑ | ↑↑↑ | ↑↑↑ | ↑↑↑ |
| | Ketones, fasted (plasma) | ↓ | ↓ | ↓ | ↓ | ↓ |
| | Ketones, fasted (urine) | ↓ | ↓ | ↓ | ↓ | ↓ |
| | Lactate, fasted (plasma) | ↑ | ↑ | ↑ | ↑ | ↑ |
| | Lactate, fasted (urine) | ↑ | ↑ | ↑ | ↑ | ↑ |
| | Triglyceride (serum) | ↑ | ↑ | ↑ | ↑ | ↑ |
| | Uric acid (plasma) | ↑ | ↑ | ↑ | ↑ | ↑ |
| | Uric acid (urine) | ↑ | ↑ | ↑ | ↑ | ↑ |

**Table 39.46** Glucose-6-phosphatase catalytic subunit 3 deficiency

| System | Symptoms and biomarkers | Neonatal (birth–1 month) | Infancy (1–18 months) | Childhood (1.5–11 years) | Adolescence (11–16 years) | Adulthood (>16 years) |
|---|---|---|---|---|---|---|
| Digestive | Diarrhea | ± | ± | ± | ± | ± |
| | **Inflammatory bowel disease** | ± | ± | ± | ± | ± |
| | **Oral ulcerations** | ± | ± | ± | ± | ± |
| Haematological | Anaemia | ± | ± | ± | ± | ± |
| | **Leukocyte function impaired** | + | + | + | + | + |
| | **Neutropenia** | + | + | + | + | + |
| Other | Failure to thrive | ± | ± | ± | ± | ± |
| | **Recurrent infections** | + | + | + | + | + |
| Laboratory findings | 1,5-Anhydroglucitol-6-phosphate (plasma, urine) | ↑-↑↑↑ | ↑-↑↑↑ | ↑-↑↑↑ | ↑-↑↑↑ | ↑-↑↑↑ |
| | Neutrophil count | ↓ | ↓ | ↓ | ↓ | ↓ |
| | Neutrophil function | ↓ | ↓ | ↓ | ↓ | ↓ |

**Table 39.47** Glycogen storage disease type I *non*-a (Glucose-6-phosphate translocase deficiency) (*see also* Visser et al. 2002)

| System | Symptoms and biomarkers | Neonatal (birth–1 month) | Infancy (1–18 months) | Childhood (1.5–11 years) | Adolescence (11–16 years) | Adulthood (>16 years) |
|---|---|---|---|---|---|---|
| Digestive | **Diarrhea** | ± | ± | ± | ± | ± |
| | **Hepatomegaly** | | ± | ++ | + | + |
| | **Inflammatory bowel disease** | + | + | + | + | + |
| | Liver adenoma | | ± | ++ | + | + |
| | Liver carcinoma | | ± | ++ | + | + |
| | **Oral ulcerations** | + | + | + | + | + |
| | Pancreatitis | | | | | ± |
| Haematological | Anaemia | | + | + | + | + |
| | Bleeding tendency | ± | ± | ± | ± | ± |
| | **Leukocyte function impaired** | + | + | + | + | + |
| | **Neutropenia** | + | + | + | + | + |
| Metabolic | **Hypoglycaemia** | + | + | + | + | + |
| Musculoskeletal | Osteopenia | ± | ± | ± | ± | ± |
| | Short stature | | ± | + | + | + |
| Other | Adiposity (doll-like facies) | | ± | + | + | + |
| | **Recurrent infections** | + | + | + | + | + |
| Renal | Glomerulosclerosis | | | | ± | + |
| | Hyperfiltration | | | | ± | + |
| Respiratory | Tachypnea | + | + | + | | |
| Laboratory findings | 1,5-Anhydroglucitol-6-phosphate (plasma, urine) | ↑-↑↑↑ | ↑-↑↑↑ | ↑-↑↑↑ | ↑-↑↑↑ | ↑-↑↑↑ |
| | ASAT/ALAT (plasma) | n-↑ | n-↑ | n-↑ | n-↑ | n-↑ |
| | Biotinidase (plasma) | n-↑ | ↑-↑↑↑ | ↑-↑↑↑ | ↑-↑↑ | n-↑ |
| | Cholesterol (serum) | ↑ | ↑ | ↑ | ↑ | ↑ |
| | Glucose, fasted (plasma) | ↓ | ↓ | ↓ | ↓ | ↓ |
| | Glucose-6-phosphatase (liver, frozen) | n | n | n | n | n |
| | Glucose-6-phosphatase (liver, unfrozen) | ↓ | ↓ | ↓ | ↓ | ↓ |
| | Glycogen (liver) | n-↑↑↑ | ↑↑↑ | ↑↑↑ | ↑↑↑ | ↑↑↑ |
| | Ketones, fasted (plasma) | ↓ | ↓ | ↓ | ↓ | ↓ |
| | Ketones, fasted (urine) | ↓ | ↓ | ↓ | ↓ | ↓ |
| | Lactate, fasted (plasma) | ↑ | ↑ | ↑ | ↑ | ↑ |
| | Lactate, fasted (urine) | ↑ | ↑ | ↑ | ↑ | ↑ |
| | Neutrophil count | ↓ | ↓ | ↓ | ↓ | ↓ |
| | Triglyceride (serum) | ↑ | ↑ | ↑ | ↑ | ↑ |
| | Uric acid (plasma) | ↑ | ↑ | ↑ | ↑ | ↑ |
| | Uric acid (urine) | ↑ | ↑ | ↑ | ↑ | ↑ |

**Table 39.48** HOIL1 deficiency

| System | Symptoms and biomarkers | Neonatal (birth–1 month) | Infancy (1–18 months) | Childhood (1.5–11 years) | Adolescence (11–16 years) | Adulthood (>16 years) |
|---|---|---|---|---|---|---|
| Cardiovascular | Amylopectinosis (biopsy) | + | + | | | |
| | **Cardiomyopathy, dilated** | + | + | | | |
| Dermatological | Rash, eczematous | ± | ± | | | |
| Digestive | Hepatomegaly | ± | ± | | | |
| Eye | Ptosis of eyelid | ± | ± | | | |
| Haematological | Immunodeficiency | ± | ± | | | |
| Musculoskeletal | **Growth retardation** | + | + | | | |
| | **Muscle weakness, proximal** | + | + | | | |
| | **Myalgia** | + | + | | | |
| | Scoliosis | ± | ± | | | |
| Other | Failure to thrive | + | + | | | |
| | Recurrent infections | ± | ± | | | |
| Laboratory findings | ASAT/ALAT (plasma) | n-↑ | n-↑ | | | |
| | Creatine kinase (plasma) | ↑ | ↑ | | | |
| | IgA (serum) | n-↑ | n-↑ | | | |

**Table 39.49** HOIL1 interacting protein deficiency

| System | Symptoms and biomarkers | Neonatal (birth–1 month) | Infancy (1–18 months) | Childhood (1.5–11 years) | Adolescence (11–16 years) | Adulthood (>16 years) |
|---|---|---|---|---|---|---|
| Haematological | Anaemia | | | + | | |
| | **Autoinflammation** | | | + | | |
| | Immunodeficiency | | | + | | |
| | Immunodeficiency | | | + | | |
| | **Lymphadenopathy** | | | + | | |
| | Lymphangiectasia | | | + | | |
| Respiratory | **Respiratory distress** | | | + | | |
| Laboratory findings | Albumin (serum) | | | ↓ | | |
| | Amylopectin (liver) | | | + | | |
| | IgG (serum) | | | ↓ | | |
| | Iron (serum) | | | ↓ | | |
| | Potassium (plasma) | | | ↓ | | |
| | Vitamin D (plasma) | | | ↓ | | |

**Table 39.50** Laforin deficiency

| System | Symptoms and biomarkers | Neonatal (birth–1 month) | Infancy (1–18 months) | Childhood (1.5–11 years) | Adolescence (11–16 years) | Adulthood (>16 years) |
|---|---|---|---|---|---|---|
| CNS | Dementia | | | | + | + |
| | EEG abnormalities | | | | + | + |
| | Gait disturbances | | | | + | + |
| | Hallucinations | | | | ± | ± |
| | Mental retardation | | | | + | + |
| | **Myoclonic epilepsy, progressive** | | | | + | + |
| | Myoclonus | | | | ± | ± |
| | Seizures, tonic-clonic, generalized | | | | ± | ± |
| | Seizures, absence | | | | ± | ± |
| | Seizures, partial | | | | ± | ± |
| Other | PAS positive polyglucosan inclusions in brain, liver, muscle, heart, skin | n | n | | + | |
| | Rapidly progressive | | | | + | + |
| | Short survival (<10 years) | | | | + | + |
| Psychiatric | Psychiatric symptoms | | | | ± | ± |

**Table 39.51** Malin deficiency

| System | Symptoms and biomarkers | Neonatal (birth–1 month) | Infancy (1–18 months) | Childhood (1.5–11 years) | Adolescence (11–16 years) | Adulthood (>16 years) |
|---|---|---|---|---|---|---|
| CNS | Demetia | | | | + | + |
| | EEG abnormalities | | | | + | + |
| | Gait disturbances | | | | + | + |
| | Mental retardation | | | | + | + |
| | **Myoclonic epilepsy, progressive** | | | | + | + |
| | Myoclonus | | | | ± | ± |
| | Seizures, tonic-clonic, generalized | | | | ± | ± |
| | Seizures, absence | | | | ± | ± |
| | Seizures, partial | | | | ± | ± |
| Other | PAS positive polyglucosan inclusions in brain, liver, muscle, heart, skin | n | n | | + | |
| | Rapidly progressive | | | | + | + |
| | Short survival (<15 years) | | | | + | + |
| Psychiatric | Hallucinations | | | | ± | ± |
| | Psychiatric symptoms | | | | ± | ± |

**Table 39.52** Glycogen storage disease type IIa (Lysosomal α-1,4-glucosidase deficiency) (*see also* Kishnani et al. 2006; van der Ploeg et al. 2017)

| System | Symptoms and biomarkers | Neonatal (birth–1 month) | Infancy (1–18 months) | Childhood (1.5–11 years) | Adolescence (11–16 years) | Adulthood (>16 years) |
|---|---|---|---|---|---|---|
| Cardiovascular | **Cardiac failure** | + | + | + | | |
| | **Cardiac preexcitation syndrome** | + | + | | | |
| | **Cardiomyopathy, dilated** | ++ | ++ | | | |
| | **Cardiomyopathy, hypertrophic** | ++ | ++ | | | |
| CNS | EEG, abnormal | + | + | | | |
| | Intellectual disability | | + | + | | |
| | Neuropathy, peripheral | | + | ± | ± | ± |
| Digestive | Hepatomegaly | ± | ± | | | |
| | Macroglossia | + | + | | | |
| Ear | Hearing loss, sensorineural | | | + | + | + |
| Haematological | **Vacuolated lymphocytes** | + | + | | | |
| Musculoskeletal | **Hypotonia, muscular-axial** | ++ | ++ | ++ | ++ | ++ |
| Other | **Early death** | ± | ± | | | |
| Respiratory | Orthopnea | | | + | + | + |
| | Sleep apnea | | | + | + | + |
| Laboratory findings | Alpha-1,4-glucosidase (dried blood spot) | ↓ | ↓ | ↓ | ↓ | ↓ |
| | Alpha-1,4-glucosidase (fibroblasts) | ↓ | ↓ | ↓ | ↓ | ↓ |
| | Alpha-1,4-glucosidase (muscle) | ↓ | ↓ | ↓ | ↓ | ↓ |
| | ASAT/ALAT (plasma) | ↑ | ↑ | ↑ | ↑ | ↑ |
| | Creatine kinase (plasma) | ↑ | ↑ | ↑ | ↑ | ↑ |
| | Glucotetrasaccharide (urine) | ↑ | ↑ | ↑ | ↑ | ↑ |
| | Glycogen (all tissues) | ↑ | ↑ | n-↑ | n-↑ | n-↑ |
| | Lymphocytes, vacuolated | | n-↑ | n-↑ | n-↑ | n-↑ |
| | Myocytes, vacuolated | | | n-↑ | n-↑ | n-↑ |

**Table 39.53** Glycogen storage disease type IIb (Lysosome-associated membrane protein 2 deficiency)

| System | Symptoms and biomarkers | Neonatal (birth–1 month) | Infancy (1–18 months) | Childhood (1.5–11 years) | Adolescence (11–16 years) | Adulthood (>16 years) |
|---|---|---|---|---|---|---|
| Cardiovascular | **Cardiac failure** | | | ++ | ++ | |
| | **Cardiac preexcitation syndrome** | | | + | + | + |
| | **Cardiomyopathy, dilated** | | | ++ | ++ | |
| | **Cardiomyopathy, hypertrophic** | | | ++ | ++ | |
| CNS | EEG, abnormal | | | + | + | + |
| | **Intellectual disability** | | | + | ++ | ++ |
| Eye | **Lens changes** | | | + | + | + |
| | Loss of central vision | | | + | + | + |
| | **Loss of peripheral retinal pigment** | | | + | + | + |
| | Myopia | | | + | + | + |
| Musculoskeletal | **Hypotonia, muscular-axial** | | | + | + | + |
| | **Muscle cramps** | | | + | + | + |
| Other | **Sudden death** | | | | + | + |
| Laboratory findings | Alpha-1,4-glucosidase (dried blood spot) | n | n | n | n | n |
| | Alpha-1,4-glucosidase (fibroblasts) | n | n | n | n | n |
| | Alpha-1,4-glucosidase (muscle) | n | n | n | n | n |
| | ASAT/ALAT (plasma) | | | ↑ | ↑ | ↑ |
| | Creatine kinase (plasma) | | | ↑ | ↑ | ↑ |
| | Glycogen (heart) | | | ↑ | ↑ | ↑ |
| | Glycogen (muscle) | | | ↑ | ↑ | ↑ |
| | Lymphocytes, vacuolated | | | + | + | + |
| | Myocytes, vacuolated | | | + | + | + |

**Table 39.54** Pyruvate carboxylase deficiency

| System | Symptoms and biomarkers | Neonatal (birth–1 month) | Infancy (1–18 months) | Childhood (1.5–11 years) | Adolescence (11–16 years) | Adulthood (>16 years) |
|---|---|---|---|---|---|---|
| CNS | **Basal ganglia disease** | + | + | + | + | + |
| | **Global developmental retardation** | + | + | + | + | + |
| | **Hypoglycaemia** | + | + | + | + | + |
| | Impaired myelination | + | + | + | + | + |
| | Leukodystrophy | + | + | + | + | + |
| | Muscular hypotonia | + | + | + | + | + |
| | Seizures | + | + | + | + | + |
| Digestive | Liver dysfunction | + | + | + | + | + |
| | Liver, fatty | + | + | + | + | + |
| | Renal tubular acidosis | + | + | + | + | + |
| Metabolic | Hepatomegaly | + | + | + | + | + |
| Renal | pH | ↓ - ↓↓↓ | ↓ - ↓↓↓ | ↓ - ↓↓↓ | ↓ - ↓↓ | ↓ |
| Laboratory findings | Acetoacetate/β-hydroxybutyrate ratio | ↑ | ↑ | ↑ | ↑ | ↑ |
| | Alanine (plasma) | ↑ | ↑ | ↑ | ↑ | ↑ |
| | Ammonia (plasma) | ↑ | ↑ | n - ↑ | n - ↑ | n - ↑ |
| | Citrullin (plasma) | ↑ | ↑ | n - ↑ | n - ↑ | n - ↑ |
| | Glucose (plasma) | ↓ | ↓ | ↓ | ↓ | ↓ |
| | Ketones (blood) | ↑ | ↑ | ↑ | ↑ | ↑ |
| | Ketones (urine) | ↑ | ↑ | ↑ | ↑ | ↑ |
| | Lactate (plasma) | ↑ - ↑↑↑ | ↑ - ↑↑↑ | ↑ - ↑↑↑ | ↑ - ↑↑ | ↑ |
| | Lactate: pyruvate ratio | ↑ | ↑ | ↑ | ↑ | ↑ |
| | Lysine (plasma) | ↑ | ↑ | n - ↑ | n - ↑ | n - ↑ |
| | Pyruvate carboxylase (fibroblasts) | ↓ | ↓ | ↓ | ↓ | ↓ |

**Table 39.55** Mitochondrial phosphoenolpyruvate carboxykinase deficiency

| System | Symptoms and biomarkers | Neonatal (birth–1 month) | Infancy (1–18 months) | Childhood (1.5–11 years) | Adolescence (11–16 years) | Adulthood (>16 years) |
|---|---|---|---|---|---|---|
| Metabolic | **Hypoglycaemia** | + | | | | |
| Digestive | **Liver dysfunction** | + | | | | |
| | Liver, fatty | + | | | | |
| Laboratory findings | Glucose (plasma) | ↓ | | | | |
| | Lactate (plasma) | ↑ | | | | |

**Table 39.56** Cytosolic phosphoenolpyruvate carboxykinase deficiency

| System | Symptoms and biomarkers | Neonatal (birth–1 month) | Infancy (1–18 months) | Childhood (1.5–11 years) | Adolescence (11–16 years) | Adulthood (>16 years) |
|---|---|---|---|---|---|---|
| CNS | **Seizures** | ± | ± | ± | | |
| Dermatological | Cyanosis | + | + | + | | |
| Digestive | **Hepatomegaly** | + | + | + | | |
| | Liver failure | | | ± | | |
| Eye | **Optic nerve hypoplasia** | + | + | + | | |
| Metabolic | **Hypoglycaemia, fasting** | + | + | + | | |
| Respiratory | Apnea | ± | ± | ± | | |

**Table 39.56** (continued)

| System | Symptoms and biomarkers | Neonatal (birth–1 month) | Infancy (1–18 months) | Childhood (1.5–11 years) | Adolescence (11–16 years) | Adulthood (>16 years) |
|---|---|---|---|---|---|---|
| Laboratory findings | ALAT (plasma) | ↑ | ↑ | ↑ | | |
| | Ammonia (blood) | n-↑ | n-↑ | n-↑ | | |
| | Arginine (plasma) | ↓-n | ↓-n | ↓-n | | |
| | Citrulline (plasma) | ↓-n | ↓-n | ↓-n | | |
| | Dicarboxylic acids (urine) | ↑ | ↑ | ↑ | | |
| | Glucose, fasted (plasma) | ↓ | ↓ | ↓ | | |
| | Glutamine (plasma) | n-↑ | n-↑ | n-↑ | | |
| | Ketones (urine)[a] | + | + | + | | |
| | Lactate (plasma) | ↑ | ↑ | ↑ | | |
| | Lactate (urine) | ↑ | ↑ | ↑ | | |

[a]Pronounced during crises

**Table 39.57** Fructose-1,6-bisphosphatase deficiency

| System | Symptoms and biomarkers | Neonatal (birth–1 month) | Infancy (1–18 months) | Childhood (1.5–11 years) | Adolescence (11–16 years) | Adulthood (>16 years) |
|---|---|---|---|---|---|---|
| Digestive | Hepatomegaly | + | + | ± | ± | ± |
| Respiratory | Tachypnea[a] | + | + | + | | |
| Metabolic | **Hypoglycemia[a]** | + | + | + | ± | ± |
| Laboratory findings | Alanine (plasma)[a] | ↑ | ↑ | ↑ | ↑ | |
| | Fructose-1,6-bisphosphatase (liver) | ↓ | ↓ | ↓ | ↓ | ↓ |
| | Glucose (plasma)[a] | ↓ | ↓ | ↓ | ↓-n | ↓-n |
| | Glycerol (urine)[a] | n-↑ | n-↑ | n-↑ | | |
| | Ketones (plasma)[a] | ↑ | ↑ | ↑ | | |
| | Ketones (urine)[a] | ↑ | ↑ | ↑ | | |
| | Lactate (plasma)[a] | ↑ | ↑ | ↑ | ↑ | |
| | Phosphate (plasma)[a] | ↓-n | ↓-n | ↓-n | n | n |
| | Triglyceride (serum)[a,b] | ↑ | ↑ | ↑ | n-↑ | n-↑ |
| | Uric acid (plasma)[a] | n-↑ | n-↑ | n-↑ | n | n |
| | Uric acid (urine)[a] | n-↑ | n-↑ | n-↑ | n | n |

[a]Disease features occur in the fasted state and can be exaggerated by fructose, sorbitol, or glycerol intake
[b]Pseudo(!)hypertriglyceridaemia

## Diagnosis

Like in many other metabolic disorders, clinical hypothesis-driven pattern recognition is traditionally based on information from history taking, physical examination and additional (laboratory, imaging) investigations. For several disorders of carbohydrate absorption, transmembrane transport and metabolism, the nutritional history is of utmost importance for clinical reasoning and the following questions should be addressed:

- Is there intolerance or avoidance of certain carbohydrates (lactose, fruit, or fruit juice)?
- Did symptoms occur with a change in diet?
- When do symptoms occur in relation to the patient's last meal?
- How does the patient tolerate nocturnal fasting?

The answers to these questions can lead to a new direction of thinking in which the following signs and symptoms can point to fasting intolerance:

- Tremor, perspiration (adrenergic response, effective or ineffective counterregulation)
- Drowsiness, lethargy, double vision, seizures (neuroglycopenia)
- Morning anorexia can be a sign of nocturnal counter-regulation with mobilisation of ketones that can even cause an abnormal, strong, penetrating smell in the bedroom.
- Muscle pain in the morning may indicate nocturnal counterregulatory proteolysis.

To approach the aetiology of fasting hypoglycaemia, the following information is helpful:

- The relationship between the time when the patient becomes symptomatic or hypoglycaemic and the last meal
- The presence of hepatomegaly
- The lactate concentration during hypoglycaemia
- The ketone concentrations during hypoglycaemia

Special laboratory tests (*see* Table below) to come to a diagnosis should be performed in laboratories with specific expertise. These procedures may include both in vivo clinical (loading or provocation) tests, in vitro functional studies in tissues expressing the affected protein (a transporter or an enzyme), prenatal diagnosis, and molecular genetic analysis of the relevant gene (usually in DNA samples from peripheral blood, but DNA can also be obtained from other sources, such as fibroblasts).

Since in vivo and in vitro functional studies are laborious and may be invasive, nowadays a primary molecular genetic approach may be warranted. In that case, a working hypothesis has to be formulated on the basis of clinical and non-invasive paraclinical investigations. This is an option, particularly in disorders in which the affected gene is small or when few prevalent mutations are responsible for the cases of a population (*see* Table 'Special conditions for enzymatic and/or molecular genetic diagnosis in disorders of carbohydrate metabolism').

Alternatively, genetic testing by (panel) DNA has become preferable to (invasive, laborious) enzymology and has replaced invasive in vivo testing in many situations. However, these traditional approaches may still be warranted when no definite diagnosis can be made non-invasively, or to confirm the pathogenicity of genetic variants of unknown significance found by panel, whole exome, or whole genome sequencing.

## Reference Values and Pathological Values

The reference values for metabolites whose concentrations are altered in disorders of carbohydrate metabolism are shown in Table below. Due to variable assay conditions, results of additional transport or enzymatic tests have to be interpreted in comparison to laboratory-specific reference values and can be presented as a percentage of the average of normal controls. For example, diagnostic values of monosaccharide uptake by enterocytes in SGLT1 deficiency (an autosomal recessive condition) usually fall below 10% of normal; diagnostic values of glucose uptake by erythrocytes in GLUT1 deficiency (an autosomal dominant condition) have been reported to be 46 ± 8% of controls.

Reference and pathological values for metabolites related to carbohydrate metabolism

| Metabolite | | Age group | Reference values | | Pathological values | |
|---|---|---|---|---|---|---|
| Glucose (P) | Fasting | 1 d | 2.2–3.3 mmol/L | 40–60 mg/dL | | |
| | | >1 d | 2.8–5.0 mmol/L | 50–90 mg/dL | | |
| | | Child | 3.3–5.5 mmol/L | 60–100 mg/dL | | |
| | | Adult | 3.9–5.8 mmol/L | 70–105 mg/dL | | |
| | 1 h after ingestion | Adult | 6.6–9.4 mmol/L | 120–170 mg/dL | | |
| Glucose (CSF) | Fasting | Child | 1.7–3.7 mmol/L | 32–68 mg/dL | <3.3 mmol/L | <60 mg/dL |
| | | | | | or <P10 for age for GLUT1-D[a] | |
| Glucose (CSF/P ratio) | | Child | 65–85%xyx | | | <40–60%[a] |
| Glucose (U) | | | <0.8 mmol/L | <15 mg/dL | >0.8 mmol/L | >15 mg/dL |
| | | | 0.13–0.32 g/1.73 m²/d | | >0.32 g/1.73 m²/d | |
| Reducing substances (stool) | | | *Negative* | | | *Positive* |
| Galactose (P) | Fasting | | 0–0.03 mmol/L | 0–0.5 mg/dL | | |
| | After milk ingestion | Newborn | <1.1 mmol/L | <20 mg/dL | >1.1 mmol/L | >20 mg/dL |
| | | Child | <0.5 mmol/L | <9 mg/dL | >0.5 mmol/L | >9 mg/dL |
| | | Adult | <0.24 mmol/L | <4.3 mg/dL | >0.24 mmol/L | >4.3 mg/dL |
| Galactose-1-phosphate (RBC) | | | <0.17 µmol/g Hb | | >1.70 µmol/g Hb | |
| Galactose (U) | | | <377 mmol/mol crea | | >631 mmol/mol crea | |
| Galactitol (U) | | | 2–5 mmol/mol crea | | >30 mmol/mol crea | |
| Fructose (B) | | | <0.16 mmol/L | | >0.16 mmol/L | |
| Fructose (U) | | | 10–14 mmol/mol crea | | >20 Mmol/mol crea | |
| Sorbitol (U) | | | 2–26 mmol/mol crea | | | |
| Lactic acid (P) | Fasting | Child | 0.6–1.8 mmol/L | | >3.0 mmol/L | |
| Lactic acid (CSF) | | Child | 1.1–2.6 mmol/L | | >3.0 mmol/L | |
| Lactic acid (U) | | Child | <200 mmol/mol crea | | >300 mmol/mol crea | |
| Biotinidase (P) | | | 7.0–10.6 mU/mL | | >10.6 mU/mL | |
| Glycogen (L) | | | <5.0 g/100 g wet tissue | | >5.0 g/100 g wet tissue | |
| Glycogen (M) | | | <1.0 g/100 g wet tissue | | >1.0 g/100 g wet tissue | |

*n.d.* Not detectable

[a]Lumbar punction should be performed after 4 h of fasting. For age-dependent cut-off values for CSF glucose and CSF to plasma glucose ratio *see* Leen et al. (2013)

## Functional In Vivo Tests

Functional in vivo (provocation and/or loading) tests can be helpful in certain conditions (Table below) and should only be performed by clinicians with expertise.

**Functional tests glucose monitoring (CGM)**
*Indication:*
Assessment of fasting intolerance, recurrent episodes of hypoglycaemia of unknown origin, determination of metabolic profile during hypoglycaemia, monitoring of the dietary management. Can be performed in hospital or at home.
Stable clinical condition. Instruct on documentation of the use of CGM and alarming function. For patients with ketotic fasting intolerance or ketogenic diets, parallel documentation of ketones by a specific device may be helpful.
*Caution:*
Correlation between subcutaneous glucose and blood/plasma glucose concentrations may be poor.
Thresholds for CGM-alarms and capillary blood glucose/ketone values should be discussed on an individual basis.
*Interpretation:*
Requires integration of symptoms and signs, documented diet history (including times), CGM (including the slope of the curves), and capillary blood glucose and ketone concentrations.

**Fasting test**
*Indication:*
Assessment of fasting intolerance, recurrent episodes of hypoglycaemia of unknown origin, determination of metabolic profile during hypoglycaemia.
Stable clinical condition. Plan maximal fasting time according to anamnestic tolerance.
During test measure glucose (P), blood gases, lactate (P), ketones (P, U) every hour starting with the first meal that is missed.
Terminate test in case of hypoglycaemia (<45 mg/dL, <2.5 mM) or if clinical symptoms occur *after* diagnostic blood samples were drawn for glucose (P), blood gases, lactate (P), amino acids (alanine) (P), acylcarnitines (dried blood spots), organic acids (U), ketone bodies (P,U), (FFA (P), 3-hydroxybutyrate (P)), insulin (P), cortisol (P), growth hormone (P), others.
*Caution:*
Hypoglycaemia from dangerous causes has to be excluded prior to a fasting test. For example, accumulation of metabolites from disorders of fatty acid metabolism may lead to life-threatening complications which means that fatty acid oxidation defects have to be excluded by determination of acylcarnitines prior to such a test. In general, fasting tests should only be performed in specialised centres experienced with potential differential diagnoses.
10% i.v. glucose solution should be immediately available as needed in symptomatic patients (*see* Table "Emergency treatment").
*Interpretation:*
Glucose (P) <45 mg/dL (2.5 mM) is suggestive of an abnormal response particularly when combined with typical changes of other metabolites such as ketones or lactate (*see* Sign and Symptoms Tables).

**Oral glucose loading test**
*Indication:*
1. To test for impaired intestinal uptake in SGLT1-D.
2. To test for glucose intolerance (decreased hepatic uptake in FBS and GSD-0a, decreased β-cell insulin secretion in FBS).
Fasting state: 4–12 h (depending on age).
Glucose dose: 2 g/kg as 10% solution or as an equivalent amount of oligosaccharides (maximum dose 50 g) given by mouth within 5–7 min.
*Criteria:*
ad 1. Clinical signs, abdominal pain, diarrhea, reducing substances in stool, $H_2$ breath test and glucose (P) determination at baseline and every 30 min for 3 h;
ad 2. Glucose (P) and lactic acid (P) determinations at baseline and every 30 min for 3 h.
*Caution:*
Hypovolaemia may develop in SGLT1-D.
*Interpretation:*
Pathologic increase of $H_2$ (breath test) and diminished increase of glucose (P) in SGLT1-D. Glucose (P) low or normal and lactate (P) high or normal at baseline, exaggerated increase of glucose (P) and decrease of lactate (P) after glucose load in FBS. Exaggerated increase of glucose (P) and increased lactate (P) after glucose in GSD-0a.

**Oral galactose loading test**
*Indication:*
1. To test for impaired intestinal uptake in SGLT1-D.
2. To test for galactose intolerance (decreased hepatic uptake) in FBS.
Fasting state: 4–12 h (depending on age).
Galactose dose: 1 g/kg as 20% solution given by mouth within 5–7 min.
*Criteria:*
ad 1. Clinical signs, abdominal pain, diarrhea, reducing substances in stool, $H_2$ breath test and glucose (P) determination at baseline and every 30 min for 3 h;
ad 2. Glucose (P), galactose (P) and lactic acid (P) determinations at baseline and every 30 min for 3 h.
*Caution:*
Hypovolaemia may develop in SGLT1-D.
Not indicated in galactosaemia patients who may be detected in screening programs or by typical metabolites and enzymatic studies on a galactose-containing diet.
*Interpretation:*
Pathologic increase of $H_2$ (breath test) and diminished increase of galactose (P) in SGLT1-D. Glucose low or normal and lactate high or normal at baseline, exaggerated increase of galactose after galactose load in FBS.

**Oral fructose loading test**
*Indication:*
While dangerous and obsolete in the diagnosis of HFI, the *oral* fructose loading test may serve as a reference test in the diagnosis of SGLT1-D.
Fasting state: 4–12 h (depending on age).
Fructose dose: 1 g/kg as 20% solution given by mouth within 5–7 min.
*Criteria:*
Clinical signs, abdominal pain, diarrhea, reducing substances in stool, $H_2$ breath test and glucose (P) determination at baseline and every 30 min for 2 h.
*Interpretation:*
No increase of $H_2$ (breath test) and normal increase of glucose (P) in SGLT1-D.

Functional tests (continued)

| **Intravenous fructose loading test** |
|---|
| *Indication:*<br>Diagnosis of HFI and FBP-D (FK-D) in questionable cases.<br>(Before this test, think of less dangerous ways of diagnosis. Should only be performed in experienced centres.)<br>Preparation: 2 weeks before the test a diet without sucrose and fructose is prescribed.<br>Fasting state: overnight or 6 h.<br>Fructose dose: 0.25 g/kg as 10% solution given over 1–3 min.<br>Blood samples: baseline, 10, 20, 30, 40, 50, 60 and 90 min.<br>Determinations: glucose, (fructose), lactic acid, phosphate and uric acid (P).<br>*Caution:*<br>Watch for hypoglycaemia between 20 and 50 min.<br>10% i.v. glucose solution should be immediately available as needed in symptomatic patients (*see* Table "Emergency treatment").<br>Nausea and abdominal pain are frequent in affected individuals.<br>*Interpretation:*<br>A decrease of glucose and phosphate and an increase of uric acid are typical for HFI. A decrease of glucose and an increase of lactate are characteristic for FBP-D. In FK-D a blunted increase of glucose and a rise in fructose can be detected. Oral fructose loading test is not advocated in the case of suspicion of HFI since oral administration of fructose may cause severe gastrointestinal symptoms and long-lasting hypoglycaemia.<br>*Indications:*<br>Patients with a suspicion of glycerate kinase deficiency (*see* Chap. 71).<br>Fasting state: overnight or 6 h.<br>Fructose dose: 1.0 g/kg as 10% solution given over 5–10 min.<br>Following the load, approximately 4% of the test dose is excreted as d-glycerate in a 24-h urine. A loading test with 200–300 mg/kg of the amino<br>acid l-serine may be equally effective. |

Functional tests (continued)

| **Intravenous glucagon test** |
|---|
| *Indication:*<br>Differentiation of hypoglycaemia. Today less important after development of enzymatic and molecular genetic studies. Helpful in questionable cases.<br>Application of glucagon 0.03 mg/kg (slowly iv) during spontaneous or induced hypoglycaemia.<br>Baseline glucose (P) <60 mg/dL (<3.5 mM), glucose (P) and lactate (P) at 15, 25, 35, 45, 60 min<br>*Caution:*<br>Nausea, vomiting, if given too fast; may be caused by additional formation of ketones.<br>*Interpretation:*<br>Normally, glucose (P) rises by >25 mg/dL (>1.4 mM). Insufficient response indicates depleted glycogen stores, inability to convert glycogen to glucose, or, at the end of a fasting test, impaired gluconeogenesis. Lactate (P) may rise in disorders of gluconeogenesis. X |
| **Non-ischaemic forearm test** (*see also* Hogrel et al. 2015) |
| *Indication:*<br>Diagnosis of muscular GSDs, *e.g.,* types V and VII.<br>An indwelling catheter is placed in the exercising arm.<br>Grip contraction at 70% of maximal voluntary contraction for 30 s.<br>Blood samples: baseline, 1, 2, 3, 4, 6 and 10 min after the end of the exercise<br>Determinations: ammonia (P) and lactate (P).<br>*Cautions:*<br>In case of muscle cramp, stop exercise immediately.<br>*Interpretation:*<br>No increase of lactate (P) occurs in muscle GSDs (except GSD-XI, LDH deficiency), in contrast ammonia (P) increases. |

## Specimen Collection

For specimen collection see Table below.

Specimen collection for laboratory tests in disorders of carbohydrate metabolism

| Test | Material | Preconditions | Handling | Pitfalls |
|---|---|---|---|---|
| *Metabolites* | | | | |
| Glucose | P | Fasted/*non*-fasted | NaF tubes | Bacterial contamination[a] |
| Glucose | CSF | Fasted (!)[b] | | Bacterial contamination[a], pleocytosis |
| Glucose | U | | | Bacterial contamination[a] |
| Reducing substances | U | | | Bacterial contamination[a] , medications |
| Reducing substances | Stool | | | Bacterial contamination[a] |
| Galactose | P | Fasted/*non*-fasted | Perchloric acid extract | |
| Galactose | U | | | Bacterial contamination[a] |
| Gal-1-P | RBC | | Washed | |
| Galactitol | U | | | Bacterial contamination[a] |
| Sorbitol | U | | | Bacterial contamination[a] |
| Lactic acid | P | Fasted/*non*-fasted | Perchloric acid extract or NaF tubes | Hypoxia[a] |
| Lactic acid | CSF | Fasted (!) | Perchloric acid extract or NaF tubes | [a] |
| Glycogen | Liver | | Freeze immediately, store at –70 °C[c] | |
| Glycogen | Muscle | | Freeze immediately, store at –70 °C[c] | |
| *Enzymes* | | | | |
| Lactase | Intestine | | Freeze immediately, store at –70 °C[c] | |
| Sucrase | Intestine | | Freeze immediately, store at –70 °C[c] | |

| Test | Material | Preconditions | Handling | Pitfalls |
|---|---|---|---|---|
| Isomaltase | Intestine | | Freeze immediately, store at −70 °C[c] | |
| Trehalase | Intestine | | Freeze immediately, store at −70 °C[c] | |
| Galactokinase | RBC | | Washed, frozen[c] | |
| GALT | RBC | | Washed, ship at room temperature[c] | |
| UDPGal-4-epimerase | RBC | | Washed, frozen[c] | |
| Frc-1-P aldolase (AldoB) | Liver, Intestine | | Freeze immediately, store at −70 °C[c] | |
| Frc-1,6-P biphosphatase | Liver | | Freeze immediately, store at −70 °C[c] | |
| Liver GSD enzymes | Liver | | Freeze immediately, store at −70 °C[c] | |
| Muscle GSD enzymes | Muscle | | Freeze immediately, store at −70 °C[c] | |
| *Transporter assays* | | | | |
| GLUT1 | RBC | | Assay in unfrozen EDTA sample[c] | |
| SGLT1 | Intestinal biopsy | | Assay in unfrozen tissue[c] | |
| Glucose-6-P-translocase | Liver | | Assay in unfrozen tissue[c] | |

[a]Always store samples at −20 °C if immediate processing is not possible

[b]Always use fasted samples and draw a plasma sample for determination of CSF/P ratio just *before (!)* the lumbar puncture

[c]Since assay conditions may vary with time and with different reference laboratories, you are encouraged to contact these laboratories before obtaining specimens

## DNA Testing

Table 'Special conditions for enzymatic and/or molecular genetic diagnosis in disorders of carbohydrate metabolism' refers to the question how to arrive at a definite diagnosis with minimal invasiveness and calculated costs.

Metabolites (in easily accessible samples!) can be helpful in some cases but it is not necessary, for example, to quantitate glycogen content in liver or muscle tissue in all cases with a suspicion of GSD. Likewise, it is possible to arrive at a definite diagnosis by transporter studies or measurement of enzymatic activity in biopsy samples; however, affected proteins are not always expressed in tissues that are easily available, which can make conventional diagnosis very invasive. Today, molecular genetic studies from DNA samples from peripheral blood are possible for all disorders. Targeted genetic diagnosis is warranted in cases with good clinical classification; it will depend on the size of the respective gene and the existence of common genetic variants in the population under study. DNA panel studies have become available recently for cases without high suspicion of a single gene defect, and cases with unspecific clinical signs and symptoms will be diagnosed by whole exome, genome, or transcriptome studies with increasing frequency.

Special conditions for enzymatic and/or molecular genetic diagnosis in disorders of carbohydrate metabolism (Detailed information should be retrieved from databases)

| No. | Disorder | Basis for enzyme/transporter assay (from peripheral blood) | | Basic data for molecular genetic characterisation | | |
|---|---|---|---|---|---|---|
| | | Possible | | Gene | (Gene size) | Common pathogenic variants |
| 39.1 | CL-D | | | *LCT* | (17 exons) | p.Y1390* in Finland |
| 39.2 | CSI-D | | | *SI* | (48 exons) | c.273_274delAG in Inuits;<br>p.V577G,<br>p.G1073D,<br>p.F1745C, and<br>p.R1124* responsible for 80% of cases in Greenlanders (8% homozygous) |
| 39.3 | TREH-D | | | *TREH* | (15 exons) | |
| 39.4 | SGLT1-D (GGM) | | | *SLC5A1* | (15 exons) | Common haplotype in Amish |
| 39.5 | SGLT2-D | | | *SLC5A2* | (14 exons) | c.885+5G>A mutational hotspot with variable ethnic background |
| 39.6 | MAP17-D | | | *MAP17* | (4 exons) | *Reported only in single case* |
| 39.7 | GLUT1-D | ↓ | Transport/protein in RBC | *SLC2A1* | (10 exons) | |
| 39.8 | IDDNPF | | | *SLC45A1* | (9 exons) | *Reported only in two families* |
| 39.9 | GLUT2 (FBS) | | | *SLC2A2* | (11 exons) | |
| 39.10 | GALM-D | | | *GALM* | (7 exons) | *Only recently described*[a] |
| 39.11 | GALK-D | ↓ | Enzyme act in RBC | *GALK* | (8 exons) | p.P28T in Eastern European Roma<br>p.A198V in Japanese and Koreans |
| 39.12 | GALT-D | ↓ | Enzyme act in RBC | *GALT* | (10 exons) | p.Q188R in Caucasians<br>p.K285N in Caucasians |
| 39.13 | GALE-D | ↓ | Enzyme act in RBC | *GALE* | (11 exons) | |
| 39.14 | FK-D | | | *FK* | (7 exons) | |

Enzymatic and molecular diagnosis (continued)

| | | | | | | |
|---|---|---|---|---|---|---|
| 39.15 | ALDOB-D (HFI) | | | *ALDOB* | (9 exons) | p.A150P in Caucasians<br>p.A175D in Caucasians<br>p.N335K on the Balkans<br>IVS1+1G>C in Hispanics and Afro-Americans |
| 39.16 | HK1-D | ↓ | Enzyme act in RBC | *HK1* | (18 exons) | |
| 39.17 | HK1-D (NEDVIBA) | | *Enzyme act normal !* | *HK1* | | In the N-terminal regulatory domain |
| 39.18 | HK1-D (HMSNR) | | *Enzyme act normal !* | *HK1* | | Common haplotype in Roma Gypsy |
| 39.19 | HK1-D (RP79) | | *Enzyme act normal !* | *HK1* | | p.E847K in all patients |
| 39.20 | GCK-D (MODY2) | | | *GCK* | (11 exons) | |
| 39.21 | GCK-HI (HHF3) | | | *GCK* | | Activating variants, frequently in exon 11 |
| 39.22 | G6PI-D | ↓ | Enzyme act in RBC, WBC | *GPI* | (18 exons) | |
| 39.23 | GSD-VII | ↓ | Enzyme act in RBC | *PFKM* | (24 exons) | IVS5+1G>A in Ashkenazi Jews |
| 39.24 | ALDOA-D | ↓ | Enzyme act in RBC | *ALDOA* | (12 exons) | |
| 39.25 | TPI-D | ↓ | Enzyme act in RBC | *TPI1* | (7 exons) | p.E104D in Caucasians |
| 39.26 | PGK-D | ↓ | Enzyme act in RBC | *PGK1* | (11 exons) | |
| 39.27 | GSD-X | | | *PGAM2* | (3 exons) | p.W78* in Afro-Americans (?)[b] |
| 39.28 | GSD-XIII | | | *ENO3* | (12 exons) | |
| 39.29 | PK-D | ↓ | Enzyme act in RBC | *PKLR* | (11 exons) | p.R486W and p.R479H in Indians<br>p.R510Q in Central Europe |
| 39.30 | LDHA-D (GSD-XI) | + | Enzyme act in RBC | *LDHA* | (7 exons) | ex6 del20bp in Japanese (?)[b] |
| 39.31 | LDHB-D | ↓ | Enzyme act in RBC, serum | *LDHB* | (8 exons) | *Non-disease* |
| 39.32 | D-LDH-D | | | *DLDH* | (11 exons) | *Reported only in two families* |
| 39.33 | GSD-XV (PGBM2) | | | *GYG1* | (8 exons) | |
| 39.34 | GSD-0b | | | *GYS1* | (16 exons) | |
| 39.35 | GSD-0a | | | *GYS2* | (16 exons) | |
| 39.36 | GSD-IV | ↓ | Enzyme act in WBC, RBC | *GBE1* | (16 exons) | |
| 39.37 | GSD-IXd | | | *PHKA1* | (31 exons) | |
| 39.38 | GSD-IXa | ↓[c] | Enzyme act in RBC, WBC | *PHKA2* | (33 exons) | p.P1205L in Dutch |
| 39.39 | GSD-IXb | ↓ | Enzyme act in RBC, WBC | *PHKB* | (33 exons) | |
| 39.40 | GSD-IXc | ↓ | Enzyme act in RBC, WBC | *PHKG2* | (10 exons) | |
| 39.41 | AMPK-A | | | *PRKAG2* | (12 exons[d]) | p.R302Q (?)[b,e]<br>p.R531Q (?)[b,f] |
| 39.42 | GSD-V | | | *PYGM* | (20 exons) | p.R50* in Japanese and Caucasians<br>p.G205S in Japanese and Spanish<br>p.L542T in Japanese |
| 39.43 | GSD-VI | | | *PYGL* | (20 exons) | c.1620+1G>A (heterozygosity in ~ 3% of the Mennonite population) |
| 39.44 | GSD-III | ↓ | Enzyme act in WBC | *AGL* | (35 exons) | c.16C>T [p.R6*][g]<br>c.17_18delAG[f]<br>p.R408* in Norwegians and Faroese<br>c.2039G>A (p.Trp680*) in Arubans<br>c.4455delT in North African Jews |
| 39.45 | GSD-Ia | | | *G6PC* | (5 exons) | p.R83C in Caucasians, Turks, Ashkenazi Jews<br>p.Q347* in Caucasians<br>c.648G>T [p.=] in Japanese, Chinese<br>c.380insTA in Hispanics<br>c.648G>T in Koreans |
| 39.46 | G6PC3-D | ↓ | Enzyme act in WBC | *G6PC3* | (5 exons) | p.R235H in Turks and Arabs |
| 39.47 | GSD-Ib | ↓<br>↓ | Transport act in WBC[h]<br>G6Pase act in WBC[h] | *G6PT* | (9 exons) | p.W118R in Japanese<br>p.G339C in Caucasians<br>c.1042_3delCT in Caucasians |
| 39.48 | HOIL1-D (PGBM1) | | | *RBCK1* | (11 exons) | |
| 39.49 | HOIL1-IP-D | | | *RNF31* | (21 exons) | *Reported only in two families* |

Enzymatic and molecular diagnosis (continued)

| | | | | | | |
|---|---|---|---|---|---|---|
| 39.50 | EPM2A-D (Laforin-D) | | | *EPM2A* | (5 exons) | |
| 39.51 | EPM2B-D (Malin-D) | | | *NHLRC1* | (1 exon) | p.C26S, p.P69A in Canadians |
| 39.52 | GSD-IIa | ↓ | Enzyme act in WBC, dried blood spots | *GAA* | (20 exons) | IVS1-13T>G in Caucasians[i]<br>c.525delT in Caucasians<br>ex18del in Caucasians<br>p.D645E in Chinese and Taiwanese |
| 39.53 | GSD-IIb | | | *LAMP2* | (10 exons) | IVS5+1G>A (?)[b] in Japanese, Caucasians |
| 39.54 | PC-D | | | *PC* | (19 exons) | |
| 39.55 | mtPCK-D | | | *PCK2* | (10 exons) | |
| 39.56 | cPCK-D | | | *PCK1* | (10 exons) | |
| 39.57 | FBP-D | | | *FBP1* | (7 exons) | 1del in Turkey and Armenia[j] c.960insG in Japan |

[a] Wada et al. (2019)
[b] Question mark refers to a small number of cases
[c] Phosphorylase kinase activity in blood cells is diminished in types IXb and IXc but only in about 50% of GSD-IXa cases (=GSD-IXa-1 = XLG-1)
[d] For *PRKAG2b*
[e] In lethal congenital GSD of the heart
[f] In hypertrophic cardiomyopathy and WPW syndrome
[g] In GSD-IIIb patients
[h] In unfrozen sample
[i] With an adult-type variant of the disease
[k] *See* Santer et al. (2016)

### Prenatal Diagnosis

In principle, prenatal diagnosis is possible for all disorders by molecular genetic techniques with DNA samples from chorionic villi or amniotic fluid cells. For some disorders, prenatal enzymatic studies in amniotic fluid cells have been reported.

## Treatment Summary

Treatment depends on the underlying disorder and, for some disorders (*highlighted in bold in* Table 'Principles and measures of long-term treatment'), guidelines are published. In many of these disorders with symptomatic hypoglycaemia as part of the acute presentation, a rapid normalisation of blood glucose is important (*see* Table 'Initial treatment'). Long-term treatment aims and measures are summarised in Table 'Principles and measures of long-term treatment'; specific treatment in certain groups of disorders are given below. Many patients require personalised dietary measures prescribed by specialised dietitians, familiar with age-specific requirements, from the newborn period until late adulthood.

### Emergency Treatment

In some disorders, episodes of metabolic emergencies can be triggered by catabolism, evoked by combinations of fever, decreased enteral intake and increased enteral losses by vomiting and/or diarrhea. To ensure safe shared care for patients with fasting intolerance in a subset of the disorders of carbohydrate absorption, transmembrane transport and metabolism, a written emergency protocol is warranted and should be personalised based on the age/body weight and specific disorder. If possible, the responsible metabolic centre should be contacted in advance in the case of a surgical procedure, to provide perioperative recommendations.

Initial treatment of acute, symptomatic hypoglycaemia in patients with a disorder affecting endogenous glucose production[a]

| Age | | Immediate bolus (within 5–10 min) | | Followed by continuous glucose infusion[b] |
|---|---|---|---|---|
| | | mg Glc/kg b.w. | mL (Glc 10%)/kg b.w. | mg glucose/kg b.w.per min |
| 0–1 | Years | 500 | 5 | 7–9 |
| 1–6 | Years | 400 | 4 | 6–8 |
| 6–12 | Years | 350 | 3.5 | 5–7 |
| Adolescents | | 300 | 3 | 4–6 |
| Adults | | 250 | 2.5 | 2–4 |

[a] In patients with a confirmed metabolic disorder causing hypoglycaemia, treatment is challenged by (a) the risk of rebound hypoglycaemia due to hyperinsulinism, (b) the necessity of continuation of iv glucose, and/or (c) the careful reintroduction of enteral feeds. If possible, oral treatment is preferable to manage both symptomatic and asymptomatic hypoglycaemia, under clinical supervision. Based on symptoms and signs, the exogenous glucose intake should be titrated based on blood glucose values and secondary metabolic parameters, such as lactate concentrations and blood gas analyses in GSD-I patients.
[b] Consider to adapt rate of glucose in case of fever

If galactose-1-phosphate uridyltransferase deficiency is suspected, for instance after positive newborn screening tests, a galactose-restricted diet should be started immediately, without waiting for confirmation of the diagnosis. Likewise, severe liver problems (*e.g.* a coagulation disorder) and a suitable dietary history justify to stop fructose intake with the diet. Severe postnatal osmotic diarrhoea and hypovolaemia should be treated by intravenous rehydration and omitting enteral carbohydrates prior to a definite diagnosis.

## Standard Treatment

Principles and measures of long-term treatment of disorders of carbohydrate metabolism[a]

| No. | Disorder | Principle | Measures |
|---|---|---|---|
| 39.1 | CL-D | Avoid *non*-absorbable lactose | Lac-free diet for life |
| 39.2 | CSI-D | Avoid *non*-absorbable disaccharides, starch | Sac-restricted diet, sucrase replacement with feeds |
| 39.3 | TREH-D | Avoid *non*-absorbable disaccharide | Treh-restricted diet |
| 39.4 | SGLT1-D (GGM) | Avoid *non*-absorbable monosaccharides | Glc- and Gal-restricted diet for life |
| 39.5 | SGLT2-D | | *No specific Tx necessary* |
| 39.6 | MAP17-D | | *No specific Tx necessary* |
| 39.7 | **GLUT1-D** | Improve energy supply to the brain:<br>Use ketone bodies (transported by MCT1 at the BBB) as an alternative substrate | Avoid fasting, avoid valproic acid; low CH, high-fat (modified Atkins) diet, ketogenic diet |
| 39.8 | IDDNPF | *as for* 39.7 (?) | *as for* 39.7 (?) |
| 39.9 | GLUT2-D (FBS) | Compensate for impaired hepatic Glc uptake and release<br>Compensate for impaired hepatic Gal uptake<br>Compensate for generalised impairment of proximal renal tubular cells secondary to Glc and glycogen overload | Continuous enteral supply of slowly released CH to stabilise blood Glc and suppress gluconeogenesis<br>Gal restriction<br>Symptomatic Tx of renal Fanconi syndrome |
| 39.10 | GALM-D | Prevent accumulation of toxic galactitol in eye lens | Gal-restricted diet for life |
| 39.11 | GALK-D | Prevent accumulation of toxic galactitol in eye lens | Gal-restricted diet for life |
| 39.12 | **GALT-D** | Prevent accumulation of toxic Gal-1-P | Gal-restricted diet for life |
| 39.13 | GALE-D | Prevent accumulation of toxic Gal-1-P | Gal-restricted diet for life |
| 39.14 | FK-D | | *No specific Tx necessary* |
| 39.15 | ALDOB-D (HFI) | Prevent accumulation of toxic Frc-1-P | Strict Frc-restriction for life, avoid iv Frc/sorbitol |
| 39.16 | HK1-D | | |
| 39.17 | HK1 (NEDVIBA) | | |
| 39.18 | HK1 (HMSNR) | | |
| 39.19 | HK1 (RP79) | | |
| 39.20 | **GCK-D** (MODY2) | Normalise blood glucose | Diet, antidiabetic drugs, insulin |
| 39.21 | GCK-HI (HHF3) | Normalise blood glucose | Diet, diazoxide |
| 39.22 | G6PI-D | | |
| 39.23 | GSD-VII | Compensate for diminished access to glycogen (M) | Symptoms can worsen if carbohydrates are taken before exercise |
| 39.24 | ALDOA-D | Compensate for diminished access to glycogen (M) | |
| 39.25 | TPI-D | | |
| 39.26 | PGK-D | Compensate for diminished access to glycogen (M) | |
| 39.27 | GSD-X | Compensate for diminished access to glycogen (M) | |
| 39.28 | GSD-XIII | Compensate for diminished access to glycogen (M) | |
| 39.29 | **PK-D** | | |
| 39.30 | LDHA-D (GSD-XI) | Compensate for diminished access to glycogen (M) | |
| 39.31 | LDHB-D | | *No specific Tx necessary* |
| 39.32 | D-LDH-D | Avoid accumulation of uric acid | Allopurinol |
| 39.33 | GSD-XV (PGBM2) | Compensate for diminished glycogen stores (M) | |
| 39.34 | GSD-0b | Compensate for diminished glycogen stores (M) | |
| 39.35 | GSD-0a | Provide exogenous CH that can compensate for diminished glycogen stores (L) | Avoid fasting, frequent CH-rich feeds, continuous enteral supply of slowly released CH |
| 39.36 | GSD-IV | Treat cirrhosis induced by abnormal glycogen (L) | Symptomatic Tx (… liver Tpx) |
| 39.37 | GSD-IXd | Compensate for diminished access to glycogen (M) | |
| 39.38 | **GSD-IXa** | Provide exogenous CH that can be metabolised despite impairment of glycogenolysis (L) | Avoid fasting, frequent CH-rich feeds, continuous enteral supply of slowly released CH |
| 39.39 | **GSD-IXb** | *See* 39.38 | *See* 39.38 |
| 39.40 | **GSD-IXc** | *See* 39.38, treat cirrhosis | *See* 39.38, symptomatic Tx of cirrhosis (… liver Tpx) |
| 39.41 | AMPK-A | | *No specific Tx available,* symptomatic Tx (… heart Tpx) |
| 39.42 | **GSD-V** | Compensate for diminished access to glycogen (M) | Diet rich in complex carbohydrates, exercise program |

Standard Treatment (continued)

| No. | Disorder | Principle | Measures |
|---|---|---|---|
| 39.43 | **GSD-VI** | Provide exogenous CH that can be metabolised despite impairment of glycogenolysis (L) | Avoid fasting, frequent CH-rich feeds, continuous enteral supply of slowly released CH |
| 39.44 | **GSD-III** | Provide exogenous CH that can be metabolised despite impairment of glycogenolysis (L)<br>Treat cirrhosis | Avoid fasting, frequent CH-rich feeds, continuous enteral supply of slowly released CH<br>Symptomatic Tx (… liver Tpx) |
| 39.45 | **GSD-Ia** | Provide exogenous CH that can be metabolised despite impairment of glycogenolysis and gluconeogenesis (L)<br>Avoid accumulation of uric acid<br>Correct primary defect<br>Treat adenoma complications (anaemia, tumour)<br>Treat renal complications | Avoid fasting, frequent CH-rich feeds, continuous enteral supply of slowly released CH, Gal- and Frc-restriction<br>Allopurinol<br>L-Tpx (?)<br>L-Tpx<br>Symptomatic Tx (… kidney Tpx) |
| 39.46 | G6PC3-D | | |
| 39.47 | **GSD-Ib** | *See* 39.45 *plus*<br>Prophylaxis and Tx of bacterial infections | *See* 39.45 *plus*<br>Antibiotic prophylaxis, G-CSF |
| 39.48 | HOIL1-D (PGBM1) | | *No specific Tx available,* symptomatic |
| 39.49 | HOIL1-IP-D | | *No specific Tx available,* symptomatic |
| 39.50 | EPM2A-D (Laforin-D) | | *No specific Tx available,* symptomatic |
| 39.51 | EPM2B-D (Malin-D) | | *No specific Tx available,* symptomatic |
| 39.52 | **GSD-IIa** | Replace missing enzyme in lysosomes | Enzyme replacement therapy |
| 39.53 | GSD-IIb | | *No specific Tx available,* symptomatic (… heart Tpx) |
| 39.54 | PC-D | Circumvent impaired gluconeogenesis, Anaplerosis; stimulate residual enzyme activity | Avoid fasting,<br>supply citrate, triheptanoate; biotin, (… liver Tpx?) |
| 39.55 | mtPCK-D | Circumvent impaired gluconeogenesis | Avoid fasting |
| 39.56 | cPCK-D | Circumvent impaired gluconeogenesis | Avoid fasting |
| 39.57 | FBP-D | Circumvent impaired gluconeogenesis<br>Avoid additional inhibition of glycogenolytic enzymes by accumulating Frc-1-P | Avoid fasting,<br>Frc-restricted diet for life, particularly during fasting |

(L), in liver; (M) in muscle; *Tx* Treatment, *CH* Carbohydrates, *BBB* Blood brain barrier, *Tpx* Transplantation, *G-CSF* Granulocyte-colony stimulating factor

aFor disorders presented in bold an international treatment guideline exists (*see* Kossoff et al. 2018; Welling et al. 2017; Rubio-Cabezas et al. 2014; Bianchi et al. 2019; Kishnani et al. 2019; Quinlivan et al. 2014; Rake et al. 2002; Kishnani et al. 2010; Kishnani et al. 2014; Visser et al. 2002; Kishnani et al. 2006; van der Ploeg et al. 2017)

## Intestinal Carbohydrate Malabsorption

Neonatal hypertonic dehydration frequently requires intravenous fluid therapy for which glucose-containing solutions with electrolytes can be used. Long-term enteral nutrition has to avoid the offending sugars: both glucose and galactose as monomers, as well as disaccharides and polymers of these sugars in GGM, and lactose in CL-D. Specialised commercial infant formulas containing fat and protein but free of a carbohydrate component can be used in GGM and fructose should be added according to the dietary allowances for carbohydrates to meet caloric needs. Small amounts of glucose and galactose are usually tolerated later in life. Patients with CL-D tolerate mono- and oligosaccharides. High fluid intake is recommended to prevent renal stone formation, which has repeatedly been reported in both conditions.

*Follow-up:* Clinical monitoring (nutrient intake, growth, nutritional status, general health), biochemical and paraclinical monitoring (haemoglobin, total protein, general parameters of liver and kidney function, plasma osmolarity and electrolytes, urinary glucose, renal ultrasound) should be planned depending on age, severity of initial decompensation and compliance.

## Renal Glucosuria

Allow free access to fluid. Caloric intake should compensate for renal losses in the severe cases. No specific treatment is necessary.

*Follow-up:* Only the severe recessive types need systematic follow-up.

## Glucose Transporter-1 Deficiency

For most patients, an effective treatment is available by means of a modified Atkins diet or a ketogenic diet, both providing ketones as an alternative fuel for the brain. Ketones enter the brain via the facilitative MCT1 transporter. The diet should be introduced in a clinical setting and requires an experienced pediatrician and a dietitian. The classic ketogenic diet, with a

3:1 ratio (fat vs *non*-fat intake in grams) using long-chain triglycerides is used for seizure control in infantile cases and preschool children. A modified Atkins diet, which is less restrictive, may be sufficient in milder cases with an isolated movement disorder. It can be considered in school-age children, adolescents and adults when the classic ketogenic diet is not tolerated. Fluids and calories are not restricted. Supplements (multivitamins, calcium and often carnitine) are required. Certain anticonvulsive drugs are relatively contraindicated: chloralhydrate, valproate and topiramate interfere with the diet, while others (phenobarbital, methylxanthines (caffeine), ethanol) have been shown to affect GLUT1 function.

*Experimental treatment:* In individual patients, acetazolamide has shown good responses in movement disorders caused by GLUT1-D. However, when acetazolamide is given in combination with a ketogenic diet, there is an increased risk of nephrolithiasis and it may potentiate metabolic acidosis. *Alpha*-lipoic acid, an antioxidant, has been shown to increase glucose transport in cultured muscle cells but *in vivo* data is not available. Oral triheptanoin, an artificial triglyceride composed of three seven-carbon fatty acids and potentially providing additional fuel for brain energy metabolism, is currently on clinical trial.

Pitfalls/dangers of a ketogenic diet

1. Incorrect calculations: *Note* that the ratio of the ketogenic diet is defined in grams, not in calories or percentages! A 3:1 ratio means that, for 3 g of ingested fat, only 1 g of protein and carbohydrates is allowed. Thus, on a 3:1 ketogenic diet, 87% of kilocalories per day are supplied by fat. Percentages of protein and carbohydrates vary due to age-dependent protein requirements.
2. Non-compliance: *Assess* ketones in blood and urine. If ketones are inappropriately low, intensify dietary instructions and be aware that many medications have a high carbohydrate content!
3. Contraindications: β-oxidation defects, disorders of gluconeogenesis, ketolysis defects, porphyria, long QTc syndrome, relative contraindication concomitant use of propofol or pentobarbital coma
4. During intercurrent illness there is a risk of ketoacidosis and/or hypoglycaemia, provide an emergency protocol for these situations. Include a perioperative plan regarding intravenous fluids and monitoring of glucose/ketones in case surgery is necessary.

Nutritional requirements on a ketogenic diet

| Age | | Fat requirements (g/kg bw per day) | Protein requirements[a] (g/kg bw per day) | Carbohydrates (g/kg bw per day) | Energy demand[b] (g/kg bw per day) |
|---|---|---|---|---|---|
| 0–4 | months | 9.0 | 2.2 | 0.8 | 93 |
| 4–12 | months | 9.0 | 1.6 | 1.4 | 91 |
| 1–3 | years | 8.7 | 1.2 | 1.7 | 90 |
| 4–6 | years | 7.8 | 1.1 | 1.5 | 80 |
| 7–9 | years | 7.0 | 1.0 | 1.3 | 72 |
| 10–12 | years | 5.8 | 1.0 | 0.9 | 60 |
| 13–15 | years | 5.0 | 1.0 | 0.7 | 52 |
| Adults | | 5.0 | 1.0 | 0.7 | 52 |

[a]Recommendations from the German Society for Nutrition (DGE; 1991)
[b]German-Austrian-Swiss (DACH) recommendations (2000)

Investigations on introduction and follow-up of a ketogenic diet

| On admission | Initiation of diet | On discharge | Follow-up every 2–3(–6) months |
|---|---|---|---|
| Clinical[a]<br>Paraclinical<br>Glucose (P), OHB, BGA<br>Electrolytes<br>Liver/kidney parameters<br>Blood count, CRP<br>Fasting lipid profile<br>Essential fatty acids<br>Vitamin D level<br>Acylcarnitine profile<br>Serum amino acids and Urine organic acids (If diagnosis unclear)<br>Urine sediment and calcium/creatinin ratio<br>Drug monitoring<br>EEG, EKG<br>Abdominal sonography on Indication when there is A risk of nephrolithiasis | Clinical[a]<br>Paraclinical<br>Glucose (P), OHB, BGA<br>Preferably bedside 2–4×/day;<br>If not possible, Ketones in urine | Clinical[a]<br>Paraclinical<br>Glucose (P), OHB, BGA<br>Electrolytes<br>Liver/kidney parameters<br>EEG<br>Abdominal sonography | Clinical[a]<br>Paraclinical<br>Glucose (P), OHB, BGA<br>Electrolytes<br>Liver/kidney parameters<br>Blood count, CRP<br>Acylcarnitine profile<br>Fasting lipid profile<br>Essential fatty acids<br>Vitamin D level<br>Selenium level<br>Urine sediment and Calcium/creatinin ratio<br>Drug monitoring<br>EEG (seizure control?)<br>EKG (long QT?)<br>Abdominal sonography (Nephrolithiasis?)<br>DXA scan after 2 years |

[a]Nutrient intake, growth, nutritional status, somatic findings, review medication for carbohydrate content

Monitoring of ketosis on a ketogenic diet

| Sample | Ketone body | Test | Target value |
|---|---|---|---|
| Urine | Acetoacetate | Test strips | 80 (++)–160 (+++) mg/dL |
| Blood | Hydroxybutyrate | Test strips (hand devices) | >2 mmol/L |
| Serum/plasma | Total ketone bodies | Enzymatic | 3–5 mmol/L |

### Fanconi-Bickel syndrome

Patients with FBS show signs of a hepatic GSD with impaired glycogenolysis and gluconeogenesis. Therefore, treatment should be similar to GSD-1 (*see below*) with frequent feeds and the use of slowly absorbed carbohydrates. Continuous nocturnal enteral nutrition may rescue growth failure (Pennisi et al. 2020). Blood glucose concentrations should be in a range, so that gluconeogenesis is suppressed in order to avoid glycogen accumulation. This can be accomplished by a constant supply of slow release carbohydrates (frequent feeds, corn starch, nasogastric oligosaccharide drip feeding). In contrast to GSD-1, there is no evidence that a fructose-/sucrose-restricted diet is beneficial to FBS patients. Likewise, there are patients with FBS that have ingested high amounts of galactose/lactose without developing cataracts. Therefore, galactose restriction is not generally recommended, but galactose and galactose-1-phosphate levels should be monitored.

Due to the propensity to hypoglycaemia of FBS patients, the use of insulin for impaired glucose tolerance has to be considered with extreme caution and only after dietary measures have failed.

There is no specific treatment for the Fanconi-type nephropathy. Symptomatic treatment is recommended to compensate for losses of water, sodium, potassium, calcium, phosphate, vitamin D and bicarbonate. Maintenance therapy should be monitored by urinary calcium excretion. Carnitine supplementation should only be performed at low plasma levels or when signs and symptoms of a secondary mitochondrial disorder are observed.

### Disorders of Galactose Metabolism

If a disorder of galactose metabolism is suspected in a newborn, dietary treatment consisting of a lactose-/galactose-free feeding regimen should be initiated without delay, even before the diagnosis has been confirmed enzymatically or by DNA analysis. In classical galactosaemia, supportive care depends on the severity of liver, renal and central nervous system disease and comprises intravenous fluids, plasma and vitamin K. Initiate treatment with broad-spectrum antibiotics without delay if suspicion of sepsis arises, since, in the event of acute metabolic derangement, patients are at risk of infections due to the compromised response of the immune system.

Long-term treatment requires a galactose-restricted diet for life in all four conditions. There is increasing evidence that small amounts of galactose are acceptable in GALK-D and GALT-D as long as it is in the range of endogenous galactose production. In the severe forms of GALE-D, some dietary galactose (1–2 g/d) and also N-acetyl-galactosamine intake is even necessary for the biosynthesis of complex carbohydrates and galactolipids. Excess, however, should be avoided, as this leads to accumulation of galactose-1-phosphate. Sufficient calcium intake and if necessary supplementation of vitamin D should be guaranteed to protect patients from osteoporosis.

Ovarian dysfunction with hypergonadotropic hypogonadism is observed in almost all female patients with GALT-D. Start ethinyl estradiol therapy from age 12–13 years, when gonadotropin levels are high and estradiol levels are low (first 6 months 2 μg daily; 6–12 months 2–5 μg daily; 12–24 months 5 μg daily; 24–36 months 10 μg daily; after 3 years, followed by an oral contraceptive preparation containing ethinyl estradiol and a progestagen daily for 21 days, 7 days abstinence) (Berry et al. 2016, Welling et al. 2017).

Follow-up in patients with disorders of galactose and fructose metabolism

| Disorder | Investigations | Frequency |
|---|---|---|
| GALM-D | Ophthalmological investigation<br>Paraclinical<br>Calcium metabolism, 25-OH-vitamin D<br>Galactose (P,U)<br>Galactitol (P,U) | <18 years: annually<br>>18 years: biannually |
| GALK-D | Ophthalmological investigation<br>Paraclinical<br>Calcium metabolism, 25-OH-vitamin D<br>Galactose (P,U)<br>Galactitol (P,U) | <18 years: annually<br>>18 years: biannually |
| GALT-D | Clinical[a,b]<br>Ophthalmological investigations<br>Paraclinical<br>Liver/kidney parameters<br>Calcium metabolism, 25-OH-vitamin D<br>Gal-1-P (RBC)<br>Galactitol (P,U)<br>CDT[d]<br>LH, FSH, estradiol (in females, starting around 12 years)<br>Pelvic ultrasound (in females)[e]<br>X-ray (left hand for bone age)[f]<br>Bone mineral density assessment[g] | <1 year: 3 monthly<br>1–4 years: 4 monthly<br>4–8 years: 6 monthly[c]<br>>18 years: annually[c] |

| Disorder | Investigations | Frequency |
|---|---|---|
| GALE-D | Clinical[a,b]<br>Ophthalmological investigations<br>Paraclinical<br>Liver/kidney parameters<br>Gal-1-P (RBC)<br>UDP-Gal (RBC)<br>Galactitol (U)<br>X-ray (left hand for bone age)[f]<br>Bone mineral density assessment[g] | <1 year: 3 monthly[h]<br>1–4 years: 4 monthly[h]<br>4–18 years: 6 monthly[h]<br>>18 years: annually[h] |
| FK-D | *None* | |
| HFI | Clinical[a]<br>Paraclinical<br>Liver/kidney parameters<br>CDT[d]<br>Folic acid (P), vitamin C (P)<br>Liver ultrasound | <12 years: 6 monthly<br>12–18 years: annually<br>>18 years: biannually |
| FBP-D | Clinical[a]<br>Paraclinical<br>Liver parameters<br>Glucose (P), Lactate (P) during infections | |

[a]Nutrient intake, growth, nutritional status, somatic findings (liver size)
[b]Neurological, psychological, cognitive functions, speech and language development
[c]Follow-up of female GALT-D patients on hormone treatment should be done on a more regular interval
[d]CDT, carbohydrate-deficient transferrin (abnormal glycosylation of transferrin)
[e]Not routinely recommended
[f]Depending on growth
[g]Start at age 8–10 years, repeat at puberty with follow-ups every 5 years
[h]In milder forms of GALE-D, follow-up can be less extensive

## Disorders of Fructose Metabolism

If HFI or FBP-D is suspected, dietary treatment consisting of a sucrose-, fructose-, and sorbitol-free feeding regimen should be initiated without delay, even before the diagnosis has been confirmed enzymatically or by DNA analysis (Steinmann and Santer 2016). Supportive care depends on the severity of liver and renal disease and comprises intravenous fluids, plasma and vitamin K.

In the long term, fructose tolerance in HFI is highly variable. At least in infancy, fructose should be maximally restricted and intake should not be determined by subjective tolerance.

For the maintenance of normal blood glucose concentrations, patients with FBP-D depend on glycogen breakdown and on exogenous glucose from intestinal absorption. Especially in young children, the relative amount of hepatic glycogen is limited. Only after a short period of fasting, patients may develop hypoglycaemia accompanied by accumulation of lactate. The most important aim of the dietary treatment is therefore maintenance of normoglycaemia by avoidance of fasting. In FBP-D, fructose intake should therefore be limited during periods of acute illness because accumulating fructose-1-phosphate inhibits liver phosphorylase. Certain amounts of fructose, particularly when taken with other carbohydrates, are generally tolerated in *non*-catabolic periods.

In patients on a fructose-restricted diet, vitamin C and folic acid should be supplemented.

## Glycogen Storage Diseases—Mainly Affecting Liver

Patients with defects in hepatic glycogenolysis (FBS, GSD-I, GSD-III, GSD-VI, GSD-IXa-c) but also with diminished hepatic glycogen formation (GSD-0a) may develop hypoglycaemia after only a short period of fasting. This holds especially true for younger patients and patients with GSD-I. A guideline for acute treatment of hypoglycaemia is given in Table 'Initial treatment of acute, symptomatic hypoglycaemia in patients with a disorder affecting endogenous glucose production', but amounts should be interpreted with caution because of the risk of overtreatment and iatrogenic hypoglycaemias. Hypoglycaemia may be accompanied by metabolic acidosis caused by accumulation of lactate (fasted in GSD-I, postprandial in so-called 'ketotic' GSDs) or ketones (GSD-III, GSD-VI, GSD-IXa-c, GSD-0, FBS). While lactic acidaemia will improve upon glucose administration in GSD I patients, in patients with a disorder affecting endogenous glucose production application of an excess of glucose in GSD-0a patients may lead to hyperglycaemia and/or lactacidaemia.

The aim of long-term treatment in hepatic GSDs is the stabilisation of blood glucose with concentrations at which gluconeogenesis and secondary metabolic perturbations are suppressed as much as possible, in order to prevent long-term complications and maximise quality of life. No consensus exists about the extent of avoiding lactate production in GSD-I from galactose, fructose and sucrose. Moderate hyperlactacidaemia may prevent cerebral symptoms if blood glucose concentration is low, as lactate may serve as an alternative fuel for the brain. On the other hand, some evidence exists that avoiding lactate production from endogenous sources or from galactose and fructose intake may favor long-term outcome.

Since glycogenolysis is impaired in hepatic GSDs (with the additional involvement of gluconeogenesis in GSD-I), these patients depend on exogenous glucose from intestinal absorption for the maintenance of a normal blood glucose concentration. After a short period of fasting, especially younger patients and patients with GSD-I may develop hypoglycaemia. There is evidence that both the *G6PC* genotype and alternative pathways of glycogenolysis define the GSD-Ia phenotype severity. The most important aim of dietary treatment is avoidance of fasting. Intensive dietary treatment induces catch-up growth, reduces liver size and ameliorates secondary biochemical abnormalities. In GSD-I, life-long dietary treatment is necessary. In GSD-III, dietary treatment is often less demanding and in general, in types VI and IX therapy is markedly easier with only about 50% of patients being prone to hypoglycaemia. In the latter types, dietary treatment is generally limited to younger children. In GSD-IV, dietary treatment may improve fasting intolerance related symptoms and signs, improve growth, normalize serum aminotransferases, and delay or prevent liver transplantation in a subset of patients (Derks et al. 2020).

Intensive dietary treatment with carbohydrates slowly absorbed from the intestine and dietary protein enrichment may also ameliorate secondary myogenic symptoms in the group of hepatic GSDs by counteracting increased gluconeogenesis and avoiding a drain from muscle protein.

Dietary treatment is based on frequent feedings during daytime depending on GSD type and individual fasting tolerance. For type I patients, the entire estimated endogenous glucose production has to be replaced by enteral feedings. The numbers given in the right column of Table 'Initial treatment of acute, symptomatic hypoglycaemia in patients with a disorder affecting endogenous glucose production' can serve as an orientation for a dietary prescription and have to be adapted individually and throughout life based on the age-specific requirements. Fasting tolerance during daytime can be prolonged by using uncooked cornstarch from which glucose is only slowly released to the blood stream. During the night and at a younger age (especially in GSD-I and III), continuous gastric drip-feeding may be necessary for 8–12 h. Uncooked cornstarch should not be started in children less than 6 months and may be carefully introduced after the age of 6-12 months, when pancreatic amylase activity maturates. Alternatively, but only at a later age, uncooked cornstarch may be given during the night at 4- to 6-h intervals, in late adolescence or adulthood at 6- to 8-h intervals, depending on parameters of metabolic control (Chen 2001).

In general, it is not necessary to replace breast milk in infants, except for those with GSD-I who may benefit from glucose-enriched lactose-/sucrose-free feedings or an oligosaccharide-based formula. In GSD-I for continuous gastric drip-feeding, a glucose/glucose polymer solution should be used; formulas enriched with maltodextrin are not recommended due to their high energy content.

Dietary manipulations in hepatic glycogen storage diseases

| Disorder | |
|---|---|
| GSD-0a | Frequent feeds, prevention of fasting[a]<br>Protein enriched diet (20%) |
| GSD-Ia<br>GSD-Ib | Frequent feeds, prevention of fasting[a]<br>High carbohydrate intake (55–70% of energy)<br>Moderate fat restriction (20–30%)<br>Predominantly polyunsaturated fatty acids<br>Moderate protein restriction (10-15%)<br>Sodium restriction<br>Galactose/fructose restriction |
| GSD-III | Frequent feeds, prevention of fasting[a]<br>Carbohydrate enriched diet (50–55% of energy)<br>Moderate fat restriction (20–30%)<br>Predominantly polyunsaturated fatty acids<br>Protein enriched diet (20%)[b] |
| All | Frequent feeds, prevention of fasting[a] |

[a]Depending on GSD type, individual fasting tolerance and age consider frequent snacks or corn starch during daytime and continuous gastric drip feeding and use of corn starch during the night (*see* text)
[b]In type IIIa with muscle involvement

In adolescent patients with GSD-I, in analogy to proteinuric insulin-dependent diabetic mellitus, reduction of protein intake should be considered. Furthermore, a reduction in sodium intake may enhance the beneficial effects of angiotensin-converting enzyme inhibitors.

Renoprotective treatment with an ACE inhibitor should be started in GSD-I patients as soon as microalbuminuria persists and before hypertension develops. Angiotensin II antagonists may elicit comparable results; however, clinical experience in GSD-I is more limited.

In order to prevent urate nephropathy in patients with hepatic glycogenosis, allopurinol (10 mg/kg/d in 3 doses, max 900 mg/d) should be started if serum uric acid concentration exceeds the upper normal level for age despite optimal dietary treatment. As uric acid is regarded to be a potent radical scavenger (with a possible protective role against premature atherosclerosis), the targeted uric acid concentration is in the high normal range.

Supplementation of vitamins should commence when WHO recommendations are not met. Furthermore, supplementation of calcium and vitamin D is important when intake of milk and milk-derived products is limited (GSD-I). Special attention is also needed regarding vitamin $B_1$ intake as increased metabolism of carbohydrates needs sufficient vitamin $B_1$.

If GSD-I patients show persistence of a deficit of bases (base excess <−5 mmol/L) or a low blood bicarbonate concentration (<20 mmol/L) despite intensive dietary treatment, it is recommended to correct lactacidaemia with (sodium) bicarbonate or (potassium) citrate. In addition to correcting acidosis, this will result in alkalinisation of the urine, which reduces the risk for urolithiasis and nephrocalcinosis. Citrate (initial dosage 1–2 mEq/kg/d in 3–4 doses) is preferred since it also corrects hypocitraturia, another risk factor for urolithiasis. Hypocitraturia is more often seen with increasing age of the patients.

A percutaneous endoscopic gastrostomy (PEG) tube should be placed only under the protection of granulocyte colony-stimulating factor (G-CSF; Neupogen) if a patient has neutropenia.

In GSD-Ib, prophylactic oral antibiotic treatment may be beneficial in patients with neutropenia but the effect has not been systematically studied. Cotrimoxazol has been recommended in symptomatic patients or those with an absolute neutrophil count below 500/nL.

For more than 25 years, GSD-Ib patients have been treated with G-CSF. The use of G-CSF should be restricted to the following indications: (1) persistent neutrophil count <$0.2 \times 10^9$/L; (2) a life-threatening infection requiring intravenous antibiotics; (3) complaints of inflammatory bowel disease, including oral or perianal infections, or severe diarrhoea. The clinical benefits (bacterial infections, enterocolitis) should be carefully balanced against the drawbacks (invasiveness, increased spleen size, risk of myelodysplasia or acute myeloid leukaemia) and the indication of haematopoietic stem cell transplantation, in severe cases.

A recent study enrolled 103 patients with a median G-CSF dose of 3.0 μg/kg/day. GSD-Ib patients seem to respond to low doses of G-CSF: a starting dose of 1.0 μg/kg sc daily or every other day is therefore recommended. Determine neutrophil count frequently and adjust the dose in steps of 2.5–5 μg/kg/d (maximum 25 μg/kg) based on symptoms and signs and target ANC of 0.5–1.0 × $10^9$/L. However, symptoms and signs do not seem to correlate strongly with ANC. In many cases, G-CSF decreases bacterial infections and ameliorates enterocolitis, but in some cases, conservative treatment (for instance, with 5-aminosalicylic acid, Mesalazin) might be of additional benefit.

Empagliflozin may develop into a promising treatment for neutropenia and neutrophil-dysfunction-related symptoms and signs in GSD-Ib patients (Santer et al. 2010, Wortmann et al. 2020).

Fibrates are indicated if triglyceride concentration in patients with hepatic GSDs remain above 10.0 mmol/l despite maximal dietary efforts. Fish oil treatment of hyperlipidaemia has a limited and temporary effect; use of medium-chain triglycerides has been advocated but remains controversial. Statins may be indicated in adult GSD-I patients with massive hypercholesterolaemia.

Treatment with growth hormones in patients with hepatic GSDs and growth retardation is not advocated, since the effect on final height is negligible.

Liver transplantation is considered with increasing frequency in patients with hepatic GSDs. It can be an option in GSD-Ia to correct the basic defect in liver. Also, patients with hepcidin-producing adenoma and severe anaemia and proven or suspected hepatocellular carcinoma within an adenoma (mainly GSD-I) may benefit. Finally, patients with cirrhosis, observed in disorders associated with an abnormal glycogen structure (GSD-III, GSD-IV) but also in GSD-IXc, will require this procedure.

A rather unique development regarding the definition of research priorities has been the international priority-setting partnership for liver GSDs. From these activities, there is now a list of 11 top research priorities (Table 'Research priorities for liver glycogen storage disease'), among which are novel treatment modalities (*see* Table 'Novel treatments in disorders of carbohydrate absorption, transmembrane transport and metabolism').

Research priorities for liver glycogen storage disease (from Peeks et al. 2020)

| Rank | Priority |
|---|---|
| 1 | What are the best options (*e.g.* gene therapy or enzyme replacement therapy) for achieving sufficient amount of working enzyme in patients with liver GSDs? |
| 2 | Can consensus guidelines (for management) be achieved for patients with liver GSD? |
| 3 | How should optimal metabolic control both clinically and biochemically (like lactate, ketones and/or lipids) be achieved in liver GSD? |
| 4 | How should sickness and emergency situations be managed for patients with liver GSD? |
| 5 | What is the best way to start dietary treatment, finding the optimal doses, and to administer the diet for patients with liver GSD? |
| 6 | How can existing cornstarch preparations be modified or alternative treatments be implemented that are easier to administer and/or keep blood sugar levels more stable for patients with liver GSD? |
| 7 | What is the role for new methods for monitoring metabolic control (like non-invasive continuous glucose and lactate measurements, new biomarkers) for patients with liver GSD? |
| 8 | How to manage diet regimen in relation to 'before, during and after' physical exercise (sport, playing) for patients with liver GSD? |
| 9 | What are the long-term complications (liver, renal, gut) of a diet rich in uncooked cornstarch and/or high protein and should the diet be adjusted to prevent complications in liver GSD? |
| 10 | What are the risks and benefits of different options for overnight treatment for patients with liver GSD and how can we maximise safety? |
| 11 | How to prevent and/or treat muscle problems in patients with liver GSD? |

## Follow-Up and Monitoring

Follow-up in patients with hepatic glycogen storage diseases

| Disorder | Investigations | Frequency/ Remarks |
|---|---|---|
| FBS | *See* GSD-I plus<br>Ophthalmologic examination (cataract?) | |
| | Glucose (P) (postprandial target conc <10.0 mM)<br>Gal, Gal-1-P<br>Carnitine | Depending on age, symptoms and medication |
| GSD-I | Clinical[a,b,c,•] | 0–3 years: 2 monthly<br>3–20 years: 3 monthly<br>>18 years: 6 monthly |
| | Paraclinical<br>Haematological parameters•<br>Electrolytes<br>Blood gases, lactate<br>Lactate (U)<br>(target conc <0.6 mmol/L or <0.06 mmol/mmol crea)<br>Liver parameters•<br>Kidney function (creatinine, GFR)<br>Uric acid (P)•<br>Calcium, phosphate, AP, PTH, vitamin D<br>Cholesterol, triglycerides, amylase, lipase<br>Home blood glucose profile[d,•]<br>(preprandial target conc >3.5–4.0 mM)<br>Microalbumin (U), protein (U)<br>α-fetoprotein•<br>Ultrasound (liver•, pancreas, ovaries)<br>Bone density<br>EEGc | Depending on age, symptoms and medication |
| GSD Ib | *See* GSD-I plus | |
| | CRP, ESR<br>Fecal $\alpha_1$-antitrypsin, calprotectin<br>Total blood count with differential<br>Bone marrow | Depending on age, symptoms and medication |
| GSD IIIa | *See* GSD-I plus | |

| Disorder | Investigations | Frequency/ Remarks |
|---|---|---|
| | Creatine kinase (P), pre-albumin<br>BNP<br>EKG, echocardiography<br>Muscle function<br>Lung function | Depending on age, symptoms and medication (in general less often than in GSD I) |
| GSD VI, GSD IXa-c | *See* GSD-I | Depending on age, symptoms, and medication (in general markedly less often than in GSD I) and restricted to investigations marked by •. |

Urinary tetrasaccharide is an important biomarker for follow-up of GSD-II patients, but not specific, and it can be increased in patients with hepatic GSDs, especially GSD-III. The role in single-patient follow up after (novel) treatment needs to be considered

[a]Nutrient intake, growth, sexual maturation, nutritional status, somatic findings (liver size)

[b]Neurological, psychological, cognitive functions, developmental investigations on demand

[c]Particular in cases with frequent hypoglycaemia

[d]Consider subcutaneous continuous monitoring

## Glycogen Storage Diseases—Mainly Affecting (Skeletal and Cardiac) Muscle

Patients with GSD-0b, GSD-XV, GSD-XIV, GSD-III, GSD-V, GSD-IXb and d, GSD VII, ALDOA-D, PGK-D, GSD-X, GSD-XIII and LDHA-D may have primary muscle weakness; in GSD-V and GSD-VII and the rare types GSD-XIV, ALDOA-D, PGK-D, GSD-X, GSD-XIII, LDHA-D, severe rhabdomyolysis, which sometimes results in acute renal failure, may additionally occur after (short-term) intensive exertion (Tarnopolsky 2018). These patients benefit from regular physical exercise at a submaximal level.

A carbohydrate-enriched diet (55-65% of energy) and sucrose, ribose or glucose ingestion before exercise may improve aerobic exertion tolerance in patients with GSD-V. However, it may also lead to overweight and to increased insulin secretion, potentially inhibiting the use of fatty acids. The benefits of using uncooked cornstarch in these patients to guarantee a constant glucose source from blood to muscle as oxidative substrate for glycolysis needs further investigation. Supplementation with branched-chain amino acids, vitamin $B_6$ (50–100 mg/kg/d) and creatine (10–20 g/d) has been recommended; however, there is a lack of evidence for these supplements.

Patients with GSD-VII depend on fatty acid oxidation in muscle as the main energy substrate. Therefore, in these patients, a surplus of dietary carbohydrates should be avoided, since it would enhance the metabolic muscle problems by decreasing the availability of fatty acids for oxidation. The diet should be rich in fat (30–40%) and proteins (15–20% of energy).

### GSD-IIa

A special role among GSDs with muscular (and cardiomuscular) symptoms is taken by GSD-IIa, a lysosomal disorder. Symptomatic treatment with regular physical exercise and physiotherapy, and a protein-enriched diet (20% of energy) still are important to maintain a range of motions and assist in ambulation in all affected age groups. Furthermore, individualised care of cardiomyopathy is important as standard drugs may be contraindicated and risk for tachyarrhythmia and sudden death is high. Respiratory support may include CPAP and/or tracheostomy. Surgery for contractures may be needed.

Enzyme replacement therapy (ERT) with alglucosidase-α (Myozyme® or Lumizyme®, at a dosage of 20 mg/kg every other week but also higher (Khan et al. 2020)) has been available for a few years now and should be started as soon as the diagnosis is established. In some countries, newborn screening for GSD-IIa exists and ERT can be started within the first days of life. A majority of infants in whom ERT was initiated before the age of six months and before the need for ventilatory assistance demonstrated improved survival, ventilator-independent survival, acquisition of motor skills, and reduced cardiac mass compared to untreated controls.

In patients with late-onset disease, ERT may stabilise ventilatory function and motor ability, measured by a six-minute walk and pulmonary function testing. ERT can be accompanied by treatable infusion reactions as well as anaphylaxis. Prevention of secondary complications includes aggressive management of infections; keeping immunisations up to date; annual influenza vaccination of the patient and household members; respiratory syncytial virus (RSV) prophylaxis (palivizumab) in the first two years of life; and use of anesthaesia only when absolutely necessary.

Follow-up in patients with muscle glycogen storage diseases

| Disorder | Investigations | Frequency/ Remarks |
|---|---|---|
| GSD-IIa<br>GSD-V<br>GSD-VII | Clinical[a,b]<br>Paraclinical<br>Creatine kinase (P)<br>Urinary glucose tetrasaccharide[c]<br>Uric acid (P)<br>Kidney function<br>Myoglobin (U)<br>BNP<br>Antibodies (in ERT)[c]<br>EKG, echocardiography<br>Muscle function<br>Lung function<br>Sleep evaluation, oximetry, capnometry<br>Hearing evaluation[c]<br>Haematology parameters (haemolysis)[d] | depending on underlying disorder, age, symptoms and medication |

[a]Nutrient intake, growth, sexual maturation, nutritional status, somatic findings (muscle strength, trophic, tone)

[b]Neurological, psychological, cognitive functions, developmental investigations

[c]In GSD-IIa

[d]In GSD-VII

## Novel Treatments

Reimbursement of (novel) treatments is a general matter of concern for rare diseases and exemplified in patients with disorders of carbohydrate absorption, transmembrane transport and metabolism. For several disorders, novel treatment options are available, either off-label or registered in controlled clinical trials. Examples include dietary interventions, drugs (repurposing), enzyme replacement therapies and gene therapy. In the process of novel treatment development, many companies act as either sponsor or collaborator.

Novel treatments in disorders of carbohydrate absorption, transmembrane transport and metabolism

| Number | Disorder | Intervention/Treatment | Sponsor | Phase | ClinicalTrials.gov Identifier or EudraCT number |
|---|---|---|---|---|---|
| 39.7 | GLUT1-D | Other: Red Blood Cell Transfusion | University of Texas Southwestern Medical Center, USA | 1 | NCT04137692 |
| | | Other: sodium lactate | Radboud University, The Netherlands | 2 | NCT04112862 |
| | | Drug: Triheptanoin | University of Texas Southwestern Medical Center | 1 | NCT03301532 |
| | | Drug: Triheptanoin | Cook Children's Health Care System, USA | 2 | NCT02036853 |
| | | Drug: Triheptanoin | University of Texas Southwestern Medical Center | 1 | NCT03041363 |
| | | Drug: Triheptanoin | University of Texas Southwestern Medical Center | 2 | NCT03181399 |
| | | Drug: UX007 (triheptanoin) | Ultragenyx Pharmaceutical Inc | 2 | NCT01993186<br>2013-003771-35 |
| | | Drug: UX007 (triheptanoin) | Ultragenyx Pharmaceutical Inc | 2 | NCT02599961[a]<br>2015-000389-69 |
| | | Drug: UX007 (triheptanoin) | Ultragenyx Pharmaceutical Inc | 3 | NCT02960217[a]<br>2015-005536-17 |
| 39.12 | GALT-D | Drug: AT-007 (aldose reductase inhibitor) | Applied Therapeutics, Inc. | 1/2 | NCT04117711 |
| | | Behavioral: Babble Boot Camp | Arizona State University, USA | n/a | NCT03838016 |
| | | Drug: arginine aspartate | Academisch Ziekenhuis Maastricht, The Netherlands | 2 | NCT03580122[a]<br>2014-002674-36 |
| 39.15 | HFI | Dietary Supplement: Alanine | Augusta University, USA | n/a | NCT04022434<br>NCT01185210 |
| 39.23<br>39.33<br>39.44 | GSD-VII<br>GSD-XV<br>GSD-IV | Drug: Triheptanoin | Rigshospitalet, Denmark | 2 | NCT03642860<br>2017-004153-17 |
| 39.23<br>39.26<br>39.27<br>39.28<br>39.30<br>39.33<br>39.34<br>39.36<br>39.37<br>39.42<br>39.43<br>39.52 | GSD-VII<br>PGK-D<br>GSD-X<br>GSD-XIII<br>LDHA-D<br>GSD-XV<br>GSD-0b<br>GSD-IV<br>GSD-IXd<br>GSD-V<br>GSD-III<br>GSD-IIa | Other: Sugar | Rigshospitalet, Denmark | n/a | NCT02635269 |
| 39.29 | PK-D | Drug: AG-348 | Agios Pharmaceuticals, Inc. | 2 | NCT02476916<br>2015-000484-13 |
| | | Drug: AG-348 | Agios Pharmaceuticals, Inc. | 3 | NCT03853798<br>NCT03559699<br>NCT03548220<br>2017-003803-22<br>2018-003459-39<br>2017-003823-31 |
| | | Biological: RP-L301 (Autologous CD34+ Cells Transduced With a Lentiviral Vector) | Rocket Pharmaceuticals Inc. | 1 | NCT04105166<br>2019-001656-19 |
| 39.36 | GSD-IV | Drug: Triheptanoin | Baylor Research Institute, USA | 2 | NCT00947960 |

| Number | Disorder | Intervention/Treatment | Sponsor | Phase | ClinicalTrials.gov Identifier or EudraCT number |
|---|---|---|---|---|---|
| 39.37<br>39.39<br>39.40<br>39.43<br>39.44<br>39.45<br>39.47 | GSD-IXa<br>GSD-IXb<br>GSD-IXc<br>GSD-VI<br>GSD-III<br>GSD-Ia<br>GSD-Ib | Dietary: Glycosade | Vitaflo International, Ltd | n/a | NCT02318966 |
| 39.42 | GSD-V | Drug: Triheptanoin | Rigshospitalet, Denmark | 2 | NCT02432768<br>2014-003644-12 |
| | | Drug: Sodium Valproate | University College, London, UK | 2 | NCT03112889<br>2014-001637-88 |
| | | Drug: REN001 (selective PPAR delta agonist) | Reneo Pharma Ltd | 1 | NCT04226274 |
| | | Dietary: Ketocal 4:1 liquid Nutricia (intervention) | Rigshospitalet, Denmark | n/a | NCT04044508 |
| | | Dietary: β-hydroxybuturate esters | Rigshospitalet, Denmark | n/a | NCT03945370 |
| | | Other: Modified ketogenic diets | | n/a | NCT03843606 |
| 39.44 | GSD-III | Dietary: Ketone-ester drink | University Medical Center Groningen, The Netherlands | n/a | NCT03011203 |
| 39.45 | GSD-Ia | Dietary: sweet polvilho | Hospital de Clinicas de Porto Alegre, Brazil | n/a | NCT03871673 |
| | | Drug: Triheptanoin | Duke University, USA | 1 | NCT03665636 |
| | | Genetic: DTX401 (AAV8-mediated gene therapy | Ultragenyx Pharmaceutical Inc | ½ | NCT03517085<br>2016-003023-30 |
| | | Genetic: DTX401 (AAV8-mediated gene therapy | Ultragenyx Pharmaceutical Inc | n/a | NCT03970278 |
| 39.45<br>39.47 | GSD-Ia<br>GSD-Ib | Drug: Triheptanoin | Duke University, USA | 1 | NCT03665636 |
| 39.46<br>39.47 | G6PC3-D<br>GSD-Ib | Drug: Empagliflozin | Université Catholique de Louvain, Belgium | 2 | NCT04138251<br>2018-004191-35 |
| 39.45<br>39.47 | GSD-Ia<br>GSD-Ib | Drug: ACRE inhibitors | Dipartimento di Pediatria, Italia[b] | 3 | 2006-005449-12 |
| 39.52 | GSD-IIa (late-onset) | Other: Lingual Muscle Training | Duke University, USA | n/a | NCT03255213 |
| 39.52 | GSD-IIa (late-onset) | Device: Respiratory muscle training using modified RMT device | Duke University, USA | n/a | NCT02801539 |
| 39.52 | GSD-IIa | Drug: alglucosidase alfa (Myozyme) | Sanofi | 4 | NCT03687333 |
| 39.52 | GSD-IIa (late-onset) | Drug: avalglucosidase alfa GZ402666 | Sanofi | 3 | NCT02782741<br>2016-000942-77 |
| 39.52 | GSD-IIa (infantile-onset) | Drug: avalglucosidase alfa GZ402666 | Sanofi | 2 | NCT03019406<br>2013-003321-28<br>2016-003475-21 |
| | | Drug: avalglucosidase alfa(GZ402666) | Sanofi | 2/3 | NCT02032524 |
| 39.52 | GSD-IIa (late-onset) | Biological: alglucosidase alfa | Sanofi | 4 | NCT01410890<br>NCT00701701<br>NCT00701129<br>2006-003644-31<br>2010-022231-11<br>2011-005595-42<br>2015-000583-34<br>2015-000584-14<br>2015-000582-31 |
| | GSD-IIa | Other: Diet and Exercise | University of Florida, USA | n/a | NCT02363153 |
| | GSD-IIa | Drug: rAAV1-CMV-GAA (AAV1-mediated gene therapy) | University of Florida, USA | 1/2 | NCT00976352 |
| 39.52 | GSD-IIa (late-onset) | Drug: VAL-1221<br>Drug: RhGAA | Valerion Therapeutics, LLC | 1<br>2 | NCT02898753<br>2016-004578-16 |

| Number | Disorder | Intervention/Treatment | Sponsor | Phase | ClinicalTrials.gov Identifier or EudraCT number |
|---|---|---|---|---|---|
| | | Drug: Clenbuterol | Duke University, USA | 1/2 | NCT01942590 |
| | GSD-IIa (late-onset) | Drug: Clenbuterol | Duke University, USA | 2 | NCT04094948 |
| | GSD-IIa (late-onset) | Genetic: AT845 (AAV8-mediated gene therapy) | Audentes Therapeutics | 1/2 | NCT04174105 |
| | GSD-IIa (late-onset) | Biological: AAV2/8LSPhGAA (AAV8-mediated gene therapy) | Asklepios Biopharmaceutical, Inc. | 1/2 | NCT03533673 |
| | GSD-IIa | Device: NeuDx Diaphragm pacer (DPS) | University of Florida, USA | n/a | NCT02354651 |
| | GSD-IIa | Genetic: Recombinant Adeno-Associated Virus Acid Alpha-Glucosidase (re-administration of AAV9-mediated gene therapy) | University of Florida, USA | 1 | NCT02240407 |
| | GSD-IIa (late-onset) on ERT | Drug: Albuterol | Duke University, USA | 1/2 | NCT01885936 |
| | GSD-IIa (late-onset) | Drug: Albuterol | Duke University, | 1 | NCT01859624 |
| | GSD-IIa (late-onset) | Biological: ATB200<br>Drug: AT2221 | Amicus Therapeutics | n/a | NCT03865836 |
| | | Drug: ATB200<br>Drug: AT2221 | Amicus Therapeutics | 1/2 | NCT02675465<br>2008-002302-18<br>2011-002154-32<br>2015-004798-34 |
| | GSD-IIa (late-onset) | Drug: AT2221<br>Biological: ATB200 | Amicus Therapeutics | 3 | NCT04138277 |
| | GSD-IIa (late-onset) | Biological: ATB200<br>Drug: AT2221 | Amicus Therapeutics | 3 | NCT03911505 |
| | GSD-IIa (late-onset) | Biological: ATB200<br>Drug: AT2221 | Amicus Therapeutics | 3 | NCT03729362 |
| | GSD-IIa (late-onset) | Genetic: SPK-3006 (AAV-mediated gene therapy) | Spark Therapeutics | 1/2 | NCT04093349 |
| | GSD-IIa (late-onset) | Drug: BMN 701 | BioMarin Pharmaceutical | 2<br>3 | 2011-001805-28<br>2014-002158-38<br>NCT01924845<br>2013-001768-48 |
| | GSD-IIa (late-onset) | Drug: glucosidase alfa | University of Munich, Germany | n/a | NCT02824068 |
| | GSD-IIa (late-onset) | Drug: Miglustat in co-administration with ERT | Universita degli studi di Napoli Federico II, Italy | 2 | 2010-024647-32 |
| 39.53 | GSD-IIb | Biological: RP-A501 (AAV9-mediated gene therapy) | Rocket Pharmaceuticals Inc. | 1 | NCT03882437 |
| 39.54 | PC-D | Drug: triheptanoin | University of Pittsburgh, USA | n/a | NCT01461304 |

Only active (recruiting and not recruiting) interventional clinical trials with recent (<2 years) updates were included
*ERT* Enzyme replacement treatment
[a]This study was halted prematurely due to lack of efficacy
[b]Not specified

## Online Resources

As described throughout the chapter, online resources are available for

Clinical and genetic information

- Online Mendelian Inheritance in Man (OMIM): https://www.ncbi.nlm.nih.gov/omim
- GenBank: https://www.ncbi.nlm.nih.gov/genbank/
- GeneReviews: https://www.ncbi.nlm.nih.gov/books/NBK1116/
- Orphanet: https://www.orpha.net/consor/cgi-bin/index.php?lng=EN
- IEMbase: http://www.iembase.org/

Registered clinical trials

- Clinicaltrials.gov: https://clinicaltrials.gov/
- EU Clinical Trials Register: https://www.clinicaltrialsregister.eu/

Clinical guidelines for specific disorders (*see* Table 'Pitfalls/dangers of a ketogenic diet') International Liver GSD Priority Setting Partnership: https://igsdpsp.com/

## References


Berry GT, Walter J, Fridovich-Keil JL. Disorders of galactose metabolism. In: Saudubray JM, Baumgartner M, Walter JH, editors. Inborn metabolic diseases: diagnosis and treatment. 6th ed. Heidelberg: Springer-Verlag; 2016. p. 139–48.

Bianchi P, Fermo E, Glader B, Kanno H, Agarwal A, Barcellini W, et al. Addressing the diagnostic gaps in pyruvate kinase deficiency: consensus recommendations on the diagnosis of pyruvate kinase deficiency. Am J Hematol. 2019;94:149–61.

Chen YT. Glycogen storage diseases. In: Scriver CR, Beaudet AL, Sly WS, Valle D, editors. The metabolic and molecular bases of inherited disease. New York: McGraw-Hill; 2001. p. 1521–51.

Coady MJ, El Tarazi A, Santer R, Bissonnette P, Sasseville LJ, Calado J, et al. MAP17 is a necessary activator of renal Na+/glucose cotransporter SGLT2. J Am Soc Nephrol. 2016;28:85–93.

Cortese A, Zhu Y, Rebelo AP, Negri S, Courel S, Abreu L, et al. Biallelic mutations in SORD cause a common and potentially treatable hereditary neuropathy with implications for diabetes. Nat Genet. 2020;52:473–81.

Derks TGJ, Peeks F, de Boer F, Fokkert-Wilts M, van der Doef HPJ, van den Heuvel MC, et al. The potential of dietary treatment in patients with glycogen storage disease type IV. J Inherit Metab Dis. 2020. https://doi.org/10.1002/jimd.12339. Epub ahead of print.

Fermo E, Vercellati C, Marcello AP, Zaninoni A, Aytac S, Cetin M, et al. Clinical and molecular spectrum of glucose-6-phosphate isomerase deficiency. Report of 12 new cases. Front Physiol. 2019;10:467.

Ghezzi C, Loo DDF, Wright EM. Physiology of renal glucose handling via SGLT1, SGLT2 and GLUT2. Diabetologia. 2018;61:2087–97.

Hogrel JY, van den Bogaart F, Ledoux I, Ollivier G, Petit F, Koujah N, et al. Diagnostic power of the non-ischaemic forearm exercise test in detecting glycogenosis type V. Eur J Neurol. 2015;22: 933–40.

Jamwal M, Aggarwal A, Palodi A, Sharma P, Bansal D, Maitra A, et al. A nonsense variant in the hexokinase 1 gene (HK1) causing severe non-spherocytic haemolytic anaemia: genetic analysis exemplifies ambiguity due to multiple isoforms. Br J Haematol. 2019;186:e142–5.

Khan AA, Case LE, Herbert M, DeArmey S, Jones H, Crisp K, et al. Higher dosing of alglucosidase alfa improves outcomes in children with Pompe disease: a clinical study and review of the literature. Genet Med. 2020;22:898–907.

Kishnani PS, Steiner RD, Bali D, Berger K, Byrne BJ, Case LE, et al. Pompe disease diagnosis and management guideline. Genet Med. 2006;8:267–88.

Kishnani PS, Austin SL, Arn P, Bali DS, Boney A, Case LE, et al. Glycogen storage disease type III diagnosis and management guidelines. Genet Med. 2010;12:446–63.

Kishnani PS, Austin SL, Abdenur JE, Arn P, Bali DS, Boney A, et al. Diagnosis and management of glycogen storage disease type I: a practice guideline of the American College of Medical Genetics and Genomics. Genet Med. 2014;16:e1.

Kishnani PS, Goldstein J, Austin SL, Arn P, Bachrach B, Bali DS, et al. Diagnosis and management of glycogen storage diseases type VI and IX: a clinical practice resource of the American College of Medical Genetics and Genomics (ACMG). Genet Med. 2019;21:772–89.

Kossoff EH, Zupec-Kania BA, Auvin S, Ballaban-Gil KR, Christina Bergqvist AG, Blackford R, et al. Optimal clinical management of children receiving dietary therapies for epilepsy: updated recommendations of the International Ketogenic Diet Study Group. Epilepsia Open. 2018;3:175–92.

Leen WG, Wevers RA, Kamsteeg EJ, Scheffer H, Verbeek MM, Willemsen MA. Cerebrospinal fluid analysis in the workup of GLUT1 deficiency syndrome: a systematic review. JAMA Neurol. 2013;70:1440–4.

Monroe GR, van Eerde AM, Tessadori F, Duran KJ, Savelberg SMC, van Alfen JC, et al. Identification of Human D lactate dehydrogenase deficiency. Nat Commun. 2019;10:1477.

Okur V, Cho MT, van Wijk R, van Oirschot B, Picker J, Coury SA, et al. De novo variants in HK1 associated with neurodevelopmental abnormalities and visual impairment. Eur J Hum Genet. 2019;27:1081–9.

Peeks F, Boonstra WF, de Baere L, Carøe C, Casswall T, Cohen D, et al. Research priorities for liver glycogen storage disease: an international priority setting partnership with the James Lind Alliance. J Inherit Metab Dis. 2020;43:279–89.

Pennisi A, Maranda B, Benoist JF, Baudouin V, Rigal O, Pichard S, et al. Nocturnal enteral nutrition is therapeutic for growth failure in Fanconi-Bickel syndrome. J Inherit Metab Dis. 2020;43:540–8.

Quinlivan R, Martinuzzi A, Schoser B. Pharmacological and nutritional treatment for McArdle disease (glycogen storage disease type V). Cochrane Database Syst Rev. 2014:CD003458. https://doi.org/10.1002/14651858.CD003458.pub5.

Rake JP, Visser G, Labrune P, Leonard JV, Ullrich K, Smit GP, et al. Guidelines for management of glycogen storage disease type I—European study on glycogen storage disease type I (ESGSD I). Eur J Pediatr. 2002;161(suppl 1):S112–9.

Rubio-Cabezas O, Hattersley AT, Njølstad PR, Mlynarski W, Ellard S, White N, et al. ISPAD clinical practice consensus guidelines 2014. The diagnosis and management of monogenic diabetes in children and adolescents. Pediatr Diabetes. 2014;15(suppl 20):47–64.

Santer R, Calado J. Familial renal glucosuria and SGLT2: from a Mendelian trait to a therapeutic target. Clin J Am Soc Nephrol. 2010;5:133–41.

Santer R, du Moulin M, Shahinyan T, Vater I, Maier E, Muntau AC, et al. A summary of molecular genetic findings in fructose-1,6-bisphosphatase deficiency with a focus on a common long-range deletion and the role of MLPA analysis. Orphanet J Rare Dis. 2016;11:44.

Sentner CP, Hoogeveen IJ, Weinstein DA, Santer R, Murphy E, McKiernan PJ, et al. Glycogen storage disease type III: diagnosis, genotype, management, clinical course and outcome. J Inherit Metab Dis. 2016;39:697–704.

Steinmann B, Santer R. Disorders of fructose metabolism. In: Saudubray JM, Baumgartner M, Walter JH, editors. Inborn metabolic diseases: diagnosis and treatment. 6th ed. Heidelberg: Springer-Verlag; 2016. p. 161–8.

Srour M, Shimokawa N, Hamdan FF, Nassif C, Poulin C, Al Gazali L. Dysfunction of the cerebral glucose transporter SLC45A1 in individuals with intellectual disability and epilepsy. Am J Hum Genet. 2017;100:824–30.

Sullivan MA, Nitschke S, Steup M, Minassian BA, Nitschke F, Sullivan MA, et al. Pathogenesis of Lafora disease: transition of soluble glycogen to insoluble polyglucosan. Int J Mol Sci. 2017;18:1743.

Tarnopolsky MA. Myopathies related to glycogen metabolism disorders. Neurotherapeutics. 2018;15:915–27.

Visser G, Rake JP, Labrune P, Leonard JV, Moses S, Ullrich K, et al. Consensus guidelines for management of glycogen storage disease type 1b—European study on glycogen storage disease type 1. Eur J Pediatr. 2002;161(suppl 1):S120–3.

van der Ploeg AT, Kruijshaar ME, Toscano A, Laforêt P, Angelini C, Lachmann RH, et al. European consensus for starting and stopping enzyme replacement therapy in adult patients with Pompe disease: a 10-year experience. Eur J Neurol. 2017;24:768–e31.

Wada Y, Kikuchi A, Arai-Ichinoi N, Sakamoto O, Takezawa Y, Iwasawa S, et al. Biallelic GALM pathogenic variants cause a novel type of galactosemia. Genet Med. 2019;21:1286–94.

Wanes D, Husein DM, Naim HY. Congenital lactase deficiency: mutations, functional and biochemical Implications, and future perspectives. Nutrients. 2019;11:461.

Welling L, Bernstein LE, Berry GT, Burlina AB, Eyskens F, Gautschi M, et al. International clinical guideline for the management of classical galactosemia: diagnosis, treatment, and follow-up. J Inherit Metab Dis. 2017;40:171–6.

Wortmann SB, van Hove JLK, Derks TGJ, Chevalier N, Knight V, Koller A, et al. Treating neutropenia and neutrophil dysfunction in glycogen storage disease IB with an SGLT2-inhibitor. Blood. 2020; https://doi.org/10.1182/blood.2019004465. Epub ahead of print.

# Disorders of the Pentose Phosphate Pathway and Polyol Metabolism

40

Mirjam M. C. Wamelink and Monique Williams

## Contents



## Summary

Five inborn errors in the pentose phosphate pathway (PPP) have been described of which *Glucose-6-phosphate dehydrogenase (G6PD) deficiency* is a defect in the first, irreversible step of the pathway. As a consequence, nicotinamide adenine dinucleotide phosphate (NADPH) production is decreased, making erythrocytes vulnerable to oxidative stress. Drug- and fava bean-induced haemolytic anaemia is the main presenting symptom of this defect. G6PD deficiency is an X-linked disorder. This haematological disorder is not further discussed.

Three other defects with associated clinical pictures are:

*Deficiency of ribose-5-phosphate isomerase* has to date been described in three cases, who presented with psychomotor developmental delay, visual impairment, spasticity and leukoencephalopathy.

*Transaldolase deficiency* presents with hepato- and splenomegaly, cardiac abnormalities, liver function problems, anaemia, thrombocytopenia and abnormal skin (e.g. cutis laxa) in most patients.

*Transketolase deficiency* was identified by whole exome sequencing (WES) in five patients of three

M. M. C. Wamelink (✉) · M. Williams
Metabolic Unit, Department of Clinical Chemistry, Amsterdam UMC, Vrije Universiteit Amsterdam, Amsterdam, The Netherlands
e-mail: m.wamelink@amsterdamumc.nl; m.williams@erasmusmc.nl


N. Blau et al. (eds.), *Physician's Guide to the Diagnosis, Treatment, and Follow-Up of Inherited Metabolic Diseases*,
https://doi.org/10.1007/978-3-030-67727-5_40

families with common clinical findings: short stature, developmental delay and congenital heart defects.

Four other inborn errors with polyol abnormalities without a clear suspected clinical phenotype are:

*Sedoheptulokinase deficiency* results in urinary accumulation of sedoheptulose and erythritol and is the result of mutations in the *SHPK* gene. A 57-kb-deletion, the most common cause of nephropathic cystinosis, also results in SHPK deficiency. Two unrelated patients with isolated SHPK deficiency have been described with completely different clinical pictures suggesting the clinical phenotype may not be related to sedoheptulokinase deficiency.

l-*xylulose reductase deficiency,* a defect of the glucuronic oxidation pathway with the biochemical feature of pentosuria, is a benign condition.

l-*arabinosuria* has been documented in only one patient. The defect has not been fully elucidated in humans.

*Sorbitol dehydrogenase* is an enzyme that participates in fructose and mannose metabolism. Deficiency is associated with cataract, although no direct relation has been confirmed of this enzyme deficiency and (congenital) cataract.

## Introduction

The pentose phosphate pathway (PPP), also known as the hexose monophosphate shunt, provides an alternative pathway for glucose oxidation. It is present in the cytosol of all cells and has two major functions: production of NADPH, and synthesis of ribose-5-phosphate. The pathway can be divided into two branches. The oxidative branch consists of three irreversible reactions, which result in NADPH and pentose phosphate production. The non-oxidative branch of the pathway reconverts pentose phosphates into glucose-6-phosphate (glucose-6P), and two of the intermediates, fructose-6P and glyceraldehyde-3P, are also glycolytic intermediates. The reactions in the non-oxidative branch are reversible. The flow of glucose-6P through the PPP or glycolysis is dependent upon the cellular requirement for NADPH, ribose-5P and ATP. The PPP is linked to the glucuronic oxidation pathway through xylulose-5P (Fig. 40.1).

*Ribose-5-phosphate isomerase (RPI) deficiency* was first described in a patient with a slowly progressive leukoencephalopathy with accumulation of the pentitols ribitol and arabitol in brain and body fluids (van der Knaap et al. 1999; Huck et al. 2004). Since then, two additional patients with RPI deficiency have been described. The first patient with RPI deficiency presented with impaired psychomotor development and epilepsy followed by neurological regression with cerebellar ataxia and peripheral neuropathy. At diagnosis, he suffered from serious intellectual disability, but somatic examination was normal. The second patient was similar to the first patient but lacked peripheral neuropathy (Naik et al. 2017). The 6-year-old patient described by Brooks et al. (2018) presented similarly as the first patient, showed dysmorphic features (resembling Allan-Hernon-Dudley syndrome), but has not developed epilepsy or regression yet. MRI showed extensive abnormalities of the cerebral white matter. Magnetic resonance spectroscopy (MRS) revealed abnormal resonances, corresponding to arabitol and ribitol. The diagnosis of RPI deficiency can be made by the analysis of sugars and polyols in urine, plasma or CSF. Urinary ribitol and arabitol, as well as xylulose, are elevated. High concentrations of the pentitols are also observed in CSF (see Table 40.1).

*Transaldolase (TALDO) deficiency* was first described in 2001 (Verhoeven et al. 2001) in a single patient presenting with cirrhosis, with to date more than 35 additional patients diagnosed from 22 different families (Williams et al. 2019, personal communication). A great phenotypic variability has been reported in TALDO patients. Most patients displayed the first symptoms of the disease in the neonatal or antenatal period when intra-uterine growth retardation, oligohydramnios and hydrops foetalis with dysmorphic features, and congenital heart defects have been described (Valayannopoulos et al. 2006). Neonates reveal hepatosplenomegaly, bleeding, abnormal liver function tests, cholestatic jaundice and elevated liver enzymes. Hepatic fibrosis or cirrhosis is the pathological liver hallmark in older patients. An asymptomatic sibling was diagnosed at 9 years of age, only then hepatomegaly was noted (LeDuc et al. 2014). Liver pathology includes hepatocellular damage and degeneration of hepatocytes or hyperplastic and enlarged hepatocytes with fibrosis and cirrhosis. In one patient, development of liver carcinoma occurred. Another frequent finding (in 76% of cases) is anaemia. Renal manifestations and endocrine disorders are seen in about 30% of patients. Mild transient hypotonia was described in several patients but mental and motor development were normal in the majority. Brain MRI and MRS did not reveal abnormalities in patients with TALDO deficiency. Death in TALDO deficiency occurs due to liver failure and consequences of liver complications later in life. TALDO deficiency results in the accumulation of seven-carbon sugars from sedoheptulose-7P and polyols derived from the pathway intermediates (see Table 40.2) (Wamelink et al. 2008). Citric acid cycle intermediates have been detected, indicating a possible disturbed mitochondrial metabolism in TALDO deficiency (Engelke et al. 2010).

*Transketolase (TKT) deficiency* was identified as disease causing when performing whole exome sequencing (WES) in five patients of three families with common clinical findings: short stature, developmental delay and congenital heart defects. Additional features can be found in Table 40.3. Elevated excretion of erythritol, arabitol, ribitol, and pent(ul)ose-5P, as well as elevated plasma levels of erythritol, arabitol and ribitol, are found in affected patients. TKT activity in lymphoblasts, fibroblasts or erythrocytes from all five individuals showed complete absence or low residual enzyme activity (Boyle et al. 2016).

*Sedoheptulokinase (SHPK) deficiency*: The two patients described with SHPK deficiency excreted increased amounts of erythritol and sedoheptulose (Wamelink et al. 2015). The finding of erythritol is likely the result of phosphorylation of sedoheptulose by fructokinase to sedoheptulose-1P and cleavage of the latter by aldolase B to the formation of erythrose, and further reduction to erythritol (Kardon et al. 2008). Their clinical phenotype however was diverse, so a causal relationship seems doubtful. The phenotype ranged from neonatal cholestasis, hypoglycaemia, anaemia and cerebral abnormalities with facial dysmorphisms to congenital arthrogryposis with facial dysmorphisms (see Table 40.4).

1-*xylulose reductase deficiency* is associated with pentosuria, first shown in 1892 by Salkowski and Jastrowitz and was suggested an inborn error of metabolism in 1908. The defective enzyme in humans was found by Wang and Van Eys (1970). In 1981, in a group of 1117 patients with a suspected inherited disease, 20 patients (2%) with pentosuria were found (Vaca et al. 1981). Not only L-xylulose was found in urine but also increased levels in plasma were found. Touster and Harwell (1958) reported finding only L-arabitol in pentosuric urine compared to both D/L-arabitol in normal urine. The pentose sugar was identified as L-xylulose and mutations in *DCXR* leading to enzyme deficiency were found in 2011 in the persons with pentosuria that had been studied by Margaret Lasker (xyloketosuria) in 1936. It is an autosomal recessive phenomenon and a benign condition (Pierce et al. 2011) (see Table 40.5).

1-*arabinosuria*, detected in one patient with delayed motor development and facial dysmorphism (Onkenhout et al. 2002), possibly due to L-arabitol dehydrogenase, leads to strongly elevated excretion of L-arabitol and arabinose after ingestion of fruit. Additionally, high levels of arabinose and L-arabitol were also found in plasma and CSF (see Table 40.6). L-arabitol dehydrogenase has been detected in yeast and fungi. The enzyme has been purified from fungus and the gene cloned. This has not yet been established in human (Onkenhout et al. 2002). It is unclear whether this biochemical finding is disease related. However, it was speculated that accumulation of L-arabitol over time could be toxic to the brain.

*Sorbitol dehydrogenase (SORD) deficiency* was found in predominantly male patients of two families with congenital cataract (Vaca et al. 1981; Shin et al. 1984). SORD deficiency is also thought to play a role in diabetic complications (cataract) where at high glucose levels it is believed that the polyol pathway is very active, and that enzyme activity is high in kidney and lens (Carr and Markham 1995). Sorbitol dehydrogenase converts D-sorbitol to D-fructose in the fructose and mannose metabolism and xylitol to D-xylulose in the glucuronic oxidation pathway resulting in elevated sorbitol and xylitol in urine and plasma (see Table 40.7).

## Nomenclature

| No. | Disorder | Alternative name | Abreviation | Gene symbol | Chromosomal location | Mode of Inheritance | Affected protein | OMIM |
|---|---|---|---|---|---|---|---|---|
| 40.1 | Ribose-5-phosphate isomerase deficiency | RPI deficiency | RPI | *RPIA* | 2p11.2 | AR | Ribose-5-phosphate isomerase | 608611 |
| 40.2 | Transaldolase deficiency | TALDO deficiency | TALDO | *TALDO1* | 11p15.5 | AR | Transaldolase | 606003 |
| 40.3 | Transketolase deficiency | TKT deficiency; Short stature, developmental delay, and congenital heart defects | TKT, SDDHD | *TKT* | 3p21.1 | AR | Transketolase | 617044 |
| 40.4 | Sedoheptulokinase deficiency | SHPK deficiency | SHPK | *SHPK* | 17p13.2 | AR | Sedoheptulokinase | 617213 |
| 40.5 | L-xylulose reductase deficiency | Pentosuria, Xylitol dehydrogenase deficiency; L-Xylulosuria | PNTSU, DCXR | *DCXR* | 17q25.3 | AR | Dicarbonyl (diacetyl)/L-Xylulose reductase | 260800 |
| 40.6 | L-arabinosuria | | | To be determined | Unknown | AR **(presumed)** | L-arabitol dehydrogenase (presumed) | |
| 40.7 | Sorbitol dehydrogenase deficiency | | SORD | *SORD* | 15q21.1 | | Sorbitol dehydrogenase | 182500 |

## Metabolic Pathways

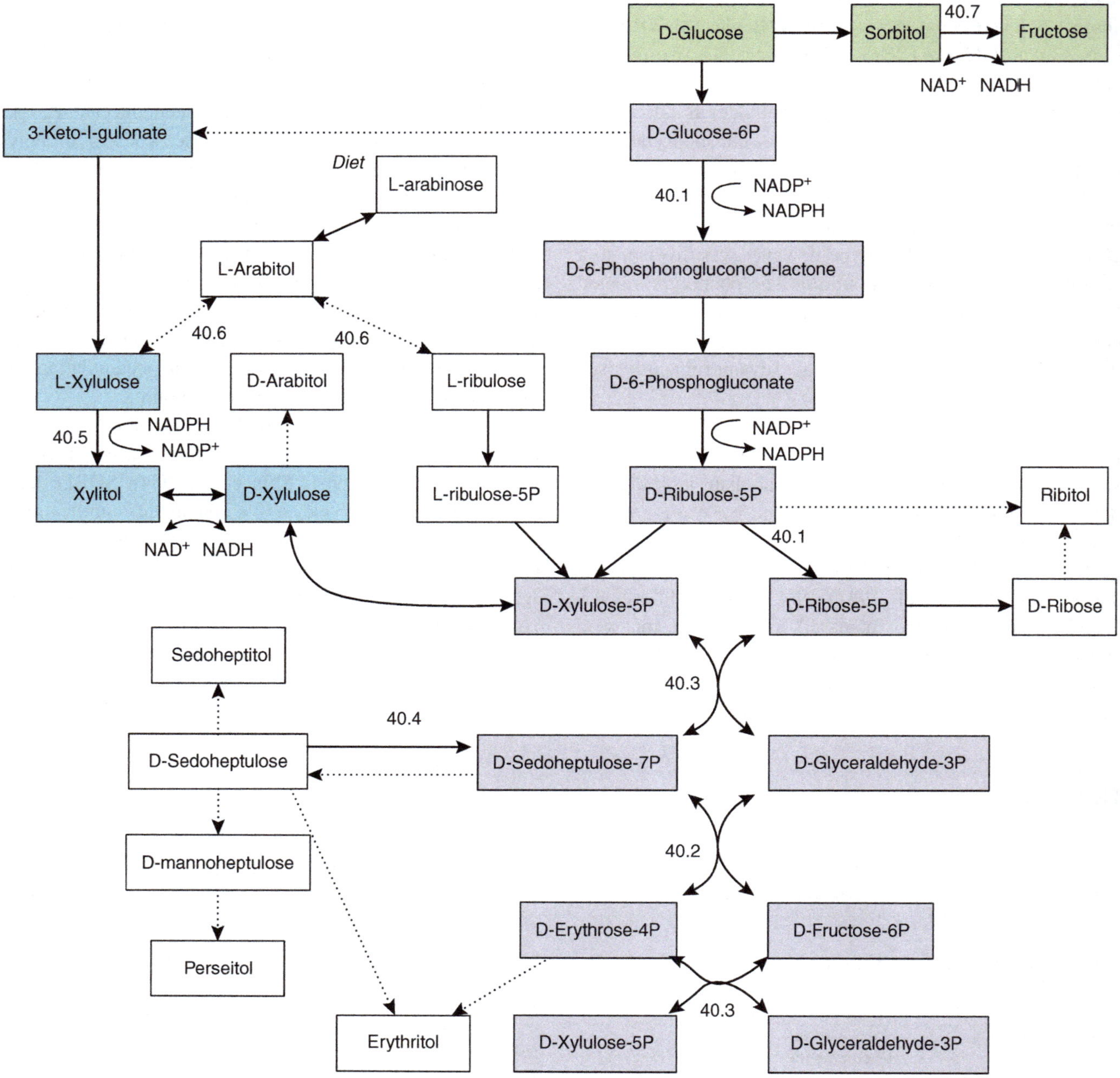


**Fig. 40.1** The pentose phosphate pathway in purple, the glucuronic (uronic) acid pathway in blue and the polyol pathway in green. The conversions displayed with the dotted arrow have not been proven in humans. 40.1: Glucose-6-phosphate dehydrogenase; 40.1: Ribose-5-phosphate isomerase; 40.2: Transaldolase; 40.3: Transketolase; 40.4: Sedoheptulokinase; 40.5: L-xylulose reductase; 40.6: Presumed L-arabitol dehydrogenase with conversion to either L-xylulose or L-ribulose; 40.7: Sorbitol dehydrogenase, P phosphate

## Signs and Symptoms

**Table 40.1** Ribose-5-phosphate isomerase deficiency

| System | Symptoms and biomarkers | Neonatal (birth–1 month) | Infancy (1–18 months) | Childhood (1.5–11 years) | Adolescence (11–16 years) | Adulthood (>16 years) |
|---|---|---|---|---|---|---|
| CNS | Ataxia, cerebellar | | | + | + | |
| | **Brain, abnormal (MRI)** | | + | + | + | + |
| | **Epilepsy** | | – | ++ | ++ | ++ |
| | **Leukoencephalopathy** | | + | ++ | ++ | ++ |
| | **Neuropathy** | | | + | ++ | ++ |
| | Regression, psychomotor | | | + | + | |
| | **Retardation, psychomotor** | | ++ | ++ | ++ | ++ |
| | **Spasticity** | | | + | + | + |
| | Hypotonia | ± | ± | ± | | |
| Dermatological | Hyperpigmentation | | | ± | | |
| Ear | Hearing loss | | | ± | ± | ± |
| Eye | Nystagmus | ± | ± | ± | ± | ± |
| | Optic atrophy | | | + | + | + |
| | Retinitis pigmentosa | | | | | ± |
| | Visual impairment | | | ± | ± | ± |
| Other | Dysmorphism | ± | ± | ± | | |
| Psychiatric | Behavioral abnormalities | | | ± | ± | ± |
| Laboratory findings | **Arabitol (cerebrospinal fluid)** | | | ↑↑↑ | ↑↑↑ | ↑↑↑ |
| | **Arabitol (plasma)** | | | ↑↑↑ | ↑↑↑ | ↑↑↑ |
| | **Arabitol (urine)** | | | ↑↑↑ | ↑↑↑ | ↑↑↑ |
| | **Polyols (MRI)** | | | ↑↑ | ↑↑ | ↑↑ |
| | **Ribitol (cerebrospinal fluid)** | | | ↑↑↑ | ↑↑↑ | ↑↑↑ |
| | **Ribitol (plasma)** | | | ↑↑↑ | ↑↑↑ | ↑↑↑ |
| | **Ribitol (urine)** | | | ↑↑↑ | ↑↑↑ | ↑↑↑ |
| | **Xylulose (urine)** | | | ↑↑ | ↑↑ | ↑↑ |

**Table 40.2** Transaldolase deficiency

| System | Symptoms and biomarkers | Neonatal (birth–1 month) | Infancy (1–18 months) | Childhood (1.5–11 years) | Adolescence (11–16 years) | Adulthood (>16 years) |
|---|---|---|---|---|---|---|
| Cardiovascular | **Cardiac, anomalies, malformations** | + | + | + | ± | ± |
| | Patent ductus arteriosus | ± | ± | ± | | |
| CNS | Hypotonia | ± | ± | | | |
| | Intellectual disability | ± | ± | ± | ± | ± |
| Dermatological | **Abnormal skin** | ± | ± | ± | | |
| | **Cutis laxa** | ± | ± | ± | | |
| Digestive | Cholestasis | ± | ± | | | |
| | **Hepatomegaly** | + | + | + | ± | ± |
| | **Liver cirrhosis** | ± | ± | ± | ± | ± |
| | Liver failure, acute | ± | ± | ± | | |
| | Liver failure, progressive | ± | ± | ± | ± | ± |
| | **Liver fibrosis** | ± | ± | ± | ± | ± |
| | Splenomegaly | + | + | + | ± | ± |
| Endocrine | Hypogonadotropic hypogonadism | ± | ± | ± | ± | ± |
| Genitourinary | Clitoral hypertrophy | ± | ± | | | |
| | Cryptorchidism | ± | ± | ± | | |
| | Micropenis | ± | ± | ± | | |
| | **Oligohydramnios, prenatally** | ± | | | | |
| Hematological | **Anemia** | + | + | + | + | + |
| | Leukopenia | | | ± | ± | ± |
| | **Thrombocytopenia** | ± | ± | ± | ± | ± |
| Musculoskeletal | Dysmorphic features | ++ | + | ± | | |

(continued)

Table 40.2 (continued)

| System | Symptoms and biomarkers | Neonatal (birth–1 month) | Infancy (1–18 months) | Childhood (1.5–11 years) | Adolescence (11–16 years) | Adulthood (>16 years) |
|---|---|---|---|---|---|---|
| Other | Early death | ± | ± | | ± | ± |
| | **Fetal hydrops** | ± | | | | |
| | Intrauterine growth retardation | ± | | | | |
| Renal | Nephrocalcinosis | ± | ± | ± | | |
| | Renal failure, chronic | ± | ± | ± | ± | ± |
| | Renal tubulopathy | ± | ± | ± | ± | ± |
| Laboratory findings | Albumin (serum) | ↓-n | ↓-n | ↓-n | ↓-n | ↓-n |
| | Alkaline phosphatase (plasma) | n-↑ | n-↑ | n-↑ | n | |
| | **Arabitol (urine)** | ↑ | ↑ | ↑ | ↑ | ↑ |
| | **ASAT/ALAT (plasma)** | ↑ | ↑ | **n-↑** | **n-↑** | **n-↑** |
| | Bilirubin (plasma) | n-↑ | n-↑ | n-↑ | n-↑ | n-↑ |
| | **Erythritol (urine)** | ↑↑ | ↑↑ | ↑ | **n** | **n** |
| | **Erythronic acid (urine)** | ↑↑ | ↑↑ | ↑↑ | ↑↑ | ↑↑ |
| | Ferritin (serum) | n-↑ | n-↑ | n-↑ | n-↑ | |
| | Gamma-glutamyl transpeptidase, GGT (plasma) | n-↑ | n-↑ | n-↑ | n-↑ | n |
| | Glucose (plasma) | ↓-n | ↓-n | | | |
| | **Hemoglobin (blood)** | ↓↓ | **↓-n** | **↓-n** | **↓-n** | **↓-n** |
| | **Mannoheptulose (urine)** | ↑ | ↑ | ↑ | ↑ | ↑ |
| | **Perseitol (urine)** | ↑ | ↑ | ↑ | ↑ | ↑ |
| | **Prothrombin time** | ↑ | ↑ | ↑ | **n-↑** | **n-↑** |
| | Respiratory chain activity (muscle) | ↓-n | ↓-n | ↓-n | | |
| | **Ribitol (urine)** | ↑↑ | ↑↑ | ↑↑ | ↑↑ | ↑↑ |
| | **Sedoheptitol (urine)** | ↑ | ↑ | ↑ | ↑ | ↑ |
| | **Sedoheptulose (urine)** | ↑↑ | ↑↑ | ↑↑ | ↑↑ | ↑↑ |
| | **Sedoheptulose-7-P (urine)** | ↑↑ | ↑↑ | ↑↑ | ↑↑ | ↑↑ |

Table 40.3 Transketolase deficiency

| System | Symptoms and biomarkers | Neonatal (birth–1 month) | Infancy (1–18 months) | Childhood (1.5–11 years) | Adolescence (11–16 years) | Adulthood (>16 years) |
|---|---|---|---|---|---|---|
| Cardiovascular | **Congenital heart defects** | + | + | + | + | + |
| CNS | **Developmental delay** | | + | + | + | + |
| | Hypotonia | | | | ± | ± |
| | Self injury | | | ± | ± | ± |
| | **Speech delay** | | + | + | + | + |
| | Stereotyped hand movements | | | ± | ± | ± |
| Digestive | Loose stools | | | | | |
| Eye | Cataract | | | | ± | ± |
| | Conjunctivitis | | | | ± | ± |
| | Strabismus | | | | ± | ± |
| | Uveitis | | | | ± | ± |
| Musculoskeletal | Dysmorphic features | | | ± | ± | ± |
| | **Growth retardation** | + | + | + | + | + |
| | **Microcephaly** | + | + | + | + | + |
| Psychiatric | Behavioral abnormalities | | | ± | ± | ± |
| | Obsessive-Compulsive Disorder (OCD) | | | ± | ± | ± |
| Laboratory findings | **Arabitol (plasma)** | | | ↑ | ↑ | ↑ |
| | **Arabitol (urine)** | | | ↑ | ↑ | ↑ |
| | **Erythritol (plasma)** | | | ↑↑ | ↑↑ | ↑↑ |
| | **Erythritol (urine)** | | | ↑↑ | ↑↑ | ↑↑ |
| | **Pent(ul)ose 5 phophates (urine)** | | | ↑ | ↑ | ↑ |
| | **Ribitol (plasma)** | | | ↑↑ | ↑↑ | ↑↑ |
| | **Ribitol (urine)** | | | ↑↑ | ↑↑ | ↑↑ |

**Table 40.4** Sedoheptulose kinase deficiency

| System | Symptoms and biomarkers | Neonatal (birth–1 month) | Infancy (1–18 months) | Childhood (1.5–11 years) | Adolescence (11–16 years) | Adulthood (>16 years) |
|---|---|---|---|---|---|---|
| Musculoskeletal | Dysmorphic features | ± | ± | ± | | |
| Other | No clinical significance | + | + | + | + | + |
| Laboratory findings | **Erythritol (urine)** | | ↑↑ | ↑↑ | | |
| | **Sedoheptulose (urine)** | | ↑↑ | ↑↑ | | |

**Table 40.5** L-xylulose reductase deficiency

| System | Symptoms and biomarkers | Neonatal (birth–1 month) | Infancy (1–18 months) | Childhood (1.5–11 years) | Adolescence (11–16 years) | Adulthood (>16 years) |
|---|---|---|---|---|---|---|
| Other | No clinical significance | + | + | + | + | + |
| Laboratory findings | Arabitol (urine) | | ↑ | ↑ | ↑ | ↑ |
| | **L-Xylulose (plasma)** | ↑↑ | ↑↑ | ↑↑ | ↑↑ | ↑↑ |
| | **L-Xylulose (urine)** | ↑↑ | ↑↑ | ↑↑ | ↑↑ | ↑↑ |
| | **Reducing substances (urine)** | ↑ | ↑ | ↑ | ↑ | ↑ |

**Table 40.6** L-arabinosuria

| System | Symptoms and biomarkers | Neonatal (birth–1 month) | Infancy (1–18 months) | Childhood (1.5–11 years) | Adolescence (11–16 years) | Adulthood (>16 years) |
|---|---|---|---|---|---|---|
| Other | Unclear clinical features-possibly benign | + | + | + | + | + |
| Laboratory findings | L-Arabinose (cerebrospinal fluid) | | ↑↑ | ↑↑ | | |
| | L-Arabinose (plasma) | | ↑↑ | ↑↑ | | |
| | L-Arabinose (urine) | | ↑↑ | ↑↑ | | |
| | L-Arabitol (cerebrospinal fluid) | | ↑↑ | ↑↑ | | |
| | L-Arabitol (plasma) | | ↑↑ | ↑↑ | | |
| | L-Arabitol (urine) | | ↑↑ | ↑↑ | | |

**Table 40.7** Sorbitol dehydrogenase deficiency

| System | Symptoms and biomarkers | Neonatal (birth–1 month) | Infancy (1–18 months) | Childhood (1.5–11 years) | Adolescence (11–16 years) | Adulthood (>16 years) |
|---|---|---|---|---|---|---|
| Eye | Cataract | ± | | | | |
| | Cataract risk in dysregulated Diabetes Mellitus | | | | | ± |
| Other | Unclear clinical significance: | + | + | + | + | + |
| Laboratory findings | **Sorbitol (plasma)** | ↑↑ | ↑↑ | ↑↑ | ↑↑ | ↑↑ |
| | **Sorbitol (urine)** | ↑↑ | ↑↑ | ↑↑ | ↑↑ | ↑↑ |
| | **Xylitol (plasma)** | ↑↑ | ↑↑ | ↑↑ | ↑↑ | ↑↑ |
| | **Xylitol (urine)** | ↑↑ | ↑↑ | ↑↑ | ↑↑ | ↑↑ |

## Reference Values

### Urine (mmol/mol creatinine)

| Carbohydrate | Age | Reference values |
|---|---|---|
| Erythritol[a] | 0–4 months | 89–209 |
| | 4 month–5 years | 38–148 |
| | 5–80 years | 14–88 |
| Ribitol[a] | 0–4 months | 0–25 |
| | 4 months–5 years | 1–14 |
| | 5–80 years | 0–7 |
| Arabitol[a] | 0–4 months | 30–151 |
| | 4 months–5 years | 22–103 |
| | 5–80 years | 6–60 |
| Xylitol[a] | 0–5 years | 3–13 |
| | 5–80 years | 0–12 |
| Xylulose[b] | 0–80 years | <5 |
| Arabinose[b] | 1–6 years | 16–81 |
| Sorbitol[a] | 0–4 months | 2–12 |
| | 4 months-5 years | 0–28 |
| | 5–80 years | 0–15 |
| Sedoheptulose[a] | 0–1 month | <40 |
| | 1 month–80 years | <9 |
| Mannoheptulose[a] | 0–80 years | <3 |
| Sedoheptitol[a] | 0–80 years | <1 |
| Perseitol[a] | 0–80 years | <1 |
| Sedoheptulose-7-P[a] | 0–1 year | <0.07 |
| | 1–10 years | <0.06 |
| | 10–80 years | n.d. |
| Erythronic acid[c] | 0–3 months | <120 |
| | 3 months–80 years | <50 |

[a]Liquid chromatography tandem mass spectrometry (LC-MS/MS; Wamelink et al. 2008)
[b]Gas chromatography-flame ionisation detection (Jansen et al. 1986)
[c]$^1$H-NMR (Engelke et al. 2010)

### Plasma (μmol/l)[a]

| Carbohydrate | Reference values |
|---|---|
| Erythritol | <5 |
| Ribitol | <5 |
| Arabitol | <5 |
| Arabinose | <5 |
| Xylitol | <5 |
| Xylulose | <5 |
| Sorbitol | <5 |

[a]Gas chromatography-flame ionisation detection (Jansen et al. 1986)

### CSF (μmol/l)[a]

| Carbohydrate | Reference values |
|---|---|
| Erythritol | 12–33 |
| Ribitol | <5 |
| Arabitol | 9–39 |
| Arabinose | 6–23 |

[a]Gas chromatography-flame ionisation detection (Jansen et al. 1986)

## Pathological Values

### Urine (mmol/mol creatinine)

| Carbohydrate | Age | 40.2 | 40.3 | 40.4 | 40.5 | 40.6 | 40.7 ($n = 1$)[a] | 40.8 |
|---|---|---|---|---|---|---|---|---|
| Erythritol[b] | 0–4 months | | 427–976 | 466–716 | 2753 | | | |
| | 4 months–5 years | | 139–1131 | | 1045 | | | |
| | 5–80 years | N–↓ | 90–629 | | | | | |
| Ribitol[b] | 0–4 months | | 233–722 | 244–506 | N–↑ | | | |
| | 4 months–5 years | | 63–432 | | | | | |
| | 5–80 years | 123–516 | 43–313 | | | | | |
| Arabitol[b] | 0–4 months | | 216–588 | 202–509 | N–↑ | ↑[c] | 583–2704[c] | |
| | 4 months–5 years | | 163–588 | | | | | |
| | 5–80 years | 1021-3609[d] | 99–583 | | | | | |
| Arabinose[e] | 1–6 years | N | | N-↓ | | | 763–12,862[c] | |
| Xylitol[b] | 0–80 years | 15–34 | | N | | | N | ↑↑ |
| Xylulose[e] | 0–80 years | 39–52 | | N | | ↑↑[c] | | |
| Sorbitol[b] | 0–80 years | | | | | | | ↑↑ |
| Sedoheptulose[b] | 0–1 months | N | 1361 | N | 253 | | | |
| | 1 months–80 year | | 70–5300 | | 576 | | | |
| Mannoheptulose[b] | 0–80 years | N | 6–112 | N | | | | |
| Sedoheptitol[b] | 0–80 years | N | 2–27 | N | | | | |
| Perseitol[b] | 0–80 years | N | 3–67 | N | | | | |
| Sedoheptulose-7-P[b] | 0–1 year | N | 2.5–8.3 | N | N | | | |
| | 1–10 years | | 0.5–23.8 | | | | | |
| | 10–80 years | | 1.8–8.5 | | | | | |
| Pen(tu)lose-5-P[b,f] | 0–80 years | | | ↑ | | | | |
| Erythronic acid[f] | 0–3 months | | 2900 | | | | | |
| | 3 months-80 years | | 350–770 | | | | | |

*N* Normal
[a]Diet with fruit
[b]Liquid chromatography tandem mass spectrometry (LC-MS/MS; Wamelink et al. 2008)
[c]Predominantly the L-isomer was found

[d]Predominantly the D-isomer was found
[e]Gas chromatography-flame ionisation detection (Jansen et al. 1986)
[f]1H-NMR (Engelke et al. 2010)

### Plasma (μmol/l)[a]

| Carbohydrate | 40.2 | 40.3 | 40.4 | 40.6 | 40.7 ($n$ = 1)[b] | 40.8 |
|---|---|---|---|---|---|---|
| Erythritol | N | 10–18 | 28–60 | | | |
| Ribitol | 14–30 | 6–12 | 13–80 | | | |
| Arabitol | 90–163[c] | 15–32 | 18–111 | | 12–49[d] | |
| Arabinose | | | | | 11–106[d] | |
| Xylitol | | | N | | | ↑ |
| Xylulose | | | | ↑[c] | | |
| Sorbitol | | | | | | ↑ |

*N* Normal
[a]Gas chromatography-flame ionisation detection (Jansen et al. 1986)
[b]Diet with fruit
[c]Predominantly the D-isomer was found
[d]Predominantly the L-isomer was found

### CSF (μmol/l)[a]

| Carbohydrate | 40.2 ($n$ = 1) | 40.3 ($n$ = 1) | 40.7 ($n$ = 1)[b] |
|---|---|---|---|
| Erythritol | <5 | N | |
| Ribitol | 891–1249 | 19 | |
| Arabitol | 5234–5535 | N | 225 |
| Arabinose | | | 65[c] |

*N* Normal
[a]Gas chromatography-flame ionisation detection (Jansen et al. 1986)
[b]Diet with fruit
[c]Predominantly the L-isomer was found

## Diagnostic Flowcharts

(See Fig. 40.2)

## Loading Test

In the case of L-arabinosuria, when the diet contains fruit, large amounts of L-arabinose and L-arabitol are detected. Without the ingestion of fruit arabinose and arabitol normalise. For the other defects loading tests are not applicable.

## Specimen Collection

| Investigation | Specimen | Storage |
|---|---|---|
| Sugars and polyols[a] | U, P, CSF | Frozen |
| C7-carbohydrates | U, BSP | Frozen |
| Transaldolase activity | FIB, LYB, ERY<br>Liver | Room temperature<br>Frozen |
| Ribose-5-phosphate isomerase activity | FIB, LYB | Room temperature |
| Transketolase activity | FIB, LYB | Room temperature |
| Sedoheptulokinase activity | FIB | Room temperature |
| Sorbitol dehydrogenase activity | SER, RBC | Room temperature |

[a]Urine can be spotted on filter paper and sent at room temperature for analysis of polyols (sugars are not stable in spotted urine and therefore unreliable for diagnosis)

## Prenatal Diagnosis

| Disorder | | Material | Testing | Trimester |
|---|---|---|---|---|
| 40.1 | RPI deficiency | CV, AMN | DNA | I, II |
| 40.2 | Transaldolase deficiency | CV, AMN<br>Cell free amniotic fluid | DNA<br>Metabolite | I, II<br>(II), III (performed only ones at 28 weeks gestation) |
| 40.3 | Transketolase deficiency | CV, AMN | DNA | I, II |
| 40.4 [a] | Sedoheptulose kinase deficiency | CV, AMN | DNA | I, II |
| 40.5 [a] | L-xylulose reductase deficiency | CV, AMN | DNA | I, II |
| 40.6 [a] | L-arabinosuria | – | – | – |
| 40.7 [a] | Sorbitol dehydrogenase deficiency | CV, AMN | DNA | I, II |

[a]Presumable benign disorder, prenatal diagnostics is not recommended

## DNA Testing

| Disorder | | Material | Gene locus |
|---|---|---|---|
| 40.1 | RPI deficiency | Any DNA source (WBC, FB, CV, AMN) | 2p11 |
| 40.2 | Transaldolase deficiency | Any DNA source (WBC, FB, CV, AMN) | 11p15 |
| 40.3 | Transketolase deficiency | Any DNA source (WBC, FB, CV, AMN) | 3p21 |
| 40.4 | Sedoheptulose kinase deficiency | Any DNA source (WBC, FB, CV, AMN) | 17p13.2 |
| 40.5 | L-xylulose reductase deficiency | Any DNA source (WBC, FB, CV, AMN) | 17q25.3 |
| 40.7 | Sorbitol dehydrogenase deficiency | Any DNA source (WBC, FB, CV, AMN) | 15q21.1 |

## Treatment Summary

For all disorders in polyol metabolism described in this chapter there is no specific treatment. For some clinical significance is still unclear, for example, SHPK deficiency, L-arabinosuria and SORD deficiency. L-xylulose reductase deficiency is a benign disorder and needs no treatment.

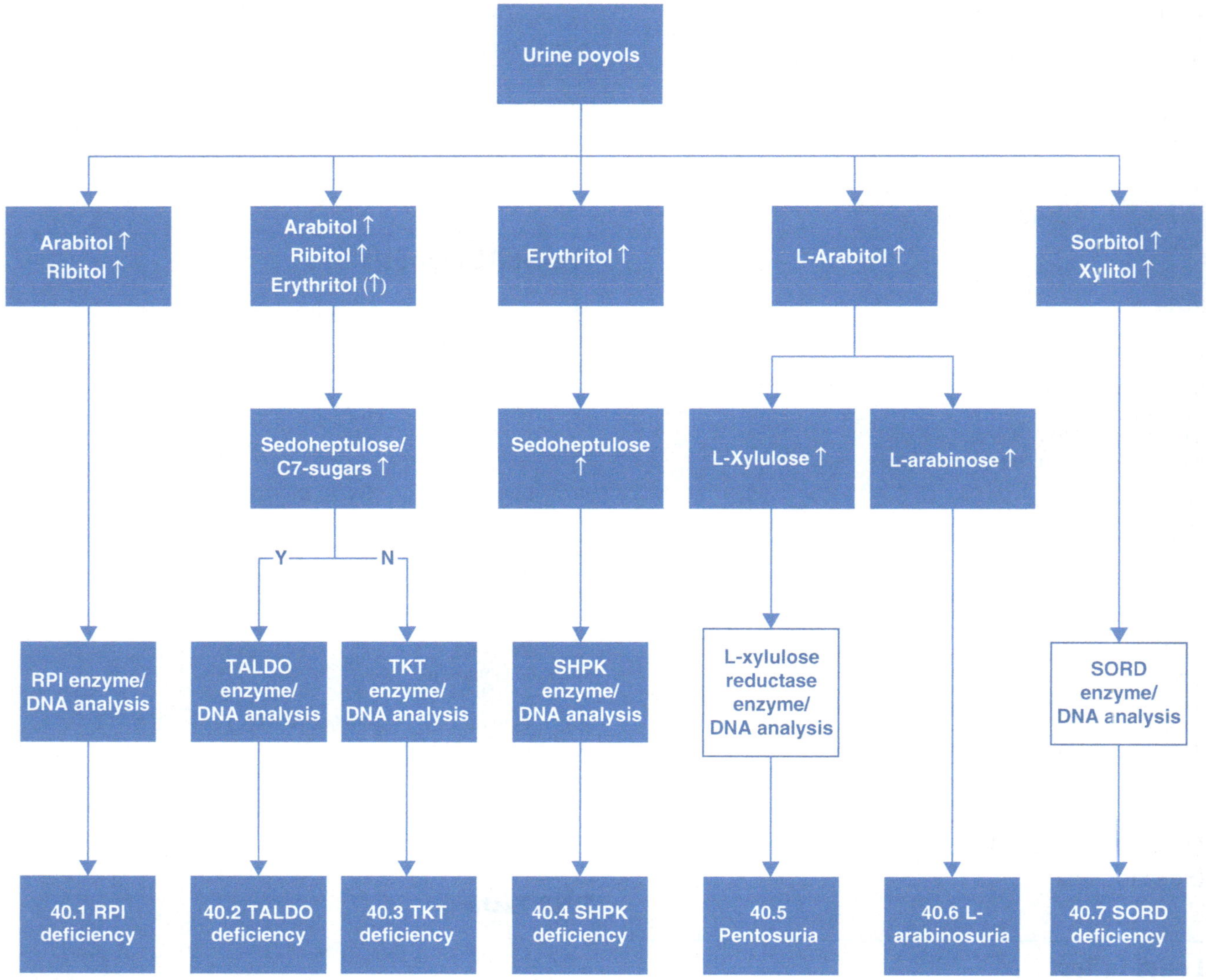


**Fig. 40.2** Diagnostic flowchart in case of abnormally elevated urinary polyols

In RPI, and TKT deficiency supportive therapy for their symptoms are indicated.

For TALDO deficiency treatment is symptomatic and focused on liver disease, which is the main cause of morbidity and mortality of this condition. Medication with a possible liver toxic effect should be used with care and (possibly) adjusted in dosage. Liver transplantation, according to literature, has been performed in three affected patients before the age of 1 year (Williams et al. 2019). Two of the patients were stable at 7 and 3 years, the other died in the course of the liver transplantation. Correction of anaemia and low clotting factors may require transfusions of packed red cells and fresh frozen plasma, respectively. Surgical correction of heart septal defects and medical treatment of tubulopathy, arterial hypertension and endocrine disorders may be required.

The only patient described with L-arabinosuria has been treated with a fruit restricted diet; this resulted in a decrease in excretion of the metabolites concerned.

## Emergency Treatment

There is currently no known emergency treatment for any of the disorders of polyol metabolism described in this chapter.

In TALDO deficiency, especially when liver dysfunction has been observed, care with respect to medications metabolised by the liver should be given. Dosing of medications might need to be reconsidered and acetaminophen even at normal dosage could be toxic. With the suggested positive effect of N-acetylcysteine on the prevention of liver failure and carcinogenesis of the liver in the mouse, treatment with N-acetylcysteine can be considered in case of fulminant liver failure (replenishment of glutathione).

## Experimental Treatment

In the TALDO knockout mouse model lifelong administration of the potent antioxidant N-acetylcysteine (NAC) prevented acetaminophen-induced liver failure, and blocked hepatocarcinogenesis in Taldo1−/− mice. (Hanczko et al. 2009). Rodan and Berry (2017) concluded that supplementation of NAC probably helped a TALDO-deficient patient, since NAC normalized AFP levels and could have resulted in decreased hepatocyte injury. The data from the long-term follow-up of Polish patients show that AFP levels however normalized with age (Limpinski et al. 2018)

In animal studies it has been shown that benfotiamine, a lipid-soluble thiamine derivative, can activate TKT and prevent retinopathy and vascular damage due to accumulation of glycolytic metabolites in diabetic rats. It is possible that benfotiamine could be used therapeutically in individuals with TKT deficiency with some residual activity, and this should of course be investigated (Hammes 2003).

For all other disorders in polyol metabolism no experimental treatment has been suggested.

## Follow-Up and Monitoring

For TALDO deficiency the advice is to follow haematological parameters to evaluate anaemia (blood count, including reticulocyte, LDH, haptoglobin and erythropoietin), liver function (clotting factors, transaminases, bilirubin, conjugated bilirubin, gamma-glutamyl transpeptidase (GGT), alkaline phosphatase) and AFP for evaluation of liver carcinogenesis every 3–6 months, and kidney function (glomerular and tubular). Decreased tubular function also warrants evaluation of bone mineral content (dual-energy X-ray absorptiometry (DXA) scans). Regular visceral imaging studies (US, computed tomography, magnetic resonance imaging) should be performed according to local protocols for patients with chronic liver disease at risk for cirrhosis. Follow-up of height, weight and puberty, including Tanner staging, is important. Gonadal function should be assessed based on clinical symptoms such as cryptorchidism, microphallus, delayed puberty or infertility. We advise a low-threshold for assessment of thyroid function (Williams et al. 2019). Referral to a clinical geneticist and cardiologist when the diagnosis has been made is further suggested.

For RPI or TKT deficiency, follow-up programmes/guidelines for neurological and/or developmental impairment are most likely applicable. No specific advice for these diseases can be given, yet this is also determined by disease progression.

## References


Boyle L, Wamelink MMC, Salomons GS, et al. Mutations in TKT are the cause of a syndrome including short stature, developmental delay, and congenital heart defects. Am J Human Genetics. 2016;98:1235–42.

Brooks SS, Anderson S, Bhise V, et al. Further delineation of ribose-5-phosphate isomerase deficiency: report of a third case. J Child Neurol. 2018;33:784–7.

Carr IM, Markham AF. Molecular genetic analysis of the human sorbitol dehydrogenase gene. Mamm Genome. 1995;6:645–52.

Engelke UFH, Zijlstra FSM, Mochel F, et al. Mitochondrial involvement and erythronic acid as a novel biomarker in transaldolase deficiency. Biochim Biophys Acta. 2010;1802:1028–35.

Hammes HP. Pathophysiological mechanisms of diabetic angiopathy. J Diabetes Complicat. 2003;17:16–9.

Hanczko R, Fernandez DR, Doherty E, et al. Prevention of hepatocarcinogenesis and increased susceptibility to acetaminophen-induced liver failure in transaldolase-deficient mice by N-acetylcysteine. J Clin Invest. 2009;119:1546–57.

Huck JHJ, Verhoeven NM, Struys EA, et al. Ribose-5-phosphate isomerase deficiency: new inborn error in the pentose phosphate pathway associated with a slowly progressive leukoencephalopathy. Am J Hum Genet. 2004;74:745–51.

Jansen G, Muskiet FA, Schierbeek H, et al. Capillary gas chromatographic profiling of urinary, plasma and erythrocyte sugars and polyols as their trimethylsilyl derivatives, preceded by a simple and rapid prepurification method. Clin Chim Acta. 1986;157:277–93.

Kardon T, Stroobant V, Veiga-da-Cunha M, et al. Characterization of mammalian sedoheptulokinase and mechanism of formation of erythritol in sedoheptulokinase deficiency. FEBS Lett. 2008;582:3330–4.

LeDuc CA, Crouch EE, Wilson A, et al. Novel association of early onset hepatocellular carcinoma with transaldolase deficiency. JIMD Reports. 2014;12:121–7.

Limpinski P, Pawlowska J, Stradomska T, et al. Long-term systematic monitoring of four Polish transaldolase deficient patients. J Inherit Metab Dis Reports. 2018;42:79–87.

Naik N, Shah A, Wamelink MMC, et al. Rare case of ribose 5 phosphate isomerase deficiency with slowly progressive leukoencephalopathy. Neurology. 2017;89:1195–6.

Onkenhout W, Groener JE, Verhoeven NM, et al. L-Arabinosuria: a new defect in human pentose metabolism. Mol Genet Metab. 2002;77:80–5.

Pierce SB, Spurrell CH, Mandell JB, et al. Garrod's fourth inborn error of metabolism solved by the identification of mutations causing pentosuria. PNAS. 2011;108:18313–7.

Rodan LH, Berry GT. N-acetylcysteine therapy in an infant with transaldolase deficiency is well tolerated and associated with normalization of alpha fetoprotein levels. J Inherit Metab Dis Reports. 2017;31:73–7.

Shin YS, Rieth M, Endres W, et al. Sorbitol dehydrogenase deficiency in a family with congenital cataracts. J Inherit Metab Dis. 1984;7(suppl 2):151–2.

Touster O, Harwell SO. The isolation of L-arabitol from pentosuric urine. J Biol Chem. 1958;230:1031–41.

Vaca G, Hernandez A, Ibarra B. Detection of inborn errors of metabolism in 1,117 patients studied because of suspected inherited disease. Arch Invest Med (Mex). 1981;12:341–8.

Valayannopoulos V, Verhoeven N, Mention K, et al. Transaldolase deficiency: a new cause of hydrops fetalis and neonatal multi-organ disease. J Pediatr. 2006;149:713–7.

van der Knaap MS, Wevers RA, Struys EA, et al. Leukoencephalopathy associated with a disturbance in the metabolism of polyols. Ann Neurol. 1999;46:925–8.

Verhoeven NM, Huck JH, Roos B, et al. Transaldolase deficiency: liver cirrhosis associated with a new inborn error in the pentose phosphate pathway. Am J Hum Genet. 2001;68:1086–92.

Wang YM, Van Eys J. The enzymatic defect in essential pentosuria. N Engl J Med. 1970;282:892–6.

Wamelink MMC, Struys EA, Jakobs C. The biochemistry, metabolism and inherited defect of the pentose phosphate pathway: a review. J Inherit Metab Dis. 2008;31:703–17.

Wamelink MMC, Ramos RJJF, van den Elzen APM, et al. First two unrelated cases of isolated sedoheptulokinase deficiency: a benign disorder? J Inherit Metab Dis. 2015;38:889–94.

Williams M, Valayannopoulos V, Altassan R, et al. Clinical, biochemical, and molecular overview of transaldolase deficiency and evaluation of the endocrine function: update of 34 patients. J Inherit Metab Dis. 2019;42:147–58.

# Congenital Hyperinsulinism

# 41

Jean-Baptiste Arnoux, Arianna Maiorana, Marlène Rio, and Pascale de Lonlay

## Contents



Jean-Baptiste Arnoux and Arianna Maiorana are equally contributed to this work.

J.-B. Arnoux (✉)
French Metabolic Network G2M, Necker-Enfants Malades Hospital, APHP, Paris, France
e-mail: Jean-baptiste.arnoux@aphp.fr

A. Maiorana
Division of Metabolism, Department of Pediatric Subspecialties, Bambino Gesù Children's Hospital, Rome, Italy
e-mail: arianna.maiorana@opbg.net

M. Rio
Genetic Department, Necker-Enfants Malades Hospital, APHP, Paris, France
e-mail: Marlene.rio@aphp.fr

P. de Lonlay
French Metabolic Network G2M, Necker-Enfants Malades Hospital, APHP, Paris, France
e-mail: Pascale.delonlay@aphp.fr


N. Blau et al. (eds.), *Physician's Guide to the Diagnosis, Treatment, and Follow-Up of Inherited Metabolic Diseases*,
https://doi.org/10.1007/978-3-030-67727-5_41

**Summary**

Hyperinsulinemic hypoglycaemia (HI) includes all conditions in which inappropriate high plasma insulin levels are observed during hypoglycaemia, regardless of whether the cause is related to a perinatal stress, to a genetic disorder (specific to the ß-cell or syndromic), drug-induced or else. In this chapter, we will consider genetic causes of HI, and discuss transient and syndromic aetiologies. Recently, exceptional causes of non-ketotic hypoglycaemia related to disorders of the insulin receptor pathway were added to the spectrum of HI. Congenital hyperinsulinism (CHI) is per se limited to all genetic defects of the pancreatic ß-cell leading to HI. CHI can present throughout life but is most common in infancy. CHI is responsible for recurrent severe hypoglycaemia in neonates, in whom delayed diagnosis or improper medical management is responsible for brain damage in about 1/3 of them. Most CHI patients are responsive to a first line oral treatment with diazoxide. When unresponsive, the treatment also includes somatostatin analogues and/or dietetic treatment. Further exploration of the histopathological form of CHI is a crucial point. Indeed, two main histopathological forms of CHI exist: a diffuse form, where all the ß-cells throughout the pancreas are involved, and a focal form, where hypersecreting ß-cells are restricted to a small region of the pancreas. The severity of CHI improves with time, allowing a progressive weaning of all therapies. Focal forms can also be immediately and definitively cured after a partial pancreatectomy, whereas alternative strategies for diffuse forms of CHI aim at avoiding a near-total pancreatectomy since surgery does not guarantee the achievement of normoglycaemia and leads to insulin-dependent diabetes in most cases. Developments of several new medical treatments are in process to ease the conservative medical treatment in order to limit the need of a near-total pancreatectomy.

## Introduction

In adults and children, hyperinsulinemic hypoglycaemia (HI) is revealed by autonomic (pallor, sweating, tachycardia, tremor, paresthesias) and neuroglucopenic symptoms (drowsiness, faint, seizures, hallucinations, coma). In some patients, symptoms may be mistaken for epilepsy (unless glycaemia is sampled during/after seizures) or, in some others, hypoglycaemia can be asymptomatic. The hypoglycaemic events may happen after a meal or at fast, several times a day or occasionally. Some family history of hypoglycaemia or MODY diabetes can be found. Rarely, CHI can be induced by a strenuous physical exercise (MCT1, *SLC16A1* gene mutation). When the age at onset of HI is beyond 4 years, screening for insulinoma is recommended (Arnoux et al. 2014).

In newborns, HI is the most prevalent cause of hypoglycaemia. Hypoglycaemia may be screened by a routine capillary glycaemia which is recommended in all neonates *except* those born full-term, with normal birth weight and without pathological context (perinatal stress, sepsis, dysmorphisms, family history of hypoglycaemic disorder). Actually, half patients are still diagnosed following an episode of seizure or coma. In affected newborns, hypoglycaemia is almost permanent and a high rate of continuous glucose infusion (GIR) or feedings (>10 mg/kg/min; physiological requirements in newborns 4–8 mg/kg/min) is required to normalize glycaemia. Associated features may be a transient hypertrophic cardiomyopathy and a transient inadequate cortisol response to hypoglycaemia (Hussain et al. 2003). Because of late diagnosis or insufficient medical management, the neurological outcome is unsatisfactory in almost half of the patients. Thus, it is recommended to check glycemia in all newborns with risk factors of hypoglycaemia, because an early diagnosis and a prompt treatment of hypoglycemia are essential to avoid hypoglycemia-induced brain damage (Ludwig et al. 2018; Yorifuji et al. 2017).

In neonates, HI can be related to three clinical pictures:

1. **Transient neonatal HI** can occur in newborns from diabetic mothers, large or small for gestational age or as a consequence of perinatal stress (foetal distress, birth asphyxia, maternal eclampsia, meconium aspiration syndrome, hypothermia, foetal erythroblastosis). Although hypoglycaemia can be severe, it usually resolves within a few weeks (max 3 months). However, it may require a transient treatment (glucose enriched feeds and/or diazoxide).
2. **Syndromic HI** is a condition in which HI is included in a developmental syndrome. Hypoglycaemia can be the revealing sign during the neonatal period (Beckwith-Wiedemann, Perlman, Simpson-Golabi, Kabuki, Sotos, Costello, Turner syndrome, Congenital Disorder of Glycosylation type I, etc.) or be discovered later during the follow-up (e.g. Ondine syndrome). In various series, about 10% of neonates with HI presented an underlying syndrome. Subsequently, an oriented clinical examination and imaging procedures (abdominal US, heart US, spine X-ray) are systematically recommended in newborns diagnosed with HI. Syndromic HI is usually responsive to diazoxide and shows HI resolution within months or a few years. HI was also occasionally described in patients with Moebius, Cowden, Nager, Usher type C,

Poland, CHARGE syndrome, trisomy 13 and tyrosinemia type I (Galcheva et al. 2019).

3. **"Isolated" congenital HI** occurs when HI is inherited and is mostly considered as an isolated symptom. However, despite isolated CHI is described as non-syndromic, patients may present with additional features (Arnoux et al. 2014):

   Mutations in known genes account for 50% of diazoxide-responsive cases: *ABCC8*, *KCNJ11*, *GCK*, *HK1*, *GLUD1*, *HADH*, *HNF4A*, *HNF1A*, *SLC16A1*, *UCP2*, *INSR*. Hypoglycaemia can start at any age. The familial history may disclose members with hypoglycaemia and/or maturity-onset diabetes of youth (*ABCC8*, *KCNJ11*, *GCK*, *HNF1A*, *HNF4A* genes), or with mild hyperammonemia, mental retardation and/or epilepsy (*GLUD1* gene). In neonates, the revealing symptom is seizures in half patients. The age at presentation is earlier in *HNF4A* mutation (1 day), variable in $K_{ATP}$ genes mutation (1 day to 1 year, mean: 27.4 days), and delayed in *GLUD1* and *HADH* mutation (157 and 125 days) (Snider et al. 2013). Hypoglycaemia can occur in the fasting and the post-prandial states.

   CHI severity is classified as diazoxide responsive, in whom the genetic cause is identified in 47% of patients vs. diazoxide unresponsive patients, in whom almost 90% of patients display mutations in *ABCC8*, *KCNJ11* or *GCK* genes (Lord et al. 2013).

   CHI is a rare condition, involving 1/20,000–50,000 newborns in the Caucasian population (up to 1/2500 in countries with substantial inbreeding) and usually present from the neonatal period. In the ***diffuse form***, the disease involves the whole pancreas with presence of enlarged nuclei in the Langerhans islets β-cells throughout the pancreas, whereas in the ***focal form*** an adenomatous hyperplasia of the islets is limited to a small portion of the pancreas, and only the combination of genetics and pancreatic $^{18}$F-DOPA PET/TC scan can distinguish between the two forms, which even share almost the same prevalence. Mutations in *ABCC8* and *KCNJ11* genes, which respectively encode for the SUR1 and Kir6.2 subunits of the $K_{ATP}$ channel, have been associated with diffuse and focal forms. Particularly, diffuse forms of CHI are inherited as either autosomal recessive or dominant trait, whereas the focal form results from the combination of a paternally inherited germinal mutation, a somatic loss of heterozygosity of the maternal allele in a restricted group of β-cells, and a paternal disomy of the 11p15 chromosomal region in these cells (De Lonlay et al. 1997). Besides these two classical histopathological forms, ***atypical forms*** exist with negative genetics in blood leukocytes, and a particular one called LINE (localized islets cells nuclear enlargement), displays, in some cases, a somatic dominant mutation in the *ABCC8* or *GCK* genes, found after a genetic study on the abnormal pancreatic tissue. These forms lead to a "diffuse type histology" but restricted to a variable portion of the pancreas as segmental mosaic forms or extensive focal forms (Sempoux et al. 2011; Capito et al. 2011).

   Mutations in all the other known genes cause diffuse forms. Some forms exhibit peculiar characteristics: protein-sensitivity ($K_{ATP}$ genes, *GLUD1*, *HADH*), leucine-sensitivity (*GLUD1*), hyperammonemia (*GLUD1*), increased urinary excretion of α-ketoglutarate (*GLUD1*), increased risk of neurological symptoms, atypical absence, myoclonia, ADHD, pyramidal syndrome, dystonia (*GLUD*1), increased hydroxybutirylcarnitine and urinary 3-hydroxyglutaric acid (*HADH*), family history of MODY (*HNF4A*, *HNF1A*), hepatomegaly and renal Fanconi syndrome (*HNF4A*), liver adenomatosis (*HNF1A*), exercise-sensitivity (*SLC16A1*, *HADH*), hypersensitivity to glucose-induced hypoglycaemia (*UCP2*).

## Nomenclature

| No. | Disease name | Alternative name | Disease Abreviation | Gene symbols | Chromosomal localization | Inheritance | Affected protein | OMIM# | HI form |
|---|---|---|---|---|---|---|---|---|---|
| *Isolated CHI* | | | | | | | | | |
| 41.1 | ATP-sensitive potassium channel regulatory subunit deficiency | Familial hyperinsulinemic hypoglycaemia type 1 | KATP-HI | *ABCC8* | 11p15.1 | AD, AR, somatic | SUR1 | 600509 | Focal, diffuse, LINE |
| 41.2 | ATP-sensitive potassium channel pore-forming subunit deficiency | Familial hyperinsulinemic hypoglycaemia type 2 | KATP-HI | *KCNJ11* | 11p15.1 | AD, AR | Kir6.2 | 600937 | Focal, diffuse |
| 41.3 | Glucokinase superactivity | Familial hyperinsulinemic hypoglycaemia type 3 | GCK-HI | *GCK* | 7p13 | AD, somatic | Glucokinase | 138079 | Diffuse, LINE |
| 41.4 | Short-chain 3-hydroxyacyl-CoA dehydrogenase deficiency | Familial hyperinsulinemic hypoglycaemia type 4 | SCHAD-HI | *HADH* | 4q25 | AR | Short chain hydroxyacyl-CoA dehydrogenase | 601609 | Diffuse |
| 41.5 | Insulin receptor dysregulation | Familial hyperinsulinemic hypoglycaemia type 5 | | *INSR* | 19p13.2 | AD | InsR | 147670 | Diffuse |
| 41.6 | Glutamate dehydrogenase superactivity | Hyperinsulinism-hyperammonemia syndrome; familial hyperinsulinemic hypoglycaemia type 6 | HIHA syndrome | *GLUD1* | 10q23.2 | AD | Glutamate dehydrogenase | 138130 | Diffuse |
| 41.7 | Exercise induced hyperinsulinemic hypoglycaemia | Familial hyperinsulinemic hypoglycaemia type 7 | EI-HI | *SLC16A1* | 1p13.2 | AD | MCT1 | 610021 | Diffuse |
| 41.8 | Hepatocyte nuclear factor-4α deficiency | MODY1 | MODY1 | *HNF4A* | 20q13.12 | AD | HNF4A | 600281 | Diffuse |
| 41.9 | Hepatocyte nuclear factor-1α deficiency | MODY3 | MODY3 | *HNF1A* | 12q24.31 | AD | HNF1A | 142410 | Diffuse |
| 41.10 | Hexokinase 1 mutation | | | *HK1* | 10q22.1 | AD, somatic | Hexokinase 1 | 142600 | Diffuse |
| 41.11 | Uncoupling protein 2 deficiency | | UCP2-HI | *UCP2* | 11q13.4 | AD | UCP2 | 601693 | Diffuse |
| *Syndromic CHI* | | | | | | | | | |
| 41.12 | Beckwith-Wiedemann syndrome | Exomphalos–macroglossia–Gogantism syndrome | BWS | Genetic or epigenetic changes of imprinted region 11p15.5. IGF2/H19/CDKN1C/KCNQ1 | 11p15.4 | Sporadic, AD, mosaic, genomic imprinting | IGF2, H19, p57(KIP2)/KCNQ1OT1 | 130650 | Diffuse, focal, atypical |

| | | | | | | | | | |
|---|---|---|---|---|---|---|---|---|---|
| 41.13 | Kabuki syndrome | Niikawa-Kuroki syndrome | KS | *KMT2D/ KDM6A* | 12q13.12/Xp11.3 | AD/sporadic XLD | Lysine specific methyltransferase 2D/ H3K27me3-specific demethylase | 602113/300867 | Diffuse |
| 41.14 | Turner syndrome | 45,X syndrome | TS | Partial or complete X chromosome monosomy | X | Sporadic, mosaic | / | / | Diffuse |
| 41.15 | Adenosine kinase deficiency | Hypermethioninemia due to adenosine kinase deficiency | ADK deficiency | *ADK* | 10q22.2 | AR | ADK | 614300 | Diffuse |
| 41.16 | Phosphomannomutase 2 deficiency | PMM2-CDG | CDG1a | *PMM2* | 16p13.2 | AR | Phosphomannomutase 2 | 601785 | Diffuse |
| 41.17 | Mannosephosphate isomerase deficiency | MPI-CDG | CDG1b | *MPI* | 15q24.1 | AR | Phosphomanno-isomerase | 154550 | Diffuse |
| 41.18 | ALG3 α-1,3-mannosyltransferase deficiency | ALG3-CDG | CDG1d | *ALG3* | 3q27.1 | AR | α-1,3-mannosyltransferase | 608750 | Diffuse |
| 41.19 | ALG6 α-1,3-glucosyltransferase deficiency | ALG6-CDG | CDG1c | *ALG6* | 1p31.3 | AR | α-1,3-glucosyltransferase | 604566 | Diffuse |
| 41.20 | Phosphoglucomutase 1 deficiency | PGM1-CDG; glycogen storage disease type 14 | CDG1t | *PGM1* | 1p31.3 | AR | Phosphoglucomutase | 171900 | Diffuse |
| 41.21 | Sotos syndrome | Cerebral gigantism | | *NSD1/5q35 deletion/NFIX* | 5q35.3/5q35.3/19p13.3 | AD/AR/ sporadic | Histone methyltransferase/ transcription factor | 117550/617169 | Diffuse |
| 41.22 | Timothy syndrome | Long QT syndrome with syndactily | TS | *CACNA1C* | 12p13.33 | AD, sporadic | CACNA1C (voltage-dependent L-type calcium channel subunit alpha-1C) | 601005 | Diffuse |
| 41.23 | PASNA: Primary aldosteronism, seizures, and neurologic abnormalities | | PASNA | *CACNA1D* | 3p21.1 | AD, AR | CACNA1D (voltage-dependent L-type calcium channel subunit alpha-1D) | 615474 | Diffuse |
| 41.24 | MSSGM1 | Microcephaly, short stature, and impaired glucose metabolism 1 | MSSGM1 | *TRMT10A* | 4q23 | AR | TRMT10A (tRNA methyltransferase 10) | 616013 | Diffuse |
| 41.25 | Costello syndrome | Facio-cutaneo-skeletal syndrome | FCS syndrome | *HRAS* | 11p15.5 | AD, sporadic | GTPase HRas | 218040 | Diffuse |
| 41.26 | Perlman syndrome | | PRLMNS | DIS3L2 | 2q37.1 | AR | DIS3-like exonuclease 2 | 267000 | Diffuse |

(continued)

| No. | Disease name | Alternative name | Disease Abreviation | Gene symbols | Chromosomal localization | Inheritance | Affected protein | OMIM# | HI form |
|---|---|---|---|---|---|---|---|---|---|
| 41.27 | Simpson-Golabi-Behmel syndrome | | SGBS | GPC3 | Xq26.2 | XLR | Glypican-3 | 312870 | Diffuse |
| 41.28 | FOXA2 | HNF3B | FOXA2 | *FOXA2* | 20p11.21 | AD | Forkhead box A2 | 600288 | Diffuse |
| 41.29 | Ondine syndrome | Congenital central hypoventilation syndrome | CCHS | PHOX2B | 4p13 | AD, sporadic | Paired mesoderm homeobox protein 2B | 209880 | Diffuse |
| 41.30 | Rubinstein-Taybi | | | | | AD, sporadic | CREBBP, EP300 | 600140 | Diffuse |
| *CHI-like hypoglycaemia (genetic, hypoinsulinemic)* | | | | | | | | | |
| 41.31 | AKT2 superactivity | Hypoinsulinemic hypoglycaemia with hemihypertrophy | | *AKT2* | 19q13.2 | AD, sporadic, mosaic | RAC-beta serine/ threonine-protein kinase | 164731 | Diffuse |
| 41.32 | AKT3 superactivity | Megalencephaly-micropolygyria-polydactily-hydrocephalus syndrome | MPPH2 | AKT3 | 1q43-44 | AD, sporadic, mosaic | RAC-gamma serine/ threonine-protein kinase | 611223 | Diffuse |
| 41.32 | Catalytic phosphatidylinositol 3-kinase α subunit superactivity | | CLOVE syndrome, MCAP syndrome | *PIK3CA* | 3q26-32 | Somatic, mosaic | Phosphatidylinositol 4,5-bisphosphate 3-kinase catalytic subunit alpha isoform | 612918/602501 | Diffuse |

## Metabolic Pathways

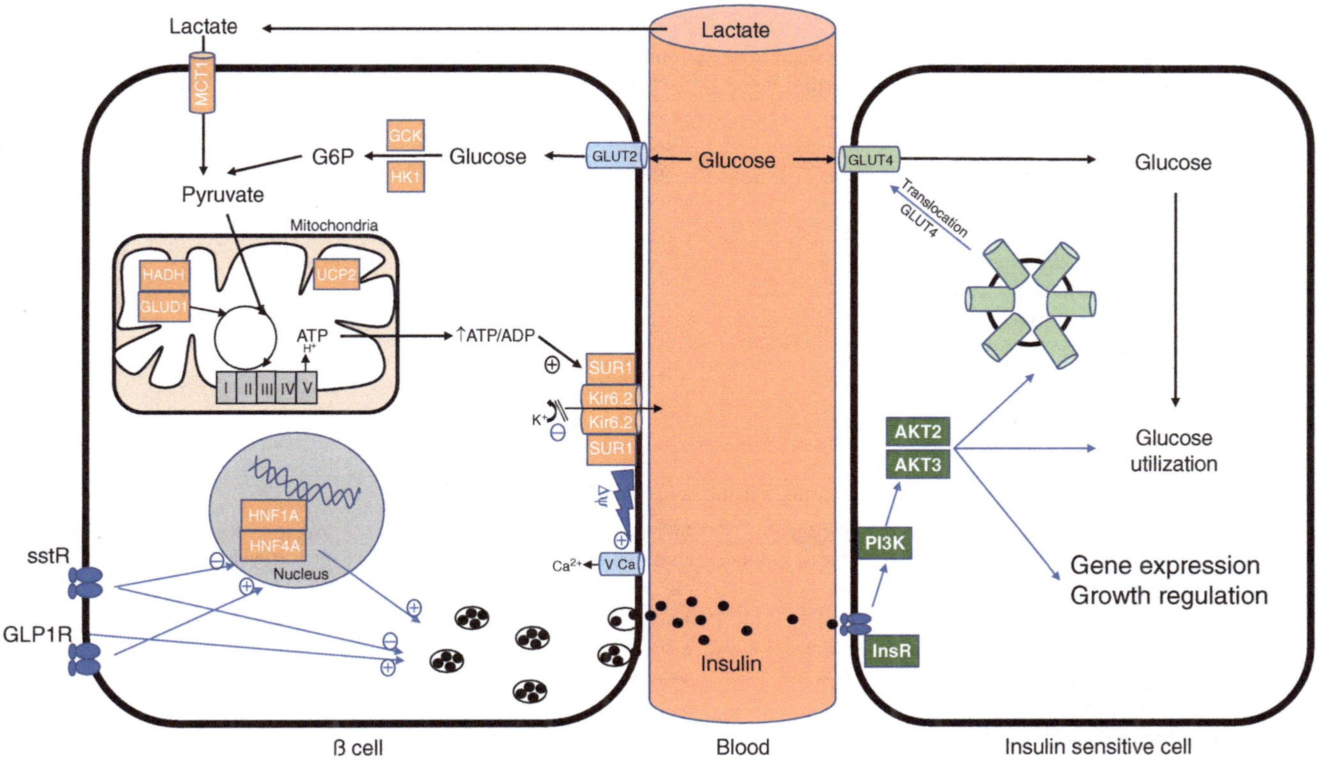


**Fig. 41.1** Insulin secretion and action
Schematic representation of a ß-cell and of an insulin-sensitive cell (i.e. striated muscle). For simplicity not all the substrates and products of each reaction are shown. Black arrows: metabolic pathways. Blue arrows: signalling pathways. Red boxes: proteins involved in the GSIS, and responsible for isolated CHI: SUR1 and Kir6.2 (subunits of the $K_{ATP}$ channel encoded respectively by *ABCC8* and *KCNJ11*); GCK; HK1, MCT1 (encoded by *SLC16A1*); HADH; GDH (encoded by *GLUD1*); HNF1A and HNF4A; UCP2. Glucose enters into the ß-cells through GLUT2 channels, is phosphorylated to glucose-6-phophate (G6P) then undergoes glycolysis to produce pyruvate. This latter will be oxidized in the Krebs cycle leading to the production of ATP. At the cell membrane, the ATP-dependent potassium channel ($K_{ATP}$ channel) closes when the ATP/ADP ratio increases, stopping a potassium efflux, which leads to membrane depolarization and activation of the voltage-dependent calcium channels. The influx of calcium into the ß-cells will stimulate the exocytosis of insulin containing secretory granules and the transcription of new insulin. Therefore, all the mechanisms which lead to an increased ATP production will cause hyperinsulinism ("metabolic HI"): glucokinase or glutamate dehydrogenase hyperactivity, UCP2 or HAHD deficiency, improper MCT1 expression. Mutations of the $K_{ATP}$ channel causing a permanent/predominant closed state of the channel are the most frequent cause of HI ("$K_{ATP}$ HI"). Finally, some transcription factors, also involved in monogenic diabetes, can inversely lead to CHI during childhood: HNF1A, HNF4A ("Transcription factor CHI")

Green boxes: proteins involved in hypoketotic hypoinsulinemic hypoglycaemia related to a genetic defect of the insulin receptor pathway: PI3KCA, AKT2 and AKT3. When insulin binds the insulin receptor of an insulin-sensitive cell, it will activate the mTOR pathway, with consequences such as: externalization of GLUT4 glucose transporter; raise of the cell glucose uptake; activation of metabolic pathways involved in glucose utilization or storage; activation of the cellular growth

## Signs and Symptoms

**Table 41.1** ATP-sensitive potassium channel regulatory subunit deficiency (ABCC8-HI)

| System | Symptoms and biomarkers | Neonatal (birth–1 month) | Infancy (1–18 months) | Childhood (1.5–11 years) | Adolescence (11–16 years) | Adulthood (>16 years) |
|---|---|---|---|---|---|---|
| CNS | **Convulsions** | ++ | ++ | + | ± | ± |
| Endocrine | Diabetes mellitus | | ± | ± | ± | ± |
| | **Hyperinsulinism** | ++ | ++ | ++ | + | ± |
| Metabolic | **hypoglycaemia, hypoketotic** | +++ | +++ | ++ | + | ± |
| Other | Macrosomia | ± | | | | |
| Laboratory findings | Free fatty acids (serum), during hypoglycaemia | ↓↓↓ | ↓↓↓ | ↓↓ | ↓↓ | ± |
| | Glucose (plasma) | ↓ | ↓ | ↓ | ↓ | ± |
| | Insulin, durig hypoglycaemia | ↑ | ↑ | ↑ | ↑ | ↑ |
| | Ketones, during hypoglycaemia | ↓↓↓ | ↓↓↓ | ↓↓ | ↓ | ± |

**Table 41.2** ATP-sensitive potassium channel pore-forming subunit deficiency (KCNJ11-HI)

| System | Symptoms and biomarkers | Neonatal (birth–1 month) | Infancy (1–18 months) | Childhood (1.5–11 years) | Adolescence (11–16 years) | Adulthood (>16 years) |
|---|---|---|---|---|---|---|
| CNS | **Convulsions** | ++ | ++ | + | ± | ± |
| Endocrine | Diabetes mellitusf | ++ | ++ | ++ | + | ± |
| | **Hyperinsulinism** | | ± | ± | ± | ± |
| Metabolic | **hypoglycaemia, hypoketotic** | +++ | +++ | ++ | + | ± |
| Other | Macrosomia | ± | | | | |
| Laboratory findings | Free fatty acids (serum) | ↓↓↓ | ↓↓↓ | ↓↓ | ↓↓ | ± |
| | Glucose (plasma) | ↓ | ↓ | ↓ | ↓ | ± |
| | Insulin, durig hypoglycaemia | ↑ | ↑ | ↑ | ↑ | ↑ |
| | Ketones, during hypoglycaemia | ↓↓↓ | ↓↓↓ | ↓↓ | ↓ | ± |

**Table 41.3** Glucokinase superactivity (GCK-HI)

| System | Symptoms and biomarkers | Neonatal (birth–1 month) | Infancy (1–18 months) | Childhood (1.5–11 years) | Adolescence (11–16 years) | Adulthood (>16 years) |
|---|---|---|---|---|---|---|
| CNS | Convulsions | ± | ± | | | |
| | Intellectual disability | ± | ± | ± | ± | ± |
| Endocrine | Diabetes, neonatal/monogenic | ++ | ++ | ++ | ++ | ± |
| | **Hyperinsulinism** | ± | ± | ± | ± | ± |
| Metabolic | Hypoglycaemia | ++ | ++ | ++ | ++ | ± |
| | **Hypoglycaemia, hypoketotic** | ++ | ++ | ++ | ++ | ± |
| Laboratory findings | Free fatty acids (serum) | ↓ | ↓ | ↓ | ↓ | ↓ |
| | Glucose (plasma) | ↓ | ↓ | ↓ | ↓ | ↓ |
| | Insulin, durig hypoglycaemia | ↑ | ↑ | ↑ | ↑ | ↑ |
| | Ketones, during hypoglycaemia | ↓ | ↓ | ↓ | ↓ | |

**Table 41.4** Hyperinsulinemic hypoglycaemia-4 (SCHAD_HI)

| System | Symptoms and biomarkers | Neonatal (birth–1 month) | Infancy (1–18 months) | Childhood (1.5–11 years) | Adolescence (11–16 years) | Adulthood (>16 years) |
|---|---|---|---|---|---|---|
| Cardiovascular | Cardiomyopathy | ± | | | | |
| CNS | Intellectual disability | ± | ± | ± | ± | ± |
| | Seizures | ± | ± | | | |
| Digestive | Liver failure, Reye-like | | + | + | | |
| Endocrine | **Hyperinsulinism** | + | + | + | | |
| | Protein sensitivity | + | ++ | ++ | ++ | |
| Metabolic | **Hypoglycaemia, hypoketotic** | + | + | + | | |

**Table 41.4** (continued)

| System | Symptoms and biomarkers | Neonatal (birth–1 month) | Infancy (1–18 months) | Childhood (1.5–11 years) | Adolescence (11–16 years) | Adulthood (>16 years) |
|---|---|---|---|---|---|---|
| Laboratory findings | 3-Hydroxydicarboxylic acid (urine) | (↑) | (↑) | (↑) | | |
| | 3-Hydroxyglutarate (urine) | ↑ | ↑ | ↑ | | |
| | Ammonia (blood) | | ↑ | ↑ | ↑ | |
| | C4-OH Hydroxybutyrylcarnitine (dried blood spot) | ↑ | ↑ | ↑ | | |
| | C4-OH Hydroxybutyrylcarnitine (plasma) | ↑ | ↑ | ↑ | | |
| | Glucose (plasma) | ↓ | ↓ | | | |
| | Insulin, durig hypoglycaemia | ↑ | ↑ | ↑ | ↑ | ↑ |
| | Ketones (urine) | ↓ | ↓ | | | |
| | Medium chain dicarboxylic acids (urine) | (↑) | (↑) | (↑) | | |

**Table 41.5** Hyperinsulinemic hypoglycaemia-5 (INSR)

| System | Symptoms and biomarkers | Neonatal (birth–1 month) | Infancy (1–18 months) | Childhood (1.5–11 years) | Adolescence (11–16 years) | Adulthood (>16 years) |
|---|---|---|---|---|---|---|
| CNS | **Seizures** | | | + | + | + |
| Dermatological | Hyperpigmentation | | | | | ± |
| Endocrine | Hyperinsulinism | + | + | | | |
| Metabolic | **Hypoglycaemia, hypoketotic** | + | + | | | |
| Laboratory findings | Free fatty acids (serum) | ↓ | ↓ | | | |
| | Glucose (plasma) | ↓ | ↓ | | | |
| | Insulin, durig hypoglycaemia | ↑ | ↑ | ↑ | ↑ | ↑ |
| | Ketones, during hypoglycaemia | ↓ | ↓ | | | |

**Table 41.6** Glutamate dehydrogenase superactivity (HIHA syndrome)

| System | Symptoms and biomarkers | Neonatal (birth–1 month) | Infancy (1–18 months) | Childhood (1.5–11 years) | Adolescence (11–16 years) | Adulthood (>16 years) |
|---|---|---|---|---|---|---|
| CNS | Convulsions | ± | ± | ± | ± | ± |
| | EEG, abnormal | + | + | + | ± | ± |
| | **Epilepsy, generalized** | + | ++ | ++ | ± | ± |
| | Intellectual disability | | ± | ± | ± | ± |
| | Seizures | ± | ± | ± | ± | ± |
| Endocrine | **Hyperinsulinism** | + | ++ | ++ | + | + |
| Metabolic | **Hypoglycaemia** | ++ | ++ | + | + | + |
| | **Hypoglycaemia, hypoketotic** | ++ | ++ | + | + | + |
| | **Leucine sensitivity causing hypoglycaemia** | ++ | ++ | ++ | ++ | ++ |
| Laboratory findings | Alpha-ketoglutarate (urine) | n-↑ | n-↑ | n-↑ | n-↑ | n-↑ |
| | Ammonia, fasting (blood and plasma) | ↑ | ↑ | ↑ | ↑ | ↑ |
| | Free fatty acids (serum) | ↓ | ↓ | ↓ | ↓ | |
| | Glucose (plasma) | ↓ | ↓ | ↓ | ↓ | ↓ |
| | Insulin (plasma) | ↑ | ↑ | ↑ | ↑ | ↑ |
| | Ketones (plasma) | ↓ | ↓ | ↓ | ↓ | ↓ |
| | Ketones (urine) | ↓ | ↓ | ↓ | ↓ | ↓ |

**Table 41.7** Exercise induced hyperinsulinemic hypoglycaemia (SLC16A1-HI)

| System | Symptoms and biomarkers | Neonatal (birth–1 month) | Infancy (1–18 months) | Childhood (1.5–11 years) | Adolescence (11–16 years) | Adulthood (>16 years) |
|---|---|---|---|---|---|---|
| Endocrine | Hyperinsulinism | | | | ++ | +++ |
| Metabolic | Hypoglycaemia, exercise induced | | | | ++ | ++ |
| Laboratory findings | Ammonia (plasma) | | | | n | |
| | Free fatty acids (serum) | | | | ↓ | ↓↓ |
| | Glucose (plasma) | | | | ↓ | ↓↓ |
| | Ketones (plasma) | | | | ↓ | ↓ |
| | Ketones (urine) | | | | ↓ | ↓ |
| | Ketones, during hypoglycaemia | | | | ↓ | ↓↓ |
| | Pyruvate test | | | ++ | +++ | +++ |

**Table 41.8** Hepatocyte nuclear factor 4-alpha loss-of-function mutations (HNF4A-HI)

| System | Symptoms and biomarkers | Neonatal (birth–1 month) | Infancy (1–18 months) | Childhood (1.5–11 years) | Adolescence (11–16 years) | Adulthood (>16 years) |
|---|---|---|---|---|---|---|
| Endocrine | **Diabetes type MODY** | | | + | ++ | ++ |
| | **Hyperinsulinism** | + | + | + | | |
| Metabolic | Hypoglycaemia | + | + | + | | |
| | **Hypoglycaemia, hypoketotic** | + | + | + | | |
| Other | **Macrosomia** | +++ | | | | |
| Laboratory findings | Free fatty acids (serum), during hypoglycaemia | ↓ | ↓ | ↓ | | |
| | Glucose (plasma) | ↓ | ↓ | ↓ | | |
| | Insulin, durig hypoglycaemia | ↑ | ↑ | ↑ | ↑ | ↑ |
| | Ketones, during hypoglycaemia | ↓ | ↓ | ↓ | | |

**Table 41.9** HNF1a deficiency

| System | Symptoms and biomarkers | Neonatal (birth–1 month) | Infancy (1–18 months) | Childhood (1.5–11 years) | Adolescence (11–16 years) | Adulthood (>16 years) |
|---|---|---|---|---|---|---|
| Endocrine | **Diabetes type MODY** | | | + | ++ | +++ |
| | **Hyperinsulinism** | + | + | | | |
| Metabolic | **hypoglycaemia, hypoketotic** | + | + | | | |
| Laboratory findings | Free fatty acids (serum), during hypoglycaemia | ↓ | ↓ | | | |
| | Glucose (plasma) | ↓ | ↓ | | | |
| | Insulin, durig hypoglycaemia | ↑ | ↑ | ↑ | ↑ | ↑ |
| | Ketones, during hypoglycaemia | ↓ | ↓ | | | |

**Table 41.10** Uncoupling protein 2 deficiency (UCP2-HI)

| System | Symptoms and biomarkers | Neonatal (birth–1 month) | Infancy (1–18 months) | Childhood (1.5–11 years) | Adolescence (11–16 years) | Adulthood (>16 years) |
|---|---|---|---|---|---|---|
| Endocrine | **Hyperinsulinism** | + | + | + | | |
| Metabolic | **hypoglycaemia, hypoketotic** | + | + | + | | |
| Laboratory findings | Free fatty acids (serum), during hypoglycaemia | ↓ | ↓ | ↓ | | |
| | Glucose (plasma) | ↓ | ↓ | ↓ | | |
| | Insulin, during hypoglycaemia | n-↑ | n-↑ | n-↑ | | |
| | Ketones, during hypoglycaemia | ↓ | ↓ | ↓ | | |

**Table 41.11** Beckwith-Wiedemann syndrome

| System | Symptoms and biomarkers | Neonatal (birth–1 month) | Infancy (1–18 months) | Childhood (1.5–11 years) | Adolescence (11–16 years) | Adulthood (>16 years) |
|---|---|---|---|---|---|---|
| Digestive | **Macroglossia** | + | ± | ± | | |
| Ear | **Ear creases and/or pits** | + | | | | |
| Endocrine | Hyperinsulinism | + | ± | ± | ± | ± |
| Musculoskeletal | **Exomphalos** | ± | | | | |
| | **Facial naevus simplex** | ± | ± | ± | | |
| | **Umbilical hernia** | ± | | | | |
| Other | **Lateralized overgrowth** | ± | + | + | ± | ± |
| | **Macrosomia** | +++ | | | | |
| | **Tumors (Wilms, nephroblastomatosis, neuroblastoma…)** | + | + | + | ± | ± |
| Laboratory findings | Free fatty acids (serum), during hypoglycaemia | ↓↓↓ | ↓↓↓ | ↓↓↓ | ↓↓↓ | ↓↓↓ |
| | Glucose (plasma) | ↓-↓↓-↓↓↓ | ↓-↓↓-↓↓↓ | ↓-↓↓ | ↓-↓↓ | ↓-↓↓ |
| | Insulin, during hypoglycaemia | n-↑ | n-↑ | n-↑ | n-↑ | n-↑ |
| | Ketones, during hypoglycaemia | ↓↓↓ | ↓↓↓ | ↓↓↓ | ↓↓↓ | ↓↓↓ |

**Table 41.12** Kabuki Syndrome

| System | Symptoms and biomarkers | Neonatal (birth–1 month) | Infancy (1–18 months) | Childhood (1.5–11 years) | Adolescence (11–16 years) | Adulthood (>16 years) |
|---|---|---|---|---|---|---|
| Cardiovascular | **Heart septal defect** | ± | | | | |
| Endocrine | **Hyperinsulinism** | + | + | | | |
| Musculoskeletal | **Eversion of the external third of the lower lid** | ± | ± | ++ | ++ | ++ |
| | **Facial dysmorphism** | ± | + | ++ | ++ | ++ |
| | **Fetal pads** | ++ | ++ | ++ | ++ | ++ |
| | **Small for gestationnal age** | ± | | | | |
| | **Vertebral/costal malformation** | ± | ± | ± | ± | ± |
| Other | **Failure to thrive** | ++ | ++ | ± | | |
| Laboratory findings | **Overweight** | | | + | ++ | + |
| | Free fatty acids (serum), during hypoglycaemia | ↓↓↓ | ↓↓↓ | | | |
| | Glucose (plasma) | ↓↓ | ↓ | | | |
| | Growth hormone deficiency? | | | | | |
| | Insulin, during hypoglycaemia | n-↑ | n-↑ | | | |
| | Ketones, during hypoglycaemia | ↓↓↓ | ↓↓↓ | | | |

**Table 41.13** Turner syndrome

| System | Symptoms and biomarkers | Neonatal (birth–1 month) | Infancy (1–18 months) | Childhood (1.5–11 years) | Adolescence (11–16 years) | Adulthood (>16 years) |
|---|---|---|---|---|---|---|
| Cardiovascular | **Heart, aortic malformation** | + | + | | | |
| Dermatological | **Hand and feet edema** | + | | | | |
| Endocrine | **Diabetes** | | | | + | + |
| | **Hyperinsulinism** | + | + | | | |
| | **Hypothyroidism** | | | | ++ | ++ |
| Genitourinary | **Ovarian dysgenesis** | ± | ± | + | + | + |
| Metabolic | hypoglycaemia | ↓↓ | ↓ | ↓ | | |
| Musculoskeletal | **Short stature** | ++ | + | + | + | + |
| | **Small for gestational age** | + | | | | |
| | **Webbed neck** | + | + | + | + | + |
| Laboratory findings | Free fatty acids (serum), during hypoglycaemia | ↓↓↓ | ↓↓↓ | ↓↓↓ | | |
| | Insulin, during hypoglycaemia | n-↑ | n-↑ | n-↑ | | |
| | Ketones, during hypoglycaemia | ↓↓↓ | ↓↓↓ | ↓↓↓ | | |

**Table 41.14** Adenosine kinase deficiency

| System | Symptoms and biomarkers | Neonatal (birth–1 month) | Infancy (1–18 months) | Childhood (1.5–11 years) | Adolescence (11–16 years) | Adulthood (>16 years) |
|---|---|---|---|---|---|---|
| Cardiovascular | Cardiac anomalies, malformations | ± | ± | ± | ± | ± |
| CNS | **Developmental delay** | | ++-+++ | ++-+++ | ++-+++ | ++-+++ |
| | Epilepsy | | ± | ±-++ | ±-++ | ±-++ |
| | **Hypotonia** | ±-++ | +-++ | + -++ | +-++ | +-++ |
| | Thin corpus callosum | ± | ± | ± | ± | ± |
| Digestive | Cholestasis | ± | ± | ± | ± | ± |
| | Liver dysfunction | ± | ± | ± | ± | ± |
| | Liver steatosis | ± | + | + | + | + |
| Ear | Hearing loss, sensorineural | – | ±-++ | ±-++ | ±-++ | ±-++ |
| Metabolic | hypoglycaemia | ± | ± | ± | ± | ± |
| Musculoskeletal | **Frontal bossing** | | + | + | + | + |
| | Macrocephaly | | ±-++ | ±-++ | ±-++ | ±-++ |
| | Muscle weakness, progressive | | ±-+ | ±-++ | ±-++ | ±-++ |
| | Short stature | ± | ± | ± | ± | ± |
| | Slender hands and feet | ± | ± | ± | ± | ± |
| Other | Failure to thrive | ± | ± | ± | ± | ± |
| Laboratory findings | Adenosine (dried blood spots) | | | n-↑ | n-↑ | n-↑ |
| | Adenosine (urine) | | | n-↑ | n-↑ | n-↑ |
| | ALAT (plasma) | ↑-↑↑ | n-↑↑ | n-↑↑ | n-↑↑ | n-↑↑ |
| | Bilirubin, conjugated (plasma) | ↑ | ↑ | | | |
| | Creatine kinase (plasma) | n-↑ | n-↑ | n-↑ | n-↑ | n-↑ |
| | Glucose (plasma) | n-↓ | n-↓ | n-↓ | n-↓ | |
| | Homocysteine, total (plasma) | n-↑ | n-↑ | n-↑ | n-↑ | n-↑ |
| | Methionine (plasma and urine) | n-↑↑↑ | n-↑↑↑ | n-↑↑↑ | n-↑↑↑ | n-↑↑↑ |
| | Prothrombin time | n-↑ | n-↑ | n-↑ | n-↑ | n-↑ |
| | S-Adenosylhomocysteine (plasma) | | | ↑-↑↑ | ↑-↑↑ | ↑-↑↑ |
| | S-Adenosylmethionine (plasma) | | | ↑-↑↑ | ↑-↑↑ | ↑-↑↑ |
| | Uric acid (plasma) | | n-↑ | n-↑↑ | n-↑↑ | n-↑ |

**Table 41.15** Phosphomannomutase 2 deficiency PMM2-CDG

| System | Symptoms and biomarkers | Neonatal (birth–1 month) | Infancy (1–18 months) | Childhood (1.5–11 years) | Adolescence (11–16 years) | Adulthood (>16 years) |
|---|---|---|---|---|---|---|
| Cardiovascular | Cardiomyopathy | ± | ± | ± | ± | ± |
| | Pericardial effusion | ± | ± | ± | ± | ± |
| CNS | **Cerebellar hypoplasia** | + | ++ | ++ | ++ | ++ |
| | **Demyelination** | + | + | + | + | + |
| | **Epilepsy** | ± | ± | + | ± | ± |
| | Hypotonia | ++ | ++ | + | + | + |
| | **Retardation, psychomotor** | ++ | ++ | ++ | ++ | ++ |
| | Stroke-like episodes | ± | ± | ± | ± | ± |
| | **Tendon reflexes, decreased** | ± | + | + | + | + |
| Dermatological | Inverted nipples | + | + | + | | |
| | Subcutaneous fat distribution, abnormal | ± | ± | ± | ± | ± |
| Digestive | Anorexia | ± | ± | ± | ± | ± |
| | Ascites | ± | ± | ± | ± | ± |
| | Diarrhea | ± | ± | ± | ± | ± |
| | **Liver dysfunction** | + | + | + | ± | ± |
| | Vomiting | ± | ± | ± | | |

**Table 41.15** (continued)

| System | Symptoms and biomarkers | Neonatal (birth–1 month) | Infancy (1–18 months) | Childhood (1.5–11 years) | Adolescence (11–16 years) | Adulthood (>16 years) |
|---|---|---|---|---|---|---|
| Endocrine | Hypergonadotropic hypogonadism, female | | | | + | + |
| | **Hyperinsulinism** | ± | ± | ± | | |
| Eye | **Pigmentary retinopathy** | ± | + | + | + | + |
| | Strabismus | ± | ± | ± | ± | ± |
| Metabolic | **Hypoglycaemia, hypoketotic** | ± | ± | ± | | |
| Musculoskeletal | Cervical compressive myelopathy | | – | ± | ± | ± |
| | Dysmorphic features | ± | ± | ± | ± | ± |
| | Dysostosis multiplex | ± | ± | ± | ± | ± |
| | Joint contractures | | | ± | ± | ± |
| | **Osteopenia** | | ± | + | + | + |
| | Vertebral anomalies | ± | ± | ± | ± | ± |
| Renal | Proteinuria | ± | ± | ± | ± | ± |
| | Renal enlargement | ± | ± | ± | ± | ± |
| Other | Failure to thrive | ± | ± | ± | ± | ± |
| | Fetal hydrops | ± | | | | |
| Laboratory findings | Albumin (serum) | ↑ | ↑ | ↑ | ↑ | ↑ |
| | Antithrombin III (plasma) | ↓ | ↓ | ↓ | ↓ | |
| | Arylsulfatase A (serum) | ↑ | ↑ | ↑ | n-↑ | n-↑ |
| | Asialotransferrin (serum) | ↑ | ↑ | ↑ | | |
| | Cholesterol (serum) | ↓ | ↓ | ↓ | ↓ | ↓ |
| | Cholesterol (serum) | ↓ | ↓ | ↓ | ↓ | |
| | Cholinesterase (plasma) | ↓ | ↓ | ↓ | ↓ | |
| | Disialotransferrin (serum) | ↑ | ↑ | ↑ | | |
| | Factor XI (blood) | ↓ | ↓ | ↓ | ↓ | ↓ |
| | Free fatty acids (serum), during hypoglycaemia | ↓↓↓ | ↓↓↓ | ↓↓ | | |
| | Glucose (plasma) | ↓ | ↓ | ↓ | | |
| | Insulin, durig hypoglycaemia | ↑ | ↑ | ↑ | ↑ | ↑ |
| | Ketones, during hypoglycaemia | ↓↓↓ | ↓↓↓ | ↓↓ | | |
| | Protein C (serum) | ↓ | ↓ | ↓ | ↓ | |
| | Sialotransferrins, type 1 pattern (serum) | ++ | ++ | ++ | + | ± |
| | Tetrasialotransferrin (serum) | ↓ | ↓ | ↓ | | |
| | Thyroxin-binding globulin (serum) | ↓ | ↓ | ↓ | ↓-n | ↓-n |
| | Transaminase (plasma) | ↑ | ↑ | ↑ | n-↑ | n-↑ |

**Table 41.16** Phosphomannose isomerase deficiency MPI-CDG

| System | Symptoms and biomarkers | Neonatal (birth–1 month) | Infancy (1–18 months) | Childhood (1.5–11 years) | Adolescence (11–16 years) | Adulthood (>16 years) |
|---|---|---|---|---|---|---|
| CNS | Hypotonia | ± | ± | ± | ± | ± |
| | Retardation, psychomotor | ± | ± | ± | ± | ± |
| Digestive | Diarrhea | | +/++ | +/++ | ± | ± |
| | **Liver fibrosis** | | + | + | + | + |
| | **Protein-losing enteropathy** | | +/++ | +/++ | ± | ± |
| Endocrine | **Hyperinsulinism** | ± | ± | ± | | |
| Hematological | Thrombosis | | ± | ± | ± | ± |
| Metabolic | **Hypoglycaemia, hypoketotic** | ± | ± | ± | | |

(continued)

**Table 41.16** (continued)

| System | Symptoms and biomarkers | Neonatal (birth–1 month) | Infancy (1–18 months) | Childhood (1.5–11 years) | Adolescence (11–16 years) | Adulthood (>16 years) |
|---|---|---|---|---|---|---|
| Laboratory findings | Albumin (serum) | ↓ | ↓ | ↓ | ↓ | ↓ |
| | Antithrombin III (plasma) | ↓ | ↓ | ↓ | | |
| | Arylsulfatase A (serum) | ↑ | ↑ | ↑ | n-↑ | n-↑ |
| | Asialotransferrin (serum) | ↑ | ↑ | ↑ | | |
| | Cholesterol (serum) | ↓ | ↓ | ↓ | ↓ | ↓ |
| | Cholesterol (serum) | ↓ | ↓ | ↓ | | |
| | Cholinesterase (plasma) | ↓ | ↓ | ↓ | | |
| | Disialotransferrin (serum) | ↑ | ↑ | ↑ | | |
| | Factor XI (blood) | ↓ | ↓ | ↓ | ↓ | ↓ |
| | Free fatty acids (serum), during hypoglycaemia | ↓↓↓ | ↓↓↓ | ↓↓ | | |
| | Glucose (plasma) | ↓ | ↓ | ↓ | | |
| | Insulin, during hypoglycaemia | ↑ | ↑ | ↑ | ↑ | ↑ |
| | Ketones, during hypoglycaemia | ↓↓↓ | ↓↓↓ | ↓↓ | | |
| | Protein C (serum) | ↓ | ↓ | ↓ | | |
| | Sialotransferrins, type 1 pattern (serum) | ++ | ++ | ++ | + | −/+ |
| | Tetrasialotransferrin (serum) | ↓ | ↓ | ↓ | | |
| | Thyroxin-binding globulin (serum) | ↓ | ↓ | ↓ | ↓-n | ↓-n |
| | Transaminase (plasma) | ↑ | ↑ | ↑ | n-↑ | n-↑ |

**Table 41.17** Mannosyltransferase 6 deficiency ALG3-CDG

| System | Symptoms and biomarkers | Neonatal (birth–1 month) | Infancy (1–18 months) | Childhood (1.5–11 years) | Adolescence (11–16 years) | Adulthood (>16 years) |
|---|---|---|---|---|---|---|
| Cardiovascular | **Congenital heart defects** | ± | ± | ± | ± | ± |
| CNS | **Axial hypotonia** | + | ++ | ++ | + | + |
| | Cerebral atrophy (MRI) | ± | ± | ± | + | + |
| | **Epilepsy** | ++ | ++ | ++ | ++ | ++ |
| | **Hypertonia, extremities** | + | + | + | + | + |
| | **Hypsarrhythmia (EEG)** | + | + | + | + | + |
| | **Microcephaly** | + | + | + | + | + |
| | **Retardation, psychomotor** | +++ | +++ | +++ | +++ | +++ |
| Digestive | Feeding difficulties | ± | ± | ± | ± | ± |
| Eye | Optic atrophy | ± | ± | ± | ± | |
| | Strabismus | ± | ± | ± | ± | ± |
| Musculoskeletal | **Arachnodactyly** | ± | ± | ± | ± | ± |
| | **Club foot** | ± | ± | ± | ± | ± |
| | **Facial dysmorphism** | ± | + | + | + | + |
| | Microcephaly | ± | + | ++ | + | |
| | Micrognathia | ± | ± | ± | ± | ± |
| | **Skeletal dysplasia** | ± | ± | ± | ± | ± |
| Laboratory findings | Antithrombin III (plasma) | ↓ | ↓ | ↓ | | |
| | Apolipoprotein B (serum) | ↓ | ↓ | ↓ | | |
| | Asialotransferrin (serum) | ↑ | ↑ | ↑ | ↑ | ↑ |
| | Disialotransferrin (serum) | ↑ | ↑ | ↑ | ↑ | ↑ |
| | Free fatty acids (serum), during hypoglycaemia | ↓↓↓ | ↓↓↓ | | | |
| | Glucose (plasma) | ↓ | ↓ | | | |
| | Insulin, durig hypoglycaemia | ↑ | ↑ | | | |
| | Ketones, during hypoglycaemia | ↓↓↓ | ↓↓↓ | | | |
| | Lipid-linked Man5GlcNAc2 (fibroblasts) | ↑↑ | ↑↑ | ↑↑ | ↑↑ | ↑↑ |
| | Protein S (serum) | ↓ | ↓ | ↓ | | |
| | Sialotransferrins, type 1 pattern (serum) | + | + | + | + | + |
| | Tetrasialotransferrin (serum) | ↓ | ↓ | ↓ | ↓ | ↓ |

**Table 41.18** Glucosyltransferase 1 deficiency ALG6-CDG

| System | Symptoms and biomarkers | Neonatal (birth–1 month) | Infancy (1–18 months) | Childhood (1.5–11 years) | Adolescence (11–16 years) | Adulthood (>16 years) |
|---|---|---|---|---|---|---|
| CNS | **Ataxia** | ± | ± | ± | ± | ± |
| | **Axial hypotonia** | ++ | ++ | + | ± | − |
| | **Epileptic seizures** | + | ++ | + | ± | ± |
| | **Retardation, psychomotor** | ++ | ++ | ++ | ++ | ++ |
| Eye | **Nystagmus** | ± | ± | ± | ± | ± |
| | **Strabismus** | ++ | ++ | ++ | ++ | ++ |
| Musculoskeletal | **Skeletal abnormalities** | ± | ± | ± | ± | ± |
| Psychiatric | **Behaviour difficulties** | ± | ± | ± | ± | ± |
| Laboratory findings | Antithrombin III (plasma) | ↓ | ↓ | ↓ | | |
| | Arylsulfatase A (serum) | ↑ | ↑ | ↑ | n-↑ | n-↑ |
| | Asialotransferrin (serum) | ↑ | ↑ | ↑ | | |
| | Cholesterol (serum) | ↓↓ | ↓↓ | ↓↓ | ↓↓ | ↓↓ |
| | Disialotransferrin (serum) | ↑ | ↑ | ↑ | | |
| | Dolichol-linked Man9GlcNAc2 (serum) | ↑ | ↑ | ↑ | | |
| | Factor XI (blood) | ↓ | ↓ | ↓ | ↓ | ↓ |
| | Factor XI (blood) | ↓ | ↓ | ↓ | | |
| | Free fatty acids (serum), during hypoglycaemia | ↓↓↓ | ↓↓↓ | ↓↓ | ↓↓ | ↓↓ |
| | Glucose (plasma) | ↓ | ↓ | ↓ | ↓ | ↓ |
| | Insulin, during hypoglycaemia | ↑ | ↑ | ↑ | ↑ | ↑ |
| | Ketones, during hypoglycaemia | ↓↓↓ | ↓↓↓ | ↓↓ | ↓↓ | ↓↓ |
| | Lipid-linked Man9GlcNAc2 (fibroblasts) | ↑ | ↑ | ↑ | ↑ | ↑ |
| | Sialotransferrins, type 1 pattern (serum) | + | + | + | + | ± |
| | Tetrasialotransferrin (serum) | ↓ | ↓ | ↓ | | |
| | Thyroxin-binding globulin (serum) | ↓ | ↓ | ↓ | ↓-n | ↓-n |
| | Transaminase (plasma) | ↑ | ↑ | ↑ | n-↑ | n-↑ |

**Table 41.19** Phosphoglucomutase 1 deficiency PGM1-CDG

| System | Symptoms and biomarkers | Neonatal (birth–1 month) | Infancy (1–18 months) | Childhood (1.5–11 years) | Adolescence (11–16 years) | Adulthood (>16 years) |
|---|---|---|---|---|---|---|
| Cardiovascular | Cardiomyopathy, dilated | + | | | | |
| | Tachycardia | | + | + | | |
| CNS | Fatigue | | + | + | | |
| | **Thrombosis, cerebral** | + | | | | |
| Digestive | **Bifid uvula** | + | | | | |
| | Hepatitis, chronic | | + | + | | |
| | Hepatopathy | + | | | | |
| Endocrine | **Growth hormone deficiency** | + | | | | |
| | Hyperinsulinism | ± | ± | | | |
| | Hypogonadotropic hypogonadism | ± | ± | ± | ± | ± |
| Metabolic | Hypoglycaemia | + | + | | | |
| | Hypoglycaemia, hypoketotic | ± | ± | | | |
| Musculoskeletal | **Cleft palate** | | + | + | | |
| | **First arch syndrome** | + | | | | |
| | Muscle weakness | + | | | | |
| | Rhabdomyolysis | ± | ± | ± | ± | ± |
| | **Short stature** | + | + | + | | |

(continued)

**Table 41.19** (continued)

| System | Symptoms and biomarkers | Neonatal (birth–1 month) | Infancy (1–18 months) | Childhood (1.5–11 years) | Adolescence (11–16 years) | Adulthood (>16 years) |
|---|---|---|---|---|---|---|
| Respiratory | Dyspnea | | + | + | | |
| Other | Ammonia (blood) | ↑ | | | | |
| | Increased susceptibility to malignant hyperthermia | ± | ± | ± | ± | ± |
| Laboratory findings | Antithrombin III (plasma) | ↓ | | | | |
| | Asialotransferrin (serum) | ↑ | | | | |
| | Creatine kinase (plasma) | ↑ | | | | |
| | Disialotransferrin (serum) | ↑ | | | | |
| | Free fatty acids (serum), during hypoglycaemia | ↓↓↓ | ↓↓↓ | | | |
| | Glucose (plasma) | ↓ | ↓ | | | |
| | Insulin, durig hypoglycaemia | ↑ | ↑ | ↑ | ↑ | ↑ |
| | Ketones, during hypoglycaemia | ↓↓↓ | ↓↓↓ | | | |
| | Monosialotransferrin (serum) | ↑ | | | | |
| | Tetrasialotransferrin (serum) | ↓ | | | | |
| | Transaminase (plasma) | ↑ | | | | |
| | Trisialotransferrin (serum) | ↑ | | | | |

**Table 41.20** AKT2 superactivity

| System | Symptoms and biomarkers | Neonatal (birth–1 month) | Infancy (1–18 months) | Childhood (1.5–11 years) | Adolescence (11–16 years) | Adulthood (>16 years) |
|---|---|---|---|---|---|---|
| CNS | **Hemihypertrophy, left side** | | +++ | +++ | +++ | +++ |
| | **Seizures** | ++ | ++ | ± | ± | ± |
| Metabolic | **Hypoglycaemia** | +++ | +++ | +++ | +++ | +++ |
| Musculoskeletal | **Gynecomastia** | | | | ++ | ++ |
| Other | **Macrosomia** | ++ | | | | |
| Laboratory findings | Free fatty acids (serum), during hypoglycaemia | ↓↓↓ | ↓↓↓ | ↓↓ | ↓↓ | ↓↓ |
| | Glucose (plasma) | ↓ | ↓ | ↓ | ↓ | ↓ |
| | Insulin, durig hypoglycaemia | ↓↓↓ | ↓↓↓ | ↓↓ | ↓↓ | ↓↓ |
| | Ketones, during hypoglycaemia | ↓↓↓ | ↓↓↓ | ↓↓ | ↓↓ | ↓↓ |

**Table 41.21** AKT3 superactivity

| System | Symptoms and biomarkers | Neonatal (birth–1 month) | Infancy (1–18 months) | Childhood (1.5–11 years) | Adolescence (11–16 years) | Adulthood (>16 years) |
|---|---|---|---|---|---|---|
| Metabolic | **Hypoglycaemia** | + | + | + | + | + |
| Laboratory findings | Glucose (plasma) | ↓ | ↓ | ↓ | ↓ | ↓ |
| | Insulin, durig hypoglycaemia | ↓↓↓ | ↓↓↓ | ↓↓ | ↓↓ | ↓↓ |
| | Ketones, during hypoglycaemia | ↓ | ↓ | ↓ | ↓ | ↓ |

**Table 41.22** Catalytic phosphatidylinositol 3-kinase α subunit superactivity (PIK3CA)

| System | Symptoms and biomarkers | Neonatal (birth–1 month) | Infancy (1–18 months) | Childhood (1.5–11 years) | Adolescence (11–16 years) | Adulthood (>16 years) |
|---|---|---|---|---|---|---|
| CNS | Hemihyperplasia | + | + | + | + | + |
| | Intellectual disability | + | + | + | + | + |
| | Intellectual disability | + | + | + | + | + |
| | Seizures | + | + | + | + | + |
| Metabolic | Hypoglycaemia | + | + | + | + | + |
| Musculoskeletal | Gynecomastia | + | + | + | + | + |
| | Syndactyly, polydactyly | + | + | + | + | + |
| Other | Increased risk of tumors | | | | + | + |
| | Macrosomia | + | + | + | + | + |
| Laboratory findings | Free fatty acids (serum), during hypoglycaemia | ↓↓↓ | ↓↓↓ | ↓↓ | ↓↓ | ↓↓ |
| | Glucose (plasma) | ↓ | ↓ | ↓ | ↓ | ↓ |
| | Insulin, durig hypoglycaemia | ↓↓↓ | ↓↓↓ | ↓↓ | ↓↓ | ↓↓ |
| | Ketones, during hypoglycaemia | ↓↓↓ | ↓↓↓ | ↓↓ | ↓↓ | ↓↓ |

## Reference Values

| Age | <48 h | >48 h |
|---|---|---|
| Plasma | | |
| Glucose (mmol/L) | 3–3.6 | 3.9–5.5 |
| Insulin (µUI/mL) | | <2[a]/0.8–10 |
| C-peptide (ng/mL) | | <0.5[a]/0.25–1.2 |
| 3 Hydroxybutyrate (mmol/L) | | >1.8[a]/0.1–0.3 |
| Free fatty acids (mmol/L) | | >1.7[a]/0.02–0.6 |
| C4-OH | 0 | 0 |
| Ammonemia (µmol/L) | <100 | <50[b] |
| Urines | | |
| 3OH glutarate | 0 | 0 |

[a]During hypoglycaemia
[b]<50 µM until 1 month old, then <100 µM

## Pathological Values (Ferrara et al. 2016)

| Age | <48 h | >48 h | <1 month | >1 month |
|---|---|---|---|---|
| Plasma | | | | |
| Glucose (mmol/L) | <2.7 | <3.3 | <3.3 | <3.3 |
| Insulin (µUI/mL)[a] | ≥2 | ≥2 | ≥2 | ≥2 |
| C-peptide (ng/mL)[a] | >0.2 | >0.2 | >0.2 | >0.2 |
| 3 Hydroxybutyrate (mmol/L)[a] | <1.8 | <1.8 | <1.8 | <1.8 |
| Free fatty acids (mmol/L)[a] | <1.7 | <1.7 | <1.7 | <1.7 |
| C4-OH (µmol/L)[a,b] | ↑ | ↑ | ↑ | ↑ |
| Ammonemia (µmol/L)[a] | <100 | <100 | <100 | <50 |
| Urines | | | | |
| 3OH glutarate (µmol/mmol c.)[c] | ↑ | ↑ | ↑ | ↑ |

[a]During hypoglycaemia
[b]C4-OH appears also during prolonged fasting with ketosis. In hyperinsulinemic hypoglycaemia, this marker is associated with a low/absent ketosis
[c]µmol/mmol creatinine

## Diagnostic Flowchart

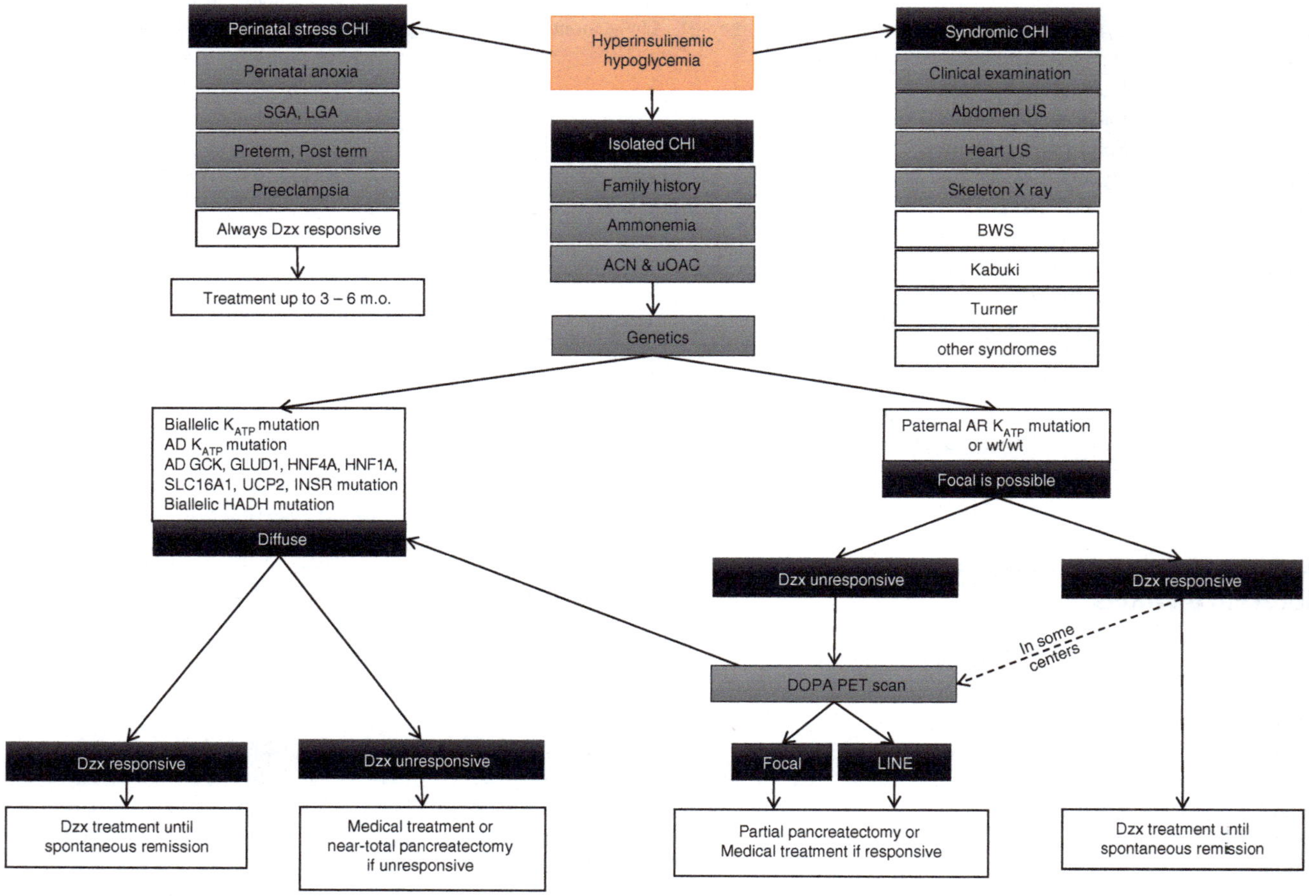


*Dzx* Diazoxide, *SGA* Small for gestational age, *LGA* Large for gestational age, $K_{ATP}$ ATP-dependent potassium channel, *AD* Autosomal dominant, *ACN* Acylcarnitine (plasma or dried blood spot), *uOAC* Urine organic acid chromatography, *LINE* Localized islets nuclear enlargement, *US* Ultrasound, *BWS* Beckwith-Wiedemann syndrome.

## Loading Test

- Glucagon loading test. This test can be performed for diagnostic purpose at the time of hypoglycaemia. An increase in blood glucose greater than 1.7 mmol/L (30 mg/dL) within 30–40 min after IM or IV administration of glucagon 1 mg proves the paradoxical hepatic glycogen content despite hypoglycaemia.
- Oral protein tolerance test. This test can be performed to investigate protein sensitivity. Patients are administered with protein powder 1 g/kg. Plasma glucose and insulin are measured every 30 min for 3 h. The test is positive if glycaemia <3.8 mmol/L (70 mg/dL) in response to the protein load.

## Prenatal Diagnosis

| Disorder | | | Test recommended |
|---|---|---|---|
| Disease Name | Disease Abbreviation | Gene symbols | |
| ATP-sensitive potassium channel regulatory subunit deficiency | KATP-HI | *ABCC8* | Diffuse form: Mutation analysis on DNA from CVS or AFC<br>Focal form: Not applicable |
| ATP-sensitive potassium channel pore-forming subunit deficiency | KATP-HI | *KCNJ11* | Diffuse form: Mutation analysis on DNA from CVS or AFC<br>Focal form: Not applicable |
| Glucokinase superactivity | GCK-HI | *GCK* | Mutation analysis on DNA from CVS or AFC |
| Short-chain 3-hydroxyacyl-CoA dehydrogenase deficiency | SCHAD-HI | *HADH* | Mutation analysis on DNA from CVS or AFC |
| Insulin receptor dysregulation | | *INSR* | Mutation analysis on DNA from CVS or AFC |
| Glutamate dehydrogenase superactivity | HIHA syndrome | *GLUD1* | Mutation analysis on DNA from CVS or AFC |
| Exercise induced hyperinsulinemic hypoglycaemia | EI-HI | *SLC16A1* | Mutation analysis on DNA from CVS or AFC[a] |
| Hepatocyte nuclear factor-4α deficiency | MODY1 | *HNF4A* | Mutation analysis on DNA from CVS or AFC[a] |
| Hepatocyte nuclear factor-1α deficiency | MODY3 | *HNF1A* | Mutation analysis on DNA from CVS or AFC[a] |
| Uncoupling protein 2 deficiency | UCP2-HI | *UCP2* | Mutation analysis on DNA from CVS or AFC[a] |
| Beckwith-Wiedemann syndrome | BWS | Genetic or epigenetic changes of imprinted region 11p15.5 | Prenatal testing may be requested occasionally in cases of familial chromosomal rearrangements affecting chromosomes 11p15 or in case of familial CDKN1C point mutation |
| Kabuki syndrome | KS | *KMT2D / KDM6A* | Mutation analysis on DNA from CVS or AFC |
| Turner syndrome | TS | Partial or complete X chromosome monosomy | Karyotype from CVS or AFC |
| Adenosine kinase deficiency | ADK deficiency | *ADK* | Mutation analysis on DNA from CVS or AFC |
| PMM2-CDG | CDG1a | *PMM2* | Mutation analysis on DNA from CVS or AFC |
| MPI-CDG | CDG1b | *MPI* | Mutation analysis on DNA from CVS or AFC |
| ALG3-CDG | CDG1d | *ALG3* | Mutation analysis on DNA from CVS or AFC |
| ALG6-CDG | CDG1c | *ALG6* | Mutation analysis on DNA from CVS or AFC |
| PGM1-CDG; glycogen storage disease type 14 | CDG1t | *PGM1* | Mutation analysis on DNA from CVS or AFC |
| Sotos syndrome | | *NSD1 / 5q35 deletion* | Mutation analysis on DNA from CVS or AFC |
| Thimothy syndrome | TS | *CACNA1C* | Mutation analysis on DNA from CVS or AFC |
| PASNA syndrome | PASNA | *CACNA1D* | Mutation analysis on DNA from CVS or AFC |
| MSSGM1 syndrome | MSSGM1 | *TRMT10A* | Mutation analysis on DNA from CVS or AFC |
| Costello syndrome | FCS syndrome | *HRAS* | Mutation analysis on DNA from CVS or AFC |
| Perlmann syndrome | PRLMNS | DIS3L2 | Mutation analysis on DNA from CVS or AFC |
| Simpson-Golabi-Behmel syndrome | SGBS | GPC3 | Mutation analysis on DNA from CVS or AFC |
| FOXA2 / HNF3β | FOXA2 | *FOXA2* | Mutation analysis on DNA from CVS or AFC |
| Ondine syndrome | CCHS | PHOX2B | Mutation analysis on DNA from CVS or AFC |
| Rubinstein-Taybi syndrome | RSTS1/2 | CREBBP/EP300 | Mutation analysis on DNA from CVS or AFC |
| AKT2 superactivity | | *AKT2* | Mutation analysis on DNA from CVS or AFC |
| AKT3 superactivity | MPPH2 | *AKT3* | Mutation analysis on DNA from CVS or AFC |
| CLOVE syndrome, MCAP syndrome | CLOVE syndrome, MCAP syndrome | *PIK3CA* | Not applicable (somatic mosaicism for postzygotic activating mutations in the PIK3CA gene) |

Recommended analyses and sample requirements for prenatal diagnosis
*CVS* chorionic villous sampling, *AFC* amniotic fluid cells
[a]Is not a severe disorder. Prenatal diagnosis might not be appropriate in most cases

## DNA Testing

| Disorder | | | |
|---|---|---|---|
| Disease name | Disease abbreviation | Gene symbols | Sample and test recommended |
| Perinatal stress HI | / | / | Not applicable |
| ATP-sensitive potassium channel regulatory subunit deficiency | KATP-HI | *ABCC8* | Diffuse form: Mutation analysis on DNA from blood leukocytes |
| | | | Focal form: Mutation analysis on DNA from blood leukocytes |
| | | | LINE: Mutation analysis on DNA from the pancreatic lesion |
| ATP-sensitive potassium channel pore-forming subunit deficiency | KATP-HI | *KCNJ11* | Diffuse form: Mutation analysis on DNA from blood leukocytes |
| | | | Focal form: Mutation analysis on DNA from blood leukocytes |
| Glucokinase superactivity | GCK-HI | *GCK* | Diffuse form: Mutation analysis on DNA from blood leukocytes |
| | | | LINE: Mutation analysis on DNA from the pancreatic lesion |
| Short-chain 3-hydroxyacyl-CoA dehydrogenase deficiency | SCHAD-HI | *HADH* | Mutation analysis on DNA from blood leukocytes |
| Insulin receptor dysregulation | | *INSR* | Mutation analysis on DNA from blood leukocytes |
| Glutamate dehydrogenase superactivity | HIHA syndrome | *GLUD1* | Mutation analysis on DNA from blood leukocytes |
| Exercise induced hyperinsulinemic hypoglycaemia | EI-HI | *SLC16A1* | Mutation analysis on DNA from blood leukocytes |
| Hepatocyte nuclear factor-4α deficiency | MODY1 | *HNF4A* | Mutation analysis on DNA from blood leukocytes |
| Hepatocyte nuclear factor-1α deficiency | MODY3 | *HNF1A* | Mutation analysis on DNA from blood leukocytes |
| Uncoupling protein 2 deficiency | UCP2-HI | *UCP2* | Mutation analysis on DNA from blood leukocytes |
| Beckwith-Wiedemann syndrome | BWS | Genetic or epigenetic changes of imprinted region 11p15.5, pathogenic variant in CDKN1C gene | Karyotype, methylation analysis at 11p15.5 locus, CDKN1C testing |
| Kabuki syndrome | KS | *KMT2D / KDM6A* | Mutation analysis on DNA from blood leukocytes |
| Turner syndrome | TS | Partial or complete X chromosome monosomy | Karyotype, CGH-array from blood leukocytes. |
| Adenosine kinase deficiency | ADK deficiency | *ADK* | Mutation analysis on DNA from blood leukocytes |
| PMM2-CDG | CDG1a | *PMM2* | Mutation analysis on DNA from blood leukocytes |
| MPI-CDG | CDG1b | *MPI* | Mutation analysis on DNA from blood leukocytes |
| ALG3-CDG | CDG1d | *ALG3* | Mutation analysis on DNA from blood leukocytes |
| ALG6-CDG | CDG1c | *ALG6* | Mutation analysis on DNA from blood leukocytes |
| PGM1-CDG; glycogen storage disease type 14 | CDG1t | *PGM1* | Mutation analysis on DNA from blood leukocytes |
| Sotos syndrome | | *NSD1 / 5q35 deletion* | Mutation analysis on DNA from blood leucocytes / array CGH |
| Timothy syndrome | TS | *CACNA1C* | Mutation analysis on DNA from blood leukocytes |
| PASNA syndrome | PASNA | *CACNA1D* | Mutation analysis on DNA from blood leukocytes |

| Disorder | | | |
| --- | --- | --- | --- |
| Disease name | Disease abbreviation | Gene symbols | Sample and test recommended |
| MSSGM1 syndrome | MSSGM1 | *TRMT10A* | Mutation analysis on DNA from blood leukocytes |
| Costello syndrome | CSTLO | *HRAS* | Mutation analysis on DNA from blood leukocytes |
| Perlmann syndrome | PRLMNS | DIS3L2 | Mutation analysis on DNA from blood leukocytes |
| Simpson-Golabi-Behmel syndrome | SGBS | GPC3 | Mutation analysis on DNA from blood leukocytes |
| FOXA2 / HNF3β | FOXA2 | *FOXA2* | Mutation analysis on DNA from blood leukocytes |
| Ondine syndrome | CCHS | PHOX2B | Mutation analysis on DNA from blood leukocytes |
| Rubinstein-Taybi syndrome | RSTS1/2 | CREBBP/EP300 | Mutation analysis on DNA from blood leukocytes / array CGH |
| AKT2 superactivity | | *AKT2* | Mutation analysis on DNA from blood leukocytes |
| Megalencephaly-polymicrogyria-polydactyly-hydrocephalus syndrome | MPPH2 | AKT3 | Mutation analysis on DNA from blood leukocytes |
| CLOVE syndrome, MCAP syndrome | CLOVE syndrome, MCAP syndrome | *PIK3CA* | Mutation analysis on DNA from affected tissus |

## Treatment

In neonates, treatment should be intensively performed to prevent irreversible brain damage. In case of severe hypoglycaemia, patients should be urgently treated with 2 mL/kg 10% dextrose IV (200 mg/kg), followed by continuous 10% dextrose until glycemia >3.9 mmol/L (>70 mg/dL). Central lines are frequently required. After stabilization, patients should be transitioned to an enteral nutrition scheme by mouth or nasogastric tube. Glucagon IM, IV can also be used as emergency treatment, then can be maintained continuously IV or SQ when GIR is higher than 12 mg/kg/min or in case of diazoxide-unresponsiveness (Hawkes et al. 2019).

Unresponsive patients to diazoxide after 5 days of trial at maximum dosage should be screened for a focal form by performing a prompt genetic testing and a pancreatic $^{18}$F DOPA PET scan (Blomberg et al. 2013). When a focal form is localized, it can be removed by a selective partial pancreatectomy, which is usually curative (Laje et al. 2012). However, in case of diffuse form, a near-total pancreatectomy is performed only if all conservative medical treatments fail, because of the high risk of insulin-dependent diabetes within 15 years after the surgery (Beltrand et al. 2012). Conservative medical treatment include: glucose-enriched feedings or enteral feeding, somatostatin analogues, nifedipine (Le Quan Sang et al. 2012; Modan-Moses et al. 2011; McMahon et al. 2017; Thornton et al. 2019) and/or experimental therapies: sirolimus (Maria et al. 2019), exendin (Ng et al. 2018), anti-insulin receptor antibodies (Patel et al. 2018), pasireotide (Schwetz et al. 2016). A case of GCK-HI with epilepsy and mild intellectual disability was successfully treated with a ketogenic diet, providing cerebral energy fuel alternative to glucose (Maiorana et al. 2015).

The long-term glycaemic control progressively improves, leading to wean sequentially the treatment. Rarely, some patients may evolve toward a diabetes.

A careful cognitive follow-up is also mandatory since one-third to half patients suffer from cognitive impairment and will need supportive therapies and rehabilitation (Ludwig et al. 2018).

## Emergency Treatment

| | Route | Neonate | Children/adults | Pitfalls | Important information |
|---|---|---|---|---|---|
| Dextrose | PO or IV | 10% dextrose 2 mL/kg | 30% dextrose 10 mL/20 kg (max 30 mL) | | To be repeated every 5 min until glycemia reaches normal values |
| 10% dextrose[a] | Continuous IV infusion | As needed to normalize glycemia. | As needed to normalize glycemia. | In severe neonates, the precocious insertion of a central IV line is recommended. | Normal GIR needs of neonates is <8 mg/kg/min. Needs over this threshold is pathognomonic for an insulin related hypoglycaemia. In HI neonates, the average GIR needed is 16 mg/kg/min. |
| Enteral feeding[a] | Continuous enteral feeding | Carbohydrate enriched feedings¥. | As needed to normalize glycemia. | Risk of enterocolitis if hyperosmolar feedings in neonates. | MCT supplements are useless, because HI inhibits gluconeogenesis. |
| Glucagon | IV | 0.3 mg/kg (max 2 mg) | 1 mg | Vomiting. | Emergency treatment of severe hypoglycaemia in HI. Give time to set a IV line. |
| Glucagon | Continuous IV, SQ | 2.5–10 µg/kg/h | 1–2 mg/24 h | Necrolytic migratory erythema. IV line and pump occlusion. | Not a long term treatment due to frequent catheter obstruction. |

*GIR* Glucose infusion rate, *MCT* Medium chain triglycerides

[a]In neonates, glucose intake required to avoid hypoglycaemia may exceed the gut tolerance. Therefore, hyperosmolar feeding mixtures and fluids overloads should be avoided

## Standard Treatment

| | Route | Dose | Pitfalls | Important informations |
|---|---|---|---|---|
| **Diazoxide** | Orally | 5–15 mg/kg/d | • Risk of PHT until 4 months old<br>• Heart ultrasound mandatory before treatment and within 1 month after initiation<br>• Risk of PHT stronger in premature, persistent ductus arteriosus, heart malformation<br>• Risk of sodium and fluid retention,edema, PHT, thrombocytopenia, neutropenia | • At least 5 days of diazoxide treatment at maximum dosage are needed to evaluate its efficiency<br>• Start with lower doses in premature babies<br>• Hypertrichosis is a usual side effect |
| **Octreotide** | SQ q 6–8 h or continuous IV infusion or continuous SQ infusion with an insulin pump | 5–30 µg/kg/d | • Risk of NEC in neonates contraindication in case of enteropathy, severe infection, hemodynamic distress<br>• Risk of drug induced hepatitis<br>• Risk of cholelithiasis | • Start with 5-10 µg/kg/d, then titrate up every 2–3 days by +5-10 µg/kg/d because of tachyphylaxis and to assess tolerance<br>• Abdominal US to screen for gallblader stones<br>• Injection site rotation is recommended to avoid nodule formation |
| **Octreotide LAR** | IM | Idem (cumulative dose) or 10–30 mg q4–6 weeks | • If somatostatin analogue were proven efficient with SQ octreotide | • Idem |
| **Lanreotide** | Deep SQ | Idem (cumulative dose) or 30–120 mg q4–6 weeks | • Idem | • Idem |

| | Route | Dose | Pitfalls | Important informations |
|---|---|---|---|---|
| **Feeding** | Oral, enteral | • Carbohydrate enriched diet additioned with maltodextridine or uncoocked cornstarch<br>• Ketogenic diet can be discussed in unresponsive GCK-HI | • In neonates, risk of enterocolitis if hyperosmolar feedings.<br>• Ketogenogenic diet: Risk of symptomatic hypoglycaemia in the phase of induction | • Risk of overweight in hypercaloric diet. Prefer carbohydrate enriched food without fat (maltodextridine, row corn starch from 12 month old)<br>• Ketogenic diet: Risk of metabolic acidosis, hyperuricemia, dyslipidemia.<br>• Ketogenic diet: Need of supplementation with multivitaminic, vitamin D and eventually calcium |

Co-med diuretics at initiation of Dzx. Outside neonatal period, do not systematically readapt dose to the weight. Most patients are Dzx-responsive

*PHT* Pulmonary hypertension, *NEC* Necrotizing enterocolitis

*Note:* Patients with an insulin receptor pathway disorder (e.g. AKT2 hyperactivity) have an increased uptake of glucose in their insulin-sensitive tissues. Thus medications aiming at decreasing the pancreatic insulin secretion will not be effective

## Experimental Treatments

Patients with a diffuse disease unresponsive to the standard treatment, thus requiring an enteral feeding, can be discussed for near-total pancreatectomy. Alternatively, if available, the patient can join a research program. Several experimental treatments are actually under investigation:

– Repositioning of drugs marketed in other indications: mTOR inhibitor (sirolimus, everolimus), somatostatin analogues.
– New therapies specific to hyperinsulinemic hypoglycaemia: GLP1 receptor inhibitor (Exendin (9–39), allosteric inhibitor of the insulin receptor (XMetD), soluble formulation of glucagon analogues (Dasiglucagon).

## References


Arnoux JB, Saint-Martin C, Montravers F, Verkarre V, Galmiche L, Télion C, Capito C, Robert JJ, Hussain K, Aigrain Y, Bellanné-Chantelot C, de Lonlay P. An update on congenital hyperinsulinism: advances in diagnosis and management. Expert Opin Orphan Drugs. 2014;2(8):779–95.

Beltrand J, Caquard M, Arnoux JB, Laborde K, Velho G, Verkarre V, Rahier J, Brunelle F, Nihoul-Fékété C, Saudubray JM, Robert JJ, de Lonlay P. Glucose metabolism in 105 children and adolescents after pancreatectomy for congenital hyperinsulinism. Diabetes Care. 2012;35(2):198–203.

Blomberg BA, Moghbel MC, Saboury B, Stanley CA, Alavi A. The value of radiologic interventions and (18)F-DOPA PET in diagnosing and localizing focal congenital hyperinsulinism: systematic review and meta-analysis. Mol Imaging Biol. 2013;15(1):97–105.

Capito C, de Lonlay P, Verkarre V, et al. The surgical management of atypical forms of congenital hyperinsulinism. Semin Pediatr Surg. 2011;20:54–5.

De Lonlay P, Fournet JC, Rahier J, et al. Somatic deletion of the imprinted 11p15 region in sporadic persistent hyperinsulinemic hypoglycemia of infancy is specific of focal adenomatous hyperplasia and endorses partial pancreatectomy. J Clin Invest. 1997;100:802–7.

Ferrara C, Patel P, Becker S, Stanley CA, Kelly A. Biomarkers of Insulin for the Diagnosis of Hyperinsulinemic Hypoglycemia in Infants and Children. J Pediatr. 2016;168:212–9.

Galcheva S, Demirbilek H, Al-Khawaga S, Hussain K. The genetic and molecular mechanisms of congenital hyperinsulinism. Front Endocrinol (Lausanne). 2019;10:111.

Hawkes CP, Lado JJ, Givler S, De Leon DD. The Effect of Continuous Intravenous Glucagon on Glucose Requirements in Infants with Congenital Hyperinsulinism. JIMD Rep. 2019;45:45–50.

Hussain K, Hindmarsh P, Aynsley-Green A. Neonates with symptomatic hyperinsulinemic hypoglycemia generate inappropriately low serum cortisol counterregulatory hormonal responses. J Clin Endocrinol Metab. 2003;88(9):4342–7.

Laje P, Stanley CA, Palladino AA, Becker SA, Adzick NS. (2012) Pancreatic head resection and Roux-en-Y pancreaticojejunostomy for the treatment of the focal form of congenital hyperinsulinism. J Pediatr Surg. 2012;47(1):130–5.

Le Quan Sang KH, Arnoux JB, Mamoune A, Saint-Martin C, Bellanné-Chantelot C, Valayannopoulos V, Brassier A, Kayirangwa H, Barbier V, Broissand C, Fabreguettes JR, Charron B, Thalabard JC, de Lonlay P. Successful treatment of congenital hyperinsulinism with long-acting release octreotide. Eur J Endocrinol. 2012;166(2):333–9.

Lord K, Dzata E, Snider KE, Gallagher PR, De León DD. Clinical presentation and management of children with diffuse and focal hyperinsulinism: a review of 223 cases. J Clin Endocrinol Metab. 2013;98(11):E1786–9.

Ludwig A, Enke S, Heindorf J, Empting S, Meissner T, Mohnike K. Formal Neurocognitive Testing in 60 Patients with Congenital Hyperinsulinism. Horm Res Paediatr. 2018;89(1):1–6.

Maiorana A, Manganozzi L, Barbetti F, et al. Ketogenic diet in a patient with congenital hyperinsulinism: a novel approach to prevent brain damage. Orphanet J Rare Dis. 2015;10:120.

Maria G, Antonia D, Michael A, Kate M, Sian E, Sarah FE, Mehul D, Pratik S. Sirolimus: efficacy and complications in children with hyperinsulinemic hypoglycemia: a 5-year follow-up study. J Endocr Soc. 2019;3:699–713.

Modan-Moses D, Koren I, Mazor-Aronovitch K, Pinhas-Hamiel O, Landau H. Treatment of congenital hyperinsulinism with lanreotide acetate (Somatuline Autogel). J Clin Endocrinol Metab. 2011;96(8):2312–7.

McMahon AW, Wharton GT, Thornton P, De Leon DD. Octreotide use and safety in infants with hyperinsulinism. Pharmacoepidemiol Drug Saf. 2017;26(1):26–31.

Ng CM, Tang F, Seeholzer SH, Zou Y, De León DD. Population pharmacokinetics of exendin-(9–39) and clinical dose selection in patients with congenital hyperinsulinism. Br J Clin Pharmacol. 2018;84(3):520–32.

Patel P, Charles L, Corbin J, Goldfine ID, Johnson K, Rubin P, De León DD. A unique allosteric insulin receptor monoclonal antibody that prevents hypoglycemia in the SUR-1−/− mouse model of KATP hyperinsulinism. MAbs. 2018;10(5):796–802.

Snider KE, Becker S, Boyajian L, Shyng SL, MacMullen C, Hughes N, Ganapathy K, Bhatti T, Stanley CA, Ganguly A. Genotype and phenotype correlations in 417 children with congenital hyperinsulinism. J Clin Endocrinol Metab. 2013;98(2):E355–63.

Schwetz V, Horvath K, Kump P, Lackner C, Perren A, Forrer F, Pieber TR, Treiber G, Sourij H, Mader JK. Successful medical treatment of adult nesidioblastosis with pasireotide over 3 years: a case report. Medicine (Baltimore). 2016;95(14):e3272.

Sempoux C, Capito C, Bellanne-Chantelot C, et al. Morphological mosaicism of the pancreatic islets: a novel anatomopathological form of persistent hyperinsulinemic hypoglycemia of infancy. J Clin Endocrinol Metab. 2011;96:3785–93.

Thornton P, Truong L, Reynolds C, Hamby T, Nedrelow J. Rate of Serious Adverse Events Associated with Diazoxide Treatment of Patients with Hyperinsulinism. Horm Res Paediatr. 2019;19:1–8.

Yorifuji T, Horikawa R, Hasegawa T, et al. Clinical practice guidelines for congenital hyperinsulinism. Clin Pediatr Endocrinol. 2017;26(3):127–52.

GPSR Compliance

*The European Union's (EU) General Product Safety Regulation (GPSR) is a set of rules that requires consumer products to be safe and our obligations to ensure this.*

*If you have any concerns about our products, you can contact us on ProductSafety@springernature.com*

In case Publisher is established outside the EU, the EU authorized representative is:

Springer Nature Customer Service Center GmbH
Europaplatz 3
69115 Heidelberg, Germany

**Batch number: 10777741**

Printed by Printforce, the Netherlands

Physician's Guide to the Diagnosis, Treatment, and Follow-Up of Inherited Metabolic Diseases

Nenad Blau • Carlo Dionisi Vici
Carlos R. Ferreira • Christine Vianey-Saban
Clara D. M. van Karnebeek
Editors

# Physician's Guide to the Diagnosis, Treatment, and Follow-Up of Inherited Metabolic Diseases

Second Edition

Volume II

Springer

*Editors*
Nenad Blau
Division of Metabolism
University Children's Hospital
Zürich
Switzerland

Carlos R. Ferreira
Division of Genetics and Metabolism
Children's National Health System
Washington, DC
USA

Clara D. M. van Karnebeek
Departments of Pediatrics and Human Genetics
Emma Children's Hospital, Amsterdam
University Medical Centers
Amsterdam
The Netherlands

Carlo Dionisi Vici
Division of Metabolic Disease, Department
of Pediatric Subspecialties
Bambino Gesù Children's Hospital-IRCCS
Rome
Italy

Christine Vianey-Saban
Department of Inborn Errors of Metabolism
and Newborn Screening
CHU Lyon, Centre de Biologie et de Pathologie
Est
Bron Cedex
France

ISBN 978-3-030-67729-9 ISBN 978-3-030-67727-5 (eBook)
https://doi.org/10.1007/978-3-030-67727-5



This Springer imprint is published by the registered company Springer Nature Switzerland AG
The registered company address is: Gewerbestrasse 11, 6330 Cham, Switzerland

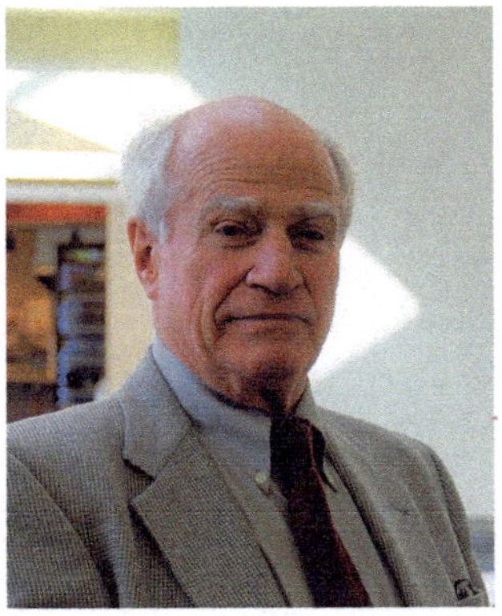

**Stephen Irwin Goodman (1938–2020)**

*The Editors take this opportunity to acknowledge Stephen Irwin Goodman, MD—one of the pioneers in the field of diagnosis and treatment of inborn errors of metabolism, who passed away while this book was in press, on October 30, 2020—for his longstanding efforts and contributions to our series Physician's Guide in Inherited Metabolic Disease. A founding member of both the Society for Inherited Metabolic Disorders and the American College of Medical Genetics (and Genomics), Steve spent his entire professional career at the University of Colorado in Denver with his wife, Patricia, their daughters Michelle and Karen, and their families.*

*Steve is remembered for his role in establishing the diagnostic methods for organic acidemias, for writing a seminal text on use of GC-MS for analysis of organic acids (with Sanford Markey), defining and characterizing glutaric acidurias type I and II, and contributing knowledge to the diagnosis and management of many other inborn errors of metabolism.*

*In recognition of his constant guidance and valuable contributions (see Chap. 71), we wish to dedicate this edition of the Physician's Guide to the Diagnosis, Treatment, and Follow-Up of Inherited Metabolic Diseases to his memory.*

*Nenad Blau*
*Carlo Dionisi Vici*
*Carlos R. Ferreira*
*Christine Vianey-Saban*
*Clara D.M. van Karnebeek*

# Foreword

A new edition for an old subject

The study of inborn errors of metabolism arguably began with Garrod's seminal 1902 paper on alkaptonuria (Garrod 1902). At the time, the diagnosis of this disorder was achieved using state-of-the-art technology: visual inspection of recently voided urine. Garrod's genius was to use this method to identify and collect a large number of individuals with this rare disorder and to recognize, with input from Bateson, that the familial clustering and distribution of affected individuals (19 affected of 48 individuals in 9 sibships) was consistent with observations made by Gregor Mendel in pea plants some 37 years earlier. An additional feature of alkaptonuria, crucial for Garrod's study, is that, at the phenotypic level, it is a relatively mild disorder with minimal, if any, effect on life span. To quote Garrod, "an alternative course of metabolism, harmless and usually congenital and lifelong." Thus, it was possible for Garrod to collect affected individuals, many of whom were adults at the time of diagnosis.

From this modest beginning, Garrod not only demonstrated that Mendelism held true in humans, but also suggested that alkaptonuria and a handful of similar disorders (cystinuria, pentosuria, and albinism) were "merely extreme examples of variations in chemical behavior which are probably everywhere present in minor degree" so that "just as no two individuals of a species are absolutely identical in bodily structure neither are their chemical processes carried out on exactly the same lines." First stated in 1902, these ideas lead to Garrod's definition in 1931 (Garrod 1931) of "chemical individuality" as genetically determined biochemical characteristics and capabilities which confer "predisposition to and immunities from the various mishaps which are spoken of as diseases." We are only now beginning to put meat on the bones of these prescient predictions.

From Garrod's time to the present, progress in identifying specific inborn errors of metabolism has been dependent on technological advances. Thus, in the early 1950s following the development of the first amino acid analyzer, a host of "new" (really "newly recognized") disorders were described on the basis of abnormal patterns of amino acids in plasma and/or urine. Similarly, the development of GC/MS technology leads to the recognition of many organic acidemias, and the development of tissue culture and somatic cell genetic techniques leads to a burst of newly recognized lysosomal storage diseases.

Currently, we are experiencing at least two technologic revolutions: genomic sequencing methods that began with the seminal 2009 paper of Ng et al. (2009) showing that the cause of rare Mendelian disorders could be identified by applying genomic methods to well-phenotyped patients and, more recently, the development of unstructured metabolomic methods that measure thousands of metabolites not previously examined by classical biochemical methods. Application of genomic methods has already had a profound effect on our identification and diagnosis of patients with inborn errors (Posey et al. 2019; Bamshad et al. 2019). Advances and widespread application of metabolomics seems likely to have a similar effect (Burrage et al. 2019; Miller et al. 2015). Moreover, the two technologies are synergistic in their power to identify newly recognized monogenic disorders and to expose their pathophysiology.

While exciting and gratifying, this rapid expansion of the number of recognizable inborn errors is a daunting challenge to the beleaguered clinicians who take care of these patients; one can never know what the next patient who comes to clinic will have: a defect in purine metabolism; a problem in lysosomal function; a peroxisome biogenesis disorder; or some tRNA charging abnormality impairing translation. The possibilities are as broad as all biology and hence justify newly revised editions of this text and associated online resources.

A salient challenge derived from the rapid expansion of our field and any such effort to describe it, is how to modernize the definition of inborn errors of metabolism, a term, after all, that has been in use since 1908 when Garrod coined it in his Croonian lectures (Garrod 1908). Recent efforts to update the definition have included inclusion of phenotypic features, diagnostic technologies, and limitations to specific biological systems (Morava et al. 2015; Ferreira et al. 2019). While useful, phenotypic features for any disorder are always variable and typically overlap with those of other disorders. Diagnostic technology changes over time and will continue to do so. A focus on biologic systems is useful for understanding pathophysiology, but the margins of any particular system often overlap with those of others and, currently, we do not have a well-defined list of all biological systems.

Based on these considerations, I argue that we consider all monogenic disorders as Garrodian inborn errors of metabolism. This gene-based definition is enriched by a foundation built on genetic principles and emphasizes the discrete monogenic cause of these disorders. It also benefits from the fact that it is easier to enumerate and designate all the genes in the genome than all the phenotypes that bring patients to our clinics. For example, at the time I write this (25 November 2020), OMIM lists 4355 genes with variants that cause monogenic disease (OMIM® n.d.). This number is increasing steadily with no asymptote in sight (Posey et al. 2019; Bamshad et al. 2019). Moreover, all monogenic disorders have an associated biochemical phenotype increasingly recognized by standard or newly developed technologies such as metabolomics or proteomics. Identification of the biochemical abnormalities associated with each monogenic disease is sometimes challenging but feasible and leads to improved understanding of the pathophysiology of each disorder, a necessary step on the path to rational development of treatment.

One possible concern of a gene-based definition of IEM is that for some genes, allelic heterogeneity produces phenotypic variation which in some instances is so extreme that we do not a priori expect variants in the same gene to underlie the apparently discrete phenotypes. For example, variants in *FBN1* can cause either Marfan syndrome (OMIM 154700) with tall stature, arachnodactyly, loose joints, ectopia lentis and aortic root aneurysms or stiff skin syndrome (OMIM 184900) with short stature, no arachnodactyly, limited range of joint mobility, and no ocular nor aortic symptoms. In fact, about a third of disease genes listed in OMIM are responsible for two or more clinically discrete phenotypes (OMIM® n.d.). A gene-based definition of IEM would, however, anticipate this biologic complexity and incorporate it so that each gene would be linked to a specific phenotype or set of phenotypes, with the benefit that we would expect these genotype–phenotype relationships as a part of disease biology and use them to inform our understanding of the disorders and the function of the protein(s) encoded by each gene.

Using this definition, the ultimate number of IEMs depends on how many genes are found to house variants of major effect, sufficient to produce a phenotype. The fact that evolution seems to care about (conserve) the vast majority of protein-coding genes in the genome suggests that certain variants in nearly all protein-coding genes will ultimately be found to be capable of producing a monogenic phenotype (and thus, by this definition, be considered an inborn error of metabolism or, perhaps better, simply an inborn error). This logic suggests that long non-coding RNA genes, which are less well conserved, may play a much smaller role in monogenic disease. How this will end up in the future is an uncertain but exciting prospect.

One thing for sure is that new resources for clinicians and investigators such as this new edition of a *Physician's Guide to the Diagnosis, Treatment, and Follow-Up of Inherited Metabolic Diseases* will be much needed and appreciated.

David Valle
McKusick-Nathans Department of Genetic Medicine
The Johns Hopkins University School of Medicine
Baltimore, MD, USA

## References

Bamshad MJ, et al. Mendelian gene discovery: fast and furious with no end in sight. Am J Hum Genet. 2019;105:448–55.

Burrage LC, et al. Untargeted metabolomic profiling reveals multiple pathway perturbations and new clinical biomarkers in urea cycle disorders. Genet Med. 2019;21:1977–86.

Ferreira CR, et al. A proposed nosology of inborn errors of metabolism. Genet Med. 2019;21:102–6.

Garrod AE. The incidence of alkaptonuria: a study in chemical individuality. The Lancet. 1902;2:1616–20.

Garrod AE. The Croonian Lectures on inborn errors of metabolism. The Lancet. 1908;2:1–7, 73–9, 142–8, 214–20.

Garrod AE. Inborn factors in disease. Oxford University Press; 1931.

Miller MJ, et al. Untargeted metabolomic analysis for the clinical screening of inborn errors of metabolism. J Inherit Metab Dis. 2015;38:1029–39.

Morava E, et al. Quo vadis: the re-definition of inborn metabolic diseases. J Inherit Metab Dis. 2015;38:1003–6.

Ng SB, et al. Targeted capture and massively parallel sequencing of 12 human exomes. Nature. 2009;461:272–6.

Online Mendelian Inheritance in Man, OMIM®. McKusick-Nathans Department of Genetic Medicine, Johns Hopkins University (Baltimore, MD), 24 November 2020. https://omim.org/

Posey JE, et al., Insights into genetics, human biology, and disease gleaned from family based genomic studies. Genet Med. 2019;21:798–812.

# Preface

Our expert faculty of more than 170 recognized authorities has broadened the scope and content of this book, the fourth edition of the Physician's Guide series. We overhauled the structure of the book to accommodate 18 new chapters: 73 chapters now address almost 1200 inherited metabolic disorders. The original edition, published in 1996, focused on diagnosis only and was translated into Chinese in 2001. Today, along with a comprehensive update to this vital aspect of care, the current edition presents the state of the art on the treatment and follow-up, providing insight into the full clinical course of these rare diseases.

Based upon their experience, our expert faculty have created flowcharts and diagnostic algorithms for each disorder. Initially, recommendations on confirmatory tests and initial treatment regimens are provided for practitioners who lack extensive experience in the management of inborn errors of metabolism. The second part of each chapter describes the treatment of groups of disorders in more detail. The book presents the signs and symptoms of most of the recognized inborn errors of metabolism in relation to age, with a chronological sequence of signs and symptoms from infancy through childhood, adolescence, and adulthood. In addition, reference and pathological values are provided for each of the disorders to simplify and facilitate the interpretation of the results of laboratory tests.

The guide will also be available in an eBook format that will allow the user to locate a disorder rapidly, using standard searches with keywords. Additionally, the entire content of this edition is stored in a single database, IEMbase (http://www.iembase.org). This comprehensive online resource provides the foundation for the current and future knowledge base of inborn errors of metabolism.

While the major goals of this edition remain comparable to those of earlier editions, we, the Editors, feel that this new edition takes clinical practice in rare metabolic disorders to the next level. We hope that our readers will find this edition helpful, both now and in the future, for the treatment and care of patients with inborn errors of metabolism.

Finally, we acknowledge the former Editors, Dr. Marinus Duran and Dr. K. Michael Gibson in supporting this book project.


Zürich, Switzerland — Nenad Blau
Rome, Italy — Carlo Dionisi Vici
Washington, DC, USA — Carlos R. Ferreira
Lyon, France — Christine Vianey-Saban
Amsterdam, The Netherlands — Clara D. M. van Karnebeek


The original version of this book has been updated: fifth Editor Dr. Clara D. M. van Karnebeek's affiliation has been updated. A Correction to this book is available at https://doi.org/10.1007/978-3-030-67727-5_74

# How to Use This Book

This book is meant to supply clinicians and clinical biochemists with data that should facilitate the diagnosis of an inherited metabolic disorder. No information about detailed laboratory methods is given; rather, the relationship between laboratory data and clinical signs and symptoms is highlighted. Furthermore the current knowledge on the immediate emergency intervention, standard treatment, and experimental options is given. Entry to the book is achieved by scanning either of the indices, i.e., the signs and symptoms index, the tests index, or the disorders index. Due to the great clinical variability of inherited metabolic diseases, one should not restrict oneself to one disorder when observing a given symptom or sign. Most chapters have a uniform layout as given below. In a few chapters, however, this was not possible, and information is given for the entire related group of disorders in the chapter.

## Introduction

The introduction gives a brief overview of the clinical conditions described in the chapter and relates them to the biochemical abnormalities. Key references for further reading are provided.

## Nomenclature

Disorders in each chapter are numbered in accordance with the corresponding OMIM number, gene symbols and gene products, and chromosomal localization if known.

## Metabolic Pathway

Disorders are identified by corresponding reference numbers at the step where the defect is localized. Pathological metabolites ("markers") are given in most chapters.

## Signs and Symptoms

The tables describe most, if not all, of the signs and symptoms for each disorder, including its reference number, and the most important laboratory tests, in relation to age. In all instances, the signs and symptoms are found in the untreated patients. The signs written in **bold** represent characteristic features of the particular disease.

± indicates that a sign or symptom *may* occur but is not inevitably present.

+ indicates that a sign or symptom is always or nearly always present. If there are significant clinical signs and symptoms which exceed the usual, or if changes occur, this is indicated with + to + + +, etc.

n (normal) is used only when it is significant and may be useful in distinguishing one condition from another.

Relative increases or decreases of substances, compounds, metabolites, etc., are indicated with the use of arrows; for example, metabolite X ↑ to ↓↓↓. Where metabolite X *may* change, it would be indicated by n-↑ for a possible increase or ↓-n for a possible decrease, whichever the case.

In all tables, the test substance, material, compound, metabolite, etc., are listed and the source—(U), (B), (CSF), (P), (RBC), etc.—is given in parentheses, with an arrow or arrows indicating increase/decrease or relative increase/decrease.

Body fluids, cells, tissues, etc., are defined as:

| | | | |
|---|---|---|---|
| P | Plasma | CV | Chorionic villi |
| S | Serum | AF | Amniotic fluid |
| B | Blood | AFC | Amniocytes |
| U | Urine | CCV | Cultured chorionic villi |
| CSF | Cerebrospinal fluid | PLT | Platelets |
| RBC | Red blood cells | WBC | White blood cells |
| LYM | Lymphocytes | Hb | Hemoglobin |
| FB | Fibroblasts | creat | Creatinine |
| BM | Bone marrow | | |

Age groups are defined as:

| | |
|---|---|
| Neonatal | Birth to 1 month |
| Infancy | 1–18 months |
| Childhood | 1.5–11 years |
| Adolescence | 11–16 years |
| Adulthood | >16 years |

## Reference Values/Pathological Values/Differential Diagnosis

Reference and pathological values are listed for all parameters relevant to the diagnosis according to the specimen (e.g., P, U, CSF) and age. For some parameters, reference values depend on methodology and may differ from chapter to chapter. Methods are specified where necessary.

Pathological values are listed either as absolute values or with symbols (e.g., ↑, ↓) according to the disorder. Values are limited to the analyses which can be performed in a laboratory experienced in selective screening. Data on enzyme studies are not given in most cases, but can be found in the pertinent literature.

## Loading Tests

There is a brief description of the tests, with a table or figure to illustrate the interpretation.

## Diagnostic Flow Chart

The flow charts use simple yes/no algorithms to demonstrate the sequence for differential diagnosis, starting with clinical symptoms or general tests and proceeding to specific tests and a final diagnosis.

## Specimen Collection

This table lists preconditions, material, handling, and pitfalls for each parameter used in the diagnosis.

## Prenatal Diagnosis

This table lists the tissue or specimen, timing, and pitfalls for each disorder.

## DNA Analysis

This table lists the tissue or specimen and methodology for each disorder.

## Treatment and Follow-Up

This section outlines urgent treatment to consider before a definitive diagnosis is established for each (or each group of) disorder(s). Long-term treatment and alternative therapeutic options are highlighted in this book.

## Indices

Three indices are included: (1) disorders, (2) signs and symptoms, and (3) tests and medications. Each entry is linked to the corresponding disorder or page.

# Contents

# Contributors


**Cécile Acquaviva** CHU de Lyon, Department of Biochemistry & Molecular Biology, Division of Inborn Errors of Metabolism, Lyon University Hospital Centre, Bron, France

**Majid Alfadhel** King Abdullah International Medical Research Centre, King Saud bin Abdulaziz University for Health Sciences, Riyadh, Saudi Arabia

**Anna Ardissone** Unit of Child Neurology, Fondazione IRCCS Istituto Neurologico Carlo Besta, Milan, Italy

**Jean-Baptiste Arnoux** French Metabolic Network G2M, Necker-Enfants Malades Hospital, APHP, Paris, France

**Rafael Artuch** CIBERER, Instituto de Salud Carlos III, Madrid, Spain

Clinical Chemistry Department, Institut de Recerca Sant Joan de Déu, Barcelona, Spain

Pathology Department, Institut de Recerca Sant Joan de Déu, Barcelona, Spain

**Tamar V. Av-Shalom** Department of Medical Genetics, Centre for Molecular Medicine and Therapeutics, BC Children's Hospital Research Institute, University of British Columbia, Vancouver, BC, Canada

**Ivo Barić** Division for Genetics and Metabolic Diseases, Department of Pediatrics, University Hospital Center Zagreb and University of Zagreb, School of Medicine, Zagreb, Croatia

**Bruce A. Barshop** Department of Pediatrics, University of California San Diego, La Jolla, CA, USA

**Matthias R. Baumgartner** Division of Metabolism and Children's Research Center, University Children's Hospital Zürich, University of Zürich, Zürich, Switzerland

**Bodo B. Beck** Department of Human Genetics, University Hospital Cologne, Cologne, Germany

**Michael Beck** SphinCS GmbH–Clinical Science for LSD, Hochheim, Germany

**Cinzia Maria Bellettato** Regional Coordinating Center for Rare Diseases, Udine University Hospital, Udine, Italy

**Jean-François Benoist** APHP, Reference Center for Inborn Error of Metabolism and Filiere G2M, Pediatrics Department, Necker Univ Hospital, Paris, France

**Anna Biason-Lauber** Division of Medicine, University of Fribourg, Fribourg, Switzerland

**Jörgen Bierau** Department of Clinical Genetics, Erasmus MC, Rotterdam, The Netherlands

**Nenad Blau** Division of Metabolism, University Children's Hospital, Zürich, Switzerland

**Annet M. Bosch** Department of Pediatrics, Emma Children's Hospital, Amsterdam University Medical Centers, Amsterdam, The Netherlands

**Olivier Braissant** Service of Clinical Chemistry, Department of Laboratories, University Hospital and University of Lausanne, Lausanne, Switzerland

**Anaïs Brassier** APHP, Reference Center for Inborn Error of Metabolism and Filiere G2M, Pediatrics Department, Necker Univ Hospital, Paris, France

**Stefan Bröer** Research School of Biology, The Australian National University, Canberra, ACT, Australia

**Alberto Burlina** Division of Inherited Metabolic Diseases, Reference Centre Expanded Newborn Screening, Department of Woman's and Child's Health, University Hospital, Padova, Italy

**John R. Burnett** Department of Clinical Biochemistry, Royal Perth Hospital and Fiona Stanley Hospital, PathWest Laboratory Medicine WA, Perth, WA, Australia

School of Medicine, University of Western Australia, Perth, WA, Australia

**Maria Domenica Cappellini** Fondazione Ca Granda Policlinico IRCCS, Università di Milano, Milan, Spain

**Rosalba Carrozzo** Molecular Genetic, Bambino Gesù Children's Hospital, Rome, Italy

**Rita Carsetti** Diagnostic Immunology Clinical Unit, Bambino Gesù Children's Hospital IRCCS, Rome, Italy

**David Cassiman** Center for Metabolic Diseases, University of Leuven, Leuven, Belgium

**Peter T. Clayton** UCL GOS Institute of Child Health, University College, London, UK

**Karlien L. M. Coene** Translational Metabolic Laboratory, Department Laboratory Medicine, Radboud University Medical Centre, Nijmegen, The Netherlands

**Curtis R. Coughlin II** Section of Clinical Genetics and Metabolism, Department of Pediatrics, University of Colorado, Children's Hospital Colorado, Aurora, CO, USA

**James Davison** Metabolic Unit, Great Ormond Street Hospital for Children, NHS Foundation Trust and Institute for Child Health, London, UK

**Lonneke de Boer** Department of Pediatrics, Radboud Center for Mitochondrial Medicine, Radboud University Medical Centre (Radboudumc), Nijmegen, The Netherlands

**Tom J. de Koning** Department of Clinical Sciences, Lund University, Lund, Sweden

**Pascale de Lonlay** French Metabolic Network G2M, Necker-Enfants Malades Hospital, APHP, Paris, France

**Linda de Meirleir** Department of Pediatric Neurology, UZ-Brussel, Brussels, Belgium

**Terry G. J. Derks** Section of Metabolic Diseases, Beatrix Children's Hospital, University Medical Center Groningen, Groningen, The Netherlands

**Maaike C. de Vries** Department of Pediatrics, Radboud Center for Mitochondrial Medicine, Radboud University Medical Centre (Radboudumc), Nijmegen, The Netherlands

**Ivano Di Meo** Unit of Medical Genetics and Neurogenetics, Fondazione IRCCS Istituto Neurologico Carlo Besta, Milan, Italy

**Daria Diodato** Neuromuscular and Neurodegenerative Disease Unit, Children Hospital Bambino Gesù, Rome, Italy

**Carlo Dionisi Vici** Division of Metabolism, Department of Pediatric Medicine, Bambino Gesù Children's Research Hospital, IRCCS, Rome, Italy

**Katrina M. Dipple** Division of Genetic Medicine, Department of Pediatrics, University of Washington School of Medicine and Seattle Children's Hospital, Seattle, WA, USA

**Francesco Emma** Department of Pediatric Subspecialties, Division of Nephrology and Dialysis, Bambino Gesù Children's Hospital, IRCCS, Rome, Italy

**Marc Engelen** Departments of Pediatric Neurology, Emma Children's Hospital, Amsterdam University Medical Centers, Academic Medical Center, Amsterdam, The Netherlands

**Udo F. H. Engelke** Translational Metabolic Laboratory, Department Laboratory Medicine, Radboud University Medical Centre, Nijmegen, The Netherlands

**Sacha Ferdinandusse** Laboratory Genetic Metabolic Diseases, Amsterdam UMC, Amsterdam, The Netherlands

**Carlos R. Ferreira** Division of Genetics and Metabolism, Children's National Health System, Washington, DC, USA

**Ralph Fingerhut** SYNLAB MVZ Weiden, Weiden, Germany

**Janice Fletcher** SA Pathology (at Women's and Children's Hospital), Adelaide, SA, Australia

**Brian Fowler** Division for Metabolic Diseases, University Children's Hospital, Zürich, Switzerland

**D. Sean Froese** Division of Metabolism and Children's Research Center, University Children's Hospital Zürich, University of Zürich, Zürich, Switzerland

**Silvia Funghini** Newborn Screening, Clinical Chemistry and Pharmacology Lab, Meyer Children's University Hospital, Florence, Italy

**Roberto Giugliani** Department of Genetics, Federal University of Rio Grande do Sul, Porto Alegre, RS, Brazil

Medical Genetics Service, Hospital de Clinicas de Porto Alegre, Porto Alegre, RS, Brazil

**Stephen I. Goodman** University of Colorado Denver School of Medicine, Aurora, CO, USA

**Andrea Gropman** Department of Neurology, Children's National Health System, Washington, DC, USA

**Sarah C. Grünert** Zentrum für Kinder- und Jugendmedizin, Universitätsklinikum Freiburg, Freiburg, Germany

**Stephanie Grünewald** Metabolic Unit, Great Ormond Street Hospital for Children, NHS Foundation Trust and Institute for Child Health, London, UK

**Chandan Guha** Marion Bessin Liver Research Center, Albert Einstein College of Medicine, Bronx, NY, USA

Departments of Radiation Oncology and Pathology, Albert Einstein College of Medicine, Bronx, NY, USA

**Johannes Häberle** Division of Metabolism and Children's Research Center, University Children's Hospital, Zürich, Switzerland

**Robert A. Hegele** Schulich School of Medicine and Dentistry, University of Western Ontario, London, ON, Canada

**Georg F. Hoffmann** University Children's Hospital, Heidelberg, Germany

**Carla Hollak** Division of Endocrinology and Metabolism, Department of Internal Medicine, Academic Medical Center, University of Amsterdam, Amsterdam, The Netherlands

**Ian J. Holt** Biodonostia Health Research Institute, San Sebastián, Spain

IKERBASQUE, Basque Foundation for Science, Bilbao, Spain

CIBERNED (Center for Networked Biomedical Research on Neurodegenerative Diseases, Ministry of Economy and Competitiveness Institute Carlos III), Madrid, Spain

**Amanda J. Hooper** Department of Clinical Biochemistry, Royal Perth Hospital and Fiona Stanley Hospital, PathWest Laboratory Medicine WA, Perth, WA, Australia

School of Medicine, University of Western Australia, Perth, WA, Australia

**Bernd Hoppe** Hyperoxaluria Center, German Hyperoxaluria Center, Bonn, Germany

**Hidde H. Huidekoper** Center for Lysosomal and Metabolic diseases, Department of Pediatrics, Erasmus MC University Medical Center, Rotterdam, The Netherlands

**Jaak Jaeken** Center for Metabolic Disease, University Hospital Gasthuisberg, Leuven, Belgium

**Judith J. M. Jans** Translational Metabolic Laboratory, Department Laboratory Medicine, Radboud University Medical Centre, Nijmegen, The Netherlands

**Mirian C. H. Janssen** Department of Internal Medicine, Radboud Center for Mitochondrial Medicine, Nijmegen, The Netherlands

**Heinz Jungbluth** Department of Paediatric Neurology, Evelina Children's Hospital, Guy's and St Thomas' Hospital NHS Foundation Trust, London, UK

**Richard I. Kelley** Central Pennsylvania Clinic, Belleville, PA, USA

**Femke C. C. Klouwer** Departments of Neurology and Pediatric Neurology, Emma Children's Hospital, Amsterdam University Medical Centers, Amsterdam, The Netherlands

**Stefan Kölker** Division of Pediatric Neurology and Metabolic Medicine, Clinic I, Center for Pediatric and Adolescent Medicine, Heidelberg, Germany

**Werner J. H. Koopman** Department of Biochemistry, Radboud Institute for Molecular Life Sciences (RIMLS), Radboud Center for Mitochondrial Medicine, Radboud University Medical Centre (Radboudumc), Nijmegen, The Netherlands

**Viktor Kožich** Department of Pediatrics and Inherited Metabolic Diseases, Charles University-First Faculty of Medicine and General University Hospital in Prague, Praha, Czech Republic

**Lisa E. Kratz** Department of Neurogenetics, Kennedy Krieger Institute, Baltimore, MD, USA

**Ilja Kubisch** Center of Internal Medicine II, Gastroenterology, Hepatology, Endocrinology, Metabolic Disorders, Oncology, Saxony Porphyria Center, Klinikum Chemnitz gGmbH, Chemnitz, Germany

**Martina Kutmon** Department of Bioinformatics—BiGCaT, NUTRIM, Maastricht University, Maastricht, The Netherlands

Maastricht Centre for Systems Biology—MaCSBio, Maastricht University, Maastricht, The Netherlands

**Giancarlo la Marca** Newborn Screening, Clinical Chemistry and Pharmacology Lab, Meyer Children's University Hospital, Florence, Italy

Department of Experimental and Clinical Biomedical Sciences, University of Florence, Florence, Italy

**Jessica J. Y. Lee** Department of Medical Genetics, Centre for Molecular Medicine and Therapeutics, BC Children's Hospital Research Institute, University of British Columbia, Vancouver, BC, Canada

**Min Ae Lee-Kirsch** Department of Pediatrics, Medizinische Fakultät Carl Gustav Carus, Technische Universität Dresden, Dresden, Germany

**Elena Levtchenko** Department of Pediatric Nephrology, University Hospitals Leuven, Catholic University of Leuven, Leuven, Belgium

**Nicola Longo** University of Utah and ARUP Laboratories, Salt Lake City, UT, USA

**Charlotte M. A. Lubout** Section of Metabolic Diseases, Beatrix Children's Hospital, University Medical Center Groningen, Groningen, The Netherlands

**Zoltan Lukacs** Newborn Screening and Metabolic Diagnostics Unit, Hamburg University Medical Center, Hamburg, Germany

**Arianna Maiorana** Division of Metabolism, Department of Pediatric Subspecialties, Bambino Gesù Children's Hospital, Rome, Italy

**Sabrina Malvagia** Newborn Screening, Clinical Chemistry and Pharmacology Lab, Meyer Children's University Hospital, Florence, Italy

**Diego Martinelli** Division of Metabolism, Department of Pediatric Medicine, Bambino Gesù Children's Research Hospital, Rome, Italy

Division of Metabolic Diseases, Bambino Gesù Children's Hospital, IRCCS, Rome, Italy

**Cristina Martin-Higueras** Department of Pediatrics, Division of Pediatric Nephrology, University Hospital Bonn, Bonn, Germany

Department of Basic Medical Science, Faculty of Medicine, University of La Laguna, La Laguna, Spain

**Dietrich Matern** Biochemical Genetics Laboratory, Department of Laboratory Medicine and Pathology, Mayo Clinic, Rochester, MN, USA

**Ertan Mayatepek** Department of General Pediatrics, Neonatology and Pediatric Cardiology, University Children's Hospital, Heinrich-Heine University Düsseldorf, Düsseldorf, Germany

**Johannes A. Mayr** University Children's Hospital, Paracelsus Medical University, Salzburg, Austria

**Philippa B. Mills** UCL GOS Institute of Child Health, University College, London, UK

**Fanny Mochel** Reference Center for Adult Neurometabolic diseases, La Pitié-Salpêtrière University Hospital, Paris, France

**Eva Morava** Department of Medical Genetics, Mayo Clinic, Rochester, MN, USA

**Marwan Nashabat** King Abdulaziz Medical City, Riyadh, Saudi Arabia

**Gaia Novarino** Institute of Science and Technology (IST) Austria, Klosterneuburg, Austria

**Thomas Opladen** Division of Neuropediatrics and Metabolic Medicine, Department of Pediatrics, University Children's Hospital, Heidelberg, Germany

**Simona Orcesi** Unit of Child Neurology and Psychiatry, IRCCS Mondino Foundation, Pavia, Italy

**Esmee Oussoren** Center for Lysosomal and Metabolic diseases, Department of Pediatrics, Erasmus MC University Medical Center, Rotterdam, The Netherlands

**Manuel Palacín** Institute for Research in Biomedicine (IRB Barcelona), Barcelona Institute of Science and Technology, Barcelona, Spain

Barcelona, Centro de Investigación Biomédica en Red de Enfermedades Raras (CIBERER), Spain

Department of Biochemistry and Molecular Biomedicine, Faculty of Biology, University of Barcelona, Barcelona, Spain

**Giancarlo Parenti** Department of Translational Medical Sciences, Federico II University, Naples, Italy

Telethon Institute of Genetics and Medicine, Pozzuoli, Italy

**Marzia Pasquali** University of Utah and ARUP Laboratories, Salt Lake City, UT, USA

**Phillip L. Pearl** Department of Neurology, Boston Children's Hospital, Harvard Medical School, Boston, MA, USA

**Verena Peters** Centre for Pediatric and Adolescent Medicine, University of Heidelberg, Heidelberg, Germany

**Barbara Plecko** Department of Pediatrics and Adolescent Medicine, Division of General Pediatrics, Medical University of Graz, Graz, Austria

**Giulia Polo** Division of Inherited Metabolic Diseases, Department of Women and Children's Health, Regional Center for Expanded Neonatal Screening, University Hospital of Padova, Padova, Italy

**Holger Prokisch** Institute of Human Genetics, Technische Universität München, Munich, Germany

Institute of Neurogenomics, Helmholtz Zentrum München, Munich, Germany

**Enzo Ranieri** SA Pathology (at Women's and Children's Hospital), Adelaide, SA, Australia

**Antonia Ribes** Section of Inborn Errors of Metabolism, Department of Biochemistry and Molecular Genetics, Hospital Clinic de Barcelona, IDIBAPS, CIBERER, Barcelona, Spain

**Marlène Rio** Genetic Department, Necker-Enfants Malades Hospital, APHP, Paris, France

**Lance Rodan** Department of Neurology, Boston Children's Hospital, Harvard Medical School, Boston, MA, USA

**Richard J. Rodenburg** Department of Paediatrics, Translational Metabolic Laboratory, Radboud Center for Mitochondrial Medicine, Nijmegen, The Netherlands

**Jayanta Roy-Chowdhury** Depatments of Medicine and Genetics, Albert Einstein College of Medicine, Bronx, NY, USA

Marion Bessin Liver Research Center, Albert Einstein College of Medicine, Bronx, NY, USA

**Namita Roy-Chowdhury** Depatments of Medicine and Genetics, Albert Einstein College of Medicine, Bronx, NY, USA

Marion Bessin Liver Research Center, Albert Einstein College of Medicine, Bronx, NY, USA

**Vicente Rubio** Structural Enzymopathology Unit, Department of Genomics and Proteomics, Instituto de Biomedicina de Valencia of the Spanish National Research Council (CSIC) and Centre for Biomedical Network Research on Rare Diseases (CIBERER-ISCIII), Valencia, Spain

**Frans G. M. Russel** Department of Pharmacology and Toxicology, Radboud Center for Mitochondrial Medicine, Radboud Institute for Molecular Life Sciences, Radboud University Medical Center, Nijmegen, The Netherlands

**Gajja Salomons** Department of Genetic Metabolic Diseases, Amsterdam University Medical Centers, Amsterdam, The Netherlands

**Leonardo Salviati** Clinical Genetics Unit, Department of Women and Children's Health, University of Padova and IRP Città della Speranza, Padova, Italy

**René Santer** Department of Paediatrics, University Medical Center Eppendorf, Hamburg, Germany

**Jörn Oliver Sass** Research Group Inborn Errors of Metabolism, Department of Natural Sciences & Institute for Functional Gene Analytics (IFGA), Bonn-Rhein-Sieg University of Applied Sciences, Rheinbach, Germany

**Maurizio Scarpa** Regional Coordinating Center for Rare Diseases, Udine University Hospital, Udine, Italy

**Manuel Schiff** APHP, Reference Center for Inborn Error of Metabolism and Filière G2M, Pediatrics Department, Necker Univ Hospital, Paris, France

**Tom J. J. Schirris** Department of Pharmacology and Toxicology, Radboud Center for Mitochondrial Medicine, Radboud Institute for Molecular Life Sciences, Radboud University Medical Center, Nijmegen, The Netherlands

**Andreas Schulze** Division of Clinical and Metabolic Genetics, The Hospital for Sick Children, Toronto, ON, Canada

Departments of Pediatrics and Biochemistry, University of Toronto, Toronto, ON, Canada

**Detlef Schuppan** Institute of Translational Immunology and Research Center for Immune Therapy, University Medical Center, Johannes Gutenberg University, Mainz, Germany

Division of Gastroenterology, Beth Israel Deaconess Medical Center, Harvard Medical School, Boston, MA, USA

**Bernd C. Schwahn** Willink Metabolic Unit, Manchester Centre for Genomic Medicine, Manchester University Hospitals NHS Foundation Trust, Saint Mary's Hospital, Manchester, UK

**Guenter Schwarz** Department of Chemistry, Center for Molecular Medicine, Institute of Biochemistry, University of Cologne, Koeln, Germany

**Ivan Šebesta** Institute of Medical Biochemistry and Laboratory Medicine, Institute of Inherited Metabolic Disorders, First Faculty of Medicine, Charles University, Prague 2, Czech Republic

**Annalisa Sechi** Regional Coordinating Center for Rare Diseases, Udine University Hospital, Udine, Italy

**Denise N. Slenter** Department of Bioinformatics—BiGCaT, NUTRIM, Maastricht University, Maastricht, The Netherlands

**Jan A. M. Smeitink** Department of Pediatrics, Radboud Center for Mitochondrial Medicine, Radboud University Medical Center, Nijmegen, The Netherlands

**Johannes N. Spelbrink** Department of Paediatrics, Radboud Center for Mitochondrial Medicine, Nijmegen, The Netherlands

**Ute Spiekerkoetter** Department of Pediatrics and Adolescent Medicine, University Children's Hospital, Albert Ludwigs University, Freiburg, Germany

**Antonella Spinazzola** MRC Centre for Neuromuscular Diseases, UCL Queen Square Institute of Neurology and National Hospital for Neurology and Neurosurgery, London, UK

Department of Clinical and Movement Neurosciences, UCL Queen Square Institute of Neurology, London, UK

**Thomas Stauch** Department of Clinical Chemistry and Toxicology, German Competence Center for Porphyria Diagnosis and Consultation, MVZ Labor PD Dr. Volkmann und Kollegen GbR, Karlsruhe, Germany

**Robert Steinfeld** Division of Pediatric Neurology, University Children's Hospital Zürich, Zürich, Switzerland

**Sarah L. Stenton** Institute of Human Genetics, Technische Universität München, Munich, Germany

Institute of Neurogenomics, Helmholtz Zentrum München, Munich, Germany

**Sylvia Stöckler-Ipsiroglu** Division of Biochemical Genetics, BC Children's Hospital, Vancouver, BC, Canada

Department of Pediatrics, University of British Columbia, Vancouver, BC, Canada

**Ulrich Stölzel** Center of Internal Medicine II, Gastroenterology, Hepatology, Endocrinology, Metabolic Disorders, Oncology, Saxony Porphyria Center, Klinikum Chemnitz gGmbH, Chemnitz, Germany

**Eduard A. Struys** Metabolic Unit, Clinical Chemistry, VUmc Medical Center, Amsterdam, The Netherlands

**Michael A. Swanson** Section of Clinical Genetics and Metabolism, Department of Pediatrics, University of Colorado, Children's Hospital Colorado, Aurora, CO, USA

**Isabel Tavares de Almeida** Metabolism and Genetics, iMed.UL, Faculdade de Farmácia da Universidade de Lisboa, Lisboa, Portugal

**Valeria Tiranti** Unit of Medical Genetics and Neurogenetics, Fondazione IRCCS Istituto Neurologico Carlo Besta, Milan, Italy

**Davide Tonduti** Child Neurology Unit, COALA (Center for Diagnosis and Treatment of Leukodystrophy)—V. Buzzi Children's Hospital, Milano, Italy

**Frederic Tort** Section of Inborn Errors of Metabolism-IBC, Department of Biochemistry and Molecular Genetics, Hospital Clínic de Barcelona, CIBERER, Barcelona, Spain

**Victoria Tüngler** Department of Pediatrics, Medizinische Fakultät Carl Gustav Carus, Technische Universität Dresden, Dresden, Germany

**Karin Tuschl** Department of Developmental Neurobiology, Kings College, London, UK

Department of Cell and Developmental Biology, University College, London, UK

UCL GOS Institute of Child Health, University College, London, UK

**Lambert van den Heuvel** Institute for Genetic and Metabolic Disease, Nijmegen Medical Centre, Radboud University, Nijmegen, The Netherlands

**Johan L. K. Van Hove** Section of Clinical Genetics and Metabolism, Department of Pediatrics, University of Colorado, Children's Hospital Colorado, Aurora, CO, USA

**Clara D. M. van Karnebeek** Departments of Pediatrics and Human Genetics, Emma Children's Hospital, Amsterdam University Medical Centers, Amsterdam, The Netherlands

**Francjan J. van Spronsen** Division of Metabolic Diseases, University of Groningen, University Medical Center Groningen, Beatrix Children's Hospital, Groningen, The Netherlands

**Frédéric M. Vaz** Laboratory Genetic Metabolic Diseases, Amsterdam UMC, Amsterdam, The Netherlands

**Nanda Verhoeven-Duif** Section Metabolic Diagnostics, Department of Genetics, University Medical Center Utrecht, Utrecht, The Netherlands

**Christine Vianey-Saban** CHU de Lyon, Department of Biochemistry & Molecular Biology, Division of Inborn Errors of Metabolism, Lyon University Hospital Centre, Bron, France

**Jerry Vockley** Children's Hospital of Pittsburgh, University of Pittsburgh Medical Center, University of Pittsburgh, Pittsburgh, PA, USA

**Mirjam M. C. Wamelink** Metabolic Unit, Department of Clinical Chemistry, Amsterdam UMC, Vrije Universiteit Amsterdam, Amsterdam, The Netherlands

**Ronald J. A. Wanders** Departments of Pediatrics, Emma Children's Hospital, and Laboratory Medicine, Amsterdam University Medical Centers, Academic Medical Center, Amsterdam, The Netherlands

**Wyeth W. Wasserman** Department of Medical Genetics, Centre for Molecular Medicine and Therapeutics, BC Children's Hospital Research Institute, University of British Columbia, Vancouver, BC, Canada

**Hans R. Waterham** Departments of Pediatrics, Emma Children's Hospital, and Laboratory Medicine, Amsterdam University Medical Centers, Academic Medical Center, Amsterdam, The Netherlands

**Ron A. Wevers** Translational Metabolic Laboratory, Department Laboratory Medicine, Radboud University Medical Centre, Nijmegen, The Netherlands

**Matthew T. Whitehead** Department of Radiology, Children's National Health System, Washington, DC, USA

**Monique Williams** Metabolic Unit, Department of Clinical Chemistry, Amsterdam UMC, Vrije Universiteit Amsterdam, Amsterdam, The Netherlands

**Egon L. Willighagen** Department of Bioinformatics—BiGCaT, NUTRIM, Maastricht University, Maastricht, The Netherlands

**Mathias Woidy** Department of Paediatrics, University Medical Center Eppendorf, Hamburg, Germany

**Saskia B. Wortmann** Institute of Human Genetics, Academic Medical Center, Munich, Germany

Institute of Neurogenomics, Helmholtz Zentrum München, Munich, Germany

University Children's Hospital, Paracelsus Medical University, Salzburg, Austria

Radboud Centre for Mitochondrial Medicine, Amalia Children's Hospital, Radboudumc, Nijmegen, The Netherlands

**Johannes Zschocke** Institute of Human Genetics, Medical University Innsbruck, Innsbruck, Austria

# Part V

# Mitochondrial Disorders of Energy Metabolism

# Disorders of the Pyruvate Metabolism and the Krebs Cycle

# 42

Eva Morava, Linda de Meirleir, and Rosalba Carrozzo

## Contents




**Summary**

This chapter focuses on pyruvate metabolism disorders, two classic Krebs cycle disorders (2-oxoglutaric aciduria and fumarase deficiency) and two other disorders of the Krebs cycle, severely affecting mitochondrial function and mitochondrial maintenance (succinyl-CoA synthetase—SCS—deficiencies, caused by mutations in *SUCLA2* and *SUCLG1* genes). Pyruvate carboxylase and pyruvate dehydrogenase deficiency are the most common disorders in pyruvate metabolism and almost always affect the central nervous system. The severity and the clinical phenotypes vary, with a range from severe neonatal lactic acidosis and early death to milder presentations. Pyruvate carboxylase (PC) deficiency constitutes a defect both in the Krebs cycle and in gluconeogenesis and


Linda de Meirleir was deceased at the time of publication.


E. Morava (✉)
Department of Medical Genetics, Mayo Clinic, Rochester, MN, USA
e-mail: Morava-Kozicz.Eva@Mayo.edu

L. de Meirleir
Department of Pediatric Neurology, UZ-Brussel, Brussels, Belgium

R. Carrozzo
Molecular Genetic, Bambino Gesù Children's Hospital, Rome, Italy
e-mail: rosalba.carrozzo@opbg.net






N. Blau et al. (eds.), *Physician's Guide to the Diagnosis, Treatment, and Follow-Up of Inherited Metabolic Diseases*,
https://doi.org/10.1007/978-3-030-67727-5_42

generally presents with severe neurologic dysfunction and lactic acidosis more frequently than with fasting hypoglycemia. Pyruvate dehydrogenase deficiency (PDH) is most common due to deficiency in the X-linked PDH E1 alpha, but defects in other subunits of the PDH complex have been described. Secondary PDH deficiency and profound neurodegeneration was described in LONP1 deficiency. Neonatal lactic acidosis and Leigh's encephalopathy occur more frequently in boys; girls can present with severe seizures and microcephaly. Fumarase deficiency and 2-oxoglutaric aciduria are rare disorders with global developmental delay and severe neurologic problems in infants. Patients with oxoglutaric aciduria have a variable severity of neurological involvement and metabolic acidosis and develop severe microcephaly and intellectual disability. Some patients with oxoglutaric aciduria present with DOORS syndrome (deafness, onychodystrophy, osteodystrophy, mental retardation, seizures). New disorders, like LIPT1 deficiency are known in the lipoic pathway leading to combined oxoglutaric aciduria and PDHc deficiency. Patients with fumarase deficiency present with either a fulminant course associated with fatal outcome within the first 2 years of life or a subacute encephalopathy with profound speech delay without metabolic crises. Hereditary leiomyomatosis and renal cell carcinoma (HLRCC) syndrome secondary to heterozygous germline fumarate hydratase (FH) mutations is an autosomal dominant condition and presents in young adults with cutaneous and uterine leiomyomas, and a distinctive aggressive renal carcinoma.

SUCLA2 and SUCLG1 defects have the clinical presentation of mitochondrial depletion syndromes with profound hypotonia, progressive dystonia, and muscular atrophy, in addition to severe sensorineural hearing impairment, which has been specifically associated with SUCLA2 defect. SUCLG1 defect has been also associated with congenital malformations (El-Hattab and Scaglia 2009).

In disorders of the pyruvate metabolism the diagnosis is suspected with lactic acidemia and hypoglycemia, in PDH deficiency, when lactate and pyruvate are elevated, with a normal pyruvate to lactate ratio. Further confirmation is done biochemically on fibroblasts, lymphocytes, muscle, and the different genes can be investigated.

The most important clues for the diagnosis in all the Krebs cycle disorders rely on urine organic analysis. 2-Oxoglutaric aciduria leads to chronic metabolic acidosis and variable urinary excretion of 2-oxoglutarate, while fumarase deficiency occurs with an increased excretion of fumarate associated with succinate and lactate excretion with eventual 2-oxoglutaric aciduria. A normal excretion of fumaric acid and a relative high fumarase residual activity do not rule out fumarase deficiency. In questionable cases, mutation analysis is needed to confirm the diagnosis. In SCS defects, mild methylmalonic aciduria with abnormal urine carnitine-ester profile is associated with only subtle abnormalities of the Krebs cycle intermediates. Due to the recognizable pattern of dystonia/±deafness syndrome and mild methylmalonic aciduria in SCS defects, direct genetic testing is a possible approach in the diagnosis of SUCLA2 and SUCLG1 defects. Carrier screening in fumarase deficiency is important due to the possible increased risk for certain malignancies.

## Introduction

Pyruvate carboxylase is a biotin-containing nuclear-encoded mitochondrial enzyme, responsible for the carboxylation of pyruvate to oxaloacetate. The reaction covers for the replenishment of pools of intermediates of the citric acid cycle, a process called anaplerosis. Pyruvate carboxylase is also involved in several metabolic pathways that depend on the availability of oxaloacetate such as gluconeogenesis, glycogen synthesis, lipogenesis, glycerogenesis, and synthesis of amino acids and neurotransmitters.

Pyruvate carboxylase deficiency is associated with metabolic acidosis, failure to thrive, and developmental delay. Three phenotypes are associated with pyruvate carboxylase deficiency. In type A infantile North American phenotype, patients are severely ill between 2 and 5 months of age with progressive hypotonia. Episodes of acute vomiting, dehydration, tachypnea, facial pallor, cold cyanotic extremities, and metabolic acidosis, characteristically precipitated by metabolic or infectious stress, occur. Clinical examination includes pyramidal tract signs, ataxia, and nystagmus. All patients are severely mentally retarded and most of them have convulsions. In type B (French phenotype), patients become acutely ill 3–48 h after birth with hypothermia, hypotonia, lethargy, and vomiting. There is a rapid deterioration with rigidity, hypokinesia, and tremor (resembling infantile Parkinson) and abnormal ocular movements. Most die in the neonatal period. Some survive but remain unresponsive and severely hypotonic, often with death due to respiratory infection before the age of 5 months. Type C is a more benign phenotype, only reported in a few patients. The clinical course consists of acute episodes of lactic acidosis and ketoacidosis, usually responding rapidly to hydration and bicarbonate therapy. Despite the important enzymatic deficiency on testing in fibroblasts, the patients have a nearly normal cognitive and neuromotor development (Barnerias et al. 2010; De Meirleir 2013).

Pyruvate dehydrogenase (PDHC) is composed of three components: E1; E2, dihydrolipoamide acyl-transferase; and E3, dihydrolipoamide dehydrogenase. E1 utilizes thiamine pyrophosphate and is composed of two different subunits, E1α and E1β. The E1 reaction results in decarboxylation of the specific α-ketoacid.

For the PDHC, the E1 component is the rate-limiting step and is regulated by phosphorylation/dephosphorylation catalyzed by two enzymes, E1 kinase (inactivation) and E1 phosphatase (activation). E2 is a transacetylase that utilizes lipoic acid. E3 is a flavoprotein common to all three 2-ketoacid dehydrogenases. Another important structural component of the PDHC is E3BP, E3 binding protein, formerly protein X. This component has its role in attaching E3 subunits to the core of E2.

PDHE1α deficiency is most commonly present with features of delayed development, hypotonia, seizures, and ataxia. In males, there are three presentations: neonatal lactic acidosis, Leigh's encephalopathy, and intermittent ataxia. In the first presentation, neonatal lactic acidosis is often associated with brain dysgenesis, such as agenesis of the corpus callosum. In Leigh's encephalopathy, the initial presentation is usually within the first 5 years of life and includes respiratory disturbances or episodic weakness and ataxia with absence of tendon reflexes. Respiratory disturbances may lead to apnea, dependence on assisted ventilation, or sudden unexpected death. Intermittent dystonic posturing of the lower limbs occurs frequently. A moderate to severe developmental delay becomes evident within the next years. A very small subset of male patients is initially much less severely affected, with intermittent episodic ataxia after carbohydrate-rich meals, progressing slowly over years into a mild Leigh's encephalopathy. A number of patients have developed an acute peripheral neuropathy during infancy or an acute episodic ataxia. In females with PDHE1α deficiency, there is a more uniform clinical presentation, although with variable severity. This includes dysmorphic features, microcephaly, moderate to severe mental retardation, and spastic di- or quadriplegia, resembling nonprogressive encephalopathy. Dysmorphism comprises a narrow head with frontal bossing, wide nasal bridge, upturned nose, long philtrum, and flared nostrils. Seizures are encountered in almost all female patients. These appear within the first 6 months of life and are diagnosed as infantile spasms (flexor and extensor) or severe myoclonic seizures. Brain MRI frequently reveals severe cortical/subcortical atrophy, dilated ventricles, and partial to complete corpus callosum agenesis. Severe neonatal lactic acidosis can be present.

Few cases have been reported with PDH E1beta deficiency with early-onset lactic acidosis and severe developmental delay. A moderate clinical course with slowly progressive neurological features reflecting basal ganglia and brain stem involvement associated with typical findings of Leigh syndrome has also been reported.

A few cases of PDH E2 (dihydrolipoamide transacetylase) deficiency have been reported recently with developmental delay and lactic acidosis.

PDH E3 is an enzyme, common to all the 2-ketoacid dehydrogenases; E3 deficiency results in multiple 2-ketoacid dehydrogenase deficiency and should be thought of as a combined PDHC and TCA cycle defect. E3 deficiency presents with severe and progressive hypotonia and failure to thrive, starting in the first months of life. Metabolic decompensations are triggered by infections. Progressively hypotonia, psychomotor retardation, microcephaly, and spasticity occur. Some patients develop a typical picture of Leigh's encephalopathy. A Reye-like picture with liver involvement and myopathy with myoglobinuria without intellectual disability is seen in the Ashkenazi Jewish population. Increased blood lactate and pyruvate, elevated plasma alanine, glutamate, glutamine, and branched-chain amino acids (leucine, isoleucine, and valine) and increased urinary lactic, pyruvic, 2-ketoglutaric, and branched-chain 2-hydroxy and 2-keto acids are characteristic.

The main clinical manifestations of E3BP (formerly protein X) deficiency are hypotonia, delayed psychomotor development, and prolonged survival. Often more slowly progressive, it also comprises early-onset neonatal lactic acidosis associated with subependymal cysts and thin corpus callosum.

E1-phosphatase deficiency has been identified in two brothers with hypotonia, feeding difficulties, and delayed psychomotor development. A lethal infantile phenotype has also been described (Lissens et al. 2000; Grafakou et al. 2003; Brown et al. 2006; Willemsen et al. 2006; De Meirleir 2013).

PDH deficiency was also described due to LonP1 deficiency in association with neurologic regression during infancy, profound hypotonia and muscle weakness, severe intellectual disability and normal plasma lactate:pyruvate ratios. PDH dysfunction was caused by increased levels of the phosphorylated E1α subunit of PDH, which inhibits enzyme activity (Nimmo et al. 2019).

The Krebs cycle disorders 2-oxoglutaric aciduria and fumarase deficiency are clinically similar disorders of hypotonia, spasticity, developmental delay, and extrapyramidal symptoms of variable severity. These very rare disorders present with episodes of acute metabolic acidosis and eventually hypoketotic hypoglycemia in stress situations. Krebs cycle disorders have recurrent episodes of severe decompensations, related mostly to acute, intercurrent infections. Lactic acidosis can be significant in acute episodes, and the disorder might imitate a mitochondrial disorder both based on the clinical and metabolic presentation. Most cases are lethal in the first 10 years of life.

The 2-KGD complex is composed of three separate enzymes: E1, E2, and E3. It has been postulated that in most patients, the E2 component could be responsible for the "classic metabolic" presentation of the defect (Bonnefont et al. 1992; Guffon et al. 1993). In occasional cases the disease appears only after infancy, with progressive extrapyramidal and psychiatric symptoms (Kohlschutter et al. 1982).

There are two distinct phenotypes in 2-oxoglutaric aciduria, an encephalopathic form related to E2 subunit deficiency and a clinically recognizable form of deafness, onycho-osteodystrophy, short terminal phalanges, intellectual disability and seizures, also labeled as DOORS syndrome, due to a defect of the E1 subunit of the enzyme complex (Surendran et al. 2002). DOORS syndrome is genetically heterogenous, also caused by *TBC1D24*, *SMARCB1*, and *PIGB* defects. The diagnosis in 2-oxoglutaric acidemia might remain uncertain in some cases, due to relatively high residual activity of the 2-oxoglutarate dehydrogenase in homogenates of cultured skin fibroblasts, which can be found in some patients with a proven E2 subunit deficiency.

Lipoate serves as a cofactor for both α-oxoglutarate dehydrogenase and pyruvate dehydrogenase [PDHc]). Mutations in the mitochondrial lipoate synthesis involving lipoyltransferase 1 (LIPT1) have been associated with nonketotic hyperglycinemia-like early-onset convulsions and encephalopathy combined with a defect in *LIPT1*-related mitochondrial energy metabolism, reduced leucine catabolic flux, and decreased protein lipoylation (Habarou et al. 2017).

Fumarase is a dual-targeted enzyme, detected in both the mitochondrial and cytosolic/nuclear compartments of all the eukaryotic organisms. Fumarase deficiency has been described in less than 50 cases with severe infantile encephalopathy (De Meirleir et al. 2006; Zinn et al. 1986; Zeman et al. 2000). The disorder is lethal in one-third of the patients in early childhood and leads to severe intellectual disability. Fumarase deficiency has been reported with intrauterine complications such as brain malformations and intrauterine growth retardation. Some of the children are dysmorphic (Maradin et al. 2006). Severe visual disturbance, Dandy–Walker malformation, and polymicrogyria have been observed in a few cases. The oldest reported patient survived to the second decade of life (Allegri et al. 2010).

The human fumarate hydratase (*FH*) gene consists of 10 exons encoding 510 amino acids. The first exon (exon 0) encodes a mitochondrial localization signal peptide of 43 amino acids. The 3-bp AAA duplication (c.1431_1433dupAAA) coding for an additional lysine amino acid is detected in approximately one-third of cases and is the most frequent abnormal allele in patients. All affected individuals with this allele are compound heterozygous with a different mutation on the other allele. Other mutations in the *FH* gene are private, although, interestingly, most mutations are clustered at the C-terminus (Picaud et al. 2011).

Most heterozygous relatives of patients with fumarase defect are normal. However, the finding of cutaneous leiomyomata without uterine fibroids in the mother of an affected child, a report of a mother with uterine myomas, and the death of the mother of an affected child from renal cell carcinoma led to the definition of a new hereditary condition with increased risk for tumor genesis (hereditary leiomyomatosis and renal cell carcinoma (HLRCC) syndrome) in carriers for fumarate hydratase deficiency (Bhola et al. 2018).

Mutations on *SUCLA2* and *SUCLG1* genes are associated to unique disorders due to the involvement of both the citric acid cycle, due to abnormal succinate metabolism, and the mitochondrial DNA (mtDNA) maintenance, manifesting with low mtDNA content in most patients. So far more than 50 patients have been reported with SUCLA2 and less than 25 with SUCLG1 defect.

Succinyl-CoA synthetase (SCS), which catalyzes the reversible conversion of succinyl-CoA and ADP or GDP to succinate and ATP or GTP, is part of the Krebs cycle. Deficient SCS activity has been associated with mutations in two out of the three subunits making up the enzyme: *SUCLA2* and *SUCLG1*, respectively. These genes encode the β-subunit of the ADP-forming SCS and the α-subunit of SCS. In multicellular eukaryotes, two different isoforms exist, consisting of the common α-subunit and a different β-subunit, one specific for ATP (A-SCS) and the other specific for GTP (G-SCS) (Johnson et al. 1998). Therefore, the β-subunits determine the substrate specificity of the two forms of the enzyme. Both enzymes are located in the mitochondrial matrix, where A-SCS, and probably also G-SCS, participates in the citric acid cycle. Several studies have indicated that SCS forms a complex with nucleoside diphosphate kinase (NDPK), which is important for the salvage of deoxyribonucleotides for mtDNA synthesis and for its integrity (Kadrmas et al. 1991; Kavanaugh-Black et al. 1994; Kowluru et al. 2002).

Mutations in *SUCLA2*, the gene encoding the β-subunit of ADP-forming SCS (Elpeleg et al. 2005), have been reported in several ethnicities and are associated with a distinct clinical phenotype consisting of a Leigh-like syndrome, dystonia, deafness, and feeding difficulties. Other, less frequent, features include distinctive facial features, contractures, kyphoscoliosis, gastroesophageal reflux, ptosis, choreoathetosis, ophthalmoplegia, and epilepsy (infantile spasms or generalized convulsions) (El-Hattab and Scaglia 2017). Normal cognition has been also observed. There is a mild lactic acidosis, and a variable degree of deficiency of the respiratory chain enzyme complexes (complex I and IV) in muscle, a mild-to-moderate mtDNA depletion, and mild elevation of methylmalonic acid in body fluids (Carrozzo et al. 2007; Ostergaard et al. 2007a, b; Morava et al. 2009; Carrozzo et al. 2016). A founder effect has been found underlying the common mutation in the Faroese and Scandinavian population.

Patients with mutations in *SUCLG1*, the gene coding for the α-subunit of SCS, might present with either a severe, fatal form of mitochondrial encephalomyopathy (Ostergaard et al. 2007a, b) with severe lactic acidosis, hepathopathy, seizures, microcephaly, and multiple congenital anomalies including renal and cardiac defects (El-Hattab and Scaglia 2017), or a somewhat milder clinical syndrome highly reminiscent of that seen in children with mutations in *SUCLA2* (Ostergaard et al. 2009; Rouzier et al. 2010; Landsverk et al. 2014). Some affected individuals present with hypertrophic cardiomyopathy, myoclonus, sleep disturbance, rhabdomyolysis, contractures, hypothermia, and/or hypoglycemia. *SUCLG1* mutations that lead to complete absence of SUCLG1 protein are responsible for a very severe disorder with antenatal manifestations (malformations), and profound CNS involvement, whereas a SUCLA2-like phenotype is found in patients with residual SUCLG1 protein. Furthermore, it has been shown that in the absence of SUCLG1 protein, no SUCLA2 protein is found in fibroblasts by western blot analysis. This result is consistent with a degradation of SUCLA2 when its heterodimer partner, SUCLG1, is absent.

The outcome for the two disorders is quite different. The median onset of symptoms has been 2 months for patients with *SUCLA2* mutations and at birth for SUCLG1-deficient patients. Median survival has been 20 years for patients with SUCLA2 deficiency and 20 months for patients with SUCLG1 deficiency (Carrozzo et al. 2016).

## Nomenclature

| No. | Disorder | Alternative name | Abbreviation | Gene | Chromosomal location | Mode of inheritance | Affected protein | OMIM |
|---|---|---|---|---|---|---|---|---|
| 42.1 | Pyruvate carboxylase deficiency | Leigh syndrome due to PC deficiency and ataxia with lactic acidosis II | PCD | *PC* | 11q13.2 | AR | Pyruvate carboxylase | 266150 |
| 42.2 | Pyruvate dehydrogenase E1-α deficiency | Pyruvate decarboxylase deficiency, ataxia, intermittent with abnormal pyruvate metabolism and ataxia with lactic acidosis I | PDHAD | *PDHA1* | Xp22.12 | XLD | Pyruvate dehydrogenase E1-α | 312170 |
| 42.3 | Pyruvate dehydrogenase E1-β deficiency | | PDHBD | *PDHB* | 3p14.3 | AR | Pyruvate dehydrogenase E1-β | 614111 |
| 42.4 | Dihydrolipoamide acetyltransferase deficiency | Pyruvate dehydrogenase complex E2 subunit | PDHDD | *DLAT* | 11q23.1 | AR | Dihydrolipoamide acetyltransferase | 608770 |
| 42.5 | Pyruvate dehydrogenase E3-binding protein deficiency | Lactic acidemia due to defect in lipoyl-containing component X of the pyruvate dehydrogenase-complex | PDHXD | *PDHX* | 11.p13 | AR | Pyruvate dehydrogenase E3-binding protein | 245349 |
| 42.6 | Pyruvate dehydrogenase phosphatase deficiency | Lactic Acidemia with pyruvate dehydrogenase phosphatase deficiency | PDHPD | *PDP1* | 8q22.1 | AR | Pyruvate dehydrogenase phosphatase | 608782 |
| 42.7 | Mitochondrial pyruvate carrier deficiency | | MPYCD | *MPC1* | 6q27 | AR | Mitochondrial pyruvate carrier | 614741 |
| 42.8 | Pyruvate dehydrogenase kinase isoenzyme 3 superactivity | Charcot Matie tooth disease X-linked dominant | CMTX6 | *PDK3* | Xp22.11 | XLD | Pyruvate dehydrogenase kinase isoenzyme 3 | 300905 |
| 42.9 | Dihydrolipoamide dehydrogenase deficiency | DLD deficiency, lactic acidosis due to, E3 deficiency, maple syrup urine disease type 3 | DLDD | *DLD* | 7q31.1 | AR | Dihydrolipoamide dehydrogenase | 246900 |
| 42.10 | Mitochondrial aconitase deficiency | Myopathy with lactic acidosis, hereditary, myopathy with exercise intolerance, Swedish type and myopathy with deficiency of succinate dehydrogenase and aconitase | HML | *ISCU* | 12q23.3 | AR | Iron-sulfur cluster scaffold protein | 255125 |
| 42.11 | Mitochondrial NADH-dependent isocitrate dehydrogenase 2 superactivity | D-2-hydroxy-glutaric aciduria 2 | D2HGA2 | *IDH2* | 15q26.1 | (AD) | Mitochondrial NADH-dependent isocitrate dehydrogenase 2 | 613657 |
| 42.12 | Mitochondrial NADPH-dependent isocitrate dehydrogenase 3 β subunit deficiency | Retinitis pigmentosa 46, retinitis pigmentosa AR, IDH3B-related | RP46 | *IDH3B* | 20p13 | AR | Mitochondrial NADPH-dependent isocitrate dehydrogenase 3 β subunit | 612572 |
| 42.13 | α-Ketoglutarate dehydrogenase deficiency | 2-Ketoglutarate dehydrogenase deficiency, Oxoglutaric Aciduria | N/A | *OGDH* | 7p13 | AR | α-Ketoglutarate dehydrogenase | 203740 |
| 42.14 | ATP-specific succinyl-CoA ligase β subunit deficiency | Mitochondrial DNA depletion syndrome 5 (encephalomyopathic with or without methylmalonic aciduria), AR, SUCLA2-related | MTDPS5 | *SUCLA2* | 13q14.2 | AR | ATP-specific succinyl-CoA ligase β subunit | 612073 |
| 42.15 | GTP-specific succinyl-CoA ligase α subunit deficiency | Mitochondrial DNA depletion syndrome 9 (encephalomyopathic type with methylmalonic aciduria) | MTDPS9 | *SUCLG1* | 2p11.2 | AR | GTP-specific succinyl-CoA ligase α subunit | 245400 |

| | | | | | | | | |
|---|---|---|---|---|---|---|---|---|
| 42.16 | Succinate dehydrogenase subunit A deficiency | Mitochondrial respiratory chain complex II deficiency | N/A | *SDHA* | 5p15.33 | AR | Succinate dehydrogenase subunit A | 252011 |
| 42.17 | Succinate dehydrogenase subunit A deficiency, tumoral phenotype | Paragangliomas 5 | PGL5 | *SDHA* | 5p15.33 | AD | Succinate dehydrogenase subunit A | 614165 |
| 42.18 | Succinate dehydrogenase subunit B deficiency | | N/A | *SDHB* | 1p36.13 | AR | Succinate dehydrogenase subunit B | Non |
| 42.19 | Succinate dehydrogenase subunit B deficiency, tumoral phenotype | Paragangliomas 4, and pheochromocytoma, familial extraadrenal, and pheochromocytoma, extraadrenal and cervical paraganglioma | PGL4 | *SDHB* | 1p36.13 | AD | Succinate dehydrogenase subunit B | 115310 |
| 42.20 | Succinate dehydrogenase subunit C deficiency, tumoral phenotype | Paragangliomas 3 and glomus tumors, familial | PGL3 | *SDHC* | 1q23.3 | AD | Succinate dehydrogenase subunit C | 605373 |
| 42.21 | Succinate dehydrogenase subunit D deficiency | Mitochondrial complex II deficiency | N/A | *SDHD* | 11q23.1 | AR | Succinate dehydrogenase subunit D | 252011 |
| 42.22 | Succinate dehydrogenase subunit D deficiency, tumoral phenotype | Paragangliomas 1 | PGL1 | *SDHD* | 11q23.1 | AD | Succinate dehydrogenase subunit D | 168000 |
| 42.23 | Fumarate hydratase deficiency | Fumarase deficiency or fumaric aciduria | FMRD | *FH* | 1q43 | AR | Fumarate hydratase | 606812 |
| 42.24 | Fumarate hydratase deficiency, tumoral phenotype | Hereditery Leiomyomatosis and renal cell cancer | HLRCC | *FH* | 1q43 | AD | Fumarate hydratase | 150800 |
| 42.25 | Mitochondrial malate dehydrogenase deficiency | Epileptic encephalopathy, early infantile, 51 | EIEE51 | *MDH2* | 7q11.23 | AR | Mitochondrial malate dehydrogenase | 617339 |
| 42.26 | Mitochondrial malate dehydrogenase deficiency, tumoral phenotype | | N/A | *MDH2* | 7q11.23 | AD | Mitochondrial malate dehydrogenase | Non |

## Metabolic Pathways

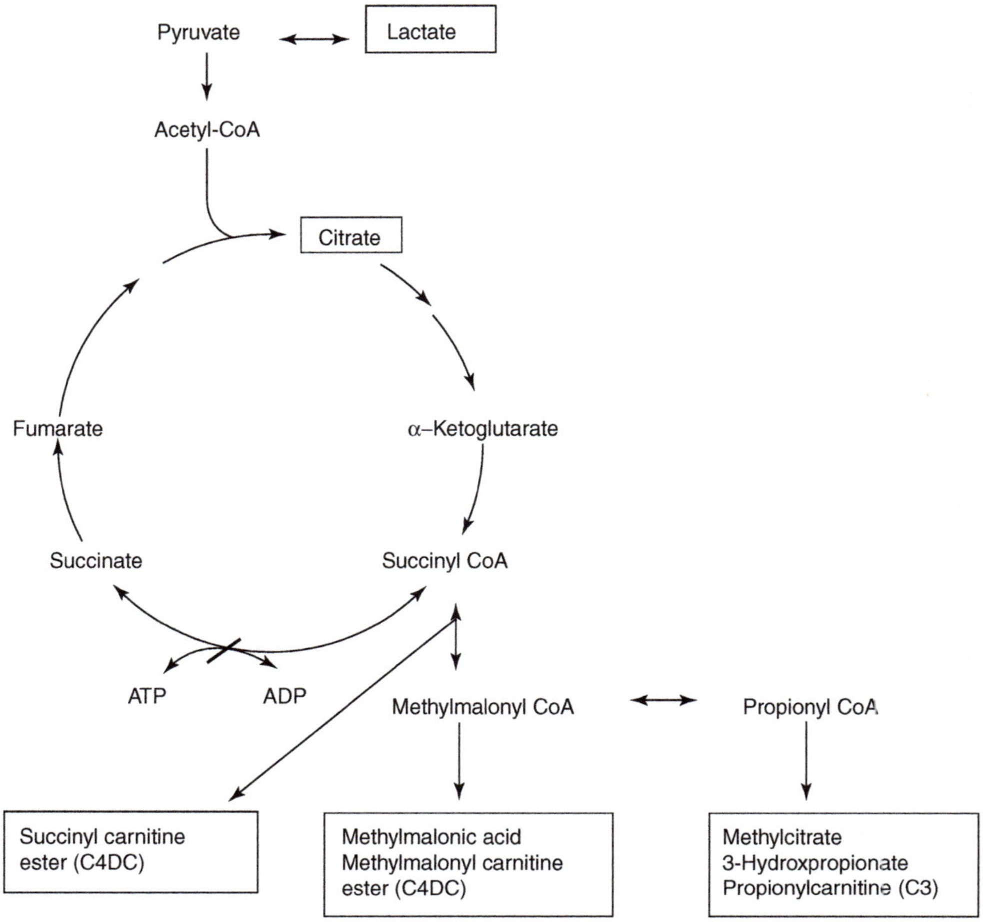


**Fig. 42.1** Relevant metabolic pathways illustrating the metabolic effects of succinyl-CoA synthetase deficiency

## Signs and Symptoms

**Table 42.1** Pyruvate carboxylase deficiency

| System | Symptoms and biomarkers | Neonatal (birth–1 month) | Infancy (1–18 months) | Childhood (1.5–11 years) | Adolescence (11–16 years) | Adulthood (>16 years) |
|---|---|---|---|---|---|---|
| CNS | Developmental delay | +++ | v+++ | +++ | | |
| | Hypokinesia | ++ | + | | | |
| | **Hypotonia** | +++ | +++ | +++ | | |
| | Parkinsonism, hypokinetic features | ++ | n | n | | |
| | Pyramidal signs | ++ | ++ | ++ | | |
| | **Seizures** | +++ | +++ | +++ | | |
| Digestive | **Vomiting** | +++ | +++ | ++ | | |
| Metabolic | Hypoglycemia | ± | ± | ± | ± | |
| Other | **Failure to thrive** | +++ | +++ | +++ | | |
| Laboratory findings | 3-OH-butyrate/acetoacetate ratio (plasma) | ↓ | | | | |
| | Alanine (plasma) | ↑ | ↑ | ↑ | | |
| | Ammonia (blood) | n-↑ | n-↑ | n-↑ | | |
| | Citrulline (plasma) | ↑ | ↑ | ↑ | | |
| | Glucose (plasma) | ↓-n | ↓-n | ↓-n | ↓-n | |
| | Ketones (plasma) | ↑ | ↑ | ↑ | | |
| | Ketones (urine) | ↑ | ↑ | ↑ | | |
| | Lactate (plasma) | ↑↑ | ↑ | ↑ | | |
| | Lactate/pyruvate ratio | ↑↑ | n | n | | |
| | Pyruvate (plasma) | ↑↑ | ↑ | ↑ | | |

**Table 42.2** Pyruvate dehydrogenase complex deficiency E1α

| System | Symptoms and biomarkers | Neonatal (birth–1 month) | Infancy (1–18 months) | Childhood (1.5–11 years) | Adolescence (11–16 years) | Adulthood (>16 years) |
|---|---|---|---|---|---|---|
| CNS | **Agenesis, corpus callosum (MRI)** | + | + | + | + | + |
| | Developmental delay | +++ | +++ | +++ | | |
| | Hypotonia | +++ | +++ | +++ | | |
| | Leigh syndrome | ± | ++ | ++ | ++ | ++ |
| | Neuropathy, peripheral | | + | ++ | ++ | ++ |
| | Pyramidal signs | ++ | ++ | ++ | | |
| | Seizures | +++ | +++ | +++ | | |
| Metabolic | **Lactic acidosis** | ++ | ++ | ++ | ++ | ++ |
| Musculoskeletal | **Dysmorphic features** | + | + | + | + | + |
| | **Microcephaly** | + | + | + | + | + |
| Other | **Failure to thrive** | +++ | +++ | +++ | | |
| Laboratory findings | Alanine (plasma) | ↑ | ↑ | ↑ | ↑ | ↑ |
| | Glucose (plasma) | n | n | n | n | n |
| | Ketones (plasma) | ↑ | ↑ | ↑ | ↑ | ↑ |
| | Ketones (urine) | ↑ | ↑ | ↑ | ↑ | ↑ |
| | Lactate (plasma) | ↑↑ | ↑↑ | ↑↑ | ↑↑ | ↑↑ |
| | Lactate/pyruvate ratio | n | n | n | n | n |
| | Pyruvate (plasma) | ↑↑ | ↑↑ | ↑↑ | ↑↑ | ↑↑ |

**Table 42.3** Pyruvate dehydrogenase complex deficiency E1β

| System | Symptoms and biomarkers | Neonatal (birth–1 month) | Infancy (1–18 months) | Childhood (1.5–11 years) | Adolescence (11–16 years) | Adulthood (>16 years) |
|---|---|---|---|---|---|---|
| CNS | Agenesis, corpus callosum (MRI) | + | + | (↑) | | |
| | **Developmental delay** | +++ | +++ | +++ | | |
| | Hypogenesis, corpus callosum | + | + | (↑) | | |
| | **Hypotonia** | +++ | +++ | +++ | | |
| | **Leigh syndrome** | ± | ++ | ++ | ++ | ++ |
| | Pyramidal signs | ++ | ++ | ++ | | |
| Metabolic | **Lactic acidosis** | ++ | ++ | ++ | ++ | ++ |
| Musculoskeletal | Microcephaly | + | + | + | + | + |
| Other | Failure to thrive | +++ | +++ | +++ | | |
| Laboratory findings | Alanine (plasma) | ↑ | ↑ | ↑ | ↑ | ↑ |
| | Glucose (plasma) | n | n | n | n | |
| | Ketones (plasma) | ↑ | ↑ | ↑ | | |
| | Ketones (urine) | ↑ | ↑ | ↑ | | |
| | Lactate (plasma) | ↑↑ | ↑↑ | ↑↑ | ↑↑ | ↑↑ |
| | Lactate/pyruvate ratio | n | n | n | n | n |
| | Pyruvate (plasma) | ↑↑ | ↑↑ | ↑↑ | ↑↑ | ↑↑ |

**Table 42.4** Dihydrolipoamide acetyltransferase deficiency

| System | Symptoms and biomarkers | Neonatal (birth–1 month) | Infancy (1–18 months) | Childhood (1.5–11 years) | Adolescence (11–16 years) | Adulthood (>16 years) |
|---|---|---|---|---|---|---|
| CNS | Developmental delay | +++ | +++ | +++ | | |
| | Dystonia | | +++ | +++ | +++ | |
| | **Hypotonia** | +++ | +++ | +++ | | |
| Metabolic | **Lactic acidosis** | ++ | ++ | ++ | ++ | ++ |
| Laboratory findings | Alanine (plasma) | ↑ | ↑ | ↑ | ↑ | ↑ |
| | Glucose (plasma) | n | n | n | n | |
| | Ketones (plasma) | ↑ | ↑ | ↑ | | |
| | Ketones (urine) | ↑ | ↑ | ↑ | | |
| | Lactate (plasma) | ↑↑ | ↑↑ | ↑↑ | ↑↑ | ↑↑ |
| | Lactate/pyruvate ratio | n | n | n | n | n |
| | Pyruvate (plasma) | ↑↑ | ↑↑ | ↑↑ | ↑↑ | ↑↑ |

**Table 42.5** Pyruvate dehydrogenase E3-binding protein deficiency

| System | Symptoms and biomarkers | Neonatal (birth–1 month) | Infancy (1–18 months) | Childhood (1.5–11 years) | Adolescence (11–16 years) | Adulthood (>16 years) |
|---|---|---|---|---|---|---|
| CNS | **Agenesis, corpus callosum (MRI)** | + | + | + | + | + |
| | Developmental delay | +++ | +++ | +++ | | |
| | Hypotonia | +++ | +++ | +++ | | |
| | Seizures | | + | + | | |
| Metabolic | **Lactic acidosis** | ++ | ++ | ++ | ++ | ++ |
| Musculoskeletal | **Microcephaly** | + | + | + | + | + |
| Other | **Failure to thrive** | +++ | +++ | +++ | | |
| Laboratory findings | Alanine (plasma) | ↑ | ↑ | ↑ | ↑ | ↑ |
| | Glucose (plasma) | n | n | n | n | n |
| | Ketones (plasma) | ↑ | ↑ | ↑ | ↑ | ↑ |
| | Ketones (urine) | ↑ | ↑ | ↑ | ↑ | ↑ |
| | Lactate (plasma) | ↑↑ | ↑↑ | ↑↑ | ↑↑ | ↑↑ |
| | Lactate/pyruvate ratio | n | n | n | n | n |
| | Pyruvate (plasma) | ↑↑ | ↑↑ | ↑↑ | ↑↑ | ↑↑ |

**Table 42.6** Pyruvate dehydrogenase phosphatase deficiency

| System | Symptoms and biomarkers | Neonatal (birth–1 month) | Infancy (1–18 months) | Childhood (1.5–11 years) | Adolescence (11–16 years) | Adulthood (>16 years) |
|---|---|---|---|---|---|---|
| CNS | Developmental delay | +++ | +++ | +++ | +++ | |
| | Hypotonia | +++ | +++ | +++ | | |
| | **Seizures** | +++ | +++ | +++ | | |
| Metabolic | **Lactic acidosis** | ++ | ++ | ++ | ++ | ++ |
| Other | **Failure to thrive** | +++ | +++ | +++ | | |
| Laboratory findings | Alanine (plasma) | ↑ | ↑ | ↑ | ↑ | ↑ |
| | Glucose (plasma) | n | n | n | n | n |
| | Ketones (plasma) | ↑ | ↑ | ↑ | ↑ | ↑ |
| | Ketones (urine) | ↑ | ↑ | ↑ | ↑ | ↑ |
| | Lactate (plasma) | ↑↑ | ↑↑ | ↑↑ | ↑↑ | ↑↑ |
| | Lactate/pyruvate ratio | n | n | n | n | n |
| | Pyruvate (plasma) | ↑↑ | ↑↑ | ↑↑ | ↑↑ | ↑↑ |

**Table 42.7** Mitochondrial pyruvate carrier deficiency

| System | Symptoms and biomarkers | Neonatal (birth–1 month) | Infancy (1–18 months) | Childhood (1.5–11 years) | Adolescence (11–16 years) | Adulthood (>16 years) |
|---|---|---|---|---|---|---|
| CNS | **Hypotonia** | + | + | + | | |
| | Neuropathy, peripheral | | + | + | | |
| | Retardation, psychomotor | | + | + | | |
| | Seizures | | ± | ± | | |
| Digestive | Hepatomegaly | | + | + | | |
| Eye | Nystagmus | | ± | | | |
| Metabolic | **Hypoglycemia** | + | + | + | | |
| | **Lactic acidosis** | + | + | + | | |
| Musculoskeletal | Growth retardation | | + | + | | |
| | Microcephaly | ± | | | | |
| | Tin upper lips | | ± | | | |
| Other | Epicanthal folds | | ± | | | |
| Respiratory | Respiratory distress | | ± | | | |
| Laboratory findings | 3-Hydroxybutyric acid (U) | ↑ | | | | |
| | 4-Hydroxyphenyllactate (U) | ↑ | | | | |
| | 4-Hydroxyphenylpyruvate (U) | ↑ | | | | |
| | Alpha-ketoglutarate (U) | ↑ | | | | |
| | Glucose (P) | ↓ | | | | |
| | Lactate/Pyruvate (ratio) | | n | n | | |
| | Pyruvate (P) | ↑ | | | | |

**Table 42.8** Pyruvate dehydrogenase kinase isoenzyme 3 superactivity

| System | Symptoms and biomarkers | Neonatal (birth–1 month) | Infancy (1–18 months) | Childhood (1.5–11 years) | Adolescence (11–16 years) | Adulthood (>16 years) |
|---|---|---|---|---|---|---|
| CNS | **Auditory brainstem potential, abnormal** | | | | | + |
| | **Axonal sensorimotor polyneuropathy** | | | | ± | + |
| | Hand tremor (females) | | | | | + |
| Ear | Hearing loss, sensorineural | | | | **n** | **n** |
| Musculoskeletal | **Muscle weakness, distal** | | | | ± | + |
| | **Pes Cavus** | | | | ± | + |

**Table 42.9** Dihydrolipoamide dehydrogenase deficiency

| System | Symptoms and biomarkers | Neonatal (birth–1 month) | Infancy (1–18 months) | Childhood (1.5–11 years) | Adolescence (11–16 years) | Adulthood (>16 years) |
|---|---|---|---|---|---|---|
| CNS | Agenesis, corpus callosum (MRI) | + | + | + | | |
| | Developmental delay | ++ | ++ | ++ | | |
| | Hypogenesis, corpus callosum | + | + | + | | |
| | **Hypotonia, progressive generalized** | ++ | ++ | ++ | | |
| | Leigh syndrome | ± | ++ | ++ | | |
| | Spasticity | ± | ++ | ++ | | |
| Digestive | **Liver failure, acute recurrent** | + | + | + | + | + |
| Musculoskeletal | **Microcephaly** | + | ++ | ++ | | |
| | Myoglobinuria | | | | ↑ | ↑ |
| | **Myopathy** | **n** | **n** | **n** | ↑ | ↑ |
| Laboratory findings | 2-Oxoadipate (urine) | ↑ | ↑ | ↑ | ↑ | ↑ |
| | 2-Oxoglutaric acid (urine) | ↑ | ↑ | ↑ | ↑ | ↑ |
| | Isoleucine (plasma) | ↑ | ↑ | ↑ | ↑ | ↑ |
| | Lactate (urine) | ↑ | ↑ | ↑ | ↑ | ↑ |
| | Lactate/pyruvate ratio | n | n | n | n | n |
| | Leucine (plasma) | ↑ | ↑ | ↑ | ↑ | ↑ |
| | Valine (plasma) | ↑ | ↑ | ↑ | ↑ | ↑ |

**Table 42.10** Mitochondrial aconitase deficiency

| System | Symptoms and biomarkers | Neonatal (birth–1 month) | Infancy (1–18 months) | Childhood (1.5–11 years) | Adolescence (11–16 years) | Adulthood (>16 years) |
|---|---|---|---|---|---|---|
| CNS | Areflexia | | | | | |
| | **Ataxia** | | + | | | |
| | **Athetosis** | | + | | | |
| | **Cerebellar atrophy** | ± | + | + | | |
| | **Cerebral atrophy** | ± | + | | | |
| | **Delayed psychomotor development, severe** | | + | + | | |
| | **Hyporeflexia** | | | | | |
| | **Hypotonia** | ± | + | | | |
| | **Intellectual disability, severe to profound** | | + | + | | |
| | **Peripheral demyelinating neuropathy** | | ± | | | |
| | **Seizures** | | + | | | |
| | White matter disease | | ± | | | |
| Ear | Hearing loss, sensorineural | | ± | | | |
| Eye | **Nystagmus** | ± | + | + | | |
| | Optic atrophy | | ± | + | | |
| | **Retinal dystrophy** | ± | + | | | |
| | **Strabismus** | ± | + | | | |
| Metabolic | Metabolic acidosis | | ± | | | |
| Musculoskeletal | **Microcephaly** | | ± | + | | |
| Other | **Failure to thrive** | | ± | + | | |
| Laboratory findings | Glucose (plasma) | | ↑ | | | |
| | Glutamate oxidation | | ↓ | | | |
| | Lactate (plasma) | | ± | | | |

**Table 42.11** Mitochondrial NADP+-dependent isocitrate dehydrogenase 2 superactivity

| System | Symptoms and biomarkers | Neonatal (birth–1 month) | Infancy (1–18 months) | Childhood (1.5–11 years) | Adolescence (11–16 years) | Adulthood (>16 years) |
|---|---|---|---|---|---|---|
| Cardiovascular | **Cardiomyopathy** | ± | ± | ± | ± | ± |
| CNS | **Developmental delay** | + | + | + | + | + |
| | Epilepsy | ± | ± | ± | ± | ± |
| | **Hypotonia** | + | + | + | + | + |
| Laboratory findings | D-2-Hydroxyglutaric acid (CSF) | ↑ | ↑ | ↑ | ↑ | ↑ |
| | D-2-Hydroxyglutaric acid (P) | ↑ | ↑ | ↑ | ↑ | ↑ |
| | D-2-Hydroxyglutaric acid (U) | ↑ | ↑ | ↑ | ↑ | ↑ |

**Table 42.12** Mitochondrial NADPH-dependent isocitrate dehydrogenase 3 β subunit deficiency

| System | Symptoms and biomarkers | Neonatal (birth–1 month) | Infancy (1–18 months) | Childhood (1.5–11 years) | Adolescence (11–16 years) | Adulthood (>16 years) |
|---|---|---|---|---|---|---|
| Eye | **Retinitis pigmentosa** | | | | | + |

**Table 42.13** α-Ketoglutarate dehydrogenase deficiency

| System | Symptoms and biomarkers | Neonatal (birth-1 month) | Infancy (1–18 months) | Childhood (1.5–11 years) | Adolescence (11–16 years) | Adulthood (>16 years) |
|---|---|---|---|---|---|---|
| CNS | Ataxia | | ± | ± | ± | ± |
| | Dystonia | | ± | ± | ± | ± |
| | **Global developmental delay** | ± | + | + | + | + |
| | **Hypotonia** | ± | + | + | + | + |
| | Seizures | | | | | ± |
| Laboratory findings | Alpha-ketoglutarate (urine) | n-↑ | n-↑ | n-↑ | n-↑ | |
| | Lactate (plasma) | ↑ | ↑ | ↑ | ↑ | |

**Table 42.14** ATP-specific succinyl-CoA ligase β subunit deficiency

| System | Symptoms and biomarkers | Neonatal (birth–1 month) | Infancy (1–18 months) | Childhood (1.5–11 years) | Adolescence (11–16 years) | Adulthood (>16 years) |
|---|---|---|---|---|---|---|
| CNS | **Axial hypotonia** | + | ++ | ++ | + | + |
| | Choreoathetosis | ± | ± | ± | ± | ± |
| | Dystonia | – | ± | + | ++ | ++ |
| | Leigh syndrome | – | ± | + | ++ | ++ |
| | **Neurological symptoms** | ++ | ++ | ++ | ++ | ++ |
| | Neuropathy, peripheral | – | – | ± | ± | ± |
| | Pyramidal signs | – | ± | + | ++ | ++ |
| | **Retardation, psychomotor** | ± | ++ | ++ | ++ | ++ |
| Digestive | Feeding difficulties | ± | ± | ± | + | + |
| Ear | Deafness, sensorineural | ± | ++ | ++ | ++ | ++ |
| Metabolic | Lactic acidosis | + | + | + | + | + |
| Other | Failure to thrive | + | + | + | + | + |
| Laboratory findings | ASAT/ALAT (plasma) | n-↑ | n-↑ | n-↑ | n-↑ | n-↑ |
| | C4-DC Methylmalonylcarnitine (urine) | ↑ | ↑ | ↑ | ↑ | ↑ |
| | C4-DC Succinylcarnitine (urine) | ↑ | ↑ | ↑ | ↑ | ↑ |
| | Lactate (plasma) | ↑ | ↑ | ↑ | ↑ | ↑ |
| | Lactate/pyruvate ratio | ↑ | ↑ | ↑ | ↑ | ↑ |
| | Methylmalonic acid (urine) | ↑ | ↑ | ↑ | ↑ | ↑ |
| | mtDNA levels | ↓ | ↓ | ↓ | | |
| | Respiratory chain enzyme deficiencies (muscle) | | ↓ | ↓ | | |

**Table 42.15** GTP-specific succinyl-CoA ligase α subunit deficiency

| System | Symptoms and biomarkers | Neonatal (birth–1 month) | Infancy (1–18 months) | Childhood (1.5–11 years) | Adolescence (11–16 years) | Adulthood (>16 years) |
|---|---|---|---|---|---|---|
| Cardiovascular | Congenital heart defects | ± | ± | ± | ± | ± |
| CNS | Ataxia | | ± | ± | ± | |
| | Axial hypotonia | + | ++ | ++ | + | + |
| | Choreoathetosis | ± | ± | ± | ± | ± |
| | Dystonia | | ± | + | ++ | ++ |
| | **Encephalopathy, necrotizing** | | ++ | ++ | | |
| | **Hypotonia** | | ++ | ++ | ++ | |
| | Leigh syndrome | | ± | + | ++ | ++ |
| | Neurological symptoms | ++ | ++ | ++ | ++ | ++ |
| | Neuropathy, peripheral | | | ± | ± | ± |
| | Pyramidal signs | | ± | + | ++ | ++ |
| | Retardation, psychomotor | ± | ++ | ++ | ++ | ++ |
| | Seizures | | ± | ± | ± | |
| Digestive | **Feeding difficulties** | ++ | ++ | ++ | ++ | ++ |
| | Liver dysfunction | ± | ± | ± | + | + |
| Ear | Deafness, sensorineural | ± | ± | ± | ± | ± |
| Metabolic | **Lactic acidosis** | + | + | + | + | + |
| Other | Death | | + | + | + | |
| | Failure to thrive | ++ | ++ | ++ | ++ | ++ |
| Laboratory findings | ASAT/ALAT (plasma) | n-↑ | n-↑ | n-↑ | n-↑ | n-↑ |
| | C4-DC Methylmalonylcarnitine (urine) | ↑ | ↑ | ↑ | ↑ | ↑ |
| | C4-DC Succinylcarnitine (urine) | ↑ | ↑ | ↑ | ↑ | ↑ |
| | Lactate (plasma) | ↑ | ↑ | ↑ | ↑ | ↑ |
| | Lactate/pyruvate ratio | ↑ | ↑ | ↑ | ↑ | ↑ |
| | Methylmalonic acid (urine) | ↑ | ↑ | ↑ | ↑ | ↑ |
| | mtDNA levels | ↓ | ↓ | ↓ | | |
| | Respiratory chain enzymes (muscle) | ↓ | ↓ | ↓ | | |

**Table 42.16** Succinate dehydrogenase subunit A deficiency

| System | Symptoms and biomarkers | Neonatal (birth–1 month) | Infancy (1–18 months) | Childhood (1.5–11 years) | Adolescence (11–16 years) | Adulthood (>16 years) |
|---|---|---|---|---|---|---|
| Cardiovascular | **Cardiomyopathy, hypertrophic** | | + | + | + | + |
| CNS | **Encephalopathy** | | + | + | + | + |
| | **Dementia** | | | + | + | + |
| | Kearns-Sayre Syndrome | | | | | + |
| | Leigh syndrome | | + | + | | |
| Musculoskeletal | **Myopathy** | | + | + | + | + |
| | **Short stature** | | + | + | + | + |
| Laboratory findings | Complex II activity | ↓ | ↓ | ↓ | ↓ | ↓ |
| | Lactate (plasma) | ↑ | ↑ | ↑ | ↑ | ↑ |

**Table 42.17** Succinate dehydrogenase subunit A deficiency, tumoral phenotype

| System | Symptoms and biomarkers | Neonatal (birth–1 month) | Infancy (1–18 months) | Childhood (1.5–11 years) | Adolescence (11–16 years) | Adulthood (>16 years) |
|---|---|---|---|---|---|---|
| Autonomic system | **Hypertension** | | | | | + |
| Endocrine | **Hyperadrenergic** | | | | | + |
| Other | **Paraganglioma** | | | | | + |
| Laboratory findings | Norepinephrine (U) | | | | | ↑ |
| | Normetanephrine (U) | | | | | ↑ |

**Table 42.18** Succinate dehydrogenase subunit B deficiency

| System | Symptoms and biomarkers | Neonatal (birth–1 month) | Infancy (1–18 months) | Childhood (1.5–11 years) | Adolescence (11–16 years) | Adulthood (>16 years) |
|---|---|---|---|---|---|---|
| CNS | Ataxia | | ± | ± | ± | ± |
| | **Developmental regression** | | + | + | + | + |
| | Hypotonia | | + | + | + | + |
| | Irritability | | ± | ± | ± | ± |
| | **Leukodystrophy** | | + | + | + | + |
| | **Leukoencephalopathy** | | + | + | + | + |
| | Spasticity | | ± | ± | ± | ± |
| Eye | Optic atrophy | | ± | ± | ± | ± |
| Laboratory findings | 2-Ketoglutarate (U) | | ↑ | ↑ | ↑ | ↑ |
| | Lactate (P) | | ↑ | ↑ | ↑ | ↑ |

**Table 42.19** Succinate dehydrogenase subunit B deficiency, tumoral phenotype

| System | Symptoms and biomarkers | Neonatal (birth–1 month) | Infancy (1–18 months) | Childhood (1.5–11 years) | Adolescence (11–16 years) | Adulthood (>16 years) |
|---|---|---|---|---|---|---|
| Other | Paraganglioma | | | | | ± |
| | Pheochromocytoma | | | | | ± |
| Digestive | Gastrointestinal stromal tumor | | | | | ± |
| Renal | Renal cancer | | | | + | + |

**Table 42.20** Succinate dehydrogenase subunit C deficiency, tumoral phenotype

| System | Symptoms and biomarkers | Neonatal (birth–1 month) | Infancy (1–18 months) | Childhood (1.5–11 years) | Adolescence (11–16 years) | Adulthood (>16 years) |
|---|---|---|---|---|---|---|
| Other | Carotid body tumors | | | | | ± |
| | Chemodectomas | | | | | ± |
| | Glomus jugular tumors | | | | | ± |
| | **Paraganglioma** | | | | | + |
| | **Pheochromocytoma** | | | | | + |
| Laboratory findings | Catecholamine (urine) | | | | | ± |

**Table 42.21** Succinate dehydrogenase subunit D deficiency

| System | Symptoms and biomarkers | Neonatal (birth–1 month) | Infancy (1–18 months) | Childhood (1.5–11 years) | Adolescence (11–16 years) | Adulthood (>16 years) |
|---|---|---|---|---|---|---|
| Cardiovascular | Dilated cardiomyopathy | | | | | ± |
| | **Hypertrophic cardiomyopathy** | | | | | ± |
| | Left ventricular noncompaction | | | | | ± |
| CNS | Ataxia | | | ± | ± | ± |
| | **Cognitive impairment** | ± | ± | + | ± | ± |
| | Dystonia | ± | ± | ± | ± | ± |
| | Hyperreflexia | | | + | + | + |
| | **Hypotonia** | ± | ± | + | | |
| | Kearns-Sayre syndrome | | | ± | ± | ± |
| | Leigh syndrome | ± | ± | ± | ± | ± |
| | Leukoencephalopathy, progressive | ± | ± | ± | ± | ± |
| | Myoclonus | ± | ± | ± | ± | ± |
| | Psychomotor regression | | + | + | + | + |
| | **Seizures** | ± | ± | ± | ± | ± |
| | Spasticity | | | + | + | + |
| | Spongiform encephalomyelopathy | ± | ± | ± | ± | ± |
| Eye | **Impaired vision** | ± | ± | ± | ± | ± |
| | Nystagmus | ± | ± | ± | ± | ± |
| | Ophthalmoplegia | | | | | ± |
| | Optic atrophy | ± | ± | ± | ± | ± |
| | Pigmentary retinopathy | ± | ± | + | ? | ± |
| | **Ptosis** | | | ± | ± | ± |
| Metabolic | Metabolic acidosis | ± | ± | ± | ± | ± |
| Musculoskeletal | Exercise intolerance | | | + | + | + |
| | Joint contractures | ± | ± | ± | ± | ± |
| | **Muscle weakness** | | | + | + | + |
| | **Short stature** | ± | ± | + | + | + |
| Other | Abnormal mitochondria with paracrystalline inclusions (muscle biopsy) | ± | ± | ± | ± | ± |
| | **Accumulated lipid droplets (muscle biopsy)** | ± | ± | ± | ± | ± |
| | **Failure to thrive** | ± | ± | + | + | + |
| | Ragged red fibers seen on muscle biopsy | ± | ± | ± | ± | ± |
| Laboratory findings | Lactate (serum) | n-↑ | n-↑ | n-↑ | n-↑ | n-↑ |
| | Succinate dehydrogenase (plasma) | ↓↓ | ↓↓ | ↓↓ | ↓↓ | ↓↓ |

**Table 42.22** Succinate dehydrogenase subunit D deficiency, tumoral phenotype

| System | Symptoms and biomarkers | Neonatal (birth–1 month) | Infancy (1–18 months) | Childhood (1.5–11 years) | Adolescence (11–16 years) | Adulthood (>16 years) |
|---|---|---|---|---|---|---|
| Other | **Paraganglioma** | | | | | + |
| | **Pheochromocytoma** | | | | | + |
| Laboratory findings | Norepinephrine (U) | | | | | ↑ |
| | Normetanephrine (U) | | | | | ↑ |

**Table 42.23** Fumarate hydratase deficiency

| System | Symptoms and biomarkers | Neonatal (birth–1 month) | Infancy (1–18 months) | Childhood (1.5–11 years) | Adolescence (11–16 years) | Adulthood (>16 years) |
|---|---|---|---|---|---|---|
| CNS | Altered consciousness | ++ | ++ | ++ | | |
| | Athetosis | ++ | ++ | ++ | | |
| | Autism | | ± | ± | | |
| | **Cerebral palsy** | + | ++ | +++ | | |
| | Dystonia | ± | ± | ± | | |
| | EEG, abnormal | ± | ± | ± | | |
| | **Hypotonia** | +++ | ++ | + | | |
| | **Irritability** | +++ | +++ | +++ | | |
| | **Neurological symptoms** | +++ | +++ | +++ | | |
| | Pyramidal signs | + | ++ | ++ | | |
| | Regression, motor | ± | ++ | ++ | | |
| | **Retardation, psychomotor** | +++ | +++ | +++ | | |
| | Seizures | ++ | ++ | ++ | | |
| | Speech delay | | +++ | +++ | | |
| Digestive | **Feeding difficulties** | +++ | +++ | +++ | | |
| | **Gastroesophageal reflux** | ++ | ++ | | | |
| | Hepatosplenomegaly | ± | ± | ± | | |
| | **Malnutrition, chronic** | ++ | ++ | ++ | | |
| Eye | Optic atrophy | ± | ± | ± | | |
| | Vision, impaired | ± | ± | ± | | |
| Hematological | Neutropenia | ± | ± | ± | | |
| Metabolic | Lactic acidosis | ± | ± | ± | | |
| | **Metabolic acidosis** | + | + | + | | |
| Musculoskeletal | Coarse facial features | ± | ± | ± | | |
| | Dysmorphic features | ± | ± | ± | | |
| | Hypertelorism | ± | ± | ± | | |
| | Microcephaly | ± | ± | ± | | |
| Other | **Course, episodic** | + | + | + | | |
| | **Failure to thrive** | ++ | ++ | + | | |
| | Fetal hydrops | ± | | | | |
| | **Sudden death** | ++ | ++ | + | | |
| Laboratory findings | 2-Oxoglutaric acid (urine) | n-↑ | n-↑ | n-↑ | | |
| | ASAT/ALAT (plasma) | n-↑ | n-↑ | n-↑ | | |
| | Bilirubin (plasma) | n-↑ | n-↑ | | | |
| | Fumaric acid (urine) | ↑↑ | ↑↑ | ↑↑ | | |
| | Lactate (cerebrospinal fluid) | n-↑ | n-↑ | n-↑ | | |
| | Lactate (plasma) | ↑ | ↑ | ↑ | | |
| | Succinic acid (urine) | n-↑ | n-↑ | n-↑ | | |

**Table 42.24** Fumarate hydratase deficiency, tumoral phenotype

| System | Symptom name | Neonatal (birth–1 month) | Infancy (1–18 months) | Childhood (1.5–11 years) | Adolescence (11–16 years) | Adulthood (>16 years) |
|---|---|---|---|---|---|---|
| Other | Cutaneous leiomyomata | | | ± | + | + |
| | Uterine leiomyomata/fibroids | | | | | + |
| | Renal cell carcinoma | | | | | + |
| | Pheochromocytoma | | | | | + |

**Table 42.25** Mitochondrial malate dehydrogenase deficiency

| System | Symptoms and biomarkers | Neonatal (birth–1 month) | Infancy (1–18 months) | Childhood (1.5–11 years) | Adolescence (11–16 years) | Adulthood (>16 years) |
|---|---|---|---|---|---|---|
| CNS | **Dystonia** | ± | ± | | | |
| | **Encephalopathy** | ± | + | | | |
| | **Hyperreflexia** | | + | | | |
| | **Hypotonia** | + | + | | | |
| | **Myoclonus** | ± | + | | | |
| | **Seizures** | + | + | | | |
| Digestive | **Constipation** | ± | ± | | | |
| | **Feeding difficulties** | + | + | | | |
| Eye | **Pigmentary retinopathy** | ± | ± | | | |
| | **Strabismus** | + | + | | | |
| Musculoskeletal | **Absent speech** | ± | ± | | | |
| | Cerebellar atrophy | ± | ± | | | |
| | Corpus callosum hypoplasia | ± | ± | | | |
| | Delayed myelinisation | ± | ± | | | |
| | **Muscle weakness** | + | + | | | |
| | **Psychomotor delay** | | + | | | |
| | **Spasticity** | | + | | | |
| | Supernumery nipples | ± | ± | | | |
| Other | **Failure to thrive** | ± | + | | | |
| Laboratory findings | Fumarate (urine) | ± | ± | | | |
| | Lactate (blood) | ↑↑ | ↑↑ | | | |
| | Lactate (CSF) | ↑↑ | ↑↑ | | | |
| | Malate (urine) | ± | ± | | | |
| | OXPHOS enzyme activity (muscle, liver) | ↓↓ | ↓↓ | | | |

**Table 42.26** Mitochondrial malate dehydrogenase deficiency, tumoral phenotype

| System | Symptoms and biomarkers | Neonatal (birth–1 month) | Infancy (1–18 months) | Childhood (1.5–11 years) | Adolescence (11–16 years) | Adulthood (>16 years) |
|---|---|---|---|---|---|---|
| Other | **Paraganglioma** | | | | | ± |

## Reference Values

| Metabolite | Normal range | Sample |
|---|---|---|
| Fumaric acid (FA) | 0–20 µmol/mmol creat | Urine |
| Succinic acid (SA) | 0–50 µmol/mmol creat | Urine |
| 2-Oxoglutaric acid (2OGA) | 0–50 µmol/mmol creat | Urine |
| Methylmalonic acid (MMA) | 0–5.0 µmol/mmol creat | Urine |
| Lactic acid (LA) | 0.5–2.1 mmol/L | Blood |
| Lactic acid (LA) | 0.4–1.4 mmol/L | CSF |
| Glucose | 3.4–6.4 mmol/L | Blood |

## Pathological Values

| | Differential diagnosis in PDHc deficiency |
|---|---|
| PC type A | Normal lactate/pyruvate ratio. Lactate 2–10 mmol/L; increased alanine and proline; normal citrulline and lysine. Hypoglycemia; ketosis |
| PC type B | Increased lactate/pyruvate ratio; increased acetoacetate to 3-OH-butyrate ratio; elevated concentrations of citrulline (100–400 µM, normal <40), lysine, and ammonia (100–600 µM, normal <60); low concentration of glutamine; lactate >10 mmol/L; pyruvate in type B 0.14–0.90 mmol/L; normal range 0.04–0.13, resulting in increased lactate/pyruvate ratio >20, hypoglycemia and ketosis |
| PC type C | Episodic metabolic acidosis with normal citrulline plasma concentrations and elevated lysine and proline plasma concentration. Lactate 2–5 mmol/L, lactate/pyruvate ratio normal, ketosis during metabolic stress |
| PDHC CSF | Elevated lactate and pyruvate. Marked reduced glutamine. Elevated glutamic acid and proline |
| PDHC urine | Organic acid profile shows, besides large amounts of lactate, pyruvate, and 3-OH-butyrate, an increase of 2-oxoglutarate |

| Disorder | Definition | Sample |
|---|---|---|
| 20.1 2-Oxoglutaric aciduria | 2OGA 5–1700 µmol/mmol creat | Urine |
| | LA 2.5–8.0 mmol/L | Blood |
| 20.2 Fumarase deficiency | FA 20–3828 µmol/mmol creat | Urine |
| | SA 50–800 µmol/mmol creat | Urine |
| | 2OGA 5–800 µmol/mmol creat | Urine |
| | LA 2.1–3.0 mmol/L | Blood |
| 20.3 SUCLA2 deficiency | MMA 16–80 µmol/mmol creat | Urine |
| 20.3 SUCLG1 deficiency | MMA 24–2400 µmol/mmol creat | Urine |

## Diagnostic Flowchart (see Fig. 42.2)

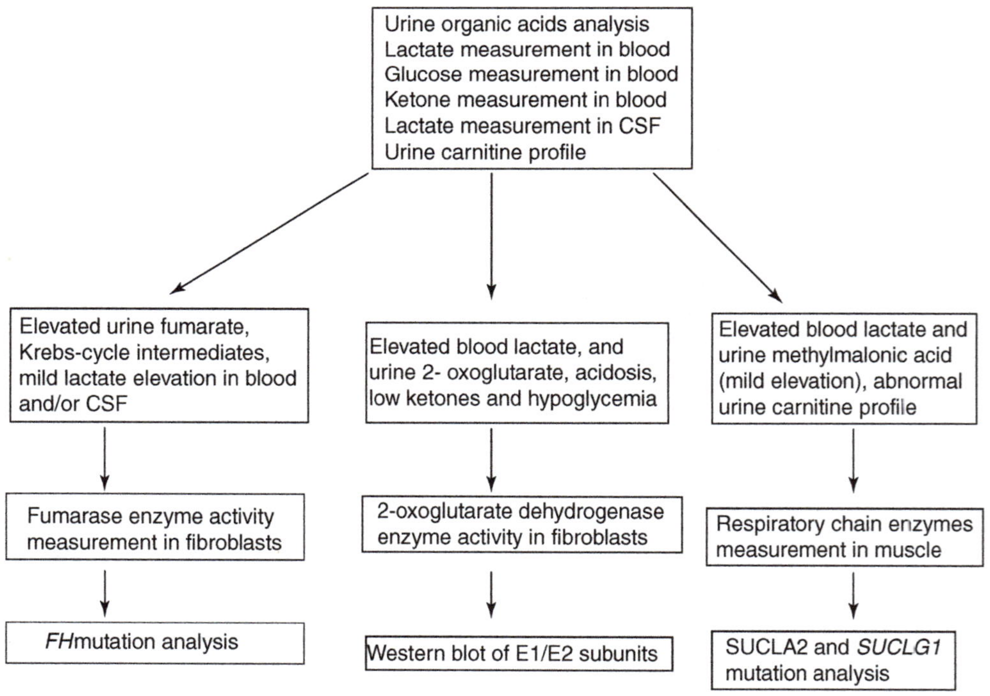


**Fig. 42.2** Diagnostic flowchart. *Note*: direct sequencing can be performed without functional studies based on the clinical/metabolic phenotype

## Specimen Collection and Pitfalls

The diagnosis of PC and PDHc deficiency is based on the collection of metabolic data during acute presentation including blood lactate, pyruvate, ketones and glucose, organic acids and amino acids in urine, and.

CSF measurements for lactate and pyruvate (see also Tables 42.5 and 42.6). While the diagnosis is highly challenging for PC deficiency, because of the variable clinical and metabolic phenotype, PDHc deficiency is mostly recognizable based on the normal lactate/pyruvate ratio and cerebral lactic academia. The confirmation of the diagnosis is typically possible in cultured fibroblasts or liver. PC enzyme assay in fibroblast shows a PC enzyme activity <5% of controls in type B and 5–23% in type A and <10% in type C; similar in lymphocytes. Assays can also be performed in postmortem liver, in which the activity of PC is tenfold higher than in fibroblasts but must be interpreted with caution because of rapid postmortem degradation of the enzyme. DNA testing is less invasive.

Total PDH activity, subunits, and DCA activation can be measured using spectrophotometric methods on cultured fibroblasts, lymphocytes, and muscle. Western blot for E3BP DNA testing is possible; most frequently PDH E1alpha on X chromosome (Willemsen et al. 2006).

Lipoic acid (LA) is an essential cofactor required for the activity of both pyruvate dehydrogenase (PDH), and 2-oxoglutarate dehydrogenase. LA is synthesized in a complex multistep process. Disease-causing mutations in genes encoding for proteins involved in LA metabolism have been reported in *NFU1*, *BOLA3*, *IBA57*, *LIAS*, *GLRX5*, *LIPT1*, *ISCA2*, and *LIPT2* (Tort et al. 2016).

The diagnosis of 2-oxoglutaric aciduria and fumarase deficiency is established by combining the clinical features, the metabolic findings, and the biochemical enzyme activity and should be validated by molecular genetic testing.

### Metabolic Findings in Urine

The massive excretion of 2-oxoglutaric acid and fumaric acid in urine is, respectively, diagnostic in almost all patients. The excretion of 2-oxoglutaric or fumaric acid in the two different disorders is, respectively, 15- to 1000-fold elevated when compared to the normal control range.

DOORS syndrome is a severe form of 2-oxoglutaric aciduria. In case of mild increase of 2-oxoglutaric acid one should consider genetic heterogeneity in DOORS. *TBC1D24 and SMARCB1* mutations might lead to the same phenotype with normal 2-oxoglutarate excretion (Campeau et al. 2014). *PIGB* mutations cause a GPI biosynthesis defect with axonal neuropathy, DOORS syndrome, and 2-oxoglutaric aciduria (Murakami et al. 2019).

2-Oxoglutaric acid might be elevated in fumarase deficiency, but less pronounced. Unfortunately, fumarate is not at all times present in excessive amounts in the urine in children with fumarase deficiency, and the concentration is not always corresponding with the measured residual fumarase activity (Ottolenghi et al. 2011). High residual activity has been found in some of the patients with 2-oxoglutaric aciduria as well. The presence of Krebs cycle intermediates in fumarase deficiency is probably due to secondary enzymatic inhibition of succinate dehydrogenase (SDH). Other metabolites have been detected as well in the urine, without a consistent pattern.

2-Oxoglutaric acid excretion is also elevated in mitochondrial ribosomal protein MRPS2 deficiency. This shows an overlapping phenotype with motor developmental delay hearing loss, hypoglycemia, and OXPHOS complex deficiencies (Gardeitchik et al. 2018).

Mild methylmalonic aciduria, Leigh-like encephalomyopathy, dystonia, and deafness characterize the group of patients with *SUCLA2* gene mutations, in whom the key diagnostic features are represented by mild methylmalonic acid excretion combined with an abnormal profile of carnitine esters (specifically succinyl carnitine). Most of the patients present with early onset hypotonia, severe developmental delay or early neurological deterioration, slowly progressive dystonic/athetoid movements, and sensorineural deafness. In the course of the first year of life, no abnormalities or mild cerebral atrophy with enlarged subarachnoid spaces and widening of the ventricular system is observed. Later on basal ganglia involvement becomes obvious. At first putamen and caudate seem to be specifically affected, but after infancy also the other parts of the basal ganglia show abnormalities on the MRI. Unlike classical methylmalonic acid (MMA) (Trinh et al. 2001), the globus pallidus can be spared or seems to be the least affected. In the end stage of the disease, as observed postmortem in one case, only a very small residual volume of the nucleus caudatus remained intact. The increase of methylmalonic acid in body fluids is considerably less pronounced in these patients compared to classical MMA patients (Deodato et al. 2006). Abnormal activity of respiratory chain enzymes and mtDNA depletion, together with methylmalonic aciduria, are the biochemical hallmarks of this disorder.

In addition, in a subgroup of patients, all presenting with mild methylmalonic aciduria, Leigh-like encephalomyopathy, and dystonia, clinical features closely resembling those seen in patients with *SUCLA2* mutations (Carrozzo et al. 2007; Morava et al. 2009), but without sensorineural deafness in the vast majority of the cases, mutations in *SUCLG1* were discovered.

### Metabolic Findings in Plasma and Cerebral Spinal Fluid

Increased plasma concentrations of 2-oxogutarate and significant elevation of lactate with increased L/P ratio and hypoketosis have been detected in 2-oxoglutaric aciduria. Increased plasma concentrations of fumarate, lactate, and pyruvic acid have been detected in fumarase deficiency. These metabolites are also abnormally elevated in the cerebrospinal fluid (CSF), especially lactic acid. In one patient with fumarase deficiency, additionally, two succinylpurine derivatives were found in CSF. These two metabolites, 5-aminoimidazole-*N*-succinyl-carboxamide ribotide (SAICAR) and adenylosuccinate, have a potential neurotoxic effect.

Mutations in *SUCLA2* and *SUCLG1* are associated with mild methylmalonic acidemia with normal homocysteine and the increased C4-dicarboxylic-carnitine level in plasma and even more in urine. As expected in a TCA cycle defect, variable lactic acidemia and consistent lactate increase in CSF are accompanying characteristics in patients with these defects. TCA cycle intermediates were found increased to a variable extent in the urine of the patients. The increase of methylmalonic acid in body fluids that is considerably less pronounced in patients with SCS defect than in classical MMA (Deodato et al. 2006) may be explained by the impaired conversion of succinyl-CoA to succinate, resulting in metabolite accumulation proximal to the enzymatic block.

### Enzyme Measurements

The activity of 2-oxoglutarate dehydrogenase in homogenates of cultured skin fibroblasts can be as high as 25% of control values in patients. Additional Western blot analysis of the E1 and E2 subunits might be needed to confirm the diagnosis.

The residual enzyme activity of fumarate hydratase deficiency shows no clear correlation with either the metabolic derangement or the clinical severity. The enzyme activity can be measured in fibroblasts, lymphoblasts, and white blood cells. Different tissues show different residual activities, and although most patients show an activity below 10%, the FH activity can range from undetectable to 35% compared to the activity measured in healthy controls. Enzyme measurements therefore might be insufficient to confirm the diagnosis, since the FH activity in healthy heterozygous parents ranges from 22% to 74% of controls.

Fumarase deficiency can lead to mitochondrial dysfunction, including variable degree of complex I and II deficiency (Tyrakis et al. 2017).

The SCS-A activity in muscle mitochondria from a *SUCLA2*-mutated patient has been demonstrated to be reduced compared to controls (Carrozzo et al. 2007), as well as the *SUCLA2* and *SUCLG1* gene products measured through Western blotting in muscle homogenate and in fibroblasts mitochondria, respectively (Carrozzo et al. 2007; Ostergaard et al. 2007a, b). Analysis of respiratory chain enzyme activities in muscle generally shows a combined deficiency of complexes I and IV, but normal histological and biochemical findings in muscle did not preclude a diagnosis of succinate-CoA ligase deficiency (Carrozzo et al. 2016).

## Prenatal Diagnosis

Prenatal diagnosis is the most frequently based on mutation analysis in familial cases of PDHC and PC deficiency. Measurement of PC or PDH activity in cultured amniotic fluid cells, or direct measurement in chorionic villi biopsy specimens are alternatives to DNA analysis, when the familial mutations are not known.

Molecular genetic testing is possible in fumarase deficiency and can be started with targeted mutation analysis of *FH* for the common 3-bp AAA duplication (c.1431_1433dupAAA), as the first genetic screening test. Due to compound heterozygosity of the mutation, further analysis of the whole *FH* gene is required to fully confirm the genetic defect. Prenatal diagnosis and preimplantation genetic diagnosis for at-risk pregnancies require prior identification of the disease-causing mutations in the family, although prenatal diagnosis of fumarase deficiency has even been successfully performed by enzyme activity measurements (Coughlin et al. 1998; Manning et al. 2000). In SUCLA2 and SUCLG1 defects, prenatal diagnosis is also possible in chorionic samples by sequence analysis in at-risk pregnancies.

| Disorder | Prenatal diagnosis |
|---|---|
| PDH, PC, and fumarase deficiency | Mutation analysis in chorionic sample |
| | FH enzyme measurement in amniocytes |
| SUCLA2and SUCLG1 defects | Mutation analysis in chorionic sample |

## Treatment and Prognosis

Patients with PC and PDHc deficiency should be treated for their acute hypoglycemic and acidotic episodes. One should monitor lactate levels regularly, since high glucose intake increases lactic acidosis.

Neither biotin, thiamine, dichloroacetate, nor a high-fat or high-carbohydrate diet has been shown to provide clinical benefit.

The general prognosis for individuals with PDHC deficiency is poor, and treatment is not very effective. Best strategy for treating PDHC deficiency is the use of a ketogenic diet (Scholl-Bürgi et al. 2015). Thiamine has been given in variable doses (500–2000 mg/day), with lowering of blood lactate and clinical improvement in some patients. DL-lipoic acid has been tried, but its efficacy remains controversial in PDHE3.

So far there is no curative treatment, and there are no known distinctive clinical symptoms and biochemical or genetic findings that can be used for prognosis assessment and prediction of the course of 2-oxoglutaric aciduria and fumarase deficiency. In 2-oxoglutaric aciduria, bicarbonate supplementation might be needed due to the chronic metabolic acidosis, and dietary intervention should be applied in patients with recurrent hypoketotic hypoglycemia. The outcome of both disorders appears to depend on the progression of the central nervous system symptoms and how effectively these symptoms are treatable. The prognosis ranges from death within the first year of life to survival to puberty or adulthood. The oldest patient with fumarase deficiency described was 25 years old at time of the case report.

In patients with SCS defects, most patients have a slowly progressive neurodegenerative course with possible survival to adulthood. Most of the SUCLG1-deficient patients have a neonatal, or early pediatric fatal outcome.

Fumarate is a positive regulator of genome stability (its absence supports genome instability and tumorigenesis) and its accumulation drives angiogenesis and proliferation (thereby supporting tumor establishment). If the fumarate hydratase-causing mutations are known in the family, it is appropriate to consider offering molecular genetic testing to relatives who might be at risk of developing multiple cutaneous and uterine leiomyomas (MCUL) or papillary renal cell carcinoma with leiomyomatosis (HLRCC) (Tomlinson et al. 2000).

| Disorder | Specific treatment |
|---|---|
| PDHc deficiency | Ketogenic diet |
| 2-Oxoglutaric aciduria | Bicarbonate supplementation |
| | Frequent feedings |
| | Avoidance of high CH intake |
| Fumarase deficiency | None |
| SUCLA2 and SUCLG1 defects | Protein restriction was not proved to be effective |

## Alternative Therapies

An orthotopic hepatic transplantation reversed ketoacidosis and renal tubular abnormalities, and decreased lactic acidemia in a patient with a severe PDHc phenotype. A patient with the French phenotype was started on early.

treatment with triheptanoin in order to restore anaplerosis. Although there was a clinical improvement without evidence of neurodegeneration, the patient died during an episode of acute decompensation at 8 months of age.

Phenylbutyrate has been shown beneficial effect in increasing enzyme activity (Ferriero et al. 2014).

| Disorder | Alternative therapies |
|---|---|
| 2-Oxoglutaric aciduria | Not successful |
| Fumarase deficiency | Not successful |
| SUCLA2 and SUCLG1 defects | Anaplerosis |

## References


Allegri G, Fernandes MJ, Scalco FB, et al. Fumaric aciduria: an overview and the first Brazilian case report. J Inherit Metab Dis. 2010;33:411–9.

Barnerias C, Saudubray JM, Touati G, et al. Pyruvate dehydrogenase complex defi ciency: four neurological phenotypes with differing pathogenesis. Dev Med Child Neurol. 2010;52(2):e1–9.

Brown RM, Head R, Morris AA, Raiman JA, et al. Pyruvate dehydrogenase E3 binding protein (protein X) defi ciency. Dev Med Child Neurol. 2006;48:756–60.

Bhola PT, Gilpin C, Smith A, Graham GE. A retrospective review of 48 individuals, including 12 families, molecularly diagnosed with hereditary leiomyomatosis and renal cell cancer (HLRCC). Familial Cancer. 2018;17(4):615–20.

Bonnefont JP, Chretien D, Rustin P, et al. Alpha-ketoglutarate dehydrogenase deficiency presenting as congenital lactic acidosis. J Pediatr. 1992;121:255–8.

Campeau PM, Hennekam RC, DOORS Syndrome Collaborative Group. DOORS syndrome: phenotype, genotype and comparison with coffin-Siris syndrome. Am J Med Genet C Semin Med Genet. 2014;166C(3):327–32.

Carrozzo R, Dionisi-Vici C, Steuerwald U, et al. SUCLA2 mutations are associated with mild methylmalonic aciduria, Leigh-like encephalomyopathy, dystonia and deafness. Brain. 2007;130:862–74.

Carrozzo R, Verrigni D, Rasmussen M, de Coo R, Amartino H, Bianchi M, Buhas D, Mesli S, Naess K, Born AP, Woldseth B, Prontera P, Batbayli M, Ravn K, Joensen F, Cordelli DM, Santorelli FM, Tulinius M, Darin N, Duno M, Jouvencel P, Burlina A, Stangoni G, Bertini E, Redonnet-Vernhet I, Wibrand F, Dionisi-Vici C, Uusimaa J, Vieira P, Osorio AN, McFarland R, Taylor RW, Holme E, Ostergaard E. Succinate-CoA ligase deficiency due to mutations in SUCLA2 and SUCLG1: phenotype and genotype correlations in 71 patients. J Inherit Metab Dis. 2016;39(2):243–52.

Coughlin EM, Christensen E, Kunz PL, et al. Molecular analysis and prenatal diagnosis of human fumarase deficiency. Mol Genet Metab. 1998;63:254–62.

De Meirleir L, Hansikova H, Zeman J, et al. Fumarate hydratase deficiency—a rare cause of development delay and seizures. J Inherit Metab Dis. 2006;29:106–8.

De Meirleir L. Disorders of pyruvate metabolism. Handb Clin Neurol. 2013;113:1667–73.

Deodato F, Boenzi S, Santorelli FM, Dionisi-Vici C. Methylmalonic and propionic aciduria. Am J Med Genet C Semin Med Genet. 2006;142:104–12.

Elpeleg O, Miller C, Hershkovitz E, et al. Deficiency of the ADP-forming succinyl-CoA synthase activity is associated with encephalomyopathy and mitochondrial DNA depletion. Am J Hum Genet. 2005;76:1081–6.

El-Hattab AW, Scaglia F. SUCLA2-related mitochondrial DNA depletion syndrome, encephalomyopathic form with methylmalonic aciduria. In: Adam MP, Ardinger HH, Pagon RA, Wallace SE, LJH B, Stephens K, Amemiya A, editors. GeneReviews® [Internet]. Seattle, WA: University of Washington, Seattle; 1993–2018; 2009; [updated 2017 May 18].

El-Hattab AW, Scaglia F. SUCLG1-related mitochondrial DNA depletion syndrome, Encephalomyopathic form with Methylmalonic Aciduria. 2017 mar 30. In: Adam MP, Ardinger HH, Pagon RA, Wallace SE, LJH B, Stephens K, Amemiya A, editors. GeneReviews® [internet]. Seattle, WA: University of Washington, Seattle; 1993–2018; 2017.

Ferriero R, Boutron A, Brivet M, Kerr D, Morava E, Rodenburg RJ, Bonafé L, Baumgartner MR, Anikster Y, Braverman NE, Brunetti-Pierri N. Phenylbutyrate increases pyruvate dehydrogenase complex activity in cells harboring a variety of defects. Ann Clin Transl Neurol. 2014;1(7):462–70.

Gardeitchik T, Mohamed M, Ruzzenente B, Karall D, Guerrero-Castillo S, Dalloyaux D, van den Brand M, van Kraaij S, van Asbeck E, Assouline Z, Rio M, de Lonlay P, Scholl-Buergi S, DFGJ W, Hoischen A, Rodenburg RJ, Sperl W, Urban Z, Brandt U, Mayr JA, Wong S, de Brouwer APM, Nijtmans L, Munnich A, Rötig A, Wevers RA, Metodiev MD, Morava E. Bi-allelic mutations in the mitochondrial ribosomal protein MRPS2 cause sensorineural hearing loss, hypoglycemia, and multiple OXPHOS complex deficiencies. Am J Hum Genet. 2018;102(4):685–95.

Grafakou O, Oexle K, van den Heuvel L, et al. Leigh syndrome due to compound heterozygosity of dihydrolipoamide dehydrogenase gene mutations. Description of the fi rst E3 splice site mutation. Eur J Pediatr. 2003;162:714–8.

Guffon N, Lopez-Mediavilla C, Dumoulin R, et al. 2-Ketoglutarate dehydrogenase deficiency, a rare cause of primary hyperlactataemia: report of a new case. J Inherit Metab Dis. 1993;16:821–30.

Habarou F, Hamel Y, Haack TB, Feichtinger RG, Lebigot E, Marquardt I, Busiah K, Laroche C, Madrange M, Grisel C, Pontoizeau C, Eisermann M, Boutron A, Chrétien D, Chadefaux-Vekemans B, Barouki R, Bole-Feysot C, Nitschke P, Goudin N, Boddaert N, Nemazanyy I, Delahodde A, Kölker S, Rodenburg RJ, Korenke GC, Meitinger T, Strom TM, Prokisch H, Rotig A, Ottolenghi C, Mayr JA, de Lonlay P. Biallelic mutations in LIPT2 cause a mitochondrial lipoylation defect associated with severe neonatal encephalopathy. Am J Hum Genet. 2017;101(2):283–90.

Johnson JD, Muhonen WW, Lambeth DO. Characterization of the ATP- and GTP-specific succinyl-CoA synthetases in pigeon. The enzymes incorporate the same alpha-subunit. J Biol Chem. 1998;273:27573–9.

Kadrmas EF, Ray PD, Lambeth DO. Apparent ATP-linked succinate thiokinase activity and its relation to nucleoside diphosphate kinase in mitochondrial matrix preparations from rabbit. Biochim Biophys Acta. 1991;1074:339–46.

Kavanaugh-Black A, Connolly DM, Chugani SA, Chakrabarty AM. Characterization of nucleoside-diphosphate kinase from Pseudomonas aeruginosa: complex formation with succinyl-CoA synthetase. Proc Natl Acad Sci U S A. 1994;91:5883–7.

Kohlschutter A, Behbehani A, Langenbeck U, et al. A familial progressive neurodegenerative disease with 2-oxoglutaric aciduria. Europ J Pediatr. 1982;138:32–7.

Kowluru A, Tannous M, Chen HQ. Localization and characterization of the mitochondrial isoform of the nucleoside diphosphate kinase in the pancreatic beta cell: evidence for its complexation with mitochondrial succinyl-CoA synthetase. Arch Biochem Biophys. 2002;398:160–9.

Landsverk ML, Zhang VW, Wong LC, Andersson HC. A SUCLG1 mutation in a patient with mitochondrial DNA depletion and congenital anomalies. Mol Genet Metab Rep. 2014;1:451–4.

Lissens W, De Meirleir L, Seneca S, et al. Mutations in the X-linked pyruvate dehydrogenase (E1) α sububit gene (PDHA1) in patients with a pyruvate dehydrogenase complex defi ciency. Hum Mutat. 2000;15:209–19.

Manning NJ, Olpin SE, Pollitt RJ, et al. Fumarate hydratase deficiency: increased fumaric acid in amniotic fluid of two affected pregnancies. J Inherit Metab Dis. 2000;23:757–9.

Maradin M, Fumić K, Hansikova H, et al. Fumaric aciduria: mild phenotype in a 8-year-old girl with novel mutations. J Inherit Metab Dis. 2006;29:683.

Morava E, Steuerwald U, Carrozzo R, et al. Dystonia and deafness due to SUCLA2 defect; clinical course and biochemical markers in 16 children. Mitochondrion. 2009; https://doi.org/10.1016/j.mito.2009.08.003.

Nimmo GAM, Venkatesh S, Pandey AK, Marshall CR, Hazrati LN, Blaser S, Ahmed S, Cameron J, Singh K, Ray PN, Suzuki CK, Yoon G. Bi-allelic mutations of LONP1 encoding the mitochondrial LonP1 protease cause pyruvate dehydrogenase deficiency and profound neurodegeneration with progressive cerebellar atrophy. Hum Mol Genet. 2019;28(2):290–306.

Ostergaard E, Hansen FJ, Sorensen N, et al. Mitochondrial encephalomyopathy with elevated methylmalonic acid is caused by SUCLA2 mutations. Brain. 2007a;130:853–61.

Ostergaard E, Christensen E, Kristensen E, et al. Deficiency of the alpha subunit of succinate-coenzyme A ligase causes fatal infantile lactic acidosis with mitochondrial DNA depletion. Am J Hum Genet. 2007b;81:383–7.

Ostergaard E, Schwartz M, Batbayli M, et al. A novel missense mutation in SUCLG1 associated with mitochondrial DNA depletion, encephalomyopathic form, with methylmalonic aciduria. Eur J Pediatr. 2009; https://doi.org/10.1007/s00431-009-1007-z.

Ottolenghi C, Hubert L, Allanore Y, et al. Clinical and biochemical heterogeneity associated with fumarase deficiency. Hum Mutat. 2011; https://doi.org/10.1002/humu.21534.

Picaud S, Kavanagh KL, Yue WW, et al. Structural basis of fumarate hydratase deficiency. J Inherit Metab Dis. 2011;34:671–6.

Rouzier C, Le Guédard-Méreuze S, Fragaki K, et al. The severity of phenotype linked to SUCLG1 mutations could be correlated with residual amount of SUCLG1 protein. J Med Genet. 2010;47(10):670–6.

Scholl-Bürgi S, Höller A, Pichler K, Michel M, Haberlandt E, Karall D. Ketogenic diets in patients with inherited metabolic disorders. J Inherit Metab Dis. 2015;38(4):765–73.

Surendran S, Michals-Matalon K, Krywawych S. DOOR syndrome: deficiency of E1 component of the 2-oxoglutarate dehydrogenase complex. Am J Med Genet. 2002;113(4):371–4.

Tomlinson IP, Alam NA, Rowan AJ. Multiple leiomyoma consortium. Germline mutations in FH predispose to dominantly inherited uterine fibroids, skin leiomyomata and papillary renal cell cancer. Nat Genet. 2000;30:406–10.

Tort F, Ferrer-Cortes X, Ribes A. Differential diagnosis of lipoic acid synthesis defects. J Inherit Metab Dis. 2016;39(6):781–93.

Tyrakis PA, Yurkovich ME, Sciacovelli M, Papachristou EK, Bridges HR, Gaude E, Schreiner A, D'Santos C, Hirst J, Hernandez-Fernaud J, Springett R, Griffiths JR, Frezza C. Fumarate Hydratase loss causes combined respiratory chain defects. Cell Rep. 2017;21(4):1036–47.

Trinh BC, Melhem ER, Barker PB. Multi-slice proton MR spectroscopy and diffusion weighted imaging in methylmalonic acidemia: report of two cases and review of the literature. Am J Neuroradiol. 2001;22:831–3.

Willemsen M, Rodenburg RJT, Teszas A, et al. Females with PDHA1 gene mutations: a diagnostic challenge. Mitochondrion. 2006;6:155–9.

Murakami Y, Nguyen TTM, Baratang N, Raju PK. Mutations in PIGB cause an inherited GPI biosynthesis defect with an axonal neuropathy and metabolic abnormality in severe cases. Am J Hum Genet. 2019;105(2):384–94.

Zeman J, Krijt J, Stratilová L, et al. Abnormalities in succinylpurines in fumarase deficiency: possible role in pathogenesis of CNS impairment. J Inherit Metab Dis. 2000;23:371–4.

Zinn AB, Kerr DS, Hoppel CL. Fumarase deficiency: a new cause of mitochondrial encephalomyopathy. N Engl J Med. 1986;315:469–75.

# Disorders of Mitochondrial Carriers

# 43

Tom J. J. Schirris, Jan A. M. Smeitink,
and Frans G. M. Russel

## Contents



T. J. J. Schirris (✉) · F. G. M. Russel
Department of Pharmacology and Toxicology, Radboud Center for Mitochondrial Medicine, Radboud Institute for Molecular Life Sciences, Radboud University Medical Center, Nijmegen, The Netherlands
e-mail: Tom.Schirris@radboudumc.nl; Frans.Russel@radboudumc.nl

J. A. M. Smeitink
Department of Pediatrics, Radboud Center for Mitochondrial Medicine, Radboud University Medical Center, Nijmegen, The Netherlands
e-mail: Jan.Smeitink@radboudumc.nl

**Summary**

Most mitochondrial metabolic pathways are heavily interconnected and dependent on cytosolic metabolic routes. To allow such a cooperative action, a large variety of metabolites need to be exchanged between both compartments. This is mediated by transport proteins embedded in the mitochondrial inner membrane. Most of these transporters belong to the mitochondrial carrier family, consisting of 53 members that are encoded by genes of the solute carrier family 25, which are distributed equally over most chromosomes. Expression patterns differ largely between different carriers ranging from ubiquitous expression in all organs up to organ-


N. Blau et al. (eds.), *Physician's Guide to the Diagnosis, Treatment, and Follow-Up of Inherited Metabolic Diseases*,
https://doi.org/10.1007/978-3-030-67727-5_43

specific expression, or even related to specific metabolic states. Although these carriers are involved in the import and export of a large variety of chemically distinct cellular metabolic substrates, they are expected to act via a similar structural transport mechanism, which preserves the mitochondrial membrane potential during transport. Up to now, 15 mitochondrial carriers have been linked to various rare inherited metabolic diseases. This chapter provides an overview of the wide variety of clinical phenotypes associated with mitochondrial carrier deficiencies, including carnitine/acylcarnitine deficiency, HHH syndrome, epileptic encephalomyopathy, transient infantile hypertriglyceridemia, citrullinemia, sideroblastic anemia, Amish microcephaly, Gorlin–Chaudhry–Moss syndrome, Fontaine syndrome and neonatal myoclonic epilepsy. Both clinical and molecular phenotypes largely depend on the metabolites being transported, leading to a decreased function of one but often multiple metabolic pathways located in the mitochondrial matrix or the cytosol. This, however, most often causes a characteristic pattern of metabolite changes, which can be used for diagnostic purposes. A vast number of carrier deficiencies result in a decreased mitochondrial ATP production and oxidative phosphorylation (OXPHOS) function, whereas other deficiencies are characterized by deficient amino acid, galactose, or fatty acid metabolism. Although therapeutic strategies are lacking for most carrier deficiencies, some dietary alterations like a ketogenic diet or supplementation (i.e., riboflavin, citrate) have shown promising effects.

## Introduction

Most mitochondrial metabolic pathways are heavily interconnected and dependent on cytosolic metabolic routes. To allow such a cooperative action, a large variety of metabolites need to be exchanged between both compartments. Although polar substrates can easily pass the mitochondrial outer membrane, which is permeable to molecules up to 5000 Da, they need an active transport step to cross the largely impermeable mitochondrial inner membrane. This transport is mediated by transport proteins embedded in the mitochondrial inner membrane. Most of these transporters belong to the mitochondrial carrier family, consisting of 53 members that enable import and efflux of a wide variety of metabolites (Ruprecht and Kunji 2020). Other type of transport proteins that are embedded in the mitochondrial inner membrane include six ATP-binding cassette (ABC) transporters (Schaedler et al. 2015), various ion channels, the mitochondrial pyruvate carrier (Bender and Martinou 2016), and five sideroflexins (Paul et al. 2019; Sofou et al. 2019).

The mitochondrial carrier family comprises proteins that are encoded by genes of the solute carrier (SLC) family 25, which are distributed equally over most chromosomes (Palmieri and Monné 2016). Expression patterns vary largely between different carriers ranging from ubiquitous expression in all organs up to organ-specific expression, or even related to specific metabolic states, like association of the glycolytic rate with ADP/ATP carrier isoform 2 expression (Palmieri and Monné 2016). These expression patterns are most likely due to the specialized function of the carrier proteins and their different isoforms.

Although mitochondrial carriers are involved in the import and export of a large variety of chemically distinct cellular metabolic substrates via different operating modes (e.g., uniporter, symporter, antiporter), they are expected to act via a similar structural transport mechanism, which has recently been clarified for the ADP/ATP carrier (Ruprecht and Kunji 2019). This is also evident from a highly conserved sequence similarity of the functional motives, which are essential for carrier function (Robinson et al. 2008). All carriers consist of three homologous sequence repeats of approximately 100 amino acids. Each repeat consists of an odd numbered helix (H1, H3, or H5), which penetrates the membrane, a matrix helix (h12, h34, h56), which is positioned parallel to the membrane, and an even numbered helix (H2, H4, H6), which also penetrates the membrane. Characteristic amino acid sequences in the cytoplasmic and matrix regions contribute to the formation of salt-bridge networks that form the cytoplasmic and mitochondrial brace, respectively. Upon binding of the carrier substrate, these salt-bridge networks and braces are formed and bring the carrier either in the matrix-open (m-state) or cytosolic-open (c-state) state. In both conditions, the central substrate binding cavity is protected by a ~15 Å wide gate, which is structurally unique for mitochondrial carrier proteins and is expected to prevent proton leak (Ruprecht et al. 2019). In contrast to the conserved regions required for the transport mechanism, the carriers contain a highly variable central region that determine substrate specificity (Robinson et al. 2008).

Since the first observation mentioning that mitochondrial carriers might cause mitochondrial disease, 15 mitochondrial carrier proteins have been linked to various rare inherited metabolic diseases (Trijbels et al. 1998; Palmieri and Monné 2016). The clinical phenotypes are very heterogenous and largely depend on the metabolic pathway in which the metabolic substrates are involved. Deficiencies of mitochondrial ADP/ATP and phosphate carries are, for example, associated with a decreased mitochondrial ATP production, as they facilitate the mitochondrial import of two main substrates for the oxidative phosphorylation (OXPHOS) (i.e., ADP and phosphate). Deficiencies of other carriers are associated with a disturbed fatty acid biosynthesis and oxidation, deficient urea cycle metabolism, decreased amino acid synthesis, or disturbed heme synthesis. Clinically, this results in a whole gamut of different symptoms and diseases associated with carrier deficiencies, including carnitine/acylcarnitine deficiency, HHH syndrome, epileptic encephalomyopathy, transient infantile hypertriglyceridemia, citrullinemia, sideroblastic anemia, Amish microcephaly, Gorlin–Chaudhry–Moss syndrome, Fontaine syndrome and neonatal myoclonic epilepsy.

## Nomenclature

| No. | Disease name | Alternative names | Disease abbreviation | Gene symbol | Chromosomal location | Mode of Inheritance | Affected protein | Disease OMIM |
|---|---|---|---|---|---|---|---|---|
| 43.1 | Adenine nucleotide translocator deficiency | Mitochondrial DNA depletion syndrome type 12 (cardiomyopathic type) | | *SLC25A4* | 4q35.1 | AR | Adenine nucleotide translocator 1 | 615,418 |
| 43.2 | Adenine nucleotide translocator deficiency | adPEO with mitochondrial DNA deletions type 2 | | *SLC25A4* | 4q35.1 | AD | Adenine nucleotide translocator 1 | 609,283 |
| 43.3 | Mitochondrial phosphate carrier deficiency | | | *SLC25A3* | 12q23 | AR | SLC25A3 | 610,773 |
| 43.4 | Aspartate-glutamate carrier 1 deficiency | Early infantile epileptic encephalopathy type 39 | EIEE39 | *SLC25A12* | 2q31.1 | AR | Neuronal- and muscle-specific mitochondrial aspartate/glutamate transporter 1 (AGC1; Aralar) | 612,949 |
| 43.5 | Cytosolic glycerol-3-phosphate dehydrogenase deficiency | Transient infantile hypertriglyceridemia | HTGTI | *GPD1* | 12q13.12 | AR | Glycerol-3-phosphate dehydrogenase | 614,480 |
| 43.6 | Combined oxidative phosphorylation deficiency-28 | SAM transporter deficiency | COXPD28 | *SLC25A26* | 3p14.1 | AR | S-adenosylmethionine (SAM) carrier protein | 616,794 |
| 43.7 | Mitochondrial citrate carrier deficiency | Combined d-2- and l-2-hydroxyglutaric aciduria | D2L2AD | *SLC25A1* | 22q11.21 | AR | Mitochondrial tricarboxylate transporter | 615,182 |
| 43.8 | Mitochondrial ATP-$Mg^{2+}$/phosphate transporter deficiency | Gorlin–Chaudhry–Moss syndrome; Fontaine syndrome | FPS | *SLC25A24* | 1p13.3 | AD | Calcium-binding carrier | 612,289 |
| 43.9 | Mitochondrial aspartate aminotransferase deficiency | | | *GOT2* | 16q21 | AR | Glutamate oxaloacetate transaminase, mitochondrial | 138,150 |
| 43.10 | Mitochondrial dicarboxylate transporter deficiency | | | *SLC25A10* | 17q25.3 | AR | Solute carrier family 25 (mitochondrial carrier), member 10 | 606,794 |
| 43.11 | Mitochondrial ornithine transporter deficiency | Hyperammonemia–hyperornithinemia–homocitrullinuria syndrome; HHH syndrome | HHH | *SLC25A15* | 13q14.11 | AR | Mitochondrial ornithine transporter (ORNT1) SLC25A15 | 238,970 |
| 43.12 | Citrin deficiency | Citrullinemia type II | CTLN2 | *SLC25A13* | 7q21.3 | AR | Aspartate glutamate carrier (SLC25A13) | 605,814;603,471 |

(continued)

| No. | Disease name | Alternative names | Disease abbreviation | Gene symbol | Chromosomal location | Mode of Inheritance | Affected protein | Disease OMIM |
|---|---|---|---|---|---|---|---|---|
| 43.13 | Mitochondrial glutamate carrier 1 deficiency | Early infantile epileptic encephalopathy-3 | EIEE3 | *SLC25A22* | 11p15.5 | AR | Mitochondrial glutamate/$H^+$ symporter 1 (glutamate carrier 1, GC1) | 609,304 |
| 43.14 | Mitochondrial glycine transporter deficiency | Pyridoxine-refractory sideroblastic anemia type 2 | | *SLC25A38* | 3p22.1 | AR | Solute carrier family 25, member 38 | 205,950 |
| 43.15 | Bilateral striatal necrosis (SLC25A19) | Mitochondrial thiamine pyrophosphate carrier deficiency; Amish microcephaly | | *SLC25A19* | | AR | Amish microcephaly | 606,521 |
| 43.16 | Mitochondrial flavin adenine dinucleotide transporter deficiency | Riboflavin-responsive exercise intolerance | RREI | *SLC25A32* | 8q22.3 | AR | Mitochondrial flavin adenine dinucleotide transporter | 616,839 |
| 43.17 | Mitochondrial coenzyme A transporter deficiency | | | *SLC25A42* | 19p13.11 | AR | Solute carrier family 25, member 42 | 610,823 |

## Metabolic Pathways

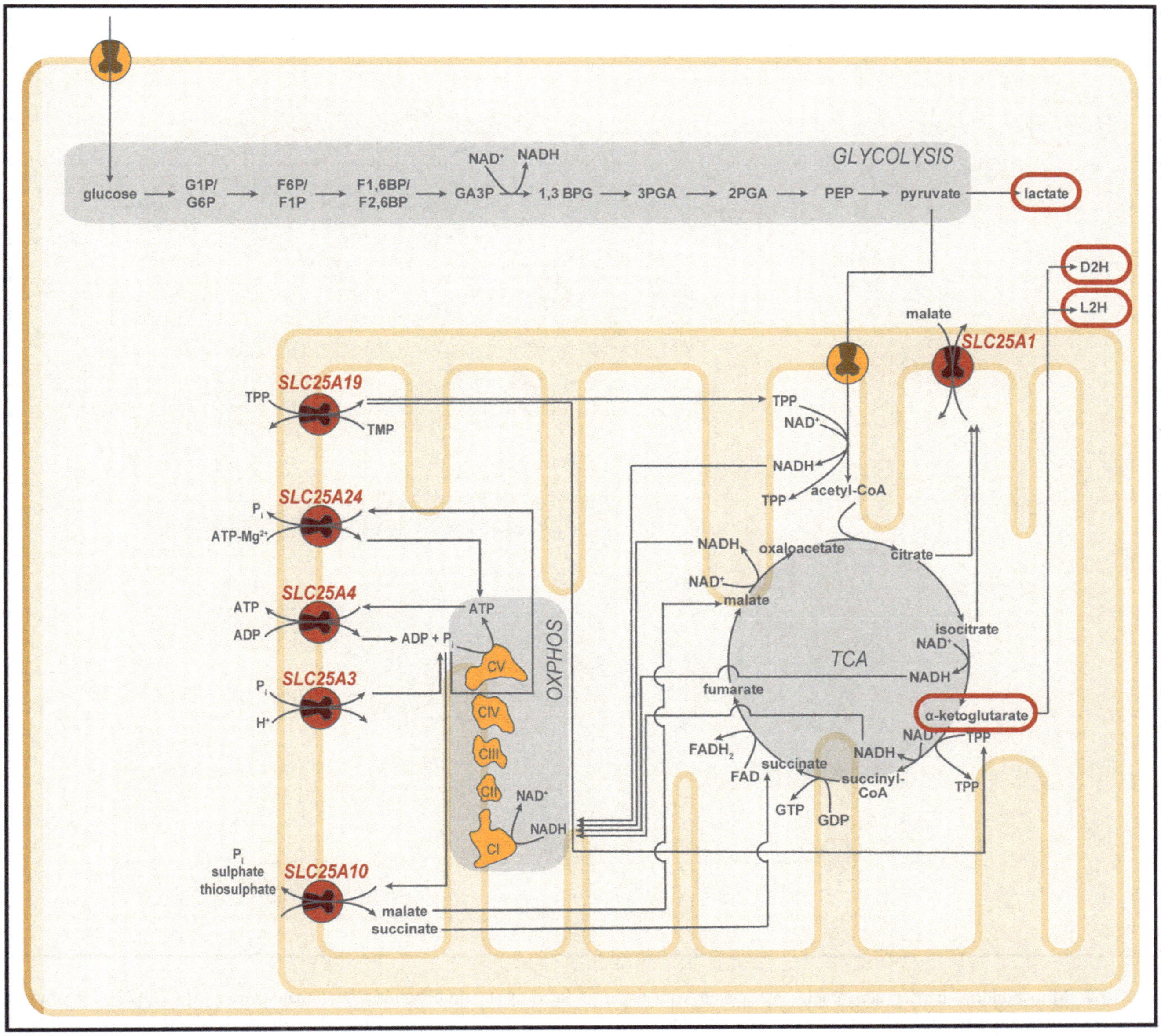


**Fig. 43.1** Mitochondrial carrier deficiencies associated with a decreased TCA or OXPHOS capacity. Classically, mitochondrial ADP/ATP carrier (*SLC25A4*) and phosphate carrier (*SLC25A3*) deficiencies have been directly linked to an impaired OXPHOS capacity (Palmieri and Monné 2016), which is obvious as they facilitate the mitochondrial import of both substrates for ATP generation by the fifth OXPHOS complex (i.e., $F_oF_1$-ATP-synthase). The concurrent inhibition of the entire OXPHOS capacity results in a decreased mitochondrial respiration, which leads to the conversion of pyruvate to lactate. In addition to the ADP/ATP carrier, ADP and ATP can also be transported bidirectionally by the ATP-$Mg^{2+}$/phosphate carrier (*SLC25A24*). In contrast to the ADP/ATP carriers, this transport is not equimolar, which allows this carrier to regulate the size of the mitochondrial and cytosolic nucleotide pools (Palmieri and Monné 2016). Decreased OXPHOS capacity also occurs secondary to inhibition of the TCA cycle, which can result from deficiencies of the citrate carrier (*SLC25A1*), dicarboxylate carrier (*SLC25A10*), and thiamine pyrophosphate carrier (*SLC25A19*). Although most consequences of citrate carrier deficiencies are due to low cytosolic citrate availability to processes like cholesterol, fatty acid, and coenzyme Q synthesis, it also hampers the mitochondrial import of malate. On the other hand, increased matrix citrate concentrations lead to increased concentrations of downstream TCA metabolites, most prominently observed with α-ketoglutarate, which leads to increased levels of two enantiomers of 2-hydroxyglutarate (D2H, L2H) (Nota et al. 2013). Malate supply for the TCA cycle can, however, also be facilitated by the dicarboxylate carrier. This carrier also imports succinate into the mitochondrial matrix, and deficiencies are consequently associated with TCA cycle defects. Finally, the thiamine pyrophosphate carrier facilitates mitochondrial thiamine pyrophosphate import, which is an important cofactor for pyruvate dehydrogenase, but also for α-ketoglutarate dehydrogenase that converts α-ketoglutarate to succinyl-CoA. The latter gives rise to increased α-ketoglutarate levels. Abbreviations: *1,3 BPG* 1,3-biphosphoglycerate, *CI-V* mitochondrial OXPHOS complex I–V, *D2H* D-2-hydroxyglutaric acid, *F1P* fructose-1-phosphate, *F1,6BP* fructose-1,6-biphosphate, *F2,6BP* fructose-2,6-biphosphate, *F6P* fructose-6-phosphate, *G1P* glucose-1-phosphate, *G6P* glucose-6-phosphate, *GA3P* glyceraldehyde 3-phosphate, *3PGA* 3-phosphoglycerate, *L2H* L-2-hydroglutaric acid, *PEP* phosphoenolpyruvate, *2PGA* 2-phosphoglycerate, *TCA* tricarboxylic acid cycle, *TMP* thiamine monophosphate, *TPP* thiamine pyrophosphate

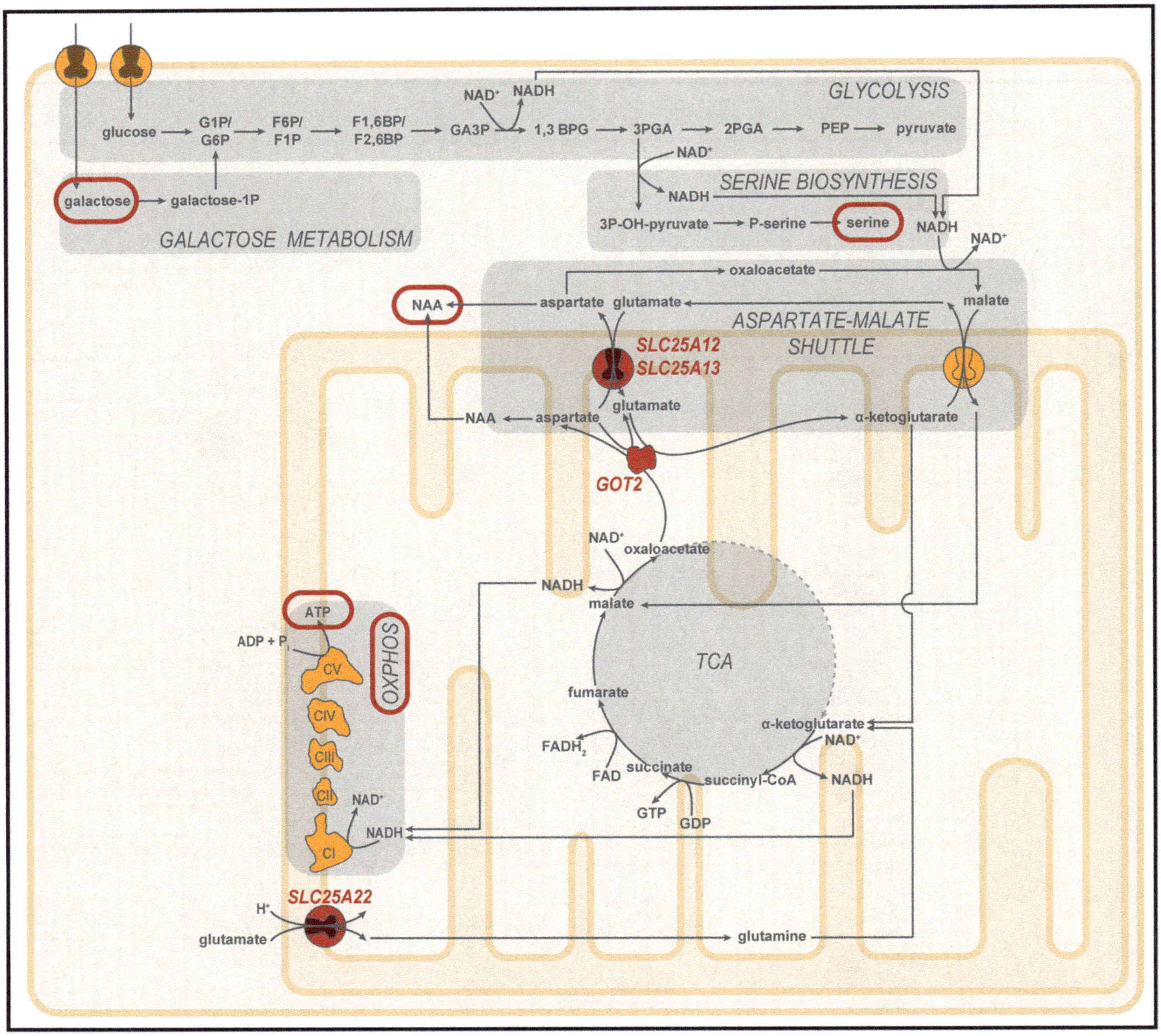


**Fig. 43.2** Mitochondrial carrier deficiencies associated with aspartate–malate shuttle disturbance. The malate–aspartate shuttle is one of the mitochondrial shuttles that transfer reducing equivalents from cytosolic NADH to mitochondrial matrix NADH. Consequently, inhibition of this shuttle by deficiencies of the aspartate–glutamate carrier (*SLC25A12/A13*) leads to high cytosolic NADH levels. This will subsequently inhibit glycolysis, which also results in a decreased galactose utilization. In neurons, which mainly express *SLC25A12*, reduced activity of this carrier leads to decreased *N*-acetyl aspartate (NAA) levels, as cytosolic aspartate is the main precursor for this metabolite. In liver mitochondria, which predominantly express *SLC25A13*, deficiency of this carrier is mainly characterized by increased galactose levels as described above, and a disturbed urea cycle and amino acid metabolism as described in Fig. 43.3. The glycolytic inhibition will also lead to a decreased pyruvate production, simultaneously less glutamate will enter the mitochondrial matrix. Therefore, α-ketoglutarate production from glutamate will limit the potential of this compensatory mechanism to correct for the reduced pyruvate availability, consequently *SLC25A12* deficiencies result in a decreased mitochondrial OXPHOS capacity and ATP-production. Matrix glutamate levels are also regulated by the mitochondrial glutamate carrier (*SLC25A22*), for which a net efflux of glutamate (i.e., matrix to cytosol transport) was postulated based on deficiencies of this carrier (Reid et al. 2017). The resulting high glutamate concentrations also drive amino acid metabolism toward proline synthesis, as described in Fig. 43.3. Next to the aspartate–glutamate carrier deficiencies, inhibition of the malate–aspartate shuttle can result from *GOT2* deficiency, which is closely involved in this shuttle by the interconversion of aspartate to glutamate and glutamate to α-ketoglutarate. In analogy with SLC25A12/13 deficiencies this results in increased cytosolic NADH levels, which inhibits serine biosynthesis. Abbreviations: *1,3 BPG* 1,3-biphosphoglycerate, *CI-V* mitochondrial OXPHOS complex I–V, *F1P* fructose-1-phosphate, *F1,6BP* fructose-1,6-biphosphate, *F2,6BP* fructose-2,6-biphosphate, *F6P* fructose-6-phosphate, *G1P* glucose-1-phosphate, *G6P* glucose-6-phosphate, *galactose-1P* galactose-1-phosphate, *GA3P* glyceraldehyde 3-phosphate, *3PGA* 3-phosphoglycerate, *NAA N*-acetyl aspartate, *PEP* phosphoenolpyruvate, *2PGA* 2-phosphoglycerate, *3P-OH-pyruvate* 3-phosphohydroxypyruvate, *P-serine* phosphoserine, *TCA* tricarboxylic acid cycle

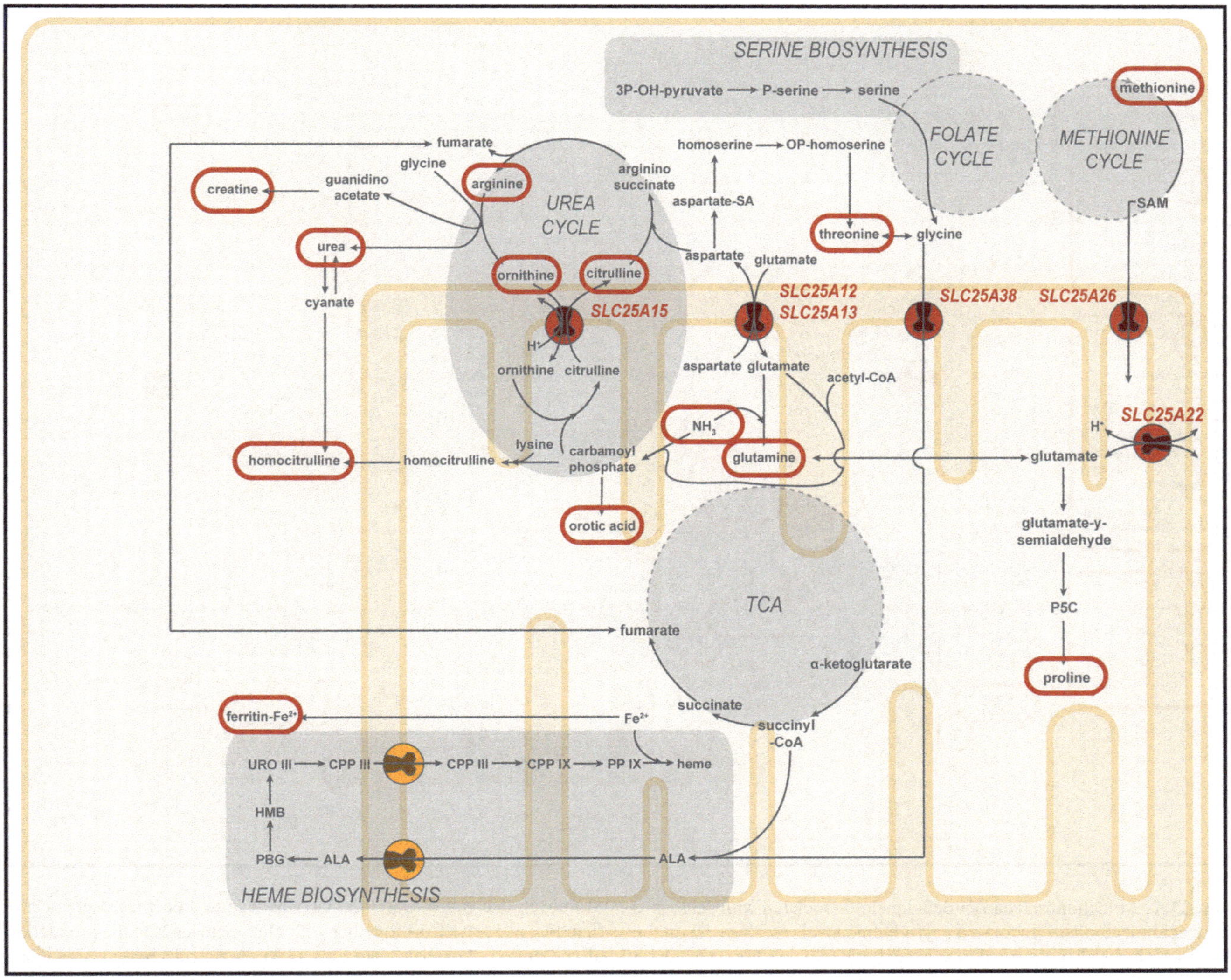


**Fig. 43.3** Mitochondrial carrier deficiencies associated with disturbed amino acid metabolism. Various mitochondrial carrier deficiencies result in a disturbed amino acid metabolism, which is also reflected in amino acids plasma levels. For the majority of amino acid alterations this is due to interference with the urea cycle, which is partially located in the mitochondrial matrix and partially in the cytosol. Most obvious are ornithine carrier (*SLC25A15*) deficiencies, as this carrier exchanges ornithine for citrulline, and is therefore central in the coupling of the cytosolic and matrix steps of the urea cycle. Consequently, this results in increased cytosolic ornithine and (homo)citrulline levels, which is also reflected in high plasma levels of both amino acids. In contrast to these levels in the cytosol, mitochondrial levels are low. The urea cycle can also be disturbed by aspartate–glutamate carrier (*SLC25A12/13*) deficiencies, which is due to a shortage of cytosolic aspartate. These low aspartate concentrations also inhibit synthesis of threonine. In addition to disturbed amino acid patterns, this also leads to increased orotic acid levels and decreased synthesis of urea, which is directly generated by the urea cycle, and decreased levels of creatine formed from guanidinoacetate (i.e., a urea cycle product). Finally, urea cycle defects are characterized by increased ammonia and glutamine levels, the latter also being characteristic for hepatic aspartate-glutamate carrier (i.e., *SLC25A13*) deficiencies. Glutamine is interconverted with mitochondrial glutamate, which is mainly transported out of the matrix by the mitochondrial glutamate carrier (*SLC25A22*), as described in Fig. 43.2. Although deficiencies of this carrier result in high glutamate levels, glutamine levels are not increased. The high glutamate levels are, however, expected to promote proline synthesis (Reid et al. 2017), as apparent from the hyperprolinemia observed in glutamate carrier-deficient patients. Other amino acid disturbances associated with mitochondrial carrier deficiencies include increased cytosolic methionine levels, as its downstream product *S*-adenosylmethionine is not imported into the mitochondrial matrix by the *S*-adenosylmethionine carrier (*SLC25A26*). Finally, as a result of glycine carrier (*SLC25A38*) deficiencies matrix glycine concentrations are decreased, leading to an inhibited heme synthesis, as glycine is one of its primary metabolic building blocks. The decreased heme biosynthesis gives rise to a lower incorporation of iron, which then binds to ferritin in the cytosol. Consequently, increased ferritin concentrations are observed with glycine carrier deficiencies (Kannengiesser et al. 2011). Abbreviations: *ALA* Delta aminolevulinic acid, *aspartate-SA* Aspartate semialdehyde, *CPPIII* Coproporphyrinogen III, *CPP IX* Protoporphyrinogen IX, *PP IX* Protoporphyrin IX, *HMB* Hydroxymethylbilane, *OP-homoserine* *O*-phospho-homoserine, *3P-OH-pyruvate* 3-Phosphohydroxypyruvate, *P5C* Pyrroline-5-carboxylate, *PBG* Porphobilinogen, *P-serine* Phospho-serine, *SAM* *S*-adenosylmethionine, *TCA* Tricarboxylic acid cycle, *URO III* Uroporphyrinogen III

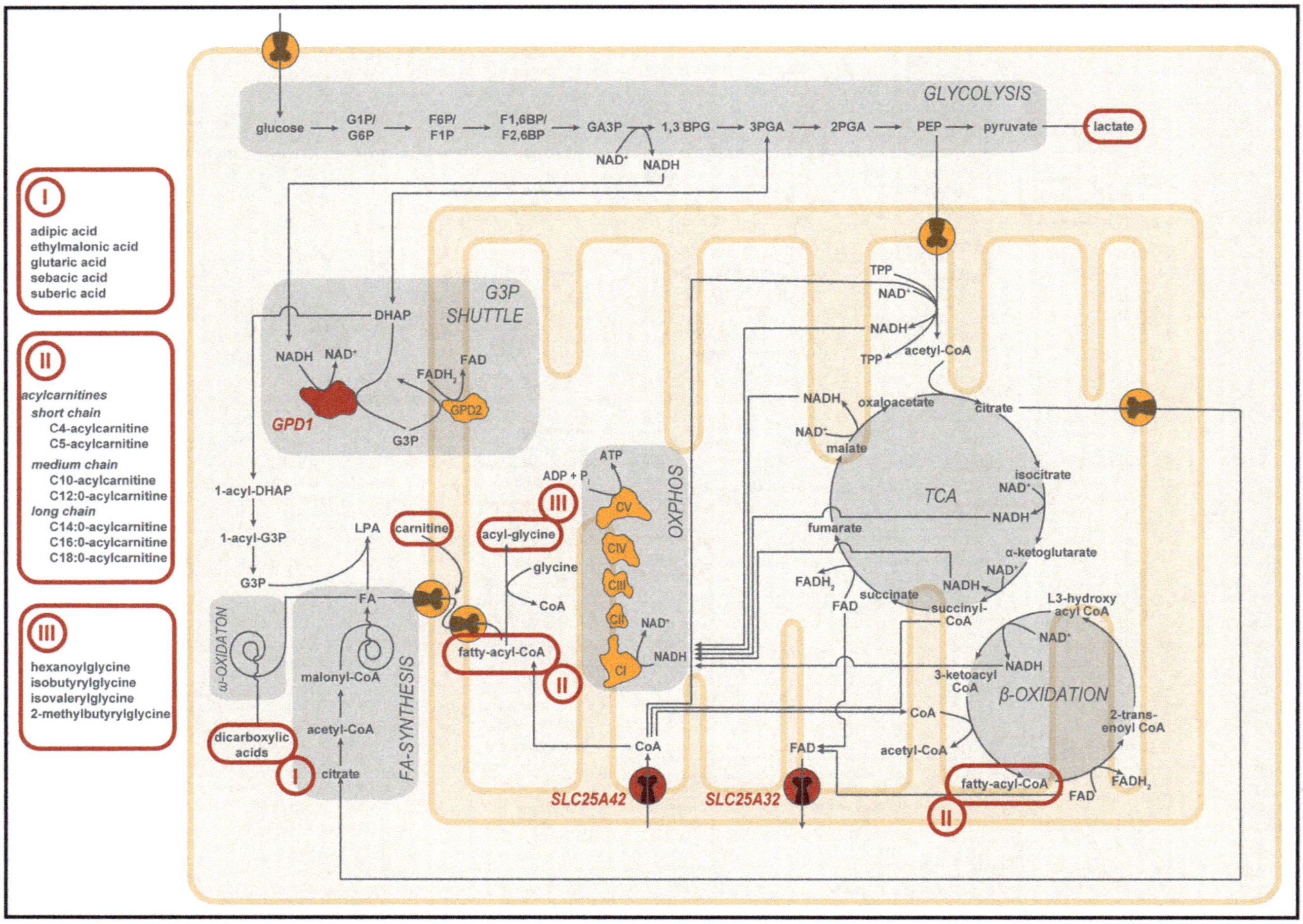


**Fig. 43.4** Mitochondrial carrier deficiencies associated with decreased fatty acid metabolism. Increased acyl-glycine levels (see box III on the left), which are also observed in various fatty acid and branched chain amino acid oxidation disorders, are associated with mitochondrial folate carrier (*SLC25A32*) and coenzyme A (*SLC25A42*) carrier deficiencies. For folate carrier deficiencies, this phenotype results from a decreased fatty acid β-oxidation due to decreased mitochondrial flavin adenine dinucleotide (FAD) levels, which drive the first enzymatic conversion of this pathway and FAD is imported into the matrix by *SLC25A32* (Schiff et al. 2016). More severe deficiencies, also result in a decreased activity of the second OXPHOS complex (i.e., complex II), which similarly uses FAD as cofactor (Hellebrekers et al. 2017). This subsequently leads to a decreased ATP production capacity. The decreased fatty acid oxidation in these deficiencies also leads to increased cytosolic fatty acid levels that give rise to an increased peroxisomal fatty acid ω-oxidation, which results in increased dicarboxylic acid concentrations (see box I on the left). Increased acyl-glycine levels are also characteristic for coenzyme A carrier deficiencies, as coenzyme A (CoA) is vital for mitochondrial uptake of medium and long-chain fatty acids (see box II on the left). Moreover, this leads to increased carnitine levels that are used for mitochondrial fatty acid import. As CoA is essential for many other mitochondrial metabolic pathways, these deficiencies are also characterized by increased lactate levels, as the conversion of pyruvate to acetyl-CoA is inhibited. Moreover, decreased acetyl-CoA levels lead to a decreased urea cycle function, as acetyl-CoA together with glutamate leads to the production of carbamoyl phosphate (see Fig. 43.3). Such a decreased urea cycle function explains the increased ammonia levels in coenzyme A carrier deficiencies. Cytosolic glycerol-3-phosphate dehydrogenase deficiencies are characterized by an enhanced triglyceride synthesis, which can most likely be explained by an increased concentration of dihydroxyacetone phosphate (DHAP), which can alternatively be converted into glycerol-3-phosphate (G3P) by dihydroxyacetone phosphate acyltransferase (Hebestreit et al. 1996). The produced glycerol-3-phosphate can together with fatty acids be used for the production of triglycerides. This link with fatty acid metabolism is emphasized by increased dicarboxylic acid levels, indicative of an increased peroxisomal fatty acid ω-oxidation, as described above. Abbreviations: *1,3 BPG* 1,3-Biphosphoglycerate, *CI-V* Mitochondrial OXPHOS complex I–V, *DHAP* Dihydroxyacetone phosphate, *F1P* Fructose-1-phosphate, *F1,6BP* Fructose-1,6-biphosphate, *F2,6BP* Fructose-2,6-biphosphate, *F6P* Fructose-6-phosphate, *FA* Fatty acid, *G1P* Glucose-1-phosphate, *G3P* Glycerol-3-phosphate, *G6P* Glucose-6-phosphate, *GA3P* Glyceraldehyde 3-phosphate, *GPD1* Glycerol-3-phosphate dehydrogenase 1, *GPD2* Glycerol-3-phosphate dehydrogenase 2, *LPA* Lysophosphatidic acid, *3PGA* 3-Phosphoglycerate, *PEP* phosphoenolpyruvate, *2PGA* 2-Phosphoglycerate, *TCA* Tricarboxylic acid cycle, *TPP* Thiamine pyrophosphate

## Signs and Symptoms

**Table 43.1** Adenine nucleotide translocator deficiency

| System | Symptom | Neonatal (birth–1 month) | Infancy (1–18 months) | Childhood (1.5–11 years) | Adolescence (11–16 years) | Adulthood (>16 years) |
|---|---|---|---|---|---|---|
| Cardiovascular | **Cardiomyopathy, hypertrophic** | | | + | + | |
| CNS | Retardation, psychomotor | | | ± | ± | |
| Ear | Hearing loss, sensorineural | | | | | ± |
| Eye | Cataract | | | ± | ± | |
| | **Ophthalmoplegia** | | | | | ++ |
| | **Ptosis** | | | | | ++ |
| Musculoskeletal | **Exercise intolerance** | | | + | + | |
| | Muscle atrophy | | | ± | ± | |
| | Muscle weakness | | | ± | ± | |
| Routine laboratory | Lactate (*P*) | | | ↑ | ↑ | |
| | Lactate (*CSF*) | | | ↑ | ↑ | |

*CSF* Cerebrospinal fluid, *P* Plasma

**Table 43.2** Adenine nucleotide translocator deficiency

| System | Symptom | Neonatal (birth–1 month) | Infancy (1–18 months) | Childhood (1.5–11 years) | Adolescence (11–16 years) | Adulthood (>16 years) |
|---|---|---|---|---|---|---|
| CNS | Dementia | | | | | ± |
| Ear | Hearing loss | | | | | + |
| | Ophthalmoplegia | | | | | + |
| Musculoskeletal | **Exercise intolerance** | | | | | + |
| | Muscle weakness | | | | | + |
| Routine laboratory | Lactate (*P*) | | | | | *n*-↑ |

*P* Plasma

**Table 43.3** Mitochondrial phosphate carrier deficiency

| System | Symptoms and biomarkers | Neonatal (birth–1 month) | Infancy (1–18 months) | Childhood (1.5–11 years) | Adolescence (11–16 years) | Adulthood (>16 years) |
|---|---|---|---|---|---|---|
| Cardiovascular | Cardiomyopathy, hypertrophic | +++ | +++ | ± | | + |
| CNS | Developmental delay, motor | | +++ | + | | |
| | Hypotonia | +++ | +++ | | | |
| Musculoskeletal | Exercise intolerance | | | + | | + |
| | Myopathy | | +++ | + | | + |
| Other | Death | | +++ | | | |
| | Failure to thrive | +++ | +++ | | | |
| Laboratory findings | Lactate (*P*) | ↑↑ | ↑↑ | | | |

*P* Plasma

**Table 43.4** Aspartate-glutamate carrier 1 deficiency

| System | Symptom | Neonatal (birth–1 month) | Infancy (1–18 months) | Childhood (1.5–11 years) | Adolescence (11–16 years) | Adulthood (>16 years) |
|---|---|---|---|---|---|---|
| CNS | Apnea | | | + | | |
| | Cerebral hypomyelination | + | + | + | | |
| | Cerebrum volume | | | ↓ | | |
| | Hypotonia, muscular-axial | + | + | ++ | | |
| | Hypomyelination, global | | | ++ | | |
| | **Retardation, psychomotor** | | ++ | ++ | | |
| | Spasticity | | | ++ | | |
| | **Sporadic tonic seizures** | | + | + | | |
| | Tendon reflexes, increased | | | ++ | | |
| Routine laboratory | **Lactate (*P*)** | ↑↑ | ↑↑ | ↑↑ | | |
| Special laboratory | **ATP production (*M*)** | | | ↓↓ | | |
| | *MRS*: *N*-acetyl aspartate (*CNS*) | | | ↓↓ | | |
| | Respiratory chain activity (*M*) | | | *n* | | |

*MRS* Magnetic resonance spectroscopy, *M* Muscle, *P* Plasma

**Table 43.5** Cytosolic glycerol-3-phosphate dehydrogenase deficiency

| System | Symptom | Neonatal (birth–1 month) | Infancy (1–18 months) | Childhood (1.5–11 years) | Adolescence (11–16 years) | Adulthood (>16 years) |
|---|---|---|---|---|---|---|
| Digestive | Hepatomegaly | + | + | + | | |
| | Liver fibrosis | + | + | + | | |
| | Liver steatosis | + | + | + | | |
| Hematological | Splenomegaly | ± | ± | ± | | |
| Musculoskeletal | Short stature | + | + | + | | |
| Routine laboratory | ASAT/ALAT (*P*) | ↑ | ↑ | ↑ | | |
| | Cholesterol (*S*) | *n*-↑ | *n*-↑ | *n*-↑ | | |
| | Lipoprotein (a) (*P*) | *n*-↑ | *n*-↑ | *n*-↑ | | |
| | Triglyceride (*S*) | ↑ | ↑ | *n*-↑ | | |
| Special laboratory | Dicarboxylic acids (*U*) | ↑ | ↑ | | | |

*P* Plasma, *S* Serum, *U* Urine

**Table 43.6** Combined oxidative phosphorylation deficiency-28

| System | Symptom | Neonatal (birth–1 month) | Infancy (1–18 months) | Childhood (1.5–11 years) | Adolescence (11–16 years) | Adulthood (>16 years) |
|---|---|---|---|---|---|---|
| Cardiovascular | Cardiopulmonary failure | + | + | | | |
| Musculoskeletal | Hydrops | ± | ± | | | |
| | **Muscle weakness** | + | + | | | |
| Other | Death | ± | ± | | | |
| | Developmental delay | + | + | | | |
| | **Lactic acidosis** | + | + | | | |
| Routine laboratory | **Pyruvate (*P*)** | ↑ | ↑ | | | |
| Special laboratory | Respiratory chain activity (*M*) | ↓ | ↓ | | | |

*M* Muscle, *P* Plasma

**Table 43.7** Mitochondrial citrate carrier deficiency

| System | Symptom | Neonatal (birth–1 month) | Infancy (1–18 months) | Childhood (1.5–11 years) | Adolescence (11–16 years) | Adulthood (>16 years) |
|---|---|---|---|---|---|---|
| CNS | **Cerebellar hypoplasia** | + | + | + | | |
| | Delayed gyration | + | + | + | | |
| | **Delayed myelination** | + | + | + | | |
| | **Encephalopathy** | + | + | + | | |
| | Irritability | + | + | + | | |
| | Lateral ventricular enlargement | + | + | + | | |
| | Microcephaly | ± | ± | ± | | |
| | **Seizures** | + | + | + | | |
| Digestive | **Feeding difficulties** | + | + | + | | |
| | Hepatomegaly | ± | ± | ± | | |
| Eye | Blindness, cortical | ± | ± | ± | | |
| | **Poor visual fixation** | + | + | + | | |
| Musculoskeletal | Hypotonia | ++ | ++ | ++ | | |
| | Regression, psychomotor | | + | + | | |
| Respiratory | Dyspnea | + | + | + | | |
| | **Respiratory insufficiency** | + | + | + | | |
| | Stridor, inspiratory | + | + | + | | |
| Other | Death | | + | + | | |
| Routine laboratory | Alpha-ketoglutaric acid (*U*) | ↑ | ↑ | ↑ | | |
| | d-2-Hydroxyglutaric acid (*CSF*) | ↑ | ↑ | ↑ | | |
| | d-2-Hydroxyglutaric acid (*P*) | ↑ | ↑ | ↑ | | |
| | d-2-Hydroxyglutaric acid (*U*) | ↑ | ↑ | ↑ | | |
| | l-2-Hydroxyglutaric acid (*CSF*) | ↑ | ↑ | ↑ | | |
| | l-2-Hydroxyglutaric acid (*P*) | ↑ | ↑ | ↑ | | |
| | l-2-Hydroxyglutaric acid (*U*) | ↑ | ↑ | ↑ | | |

*CSF* Cerebrospinal fluid, *P* Plasma, *U* Urine

**Table 43.8** Mitochondrial ATP-$Mg^{2+}$/phosphate transporter deficiency

| System | Symptom | Neonatal (birth–1 month) | Infancy (1–18 months) | Childhood (1.5–11 years) | Adolescence (11–16 years) | Adulthood (>16 years) |
|---|---|---|---|---|---|---|
| Cardiovascular | Aortic ectasia | + | + | + | + | |
| | **Atrial septal defect** | + | + | + | + | |
| | Bicuspid aortic valve | + | + | + | | |
| | Left ventricular hypertrophy | + | + | + | + | |
| | **Patent ductus arteriosus** | + | + | + | + | |
| | **Pulmonary arterial hypertension** | + | + | + | + | |
| | **Tricuspid insufficiency** | + | + | + | + | |
| CNS | **Brachycephaly** | + | + | + | + | + |
| | Cerebellar hypoplasia | + | + | + | + | |
| | Lateral ventricular enlargement | + | + | + | | |
| | Microcephaly | ± | ± | ± | ± | |
| | Posterior fossa anomalies (*MRI*) | + | + | + | | |
| | **Thin corpus callosum** | + | + | + | | |
| | Turricephaly | + | + | + | + | + |
| Dermatological | Coarse scalp hair | | + | + | + | |
| | Dermal translucency | + | + | + | + | |
| | Nail abnormalities | + | + | + | + | |
| | **Wrinkly skin** | + | + | + | | |
| Digestive | Feeding difficulties | + | + | + | | |
| | **Gastroesophageal reflux** | + | + | + | + | |
| Ear | **Dysplastic ears** | + | + | + | + | |
| | Hearing loss, conductive | | ± | ± | ± | |
| | **Low-set ears** | + | + | + | + | |
| | **Posteriorly rotated ears** | + | + | + | + | |
| Eye | **Deeply set eyes** | + | + | + | + | |
| | **Downslanting palpebral fissures** | + | + | + | + | |
| | **Hyperopia** | + | + | + | + | |
| | Hypertelorism | + | + | + | + | |
| | Laterally upslanting eyebrows | + | + | + | + | |
| | Short palpebral fissures | + | + | + | + | |
| Genitourinary | Cryptorchidism | + | + | + | | |
| | Hypoplastic labia majora | + | + | + | | |
| | Micropenis | | + | + | + | |
| Hair | **Hypertrichosis** | | + | + | + | |
| | Hypertrichosis | + | + | + | + | |
| | **Low frontal hairline** | | + | + | + | + |
| Musculoskeletal | **Flat philtrum** | + | + | + | + | |
| | Hydrocephalus | + | + | | | |
| | Hypotonia | + | + | + | + | |
| | **Long philtrum** | + | + | + | + | |
| | **Micrognathia** | + | + | + | + | |
| | Midface hypoplasia | + | + | + | + | |
| | Muscle weakness | | ± | ± | ± | |
| | Prognathia | + | + | + | + | |
| | Regression, psychomotor | | + | + | + | |
| | **Retrognathia** | + | + | + | + | |
| | **Short stature** | | + | + | + | + |
| | **Triangular face** | + | + | + | + | + |

(continued)

**Table 43.8** (continued)

| System | Symptom | Neonatal (birth–1 month) | Infancy (1–18 months) | Childhood (1.5–11 years) | Adolescence (11–16 years) | Adulthood (>16 years) |
|---|---|---|---|---|---|---|
| Respiratory | **Pulmonary hypoplasia** | + | + | + | + | |
| | Respiratory insufficiency | + | + | + | + | |
| Other | Arched palate, high | + | + | + | + | |
| | Death | ± | ± | | | |
| | Failure to thrive | + | + | | | |
| | Intrauterine growth retardation | + | | | | |
| | Large anterior fontanel | + | + | | | |
| | **Microdontia** | | + | + | + | |
| | **Oligodontia** | | + | + | + | |
| | Progeroid appearance | + | + | + | + | |
| | Protruding tongue | + | + | + | + | |
| | **Small nipples** | + | + | + | | |
| | Small nose | + | + | + | + | |
| | **Synophrys** | + | + | + | + | |
| | **Thin upper lips** | + | + | + | + | |
| | Umbilical hernia | + | + | + | | |
| | Widely spaced nipples | + | + | + | | |

*MRI* Magnetic resonance imaging

**Table 43.9** Mitochondrial aspartate aminotransferase deficiency

| System | Symptom | Neonatal (birth–1 month) | Infancy (1–18 months) | Childhood (1.5–11 years) | Adolescence (11–16 years) | Adulthood (>16 years) |
|---|---|---|---|---|---|---|
| CNS | **Microcephaly** | | | + | | |
| | **Seizures** | | | + | | |
| | Sleep disturbances | | | + | | |
| | **Spasticity** | | | + | | |
| Digestive | Abdominal pain | | | + | | |
| Special laboratory | Serine (*CSF*) | | | ↓ | | |

*CSF* Cerebrospinal fluid

**Table 43.10** Mitochondrial dicarboxylate transporter deficiency

| System | Symptom | Neonatal (birth–1 month) | Infancy (1–18 months) | Childhood (1.5–11 years) | Adolescence (11–16 years) | Adulthood (>16 years) |
|---|---|---|---|---|---|---|
| CNS | EEG, abnormal | | | + | | |
| | **Infantile spasms** | | | + | | |
| | **Quadriparesis** | | | + | | |
| | **Seizures** | | | + | | |
| Hematological | Anemia, microcytic, hypochromic | | | | | |
| Musculoskeletal | **Hypotonia** | | | + | | |

**Table 43.11** Mitochondrial ornithine transporter deficiency

| System | Symptom | Neonatal (birth–1 month) | Infancy (1–18 months) | Childhood (1.5–11 years) | Adolescence (11–16 years) | Adulthood (>16 years) |
|---|---|---|---|---|---|---|
| Autonomic system | Temperature instability | ± | | | | |
| CNS | Asterixis | | | | | ± |
| | Ataxia | | | ± | ± | ± |
| | **Coma** | ± | ± | ± | ± | ± |
| | Confusion, episodic | | | ± | ± | ± |
| | **Developmental delay** | | + | + | + | + |
| | **Encephalopathy** | ± | ± | ± | ± | ± |
| | **Pyramidal signs** | | | ± | ± | ± |
| | Seizures | ± | ± | ± | ± | ± |
| | **Spastic paresis** | | | ± | ± | ± |
| | **Stroke-like episodes** | ± | ± | ± | ± | ± |

Table 43.11 (continued)

| System | Symptom | Neonatal (birth–1 month) | Infancy (1–18 months) | Childhood (1.5–11 years) | Adolescence (11–16 years) | Adulthood (>16 years) |
|---|---|---|---|---|---|---|
| Digestive | Feeding, protein aversion | ± | ± | ± | ± | ± |
| | Liver dysfunction | ± | ± | ± | ± | ± |
| | Liver failure, acute | | ± | ± | | |
| | **Vomiting** | ± | ± | ± | ± | ± |
| Eye | Vision, impairment | | | | ± | ± |
| Other | Failure to thrive | *n* | ± | ± | ± | ± |
| Routine laboratory | ASAT/ALAT (*P*) | ↑ | ↑ | ↑ | ↑ | ↑ |
| | **Ammonia (*B*)** | ↑↑ | ↑↑ | ↑↑ | ↑↑ | ↑↑ |
| | Urea (*P*) | ↓-*n* | ↓-*n* | ↓-*n* | ↓-*n* | ↓-*n* |
| Special laboratory | Arginine (*P*) | n | n | n | n | n |
| | Citrulline (*P*) | n | n | n | n | n |
| | Creatine (*P*) | n | ↓-*n* | ↓-*n* | ↓-*n* | ↓-*n* |
| | Factor VII | ↓-*n* | ↓-*n* | ↓-*n* | ↓-*n* | ↓-*n* |
| | Factor X | ↓-*n* | ↓-*n* | ↓-*n* | ↓-*n* | ↓-*n* |
| | Glutamine (*P*) | *n*-↑ | *n*-↑ | *n*-↑ | *n*-↑ | *n*-↑ |
| | **Homocitrulline (*U*)** | ↑↑ | ↑↑ | ↑↑ | ↑↑ | ↑↑ |
| | **Ornithine (*P*)** | *n*-↑ | ↑↑ | ↑↑ | ↑↑ | ↑↑ |
| | $^{14}$C-Ornitine incorporation (*F*) | ↓ | ↓ | ↓ | ↓ | ↓ |
| | Orotic acid (*U*) | *n*-↑ | *n*-↑ | *n*-↑ | *n*-↑ | *n*-↑ |

*B* Blood, *F* Fibroblasts, *P* Plasma, *U* Urine

Table 43.12 Citrin deficiency

| System | Symptoms and biomarkers | Neonatal (birth–1 month) | Infancy (1–18 months) | Childhood (1.5–11 years) | Adolescence (11–16 years) | Adulthood (>16 years) |
|---|---|---|---|---|---|---|
| CNS | Ataxia | | | | ± | ± |
| | **Coma** | | | | + | + |
| | Confusion, episodic | | | | ± | ± |
| | Consciousness disturbance | | | | ± | ± |
| | **Developmental delay** | | | | ± | ± |
| | **Encephalopathy** | | | | + | + |
| | Fatigue | | | ± | | |
| Digestive | **Cholestasis, intrahepatic** | ++ | + | | | |
| | Hepatomegaly | + | + | | | |
| | **Jaundice** | ++ | + | | | |
| | Liver dysfunction | ++ | + | | | |
| | Liver steatosis | ± | ± | | ± | ± |
| | **Low carbohydrate, high protein and high fat intake** | | | + | + | + |
| | Pancreatitis, recurrent | | | ± | | ± |
| Hematological | Anemia | ++ | + | | | |
| | Impaired coagulation | + | + | | | |
| Musculoskeletal | Growth retardation | ± | ± | ± | | |
| Other | Failure to thrive | ++ | + | ± | | |
| Psychiatric | **Neuropsychiatric manifestations, sudden onset** | | | | ± | ± |

(continued)

**Table 43.12** (continued)

| System | Symptoms and biomarkers | Neonatal (birth–1 month) | Infancy (1–18 months) | Childhood (1.5–11 years) | Adolescence (11–16 years) | Adulthood (>16 years) |
|---|---|---|---|---|---|---|
| Laboratory findings | Albumin (*P*) | ↓↓ | ↓ | n | n | n |
| | Alpha-fetoprotein (*S*) | ↑↑ | ↑ | n | n | n |
| | Ammonia (*B* and *P*) | n-↑ | n-↑ | n | n-↑↑ | ↑↑ |
| | Arginine (*P*) | n-↑ | n-↑ | n | n | n-↑ |
| | ASAT/ALAT (*P*) | n-↑ | n-↑ | n | n | n |
| | Bilirubin, total/direct (*P*) | ↑↑ | ↑ | n | n | n |
| | Citrulline (*P*) | ↑-↑↑ | ↑-↑↑ | n-↑ | n-↑ | ↑↑ |
| | Erythrocyte count (*B*) | ↓↓ | ↓ | n | n | n |
| | Galactose (*P*) | ↑ | ↑ | n | n | n |
| | Galactose (*U*) | ↑↑ | ↑ | n | n | n |
| | Gamma-glutamyltransferase GGT (*P*) | ↑↑ | ↑-n | n | n | n |
| | Glucose (*P*) | n-↓ | n-↓ | n | n | n |
| | Glutamine (*P*) | n-↑ | n-↑ | n | n | n-↑ |
| | HDL cholesterol (*P*) | n | n | n-↑ | n | n |
| | LDL cholesterol (*P*) | n | n | n-↑ | n | n |
| | Methionine (*P*) | ↑ | ↑ | n | n | ↑ |
| | Phenylalanine (*P*) | ↑ | ↑ | n | n | ↑ |
| | Prothrombin time | n-↑ | n-↑ | n | n | n |
| | Succinylacetone (*P*) | n | n | n | n | n |
| | Threonine (*P*) | ↑ | ↑ | n | n | ↑ |
| | Total protein (*P*) | ↓↓ | ↓ | n | n | n |
| | Tyrosine (*P*) | ↑ | ↑ | n | n | ↑ |

Two forms, neonatal and later form, are distinguished. The neonatal form is dominated by intrahepatic cholestasis and jaundice, generally waning out with carbohydrate-devoid formula. The adult form is dominated by the symptoms and signs of hyperammonemia. Both forms are caused by mutations in the same gene
*B* Blood, *P* Plasma, *S* Serum, *U* Urine

**Table 43.13** Mitochondrial glutamate carrier 1 deficiency

| System | Symptom | Neonatal (birth–1 month) | Infancy (1–18 months) | Childhood (1.5–11 years) | Adolescence (11–16 years) | Adulthood (>16 years) |
|---|---|---|---|---|---|---|
| CNS | **Cerebral atrophy (*MRI*)** | + | + | + | + | |
| | **CNS, abnormal (*MRI*)** | | | ++ | | |
| | ERG, abnormal | | | ± | | |
| | **EEG, abnormal** | ++ | ++ | ++ | | |
| | **Encephalopathy, progressive** | + | + | ++ | + | |
| | **Hypotonia** | ++ | ++ | ++ | ++ | |
| | Microcephaly | - | – | + | | |
| | **Myoclonic epilepsy** | ++ | ++ | ++ | ++ | |
| | Retardation, psychomotor | + | ++ | ++ | +++ | |
| | Spasticity | | | ± | | |
| | Vegetative state | | | ± | | |
| Routine laboratory | **Proline (*P*)** | ↑ | ↑ | ↑ | | |
| Special laboratory | **Glutamate oxidation (*F*)** | | | ↓↓ | | |

*F* Fibroblasts, *MRI* Magnetic resonance imaging, *P* Plasma

**Table 43.14** Mitochondrial glycine transporter deficiency

| System | Symptom | Neonatal (birth–1 month) | Infancy (1–18 months) | Childhood (1.5–11 years) | Adolescence (11–16 years) | Adulthood (>16 years) |
|---|---|---|---|---|---|---|
| Hematological | **Anemia, microcytic, hypochromic** | ++ | ++ | ++ | ++ | ++ |
| | **Anemia, sideroblastic** | ++ | ++ | ++ | ++ | ++ |
| | **Hepatosplenomegaly** | | + | + | + | + |
| Special laboratory | **Ferritin (*S*)** | | ↑ | ↑ | ↑ | ↑ |

*S* Serum

**Table 43.15** Bilateral striatal necrosis (SLC25A19)

| System | Symptom | Neonatal (birth–1 month) | Infancy (1–18 months) | Childhood (1.5–11 years) | Adolescence (11–16 years) | Adulthood (>16 years) |
|---|---|---|---|---|---|---|
| CNS | **Basal ganglia lesions (*MRI*)** | | | +++ | +++ | +++ |
| | **Dystonia** | | | ++ | ++ | ++ |
| | **Encephalopathy acute, precipitated by infection** | | | +++ | +++ | +++ |
| | **Polyneuropathy** | | | +++ | +++ | +++ |
| Routine laboratory | **Lactate (*CSF*)** | | | *n*-↑ | *n*-↑ | *n*-↑ |
| Special laboratory | Alpha-ketoglutarate (*U*) | | | ↑ | ↑ | ↑ |

*CSF* Cerebrospinal fluid, *MRI* Magnetic resonance imaging, *U* Urine

**Table 43.16** Mitochondrial flavin adenine dinucleotide transporter (MFT) deficiency

| System | Symptoms and biomarkers | Neonatal (birth–1 month) | Infancy (1–18 months) | Childhood (1.5–11 years) | Adolescence (11–16 years) | Adulthood (>16 years) |
|---|---|---|---|---|---|---|
| CNS | Dysarthria | | | | | ± |
| | Swallowing difficulties | | | | | ± |
| Musculoskeletal | **Exercise intolerance** with nausea or vomiting during excercise | | | | + | + |
| | **Lipid storage myopathy with ragged-red fibres** | | | | + | + |
| | Muscle weakness | | | ± | ± | ± |
| Other | **Riboflavin responsiveness** | | | ++ | ++ | ++ |
| Laboratory findings | 2-Hydroxyglutaric acid (*U*) | | | | n to ↑ | n-↑ |
| | **2-Methylbutyrylglycine (*U*)** | | | | ↑ | ↑ |
| | **C4-C10 acylcarnitines (*P*, *DBS*)** | | | | ↑↑ | ↑↑ |
| | **Ethylmalonic acid (*U*)** | | | | ↑↑ | ↑↑ |
| | Glutaric acid (*U*) | | | | n to ↑↑ | n-↑ |
| | Glutarylcarnitine (*P*, *DBS*) | | | | ↑ | ↑ |
| | Hexanoylglycine (*U*) | | | | n | n |
| | **Isobutyrylglycine (*U*)** | | | | ↑ | ↑ |
| | **Isovalerylglycine (*U*)** | | | | ↑ | ↑ |
| | Lactate (*B*) | | | | ↑ | ↑ |
| | Suberylglycine (*U*) | | | | n | n |

*B* Blood, *DBS* Dried blood spot, *P* Plasma, *U* Urine

**Table 43.17** Mitochondrial coenzyme A transporter deficiency

| System | Symptom | Neonatal (birth–1 month) | Infancy (1–18 months) | Childhood (1.5–11 years) | Adolescence (11–16 years) | Adulthood (>16 years) |
|---|---|---|---|---|---|---|
| CNS | **Basal ganglia abnormalities (*MRI*)** | ± | ± | ± | + | + |
| | Intellectual disability | + | + | + | ± | ± |
| Cardiovascular | Cardiomegaly | ± | ± | ± | ± | ± |
| Musculoskeletal | Movement disorder | ± | ± | ± | ± | ± |
| | **Myopathy** | + | + | + | + | + |
| Other | Developmental delay | + | + | + | ± | ± |
| Routine laboratory | Ammonia (*P*) | *n*-↑ | *n*-↑ | *n*-↑ | *n*-↑ | |
| | Carnitine, free | ↓-*n* | ↓-*n* | ↓-*n* | ↓-*n* | |
| | Creatine kinase (*P*) | *n*-↑ | *n*-↑ | *n*-↑ | *n*-↑ | |
| | Lactate (*P*) | ↑ | ↑ | ↑ | ↑ | |
| | Long-chain acylcarnitine | *n*-↑ | *n*-↑ | *n*-↑ | *n*-↑ | |
| | Medium-chain acylcarnitine | *n*-↑ | *n*-↑ | *n*-↑ | *n*-↑ | |

*MRI* Magnetic resonance imaging, *P* Plasma

## Reference Values

Important note: reference values may vary between laboratories, and the values listed in this chapter should only be used as a guideline.

| Parameter | Method | Neonatal | Infancy | Childhood | Adolescence | Adulthood |
|---|---|---|---|---|---|---|
| Adipic acid (*U*) (mmol/mol creatinine)[a] | GC–MS | 2–27 | 0–25 | 2–10 | 1–7 | 1–7 |
| Alpha-ketoglutarate (*U*) (mmol/mol creatinine)[b] | GC–MS | <150 | <150 | <150 | <150 | <150 |
| Ammonia (*P, B*) (μmol/L)[a] | Enzymatic-UV | 0–60 | 0–60 | 0–60 | 0–60 | 0–60 |
| Arginine (*P*) (μmol/L)[a] | LC–MS/MS | 29–134 | 29–134 | 31–132 | 31–132 | 32–120 |
| ALAT (*P*) (IU/L)[a] | Enzymatic–fluorometric | 10–50 | 10–40 | 10–40 | 10–40 | 10–40 |
| ASAT (*P*) (IU/L)[a] | Enzymatic–fluorometric | 20–80 | 15–60 | 10–40 | 10–40 | 10–40 |
| Carnitine, free (nmol/mL)[a] | FIA-MS/MS | 10–49 | 24–63 | 22–66 | 22–65 | 25–54 |
| C4 acylcarnitine (*P*) (nmol/mL)[a] | FIA-MS/MS | <0.46 | <1.06 | <1.06 | <0.83 | <0.83 |
| C5 acylcarnitine (*P*) (nmol/mL)[a] | FIA-MS/MS | <0.38 | <0.38 | <0.63 | <0.51 | <0.51 |
| C10-acylcarnitine (*P*) (nmol/mL)[a] | FIA-MS/MS | <0.27 | <0.27 | <0.91 | <0.88 | <0.88 |
| C12:0-acylcarnitine (*P*) (nmol/mL)[a] | FIA-MS/MS | <0.18 | <0.18 | <0.35 | <0.26 | <0.26 |
| C14:0-acylcarnitine (*S*) (nmol/mL)[a] | FIA-MS/MS | <0.11 | <0.11 | <0.15 | <0.12 | <0.12 |
| C16:0-acylcarnitine (*P*) (nmol/mL)[a] | FIA-MS/MS | <0.36 | <0.36 | <0.52 | <0.23 | <0.23 |
| C18:0-acylcarnitine (*P*) (nmol/mL)[a] | FIA-MS/MS | <0.10 | <0.10 | <0.12 | <0.14 | <0.14 |
| Cholesterol (*S*) (mg/dL)[a] | Enzymatic–colorimetric | ≤199 | ≤199 | ≤199 | ≤199 | ≤199 |
| Citrulline (*P*) (μmol/L)[a] | LC–MS/MS | 9–38 | 9–45 | 11–45 | 11–45 | 17–46 |
| Creatine (*P*) (μmol/L)[c] | LC–MS/MS | 17–109 | 17–109 | 17–109 | 6–50 | 6–50 |
| Creatine kinase (*P*) (U/L)[a] | Enzymatic-UV | **M** 30–225<br>**F** 20–175 | **M** 30–225<br>**F** 20–175 | **M** 30–225<br>**F** 20–175 | **M** 30–225<br>**F** 20–175 | **M** 30–225<br>**F** 20–175 |
| D-2-Hydroxyglutaric acid (*CSF*) (μmol/L)[b] | GC–MS | 0.07–0.34 | 0.07–0.34 | 0.07–0.34 | 0.07–0.34 | 0.07–0.34 |
| D-2-Hydroxyglutaric acid (*P*) (μmol/L)[b] | GC–MS | 0.28–0.93 | 0.28–0.93 | 0.28–0.93 | 0.28–0.93 | 0.28–0.93 |
| D-2-Hydroxyglutaric acid (*U*) (mmol/mol creatinine)[b] | GC–MS | 2.8–17 | 2.8–17 | 2.8–17 | 2.8–17 | 2.8–17 |
| Dicarboxylic acids (*U*) (mmol/mol creatinine)[d] | GC–MS | See sebacid and suberic acid below, as examples of urinary dicarboxylic acids | | | | |
| Ethylmalonic acid (*U*) (mg/g creatinine)[a] | GC–MS | 0.5–20.2 | 0.5–20.2 | 0.5–20.2 | 0.5–20.2 | 0.5–20.2 |
| Factor VII (% of normal activity)[e] | Enzymatic–colorimetric | 58–150 | 58–150 | 58–150 | 58–150 | 58–150 |
| Factor X (% of normal activity)[e] | Enzymatic–colorimetric | 65–142 | 65–142 | 65–142 | 65–142 | 65–142 |
| Ferritin (*S*) (μg/L)[a] | Immunoturbidimetric | 25–200 | **1–2 months**<br>200–600<br>**2–6 months**<br>50–200<br>**6–48 months**<br>7–142 | 7–142 | 7–142 | **M** 24–336<br>**F** 11–307 |
| Galactose (*P*) (mg/dL)[a] | Spectrophotometric, kinetic | **≤7 days** < 5.4<br>**8–14 days** < 3.6<br>**≥15 days** < 2.0 | <2.0 | <2.0 | <2.0 | <2.0 |
| Galactose (*U*) (mg/dL)[a] | TLC | 0 | 0 | 0 | 0 | 0 |
| Glutamine (*P*) (μmol/L)[a] | LC–MS/MS | 316–1020 | 316–976 | 329–976 | 329–976 | 317–957 |
| Glutamine (*CSF*) (μmol/L)[a] | LC–MS/MS | 467–1832 | 301–1128 | 326–1092 | 326–1092 | 380–1348 |
| Glutaric acid (*U*) (mg/g creatinine)[a] | GC–MS | 0.6–15.2 | 0.6–15.2 | 0.6–15.2 | 0.6–15.2 | 0.6–15.2 |
| Hexanoylglycine (*U*) (mg/g creatinine)[a] | GC–MS | 0.2–1.9 | 0.2–1.9 | 0.2–1.9 | 0.2–1.9 | 0.2–1.9 |
| Homocitrulline (*U*) (μmol/L)[a] | LC–MS/MS | <5 | <5 | <2 | <2 | <2 |
| Isobutyrylglycine (*U*) (mg/g creatinine)[a] | GC–MS | 0–11 | 0–11 | 0–11 | 0–11 | 0–11 |

(continued)

| Parameter | Method | Neonatal | Infancy | Childhood | Adolescence | Adulthood |
|---|---|---|---|---|---|---|
| Isovalerylglycine (*U*) (mg/g creatinine)[a] | GC–MS | 0.3–14.3 | 0.3–14.3 | 0.3–14.3 | 0.3–14.3 | 0.3–14.3 |
| L-2-Hydroxyglutaric acid (*CSF*) (μmol/L)[b] | GC–MS | 0.25–2.3 | 0.25–2.3 | 0.25–2.3 | 0.25–2.3 | 0.25–2.3 |
| L-2-Hydroxyglutaric acid (*P*) (μmol/L)[b] | GC–MS | 0.45–1.0 | 0.45–1.0 | 0.45–1.0 | 0.45–1.0 | 0.45–1.0 |
| L-2-Hydroxyglutaric acid (*U*) (mmol/mol creatinine)[b] | GC–MS | 1.3–19 | 1.3–19 | 1.3–19 | 1.3–19 | 1.3–19 |
| Lactate (*P*) (mmol/L)[a] | Enzymatic–colorimetric | 0–2 | 0–2 | 0–2 | 0–2 | 0–2 |
| Lactate (*CSF*) (mmol/L)[a] | Enzymatic–colorimetric | 0–2 | 0–2 | 0–2 | 0–2 | 0–2 |
| Lipoprotein (a) (*P*) (mg/dL)[a] | Immunoturbidimetric | <30 | <30 | <30 | <30 | <30 |
| Long-chain acylcarnitine (*P*) (μmol/L)[a] | FIA–MS/MS | See C12:0, C14:0, C16:0, and C16-acycarnitine above as examples of long-chain acylcarnitine | | | | |
| Medium-chain acylcarnitine (*P*) (μmol/L)[a] | FIA–MS/MS | See C10-acycarnitine above as an example of medium-chain acylcarnitine | | | | |
| Methionine (*P*) (μmol/L)[a] | LC–MS/MS | 11–35 | 11–37 | 11–37 | 11–37 | 4–44 |
| 2-Methylbutyrylglycine (*U*) (mg/g creatinine)[a] | GC–MS | 0.3–7.5 | 0.3–7.5 | 0.3–7.5 | 0.3–7.5 | 0.3–7.5 |
| Ornithine (*P*) (μmol/L)[a] | LC–MS/MS | 20–130 | 20–130 | 22–97 | 22–97 | 38–130 |
| Orotic acid (*U*) (mmol/mol creatinine)[a] | Enzymatic–colorimetric | **<2 weeks** 1.4–5.3<br>**1–4 weeks** 1–3.2 | 1.0–3.2 | 0.5–3.3 | 0.4–1.2 | 0.4–1.2 |
| Proline (μmol/L)[a] | LC–MS/MS | 85–303 | 85–303 | 80–357 | 80–357 | 97–368 |
| Pyruvate (*P*) (mmol/L)[a] | Enzymatic–colorimetric | 0.03–0.15 | 0.03–0.15 | 0.03–0.15 | 0.03–0.15 | 0.03–0.15 |
| Sebacic acid (*U*) (mmol/mol creatinine)[d] | GC–MS | 3–16 | 3–16 | <8 | <8 | <8 |
| Serine (*CSF*) (μmol/L)[a] | LC–MS/MS | 69–271 | 69–271 | 71–208 | 71–208 | 63–187 |
| Suberic acid (*U*) (mmol/mol creatinine)[d] | GC–MS | 4–20 | 4–20 | <8 | <8 | <8 |
| Threonine (*P*) (μmol/L)[a] | LC–MS/MS | 47–237 | 47–237 | 58–195 | 58–195 | 85–231 |
| Triglyceride (*S*) (mmol/L)[a] | Enzymatic–colorimetric | <150 | <150 | <150 | <150 | <150 |
| Tyrosine (*P*) (μmol/L)[a] | LC-MS/MS | 26–115 | 26–115 | 31–106 | 31–106 | 31–90 |
| Urea (*P*) (mg/dL)[a] | Enzymatic–colorimetric | 4–16 | **2-3 months**<br>4–16<br>**3–48 months**<br>6–18 | 6–18 | 6–18 | 8–20 |

Abbreviations: *CSF* Cerebrospinal fluid, *FIA-MS/MS* Flow injection analysis–tandem mass spectrometry, *GC–MS* Gas chromatography–mass Spectrometry, *LC–MS/MS* Liquid chromatography–tandem mass spectrometry, *P* Plasma, *S* Serum, *TLC* Thin-layer chromatography, *U* Urine, *UV* Ultraviolet

[a]Reference values obtained from Spectrum Health's Laboratory Test Directory (spectrumhealth.testcatalog.org)

[b]Reference values obtained from Muntau et al. (2000)

[c]Reference values obtained from Halbach et al. (2011)

[d]Reference values obtained from Rinaldo (2008)

[e]Reference values obtained from Andropoulos (2012)

## Pathological Values

| Parameter | Disease | Neonatal | Infancy | Childhood | Adolescence | Adulthood |
|---|---|---|---|---|---|---|
| Adipic acid (*U*) | 43.16 | | | ↑ | | |
| Alpha-ketoglutarate (*U*) | 43.7 | ↑ | ↑ | ↑ | | |
| | 43.15 | | | ↑ | ↑ | ↑ |
| Ammonia (*B*) | 43.11 | ↑↑ | ↑↑ | ↑↑ | ↑↑ | ↑↑ |
| | 43.12 | *n*–↑ | *n*–↑ | *n*–↑ | ↑ | ↑ |
| Ammonia (*P*) | 43.17 | *n*–↑ | *n*–↑ | *n*–↑ | *n*–↑ | |
| Arginine (*P*) | 43.11 | *n* | *n* | *n* | *n* | *n* |
| | 43.12 | ↑ | ↑ | ↑ | (↑) | (↑) |

| Parameter | Disease | Neonatal | Infancy | Childhood | Adolescence | Adulthood |
|---|---|---|---|---|---|---|
| ALAT (*P*) (IU/L) | 43.5 | ↑ | ↑ | ↑ | | |
| | 43.11 | ↑ | ↑ | ↑ | ↑ | ↑ |
| | 43.12 | *n*–↑ | *n*–↑ | *n*–↑ | *n* | *n* |
| ASAT (*P*) (IU/L) | 43.5 | ↑ | ↑ | ↑ | | |
| | 43.11 | ↑ | ↑ | ↑ | ↑ | ↑ |
| | 43.12 | *n*–↑ | *n*–↑ | *n*–↑ | *n* | *n* |
| Carnitine, free | 43.17 | ↓–*n* | ↓–*n* | ↓–*n* | ↓–*n* | |
| C4 acylcarnitine | 43.16 | | | ↑ | | |
| C5 acylcarnitine (*P*) | 43.16 | | | ↑ | | |
| C10-acylcarnitine (*P*) | 43.16 | | | ↑ | | |
| C12:0-acylcarnitine (*P*) | 43.16 | | | ↑ | | |
| C14:0-acylcarnitine (*S*) | 43.16 | | | ↑ | | |
| C16:0-acylcarnitine (*P*) | 43.16 | | | ↑ | | |
| C18:0-acylcarnitine (*P*) | 43.16 | | | ↑ | | |
| Cholesterol (*S*) | 43.5 | *n*–↑ | *n*–↑ | *n*–↑ | | |
| Citrulline (*P*) | 43.11 | *n* | *n* | *n* | *n* | *n* |
| | 43.12 | *n*–↑↑ | *n*–↑↑ | *n*–↑↑ | ↑↑ | ↑↑ |
| Creatine (*P*) | 43.11 | *n* | ↓–*n* | ↓–*n* | ↓–*n* | ↓–*n* |
| Creatine kinase (*P*) | 43.17 | *n*–↑ | *n*–↑ | *n*–↑ | *n*–↑ | |
| D-2-hydroxyglutaric acid (*CSF*) | 43.7 | ↑ | ↑ | ↑ | | |
| D-2-Hydroxyglutaric acid (*P*) | 43.7 | ↑ | ↑ | ↑ | | |
| D-2-Hydroxyglutaric acid (*U*) | 43.7 | ↑ | ↑ | ↑ | | |
| Dicarboxylic acids (*U*) | 43.5 | ↑ | ↑ | | | |
| Ethylmalonic acid (*U*) | 43.16 | | | ↑ | | |
| Factor VII | 43.11 | ↓–*n* | ↓–*n* | ↓–*n* | ↓–*n* | ↓–*n* |
| Factor X | 43.11 | ↓–*n* | ↓–*n* | ↓–*n* | ↓–*n* | ↓–*n* |
| Ferritin (*S*) (μmol/L) | 43.14 | | ↑ | ↑ | ↑ | ↑ |
| Galactose (*P*) | 43.12 | ↑ | ↑ | *n* | *n* | *n* |
| Galactose (*U*) | 43.12 | ↑↑ | ↑ | *n* | *n* | *n* |
| Glutamine (*P*) | 43.11 | *n*–↑ | *n*–↑ | *n*–↑ | *n*–↑ | *n*–↑ |
| | 43.12 | *n*–↑ | *n*–↑ | *n*–↑ | *n*–↑ | *n*–↑ |
| Glutamine (*CSF*) | 43.12 | *n*–↑ | *n*–↑ | *n*–↑ | ↑ | ↑ |
| Glutaric acid (*U*) | 43.16 | | | ↑ | | |
| Hexanoylglycine (*U*) | 43.16 | | | ↑ | | |
| Homocitrulline (*U*) | 43.11 | ↑↑ | ↑↑ | ↑↑ | ↑↑ | ↑↑ |
| Isobutyrylglycine (*U*) | 43.16 | | | ↑ | | |
| Isovalerylglycine (*U*) | 43.16 | | | ↑ | | |
| L-2-Hydroxyglutaric acid (*CSF*) | 43.7 | ↑ | ↑ | ↑ | | |
| L-2-Hydroxyglutaric acid (*P*) | 43.7 | ↑ | ↑ | ↑ | | |
| L-2-Hydroxyglutaric acid (*U*) | 43.7 | ↑ | ↑ | ↑ | | |
| Lactate (*P*) | 43.1 | | | ↑ | ↑ | |
| | 43.2 | | | | | *n*–↑ |
| | 43.3 | ↑↑↑ | ↑↑↑ | | | |
| | 43.4 | ↑↑ | ↑↑ | ↑↑ | | |
| | 43.17 | ↑ | ↑ | ↑ | ↑ | |
| Lactate (*CSF*) | 43.1 | | | ↑ | ↑ | |
| | 43.15 | | | *n*–↑ | *n*–↑ | *n*–↑ |
| Lipoprotein (a) (*P*) | 43.5 | *n*–↑ | *n*–↑ | *n*–↑ | | |
| Long-chain acylcarnitine | 43.17 | *n*–↑ | *n*–↑ | *n*–↑ | *n*–↑ | |
| Medium-chain acylcarnitine | 43.17 | *n*–↑ | *n*–↑ | *n*–↑ | *n*–↑ | |
| Methionine (*P*) (μmol/L) | 43.12 | ↑ | ↑ | ↑ | ↑ | ↑ |
| 2-Methylbutyrylglycine (*U*) | 43.16 | | | ↑ | | |
| Ornithine (*P*) | 43.11 | *n*–↑ | ↑↑ | ↑↑ | ↑↑ | ↑↑ |
| Orotic acid (*U*) | 43.11 | *n*–↑ | *n*–↑ | *n*–↑ | *n*–↑ | *n*–↑ |
| Proline | 43.13 | ↑ | ↑ | ↑ | | |
| Pyruvate (*P*) | 43.6 | ↑ | ↑ | | | |

(continued)

| Parameter | Disease | Neonatal | Infancy | Childhood | Adolescence | Adulthood |
|---|---|---|---|---|---|---|
| Sebacic acid (*U*) | 43.16 | | | ↑ | | |
| Serine (*CSF*) | 43.9 | | | ↓ | | |
| Suberic acid (*U*) | 43.16 | | | ↑ | | |
| Threonine (*P*) | 43.12 | ↑ | ↑ | ↑ | ↑ | ↑ |
| Triglyceride (*S*) | 43.5 | ↑ | ↑ | *n*–↑ | | |
| Tyrosine (*P*) | 43.12 | ↑ | ↑ | ↑ | ↑ | ↑ |
| Urea (*P*) | 43.11 | ↓–*n* | ↓–*n* | ↓–*n* | ↓–*n* | ↓–*n* |

Abbreviations: *CSF* Cerebrospinal fluid, *P* Plasma, *S* Serum, *U* Urine

## Diagnostic Flowchart

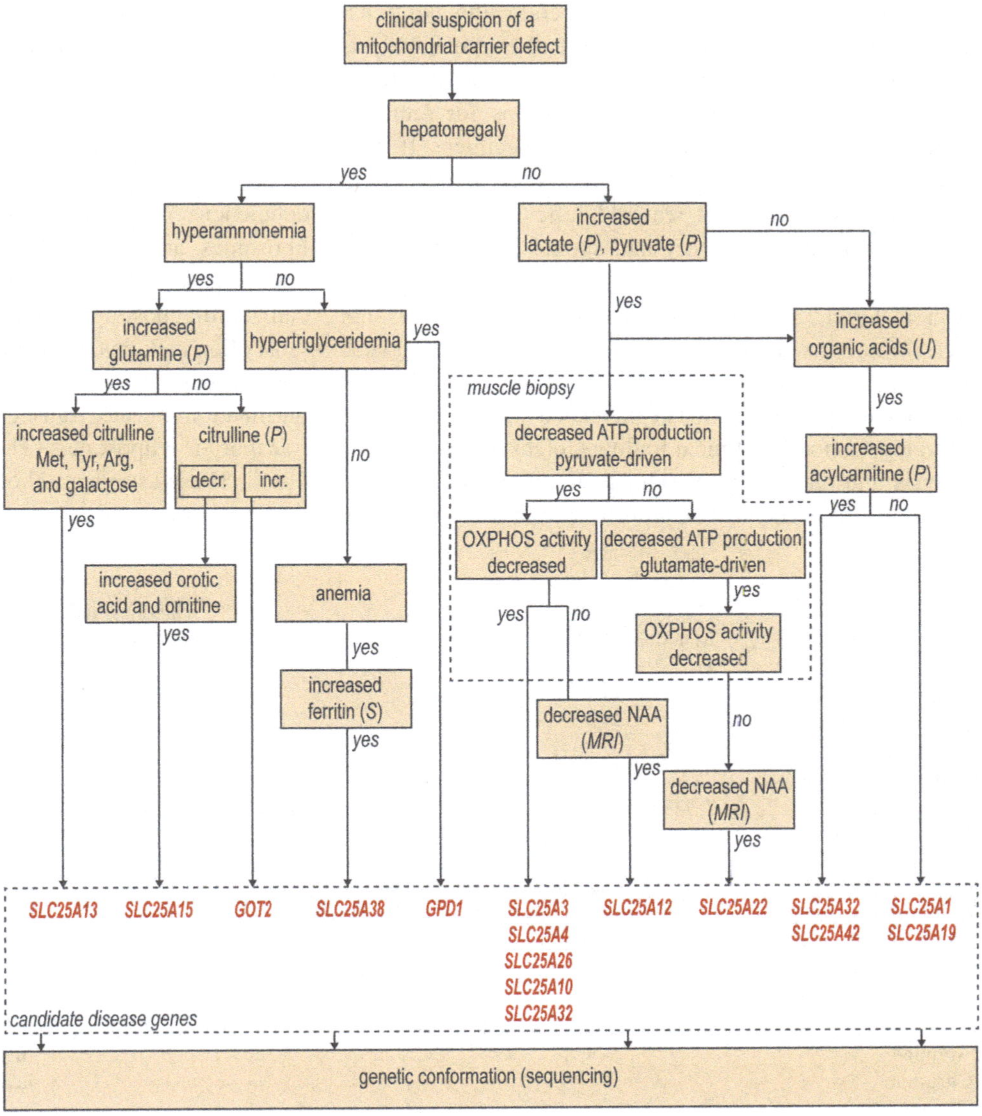


**Fig. 43.5** Diagnostic flow chart of mitochondrial carrier deficiencies. If only one option (i.e., yes or no) is indicated, the other is associated with a disease not related to a mitochondrial carrier deficiency. Besides, nowadays hardly any single candidate gene approach is done, but instead direct whole exome sequencing (WES) or even whole genome sequencing (WGS). Abbreviations: *decr* Decreased, *incr* Increased, *MRI* Magnetic resonance imaging, *NAA* *N*-acetyl aspartate, *OXPHOS* Oxidative phosphorylation, *P* Plasma, *S* Serum, *U* Urine

## Specimen Collection

The diagnostic workflow is initiated by a metabolic screening, as indicated in the above flow chart. Most often, whole exome sequencing or whole genome sequencing will subsequently be performed, which could identify a pathogenic gene defect. For others, a definite diagnosis can only be reached by biochemical examination of a tissue specimen, for example, when the genomic approaches identify a variant of uncertain significance. As a rule, the patient under investigation should not be on treatments that could mask possible enzyme deficiencies (e.g., vitamins, carnitine, certain drugs). For most biochemical determinations, one should ask the diagnostic center for information about specific requirements as to the practice of collecting and transporting material. Especially in the case of enzyme analysis in tissues or cells, it is important to consult the diagnostic laboratory in advance about the conditions for removal, preparation, storage, and transport of the specimens. If fresh tissue (e.g., a muscle biopsy) is to be studied, samples have to be collected in a special, ice-cold buffer and immediately transported to the laboratory and should preferentially be examined biochemically within 2 h after collection. In this fresh material, in which mitochondrial integrity has not been compromised, mitochondrial flux measurements, such as oxygen consumption, substrate oxidation, and ATP production can be performed. The physician should inform the laboratory about the clinical findings to ensure an adequate analysis and data interpretation. It is important to discuss which type of tissue or cell is preferable in each individual case, thereby causing the patient as little inconvenience as possible. Tissue-specific expression of mitochondrial deficiencies renders fibroblasts and lymphocytes less appropriate for general purposes than skeletal muscle, although fibroblast analysis does have an added diagnostic value when combined with a muscle sample examination. In the case of unexpected death, blood and urine specimens need to be collected as soon as possible after the patient has passed away. They should be snap frozen (not fixed) immediately after collection using liquid nitrogen and stored for possible additional studies. For enzymatic purposes, tissues must be removed within 1–2 h after death and should be frozen immediately in liquid nitrogen. Skin biopsies can be performed as late as 48 h after death and must be collected at room temperature in cell culture medium, after which the sample can be transported at room temperature to the cell culture laboratory. Because few reference values are generally available for neonates, it is recommended to perform a muscle biopsy beyond the first month of life, unless a life-threatening situation exists. To assess the effect of genetic deficiencies on functional transport, radiolabeled assays in liposomes are still considered as the 'golden standard' assay. These methods are, however, only performed in specialized diagnostic or research laboratories. This approach most often includes the overexpression of the human codon-optimized transporter in *E. coli* or *L. lactis*, followed by purification of the transporter and reconstitution of the transporter in liposomes (Thompson et al. 2016; Punzi et al. 2018). These assays are though not available in most diagnostic laboratories.

| Test | Material | Collection and transport | Handling and storage | Pitfalls |
|---|---|---|---|---|
| *Acylglycines*<br>Hexanoylglycine<br>Isobutyrylglycine<br>Isovalerylglycine<br>2-Methylbutyrylglycine | *U* | – | −20 °C | – |
| *Acylcarnitines*<br>C4 acylcarnitine<br>C5 acylcarnitine<br>C10-acylcarnitine<br>C12:0-acylcarnitine<br>C14:0-acylcarnitine<br>C16:0-acylcarnitine<br>C18:0-acylcarnitine | *P, DBS* | Heparinized or EDTA blood (or serum) supernatant from clinical centrifugation (within 20 min), fresh or promptly frozen and shipped frozen (packed with dry ice) or lyophilized and shipped at room temperature with original volume specified. | *P*: 20 °C<br>*DBS*: Ambient temp. | During anabolism eventually normal values, different profile with MCT diet, long-chain acylcarnitine accumulation also in healthy individuals during catabolism |
| *Amino acids*<br>Arginine<br>Citrulline<br>Glutamine<br>Methionine<br>Ornithine<br>Proline<br>Serine<br>Threonine<br>Tyrosine | *P, CSF* | Heparinized blood sample. | −20 °C | *General*: Draw blood 3 – 4 h after a meal; harvest plasma promptly; avoid hemolysis. *Glutamine*: Freeze quickly since glutamine is unstable. *Methionine*: Liver disease, any cause. Immediate separation from plasma essential. *Citrulline*: Watermelon contains citrulline and can increase its level. *Proline*: Obtain fasting. *Tyrosine*: Liver disease, any cause; false negatives in diet - treated patients. |

(continued)

| Test | Material | Collection and transport | Handling and storage | Pitfalls |
|---|---|---|---|---|
| Ammonia | *B*, *P* | Analyze within 30 min of blood drawing. Transport blood refrigerated. Arterial blood preferable, use tourniquets minimally, do not request muscular contractions. | No storage allowed | |
| ALAT | *P* | Blood sample should be processed (centrifuged) within 2 h. Avoid hemolysis. | −20 °C (up to 72 h) | |
| ASAT | *P* | Blood sample should be processed (centrifuged) within 2 h. Avoid hemolysis. | −20 °C (up to 72 h) | |
| ATP production | *M*, *FB* | | No storage allowed | Maintain at 0 °C during analysis. |
| Carnitine, free | *P*, *DBS* | | *P*: 20 °C<br>*DBS*: Ambient temp. | |
| Cholesterol | *S* | Blood sample should be processed (centrifuged) within 2 h. transport at 4 °C. | Process and store up to 72 h at 4 °C | |
| Creatine | *P* | | | |
| Creatine kinase | *P* | | −20 °C | |
| 2-Hydroxyglutaric acid (D- and L-enantiomers) | *CSF*, *P*, *U* | | −20 °C | For specific quantification of L2HG enantiomeric separation, hyphenated to mass spectrometry is required. |
| Organic acids<br>Adipic acid<br>Alpha-ketoglutarate<br>Ethylmalonic acid<br>Glutaric acid<br>Orotic acid<br>Sebacic acid<br>Suberic acid | *U* | Fresh or frozen without preservatives and shipped frozen (packed in dry-ice) or lyophilized and shipped at room temperature with original volume specified or shipped as fresh sample with 1–2 drops of chloroform for preservation | −20 °C | If urine is refrigerated or frozen, it can precipitate out; heat urine at 37 °C until precipitate is dissolved. |
| Factor VII | *P* | Transport at ambient temperature. | Ambient temperature | Avoid hemolysis. |
| Factor X | *P* | Transport at ambient temperature. | Ambient temperature | Avoid hemolysis. |
| Ferritin | *S* | Blood sample should be processed (centrifuged) within 2 h. transport at 4 °C. | −20 °C | |
| Galactose | *P*, *U* | | Analyze perchloric acid extract, −20 °C | For urinary samples: Bacterial contamination |
| Homocitrulline | *U* | | −70 °C | Antiepileptic drugs or antibiotic artifacts may arise. |
| Lactate | *B*, *CSF*, *U* | | −20 °C | Prevent glycolysis, collect CSF samples fasted. |
| Lipoprotein (a) | *P* | | −20 °C | |
| $^{14}$C-ornithine incorporation | *FB*, *L* | | No storage allowed | |
| Oxygen consumption | *M*, *FB*, *BrF* | | No storage allowed | Maintain at 0 °C |
| Pyruvate | *B*, *CSF* | | −20 °C | Prevent glycolysis and LDH activity |
| Respiratory chain enzymes | *M*, *FB*, *L*, *CV* | | −70 °C | |
| Serine | *CSF* | Tap without blood or protein. | −20 °C | |
| Triglyceride | *S* | Blood sample should be processed (centrifuged) within 2 h. transport at 4 °C. | Process and store up to 72 h at 4 °C | Collect fasted |
| Urea | *P* | | Process and store up to 72 h at 4 °C | |

*B* Blood, *BrF* Brain (fresh), *CSF* Cerebrospinal fluid, *CV* Chorionic villi, *DBS* Dried blood spot, *FB* Fibroblasts, *L* Liver, *M* Muscle, *P* Plasma, *S* Serum, *U* Urine

## Prenatal Diagnosis

Prenatal diagnosis for mitochondrial carrier defects is indicated if mutations of mitochondrial carriers have been identified in family members. For such at-risk pregnancies, prenatal genetic testing is performed in chorionic villi, amniotic fluid cells, or cultured amniocytes.

## DNA Testing

If a there is a clinical suspicion of a mitochondrial carrier deficiency, genetic variants of mitochondrial carriers can be determined using conventional sequencing techniques (e.g., whole exome sequencing, Sanger sequencing, whole genome sequencing). This can be accomplished in all DNA containing samples, but preferably in a non-invasive sample like peripheral blood mononuclear cells (PBMCs) or buccal swabs. When variants of uncertain significance are found, their pathogenic role should be investigated using functional (transport) assays described above.

## Treatment

Depending on the specific clinical phenotype associated with mitochondrial carrier deficiencies, emergency treatments mainly focus on seizure control or the control of hyperammonemia and/or lactic acidosis. Although drug treatments are lacking for the 7 out of 16 carrier deficiencies, strategies for symptom alleviation have shown therapeutic potential for other carrier deficiencies. Confirmation of the therapeutic value in a more controlled setting is, however, warranted. These therapies comprise a switch to a diet with low carbohydrates and high fat and protein intake (i.e., ketogenic diet), which has mainly proven to be beneficial for carrier deficiencies that result in a defective aspartate malate shuttle (i.e., aspartate–glutamate carriers and mitochondrial aspartate aminotransferase). In contrast, protein-restricted diets are beneficial for ornithine carrier-deficient patients. Alternatively, carrier substrates or their precursors can be supplemented to compensate for the carrier defect. This has shown to be a promising option for defects in the citrate carrier (i.e., using citrate), thiamine pyrophosphate carrier (i.e., using thiamine), and flavin adenine dinucleotide carrier (i.e., using riboflavin). A similar approach is also applied in several experimental treatments that use folate and glycine or pantethine for glycine or coenzyme A carrier deficiencies, respectively. Interestingly, carrier deficiencies for which no treatment is available yet, all directly provide substrates or cofactors that are essential for proper OXPHOS function. Currently, therapeutic options for these patients are though limited to supportive care.

## Emergency Treatment

| No. | Disease name | Disease management and treatment |
|---|---|---|
| 43.1 | Adenine nucleotide translocator deficiency | Most patients reported to date demonstrate severely elevated plasma lactate levels. Buffering of these lactate levels by bicarbonate is of immediate significance to correct the lactic acidosis (Thompson et al. 2016). Moreover, most patients require mechanical ventilation. |
| 43.2 | Adenine nucleotide translocator deficiency | Most patients reported to date demonstrate severely elevated plasma lactate levels. Buffering of these lactate levels by bicarbonate is of immediate significance to correct the lactic acidosis (Thompson et al. 2016). Moreover, most patients require mechanical ventilation. |
| 43.3 | Mitochondrial phosphate carrier deficiency | Although the disease severity and associated progression differ largely between patients, most patients reported (i.e., five out of six) demonstrate severely elevated plasma lactate levels (Bhoj et al. 2014). Buffering of these lactate levels by bicarbonate was unsuccessful in one case and is not reported in all other cases. All patients demonstrate a characteristic cardiomyopathy. In one patient heart failure was treated with anticongestive therapy (e.g., digoxin and diuretics). Although clinically stabilized, cardiac hypertrophy was progressive in this patient who died at the age of 4 months (Mayr et al. 2007). Moreover, most patients require mechanical ventilation. |
| 43.4 | Aspartate-glutamate carrier 1 deficiency | Seizure episodes are experienced by all reported aspartate-glutamate carrier 1-deficient patients and should be treated with antiepileptic drugs or a combination thereof, like oxcarbazepine, levetiracetam, topiramate and phenobarbital (Kavanaugh et al. 2019). Moreover, most patients require mechanical ventilation. |
| 43.5 | Cytosolic glycerol-3-phosphate dehydrogenase deficiency | No specific emergency treatments have been reported for cytosolic glycerol-3-phosphate dehydrogenase-deficient patients. |
| 43.6 | Combined oxidative phosphorylation deficiency-28 | Most patients reported to date demonstrate severely elevated plasma lactate levels. Buffering of these lactate levels by bicarbonate is of immediate significance to correct the lactic acidosis (Kishita et al. 2015). Moreover, most patients require mechanical ventilation. |

(continued)

| No. | Disease name | Disease management and treatment |
|---|---|---|
| 43.7 | Mitochondrial citrate carrier deficiency | Patients with citrate carrier deficiencies experience epileptic seizures, which often increase in frequency and severity over the disease course (Mühlhausen et al. 2014; Pop et al. 2018). These epileptic seizures should be treated with antiepileptic drugs, such as levetiracetam (Mühlhausen et al. 2014). |
| 43.8 | Mitochondrial ATP-$Mg^{2+}$/ phosphate transporter deficiency | No specific emergency treatments have been reported for ATP-$Mg^{2+}$/phosphate carrier-deficient patients (Writzl et al. 2017). |
| 43.9 | Mitochondrial aspartate aminotransferase deficiency | In analogy with other aspartate-malate shuttle deficiencies (i.e., aspartate-glutamate carrier deficiency) seizure episodes are frequently reported in mitochondrial aspartate aminotransferase deficient patients (van Karnebeek et al. 2019). These seizures should be treated with antiepileptic drugs or a combination thereof (van Karnebeek et al. 2019), like carbamazepine, oxcarbazepine, lamotrigine, levetiracetam, topiramate, phenobarbital, and sodium valproate. GOT2-deficient patients, however, did not respond to antiepileptic drugs in all cases. |
| 43.10 | Mitochondrial dicarboxylate transporter deficiency | Seizure episodes are experienced by dicarboxylate carrier-deficient patients, and should be treated with antiepileptic drugs or a combination thereof, like clonazepam, levetiracetam, pyridoxine, and sodium valproate. It has, however, to be noted that seizures experienced by these patients are not always responsive to antiepileptic drugs. |
| 43.11 | Mitochondrial ornithine transporter deficiency | Rapid control of hyperammonemic episodes is of primary importance (Häberle et al. 2019). Therefore, protein intake should immediately be discontinued, accompanied by intravenous infusion of glucose. If needed, infusion of supplemental arginine can be added. Moreover, ammonia removal drugs like sodium benzoate and sodium phenylacetate can be used to control hyperammonemic episodes. However, if hyperammonemia persists and/or the neurologic status deteriorates hemodialysis/filtration is indicated. |
| 43.12 | Citrin deficiency | No specific emergency treatments have been reported for citrin-deficient patients. However, acute treatment of hyperammonemia may be required, using ammonia removal drugs like sodium benzoate and sodium phenylacetate. To prevent hyperammonemia on the long-term dietary adaptations should be made as described in Sect. 43.13. |
| 43.13 | Mitochondrial glutamate carrier 1 deficiency | Seizure episodes are experienced by all reported glutamate carrier-deficient patients, and should be treated with antiepileptic drugs or a combination thereof, like clonazepam, levetiracetam, pyridoxine, and sodium valproate (Reid et al. 2017). |
| 43.14 | Mitochondrial glycine transporter deficiency | Sideroblastic anemia in these patients should be treated by chronic blood transfusion with oral iron chelation therapy (Fernández-Murray et al. 2016). |
| 43.15 | Bilateral striatal necrosis (SLC25A19) | No specific emergency treatments have been reported for mitochondrial thiamine pyrophosphate carrier-deficient patients. |
| 43.16 | Mitochondrial flavin adenine dinucleotide transporter deficiency | No specific emergency treatments have been reported for mitochondrial flavin adenine dinucleotide carrier-deficient patients. |
| 43.17 | Mitochondrial coenzyme A transporter deficiency | Most patients reported to date demonstrate profoundly elevated plasma lactate levels (Almannai et al. 2018; Iuso et al. 2018a). Buffering of these lactate levels by bicarbonate is of immediate significance to correct the lactic acidosis. Moreover, hyperammonemia is observed in many coenzyme A carrier deficient patients (Almannai et al. 2018; Iuso et al. 2018a). To control hyperammonemia protein intake should be limited. Moreover, ammonia removal drugs like sodium benzoate and sodium phenylacetate can be used to control hyperammonemia. |

## Standard Treatment

| No. | Disease name | Disease management and treatment |
|---|---|---|
| 43.1 | Adenine nucleotide translocator deficiency | Up to now, no treatments are available for childhood muscle and cardiomyopathy associated with adenine nucleotide translocator deficiencies. Consequently, supportive care should be provided to these patients, as described below (Sect. 43.15). |
| 43.2 | Adenine nucleotide translocator deficiency | Up to now, no treatments are available for autosomal dominant progressive external ophthalmoplegia (adPEO) associated with adenine nucleotide translocator deficiencies in adults. Consequently, supportive care should be provided to these patients, as described below (Sect. 43.15). |

| No. | Disease name | Disease management and treatment |
|---|---|---|
| 43.3 | Mitochondrial phosphate carrier deficiency | Although disease severity and progression differ significantly, patients with a less progressive and severe phenotype could benefit from symptomatic treatment as described in one of the patients reported. This treatment strategy consisted of carvedilol, sodium bicarbonate and vitamin D (Bhoj et al. 2014), but was only described for this one patient. |
| 43.4 | Aspartate-glutamate carrier 1 deficiency | Up to now, one patient with aspartate-glutamate carrier deficiency has benefited substantially from the introduction of a ketogenic diet. Initiation of the diet in this 6-year-old girl, significantly improved psychomotor development and demyelination was reversed (Dahlin et al. 2015). The diet was based on a modified Johns Hopkins diet, with an initial ketogenic ratio of 1:1 (fat to protein and carbohydrates). This was increased to 3:1 (10 days), 3.5:1 (8 months) and 4:1 (13.5 months). The therapeutic potential of a ketogenic diet has, up to now, not been investigated in four other cases reported (Kavanaugh et al. 2019). Consequently, the therapeutic value of ketogenic diet for aspartate-glutamate carrier deficient patients should be further evaluated. |
| 43.5 | Cytosolic glycerol-3-phosphate dehydrogenase deficiency | So far, 16 patients have been described with a mutation in cytosolic glycerol-3-phosphate dehydrogenase (Li et al. 2018). Most of these affected individuals present with liver fibrosis in early infancy, but because they have a good prognosis liver transplantation is not recommended. High plasma triglyceride levels can, however, require lipoprotein apheresis, but this is only recommended for patients with severe hyperlipidemia. |
| 43.6 | Combined oxidative phosphorylation deficiency-28 | Up to now, no treatments are available for *S*-adenosylmethionine (SAM) carrier-deficient patients. Consequently, supportive care should be provided to these patients, as described below (Sect. 43.15). |
| 43.7 | Mitochondrial citrate carrier deficiency | Several patients with citrate carrier deficiencies, characterized by a combined D2–/L2-hydroxyglutaric aciduria, experienced beneficial effects of off-label citrate use. The first case included a 5-month-old girl, who received increasing citrate doses up to 1500 mg/kg/day (Mühlhausen et al. 2014). This led to decreased concentrations of the toxic metabolites D2- and L2-hydroxyglutaric acid, and increased urinary TCA metabolites. Clinically, seizure frequency and severity were decreased upon citrate treatment. Similar effects were observed in two patients, who upon citrate treatment (800 mg/kg/day or 1500 mg/kg/day) had less cerebral attacks and showed developmental gains, increased muscle tone and the absence of clinical seizures and apneic events (Pop et al. 2018). However, therapy in these cases (3 months and 9 months old) as well as the first case was initiated well into the disease course (Pop et al. 2018). Consequently, the effect of earlier therapy initiation should be investigated, and especially whether it can so attenuate the other clinical phenotypes associated with citrate carrier deficiencies (e.g., developmental delay, microcephaly, structural brain malformations). Besides the need for systemic prospective studies to investigate these effects, it has to be noted that all patients treated showed a mild clinical phenotype. Therefore, it also needs to be explored whether patients with a severe phenotype, and poorer prognosis, can benefit from citrate therapy. Promising results have been observed in one patient with a severe neonatal phenotype. Treatment with a low citrate dose (3 mg/kg/day) at 33 months of age resulted in an improvement of apneic events and increased the spontaneous respiratory drive (Smith et al. 2015). Although blood lactate levels were decreased, urinary hydroxyglutaric acids remained increased. |
| 43.8 | Mitochondrial ATP-$Mg^{2+}$/phosphate transporter deficiency | Up to now, no treatments are available for ATP-$Mg^{2+}$/phosphate carrier-deficient patients. Consequently, supportive care should be provided to these patients, as described below (Sect. 43.15). |
| 43.9 | Mitochondrial aspartate aminotransferase deficiency | Recently, two mitochondrial aspartate aminotransferase (GOT2)-deficient patients (i.e., a 17 months old boy and a 5-year-old boy) have demonstrated benefit from serine (300 mg/kg/day) and pyridoxine (20 mg/kg/day) supplementation, which was apparent from full seizure control and increased cognitive functions (van Karnebeek et al. 2019). Interestingly, single serine supplementation also showed beneficial effects, but addition of pyridoxine (vitamin B6), an essential precursor for *de novo* serine biosynthesis (Ramos et al. 2017), significantly enhanced these effects. The decreased serine biosynthesis in GOT2-deficient patients is most likely due to high cytosolic NADH levels arising from a decreased aspartate-malate shuttle function (Fig. 43.3). The reduction of these levels by pyruvate supplementation restored serine biosynthesis in GOT-2 deficient cells. Consequently, the authors suggest a diet low in carbohydrates, high in fat and supplemented with ketone bodies, the latter to circumvent lactate-induced acidification (van Karnebeek et al. 2019). |
| 43.10 | Mitochondrial dicarboxylate transporter deficiency | Up to now, no treatments are available for mitochondrial dicarboxylate carrier-deficient patients. Consequently, supportive care should be provided to these patients, as described below (Sect. 43.15). |
| 43.11 | Mitochondrial ornithine transporter deficiency | After emergency measures described above (Sect. 43.12), an age-appropriate protein-restricted diet should be maintained and supplemented with citrulline and sodium phenylbutyrate to maintain plasma concentrations of ammonia, glutamine, arginine, and essential amino acids within normal range (Häberle et al. 2019). |

(continued)

| No. | Disease name | Disease management and treatment |
|---|---|---|
| 43.12 | Citrin deficiency | Glutamate aspartate carrier (SLC25A13) deficiencies are associated with neonatal intrahepatic cholestasis (NICCD) and adult-onset type II citrullinemia (CTLN2). For both clinical manifestations therapies are aimed at the preventions of cholestasis and the need for liver transplantation (Okano et al. 2019). For NICCD, positive effects were found by treatment with medium chain triglycerides (MCT) milk and lactose (galactose)-free milk (Hayasaka et al. 2011; Okano et al. 2019). These formulations need to be supplemented with vitamins, which are not absorbed due to cholestasis (i.e., vitamin K2 and lipid-soluble vitamins) and ursodeoxycholic acid to treat cholestasis (Okano et al. 2019). Around the age of one, many NICCD patients experience a spontaneous remission. Dietary therapy is the key in the adaptation/compensation stage that follows after the remission. Such dietary adaptations include a protein- and fat-rich diet with a protein: fat: carbohydrate ratio being 15–25%: 40–50%: 30–40%, along with the appropriate energy intake. The use of MCT oil and sodium pyruvate is also effective (Okano et al. 2019). These therapies, which aim to decrease cytosolic NADH levels and provide mitochondrial energy sources, have also shown to be promising as a treatment for CTLN2 (Hayasaka et al. 2014). However, continuous intravenous hyperalimentation with high glucose concentration or administration of Glyceol® is contraindicated (Okano et al. 2019). Commonly, NICCD patients develop CTLN2 at an older age, however, with the above dietary therapy and appropriate medical support no NICCD patients have shown to develop CTLN2 up to now (Okano et al. 2019). |
| 43.13 | Mitochondrial glutamate carrier 1 deficiency | Up to now, no treatments are available for mitochondrial glutamate carrier-deficient patients. Consequently, supportive care should be provided to these patients, as described below (Sect. 43.15). |
| 43.14 | Mitochondrial glycine transporter deficiency | Up to now, no treatments are available for mitochondrial glycine carrier-deficient patients. Consequently, supportive care should be provided to these patients, as described below (Sect. 43.15). More specifically, the sideroblastic anemia in these patients should be treated by chronic blood transfusion with oral iron chelation therapy (Fernández-Murray et al. 2016). |
| 43.15 | Bilateral striatal necrosis (SLC25A19) | Mitochondrial thiamine pyrophosphate carrier deficiencies are associated with Amish lethal microcephaly. This is characterized by severe congenital microcephaly, death before the age of one and severe 2-oxoglutaric aciduria. Patients with this phenotype all have a homozygous p.G177A mutation in the *SLC25A19* gene, and unfortunately do not respond to thiamine or biotin supplementation (Gowda et al. 2019). As a consequence, supportive care should be provided to these patients, as described below (Sect. 43.15). More recently, patients with other mitochondrial thiamine pyrophosphate carrier mutations have responded positively to thiamine supplementation. Three out of five patients with homozygous *SLC25A19* mutations (i.e., p.G125S and p. S194P) described by Ortigoza-Escobar et al, showed substantial improvement in peripheral neuropathy and gait after thiamin treatment (400–600 mg/day) (Ortigoza-Escobar et al. 2017). The absence of an effect in the other two patients may be explained by the age after onset at which therapy was initiated, which was significantly higher in these two (i.e., 9 and 12 years), compared to the other patients (i.e., 3 years). Interestingly, beneficial effects were reported after acute high dose (1500 mg/kg/day) thiamine in one of these patients to treat a severe episode of flaccid paralysis that occurred with fever. Two other patients with a p.E304K and p.L290G mutation experienced no recurring encephalopathy episodes over a 2-year follow-up (400–600 mg/day). The beneficial effects of thiamin supplementation thus seem to depend on the mutation and resulting severity of the clinical phenotype. This was also suggested by a recent report that described another mutation (p.Q192H), which did not respond on thiamin treatment (400 mg/day) (Bottega et al. 2019). |
| 43.16 | Mitochondrial flavin adenine dinucleotide transporter deficiency | Mitochondrial flavin adenine dinucleotide (FAD) carrier deficiencies are predominantly associated with exercise intolerance. Riboflavin, a FAD precursor, treatment has, however, been shown to dramatically improve these symptoms, as described for a 14-year-old girl administered 10 mg/kg/day (Schiff et al. 2016), and 51-year-old man administered 30 mg/day (Hellebrekers et al. 2017). |
| 43.17 | Mitochondrial coenzyme A transporter deficiency | Vitamins and cofactors, like thiamine, biotin, riboflavin, and carnitine, were tried in several subjects with no evidence of response or correlation to disease severity (Almannai et al. 2018). Consequently, supportive care should be provided to these patients, as described below (Sect. 43.15). |

## Experimental Treatment

For several mitochondrial carrier deficiencies, for which currently no therapy exists, experimental treatments have demonstrated positive effects. Conformation of their therapeutic potential in a more controlled setting is though warranted. This includes the supplementation of glycine and folate for glycine carrier deficiencies. Although beneficial effects of this combination were observed in yeast and zebrafish *SLC25A38*-deficient models (Fernández-Murray et al. 2016), no impact could be observed on transfusion requirements or hematological parameters in three *SLC25A38* patients (LeBlanc et al. 2016). It is though, unknown what may have caused this different response between zebrafish and humans, which could be related to a species difference in pathophysiology and/or pharmacokinetics. Currently, several efforts are attempting to elucidate these differences, which include the generation of a *SLC25A38*-deficient mouse model (LeBlanc et al. 2016). In addition to glycine carrier deficiencies, experimental studies have demonstrated therapeutic potential of pantethine for coenzyme A carrier deficiencies (Iuso et al. 2018a).

Pantethine replenishes the cellular CoA levels, and its supplementation increased the viability of Drosophila disease models also characterized by decreased CoA levels (i.e., *PKAN* (Iuso et al. 2018a); and *PPCS* (Iuso et al. 2018b)).

## Follow-Up and Monitoring

For treatable carrier deficiencies described above, a careful clinical evaluation of the disease phenotype is essential. Moreover, supportive care is vital for most carrier-deficient patients, in particular if no treatment is available yet. Due to the multiple cellular metabolic pathways affected by carrier deficiencies (Figs. 43.1, 43.2, 43.3, 43.4), patients mostly present with a combination of various symptoms (see Sect. 43.4). Consequently, it is important to focus on symptom relief or adjustment of living environment (e.g., wheelchairs, splints, adjusted furniture). For patients with a cytosolic glycerol-3-phosphate dehydrogenase deficiency, specific follow-up measures should be considered, including evaluation of growth and development, liver function, total cholesterol, triglycerides, abdominal ultrasound, and FibroScan (Li et al. 2018). In addition, it is necessary in the long-term follow up to pay attention to coronary artery disease and pancreatitis, which is associated with hypertriglyceridemia (Li et al. 2018).

## Online Resources

International laboratories with an outstanding track record on the functional characterization of mitochondrial disorders, and in particularly of mitochondrial carriers and deficiencies thereof:

- Prof. Dr. Edmund Kunji group. (http://www.mrc-mbu.cam.ac.uk/people/edmund-kunji)
- Prof. Dr. Luigi Palmieri group. (https://www.uniba.it/ricerca/dipartimenti/bioscienze-biotecnologie)
- Raboud Center for Mitochondrial Medicine. (https://www.radboudumc.nl/expertisecentra/zeldzame-aandoeningen/radboud-center-for-mitochondrial-medicine)

## References


Almannai M, Alsamri A, Alqasmi A, et al. Expanding the phenotype of SLC25A42-associated mitochondrial encephalomyopathy. Clin Genet. 2018;98:1097–102.

Andropoulos DB. Appendix B: pediatric normal laboratory values. Greg Pediatr Anesth. 2012:1300–14.

Bender T, Martinou JC. The mitochondrial pyruvate carrier in health and disease: to carry or not to carry? Biochim Biophys Acta, Mol Cell Res. 2016;1863:2436–42.

Bhoj EJ, Li M, Ahrens-Nicklas R, et al. Pathologic variants of the mitochondrial phosphate carrier SLC25A3: two new patients and expansion of the cardiomyopathy/skeletal myopathy phenotype with and without lactic acidosis. JIMD Rep. 2014;1:73–8.

Bottega R, Perrone MD, Vecchiato K, et al. Functional analysis of the third identified SLC25A19 mutation causative for the thiamine metabolism dysfunction syndrome 4 Roberta. J Hum Genet. 2019;64:1075–81.

Dahlin M, Martin DA, Hedlund Z, et al. The ketogenic diet compensates for AGC1 deficiency and improves myelination. Epilepsia. 2015;56:e176–81. https://doi.org/10.1111/epi.13193.

Fernández-Murray JP, Prykhozhij SV, Dufay JN, et al. Glycine and folate ameliorate models of congenital Sideroblastic Anemia. PLoS Genet. 2016;12.

Gowda VK, Srinivasan VM, Jehta K, Bhat MD. Bilateral striatal necrosis with polyneuropathy with a novel SLC25A19 (mitochondrial thiamine pyrophosphate carrier OMIMI*606521) mutation: treatable thiamine metabolic disorder-a report of two Indian cases. Neuropediatrics. 2019;50:313–7.

Häberle J, Burlina A, Chakrapani A, et al. Suggested guidelines for the diagnosis and management of urea cycle disorders: first revision. J Inherit Metab Dis. 2019;42:1192–230.

Halbach NSJ, Smeets EEJ, Bierau J, et al. Altered carbon dioxide metabolism and creatine abnormalities in Rett syndrome. JIMD Rep. 2011;1:73–8.

Hayasaka K, Numakura C, Toyota K, et al. Medium-chain triglyceride supplementation under a low-carbohydrate formula is a promising therapy for adult-onset type II citrullinemia. Mol Genet Metab Rep. 2014;1:42–50.

Hayasaka K, Numakura C, Toyota K, Kimura T. Treatment with lactose (galactose)-restricted and medium-chain triglyceride-supplemented formula for neonatal intrahepatic cholestasis caused by Citrin deficiency. JIMD Rep. 2011;1:37–44.

Hebestreit H, Wanders RJA, Schutgens RBH, et al. Isolated dihydroxyacetonephosphate-acyl-transferase deficiency in rhizomelic chondrodysplasia punctata: clinical presentation, metabolic and histological findings. Eur J Pediatr. 1996;155:1035–9.

Hellebrekers DMEI, Sallevelt SCEH, Theunissen TEJ, et al. Novel SLC25A32 mutation in a patient with a severe neuromuscular phenotype. Eur J Hum Genet. 2017;25:886–8.

Iuso A, Alhaddad B, Weigel C, et al. A homozygous splice site mutation in SLC25A42, encoding the mitochondrial transporter of coenzyme A, causes metabolic crises and epileptic encephalopathy. JIMD Rep. 2018a:1–7.

Iuso A, Wiersma M, Schüller HJ, et al. Mutations in PPCS, encoding phosphopantothenoylcysteine synthetase, cause autosomal-recessive dilated cardiomyopathy. Am J Hum Genet. 2018b;102:1018–30.

Kannengiesser C, Sanchez M, Sweeney M, et al. Missense SLC25A38 variations play an important role in autosomal recessive inherited sideroblastic anemia. Haematologica. 2011;96:808–13.

Kavanaugh BC, Warren EB, Baytas O, et al. Longitudinal MRI findings in patient with SLC25A12 pathogenic variants inform disease progression and classification. Am J Med Genet Part A. 2019;179:2284–91.

Kishita Y, Pajak A, Bolar NA, et al. Intra-mitochondrial methylation deficiency due to mutations in SLC25A26. Am J Hum Genet. 2015;97:761–8.

LeBlanc MA, Bettle A, Berman JN, et al. Study of glycine and folic acid supplementation to ameliorate transfusion dependence in congenital SLC25A38 mutated sideroblastic anemia. Pediatr Blood Cancer. 2016;63:1307–9.

Li JQ, Xie XB, Feng JY, et al. A novel homozygous mutation in the glycerol-3-phosphate dehydrogenase 1 gene in a Chinese patient

with transient infantile hypertriglyceridemia: a case report. BMC Gastroenterol. 2018;18 https://doi.org/10.1186/s12876-018-0827-6.
Mayr JA, Merkel O, Kohlwein SD, et al. Mitochondrial phosphate-carrier deficiency: a novel disorder of oxidative phosphorylation. Am J Hum Genet. 2007;80:478–84.
Mühlhausen C, Salomons GS, Lukacs Z, et al. Combined D2−/L2-hydroxyglutaric aciduria (SLC25A1 deficiency): clinical course and effects of citrate treatment. J Inherit Metab Dis. 2014;37:775–81.
Muntau AC, Röschinger W, Merkenschlager A, et al. Combined D-2- and L-2-hydroxyglutaric aciduria with neonatal onset encephalopathy: a third biochemical variant of 2-hydroxyglutaric aciduria? Neuropediatrics. 2000;31:137–40.
Nota B, Struys EA, Pop A, et al. Deficiency in SLC25A1, encoding the mitochondrial citrate carrier, causes combined D-2- and L-2-hydroxyglutaric aciduria. Am J Hum Genet. 2013;92:627–31.
Okano Y, Ohura T, Sakamoto O, Inui A. Current treatment for citrin deficiency during NICCD and adaptation/compensation stages: strategy to prevent CTLN2. Mol Genet Metab. 2019;127:175–83.
Ortigoza-Escobar JD, Alfadhel M, Molero-Luis M, et al. Thiamine deficiency in childhood with attention to genetic causes: survival and outcome predictors. Ann Neurol. 2017;82:317–30.
Palmieri F, Monné M. Discoveries, metabolic roles and diseases of mitochondrial carriers: a review. Biochim Biophys Acta, Mol Cell Res. 2016;1863:2362–78.
Paul BT, Tesfay L, Winkler CR, et al. Sideroflexin 4 affects Fe-S cluster biogenesis, iron metabolism, mitochondrial respiration and heme biosynthetic enzymes. Sci Rep. 2019;9:1–13.
Pop A, Williams M, Struys EA, et al. An overview of combined D-2- and L-2-hydroxyglutaric aciduria: functional analysis of CIC variants. J Inherit Metab Dis. 2018;41:169–80.
Punzi G, Porcelli V, Ruggiu M, et al. SLC25A10 biallelic mutations in intractable epileptic encephalopathy with complex I deficiency. Hum Mol Genet. 2018;27:499–504.
Ramos RJ, Pras-Raves ML, Gerrits J, et al. Vitamin B6 is essential for serine de novo biosynthesis. J Inherit Metab Dis. 2017;40:883–91.
Reid ES, Williams H, Anderson G, et al. Mutations in SLC25A22: hyperprolinaemia, vacuolated fibroblasts and presentation with developmental delay. J Inherit Metab Dis. 2017;40:385–94.
Rinaldo P. Organic acids. In: Blau N, Duran M, editors. Laboratory guide to the methods in biochemical genetics. Berlin: Springer; 2008. p. 85–97.
Robinson AJ, Overy C, Kunji ERS. The mechanism of transport by mitochondrial carriers based on analysis of symmetry (supplementary information). Proc Natl Acad Sci U S A. 2008;105:17,766–71.
Ruprecht JJ, King MS, Zögg T, et al. The molecular mechanism of transport by the mitochondrial ADP/ATP carrier. Cell. 2019;176:435–447.e15.
Ruprecht JJ, Kunji ER. Structural changes in the transport cycle of the mitochondrial ADP/ATP carrier. Curr Opin Struct Biol. 2019;57:135–44.
Ruprecht JJ, Kunji ERS. The SLC25 mitochondrial carrier family: structure and mechanism. Trends Biochem Sci. 2020;45:244–58.
Schaedler TA, Faust B, Shintre CA, et al. Structures and functions of mitochondrial ABC transporters. Biochem Soc Trans. 2015;43:943–51.
Schiff M, Veauville-Merllié A, Hsien Su C, et al. SLC25A32 mutations and riboflavin-responsive exercise intolerance. N Engl J Med. 2016;374:793.
Smith A, McBride S, Marcadier JL, et al. Severe neonatal presentation of mitochondrial citrate carrier (SLC25A1) deficiency. JIMD Rep. 2015:73–8.
Sofou K, Hedberg-Oldfors C, Kollberg G, et al. Prenatal onset of mitochondrial disease is associated with sideroflexin 4 deficiency. Mitochondrion. 2019;47:76–81.
Thompson K, Majd H, Dallabona C, et al. Recurrent de novo dominant mutations in SLC25A4 cause severe early-onset mitochondrial disease and loss of mitochondrial DNA copy number. Am J Hum Genet. 2016;99:860–76.
Trijbels F, Huizing M, Ruitenbeek W, et al. Disturbances in mitochondrial transport systems leading to encephalomyopathies. Biofactors. 1998;7:225–7.
van Karnebeek CDM, Ramos RJ, Wen XY, et al. Bi-allelic GOT2 mutations cause a treatable malate-aspartate shuttle-related encephalopathy. Am J Hum Genet. 2019;105:534–48.
Writzl K, Maver A, Kovačič L, et al. De novo mutations in SLC25A24 cause a disorder characterized by early aging, bone dysplasia, characteristic face, and early demise. Am J Hum Genet. 2017;101:844–55.

# Isolated Mitochondrial Complex Deficiencies

# 44

Mirian C. H. Janssen, Maaike C. de Vries, Lonneke de Boer, and Richard J. Rodenburg

## Contents




M. C. H. Janssen
Department of Internal Medicine, Radboud Center for Mitochondrial Medicine, Nijmegen, The Netherlands
e-mail: mirian.janssen@radboudumc.nl

M. C. de Vries · L. de Boer
Department of Paediatrics, Radboud Center for Mitochondrial Medicine, Nijmegen, The Netherlands

R. J. Rodenburg (✉)
Department of Paediatrics, Translational Metabolic Laboratory, Radboud Center for Mitochondrial Medicine, Nijmegen, The Netherlands
e-mail: richard.rodenburg@radboudumc.nl



### Summary

Mitochondrial disorders belong to the most frequently encountered inborn errors of metabolism. Most affected mitochondrial disease patients harbour a defect in the oxidative phosphorylation system (OXPHOS) of which the incidence is estimated to be over one in 5000 live births. The OXPHOS performs the final step in the aerobic production of adenosine triphosphate (ATP) in mitochondria. Defects in OXPHOS can be caused by mutations in either the mitochondrial DNA (mtDNA) or nuclear DNA (nDNA). Most patients with mitochondrial disorders present with a multisystem disorder. The organs requiring the most energy, such as the brain, retina, heart, kidney and skeletal muscle, are most commonly and severely affected. Onset of disease can be at any age and the symptoms are almost always progressive. A definitive diagnosis solely based on clinical signs and symptoms is very unlikely. Whole exome/



N. Blau et al. (eds.), *Physician's Guide to the Diagnosis, Treatment, and Follow-Up of Inherited Metabolic Diseases*,
https://doi.org/10.1007/978-3-030-67727-5_44

genome sequencing (WES/WGS) has greatly improved disease diagnosis and often simplified it, although in some cases has also resulted in new diagnostic challenges. Nonetheless, clinical diagnostic criteria, combined with brain imaging, metabolic, biochemical and other functional tests are still needed. Since specific treatment options are still limited, the management of mitochondrial disorders is largely supportive. For diagnosis and treatment, patients should be referred to a specialized centre.

## Introduction

### Physiology of the Oxidative Phosphorylation

The condensation of energy in the form of ATP by mitochondria is a stepwise process, of which the oxidative phosphorylation (OXPHOS) constitutes the final step. The metabolic pathways preceding the oxidative phosphorylation are fatty acid oxidation, glycolysis, pyruvate dehydrogenase and Krebs cycle. During the aerobic conversion of substrates, such as glucose and fatty acids, into ATP, the formation of the reduction equivalents NADH and $FADH_2$ takes place in the tricarboxylic acid cycle and the beta-oxidation. These reduction equivalents are oxidized by the respiratory chain complexes I and II, respectively. The electrons that are released during this conversion flow through the electron transport chain via coenzyme Q10 and cytochrome c and finally to molecular oxygen, which results in the formation of water. These subsequent conversions are catalyzed by the respiratory chain enzymes complex I, II, III and IV. The oxidation–reduction reactions are accompanied by the pumping of protons from the mitochondrial matrix to the cellular environment by complex I, III and IV. This results in a proton gradient (and membrane potential) over the inner mitochondrial membrane. This proton gradient is used by complex V (ATP synthase) to convert ADP and $P_i$ into ATP. This results in an increase in the ATP/ADP ratio within the mitochondrial matrix, which is balanced by the export of ATP by the adenine nucleotide transporter (ANT), which in turn is accompanied by the import of equimolar amounts ADP.

### Mitochondrial Function

The proteins that make up the OXPHOS, as well as the proteins and RNA molecules necessary for proper production, assembly, and functioning of the OXPHOS, are encoded by hundreds of genes distributed over the nuclear DNA (nDNA) and mitochondrial DNA (mtDNA). The mtDNA encodes 37 genes, 22 code for tRNAs, 2 for rRNAs and 13 code for subunits of the OXPHOS complexes I, III, IV and V. Mitochondria are not self-supporting entities, but require imported nDNA-encoded proteins and other imported molecules in order to function properly. In addition to the OXHPOS genes, the mtDNA also encodes the RNA molecules required for the translation of these mtDNA-encoded OXPHOS genes. The mtDNA encoded ribosomal RNAs, together with nuclear encoded ribosomal proteins, form mitoribosomes. The mtDNA encoded tRNAs are charged with amino acids by their corresponding (nDNA-encoded) aminoacyl tRNA synthases. The mitoribosomes and charged tRNAs, with the help of nuclear encoded translation initiation and elongation factors, synthesize the 13 polypeptides of the OXPHOS system encoded by the mtDNA. Replication of mtDNA, under the control of nuclear DNA-encoded products, involves the unwinding of the double-stranded mtDNA and the polymerization of new mtDNA strands. Factors involved include polymerase gamma (POLG), the helicase Twinkle (C10orf2 or TWNK), single stranded binding protein 1 (SSBP1) and several other proteins.

### Mitochondrial Dysfunction

Mitochondrial dysfunction can be a result of a primary defect in the OXPHOS system or a defect in the regulation, organisation or maintenance of mitochondria, caused by a mutation in the nDNA or mtDNA. Secondary causes of mitochondrial dysfunction include aging, cellular stress and inactivity. Also other inherited metabolic diseases (e.g. creatine biosynthesis defects and organic acidurias) can cause secondary mitochondrial dysfunction. As this chapter is about isolated mitochondrial complex deficiencies, we will focus on primary mitochondrial dysfunction. The incidence of primary mitochondrial dysfunction, based on an OXPHOS defects is over 1:5000 of all live births. Mutations in the mtDNA genes encoding structural components of the OXPHOS enzymes theoretically cause isolated deficiencies of the complexes that contain these mtDNA-encoded subunits, complex I, III, IV and V. A mutation in one of the mtDNA-encoded tRNAs or rRNAs causes a combined deficiency of the complexes that contain mtDNA-encoded subunits. Mutations in nuclear genes encoding proteins involved in the OXPHOS system may cause single or multi-complex deficiencies.

### Clinical Signs and Symptoms

Mitochondrial dysfunction causes a wide variety of symptoms, in many different organ systems. The disease course is often progressive, although the rate of deterioration is highly variable between different patients. The onset of symptoms can be at any age. The organs requiring the most energy, such as the brain, retina, heart, kidney and skeletal muscle, are most commonly and severely affected. A mitochondrial disease should therefore be suspected in patients with progressive multisystem involvement, although mitochondrial disorders may present with *'Any symptom of any organ at any age'*. In general, symptoms present in mitochondrial disorders can also be seen in a variety of other diseases. Mitochondrial disorders should be first and foremost considered in the differential diagnosis of patients with signs and symptoms including combinations of encephalopathy and hepatopathy, myoclonic epilepsy, developmental regression, stroke-like episodes, ophthalmoplegia, optic nerve atrophy, retinal degeneration, early onset hearing loss and ataxia.

## Approach to Diagnosis

Because of the clinical and genetic heterogeneity of mitochondrial diseases, there is no single diagnostic test. Instead, a range of multimodality testing needs to be performed in order to achieve a precise diagnosis. Currently, exome- or genome sequencing is often used in order to establish a molecular diagnosis. However, in many cases the biochemical examination of tissue specimens could be required, either to obtain biochemical information to guide the analysis of exome/genome data or to validate the possible pathogenicity of genetic variants of unknown clinical significance. When collecting tissue samples for functional/biochemical diagnostic tests, as a rule, the patient under investigation should not be on vitamin therapy, in order to avoid masking of possible enzyme deficiencies.

### Metabolic Investigations

Although lactic acidosis is generally thought of as a cardinal feature of mitochondrial disease, plasma lactate might also be normal or only mildly elevated in patients with mitochondrial dysfunction. Post-exercise lactates are more consistently elevated, and the presence of raised alanine levels in the plasma amino acid profile is suggestive of intermittent lactic acidosis. Creatine kinase is often normal or only mildly elevated in patients with mitochondrial myopathies.

### Imaging

Magnetic resonance imaging (MRI) brain is normal in many patients with mitochondrial disease, particularly in those patients with a predominantly neuromuscular clinical presentation. However, MRI can be very helpful in the differential diagnosis of patients with mitochondrial encephalomyopathies. Patients with MELAS syndrome may have parietooccipital lesions (not confined to vascular territories) during acute episodes, which subsequently resolve. Patients with Leigh syndrome present bilateral symmetrical lesions involving basal ganglia structures and brainstem nuclei. These lesions appear hyperintense on T2-weighted or Fluid-attenuated inversion recovery (FLAIR) sequences.

### Neurophysiology

Electromyography reveals myopathy in approximately 50% of patients with mitochondrial disorders. Peripheral neuropathy is increasingly recognized in adults with mitochondrial diseases; a recent study showed evidence of axonal sensorimotor polyneuropathy in 36% of patients.

### Muscle Histology

Muscle histology is frequently abnormal in patients presenting with mitochondrial disease. The morphological hallmarks of mitochondrial disease are ragged-red fibers (RRF), best observed in the modified Gomori trichrome stain and cytochrome *c* oxidase (COX) negative fibres. RRF often show increased mitochondrial numbers, with marked subsarcolemmal accumulation of mitochondria. COX-negative fibres are most easily demonstrated using the combined COX-SDH stain, in which they appear blue. The presence of small numbers of RRF and COX-negative fibres is normal in elderly individuals; for example, up to one RRF is normal in adults up to 40 years of age, while up to five RRF may be normal above 60 years of age. Electron microscopy may reveal increased mitochondrial numbers or size, abnormal morphology of cristae, such as whorling or electron-dense crystalline inclusions.

### Muscle Biochemistry

For most biochemical determinations in tissue biopsy material one should ask the diagnostic centre for information about specific requirements as to the practice of collecting and transporting material. Especially in the case of enzyme analysis in tissues or cells, one must consult the diagnostic laboratory in advance about the conditions for removal, preparation, storage (usually at −70 °C) and transport of the specimens. If freshly collected tissue needs to be studied, samples have to be collected in a special, ice-cold but not frozen buffer and immediately transported to the laboratory. The biochemical tests of mitochondrial flux measurements, such as oxygen consumption, substrate oxidation and ATP production should be performed within 2 h of collection. Frozen tissue samples are suitable for the analysis of individual mitochondrial enzymes, and histochemical tests, and can be stored for many years.

The physician should inform the laboratory about the clinical findings to ensure an adequate analysis and to aid data interpretation. It is important to discuss which type of tissue or cell is preferable in each case, thereby causing the patient as little inconvenience as possible. Tissue-specific expression of mitochondrial deficiencies renders fibroblasts and lymphocytes less universally appropriate than skeletal muscle, although fibroblast analysis does have an added diagnostic value when combined with a muscle sample examination and it is surprising how often mitochondrial abnormalities are evident in cells cultured in the laboratory.

In the case of unexpected death, tissue, blood and urine specimens should be collected as soon as possible after death. They should be snap frozen (not fixed) immediately after collection using liquid nitrogen, and stored for possible additional studies. For enzymatic purposes tissues must be removed within 1–2 h after death and should be frozen immediately in liquid nitrogen. Skin biopsies can be performed as late as 48 h after death, and must be collected at room temperature in cell culture medium, after which the biopsy can be transported at room temperature to the cell culture laboratory.

Because few reference values are generally available for neonates, it is recommended to perform a muscle biopsy beyond the first month of life, unless a life-threatening situation exists.

### Genetic Testing

For most patients initial genetic testing should be directed towards the mitochondrial genome. Patients with suspected MIDD or MELAS should be screened for the common m.3243A>G mtDNA mutation in the *MT-TL1* gene, and those with suspected MERRF for the m.8344 mutation in *MT-TK*. Patients with LHON have one of three common mtDNA mutations in complex I subunits, while those with NARP usually have a mutation in the ATP6 subunit of complex V (most commonly m.8993T>G/C). These mutations are usually present in DNA extracted from blood or urinary epithelial cells, so a muscle biopsy is often not needed to secure a diagnosis for these syndromes. Large-scale mtDNA rearrangements are typically absent in the blood after the age of 20 years, and so a muscle sample is needed for genetic diagnosis of patients with progressive external ophthalmoplegia (PEO). Patients with Kearns–Sayre syndrome (KSS) typically present at an earlier age than those with isolated PEO, and in these patients screening for mtDNA deletions can be performed in blood or urinary epithelial cells. If this testing is negative, a muscle biopsy is indicated for further genetic (mtDNA) investigations. Sequence analysis of muscle DNA is needed to diagnose other mtDNA point mutations.

Some nuclear-encoded mitochondrial syndromes are associated with specific gene defects. If one of these syndromes is clinically suspected, then a sequence analysis of the relevant gene may be the appropriate first-line test, for example *SURF1* in classical Leigh syndrome with hypertrichosis, bypassing the need for muscle biopsy. Although in these cases, exome sequencing will most probably also result in the identification of the SURF1 defect, this approach does have a small chance of unsolicited genetic findings, and therefore specific gene sequencing is preferred over exome sequencing in the case of a strong clinical suspicion for such a specific gene defect. Patients with multiple mtDNA deletions in muscle may have mutations in one of 11 genes, which may be screened simultaneously using a next-generation sequencing gene panel approach. If a genetic diagnosis has not been achieved after screening the mtDNA for large-scale rearrangements and point mutations (using long-range PCR and sequence analysis respectively) whole exome sequence analysis is the most efficient method for identifying the causative nuclear gene defect. However, functional testing will still be needed in several situations, for example to verify the pathogenicity of genetic variants identified by sequencing.

### Scoring Systems

Several scoring systems have been proposed to help in the diagnosis of mitochondrial disease. However, these tend to be complicated and cumbersome to use and may just indicate the relative likelihood of a mitochondrial disorder being present, rather than definitively establishing a diagnosis. Such scoring systems are likely to play a minor role in the future as genetic diagnosis becomes more widespread with the use of increasingly sophisticated diagnostic tools such as whole exome and whole genome sequencing. Besides a diagnostic tool, scoring systems are useful tools for evaluation of the disease course.

## Nomenclature

| No. | Disorder | Alternative name | Abbreviation | Gene symbol | Chromosomal localisation | Inheritance | Affected protein | OMIM no. |
|---|---|---|---|---|---|---|---|---|
| 44.1 | Mitochondrial complex I subunit deficiency (NDUFV1) | NDUFV1 deficiency | NDUFV1 | *NDUFV1* | 11q13.2 | AR | NADH:ubiquinone oxidoreductase flavoprotein 1 | 252010 |
| 44.2 | Mitochondrial complex I subunit deficiency (NDUFV2) | NDUFV2 deficiency | NDUFV2 | *NDUFV2* | 18p11.22 | AR | NADH:ubiquinone oxidoreductase flavoprotein 2 | 252010 |
| 44.3 | Mitochondrial complex I subunit deficiency (NDUFS1) | NDUFS1 deficiency | NDUFS1 | *NDUFS1* | 2q33.3 | AR | NADH:ubiquinone oxidoreductase Fe-S protein 1 | 252010 |
| 44.4 | Mitochondrial complex I subunit deficiency (NDUFS2) | NDUFS2 deficiency | NDUFS2 | *NDUFS2* | 1q23.3 | AR | NADH:ubiquinone oxidoreductase Fe-S protein 2 | 252010 |
| 44.5 | Mitochondrial complex I subunit deficiency (NDUFS3) | NDUFS3 deficiency | NDUFS3 | *NDUFS3* | 11p11.2 | AR | NADH:ubiquinone oxidoreductase Fe-S protein 3 | 256000; 252010 |
| 44.6 | Mitochondrial complex I subunit deficiency (NDUFS7) | NDUFS7 deficiency | NDUFS7 | *NDUFS7* | 19p13.3 | AR | NADH:ubiquinone oxidoreductase Fe-S protein 7 | 256000 |
| 44.7 | Mitochondrial complex I subunit deficiency (NDUFS8) | NDUFS8 deficiency | NDUFS8 | *NDUFS8* | 11q13.2 | AR | NADH:ubiquinone oxidoreductase Fe-S protein 8 | 256000 |
| 44.8 | Mitochondrial complex I subunit deficiency (NDUFS4) | NDUFS4 deficiency | NDUFS4 | *NDUFS4* | 5q11.2 | AR | NADH:ubiquinone oxidoreductase Fe-S protein 4 | 256000; 252010 |
| 44.9 | Mitochondrial complex I subunit deficiency (NDUFS6) | NDUFS6 deficiency | NDUFS6 | *NDUFS6* | 5p15.33 | AR | NADH:ubiquinone oxidoreductase Fe-S protein 6 | 252010 |
| 44.10 | Mitochondrial complex I subunit deficiency (NDUFA1) | NDUFA1 deficiency | NDUFA1 | *NDUFA1* | Xq24 | X-linked | NADH:ubiquinone oxidoreductase 1 alpha subcomplex 1 | 252010 |
| 44.11 | Mitochondrial complex I subunit deficiency (NDUFA2) | NDUFA2 deficiency | NDUFA2 | *NDUFA2* | 5q31.3 | AR | NADH:ubiquinone oxidoreductase 1 alpha subcomplex 2 | 256000 |
| 44.12 | Mitochondrial complex I subunit deficiency (NDUFA9) | NDUFA9 deficiency | NDUFA9 | *NDUFA9* | 12p13.32 | AR | NADH:ubiquinone oxidoreductase 1 alpha subcomplex 9 | 256000 |
| 44.13 | Mitochondrial complex I subunit deficiency (NDUFA10) | NDUFA10 deficiency | NDUFA10 | *NDUFA10* | 2q37.3 | AR | NADH:ubiquinone oxidoreductase 1 alpha subcomplex 10 | 256000 |
| 44.14 | Mitochondrial complex I subunit deficiency (NDUFA11) | NDUFA11 deficiency | NDUFA11 | *NDUFA11* | 19p13.3 | AR | NADH:ubiquinone oxidoreductase 1 alpha subcomplex 11 | 252010 |

(continued)

| No. | Disorder | Alternative name | Abbreviation | Gene symbol | Chromosomal localisation | Inheritance | Affected protein | OMIM no. |
|---|---|---|---|---|---|---|---|---|
| 44.15 | Mitochondrial complex I subunit deficiency (NDUFA12) | NDUFA12 deficiency | NDUFA12 | *NDUFA12* | 12q22 | AR | NADH:ubiquinone oxidoreductase 1 alpha subcomplex 12 | 256000 |
| 44.16 | Mitochondrial complex I subunit deficiency (NDUFA13) | NDUFA13 deficiency | NDUFA13 | *NDUFA13* | 19p13.11 | AR | NADH:ubiquinone oxidoreductase 1 alpha subcomplex 13 | 618249 |
| 44.17 | Mitochondrial complex I subunit deficiency (NDUFB3) | NDUFB3 deficiency | NDUFB3 | *NDUFB3* | 2q33.1 | AR | NADH:ubiquinone oxidoreductase 1 beta subcomplex 3 | 252010 |
| 44.18 | NADH dehydrogenase β subcomplex subunit 8 deficiency | NDUFB8 deficiency | NDUFB8 | *NDUFB8* | 10q24.31 | AR | NADH dehydrogenase β subcomplex subunit 8 | 602140 |
| 44.19 | Mitochondrial complex I subunit deficiency (NDUFB9) | NDUFB9 deficiency | NDUFB9 | *NDUFB9* | 8q24.13 | AR | NADH:ubiquinone oxidoreductase 1 beta subcomplex 9 | 252010 |
| 44.20 | Mitochondrial complex I subunit deficiency (NDUFB11) | NDUFB11 deficiency | NDUFB11 | *NDUFB11* | Xp11.3 | X-linked | NADH dehydrogenase 1 beta subcomplex 11 | 252010 |
| 44.21 | Mitochondrial complex I subunit deficiency (MTND1) | MTND1 deficiency | MTND1 | *MTND1* | mtDNA | Mitochondrial | NADH:ubiquinone oxidoreductase subunit ND1 | 252010 |
| 44.22 | Mitochondrial complex I subunit deficiency (MTND2) | MTND2 deficiency | MTND2 | *MTND2* | mtDNA | Mitochondrial | NADH:ubiquinone oxidoreductase subunit ND2 | 252010 |
| 44.23 | Mitochondrial complex I subunit deficiency (MTND3) | MTND3 deficiency | MTND3 | *MTND3* | mtDNA | Mitochondrial | NADH:ubiquinone oxidoreductase subunit ND3 | 252010 |
| 44.24 | Mitochondrial complex I subunit deficiency (MTND4) | MTND4 deficiency | MTND4 | *MTND4* | mtDNA | Mitochondrial | NADH:ubiquinone oxidoreductase subunit ND4 | 252010 |
| 44.25 | Mitochondrial complex I subunit deficiency (MTND4L) | MTND4L deficiency | MTND4L | *MTND4L* | mtDNA | Mitochondrial | NADH:ubiquinone oxidoreductase subunit ND4L | 252010 |
| 44.26 | Mitochondrial complex I subunit deficiency (MTND5) | MTND5 deficiency | MTND5 | *MTND5* | mtDNA | Mitochondrial | NADH:ubiquinone oxidoreductase subunit ND5 | 252010 |
| 44.27 | Mitochondrial complex I subunit deficiency (MTND6) | MTND6 deficiency | MTND6 | *MTND6* | mtDNA | Mitochondrial | NADH:ubiquinone oxidoreductase subunit ND6 | 252010 |
| 44.28 | Mitochondrial complex I assembly deficiency (NDUFAF1) | NDUFAF1 deficiency | NDUFAF1 | *NDUFAF1* | 15q15.1 | AR | NADH dehydrogenase (ubiquinone) complex I, assembly factor 1 | 252010 |
| 44.29 | Mitochondrial complex I assembly deficiency (NDUFAF2) | NDUFAF2 deficiency | NDUFAF2 | *NDUFAF2* | 5q12.1 | AR | NADH dehydrogenase (ubiquinone) complex I, assembly factor 2 | 252010 |

| | | | | | | | | |
|---|---|---|---|---|---|---|---|---|
| 44.30 | Mitochondrial complex I assembly deficiency (NDUFAF3) | NDUFAF3 deficiency | NDUFAF3 | *NDUFAF3* | 3p21.31 | x-linked | NADH dehydrogenase (ubiquinone) complex I, assembly factor 3 | 252010 |
| 44.31 | Mitochondrial complex I assembly deficiency (NDUFAF4) | NDUFAF4 deficiency | NDUFAF4 | *NDUFAF4* | 6q16.1 | AR | NADH dehydrogenase (ubiquinone) complex I, assembly factor 4 | 252010 |
| 44.32 | Mitochondrial complex I assembly deficiency (NDUFAF5) | NDUFAF5 deficiency | NDUFAF5 | *NDUFAF5* | 20p12.1 | AR | NADH dehydrogenase (ubiquinone) complex I, assembly factor 5 | 252010 |
| 44.33 | Mitochondrial complex I assembly deficiency (NDUFAF6) | NDUFAF6 deficiency | NDUFAF6 | *NDUFAF6* | 8q22.1 | AR | NADH dehydrogenase (ubiquinone) complex I, assembly factor 6 | 256000; 612392 |
| 44.34 | Mitochondrial complex I assembly deficiency (FOXRED1) | FOXRED1 deficiency | FOXRED1 | *FOXRED1* | 11q24.2 | AR | FAD-dependent oxidoreductese domain-containing protein 1 | 252010; 256000 |
| 44.35 | NUBPL deficiency | NUBPL deficiency | NUBPL | *NUBPL* | 14q12 | AR | Nucleotide-binding protein-like protein | 252010 |
| 44.36 | Acyl-CoA Dehydrogenase 9 deficiency | Complex I assembly disorder ACAD9 Deficiency | ACAD9D | *ACAD9D* | 3q26 | AR | Acyl-CoA dehydrogenase 9 | 611126 |
| 44.37 | Mitochondrial complex I assembly deficiency (TMEM126B) | TMEM126B deficiency | TMEM126B | *TMEM126B* | 11q14.1 | AR | Transmembrane protein 126B | 252010 |
| 44.38 | Succinate dehydrogenase subunit A deficiency | Mitochondrial complex II deficiency, nuclear type 1 | SDHA | *SDHA* | 5p15.33 | AR | Succinate dehydrogenase complex, subunit a, flavoprotein | 252011 |
| 44.39 | Succinate dehydrogenase subunit A deficiency, tumoral phenotype | Hereditary paraganglioma syndrome type 5 | **PGL5** | *SDHA* | 5p15.33 | AD | Succinate dehydrogenase complex, subunit a, flavoprotein | 614165 |
| 44.40 | Succinate dehydrogenase subunit B deficiency | | | *SDHB* | 1p36.13 | AR | Succinate dehydrogenase subunit B | 185470 |
| 44.41 | Succinate dehydrogenase subunit B deficiency, tumoral phenotype | Hereditary paraganglioma syndrome type Cowden syndrome type 2 | | *SDHB* | 1p36.13 | AD | Succinate dehydrogenase subunit B | 115310; 612359 |
| 44.42 | Succinate dehydrogenase subunit C deficiency, tumoral phenotype | Hereditary paraganglioma syndrome type 3 | PGL3 | *SDHC* | 1q23.3 | AD | Succinate dehydrogenase subunit C | 605373 |
| 44.43 | Succinate dehydrogenase subunit D deficiency | | | *SDHD* | 11q23.1 | AR | Succinate dehydrogenase subunit D | 252011 |

(continued)

| No. | Disorder | Alternative name | Abbreviation | Gene symbol | Chromosomal localisation | Inheritance | Affected protein | OMIM no. |
|---|---|---|---|---|---|---|---|---|
| 44.44 | Succinate dehydrogenase subunit D deficiency, tumoral phenotype | Hereditary paraganglioma syndrome type 1 Cowden syndrome type 3 | | *SDHD* | 11q23.1 | AD | Succinate dehydrogenase subunit D | 615106; 168000 |
| 44.45 | Succinate dehydrogenase complex assembly factor 1 deficiency | Mitochondrial complex II deficiency, nuclear type 2 | | *SDHAF1* | 19q13.12 | AR | Succinate dehydrogenase complex assembly factor 1 | 252011 |
| 44.46 | Succinate dehydrogenase complex assembly factor 2 deficiency, tumoral phenotype | Hereditary paraganglioma syndrome type 2 | PGL2 | *SDHAF2* | 11q12.2 | AD | Succinate dehydrogenase 5 | 601650 |
| 44.47 | Mitochondrial complex III subunit deficiency (UQCRB) | UQCRB deficiency Mitochondrial complex III deficiency, nuclear type 3 | UQCRB | *UQCRB* | 8q22.1 | AR | Ubiquinol-cytochrome c oxidoreductase-binding protein | 615158 |
| 44.48 | Mitochondrial complex III subunit deficiency (UQCRC2) | UQCRC2 deficiency Mitochondrial complex III deficiency, nuclear type 5 | MC3DN5 | *UQCRC2* | 16p12.2 | AR | Ubiquinol-cytochrome C reductase core protein II | 615160 |
| 44.49 | Mitochondrial complex III subunit deficiency (UQCRQ) | UQCRQ deficiency Mitochondrial complex III deficiency, nuclear type 4 | UQCRQ | *UQCRQ* | 5q31.1 | AR | Ubiquinol-cytochrome C reductase complex III subunit VII | 615159 |
| 44.50 | Mitochondrial complex III assembly deficiency (UQCC3) | UQCC3 deficiency Mitochondrial complex III deficiency, nuclear type 9 | UQCC3 | *UQCC3* | 11q12.3 | AR | Ubiquinol-cytochrome C reductase complex assembly factor 3 | 616111 |
| 44.51 | GRACILE syndrome; | Fellman disease; Björnstad syndrome Growth Retardation, Aminoaciduria, Cholestasis, Iron overload, Lactic acidosis and Early death syndrome | GRACILE | *BCS1L* | 2q35 | AR | BCS1L assembly of complex III of the mitochondrial respiratory chain. | 603358 |

| | | | | | | | | |
|---|---|---|---|---|---|---|---|---|
| 44.52 | Mitochondrial complex III subunit deficiency (TTC19) | TTC19 deficiency Mitochondrial complex III deficiency, nuclear type 2 | TTC19 | *TTC19* | 17p12 | AR | Tetratricopeptide repeat domain-containing protein 19 | 615157 |
| 44.53 | Mitochondrial complex III assembly deficiency (UQCC2) | UQCC2 deficiency Mitochondrial complex III deficiency, nuclear type 7 | UQCC2 | *UQCC2* | 6p21.31 | AR | Ubiquinol-cytochrome C reductase complex assembly factor 2 | 615824 |
| 44.54 | Mitochondrial complex III assembly deficiency (LYRM7) | LYRM7 deficiency Mitochondrial complex III deficiency, nuclear type 8 | LYRM7 | *LYRM7* | 5q23.3-q31.1 | AR | LYR motif-containing protein 7 | 615838 |
| 44.55 | Mitochondrial complex IV subunit deficiency (MTCO1) | MTCO1 deficiency | MTCO1 | *MTCO1* | mtDNA | mitochondrial | Complex IV cytochrome C oxidase subunit 1 | 516030 |
| 44.56 | Mitochondrial complex IV subunit deficiency (MTCO2) | MTCO2 deficiency | MTCO2 | *MTCO2* | mtDNA | Mitochondrial | Complex IV cytochrome C oxidase subunit 2 | 516040 |
| 44.57 | Mitochondrial complex IV subunit deficiency (MTCO3) | MTCO3 deficiency | MTCO3 | *MTCO3* | mtDNA | Mitochondrial | Complex IV cytochrome C oxidase subunit 3 | 516050 |
| 44.58 | Mitochondrial complex IV subunit deficiency (COX4I2) | COX4I2 deficiency, Exocrine pancreatic insufficiency, dyserythropoietic anemia, and calvarial hyperostosis | COX4I2 | *COX4I2* | 20q11.21 | AR | Cytochrome C oxidase subunit 4I2 | 612714 |
| 44.59 | Mitochondrial complex IV subunit deficiency (COX6A1) | COX6A1 deficiency, Charcot-Marie-Tooth disease, recessive intermediate D | COX6A1 | *COX6A1* | 12q24.31 | AR | Cytochrome C oxidase subunit 6A1 | 616039 |
| 44.60 | Mitochondrial complex IV subunit deficiency (COX6B1) | COX6B1 deficiency | COX6B1 | *COX6B1* | 19q13.12 | AR | Cytochrome C oxidase subunit 6B1 | 220110 |
| 44.61 | Mitochondrial complex IV subunit deficiency (COX7B) | COX7B deficiency linear skin defects with multiple congenital anomalies 2 | COX7B | *COX7B* | Xq21.1 | X-linked | Cytochrome C oxidase subunit 7B | 300887 |
| 44.62 | Mitochondrial complex IV subunit deficiency (COX8A) | COX8A deficiency | COX8A | *COX8A* | 11q13.1 | Mitochondrial | Cytochrome C oxidase subunit 8A | 220110 |
| 44.63 | Mitochondrial complex IV assembly deficiency (COA3) | COA3 deficiency | COA3 | *COA3* | 17q21.2 | AR | Cytochrome C oxidase assembly factor 3 (CCDC56) | 614775 |

(continued)

| No. | Disorder | Alternative name | Abbreviation | Gene symbol | Chromosomal localisation | Inheritance | Affected protein | OMIM no. |
|---|---|---|---|---|---|---|---|---|
| 44.64 | Mitochondrial complex IV assembly deficiency (COA5) | COA5 deficiency, Cardioencephalomyopathy, fatal infantile, due to cytochrome c oxidase deficiency 3 | COA5 | *COA5* | 2q11.2 | AR | Cytochrome C oxidase assembly factor 5 | 616500 |
| 44.65 | Mitochondrial complex IV assembly deficiency (COA6) | COA6 deficiency, cardioencephalomyopathy, fatal infantile, due to cytochrome c oxidase deficiency 4 | COA6 | *COA6* | 1q42.2 | AR | Cytochrome C oxidase assembly factor 6 | 616501 |
| 44.66 | Mitochondrial complex IV assembly deficiency (COA7) | COA7 deficiency | COA7 | *COA7* | 1p32.3 | AR | Cytochrome C oxidase assembly factor 7 | 220110 |
| 44.67 | Mitochondrial complex IV assembly deficiency (COX14) | COX14 deficiency | COX14 | *COX14* | 12q13.12 | AR | Cytochrome C oxidase assembly factor 14 | 220110 |
| 44.68 | Mitochondrial complex IV assembly deficiency (COX10) | COX10 deficiency, Leigh syndrome due to mitochondrial COX4 deficiency | COX10 | *COX10* | 17p12 | AR | Cytochrome C oxidase assembly factor 10 | 220110; 256000 |
| 44.69 | Mitochondrial complex IV assembly deficiency (COX15) | Leigh syndrome due to cytochrome c oxidase deficiency, Cardioencephalomyopathy, fatal infantile, due to cytochrome c oxidase deficiency 2 | COX15 | *COX15* | 10q24.2 | AR | Cytochrome C oxidase assembly factor 15 | 615119; 256000 |
| 44.70 | Mitochondrial complex IV assembly deficiency (COX20) | COX20 deficiency | COX20 | *COX20* | 1q44 | AR | Cytochrome C oxidase assembly factor 20 | 220110 |
| 44.71 | Mitochondrial complex IV assembly deficiency (SCO1) | SCO1 deficiency | SCO1 | *SCO1* | 17p13.1 | AR | Copper-binding cytochrome C oxidase assembly protein 1 | 220110 |
| 44.72 | Mitochondrial complex IV assembly deficiency (SCO2) | Myopia 6, cardioencephalomyopathy, fatal infantile, due to cytochrome c oxidase deficiency 1 | SCO2 | *SCO2* | 22q13.33 | AR | SCO2 cytochrome C oxidase assembly protein | 604377; 608908 |

| | | | | | | | | |
|---|---|---|---|---|---|---|---|---|
| 44.73 | Mitochondrial complex IV subunit deficiency (COXFA4) | COXFA4 deficiency, NDUFA4 deficiency, mitochondrial complex IV deficiency, nuclear type 21 | COXFA4 | *COXFA4* | 7p21.3 | AR | Cytochrome c oxidase subunit FA4 | 603833 |
| 44.74 | CEP89 deficiency | | CEP89 | *CEP89* | 19q13.11 | AR | Centrosomal protein, 89-KD | 615470 |
| 44.75 | Mitochondrial complex IV assembly deficiency (SURF1) | Leigh syndrome, due to COX IV deficiency, Charcot-Marie-Tooth disease, type 4K | SURF1 | *SURF1* | 9q34.2 | AR | Surfeit 1 | 256000; 616684 |
| 44.76 | Leigh Syndrome with French-Canadian Ethnicity | Mitochondrial complex IV deficiency, nuclear type 5 | LSFC | *LRPPRC* | 2p21-p16 | AR | Leucine-rich PPR Motif-containing protein | 220111 |
| 44.77 | TACO1 deficiency | Mitochondrial complex IV deficiency, nuclear type 8 | TACO1 | *TACO1* | 17q23.3 | AR | Mitochondrial translational activator | 220110 |
| 44.78 | PET100 deficiency | Mitochondrial complex IV deficiency, nuclear type 12 | | *PET100* | 19p13.2 | AR | PET100 protein involved in the biogenesis of mitochondrial complex IV | 220110 |
| 44.79 | FASTKD2 deficiency | | | *FASTKD2* | 2q33.3 | AR | Fast kinase domain-containing protein 3 | 220110 |
| 44.80 | APOPT1 deficiency | Mitochondrial complex IV deficiency, nuclear type 17 | | *APOPT1* | 14q32.33 | AR | Apoptogenic protein 1 | 220110 |
| 44.81 | Mitochondrial phosphate carrier deficiency | | | *SLC25A3* | 12q23 | AR | SLC25A3 | 610773 |
| 44.82 | Mitochondrial ATP synthase F1 subunit a deficiency | Combined oxidative phosphorylation deficiency 22, mitochondrial complex (ATP synthase) deficiency, nuclear type 4 | ATP5A1 | *ATP5F1A* | 18q21.1 | AR | ATP synthase F1 complex H+ transporter subunit 1 | 616045; 615228 |
| 44.83 | Mitochondrial ATP synthase F1 subunit δ deficiency | | | *ATP5F1D* | 19p13.3 | AR | Mitochondrial F1Fo-ATP synthase complex delta subunit | 603150 |

(continued)

| No. | Disorder | Alternative name | Abbreviation | Gene symbol | Chromosomal localisation | Inheritance | Affected protein | OMIM no. |
|---|---|---|---|---|---|---|---|---|
| 44.84 | Mitochondrial ATP synthase F1 subunit e deficiency | ATP5E deficiency, mitochondrial complex V (ATP synthase) deficiency, nuclear type 3 | ATP5E | *ATP5F1E* | 20q13.32 | AR | ATP synthase F1 complex H+ transporter epsilon subunit | 614053 |
| 44.85 | Mitochondrial complex V subunit deficiency (MTATP6) | MTATP6 deficiency | MTATP6 | *MTATP6* | mtDNA | Mitochondrial | ATP synthase (complex V) subunit 6 | 516060 |
| 44.86 | Mitochondrial complex V subunit deficiency (MTATP8) | MTATP8 deficiency | MTATP8 | *MTATP8* | mtDNA | Mitochondrial | ATP synthase (complex V) subunit 8 | 516070 |
| 44.87 | Transmembrane protein 70 deficiency | Neonatal mitochondrial encephalocardiomyopathy | NME | *TMEM70* | 8q21.11 | AR | Complex V assembly protein | 614052 |
| 44.88 | Mitochondrial complex V assembly deficiency (ATPAF2) | ATPAF2 deficiency, Mitochondrial complex V (ATP synthase) deficiency, nuclear type 1 | ATPAF2 | *ATPAF2* | 17p11.2 | AR | ATP synthase F1 complex assembly factor 1 | 604273 |
| 44.89 | DAPIT deficiency | Diabetes-associated protein deficiency | | *ATP5MD* | 10q24.33 | AR | Diabetes-associated protein in insulin-sensitive tissues | 615204 |
| 44.90 | Mitochondrial cytochrome b deficiency | | MT-CYB | *MTCYB* | mtDNA | Mitochondrial | Cytochrome b complex III | 516020 |
| 44.91.1 | Mitochondrial cytochrome c1 deficiency | Mitochondrial complex III deficiency, nuclear type 6 | CYC1 | *CYC1* | 8q24.3 | AR | Cytochrome c1 | 615453 |
| 44.91.2 | Mitochondrial cytochrome c deficiency | Thrombocytopenia type 4 | CYCS | *CYCS* | 7p15.3 | AD | Cytochrome c, somatic | 612004 |
| 44.92 | Holocytochrome c synthase deficiency | Linear skin defects with multiple congenital anomalies type 1 | HCCS | *HCCS* | Xp22.2 | X-linked | Holocytochrome c synthase | 309801 |

## Metabolic Pathway

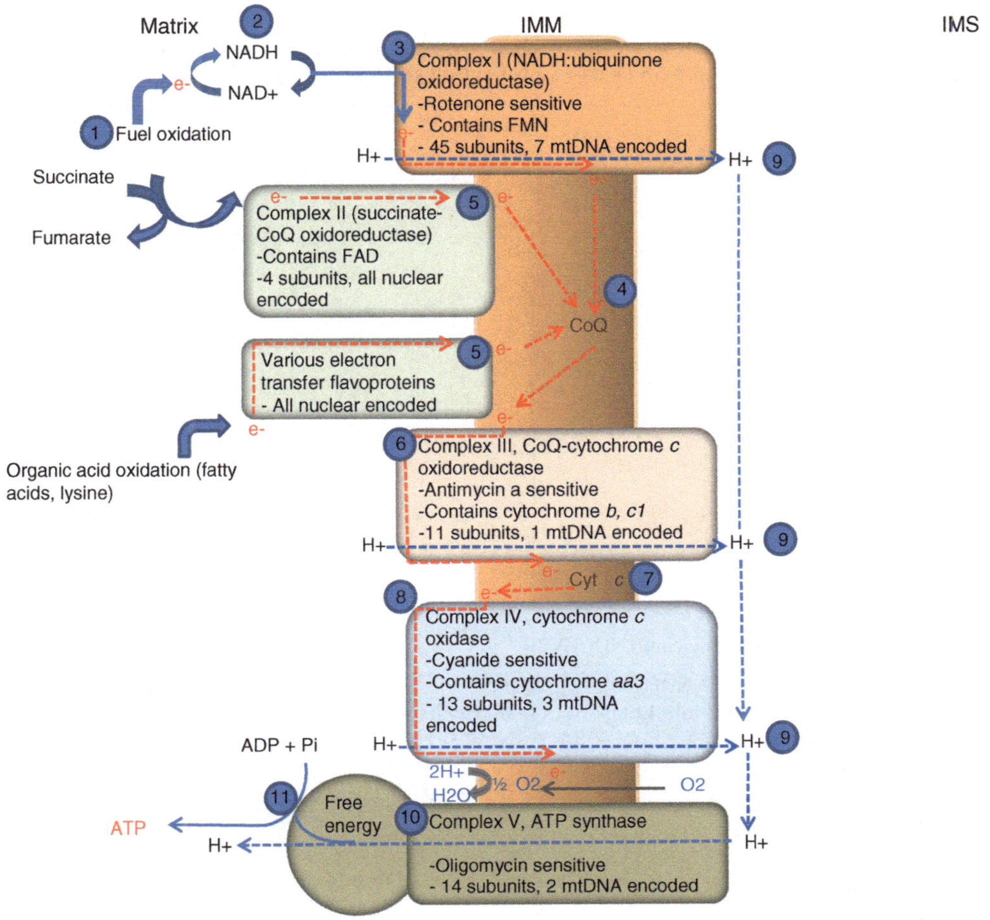


**Fig. 44.1** Oxidative phosphorylation (OXPHOS) system in mammalian mitochondria. Electrons ($e^-$) from carbon oxidations (step 1 and red dotted lines) are transferred via NADH (step 2) into OXPHOS complex I (step 3), which is embedded in the inner mitochondrial membrane (IMM), then transported to coenzyme Q (CoQ) (step 4). Some electrons from organic-acid oxidations are transferred via other flavin-containing enzyme complexes (step 5) directly to CoQ. CoQ delivers electrons via complex III (step 6) and cytochrome c (Cyt *c*) to the final electron acceptor complex IV (step 8). Here, oxygen is reduced to water. The electrons lose free energy at each transfer step, and in complexes I, III and IV. The energy is harnessed and coupled to the movement of $H^+$ (step 9 and blue dashed lines) from the mitochondrial matrix to the intermembrane space (IMS). The proton-gradient thus generated is used for the production of ATP by complex V (steps 10 and 11). Except for complex II, all complexes contain some proteins encoded by the mitochondrial genome and others encoded by the nuclear genome. The number of subunits for each complex is indicated (FMN, flavin mononucleotide; mt, mitochondrial)

## Signs and Symptoms

**Table 44.1** Mitochondrial complex I subunit deficiency (NDUFV1)

| System | Symptoms and biomarkers | Neonatal (birth–1 month) | Infancy (1–18 months) | Childhood (1.5–11 years) | Adolescence (11–16 years) | Adulthood (>16 years) |
|---|---|---|---|---|---|---|
| Cardiovascular | **Cardiomyopathy, hypertrophic** | + | + | + | + | |
| CNS | **Ataxia** | + | + | + | + | |
| | Basal ganglia abnormalities (MRI) | + | + | + | + | |
| | Brain stem lesions (MRI) | | | | | |
| | **Encephalopathy** | + | + | + | + | |
| | **Leigh syndrome** | + | + | + | | |
| | Microcephaly | + | + | + | + | |
| | Regression, psychomotor | + | + | + | + | |
| Eye | **Ophthalmoplegia** | | + | + | + | |
| Metabolic | Lactic acidosis | + | + | + | + | |
| Other | Failure to thrive | + | + | + | + | |
| Laboratory findings | Decreased complexI activity | ↓ | ↓ | ↓ | ↓ | |
| | Lactate (serum) | ↑ | ↑ | ↑ | ↑ | |

**Table 44.2** Mitochondrial complex I subunit deficiency (NDUFV2)

| System | Symptoms and biomarkers | Neonatal (birth–1 month) | Infancy (1–18 months) | Childhood (1.5–11 years) | Adolescence (11–16 years) | Adulthood (>16 years) |
|---|---|---|---|---|---|---|
| Cardiovascular | **Cardiomyopathy, hypertrophic** | + | + | + | + | + |
| CNS | **Leigh syndrome** | + | + | + | + | + |
| | **Leukodystrophy** | + | + | + | + | + |
| | Parkinsonism | | | + | + | + |
| Digestive | **Liver dysfunction** | + | + | + | + | + |
| Eye | **Optic neuropathy** | | + | + | + | + |
| Musculoskeletal | **Myopathy** | + | + | + | + | + |
| Laboratory findings | Decreased complex I activity | ↓ | ↓ | ↓ | ↓ | ↓ |

**Table 44.3** Mitochondrial complex I subunit deficiency (NDUFS1)

| System | Symptoms and biomarkers | Neonatal (birth–1 month) | Infancy (1–18 months) | Childhood (1.5–11 years) | Adolescence (11–16 years) | Adulthood (>16 years) |
|---|---|---|---|---|---|---|
| Cardiovascular | **Cardiomyopathy, hypertrophic** | | + | + | + | + |
| CNS | **Encephalopathy** | + | + | + | + | + |
| | Hypotonia | + | + | + | + | + |
| | **Leukodystrophy** | + | + | + | + | + |
| Digestive | **Liver dysfunction** | + | + | + | + | + |
| Eye | **Optic neuropathy** | | + | + | + | + |
| Musculoskeletal | **Myopathy** | + | + | + | + | + |
| Laboratory findings | Decreased complex I activity | ↓ | ↓ | ↓ | ↓ | ↓ |
| | Lactate (plasma) | ↑ | ↑ | ↑ | ↑ | ↑ |

**Table 44.4** Mitochondrial complex I subunit deficiency (NDUFS2)

| System | Symptoms and biomarkers | Neonatal (birth–1 month) | Infancy (1–18 months) | Childhood (1.5–11 years) | Adolescence (11–16 years) | Adulthood (>16 years) |
|---|---|---|---|---|---|---|
| Cardiovascular | **Cardiomyopathy, hypertrophic** | | + | + | + | + |
| CNS | **Encephalopathy** | + | + | + | + | + |
| | **Hypotonia** | + | + | + | + | + |
| | **Leigh syndrome** | + | + | + | + | + |
| | **Parkinsonism** | | + | + | + | + |
| Digestive | **Liver dysfunction** | + | + | + | + | + |
| Musculoskeletal | **Myopathy** | + | + | + | + | + |
| Laboratory findings | Decreased complex I activity | ↓ | ↓ | ↓ | ↓ | ↓ |
| | Lactate (plasma) | ↑ | ↑ | ↑ | ↑ | ↑ |

**Table 44.5** Mitochondrial complex I subunit deficiency (NDUFS3)

| System | Symptoms and biomarkers | Neonatal (birth–1 month) | Infancy (1–18 months) | Childhood (1.5–11 years) | Adolescence (11–16 years) | Adulthood (>16 years) |
|---|---|---|---|---|---|---|
| CNS | **Developmental delay** | + | + | + | + | |
| | **Encephalopathy** | + | + | + | + | |
| | **Leigh syndrome** | + | + | + | + | |
| Musculoskeletal | **Myopathy** | + | + | + | + | |
| Laboratory findings | Decreased complex I activity | ↓ | ↓ | ↓ | | |
| | Lactate (plasma) | ↑ | ↑ | ↑ | | |

**Table 44.6** Mitochondrial complex I subunit deficiency (NDUFS7)

| System | Symptoms and biomarkers | Neonatal (birth–1 month) | Infancy (1–18 months) | Childhood (1.5–11 years) | Adolescence (11–16 years) | Adulthood (>16 years) |
|---|---|---|---|---|---|---|
| Cardiovascular | **Cardiomyopathy** | + | + | + | | |
| CNS | **Ataxia** | + | + | + | | |
| | **Encephalopathy** | + | + | + | | |
| | **Epilepsy** | + | + | + | | |
| | **Leigh syndrome** | + | + | + | | |
| Digestive | **Feeding difficulties** | + | + | + | | |
| | **Liver dysfunction** | + | + | + | | |
| Metabolic | Lactic acidosis | + | + | + | | |
| Musculoskeletal | Myopathy | + | + | + | | |
| Laboratory findings | Complex I activity | ↓ | ↓ | ↓ | | |
| | Lactate (plasma) | ↑ | ↑ | ↑ | | |

**Table 44.7** Mitochondrial complex I subunit deficiency (NDUFS8)

| System | Symptoms and biomarkers | Neonatal (birth–1 month) | Infancy (1–18 months) | Childhood (1.5–11 years) | Adolescence (11–16 years) | Adulthood (>16 years) |
|---|---|---|---|---|---|---|
| Cardiovascular | **Cardiomyopathy, hypertrophic** | | + | + | + | |
| CNS | **Ataxia** | | + | + | + | |
| | **Dysarthria** | | + | + | + | |
| | **Hypotonia** | | + | + | + | |
| | **Leigh syndrome** | + | + | + | + | |
| Eye | **Ophthalmoplegia, progressive external** | | + | + | + | |
| Musculoskeletal | **Myopathy** | | + | + | + | |
| Laboratory findings | Complex I activity | ↓ | ↓ | ↓ | ↓ | ↓ |

**Table 44.8** Mitochondrial complex I subunit deficiency (NDUFS4)

| System | Symptoms and biomarkers | Neonatal (birth–1 month) | Infancy (1–18 months) | Childhood (1.5–11 years) | Adolescence (11–16 years) | Adulthood (>16 years) |
|---|---|---|---|---|---|---|
| Cardiovascular | **Cardiomyopathy, hypertrophic** | + | + | + | + | |
| CNS | **Basal ganglia abnormalities (MRI)** | + | + | + | + | |
| | **Hypotonia** | + | + | + | + | |
| | **Leigh syndrome** | + | + | + | + | |
| Metabolic | **Lactic acidosis** | + | + | + | + | |
| Other | **Failure to thrive** | + | + | + | + | |
| Laboratory findings | Complex I activity | ↓ | ↓ | ↓ | ↓ | |
| | Complex III activity | ↓ | ↓ | ↓ | ↓ | |
| | Lactate (plasma) | ↑ | ↑ | ↑ | ↑ | |

**Table 44.9** Mitochondrial complex I subunit deficiency (NDUFS6)

| System | Symptoms and biomarkers | Neonatal (birth–1 month) | Infancy (1–18 months) | Childhood (1.5–11 years) | Adolescence (11–16 years) | Adulthood (>16 years) |
|---|---|---|---|---|---|---|
| Cardiovascular | **Cardiomyopathy, hypertrophic** | + | + | + | + | |
| CNS | **Basal ganglia abnormalities (MRI)** | + | + | + | + | |
| | **Hypotonia** | + | + | + | + | |
| | **Leigh syndrome** | + | + | + | + | |
| Metabolic | Lactic acidosis | + | + | + | | |
| Other | Failure to thrive | + | + | + | + | |
| | **Severe multisystem disease** | + | + | | | |
| Laboratory findings | Complex I activity | ↓ | ↓ | ↓ | | |
| | Lactate (plasma) | ↑ | ↑ | ↑ | | |

**Table 44.10** Mitochondrial complex I subunit deficiency (NDUFA1)

| System | Symptoms and biomarkers | Neonatal (birth–1 month) | Infancy (1–18 months) | Childhood (1.5–11 years) | Adolescence (11–16 years) | Adulthood (>16 years) |
|---|---|---|---|---|---|---|
| CNS | **Basal ganglia abnormalities (MRI)** | + | + | + | + | |
| | **Epilepsy** | + | + | + | + | |
| | Hypotonia | + | + | + | + | |
| | **Leigh syndrome** | + | + | + | + | |
| | **Retardation, psychomotor** | + | + | + | + | |
| Metabolic | **Lactic acidosis** | + | + | + | + | |
| Laboratory findings | Complex I activity | ↓ | ↓ | ↓ | ↓ | |
| | Lactate (plasma) | ↑ | ↑ | ↑ | ↑ | |

**Table 44.11** Mitochondrial complex I subunit deficiency (NDUFA2)

| System | Symptoms and biomarkers | Neonatal (birth–1 month) | Infancy (1–18 months) | Childhood (1.5–11 years) | Adolescence (11–16 years) | Adulthood (>16 years) |
|---|---|---|---|---|---|---|
| CNS | **Leigh syndrome** | + | + | + | | |
| | **Leukoencephalopathy** | + | + | + | | |
| Metabolic | **Lactic acidosis** | + | + | + | | |
| Laboratory findings | Complex I deficiency | ↓ | ↓ | ↓ | | |
| | Lactate (plasma) | ↑ | ↑ | ↑ | | |

**Table 44.12** Mitochondrial complex I subunit deficiency (NDUFA9)

| System | Symptoms and biomarkers | Neonatal (birth–1 month) | Infancy (1–18 months) | Childhood (1.5–11 years) | Adolescence (11–16 years) | Adulthood (>16 years) |
|---|---|---|---|---|---|---|
| CNS | **Brainstem abnormal (MRI)** | + | + | + | | |
| | Dysarthria | | + | + | | |
| | Dystonia | | + | + | | |
| | **Leigh syndrome** | + | + | + | | |
| Digestive | Dysphagia | | + | + | | |
| Eye | **Retinitis pigmentosa** | + | + | + | | |
| Metabolic | **Lactic acidosis** | + | + | + | | |
| Laboratory findings | Complex I activity | ↓ | ↓ | ↓ | | |
| | Lactate (plasma) | ↑ | ↑ | ↑ | | |

**Table 44.13** Mitochondrial complex I subunit deficiency (NDUFA10)

| System | Symptoms and biomarkers | Neonatal (birth–1 month) | Infancy (1–18 months) | Childhood (1.5–11 years) | Adolescence (11–16 years) | Adulthood (>16 years) |
|---|---|---|---|---|---|---|
| Cardiovascular | **Cardiomyopathy, hypertrophic** | + | + | | | |
| CNS | **Basal ganglia abnormalities (MRI)** | + | + | | | |
| | **Hypotonia** | + | + | | | |
| | **Leigh syndrome** | + | + | | | |
| | **Retardation, psychomotor** | + | + | | | |
| Metabolic | **Lactic acidosis** | + | + | | | |
| Laboratory findings | Complex I deficiency | ↓ | ↓ | | | |
| | Lactate (plasma) | ↑ | ↑ | | | |

**Table 44.14** Mitochondrial complex I subunit deficiency (NDUFA11)

| System | Symptoms and biomarkers | Neonatal (birth–1 month) | Infancy (1–18 months) | Childhood (1.5–11 years) | Adolescence (11–16 years) | Adulthood (>16 years) |
|---|---|---|---|---|---|---|
| Cardiovascular | **Cardiomyopathy** | + | + | | | |
| CNS | **Encephalopathy** | + | + | | | |
| Metabolic | **Lactic acidosis** | + | + | | | |
| Laboratory findings | Complex I deficiency | ↓ | ↓ | | | |
| | Lactate (plasma) | ↑ | ↑ | | | |

**Table 44.15** Mitochondrial complex I subunit deficiency (NDUFA12)

| System | Symptoms and biomarkers | Neonatal (birth–1 month) | Infancy (1–18 months) | Childhood (1.5–11 years) | Adolescence (11–16 years) | Adulthood (>16 years) |
|---|---|---|---|---|---|---|
| CNS | Dystonia | | + | + | | |
| | Hypotonia | | + | + | | |
| | **Leigh syndrome** | + | + | + | | |
| | Retardation, psychomotor | | + | + | | |
| Musculoskeletal | Growth retardation | | + | + | | |
| Laboratory findings | Complex I activity | ↓ | ↓ | ↓ | | |

**Table 44.16** Mitochondrial complex I subunit deficiency (NDUFA13)

| System | Symptoms and biomarkers | Neonatal (birth–1 month) | Infancy (1–18 months) | Childhood (1.5–11 years) | Adolescence (11–16 years) | Adulthood (>16 years) |
|---|---|---|---|---|---|---|
| CNS | **Cerebellar atrophy (MRI)** | + | + | + | | |
| | **Developmental delay** | + | + | + | | |
| | **Encephalopathy** | + | + | + | | |
| | **Hypotonia** | + | + | + | | |
| Digestive | **Feeding difficulties** | + | + | + | | |
| Metabolic | Lactic acidosis | + | + | + | | |
| Laboratory findings | Complex I activity | ↓ | ↓ | ↓ | | |
| | Lactate (plasma) | ↑ | ↑ | ↑ | | |

**Table 44.17** Mitochondrial complex I subunit deficiency (NDUFB3)

| System | Symptoms and biomarkers | Neonatal (birth–1 month) | Infancy (1–18 months) | Childhood (1.5–11 years) | Adolescence (11–16 years) | Adulthood (>16 years) |
|---|---|---|---|---|---|---|
| CNS | **Developmental delay** | + | + | + | | |
| | **Encephalopathy** | + | + | + | | |
| | Hypotonia | + | + | + | | |
| Metabolic | **Lactic acidosis** | + | + | + | | |
| Musculoskeletal | **Myopathy** | + | + | + | | |
| Laboratory findings | Complex I activity | ↓ | ↓ | ↓ | | |
| | Lactate (plasma) | ↑ | ↑ | ↑ | | |

**Table 44.18** NADH dehydrogenase β subcomplex subunit 8 deficiency

| System | Symptoms and biomarkers | Neonatal (birth–1 month) | Infancy (1–18 months) | Childhood (1.5–11 years) | Adolescence (11–16 years) | Adulthood (>16 years) |
|---|---|---|---|---|---|---|
| Cardiovascular | **Cardiomyopathy, hypertrophic** | | + | + | | |
| CNS | **Epilepsy** | | + | + | | |
| | Hypotonia | + | + | + | | |
| | **Leigh syndrome** | + | + | + | | |
| | **Retardation, psychomotor** | + | + | + | | |
| Metabolic | **Lactic acidosis** | + | + | + | | |
| Other | Failure to thrive | + | + | + | | |
| Laboratory findings | Complex I activity | ↓ | ↓ | ↓ | | |
| | Lactate (plasma) | ↑ | ↑ | ↑ | | |

**Table 44.19** Mitochondrial complex I subunit deficiency (NDUFB9)

| System | Symptoms and biomarkers | Neonatal (birth–1 month) | Infancy (1–18 months) | Childhood (1.5–11 years) | Adolescence (11–16 years) | Adulthood (>16 years) |
|---|---|---|---|---|---|---|
| CNS | **Hypotonia** | + | + | | | |
| Metabolic | **Lactic acidosis** | + | + | | | |
| Other | Death | + | + | | | |
| Laboratory findings | Complex I activity | ↓ | ↓ | | | |
| | Lactate (plasma) | ↑ | ↑ | | | |

**Table 44.20** Mitochondrial complex I subunit deficiency (NDUFB11)

| System | Symptoms and biomarkers | Neonatal (birth–1 month) | Infancy (1–18 months) | Childhood (1.5–11 years) | Adolescence (11–16 years) | Adulthood (>16 years) |
|---|---|---|---|---|---|---|
| Cardiovascular | **Cardiomyopathy** | | + | + | | |
| Eye | **Microphthalmia** | + | + | + | | |
| Hematological | **Anemia, sideroblastic** | + | + | + | | |
| Metabolic | **Lactic acidosis** | + | + | + | | |
| Other | Death | | + | + | | |
| Laboratory findings | Complex I activity | ↓ | ↓ | ↓ | | |
| | Lactate (plasma) | ↑ | ↑ | ↑ | | |

**Table 44.21** Mitochondrial complex I subunit deficiency (MTND1)

| System | Symptoms and biomarkers | Neonatal (birth–1 month) | Infancy (1–18 months) | Childhood (1.5–11 years) | Adolescence (11–16 years) | Adulthood (>16 years) |
|---|---|---|---|---|---|---|
| Cardiovascular | **Cardiomyopathy, hypertrophic** | + | + | + | + | + |
| CNS | **Dystonia** | | + | + | + | + |
| | **Spasticity** | | + | + | + | + |
| Eye | Leber hereditary optic neuropathy | | | | + | + |
| Musculoskeletal | Exercise intolerance | | | + | + | + |
| | **Myopathy** | + | + | + | + | + |
| Other | **MELAS syndrome** | | + | + | + | + |
| Laboratory findings | Complex I activity | ↓ | ↓ | ↓ | ↓ | ↓ |
| | Lactate (plasma) | ↑ | ↑ | ↑ | ↑ | ↑ |

**Table 44.22** Mitochondrial complex I subunit deficiency (MTND2)

| System | Symptoms and biomarkers | Neonatal (birth–1 month) | Infancy (1–18 months) | Childhood (1.5–11 years) | Adolescence (11–16 years) | Adulthood (>16 years) |
|---|---|---|---|---|---|---|
| CNS | **Leigh syndrome** | + | + | + | | |
| Eye | Leber hereditary optic neuropathy | | | | + | + |
| Metabolic | **Ragged red fibers** | + | + | + | + | + |
| Musculoskeletal | Exercise intolerance | | + | + | + | + |
| Laboratory findings | Complex I activity | ↓ | ↓ | ↓ | ↓ | ↓ |
| | Lactate (plasma) | ↑ | ↑ | ↑ | ↑ | ↑ |

**Table 44.23** Mitochondrial complex I subunit deficiency (MTND3)

| System | Symptoms and biomarkers | Neonatal (birth–1 month) | Infancy (1–18 months) | Childhood (1.5–11 years) | Adolescence (11–16 years) | Adulthood (>16 years) |
|---|---|---|---|---|---|---|
| CNS | Dystonia | | + | + | + | + |
| | **Encephalopathy** | + | + | + | + | + |
| | **Epilepsy** | + | + | + | + | + |
| | **Leigh syndrome** | + | + | + | + | |
| | Neuropathy | | + | + | + | + |
| Eye | **Eye movements, abnormal** | | + | + | + | + |
| | Leber hereditary optic neuropathy | | | | + | + |
| | **Optic atrophy** | | + | + | + | + |
| Musculoskeletal | **Myopathy** | | + | + | + | + |
| Laboratory findings | Complex I activity | ↓ | ↓ | ↓ | ↓ | ↓ |
| | Lactate (plasma) | ↑ | ↑ | ↑ | ↑ | ↑ |

**Table 44.24** Mitochondrial complex I subunit deficiency (MTND4)

| System | Symptoms and biomarkers | Neonatal (birth–1 month) | Infancy (1–18 months) | Childhood (1.5–11 years) | Adolescence (11–16 years) | Adulthood (>15 years) |
|---|---|---|---|---|---|---|
| CNS | Dystonia | | | + | + | + |
| | **Leigh syndrome** | + | + | + | + | + |
| Eye | Leber hereditary optic neuropathy | | | | + | + |
| Other | MELAS syndrome | | | | | + |
| Laboratory findings | Complex I activity | ↓ | ↓ | ↓ | ↓ | ↓ |
| | Lactate (plasma) | ↑ | ↑ | ↑ | ↑ | ↑ |

**Table 44.25** Mitochondrial complex I subunit deficiency (MTND4L)

| System | Symptoms and biomarkers | Neonatal (birth–1 month) | Infancy (1–18 months) | Childhood (1.5–11 years) | Adolescence (11–16 years) | Adulthood (>16 years) |
|---|---|---|---|---|---|---|
| Eye | Leber hereditary optic neuropathy | | | | + | + |
| Laboratory findings | Complex I activity | ↓ | ↓ | ↓ | ↓ | ↓ |

**Table 44.26** Mitochondrial complex I subunit deficiency (MTND5)

| System | Symptoms and biomarkers | Neonatal (birth–1 month) | Infancy (1–18 months) | Childhood (1.5–11 years) | Adolescence (11–16 years) | Adulthood (>16 years) |
|---|---|---|---|---|---|---|
| CNS | Leigh syndrome | | + | + | + | + |
| Eye | Leber hereditary optic neuropathy | | | + | + | + |
| Musculoskeletal | **Myopathy** | | + | + | + | + |
| Renal | Renal failure | | | + | + | + |
| Other | MELAS syndrome | | + | + | + | + |
| | MERFF syndrome | | + | + | + | + |
| Laboratory findings | Complex I activity | ↓ | ↓ | ↓ | ↓ | ↓ |
| | Lactate (plasma) | ↑ | ↑ | ↑ | ↑ | ↑ |

**Table 44.27** Mitochondrial complex I subunit deficiency (MTND6)

| System | Symptoms and biomarkers | Neonatal (birth–1 month) | Infancy (1–18 months) | Childhood (1.5–11 years) | Adolescence (11–16 years) | Adulthood (>16 years) |
|---|---|---|---|---|---|---|
| CNS | Dystonia | | + | + | + | + |
| | **Epilepsy** | + | + | + | + | + |
| | **Leigh syndrome** | + | + | + | + | + |
| | Stroke-like episodes | | + | + | + | + |
| Eye | Leber hereditary optic neuropathy | | | + | + | + |
| | **Optic atrophy** | | + | + | + | + |
| Metabolic | Lactic acidosis | + | + | + | + | + |
| Other | MELAS syndrome | + | + | + | + | + |
| Laboratory findings | Complex I activity | ↓ | ↓ | ↓ | ↓ | ↓ |
| | Lactate (plasma) | ↑ | ↑ | ↑ | ↑ | ↑ |

**Table 44.28** Mitochondrial complex I assembly deficiency (NDUFAF1)

| System | Symptoms and biomarkers | Neonatal (birth–1 month) | Infancy (1–18 months) | Childhood (1.5–11 years) | Adolescence (11–16 years) | Adulthood (>16 years) |
|---|---|---|---|---|---|---|
| Cardiovascular | **Cardiomyopathy** | + | + | + | + | |
| CNS | Hypotonia | + | + | + | + | |
| Metabolic | **Lactic acidosis** | + | + | + | + | |
| Other | Failure to thrive | + | + | | | |
| | **MELAS syndrome** | + | + | + | + | |
| Laboratory findings | Complex I activity | ↓ | ↓ | ↓ | ↓ | |
| | Lactate (plasma) | ↑ | ↑ | ↑ | ↑ | |

**Table 44.29** Mitochondrial complex I assembly deficiency (NDUFAF2)

| System | Symptoms and biomarkers | Neonatal (birth–1 month) | Infancy (1–18 months) | Childhood (1.5–11 years) | Adolescence (11–16 years) | Adulthood (>16 years) |
|---|---|---|---|---|---|---|
| CNS | Ataxia | | + | + | + | |
| | **Basal ganglia abnormalities (MRI)** | + | + | + | + | |
| | **Encephalopathy** | + | + | + | + | |
| | Hypotonia | + | + | + | + | |
| Eye | **Nystagmus** | + | + | + | + | |
| | **Optic atrophy** | + | + | + | + | |
| Renal | Renal tubular acidosis | | + | + | + | |
| Respiratory | Respiratory insufficiency | ± | ± | ± | ± | |
| Laboratory findings | Complex I activity | ↓ | ↓ | ↓ | ↓ | |
| | Lactate (plasma) | ↑ | ↑ | ↑ | ↑ | |

**Table 44.30** Mitochondrial complex I assembly deficiency (NDUFAF3)

| System | Symptoms and biomarkers | Neonatal (birth–1 month) | Infancy (1–18 months) | Childhood (1.5–11 years) | Adolescence (11–16 years) | Adulthood (>16 years) |
|---|---|---|---|---|---|---|
| CNS | **Hypotonia** | + | + | | | |
| | **Leukomalacia, diffuse** | + | + | | | |
| Eye | **Optic atrophy** | + | + | | | |
| Respiratory | **Respiratory failure** | + | + | | | |
| Other | Death | + | + | | | |
| Laboratory findings | Complex I activity | ↓ | ↓ | | | |
| | Lactate (plasma) | ↑ | ↑ | | | |

**Table 44.31** Mitochondrial complex I assembly deficiency (NDUFAF4)

| System | Symptoms and biomarkers | Neonatal (birth–1 month) | Infancy (1–18 months) | Childhood (1.5–11 years) | Adolescence (11–16 years) | Adulthood (>16 years) |
|---|---|---|---|---|---|---|
| Cardiovascular | Cardiomyopathy | + | + | | | |
| CNS | Encephalomyopathy | + | + | | | |
| | Leigh syndrome | + | + | | | |
| Laboratory findings | Decreased complex I activity | ↓ | ↓ | | | |
| | Lactate (plasma) | ↑ | ↑ | | | |

**Table 44.32** Mitochondrial complex I assembly deficiency (NDUFAF5)

| System | Symptoms and biomarkers | Neonatal (birth–1 month) | Infancy (1–18 months) | Childhood (1.5–11 years) | Adolescence (11–16 years) | Adulthood (>16 years) |
|---|---|---|---|---|---|---|
| CNS | Basal ganglia abnormalities (MRI) | + | + | + | + | + |
| | Dystonia | | | + | + | + |
| | Epilepsy | | + | + | | |
| | Hypotonia | | + | + | + | + |
| | Intellectual disability | | + | + | + | + |
| | Spasticity | | | + | + | + |
| Metabolic | Lactic acidosis | + | + | + | + | + |
| Other | Leigh syndrome | + | + | + | | |
| Laboratory findings | Complex I activity | ↓ | ↓ | ↓ | ↓ | ↓ |
| | Lactate (plasma) | ↑ | ↑ | ↑ | ↑ | ↑ |

**Table 44.33** Mitochondrial complex I assembly deficiency (NDUFAF6)

| System | Symptoms and biomarkers | Neonatal (birth–1 month) | Infancy (1–18 months) | Childhood (1.5–11 years) | Adolescence (11–16 years) | Adulthood (>16 years) |
|---|---|---|---|---|---|---|
| CNS | Ataxia | | + | + | + | |
| | **Basal ganglia abnormalities (MRI)** | + | + | + | + | |
| | Dystonia | | + | + | + | |
| | **Epilepsy** | + | + | + | + | |
| | **Leigh syndrome** | + | + | + | | |
| | Retardation, psychomotor | | + | + | + | |
| | **Striatal necrosis, isolated bilateral** | + | + | + | + | |
| Metabolic | **Lactic acidosis** | + | + | + | + | |
| Laboratory findings | Complex I activity | ↓ | ↓ | ↓ | ↓ | |
| | Lactate (plasma) | ↑ | ↑ | ↑ | ↑ | |

**Table 44.34** Mitochondrial complex I assembly deficiency (FOXRED1)

| System | Symptoms and biomarkers | Neonatal (birth–1 month) | Infancy (1–18 months) | Childhood (1.5–11 years) | Adolescence (11–16 years) | Adulthood (>16 years) |
|---|---|---|---|---|---|---|
| Cardiovascular | **Cardiomyopathy, hypertrophic** | | + | + | | |
| CNS | Cerebellar atrophy (MRI) | + | + | + | + | + |
| | Epilepsy | + | + | + | + | + |
| | Hypotonia | + | + | + | + | + |
| | Leigh syndrome | + | + | + | + | + |
| Pulmonary | **Pulmonary hypertension** | | + | + | + | |
| Laboratory findings | Complex I activity | ↓ | ↓ | ↓ | ↓ | ↓ |
| | Lactate (plasma) | ↑ | ↑ | ↑ | ↑ | ↑ |

**Table 44.35** NUBPL deficiency

| System | Symptoms and biomarkers | Neonatal (birth–1 month) | Infancy (1–18 months) | Childhood (1.5–11 years) | Adolescence (11–16 years) | Adulthood (>16 years) |
|---|---|---|---|---|---|---|
| CNS | Ataxia | | + | + | | |
| | Developmental delay | | + | + | | |
| | Dystonia | | + | + | | |
| | **Leukodystrophy** | + | + | + | | |
| | Pyramidal signs | | + | + | | |
| Eye | Nystagmus | | + | + | | |
| Musculoskeletal | Myopathy | + | + | + | | |
| Laboratory findings | Complex I acivity | ↓ | ↓ | ↓ | | |
| | Lactate (plasma) | ↑ | ↑ | ↑ | | |

Table 44.36 Acyl-CoA Dehydrogenase 9 deficiency

| System | Symptoms and biomarkers | Neonatal (birth–1 month) | Infancy (1–18 months) | Childhood (1.5–11 years) | Adolescence (11–16 years) | Adulthood (>16 years) |
|---|---|---|---|---|---|---|
| Cardiovascular | **Cardiomyopathy, dilated** | | + | + | | |
| CNS | **Encephalopathy** | | + | | | |
| | **Neurologic dysfunction** | | + | + | | |
| Digestive | **Liver dysfunction** | | + | + | | |
| | **Liver failure** | | + | + | | |
| | **Liver failure, Reye-like** | | | | + | |
| Ear | **Hearing loss** | | + | + | | |
| Metabolic | Hypoglycemia | | + | + | | |
| | Lactic acidosis | | + | + | | |
| Musculoskeletal | **Exercise Intolerance** | | + | + | | |
| | **Hypotonia, muscular-axial** | | + | + | | |
| | **Rhabdomyolysis** | | + | + | | |
| | **Skeletal myopathy** | | + | + | | |
| Other | Complex I assembly disorder | | + | + | | |
| | **Failure to thrive** | | + | + | | |
| Laboratory findings | Adipic acid (urine) | | ↑ | ↑ | | |
| | Alanine (plasma) | | ↑ | ↑ | | |
| | Alanine (urine) | | ↑ | ↑ | | |
| | Ammonia (blood) | | (↑) | (↑) | (↑) | |
| | Beta-hydroxybutyrate (urine) | | ↑ | | | |
| | C14:0-Acylcarnitine (dried blood spot) | | ↑ | ↑ | | |
| | C14:0-Acylcarnitine (serum) | | ↑ | ↑ | | |
| | C16:0-Acylcarnitine (dried blood spot) | | ↑ | ↑ | | |
| | C16:0-Acylcarnitine (plasma) | | ↑ | ↑ | | |
| | C16:1-Acylcarnitine (dried blood spot) | | ↑ | ↑ | | |
| | C16:1-Acylcarnitine (plasma) | | ↑ | ↑ | | |
| | C18:0-Acylcarnitine (dried blood spot) | | ↑ | ↑ | | |
| | C18:0-Acylcarnitine (plasma) | | ↑ | ↑ | | |
| | C18:1-Acylcarnitine (dried blood spot) | | ↑ | ↑ | | |
| | C18:1-Acylcarnitine (plasma) | | ↑ | ↑ | | |
| | C18:2-Acylcarnitine (dried blood spot) | | ↑ | ↑ | | |
| | C18:2-Acylcarnitine (plasma) | | ↑ | ↑ | | |
| | Carnitine, free (dried blood spot) | | ↓ | ↓ | | |
| | Carnitine, free (plasma) | | ↓ | ↓ | | |
| | Creatine kinase (plasma) | | ↑ | ↑ | | |
| | Glucose (plasma) | ↓ | ↓ | ↓ | | |
| | Lactate (plasma) | ↑ | ↑ | | | |
| | Lactate (urine) | ↑ | ↑ | ↑ | | |
| | Lactate/Pyruvate ratio | ↑ | ↑ | ↑ | ↑ | |
| | Long-chain acylcarnitine (dried blood spot) | | ↑ | ↑ | | |
| | Long-chain acylcarnitine (plasma) | | ↑ | ↑ | | |
| | Sebacic acid (urine) | | ↑ | ↑ | | |
| | Sebacic acid, unsaturated (urine) | | ↑ | ↑ | | |
| | Suberic acid (urine) | | ↑ | ↑ | | |
| | Suberic acid, unsaturated (urine) | | ↑ | ↑ | | |
| | Transaminase (plasma) | | ↑↑ | ↑↑ | | |

**Table 44.37** Mitochondrial complex I assembly deficiency (TMEM126B)

| System | Symptoms and biomarkers | Neonatal (birth–1 month) | Infancy (1–18 months) | Childhood (1.5–11 years) | Adolescence (11–16 years) | Adulthood (>16 years) |
|---|---|---|---|---|---|---|
| Cardiovascular | **Cardiomyopathy, hypertrophic** | | + | + | + | + |
| Musculoskeletal | **Exercise intolerance** | | + | + | + | + |
| | **Myopathy** | | + | + | + | + |
| Renal | Renal tubular acidosis | | + | + | + | + |
| Laboratory findings | Complex I activity | ↓ | ↓ | ↓ | ↓ | ↓ |

**Table 44.38** Succinate dehydrogenase subunit A deficiency

| System | Symptoms and biomarkers | Neonatal (birth–1 month) | Infancy (1–18 months) | Childhood (1.5–11 years) | Adolescence (11–16 years) | Adulthood (>16 years) |
|---|---|---|---|---|---|---|
| Cardiovascular | **Cardiomyopathy, hypertrophic** | | + | + | + | + |
| CNS | **Dementia** | | | + | + | + |
| | **Encephalopathy** | | + | + | + | + |
| | Kearns-Sayre Syndrome | | | | | + |
| | Leigh syndrome | | + | + | | |
| Musculoskeletal | **Myopathy** | | + | + | + | + |
| | **Short stature** | | + | + | + | + |
| Laboratory findings | Complex II activity | ↓ | ↓ | ↓ | ↓ | ↓ |
| | Lactate (plasma) | ↑ | ↑ | ↑ | ↑ | ↑ |

**Table 44.39** Succinate dehydrogenase subunit A deficiency, tumoral phenotype

| System | Symptoms and biomarkers | Neonatal (birth–1 month) | Infancy (1–18 months) | Childhood (1.5–11 years) | Adolescence (11–16 years) | Adulthood (>16 years) |
|---|---|---|---|---|---|---|
| Cardiovascular | **Cardiomyopathy, hypertrophic** | | + | + | + | + |
| CNS | **Dementia** | | | + | + | + |
| | **Encephalopathy** | | + | + | + | + |
| | Kearns-Sayre Syndrome | | | | | + |
| | Leigh syndrome | | + | + | | |
| Musculoskeletal | **Myopathy** | | + | + | + | + |
| | **Short stature** | | + | + | + | + |
| Laboratory findings | Complex II activty | | ↓ | ↓ | ↓ | ↓ |

**Table 44.40** Succinate dehydrogenase subunit B deficiency

| System | Symptoms and biomarkers | Neonatal (birth–1 month) | Infancy (1–18 months) | Childhood (1.5–11 years) | Adolescence (11–16 years) | Adulthood (>16 years) |
|---|---|---|---|---|---|---|
| CNS | Paraganglioma | | | | + | + |
| | Pheochromocytoma | | | | + | + |
| Digestive | Gastro intestinal stromal tumor | | | | + | + |
| Renal | Renal cancer | | | | + | + |

**Table 44.41** Succinate dehydrogenase subunit B deficiency, tumoral phenotype

| System | Symptoms and biomarkers | Neonatal (birth–1 month) | Infancy (1–18 months) | Childhood (1.5–11 years) | Adolescence (11–16 years) | Adulthood (>16 years) |
|---|---|---|---|---|---|---|
| Musculoskeletal | Dysmorphic features | | | | | + |
| | Macrocephaly | | | | | + |
| Other | Malignancies | | | | | + |
| | Papilloma | | | | | + |

**Table 44.42** Succinate dehydrogenase subunit C deficiency, tumoral phenotype

| System | Symptoms and biomarkers | Neonatal (birth–1 month) | Infancy (1–18 months) | Childhood (1.5–11 years) | Adolescence (11–16 years) | Adulthood (>16 years) |
|---|---|---|---|---|---|---|
| Other | Carotid body tumors | | | | | ± |
| | Chemodectomas | | | | | ± |
| | Paraganglioma | | | | | + |
| | Pheochromocytoma | | | | | + |
| Laboratory findings | Catecholamines (urine) | | | | | ↑ |

**Table 44.43** Succinate dehydrogenase subunit D deficiency

| System | Symptoms and biomarkers | Neonatal (birth–1 month) | Infancy (1–18 months) | Childhood (1.5–11 years) | Adolescence (11–16 years) | Adulthood (>16 years) |
|---|---|---|---|---|---|---|
| Cardiovascular | Cardiomyopathy, dilated | | | | | ± |
| | **Cardiomyopathy, hypertrophic** | | | | | ± |
| | Left ventricular non-compaction | | | | | ± |
| CNS | Ataxia | | | ± | ± | ± |
| | Cognitive impairment | ± | ± | + | ± | ± |
| | Dystonia | ± | ± | ± | ± | ± |
| | Hyperreflexia | | | + | + | + |
| | Hypotonia | ± | ± | + | | |
| | Kearns-Sayre Syndrome | | | ± | ± | ± |
| | Leigh syndrome | ± | ± | ± | ± | ± |
| | Myoclonus | ± | ± | ± | ± | ± |
| | Regression, psychomotor | | + | + | + | + |
| | Seizures | ± | ± | ± | ± | ± |
| | Spasticity | | | + | + | + |
| Eye | Nystagmus | ± | ± | ± | ± | ± |
| | **Ophthalmoplegia** | | | | | ± |
| | Optic atrophy | ± | ± | ± | ± | ± |
| | Pigmentary retinopathy | ± | ± | + | ± | ± |
| | Vision, impaired | ± | ± | ± | ± | ± |
| Metabolic | Metabolic acidosis | ± | ± | ± | ± | ± |
| Musculoskeletal | Exercise intolerance | | | + | + | + |
| | Joint contractures | ± | ± | ± | ± | ± |
| | Muscle weakness | | | + | + | + |
| | **Short stature** | ± | ± | + | + | + |
| Other | Failure to thrive | ± | ± | + | + | + |
| Laboratory findings | Lactate (plasma) | n-↑ | n-↑ | n-↑ | n-↑ | n-↑ |

**Table 44.44** Succinate dehydrogenase subunit D deficiency, tumoral phenotype

| System | Symptoms and biomarkers | Neonatal (birth–1 month) | Infancy (1–18 months) | Childhood (1.5–11 years) | Adolescence (11–16 years) | Adulthood (>16 years) |
|---|---|---|---|---|---|---|
| Other | Paraganglioma | | | | | + |
| | Pheochromocytoma | | | | | + |
| Musculoskeletal | Macrocephaly | | | | | + |

**Table 44.45** Succinate dehydrogenase complex assembly factor 1 deficiency

| System | Symptoms and biomarkers | Neonatal (birth–1 month) | Infancy (1–18 months) | Childhood (1.5–11 years) | Adolescence (11–16 years) | Adulthood (>16 years) |
|---|---|---|---|---|---|---|
| Cardiovascular | **Cardiomyopathy** | + | + | + | | |
| CNS | Dystonia | | + | + | | |
| | **Encephalopathy** | + | + | + | | |
| | Kearns Sayre syndrome | | + | + | | |
| | Leigh syndrome | + | + | + | | |
| | **Leukodystrophy** | + | + | + | | |
| | Retardation, psychomotor | | + | + | | |
| | Spastic quadriplegia | | + | + | | |
| Musculoskeletal | Exercise intolerance | | + | + | | |
| | Myopathy | + | + | + | | |
| Laboratory findings | Complex II activity | ↓ | ↓ | ↓ | | |

**Table 44.46** Succinate dehydrogenase complex assembly factor 2 deficiency, tumoral phenotype

| System | Symptoms and biomarkers | Neonatal (birth–1 month) | Infancy (1–18 months) | Childhood (1.5–11 years) | Adolescence (11–16 years) | Adulthood (>16 years) |
|---|---|---|---|---|---|---|
| Other | Paraganglioma | | | | | + |
| | Pheochromocytoma | | | | | + |
| Laboratory findings | Catecholamines (urine) | | | | | ↑ |

**Table 44.47** Mitochondrial complex III subunit deficiency (UQCRB)

| System | Symptoms and biomarkers | Neonatal (birth–1 month) | Infancy (1–18 months) | Childhood (1.5–11 years) | Adolescence (11–16 years) | Adulthood (>16 years) |
|---|---|---|---|---|---|---|
| Cardiovascular | **Cardiomyopathy** | + | + | + | + | + |
| CNS | **Encephalopathy** | + | + | + | + | + |
| | **Epilepsy** | + | + | + | + | + |
| | Intellectual disability | | + | + | + | + |
| Metabolic | Lactic acidosis | + | + | + | + | + |
| Musculoskeletal | Exercise intolerance | | + | + | + | + |
| | Growth retardation | + | + | + | + | + |
| | **Myopathy** | | + | + | + | + |
| Laboratory findings | Complex III activity | ↓ | ↓ | ↓ | ↓ | ↓ |
| | Lactate (plasma) | ↑ | ↑ | ↑ | ↑ | ↑ |

**Table 44.48** Mitochondrial complex III subunit deficiency (UQCRC2)

| System | Symptoms and biomarkers | Neonatal (birth–1 month) | Infancy (1–18 months) | Childhood (1.5–11 years) | Adolescence (11–16 years) | Adulthood (>16 years) |
|---|---|---|---|---|---|---|
| CNS | Developmental delay | | ± | | | |
| Metabolic | **Hypoglycemia** | + | | | | |
| | **Metabolic acidosis** | + | | | | |
| Laboratory findings | Ammonia (blood) | ↑ | | | | |
| | Glucose (plasma) | ↓ | | | | |
| | Lactate (plasma) | ↑ | | | | |
| | Transaminase (plasma) | ↑ | | | | |

**Table 44.49** Mitochondrial complex III subunit deficiency (UQCRQ)

| System | Symptoms and biomarkers | Neonatal (birth–1 month) | Infancy (1–18 months) | Childhood (1.5–11 years) | Adolescence (11–16 years) | Adulthood (>16 years) |
|---|---|---|---|---|---|---|
| CNS | Basal ganglia abnormalities (MRI) | | ± | ± | ± | ± |
| | Extrapyramidal signs | | + | + | + | + |
| | Intellectual disability | | + | + | + | + |
| | Loss of speech | | + | + | + | + |
| Other | Non ambulant | | + | + | + | + |
| Laboratory findings | Lactate (plasma) | ↑ | ↑ | ↑ | ↑ | ↑ |

**Table 44.50** Mitochondrial complex III assembly deficiency (UQCC3)

| System | Symptoms and biomarkers | Neonatal (birth–1 month) | Infancy (1–18 months) | Childhood (1.5–11 years) | Adolescence (11–16 years) | Adulthood (>16 years) |
|---|---|---|---|---|---|---|
| CNS | Developmental delay | | + | + | | |
| Musculoskeletal | Short stature | | + | + | | |
| Laboratory findings | Lactate (plasma) | ↑ | ↑ | ↑ | | |

**Table 44.51** GRACILE syndrome

| System | Symptoms and biomarkers | Neonatal (birth–1 month) | Infancy (1–18 months) | Childhood (1.5–11 years) | Adolescence (11–16 years) | Adulthood (>16 years) |
|---|---|---|---|---|---|---|
| CNS | Developmental delay | ++ | ++ | ++ | | |
| | Hypotonia | ++ | ++ | ++ | | |
| Digestive | Cholestasis | +++ | ± | | | |
| | **Hemosiderosis** | ++ | ++ | | | |
| Ear | **Deafness, sensorineural** | | ++ | ++ | | |
| Hair | Pili torti | | ++ | ++ | | |
| Metabolic | **Intrauterine growth retardation** | +++ | | | | |
| | **Lactic acidosis** | +++ | ± | | | |
| Renal | **Renal Fanconi Syndrome** | ++ | ++ | | | |
| | **Renal tubulopathy, proximal** | +++ | ± | | | |
| Other | **Early death** | +++ | ++ | | | |
| Laboratory findings | Iron (serum) | ↑↑↑ | ↑ | | | |
| | Lactate (plasma) | ↑↑↑ | ↑ | | | |

**Table 44.52** Mitochondrial complex III subunit deficiency (TTC19)

| System | Symptoms and biomarkers | Neonatal (birth–1 month) | Infancy (1–18 months) | Childhood (1.5–11 years) | Adolescence (11–16 years) | Adulthood (>16 years) |
|---|---|---|---|---|---|---|
| CNS | Basal ganglia abnormalities (MRI) | | ± | ± | ± | ± |
| | Developmental delay | | ± | ± | ± | ± |
| | **Gait ataxia** | | + | + | + | + |
| Metabolic | Hypoglycemia | ± | | | | |
| | **Metabolic acidosis** | + | | | | |
| Laboratory findings | Glucose (plasma) | n-↓ | | | | |
| | Lactate (plasma) | ↑ | ↑ | ↑ | | |

**Table 44.53** Mitochondrial complex III assembly deficiency (UQCC2)

| System | Symptoms and biomarkers | Neonatal (birth–1 month) | Infancy (1–18 months) | Childhood (1.5–11 years) | Adolescence (11–16 years) | Adulthood (>16 years) |
|---|---|---|---|---|---|---|
| CNS | Epilepsy | ± | | | | |
| Metabolic | Lactic acidosis | ++ | | | | |
| Renal | Renal tubulopathy | + | | | | |
| Other | Intrauterine growth retardation | ++ | | | | |
| Laboratory findings | Lactate (plasma) | ↑↑ | | | | |

**Table 44.54** Mitochondrial complex III assembly deficiency (LYRM7)

| System | Symptoms and biomarkers | Neonatal (birth–1 month) | Infancy (1–18 months) | Childhood (1.5–11 years) | Adolescence (11–16 years) | Adulthood (>16 years) |
|---|---|---|---|---|---|---|
| CNS | Cavitating leucodystrophia (MRI) | | + | ++ | | |
| | Developmental delay | | ++ | | | |
| | Hypotonia | | + | ++ | | |
| | Recurrent encephalopatic periods | | ++ | ++ | | |
| Other | Death | | | ± | | |
| Laboratory findings | Lactate (plasma) | | ↑ | ↑ | | |

**Table 44.55** Mitochondrial complex IV subunit deficiency (MTCO1)

| System | Symptoms and biomarkers | Neonatal (birth–1 month) | Infancy (1–18 months) | Childhood (1.5–11 years) | Adolescence (11–16 years) | Adulthood (>16 years) |
|---|---|---|---|---|---|---|
| CNS | **Epilepsy** | | | | ± | + |
| | Stroke-like episodes | | | | ± | + |
| Musculoskeletal | **Muscle weakness** | | | | | + |
| | rhabdomyolysis | | | | | + |
| Laboratory findings | Alanine (plasma) | | | | | n-↑ |

**Table 44.56** Mitochondrial complex IV subunit deficiency (MTCO2)

| System | Symptoms and biomarkers | Neonatal (birth–1 month) | Infancy (1–18 months) | Childhood (1.5–11 years) | Adolescence (11–16 years) | Adulthood (>16 years) |
|---|---|---|---|---|---|---|
| Cardiovascular | Cardiomyopathy | | | ± | | |
| CNS | Developmental delay | | | ± | | |
| Eye | Retinopathy | | | ± | | |
| Musculoskeletal | **Muscle weakness** | + | + | + | + | + |
| | Myopathy | | + | + | + | + |
| Laboratory findings | Lactate (plasma) | ↑ | ↑ | ↑ | ↑ | ↑ |

**Table 44.57** Mitochondrial complex IV subunit deficiency (MTCO3)

| System | Symptoms and biomarkers | Neonatal (birth–1 month) | Infancy (1–18 months) | Childhood (1.5–11 years) | Adolescence (11–16 years) | Adulthood (>16 years) |
|---|---|---|---|---|---|---|
| CNS | Leigh syndrome | | | ± | | |
| | Retardation, psychomotor | | ± | ± | ± | |
| Musculoskeletal | **Muscle weakness** | | | + | + | + |
| | Myopathy | | | + | + | + |
| Laboratory findings | Lactate (plasma) | | ↑ | ↑ | ↑ | ↑ |

**Table 44.58** Mitochondrial complex IV subunit deficiency (COX4I2)

| System | Symptoms and biomarkers | Neonatal (birth–1 month) | Infancy (1–18 months) | Childhood (1.5–11 years) | Adolescence (11–16 years) | Adulthood (>16 years) |
|---|---|---|---|---|---|---|
| Digestive | Exocrine pancreas insufficiency | + | + | + | | |
| | Hepatomegaly | + | + | + | | |
| | Splenomegaly | + | + | + | | |
| Other | **Failure to thrive** | + | + | + | | |

**Table 44.59** Mitochondrial complex IV subunit deficiency (COX6A1)

| System | Symptoms and biomarkers | Neonatal (birth–1 month) | Infancy (1–18 months) | Childhood (1.5–11 years) | Adolescence (11–16 years) | Adulthood (>16 years) |
|---|---|---|---|---|---|---|
| CNS | **Polyneuropathy** | | | + | ++ | +++ |
| Ear | Hearing loss | | | | | + |

**Table 44.60** Mitochondrial complex IV subunit deficiency (COX6B1)

| System | Symptoms and biomarkers | Neonatal (birth–1 month) | Infancy (1–18 months) | Childhood (1.5–11 years) | Adolescence (11–16 years) | Adulthood (>16 years) |
|---|---|---|---|---|---|---|
| Cardiovascular | Cardiomyopathy | ± | ± | ± | | |
| CNS | Encephalopathy | ± | ± | ± | | |
| | Epilepsy | | | ± | | |
| | Leukodystrophy | | | + | | |
| Musculoskeletal | Myopathy | | | ++ | ++ | |
| Laboratory findings | Lactate (plasma) | ↑ | ↑ | ↑ | ↑ | ↑ |

**Table 44.61** Mitochondrial complex IV subunit deficiency (COX7B)

| System | Symptoms and biomarkers | Neonatal (birth–1 month) | Infancy (1–18 months) | Childhood (1.5–11 years) | Adolescence (11–16 years) | Adulthood (>16 years) |
|---|---|---|---|---|---|---|
| CNS | Microcephaly | ± | ± | ± | | |
| Musculoskeletal | Short stature | | ± | ± | | |
| Skin | **Linear skin defect** | ++ | ++ | ++ | | |

**Table 44.62** Mitochondrial complex IV subunit deficiency (COX8A)

| System | Symptoms and biomarkers | Neonatal (birth–1 month) | Infancy (1–18 months) | Childhood (1.5–11 years) | Adolescence (11–16 years) | Adulthood (>16 years) |
|---|---|---|---|---|---|---|
| CNS | **Developmental delay** | +++ | +++ | +++ | +++ | |
| | Epilepsy | | | + | + | |
| | Microcephaly | + | + | + | + | |
| Respiratory | Pulmonary hypertension | + | + | | | |

**Table 44.63** Mitochondrial complex IV assembly deficiency (COA3)

| System | Symptoms and biomarkers | Neonatal (birth–1 month) | Infancy (1–18 months) | Childhood (1.5–11 years) | Adolescence (11–16 years) | Adulthood (>16 years) |
|---|---|---|---|---|---|---|
| CNS | **Developmental delay** | + | + | + | + | + |
| | Neuropathy | | | | + | + |
| Digestive | Obesity | | | | + | + |
| Musculoskeletal | Exercise intolerance | | | | + | + |
| | **Short stature** | | + | + | + | + |

**Table 44.64** Mitochondrial complex IV assembly deficiency (COA5)

| System | Symptoms and biomarkers | Neonatal (birth–1 month) | Infancy (1–18 months) | Childhood (1.5–11 years) | Adolescence (11–16 years) | Adulthood (>16 years) |
|---|---|---|---|---|---|---|
| Cardiovascular | Cardiomyopathy | + | | | | |
| Other | Death | + | | | | |

**Table 44.65** Mitochondrial complex IV assembly deficiency (COA6)

| System | Symptoms and biomarkers | Neonatal (birth–1 month) | Infancy (1–18 months) | Childhood (1.5–11 years) | Adolescence (11–16 years) | Adulthood (>16 years) |
|---|---|---|---|---|---|---|
| Cardiovascular | Cardiomyopathy | + | + | | | |
| Other | Death | + | + | | | |
| Laboratory findings | Lactate (plasma) | ↑ | ↑ | | | |

**Table 44.66** Mitochondrial complex IV assembly deficiency (COA7)

| System | Symptoms and biomarkers | Neonatal (birth–1 month) | Infancy (1–18 months) | Childhood (1.5–11 years) | Adolescence (11–16 years) | Adulthood (>16 years) |
|---|---|---|---|---|---|---|
| CNS | Ataxia | | | + | | |
| | Developmental delay | | + | | | |
| | Leukodystrophy | | | + | | |
| | Neuropathy, peripheral | | | + | | |

**Table 44.67** Mitochondrial complex IV assembly deficiency (COX14)

| System | Symptoms and biomarkers | Neonatal (birth–1 month) | Infancy (1–18 months) | Childhood (1.5–11 years) | Adolescence (11–16 years) | Adulthood (>16 years) |
|---|---|---|---|---|---|---|
| Cardiovascular | Cardiomyopathy | + | | | | |
| Metabolic | Lactic acidosis | + | | | | |
| Other | Death | + | | | | |
| Laboratory findings | Lactate (plasma) | ↑ | ↑ | | | |

**Table 44.68** Mitochondrial complex IV assembly deficiency (COX10)

| System | Symptoms and biomarkers | Neonatal (birth–1 month) | Infancy (1–18 months) | Childhood (1.5–11 years) | Adolescence (11–16 years) | Adulthood (>16 years) |
|---|---|---|---|---|---|---|
| Cardiovascular | Cardiomyopathy | ± | ± | | | |
| CNS | Developmental delay | | + | | | |
| | Hypotonia | | + | | | |
| | Leigh syndrome | | ± | | | |
| Hematological | Anemia, transfusion dependent | ± | ± | | | |
| Other | Death | | + | | | |
| Laboratory findings | Hemoglobin (blood) | ↓ | | | | |
| | Lactate (plasma) | ↑ | ↑ | | | |

**Table 44.69** Mitochondrial complex IV assembly deficiency (COX15)

| System | Symptoms and biomarkers | Neonatal (birth–1 month) | Infancy (1–18 months) | Childhood (1.5–11 years) | Adolescence (11–16 years) | Adulthood (>16 years) |
|---|---|---|---|---|---|---|
| Cardiovascular | Cardiomyopathy, hypertrophic | ± | | | | |
| CNS | Basal ganglia abnormalities (MRI) | | ± | ± | ± | |
| | **Developmental delay** | | +++ | +++ | +++ | |
| | Epilepsy | ± | | | | |
| | Hypotonia | ± | + | + | + | |
| | Leigh syndrome | | ± | ± | ± | |
| Other | Death | ± | | ± | | |
| Laboratory findings | Lactate (plasma) | ↑ | ↑ | ↑ | ↑ | |

Table 44.70 Mitochondrial complex IV assembly deficiency (COX20)

| System | Symptoms and biomarkers | Neonatal (birth–1 month) | Infancy (1–18 months) | Childhood (1.5–11 years) | Adolescence (11–16 years) | Adulthood (>16 years) |
|---|---|---|---|---|---|---|
| CNS | Cerebellar ataxia | | ± | + | ++ | ++ |
| | Dystonia | | | ± | ± | ± |
| | Hypotonia | | ± | ± | | |
| Laboratory findings | Lactate (plasma) | | n-↑ | n-↑ | n-↑ | n-↑ |

Table 44.71 Mitochondrial complex IV assembly deficiency (SCO1)

| System | Symptoms and biomarkers | Neonatal (birth–1 month) | Infancy (1–18 months) | Childhood (1.5–11 years) | Adolescence (11–16 years) | Adulthood (>16 years) |
|---|---|---|---|---|---|---|
| Cardiovascular | Cardiomyopathy, hypertrophic | | +/– | | | |
| CNS | Brain atrophy (MRI) | + | + | | | |
| | Epilepsy | | + | | | |
| | Hypotonia | + | + | | | |
| | Lethargy | + | + | | | |
| | Retardation, psychomotor | | + | | | |
| Digestive | **Feeding difficulties** | + | + | | | |
| | Hepatomegaly | + | + | | | |
| Musculoskeletal | **Muscle weakness** | + | + | | | |
| Respiratory | Respiratory distress | + | | | | |
| Other | Death | | + | | | |
| | Failure to thrive | | + | | | |
| Laboratory findings | Alanine (plasma) | | ↑ | | | |
| | Citric acid cycle intermediates | ↑ | ↑ | | | |
| | Lactate (cerebrospinal fluid) | ↑ | | | | |
| | Lactate (plasma) | ↑ | ↑ | | ↑ | ↑ |
| | Lactate (urine) | ↑ | ↑ | | | |

Table 44.72 Mitochondrial complex IV assembly deficiency (SCO2)

| System | Symptoms and biomarkers | Neonatal (birth–1 month) | Infancy (1–18 months) | Childhood (1.5–11 years) | Adolescence (11–16 years) | Adulthood (>16 years) |
|---|---|---|---|---|---|---|
| Cardiovascular | Cardiomyopathy, hypertrophic | + | + | + | | |
| CNS | Dystonia | | + | + | | |
| | Epilepsy | | + | | | |
| | Hypotonia | + | + | ± | | |
| | Leigh syndrome | | + | | | |
| | Neuropathy, peripheral | + | + | + | + | + |
| | Retardation, psychomotor | | + | + | | |
| Eye | Nystagmus | | + | | | |
| | Ptosis of eyelid | | | + | | |
| Musculoskeletal | **Muscle weakness** | + | + | + | + | + |
| | Muscular atrophy, distal | | | + | | + |
| Respiratory | Respiratory failure | + | + | | | |
| Other | Death | | + | + | | |
| Laboratory findings | Lactate (cerebrospinal fluid) | ↑ | ↑ | ↑ | | |
| | Lactate (plasma) | ↑ | ↑ | ↑ | | |

**Table 44.73** Mitochondrial complex I subunit deficiency (COXFA4)

| System | Symptoms and biomarkers | Neonatal (birth–1 month) | Infancy (1–18 months) | Childhood (1.5–11 years) | Adolescence (11–16 years) | Adulthood (>16 years) |
|---|---|---|---|---|---|---|
| Autonomic system | Hypertension | | | | | + |
| CNS | Developmental delay, mild- moderate | | + | + | | |
| | Diffuse hyperintense brain lesions (MRI) | | + | + | | + |
| | Dystonia | | | + | | |
| | Peripheral neuropathy, mainly lower extremities | | + | + | | |
| Eye | Nystagmus | | | + | | |
| | Optic atrophy | | | + | | |
| Renal | Proximal tubular acidosis, renal | | + | | | |
| Respiratory | Respiratory failure | | | | | + |
| Other | Failure to thrive | + | + | + | | |
| | Loss of skills | | | + | | |
| Laboratory findings | Alanine (plasma) | | ↑ | | | |
| | Lactate (cerebrospinal fluid) | | ↑ | | | |
| | Lactate (plasma) | ↑ | ↑ | ↑ | | |

**Table 44.74** CEP89 deficiency

| System | Symptoms and biomarkers | Neonatal (birth–1 month) | Infancy (1–18 months) | Childhood (1.5–11 years) | Adolescence (11–16 years) | Adulthood (>16 years) |
|---|---|---|---|---|---|---|
| CNS | Ataxia | | | | + | + |
| | Developmental delay | | + | | | |
| | Intellectual disability | | | | + | + |
| Ear | Cataract | | + | | | + |
| | Deafness, sensorineural | | + | | + | |
| Musculoskeletal | Myopathy | | + | | + | + |
| | Short stature | | | | | + |
| Psychiatric | Behaviour difficulties | | | | | + |
| Laboratory findings | Cystine (urine) | | ↑ | | | |
| | Lactate (plasma) | | ↑ | | | |

**Table 44.75** Mitochondrial complex IV assembly deficiency (SURF1)

| System | Symptoms and biomarkers | Neonatal (birth–1 month) | Infancy (1–18 months) | Childhood (1.5–11 years) | Adolescence (11–16 years) | Adulthood (>16 years) |
|---|---|---|---|---|---|---|
| Cardiovascular | Cardiomyopathy, hypertrophic | | | ± | | |
| CNS | Ataxia | | + | + | + | + |
| | Basal ganglia abnormalities (MRI) | | + | + | | |
| | Brainstem lesions (MRI) | | + | + | | |
| | Epilepsy | | | ± | | |
| | Hypotonia | | + | + | + | + |
| | Leigh syndrome | | + | + | | |
| | Retardation, psychomotor | | + | + | + | + |
| | Tremor, intentional | | + | + | + | + |
| Digestive | Feeding difficulties | | + | | + | |
| | Vomiting | | | | | |
| Eye | Nystagmus | | + | + | + | + |
| | Ophthalmoplegia | | | + | + | + |
| | Optic atrophy | | | | ± | |
| Hair | Hypertrichosis | | + | + | + | + |
| Musculoskeletal | Short stature | | + | + | + | |
| Respiratory | Respiratory failure | | | | ± | |
| Other | Death | | | + | ± | ± |
| | Failure to thrive | | + | + | + | + |
| | Loss of skills, regression | | + | + | | |
| Laboratory findings | Lactate (cerebrospinal fluid) | | ↑ | ↑ | | |
| | Lactate (plasma) | | ↑ | ↑ | ↑ | ↑ |

**Table 44.76** Leigh Syndrome with French-Canadian Ethnicity

| System | Symptoms and biomarkers | Neonatal (birth–1 month) | Infancy (1–18 months) | Childhood (1.5–11 years) | Adolescence (11–16 years) | Adulthood (>16 years) |
|---|---|---|---|---|---|---|
| CNS | Ataxia | | + | + | + | |
| | Developmental delay | | ++ | ++ | ++ | |
| | Hypotonia | ± | ++ | ++ | ++ | |
| | Leigh-like lesions (MRI) | | ++ | ++ | ++ | |
| | Retardation, psychomotor | | ++ | ++ | ++ | |
| | Tremor, intentional | | + | + | + | |
| Digestive | Feeding difficulties | + | + | | | |
| | Steatosis liver, microvesicular | | ++ | ++ | ++ | |
| Musculoskeletal | Facial dysmorphism, mild | | + | + | + | |
| Other | Death | | ++ | +++ | + | |
| | Failure to thrive | | + | | | |
| | Hirsutism, mild | | + | + | + | |
| Laboratory findings | Lactate (plasma) | ↑↑ | ↑↑↑ | ↑↑↑ | ↑↑↑ | |

**Table 44.77** TACO1 deficiency

| System | Symptoms and biomarkers | Neonatal (birth–1 month) | Infancy (1–18 months) | Childhood (1.5–11 years) | Adolescence (11–16 years) | Adulthood (>16 years) |
|---|---|---|---|---|---|---|
| CNS | Bilateral hyperintensities of basal ganglia (MRI) | | | + | + | + |
| | Developmental delay | | | + | | |
| | Dysarthria | | | + | + | + |
| | Dystonia | | | + | + | + |
| | Intellectual disability | | | + | + | + |
| | Spasticity | | | + | + | + |
| | Speech delay | | | | | |
| Eye | Optic atrophy | | | + | | + |
| Renal | Renal tubular dysfunction | | | ± | | |
| Other | Failure to thrive | | | + | + | + |
| Laboratory findings | Lactate (cerebrospinal fluid) | | | ↑ | | |
| | Lactate (plasma) | | | ↑ | | |

**Table 44.78** PET100 deficiency

| System | Symptoms and biomarkers | Neonatal (birth–1 month) | Infancy (1–18 months) | Childhood (1.5–11 years) | Adolescence (11–16 years) | Adulthood (>16 years) |
|---|---|---|---|---|---|---|
| CNS | Absent spontanous movements | | + | | + | |
| | Developmental delay | | + | + | + | |
| | Epilepsy | + | + | + | + | |
| | Hypotonia, axial | | + | | | |
| | Irritability | + | | | | |
| | Leigh-like lesions (MRI) | | + | | | |
| | Spasticity | | + | + | + | |
| Digestive | Feeding difficulties | | + | | + | |
| Eye | Cataract | | | + | | |
| | Visual impairment | | + | + | + | |
| Other | Death | + | + | | + | |
| | Failure to thrive | | + | + | | |
| Laboratory findings | Lactate (cerebrospinal fluid) | | ↑ | ↑ | | |
| | Lactate (plasma) | ↑↑↑ | n-↑ | n-↑ | | |

**Table 44.79** FASTKD2 deficiency

| System | Symptoms and biomarkers | Neonatal (birth–1 month) | Infancy (1–18 months) | Childhood (1.5–11 years) | Adolescence (11–16 years) | Adulthood (>16 years) |
|---|---|---|---|---|---|---|
| CNS | Brain atrophy, hemispheral (CT) | | | + | | |
| | Developmental delay | | | + | + | |
| | Dystonia | | | + | | |
| | Epilepsy | | + | + | + | |
| | Hemiplegia | | | + | | |
| | Irritability | + | | | | |
| | Stroke-like episode | | | | | + |
| Eye | Optic atrophy | | | | + | + |
| Other | No voluntary activity | | | + | | |
| Laboratory findings | Lactate (plasma) | | | ↑ | | ↑ |

**Table 44.80** APOPT1 deficiency

| System | Symptoms and biomarkers | Neonatal (birth–1 month) | Infancy (1–18 months) | Childhood (1.5–11 years) | Adolescence (11–16 years) | Adulthood (>16 years) |
|---|---|---|---|---|---|---|
| CNS | Ataxia | | | + | | + |
| | Cavitating leukodystrophy (MRI) | | | + | | |
| | Cognitive impairment | | | ± | | |
| | Dysarthria | | | + | | + |
| | Dysmetria | | | | | + |
| | Epilepsy | | | + | | |
| | Loss of skills, regression | | | + | | |
| | Polyneuropathy | | | + | | |
| | Spasticity | | | + | | + |
| Ear | Hearing loss | | | ± | | |
| Eye | Nystagmus | | | | | + |
| | Visual loss | | | ± | | |
| Musculoskeletal | Muscle weakness, lower extremities | | | + | | + |

**Table 44.81** Mitochondrial phosphate carrier deficiency

| System | Symptoms and biomarkers | Neonatal (birth–1 month) | Infancy (1–18 months) | Childhood (1.5–11 years) | Adolescence (11–16 years) | Adulthood (>16 years) |
|---|---|---|---|---|---|---|
| Cardiovascular | Cardiomyopathy, hypertrophic | +++ | +++ | ± | | + |
| CNS | Developmental delay, motor | | +++ | + | | |
| | Hypotonia | +++ | +++ | | | |
| Musculoskeletal | Exercise intolerance | | | + | | + |
| | Myopathy | | +++ | + | | + |
| Other | Death | | +++ | | | |
| | Failure to thrive | +++ | +++ | | | |
| Laboratory findings | Lactate (plasma) | ↑↑ | ↑↑ | | | |

**Table 44.82** Mitochondrial ATP synthase F1 subunit a deficiency

| System | Symptoms and biomarkers | Neonatal (birth–1 month) | Infancy (1–18 months) | Childhood (1.5–11 years) | Adolescence (11–16 years) | Adulthood (>16 years) |
|---|---|---|---|---|---|---|
| CNS | Asymmetric white matter lesions (MRI) | + | | | | |
| | Hypotonia | + | + | | | |
| | Irritability | + | | | | |
| | Microcephaly | + | + | | | |
| Eye | Nystagmus | + | | | | |
| Other | Death | | + | | | |
| Laboratory findings | Alanine (plasma) | ↑ | | | | |

**Table 44.83** Mitochondrial ATP synthase F1 subunit δ deficiency

| System | Symptoms and biomarkers | Neonatal (birth–1 month) | Infancy (1–18 months) | Childhood (1.5–11 years) | Adolescence (11–16 years) | Adulthood (>16 years) |
|---|---|---|---|---|---|---|
| Cardiovascular | Cardiomyopathy, dilated | | + | + | | |
| CNS | Developmental delay, mild | | + | + | | |
| | Lethargy | + | | | | |
| | Neuropathy | | | + | | |
| Metabolic | Episodic decompensation | | | + | | |
| | Hyperammonemia | | | | | |
| Musculoskeletal | Exercise intolerance | | | + | | |
| | Proximal weakness, mild | | | + | | |
| | Rhabdomyolysis | | | | | |
| | Short stature | | | + | | |
| Laboratory findings | 3-Methylglutaconic acid (urine) | ↑ | | ↑ | | |
| | Ammonia (plasma) | ↑ | | | | |
| | Citric acid cycle intermediates (urine) | ↑ | | | | |
| | Lactate (plasma) | ↑ | | n-↑ | | |

**Table 44.84** Mitochondrial ATP synthase F1 subunit e deficiency

| System | Symptoms and biomarkers | Neonatal (birth–1 month) | Infancy (1–18 months) | Childhood (1.5–11 years) | Adolescence (11–16 years) | Adulthood (>16 years) |
|---|---|---|---|---|---|---|
| Cardiovascular | Cardiomyopathy, hypertrophic | | | | | + |
| CNS | Hypotonia | | | | | + |
| | Polyneuropathy | | | | | + |
| | Retardation, psychomotor | | | | | + |
| Laboratory findings | Lactate (plasma) | | | | | ↑ |

**Table 44.85** Mitochondrial complex V subunit deficiency (MTATP6)

| System | Symptoms and biomarkers | Neonatal (birth–1 month) | Infancy (1–18 months) | Childhood (1.5–11 years) | Adolescence (11–16 years) | Adulthood (>16 years) |
|---|---|---|---|---|---|---|
| Cardiovascular | Cardiomyopathy, hypertrophic | | ± | | | |
| CNS | Ataxia | | + | + | + | + |
| | Cerebellar atrophy (MRI) | | | | | + |
| | Cognitive decline | | | | | + |
| | Developmental delay | | + | + | + | |
| | Dystonia | | | + | | + |
| | Epilepsy | | + | | + | + |
| | Hyperreflexia | | + | + | + | + |
| | Hypotonia | | + | | | |
| | Leigh-like lesions (MRI) | | + | + | + | |
| | Neuropathy, peripheral | | + | | + | + |
| | Spasticity | | + | | | + |
| | Stroke-like episode | | | + | | |
| Digestive | Feeding difficulties | | + | | | |
| Ear | Hearing loss, sensorineural | | | + | | |
| Eye | Blindness | | | | | + |
| | Night blindness | | | | + | |
| | Nystagmus | | ± | ± | | |
| | Ophthalmoplegia | | ± | | | + |
| | Optic atrophy | | ± | | | + |
| | Ptosis of eyelid | | | | + | + |
| | Retinitis pigmentosa | | + | + | + | + |
| Hematological | Anemia, sideroblastic | | + | | | |
| Musculoskeletal | Muscle weakness | | | + | + | + |
| Other | Death | | + | + | + | |
| | Failure to thrive | | + | + | | |
| | Loss of skills, regression | | + | + | | |
| Laboratory findings | Lactate (cerebrospinal fluid) | | ↑ | ↑ | | |
| | Lactate (plasma) | ↑ | n-↑ | n-↑ | n-↑ | n-↑ |

**Table 44.86** Mitochondrial complex V subunit deficiency (MTATP8)

| System | Symptoms and biomarkers | Neonatal (birth–1 month) | Infancy (1–18 months) | Childhood (1.5–11 years) | Adolescence (11–16 years) | Adulthood (>16 years) |
|---|---|---|---|---|---|---|
| Cardiovascular | Cardiomyopathy, hypertrophic | | | | + | |
| CNS | Ataxia | | | | + | |
| | Dysarthria | | | | + | |
| | Hyporeflexia | | | | + | |
| | Learning disabilities | | | | + | |
| | Polyneuropathy | | | | + | |
| Eye | Ophthalmoplegia | | | | + | |
| | Vision loss | | | + | | |
| Musculoskeletal | Exercise intolerance | | | + | | |
| | Muscle weakness | | | + | | |
| Laboratory findings | Lactate (cerebrospinal fluid) | | | | ↑ | |
| | Lactate (plasma) | | | | n | |

**Table 44.87** Transmembrane protein 70 deficiency

| System | Symptoms and biomarkers | Neonatal (birth–1 month) | Infancy (1–18 months) | Childhood (1.5–11 years) | Adolescence (11–16 years) | Adulthood (>16 years) |
|---|---|---|---|---|---|---|
| Cardiovascular | **Cardiomyopathy, hypertrophic** | + | + | + | + | + |
| | Wolf-Parkinson-White syndrome | ± | ± | ± | ± | ± |
| CNS | Apnea | ± | ± | ± | ± | ± |
| | Basal ganglia lesions (MRI) | ± | ± | ± | ± | ± |
| | Cerebellar hypoplasia, mild | ± | ± | ± | ± | ± |
| | Cortical atrophy (MRI) | ± | ± | ± | ± | ± |
| | **Encephalopathy** | + | + | + | + | + |
| | **Hypotonia, muscular-axial** | + | + | + | + | + |
| | Microcephaly | ± | ± | ± | ± | ± |
| | **Retardation, psychomotor** | ± | + | + | + | + |
| | Subcortical atrophy (MRI) | ± | ± | ± | ± | ± |
| Digestive | Gastrointestinal dysmotility | ± | ± | ± | ± | ± |
| | Hepatomegaly | + | + | ± | ± | ± |
| | Liver dysfunction | ± | ± | ± | ± | ± |
| Eye | Cataract | ± | ± | ± | ± | ± |
| Genitourinary | Cryptorchidism | ± | ± | ± | ± | ± |
| | Hypospadias | ± | ± | ± | ± | ± |
| Metabolic | **Hyperammonemia, during crisis** | + | + | + | + | ± |
| | **Hyperuricemia, during crisis** | + | + | + | + | ± |
| | **Ketonuria, pronounced during crisis** | + | + | + | + | + |
| | **Lactic acidosis** | + | + | ± | ± | ± |
| | **Metabolic acidosis** | + | + | + | + | ± |
| Musculoskeletal | Contractures | ± | ± | ± | ± | ± |
| | Facial dysmorphism | ± | ± | ± | ± | ± |
| Renal | Renal tubulopathy | ± | ± | ± | ± | ± |

**Table 44.87** (continued)

| System | Symptoms and biomarkers | Neonatal (birth–1 month) | Infancy (1–18 months) | Childhood (1.5–11 years) | Adolescence (11–16 years) | Adulthood (>16 years) |
|---|---|---|---|---|---|---|
| Respiratory | **Persistent pulmonary hypertension of the newborn** | ± | | | | |
| | Respiratory insufficiency | ± | ± | ± | ± | ± |
| Other | Failure to thrive | + | + | + | + | + |
| | Growth retardation, postnatal | ± | ± | ± | ± | ± |
| | Low birth weight | ± | | | | |
| Laboratory findings | 3-Methylglutaconic acid (urine) | ↑-↑↑ | ↑-↑↑ | ↑-↑↑ | ↑-↑↑ | ↑-↑↑ |
| | Alanine (plasma) | ↑-↑↑ | ↑-↑↑ | ↑-↑↑ | ↑-↑↑ | ↑-↑↑ |
| | Ammonia (blood and plasma) | n-↑↑ | n-↑↑ | n-↑↑ | n-↑↑ | n-↑↑ |
| | Anion gap | ↑ | ↑ | ↑ | ↑ | ↑ |
| | Citrulline (plasma) | n-↑ | n-↑ | n-↑ | n-↑ | n-↑ |
| | Complex V activity (skeletal muscle) | ↓ | ↓ | ↓ | ↓ | ↓ |
| | Creatine kinase (plasma) | n-↑↑ | n-↑↑ | n-↑↑ | n-↑↑ | n-↑↑ |
| | Glutamine (plasma) | n-↑ | n-↑ | n-↑ | n-↑ | n-↑ |
| | Lactate (cerebrospinal fluid) | n-↑↑ | n-↑↑ | n-↑↑ | n-↑↑ | n-↑↑ |
| | Lactate (plasma) | ↑-↑↑↑ | ↑-↑↑↑ | ↑-↑↑↑ | ↑-↑↑↑ | ↑-↑↑↑ |
| | Orotate (urine) | n-↑ | n-↑ | n-↑ | n-↑ | n-↑ |
| | Uric acid | n-↑↑ | n-↑↑ | n-↑↑ | n-↑↑ | n-↑↑ |

**Table 44.88** Mitochondrial complex V assembly deficiency (ATPAF2)

| System | Symptoms and biomarkers | Neonatal (birth–1 month) | Infancy (1–18 months) | Childhood (1.5–11 years) | Adolescence (11–16 years) | Adulthood (>16 years) |
|---|---|---|---|---|---|---|
| Digestive | Basal ganglia atrophy (MRI) | | + | | | |
| | CC dysgenesis (MRI) | + | | | | |
| | Cortical atrophy (MRI) | + | | | | |
| | Dvelopmental delay, severe | | + | | | |
| | Feeding difficulties | + | | | | |
| CNS | Hepatomegaly | + | | | | |
| | Hypertonia | + | | | | |
| | Seizures | + | + | | | |
| | Subcortical atrophy (MRI) | + | | | | |
| Musculoskeletal | Dysmorphic features | ± | | | | |
| Renal | Renal hypoplasia | + | | | | |
| Other | Death | + | + | | | |
| | Failure to thrive | | + | | | |
| Laboratory findings | 3-Methylglutaconic acid (urine) | ↑ | | | | |
| | Fumaric acid (urine) | ↑ | | | | |
| | Lactate (cerebrospinal fluid) | ↑ | | | | |
| | Lactate (plasma) | ↑-↑↑↑ | | | | |
| | Lactate (urine) | ↑ | | | | |

**Table 44.89** DAPIT deficiency

| System | Symptoms and biomarkers | Neonatal (birth–1 month) | Infancy (1–18 months) | Childhood (1.5–11 years) | Adolescence (11–16 years) | Aculthood (>16 years) |
|---|---|---|---|---|---|---|
| Cardiovascular | Cardiomyopathy, hypertrophic | | | ± | | |
| CNS | Ataxia | | | + | | |
| | Developmental delay, motor | | + | | | |
| | Encephalopathy | | | + | | |
| | Hypotonia | | | + | | |
| | Leigh syndrome | | | + | | |
| | Regression (acute) | | | + | | |
| | Spasticity | | | + | | |
| Eye | Eye movements, abnormal | | | + | | |
| Respiratory | Respiratory failure | | | + | | |
| Other | Death | | | + | | |
| Laboratory findings | Alanine (plasma) | | | ↑ | | |
| | Lactate (plasma) | | | ↑ | | |

**Table 44.90** Mitochondrial cytochrome b deficiency MTCYB

| System | Symptoms and biomarkers | Neonatal (birth–1 month) | Infancy (1–18 months) | Childhood (1.5–11 years) | Adolescence (11–16 years) | Adulthood (>16 years) |
|---|---|---|---|---|---|---|
| Cardiovascular | Cardiomyopathy | | | | | ± |
| CNS | Ataxia | | | | | + |
| | Brainstem atrophy (MRI) | | | | | ± |
| | Cerebellar atrophy (MRI) | | | | | ± |
| | Cognitive impairment, mild | | | + | | |
| | Cortical atrophy (MRI) | | | | | ± |
| | Encephalopathy, episodic | | | | | ± |
| | Hypotonia | | | | | + |
| | Polyneuropathy | | | + | | + |
| | Seizures | | | + | | + |
| | Stroke-like episodes | | | ± | | |
| Digestive | Gastrointestinal dysmotility | | | + | + | + |
| Ear | Deafness, sensorineural | | | | | ± |
| Eye | Cataract | | | | | ± |
| | Ophthalmoplegia | | | | | ± |
| | Visual impairment | | | | | ± |
| Metabolic | Hypoglycemia | | | ± | | |
| Musculoskeletal | Exercise intolerance | | | ++ | ++ | ++ |
| | Muscle cramps | | | | | ++ |
| | Muscle weakness, proximal | | | + | + | + |
| Psychiatric | Psychiatric symptoms | | | | | ± |
| Other | Weight loss | | | + | + | + |
| Laboratory findings | 3-Methylglutaconic acid (urine) | | | ↑ | | |
| | ASAT/ALAT (plasma) | | | n-↑ | | |
| | Carnitine, free (plasma) | | | ↓ | | |
| | Creatine kinase (plasma) | | | n-↑↑ | | |
| | Lactate (cerebrospinal fluid) | | | ↑ | | |
| | Lactate (MRS) | | | ↑ | | |
| | Lactate (plasma) | | | n-↑↑ | n-↑↑ | n-↑↑ |
| | Lactate (urine) | | | ↑ | | |

**Table 44.91** Mitochondrial cytochrome c1 deficiency CYC1

| System | Symptoms and biomarkers | Neonatal (birth–1 month) | Infancy (1–18 months) | Childhood (1.5–11 years) | Adolescence (11–16 years) | Adulthood (>16 years) |
|---|---|---|---|---|---|---|
| CNS | Encephalopathy, acute, episodic | | | ± | | |
| Digestive | Liver failure | | | ± | | |
| Metabolic | Hyperammonemia, episodic | | + | + | | |
| | Hyperglycemia, insuline treatment | | + | + | | |
| | Lactic acidosis, episodic | | + | + | | ± |
| Other | Failure to thrive | | | ± | | |
| Laboratory findings | Ammonia (plasma) | | n–↑ | n–↑ | | |
| | Lactate (plasma) | | n–↑↑ | ↑–↑↑ | | |

**Table 44.92** Holocytochrome c synthase deficiency HCCS

| System | Symptoms and biomarkers | Neonatal (birth–1 month) | Infancy (1–18 months) | Childhood (1.5–11 years) | Adolescence (11–16 years) | Adulthood (>16 years) |
|---|---|---|---|---|---|---|
| Cardiovascular | Arrhythmias | | ± | | | |
| | Cardiac anomalies | | | | | |
| CNS | Corpus callosal hypoplasia (MRI) | | ± | ± | | |
| | Developmental delay | | ± | ± | | |
| | Epilepsy | | | ± | | |
| | Microcephaly | ± | ± | ± | | |
| | Ventriculomegaly (MRI) | | | ± | | |
| Ear | Hearing impairment | | | ± | | |
| Eye | Anophthalmia, uni- or bilateral | + | + | + | + | + |
| | Cataracts | ± | ± | ± | ± | ± |
| | Microphthalmia, uni- or bilateral | ++ | ++ | ++ | ++ | ++ |
| | Sclerocornea | ± | ± | ± | ± | ± |
| Musculoskeletal | Short stature | | | ± | | |
| Skin | Linear skin defects, mainly in face and neck, healing with age | ++ | ± | ++ | ++ | ++ |
| Other | Death, female | ± | | | | |
| | Lethal, male | ± | | | | |
| | XXY karyotype, male | ± | | | | |

## Reference Values

| Compound | Serum/blood (μmol/L) | Urine (mmol/mol creat) | Cerebrospinal fluid (μmol/L) |
|---|---|---|---|
| Lactate | 450–1800 (B) | <270 (<2 months)<br><200 (2 months–2 years)<br><85 (>2 years) | 1100–1700 |
| Pyruvate | 60–100 (B) | | 80–140 |
| Lactate/pyruvate ratio | <15 (B) | | <15 |
| Alanine | 150–450 (P, S) | 70–250 (<6 months)<br>35–165 (6 months–1 year)<br>25–130 (1–7 years)<br>20–70 (>7 years) | 16–41 (<1 year)<br>13–31 (1–3 years)<br>13–31 (>3 years) |
| Acetoacetate | 5–50 (P) | | |
| 3-Hydroxybutyrate | 15–90 (B) | | |
| 3-Hydroxybutyrate/ acetoacetate ratio | <1.0 (B) | | |
| Ammonia | 10–50 (P) | | |
| Creatine kinase | <200 (M)(S, U/l)<br><170 (F)(S, U/l) | | |
| Protein (total) | | | 450–1100<br>(<1 month, mg/L)<br>160–650 (>1 month, mg/L) |
| Ethylmalonic acid | | <20 | |
| 3-Methylglutaconic acid | | <20 | |

## Pathologic Values

| Compound | Serum/blood (μmol/L) | Urine (mmol/mol creat) | Cerebrospinal fluid (μmol/L) |
|---|---|---|---|
| Lactate | >2000 (B) | >350 (<2 months)<br>>300 (2 months–2 years)<br>>130 (>2 years) | >2000 |
| Pyruvate | >130 (B) | | >200 |
| Lactate/pyruvate ratio | >17 (B) | | >17 |
| Alanine | >450 (P, S) | >300 (<6 months)<br>>150 (6 months–7 years)<br>>100 (>7 years) | |
| 3-Hydroxybutyrate + acetoacetate ratio | Postprandial increase (B) | | |
| Ammonia | >100 (P) | | |
| Creatine kinase | >200 (M)(S, U/l)<br>>170 (F)(S, U/l) | | |
| Protein (total) | | | >1300 (<1 month, mg/L)<br>>650 (>1 month, mg/L) |
| Ethylmalonic acid | | >25 | |
| 3-Methylglutaconic acid | | >25 | |

*B* Blood, *S* Serum, *P* Plasma, *M* Male, *F* Female, *U/l* Units/liter

## Diagnostic Flowchart

A proposed flowchart for the diagnosis of mitochondrial diseases is presented in Fig. 44.2. See also Chap. 45.

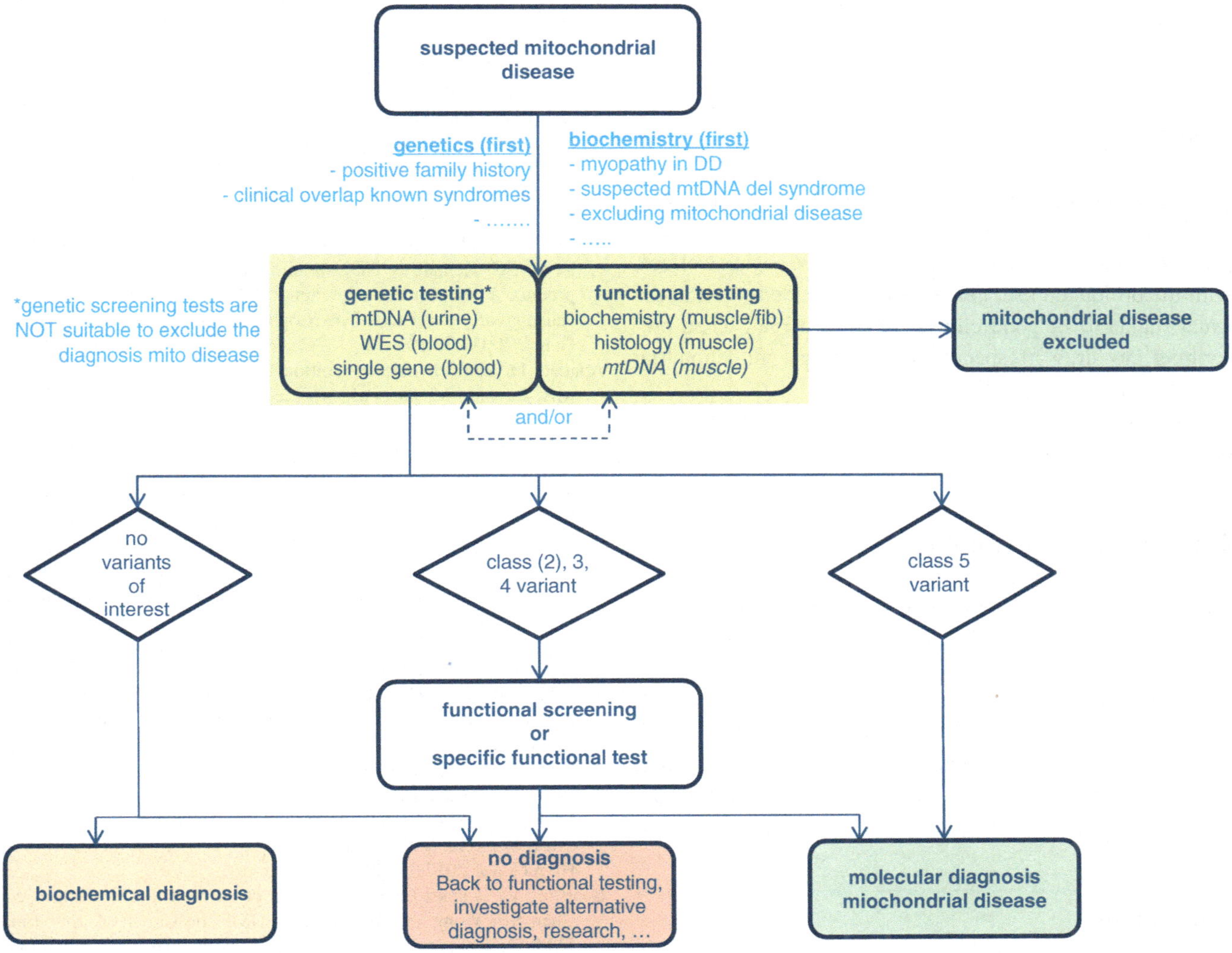


**Fig. 44.2** Flowchart for the diagnosis of mitochondrial diseases

## Specimen Collection

See Chap. 45.

## Prenatal Diagnosis

See Chap. 45.

## Treatment

Sodium valproate should never be used in patients with *POLG*-related mitochondrial disease. Certain drugs (e.g. propofol, midazolam, barbiturates) may have negative effects with the prolonged use, thus should be avoided. Overall the usual standards of good clinical practice prevail when prescribing any drug irrespective of the drug's mitochondrial toxicity potential or profile.

For more information on treatment of mitochondrial disorders, see Chap. 45.

## Experimental Treatment

Many novel approaches to treating mitochondrial disorders are currently under investigation, in cell models and in preclinical trials. These include pharmacological stimulators of mitochondrial biogenesis (such as bezafibrate, resveratrol and 5-aminoimidazole-4-carboxamide ribonucleoside), novel antioxidants, modifiers of mitochondrial dynamics, nucleoside replacement and gene therapy. Current trials are registered in clinicaltrials.gov.

## References


Abdulhag UN, Soiferman D, Schueler-Furman O, Miller C, Shaag A, Elpeleg O, Edvardson S, Saada A. Mitochondrial complex IV deficiency, caused by mutated COX6B1, is associated with encephalomyopathy, hydrocephalus and cardiomyopathy. Eur J Hum Genet. 2015;23:159–64.

Alfadhel M, Lillquist YP, Waters PJ, Sinclair G, Struys E, McFadden D, Hendson G, Hyams L, Shoffner J, Vallance HD. Infantile cardioencephalopathy due to a COX15 gene defect: report and review. Am J Med Genet. 2011;155A:840–4.

Alston CL, Morak M, Reid C, Hargreaves IP, Pope SA, Land JM, Heales SJ, Horvath R, Mundy H, Taylor RW. A novel mitochondrial MTND5 frameshift mutation causing isolated complex I deficiency, renal failure and myopathy. Neuromuscul Disord. 2010;20(2):131–5.

Alston CL, Compton AG, Formosa LE, Strecker V, Olahova M, Haack TB, Smet J, Stouffs K, Diakumis P, Ciara E, Cassiman D, Romain N, et al. Biallelic mutations in TMEM126B cause severe complex I deficiency with a variable clinical phenotype. Am J Hum Genet. 2016;99:217–27.

Anderson SL, Chung WK, Frezzo J, Papp JC, Ekstein J, DiMauro S, Rubin BY. A novel mutation in NDUFS4 causes Leigh syndrome in an Ashkenazi Jewish family. Hum Genet. 2003;112(5-6):563–6.

Andreu AL, Hanna MG, Reichmann H, Bruno C, Penn AS, Tanji K. Exercise intolerance due to mutations in the cytochrome b gene of mitochondrial DNA. N Engl J Med. 1999;341:1037–44.

Angebault C, Charif M, Guegen N, Piro-Megy C, Mousson de Camaret B, Procaccio V, Guichet PO, Hebrard M, Manes G, Leboucq N, Rivier F, Hamel CP, Lenaers G, Roubertie A. Mutation in NDUFA13/GRIM19 leads to early onset hypotonia, dyskinesia and sensorial deficiencies, and mitochondrial complex I instability. Hum Mol Genet. 2015;24(14):3948–55.

Antonicka H, Leary SC, Guercin G-H, Agar JN, Horvath R, Kennaway NG, Harding CO, Jaksch M, Shoubridge EA. Mutations in COX10 result in a defect in mitochondrial heme A biosynthesis and account for multiple, early-onset clinical phenotypes associated with isolated COX deficiency. Hum Mol Genet. 2003a;12:2693–702.

Antonicka H, Mattman A, Carlson CG, Glerum DM, Hoffbuhr KC, Leary SC, Kennaway NG, Shoubridge EA. Mutations in COX15 produce a defect in the mitochondrial heme biosynthetic pathway, causing early-onset fatal hypertrophic cardiomyopathy. Am J Hum Genet. 2003b;72:101–14.

Apatean D, Rakic B, Brunel-Guitton C, Hendson G, Bai R, Sargent MA, Lavoie PM, Patel M, Stockler-Ipsiroglu S. Congenital lactic acidosis, cerebral cysts and pulmonary hypertension in an infant with FOXRED1 related complex I deficiency. Mol Genet Metab Rep. 2019;18:32–8.

Aulbert W, Weigt-Usinger K, Thiels C, Köhler C, Vorgerd M, et al. Long survival in Leigh syndrome: new cases and review of literature. Neuropediatrics. 2014;45:346–53.

van Baars F, Cremers C, van den Broek P, Geerts S, Veldman J. Genetic aspects of nonchromaffin paraganglioma. Hum Genet. 1982;60:305–9.

Baertling F, van den Brand MAM, Hertecant JL, Al-Shamsi A, van den Heuvel LP, Distelmaier F, Mayatepek E, Smeitink JA, Nijtmans LGJ, Rodenburg RJT. Mutations in COA6 cause cytochrome c oxidase deficiency and neonatal hypertrophic cardiomyopathy. Hum Mutat. 2015;36:34–8.

Baertling F, Sanchez-Cabellero L, van den Brand MAM, Wintjes LT, Brink M, van den Brandt FA, Wilson C, Rodenburg RJT, Nijtmans LGJ. NDUFAF4 variants are associated with Leigh syndrome and cause a specific mitochondrial complex I assembly defect. Eur J Hum Genet. 2017;25:1273–7.

Baertling F, Sánchez-Caballero L, van den Brand MAM, Fung CW, Chan SH, Wong VC, Hellebrekers DME, de Coo IFM, Smeitink JAM, Rodenburg RJT, Nijtmans LGJ. NDUFA9 point mutations cause a variable mitochondrial complex I assembly defect. Clin Genet 2018;93(1):111-118.

Baide-Mairena H, Gaudó P, Marti-Sánchez L, et al. Mutations in the mitochondrial complex I assembly factor NDUFAF6 cause isolated bilateral striatal necrosis and progressive dystonia in childhood. Mol Genet Metab. 2019;126(3):250–8.

Baker RA, Priestley JRC, Wilstermann AM, Reese KJ, Mark PR. Clinical spectrum of BCS1L Mitopathies and their underlying structural relationships. Am J Med Genet A. 2019;179(3):373–80.

Balint B, Charlesworth G, Stamelou M, Carr L, Mencacci NE, Wood NW, Bhatia KP. Mitochondrial complex I NUBPL mutations cause combined dystonia with bilateral striatal necrosis and cerebellar atrophy. Eur J Neurol. 2019;

Barca E, Ganetzky RD, Potluri P, Juanola-Falgarona M, Gai X, et al. USMG5 Ashkenazi Jewish founder mutation impairs mitochondrial complex V dimerization and ATP synthesis. Hum Mol Genet. 2018;27:3305–12.

Barel O, Shorer Z, Flusser H, Ofir R, Narkis G, Finer G, Shalev H, Nasasra A, Saada A, Birk OS. Mitochondrial complex III deficiency associated with a homozygous mutation in UQCRQ. Am J Hum Genet. 2008;82:1211–6.

Barghuti F, Elian K, Gomori JM, Shaag A, Edvardson S, Saada A, Elpeleg O. The unique neuroradiology of complex I deficiency due to NDUFA12L defect. Mol Genet Metab. 2008;94:78–82.

Barletta JA, Hornick JL. Succinate dehydrogenase-deficient tumors: diagnostic advances and clinical implications. Adv Anat Pathol. 2012;19(4):193–203.

Bayley JP. Succinate dehydrogenase gene variants and their role in cowden syndrome. Am J Hum Genet. 2011;88(5):674–5.

Baysal BE, Ferrell RE, Willett-Brozick JE, Lawrence EC, Myssiorek D, Bosch A, van der Mey A, Taschner PE, Rubinstein WS, Myers EN, Richard CW 3rd, Cornelisse CJ, Devilee P, Devlin B. Mutations in SDHD, a mitochondrial complex II gene, in hereditary paraganglioma. Science. 2000;287(5454):848–51.

Bénit P, Slama A, Cartault F, Giurgea I, Chretien D, Lebon S, Marsac C, Munnich A, Rötig A, Rustin P. Mutant NDUFS3 subunit of mitochondrial complex I causes Leigh syndrome. J Med Genet. 2004;41(1):14–7.

Berger I, Hershkovitz E, Shaag A, Edvardson S, Saada A, Elpeleg O. Mitochondrial complex I deficiency caused by a deleterious NDUFA11 mutation. Ann Neurol. 2008;63(3):405–8.

Bhoj EJ, Li M, Ahrens-Nicklas R, Pyle LC, Wang J, et al. Pathologic variants of the mitochondrial phosphate carrier SLC25A3: two new patients and expansion of the cardiomyopathy/skeletal myopathy phenotype with and without lactic acidosis. JIMD Rep. 2015;19:59–66.

Bianciardi L, Imperatore V, Fernandez-Vizarra E, Lopomo A, Falabella M, Furini S, Galluzzi P, Grosso S, Zeviani M, Renieri A, Mari F, Frullanti E. Exome sequencing coupled with mRNA analysis identifies NDUFAF6 as a Leigh gene. Mol Genet Metab. 2016;119:214–22.

Blok MJ, Spruijt L, de Coo IF, Schoonderwoerd K, Hendrickx A, Smeets HJ. Mutations in the ND5 subunit of complex I of the mitochondrial DNA are a frequent cause of oxidative phosphorylation disease. J Med Genet. 2007;44(4):e74.

van den Bosch BJ, Gerards M, Sluiter W, Stegmann AP, Jongen EL, Hellebrekers DM, Oegema R, Lambrichs EH, Prokisch H, Danhauser K, Schoonderwoerd K, de Coo IF, Smeets HJ. Defective NDUFA9 as a novel cause of neonatally fatal complex I disease. J Med Genet. 2012;49(1):10–5.

Bourgeron T, Rustin P, Chretien D, Birch-Machin M, Bourgeois M, Viegas-Pequignot E, Munnich A, Rotig A. Mutation of a nuclear succinate dehydrogenase gene results in mitochondrial respiratory chain deficiency. Nat Genet. 1995;11:144–9.

Brown MD, Zhadanov S, Allen JC, Hosseini S, Newman NJ, Atamonov VV, Mikhailovskaya IE, Sukernik RI, Wallace DC. Novel mtDNA mutations and oxidative phosphorylation dysfunction in Russian LHON families. Hum Genet. 2001;109(1):33–9.

Brown MD, Starikovskaya E, Derbeneva O, Hosseini S, Allen JC, Mikhailovskaya IE, Sukernik RI, Wallace DC. The role of mtDNA background in disease expression: a new primary LHON mutation associated with Western Eurasian haplogroup. J Hum Genet. 2002;110(2):130–8.

Bruyn GW, Bots GT, Went LN, Klinkhamer PJ. Hereditary spastic dystonia with Leber's hereditary optic neuropathy: neuropathological findings. J Neurol Sci. 1992;113(1):55–61.

Budde SM, van den Heuvel LP, Janssen AJ, Smeets RJ, Buskens CA, DeMeirleir L, Van Coster R, Baethmann M, Voit T, Trijbels JM, Smeitink JA. Combined enzymatic complex I and III deficiency associated with mutations in the nuclear encoded NDUFS4 gene. Biochem Biophys Res Commun. 2000;275(1):63–8.

Bugiani M, Tiranti V, Farina L, Uziel G, Zeviani M. Novel mutations in COX15 in a long surviving Leigh syndrome patient with cytochrome c oxidase deficiency. J Med Genet. 2005;42:e28.

Calvo SE, Tucker EJ, Compton AG, Kirby DM, Crawford G, Burtt NP, Rivas M, Guiducci C, Bruno DL, Goldberger OA, Redman MC, Wiltshire E, Wilson CJ, Altshuler D, Gabriel SB, Daly MJ, Thorburn DR, Mootha VK. High-throughput, pooled sequencing identifies mutations in NUBPL and FOXRED1 in human complex I deficiency. Nat Genet. 2010;42:851–8.

Calvo SE, Compton AG, Hershman SG, Lim SC, Lieber DS, Tucker EJ, Laskowski A, Garone C, Liu S, Jaffe DB, Christodoulou J, Fletcher JM, Bruno DL, Goldblatt J, Dimauro S, Thorburn DR, Mootha VK. Molecular diagnosis of infantile mitochondrial disease with targeted next-generation sequencing. Sci Transl Med. 2012;4(118):118ra10.

Campos Y, Garcia-Redondo A, Fernandez-Moreno MA, Martinez-Pardo M, Goda G, Rubio JC, Martin MA, del Hoyo P, Cabello A, Bornstein B, Garesse R, Arenas J. Early-onset multisystem mitochondrial disorder caused by a nonsense mutation in the mitochondrial DNA cytochrome c oxidase II gene. Ann Neurol. 2001;50:409–13.

Carossa V, Ghelli A, Tropeano CV, Valentino ML, Iommarini L, Maresca A. A novel in-frame 18-bp microdeletion in MT-CYB causes a multisystem disorder with prominent exercise intolerance. Hum Mutat. 2014;35:954–8.

Catania A, Ardissone A, Verrigni D, Legati A, et al. Compound heterozygous missense and deep intronic variants in NDUFAF6 unraveled by exome sequencing and mRNA analysis. J Hum Genet. 2018;63(5):563–8.

Catteruccia M, Verrigni D, Martinelli D, Torraco A, Agovino T, et al. Persistent pulmonary arterial hypertension in the newborn (PPHN): a frequent manifestation of TMEM70 defective patients. Mol Genet Metab. 2014;111:353–9.

Cerecer-Gil NY, Figuera LE, Llamas FJ, et al. Mutation of SDHB is a cause of hypoxia-related high-altitude paraganglioma. Clin Cancer Res. 2010;16(16):4148–54.

Chinnery PF, Andrews RM, Turnbull DM, Howell NN. Leber hereditary optic neuropathy: does heteroplasmy influence the inheritance and expression of the G11778A mitochondrial DNA mutation? Am J Med Genet. 2001;98(3):235–43.

Cízková A, Stránecký V, Mayr JA, Tesarová M, Havlícková V, et al. TMEM70 mutations cause isolated ATP synthase deficiency and neonatal mitochondrial encephalocardiomyopathy. Nat Genet. 2008;40:1288–90.

Cizkova A, Stranecky V, Mayr JA, Tesarova M, Havlickova V, et al. TMEM70 mutations cause isolated ATP synthase deficiency and neonatal mitochondrial encephalocardiomyopathy. Nat Genet. 2008;40:1288–90.

Coenen MJH, van den Heuvel LP, Ugalde C, ten Brinke M, Nijtmans LGJ, Trijbels FJM, Beblo S, Maier EM, Muntau AC, Smeitink JAM. Cytochrome c oxidase biogenesis in a patient with a mutation in COX10 gene. Ann Neurol. 2004;56:560–4.

Courage C, Jackson CB, Hahn D, Euro L, Nuoffer JM, Gallati S, Schaller A. SDHA mutation with dominant transmission results in complex II deficiency with ocular, cardiac, and neurologic involvement. Am J Med Genet A. 2017 Jan;173(1):225–30.

Dallabona C, Abbink TEM, Carrozzo R, Torraco A, Legati A, van Berkel CGM, Niceta M, Langella T, Verrigni D, Rizza T, Diodato D, Piemonte F, et al. LYRM7 mutations cause a multifocal cavitating leukoencephalopathy with distinct MRI appearance. Brain. 2016;139:782–94. Note: Erratum: Brain 141: e82, 2018

De Meirleir L, Seneca S, Lissens W, De Clercq I, Eyskens F, et al. Respiratory chain complex V deficiency due to a mutation in the assembly gene ATP12. J Med Genet. 2004;41:120–4.

De Rocco D, Cerqua C, Goffrini P, Russo G, Pastore A, et al. Mutations of cytochrome c identified in patients with thrombocytopenia THC4 affect both apoptosis and cellular bioenergetics. Biochim Biophys Acta. 2014;1842:269–74.

Debray F-G, Lambert M, Lortie A, Vanasse M, Mitchell GA. Long-term outcome of Leigh syndrome caused by the NARP-T8993C mtDNA mutation. Am J Med Genet. 2007;143A:2046–51.

Debray FG, Seneca S, Gonce M, Vancampenhaut K, Bianchi E, Boemer F, Weekers L, Smet J, Van Coster R. Mitochondrial encephalomyopathy with cytochrome c oxidase deficiency caused by a novel mutation in the MTCO1 gene. Mitochondrion. 2014;17:101–5.

Doss S, Lohmann K, Seibler P, Arns B, Klopstock T, Zuhlke C, Freimann K, Winkler S, Lohnau T, Drungowski M, Nurnberg P, Wiegers K, Lohmann E, Naz S, Kasten M, Bohner G, Ramirez A, Endres M, Klein C. Recessive dystonia-ataxia syndrome in a Turkish family caused by a COX20 (FAM36A) mutation. J Neurol. 2014;261:207–12.

Dunning CJR, McKenzie M, Sugiana C, Lazarou M, Silke J, Connelly A, Fletcher JM, Kirby DM, Thorburn DR, Ryan MT. Human CIA30 is involved in the early assembly of mitochondrial complex I and mutations in its gene cause disease. EMBO J. 2007;26:3227–37.

Else T, Marvin ML, Everett JN, Gruber SB, Arts HA, Stoffel EM, Auchus RJ, Raymond VM. The clinical phenotype of *SDHC*-associated hereditary paraganglioma syndrome (PGL3). J Clin Endocrinol Metab. 2014;99(8):E1482–6.

Emmanuele V, Sotiriou E, Rios PG, Ganesh J, Ichord R, Foley AR. A novel mutation in the mitochondrial DNA cytochrome b gene (MTCYB) in a patient with mitochondrial encephalomyopathy, lactic acidosis, and strokelike episodes syndrome. J Child Neurol. 2013;28:236–42.

Fassone E, Duncan AJ, Taanman J-W, Pagnamenta AT, Sadowski MI, Holand T, Qasim W, Rutland P, Calvo SE, Mootha VK, Bitner-Glindzicz M, Rahman S. FOXRED1, encoding an FAD-dependent oxidoreductase complex-I-specific molecular chaperone, is mutated in infantile-onset mitochondrial encephalopathy. Hum Mol Genet. 2010;19:4837–47. Note: Erratum: Hum Mol Genet 24: 4183 only, 2015.

Fassone E, Taanman J-W, Hargreaves IP, Sebire NJ, Cleary MA, Burch M, Rahman S. Mutations in the mitochondrial complex I assembly factor NDUFAF1 cause fatal infantile hypertrophic cardiomyopathy. J Med Genet. 2011;48:691–7.

Feichtinger RG, Brunner-Krainz M, Alhaddad B, Wortmann SB, Kovacs-Nagy R, Stojakovic T, Erwa W, Resch B, Windischhofer W, Verheyen S, Uhrig S, Windpassinger C, Locker F, Makowski C, Strom TM, Meitinger T, Prokisch H, Sperl W, Haack TB, Mayr JA. Combined respiratory chain deficiency and UQCC2 mutations in neonatal encephalomyopathy: defective supercomplex assembly in complex III deficiencies. Oxid Med Cell Longev. 2017;2017:7202589.

Fernandez-Moreira D, Ugalde C, Smeets R, Rodenburg RJ, Lopez-Laso E, Ruiz-Falco ML, Briones P, Martin MA, Smeitink JA, Arenas J. X-linked NDUFA1 gene mutations associated with mitochondrial encephalomyopathy. Mol Genet Metab. 2011;103(4):358–61.

Fernández-Vizarra E, Zeviani M. Nuclear gene mutations as the cause of mitochondrial complex III deficiency. Front Genet. 2015 Apr 9;6:134.

Fujii T, Hattori H, Higuchi Y, Tsuji M, Mitsuyoshi I. Phenotypic differences between T-C and T-G mutations at nt 8993 of mitochondrial DNA in Leigh syndrome. Pediatr Neurol. 1998;18:275–7.

Gaignard P, Menezes M, Schiff M, Bayot A, Rak M, et al. Mutations in CYC1, encoding cytochrome c1 subunit of respiratory chain complex III, cause insulin-responsive hyperglycemia. Am J Hum Genet. 2013;93:384–9.

Gaignard P, Eyer D, Lebigot E, Oliveira C, Therond P, Boutron A, Slama A. UQCRC2 mutation in a patient with mitochondria complex III deficiency causing recurrent liver failure lactic acidosis and hypoglycemia. J Hum Genet. 2017;62:729–31.

Gerards M, Sluiter W, van den Bosch BJC, de Wit LEA, Calis CMH, Frentzen M, Akbari H, Schoonderwoerd K, Scholte HR, Jongbloed RJ, Hendrickx ATM, de Coo IFM, Smeets HJM. Defective complex I assembly due to C20orf7 mutations as a new cause of Leigh syndrome. J Med Genet. 2010;47:507–12.

Ghezzi D, Saada A, D'Adamo P, Fernandez-Vizarra E, Gasparini P, et al. FASTKD2 nonsense mutation in an infantile mitochondrial encephalomyopathy associated with cytochrome c oxidase deficiency. Am J Hum Genet. 2008;83:415–23.

Ghezzi D, Goffrini P, Uziel G, Horvath R, Klopstock T, Lochmuller H, D'Adamo P, Gasparini P, Strom TM, Prokisch H, Invernizzi F, Ferrero I, Zeviani M. SDHAF1, encoding a LYR complex-II specific assembly factor, is mutated in SDH-defective infantile leukoencephalopathy. Nat Genet. 2009;41:654–6.

Ghezzi D, Arzuffi P, Zordan M, Da Re C, Lamperti C, Benna C, D'Adamo P, Diodato D, Costa R, Mariotti C, Uziel G, Smiderle C, Zeviani M. Mutations in TTC19 cause mitochondrial complex III deficiency and neurological impairment in humans and flies. Nat Genet. 2011;43(3):259–63.

Ghosh A, Trivedi PP, Timbalia SA, Griffin AT, Rahn JJ, Chan SSL, Gohil VM. Copper supplementation restores cytochrome c oxidase assembly defect in a mitochondrial disease model of COA6 deficiency. Hum Mol Genet. 2014;23:3596–606.

Gil Borlado MC, Moreno Lastres D, Gonzalez Hoyuela M, Moran M, Blazquez A, Pello R, et al. Impact of the mitochondrial genetic background in complex III deficiency. PLOS One. 2010;5(9)

Gorman GS, Blakely EL, Hornig-Do HT, Tuppen HA, Greaves LC, He L, Baker A, Falkous G, Newman J, Trenell MI, Lecky B, Petty RK, Turnbull DM, McFarland R, Taylor RW. Novel MTND1 mutations cause isolated exercise intolerance, complex I deficiency and increased assembly factor expression. Clin Sci (Lond). 2015;128(12):895–904.

Haack TB, Haberberger B, Frisch EM, Wieland T, Iuso A, Gorza M, Strecker V, Graf E, Mayr JA, Herberg U, Hennermann JB, Klopstock T, Kuhn KA, Ahting U, Sperl W, Wilichowski E, Hoffmann GF, Tesarova M, Hansikova H, Zeman J, Plecko B, Zeviani M, Wittig I, Strom TM, Schuelke M, Freisinger P, Meitinger T, Prokisch H. Molecular diagnosis in mitochondrial complex I deficiency using exome sequencing. J Med Genet. 2012a;49(4):277–83.

Haack TB, Haberberger B, Frisch EM, Wieland T, Iuso A, Gorza M, Strecker V, Graf E, Mayr JA, Herberg U, Hennermann JB, Klopstock T, Kuhn KA, Ahting U, Sperl W, Wilichowski E, Hoffmann GF, Tesarova M, Hansikova H, Zeman J, Plecko B, Zeviani M, Wittig I, Strom TM, Schuelke M, Freisinger P, Meitinger T, Prokisch H. Molecular diagnosis in mitochondrial complex I deficiency using exome sequencing. J Med Genet. 2012b Apr;49(4):277–83.

Haack TB, Madignier F, Herzer M, Lamantea E, Danhauser K, Invernizzi F, Koch J, Freitag M, Drost R, Hillier I, Haberberger B, Mayr JA, Ahting U, Tiranti V, Rötig A, Iuso A, Horvath R, Tesarova M, Baric I, Uziel G, Rolinski B, Sperl W, Meitinger T, Zeviani M, Freisinger P, Prokisch H. Mutation screening of 75 candidate genes in 152 complex I deficiency cases identifies pathogenic variants in 16 genes including NDUFB9. J Med Genet. 2012c;49(2):83–9.

Hadzsiev K, Maasz A, Kisfali P, Kalman E, Gomori E, Pal E, Berenyi E, Komlosi K, Melegh B. Mitochondrial DNA 11777C>A mutation associated Leigh syndrome: case report with a review of the previously described pedigrees. Neuromolecular Med. 2010;12(3):277–84.

Hallmann K, Kudin AP, Zsurka G, Kornblum C, Reimann J, Stuve B, Waltz S, Hattingen E, Thiele H, Nurnberg P, Rub C, Voos W, Kopatz J, Neumann H, Kunz WS. Loss of the smallest subunit of cytochrome c oxidase, COX8A, causes Leigh-like syndrome and epilepsy. Brain. 2016;139:338–45.

Hao H-X, Khalimonchuk O, Schraders M, Dephoure N, Bayley J-P, Kunst H, Devilee P, Cremers CWRJ, Schiffman JD, Bentz BG, Gygi SP, Winge DR, Kremer H, Rutter J. SDH5, a gene required for flavination of succinate dehydrogenase, is mutated in paraganglioma. Science. 2009;325:1139–42.

Hempel M, Kremer LS, Tsiakas K, Alhaddad B, Haack TB, Löbel U, Feichtinger RG, Sperl W, Prokisch H, Mayr JA, Santer R. LYRM7—associated complex III deficiency: a clinical, molecular genetic, MR tomographic, and biochemical study. Mitochondrion. 2017;37:55–61.

Hensen EF, van Duinen N, Jansen JC, Corssmit EPM, Tops CMJ, Romijn JA, Vriends AHJT, van der Mey AGL, Cornelisse CJ, Devilee P, Bayley JP. High prevalence of founder mutations of the succinate dehydrogenase genes in the Netherlands. Clin Genet. 2012;81:284–8.

Hes FJ, Weiss MM, Woortman SA, et al. Low penetrance of a SDHB mutation in a large Dutch paraganglioma family. BMC Med Genet. 2010;11:92.

Hinttala R, Smeets R, Moilanen JS, Ugalde C, Uusimaa J, Smeitink JA, Majamaa K. Analysis of mitochondrial DNA sequences in patients with isolated or combined oxidative phosphorylation system deficiency. J Med Genet. 2006;43(11):881–6.

Hoefs SJ, Dieteren CE, Distelmaier F, Janssen RJ, Epplen A, Swarts HG, Forkink M, Rodenburg RJ, Nijtmans LG, Willems PH, Smeitink JA, van den Heuvel LP. NDUFA2 complex I mutation leads to Leigh disease. Am J Hum Genet. 2008;82(6):1306–15.

Hoefs SJG, Dieteren CEJ, Rodenburg RJ, Naess K, Bruhn H, Wibom R, Wagena E, Willems PH, Smeitink JAM, Nijtmans LG, van den Heuvel LP. Baculovirus complementation restores a novel NDUFAF2 mutation causing complex I deficiency. Hum Mutat. 2009;30:E728–36.

Hoefs SJG, van Spronsen FJ, Lenssen EWH, Nijtmans LG, Rodenburg RJ, Smeitink JAM, van den Heuvel LP. *NDUFA10* mutations cause complex I deficiency in a patient with Leigh disease. Eur J Hum Genet. 2011;19(3):270–4.

Holt IJ, Harding AE, Petty RKH, Morgan-Hughes JA. A new mitochondrial disease associated with mitochondrial DNA heteroplasmy. Am J Hum Genet. 1990;46:428–33.

Horvath R, Scharfe C, Hoeltzenbein M, Do BH, Schroder C, Warzok R, Vogelgesang S, Lochmuller H, Muller-Hocker J, Gerbitz KD, Oefner PJ, Jaksch M. Childhood onset mitochondrial myopathy and lactic acidosis caused by a stop mutation in the mitochondrial cytochrome c oxidase III gene. J Med Genet. 2002;39: 812–6.

Howell N, Oostra RJ, Bolhuis PA, Spruijt L, Clarke LA, Mackey DA, Preston G, Herrnstadt C. Sequence analysis of the mitochondrial genomes from Dutch pedigrees with Leber hereditary optic neuropathy. Am J Hum Genet. 2003 Jun;72(6):1460–9.

Huigsloot M, Nijtmans LG, Szklarczyk R, Baars MJH, van den Brand MAM, HendriksFranssen MGM, van den Heuvel LP, Smeitink JAM, Huynen MA, Rodenburg RJT. A mutation in C2orf64 causes impaired cytochrome C oxidase assembly and mitochondrial cardiomyopathy. Am J Hum Genet. 2011;88:488–93.

Indrieri A, van Rahden VA, Tiranti V, Morleo M, Iaconis D, Tammaro R, D'Amato I, Conte I, Maystadt I, Demuth S, Zvulunov A, Kutsche K, Zeviani M, Franco B. Mutations in COX7B cause microphthalmia with linear skin lesions, and unconventional mitochondrial disease. Am J Hum Genet. 2012;91:942–9.

Invernizzi F, Tigano M, Dallabona C, Donnini C, Ferrero I, Cremonte M, Ghezzi D, Lamperti C, Zeviani M. A homozygous mutation in LYRM7/MZM1L associated with early onset encephalopathy, lactic acidosis, and severe reduction of mitochondrial complex III activity. Hum Mutat. 2013;34:1619–22.

Johns DR, Neufeld MJ. Cytochrome c oxidase mutations in Leber hereditary optic neuropathy. Biochem Biophys Res Commun. 1993;196:810–5.

Jonckheere AI, Hogeveen M, Nijtmans LGJ, van den Brand MAM, Janssen AJM, et al. A novel mitochondrial ATP8 gene mutation in a patient with apical hypertrophic cardiomyopathy and neuropathy. J Med Genet. 2008;45:129–33.

Jonckheere AI, Renkema GH, Bras M, van den Heuvel LP, Hoischen A, et al. A complex V ATP5A1 defect causes fatal neonatal mitochondrial encephalopathy. Brain. 2013;136(Pt 5):1544–54.

Keightley JA, Anitori R, Burton MD, Quan F, Buist NRM, Kennaway NG. Mitochondrial encephalomyopathy and complex III deficiency associated with a stop-codon mutation in the cytochrome b gene. Am J Hum Genet. 2000;67:1400–10.

Kevelam SH, Rodenburg RJ, Wolf NI, Ferreira P, Lunsing RJ, Nijtmans LG, Mitchell A, Arroyo HA, Rating D, Vanderver A, van Berkel CGM, Abbink TEM, Heutink P, van der Knaap MS. NUBPL mutations in patients with complex I deficiency and a distinct MRI pattern. Neurology. 2013;80:1577–83.

Kirby DM, Salemi R, Sugiana C, Ohtake A, Parry L, Bell KM, Kirk EP, Boneh A, Taylor RW, Dahl HH, Ryan MT, Thorburn DR. NDUFS6 mutations are a novel cause of lethal neonatal mitochondrial complex I deficiency. J Clin Investig. 2004a;114(6):837.

Kirby DM, Salemi R, Sugiana C, Ohtake A, Parry L, Bell KM, Kirk EP, Boneh A, Taylor RW, Dahl H-HM, Ryan MT, Thorburn DR. *NDUFS6* mutations are a novel cause of lethal neonatal mitochondrial complex I deficiency. J Clin Invest. 2004b;114(6):837–45.

Koch J, Freisinger P, Feichtinger RG, Zimmermann FA, Rauscher C, Wagentristl HP, Konstantopoulou V, Seidl R, Haack TB, Prokisch H, Ahting U, Sperl W, Mayr JA, Maier EM. Mutations in TTC19: expanding the molecular, clinical and biochemical phenotype. Orphanet J Rare Dis. 2015;10:40.

Kohda M, Tokuzawa Y, Kishita Y, et al. A comprehensive genomic analysis reveals the genetic landscape of mitochondrial respiratory chain complex deficiencies. PLoS Genet. 2016a;12(1):e1005679.

Kohda M, Tokuzawa Y, Kishita Y, Nyuzuki H, Moriyama Y, Mizuno Y, et al. A comprehensive genomic analysis reveals the genetic landscape of mitochondrial respiratory chain complex deficiencies. PLoS Genet. 2016b;12(1):e1005679.

Kohda M, Tokuzawa Y, Kishita Y, Nyuzuki H, Moriyama Y, Mizuno Y, Hirata T, Yatsuka Y, Yamashita-Sugahara Y, Nakachi Y, Kato H, Okuda A, et al. A comprehensive genomic analysis reveals the genetic landscape of mitochondrial respiratory chain complex deficiencies. PLoS Genet. 2016c;12:e1005679.

Kurt YG, Çoku J, Akman HO, Naini A, Lu J, Engelstad K, Hirano M, De Vivo DC, DiMauro S. A de novo mutation in *MTND6* causes generalized dystonia in 2 unrelated children. Child Neurol Open. 2016;3:2329048X15627937.

Lassuthova P, Beharka R, Krutova M, Neupauerova J, Seeman P. COX6A1 mutation causes axonal hereditary motor and sensory neuropathy--the confirmation of the primary report. (Letter). Clin Genet. 2015;89:512–4.

Laugel V, This-Bernd V, Cormier-Daire V, Speeg-Schatz C, de Saint-Martin A, Fischbach M. Early-onset ophthalmoplegia in Leigh-like syndrome due to NDUFV1 mutations. Pediatric Neurol. 2007;36(1): 54–7.

Leary SC, Antonicka H, Sasarman F, Weraarpachai W, Cobine PA, et al. Novel mutations in SCO1 as a cause of fatal infantile encephalopathy and lactic acidosis. Hum Mutat. 2013;34:1366–70.

Lebon S, Rodriguez D, Bridoux D, Zerrad A, Rötig A, Munnich A, Legrand A, Slama A. A novel mutation in the human complex I NDUFS7 subunit associated with Leigh syndrome. Mol Genet Metab. 2007;90(4):379–82.

Levitas A, Muhammad E, Harel G, Saada A, Caspi VC, Manor E, Beck JC, Sheffield V, Parvari R. Familial neonatal isolated cardiomyopathy caused by a mutation in the flavoprotein subunit of succinate dehydrogenase. Eur J Hum Genet. 2010;18:1160–5.

Lieber DS, Calvo SE, Shanahan K, Slate NG, Liu S, Hershman SG. Targeted exome sequencing of suspected mitochondrial disorders. Neurology. 2013;80:1762–70.

Lim SC, Smith KR, Stroud DA, Compton AG, Tucker EJ, et al. A founder mutation in PET100 causes isolated complex IV deficiency in Lebanese individuals with Leigh syndrome. Am J Hum Genet. 2014;94:209–22.

Loeffen J, Smeitink J, Triepels R, Smeets R, Schuelke M, Sengers R, Trijbels F, Hamel B, Mullaart R, van den Heuvel L. The first nuclear-encoded complex I mutation in a patient with Leigh syndrome. Am J Hum Genet. 1998;63(6):1598–608.

Loeffen JL, Smeitink JA, Trijbels JM, Janssen AJ, Triepels RH, Sengers RC, van den Heuvel LP. Isolated complex I deficiency in children: clinical, biochemical and genetic aspects. Human Mutat. 2000;15(2):123–34.

Lyons M, Ardissone R, Robinson M, Ghezzi F-V, Zeviani. COA7 (C1orf163/RESA1) mutations associated with mitochondrial leukoencephalopathy and cytochrome c oxidase deficiency. J Med Genet. 2016 Dec;53(12):846–9.

Magner M, Dvorakova V, Tesarova M, Mazurova S, Hansikova H, et al. TMEM70 deficiency: long-term outcome of 48 patients. J Inherit Metab Dis. 2015;38:417–26.

Maio N, Ghezzi D, Verrigni D, Rizza T, Bertini E, Martinelli D, Zeviani M, Singh A, Carrozzo R, Rouault TA. Disease-Causing SDHAF1 Mutations Impair Transfer of Fe-S Clusters to SDHB. Cell Metab. *February 2016*;23(2):*292–302*.

Makrythanasis P, Nelis M, Santoni FA, Guipponi M, Vannier A, et al. Diagnostic exome sequencing to elucidate the genetic basis of likely recessive disorders in consanguineous families. Hum Mutat. 2014;35:1203–10.

Marina AD, Schara U, Pyle A, Möller-Hartmann C, Holinski-Feder E, Abicht A, Czermin B, Lochmüller H, Griffin H, Santibanez-Koref M, Chinnery PF, Horvath R. NDUFS8-related complex I deficiency extends phenotype from "PEO Plus" to Leigh syndrome. JIMD Rep. 2013;10:17.

Massa V, Fernandez-Vizarra E, Alshahwan S, Bakhsh E, Goffrini P, Ferrero I, Mereghetti P, D'Adamo P, Gasparini P, Zeviani M. Severe infantile encephalomyopathy caused by a mutation in COX6B1, a nucleus-encoded subunit of cytochrome c oxidase. Am J Hum Genet. 2008;82:1281–9.

Massie R, Wang J, Chen LC, Zhang VW, Collins MP, Wong LJ, Milone M. Mitochondrial myopathy due to novel missense mutation in the cytochrome c oxidase 1 gene. J Neurol Sci. 2012;319(1–2):158–63.

Mayr JA, Merkel O, Kohlwein SD, Gebhardt BR, Bohles H, et al. Mitochondrial phosphate-carrier deficiency: a novel disorder of oxidative phosphorylation. Am J Hum Genet. 2007;80:478–84.

Mayr JA, Bodamer O, Haack TB, Zimmermann FA, Madignier F, Prokisch H, Rauscher C, Koch J, Sperl W. Heterozygous mutation in the X chromosomal NDUFA1 gene in a girl with complex I deficiency. Mol Genet Metab. 2009;96(4):189–95.

Mayr JA, Havlícková V, Zimmermann F, Magler I, Kaplanová V, et al. Mitochondrial ATP synthase deficiency due to a mutation in the ATP5E gene for the F1 epsilon subunit. Hum Mol Genet. 2010;19:3430–9.

Mayr JA, Zimmermann FA, Horváth R, Schneider HC, Schoser B, et al. Deficiency of the mitochondrial phosphate carrier presenting as myopathy and cardiomyopathy in a family with three affected children. Neuromuscul Disord. 2011;21:803–8.

Mcarland R, Kirby DM, Fowler KJ, Ohtake A, Ryan MT, Amor DJ, Fletcher JM, Dixon JW, Collins FA, Turnbull DM, Taylor RW, Thorburn DR. De novo mutations in the mitochondrial ND3 gene as a cause of infantile mitochondrial encephalopathy and complex I deficiency. Ann Neurol. 2004;55(1):58–64.

Melchionda L, Haack TB, Hardy S, Abbink TE, Fernandez-Vizarra E, et al. Mutations in APOPT1, encoding a mitochondrial protein, cause cavitating leukoencephalopathy with cytochrome c oxidase deficiency. Am J Hum Genet. 2014;95:315–25.

Miryounesi M, Fardaei M, Tabei SM, Ghafouri-Fard S. Leigh syndrome associated with a novel mutation in the COX15 gene. J Pediatr Endocrinol Metab. 2016;29(6):741–4.

Miyake N, Yano S, Sakai C, Hatakeyama H, Matsushima Y, Shiina M, Watanabe Y, Bartley J, Abdenur JE, Wang RY, Chang R, Tsurusaki Y, Doi H, Nakashima M, Saitsu H, Ogata K, Goto Y, Matsumoto N. Mitochondrial complex III deficiency caused by a homozygous UQCRC2 mutation presenting with neonatal-onset recurrent metabolic decompensation. Hum Mutat. 2013;34:446–52.

Mootha VK, Lepage P, Miller K, Bunkenborg J, Reich M, et al. Identification of a gene causing human cytochrome c oxidase deficiency by integrative genomics. Proc Natl Acad Sci U S A. 2003;100:605–10.

Mordaunt DA, Jolley A, Balasubramaniam S, Thorburn DR, Mountford HS, ComptonAG NJ, Manton N, Clark D, Bratkovic D, Friend K, Yu S. Phenotypic variation of TTC19-deficient mitochondrial complex III deficiency: a case report and literature review. Am J Med Genet A. 2015;167(6):1330–6.

Mori M, Goldstein J, Young SP, Bossen EH, Shoffner J, Koeberl DD. Complex III deficiency due to an in-frame MT-CYB deletion presenting as ketotic hypoglycemia and lactic acidosis. Mol Genet Metab Rep. 2015;4:39–41.

Morin C, Mitchell G, Larochelle J, Lambert M, Ogier H, et al. Clinical, metabolic, and genetic aspects of cytochrome C oxidase deficiency in Saguenay-Lac-Saint-Jean. Am J Hum Genet. 1993;53:488–96.

Morison IM, Borde EMC, Cheesman EJ, Cheong PL, Holyoake AJ, et al. A mutation of human cytochrome c enhances the intrinsic apoptotic pathway but causes only thrombocytopenia. Nat Genet. 2008;40:387–9.

Morleo M, Franco B. Microphthalmia with linear skin defects syndrome. GeneReviews. Seattle, WA: University of Washington, Seattle; 1993–2019; 2009. [updated 2018 Jul 26].

Morleo M, Pramparo T, Perone L, Gregato G, Le Caignec C, et al. Microphthalmia with linear skin defects (MLS) syndrome: clinical, cytogenetic, and molecular characterization of 11 cases. Am J Med Genet. 2005;137A:190–8.

Mu W, Schiess N, Orthmann-Murphy JL, El-Hattab AW. The utility of whole exome sequencing in diagnosing neurological disorders in adults from a highly consanguineous population. J Neurogenet. 2019;33:21–6.

Musumeci O, Andreu AL, Shanske S, Bresolin N, Comi GP, Rothstein R, Schon EA, DiMauro S. Intragenic inversion of mtDNA: a new type of pathogenic mutation in a patient with mitochondrial myopathy. Am J Hum Genet. 2000;66(6):1900–4.

Naini AB, Lu J, Kaufmann P, Bernstein RA, Mancuso M, Bonilla E, Hirano M, DiMauro S. Novel mitochondrial DNA ND5 mutation in a patient with clinical features of MELAS and MERRF. Arch Neurol. 2005;62(3):473–6.

Nogueira C, Barros J, Sa MJ, Azevedo L, Taipa R, Torraco A, Meschini MC, Verrigni D, Nesti C, Rizza T, Teixeira J, Carrozzo R, Pires MM, Vilarinho L, Santorelli FM. Novel TTC19 mutation in a family with severe psychiatric manifestations and complex III deficiency. Neurogenetics. 2013;14:153–60.

Ogilvie I, Kennaway NG, Shoubridge EA. A molecular chaperone for mitochondrial complex I assembly is mutated in a progressive encephalopathy. J Clin Invest. 2005;115:2784–92.

Ohlenbusch A, Edvardson S, Skorpen J, Bjornstad A, Saada A, Elpeleg O, Gärtner J. *Brockmann K* "Leukoencephalopathy with accumulated succinate is indicative of SDHAF1 related complex II deficiency". Orphanet J Rare Dis. *2012*;7:*69*.

Oláhová M, Hardy SA, Hall J, Yarham JW, Haack TB, et al. LRPPRC mutations cause early-onset multisystem mitochondrial disease outside of the French-Canadian population. Brain. 2015;138(Pt 12):3503–19.

Olahova M, Haack TB, Alston CL, Houghton JAC, He L, et al. A truncating PET100 variant causing fatal infantile lactic acidosis and isolated cytochrome c oxidase deficiency. Eur J Hum Genet. 2015;23:935–9.

Oláhová M, Yoon WH, Thompson K, Jangam S, Fernandez L, et al. Biallelic mutations in ATP5F1D, which encodes a subunit of ATP synthase, cause a metabolic disorder. Am J Hum Genet. 2018;102:494–504.

Oquendo CE, Antonicka H, Shoubridge EA, Reardon W, Brown GK. Functional and genetic studies demonstrate that mutation in the COX15 gene can cause Leigh syndrome. (Letter). J Med Genet. 2004;41:540–4.

Ostergaard E, Rodenburg RJ, van den Brand M, Thomsen LL, Duno M, Batbayli M, Wibrand F, Nijtmans L. Respiratory chain complex I deficiency due to NDUFA12 mutations as a new cause of Leigh syndrome. J Med Genet. 2011;48(11):737–40.

Ostergaard E, Weraarpachai W, Ravn K, Born AP, Jonson L, Duno M, Wibrand F, Shoubridge EA, Vissing J. Mutations in COA3 cause isolated complex IV deficiency associated with neuropathy, exercise intolerance, obesity, and short stature. J Med Genet. 2015;52:203–7.

Pagliarini DJ, Calvo SE, Chang B, Sheth SA, Vafai SB, Ong S-E, Walford GA, Sugiana C, Boneh A, Chen WK, Hill DE, Vidal M, Evans JG, Thorburn DR, Carr SA, Mootha VK. A mitochondrial protein compendium elucidates complex I disease biology. Cell. 2008;134:112–23.

Papadopoulou LC, Sue CM, Davidson MM, Tanji K, Nishino I, et al. Fatal infantile cardioencephalomyopathy with COX deficiency and mutations in SCO2, a COX assembly gene. Nat Genet. 1999;23:333–7.

Parfait B, Chretien D, Rotig A, Marsac C, Munnich A, Rustin P. Compound heterozygous mutations in the flavoprotein gene of the respiratory chain complex II in a patient with Leigh syndrome. Hum Genet. 2000;106:236–43.

Perrier S, Gauquelin L, Tétreault M, Tran LT, Webb N, Srour M, Mitchell JJ, Brunel-Guitton C, Majewski J, Long V, Keller S, Gambello MJ, Simons C, Care4Rare Canada Consortium, Vanderver A, Bernard G. Recessive mutations in NDUFA2 cause mitochondrial leukoencephalopathy. Clin Genet. 2018;93(2):396–400.

Petruzzella V, Vergari R, Puzziferri I, Boffoli D, Lamantea E, Zeviani M, Papa S. A nonsense mutation in the NDUFS4 gene encoding the 18 kDa (AQDQ) subunit of complex I abolishes assembly and activity of the complex in a patient with Leigh-like syndrome. Hum Mol Genet. 2001;10(5):529–3.

Pfeffer G, Blakely EL, Alston CL, Hassani A, Boggild M, et al. Adult-onset spinocerebellar ataxia syndromes due to MTATP6 mutations. J Neurol Neurosurg Psychiatry. 2012;83:883–6.

Piekutowska-Abramczuk D, Assouline Z, Mataković L, Feichtinger RG, Koňaříková E, Jurkiewicz E, Stawiński P, Gusic M, Koller A, Pollak A, Gasperowicz P, Trubicka J, Ciara E, Iwanicka-Pronicka K, Rokicki D, Hanein S, Wortmann SB, Sperl W, Rötig A, Prokisch H, Pronicka E, Płoski R, Barcia G, Mayr JA. NDUFB8 mutations cause mitochondrial complex i deficiency in individuals with leigh-like encephalomyopathy. Am J Hum Genet. 2018;102(3):460–7.

Pitceathly RD, Murphy SM, Cottenie E, Chalasani A, Sweeney MG, et al. Genetic dysfunction of MT-ATP6 causes axonal Charcot-Marie-Tooth disease. Neurology. 2012;79:1145–54.

Pitceathly RD, Rahman S, Wedatilake Y, Polke JM, Cirak S, et al. NDUFA4 mutations underlie dysfunction of a cytochrome c oxidase subunit linked to human neurological disease. Cell Rep. 2013;3:1795–805.

Potluri P, Davila A, Ruiz-Pesini E, Mishmar D, O'Hearn S, Hancock S, Simon M, Scheffler IE, Wallace DC, Procaccio V. A novel NDUFA1 mutation leads to a progressive mitochondrial complex I-specific neurodegenerative disease. Mol Genet Metab. 2009;96:189.

Prakash SK, Cormier TA, McCall AE, Garcia JJ, Sierra R, et al. Loss of holocytochrome c-type synthetase causes the male lethality of X-linked dominant microphthalmia with linear skin defects (MLS) syndrome. Hum Mol Genet. 2002;11:3237–48.

Procaccio V, Wallace DC. Late-onset Leigh syndrome in a patient with mitochondrial complex I NDUFS8 mutations. JIMD Rep. 2013;10:17–22.

Pronicka E, Piekutowska-Abramczuk D, Szymańska-Dębińska T, Bielecka L, Kowalski P, et al. The natural history of SCO2 deficiency in 36 Polish children confirmed the genotype-phenotype correlation. Mitochondrion. 2013;13:810–6.

Pulkes T, Liolitsa D, Wills AJ, Hargreaves I, Heales S, Hanna MG. Nonsense mutations in mitochondrial DNA associated with myalgia and exercise intolerance. Neurology. 2005;64(6):1091–2.

van Rahden VA, Fernandez-Vizarra E, Alawi M, Brand K, Fellmann F, Horn D, Zeviani M, Kutsche K. Mutations in NDUFB11, encoding a complex I component of the mitochondrial respiratory chain, cause microphthalmia with linear skin defects syndrome. Am J Hum Genet. 2015 Apr 2;96(4):640–50.

Rahman S, Blok RB, Dahl H-HM, Danks DM, Kirby DM, Chow CW, Christodoulou J, Thorburn DR. Leigh syndrome: clinical features and biochemical and DNA abnormalities. Ann Neurol. 1996;39:343–51.

Rahman S, Taanman J-W, Cooper JM, Nelson I, Hargreaves I, Meunier B, Hanna MG, Garcia JJ, Capaldi RA, Lake BD, Leonard JV, Schapira AHV. A missense mutation of cytochrome oxidase subunit II causes defective assembly and myopathy. Am J Hum Genet. 1999;65:1030–9.

Ravn K, Wibrand F, Hansen FJ, Horn N, Rosenberg T, Schwartz M. An mtDNA mutation, 14453G-->A, in the NADH dehydrogenase subunit 6 associated with severe MELAS syndrome. Eur J Hum Genet. 2001 Oct;9(10):805–9.

Rebelo AP, Saade D, Pereira CV, Farooq A, Huff TC, et al. SCO2 mutations cause early-onset axonal Charcot-Marie-Tooth disease associated with cellular copper deficiency. Brain. 2018;141:662–72.

Robinson BH. Human complex I deficiency: clinical spectrum and involvement of oxygen free radicals in the pathogenicity of the defect. Biochim Biophys Acta 1998;1364 (2):271–86.

Saada A, Edvardson S, Rapoport M, Shaag A, Amry K, Miller C, Lorberboum-Galski H, Elpeleg O. C6ORF66 is an assembly factor of mitochondrial complex I. Am J Hum Genet. 2008;82:32–8.

Saada A, Vogel RO, Hoefs SJ, van den Brand MA, Wessels HJ, Willems PH, Venselaar H, Shaag A, Barghuti F, Reish O, Shohat M, Huynen MA, Smeitink JAM, van den Heuvel LP, Nijtmans LG. Mutations in NDUFAF3 (C3ORF60), encoding an NDUFAF4 (C6ORF66)-interacting complex I assembly protein, cause fatal neonatal mitochondrial disease. Am J Hum Genet. 2009;84:718–27.

Saada A, Edvardson S, Shaag A, Chung WK, Segel R, Miller C, Jalas C, Elpeleg O. Combined OXPHOS complex I and IV defect, due to mutated complex I assembly factor C20ORF7. J Inherit Metab Dis. 2012;35:125.

Sanchez-Caballero L, Ruzzenente B, Bianchi L, Assouline Z, Barcia G, Metodiev MD, Rio M, Funalot B, van den Brand MAM, Guerrero-Castillo S, Molenaar JP, Koolen D, Brandt U, Rodenburg RJ, Nijtmans LG, Rotig A. Mutations in complex I assembly factor TMEM126B result in muscle weakness and isolated complex I deficiency. Am J Hum Genet. 2016;99:208–16.

Santorelli FM, Shanske S, Macaya A, DeVivo DC, DiMauro S. The mutation at nt 8993 of mitochondrial DNA is a common cause of Leigh's syndrome. Ann Neurol. 1993;34:827–34.

Sarzi E, Brown MD, Lebon S, Chretien D, Munnich A, Rotig A, Procaccio V. A novel recurrent mitochondrial DNA mutation in ND3 gene is associated with isolated complex I deficiency causing Leigh syndrome and dystonia. Am J Med Genet A. 2007;143A(1):33–41.

Schwartz M, Vissing J. Paternal inheritance of mitochondrial DNA. N Engl J Med. 2002;347(8):576–80.

Seeger J, Schrank B, Pyle A, Stucka R, Lorcher U, et al. Clinical and neuropathological findings in patients with TACO1 mutations. Neuromuscul Disord. 2010;20:720–4.

Seifert EL, Ligeti E, Mayr JA, Sondheimer N, Hajnóczky G. The mitochondrial phosphate carrier: Role in oxidative metabolism, calcium handling and mitochondrial disease. Biochem Biophys Res Commun. 2015;464:369–75.

Sharma S, Singh P, Fernandez-Vizarra E, Zeviani M, Van der Knaap MS, et al. Cavitating leukoencephalopathy with posterior predominance caused by a deletion in the APOPT1 gene in an Indian boy. J Child Neurol. 2018;33:428–31.

Shteyer E, Saada A, Shaag A, Al-Hijawi FA, Kidess R, Revel-Vilk S, Elpeleg O. Exocrine pancreatic insufficiency, dyserythropoeitic (sic) anemia, and calvarial hyperostosis are caused by a mutation in the COX4I2 gene. Am J Hum Genet. 2009;84:412–7.

Spiegel R, Khayat M, Shalev SA, Horovitz Y, Mandel H, et al. TMEM70 mutations are a common cause of nuclear encoded ATP synthase assembly defect: further delineation of a new syndrome. J Med Genet. 2011;48:177–82.

Stiburek L, Vesela K, Hansikova H, Hulkova H, Zeman J. Loss of function of Sco1 and its interaction with cytochrome c oxidase. Am J Physiol Cell Physiol. 2009;96:C1218–26.

Sugiana C, Pagliarini DJ, McKenzie M, Kirby DM, Salemi R, Abu-Amero KK, Dahl H-HM, Hutchison WM, Vascotto KA, Smith SM, Newbold RF, Christodoulou J, Calvo S, Mootha VK, Ryan MT, Thorburn DR. Mutation of C20orf7 disrupts complex I assembly and causes lethal neonatal mitochondrial disease. Am J Hum Genet. 2008;83:468–78.

Szklarczyk R, Wanschers BFJ, Nijtmans LG, Rodenburg RJ, Zschocke J, Dikow N, van den Brand MAM, Hendriks-Franssen MGM, Gilissen C, Veltman JA, Nooteboom M, Koopman WJH, Willems PHGM, Smeitink JAM, Huynen MA, van den Heuvel LP. A mutation in the FAM36A gene, the human ortholog of COX20, impairs cytochrome c oxidase assembly and is associated with ataxia and muscle hypotonia. Hum Mol Genet. 2013;22:656–67.

Tamiya G, Makino S, Hayashi M, Abe A, Numakura C, Ueki M, Tanaka A, Ito C, Toshimori K, Ogawa N, Terashima T, Maegawa H, Yanagisawa D, Tooyama I, Tada M, Onodera O, Hayasaka K. A mutation of COX6A1 causes a recessive axonal or mixed form of Charcot-Marie-Tooth disease. Am J Hum Genet. 2014;95:294–300.

Taylor RW, Singh-Kler R, Hayes CM, Smith PE, Turnbull DM. Progressive mitochondrial disease resulting from a novel missense mutation in the mitochondrial DNA ND3 gene. Ann Neurol. 2001;50(1):104–7.

Taylor RW, Morris AA, Hutchinson M, Turnbull DM. Leigh disease associated with a novel mitochondrial DNA ND5 mutation. Eur J Hum Genet. 2002;10(2):141–4.

Torraco A, Bianchi M, Verrigni D, Gelmetti V, Riley L, Niceta M, et al. A novel mutation in NDUFB11 unveils a new clinical phenotype associated with lactic acidosis and sideroblastic anemia. Clin Genet. 2017;91(3):441–7.

Torroni A, Petrozzi M, D'Urbano L, Sellitto D, Zeviani M, Carrara F, Carducci C, Leuzzi V, Carelli V, Barboni P, De Negri A, Scozzari R. Haplotype and phylogenetic analyses suggest that one European-specific mtDNA background plays a role in the expression of Leber hereditary optic neuropathy by increasing the penetrance of the primary mutations 11778 and 14484. Am J Hum Genet. 1997;60(5):1107–21.

Triepels RH, van den Heuvel LP, Loeffen JL, Buskens CA, Smeets RJ, Rubio Gozalbo ME, Budde SM, Mariman EC, Wijburg FA, Barth PG, Trijbels JM, Smeitink JA. Leigh syndrome associated with a mutation in the NDUFS7 (PSST) nuclear encoded subunit of complex I. Am J Hum Genet. 1999;64(6):1505–10.

Triepels RH, Van Den Heuvel LP, Trijbels JM, Smeitink JA. Respiratory chain complex I deficiency. Am J Med Genet. 2001;106(1): 37–45.

Tucker EJ, Wanschers BF, Szklarczyk R, Mountford HS, Wijeyeratne XW, van den Brand MA, Leenders AM, Rodenburg RJ, Reljić B, Compton AG, Frazier AE, Bruno DL, Christodoulou J, Endo H, Ryan MT, Nijtmans LG, Huynen MA, Thorburn DR; Mutations in the UQCC1-interacting protein, UQCC2, cause human complex III deficiency associated with perturbed cytochrome b protein expression.

Tuppen HA, Hogan VE, He L, Blakely EL, Worgan L, Al-Dosary M, Saretzki G, Alston CL, Morris AA, Clarke M, Jones S, Devlin AM, Mansour S, Chrzanowska-Lightowlers ZM, Thorburn DR, McFarland R, Taylor RW. The p.M292T NDUFS2 mutation causes complex I-deficient Leigh syndrome in multiple families. Brain. 2010;133(10):2952–63.

Uchiyama Y, Yanagisawa K, Kunishima S, Shiina M, Ogawa Y, et al. A novel CYCS mutation in the alpha-helix of the CYCS C-terminal domain causes non-syndromic thrombocytopenia. Clin Genet. 2018;94:548–53.

Valnot I, Osmond S, Gigarel N, Mehaye B, Amiel J, et al. Mutations of the SCO1 gene in mitochondrial cytochrome c oxidase deficiency with neonatal-onset hepatic failure and encephalopathy. Am J Hum Genet. 2000;67:1104–9.

Van Bon BW, Oortveld MA, Nijtmans LG, Fenckova M, Nijhof B, et al. CEP89 is required for mitochondrial metabolism and neuronal function in man and fly. Hum Mol Genet. 2013;22:3138–51.

Van Coster R, Seneca S, Smet J, Van Hecke R, Gerlo E, Devreese B, Van Beeumen J, Leroy JG, De Meirleir L, Lissens W. Homozygous gly555-to-glu mutation in the nuclear-encoded 70 kDa flavoprotein gene causes instability of the respiratory chain complex II. Am J Med Genet. 2003;120A:13–8.

Van Rahden VA, Rau I, Fuchs S, Kosyna FK, de Almeida HL Jr, et al. Clinical spectrum of females with HCCS mutation: from no clinical signs to a neonatal lethal form of the microphthalmia with linear skin defects (MLS) syndrome. Orphanet J Rare Dis. 2014;9:53.

Vilain C, Rens C, Aeby A, Balériaux D, Van Bogaert P, Remiche G, Smet J, Van Coster R, Abramowicz M. Pirson A novel NDUFV1 gene mutation in complex I deficiency in consanguineous siblings with brainstem lesions and Leigh syndrome. Clin Genet. 2012;82(3):264–70.

Vulto-van Silfhout AT, Hehir-Kwa JY, van Bon BW, Schuurs-Hoeijmakers JH, Meader S, et al. Clinical significance of de novo and inherited copy-number variation. Hum Mutat. 2013;34: 1679–87.

Wanschers BFJ, Szklarczyk R, van den Brand MAM, Jonckheere A, Suijskens J, Smeets R, Rodenburg RJ, Stephan K, Helland IB, Elkamil A, Rootwelt T, Ott M, van den Heuvel L, Nijtmans LG, Huynen MA. A mutation in the human CBP4 ortholog UQCC3 impairs complex III assembly, activity and cytochrome b stability. Hum Mol Genet. 2014;23:6356–65.

Wedatilake Y, Brown RM, McFarland R, Yaplito-Lee J, Morris AA, et al. SURF1 deficiency: a multi-centre natural history study. Orphanet J Rare Dis. 2013;8:96.

Weraarpachai W, Antonicka H, Sasarman F, Seeger J, Schrank B, et al. Mutation in TACO1, encoding a translational inactivator of COX I, results in cytochrome c oxidase deficiency and late-onset Leigh syndrome. Nat Genet. 2009;41:833–7.

Weraarpachai W, Sasarman F, Nishimura T, Antonicka H, Aure K, Rotig A, Lombes A, Shoubridge EA. Mutations in C12orf62, a factor that couples COX I synthesis with cytochrome c oxidase assembly, cause fatal neonatal lactic acidosis. Am J Hum Genet. 2012;90:142–51.

Wimplinger I, Morleo M, Rosenberger G, Iaconis D, et al. Mutations of the mitochondrial holocytochrome c-type synthase in X-linked dominant microphthalmia with linear skin defects syndrome. Am J Hum Genet. 2006;79:878–89.

Wimplinger I, Shaw GM, Kutsche K. HCCS loss-of-function missense mutation in a female with bilateral microphthalmia and sclerocornea: a novel gene for severe ocular malformations? Mol Vis. 2007;13:1475–82.

Wong L-JC, Dai P, Tan D, Lipson M, Grix A, Sifry-Platt M, Gropman A, Chen T-J. Severe lactic acidosis caused by a novel frame-shift

mutation in mitochondrial-encoded cytochrome c oxidase subunit II. Am J Med Genet. 2001;102:95–9.
Yoo DH, Choi YC, Nam DE, Choi SS, Kim JW, et al. Identification of FASTKD2 compound heterozygous mutations as the underlying cause of autosomal recessive MELAS-like syndrome. Mitochondrion. 2017;35:54–8.
Zafeiriou DI, Rodenburg RJ, Scheffer H, van den Heuvel LP, Pouwels PJ, Ververi A, Athanasiadou-Piperopoulou F, van der Knaap MS. MR spectroscopy and serial magnetic resonance imaging in a patient with mitochondrial cystic leukoencephalopathy due to complex I deficiency and NDUFV1 mutations and mild clinical course. Neuropediatrics. 2008;39(3): 172–5.
Zhu Z, Yao J, Johns T, Fu K, De Bie I, et al. SURF1, encoding a factor involved in the biogenesis of cytochrome c oxidase, is mutated in Leigh syndrome. Nat Genet. 1998;20:337–43.

# Disorders of Replication, Transcription and Translation of Mitochondrial DNA

# 45

Ian J. Holt, Antonella Spinazzola, Mirian C. H. Janssen, and Johannes N. Spelbrink

## Contents




I. J. Holt
Biodonostia Health Research Institute, San Sebastián, Spain

IKERBASQUE, Basque Foundation for Science, Bilbao, Spain

CIBERNED (Center for Networked Biomedical Research on Neurodegenerative Diseases, Ministry of Economy and Competitiveness, Institute Carlos III), Madrid, Spain
e-mail: ian.holt@biodonostia.org

A. Spinazzola
MRC Centre for Neuromuscular Diseases, UCL Queen Square Institute of Neurology and National Hospital for Neurology and Neurosurgery, Queen Square, London, UK

Department of Clinical and Movement Neurosciences, UCL Queen Square Institute of Neurology, Royal Free Campus, London, UK
e-mail: a.spinazzola@ucl.ac.uk

M. C. H. Janssen
Department of Internal Medicine, Radboud Center for Mitochondrial Medicine, Nijmegen, The Netherlands
e-mail: mirian.janssen@radboudumc.nl

J. N. Spelbrink (✉)
Department of Paediatrics, Radboud Center for Mitochondrial Medicine, Nijmegen, The Netherlands
e-mail: hans.spelbrink@radboudumc.nl



N. Blau et al. (eds.), *Physician's Guide to the Diagnosis, Treatment, and Follow-Up of Inherited Metabolic Diseases*,
https://doi.org/10.1007/978-3-030-67727-5_45

**Summary**

Mitochondria are cellular organelles essential for ATP production and for a variety of metabolic pathways. They contain many copies of a small circular genome, which codes for 13 essential components of oxidative phosphorylation system, oxidative phosphorylation system (OXPHOS) and the RNAs needed for their synthesis. This mitochondrial DNA (mtDNA) requires a unique and specialized gene expression system for its replication, transcription and translation involving 200–300 nuclear-encoded gene-products. Therefore, mitochondrial function depends on the integration of few critical mtDNA-encoded factors together with many nuclear factors. Owing to its limited coding capacity, disorders of mitochondrial gene expression typically affect one or more enzymes of the OXPHOS system, but because of the central role of energy metabolism, the wider metabolic functions of mitochondria and tissue specific metabolic wiring, these diseases present with, and progress to a plethora of clinical manifestations.

Mitochondrial disorders form one of the largest groups of metabolic disorders with a birth prevalence of at least one in 5000. Within this group, disorders of mtDNA replication, transcription and translation form the largest category in which the OXPHOS system is affected, and these can stem from mutations in either nuclear or mitochondrial DNA. The most severe cases are fatal and usually present at, or shortly after, birth and involve multiple organ systems, although tissue-specificity is often observed and in these cases the most affected organs are the brain, skeletal muscle, heart and liver.

Whole exome/genome sequencing (WES/WGS) has in the past decade greatly improved disease diagnosis. But, given the complexity of the mitochondrial genetics and biochemistry, data from clinical phenotype, family history, imaging and laboratory findings need to be integrated to guide the diagnosis, including the best strategy for downstream gene analysis (WES vs. a more restricted mtDNA sequence or gene panel based analysis) and its interpretation. Because with very few exceptions there are no cures or effective treatments, patient care chiefly involves symptom management and the provision of genetic counselling. For diagnosis and care, patients should wherever possible be referred to a specialized centre.

## Introduction

### The Mitochondrial Genome and OXPHOS

Human mitochondrial DNA (mtDNA) is a small circular molecule of 16,569 nucleotide pairs (Andrews et al., 1999). It encodes 13 critical components of the oxidative phosphorylation system (OXPHOS) that converts the energy stored in food into a usable form of cellular energy, ATP (see Chap. 44). Hence, defects that directly affect mtDNA or its maintenance or expression impair the OXPHOS system, thus restricting cellular energy production. The two strands of mtDNA are transcribed almost in their entirety and processed to yield 11 messenger, 22 transfer and two ribosomal RNAs (Ojala et al., 1981). The ribosomal RNAs and tRNA(Val) are assembled into mitoribosomes with some 80 nuclear-encoded proteins (Amunts et al., 2015). This apparatus translates the 11 mRNAs into 13 proteins with the aid of the mitochondrial transfer RNAs that are charged with amino acids by tRNA synthetases and a range of ancillary proteins. Thus, the protein parts of the mitochondrial protein synthesis machinery are nuclear encoded, whereas the RNA elements derive from mtDNA. Consequently, mitochondrial translation disorders can be of dual genetic origin.

In contrast to nuclear genes, each consisting of one maternal and one paternal allele, mtDNA is maternally inherited and present with hundreds to thousands of copies in the cell. Thus, family history can guide to a nuclear or mitochondrial origin of the disease. As for the primary mtDNA mutations, they usually affect some but not all the mtDNA molecules, a situation known as heteroplasmy (Holt et al., 1988). Most of the mutations are recessive, and thus the phenotype manifests only when the percentage of the mutant molecules is above a certain threshold, which carries both for the mutation and tissue affected. Moreover, the levels of heteroplasmy (or mutant/wt ratio's) can be highly variable even within the same family, in part because a genetic bottleneck during germline development resets the ratio, and further segregation can occur throughout life. Although variation in heteroplasmy undoubtedly accounts for some of the considerable variation in disease penetrance, severity and progression, there are equally diverse clinical outcomes in diseases resulting from defects in nuclear-encoded factors required for mtDNA maintenance and expression, despite them following simple Mendelian rules.

## Replication of Mitochondrial DNA

There is considerable debate about the mechanisms of mtDNA replication (Pohjoismaki et al., 2018), yet overall agreement about the role of many of the proteins required for this process. These include a number of important disease genes, such as the mitochondrial DNA polymerase (POLG) and helicase (Twinkle) that were discovered almost 20 years ago (Van Goethem et al., 2001; Spelbrink et al., 2001). The mutant proteins often cause replication to stall or slow replication, which can result in multiple deleted molecules that accumulate over time or loss of mtDNA in the most severe cases. New defects of mtDNA replication continue to come to light with an RNA processing enzyme (RNASEH1) (Bugiardini et al., 2017) and a DNA topology-modifying enzyme (TOP3A) (Martin et al., 2018) being two of the most recent. Clinically, defects in mtDNA replication proteins produce features characteristic of mitochondrial disorders and overlap with those resulting from primary mtDNA mutations. Whilst the mitochondria share a number of DNA repair proteins with the nucleus, to date none of these have been unequivocally linked to mitochondrial disease.

## Nucleotide Metabolism

Deoxynucleotide triphosphates (dNTPs) are the building blocks of DNA. All four (A, G, C and T) are required to be in a sufficient amount and appropriately balanced, as either a surplus or a deficiency of nucleotide precursors is detrimental to mtDNA integrity, and thus can cause disease. Both anabolic and catabolic enzymes participate in the maintenance of the mitochondrial dNTP pools, and these are localized in mitochondria as well as in the cytosol. The first enzyme deficiency of this class found to cause mitochondrial disease was the catabolic and cytosolic enzyme thymidine phosphorylase (TP) (Nishino et al., 1999). Loss-of function of TP greatly increases plasma levels of thymidine and deoxyuridine resulting in high dTTP levels, depression of mitochondrial dCTP levels and mtDNA deletions and depletion. Other diseases were later associated with impaired nucleotide homeostasis, including defects in the mitochondrial salvage pathways enzymes, deoxyguanosine kinase and thymidine kinase and a component of the cytosolic ribonucleotide reductase, p53r2, which supports the de novo synthesis of deoxynucleotides in non-dividing cells. Complicating matters, deoxynucleotide homeostatic disorders are not restricted to anabolic and catabolic enzymes. The mitochondrial inner membrane protein MPV17 is thought to function as some sort of channel, and MPV17 deficiency disturbs mitochondrial dNTP levels, especially guanosine (Dalla Rosa et al., 2016). Similarly, mitochondrial nucleotide transporters are another potential cause of mtDNA disorders, although the only one identified to date is the ATP/ADP carrier, ANT1. Clinically and biochemically, the end points are similar in that MPV17 deficiency closely resembles defects in the guanine salvage pathway enzyme, DGUOK. Importantly, defects in the genes that impact dNTP levels can cause either mtDNA depletion or multiple deletions, with the former associated with severe tissue-specific infantile forms, whereas the latter results in milder and adult-onset phenotypes.

## Transcription and RNA Processing

Mitochondrial transcription involves a core machinery of four factors, the RNA polymerase, POLRMT, two transcription factors, TFAM and TFB2M and an elongation factor, TEFM. Both strands of mtDNA are transcribed almost in their entirety to yield two polycistronic transcripts in which the rRNAs and most of the protein-coding RNAs are flanked by tRNAs. This gene organization enables two enzymes that cut either side of the tRNA genes, RNase P and RNase Z, to process the polycistronic RNAs to individual tRNAs, mRNAs and rRNAs. Several conserved rRNA nucleotides are further modified by a number of enzymes (mostly RNA methyltranferases), prior or concurrent with assembly of the mitoribosome and mt-tRNA(Val), in a complex process of marrying scores of proteins with RNAs containing intricate and extensive secondary structure requiring a number of assembly factors (approximately 15 are currently known) (D'Souza & Minczuk, 2018). tRNAs are also heavily modified at conserved positions by various enzymes, and undergo CCA addition at their 3'-end by the CCA-adding tRNA-nucleotidyltransferase (TRNT1). The nine monocistronic and two bicistronic mRNAs, both rRNAs and mt-tRNAs can be oligo- or polyadenylated (for further details see Fig. 45.1). Polyadenylation is mediated principally by polyA polymerase and this enzyme is one of the few factors in this category to have been identified as a ′disease gene′.

## Translation

In striking contrast to transcription and RNA processing, defects in genes contributing to mitochondrial protein synthesis form the largest class of mitochondrial diseases. All of the 22 tRNA genes in the mtDNA have been linked to disease. The tRNALeu(UUR) gene alone has 12 assigned pathological variants, one of which (m.3243G) is the most frequent type of mtDNA disorder. The m.3243G point mutation produces a wide range of signs and symptoms, including two quite distinct clinical syndromes (de Laat et al., 2012; van den Ouweland et al., 1994; Goto et al., 1990). Collectively, mutations in the amino-acyl-tRNA synthetase genes (whose protein products add the appropriate amino acid to the tRNAs) are another substantial cause of mitochondrial disease, that often manifest as fatal infantile forms (Gonzalez-Serrano et al., 2019). Pathological variants in mitochondrial translation activators, recycling and elongation factors have also been identified and characterized in some detail. Mutations in the structural components of the mitoribosome are relatively rare, with only about 10% of its constituent proteins having so far been linked to disease. Likewise, defects in the mitochondrial ribosomal RNAs are an extremely rare cause of disease. An important exception is the m.1555G variant that in most cases is benign, but carriers are susceptible to antibiotic induced hearing loss, because of the strong homology between mitochondrial and bacterial ribosomes.

## Clinical Signs and Symptoms

Disorders of replication, transcription and translation of mtDNA can be of dual genetic origin, being caused either by maternally inherited mtDNA mutations or nuclear gene mutations that follow Mendelian rules. They all ultimately affect the production or quality of the 13 proteins encoded by mtDNA and that are essential for OXPHOS. Disease symptoms for all the disorders described in this chapter and Chap. 44 (oxidative phosphorylation disorders) therefore have many common denominators and often overlap. Nonetheless, and as a general rule for mitochondrial OXPHOS disorders, the clinical presentations are highly variable, ranging from very severe neonatal disease that is progressive and rapidly results in a fatal multisystem failure, to the onset of relatively mild muscle disease (e.g. ptosis and CPEO) in late adulthood. The wide spectrum of symptoms and severity in subjects with mtDNA mutants is partly explained by heteroplasmy (differences in the proportion of mutant and normal mtDNA) varying across tissues and with time. However, similar clinical variation and disease progression is also seen in secondary mtDNA disorders caused by defects in nuclear genes, such as Twinkle, p53R2 and Mpv17, because they too compromise mtDNA integrity. Whatever the causal mutations, disease penetrance, development and prognosis also can be influenced by environmental factors and additional gene modifiers, including common mtDNA variants that define different haplogroups.

Nuclear gene mutations, even when they occur in what could be considered the same pathway, show a diverse spectrum of disease manifestation. For example, defective mitochondrial aminoacyl-tRNA synthetases often result in encephalopathy, but in some cases specifically affect the kidney or the heart (Goto et al., 1990). In addition, different mutations in the same gene can cause distinct syndromes. In part these are explained by different modes of inheritance, mutation position and severity, etc., but the variable tissue involvement is not always straightforward to explain. For example, autosomal dominant mutations in the mtDNA helicase Twinkle typically cause a relatively mild late-onset muscular phenotype with progressive external ophthalmoplegia, ptosis and the accumulation of multiple mtDNA deletions in muscle as distinguishing features. Recessive mutations can cause a severe early-onset disease with liver mtDNA depletion, or a less severe mtDNA depletion syndrome largely restricted to the brain. Lastly, different recessive Twinkle mutations have been described in Perrault syndrome with neurological involvement. This may reflect Twinkle (and many other proteins) having multiple functions (e.g. (Hensen et al., 2019)), which highlights the need to carry out further detailed functional studies.

Thus, disorders of mtDNA maintenance and expression, like other mitochondrial diseases can result in a highly variable spectrum of symptoms and organ/tissue involvement. The organs requiring the most energy, such as the brain, heart, skeletal muscle, senses and endocrine systems are most commonly and severely affected, and show a progressive decline in function. Mitochondrial disease should therefore be suspected in patients with progressive multisystem involvement. Signs and symptoms where mitochondrial disorders should be first and foremost considered during differential diagnosis include combinations of encephalopathy and hepatopathy, myoclonic epilepsy, developmental regression, stroke-like episodes, ophthalmoplegia and ptosis, optic nerve atrophy, retinal degeneration, early onset hearing loss and ataxia.

In many patients, diagnosis cannot be made on clinical signs and symptoms alone. A more structured approach is needed, including blood and/or cerebrospinal fluid (CSF) lactate, pyruvate and alanine concentrations, neuroimaging, cardiac evaluation and muscle biopsy for histological and histochemical evidence of mitochondrial disease, biochemistry and molecular genetic testing. Family history is often important, especially when a pedigree is sufficiently extensive to indicate maternal inheritance, as this is the identifier of a primary mtDNA mutation. In any case, the investigation of most suspected mitochondrial disorders begins with screening the mtDNA as it is so small; however, increasingly whole genome/exome sequencing is being performed in parallel as costs continue to fall. In this case it is important to take into account that maternal relatives can again present with highly variable phenotypes due to variable heteroplasmy and disease indicators can skip a generation.

## Genotypic Confirmation of Mitochondrial Disorders

Some of the disorders presented in this chapter have characteristic clinical and biochemical phenotypes that should inform genotyping (see diagnostic flow diagram, Fig. 45.2). For example, the tRNA(Lys) 8344A>G mtDNA mutation is almost invariably associated with myoclonic epilepsy with ragged red fibers (MERRF). Likewise, patients presenting with mitochondrial neurogastrointestinal encephalopathy (MNGIE) most often have a mutation in the thymidine phosphorylase gene (TYMP). Nevertheless, as set out in the nomenclature table and discussed earlier in the introduction, different gene mutations in nuclear or mitochondrial DNA can produce similar symptoms. Since the costs of whole mitochondrial genome and whole exome/genome sequencing (WES/WGS) have fallen dramatically in recent years it is frequently cost effective to take this approach, rather than targeted gene sequencing, especially if the symptoms are compatible with many forms of mitochondrial disease. The small size of the mitochondrial genome means determining its sequence and integrity is an almost universal starting point for suspected mitochondrial diseases, particularly if the family history is compatible with maternal inheritance. Some specialist centres have developed PCR/sequencing arrays that screen the mitochondrial genome and around 100 nuclear genes linked to mitochondrial disorders, which provides an intermediate between sequencing one or a few targeted genes and WES/WGS and should have a lower false negative rate than the latter.

## Nomenclature

| No. | Disorder | Alternative name | Abbreviation | Gene symbol | Chromosomal localisation | Inheritance | Affected protein | OMIM No. |
|---|---|---|---|---|---|---|---|---|
| 45.1 | Mitochondrial depletion syndrome 4A | Alpers-Huttenlocher syndrome | MTDPS4A | *POLG* | 15q26.1 | AR | Polymerase gamma | 203700 |
| 45.2 | Mitochondrial depletion syndrome 4B | MNGIE, POLG-related | MTDPS4B | *POLG* | 15q26.1 | AR | Polymerase gamma | 613662 |
| 45.3 | Sensory ataxic neuropathy, dysarthria and ophthalmoparesis | Sensory ataxic neuropathy with mitochondrial DNA deletions | SANDO | *POLG* | 15q26.1 | AR | Polymerase gamma | 607459 |
| 45.4 | Progressive external ophthalmoplegia 1 | | PEOA1; PEOB1 | *POLG* | 15q26.1 | AD, AR | Polymerase gamma | 157640; 258450 |
| 45.5 | Progressive external ophthalmoplegia with mitochondrial DNA deletions, autosomal dominant 4 | adPEO with mitochondrial DNA deletions type 4 | PEOA4 | *POLG2* | 17q23.3 | AD | DNA polymerase gamma 2, accessory subunit | 610131 |
| 45.6 | Mitochondrial depletion syndrome 3 | Progressive external ophthalmoplegia with mitochondrial DNA deletions, autosomal recessive 4 | MTDPS3; PEOB4 | *DGUOK* | 2p13.1 | AR | Deoxyguanosine kinase | 251880; 617070 |
| 45.7 | Mitochondrial DNA depletion syndrome type 6 | MPV17 deficiency | MTDPS6 | *MPV17* | 2p23.3 | AR | MPV17 | 256810 |
| 45.8 | Progressive external ophthalmoplegia with mitochondrial DNA deletions, autosomal dominant 3 | TWINKLE mitochondrial DNA helicase deficiency | PEOA3 | *TWNK* | 10q24.31 | AD | Twinkle mtDNA helicase | 609286 |
| 45.9 | Mitochondrial DNA depletion syndrome type 7 | TWINKLE mitochondrial DNA helicase deficiency | MTDPS7 | *TWNK* | 10q24.31 | AR | Twinkle mtDNA helicase | 271245 |
| 45.10 | Perrault syndrome 5 | TWINKLE mitochondrial DNA helicase deficiency | PRLTS5 | *TWNK* | 10q24.31 | AR | Twinkle mtDNA helicase | 616138 |
| 45.11 | Mitochondrial depletion syndrome 2 | Progressive external ophthalmoplegia with mitochondrial DNA deletions, autosomal recessive 3 | MTDPS2; PEOB3 | *TK2* | 16q21 | AR | Mitochondrial thymidine kinase (TK2) | 617068; 609560 |
| 45.12 | Mitochondrial ribonucleotide reductase small subunit deficiency | Mitochondrial DNA depletion syndrome 8A & 8B | MTDPS8A; MTDPS8B | *RRM2B* | 8q22.3 | AR | Ribonucleotide reductase small subunit 2-like | 612075 |
| 45.13 | Mitochondrial depletion syndrome 1 | Mitochondrial neurogastrointestinal encephalopathy syndrome (MNGIE) | MTDPS1, MNGIE | *TYMP* | 22q13.32-qter | AR | Thymidine phosphorylase | 131222; 603041 |
| 45.14 | Progressive external ophthalmoplegia with mitochondrial DNA deletions, autosomal dominant 6 | DNA2 deficiency | PEOA6 | *DNA2* | 10q21.3 | AD | DNA replication helicase 2 | 615156 |
| 45.15 | Progressive external ophthalmoplegia with mitochondrial DNA deletions, autosomal recessive 2 | RNASEH1 defect | PEOB2 | *RNASEH1* | 2p25.3 | AR | Ribonuclease H1 | 616479 |
| 45.16 | Mitochondrial DNA depletion syndrome 11 | MGME1 deficiency | MTDPS11 | *MGME1* | 20p11.23 | AR | Mitochondrial genome maintenance exonuclease 1 | 615076 |
| 45.17 | Mitochondrial depletion syndrome 13 | FBXL4 deficiency | MTDPS13 | *FBXL4* | 6q16.1-q16.2 | AR | F-box and leucine-rich repeat protein 4 | 615471 |

(continued)

| No. | Disorder | Alternative name | Abbreviation | Gene symbol | Chromosomal localisation | Inheritance | Affected protein | OMIM No. |
|---|---|---|---|---|---|---|---|---|
| 45.18 | Progressive external ophthalmoplegia with mitochondrial DNA deletions, autosomal recessive 5 | | PEOB5 | *TOP3A* | 17p11.2 | AR | Topoisomerase 3α | 618098 |
| 45.19 | Mitochondrial depletion syndrome 5 | ATP-specific succinyl-CoA ligase β subunit deficiency | MTDPS5 | *SUCLA2* | 13q14.2 | AR | ATP-specific succinyl-CoA ligase β subunit | 603921 |
| 45.20 | Mitochondrial depletion syndrome 9 | Encephalomyopathic type with methylmalonic aciduria | MTDPS9 | *SUCLG1* | 2p11.2 | AR | GTP-specific succinyl-CoA ligase α subunit | 245400 |
| 45.21 | Progressive external ophthalmoplegia with mitochondrial DNA deletions, autosomal dominant 2 | | PEOA2 | *SLC25A4* | 4q35.1 | AD | Adenine nucleotide translocator 1 | 609283 |
| 45.22 | Mitochondrial DNA depletion syndrome type 12A (cardiomyopathic type) | | MTDPS12A | *SLC25A4* | 4q35.1 | AD | Adenine nucleotide translocator 1 | 617184 |
| 45.23 | Mitochondrial DNA depletion syndrome type 12B (cardiomyopathic type) | | MTDPS12B | *SLC25A4* | 4q35.1 | AR | Adenine nucleotide translocator 1 | 615418 |
| 45.24 | Mitochondrial RNA import protein deficiency | Combined oxidative phosphorylation deficiency type 13 | COXPD13 | *PNPT1* | 2p16.1 | AR | Polyribonucleotide nucleotidyltransferase 1 | 614932; 614934 |
| 45.25 | Combined oxidative phosphorylation deficiency 30 | Ribonuclease P 5′ tRNA processing enzyme deficiency | COXPD30 | *TRMT10C* | 3q12.3 | AR | RNA methyltransferase 10 | 616974 |
| 45.26 | Combined oxidative phosphorylation deficiency 17 | Ribonuclease Z 3′ tRNA processing enzyme deficiency | COXPD17 | *ELAC2* | 17p12 | AR | Long form of RNase Z | 615440 |
| 45.27 | Mitochondrial DNA depletion syndrome-15 | Mitochondrial transcription factor A deficiency | MTDPS15 | *TFAM* | 10q21.1 | AR | Mitochondrial transcription factor A | 617156 |
| 45.29 | Spastic ataxia 4, autosomal recessive | Mitochondrial poly(A) polymerase deficiency | SPAX4 | *MTPAP* | 10p11.23 | AR | Mitochondrial poly(A) polymerase | 613672 |
| 45.30 | CCA-adding tRNA-nucleotidyltransferase deficiency | Retinitis pigmentosa and erythrocytic microcytosis | – | *TRNT1* | 3p26.2 | AR | CCA-adding tRNA-nucleotidyltransferase | 616959; 616084 |
| 45.31 | Combined oxidative phosphorylation deficiency 15 | Mitochondrial methionyl-tRNA formyltransferase deficiency | COXPD15 | *MTFMT* | 15q22.31 | AR | Methionyl-tRNA formyltransferase | 614947 |
| 45.32 | tRNA 5-taurinomethyluridine modifier deficiency | Combined oxidative phosphorylation deficiency type 23 | COXPD23 | *GTPBP3* | 19p13.11 | AR | GTP-binding protein 3 | 616198 |
| 45.33 | tRNA 5-carboxymethylaminomethyl transferase deficiency | Combined oxidative phosphorylation deficiency type 10 | COXPD10 | *MTO1* | 6q13 | AR | Mitochondrial translation optimization 1 | 614702 |
| 45.34 | Myopathy lactic acidosis and sideroblastic anaemia | Pseudouridine synthase 1 deficiency | MLASA1 | *PUS1* | 12q24.33 | AR | Pseudouridine synthase 1 | 600462 |
| 45.35 | tRNA isopentenyl transferase deficiency | Combined oxidative phosphorylation deficiency 35 | COXPD35 | *TRIT1* | 1p34.2 | AR | tRNA isopentenyl transferase 1 | 617873 |
| 45.36 | tRNA methyltransferase 5 deficiency | Combined oxidative phosphorylation deficiency type 26 | COXPD26 | *TRMT5* | 14q23.1 | AR | tRNA methyltransferase 5 | 616539 |

| No. | Disorder | Alternative name | Abbreviation | Gene symbol | Chromosomal localisation | Inheritance | Affected protein | OMIM No. |
|---|---|---|---|---|---|---|---|---|
| 45.37 | Acute infantile liver failure | | | *TRMU* | 22q13 | AR | tRNA 5-methylaminomethyl-2-thiouridylate methyltransferase | 613070 |
| 45.38 | Mitochondrial RNA-processing endoribonuclease deficiency | Cartilage-hair hypoplasia | CHH | *RMRP* | 9p13.3 | AR | RNA component of mitochondrial RNA-processing endoribonuclease | 250250 |
| 45.39 | HSD10 mitochondrial disease | 17-beta-hydroxysteroid dehydrogenase type 10 deficiency | HSD10MD | *HSD17B10* | Xp11.2 | AR | 17-beta-hydroxysteroid dehydrogenase type 10 | 300438 |
| 45.40 | Mitochondrial ribosomal large subunit 3 deficiency | Combined oxidative phosphorylation deficiency type 9 | COXPD9 | *MRPL3* | 3q22.1 | AR | Mitochondrial ribosomal protein L3 | 614582 |
| 45.41 | Mitochondrial ribosomal large subunit 12 deficiency | | | *MRPL12* | 17q25.3 | AR | Mitochondrial ribosomal protein L12 | 602375 |
| 45.42 | Mitochondrial ribosomal large subunit 44 deficiency | Combined oxidative phosphorylation deficiency type 16 | COXPD16 | *MRPL44* | 2q36.1 | AR | Mitochondrial ribosomal protein L44 | 615395 |
| 45.43 | Combined oxidative phosphorylation deficiency 36 | Mitochondrial ribosomal small subunit 2 deficiency | COXPD36 | *MRPS2* | 9q34.3 | AR | Mitochondrial ribosomal protein S2 | 617950 |
| 45.44 | Combined oxidative phosphorylation deficiency 34 | Mitochondrial ribosomal small subunit 7 deficiency | COXPD34 | *MRPS7* | 17q25.1 | AR | Mitochondrial ribosomal protein S7 | 617872 |
| 45.45 | Combined oxidative phosphorylation defect 2 | Corpus callosum agenesis with dysmorphism and fatal lactic acidosis | COXPD2 | *MRPS16* | 10q22.1 | AR | Mitochondrial ribosomal protein S16 | 610498 |
| 45.46 | Combined oxidative phosphorylation defect 5 | | COXPD5 | *MRPS22* | 3q23 | AR | Mitochondrial ribosomal protein S22 | 611719 |
| No S&S* | Mitochondrial ribosomal small subunit 23 deficiency | | | *MRPS23* | 17q22 | AR | Mitochondrial ribosomal protein S23 | 611985 |
| 45.47 | Combined oxidative phosphorylation deficiency type 32 | Mitochondrial ribosomal small subunit 34 deficiency | COXPD32 | *MRPS34* | 16p13.3 | AR | Mitochondrial ribosomal protein S34 | 617664 |
| 45.48 | Mitochondrial ribosomal RNA 12S deficiency | Aminoglycoside-induced and nonsyndromic hearing loss | | *MTRNR1* | m.648–1601 | Maternal | n.a. | 561000 |
| 45.49 | Combined oxidative phosphorylation deficiency 11 | Infantile encephaloneuromyopathy due to mitochondrial translation defect | COXPD11 | *RMND1* | 6q25.1 | AR | Required for meiotic nuclear division 1 homolog | 614922 |
| 45.50 | Combined oxidative phosphorylation defect 1 | Early fatal progressive hepatoencephalopathy | COXPD1 | *GFM1* | 3q25.1-q26.2 | AR | Elongation factor G1 (EFG1) | 609060 |
| 45.51 | Mitochondrial elongation factor G2 deficiency (unconfirmed) | Putative Leigh-like syndrome | | *GFM2* | 5q13.3 | AR | Mitochondrial elongation factor G2 | 606544 |
| 45.52 | Combined oxidative phosphorylation defect 3 | Encephalomyopathy, respiratory failure and lactic acidosis | COXPD3 | *TSFM* | 12q14.1 | AR | Mitochondrial elongation factor Ts | 610505 |
| 45.53 | Combined oxidative phosphorylation defect 4 | Mitochondrial elongation factor Tu deficiency | COXPD4 | *TUFM* | 16p11.2 | AR | Mitochondrial elongation factor Tu | 610678 |

(continued)

| No. | Disorder | Alternative name | Abbreviation | Gene symbol | Chromosomal localisation | Inheritance | Affected protein | OMIM No. |
|---|---|---|---|---|---|---|---|---|
| 45.54 | Combined oxidative phosphorylation defect 7; spastic paraplegia 55 | C12orf65 release factor deficiency | COXPD7; SPG55 | *C12ORF65* | 12q24.31 | AR | C12orf65 release factor | 613559; 615035 |
| No S&S** | Myotonic dystrophy-like myopathy | | | *MT-TA* | m.5650G>A | Maternal | n.a. | 590000 |
| | Mitochondrial myopathy | | | *MT-TA* | m.5591G>A | Maternal | n.a. | 590000 |
| | Mitochondrial encephalomyopathy | | | *MT-TR* | m.10438A>G, m.10450A>G | Maternal | n.a. | 590005 |
| | Ophthalmoplegia | | | *MT-TN* | m.5703G>A, m.5692A>G | Maternal | n.a. | 590010 |
| | Combined CI/CIV deficiency | | | *MT-TN* | m.5728A>G | Maternal | n.a. | 590010 |
| | Chronic tubulointerstitial nephropathy | | | *MT-TN* | m.5656A>G | Maternal | n.a. | 590010 |
| | Mitochondrial myopathy | | | *MT-TD* | m.7526A>G | Maternal | n.a. | 590015 |
| | MELAS-like | | | *MT-TC* | m.5814A>G | Maternal | n.a. | 590020 |
| | Mitochondrial dystonia | | | *MT-TC* | m.5816A>G | Maternal | n.a. | 590020 |
| | Mitochondrial myopathy with diabetes mellitus | | | *MT-TE* | m.14709T>C | Maternal | n.a. | 590025 |
| | Transient infantile mitochondrial myopathy | | | *MT-TE* | m.14674T>C, m.14674T>G | Maternal | n.a. | 590025 |
| | Diabetes and deafness | | | *MT-TE* | m.14692A>G | Maternal | n.a. | 590025 |
| | Mitochondrial myopathy | | | *MT-TQ* | m.ins4366A | Maternal | n.a. | 590030 |
| | Sensorineural deafness and migraine | | | *MT-TQ* | m.4336A>G | Maternal | n.a. | 590030 |
| | MELAS-like | | | *MT-TQ* | m.m4332G>A | Maternal | n.a. | 590030 |
| | Hypertrophic cardiomyopathy | | | *MT-TG* | m.9997T>C | Maternal | n.a. | 590035 |
| | Exercise intolerance | | | *MT-TG* | m.10010T>C | Maternal | n.a. | 590035 |
| | Sudden death | | | *MT-TG* | m.10044A>G | Maternal | n.a. | 590035 |
| | Dilated cardiomyopathy | | | *MT-TH* | m.12192G>A | Maternal | n.a. | 590040 |
| | Pigmentary retinopathy and sensorineural deafness | | | *MT-TH* | m.12183G>A | Maternal | n.a. | 590040 |
| | MERRF/MELAS overlap syndrome | | | *MT-TH* | m.12147G>A | Maternal | n.a. | 590040 |
| | Sensorineural deafness | | | *MT-TH* | m.12201T>C | Maternal | n.a. | 590040 |
| | Fatal cardiomyopathy | | | *MT-TI* | m.4317A>G, m.4269A>G | Maternal | n.a. | 590045 |
| | Hypertrophic cardiomyopathy and sensorineural deafness | | | *MT-TI* | m.4295A>G | Maternal | n.a. | 590045 |
| | Hypertrophic cardiomyopathy | | | *MT-TI* | m.4300A>G | Maternal | n.a. | 590045 |
| | Multisystem disorder | | | *MT-TI* | m.4284G>A | Maternal | n.a. | 590045 |
| | Progressive necrotizing encephalopathy | | | *MT-TI* | m.4290T>C | Maternal | n.a. | 590045 |
| | Hypertension, hypercholesterolemiaand hypomagnesimia | | | *MT-TI* | m.4291T>C | Maternal | n.a. | 590045 |
| 45.55 | MELAS syndrome | | | *MT-TL1* | m.3243A>G, m.3271T>C | Maternal | n.a. | 590050 |

| No. | Disorder | Alternative name | Abbreviation | Gene symbol | Chromosomal localisation | Inheritance | Affected protein | OMIM No. |
|---|---|---|---|---|---|---|---|---|
| No S&S** | MERRF-like | | | *MT-TL1* | m.3256C>T | Maternal | n.a. | 590050 |
| | Cardiomyopathy and myopathy | | | *MT-TL1* | m.3303C>T, m.3260A>G | Maternal | n.a. | 590050 |
| | Mitochondrial encephalomyopathy | | | *MT-TL1* | m.3252T>C | Maternal | n.a. | 590050 |
| | Progressive external ophthalmoplegia, proximal myopathy and sudden death | | | *MT-TL1* | m.3251A>G | Maternal | n.a. | 590050 |
| | Mitochondrial myopathy | | | *MT-TL1* | m.3250T>C | Maternal | n.a. | 590050 |
| | Sudden infant death syndrome | | | *MT-TL1* | m.3290T>C | Maternal | n.a. | 590050 |
| | Kearns-Sayre like syndrome | | | *MT-TL1* | m.3249G>A | Maternal | n.a. | 590050 |
| | Myelodysplastic syndrome | | | *MT-TL1* | m.3242G>A | Maternal | n.a. | 590050 |
| | Mitochondrial encephalomyopathy | | | *MT-TL2* | m.12315G>A | Maternal | n.a. | 590055 |
| | Mitochondrial myopathy | | | *MT-TL2* | m.12320A>G | Maternal | n.a. | 590055 |
| | Mitochondrial cardiomyopathy | | | *MT-TL2* | m.12297T>C | Maternal | n.a. | 590055 |
| 45.56 | MERRF syndrome | | | *MT-TK* | m.8344A>G, m.8361G>A | Maternal | n.a. | 590060 |
| No S&S** | MERRF/MELAS overlap syndrome | | | *MT-TK* | m.8356T>C | Maternal | n.a. | 590060 |
| | Cardiomyopathy and deafness | | | *MT-TK* | m.8363G>A | Maternal | n.a. | 590060 |
| | Mitochondrial neurogastrointestinal encephalomyopathy syndrome | MNGIE syndrome | | *MT-TK* | m.8313G>A | Maternal | n.a. | 590060 |
| | Diabetes and deafness | | | *MT-TK* | m.8296A>G | Maternal | n.a. | 590060 |
| | Progressive external ophthalmoplegia with myoclonus | | | *MT-TK* | m.8342G>A | Maternal | n.a. | 590060 |
| | Mitochondrial myopathy | | | *MT-TM* | m.4409T>C | Maternal | n.a. | 590065 |
| | MELAS-like syndrome | | | *MT-TF* | m.583G>A | Maternal | n.a. | 590070 |
| | MERRF-like syndrome | | | *MT-TF* | m.611G>A | Maternal | n.a. | 590070 |
| | Late onset mitochondrial myopathy | | | *MT-TF* | m.622G>A | Maternal | n.a. | 590070 |
| | Mitochondrial epilepsy | | | *MT-TF* | m.616T>C, m.616T>G | Maternal | n.a. | 590070 |
| | Mitochondrial encephalopathy | | | *MT-TF* | m.586G>A | Maternal | n.a. | 590070 |
| | Tubulointerstitial nephropathy | | | *MT-TF* | m.608A>G | Maternal | n.a. | 590070 |
| | Mitochondrial myopathy | | | *MT-TP* | m.15990G>A | Maternal | n.a. | 590075 |
| | Parkinson disease | | | *MT-TP* | m.15965T>C | Maternal | n.a. | 590075 |
| | MERRF-like syndrome | | | *MT-TP* | m.15967G>A | Maternal | n.a. | 590075 |
| | MERRF/MELAS overlap syndrome | | | *MT-TS1* | m.7512T>C | Maternal | n.a. | 590080 |
| | Palmoplantar keratoderma with deafness | | | *MT-TS1* | m.7445A>G | Maternal | n.a. | 590080 |
| | Mitochondrial cytochrome *c* oxidase deficiency with sensorineural deafness | | | *MT-TS1* | m.ins7472C | Maternal | n.a. | 590080 |
| | Mitochondrial sensorineural deafness | | | *MT-TS1* | m.7510T>C, m.7511T>C, m.7445A>C, m.7505T>C | Maternal | n.a. | 590080 |

(continued)

| No. | Disorder | Alternative name | Abbreviation | Gene symbol | Chromosomal localisation | Inheritance | Affected protein | OMIM No. |
|---|---|---|---|---|---|---|---|---|
| | Aminoglycoside-induced deafness | | | *MT-TS1* | m.7444G>A | Maternal | n.a. | 590080 |
| | Exercise intolerance, muscle pain and lactic acidemia | | | *MT-TS1* | m.7497G>A | Maternal | n.a. | 590080 |
| | Cerebellar ataxia, cataract and diabetes mellitus | | | *MT-TS2* | m.12258C>A | Maternal | n.a. | 590085 |
| | MERRF/MELAS overlap syndrome | | | *MT-TS2* | m.12207G>A | Maternal | n.a. | 590085 |
| | Parkinson disease | | | *MT-TT* | m.15950G>A | Maternal | n.a. | 590090 |
| | Mitochondrial encephalopathy | | | *MT-TW* | m.5549G>A, m.ins5537T | Maternal | n.a. | 590095 |
| | Mitochondrial myopathy | | | *MT-TW* | m.5521G>A | Maternal | n.a. | 590095 |
| | Mitochondrial neurogastrointestinal syndrome | | | *MT-TW* | m.5532G>A | Maternal | n.a. | 590095 |
| | Mitochondrial encephalocardiomyopathy | | | *MT-TW* | m.5545C>T | Maternal | n.a. | 590095 |
| | Mitochondrial encephalomyopathy | | | *MT-TW* | m.5556G>A | Maternal | n.a. | 590095 |
| | Exercise intolerance and complex III deficiency | | | *MT-TY* | m.5874A>G | Maternal | n.a. | 590100 |
| | Chronic progressive external ophthalmoplegia with myopathy | | | *MT-TY* | m.del5885T, m.5877G>A | Maternal | n.a. | 590100 |
| | Focal segmental glomerulosclerosis and dilated cardiomyopathy | | | *MT-TY* | m.5843A>G | Maternal | n.a. | 590100 |
| | Ataxia, progressive seizures, mental deterioration and hearing loss | | | *MT-TV* | m.1606A>G | Maternal | n.a. | 590105 |
| | Neonatal death and Leigh syndrome | | | *MT-TV* | m.1624C>T | Maternal | n.a. | 590105 |
| 45.57 | Combined oxidative phosphorylation deficiency type 8 | Mitochondrial alanyl-tRNA synthetase deficiency | COXPD8 | *AARS2* | 6p21.1 | AR | Alanyl-tRNA synthetase 2 | 614096; 615889 |
| 45.58 | Pontocerebellar hypoplasia, type 6 | Mitochondrial arginyl-tRNA synthetase deficiency | PCH6 | *RARS2* | 6q15 | AR | Arginyl-tRNA synthetase 2 | 611523 |
| 45.59 | Combined oxidative phosphorylation deficiency 24 | Mitochondrial asparaginyl-tRNA synthetase deficiency | COXPD24 | *NARS2* | 11q14.1 | AR | Asparaginyl-tRNA synthetase 2 | 616239 |
| 45.60 | Leukoencephalopathy with brainstem and spinal cord involvement and lactate elevation | Mitochondrial aspartyl-tRNA synthetase deficiency | LBSL | *DARS2* | 1q25.1 | AR | Aspartyl-tRNA synthetase 2 | 611105 |
| 45.61 | Combined oxidative phosphorylation deficiency 27 | Mitochondrial cysteinyl-tRNA synthetase deficiency | COXPD27 | *CARS2* | 13q34 | AR | Cysteinyl-tRNA synthetase 2 | 616672 |
| 45.62 | Combined oxidative phosphorylation deficiency 12 | Mitochondrial glutamyl-tRNA synthetase deficiency | COXPD12 | *EARS2* | 16p12.2 | AR | Glutamyl-tRNA synthetase 2 | 614924 |
| 45.63 | Mitochondrial glutamyl-tRNA(Gln) amidotransferase subunit A deficiency | | | *QRSL1* | 6q21 | AR | Glutaminyl-tRNA synthase (glutamine-hydrolyzing)-like protein 1 | 617209 |
| 45.64 | Mitochondrial glutamyl-tRNA(Gln) amidotransferase subunit B deficiency | | | *GATB* | 4q31.3 | AR | Glutamyl-tRNA amidotransferase, subunit B | 603645 |

| No. | Disorder | Alternative name | Abbreviation | Gene symbol | Chromosomal localisation | Inheritance | Affected protein | OMIM No. |
|---|---|---|---|---|---|---|---|---|
| 45.65 | Mitochondrial glutamyl-tRNA(Gln) amidotransferase subunit C deficiency | | | *GATC* | 12q24.31 | AR | Glutamyl-tRNA amidotransferase, subunit C | 617210 |
| 45.66 | Perrault syndrome type 2 | Mitochondrial histidyl-tRNA synthetase deficiency | PRLTS2 | *HARS2* | 5q31.3 | AR | Histidyl-tRNA synthetase 2 | 614926 |
| 45.67 | Cataracts, growth hormone deficiency, sensory neuropathy, sensorineural hearing loss, and skeletal dysplasia | Mitochondrial isoleucyl-tRNA synthetase deficiency | CAGSSS | *IARS2* | 1q41 | AR | Isoleucyl-tRNA synthetase 2 | 616007 |
| 45.68 | Perrault syndrome 4 | Mitochondrial leucyl-tRNA synthetase deficiency | PRLTS4; HLASA(?) | *LARS2* | 3p21.31 | AR | Leucyl-tRNA synthetase 2 | 615300; 617021(?) |
| 45.69 | Autosomal recessive spastic ataxia type 3 | Mitochondrial methionyl-tRNA synthetase deficiency | SPAX3 | *MARS2* | 2q33.1 | AR | Methionyl-tRNA synthetase 2 | 611390 |
| 45.70 | Combined oxidative phosphorylation deficiency 25 | Mitochondrial methionyl-tRNA synthetase deficiency | COXPD25 | *MARS2* | 2q33.1 | AR | Methionyl-tRNA synthetase 2 | 616430 |
| 45.71 | Spastic paraplegia 77, autosomal recessive | Mitochondrial phenylalanyl-tRNA synthetase deficiency | SPG77 | *FARS2* | 6p25.1 | AR | Phenylalanyl-tRNA synthetase 2 | 617046 |
| 45.72 | Combined oxidative phosphorylation deficiency type 14 | Mitochondrial phenylalanyl-tRNA synthetase deficiency | COXPD14 | *FARS2* | 6p25.1 | AR | Phenylalanyl-tRNA synthetase 2 | 614946 |
| 45.73 | Hyperuricemia, pulmonary hypertension, renal failure, and alkalosis | Mitochondrial seryl-tRNA synthetase deficiency | HUPRA | *SARS2* | 19q13.2 | AR | Seryl-tRNA synthetase 2 | 613845 |
| 45.74 | Combined oxidative phosphorylation deficiency type 21 | Mitochondrial threonyl-tRNA synthetase deficiency | COXPD21 | *TARS2* | 1q21.2 | AR | Threonyl-tRNA synthetase 2 | 615918 |
| 45.75 | Myopathy lactic acidosis and Sideroblastic Anaemia type 2 | Mitochondrial tyrosyl-tRNA synthetase deficiency | MLASA2 | *YARS2* | 12p11.21 | AR | Tyrosyl-tRNA synthetase 2 | 613561 |
| 45.76 | Combined oxidative phosphorylation deficiency type 20 | Mitochondrial valyl-tRNA synthetase deficiency | COXPD20 | *VARS2* | 6p21.33 | AR | Valyl-tRNA synthetase 2 | 615917 |
| 45.77 | Mitochondrial neurodevelopmental disorder with abnormal movements and lactic acidosis, with or without seizures | Mitochondrial tryptophanyl-tRNA synthetase deficiency | NEMMLAS | *WARS2* | 1p12 | AR | Tryptophanyl-tRNA synthetase 2 | 617710 |
| 45.78 | Charcot-Marie-tooth disease type 2D; distal hereditary motor neuronopathy type 5A | Mitochondrial and cytoplasmic glycyl-tRNA synthetase deficiency | CMT2D; HMN5A | *GARS* | 7p14.3 | AR | Glycyl-tRNA synthetase | 601472; 600794 |
| 45.79 | Deafness, autosomal recessive 89 | Mitochondrial and cytoplasmic lysyl-tRNA synthetase deficiency | DFNB89; CMTRIB(?) | *KARS* | 16q23.1 | AR | Lysyl-tRNA synthetase | 613916; 613641(?) |
| 45.80 | Infantile-onset multisystem neurologic, endocrine, and pancreatic disease | Peptidyl-tRNA hydrolase 2 deficiency | IMNEPD | *PTRH2* | 17q23.1 | AR | Peptidyl-tRNA hydrolase 2 | 616263 |
| 45.81 | Perrault syndrome 6 | | PRLTS6 | *ERAL1* | 17q11.2 | AR | Era G-protein-like 1 | 617565 |
| 45.82 | NOP2/SUN RNA methyltransferase 3 deficiency | | | *NSUN3* | 3q11.2 | AR | NOP2/SUN RNA methyltransferase 3 | 617491 |
| 45.83 | Mitochondrial ribosomal small subunit 25 deficiency | | | *MRPS25* | 3p25.1 | AR | Mitochondrial ribosomal protein S25 | 611987 |

No S&S*: rare single case patient, for which no OMIM disease record was yet available and no Signs and Symptoms table is provided; for most mitochondrial tRNA mutations, with the exception of the tRNA (LeuUUR) 3243A>G and the tRNA(Lys) 8344A>G mutations, for the MELAS and MERRF syndromes respectively, Signs and Symptoms tables are not provided

## Metabolic Pathway

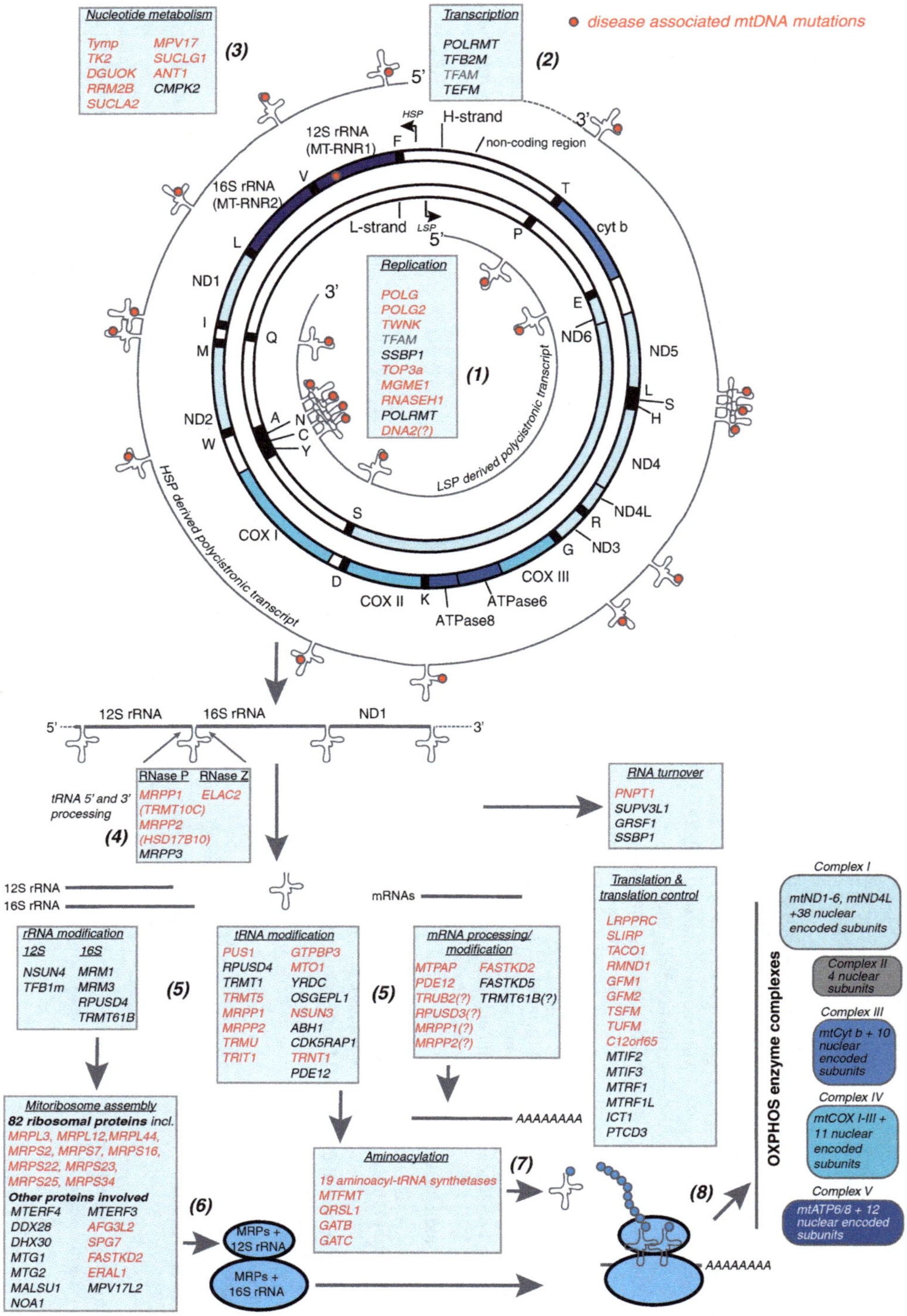

## Signs and Symptoms

**Table 45.1** Mitochondrial depletion syndrome 4A

| System | Symptoms and biomarkers | Neonatal (birth–1 month) | Infancy (1–18 months) | Childhood (1.5–11 years) | Adolescence (11–16 years) | Adulthood (>16 years) |
|---|---|---|---|---|---|---|
| CNS | Ataxia | | ++ | ++ | | |
| | Developmental delay | | ++ | ++ | | |
| | **Epilepsy, intractable** | | +++ | +++ | | |
| | Hypotonia | | ++ | ++ | | |
| | Intellectual disability | | ++ | ++ | | |
| | **Retardation, psychomotor** | | +++ | +++ | | |
| Digestive | **Liver failure, progressive** | | +++ | +++ | | |
| | Vomiting | | + | + | | |
| Eye | Vision, impaired | | + | + | | |
| Other | Death | | ++ | ++ | | |
| | Valproate induced fatal liver toxicity | | +++ | +++ | | |
| Laboratory findings | 3-Methylglutaconic acid (urine) | | ↑ | ↑ | | |
| | Lactate (plasma) | | ↑ | ↑ | | |
| | Mitochondrial DNA (liver) | | ↓↓↓ | ↓↓↓ | | |

**Table 45.2** Mitochondrial depletion syndrome 4B

| System | Symptoms and biomarkers | Neonatal (birth–1 month) | Infancy (1–18 months) | Childhood (1.5–11 years) | Adolescence (11–16 years) | Adulthood (>16 years) |
|---|---|---|---|---|---|---|
| CNS | Axonal sensory ataxic neuropathy | | | | + | |
| Digestive | **Cachexia** | + | + | ++ | +++ | |
| | **Chronic gastrointestinal dysmotility** | + | ++ | +++ | +++ | |
| | Liver failure, progressive | | ± | ± | | |
| | **Pseudo-obstruction** | + | ++ | +++ | +++ | |
| Ear | Hearing loss | ± | ± | ± | | |
| | Progressive external ophthalmoplegia | | | ± | + | |
| Musculoskeletal | **Muscle weakness** | + | ++ | ++ | ++ | |
| Other | Death | | ++ | ++ | | |
| Laboratory findings | 3-Methylglutaconic acid (urine) | | ↑ | ↑ | | |
| | Lactate (plasma) | | ↑ | ↑ | | |
| | Mitochondrial DNA (liver) | ↓-n | ↓-n | ↓-n | | |
| | Mitochondrial DNA (muscle) | ↓↓↓ | ↓↓↓ | ↓↓↓ | ↓↓↓ | |

**Fig. 45.1** Pathways and proteins involved in mitochondrial DNA replication, transcription and translation. Mitochondrial DNA (mtDNA) is a small double-stranded circular molecule that has a relatively simple machinery for its replication (*1*). Both strands serve as template for the transcription machinery (*2*) that initiates at the H-strand promoter (HSP) or the L-strand promoter (LSP), to give two large primary polycistronic transcripts here called 'HSP derived polycistronic' and 'LSP derived polycistronic' transcript. MtDNA replication requires deoxyribonucleotides provided by interconnected de novo and salvage pathways (*3*). Primary transcripts are interspersed with tRNA transcripts represented here by the standard tRNA cloverleaf structure. Endonucleolytic cleavage of the tRNAs at both ends by RNaseP and RNaseZ yields the two pre ribosomal RNAs (rRNA, 12S and 16S), pre tRNAs and pre mRNAs (*4*). These are all further processed (*5*) and in particular both rRNAs and all tRNAs are further modified at specific nucleoside positions, whilst all RNA types are also oligo/poly adenylated. Ribosomal RNAs together with mt tRNA(Val) (not indicated) are assembled into mature ribosomes (*6*) that include 82 nuclear encoded mitoribosomal proteins. This process involves approximately 15 so far identified additional 'assembly' factors, some of which have been associated with mitochondrial disease. The tRNAs after extensive modification are matured by 3′CCA addition (not indicated) and are now ready to be aminoacylated by 19 aminoacyl-tRNA synthethases (*7*), all of which have been associated with mitochondrial disease. There is no dedicated enzyme to charge the glutamine (Q)-tRNA but instead it is charged with glutamate that is converted to glutamine by the trimeric Glu-tRNA (Gln) amidotransferase complex consisting of GATA (QRSL1), GATB and GATC subunits. All these various pathways come together so that the 11 mitochondrial mRNAs that direct the synthesis of 13 essential subunits of four of the five oxidative phosphorylation complexes can be translated by the dedicated mitochondrial ribosomes and charged tRNAs (as indicated, (*8*)). A considerable number of additional nuclear encoded factors are involved in this process, for example to recycle tRNAs, and to assist in the initiation, elongation and termination of protein synthesis. Mitochondria also have a machinery to degrade dysfunctional RNA as well as long non-coding RNAs that are mostly derived from LSP initiated transcription. In total almost 200 nuclear-encoded mitochondrial proteins are here indicated to be involved in the process of mtDNA maintenance and expression, of which some 80 (here indicated in red) have so far been associated with mitochondrial disease. In addition, all mitochondrial tRNA genes have been associated with disease (indicated here with a red dot on the tRNAs of the two polycistronic transcripts), whilst one rRNA mutation [m. 1555A>G in 12S (MT-RNR1); also indicated with a red dot on mtDNA] is known principally for its association with aminoglycoside-induced hearing loss

**Table 45.3** Sensory ataxic neuropathy, dysarthria, and ophthalmoparesis (SANDO)

| System | Symptoms and biomarkers | Neonatal (birth–1 month) | Infancy (1–18 months) | Childhood (1.5–11 years) | Adolescence (11–16 years) | Adulthood (>16 years) |
|---|---|---|---|---|---|---|
| CNS | (Epileptic) seizures | | | + | + | + |
| | **Dysarthria** | | | | | +++ |
| | Headaches and/or migraine | | | + | + | + |
| | Mild cognitive impairment | | | ± | ± | ± |
| | **Sensory ataxic neuropathy** | | | | | +++ |
| Eye | **Ophthalmoparesis or ophthalmoplegia** | | | | | ++ |
| Laboratory findings | Mitochondrial DNA deletions (muscle) | | | ↑ | ↑ | ↑ |

**Table 45.4** Progressive external ophthalmoplegia 1

| System | Symptoms and biomarkers | Neonatal (birth–1 month) | Infancy (1–18 months) | Childhood (1.5–11 years) | Adolescence (11–16 years) | Adulthood (>16 years) |
|---|---|---|---|---|---|---|
| Cardiovascular | Cardiac involvement | | | | | ± |
| CNS | Ataxia | | | | | ± |
| | Parkinsonism | | | | | ± |
| | Sensory ataxic neuropathy | | | | | ± |
| Ear | Hearing loss | | | | | ± |
| Endocrine | Hypogonadism | | | | | ± |
| Eye | **Ophthalmoparesis or ophthalmoplegia** | | | | | ++ |
| Metabolic | **Ragged red fibers** | | | | | + |
| Musculoskeletal | **Muscle weakness and/or exercise intolerance** | | | | | ++ |
| Psychiatric | Depression | | | | | ± |
| Laboratory findings | Histochemical cytochrome *c* oxidase deficiency (muscle) | | | | | ↑↑ |
| | Multiple mtDNA deletions (muscle) | | | | | ↑↑ |

**Table 45.5** Mitochondrial DNA polymerase g accessory subunit deficiency ($n$ = 1)

| System | Symptoms and biomarkers | Neonatal (birth–1 month) | Infancy (1–18 months) | Childhood (1.5–11 years) | Adolescence (11–16 years) | Adulthood (>16 years) |
|---|---|---|---|---|---|---|
| Cardiovascular | **Cardiac, anomalies, malformations** | | | | | + |
| CNS | **Fatigue** | | | | | + |
| Eye | **Ophthalmoplegia** | | | | | + |
| | **Ptosis of eyelid** | | | | | + |
| Musculoskeletal | **Muscle weakness, proximal** | | | | | + |
| Laboratory findings | Histochemical cytochrome *c* oxidase deficiency (muscle) | | | | | ↑↑ |
| | Multiple mtDNA deletions (muscle) | | | | | ↑↑ |

**Table 45.6** Mitochondrial deoxyguanosine kinase deficiency

| System | Symptoms and biomarkers | Neonatal (birth–1 month) | Infancy (1–18 months) | Childhood (1.5–11 years) | Adolescence (11–16 years) | Adulthood (>16 years) |
|---|---|---|---|---|---|---|
| Autonomic system | Noncirrhotic portal hypertension | + | ± | + | | |
| CNS | Hypotonia | +++ | +++ | | | |
| | Neurologic abnormalities | +++ | +++ | | | |
| | Regression, psychomotor | +++ | +++ | | | |
| Digestive | Cholestasis | +++ | +++ | ++ | | |
| | Hepatomegaly | +++ | +++ | ++ | | |
| | Jaundice | +++ | +++ | ++ | | |
| | Liver failure | +++ | +++ | ++ | | |
| | Neonatal hemochromatosis | ± | | | | |
| Eye | Nystagmus | +++ | +++ | | | |
| | Ophthalmoplegia | | ± | | | |
| | Ptosis of eyelid | | ± | | | + |
| Musculoskeletal | Myopathy | | ± | | | |
| Other | Death | ++ | ++ | ++ | + | + |
| Laboratory findings | Activity respiratory chain complexes (I, III, IV, and V) | ↓↓↓ | ↓↓↓ | ↓↓ | | |
| | Alpha-fetoprotein (serum) | ↑↑ | ↑↑ | | | |
| | Cystathionine (urine) | | ± | | | |
| | Ferritin (serum) | ↑↑ | ↑↑ | | | |
| | Gamma-glutamyl transpeptidase, GGT (plasma) | ↑↑ | ↑↑ | | | |
| | Glucose (plasma) | ↓↓↓ | ↓↓↓ | ↓ | | |
| | Histochemical cytochrome *c* oxidase deficiency (muscle) | | | | | ↑ |
| | Histochemical mitochondrial proliferation (muscle) | | | | | ↑ |
| | Lactate (CSF) | ↑↑ | ↑↑ | | | |
| | Lactate (plasma) | ↑↑ | ↑↑ | | | |
| | mtDNA levels (liver & brain) | ↓↓↓ | ↓↓↓ | ↓↓ | | |
| | Multiple mtDNA deletions | | | | | ↑ |
| | Phenylalanine (plasma) | ↑ | ↑ | | | |
| | Succinylacetone (urine) | n | n | | | |
| | Transaminase (plasma) | ↑↑ | ↑↑ | | | |
| | Tyrosine (plasma) | ↑ | ↑ | | | |

**Table 45.7** MPV17 deficiency

| System | Symptoms and biomarkers | Neonatal (birth–1 month) | Infancy (1–18 months) | Childhood (1.5–11 years) | Adolescence (11–16 years) | Adulthood (>16 years) |
|---|---|---|---|---|---|---|
| CNS | Developmental delay | +++ | +++ | | | |
| | Hypotonia | +++ | +++ | | | |
| | Neurologic abnormalities | +++ | +++ | | | |
| | Peripheral neuropathy | | | ± | ± | ± |
| Digestive | Cholestasis | +++ | +++ | + | + | |
| | Gastrointestinal dysmotility | ± | ± | | | |
| | Hepatomegaly | +++ | +++ | + | + | |
| | Jaundice | +++ | +++ | + | + | |
| | **Liver failure** | +++ | +++ | + | + | |
| Eye | Corneal anesthesia & ulcers | | | | ± | ± |
| | Ophthalmoplegia | | | | | + |
| | Ptosis of eyelid | | | | | + |
| Musculoskeletal | Myopathy | | | | | + |
| Renal | Renal tubulopathy | ± | ± | | | |
| Other | Death | +++ | ++ | + | + | + |
| | Failure to thrive | +++ | +++ | | | |
| Laboratory findings | Activity respiratory chain complexes (I, III, IV, and V) | ↓↓↓ | ↓↓↓ | ↓↓ | | |
| | Gamma-glutamyl transpeptidase, GGT (plasma) | ↑↑ | ↑↑ | | | |
| | Glucose (plasma) | ↓↓ | ↓↓ | ↓ | | |
| | Histochemical cytochrome *c* oxidase deficiency (muscle) | | | | | ↑ |
| | Histochemical mitochondrial proliferation (muscle) | | | | | ↑ |
| | Lactate (CSF) | ↑ | ↑ | ↑ | | |
| | Lactate (plasma) | ↑ | ↑ | ↑ | | |
| | **mtDNA levels** | ↓↓↓ | ↓↓↓ | ↓↓ | | |
| | Mutiple mtDNA deletions | | | | | ↑ |
| | Transaminases (plasma) | ↑↑ | ↑↑ | | | |

**Table 45.8** Progressive external ophthalmoplegia with mitochondrial DNA deletions, autosomal dominant 3

| System | Symptoms and biomarkers | Neonatal (birth–1 month) | Infancy (1–18 months) | Childhood (1.5–11 years) | Adolescence (11–16 years) | Adulthood (>16 years) |
|---|---|---|---|---|---|---|
| Cardiovascular | Cardiac abnormalities | | | | ± | ± |
| CNS | Ataxia | | | | ± | ± |
| | Fatigue | | | | ± | ± |
| | Parkisonism | | | | ± | ± |
| | Sensory neuropathy | | | | ± | ± |
| Endocrine | Endocrine abnormalities | | | | ± | ± |
| Eye | **Ophthalmoplegia** | | | ± | ± | ++ |
| | **Ptosis of eyelid** | | | ± | ± | ++ |
| Musculoskeletal | Proximal muscle weakness | | | | ± | ± |
| Psychiatric | Depression | | | | ± | ± |
| Laboratory findings | Histochemical cytochrome *c* oxidase deficiency (muscle) | | | n-↑ | n-↑ | ↑↑ |
| | Multiple mtDNA deletions (muscle) | | | n-↑ | n-↑ | ↑↑ |

**Table 45.9** Mitochondrial DNA depletion syndrome type 7

| System | Symptoms and biomarkers | Neonatal (birth–1 month) | Infancy (1–18 months) | Childhood (1.5–11 years) | Adolescence (11–16 years) | Adulthood (>16 years) |
|---|---|---|---|---|---|---|
| CNS | **Ataxia** | | | ++ | ++ | +++ |
| | **Athetosis** | | ± | ++ | ++ | + |
| | Epileptic seizures | | ± | ± | ± | ± |
| | **Hypotonia** | ± | + | + | + | + |
| | Intellectual disability | | | | + | + |
| | **Peripheral sensory neuropathy** | | ± | ± | + | ++ |
| | **Retardation, psychomotor** | ± | + | + | + | + |
| Digestive | Liver dysfunction | ± | + | ++ | ± | ± |
| Ear | **Hearing loss** | | ± | ± | ++ | +++ |
| Endocrine | Hypogonadism | | n.a. | n.a. | + (F) | + (F) |
| Eye | Abnormal eye movements | | + | + | | |
| | **Ophthamoplegia** | | ± | ± | + | + |
| | Optic atrophy | | | | + | + |
| Other | Death | | | ± | ± | ± |
| Laboratory findings | Lactate (plasma) | | ↑ | ↑ | | |
| | Mitochondrial DNA (liver) | | ↓↓↓ | ↓↓↓ | ↓-n | ↓-n |

**Table 45.10** Perrault syndrome 5

| System | Symptoms and biomarkers | Neonatal (birth–1 month) | Infancy (1–18 months) | Childhood (1.5–11 years) | Adolescence (11–16 years) | Adulthood (>16 years) |
|---|---|---|---|---|---|---|
| CNS | **Ataxia** | | | | + | ++ |
| | **Neuropathy, sensory axonal** | | | | | ++ |
| Ear | **Hearing loss, sensorineural** | | | ++ | +++ | +++ |
| Genitourinary | **Ovarian dysgenesis** | | | | +++ | +++ |
| Laboratory findings | Estradiol (plasma) | | | | ↓ | ↓ |
| | Follicle-stimulating hormone (plasma) | | | | ↑↑ | ↑↑ |
| | Lactate (plasma) | | | | n-↑ | n-↑ |
| | Luteinizing hormone (plasma) | | | | ↑ | ↑ |

**Table 45.11** Mitochondrial thymidine kinase deficiency

| System | Symptoms and biomarkers | Neonatal (birth–1 month) | Infancy (1–18 months) | Childhood (1.5–11 years) | Adolescence (11–16 years) | Adulthood (>16 years) |
|---|---|---|---|---|---|---|
| CNS | Central nervous system manifestation | | ± | | | |
| | Hypotonia | | +++ | + | + | ± |
| | Neuropathy, peripheral | | | | ± | |
| Eye | Ophthalmoparesis | | | ± | ± | ++ |
| | Ophthalmoplegia | | | ± | ± | ++ |
| Musculoskeletal | **Myopathy** | | +++ | ++ | + | + |
| | Spinal muscle atrophy-like phenotye (type 3) | | | ± | | ± |
| Other | Death | | + | + | | + |
| Laboratory findings | Creatine kinase (plasma) | ↑↑ | ↑↑ | ↑↑ | ↑↑ | ↑↑ |
| | Histochemical cytochrome *c* oxidase deficiency (muscle) | ↑↑ | ↑ | ↑ | ↑ | ↑ |
| | Histochemical mitocondrial proliferation (muscle) | ↑ | ↑ | ↑ | ↑ | ↑ |
| | Lactate (plasma) | ↑ | ↑ | ↑ | | ↑ |
| | mtDNA deletions (muscle) | ↑ | ↑ | ↑ | ↑ | ↑ |
| | mtDNA levels (muscle) | ↓ | ↓ | ↓ | ↓ | ↓ |

**Table 45.12** Mitochondrial DNA depletion syndrome 8

| System | Symptoms and biomarkers | Neonatal (birth–1 month) | Infancy (1–18 months) | Childhood (1.5–11 years) | Adolescence (11–16 years) | Adulthood (>16 years) |
|---|---|---|---|---|---|---|
| CNS | **Encephalomyopathy** | | + | + | | ± |
| | **Hypotonia** | + | ± | + | | |
| | **Neuropathy, peripheral** | | ± | + | | ± |
| Digestive | **Gastrointestinal dysmotility** | | | | | ± |
| Ear | **Hearing loss** | | + | + | | |
| Eye | **Ophthalmoplegia** | | | | | ± |
| Renal | **Renal tubulopathy** | | + | + | | |
| Other | Death | + | +++ | + | | + |
| Laboratory findings | Histochemical cytochrome *c* oxidase deficiency (muscle) | ↑ | ↑ | | | ↑ |
| | Histochemical mitocondrial proliferation (muscle) | ↑ | ↑ | | | ↑ |
| | Lactate (P/CSF) | ↑ | ↑ | | | ↑ |
| | mtDNA deletions (muscle) | ↑ | ↑ | | | ↑ |
| | mtDNA levels (muscle) | ↓ | ↓ | | | ↓ |

**Table 45.13** Thymidine phosphorylase deficiency

| System | Symptoms and biomarkers | Neonatal (birth–1 month) | Infancy (1–18 months) | Childhood (1.5–11 years) | Adolescence (11–16 years) | Adulthood (>16 years) |
|---|---|---|---|---|---|---|
| CNS | Areflexia | | | | + | + |
| | Hypodense white matter | | | | + | + |
| | Leukoencephalopathy | | | | + | + |
| | **Neuropathy, myelinating** | | | | + | + |
| Digestive | Abdominal pain | | | | + | + |
| | **Anorexia** | | | | + | + |
| | Diarrhea | | | | + | + |
| | **Gastrointestinal dysmotility** | | | | + | + |
| | **Gastroparesis** | | | | + | + |
| | Intestinal pseudo obstruction | | | | + | + |
| | **Malabsorption** | | | | + | + |
| | **Malnutrition, chronic** | | | | + | + |
| | Vomiting | | | | + | + |
| Metabolic | **Ragged red fibers** | | | | + | + |
| Musculoskeletal | **Muscle weakness** | | | | + | + |
| | **Myopathy** | | | | + | + |
| Laboratory findings | Deoxyuridine (plasma) | | | | ↑ | ↑ |
| | Deoxyuridine (urine) | | | | ↑↑ | ↑↑ |
| | Lactate (plasma) | | | | ↑↑ | ↑↑ |
| | Thymidine (plasma) | | | | ↑ | ↑ |
| | Thymidine (urine) | | | | ↑↑ | ↑↑ |
| | Thymidine phosphorylase (white blood cells) | | | | ↓↓↓ | ↓↓↓ |

**Table 45.14** DNA2 deficiency

| System | Symptoms and biomarkers | Neonatal (birth–1 month) | Infancy (1–18 months) | Childhood (1.5–11 years) | Adolescence (11–16 years) | Adulthood (>16 years) |
|---|---|---|---|---|---|---|
| CNS | **Fatigue** | | | | ± | + |
| Eye | **Ophthalmoplegia** | | | | ± | + |
| | **Ptosis of eyelid** | | | | ± | + |
| Musculoskeletal | **Muscle weakness, proximal** | | | | ± | + |
| Respiratory | **Dyspnea** | | | | ± | + |
| Laboratory findings | Histochemical cytochrome *c* oxidase deficiency (muscle) | | | | ↑ | ↑ |
| | Histochemical mitochondrial proliferation (muscle) | | | | ↑ | ↑ |
| | Multiple mtDNA deletions (muscle) | | | | ↑ | ↑ |

**Table 45.15** RNASEH1 defect

| System | Symptoms and biomarkers | Neonatal (birth–1 month) | Infancy (1–18 months) | Childhood (1.5–11 years) | Adolescence (11–16 years) | Adulthood (>16 years) |
|---|---|---|---|---|---|---|
| CNS | **Ataxia** | | | | ± | ± |
| | Fatigue | | | | ± | ++ |
| Digestive | Dysphagia | | | | ± | ± |
| Eye | **Ophthalmoplegia** | | | ± | ± | +++ |
| | **Ptosis of eyelid** | | | ± | ± | ++ |
| Musculoskeletal | **Muscle weakness, proximal** | | | | ± | ++ |
| Respiratory | Dyspnea | | | | ± | ± |
| | Orthopnea | | | | ± | ± |
| Laboratory findings | Histochemical cytochrome *c* oxidase deficiency (muscle) | | | n-↑ | n-↑ | ↑↑ |
| | Histochemical mitochondrial proliferation (muscle) | | | ± | ± | ↑↑ |
| | Multiple mtDNA deletions (muscle) | | | ± | ± | + |

**Table 45.16** MGME1 deficiency

| System | Symptoms and biomarkers | Neonatal (birth–1 month) | Infancy (1–18 months) | Childhood (1.5–11 years) | Adolescence (11–16 years) | Adulthood (>16 years) |
|---|---|---|---|---|---|---|
| CNS | Cerebellar atrophy (MRI) | | | | ± | + |
| | Fatigue | | | | ± | ++ |
| | Intellectual disability | | | | ± | ± |
| Eye | **Ophthalmoplegia** | | | | ± | +++ |
| | **Ptosis of eyelid** | | | | ± | ++ |
| Musculoskeletal | **Muscle weakness, proximal** | | | | ± | ++ |
| Respiratory | **Dyspnea** | | | | ± | + |
| | Respiratory failure | | | | ± | + |
| Other | Death | | | | | ± |
| Laboratory findings | Histochemical cytochrome *c* oxidase deficiency (muscle) | | | | ↑ | ↑ |
| | Histochemical mitocondrial proliferation (muscle) | | | | ↑ | ↑ |
| | mtDNA levels (muscle) | | | | n-↑ | ↑ |
| | Multiple mtDNA deletions | | | | n-↑ | ↑ |

**Table 45.17** FBXL4 deficiency

| System | Symptoms and biomarkers | Neonatal (birth–1 month) | Infancy (1–18 months) | Childhood (1.5–11 years) | Adolescence (11–16 years) | Adulthood (>16 years) |
|---|---|---|---|---|---|---|
| Cardiovascular | Cardiomyopathy, hypertrophic | | + | + | | |
| CNS | Ataxia | | + | + | | |
| | Cerebellar hypoplasia | | + | + | | |
| | **Cerebral atrophy (MRI)** | | ++ | ++ | | |
| | Developmental delay | | + | + | | |
| | Encephalopathy | | + | + | | |
| | **Hypotonia** | | +++ | +++ | | |
| | **Microcephaly** | | + | + | | |
| Digestive | Gastrointestinal dysmotility | | + | + | | |
| Renal | Renal tubular acidosis | | + | + | | |
| Other | Death | | + | + | + | |
| Laboratory findings | Lactate (plasma) | | ↑ | ↑ | | |
| | mtDNA levels (muscle and fibroblasts) | | ↓↓ | ↓↓ | | |
| | Respiratory chain enzymes (muscle and cells) | | ↓ | ↓ | | |

**Table 45.18** TOP3A deficiency ($n = 1$)

| System | Symptoms and biomarkers | Neonatal (birth–1 month) | Infancy (1–18 months) | Childhood (1.5–11 years) | Adolescence (11–16 years) | Adulthood (>16 years) |
|---|---|---|---|---|---|---|
| Cardiovascular | Cardiac, anomalies, malformations | | | | | + |
| CNS | Ataxia | | | | | + |
| | Neuropathy, sensory | | | | | + |
| Ear | Hearing loss, sensorineural | | | | | + |
| Eye | Ophthalmoplegia | | | | | ++ |
| | Ptosis of eyelid | | | | | ++ |
| Musculoskeletal | Exercise intolerance | | | | | + |
| | Muscle weakness, proximal | | | | | + |
| Laboratory findings | Histochemical cytochrome *c* oxidase deficiency (muscle) | | | | | ↑↑ |
| | Multiple mtDNA deletions (muscle) | | | | | ↑↑ |
| | Ragged red fibers | | | | | ↑↑ |

**Table 45.19** ATP-specific succinyl-CoA ligase β subunit deficiency

| System | Symptoms and biomarkers | Neonatal (birth–1 month) | Infancy (1–18 months) | Childhood (1.5–11 years) | Adolescence (11–16 years) | Adulthood (>16 years) |
|---|---|---|---|---|---|---|
| CNS | **Axial hypotonia** | + | ++ | ++ | + | + |
| | Choreoathetosis | ± | ± | ± | ± | ± |
| | Dystonia | – | ± | + | ++ | ++ |
| | Leigh syndrome | – | ± | + | ++ | ++ |
| | **Neurological symptoms** | ++ | ++ | ++ | ++ | ++ |
| | Neuropathy, peripheral | – | – | ± | ± | ± |
| | Pyramidal signs | – | ± | + | ++ | ++ |
| | **Retardation, psychomotor** | ± | ++ | ++ | ++ | ++ |
| Digestive | Feeding difficulties | ± | ± | ± | + | + |
| Ear | Deafness, sensorineural | ± | ++ | ++ | ++ | ++ |

(continued)

**Table 45.19** (continued)

| System | Symptoms and biomarkers | Neonatal (birth–1 month) | Infancy (1–18 months) | Childhood (1.5–11 years) | Adolescence (11–16 years) | Adulthood (>16 years) |
|---|---|---|---|---|---|---|
| Metabolic | Lactic acidosis | + | + | + | + | + |
| Other | Failure to thrive | + | + | + | + | + |
| Laboratory findings | ASAT/ALAT (plasma) | n-↑ | n-↑ | n-↑ | n-↑ | n-↑ |
| | C4-DC Methylmalonylcarnitine (urine) | ↑ | ↑ | ↑ | ↑ | ↑ |
| | C4-DC Succinylcarnitine (urine) | ↑ | ↑ | ↑ | ↑ | ↑ |
| | Lactate (plasma) | ↑ | ↑ | ↑ | ↑ | ↑ |
| | Lactate/pyruvate ratio | ↑ | ↑ | ↑ | ↑ | ↑ |
| | Methylmalonic acid (urine) | ↑ | ↑ | ↑ | ↑ | ↑ |
| | mtDNA levels | ↓ | ↓ | ↓ | | |
| | Respiratory chain enzyme deficiencies (muscle) | | ↓ | ↓ | | |

**Table 45.20** GTP-specific succinyl-CoA ligase α subunit deficiency

| System | Symptoms and biomarkers | Neonatal (birth–1 month) | Infancy (1–18 months) | Childhood (1.5–11 years) | Adolescence (11–16 years) | Adulthood (>16 years) |
|---|---|---|---|---|---|---|
| Cardiovascular | Congenital heart defects | ± | ± | ± | ± | ± |
| CNS | Ataxia | | ± | ± | ± | |
| | Axial hypotonia | + | ++ | ++ | + | + |
| | Choreoathetosis | ± | ± | ± | ± | ± |
| | Dystonia | | ± | + | ++ | ++ |
| | **Encephalopathy, necrotizing** | | ++ | ++ | | |
| | **Hypotonia** | | ++ | ++ | ++ | |
| | Leigh syndrome | | ± | + | ++ | ++ |
| | Neurological symptoms | ++ | ++ | ++ | ++ | ++ |
| | Neuropathy, peripheral | | | ± | ± | ± |
| | Pyramidal signs | | ± | + | ++ | ++ |
| | Retardation, psychomotor | ± | ++ | ++ | ++ | ++ |
| | Seizures | | ± | ± | ± | |
| Digestive | **Feeding difficulties** | ++ | ++ | ++ | ++ | ++ |
| | Liver dysfunction | ± | ± | ± | + | + |
| Ear | Deafness, sensorineural | ± | ± | ± | ± | ± |
| Metabolic | **Lactic acidosis** | + | + | + | + | + |
| Other | Death | | + | + | + | |
| | Failure to thrive | ++ | ++ | ++ | ++ | ++ |
| Laboratory findings | ASAT/ALAT (plasma) | n-↑ | n-↑ | n-↑ | n-↑ | n-↑ |
| | C4-DC Methylmalonylcarnitine (urine) | ↑ | ↑ | ↑ | ↑ | ↑ |
| | C4-DC Succinylcarnitine (urine) | ↑ | ↑ | ↑ | ↑ | ↑ |
| | Lactate (plasma) | ↑ | ↑ | ↑ | ↑ | ↑ |
| | Lactate/pyruvate ratio | ↑ | ↑ | ↑ | ↑ | ↑ |
| | Methylmalonic acid (urine) | ↑ | ↑ | ↑ | ↑ | ↑ |
| | mtDNA levels | ↓ | ↓ | ↓ | | |
| | Respiratory chain enzymes (muscle) | ↓ | ↓ | ↓ | | |

**Table 45.21** Adenine nucleotide translocator deficiency, Ophthalmoplegia type

| System | Symptoms and biomarkers | Neonatal (birth–1 month) | Infancy (1–18 months) | Childhood (1.5–11 years) | Adolescence (11–16 years) | Adulthood (>16 years) |
|---|---|---|---|---|---|---|
| Eye | Hearing loss, sensorineural | | | | | ± |
| | **Ophthalmoplegia** | | | | | ++ |
| | **Ptosis of eyelid** | | | | | ++ |
| Laboratory findings | Histochemical cytochrome *c* oxidase deficiency (muscle) | | | | | ↑ |
| | Multiple mtDNA deletions (muscle) | | | | | ↑ |

**Table 45.22** Adenine nucleotide translocator deficiency, cardiomyopathic type

| System | Symptoms and biomarkers | Neonatal (birth–1 month) | Infancy (1–18 months) | Childhood (1.5–11 years) | Adolescence (11–16 years) | Adulthood (>16 years) |
|---|---|---|---|---|---|---|
| Cardiovascular | Cardiomyopathy, hypertrophic | ± | ± | ± | | |
| CNS | **Hyporeflexia and/or paucity of movement** | ++ | ++ | ++ | | |
| | **Hypotonia** | +++ | +++ | +++ | | |
| Musculoskeletal | Muscle weakness, proximal | | | + | | |
| Respiratory | **Respiratory dysfunction** | ++ | ++ | ++ | | |
| Other | Death | ++ | ++ | | | |
| Laboratory findings | Lactate (cerebrospinal fluid) | ↑ | ↑ | | | |
| | Lactate (plasma) | ↑↑↑ | ↑↑ | | | |
| | mtDNA levels (muscle) | ↓↓↓ | ↓↓↓ | ↓↓↓ | | |

**Table 45.23** Adenine nucleotide translocator deficiency AD

| System | Symptoms and biomarkers | Neonatal (birth–1 month) | Infancy (1–18 months) | Childhood (1.5–11 years) | Adolescence (11–16 years) | Adulthood (>16 years) |
|---|---|---|---|---|---|---|
| Cardiovascular | **Cardiomyopathy, hypertrophic** | | | | | + |
| Musculoskeletal | **Exercise intolerance** | | | | | + |
| CNS | **Fatigue** | | | + | + | + |
| Musculoskeletal | Muscle atrophy | | | | | ± |
| | Muscle weakness | | | | | ± |
| Laboratory findings | Histochemical cytochrome *c* oxidase deficiency (muscle) | | | | | ↑↑ |
| | Lactate (plasma) | | | ↑↑ | | ↑↑ |
| | Lactate (plasma) | | | ↑↑ | | |
| | Multiple mitochondrial DNA deletions (muscle) | | | | | ↑↑ |
| | Ragged red fibers | | | | | ↑↑ |

**Table 45.24** PNPT1 deficiency

| System | Symptoms and biomarkers | Neonatal (birth–1 month) | Infancy (1–18 months) | Childhood (1.5–11 years) | Adolescence (11–16 years) | Adulthood (>16 years) |
|---|---|---|---|---|---|---|
| CNS | Dystonia | | ± | ± | ± | |
| | Hypotonia | | ± | ± | ± | |
| Digestive | Dysphagia | | ± | ± | ± | |
| | Feeding difficulties | | ± | ± | ± | |
| Ear | **Deafness** | | ++ | +++ | +++ | |
| Eye | Nystagmus | | ± | ± | ± | |
| Musculoskeletal | Muscle weakness | | ± | ± | ± | |
| Other | Death | | ± | ± | | |
| | Failure to thrive | | ± | ± | ± | |
| Laboratory findings | Lactate (plasma) | | n-↑ | n-↑ | | |

**Table 45.25** Ribonuclease P 5′ tRNA processing enzyme deficiency ($n = 1$)

| System | Symptoms and biomarkers | Neonatal (birth–1 month) | Infancy (1–18 months) | Childhood (1.5–11 years) | Adolescence (11–16 years) | Adulthood (>16 years) |
|---|---|---|---|---|---|---|
| CNS | **Hypotonia** | ++ | ++ | | | |
| Digestive | **Feeding difficulties** | + | + | | | |
| Ear | **Deafness, sensorineural** | + | + | | | |
| Other | Death | | + | | | |
| | Multi organ involvement | ± | ± | | | |
| Laboratory findings | Histochemical cytochrome *c* oxidase deficiency (muscle) | | ↑↑ | | | |
| | Lactate (cerebrospinal fluid) | ↑↑ | ↑↑ | | | |
| | Lactate (plasma) | ↑↑ | ↑↑ | | | |
| | Ragged red fibers | | ↑↑ | | | |

**Table 45.26** Ribonuclease Z 3′ tRNA processing enzyme deficiency

| System | Symptoms and biomarkers | Neonatal (birth–1 month) | Infancy (1–18 months) | Childhood (1.5–11 years) | Adolescence (11–16 years) | Adulthood (>16 years) |
|---|---|---|---|---|---|---|
| Cardiovascular | **Cardiomyopathy, hypertrophic** | | +++ | +++ | +++ | |
| CNS | **Delayed psychomotor development** | | + | + | + | |
| | **Hypotonia** | | + | + | + | |
| Other | Death | | + | + | | |
| | Intrauterine growth retardation | | | | | |
| | Poor growth | | + | + | | |
| Laboratory findings | Lactate (plasma) | | ↑↑ | ↑↑ | | |

**Table 45.27** TFAM deficiency

| System | Symptoms and biomarkers | Neonatal (birth–1 month) | Infancy (1–18 months) | Childhood (1.5–11 years) | Adolescence (11–16 years) | Adulthood (>16 years) |
|---|---|---|---|---|---|---|
| Digestive | Liver failure | | + | | | |
| Other | Death | | + | | | |
| Laboratory findings | mtDNA levels (liver and muscle) | | ↓ | | | |

*Notes:* Whilst this is undoubtedly a form of mtDNA depletion syndrome it is not yet certain that the TFAM variant is pathological, as low levels of TFAM protein are a feature of all forms of MTDPS

**Table 45.28** PNPT1 deficiency

| System | Symptoms and biomarkers | Neonatal (birth–1 month) | Infancy (1–18 months) | Childhood (1.5–11 years) | Adolescence (11–16 years) | Adulthood (>16 years) |
|---|---|---|---|---|---|---|
| CNS | Encephalomyopathy | | + | | | |
| | Hypotonia | | + | | | |
| | Leukodystrophy | | | + | | |
| | Movement abnormalities | | + | | | |
| Ear | Deafness | | | + | | |
| Eye | Optic atrophy | | | + | | |
| Respiratory | Respiratory chain enzymes | | ↓ | ↓ | | |
| Other | Death | | + | ± | ± | |

**Table 45.29** Mitochondrial Poly(A) Polymerase deficiency

| System | Symptoms and biomarkers | Neonatal (birth–1 month) | Infancy (1–18 months) | Childhood (1.5–11 years) | Adolescence (11–16 years) | Adulthood (>16 years) |
|---|---|---|---|---|---|---|
| CNS | **Ataxia, cerebellar** | | | ± | + | + |
| | **Dysarthria** | | | ± | + | + |
| | **Spastic paraparesis** | | | ± | + | + |
| Eye | **Optic atrophy** | | | ± | + | + |
| Laboratory findings | Respiratory chain enzymes (I and IV) | | | ↓ | ↓ | ↓ |

**Table 45.30** CCA-adding tRNA-nucleotidyltransferase deficiency

| System | Symptoms and biomarkers | Neonatal (birth–1 month) | Infancy (1–18 months) | Childhood (1.5–11 years) | Adolescence (11–16 years) | Adulthood (>16 years) |
|---|---|---|---|---|---|---|
| CNS | Developmental delay | | ± | ± | ± | ± |
| | Intellectual disability | | ± | ± | ± | ± |
| Eye | Retinitis pigmentosa | | | | | ± |
| Hematological | Microcytosis | | | | | ± |
| | **Sideroblastic anemia (with B-cell immunodeficiency)** | ± | ± | ± | ± | ± |

**Table 45.31** Mitochondrial methionyl-tRNA formyltransferase deficiency

| System | Symptoms and biomarkers | Neonatal (birth–1 month) | Infancy (1–18 months) | Childhood (1.5–11 years) | Adolescence (11–16 years) | Adulthood (>16 years) |
|---|---|---|---|---|---|---|
| CNS | Ataxia | ± | ± | ± | ± | ± |
| | Developmental delay | | ± | ± | ± | ± |
| | Hypotonia | ± | ± | ± | ± | ± |
| | Intellectual disability | | ± | ± | ± | ± |
| | **Leigh syndrome** | ± | ± | ± | ± | ± |
| Other | Death | | ± | + | ± | + |
| Laboratory findings | Respiratory chain enzymes | ↓-n | ↓-n | ↓-n | | |

**Table 45.32** tRNA 5-taurinomethyluridine modifier deficiency

| System | Symptoms and biomarkers | Neonatal (birth–1 month) | Infancy (1–18 months) | Childhood (1.5–11 years) | Adolescence (11–16 years) | Adulthood (>16 years) |
|---|---|---|---|---|---|---|
| Cardiovascular | Cardiomyopathy, hypertrophic | | ± | ± | ± | ± |
| CNS | Hypotonia | ± | ± | ± | ± | ± |
| | Intellectual disability | | ± | ± | ± | ± |
| Metabolic | Lactic acidosis | ± | ± | ± | ± | ± |
| Laboratory findings | Lactate (plasma) | n-↑ | n-↑ | n-↑ | n-↑ | n-↑ |
| | Mitochondrial complex I and IV activity (muscle) | ↓ | ↓ | ↓ | ↓ | ↓ |
| | Protein levels of GTPBP3 in fibroblasts | ↓ | ↓ | ↓ | ↓ | ↓ |

**Table 45.33** tRNA 5-carboxymethylaminomethyl transferase deficiency

| System | Symptoms and biomarkers | Neonatal (birth–1 month) | Infancy (1–18 months) | Childhood (1.5–11 years) | Adolescence (11–16 years) | Adulthood (>16 years) |
|---|---|---|---|---|---|---|
| Cardiovascular | Cardiomyopathy, hypertrophic | | ± | ± | ± | ± |
| CNS | Ataxia | | ± | ± | ± | ± |
| | Developmental delay | | ± | ± | ± | ± |
| | Epilepsy | ± | ± | ± | ± | ± |
| Digestive | Feeding difficulties | ± | ± | ± | ± | ± |
| Eye | Optic atrophy | | ± | ± | ± | ± |
| Metabolic | Lactic acidosis | ± | ± | ± | ± | ± |
| Laboratory findings | Complex I and IV acitvity in muscle | ↓ | ↓ | ↓ | ↓ | ↓ |
| | Lactate (plasma) | n-↑ | n-↑ | n-↑ | n-↑ | n-↑ |

**Table 45.34** Pseudouridine synthase 1 deficiency

| System | Symptoms and biomarkers | Neonatal (birth–1 month) | Infancy (1–18 months) | Childhood (1.5–11 years) | Adolescence (11–16 years) | Adulthood (>16 years) |
|---|---|---|---|---|---|---|
| Cardiovascular | **Cardiomyopathy, hypertrophic** | | | + | + | + |
| Hematological | **Anemia, sideroblastic** | | | ++ | ++ | ++ |
| Musculoskeletal | Dysmorphic features | ± | ± | ± | ± | ± |
| | Exercise intolerance | | | + | + | + |
| Laboratory findings | Lactate (plasma) | | | ↑↑ | ↑↑ | ↑↑ |
| | Multiple mtDNA deletions (muscle) | ↑ | ↑ | ↑ | ↑ | ↑ |

**Table 45.35** Pseudouridine synthase 1 deficiency

| System | Symptoms and biomarkers | Neonatal (birth–1 month) | Infancy (1–18 months) | Childhood (1.5–11 years) | Adolescence (11–16 years) | Adulthood (>16 years) |
|---|---|---|---|---|---|---|
| Cardiovascular | **Cardiomyopathy, hypertrophic** | | | + | + | + |
| Hematological | **Anemia, sideroblastic** | | | ++ | ++ | ++ |
| Musculoskeletal | Dysmorphic features | ± | ± | ± | ± | ± |
| | Exercise intolerance | | | + | + | + |
| Laboratory findings | Lactate (plasma) | | | ↑↑ | ↑↑ | ↑↑ |
| | Multiple mtDNA deletions (muscle) | ↑ | ↑ | ↑ | ↑ | ↑ |

**Table 45.36** tRNA methyltransferase 5 deficiency

| System | Symptoms and biomarkers | Neonatal (birth–1 month) | Infancy (1–18 months) | Childhood (1.5–11 years) | Adolescence (11–16 years) | Adulthood (>16 years) |
|---|---|---|---|---|---|---|
| Cardiovascular | Cardiomyopathy, hypertrophic | | ± | ± | ± | ± |
| Endocrine | Glucose intolerance | | | | ± | ± |
| Metabolic | Lactic acidosis | ± | ± | ± | ± | ± |
| Musculoskeletal | Exercise intolerance | | ± | ± | ± | ± |
| Renal | Renal tubulopathy | | | | ± | ± |
| Other | Failure to thrive | ± | ± | | | |
| Laboratory findings | Lactate (plasma) | n-↑ | n-↑ | n-↑ | n-↑ | n-↑ |
| | Multiple oxidative phosphorylation enzymes (muscle) | ↓ | ↓ | ↓ | ↓ | ↓ |

**Table 45.37** Acute infantile liver failure TRMU

| System | Symptoms and biomarkers | Neonatal (birth–1 month) | Infancy (1–18 months) | Childhood (1.5–11 years) | Adolescence (11–16 years) | Adulthood (>16 years) |
|---|---|---|---|---|---|---|
| Digestive | **Hepatosplenomegaly** | ++ | +++ | **n** | **n** | |
| | Jaundice | + | + | n | n | |
| | **Liver failure** | +++ | +++ | ± | **n** | **n** |
| | **Pancreatic failure** | + | + | **n** | **n** | |
| | Vomiting | ++ | ++ | n | n | |
| Hematological | Coagulopathy | ++ | ++ | n | n | |
| Laboratory findings | Multiple oxidative phosphorylation enzymes | ↓ | ↓ | ↓ | ↓ | ↓ |

**Table 45.38** Mitochondrial RNA-processing endoribonuclease deficiency

| System | Symptoms and biomarkers | Neonatal (birth–1 month) | Infancy (1–18 months) | Childhood (1.5–11 years) | Adolescence (11–16 years) | Adulthood (>16 years) |
|---|---|---|---|---|---|---|
| Musculoskeletal | Cartilage hypoplasia | +++ | +++ | +++ | +++ | +++ |
| | Chondrodysplasia | +++ | +++ | +++ | +++ | +++ |
| Hematological | Lymphopenia | + | + | + | ± | ± |

*Notes:* Although some reports link this RNA to mtDNA replication, one study found a maximum of one molecule MRP per cell to reside in mitochondria, with the vast majority localizing to the nucleoli (PMID: 1377982). Therefore, it is not certain this is a mitochondrial disease, and the clinical features are not a good match for established mtDNA disorders.

**Table 45.39** 2-Methyl-3-hydroxybutyryl-CoA dehydrogenase deficiency

| System | Symptoms and biomarkers | Neonatal (birth–1 month) | Infancy (1–18 months) | Childhood (1.5–11 years) | Adolescence (11–16 years) | Adulthood (>16 years) |
|---|---|---|---|---|---|---|
| Cardiovascular | **Cardiomyopathy** | ± | + | + | ± | ± |
| CNS | Basal ganglia lesions (MRI) | ± | ± | ± | ± | ± |
| | Brain atrophy (MRI) | ± | ± | ± | ± | ± |
| | Choreoathetosis | ± | ± | ± | ± | ± |
| | Dysarthria | ± | ± | + | + | + |
| | **Dystonia** | ± | + | + | + | + |
| | Frontotemporal atrophy (MRI) | ± | ± | ± | ± | ± |
| | Frontotemporal atrophy (MRI) | ± | ± | + | + | + |
| | Movement disorder | ± | ± | ± | ± | ± |
| | Periventricular white matter changes | ± | ± | ± | ± | ± |
| | **Regression, psychomotor** | ± | + | + | + | + |
| | **Retardation, psychomotor** | ± | + | + | + | + |
| | **Seizures** | ± | + | + | ± | ± |
| | Spasticity | ± | ± | ± | ± | ± |
| Ear | Hearing loss, sensorineural | ± | ± | ± | ± | ± |
| Eye | Vision, decreased | ± | ± | ± | ± | ± |
| Metabolic | Hypoglycemia | ± | ± | ± | ± | ± |
| | Ketoacidosis | ± | ± | ± | ± | ± |
| | **Lactic acidosis** | ± | + | + | ± | ± |
| | Metabolic acidosis | ± | ± | ± | ± | ± |
| Musculoskeletal | Rigidity | | | ± | ± | ± |
| Other | Most patients are male | + | + | + | + | + |
| Laboratory findings | 17-Beta-hydroxysteroid dehydrogenase type 10 (fibroblasts) | ↓ | ↓ | ↓ | ↓ | ↓ |
| | 2-Methyl-3-hydroxybutyric acid (urine) | ↑ | ↑ | ↑ | ↑ | ↑ |
| | C5:1 Tiglylcarnitine (blood) | n-↑ | n-↑ | n-↑ | n-↑ | n-↑ |
| | C5:1 Tiglylcarnitine (plasma) | n-↑ | n-↑ | n-↑ | n-↑ | n-↑ |
| | C5-OH 2-Methyl-3-hydroxy-butyrylcarnitine (blood) | n-↑ | n-↑ | n-↑ | n-↑ | n-↑ |
| | C5-OH 2-Methyl-3-hydroxy-butyrylcarnitine (plasma) | n-↑ | n-↑ | n-↑ | n-↑ | n-↑ |
| | Glucose (plasma) | ↓-n | ↓-n | ↓-n | ↓-n | ↓-n |
| | Lactate (cerebrospinal fluid) | n-↑ | n-↑ | n-↑ | n-↑ | n-↑ |
| | Lactate (plasma) | n-↑ | n-↑ | n-↑ | n-↑ | n-↑ |
| | Lactate (plasma) | n-↑ | ↑ | ↑ | n-↑ | n-↑ |
| | Tiglylglycine (urine) | ↑ | ↑ | ↑ | ↑ | ↑ |

**Table 45.40** Mitochondrial ribosomal large subunit 3 deficiency MRPL3

| System | Symptoms and biomarkers | Neonatal (birth–1 month) | Infancy (1–18 months) | Childhood (1.5–11 years) | Adolescence (11–16 years) | Adulthood (>16 years) |
|---|---|---|---|---|---|---|
| Cardiovascular | Cardiomyopathy, hypertrophic | ± | ± | ± | | |
| Digestive | Liver cirrhosis | ± | ± | ± | | |
| Ear | Hearing loss, sensorineural | ± | ± | ± | | |
| Metabolic | Lactic acidosis | ± | ± | ± | | |
| Renal | Tubulointerstitial nephritis | ± | ± | ± | | |
| Laboratory findings | Lactate (plasma) | n-↑ | n-↑ | n-↑ | | |
| | Multiple oxidative phosphorylation enzymes | ↓ | ↓ | | | |

**Table 45.41** Mitochondrial ribosomal large subunit 12 deficiency MRPL12

| System | Symptoms and biomarkers | Neonatal (birth–1 month) | Infancy (1–18 months) | Childhood (1.5–11 years) | Adolescence (11–16 years) | Adulthood (>16 years) |
|---|---|---|---|---|---|---|
| CNS | Neurological deterioration | ± | ± | | | |
| Musculoskeletal | Growth retardation | ± | ± | | | |
| Laboratory findings | Multiple oxidative phosphorylation enzymes (fibroblasts) | ↓ | ↓ | | | |

**Table 45.42** Mitochondrial ribosomal large subunit 44 deficiency

| System | Symptoms and biomarkers | Neonatal (birth–1 month) | Infancy (1–18 months) | Childhood (1.5–11 years) | Adolescence (11–16 years) | Adulthood (>16 years) |
|---|---|---|---|---|---|---|
| Cardiovascular | Cardiomyopathy, hypertrophic | | ± | ± | ± | ± |
| Digestive | Liver steatosis | ± | ± | ± | ± | ± |
| Eye | Pigmentary retinopathy | ± | ± | ± | ± | ± |
| Renal | Renal insufficiency | ± | ± | ± | ± | ± |
| Laboratory findings | Mitochondrial complexes I and IV activity (heart and skeletal muscle) | ↓ | ↓ | ↓ | ↓ | ↓ |

**Table 45.43** Mitochondrial ribosomal small subunit 2 deficiency

| System | Symptoms and biomarkers | Neonatal (birth–1 month) | Infancy (1–18 months) | Childhood (1.5–11 years) | Adolescence (11–16 years) | Adulthood (>16 years) |
|---|---|---|---|---|---|---|
| CNS | Developmental delay | | ± | ± | ± | |
| | **Hypotonia** | | + | ++ | ++ | |
| Dermatological | Skin involvement | | ± | ± | ± | |
| Ear | **Hearing loss, sensorineural** | | | ++ | ++ | |
| Metabolic | **Hypoglycemia** | | | + | + | |
| Musculoskeletal | Dysmorphic features | ± | ± | ± | ± | |
| Laboratory findings | Glucose (plasma) | | | ↓ | ↓ | |
| | Lactate (plasma) | | | ↑ | ↑ | |
| | Multiple oxidative phosphorylation enzymes (liver, muscle) | | ↓↓ | ↓↓ | | |

**Table 45.44** Mitochondrial ribosomal small subunit 7 deficiency

| System | Symptoms and biomarkers | Neonatal (birth–1 month) | Infancy (1–18 months) | Childhood (1.5–11 years) | Adolescence (11–16 years) | Adulthood (>16 years) |
|---|---|---|---|---|---|---|
| Ear | **Hearing loss, sensorineural** | +++ | +++ | +++ | +++ | +++ |
| Digestive | Liver failure | | | ± | ± | ± |
| Endocrine | Hypogonadism | | | | ± | ± |
| Metabolic | Hypoglycemia | | + | + | | |
| Renal | Renal dysfunction | | | ± | ± | ± |
| Laboratory findings | Glucose (plasma) | | ↓ | ↓ | | |
| | Lactate (plasma) | | ↑ | ↑ | ↑ | |
| | Multiple oxidative phosphorylation enzymes (liver) | | ↓↓ | ↓↓ | | |

**Table 45.45** Combined oxidative phosphorylation defect 2 ($n = 1$)

| System | Symptoms and biomarkers | Neonatal (birth–1 month) | Infancy (1–18 months) | Childhood (1.5–11 years) | Adolescence (11–16 years) | Adulthood (>16 years) |
|---|---|---|---|---|---|---|
| CNS | Agenesis, corpus callosum (MRI) | ++ | | | | |
| | Hypotonia | ++ | | | | |
| | Minimal spontaneous movements | ++ | | | | |
| Musculoskeletal | Facial dysmorphism | ± | | | | |
| Other | Death | +++ | | | | |
| Laboratory findings | Lactate (plasma) | ↑↑↑ | | | | |
| | Multiple oxidative phosphorylation enzymes (liver, muscle) | ↓↓↓ | | | | |

**Table 45.46** Combined oxidative phosphorylation defect 5

| System | Symptoms and biomarkers | Neonatal (birth–1 month) | Infancy (1–18 months) | Childhood (1.5–11 years) | Adolescence (11–16 years) | Adulthood (>16 years) |
|---|---|---|---|---|---|---|
| Cardiovascular | **Cardiomyopathy, hypertrophic** | ++ | ++ | ++ | | |
| CNS | Agenesis or hypoplasia of the corpus callosum (MRI) | ++ | ++ | ++ | | |
| | **Developmental delay** | ++ | ++ | ++ | | |
| | **Hypotonia** | ++ | ++ | ++ | | |
| Dermatological | Edema, generalized | ++ | | | | |
| Digestive | Ascites | ± | | | | |
| Renal | Renal tubulopathy | ± | | | | |
| Other | Death | + | + | | | |
| Laboratory findings | Ammonia (blood) | ↑↑ | | | | |
| | Lactate (plasma) | ↑↑↑ | | | | |
| | Multiple oxidative phosphorylation enzymes (muscle, fibroblasts) | ↓↓ | ↓↓ | ↓↓ | | |

**Table 45.47** Mitochondrial ribosomal small subunit 34 deficiency

| System | Symptoms and biomarkers | Neonatal (birth–1 month) | Infancy (1–18 months) | Childhood (1.5–11 years) | Adolescence (11–16 years) | Adulthood (>16 years) |
|---|---|---|---|---|---|---|
| CNS | Developmental delay | | + | ++ | ++ | ++ |
| | **Leigh or Leigh-like syndrome** | ± | + | + | + | + |
| | Microcephaly | ± | ± | ± | ± | ± |
| Digestive | Dysphagia | | + | + | | |
| Other | Death | | + | | | |
| Laboratory findings | Lactate (plasma) | ↑↑ | ↑↑ | ↑ | ↑ | |
| | One or multiple oxidative phosphorylation enzymes (muscle, liver, fibroblasts) | ↓↓ | ↓↓ | ↓↓ | ↓↓ | |

**Table 45.48** Mitochondrial ribosomal RNA 12S deficiency

| System | Symptoms and biomarkers | Neonatal (birth–1 month) | Infancy (1–18 months) | Childhood (1.5–11 years) | Adolescence (11–16 years) | Adulthood (>16 years) |
|---|---|---|---|---|---|---|
| Ear | **Deafness** | | ± | ± | ± | ± |

**Table 45.49** Combined oxidative phosphorylation deficiency 11

| System | Symptoms and biomarkers | Neonatal (birth–1 month) | Infancy (1–18 months) | Childhood (1.5–11 years) | Adolescence (11–16 years) | Adulthood (>16 years) |
|---|---|---|---|---|---|---|
| Cardiovascular | Cardiac abnormalities | | + | | | |
| CNS | Cerebral atrophy (MRI) | | + | | | |
| | Hypotonia | + | + | | + | + |
| | Intellectual disability | | | + | + | + |
| | Seizures | + | + | | ± | ± |
| Ear | Deafness | | + | | + | + |
| Renal | Renal failure | | + | + | ++[a] | |
| Other | Death | | +++ | | | |
| | Encephalomyopathy | + | + | | | |
| Laboratory findings | Lactate (plasma) | ↑ | ↑ | | | |
| | Respiratory chain enzymes | ↓ | ↓ | | | |

[a]Two cases, kidney transplant

**Table 45.50** Mitochondrial elongation factor G1 deficiency

| System | Symptoms and biomarkers | Neonatal (birth–1 month) | Infancy (1–18 months) | Childhood (1.5–11 years) | Adolescence (11–16 years) | Adulthood (>16 years) |
|---|---|---|---|---|---|---|
| CNS | Encephalopathy | ± | ± | ± | ± | |
| Digestive | Liver failure | ± | ± | | | |
| Other | Death | + | + | ± | | |
| | Delayed growth and development | | ± | ± | ± | |
| Laboratory findings | Lactate (plasma) | ↑ | ↑ | ↑ | ↑ | |
| | Respiratory chain enzymes | ↓ | ↓ | ↓ | ↓ | |

**Table 45.51** Mitochondrial elongation factor G2 deficiency

| System | Symptoms and biomarkers | Neonatal (birth–1 month) | Infancy (1–18 months) | Childhood (1.5–11 years) | Adolescence (11–16 years) | Adulthood (>16 years) |
|---|---|---|---|---|---|---|
| CNS | Cerebellar atrophy (MRI) | ± | ± | ± | | |
| | Hypotonia | ± | | | | |
| | Microcephaly | ± | ± | ± | | |
| Endocrine | Diabetes mellitus | | | ± | | |
| Other | Death | | ± | ± | ± | |
| | Delayed growth and development | | ± | ± | | |
| Laboratory findings | Lactate (plasma) | ↑ | ↑ | ↑ | | |
| | Respiratory chain enzymes—fibroblasts | ↓ | ↓ | ↓ | | |

**Table 45.52** Mitochondrial elongation factor Ts deficiency

| System | Symptoms and biomarkers | Neonatal (birth–1 month) | Infancy (1–18 months) | Childhood (1.5–11 years) | Adolescence (11–16 years) | Adulthood (>16 years) |
|---|---|---|---|---|---|---|
| Cardiovascular | Cardiomyopathy | ± | ± | ± | ± | ± |
| CNS | Ataxia | | | ± | ± | ± |
| | Dystonia | | | | | ± |
| | Hypotonia | ± | ± | ± | | |
| Eye | Optic atrophy | | | ± | ± | ± |
| Other | Death | | + + | | | + |
| | Encephalomyopathy | ± | ± | ± | ± | ± |
| Laboratory findings | Lactate (plasma) | ↑ | ↑ | ↑ | | |
| | Respiratory chain enzymes | ↓ | ↓ | ↓ | | |

**Table 45.53** Mitochondrial elongation factor Tu deficiency

| System | Symptoms and biomarkers | Neonatal (birth–1 month) | Infancy (1–18 months) | Childhood (1.5–11 years) | Adolescence (11–16 years) | Adulthood (>16 years) |
|---|---|---|---|---|---|---|
| CNS | **Encephalopathy** | ± | ± | ± | | |
| | **Leukodystrophy** | ± | ± | ± | | |
| Other | Death | ± | ± | ± | | |
| Laboratory findings | Lactate (plasma) | ↑↑ | ↑↑ | ↑↑ | | |
| | Respiratory chain enzymes | ↓ | ↓ | ↓ | | |

**Table 45.54** Combined oxidative phosphorylation deficiency 7 C12ORF65

| System | Symptoms and biomarkers | Neonatal (birth–1 month) | Infancy (1–18 months) | Childhood (1.5–11 years) | Adolescence (11–16 years) | Adulthood (>16 years) |
|---|---|---|---|---|---|---|
| CNS | **Cerebral atrophy (MRI)** | | ± | ± | ± | ± |
| | Hypotonia | ± | ± | ± | | |
| | **Retardation, psychomotor** | | + | + | ± | ± |
| | Spastic paraplegia | ± | ± | ± | | |
| Eye | Nystagmus | ± | ± | ± | ± | ± |
| | **Optic atrophy** | ± | ± | ± | ± | ± |
| Other | Death | | | ± | | ± |
| | Encephalomyopathy | | | ± | ± | ± |
| Laboratory findings | Lactate (cerebrospinal fluid) | | | ↑ | | |
| | Respiratory chain enzymes | ↓ | ↓ | ↓ | | |

**Table 45.55** Mitochondrial tRNA(Leu) 1 deficiency

| System | Symptoms and biomarkers | Neonatal (birth–1 month) | Infancy (1–18 months) | Childhood (1.5–11 years) | Adolescence (11–16 years) | Adulthood (>16 years) |
|---|---|---|---|---|---|---|
| Cardiovascular | Cardiomyopathy | ± | | ± | ± | ± |
| CNS | Encephalopathy | ± | ± | ± | ± | ± |
| | Epilepsy | ± | ± | ± | ± | ± |
| | Stroke like episodes | | | ± | ± | ± |
| Ear | Hearing loss | | | ± | ± | ± |
| Endocrine | Diabetes mellitus | | | ± | ± | ± |
| Musculoskeletal | Exercise intolerance | | ± | ± | ± | ± |
| | Myopathy | | ± | ± | ± | ± |
| | Rhabdomyolysis | ± | ± | ± | ± | ± |
| Renal | Renal insufficiency | | ± | ± | ± | ± |
| Other | Failure to thrive | ± | ± | ± | ± | ± |
| Laboratory findings | Alanine (plasma) | ↑ | ↑ | ↑ | ↑ | ↑ |
| | Creatine kinase (plasma) | ↑ | ↑ | ↑ | ↑ | ↑ |
| | Lactate (plasma) | ↑ | ↑ | ↑ | ↑ | ↑ |

**Table 45.56** Mitochondrial tRNA(Lys) deficiency

| System | Symptoms and biomarkers | Neonatal (birth–1 month) | Infancy (1–18 months) | Childhood (1.5–11 years) | Adolescence (11–16 years) | Adulthood (>16 years) |
|---|---|---|---|---|---|---|
| Cardiovascular | Cardiomyopathy | | | | + | + |
| CNS | **Ataxia** | | | | + | + |
| | Dementia | | | | + | + |
| | **Epilepsy, generalized** | | | | + | ++ |
| | **Myoclonic epilepsy** | | | | + | +++ |
| Ear | Hearing loss | | | | + | + |
| Musculoskeletal | **Myopathy** | | | | + | ++ |
| Laboratory findings | Histochemical cytochrome *c* oxidase deficiency (muscle) | | | | ↑ | ↑↑ |
| | Lactate (cerebrospinal fluid) | | | | ↑ | ↑↑ |
| | Lactate (plasma) | | | | ↑ | ↑↑ |
| | One or multiple oxidative phosphorylation enzymes (muscle) | | | | ↓ | ↓↓ |
| | Ragged red fibers | | | | ↑ | ↑↑ |

**Table 45.57** Mitochondrial alanyl-tRNA synthetase deficiency

| System | Symptoms and biomarkers | Neonatal (birth–1 month) | Infancy (1–18 months) | Childhood (1.5–11 years) | Adolescence (11–16 years) | Adulthood (>16 years) |
|---|---|---|---|---|---|---|
| Cardiovascular | Cardiomyopathy | ++ | + | | | |
| CNS | Ataxia | | | | | |
| | Cerebellar atrophy (MRI) | | | | ± | + |
| | Developmental delay | | | ± | | |
| | **Leukoencephalopathy** | + | + | + | + | + |
| Eye | **Nystagmus** | ± | | | ± | + |
| Genitourinary | **Ovarian failure** | | | | | + |
| Other | Death | + | ++ | ± | | |
| Laboratory findings | Cytochrome c oxidase activity (skeletal muscle) | | | | | ↓ |
| | Respiratory chain enzymes (heart) | ↓ | | | | |

**Table 45.58** Mitochondrial arginine-tRNA synthetase deficiency

| System | Symptoms and biomarkers | Neonatal (birth–1 month) | Infancy (1–18 months) | Childhood (1.5–11 years) | Adolescence (11–16 years) | Adulthood (>16 years) |
|---|---|---|---|---|---|---|
| CNS | Encephalopathy | + | ± | ± | ± | |
| | Hypotonia | + | + | + | | |
| | **Intellectual disability** | | ± | ± | ± | ± |
| | Microcephaly | ± | | | | |
| | **Myoclonic epilepsy** | ± | ± | ± | ± | ± |
| | **Pontocerebellar hypoplasia (MRI)** | + + | | | | |
| | **Progressive loss of cerebral white matter** | | + | + | + | + |
| Other | Death | ++ | + | + | + | + |
| Laboratory findings | Lactate (plasma) | ↑ | ↑ | ↑ | ↑ | ↑ |
| | Respiratory chain enzymes | ↓ | ↓ | ↓ | ↓ | ↓ |

**Table 45.59** Mitochondrial asparaginyl-tRNA synthetase deficiency

| System | Symptoms and biomarkers | Neonatal (birth–1 month) | Infancy (1–18 months) | Childhood (1.5–11 years) | Adolescence (11–16 years) | Adulthood (>16 years) |
|---|---|---|---|---|---|---|
| CNS | Agenesis of the corpus callosum | ± | | | | |
| | Epilepsy | | ± | ± | ± | ± |
| | Hypomyelination of the white matter | ± | | ± | | |
| | Intellectual disability, severe | | | ± | | |
| | Microcephaly | | | ± | | |
| | Psychomotor developmental delay | | ± | | | |
| | Retardation, psychomotor | | ± | ± | | |
| Musculoskeletal | Myopathy, severe | | | | | ± |
| Other | Death | ± | ± | ± | ± | ± |
| Laboratory findings | Histochemical mitochondrial proliferation (muscle) | | | | | ↑ |
| | Lactate (plasma) | ↑ | ↑ | ↑ | ↑ | |
| | Respiratory chain enzymes | | | | | ↓ |

**Table 45.60** Mitochondrial aspartyl-tRNA synthetase deficiency

| System | Symptoms and biomarkers | Neonatal (birth–1 month) | Infancy (1–18 months) | Childhood (1.5–11 years) | Adolescence (11–16 years) | Adulthood (>16 years) |
|---|---|---|---|---|---|---|
| CNS | Ataxia, cerebellar | | | ± | ± | ± |
| | Cognitive decline | | | ± | ± | ± |
| | **Leukoencephalopathy** | | | + | + | ++ |
| | Neuropathy, axonal | | | ± | ± | ± |
| | Spasticity | | | ± | ± | ± |
| Other | Death | | | ± | ± | ± |
| Laboratory findings | Lactate (plasma) | | | ↑ | ↑ | ↑ |

**Table 45.61** Combined oxidative phosphorylation deficiency 27

| System | Symptoms and biomarkers | Neonatal (birth–1 month) | Infancy (1–18 months) | Childhood (1.5–11 years) | Adolescence (11–16 years) | Adulthood (>16 years) |
|---|---|---|---|---|---|---|
| CNS | **Brain atrophy (MRI)** | | | + | | |
| | Cognitive decline | | | + | | |
| | Delayed psychomotor development | | ± | ± | | |
| | Encephalopathy | ± | | | | |
| | Hypotonia | | ± | | | |
| | **Myoclonic and generalized tonic-clonic seizures** | | ± | + | | |
| | Tetraparesis, progressive | | | + | | |
| Ear | Hearing impairment | | | ± | | |
| Eye | Visual impairment | | | ± | | |
| Other | Death | | | ± | ± | ± |
| | Failure to thrive | | ± | | | |
| Laboratory findings | Lactate (plasma) | | ↑ | ↑ | | |
| | mtDNA levels | | | ↓ | | |
| | Respiratory chain enzymes (muscle/liver) | | ↓ | ↓ | | |

**Table 45.62** Combined oxidative phosphorylation deficiency 12

| System | Symptoms and biomarkers | Neonatal (birth–1 month) | Infancy (1–18 months) | Childhood (1.5–11 years) | Adolescence (11–16 years) | Adulthood (>16 years) |
|---|---|---|---|---|---|---|
| CNS | **Cerebellar atrophy (MRI)** | ± | ± | ± | | |
| | **Hypotonia** | ± | ± | ± | | |
| | **Psychomotor developmental delay** | | ± | ± | | |
| Other | Death | | ± | ± | ± | |
| Laboratory findings | Lactate (plasma) | ↑ | ↑ | ↑ | | |
| | Respiratory chain enzymes | ↓ | ↓ | ↓ | | |

**Table 45.63** Mitochondrial glutamyl-tRNA(Gln) amidotransferase subunit A deficiency

| System | Symptoms and biomarkers | Neonatal (birth–1 month) | Infancy (1–18 months) | Childhood (1.5–11 years) | Adolescence (11–16 years) | Adulthood (>16 years) |
|---|---|---|---|---|---|---|
| Cardiovascular | Cardiomyopathy, severe | + | + | | | |
| Metabolic | Fatal lactic acidosis | + | + | | | |
| Hematological | Anemia | + | + | | | |
| Laboratory findings | Lactate (plasma) | ↑ | ↑ | | | |

**Table 45.64** Mitochondrial glutamyl-tRNA(Gln) amidotransferase subunit B deficiency

| System | Symptoms and biomarkers | Neonatal (birth–1 month) | Infancy (1–18 months) | Childhood (1.5–11 years) | Adolescence (11–16 years) | Adulthood (>16 years) |
|---|---|---|---|---|---|---|
| Cardiovascular | Cardiomyopathy | + | + | | | |
| Hematological | Anemia | + | + | | | |
| Metabolic | Lactic acidosis | + | + | | | |
| Other | Neonatal death | + | | | | |
| Laboratory findings | Lactate (plasma) | ↑ | ↑ | | | |

**Table 45.65** Mitochondrial glutamyl-tRNA(Gln) amidotransferase subunit C deficiency

| System | Symptoms and biomarkers | Neonatal (birth–1 month) | Infancy (1–18 months) | Childhood (1.5–11 years) | Adolescence (11–16 years) | Adulthood (>16 years) |
|---|---|---|---|---|---|---|
| Cardiovascular | Cardiomyopathy | + | + | | | |
| Digestive | Hepatic dysfunction | + | + | | | |
| Hematological | Anemia | + | + | | | |
| Metabolic | Lactic acidosis | + | + | | | |
| Laboratory findings | Creatine kinase (plasma) | ↑ | ↑ | | | |
| | Lactate (plasma) | ↑ | ↑ | | | |

**Table 45.66** Mitochondrial histidyl-tRNA synthetase deficiency

| System | Symptoms and biomarkers | Neonatal (birth–1 month) | Infancy (1–18 months) | Childhood (1.5–11 years) | Adolescence (11–16 years) | Adulthood (>16 years) |
|---|---|---|---|---|---|---|
| Ear | **Hearing loss, sensorineural** | | | | + | ++ |
| Genitourinary | **Ovarian dysgenesis** | | | | + | + |

**Table 45.67** Mitochondrial isoleucyl-tRNA synthetase deficiency

| System | Symptoms and biomarkers | Neonatal (birth–1 month) | Infancy (1–18 months) | Childhood (1.5–11 years) | Adolescence (11–16 years) | Adulthood (>16 years) |
|---|---|---|---|---|---|---|
| CNS | Hypotonia | | ± | ± | ± | ± |
| | **Neuropathy, sensory** | | ± | ± | ± | ± |
| Ear | **Hearing loss, sensorineural** | | ± | ± | ± | ± |
| Endocrine | **Growth hormone deficiency** | | ± | ± | ± | ± |
| Eye | **Cataract** | | ± | ± | ± | ± |
| Musculoskeletal | **Skeletal dysplasia** | | ± | ± | ± | ± |
| Other | Death | ± | ± | ± | ± | ± |

**Table 45.68** Perrault syndrome 4

| System | Symptoms and biomarkers | Neonatal (birth–1 month) | Infancy (1–18 months) | Childhood (1.5–11 years) | Adolescence (11–16 years) | Adulthood (>16 years) |
|---|---|---|---|---|---|---|
| Ear | Hearing loss | | | | + | + |
| Endocrine | Ovarian dysfunction | | | | + | + |
| Eye | Ptosis of eyelid | | | ± | ± | ± |
| Hematological | Anemia, sideroblastic | + | | | | |
| Renal | Renal disease | ± | | | | |
| Other | Death | + | + | | | |
| | Hydrops | + | | | | |
| Laboratory findings | Lactate (plasma) | ↑↑ | ↑↑ | ↑ | ↑ | ↑ |

**Table 45.69** Mitochondrial methionyl-tRNA synthetase deficiency

| System | Symptoms and biomarkers | Neonatal (birth–1 month) | Infancy (1–18 months) | Childhood (1.5–11 years) | Adolescence (11–16 years) | Adulthood (>16 years) |
|---|---|---|---|---|---|---|
| CNS | **Ataxia** | | | ± | ± | ++ |
| | Dysarthria | | | ± | ± | ± |
| | Dystonia | | | ± | ± | ± |
| | **Hyperreflexia** | | | ± | ± | ++ |
| | Leukoencephalopathy (MRI) | | | ± | ± | ± |
| | **Spasticity** | | | ± | ± | ++ |
| Eye | Nystagmus | | | ± | ± | ± |
| Genitourinary | Neurogenic bladder | | | ± | ± | ± |
| Musculoskeletal | Scoliosis | | | ± | ± | ± |

**Table 45.70** Mitochondrial methionyl-tRNA synthetase deficiency (n = 2)

| System | Symptoms and biomarkers | Neonatal (birth–1 month) | Infancy (1–18 months) | Childhood (1.5–11 years) | Adolescence (11–16 years) | Adulthood (>16 years) |
|---|---|---|---|---|---|---|
| CNS | Hypotonia | | + | ++ | | |
| | Retardation, psychomotor | | + | + | | |
| Digestive | Constipation | | + | ++ | | |
| | Gastroesophageal reflux | | + | + | | |
| Ear | Hearing loss, sensorineural | | + | + | | |
| Musculoskeletal | Dysmorphic features | + | + | + | | |
| | Growth retardation | + | + | + | | |
| Other | Pectus carinatum | + | + | ++ | | |

**Table 45.71** Mitochondrial phenylalanyl-tRNA synthetase deficiency

| System | Symptoms and biomarkers | Neonatal (birth–1 month) | Infancy (1–18 months) | Childhood (1.5–11 years) | Adolescence (11–16 years) | Adulthood (>16 years) |
|---|---|---|---|---|---|---|
| CNS | Developmental delay | | + | + | + | |
| | Dysarthria | | | + | + | |
| | **Hyperreflexia** | | + | + | + | + |
| | **Hypotonia** | | + | + | + | + |
| | Seizures | ± | ± | ± | | |
| | **Spasticity** | | + | + | + | + |
| | Tremor | | + | + | + | |
| Genitourinary | Urinary incontinence | | | ± | ± | |
| Musculoskeletal | Scoliosis | | | ± | ± | |
| Laboratory findings | Alanine (plasma) | | ↑ | ↑ | ↑ | |
| | Lactate (plasma) | | ↑ | ↑ | ↑ | |

**Table 45.72** Mitochondrial phenylalanyl-tRNA synthetase deficiency

| System | Symptoms and biomarkers | Neonatal (birth–1 month) | Infancy (1–18 months) | Childhood (1.5–11 years) | Adolescence (11–16 years) | Adulthood (>16 years) |
|---|---|---|---|---|---|---|
| CNS | **Developmental delay** | + | ++ | ++ | ++ | |
| | **Diverse & variable CNS pathology** | | + | + | + | |
| | Hypotonia | | + | + | + | |
| | Microcephaly | ± | ± | ± | | |
| | **Retardation, psychomotor** | | ± | ± | ± | |
| | **Seizures** | ± | + | ++ | ++ | |
| Other | Death | | + | + | + | |

**Table 45.73** Mitochondrial seryl-tRNA synthetase deficiency

| System | Symptoms and biomarkers | Neonatal (birth–1 month) | Infancy (1–18 months) | Childhood (1.5–11 years) | Adolescence (11–16 years) | Adulthood (>16 years) |
|---|---|---|---|---|---|---|
| Cardiovascular | **Hypertension, pulmonary** | ++ | ++ | | | |
| Endocrine | **Diabetes mellitus** | + | + | | | |
| Hematological | Pancytopenia | ± | ± | | | |
| Metabolic | Hypochloremic metabolic alkalosis | + | ++ | | | |
| Renal | High FeMg fractional excretion | + | ++ | | | |
| | Polyuria | + | ++ | | | |
| | **Renal failure, progressive** | + | ++ | | | |
| | Salt wasting | + | ++ | | | |
| Other | **Death** | + | +++ | | | |
| | **Failure to thrive** | ++ | ++ | | | |
| | **Global developmental delay** | ++ | ++ | | | |
| | **Preterm birth** | **n.a.** | | | | |
| Laboratory findings | Creatine (plasma) | ↑↑ | ↑↑ | | | |
| | Lactate (plasma) | ↑↑ | ↑↑ | | | |
| | Magnesium (plasma) | ↓ | ↓ | | | |
| | Uric acid (plasma) | ↑↑ | ↑↑ | | | |
| | Uric acid (urine) | ↑ | ↑↑ | | | |

**Table 45.74** Mitochondrial threonyl-tRNA synthetase deficiency

| System | Symptoms and biomarkers | Neonatal (birth–1 month) | Infancy (1–18 months) | Childhood (1.5–11 years) | Adolescence (11–16 years) | Adulthood (>16 years) |
|---|---|---|---|---|---|---|
| CSF | **Delayed psychomotor development** | + | + | | | |
| | **Hypertonia, limb** | + | + | | | |
| | **Hypotonia, axial** | + | + | | | |
| Other | **Death (metabolic crisis)** | | + | | | |
| Laboratory findings | Lactate (plasma) | ↑↑ | ↑↑ | | | |
| | Multiple oxidative phosphorylation enzymes (muscle) | | ↓↓ | | | |

**Table 45.75** Mitochondrial tyrosyl-tRNA synthetase deficiency

| System | Symptoms and biomarkers | Neonatal (birth–1 month) | Infancy (1–18 months) | Childhood (1.5–11 years) | Adolescence (11–16 years) | Adulthood (>16 years) |
|---|---|---|---|---|---|---|
| Cardiovascular | **Cardiomyopathy, hypertrophic** | | | + | + | + |
| Hematological | **Anemia, sideroblastic** | | | ++ | ++ | ++ |
| Musculoskeletal | Dysmorphic features | ± | ± | ± | ± | ± |
| | Exercise intolerance | | | + | + | + |
| | **Myopathy** | | | ++ | ++ | ++ |
| Laboratory findings | Lactate (plasma) | | | ↑↑ | ↑↑ | ↑↑ |

**Table 45.76** Mitochondrial valyl-tRNA synthetase deficiency

| System | Symptoms and biomarkers | Neonatal (birth–1 month) | Infancy (1–18 months) | Childhood (1.5–11 years) | Adolescence (11–16 years) | Adulthood (>16 years) |
|---|---|---|---|---|---|---|
| Other | Encephalomyopathy | ? | ? | ? | ? | ? |

**Table 45.77** Mitochondrial tryptophanyl-tRNA synthetase deficiency

| System | Symptoms and biomarkers | Neonatal (birth–1 month) | Infancy (1–18 months) | Childhood (1.5–11 years) | Adolescence (11–16 years) | Adulthood (>16 years) |
|---|---|---|---|---|---|---|
| CNS | Ataxia | | ± | ± | ± | ± |
| | Epilepsy | ± | ± | ± | ± | ± |
| | Intellectual disability | | ± | ± | ± | ± |
| | Leukoencephalopathy | ± | ± | ± | ± | ± |
| | Retardation, psychomotor | | ± | ± | ± | ± |
| Eye | Optic atrophy | | ± | ± | ± | ± |
| Musculoskeletal | Myopathy | ± | | ± | ± | ± |
| Other | Multiorgan failure | ± | | ± | ± | ± |
| Laboratory findings | Glucose (plasma) | ↓-n | ↓-n | ↓-n | ↓-n | ↓-n |
| | Lactate (plasma) | n-↑ | n-↑ | n-↑ | n-↑ | n-↑ |

**Table 45.78** Mitochondrial and cytoplasmic glycil-tRNA synthetase deficiency

| System | Symptoms and biomarkers | Neonatal (birth–1 month) | Infancy (1–18 months) | Childhood (1.5–11 years) | Adolescence (11–16 years) | Adulthood (>16 years) |
|---|---|---|---|---|---|---|
| CNS | Charcot marie tooth disease | | ± | ± | ± | ± |
| | Distal motor neuronopathy | | ± | ± | ± | ± |

**Table 45.79** Mitochondrial and cytoplasmic lysyl-tRNA synthetase deficiency

| System | Symptoms and biomarkers | Neonatal (birth–1 month) | Infancy (1–18 months) | Childhood (1.5–11 years) | Adolescence (11–16 years) | Adulthood (>16 years) |
|---|---|---|---|---|---|---|
| CNS | Charcot marie tooth disease | | ± | ± | ± | ± |
| Ear | Deafness | | ± | ± | ± | ± |

**Table 45.80** Peptidyl-tRNA hydrolase 2 deficiency

| System | Symptoms and biomarkers | Neonatal (birth–1 month) | Infancy (1–18 months) | Childhood (1.5–11 years) | Adolescence (11–16 years) | Adulthood (>16 years) |
|---|---|---|---|---|---|---|
| CNS | **Ataxia** | | + | ++ | ++ | |
| | Cerebellar hypoplasia (progressive) | | ± | ± | ± | |
| | **Hypotonia** | ± | ± | + | + | |
| | Intellectual disability | | ± | ± | ± | |
| | Microcephaly | ± | ± | ± | ± | |
| | **Motor delay** | | + | + | + | |
| | Peripheral neuropathy | | ± | ± | ± | |
| Ear | **Hearing loss, sensorineural** | | + | ++ | ++ | |
| Endocrine | Exocrine pancreatic insufficiency | | | ± | ± | |
| | Hypothyroidism | | ± | ± | ± | |
| Musculoskeletal | Brachycephaly | ± | ± | ± | ± | |
| | Facial dysmorphism | ± | ± | ± | ± | |
| | **Growth retardation** | | + | + | + | |
| | **Hand and foot deformities** | + | + | + | + | |
| | **Muscle weakness** | ± | ± | + | + | |
| Other | **Failure to thrive** | | + | + | + | |

**Table 45.81** Perrault syndrome 6 ERAL1

| System | Symptoms and biomarkers | Neonatal (birth–1 month) | Infancy (1–18 months) | Childhood (1.5–11 years) | Adolescence (11–16 years) | Adulthood (>16 years) |
|---|---|---|---|---|---|---|
| Ear | **Hearing loss, sensorineural** | | | ++ | ++ | +++ |
| Endocrine | **Ovarian dysgenesis** | – | – | | ++ | +++ |
| Laboratory findings | Estradiol (plasma) | n.a. | n.a. | n.a. | ↓ | ↓ |
| | Follicle-stimulating hormone (FSH) | | | | ↑↑ | ↑↑ |
| | Luteinizing hormone (LH) | n.a. | n.a. | n.a. | ↑ | ↑ |

**Table 45.82** NOP2/SUN RNA methyltransferase 3 deficiency ($n = 1$)

| System | Symptoms and biomarkers | Neonatal (birth–1 month) | Infancy (1–18 months) | Childhood (1.5–11 years) | Adolescence (11–16 years) | Adulthood (>16 years) |
|---|---|---|---|---|---|---|
| CNS | Developmental delay | | + | | | |
| | Microcephaly | | + | | | |
| Eye | Nystagmus | | + | | | |
| | Ophthalmoplegia | | + | | | |
| Musculoskeletal | Muscle weakness | | + | | | |
| Laboratory findings | Lactate (plasma) | | ↑ | | | |
| | Respiratory chain enzymes (muscle) | | ↓ | | | |

**Table 45.83** Mitochondrial ribosomal small subunit 25 deficiency ($n = 1$)

| System | Symptoms and biomarkers | Neonatal (birth–1 month) | Infancy (1–18 months) | Childhood (1.5–11 years) | Adolescence (11–16 years) | Adulthood (>16 years) |
|---|---|---|---|---|---|---|
| CNS | Agenesis corpus callosum | | + | | | |
| | Dyskinetic cerebral palsy | | +++ | | | |
| | Psycomotor delay | | ++ | | | |
| Musculoskeletal | Myopathy | | | | | + |
| Laboratory findings | Activity respiratory chain complexes IV in muscle | | | | | ↓↓ |
| | Activity respiratory chain complexes (I, III, IV) in fibroblasts | | | | | ↓↓ |
| | Lactate (cerebrospinal fluid) | | n-↑ | | | |
| | Lactate (plasma) | | n-↑ | | | |
| | Mitochondrial translation | | | | | ↓↓↓ |

## Reference Values

| Compound | Serum/blood (μmol/L) | Urine (mmol/mol creat) | Cerebrospinal fluid (μmol/L) |
|---|---|---|---|
| Lactate | 450–1800 (B) | <270 (<2 months)<br><200 (2 months–2 years)<br><85 (>2 years) | 1100–1700 |
| Pyruvate | 60–100 (B) | | 80–140 |
| Lactate/pyruvate ratio | <15 (B) | | <15 |
| Alanine | 150–450 (P, S) | 70–250 (<6 months)<br>35–165 (6 months–1 year)<br>25–130 (1 year–7 year)<br>20–70 (>7 year) | 16–41 (<1 year)<br>13–31 (1–3 year)<br>13–31 (>3 year) |
| Acetoacetate | 5–50 (P) | | |
| 3-Hydroxybutyrate | 15–90 (B) | | |
| 3-Hydroxybutyrate/acetoacetate ratio | <1.0 (B) | | |
| Ammonia | 10–50 (P) | | |
| Creatine kinase | <200 (M)(S, U/l)<br><170 (F)(S, U/l) | | |
| Protein (total) | | | 450–1100<br>(<1 month, mg/L)<br>160–650<br>(>1 month, mg/L) |
| Ethylmalonic acid | | <20 | |
| 3-Methylglutaconic acid | | <20 | |

## Pathologic Values

| Compound | Serum/blood (μmol/L) | Urine (mmol/mol creat) | Cerebrospinal fluid (μmol/L) |
|---|---|---|---|
| Lactate | >2000 (B) | >350 (<2 months)<br>>300 (2 months–2 years)<br>>130 (>2 years) | >2000 |
| Pyruvate | >130 (B) | | >200 |
| Lactate/pyruvate ratio | >17 (B) | | >17 |
| Alanine | >450 (P, S) | >300 (<6 months)<br>>150 (6 months–7 years)<br>>100 (>7 years) | |
| 3-Hydroxybutyrate + acetoacetate ratio | Postprandial increase (B) | | |
| Ammonia | >100 (P) | | |
| Creatine kinase | >200 (M)(S, U/L)<br>>170 (F)(S, U/L) | | |
| Protein (total) | | | >1300 (<1 month, mg/L)<br>>650 (>1 month, mg/L) |
| Ethylmalonic acid | | >25 | |
| 3-Methylglutaconic acid | | >25 | |

*B* Blood, *S* Serum, *P* Plasma, *M* Male, *F* Female, *U/L* Units/liter

## Diagnostic Flowchart

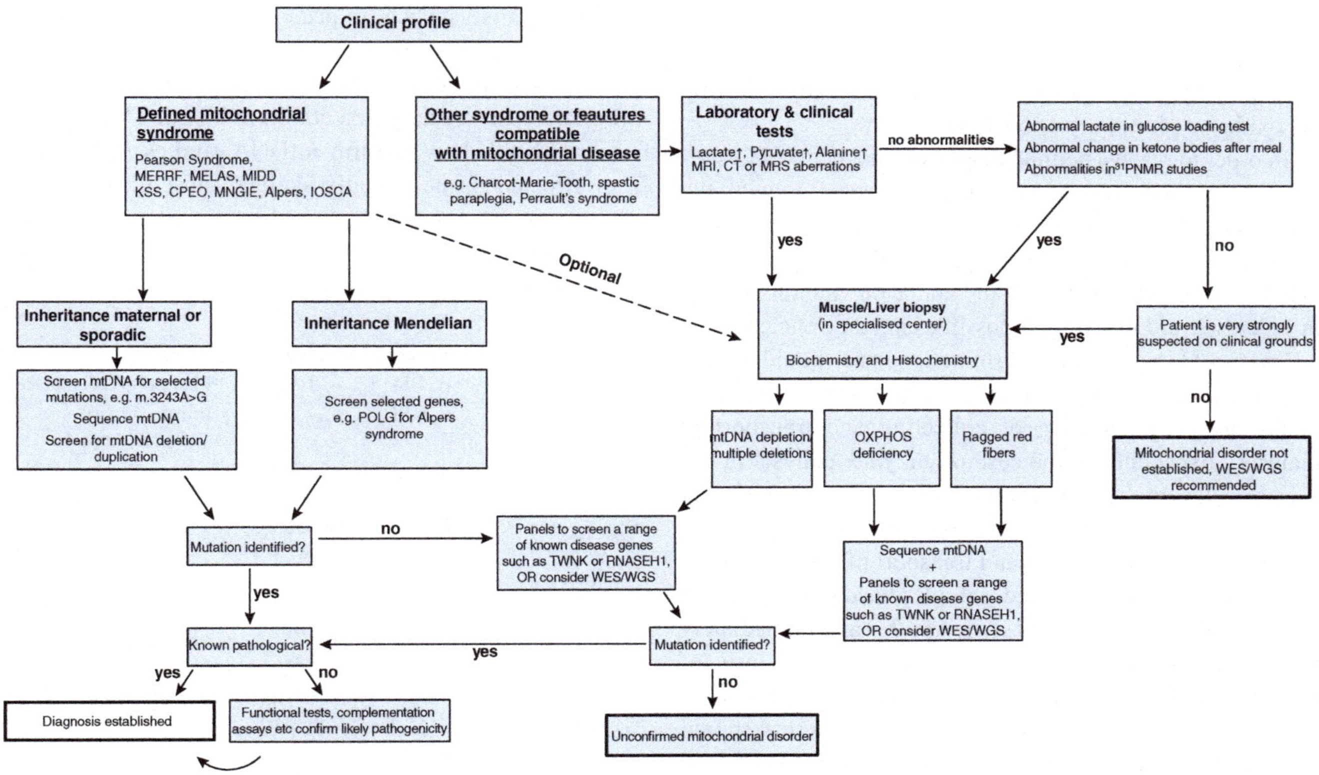


**Fig. 45.2** Common practice diagnostic flowchart for mitochondrial oxidative phosphorylation defects caused by defects in replication, transcription or translation of mtDNA

## Specimen Collection

The remainder of this Chapter reflects similar information to that found in Chap. 44, since both Chaps. 44 and 45 deal with mitochondrial diseases directly or indirectly affecting the oxidative phosphorylation system.

In order to reach a definite diagnosis, biochemical examination of tissue specimens is usually required, with the exception of a small number of well-defined mitochondrial syndromes that can be tested genetically. As a rule, the patient under investigation should not be on vitamin therapy, in order to avoid masking of possible enzyme deficiencies.

For most biochemical determinations one should ask the diagnostic centre for information about specific requirements as to the practice of collecting and transporting material. Especially in the case of enzyme analysis in tissues or cells, one must consult the diagnostic laboratory in advance about the conditions for removal, preparation, storage (usually at −70 °C) and transport of the specimens. If fresh tissue is to be studied, samples have to be collected in a special, ice-cold but not frozen buffer and immediately transported to the laboratory. The biochemical tests of mitochondrial flux measurements, such as oxygen consumption, substrate oxidation and ATP production should be performed within 2 h of collection. Frozen tissue samples are suitable for the analysis of individual mitochondrial enzymes and histochemical tests.

The physician should inform the laboratory about the clinical findings to ensure an adequate analysis and to aid data interpretation. It is important to discuss which type of tissue or cell is preferable in each case, thereby causing the patient as little inconvenience as possible. Tissue-specific expression of mitochondrial deficiencies renders fibroblasts and lymphocytes less universally appropriate than skeletal muscle, although fibroblast analysis does have an added diagnostic value when combined with a muscle sample examination, and it is surprising how often mitochondrial abnormalities are evident in cells cultured in the laboratory [e.g (Bugiardini et al. 2019)].

In the case of unexpected death, tissue, blood and urine specimens should be collected as soon as possible after death. They should be snap frozen (not fixed) immediately after collection using liquid nitrogen, and stored for possible additional studies. For enzymatic purposes tissues must be removed within 1–2 h after death and should be frozen immediately in liquid nitrogen. Skin biopsies can be performed as late as 48 h after death, and must be collected at room temperature in cell culture medium, after which the biopsy can be transported at room temperature to the cell culture laboratory.

Because few reference values are generally available for neonates, it is recommended to perform a muscle biopsy beyond the first month of life, unless a life-threatening situation exists.

MtDNA analysis can, in principle, be performed in all types of tissues or cells available. However, heteroplasmy varies from tissue to tissue, and partial deletions of mtDNA are not usually detectable in blood. Therefore, it is recommended to perform mtDNA studies in biopsies from affected tissue (usually skeletal muscle). However, some mutations can also be tested non-invasively, such as LHON mutations in blood and the MELAS/MIDD m.3243A>G mutation in urine.

| Test | Material | Storage | Pitfalls |
|---|---|---|---|
| Lactate | B, CSF, U | −20 °C | Prevent glycolysis |
| Pyruvate | B, CSF | −20 °C | Prevent glycolysis and LDH activity |
| Amino acids | S, P, U, CSF | −20 °C | – |
| Blood gases | B | No storage allowed | – |
| Creatine kinase | S | −20 °C | – |
| Acetoacetate | B | −20 °C | Feeding state is important |
| 3-Hydroxybutyrate | B | −20 °C | Feeding state is important |
| Carnitine | S, M, L, FB | −20 °C | – |
| Organic acids | U | −20 °C | – |

| Screening | Material | Storage | Pitfalls |
|---|---|---|---|
| Amino acids | U | −70 °C | Anti epileptic drugs, antibiotic artefacts |
| Pyruvate dehydrogenase | M, FB, L, CV | −70 °C | |
| 2-Oxoglutarate dehydrogenase | M, FB, L | −70 °C | |
| Fumarase | M, FB, L | −70 °C | |
| Respiratory chain enzymes | M, FB, L, CV | −70 °C | |
| ATPase | M, FB | −70 °C | |
| ATP/ ADP-translocator | M, FB, L | −70 °C | |
| Substrate oxidations | M, FB, FL | No storage allowed | Maintain at 0 °C |
| ATP production | M, FB | No storage allowed | Maintain at 0 °C |
| Oxygen consumption | M, FB, BrF | No storage allowed | Maintain at 0 °C |
| Coupling state | M, FB | No storage allowed | Maintain at 0 °C |
| DNA | | | |
| Respiratory chain enzymes | M, FB, B | −20 °C | |

*M* Muscle (fresh or frozen), *L* Liver (fresh or frozen), *MF* Fresh muscle required, *LF* Fresh liver required, *BrF* Brain (fresh), *FB* Fibroblasts, *CV* Chorionic villi

## Prenatal Diagnosis

At present prenatal diagnosis, at the enzyme level, in mitochondrial disorders can be performed in families in which the proband is suffering (or has suffered) from a complex I, complex II, succinate:cytochrome *c* oxidoreductase, complex IV or pyruvate dehydrogenase deficiency (or combinations of these enzymes), at least in our centre. A prerequisite for prenatal diagnosis at the enzyme level is that mtDNA mutations must have been excluded in the proband. In case an mtDNA mutation has been identified, preimplantation genetic diagnosis (PGD) is possible.

PGD is an IVF-based treatment that may be suitable for some women who are at risk of transmitting a mitochondrial DNA mutation to their children (Poulton et al. 2010). PGD for mtDNA disease is based on the principle that the level of mutated mitochondrial DNA can vary widely between eggs produced by a women who carries a mixture of mutated and normal mitochondrial DNA. PGD is only suitable for women who are expected to produce some eggs with low levels of mutated mitochondrial DNA.

Prenatal diagnosis at the enzyme level is preferably performed in native chorionic villi because they can be obtained earlier in pregnancy as compared with amniocytes. Moreover, it is not necessary to cultivate chorionic villi in contrast with amniocytes, thus reducing the time of the diagnostic procedure considerably. In case the investigation of chorionic villi yields no conclusive result, amniocytes can also be investigated, although in practice this is hardly ever necessary. In case causative mutations in the nuclear DNA have been identified, prenatal diagnosis is possible using conventional prenatal genetic testing for all nuclear genetic defect. Because of the expanding possibilities of molecular genetic testing of suspected mitochondrial patients, nuclear DNA-based prenatal diagnosis is expected to increase in the future. However, for those families in which it has not (yet) been possible to identify the causative genetic defect, the measurement of enzyme activities in chorionic villi provides an alternative possibility for prenatal diagnostic testing.

## Treatment

In contrast to the progress in understanding biochemical and molecular aspects of mitochondrial disease, treatment is still limited. Many potentially therapeutic agents have been used to treat mitochondrial disorders, but few of these disorders have any proven effective therapy. The management of mitochondrial disease is largely supportive, therefore clinicians must have a thorough knowledge of the potential complications of mitochondrial disorders to prevent unnecessary morbidity and mortality.

### Supportive Therapy

- *Central nervous system*: Seizures should be treated adequately, and in many cases respond well to conventional anticonvulsants. Valproic acid should be used with great caution, and has strong contraindication in, for example, Alpers-Huttenlocher syndrome.
- *Heart*: Timely placement of a pacemaker can be lifesaving in patients with cardiac conduction blocks. Cardiomyopathy can be treated with heart-failure therapy. Heart transplantation is controversial, but when cardiac involvement is the predominant problem, transplantation is justified.
- *Gastrointestinal:* Patients often have complaints of vomiting, diarrhea, constipation or abdominal pain related to dysmotility, which can be treated with prokinetics and/or laxatives. Because of these problems the diet can be inadequate, and for this reason patients should be referred to a dietician for evaluation. Exocrine pancreatic dysfunction requires replacement therapy with pancreatic enzymes.
- *Kidney:* Patients with proteinuria may be treated with ACE inhibitors. Renal tubular acidosis and Fanconi syndrome require therapy to readjust electrolyte balance. Patients with renal failure may also require dialysis or a renal transplant. Patients with a known mitochondrial disorder due to an mtDNA mutation should not be transplanted with a kidney from a maternal family member.
- *Endocrine:* Diabetes can be treated with oral medication, but as the disease progresses usually insulin is required. Hypothyroidism can be treated with thyroid hormone.
- *Eye:* Ptosis can be ameliorated by surgery, although the results of blepharoplasty are often transient. Congenital cataracts are also treated surgically.
- *Hearing*: Hearing aids are often necessary. When hearing problems are progressive, cochlear implants may be useful.
- *Muscular:* Aerobic exercise is useful in mitochondrial disease, improving work capacity, oxygen delivery to muscle (i.e. cardiac output), oxygen extraction and utilization by muscle and muscle energy metabolism. Sustained aerobic exercise is associated with mitochondrial proliferation (reflected by increased activity of citrate synthase) and improvement of respiratory chain activity (reflected by increased activity of COX) (Jeppesen et al. 2006). The specific questions that arise in those disorders associated with heteroplasmic mtDNA mutations are whether exercise preferentially promotes proliferation of normal mitochondria and, if not, whether proliferation of both normal mitochondria and abnormal mitochondria is beneficial. The former could increase ATP production, whereas the latter could increase production of reactive oxygen species. These questions have not yet been totally resolved but are being addressed in ongoing clinical trials.

## Vitamins and Cofactors

Over the last 15 years several open-label and randomized control clinical trials for potential treatments of mitochondrial diseases have been reported or are in progress. These include trials of administering dichloroacetate (an activator of PDHc), arginine or citrulline (precursors of nitric oxide), coenzyme $Q_{10}$ ($CoQ_{10}$; part of the electron transport chain and an antioxidant), idebenone (a synthetic analogue of $CoQ_{10}$), EPI-743 (a novel oral potent 2-electron redox cycling agent), creatine (a precursor of phosphocreatine) and combined administration (of creatine, α-lipoate, and $CoQ_{10}$). These trials have included patients with various mitochondrial disorders, a selected subcategory of mitochondrial disorders, or specific mitochondrial disorders (LHON, MELAS, Leigh). Trial designs varied from open-label/uncontrolled to open-label/controlled or double-blind/placebo-controlled/crossover. Primary outcomes ranged from single, clinically relevant scores to multiple measures. Eight of these trials have been well-controlled, completed trials (Glover et al. 2010). Of these only one (treatment with creatine) showed a significant change in primary outcomes, but this was not reproduced in two subsequent trials with creatine with different patients. One trial (idebenone treatment of LHON) did not show significant improvement in the primary outcome, but there was significant improvement in a subgroup of patients (Klopstock et al. 2013).

Despite the paucity of benefits found so far, well-controlled clinical trials are essential in the continuing search for more effective treatment of mitochondrial disease (Pfeffer et al. 2013), and current trials based on information gained from these prior experiences are in progress. Because of difficulties in recruiting sufficient mitochondrial disease patients and the relatively large expense of conducting such trials, advantageous strategies include crossover designs (where possible), multicentre collaboration and the selection of very few, clinically relevant, primary outcomes.

## Emergency Treatment

| Medication | Indication | Dose (route) |
|---|---|---|
| Sodium bicarbonate | Severe lactic acidosis (lactate >7 mmol/L) | (0.33 mmol/kg) × base deficit |
| L-arginine | Acute stroke like episode | 150–500 mg/kg/day (IV) |

**Funding** AS is supported by UK Medical Research Council Senior Non-clinical Fellowship (MC_PC_13029), the Muscular Dystrophy UK and the Lily Foundation. IJH is supported by grants 2018111043 and 2018222031 Departamento de Salud, Euskadi and P17/00380, Carlos III Departamento de Salud. JNS was in part supported by the "Prinses Beatrix Spierfonds" and the "Stichting Spieren voor Spieren" (W.OR15-05) and is supported by the European Union's Horizon 2020 research and innovation programme under the Marie Sklodowska-Curie grant agreement No 721757.

## References

Amunts A, Brown A, Toots J, Scheres SH, Ramakrishnan V. Ribosome. The structure of the human mitochondrial ribosome. Science. 2015;348(6230):95–8.

Andrews RM, Kubacka I, Chinnery PF, Lightowlers RN, Turnbull DM, Howell N. Reanalysis and revision of the Cambridge reference sequence for human mitochondrial DNA. Nat Genet. 1999;23(2):147.

Bugiardini E, Poole OV, Manole A, Pittman AM, Horga A, Hargreaves I, et al. Clinicopathologic and molecular spectrum of RNASEH1-related mitochondrial disease. Neurol Genet. 2017;3(3):e149.

Bugiardini E, Mitchell AL, Rosa ID, Horning-Do HT, Pitmann A, Poole OV, et al. MRPS25 mutations impair mitochondrial translation and cause encephalomyopathy. Hum Mol Genet. 2019;

Dalla Rosa I, Camara Y, Durigon R, Moss CF, Vidoni S, Akman G, et al. MPV17 loss causes deoxynucleotide insufficiency and slow DNA replication in mitochondria. PLoS Genet. 2016;12(1):e1005779.

D'Souza AR, Minczuk M. Mitochondrial transcription and translation: overview. Essays Biochem. 2018;62(3):309–20.

Glover EI, Martin J, Maher A, Thornhill RE, Moran GR, Tarnopolsky MA. A randomized trial of coenzyme Q10 in mitochondrial disorders. Muscle Nerve. 2010;42(5):739–48.

Gonzalez-Serrano LE, Chihade JW, Sissler M. When a common biological role does not imply common disease outcomes: disparate pathology linked to human mitochondrial aminoacyl-tRNA synthetases. J Biol Chem. 2019;294(14):5309–20.

Goto Y-I, Nonaka I, Horai S. A mutation in the $tRNA^{Leu(UUR)}$ gene associated with the MELAS subgroup of mitochondrial encephalomyopathies. Nature. 1990;348:651–3.

Hensen F, Potter A, van Esveld SL, Tarres-Sole A, Chakraborty A, Sola M, et al. Mitochondrial RNA granules are critically dependent on mtDNA replication factors twinkle and mtSSB. Nucleic Acids Res. 2019;47(7):3680–98.

Holt IJ, Harding AE, Morgan-Hughes JA. Deletions of muscle mitochondrial DNA in patients with mitochondrial myopathies. Nature. 1988;331(6158):717–9.

Jeppesen TD, Schwartz M, Olsen DB, Wibrand F, Krag T, Duno M, et al. Aerobic training is safe and improves exercise capacity in patients with mitochondrial myopathy. Brain. 2006;129(Pt 12):3402–12.

Klopstock T, Metz G, Yu-Wai-Man P, Buchner B, Gallenmuller C, Bailie M, et al. Persistence of the treatment effect of idebenone in Leber's hereditary optic neuropathy. Brain. 2013;136(Pt 2):e230.

de Laat P, Koene S, van den Heuvel LP, Rodenburg RJ, Janssen MC, Smeitink JA. Clinical features and heteroplasmy in blood, urine and saliva in 34 Dutch families carrying the m.3243A > G mutation. J Inherit Metab Dis. 2012;35(6):1059–69.

Martin CA, Sarlos K, Logan CV, Thakur RS, Parry DA, Bizard AH, et al. Mutations in TOP3A cause a bloom syndrome-like disorder. Am J Hum Genet. 2018;103(2):221–31.

Nishino I, Spinazzola A, Hirano M. Thymidine phosphorylase gene mutations in MNGIE, a human mitochondrial disorder. Science. 1999;283(5402):689–92.

Ojala D, Montoya J, Attardi G. tRNA punctuation model of RNA processing in human mitochondria. Nature. 1981;290:470–4.

van den Ouweland JM, Lemkes HH, Trembath RC, Ross R, Velho G, Cohen D, et al. Maternally inherited diabetes and deafness is a distinct subtype of diabetes and associates with a single point mutation in the mitochondrial tRNA(Leu(UUR)) gene. Diabetes. 1994;43(6):746–51.

Pfeffer G, Horvath R, Klopstock T, Mootha VK, Suomalainen A, Koene S, et al. New treatments for mitochondrial disease-no time to drop our standards. Nat Rev Neurol. 2013;9(8):474–81.

Pohjoismaki JLO, Forslund JME, Goffart S, Torregrosa-Munumer R, Wanrooij S. Known unknowns of mammalian mitochondrial DNA maintenance. BioEssays. 2018;40(9):e1800102.

Poulton J, Chiaratti MR, Meirelles FV, Kennedy S, Wells D, Holt IJ. Transmission of mitochondrial DNA diseases and ways to prevent them. PLoS Genet. 2010;6(8)

Spelbrink JN, Li FY, Tiranti V, Nikali K, Yuan QP, Tariq M, et al. Human mitochondrial DNA deletions associated with mutations in the gene encoding twinkle, a phage T7 gene 4-like protein localized in mitochondria. Nat Genet. 2001;28(3):223–31.

Van Goethem G, Dermaut B, Lofgren A, Martin JJ, Van Broeckhoven C. Mutation of POLG is associated with progressive external ophthalmoplegia characterized by mtDNA deletions. Nat Genet. 2001;28(3):211–2.

# Disorders of Mitochondrial Homeostasis, Dynamics, Protein Import, and Quality Control

# 46

Lonneke de Boer, Maaike C. de Vries, Jan A. M. Smeitink, and Werner J. H. Koopman

## Contents



*Potential conflict of interest:* JAMS is the founding CEO of the SME Khondrion B.V. (Nijmegen, The Netherlands). WJHK is a scientific advisor of Khondrion. This company had no involvement in this manuscript.

L. de Boer · M. C. de Vries · J. A. M. Smeitink
Department of Pediatrics, Radboud Center for Mitochondrial Medicine, Radboud University Medical Centre (Radboudumc), Nijmegen, The Netherlands
e-mail: jan.smeitink@radboudumc.nl

W. J. H. Koopman (✉)
Department of Biochemistry (286), Radboud Institute for Molecular Life Sciences (RIMLS), Radboud Center for Mitochondrial Medicine, Radboud University Medical Centre (Radboudumc), Nijmegen, The Netherlands
e-mail: Werner.Koopman@radboudumc.nl

## Summary

This chapter describes gene mutations and disorders linked to mitochondrial homeostasis, dynamics, protein import, and quality control. Although clinically highly variable, we here functionally categorized these mutations as impacting on mitochondrial biogenesis, mitochondrial morphology/motility ("mitochondrial dynamics"), and mitochondrial degradation ("mitophagy"). These three processes are described in more detail in the Introduction. In addition, several other mutations that affect mitochondrial function are presented. The gene mutations discussed in this chapter are all nuclear DNA


N. Blau et al. (eds.), *Physician's Guide to the Diagnosis, Treatment, and Follow-Up of Inherited Metabolic Diseases*,
https://doi.org/10.1007/978-3-030-67727-5_46

(nDNA) mutations. Most patients with mitochondrial disorders present with a multi-system disorder. The organs requiring the most energy, such as the brain, retina, heart, kidney, and skeletal muscle, are most commonly and severely affected. Onset of disease can be at any age and the symptoms are almost always progressive. A definitive diagnosis solely based on clinical signs and symptoms is very unlikely. Whole exome/genome sequencing (WES/WGS) has greatly improved disease diagnosis and often simplified it, although in some cases has also resulted in new diagnostic challenges. Nonetheless, clinical diagnostic criteria, combined with brain imaging, metabolic, biochemical, and other functional tests are still needed. Since specific treatment options are still limited, the management of the described mitochondrial disorders is largely supportive. For diagnosis and treatment, patients should be referred to a specialized center.

## Introduction

Mitochondria consist of a double membrane system, the mitochondrial outer membrane (MOM) and mitochondrial inner membrane (MIM), which envelops the mitochondrial matrix compartment. The MIM is highly folded to accommodate the many proteins and protein complexes required for mitochondrial ATP production and other functions (Bulthuis et al. 2019). Mitochondrial functioning requires about ~1500 proteins. Since the mitochondrial DNA (mtDNA) encodes only for 13 proteins the majority of mitochondrial proteins is encoded by the nuclear DNA (nDNA; Koopman et al. 2012). These nDNA-encoded proteins are synthesized in the cytosol and are imported into mitochondria by a dedicated machinery consisting of translocases of the mitochondrial outer membrane (TOM) and translocases of the mitochondrial inner membrane (TIM). This TOM/TIM system not only imports nDNA-encoded proteins, but also carries out posttranslational modifications and mediates the sorting of imported proteins to the correct mitochondrial subcompartment: MOM, MIM, matrix, or intermembrane space (IMS). In this sense (Fig. 46.1a), proper functioning of the TIM/TOM system is crucial for mitochondrial biogenesis and sustained mitochondrial functioning (Jackson et al. 2018). Inside cells, single mitochondria are motile and continuously fuse and divide. Although still incompletely understood, these "mitochondrial dynamics" are required for cell and organismal survival in allowing (Kluge et al. 2013): (1) individual mitochondria to reach distant parts of the cell (e.g., for their local functioning in neurons), (2) mixing of mitochondrial content (e.g., to exchange mtDNA or damaged biomolecules), (3) distribution of mitochondria between daughter cells during cell division, and (4) degradation of dysfunctional mitochondria (see below). Three main proteins are currently described to be involved in mitochondrial fusion: Mitofusin 1 (Mfn1), Mitofusin 2 (Mfn2), and Optic Atrophy Protein 1 (OPA1). With respect to mitochondrial fission, 6 main proteins were implicated: Dynamin-related protein 1 (Drp1/DNM1L), Dynamin 2 (Dyn2), Fission protein 1 (Fis1), Mitochondrial Elongation Factor 1 (MIEF1), Mitochondrial Elongation Factor 2 (MIEF2), and Mitochondrial fission factor (Mff). The function of mitochondrial fission/fusion proteins is interfaced with cellular regulatory pathways and redox signaling, primarily by posttranslational modifications like phosphorylation (Willems et al. 2015). As a consequence of mitochondrial dynamics, mitochondrial morphology can be highly heterogeneous within/between cells and ranges from "filamentous" (elongated) to fragmented phenotypes (Fig. 46.1b). Experimental evidence suggests that mitochondrial function and morphology are mutually dependent, giving rise to the concept of mitochondrial "morphofunction" (Bulthuis et al. 2019).

Following biogenesis, it is believed that individual mitochondria can accumulate damage during their life cycle. This, for instance, could be due to the presence of mitochondrial protein-encoding gene mutations, increased reactive oxygen species (ROS) levels, or external influences like environmental toxins or off-target drug effects (Koopman et al. 2012). As a homeostatic system, cells are equipped with a mitochondrial quality control mechanism that removes dysfunctional organelles by autophagy (Fig. 46.1c). The current evidence suggests that dysfunctional mitochondria are unable to maintain their trans-MIM inside-negative electrical potential ($\Delta\psi$), and that this inability can trigger mitochondria-specific autophagy ("mitophagy"). Depending on the extent of $\Delta\psi$ depolarization, mitochondrial dysfunction is associated with MOM rupture, reduced $O_2$ consumption, and blocked ATP synthesis. In the mitophagy mechanism, $\Delta\psi$ depolarization activates MOM accumulation of PTEN-induced kinase 1 (PINK1). Next, PINK recruits and activates the protein Parkin to ultimately stimulate mitochondrial recognition by the autophagy machinery (Gustaffson and Dorn 2nd 2019). In addition to this "Parkin-dependent pathway," there are also various other mechanisms to recognize and remove dysfunction mitochondria, including receptor- and lipid-mediated pathways (Yang et al. 2019).

## Nomenclature

| | Disorder | Alternative name(s) | Abbreviation | Gene symbol | Chromosomal localization | Inheritance | Affected protein | OMIM |
|---|---|---|---|---|---|---|---|---|
| 46.1 | Peroxisomal and mitochondrial fission defect | Dynamin-like protein 1 deficiency; Encephalopahty, lethal, due to defective mitochondrial peroxisomal fission | DLP1 deficiency | *DNM1L* | 12p11.21 | AR, AD | Dynamin-like protein 1 | 614388 |
| 46.2 | Mitochondrial fission factor deficiency | Encephalopathy due to defective mitochondrial and peroxisomal fission type 2 | MFF deficiency | *MFF* | 2q36.3 | AR | Mitochondrial fission factor 1 | 617086 |
| 46.3 | GDAP1 deficiency | Axonal Charcot-Marie-Tooth type 2K<br>Demyelinating Charcot-Marie-Tooth disease type 4A | CMT2K; CMT4A | *GDAP1* | 8q21.11 | AR, AD | Ganglioside-induced differentiation-associated protein 1 | 607831<br>214400 |
| 46.4 | STAT2 deficiency | Immunodeficiency type 44 | IMD44 | *STAT2* | 12q13.3 | AR | Signal transducer and activator of transcription 2 | 616636 |
| 46.5 | UGO-1 like protein deficiency | Hereditary motor and sensory neuropathy type 6B | HMSN6B | *SLC25A46* | 5q22.1 | AR | Solute carrier family 25, member 46 | 616505 |
| 46.6 | Childhood-onset optic atrophy type 1 | Juvenile Optic Atrophy | OPA1 | *OPA1* | 3q28-q29 | AD | Optic Atrophy 1 | 165500 |
| 46.7 | Optic Atrophy 1 and Deafness | Behr syndrome | – | *OPA1* | 3q28-q29 | AR, AD | Optic Atrophy 1 | 125250 |
| 46.8 | Costeff syndrome | Methylglutaconic aciduria type III | MGA3 | *OPA3* | 19q13.2-13.3 | AR, AD | Outer mitochondrial membrane lipid metabolism regulator | 258501 |
| 46.9 | Mitofusin 2 deficiency | Axonal Charcot-Marie-Tooth type 2A2A and 2A2B | CMT2A2A; CMT2A2B | *MFN2* | 1p36.22 | AR, AD | Mitofusin 2 | 609260; 617087 |
| 46.10 | MSTO1 deficiency | Mitochondrial myopathy and ataxia | MMYAT | *MSTO1* | 1q22 | AR, AD | Mitochondrial distribution and morphology regulator | 617675 |
| 46.11 | DNAJC19 deficiency | Dilated cardiomyopathy with ataxia (DCMA syndrome); 3-Methylglutaconic aciduria type 5 | MGCA5 | *DNAJC19* | 3q26.33 | AR | DNAJ/HSP40 homolog, subfamily C, member 19 | 610198 |
| 46.12 | Mohr-Tranebjaerg syndrome | Dystonia Deafness Syndrome | MTS | *TIMM8A* | Xq22.1 | X-linked | Translocase of inner mitochondrial membrane 8A | 304700 |
| 46.13 | TIMMDC1 deficiency | Mitochondrial complex I deficiency | | *TIMMDC1* | 3q13.33 | AR | Translocase of inner mitochondrial membrane domain-containing protein 1 | 252010 |
| 46.14 | Mitochondrial epileptic encephalopathy TIMM50 | Intellectual disability and seizure disorder due to TIMM50 variant | TIMM50 | *TIMM50* | 19q13.2 | AR | Translocase of inner mitochondrial membrane 50 | 607381 |
| 46.15 | GFER deficiency | Myopathy, mitochondrial progressive, with congenital cataract, hearing loss, and developmental delay | | *GFER* | 16p13.3 | AR | Growth factor, ERV1-like | 613076 |
| 46.16 | MAGMAS deficiency | Spondylometaphyseal dysplasia, Megarbane-Dagher-Melike type | SMDMDM | *PAM16* | 16p13.3 | AR | Presequence translocase-associated motor 16 | 613320 |

(continued)

| | Disorder | Alternative name(s) | Abbreviation | Gene symbol | Chromosomal localization | Inheritance | Affected protein | OMIM |
|---|---|---|---|---|---|---|---|---|
| 46.17 | Acylglycerol kinase deficiency | Sengers syndrome;<br>Cataract 38, autosomal recessive | | *AGK* | 7q34 | AR | Acylglycerol kinase | 212350; 614691 |
| 46.18 | Mitochondrial processing peptidase alpha deficiency | Autosomal recessive spinocerebellar ataxia type 2 | SCAR2 | *PMPCA* | 9q34.3 | AR | Peptidase, mitochondrial processing, alpha | 213200 |
| 46.19 | Mitochondrial processing peptidase beta deficiency | Multiple mitochondrial dysfunctions syndrome 6 | MMDS6 | *PMPCB* | 7q22.1 | AR | Peptidase, mitochondrial processing, beta | 617954 |
| 46.20 | Mitochondrial intermediate peptidase deficiency | Combined oxidative phosphorylation deficiency type 31;<br>COXPD31 | | *MIPEP* | 13q12.12 | AR | Mitochondrial intermediate peptidase | 617228 |
| 46.21 | CLPB deficiency | 3-methylglutaconic aciduria type 7, with cataracts, neurologic involvement and neutropenia | MEGCANN | *CLPB* | 11q13.4 | AR | Caseinolytic peptidase B | 616271 |
| 46.22 | CLPP deficiency | Perrault syndrome type 3 | PRLTS3 | *CLPP* | 19p13.3 | AR | Caseinolytic mitochondrial matrix peptidase proteolytic subunit | 614129 |
| 46.23 | LONP1 deficiency | Cerebral, ocular, dental, auricular, and skeletal syndrome | CODAS | *LONP1* | 19p13.3 | AR | LON peptidase 1 | 600373 |
| 46.24 | HSPA9 deficiency | Sideroblastic anemia type 4;<br>Epiphyseal, vertebral, ear, nose, plus associated malformations (EVEN-plus) syndrome | SIDBA4 | *HSPA9* | 5q31.2 | AR | Heat-shock 70-kDa protein 9 | 182170 |
| 46.25 | HSP60 deficiency | Hypomyelinating leukodystrophy type 4 (recessive);<br>Autosomal dominant spastic paraplegia type 13 | HLD4; SPG13 | *HSPD1* | 2q33.1 | AR, AD | Heat-shock 60-kDa protein 1 | 612233; 605280 |
| 46.26 | Sacsin deficiency | Autosomal recessive spastic ataxia of Charlevoix-Saguenay | SACS | *SACS* | 13q12.12 | AR | Sacsin | 270550 |
| 46.27 | m-AAA protease AFG3L2 subunit deficiency | Autosomal recessive spastic ataxia type 5;<br>Spinocerebellar ataxia type 28 | SPAX5; SCA28 | *AFG3L2* | 18p11.21 | AR | Catalytic subunit of the m-AAA protease | 614487; 610246 |
| 46.28 | Paraplegin deficiency | Spastic paraplegia type 7 | SPG7 | *SPG7* | 16q24.3 | AR, AD | Paraplegin, a component of the m-AAA protease | 607259 |
| 46.29 | HTRA2 deficiency | 3-methylglutaconic aciduria type 8 | MGCA8 | *HTRA2* | 2p13.1 | AR | HTRA serine peptidase 2 | 617248 |
| 46.30 | Parkin deficiency | Early-onset Parkinson disease type 2 | PARK2 | *PRKN* | 6q26 | AR | Parkin, a RING domain-containing E3 ubiquitin ligase | 600116 |
| 46.31 | PINK1 deficiency | Early-onset Parkinson disease type 6 | PARK6 | *PINK1* | 1p36.12 | AR | PTEN-induced putative kinase 1 | 605909 |
| 46.32 | USP9X deficiency | X-linked mental retardation type 99 | MRX99 | *USP9X* | Xp11.4 | X-linked | Ubiquitin-specific protease 9 | 300919 |
| 46.33 | Valosin-containing protein superactivity | Inclusion body myopathy with early-onset Paget disease and frontotemporal dementia type 1 | IBMPFD1 | *VCP* | 9p13.3 | AD | Valosin-containing protein | 167320 |

| | Disorder | Alternative name(s) | Abbreviation | Gene symbol | Chromosomal localization | Inheritance | Affected protein | OMIM |
|---|---|---|---|---|---|---|---|---|
| 46.34 | Pitrilysin metallopeptidase 1 deficiency | | | *PITRM1* | 10p15.2 | AR | Pitrilysin metallopeptidase 1 | 618211 |
| 46.35 | YME1L1 deficiency | Optic atrophy type 11 | OPA11 | *YME1L1* | 10p12.1 | AR | YME1-like 1 ATPase | 617302 |
| 46.36 | X-prolyl aminopeptidase 3 deficiency | Nephronophthisis-like nephropathy type 1 | NPHPL1 | *XPNPEP3* | 22q13.2 | AR | Aminopeptidase P3 | 613159 |
| 46.37 | Mitochondrial inorganic pyrophosphatase 2 deficiency | Infantile sudden cardiac failure | SCFI | *PPA2* | 4q24 | AR | Mitochondrial pyrophosphatase 2 | 617222 |
| 46.38 | Sideroflexin 4 deficiency | Combined oxidative phosphorylation deficiency type 18 | COXPD18 | *SFXN4* | 10q26.11 | AR | Sideroflexin 4 | 615578 |
| 46.39 | Combined Oxidative Phosphorylation Defect 6 | X-Linked Mitochondrial Myopathy | COXPD6 | *AIFM1* | Xq25-q26 | X-linked | Apoptosis inducing factor mitochondria associated 1 | 300816 |
| 46.40 | ATAD3A deficiency | Harel-Yoon syndrome | HAYOS | *ATAD3A* | 1p36.33 | AR, AD | ATPase family, AAA domain-containing, member 3A | 617183 |
| 46.41 | Transmembrane protein 126A deficiency | Optic atrophy type 7 | OPA7 | *TMEM126A* | 11q14.1 | AR | Transmembrane protein 126A | 612989 |
| 46.42 | C1q-binding protein deficiency | Combined oxidative phosphorylation deficiency type 33 | COXPD33 | *C1QBP* | 17p13.2 | AR | Complement C1q-binding protein | 617713 |
| 46.43 | Trafficking kinesin-binding protein 1 deficiency | – | | *TRAK1* | 3p22.1 | AR | Trafficking protein, kinesin-binding 1 | 608112 |
| 46.44 | Mitochondrial calcium uniporter deficiency | Myopathy with extrapyramidal signs | MPXPS | *MICU1* | 10q22.1 | AR | Mitochondrial calcium uptake 1 | 615673 |
| 46.45 | Reticulon 4-interacting mitochondrial protein deficiency | Optic atrophy type 10 | OPA10 | *RTN4IP1* | 6q21 | AR | Reticulon 4-interacting protein 1 | 616732 |
| 46.46 | MICOS complex subunit MIC13 deficiency | QIL1 deficiency | MIC13 | *MICOS13* | 19p13.3 | AR | Mitochondrial contact site and cristae organizing system subunit 13 | 616658 |
| 46.47 | Mitochondrial thioredoxin 2 deficiency | Combined oxidative phosphorylation deficiency type 29 | COXPD29 | *TXN2* | 22q12.3 | AR | Thioredoxin 2 | 616811 |
| 46.48 | Mitochondrial thioredoxin reductase 2 deficiency | Selenoprotein Z deficiency; Glucocorticoid deficiency type 5 | GCCD5 | *TXNRD2* | 22q11.21 | AR | Thioredoxin reductase 2 | 617825 |

All info in this table was taken from the Inborn Errors of Metabolism Knowledgebase (IEMbase; www.iembase.org) except the parts highlighted in blue, which were compiled using information from the HUGO Gene Nomenclature Committee (HGCN; www.genenames.org) and/or from Online Mendelian Inheritance in Man (OMIM; www.omim.org)

## Metabolic Pathways

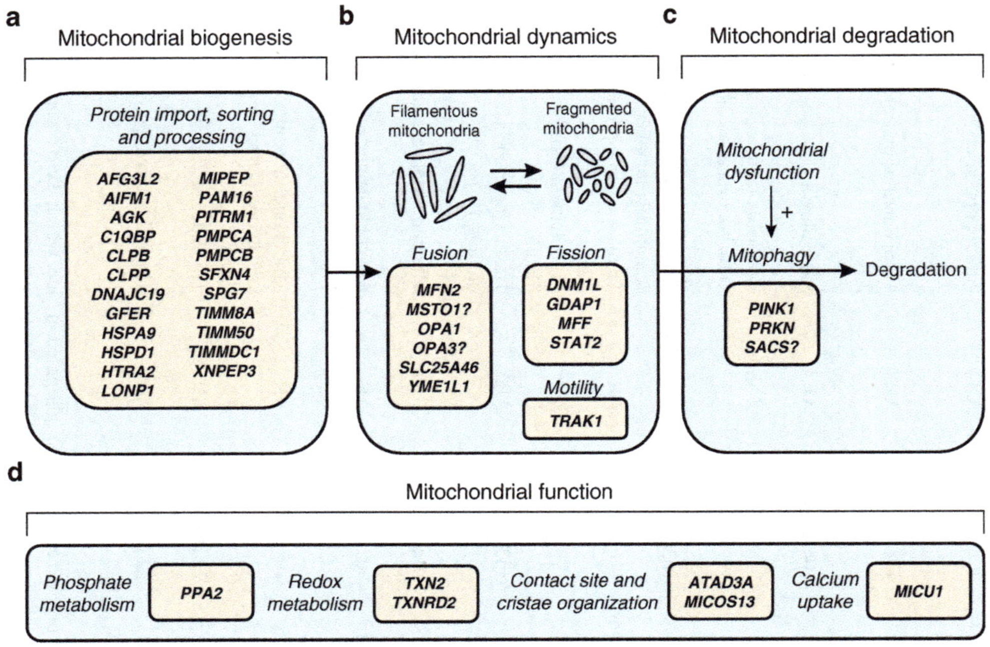


**Fig. 46.1** Mechanisms involved in disorders of mitochondrial homeostasis, dynamics, protein import, and quality control. (**a**) Biogenesis of mitochondria and their sustained functioning require import of nuclear DNA-encoded proteins, sorting of these proteins to the correct mitochondrial compartment (i.e., mitochondrial outer membrane, mitochondrial intermembrane space, mitochondrial inner membrane, and mitochondrial matrix) and posttranslational processing of these proteins. (**b**) Within cells, individual mitochondria are motile and undergo continuous fusion/fission events. Proper mitochondrial dynamics is required for mitochondrial function and is mediated by a set of dedicated mitochondrial fusion, fission, and motility proteins. (**c**) When dysfunctional, mitochondria can be removed from the cell by a mitochondria-specific autophagy process ("mitophagy"). (**d**) Aberrant mitochondrial function at the level of phosphate and redox metabolism, organization of mitochondrial contact sites, mitochondrial inner membrane folds ("cristae"), and mitochondrial calcium uptake. Within this figure, gene names linked to disease causing mutations are highlighted in bold italic. Since no exhaustive functional data was available, RTN4IP1, TMEM162A, USP9X, and VCP were not included in this figure

## Signs and Symptoms

**Table 46.1** Peroxisomal and mitochondrial fission defect

| System | Symptoms and biomarkers | Neonatal (birth–1 month) | Infancy (1–18 months) | Childhood (1.5–11 years) | Adolescence (11–16 years) | Adulthood (>16 years) |
|---|---|---|---|---|---|---|
| CNS | Abnormal gyral pattern (MRI) | + | | | | |
| | Areflexia | + | | | | |
| | Cerebral atorphy (MRI) | | + | + | | |
| | Delayed myelination (MRI) | + | + | + | | |
| | Delayed psychomotor development | | + | + | | |
| | Failure to thrive | + | + | + | | |
| | Hypotonia | + | + | + | | |
| | Microcephaly | + | + | + | | |
| | Neurologic decline | | + | + | | |
| | Pyramidal signs | | | + | | |
| | Seizures | | + | + | | |

**Table 46.1** (continued)

| System | Symptoms and biomarkers | Neonatal (birth–1 month) | Infancy (1–18 months) | Childhood (1.5–11 years) | Adolescence (11–16 years) | Adulthood (>16 years) |
|---|---|---|---|---|---|---|
| Eye | Oculomtor apraxia | | + | | | |
| | Optic atrophy | + | + | + | + | + |
| | Poor visual fixation | + | | | | |
| Musculoskeletal | Muscle weakness | + | | | | |
| Other | Death | | + | | | |
| Laboratory findings | Lactate (P) | ↑ | ↑ | ↑ | | |
| | Very-long-chain fatty acids (P) | ↑ | | | | |

**Table 46.2** Mitochondrial fission factor deficiency

| System | Symptoms and biomarkers | Neonatal (birth–1 month) | Infancy (1–18 months) | Childhood (1.5–11 years) | Adolescence (11–16 years) | Adulthood (>16 years) |
|---|---|---|---|---|---|---|
| CNS | Basal ganglia lesions (MRI) | | | + | | |
| | Cerebellar atrophy (MRI) | | + | + | | |
| | Delayed psychomotor development | | | + | | |
| | Failure to thrive | | + | | | |
| | Hypotonia | | | + | | |
| | Microcephaly | | + | + | | |
| | Neurologic decline | | | + | | |
| | Neuropathy | | + | | | |
| | Poor head and trunk control | | + | | | |
| | Seizures | | + | + | | |
| | Spasticity | | + | + | | |
| Eye | External ophthalmoparesis | | + | + | | |
| | Optic atrophy | | | + | | |
| | Visual impairment | | + | + | | |
| Other | Death | | | + | | |
| Laboratory findings | Lactate (P) | | n-↑ | n-↑ | | |
| | Very-long-chain fatty acids (P) | | | n | | |

**Table 46.3** GDAP1 deficiency

| System | Symptoms and biomarkers | Neonatal (birth–1 month) | Infancy (1–18 months) | Childhood (1.5–11 years) | Adolescence (11–16 years) | Adulthood (>16 years) |
|---|---|---|---|---|---|---|
| CNS | Areflexia | | + | + | + | + |
| | Delayed motor development | | + | + | | |
| | Distal lower limb muscle weakness/atrophy | | + | + | + | + |
| | Distal sensory impairment | | + | + | + | + |
| | Hypotonia | + | + | + | | |
| Musculoskeletal | Claw hand deformities | | | + | + | + |
| | Foot deformities | | + | + | + | + |
| | Hand/upper limb weakness | | | | + | + |
| | Kyphoscoliosis | | | + | + | + |
| | Proximal limb weakness | | | | + | + |
| | Vocal cord paresis | | | | + | + |

**Table 46.4** STAT2 deficiency

| System | Symptoms and biomarkers | Neonatal (birth–1 month) | Infancy (1–18 months) | Childhood (1.5–11 years) | Adolescence (11–16 years) | Adulthood (>16 years) |
|---|---|---|---|---|---|---|
| Hematological | Complicated viral infections | | + | + | | |
| | Deficiencies | | ± | ± | | |
| | Frequent infections | | + | + | | |
| | Post-vaccination (MMR) complications | | + | | | |
| Laboratory findings | Lactate (CSF) | | n-↑ | | | |
| | Lactate (P) | | n-↑ | | | |

**Table 46.5** UGO-1 like protein deficiency

| System | Symptoms and biomarkers | Neonatal (birth–1 month) | Infancy (1–18 months) | Childhood (1.5–11 years) | Adolescence (11–16 years) | Adulthood (>16 years) |
|---|---|---|---|---|---|---|
| CNS | Areflexia | | + | | | + |
| | Ataxia | | + | ++ | ++ | ++ |
| | Brain stem atrophy (MRI) | + | + | | | |
| | Cerebellar atrophy (MRI) | ++ | ++ | ++ | ++ | ++ |
| | Cerebellar white matter changes (MRI) | | | + | | + |
| | Developmental delay | | + | + | | |
| | Diffuse brain atrophy (MRI) | | ++ | | ++ | ++ |
| | Hypertonia | | + | + | + | + |
| | Hypotonia | ++ | | | + | + |
| | Irritability | | | ± | ± | ± |
| | Loss of skills | | | ± | | |
| | Lower limb muscle hypotrophy | | | + | + | + |
| | Myoclonus | + | + | | + | + |
| | Neuropathy | + | | ++ | ++ | ++ |
| | Thickened CC (MRI) | | | ± | | |
| | Tremor | | | | + | + |
| Ear | Deafness | | | | | + |
| Eye | Nystagmus | | + | | + | + |
| | Optic atrophy | ++ | ++ | ++ | ++ | ++ |
| | Visual impairment, progressive | | | + | + | + |
| Musculoskeletal | Flexion contractures | + | | | | |
| | Foot deformities | | | | | + |
| Other | Death | ± | ± | | | |
| | Failure to thrive | | ± | ± | ± | |
| Laboratory findings | 3-methylglutaconic acid (U) | | ↑ | ↑ | ↑ | |
| | Lactate (CSF) | | n-↑ | | | |
| | Lactate (P) | n-↑ | n-↑ | | | |
| | Pyruvate | | n-↑ | | | |

**Table 46.6** Childhood onset optic atrophy type 1

| System | Symptoms and biomarkers | Neonatal (birth–1 month) | Infancy (1–18 months) | Childhood (1.5–11 years) | Adolescence (11–16 years) | Adulthood (>16 years) |
|---|---|---|---|---|---|---|
| Eye | Color vision deficit | | | + | + | + |
| | Nystagmus | | | | ± | |
| | Optic atrophy | | | +++ | +++ | +++ |
| | Scotoma | | | + | + | + |
| | Strabismus | | | ± | | |
| | Temporal to diffuse optic nerve pallor | | | + | + | + |
| | Vision loss, onset | | | +++ | ++ | + |

**Table 46.7** Optic atrophy 1 and deafness

| System | Symptoms and biomarkers | Neonatal (birth–1 month) | Infancy (1–18 months) | Childhood (1.5–11 years) | Adolescence (11–16 years) | Adulthood (>16 years) |
|---|---|---|---|---|---|---|
| CNS | Areflexia/weak reflexes | | | ± | | + |
| | Ataxia | | | ± | | + |
| | Bilateral calcification basal ganglia (MRI) | | | | | ± |
| | Brain stem atrophy (MRI) | | | | | ± |
| | Cerebellar atrophy (MRI) | | | | | ± |
| | Cortical atrophy (MRI) | | | | | ± |
| | Developmental delay | | + | + | | |
| | Hyperreflexia | | | | | ± |
| | Migraine | | | | ± | ± |
| | Neuropathy | | | ± | | + |
| | Spasticity | | | | | ± |
| | White matter lesions (MRI) | | | | | ± |
| Digestive | Dysmotility | | | | | ± |
| Ear | Hearing loss, progressive | | | + | + | ++ |
| Endocrine | Diabetes | | | | | ± |
| | Hypothyroidism | | | | | ± |
| Eye | Color vision deficit | | | + | + | + |
| | Glaucoma | | | | | ± |
| | Ophthalmoplegia | | | ± | | + |
| | Ptosis | | | ± | | + |
| | Scotomata | | | + | + | + |
| | Temporal to diffuse optic nerve pallor | | | ++ | ++ | ++ |
| | Vision loss, onset | | | +++ | ++ | + |
| Musculoskeletal | Foot deformities | | | | | ± |
| | Myopathy | | | ± | | + |
| Laboratory findings | Lactate (P) | | | | n-↑ | n-↑ |

**Table 46.8** Costeff syndrome

| System | Symptoms and biomarkers | Neonatal (birth–1 month) | Infancy (1–18 months) | Childhood (1.5–11 years) | Adolescence (11–16 years) | Adulthood (>16 years) |
|---|---|---|---|---|---|---|
| CNS | Ataxia | | ± | + | + | + |
| | Cerebellar atrophy (MRI) | | | | | |
| | Cerebral atrophy (MRI) | | | | | ± |
| | Chorea | | | + | + | + |
| | Developmental delay/loss of skills | | + | + | | |
| | Extrapyramidal movement disorder | | ± | ± | + | + |
| | Mild intellectual disability | | | ± | + | + |
| | Movement disorder, complex, paroxysmal | | | ± | ± | ± |
| | Neuropathy | | | | | ± |
| | Non-specific white matter lesions (MRI) | | | | | ± |
| | Nystagmus | ± | + | + | + | + |
| | Spasticity | | | ± | ± | ± |
| Ear | Hearing loss | | | | | ± |
| Eye | Cataract | ± | | ± | ± | + |
| | Centrocecal scotomas | | | | ± | + |
| | Glaucoma | | | | | |
| | Optic atrophy | | + | + | + | + |
| | Visual disturbances | | ± | + | + | + |
| Laboratory findings | 3-Methylglutaconic acid (U) | ↑ | ↑ | n-↑ | ↑ | n-↑ |
| | 3-Methylglutaric acid (U) | ↑ | ↑ | ↑ | ↑ | ↑ |

**Table 46.9** Mitofusin 2 deficiency

| System | Symptoms and biomarkers | Neonatal (birth–1 month) | Infancy (1–18 months) | Childhood (1.5–11 years) | Adolescence (11–16 years) | Adulthood (>16 years) |
|---|---|---|---|---|---|---|
| CNS | Distal sensory loss | | + | + | + | + |
| | Hyperreflexia | | | | ± | ± |
| | Hypo/areflexia | | ± | | | ± |
| | Hypotonia | | ± | | | |
| | Periodic limb movement | | | ± | | ± |
| Ear | Hearing impairment | | ± | ± | | |
| Eye | Optic atrophy | | | ± | | |
| Musculoskeletal | Club foot | | + | + | + | |
| | Distal muscular atrophy | | | ± | + | + |
| | Finger contractures | | | | | ± |
| | Muscle weakness, onset in lower extremitities | | + | + | + | + |
| | Scoliosis | | | | | ± |

**Table 46.10** MSTO1 deficiency

| System | Symptoms and biomarkers | Neonatal (birth–1 month) | Infancy (1–18 months) | Childhood (1.5–11 years) | Adolescence (11–16 years) | Adulthood (>16 years) |
|---|---|---|---|---|---|---|
| CNS | Ataxia | | | + | + | + |
| | Autism spectrum disorder | | | | ± | ± |
| | Cerebellar hypotrophy (vermis) (MRI) | | ± | ± | ± | |
| | Cerebral atrophy (MRI) | | | ± | ± | ± |
| | Depression | | | | | ± |
| | Developmental delay (motor) | | + | + | + | + |
| | Dysdiadochokinesis | | | + | + | + |
| | Hyporeflexia | | | | ± | |
| | Intellectual disability | | | | | ± |
| | Non-specific white matter lesions (MRI) | | ± | ± | ± | |
| | Schizophrenia | | | | | ± |
| | Tremor | | | + | + | |
| Eye | Papillary pallor | | | | ± | |
| | Pigmentary retinopathy | | | | ± | |
| Musculoskeletal | Muscle weakness | | ± | + | + | |
| | Scoliosis | | | ± | ± | ± |
| | Thoracic deformities | | | | ± | ± |
| Other | Growth retardation | | + | + | + | |
| | Short stature | | | + | | ± |
| Laboratory findings | Citrulline (P) | | | | ↓ | |
| | Creatine kinase (P) | | | | ↑ | n-↑ |
| | Vitamin D3 | | | | | ↓ |

**Table 46.11** DNAJC19 deficiency

| System | Symptoms and biomarkers | Neonatal (birth–1 month) | Infancy (1–18 months) | Childhood (1.5–11 years) | Adolescence (11–16 years) | Adulthood (>16 years) |
|---|---|---|---|---|---|---|
| Cardiovascular | Dilated cardiomyopathy | | + | ++ | ± | ± |
| | Long QT | | | ± | | |
| CNS | Ataxia | | + | + | ± | ± |
| | Cerebellar atrophy (MRI) | | | ± | | |
| | Intellectual disability | | + | + | ± | ± |
| | Seizures | | + | + | | |
| Digestive | Microvesicular steatosis | | | ± | | |
| Eye | Optic atrophy | | ± | ± | ± | ± |
| Hematological | Anemia (microcytic, hypochrome, hemolytic) | | + | + | ± | ± |
| Other | Death | | ± | + | | |
| | Growth retardation | | ++ | ++ | | |
| | Male genital anomalies | + | + | ± | | |
| | Recuperating disease course | | | | ± | ± |
| Laboratory findings | 3-Methylglutaconic acid (U) | | ↑ | ↑ | | |
| | 3-Methylglutaric acid (U) | | ↑ | ↑ | | |
| | Lactate (CSF) | n-↑↑ | n-↑↑ | n-↑↑ | n-↑↑ | n-↑↑ |
| | Lactate (P) | ↑-↑↑↑ | ↑-↑↑↑ | ↑-↑↑↑ | ↑-↑↑↑ | ↑-↑↑↑ |

**Table 46.12** Mohr-Tranebjaerg syndrome

| System | Symptoms and biomarkers | Neonatal (birth–1 month) | Infancy (1–18 months) | Childhood (1.5–11 years) | Adolescence (11–16 years) | Adulthood (>16 years) |
|---|---|---|---|---|---|---|
| CNS | Dementia | | | | | ± |
| | Dystonia | | | + | ++ | ++ |
| | Intellectual disability | | | + | + | ++ |
| Ear | Deafness, sensorineural | + | + | + | ++ | ++ |
| Eye | Optic atrophy | | | ± | ± | + |
| | Vision, impaired | | + | + | + | + |
| Musculoskeletal | Fractures | | | | | ± |
| Other | Behavioural problems | | | | + | + |

**Table 46.13** TIMMDC1 deficiency

| System | Symptoms and biomarkers | Neonatal (birth–1 month) | Infancy (1–18 months) | Childhood (1.5–11 years) | Adolescence (11–16 years) | Adulthood (>16 years) |
|---|---|---|---|---|---|---|
| CNS | Bilateral basal ganglia hyperintensity (MRI) | | ± | | | |
| | Developmental delay | | + | + | | |
| | Dyskinesia | | ± | ± | | |
| | Dysmetria | | ± | ± | | |
| | Enlarged ventricles (MRI) | | ± | | | |
| | Hypotonia | ± | + | + | | |
| | Megacisterna magna (MRI) | | ± | | | |
| | Neuropathy | | ± | ± | | |
| | Seizures | | | ± | | |
| Ear | Deafness, sensorineural | | ± | ± | | |
| Eye | Nystagmus | | ± | ± | | |
| Other | Death | | | + | | |
| | Failure to thrive | | + | + | | |
| Laboratory findings | Lactate (P) | | n-↑ | n-↑ | | |

**Table 46.14** Mitochondrial epileptic encephalopathy TIMM50

| System | Symptoms and biomarkers | Neonatal (birth–1 month) | Infancy (1–18 months) | Childhood (1.5–11 years) | Adolescence (11–16 years) | Adulthood (>16 years) |
|---|---|---|---|---|---|---|
| CNS | Behavior, aggressive | ± | ± | ± | ± | ± |
| | Bilateral symmetric lesions globus pallidus and brain stem (MRI) | ± | ± | ± | ± | ± |
| | Brain atrophy (MRI) | ± | ± | ± | ± | ± |
| | Developmental delay | + | + | + | + | + |
| | **Epilepsy** | + | + | + | + | + |
| | Hypotonia | + | + | + | + | + |
| | Hypsarrhythmia (EEG) | + | + | + | + | + |
| Eye | **Optic atrophy** | + | + | + | + | + |
| Other | Failure to thrive | + | + | + | + | + |
| Laboratory findings | 3-Hydroxyisovaleric acid (urine) | n | n | n | n | n |
| | 3-Methylglutaconic acid (urine) | ↑↑ | ↑↑ | ↑↑ | ↑↑ | ↑↑ |
| | 3-Methylglutaric acid (urine) | ↑ | ↑ | ↑ | ↑ | ↑ |
| | Lactate (cerebrospinal fluid) | n-↑↑ | n-↑↑ | n-↑↑ | n-↑↑ | n-↑↑ |
| | Lactate (plasma) | ↑-↑↑↑ | ↑-↑↑↑ | ↑-↑↑↑ | ↑-↑↑↑ | ↑-↑↑↑ |

**Table 46.15** GFER deficiency

| System | Symptoms and biomarkers | Neonatal (birth–1 month) | Infancy (1–18 months) | Childhood (1.5–11 years) | Adolescence (11–16 years) | Adulthood (>16 years) |
|---|---|---|---|---|---|---|
| CNS | Areflexia | | | | + | + |
| | Developmental delay | | + | + | + | |
| | Epilepsy | | + | | | |
| | Hypotonia | + | + | + | + | |
| | Thin corpus callosum (MRI) | | | | + | + |
| Ear | Hearing loss, sensorineural | | + | + | + | |
| Eye | Cataract | + | + | + | | |
| | Ptosis of eyelid | | | + | + | |
| Laboratory findings | Ferritin (S) | | | n-↓ | n-↓ | n-↓ |
| | Lactate (P) | ↑ | | | n-↑ | n-↑ |

**Table 46.16** MAGMAS deficiency—*PAM16* gene

| System | Symptoms and biomarkers | Neonatal (birth–1 month) | Infancy (1–18 months) | Childhood (1.5–11 years) | Adolescence (11–16 years) | Adulthood (>16 years) |
|---|---|---|---|---|---|---|
| Cardiovascular | Cardiomegaly | + | + | | | |
| CNS | Developmental delay | + | + | | | |
| | Hypotonia, axial | | + | + | | |
| Musculoskeletal | Chrondrodysplasia | + | + | | | |
| | Enlarged fontanel | + | + | | | |
| | Facial dysmorphism | + | + | | | |
| | Narrow chest | + | + | | | |
| | Platyspondyly | + | + | | | |
| | Short nose | + | + | | | |
| Other | Death | | + | + | | |
| | Short stature | + | + | | | |

**Table 46.17** Acylglycerol kinase deficiency—*AGK* gene

| System | Symptoms and biomarkers | Neonatal (birth–1 month) | Infancy (1–18 months) | Childhood (1.5–11 years) | Adolescence (11–16 years) | Adulthood (>16 years) |
|---|---|---|---|---|---|---|
| Cardiovascular | Cardiomyopathy hypertrophic | + | + | + | + | |
| Eye | Cataract | + | + | + | | |
| Musculoskeletal | Exercise intolerance | ± | + | + | + | |
| | Myopathy | + | + | | | |
| Other | Death | ± | ± | ± | ± | ± |
| Laboratory findings | 3-Methylglutaconic acid (U) | ↑ | ↑ | ↑ | ↑ | |
| | Lactate (P) | ↑ | ↑ | ↑ | ↑ | |

**Table 46.18** Mitochondrial processing peptidase alpha (PMPCA) deficiency

| System | Symptoms and biomarkers | Neonatal (birth–1 month) | Infancy (1–18 months) | Childhood (1.5–11 years) | Adolescence (11–16 years) | Adulthood (>16 years) |
|---|---|---|---|---|---|---|
| CNS | Ataxia | | | + | + | + |
| | Cerebellar vermis atrophy (MRI) | | | ± | | |
| | Cerebral atrophy (MRI) | | | ± | | |
| | Developmental delay | | + | + | | |
| | Dysarthria | | | + | + | + |
| | Hyperreflexia | | | | | + |
| | Hypotonia | ± | ± | | | |
| | Intellectual disability | | | + | + | + |
| | Muscle weakness | ± | ± | | | |
| | Tremor | | | ± | ± | ± |
| Ear | Sensorineural hearing loss | | | ± | | |
| Eye | Cataract | | | ± | ± | ± |
| | Nystagmus | | | + | + | + |
| Other | Short stature | | ± | ± | ± | |

**Table 46.19** Mitochondrial processing peptidase beta (PMPCB) deficiency

| System | Symptoms and biomarkers | Neonatal (birth–1 month) | Infancy (1–18 months) | Childhood (1.5–11 years) | Adolescence (11–16 years) | Adulthood (>16 years) |
|---|---|---|---|---|---|---|
| CNS | Ataxia | | + | + | | |
| | Basal ganglia lesions (MRI) | | + | + | | |
| | Cerebellar atrophy (MRI) | | + | + | | |
| | Cerebral atrophy (MRI) | | + | + | | |
| | Developmental regression | | + | + | | |
| | Dystonia | | | + | | |
| | Hypotonia | | ± | ± | | |
| | Intellectual disability | | | + | | |
| | Loss of speech | | | + | | |
| | Seizures | | + | + | | |
| | Spasticity | | | + | | |
| Eye | Optic atrophy | | | + | | |
| Other | Death | | | ± | | |
| Laboratory findings | Lactate (P) | | ↑ | ↑ | | |

**Table 46.20** Mitochondrial intermediate peptidase deficiency—MIPEP gene

| System | Symptoms and biomarkers | Neonatal (birth–1 month) | Infancy (1–18 months) | Childhood (1.5–11 years) | Adolescence (11–16 years) | Adulthood (>16 years) |
|---|---|---|---|---|---|---|
| Cardiovascular | Cardiomyopathy | ± | + | | | |
| CNS | Developmental delay | | + | | | |
| | Dystonia | | | + | | |
| | Hypertonia | | | + | | |
| | Hypotonia | | + | | | |
| | Microcephaly | | ± | ± | | |
| | Seizures | ± | | + | | |
| | Symmetric hyperintense lesions in basal ganglia (MRI) | | ± | | | |
| Digestive | Intestinal dysmotility | | | + | | |
| Eye | Cataract | ± | | | | |
| Other | Death | ± | ± | ± | | |
| | Poor growth | | + | | | |
| Laboratory findings | Alanine (P) | | ↑ | ↑ | | |
| | Lactate (P) | | ↑ | ↑ | | |

**Table 46.21** CLPB deficiency

| System | Symptoms and biomarkers | Neonatal (birth–1 month) | Infancy (1–18 months) | Childhood (1.5–11 years) | Adolescence (11–16 years) | Adulthood (>16 years) |
|---|---|---|---|---|---|---|
| CNS | Ataxia | ± | ± | ± | ± | ± |
| | Cerebellar atrophy (MRI) | + | + | + | + | + |
| | Cerebral atrophy (MRI) | + | + | + | + | + |
| | Dystonia | ± | ± | ± | ± | ± |
| | Hypereckplexia | ± | | | | |
| | Hypertonia, extremities | ± | ± | + | + | + |
| | Hypotonia, muscular | + | + | ± | ± | ± |
| | Intellectual disability | + | + | + | + | + |
| | Retardation | + | + | + | + | + |
| | Seizures | ± | ± | ± | ± | ± |
| | Seizures, intra uterin | ± | | | | |
| | Spasticity | | | | | |
| | Stiffness | ± | | | | |
| Endocrine | Endocrine abnormalities | ± | ± | ± | ± | ± |
| Eye | **Cataract** | + | + | + | + | + |
| Hematological | **Neutropenia** | + | + | + | + | + |
| Other | Death | ± | | | | |
| | Intrauterine growth retardation | ± | | | | |
| | Ulcerations, oral, genital | ± | ± | ± | ± | ± |
| Laboratory findings | 3-Hydroxyisovaleric acid (urine) | n | n | n | n | n |
| | 3-Methylglutaconic acid (urine) | ↑↑ | ↑↑ | ↑↑ | ↑↑ | ↑↑ |
| | 3-Methylglutaric acid (urine) | ↑ | ↑ | ↑ | ↑ | ↑ |

**Table 46.22** CLPP deficiency

| System | Symptoms and biomarkers | Neonatal (birth–1 month) | Infancy (1–18 months) | Childhood (1.5–11 years) | Adolescence (11–16 years) | Adulthood (>16 years) |
|---|---|---|---|---|---|---|
| CNS | Ataxia | | | ± | ± | |
| | Microcephaly | | ± | ± | ± | |
| | Neuropathy | | | ± | ± | |
| | Seizures | | | ± | ± | |
| | Spasticity | | | | + | + |
| Ear | Sensorineural hearing loss | + | + | + | + | + |
| Endocrine | Hypergonadotropic hypogonadism | | | + | + | |
| | Ovarian failure | | | + | + | |
| | Secundary amenorrhoea | | | + | + | |

**Table 46.23** LONP1 deficiency

| System | Symptoms and biomarkers | Neonatal (birth–1 month) | Infancy (1–18 months) | Childhood (1.5–11 years) | Adolescence (11–16 years) | Adulthood (>16 years) |
|---|---|---|---|---|---|---|
| CNS | Developmental delay | | + | + | | |
| | Hypotonia | | | ± | ± | |
| | Intellectual disability | | ± | ± | | |
| | Microcephaly | | ± | ± | | |
| Ear | Hearing loss | | + | + | | |
| | Cataract | | + | + | | |
| Eye | Ptosis eyelid | | + | + | | |
| Musculoskeletal | Hip dysplasia, degenerative | | + | + | | |
| | Short stature | | + | + | | |
| | Teeth malposition | | ± | ± | | |
| Other | Craniofacial dysmorphias | | + | + | | |

**Table 46.24** HSPA9 deficiency

| System | Symptoms and biomarkers | Neonatal (birth–1 month) | Infancy (1–18 months) | Childhood (1.5–11 years) | Adolescence (11–16 years) | Adulthood (>16 years) |
|---|---|---|---|---|---|---|
| Cardiovascular | Heart abnormalities | | ± | + | | |
| CNS | Abnormal gait | | | ± | | |
| | Agenesis of the corpus callosum | | ± | ± | | |
| | Agenesis of the septum pellucidum | | ± | | | |
| | Developmental delay | | ± | ± | | |
| | Hypotonia | | | ± | | |
| Hematological | Anemia, sideroblastic | | | | | +++ |
| Musculoskeletal | Anal atresia | + | | | | |
| | Aplasia cutis congenita on skull vertex | ++ | | | | |
| | **Hypoplastic nose** | + | ± | +++ | | |
| | **Microtia** | + | | +++ | | |
| | **Short stature** | +++ | | +++ | | |
| | Shortened limbs | ++ | | | | |
| | **Skeletal abnormalities** | + | + | +++ | | |
| | **Synophrys** | + | | +++ | | |
| Renal | Hypoplastic kidney | | | ± | | |
| | Vesicouretral reflux | | | ± | | |
| Other | **Low weight** | +++ | | +++ | | |
| | Teeth abonormalites | | | ± | | |
| Laboratory findings | Microcytic or macrocytic red blood cells | | | | | +++ |
| | Ringed sideroblasts in bone marrow | | | | | +++ |

**Table 46.25** HSP60 deficiency

| System | Symptoms and biomarkers | Neonatal (birth–1 month) | Infancy (1–18 months) | Childhood (1.5–11 years) | Adolescence (11–16 years) | Adulthood (>16 years) |
|---|---|---|---|---|---|---|
| CNS | Apnea | ++ | | | | |
| | Head circumference | n | ↓ | ↓ | | |
| | Hypotonia | +++ | +++ | +++ | | |
| | MRI cerebrum | + | + | + | | |
| | Psychomotor retardation | +++ | +++ | +++ | | |
| | Rotator nystagmus | +++ | +++ | + | | |
| | Seizures | + | + | + | | |
| | Spastic paraplegia | | ++ | ++ | | |
| Other | Death | + | + | + | | |
| Laboratory findings | Ethylmalonic acid (U) | ↑ | ↑ | ↑ | | |
| | Lactate (P) | n-↑ | n-↑ | n-↑ | | |

**Table 46.26** Sacsin deficiency

| System | Symptoms and biomarkers | Neonatal (birth–1 month) | Infancy (1–18 months) | Childhood (1.5–11 years) | Adolescence (11–16 years) | Adulthood (>16 years) |
|---|---|---|---|---|---|---|
| CNS | Cereballar ataxia | | ++ | ++ | ++ | ++ |
| | Cerebellar vermis atrophia (MRI) | | ± | ± | + | ++ |
| | Dysarthria | | | + | ++ | ++ |
| | IQ < 70 | | – | – | – | – |
| | Peripheral neuropathy | | | | + | ++ |
| | Spasticity lower limbs | | | + | ++ | ++ |
| Digestive | Dysphagia | | | | | + |
| Eye | Demarcation retinal nerve fibres | | | | | + |
| Other | Urinary dysfunction | | | | | + |

**Table 46.27** m-AAA protease AFG3L2 subunit deficiency

| System | Symptoms and biomarkers | Neonatal (birth–1 month) | Infancy (1–18 months) | Childhood (1.5–11 years) | Adolescence (11–16 years) | Adulthood (>16 years) |
|---|---|---|---|---|---|---|
| CNS | Cerebellar ataxia | | | ± | ± | ++ |
| | Cerebellar atrophy (MRI) | | | | | + |
| | Peripheral neuropathy | | | | | + |
| | Spasticity | | | | | ± |
| Eye | Ptosis, ophtalmoplegia | | | | | ± |

**Table 46.28** Paraplegin deficiency

| System | Symptoms and biomarkers | Neonatal (birth–1 month) | Infancy (1–18 months) | Childhood (1.5–11 years) | Adolescence (11–16 years) | Adulthood (>16 years) |
|---|---|---|---|---|---|---|
| CNS | Ataxia | | | | – | – |
| | Cerebellar atrophia (MRI) | | | | | ± |
| | Peripheral neuropathy | | | | – | – |
| | Spasticity lower limbs | | | | ± | + |

**Table 46.29** HTRA2 deficiency

| System | Symptoms and biomarkers | Neonatal (birth–1 month) | Infancy (1–18 months) | Childhood (1.5–11 years) | Adolescence (11–16 years) | Adulthood (>16 years) |
|---|---|---|---|---|---|---|
| CNS | Brain atrophy (MRI) | ± | + | | | |
| | Hypertonia | + | | | | |
| | Hypotonia | + | | | | |
| | Seizures | + | | | | |
| Other | Death | ± | + | | | |
| Laboratory findings | 3-Methylglutaconic (U) | ↑ | | | | |
| | Lactate (P) | ↑ | | | | |

**Table 46.30** Parkin deficiency

| System | Symptoms and biomarkers | Neonatal (birth–1 month) | Infancy (1–18 months) | Childhood (1.5–11 years) | Adolescence (11–16 years) | Adulthood (>16 years) |
|---|---|---|---|---|---|---|
| CNS | Bradykinesia | | | | | + |
| | Dystonia | | | | + | + |
| | **Hyperreflexia** | | | | + | + |
| | **Parkinsonism, hypokinetic features** | | | | + | + |
| | **Retropulsion** | | | | + | + |
| | Tremor | | | | ± | ++ |
| Musculoskeletal | Postural instability | | | | | ± |
| | Rigidity | | | | | ± |

**Table 46.31** PINK1 deficiency

| System | Symptoms and biomarkers | Neonatal (birth–1 month) | Infancy (1–18 months) | Childhood (1.5–11 years) | Adolescence (11–16 years) | Adulthood (>16 years) |
|---|---|---|---|---|---|---|
| CNS | Anxiety | | | | ± | ± |
| | Asymmetry | | | | ± | + |
| | Autonomic instability | | | | ± | ± |
| | **Bradykinesia** | | | | ± | + |
| | Dementia | | | | ± | ± |
| | Depression | | | | ± | ± |
| | Dystonia | | | | ± | ± |
| | Gait impairment | | | | ± | + |
| | **Hyperreflexia** | | | | ± | + |
| | **Parkinsonism** | | | | ± | + |
| | Psychiatric disturbances | | | | ± | ± |
| | Sleep benefit | | | | ± | ± |
| | Tremor | | | | ± | + |
| Musculoskeletal | Postural instability | | | | ± | ± |
| | **Rigidity** | | | | ± | + |
| Genitourinary | Urinary urgency | | | | ± | ± |

**Table 46.32** USP9X deficiency

| System | Symptoms and biomarkers | Neonatal (birth–1 month) | Infancy (1–18 months) | Childhood (1.5–11 years) | Adolescence (11–16 years) | Adulthood (>16 years) |
|---|---|---|---|---|---|---|
| CNS | Hypotonia | | + | | | |
| | Intelectual disability | | + | + | | |
| Musculoskeletal | Short stature | | + | | | |

**Table 46.33** Valosin-containing protein superactivity

| System | Symptoms and biomarkers | Neonatal (birth–1 month) | Infancy (1–18 months) | Childhood (1.5–11 years) | Adolescence (11–16 years) | Adulthood (>16 years) |
|---|---|---|---|---|---|---|
| CNS | Frontotemporal dementia | | | | | ± |
| Musculoskeletal | Myopathy | | | | | + |
| | Paget bone disease | | | | | + |

**Table 46.34** Pitrilysin metallopeptidase 1 deficiency

| System | Symptoms and biomarkers | Neonatal (birth–1 month) | Infancy (1–18 months) | Childhood (1.5–11 years) | Adolescence (11–16 years) | Adulthood (>16 years) |
|---|---|---|---|---|---|---|
| CNS | Ataxia | | + | ++ | ++ | ++ |
| | Cerebellar atrophy (MRI) | | | ± | + | + |
| | Intellectual disability | | +/++ | +/++ | +/++ | + |
| Psychiatric | Psychosis | | | ± | ± | ± |
| Laboratory findings | Creatine kinase (P) | | ↑ | | | |

**Table 46.35** YME1L1 deficiency

| System | Symptoms and biomarkers | Neonatal (birth–1 month) | Infancy (1–18 months) | Childhood (1.5–11 years) | Adolescence (11–16 years) | Adulthood (>16 years) |
|---|---|---|---|---|---|---|
| CNS | Intellectual disability | | ++ | ++ | | |
| | Leukoencephalopathy (MRI) | | | + | | |
| | Motor development delay | | + | + | | |
| Eye | Optic nerve atrophy | | + | + | | |

**Table 46.36** X-prolyl aminopeptidase 3 deficiency

| System | Symptoms and biomarkers | Neonatal (birth–1 month) | Infancy (1–18 months) | Childhood (1.5–11 years) | Adolescence (11–16 years) | Adulthood (>16 years) |
|---|---|---|---|---|---|---|
| CNS | Tremor | | | ± | + | |
| Renal | Nephronophtisis | | | + | + | |
| | Renal insufficiency | | | ± | + | |

**Table 46.37** Mitochondrial inorganic pyrophosphatase 2 deficiency

| System | Symptoms and biomarkers | Neonatal (birth–1 month) | Infancy (1–18 months) | Childhood (1.5–11 years) | Adolescence (11–16 years) | Adulthood (>16 years) |
|---|---|---|---|---|---|---|
| Cardiovascular | Cardiac arrhythmia | | + | + | + | |
| CNS | Seizures | | ± | ± | | |
| Metabolic | Lactic acidosis | | + | + | + | |
| Other | Sudden death | | + | + | + | |
| Laboratory findings | Lactate (P) | | ↑ | ↑ | ↑ | |

**Table 46.38** Sideroflexin 4 deficiency

| System | Symptoms and biomarkers | Neonatal (birth–1 month) | Infancy (1–18 months) | Childhood (1.5–11 years) | Adolescence (11–16 years) | Adulthood (>16 years) |
|---|---|---|---|---|---|---|
| CNS | Microcephaly | + | + | | | |
| | Speech delay | | ± | | | |
| Hematological | Macrocytic anemia | | ± | ± | | |
| Other | IUGR | + | | | | |
| Laboratory findings | Lactate (P) | ↑ | ↑ | | | |

**Table 46.39** Combined oxidative phosphorylation defect 6

| System | Symptoms and biomarkers | Neonatal (birth–1 month) | Infancy (1–18 months) | Childhood (1.5–11 years) | Adolescence (11–16 years) | Adulthood (>16 years) |
|---|---|---|---|---|---|---|
| CNS | Areflexia | | ++ | ++ | | |
| | Hypotonia | | ++ | ++ | | |
| | Neurologic deterioration | | + | +++ | | |
| | Neuropathy | | ++ | ++ | | |
| | Regression, psychomotor | | ++ | ++ | | |
| | Seizures | | + | ++ | | |
| Other | Death | | ++ | ++ | | |
| Laboratory findings | Lactate (CSF) | | ↑ | ↑ | | |
| | Lactate (P) | | ↑ | ↑ | | |

**Table 46.40** ATAD3A deficiency

| System | Symptoms and biomarkers | Neonatal (birth–1 month) | Infancy (1–18 months) | Childhood (1.5–11 years) | Adolescence (11–16 years) | Adulthood (>16 years) |
|---|---|---|---|---|---|---|
| CNS | Developmental delay | | + | + | | |
| | Hypotonia | | + | + | + | + |
| | Seizures | ±[a] | +[a] | +[a] | +[a] | +[a] |
| Eye | Cataract | +[a] | | | | |
| | Optic atrophy | | ± | ± | | |
| Other | Death | ±[a] | | | | |

[a]Only bi-allelic mutations

**Table 46.41** Transmembrane protein 126A deficiency

| System | Symptoms and biomarkers | Neonatal (birth–1 month) | Infancy (1–18 months) | Childhood (1.5–11 years) | Adolescence (11–16 years) | Adulthood (>16 years) |
|---|---|---|---|---|---|---|
| CNS | Peripheral neuropathy | | | | | + |
| Ear | Auditory neuropathy | | ± | | | |
| Eye | Optic atrophy | | ± | ± | + | + |

**Table 46.42** C1q-binding protein deficiency

| System | Symptoms and biomarkers | Neonatal (birth–1 month) | Infancy (1–18 months) | Childhood (1.5–11 years) | Adolescence (11–16 years) | Adulthood (>16 years) |
|---|---|---|---|---|---|---|
| Cardiovascular | Cardiomyopathy | ± | ± | ± | ± | ± |
| Eye | CPEO | | | | | ± |
| Musculoskeletal | Myopathy | | | | | ± |
| Other | Death | ± | | | | ± |
| Laboratory findings | Lactate (P) | ↑ | ↑ | ↑ | n-↑ | n-↑ |

**Table 46.43** Trafficking kinesin-binding protein 1 deficiency

| System | Symptoms and biomarkers | Neonatal (birth–1 month) | Infancy (1–18 months) | Childhood (1.5–11 years) | Adolescence (11–16 years) | Adulthood (>16 years) |
|---|---|---|---|---|---|---|
| CNS | Developmental delay | | ++ | | | |
| | Encephalopathy | | ++ | | | |
| | Seizures (myoclonic) | | +++ | | | |
| Other | Death | | + | | | |

**Table 46.44** Mitochondrial calcium uniporter deficiency

| System | Symptoms and biomarkers | Neonatal (birth–1 month) | Infancy (1–18 months) | Childhood (1.5–11 years) | Adolescence (11–16 years) | Adulthood (>16 years) |
|---|---|---|---|---|---|---|
| CNS | Chorea | | ± | ± | | |
| | Learning difficulties | | + | + | + | + |
| | Motor delay | | + | + | + | + |
| Musculoskeletal | Muscle weakness | | ± | ± | ± | ± |
| Laboratory findings | Creatine kinase (P) | | ↑ | ↑ | ↑ | ↑ |

**Table 46.45** Reticulon 4-interacting mitochondrial protein deficiency

| System | Symptoms and biomarkers | Neonatal (birth–1 month) | Infancy (1–18 months) | Childhood (1.5–11 years) | Adolescence (11–16 years) | Adulthood (>16 years) |
|---|---|---|---|---|---|---|
| CNS | Learning disability | | | ± | | |
| Eyes | Optic atrophy | | ± | + | + | + |

**Table 46.46** MICOS complex subunit MIC13 deficiency

| System | Symptoms and biomarkers | Neonatal (birth–1 month) | Infancy (1–18 months) | Childhood (1.5–11 years) | Adolescence (11–16 years) | Adulthood (>16 years) |
|---|---|---|---|---|---|---|
| CNS | Cortical atrophy (MRI) | ± | ± | | | |
| | **Epilepsy** | ± | ± | | | |
| | Hypotonia, muscular | ± | ± | | | |
| | Microcephaly | ± | ± | | | |
| | Regression | ± | ± | | | |
| | Retardation, psychomotor | ± | ± | | | |
| | Subcortical atrophy (MRI) | ± | ± | | | |
| | White matter abnormalities (MRI) | ± | ± | | | |
| Digestive | **Liver dysfunction** | + | + | | | |
| | **Liver failure, acute** | + | + | | | |
| Metabolic | Hypoglycemia | ± | ± | | | |
| Other | **Death**[a] | + | + | | | |
| | Failure to thrive | ± | ± | | | |
| Laboratory findings | 3-Hydroxyisovaleric acid (urine) | n | n | | | |
| | 3-Methylglutaconic acid (urine) | ↑↑ | ↑↑ | | | |
| | 3-Methylglutaric acid (urine) | ↑ | ↑ | | | |
| | Ammonia (blood) | n | n | | | |
| | ASAT/ALAT (plasma) | ↑ | ↑ | | | |
| | Bilirubin, conjugated (plasma) | ↑ | ↑ | | | |
| | Disturbed clotting | ↑ | ↑ | | | |
| | Glucose (plasma) | ↓-n | ↓-n | | | |
| | Lactate (plasma) | ↑ | ↑ | | | |

[a]All patients died (maximum age 13 months)

**Table 46.47** Mitochondrial thioredoxin 2 deficiency

| System | Symptoms and biomarkers | Neonatal (birth–1 month) | Infancy (1–18 months) | Childhood (1.5–11 years) | Adolescence (11–16 years) | Adulthood (>16 years) |
|---|---|---|---|---|---|---|
| CNS | Developmental delay | | ++ | | | |
| | Microcephaly | + | | | | |
| | Peripheral neuropathy | | | + | | |
| | Seizures | | | + | | |
| Eye | Optic neuropathy | | | + | | |
| Laboratory findings | Lactate (P) | | ↑ | ↑ | | |

**Table 46.48** Mitochondrial thioredoxin reductase 2 deficiency

| System | Symptoms and biomarkers | Neonatal (birth–1 month) | Infancy (1–18 months) | Childhood (1.5–11 years) | Adolescence (11–16 years) | Adulthood (>16 years) |
|---|---|---|---|---|---|---|
| Endocrine | Glucocorticoid deficiency | | + | + | + | + |
| | Poor synacthen test | | + | + | + | + |

## Reference Value

| Compound | Serum/blood (μmol/L) | Urine (mmol/mol creat) | Cerebrospinal fluid (μmol/L) |
|---|---|---|---|
| Lactate | 450–1800 (B) | | 1100–1700 |
| 3-Methylglutaconic acid | | <20 (age 0–2 months)<br><15 (2 months–2 years)<br><10 (>2 years) | |
| Ferritin | | 10–150 μg/L (6 month–15 years)<br>10–200 μg/L (15–50 years female)<br>20–300 μg/L (>50 years female)<br>20–300 μg/L (>15 years male) | |
| Alanine | 150–450 (P, S) | | |

## Pathological Values

| No. | Disorder | Lactate (P) | Lactate (CSF) | Very long chain fatty acids (P) | 3-MGA (U) | 3-MG (U) | Ferritin (S) | Alanine (P) | CK (P) |
|---|---|---|---|---|---|---|---|---|---|
| 46.1 | Peroxisomal and mitochondrial fission defect | ↑ | | ↑ | | | | | |
| 46.2 | Mitochondrial fission factor deficiency | n-↑ | | n | | | | | |
| 46.3 | GDAP1 deficiency | | | | | | | | |
| 46.4 | STAT2 deficiency | n-↑ | n-↑ | | | | | | |
| 46.5 | UGO-1 like protein deficiency | n-↑ | n-↑ | | ↑ | | | | |
| 46.6 | Childhood-onset optic atrophy type 1 | | | | | | | | |
| 46.7 | Optic atrophy 1 and deafness | n-↑ | | | | | | | |
| 46.8 | Costeff syndrome | | | | n-↑ | ↑ | | | |
| 46.9 | Mitofusin 2 deficiency | | | | | | | | |
| 46.10 | MSTO1 deficiency | | | | | | | | |
| 46.11 | DNAJC19 deficiency | | | | ↑ | ↑ | | | |
| 46.12 | Mohr-Tranebjaerg syndrome | | | | | | | | |
| 46.13 | TIMMDC1 deficiency | n-↑ | | | | | | | |
| 46.14 | Mitochondrial epileptic encephalopathy TIMM50 | n-↑ | | | | n-↑ | | | |
| 46.15 | GFER deficiency | n-↑ | | | | | n-↓ | | |
| 46.16 | MAGMAS deficiency | | | | | | | | |
| 46.17 | Acylglycerol kinase deficiency | ↑ | | | | ↑ | | | |
| 46.18 | Mitochondrial processing peptidase alpha deficiency | | | | | | | | |
| 46.19 | Mitochondrial processing peptidase beta deficiency | ↑ | | | | | | | |
| 46.20 | Mitochondrial intermediate peptidase deficiency | ↑ | | | | | | ↑ | |
| 46.21 | CLPB deficiency | ↑ | ↑ | | ↑ | ↑ | | | |
| 46.22 | CLPP deficiency | | | | | | | | |
| 46.23 | LONP1 deficiency | | | | | | | | |
| 46.24 | HSPA9 deficiency | | | | | | | | |
| 46.25 | HSP60 deficiency | n-↑ | | | | | | | |

| No. | Disorder | Lactate (P) | Lactate (CSF) | Very long chain fatty acids (P) | 3-MGA (U) | 3-MG (U) | Ferritin (S) | Alanine (P) | CK (P) |
|---|---|---|---|---|---|---|---|---|---|
| 46.26 | Sacsin deficiency | | | | | | | | |
| 46.27 | m-AAA protease AFG3L2 subunit deficiency | | | | | | | | |
| 46.28 | Paraplegin deficiency | | | | | | | | |
| 46.29 | HTRA2 deficiency | ↑ | | | ↑ | ↑ | | | |
| 46.30 | Parkin deficiency | | | | | | | | |
| 46.31 | PINK1 deficiency | | | | | | | | |
| 46.32 | USP9X deficiency | | | | | | | | |
| 46.33 | Valosin-containing protein superactivity | | | | | | | | |
| 46.34 | Pitrilysin metallopeptidase 1 deficiency | | | | | | | | ↑ |
| 46.35 | YME1L1 deficiency | | | | | | | | |
| 46.36 | X-prolyl aminopeptidase 3 deficiency | | | | | | | | |
| 46.37 | Mitochondrial inorganic pyrophosphatase 2 deficiency | ↑ | | | | | | | |
| 46.38 | Sideroflexin 4 deficiency | ↑ | | | | | | | |
| 46.39 | Combined oxidative phosphorylation defect 6 | ↑ | ↑ | | | | | | |
| 46.40 | ATAD3A deficiency | | | | | | | | |
| 46.41 | Transmembrane protein 126A deficiency | | | | | | | | |
| 46.42 | C1q-binding protein deficiency | n-↑ | | | | | | | |
| 46.43 | Trafficking kinesin-binding protein 1 deficiency | | | | | | | | |
| 46.44 | Mitochondrial calcium uniporter deficiency | | | | | | | | ↑ |
| 46.45 | Reticulon 4-interacting mitochondrial protein deficiency | | | | | | | | |
| 46.46 | MICOS complex subunit MIC13 deficiency | ↑ | | | ↑ | | | | |
| 46.47 | Mitochondrial thioredoxin 2 deficiency | ↑ | | | | | | | |
| 46.48 | Mitochondrial thioredoxin reductase 2 deficiency | | | | | | | | |

*Abbreviations: 3MGA* 3-Methylglutaconic acid, *3MG* 3-Methylglutaric acid, *CK* Creatine kinase
*P* Plasma, *CSF* Cerebrospinal fluid, *U* Urine, *S* Serum

## Diagnostic Flowchart

See flowchart in Chap. 44.

## Specimen Collection

See Chap. 44.

## Prenatal Diagnosis

Prenatal DNA testing can be offered for the nDNA mutations after confirmation of parental carriage of the mutations.

## DNA Testing

If a nuclear-encoded mitochondrial syndrome is clinically suspected, then a sequence analysis of the relevant gene may be the appropriate first-line test. Although in these cases, exome sequencing will most probably also result in the identification of the defect, this approach does have a small chance of unsolicited genetic findings, and therefore specific gene sequencing is preferred over exome sequencing in the case of a strong clinical suspicion for such a specific gene defect.

## Treatment

See Chap. 44.

## References


Abrams AJ, Hufnagel RB, Rebelo A, Zanna C, Patel N, Gonzalez MA, et al. Mutations in SLC25A46, encoding a UGO1-like protein, cause an optic atrophy spectrum disorder. Nature Genet. 2015;47:926–32.

Abrams AJ, Fontanesi F, Tan NBL, Buglo E, Campeanu IJ, Rebelo AP, et al. Insights into the genotype-phenotype correlation and molecular function of SLC25A46. Hum Mutat. 2018;39:1995–2007.

Al Teneiji A, Siriwardena K, George K, Mital S, Mercimek-Mahmutoglu S. Progressive cerebellar atrophy and a novel homozygous pathogenic DNAJC19 variant as a cause of dilated cardiomyopathy ataxia syndrome. Pediatr Neurol. 2016;62:58–61.

Alcalay RN, Caccappolo E, Mejia-Santana H, Tang MX, Rosado L, Ross BM, Verbitsky M, Kisselev S, Louis ED, Comella C, Colcher A, Jennings D, et al. Frequency of known mutations in early-onset Parkinson disease: implication for genetic counseling: the consortium on risk for early onset Parkinson disease study. Arch Neurol. 2010;67:1116–22.

Alexander C, Votruba M, Pesch UEA, Thiselton DL, Mayer S, Moore A, et al. OPA1, encoding a dynamin-related GTPase, is mutated in autosomal dominant optic atrophy linked to chromosome 3q28. Nature Genet. 2000;26:211–5.

Anazi S, Maddirevula S, Salpietro V, Asi YT, Alsahli S, Alhashem A, Shamseldin HE, AlZahrani F, Patel N, Ibrahim N, Abdulwahab FM, Hashem M, et al. Expanding the genetic heterogeneity of intellectual disability. Hum Genet. 2017;136:1419–29. Note: Erratum: Hum Genet 137:105–109, 2018.

Angebault C, Guichet P-O, Talmat-Amar Y, Charif M, Gerber S, Fares-Taie L, Gueguen N, Halloy F, Moore D, Amati-Bonneau P, Manes G, Hebrard M, et al. Recessive mutations in RTN4IP1 cause isolated and syndromic optic neuropathies. Am J Hum Genet. 2015;97:754–60. Note: Erratum: Am J Hum Genet 97:769 only, 2015.

Arnoldi A, Tonelli A, Crippa F, Villani G, Pacelli C, Sironi M, Pozzoli U, D'Angelo MG, Meola G, Martinuzzi A, Crimella C, Redaelli F, Panzeri C, Renieri A, Comi GP, Turconi AC, Bresolin N, Bassi MT. A clinical, genetic, and biochemical characterization of SPG7 mutations in a large cohort of patients with hereditary spastic paraplegia. Hum Mutat. 2008;29:522–31.

Barel O, Malicdan MCV, Ben-Zeev B, Kandel J, Pri-Chen H, Stephen J, Castro IG, Metz J, Atawa O, Moshkovitz S, Ganelin E, Barshack I, et al. Deleterious variants in TRAK1 disrupt mitochondrial movement and cause fatal encephalopathy. Brain. 2017;140:568–81.

Baxter RV, Ben Othmane K, Rochelle JM, Stajich JE, Hulette C, Dew-Knight S, et al. Ganglioside-induced differentiation-associated protein-1 is mutant in Charcot-Marie-tooth disease type 4A/8q21. Nature Genet. 2002;30:21–2.

Berciano J, Combarros O, Figols J, Calleja J, Cabello A, Silos I, Coria F. Hereditary motor and sensory neuropathy type II: clinicopathological study of a family. Brain. 1986;109:897–914.

Bonifati V, Rohe CF, Breedveld GJ, Fabrizio E, De Mari M, Tassorelli C, Tavella A, Marconi R, Nicholl DJ, Chien HF, Fincati E, Abbruzzese G, et al. Early-onset parkinsonism associated with PINK1 mutations: frequency, genotypes, and phenotypes. Neurology. 2005;65:87–95.

Breckpot J, Takiyama Y, Thienpont B, Van Vooren S, Vermeesch JR, Ortibus E, Devriendt K. A novel genomic disorder: a deletion of the SACS gene leading to spastic ataxia of Charlevoix-Saguenay. Eur J Hum Genet. 2008;16:1050–4.

Brugman F, Scheffer H, Wokke JHJ, Nillesen WM, de Visser M, Aronica E, Veldink JH, van den Berg LH. Paraplegin mutations in sporadic adult-onset upper motor neuron syndromes. Neurology. 2008;71:1500–5.

Brunetti D, Torsvik J, Dallabona C, Teixeira P, Sztromwasser P, Fernandez-Vizarra E, Cerutti R, Reyes A, Preziuso C, D'Amati G, Baruffini E, Goffrini P, Viscomi C, Ferrero I, Boman H, Telstad W, Johansson S, Glaser E, Knappskog PM, Zeviani M, Bindoff LA. Defective PITRM1 mitochondrial peptidase is associated with Aβ amyloidotic neurodegeneration. EMBO Mol Med. 2016;8:176–90.

Bulthuis EP, Adjobo-Hermans MJW, Willems PHGM, Koopman WJH. Mitochondrial morphofunction in mammalian cells. Antioxid Redox Signal. 2019;30:2066–109.

Calderwood L, Holm IA, Teot LA, Anselm I. Adrenal insufficiency in mitochondrial disease: a rare case of GFER-related mitochondrial encephalomyopathy and review of the literature. J Child Neurol. 2016;31:190–4.

Cagnoli C, Stevanin G, Brussino A, Barberis M, Mancini C, Margolis RL, Holmes SE, Nobili M, Forlani S, Padovan S, Pappi P, Zaros C, Leber I, Ribai P, Pugliese L, Assalto C, Brice A, Migone N, Durr A, Brusco A. Missense mutations in the AFG3L2 proteolytic domain account for ~1.5% of European autosomal dominant cerebellar ataxias. Hum Mutat. 2010;31:1117–24.

Chung KW, Kim SB, Park KD, Choi KG, Lee JH, Eun HW, et al. Early onset severe and late-onset mild Charcot-Marie-tooth disease with mitofusin 2 (MFN2) mutations. Brain. 2006;129:2103–18.

Costeff H, Gadoth N, Apter N, Prialnic M, Savir H. A familial syndrome of infantile optic atrophy, movement disorder, and spastic paraplegia. Neurology. 1989;39:595–7.

Davey KM, Parboosingh JS, McLeod DR, Chan A, Casey R, Ferreira P, et al. Mutation of DNAJC19, a human homologue of yeast inner mitochondrial co-chaperones, causes DCMA syndrome, a novel autosomal recessive Barth syndrome-like condition. J Med Genet. 2006;43:385–93.

Demain LA, Urquhart JE, O'Sullivan J, Williams SG, Bhaskar SS, Jenkinson EM, et al. Expanding the genotypic spectrum of Perrault syndrome. Clin Genet. 2017;91:302–12.

Desir J, Coppieters F, Van Regemorter N, De Baere E, Abramowicz M. Cordonnier, M. TMEM126A mutation in a Moroccan family with autosomal recessive optic atrophy. Mol Vision. 2012;18:1849–57.

Di Bella D, Lazzaro F, Brusco A, Plumari M, Battaglia G, Pastore A, Finardi A, Cagnoli C, Tempia F, Frontali M, Veneziano L, Sacco T, et al. Mutations in the mitochondrial protease gene AFG3L2 cause dominant hereditary ataxia SCA28. Nature Genet. 2010;42:313–21.

Di Fonzo A, Ronchi D, Lodi T, Fassone E, Tigano M, Lamperti C, et al. The mitochondrial disulfide relay system protein GFER is mutated in autosomal-recessive myopathy with cataract and combined respiratory-chain deficiency. Am J Hum Genet. 2009;84:594–604.

Dikoglu E, Alfaiz A, Gorna M, Bertola D, Chae JH, Cho TJ, et al. Mutations in LONP1, a mitochondrial matrix protease, cause CODAS syndrome. Am J Med Genet. 2015;167:1501–9.

Eldomery MK, Akdemir ZC, Vogtle F-N, Charng W-L, Mulica P, Rosenfeld JA, et al. MIPEP recessive variants cause a syndrome of left ventricular non-compaction, hypotonia, and infantile death. Genome Med. 2016;8:106.

Feichtinger RG, Olahova M, Kishita Y, Garone C, Kremer LS, Yagi M, Uchiumi T, Jourdain AA, Thompson K, D'Souza AR, Kopajtich R, Alston CL, et al. Biallelic C1QBP mutations cause severe neonatal-, childhood-, or later-onset cardiomyopathy associated with combined respiratory-chain deficiencies. Am J Hum Genet. 2017;101:525–38.

Gal A, Balicza P, Weaver D, Naghdi S, Joseph SK, Varnai P, et al. MSTO1 is a cytoplasmic pro-mitochondrial fusion protein, whose mutation induces myopathy and ataxia in humans. EMBO Mol Med. 2017;9:967–84.

Ghezzi D, Sevrioukova I, Invernizzi F, Lamperti C, Mora M, D'Adamo P, Novara F, Zuffardi O, Uziel G, Zeviani M. Severe X-linked mitochondrial encephalomyopathy associated with a mutation in apoptosis-inducing factor. Am J Hum Genet. 2010;86:639–49.

Guarani V, Paulo J, Zhai B, Huttlin EL, Gygi SP, Harper JW. TIMMDC1/C3orf1 functions as a membrane-embedded mitochondrial complex I assembly factor through association with the MCIA complex. Mol Cell Biol. 2014;34:847–61.

Guarani V, Jardel C, Chretien D, Lombes A, Benit P, Labasse C, Lacene E, Bourillon A, Imbard A, Benoist J-F, Dorboz I, Gilleron M. QIL1 mutation causes MICOS disassembly and early onset fatal mitochondrial encephalopathy with liver disease. eLife. 2016;5:e17163. Note: Electronic Article.

Guimier A, Gordon CT, Godard F, Ravenscroft G, Oufadem M, Vasnier C, Rambaud C, Nitschke P, Bole-Feysot C, Masson C, Dauger S, Longman C, et al. Biallelic PPA2 mutations cause sudden unexpected cardiac arrest in infancy. Am J Hum Genet. 2016;99:666–73.

Gustaffson ÅB, Dorn GW 2nd. Evolving and expanding roles of mitophagy as a homeostatic and pathogenic process. Physiol Rev. 2019;99:853–92.

Ha AD, Parratt KL, Rendtorff ND, Lodahl M, Ng K, Rowe DB, et al. The phenotypic spectrum of dystonia in Mohr-Tranebjaerg syndrome. Mov Disord. 2012;27:1034–40.

Hambleton S, Goodbourn S, Young DF, Dickinson P, Mohamad SMB, Valappil M, et al. STAT2 deficiency and susceptibility to viral illness in humans. Proc Natl Acad Sci U S A. 2013;10:3053–8.

Hanein S, Perrault I, Roche O, Gerber S, Khadom N, Rio M, Boddaert N, Jean-Pierre M, Brahimi N, Serre V, Chretien D, Delphin N, Fares-Taie L, Lachheb S, Rotig A, Meire F, Munnich A, Dufier J-L, Kaplan J, Rozet J-M. TMEM126A, encoding a mitochondrial protein, is mutated in autosomal-recessive nonsyndromic optic atrophy. Am J Hum Genet. 2009;84:493–8.

Hansen JJ, Durr A, Cournu-Rebeix I, Georgopoulos C, Ang D, Nielsen MN, Davoine C-S, Brice A, Fontaine B, Gregersen N, Bross P. Hereditary spastic paraplegia SPG13 is associated with a mutation in the gene encoding the mitochondrial chaperonin Hsp60. Am J Hum Genet. 2002;70:1328–32.

Harel T, Yoon WH, Garone C, Gu S, Coban-Akdemir Z, Eldomery MK, Posey JE, Jhangiani SN, Rosenfeld JA, Cho MT, Fox S, Withers M, et al. Recurrent de novo and biallelic variation of ATAD3A, encoding a mitochondrial membrane protein, results in distinct neurological syndromes. Am J Hum Genet. 2016;99:831–45.

Hartmann B, Wai T, Hu H, MacVicar T, Musante L, Fischer-Zirnsak B, Stenzel W, Graf R, van den Heuvel L, Ropers H-H, Wienker TF, Hubner C, Langer T, Kaindl AM. Homozygous YME1L1 mutation causes mitochondriopathy with optic atrophy and mitochondrial network fragmentation. elife. 2016;5:e16078.

Hildick-Smith GJ, Cooney JD, Garone C, Kremer LS, Haack TB, Thon JN, Miyata N, Lieber DS, Calvo SE, Akman HO, Yien YY, Huston NC, et al. Macrocytic anemia and mitochondriopathy resulting from a defect in sideroflexin 4. Am J Hum Genet. 2013;93: 906–14.

Holzerova E, Danhauser K, Haack TB, Kremer LS, Melcher M, Ingold I, Kabayashi S, Terrile C, Wolf P, Schaper J, Mayatepek E, Baertling F, Friedmann Angeli J, Conrad M, Strom TM, Meitinger T, Prokisch H, Distelmaier F. Human thioredoxin 2 deficiency impairs mitochondrial redox homeostasis and causes early-onset neurodegeneration. Brain. 2016;139:346–54.

Homan CC, Kumar R, Nguyen LS, Haan E, Raymond FL, Abidi F, Raynaud M, Schwartz CE, Wood SA, Gecz J, Jolly LA. Mutations in USP9X are associated with X-linked intellectual disability and disrupt neuronal cell migration and growth. Am J Hum Genet. 2014;94:470–8.

Hudson G, Amati-Bonneau P, Blakely EL, Stewart JD, He L, Schaefer AM, et al. Mutation of OPA1 causes dominant optic atrophy with external ophthalmoplegia, ataxia, deafness, and multiple mitochondrial deletions: a novel disorder of mtDNA maintenance. Brain. 2008;131:329–37.

Ishihara-Paul L, Hulihan MM, Kachergus J, Upmanyu R, Warren L, Amouri R, Elango R, Prinjha RK, Soto A, Kefi M, Zouari M, Sassi SB, Yahmed SB, El Euch-Fayeche G, Matthews PM, Middleton LT, Gibson RA, Hentati F, Farrer MJ. PINK1 mutations and parkinsonism. Neurology. 2008;71:896–902.

Jackson TD, Palmer CS, Stojanovski D. Mitochondrial diseases caused by dysfunctional mitochondrial protein import. Biochem Soc Trans. 2018;46:1255–38.

Jenkinson EM, Rehman AU, Walsh T, Clayton-Smith J, Lee K, Morell RJ, et al. Perrault syndrome is caused by recessive mutations in CLPP, encoding a mitochondrial ATP-dependent chambered protease. Am J Hum Genet. 2013;92:605–13.

Jobling RK, Assoum M, Gakh O, Blaser S, Raiman JA, Mignot C, et al. PMPCA mutations cause abnormal mitochondrial protein processing in patients with non-progressive cerebellar ataxia. Brain. 2015;138:1505–17.

Kanabus M, Shahni R, Saldanha JW, Murphy E, Plagnol V, Hoff WV, Heales S, Rahman S. Bi-allelic CLPB mutations cause cataract, renal cysts, nephrocalcinosis and 3-methylglutaconic aciduria, a novel disorder of mitochondrial protein disaggregation. J Inherit Metab Dis. 2015;38:211–9.

Kennedy H, Haack TB, Hartill V, Matakovic L, Baumgartner ER, Potter H, Mackay R, Alston CL, O'Sullivan S, McFarland R, Connolly G, Gannon C, et al. Sudden cardiac death due to deficiency of the mitochondrial inorganic pyrophosphatase PPA2. Am J Hum Genet. 2016;99:674–82.

Kluge MA, Fetterman JL, Vita JA. Mitochondria and endothelial function. Circ Res. 2013;112:1171–88.

Koch J, Feichtinger RG, Freisinger P, Pies M, Schrodl F, Iuso A, et al. Disturbed mitochondrial and peroxisomal dynamics due to loss of MFF causes Leigh-like encephalopathy, optic atrophy and peripheral neuropathy. J Med Genet. 2016;53:270–8.

Koopman WJH, Willems PHGM, Smeitink JAM. Monogenic mitochondrial disorders. N Engl J Med. 2012;366:1132–41.

Kovach MJ, Waggoner B, Leal SM, Gelber D, Khardori R, Levenstien MA, Shanks CA, Gregg G, Al-Lozi MT, Miller T, Rakowica W, Lopate G, Florence J, Glosser G, Simmons Z, Morris JC, Whyte MP, Pestronk A, Kimonis VE. Clinical delineation and localization to chromosome 9p13.3-p12 of a unique dominant disorder in four families: hereditary inclusion body myopathy, Paget disease of bone, and frontotemporal dementia. Mol Genet Metab. 2001;74:458–75.

Kremer LS, Bader DM, Mertes C, Kopajtich R, Pichler G, Iuso A, et al. Genetic diagnosis of Mendelian disorders via RNA sequencing. Nat Commun. 2017;8:15,824.

Langer Y, Aran A, Gulsuner S, Abu Libdeh B, Renbaum P, Brunetti D, Teixeira PF, Walsh T, Zeligson S, Ruotolo R, Beeri R, Dweikat I, Shahrour M, Weinberg-Shukron A, Zahdeh F, Baruffini E, Glaser E, King MC, Levy-Lahad E, Zeviani M, Segel R. Mitochondrial PITRM1 peptidase loss-of-function in childhood cerebellar atrophy. J Med Genet. 2018;55:599–606.

Logan CV, Szabadkai G, Sharpe JA, Parry DA, Torelli S, Childs A-M, Kriek M, Phadke R, Johnson CA, Roberts NY, Bonthron DT, Pysden KA, et al. Loss-of-function mutations in MICU1 cause a brain and muscle disorder linked to primary alterations in mitochondrial calcium signaling. Nature Genet. 2014;46:188–93.

Li K, Jin R, Wu X. Whole-exome sequencing identifies rare compound heterozygous mutations in the MSTO1 gene associated with cerebellar ataxia and myopathy. Eur J Med Genet. 2020;63:103623.

Magen D, Georgopoulos C, Bross P, Ang D, Segev Y, Goldsher D, Nemirovski A, Shahar E, Ravid S, Luder A, Heno B, Gershoni-Baruch R, Skorecki K, Mandel H. Mitochondrial Hsp60 chaperonopathy causes an autosomal-recessive neurodegenerative disorder linked to brain hypomyelination and leukodystrophy. Am J Hum Genet. 2008;83:30–42.

Mandel H, Saita S, Edvardson S, Jalas C, Shaag A, Goldsher D, Vlodavsky E, Langer T, Elpeleg O. Deficiency of HTRA2/Omi is associated with infantile neurodegeneration and 3-methylglutaconic aciduria. J Med Genet. 2016;53:690–6.

Mayr JA, Haack TB, Graf E, Zimmermann FA, Wieland T, Haberberger B, et al. Lack of the mitochondrial protein acylglycerol kinase causes Sengers syndrome. Am J Hum Genet. 2012;90:314–20.

Megarbane A, Delague V, Salem N, Loiselet J. Autosomal recessive congenital cerebellar hypoplasia and short stature in a large inbred family. Am J Med Genet. 1999;87:88–90.

Megarbane A, Dagher R, Melki I. Sib pair with previously unreported skeletal dysplasia. Am J Med Genet. 2008;46A:2916–9.

Mehawej C, Delahodde A, Legeai-Mallet L, Delague V, Kaci N, Desvignes JP, Kibar Z. The impairment of MAGMAS function in human is responsible for a severe skeletal dysplasia. PLoS Genet. 2014;10:e1004311.

Mehta SG, Khare M, Ramani R, Watts GDJ, Simon M, Osann KE, Donkervoort S, Dec E, Nalbandian A, Platt J, Pasquali M, Wang A, Mozaffar T, Smith CD, Kimonis VE. Genotype-phenotype studies of VCP-associated inclusion body myopathy with Paget disease of bone and/or frontotemporal dementia. Clin Genet. 2013;83: 422–31.

Nasca A, Legati A, Baruffini E, Nolli C, Moroni I, Ardissone A, et al. Biallelic mutations in DNM1L are associated with a slowly progressive infantile encephalopathy. Hum Mutat. 2016;37:898–903.

Olahova M, Thompson K, Hardy SA, Barbosa IA, Besse A, Anagnostou M-E, White K, Davey T, Simpson MA, Champion M, Enns G, Schelley S, Lightowlers RN, Chrzanowska-Lightowlers ZMA, McFarland R, Deshpande C, Bonnen PE, Taylor RW. Pathogenic variants in HTRA2 cause an early-onset mitochondrial syndrome associated with 3-methylglutaconic aciduria. J Inherit Metab Dis. 2017;40:121–30.

O'Toole JF, Liu Y, Davis EE, Westlake CJ, Attanasio M, Otto EA, Seelow D, Nurnberg G, Becker C, Nuutinen M, Karppa M, et al. Individuals with mutations in XPNPEP3, which encodes a mitochondrial protein, develop a nephronophthisis-like nephropathy. J Clin Invest. 2010;120:791–802. Note: Erratum: J Clin Invest 120: 1362.

Poorkaj P, Nutt JG, James D, Gancher S, Bird TD, Steinbart E, Schellenberg GD, Payami H. Parkin mutation analysis in clinic patients with early-onset Parkinson's disease. Am. J. Med. Genet. 2004;129A:44–50. Note: Erratum: Am. J. Med. Genet. 139A: 56 only, 2005.

Prasad R, Chan LF, Hughes CR, Kaski JP, Kowalczyk JC, Savage MO, Peters CJ, Nathwani N, Clark AJL, Storr HL, Metherell LA. Thioredoxin reductase 2 (TXNRD2) mutation associated with familial glucocorticoid deficiency (FGD). J Clin Endocr Metab. 2014;99:E1556–63.

Royer-Bertrand B, Castillo-Taucher S, Moreno-Salinas R, Cho TJ, Chae JH, Choi M, et al. Mutations in the heat-shock protein A9 (HSPA9) gene cause the EVEN-PLUS syndrome of congenital malformations and skeletal dysplasia. Sci Rep. 2015;5:17,154.

Schmitz-Abe K, Ciesielski SJ, Schmidt PJ, Campagna DR, Rahimov F, Schilke BA, et al. Congenital sideroblastic anemia due to mutations in the mitochondrial HSP70 homologue HSPA9. Blood. 2015;126:2734–8.

Sengers RCA, ter Haar BGA, Trijbels JMF, Willems JL, Daniels O, Stadhouders AM. Congenital cataract and mitochondrial myopathy of skeletal and heart muscle associated with lactic acidosis after exercise. J Pediatr. 1975;86:873–80.

Shahni R, Cale CM, Anderson G, Osellame LD, Hambleton S, Jacques TS, et al. Signal transducer and activator of transcription 2 deficiency is a novel disorder of mitochondrial fission. Brain. 2015;138:2834–46.

Shahrour MA, Staretz-Chacham O, Dayan D, Stephen J, Weech A, Damseh N, et al. Mitochondrial epileptic encephalopathy, 3-methylglutaconic aciduria and variable complex V deficiency associated with TIMM50 mutations. Clin Genet. 2017;91:690–6.

Shamseldin HE, Alshammari M, Al-Sheddi T, Salih MA, Alkhalidi H, Kentab A, et al. Genomic analysis of mitochondrial diseases in a consanguineous population reveals novel candidate disease genes. J Med Genet. 2012;49:234–41.

Strauss KA, Jinks RN, Puffenberger EG, Venkatesh S, Singh K, Cheng I, et al. CODAS syndrome is associated with mutations of LONP1, encoding mitochondrial AAA+ Lon protease. Am J Hum Genet. 2015;96:121–35.

Tarpey PS, Smith R, Pleasance E, Whibley A, Edkins S, Hardy C, O'Meara S, Latimer C, Dicks E, Menzies A, Stephens P, Blow M, et al. A systematic, large-scale resequencing screen of X-chromosome coding exons in mental retardation. Nature Genet. 2009;41:535–43.

Tort F, Ugarteburu O, Texidó L, Gea-Sorlí S, García-Villoria J, Ferrer-Cortès X, et al. Mutations in TIMM50 cause severe mitochondrial dysfunction by targeting key aspects of mitochondrial physiology. Hum Mutat. 2019;40:1700–12.

Tranebjaerg L, Schwartz C, Eriksen H, Andreasson S, Ponjavic V, Dahl A, et al. A new X linked recessive deafness syndrome with blindness, dystonia, fractures, and mental deficiency is linked to Xq22. J Med Genet. 1995;32:257–63.

Vermeer S, Meijer RPP, Pijl BJ, Timmermans J, Cruysberg JRM, Bos MM, Schelhaas HJ, van de Warrenburg BPC, Knoers NVAM, Scheffer H, Kremer B. ARSACS in the Dutch population: a frequent cause of early-onset cerebellar ataxia. Neurogenetics. 2008;9:207–14. Note: Erratum: Neurogenetics 10: 87 only, 2009.

Vogtle F-N, Brandl B, Larson A, Pendziwiat M, Friederich MW, White SM, et al. Mutations in PMPCB encoding the catalytic subunit of the mitochondrial presequence protease cause neurodegeneration in early childhood. Am J Hum Genet. 2018;102:557–73.

Waterham HR, Koster J, van Roermund CWT, Mooyer PAW, Wanders RJA, Leonard JV. A lethal defect of mitochondrial and peroxisomal fission. N Eng J Med. 2007;356:1736–41.

Willems PHGM, Rossignol R, Dieteren CE, Murphy MP, Koopman WJH. Redox homeostasis and mitochondrial dynamics. Cell Metab. 2015;22:207–18.

Wortmann SB, Zietkiewicz S, Kousi M, Szklarczyk R, Haack TB, Gersting SW, et al. CLPB mutations cause 3-methylglutaconic aciduria, progressive brain atrophy, intellectual disability, congenital neutropenia, cataracts, movement disorder. Am J Hum Genet. 2015;96:245–57.

Yahalom G, Anikster Y, Huna-Baron R, Hoffmann C, Blumkin L, Lev D, et al. Costeff syndrome: clinical features and natural history. J Neurol. 2014;261:2275–82.

Yang X, Zhang R, Nakahira K, Gu Z. Mitochondrial DNA mutation, diseases, and nutrient-regulated mitophagy. Annu Rev Nutr. 2019;39:201–26.

Yu-Wai-Man P, Griffiths PG, Burke A, Sellar PW, Clarke MP, Gnanaraj L, et al. The prevalence and natural history of dominant optic atrophy due to OPA1 mutations. Ophthalmology. 2010a;117:1538–46.

Yu-Wai-Man P, Griffiths PG, Gorman GS, Lourenco CM, Wright AF, Auer-Grumbach M, et al. Multi-system neurological disease is common in patients with OPA1 mutations. Brain. 2010b;133:771–86.

Zeharia A, Friedman JR, Tobar A, Saada A, Konen O, Fellig Y, Shaag A, Nunnari J, Elpeleg O. Mitochondrial hepato-encephalopathy due to deficiency of QIL1/MIC13 (C19orf70), a MICOS complex subunit. Eur J Hum Genet. 2016;24:1778–82.

Zimon M, Baets J, Fabrizi GM, Jaakkola E, Kabzinska D, Pilch J, et al. Dominant GDAP1 mutations cause predominantly mild CMT phenotypes. Neurology. 2011;77:540–8.

# Primary Coenzyme $Q_{10}$ Deficiencies

47

Leonardo Salviati and Rafael Artuch

## Contents



**Summary**

Coenzyme $Q_{10}$($CoQ_{10}$) is a small lipophilic molecule which plays a number of crucial roles in cellular homeostasis. It is an electron carrier in the mitochondrial respiratory chain (MRC), and it is involved in other biochemical pathways such as mitochondrial fatty acid oxidation, sulfide detoxification, and pyrimidine biosynthesis. Moreover, it is modulator of the permeability transition pore, and an essential antioxidant. CoQ10 biosynthesis is still incompletely understood and involves the products of at least 12 different genes (collectively known as *COQ* genes). Mutations in these genes cause primary $CoQ_{10}$ deficiencies, a clinically and genetically heterogeneous group of conditions. To date mutations in nine genes (*PDSS1, PDSS2, COQ2, COQ4, COQ6, COQ7, COQ8A, COQ8B*, and *COQ9*) have been related to $CoQ_{10}$ deficiency in humans, while the association of two other genes (*ADCK2* and *COQ5*) must be confirmed.

The age of onset can span from birth to the 6–7th decade of life. Manifestations range from catastrophic multiorgan failure, to isolated cerebellar ataxia or steroid resistant nephrotic syndrome (SRNS). SRNS is a peculiar manifestation of $CoQ_{10}$ deficiency, since it is rarely seen in other mitochondrial disorders. Interestingly only some genetic defects cause SNRS (*PDSS1, PDSS2, COQ2, COQ6*, and *COQ8B*), while mutations in other genes (*COQ4, COQ7, COQ8A*, and *COQ9*) have never been observed in association with SRNS, but instead cause

L. Salviati (✉)
Clinical Genetics Unit, Department of Women and Children's Health, University of Padova, and IRP Città della Speranza, Padova, Italy
e-mail: leonardo.salviati@unipd.it

R. Artuch
CIBERER, Instituto de Salud Carlos III, Madrid, Spain

Clinical Chemistry Department, Institut de Recerca Sant Joan de Déu, Barcelona, Spain

Pathology Department, Institut de Recerca Sant Joan de Déu, Barcelona, Spain
e-mail: Rartuch@sjdhospitalbarcelona.org


N. Blau et al. (eds.), *Physician's Guide to the Diagnosis, Treatment, and Follow-Up of Inherited Metabolic Diseases*,
https://doi.org/10.1007/978-3-030-67727-5_47

encephalomyopathy or multisystem disorders without glomerular involvement.

$CoQ_{10}$ deficiency is one of the few treatable mitochondrial disorders. In fact, many patients (especially those with milder forms, and who are treated soon after the onset of symptoms) respond well to high-dose oral $CoQ_{10}$ supplementation. Therefore, it is essential to recognize promptly this condition to institute an appropriate treatment.

Traditionally, the diagnosis relied on biochemical analysis of $CoQ_{10}$ in muscle or cultured fibroblasts, while molecular studies were performed in a second time. Nowadays, NGS has revolutionized the diagnostic approach, and the molecular diagnosis generally precedes the biochemical one.

## Introduction

Coenzyme $Q_{10}$ ($CoQ_{10}$) is a small lipophilic molecule, comprised of a quinone group and an isoprenoid tail, which plays different crucial roles in cellular homeostasis. It is an electron carrier in the mitochondrial respiratory chain (MRC), where it shuttles electrons from respiratory complexes I and II to complex III; it is a cofactor of several other mitochondrial dehydrogenases (among which sulfide:quinone oxidoreductase which is essential for detoxification of $H_2S$), a modulator of the permeability transition pore, and an essential antioxidant (Turunen et al. 2004).

$CoQ_{10}$ biosynthesis is still incompletely understood in eukaryotic cells where it involves the products of at least 12 genes (collectively known as *COQ* genes). The precursor of the quinone group, 4-hydoxybenzoate (4HB), is derived from tyrosine through a poorly characterized set of reactions (Payet et al. 2016). The tail shares its initial biosynthetic steps with cholesterol through the cytosolic mevalonate pathway. Farnesyl-pyrophosphate is then condensed to form decaprenyl-pyrophosphate within mitochondria, by PDSS1 and PDSS2. Decaprenyl-pyrophosphate is then joined to 4HB by COQ2. The final biosynthetic steps are thought to be rate limiting and are carried out by a set of enzymes comprised of COQ3, COQ5, COQ6, and COQ7 located in the mitochondrial matrix associated to the inner membrane (Acosta et al. 2016). The proteins responsible for the decarboxylation and hydroxylation of position C1 of the ring, the first ring modifications to occur in mammals (Acosta Lopez et al. 2019), have not been identified yet. The process requires four other proteins, COQ9, which is required for the synthesis of COQ7, COQ8A, and COQ8B, which have a regulatory function, although their precise role is unclear, and COQ4, which is thought to be essential for holding together the other COQ proteins in a complex (Marbois et al. 2009).

$CoQ_{10}$ deficiency can be defined as the presence of reduced levels of $CoQ_{10}$ in tissues or cells of a patient (Acosta et al. 2016). The term primary $CoQ_{10}$ deficiency comprises a clinically and genetically heterogeneous group of disorders caused by mutations in *COQ* genes. Primary deficiencies must be distinguished from secondary forms, in which reduction of $CoQ_{10}$ is associated with mutations in genes unrelated to $CoQ_{10}$ biosynthesis (or to non-genetic factors) (Sacconi et al. 2010; Cordero et al. 2009). In this chapter, we will focus exclusively on primary forms. To date mutations in nine genes (*PDSS1, PDSS2, COQ2, COQ4, COQ6, COQ7, COQ8A, COQ8B*, and *COQ9*) have been related to primary $CoQ_{10}$ deficiency (Salviati et al. 2017), while the association with *COQ5* and *ADCK2* mutations must be confirmed.

Primary $CoQ_{10}$ deficiencies are associated with dramatically different *clinical presentations*, ranging from fatal neonatal multisystem disorders, to juvenile or adult-onset diseases with involvement of isolated organs. The genotype–phenotype correlations are only partially known. Most clinical symptoms are common to other respiratory chain disorders. However, a peculiar manifestation of $CoQ_{10}$ deficiency is renal glomerular involvement, manifesting as steroid resistant nephrotic syndrome (SRNS), which is rarely seen in other mitochondrial disorders (Emma et al. 2016).

The most severe forms are characterized by a catastrophic multiorgan failure, which leads to death at birth, or in the first days of life. Other forms may have a more subtle onset, and present in the first weeks of life with encephalomyopathic symptoms and features of Leigh syndrome on MRI. These forms are virtually indistinguishable from other severe MRC defects. Neonatal onset cases usually do not display glomerular involvement, although renal tubulopathy has been reported in patients with *COQ9* defects (Duncan et al. 2009) and renal morphological abnormalities, that did not affect function, were reported in *COQ7* patients (Kwong et al. 2019). SRNS may appear later in the course of the disease in long surviving early onset patients, or it can be the first manifestation in patients affected by intermediate forms, with disease onset occurring from the end of the first year of life through adolescence. In some cases, SRNS may be the only manifestation of $CoQ_{10}$ deficiency, while other patients develop features of neurological involvement. Curiously, SRNS has been observed in patients with mutations in *PDSS1, PDSS2, COQ2, COQ6*, and *COQ8B*, while it has never been reported in those with *COQ4, COQ7, COQ8A*, and *COQ9* mutations, which display only neuromuscular involvement (*COQ8A*) or neuromuscular involvement and multisystem dysfunction (*COQ4, COQ7*, and *COQ9*) (Acosta et al. 2016; Kwong et al. 2019). The reasons for these phenotypic differences are still unknown.

The *pathogenesis* of $CoQ_{10}$ deficiency involves deficient ATP production, increased ROS, impairment of pyrimidine metabolism (Lopez-Martin et al. 2007; Quinzii et al. 2010), and possibly impaired $H_2S$ clearance (Kleiner et al. 2018). At very low $CoQ_{10}$ concentrations, the defect in energy production prevails, while ROS are not increased, and the clinical manifestations are those of classical MRC defects. With milder $CoQ_{10}$ deficiency, ATP production is less impaired, and classical "mitochondrial" symptoms are less evident, whereas ROS production gradually increases causing the glomerular damage (Quinzii et al. 2008; Quinzii et al. 2013). For some genes, for example *COQ2*, the genotype–phenotype correlation is clear and depends on the presence of residual enzymatic activity (Desbats et al. 2016), while for others, such *COQ8B*, there is no clear genotype–phenotype correlation (Vazquez Fonseca et al. 2018).

Traditionally, the *diagnosis* was based on direct biochemical measurements of $CoQ_{10}$ in muscle biopsies or cultured fibroblasts, and then molecular genetics followed. NGS has revolutionized the diagnostic protocols, and it is simpler and cheaper to run the genetic analysis first, and then to confirm the findings with biochemical analyses on patients' tissues (Yubero et al. 2018). Measurements of plasma $CoQ_{10}$ levels are not indicated for diagnosis because they reflect dietary intake rather than tissue concentration of $CoQ_{10}$. Furthermore, in our experience, patients with later-onset forms (who present in late childhood, adolescence or even later) may display little or no reduction of $CoQ_{10}$ in fibroblasts and even in skeletal muscle, despite harboring clearly pathogenic mutations.

The suspicion of primary $CoQ_{10}$ deficiency should arise in cases of early onset mitochondrial disorders, SRNS (even isolated), and unexplained ataxia (Trevisson et al. 2011). NGS panels for these conditions routinely include *COQ* genes, but whole exome sequencing is becoming the first line investigation in these patients.

Primary $CoQ_{10}$ deficiency is one of the few treatable mitochondrial disorders. Many patients respond well to oral $CoQ_{10}$ supplementation. *Treatment* can stop the progression of the encephalopathy and reverse the nephropathy. It must however be instituted before severe tissue damage has occurred, otherwise it is largely ineffective. Severe neonatal cases often do not respond (or respond only partially) to treatment (Alcazar-Fabra et al. 2018). Doses employed range from 10 to 30 or even 50 mg/kg per day of ubiquinone (the oxidized form of $CoQ_{10}$). Ubiquinol (the reduced form) appears to be more effective than ubiquinone in animal models (Garcia-Corzo et al. 2014), but there is much less clinical experience. Moreover, long-term data about the efficacy of $CoQ_{10}$ supplementation in patients are however scarce.

Recently a novel approach, bypass therapy, has been proposed. It involves the use of specific analogues of the quinone ring which can bypass individual genetic defects (Pierrel 2017). Results are promising in cellular and animal models, but there is currently no experience in patients.

## Nomenclature

| No. | Disorder | Alternative name | Alternative name-2 | Abbreviation | Gene symbol | Chromosomal location | Affected protein | OMIM no. |
|---|---|---|---|---|---|---|---|---|
| 47.1 | Prenyl diphosphate synthase, subunit 1 (PDSS1) deficiency | Coenzyme Q10 deficiency, primary, 2 | Decaprenyl diphosphate synthase (DPS) deficiency | COQ10D2 | *PDSS1* | 10p12.1 | Prenyl diphosphate synthase subunit 1 | 614651 |
| 47.2 | Prenyl diphosphate synthase, subunit 2 (PDSS2) deficiency | Coenzyme Q10 deficiency, primary, 3 | Decaprenyl diphosphate synthase (DPS) deficiency | COQ10D3 | *PDSS2* | 6q21 | Prenyl diphosphate synthase subunit 2 | 614652 |
| 47.3 | COQ2 deficiency | Coenzyme Q10 deficiency, primary, 1 | Mitochondrial 4-hydroxybenzoate-polyprenyltransferase deficiency | COQ10D1 | *COQ2* | 4q21-q22 | 4-hydroxybenzoate-polyprenyl-transferase | 607426 |
| 47.4 | COQ4 deficiency | Coenzyme Q10 deficiency, primary, 7 | | COQ4D7 | *COQ4* | 9q34.11 | COQ4 | 616276 |
| 47.5 | COQ6 deficiency | Coenzyme Q10 deficiency, primary, 6 | Early onset steroid-resistant nephrosis with sensorineural deafness | COQ10D6 | *COQ6* | 14q24.3 | COQ6 monooxygenase | 614650 |

(continued)

| No. | Disorder | Alternative name | Alternative name-2 | Abbreviation | Gene symbol | Chromosomal location | Affected protein | OMIM no. |
|---|---|---|---|---|---|---|---|---|
| 47.6 | COQ7 deficiency | Coenzyme Q10 deficiency, primary, 8 | | COQ10D8 | *COQ7* | 16p12.3 | COQ7, di-iron oxidase | 616733 |
| 47.7 | COQ8A deficiency | Coenzyme Q10 deficiency, primary, 4 | ADCK3 deficiency | COQ10D4 | *COQ8A* | 1q42.13 | AARF DOMAIN-CONTAINING KINASE 3 | 612016 |
| 47.8 | COQ8B deficiency | Nephrotic syndrome type 9 | ADCK4 deficiency | | *COQ8B* | 19q13.2 | AARF DOMAIN-CONTAINING KINASE 4 | 615573 |
| 47.9 | COQ9 deficiency | Coenzyme Q10 deficiency, primary, 5 | | COQ10D5 | *COQ9* | 16q21 | COQ9 | 614654 |

## Metabolic Pathway

The precursors of $CoQ_{10}$, 4-hydroxybenzoate (4-HB) and farnesyl-pyrophosphate, are derived from tyrosine through a still poorly characterized set of reactions, and from acetyl-CoA, through the mevalonate pathway. Farnesyl-pyrophosphate is joined by a heterotetrameric enzyme comprised of PDSS1 and PDSS2 to form decaprenyl-pyrophosphate which is then joined to 4-HB by COQ2. The next two steps (the decarboxylation and hydroxylation of the C1 carbon) are catalyzed by still unknown enzymes, while the hydroxylation of the C5 carbon of the ring is carried out by COQ6. COQ3 then transfers a methyl group to this hydroxyl, and COQ5 transfers another methyl group directly on the C2 carbon. Last, COQ7 hydroxylates the C6 carbon and COQ3 adds the final methyl group. COQ9 is essential for the stabilization of COQ7. The precise role of COQ4, COQ8A, COQ8B, and ADCK2 is still under investigation. Gene products in red have been definitely associated to human $CoQ_{10}$ deficiency (Fig. 47.1a and b).

Besides being an electron carrier within the respiratory chain, where it shuttles electron from complex I (CI) and II (CII) to complex III (CIII), CoQ is a cofactor of electron transfer flavoprotein dehydrogenase (ETFDH) (involved in mitochondrial fatty acid oxidation), sulfide:quinone oxido-reductase (SQOR) (involved in sulfide detoxification), and dihydroorotate dehydrogenase (DHODH) involved in pyrimidine nucleotides biosynthesis. Moreover, it is a cofactor of uncoupling proteins (UCP), a modulator of the permeability transition pore (PTP) thus controlling apoptosis, and one of the most important cellular antioxidants (Fig. 47.1c).

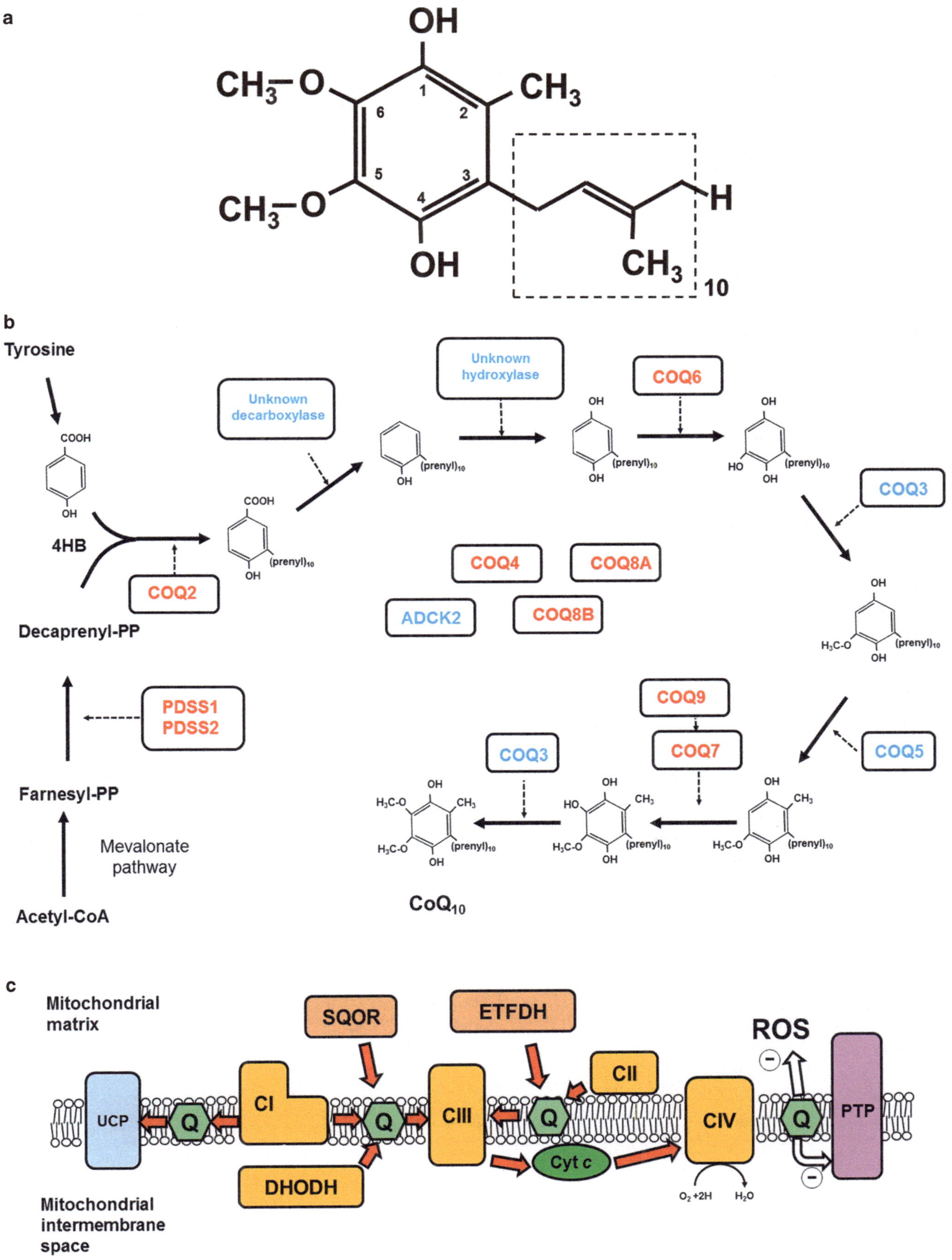


**Fig. 47.1** (**a**) Structure of the reduced form of $CoQ_{10}$. Carbons comprising the aromatic ring are numbered. (**b**) New model of the CoQ biosynthetic pathway in mammals based on the data of Acosta Lopez et al. 2019. (**c**) The central role of coenzyme $Q_{10}$ (Q) in mitochondrial homeostasis

## Signs and Symptoms

**Table 47.1** Prenyl diphosphate synthase, subunit 1 (PDSS1) deficiency

| System | Symptoms and biomarkers | Neonatal (birth–1 month) | Infancy (1–18 months) | Childhood (1.5–11 years) | Adolescence (11–16 years) | Adulthood (>16 years) |
|---|---|---|---|---|---|---|
| Cardiovascular | **Cardiomyopathy** | | | | + | + |
| CNS | Intellectual disability | | ± | + | + | + |
| | Neuropathy, peripheral | | | + | + | + |
| Digestive | Obesity | | | + | + | + |
| Ear | **Deafness** | | + | + | + | + |
| Eye | **Optic atrophy** | | | + | + | + |
| Musculoskeletal | **Macrocephaly** | | | + | + | + |
| Renal | Nephrotic syndrome | | ± | | | |
| Laboratory findings | CoQ10 (fibroblasts) | | | | ↓ | ↓ |
| | Lactate (plasma) | | ↑ | ↑ | ↑ | ↑ |

**Table 47.2** Prenyl diphosphate synthase, subunit 2 (PDSS2) deficiency

| System | Symptoms and biomarkers | Neonatal (birth–1 month) | Infancy (1–18 months) | Childhood (1.5–11 years) | Adolescence (11–16 years) | Adulthood (>16 years) |
|---|---|---|---|---|---|---|
| Cardiovascular | Cardiomyopathy | + | + | | | |
| CNS | **Epilepsy** | + | +++ | ++ | | |
| | **Leigh syndrome** | + | +++ | | | |
| | Stroke-like episodes | | + | ++ | | |
| Musculoskeletal | **Muscle weakness** | +++ | +++ | ++ | | |
| Renal | Nephrotic syndrome | | +++ | +++ | +++ | + |
| Laboratory findings | CoQ10 (fibroblasts) | ↓ | ↓ | ↓ | | |
| | CoQ10 (muscle) | ↓ | ↓ | ↓ | | |
| | Lactate (plasma) | ↑ | n-↑ | n | n | |

**Table 47.3** COQ2 deficiency

| System | Symptoms and biomarkers | Neonatal (birth–1 month) | Infancy (1–18 months) | Childhood (1.5–11 years) | Adolescence (11–16 years) | Adulthood (>16 years) |
|---|---|---|---|---|---|---|
| CNS | **Epilepsy** | + | +++ | + | + | |
| | Leigh syndrome | | ++ | | | |
| | **Multiple system atrophy-like encephalopathy** | | | | | ± |
| | Regression, psychomotor | | | ++ | | |
| | Stroke-like episodes | | | ++ | | |
| Ear | Deafness | | + | + | | |
| Eye | Retinopathy | | | ± | ± | ± |
| Musculoskeletal | Muscle weakness | | +++ | +++ | | |
| Other | **Severe multisystem disease** | +++ | | | | |
| Renal | **Nephrotic syndrome** | + | + | ++ | + | + |
| Laboratory findings | CoQ10 (fibroblasts) | ↓ | ↓ | ↓ | | |
| | CoQ10 (muscle) | ↓ | ↓ | ↓ | | |
| | Lactate (plasma) | ↑↑ | n-↑ | n | n | |

**Table 47.4** COQ4 deficiency

| System | Symptoms and biomarkers | Neonatal (birth–1 month) | Infancy (1–18 months) | Childhood (1.5–11 years) | Adolescence (11–16 years) | Adulthood (>16 years) |
|---|---|---|---|---|---|---|
| Cardiovascular | Bradycardia | ± | ± | ± | | |
| | Cardiomyopathy, hypertrophic | ± | ± | ± | | |
| | Left ventricular hypoplasia | ± | ± | ± | | |
| | Patent ductus arteriosus | ± | ± | ± | | |
| | Ataxia, cerebellar | | | + | + | + |
| | Encephalopathy, epileptic | ± | ± | ± | | |
| | Hypotonia | + | | | | |
| | Neuropathy, sensory | ± | ± | ± | | |
| | Regression, psychomotor | | ± | ± | | |
| | Seizures | ± | ± | ± | | |
| | Spasticity | | | ± | ± | ± |
| CNS | Swallowing difficulties | + | + | + | | |
| Musculoskeletal | Scoliosis | | ± | | | |
| Other | Intrauterine growth retardation | + | | | | |
| | Multiorgan failure | +++ | + | | | |
| Respiratory | **Respiratory insufficiency** | + | | | | |
| Laboratory findings | 2-Hydroxyglutarate (urine) | n-↑ | n-↑ | n-↑ | | |
| | CoQ10 (fibroblasts) | ↓ | ↓ | ↓-n | ↓-n | |
| | CoQ10 (muscle) | ↓ | ↓ | ↓-n | ↓-n | |
| | Lactate (plasma) | ↑ | ↑ | ↑ | n | n |

**Table 47.5** COQ6 deficiency

| System | Symptoms and biomarkers | Neonatal (birth–1 month) | Infancy (1–18 months) | Childhood (1.5–11 years) | Adolescence (11–16 years) | Adulthood (>16 years) |
|---|---|---|---|---|---|---|
| CNS | Ataxia | | | ± | | |
| | Epilepsy | | | ± | | |
| Ear | Deafness, sensorineural | ± | + | + | + | ± |
| Renal | **Nephrotic syndrome** | | ± | ++ | ++ | |
| Laboratory findings | CoQ10 (fibroblasts) | | | | | ↓-n |
| | Lactate (plasma) | | n | n | n | n |

**Table 47.6** COQ7 deficiency

| System | Symptoms and biomarkers | Neonatal (birth–1 month) | Infancy (1–18 months) | Childhood (1.5–11 years) | Adolescence (11–16 years) | Adulthood (>16 years) |
|---|---|---|---|---|---|---|
| Cardiovascular | Pulmonary hypertension | + | | | | |
| CNS | Axonal sensory motor polyneuropathy, chronic | | + | + | | |
| | Hypotonia | + | + | | | |
| | Retardation, motor | + | + | + | | |
| Digestive | Feeding difficulties | + | + | | | |
| Ear | **Hearing loss, sensorineural** | + | + | + | | |
| Eye | **Visual impairment** | + | + | + | | |
| Musculoskeletal | Growth retardation | + | + | + | | |
| | Joint contractures | + | + | | | |
| Other | Intrauterine growth retardation | + | | | | |
| Psychiatric | Learning disabilities | | + | + | | |
| Renal | Kidney dysplasia | + | + | + | | |
| | **Renal dysfunction** | + | | | | |
| Respiratory | Respiratory distress | + | | | | |
| Laboratory findings | CoQ10 (fibroblasts) | ↓ | ↓ | ↓ | | |
| | CoQ10 (muscle) | ↓ | ↓ | ↓ | | |
| | Fumaric acid (urine) | ↑ | ↑ | ↑ | | |
| | Lactate (cerebrospinal fluid) | ↑ | ↑ | ↑ | | |
| | Lactate (plasma) | n-↑ | n-↑ | n-↑ | | |
| | Malic acid (urine) | ↑ | ↑ | ↑ | | |

**Table 47.7** COQ8A deficiency

| System | Symptoms and biomarkers | Neonatal (birth–1 month) | Infancy (1–18 months) | Childhood (1.5–11 years) | Adolescence (11–16 years) | Adulthood (>16 years) |
|---|---|---|---|---|---|---|
| CNS | **Ataxia** | | + | ++ | ++ | ++ |
| | Cognitive dysfunction | | ± | ± | ± | ± |
| | Dystonia | | ± | ± | ± | ± |
| | **Epilepsy** | | + | + | + | + |
| | Pyramidal signs | | ± | ± | ± | ± |
| Musculoskeletal | **Muscle weakness** | | + | + | + | + |
| Laboratory findings | CoQ10 (fibroblasts) | ↓-n | ↓-n | ↓-n | ↓-n | ↓-n |
| | CoQ10 (muscle) | ↓-n | ↓-n | ↓-n | ↓-n | ↓-n |
| | Lactate (plasma) | n-↑ | n-↑ | n-↑ | n-↑ | n-↑ |

**Table 47.8** COQ8B deficiency

| System | Symptoms and biomarkers | Neonatal (birth–1 month) | Infancy (1–18 months) | Childhood (1.5–11 years) | Adolescence (11–16 years) | Adulthood (>16 years) |
|---|---|---|---|---|---|---|
| CNS | Epilepsy | | ± | ± | ± | ± |
| | Intellectual disability | | ± | ± | ± | ± |
| Musculoskeletal | **Edema** | | ± | + | + | + |
| Renal | **Nephrotic syndrome** | | ± | + | + | + |
| | Proteinuria | | ± | + | + | + |
| | **Renal failure, chronic** | | ± | + | + | + |
| | **Renal failure, end stage** | | ± | + | + | + |
| Laboratory findings | Albumin (serum) | | | ↓ | ↓ | |
| | CoQ10 (lymphoblasts or fibroblasts) | | ↓ | ↓ | ↓ | ↓ |
| | Proteins, total (urine) | | | ↑ | ↑ | |

**Table 47.9** COQ9 deficiency

| System | Symptoms and biomarkers | Neonatal (birth–1 month) | Infancy (1–18 months) | Childhood (1.5–11 years) | Adolescence (11–16 years) | Adulthood (>16 years) |
|---|---|---|---|---|---|---|
| Autonomic system | **Hypothermia** | +++ | | | | |
| Cardiovascular | Cardiomyopathy | | ++ | | | |
| CNS | Epilepsy | + | +++ | | | |
| | Regression, psychomotor | | +++ | | | |
| Digestive | **Feeding difficulties** | ++ | ++ | | | |
| Metabolic | **Lactic acidosis** | +++ | +++ | | | |
| Renal | **Renal tubulopathy** | + | + | | | |
| Laboratory findings | CoQ10 (fibroblasts) | ↓ | ↓ | | | |
| | CoQ10 (muscle) | ↓ | ↓ | | | |
| | Lactate (plasma) | ↑ | ↑ | | | |

It should be noted that relatively few patients have been described (for some genes less than 10), therefore clinical data are probably incomplete. Moreover, clinical presentations differ dramatically depending on the age of onset (see for example the case of COQ2) (Desbats et al. 2016). There are no pathognomonic manifestations, although the association of SRNS with other neurological manifestation should immediately raise the suspicion of $CoQ_{10}$ deficiency.

## Reference Values

There are currently no universally accepted reference values for $CoQ_{10}$ in muscle or fibroblasts, although most authors reported muscle CoQ10 values in a range between 110 and 580 nmol $CoQ_{10}$/g protein and in fibroblasts between 39 and 112 nmol/g protein. It is important to refer the data to a set of in-house age matched controls and it is also useful to normalize data by citrate synthase activity (Yubero et al. 2014).

## Diagnostic Flowchart

The traditional approach privileged biochemical determinations, and genetic analyses, which were more complex and expensive, were performed only in a second stage. Nowadays, NGS allows analysis of very large numbers of genes for a fraction of the cost and of the time required by traditional Sanger sequencing. Targeted NGS gene panels are commonly used for SRNS, ataxias, and mitochondrial disorders. Whole Exome Sequencing (WES) is theoretically the best option, but costs are higher and coverage is inferior to targeted panels. Moreover CNV analysis is more efficient with targeted panels. Clinical exome panels include 5–7000 genes associated with Mendelian diseases. They may be a good compromise although they may lack some critical genes (see also Chap. 9).

Fig. 47.2 Traditional versus NGS-centered approaches for the diagnosis of primary $CoQ_{10}$ deficiency

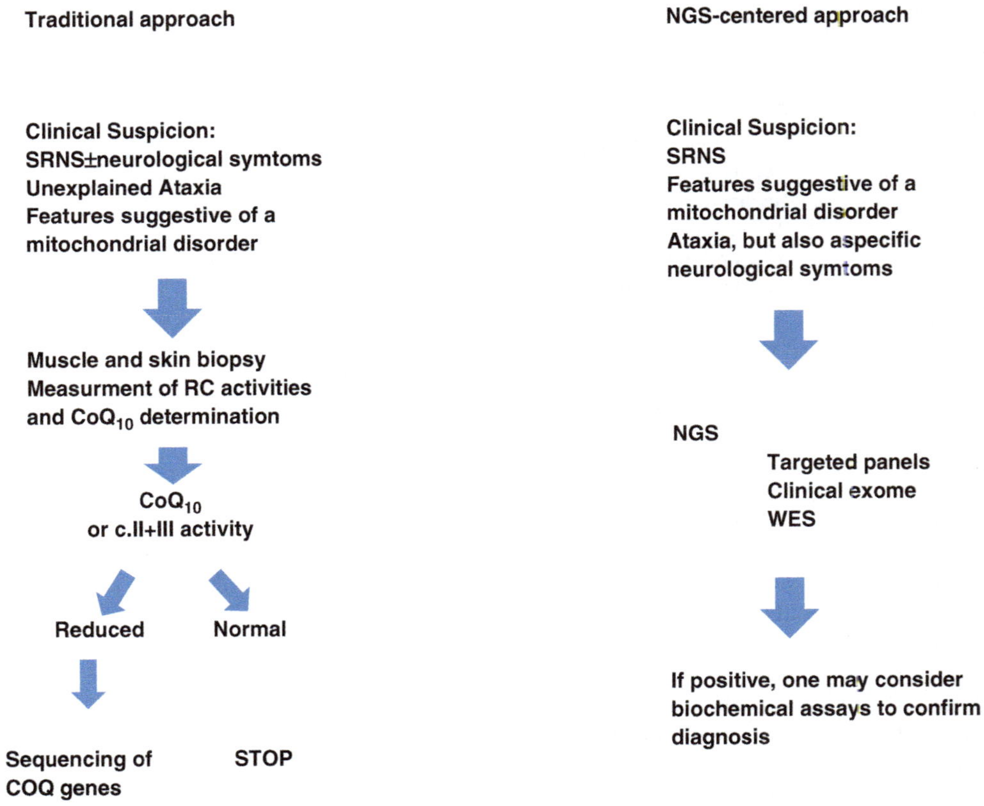


## Specimen Collection

Plasma $CoQ_{10}$ content determination is meaningless and should not be performed. Serum lactic acid should be measured with the precautions discussed for other mitochondrial disorders to avoid false positive results.

If possible $CoQ_{10}$ should be measured in muscle samples (which can be safely frozen at −80 °C or, better, in liquid nitrogen, and can be shipped in dry ice) and in cultured skin fibroblast.

## Prenatal Diagnosis

Prenatal diagnosis can be performed by molecular testing on standard chorionic villi or amniotic fluid cells, for all these forms, provided that the molecular defect in the index case has been unambiguously identified.

Biochemical tests, such as $CoQ_{10}$ determination in amniocytes, are not usually employed.

## DNA Testing

DNA testing is available for all forms of $CoQ_{10}$ deficiency. Specific strategies have been described above.

In particular cases, RNA analysis from cultured fibroblasts can be performed.

## Treatment

The mainstay of treatment is oral supplementation with high dose $CoQ_{10}$. Most reports refer to ubiquinone, the oxidized form of $CoQ_{10}$. Dosages range from 5 to 50 mg/kg/day divided in three or more doses. Several formulations are available, but in general soluble forms, soft gel caps, or oily formulations should be preferred (Desbats et al. 2015). Tablets should not be administered because of poor absorption (Bhagavan and Chopra 2007). Ubiquinol, the reduced form of $CoQ_{10}$ is also available, but there is limited experience in patients. Idebenone is not effective and should not be employed in these patients. Patients with SRNS may also benefit of treatment with ACE inhibitors. Bypass therapy using analogues of the precursor of the quinone ring has been tested in cells and model organisms, but to date there are no data in patients.

Renal transplantation is an option for patients with end-stage renal disease.

## References


Acosta Lopez MJ, Trevisson E, Canton M, Vazquez-Fonseca L, Morbidoni V, Baschiera E, Frasson C, Pelosi L, Rascalou B, Desbats MA, Alcazar-Fabra M, Rios JJ, Sanchez-Garcia A, Basso G, Navas P, Pierrel F, Brea-Calvo G, Salviati L. Vanillic acid restores coenzyme Q biosynthesis and ATP production in human cells lacking COQ6. Oxidative Med Cell Longev. 2019;2019:3904905.

Acosta MJ, Vazquez Fonseca L, Desbats MA, Cerqua C, Zordan R, Trevisson E, Salviati L. Coenzyme Q biosynthesis in health and disease. Biochim Biophys Acta. 2016;1857(8):1079–85.

Alcazar-Fabra M, Trevisson E, Brea-Calvo G. Clinical syndromes associated with coenzyme Q10 deficiency. Essays Biochem. 2018;62(3):377–98.

Bhagavan HN, Chopra RK. Plasma coenzyme Q10 response to oral ingestion of coenzyme Q10 formulations. Mitochondrion. 2007;7(Suppl):S78–88.

Cordero MD, Moreno-Fernandez AM, deMiguel M, Bonal P, Campa F, Jimenez-Jimenez LM, Ruiz-Losada A, Sanchez-Dominguez B, Sanchez Alcazar JA, Salviati L, Navas P. Coenzyme Q10 distribution in blood is altered in patients with fibromyalgia. Clin Biochem. 2009;42(7–8):732–5.

Desbats MA, Lunardi G, Doimo M, Trevisson E, Salviati L. Genetic bases and clinical manifestations of coenzyme Q10 (CoQ 10) deficiency. J Inherit Metab Dis. 2015;38(1):145–56.

Desbats MA, Morbidoni V, Silic-Benussi M, Doimo M, Ciminale V, Cassina M, Sacconi S, Hirano M, Basso G, Pierrel F, Navas P, Salviati L, Trevisson E. The COQ2 genotype predicts the severity of coenzyme Q10 deficiency. Hum Mol Genet. 2016;25(19):4256–65.

Duncan AJ, Bitner-Glindzicz M, Meunier B, Costello H, Hargreaves IP, Lopez LC, Hirano M, Quinzii CM, Sadowski MI, Hardy J, Singleton A, Clayton PT, Rahman S. A nonsense mutation in COQ9 causes autosomal-recessive neonatal-onset primary coenzyme Q10 deficiency: a potentially treatable form of mitochondrial disease. Am J Hum Genet. 2009;84(5):558–66.

Emma F, Montini G, Parikh SM, Salviati L. Mitochondrial dysfunction in inherited renal disease and acute kidney injury. Nat Rev Nephrol. 2016;12(5):267–80.

Garcia-Corzo L, Luna-Sanchez M, Doerrier C, Ortiz F, Escames G, Acuna-Castroviejo D, Lopez LC. Ubiquinol-10 ameliorates mitochondrial encephalopathy associated with CoQ deficiency. Biochim Biophys Acta. 2014;1842(7):893–901.

Kleiner G, Barca E, Ziosi M, Emmanuele V, Xu Y, Hidalgo-Gutierrez A, Qiao C, Tadesse S, Area-Gomez E, Lopez LC, Quinzii CM. CoQ10 supplementation rescues nephrotic syndrome through normalization of H2S oxidation pathway. Biochim Biophys Acta Mol basis Dis. 2018;1864(11):3708–22.

Kwong AK, Chiu AT, Tsang MH, Lun KS, Rodenburg RJT, Smeitink J, Chung BH, Fung CW. A fatal case of COQ7-associated primary coenzyme Q10 deficiency. JIMD Rep. 2019;47(1):23–9.

Lopez-Martin JM, Salviati L, Trevisson E, Montini G, DiMauro S, Quinzii C, Hirano M, Rodriguez-Hernandez A, Cordero MD, Sanchez-Alcazar JA, Santos-Ocana C, Navas P. Missense mutation of the COQ2 gene causes defects of bioenergetics and de novo pyrimidine synthesis. Hum Mol Genet. 2007;16(9):1091–7.

Marbois B, Gin P, Gulmezian M, Clarke CF. The yeast Coq4 polypeptide organizes a mitochondrial protein complex essential for coenzyme Q biosynthesis. Biochim Biophys Acta. 2009;1791(1):69–75.

Payet LA, Leroux M, Willison JC, Kihara A, Pelosi L, Pierrel F. Mechanistic details of early steps in coenzyme Q biosynthesis pathway in yeast. Cell Chem Biol. 2016;23(10):1241–50.

Pierrel F. Impact of chemical analogs of 4-hydroxybenzoic acid on coenzyme Q biosynthesis: from inhibition to bypass of coenzyme Q deficiency. Front Physiol. 2017;8:436.

Quinzii CM, Garone C, Emmanuele V, Tadesse S, Krishna S, Dorado B, Hirano M. Tissue-specific oxidative stress and loss of mitochondria in CoQ-deficient Pdss2 mutant mice. FASEB J. 2013;27(2):612–21.

Quinzii CM, Lopez LC, Gilkerson RW, Dorado B, Coku J, Naini AB, Lagier-Tourenne C, Schuelke M, Salviati L, Carrozzo R, Santorelli F, Rahman S, Tazir M, Koenig M, DiMauro S, Hirano M. Reactive oxygen species, oxidative stress, and cell death correlate with level of CoQ10 deficiency. FASEB J. 2010;24(10):3733–43.

Quinzii CM, Lopez LC, Von-Moltke J, Naini A, Krishna S, Schuelke M, Salviati L, Navas P, DiMauro S, Hirano M. Respiratory chain dysfunction and oxidative stress correlate with severity of primary CoQ10 deficiency. FASEB J. 2008;22(6):1874–85.

Sacconi S, Trevisson E, Salviati L, Ayme S, Rigal O, Redondo AG, Mancuso M, Siciliano G, Tonin P, Angelini C, Aure K, Lombes A, Desnuelle C. Coenzyme Q10 is frequently reduced in muscle of patients with mitochondrial myopathy. Neuromuscul Disord. 2010;20(1):44–8.

Salviati L, Trevisson E, Doimo M, Navas P. Primary coenzyme Q10 deficiency. In: Pagon RA, Adam MP, Ardinger HH, Wallace SE, Amemiya A, Bean LJH, Bird TD, Ledbetter N, Mefford HC, Smith RJH, Stephens K, editors. GeneReviews(R). Seattle, WA: University of Seattle; 2017.

Trevisson E, DiMauro S, Navas P, Salviati L. Coenzyme Q deficiency in muscle. Curr Opin Neurol. 2011;24(5):449–56.

Turunen M, Olsson J, Dallner G. Metabolism and function of coenzyme Q. Biochim Biophys Acta. 2004;1660(1–2):171–99.

Vazquez Fonseca L, Doimo M, Calderan C, Desbats MA, Acosta MJ, Cerqua C, Cassina M, Ashraf S, Hildebrandt F, Sartori G, Navas P, Trevisson E, Salviati L. Mutations in COQ8B (ADCK4) found in patients with steroid-resistant nephrotic syndrome alter COQ8B function. Hum Mutat. 2018;39(3):406–14.

Yubero D, Montero R, Artuch R, Land JM, Heales SJ, Hargreaves IP. Biochemical diagnosis of coenzyme q10 deficiency. Mol Syndromol. 2014;5(3–4):147–55.

Yubero D, Montero R, Santos-Ocana C, Salviati L, Navas P, Artuch R. Molecular diagnosis of coenzyme Q10 deficiency: an update. Expert Rev Mol Diagn. 2018;18(6):491–8.

# Part VI

# Disorders of Lipids

# Mitochondrial Fatty Acid Oxidation Disorders

48

Ute Spiekerkoetter and Jerry Vockley

## Contents




U. Spiekerkoetter (✉)
Department of Pediatrics and Adolescent Medicine, University Children's Hospital, Albert Ludwigs University, Freiburg, Germany
e-mail: ute.spiekerkoetter@uniklinik-freiburg.de

J. Vockley (✉)
Children's Hospital of Pittsburgh, University of Pittsburgh Medical Center, University of Pittsburgh, Pittsburgh, PA, USA
e-mail: vockleyg@upmc.edu




N. Blau et al. (eds.), *Physician's Guide to the Diagnosis, Treatment, and Follow-Up of Inherited Metabolic Diseases*,
https://doi.org/10.1007/978-3-030-67727-5_48

## Summary

Mitochondrial fatty acid oxidation disorders (FAODs) impair the ability of the body to utilize fats for energy production during times of physiologic stress such as fasting or illness, and thus can be asymptomatic and difficult to diagnose when a patient is well. Reducing equivalents from fatty acid oxidation (FAO) enzyme reactions directly enter the electron transfer chain (ETC) to support generation of adenosine triphosphate (ATP) through oxidative phosphorylation (oxphos), or by entry of its end product acetyl-coenzyme A (acetyl-CoA) into the tricarboxylic acid cycle (TCA or Krebs cycle). Acetyl-CoA from FAO can also be used to synthesize ketones, a fuel source that is used by some peripheral tissues and especially the brain during catabolic situations. Due to the ability to prevent life-threatening symptoms through early diagnosis, FAODs have been included in newborn screening (NBS) panels worldwide through tandem mass spectrometry-based screening. Acylcarnitine profiles are specific for the respective enzyme defects; however, the diagnosis should be confirmed by enzyme assay and/or molecular analysis as they may also offer insight into clinical severity. Metabolic profiles can be normal in the anabolic state and, consequently, newborn screening may miss the diagnosis when performed outside the catabolic state on days 2 and 3 of life. Mitochondrial fatty acid oxidation disorders are comprised of four groups: (1) disorders of the entry of long-chain fatty acids into mitochondria (often referred to as carnitine cycle defects), (2) intramitochondrial ß-oxidation defects of long-chain fatty acids, (3) β-oxidation defects of short- and medium-chain fatty acids affecting enzymes of the mitochondrial matrix, and (4) disorders of impaired electron transfer to the respiratory chain from mitochondrial β-oxidation. All told, more than 20 different genetic enzyme defects of FAO have now been identified, some with disease-specific characteristics that distinguish them from others in the group. The main pathophysiologic mechanism of all FAODs is an energy deficiency due to impaired fatty acid oxidation and ketone body formation. Toxic effects of accumulating acylcarnitine and acyl-CoA species may also play a role. FAODs present with heterogeneous phenotypes. Before addition of FAODs to newborn screening (NBS) panels in many countries, the commonest clinical presentations were hypoketotic hypoglycemia and sudden death, usually precipitated by an infection or fasting in the neonatal period or early childhood. With newborn screening, apparent disease incidence has significantly increased, while the proportion of milder phenotypes has grown. Newborn screening greatly reduces the morbidity and mortality, though it does not eliminate early neonatal death in severe phenotypes in some of the defects. Three major phenotypes are now recognized. Nonketotic hypoglycemia predominates in the first few years of life, but is uncommon after age 4–6 years. Cardiomyopathy and arrhythmias are seen at any time, may be of acute onset, and can also be reversible. Exercise- or illness-induced rhabdomyolysis is a common presentation in adolescents or young adults, but muscle pain and elevated creatine kinase (CK) can occur in infancy. With some disorders, patients can remain asymptomatic throughout life if they have mild defects and are not exposed to the metabolic stress. Affected asymptomatic mothers have been identified due to pathological newborn screening in their child. Correlation of genotype and/or residual enzyme activity with disease phenotype has been reported for some defects but is imperfect, suggesting an additional role for disease modifiers and environment. Treatment must be tailored to the severity of the phenotype and the specific disorder, with a focus on avoidance of fasting, mitigation of stress, and fluid and caloric support through episodes of rhabdomyolysis. New therapies are in development and may change significantly the long-term prognosis for patients.

## Introduction

Fat is an important source of energy and the body's principal fuel store. It is the main fuel for skeletal muscle during sustained exercise, and provides reducing equivalents to make ATP through oxidative phosphorylation during periods of fasting and physiologic stress. In postnatal life, fatty acids are used in preference to glucose by the heart regardless of caloric intake.

Mitochondrial fatty acid oxidation involves four processes: (1) entry of fatty acids into mitochondria (the carnitine cycle), (2) mitochondrial ß-oxidation of long-chain fatty acids via a spiral pathway utilizing membrane-bound enzymes, (3) mitochondrial β-oxidation of chain-shortened fatty acids using matrix enzymes, and (4) electron transfer to the respiratory chain.

The clinical presentation of these disorders is heterogeneous. FAODs have three characteristic clinical presentations:

1. *Acute hypoketotic hypoglycemia and encephalopathy, accompanied by hepatomegaly and liver dysfunction* precipitated by fasting or an infection, often described as the hepatic presentation or "Reye-like symptoms." Presentation generally occurs in the first weeks and months of life, and the appearance and severity can be mitigated by early identification through newborn screening by mass spectrometry. Sudden death due to a first acute episode is reduced, but not eliminated by newborn screening. Intermittent recurrence of symptoms during intercurrent illness

is common in the first few years of life, but less common after age 4–6 years.

2. *Cardiomyopathy* (usually hypertrophic, but also dilated in later stages), *arrhythmias*, or *conduction defects*. The cardiac phenotype often occurs in the first weeks and months of life, but patients are at lifelong risk for acute or chronic symptoms. Cardiomyopathy is reversible without sequelae if treated early.
3. *Myopathy*, presenting either with weakness, pain, or with acute rhabdomyolysis, precipitated by exercise or infection. The myopathic phenotype mainly occurs after the first few years of life, in later childhood and adolescence.

Since implementation of newborn screening for FAODs, milder phenotypes (including asymptomatic) associated with specific genotypes have been recognized. It is not yet clear how many of the NBS-diagnosed patients will remain asymptomatic throughout life.

Fasting hypoglycemia is due to increased peripheral glucose consumption, decreased production of glucose due to an intracellular ATP deficit, and a concomitant decreased production of glucose utilization sparing ketones (Brunengraber and Roe 2006; Herrema et al. 2008). While small amounts of ketone bodies can be synthesized, particularly in medium- or short-chain FAODs or if there is high residual enzyme activity, the plasma concentrations are lower than expected for the degree of hypoglycemia, and thus the classification as hypoketotic. Hyperammonemia occurs in some severe defects and lactic acidemia is seen particularly in long-chain 3-hydroxyacyl-CoA dehydrogenase (LCHAD), mitochondrial trifunctional protein (MTP), and multiple acyl-CoA dehydrogenase (MAD) deficiencies. Rhabdomyolysis leads to elevated creatine kinase (CK), which can exceed 100.000 U/L (normal <~150 depending on the lab). Hepatomegaly and steatosis resulting from endogenous lipolysis are reflected by increased liver transaminases (aspartate aminotransferase [AST], alanine aminotransferase [ALT]), but note that AST and ALT also are present in muscle and especially AST is elevated in rhabdomyolysis independent of hepatocellular dysfunction. The toxic effects of accumulating long-chain acylcarnitines and acyl-CoA esters are likely responsible for cardiac arrhythmias in these disorders and are especially severe in disorders of the mitochondrial trifunctional protein (MTP and LCHAD deficiencies) and carnitine acylcarnitine translocase (CACT) deficiency (Bonnet et al. 1999; Tonin et al. 2010; Tonin et al. 2014). The development of retinopathy and peripheral neuropathy in LCHAD and MTP deficiencies is associated with the accumulation of long-chain 3-hydroxyacylcarnitines, though the definite pathophysiology of these problems is unknown.

The disease-specific acylcarnitine profile determined by tandem mass spectrometry is useful as a diagnostic test and for newborn screening, but must be performed on days 2 and 3 of life for the latter as delayed blood sampling in the anabolic state may yield false negative results. The acylcarnitine profile may also normalize when a patient is well or if there is a secondary carnitine deficiency. Organic acid analysis in urine can be diagnostic with accumulation of characteristic dicarboxylic acids during a metabolic crisis; however, since they are often normal in milder phenotypes or when a patient is well, acylcarnitine analysis is typically the primary diagnostic tool. Abnormal metabolite profiles, as well as normal profiles in the context of a suggestive clinical history, should be followed by confirmatory studies such as enzyme or molecular analysis.

## Carnitine Transporter Deficiency

The organic cation carnitine transporter 2 (OCTN2) encoded by the *SLC22A5* gene is responsible for carnitine uptake across the plasma membrane, particularly in heart, muscle, and kidney. Defects of the transporter lead to primary systemic carnitine deficiency with increased renal loss of carnitine and extremely low plasma carnitine concentrations (Longo et al. 2006). Parallel measurement of carnitine in blood and urine is the first diagnostic step. On newborn screening, low carnitine concentrations may also be found in newborns of vegetarian or vegan mothers or mothers with an undiagnosed OCTN2 deficiency. Asymptomatic adults with very low plasma carnitine concentrations have been identified. Therefore, carnitine measurement in the maternal plasma and urine should be part of the diagnostic workup of a low carnitine on NBS. A common founder mutation is present in the population of the Faroe Islands. The intake of certain antibiotics such as aminoglycosides, which are eliminated as carnitine esters via the urine, may lead to an additional decrease of carnitine in affected patients and can induce life-threatening clinical symptoms in otherwise asymptomatic patients (Holme et al. 1992; Makino et al. 2007; Rasmussen et al. 2013; Nasu et al. 2014; Nakazaki et al. 2018).

## Carnitine Palmitoyltransferase I (CPTI) Deficiency

Three different genetic isoforms of CPTI have been found in liver and kidney (CPTIA), muscle and heart (CPTIB), and brain (CPTIC). CPTIA deficiency has been identified in humans presenting in infancy with hypoketotic hypoglycemia and hepatopathy, induced by fasting or illness (Longo et al. 2006). Affected patients have an extremely high level of free carnitine in their blood spot with a concomitant decrease in the long-chain acylcarnitines. Free carnitine in blood spots is generally higher than measured in plasma. A mild variant is found in First Nation peoples of North America. CPTIC deficiency presents as an autosomal dominant spastic paraplegia with heterozygous mutations in the *CPTIC* gene. It has no reported metabolic phenotype and will not be discussed further in this chapter (Carrasco et al. 2013; Rinaldi et al. 2015).

### Carnitine-Acylcarnitine Translocase (CACT) Deficiency

Most patients have presented in the neonatal period and died in infancy; however, milder variants have been reported (Longo et al. 2006). This phenotype is characterized by severe ventricular arrhythmias that are most likely triggered by accumulating toxic fatty acid metabolites during catabolism. The acylcarnitine profile is indistinguishable from that found in carnitine palmitoyltransferase II deficiency.

### Carnitine Palmitoyltransferase II (CPTII) Deficiency

The most common form of CPTII deficiency presents with recurrent episodes of rhabdomyolysis and myoglobinuria precipitated by prolonged exercise, mainly in adolescents or young adults (Longo et al. 2006). The plasma CK often normalizes between episodes but it may also remain moderately elevated, associated with chronic muscle weakness and pain. Severe neonatal onset CPTII deficiency is lethal and is associated with congenital malformations, principally renal cysts and neuronal migration defects (North et al. 1995). The adult myopathic form of CPTII deficiency, due to a common mutation that preserves partial enzyme activity, is biochemically difficult to diagnose since acylcarnitine profiles may be normal, even during metabolic derangement. This phenotype is common in the Ashkenazi Jewish population.

### Very Long-Chain Acyl-CoA Dehydrogenase (VLCAD) Deficiency

VLCAD deficiency is the second most common fatty acid oxidation disorder in Europe and the USA, with a prevalence between 1:50,000 and 1:100,000 since implementation of newborn screening, much higher than originally calculated from the incidence of clinically manifesting patients. It is characterized by episodes of hypoketotic hypoglycemia with or without hyperammonemia in the first few years of life, with recurrent rhabdomyolysis (usually without hypoglycemia) in older children and young adults. Cardiomyopathy may be acute or chronic and can appear at any age. It can also be completely reversible if diagnosed early not leaving any sequelae. Neonatal screening by tandem mass spectrometry of dried blood spots for acylcarnitine profile has identified milder phenotypes with different genotypes and higher residual activities (Spiekerkoetter et al. 2010; Pena et al. 2016). Some of these patients remained asymptomatic from diagnosis to follow-up of over 10 years. Blood acylcarnitine and urine organic acid profiles can make the diagnosis but may normalize when patient is well. Thus, functional enzyme and molecular testing are critical to make or confirm the diagnosis in a suspected patient.

### Mitochondrial Trifunctional Protein (MTP), LKAT, and LCHAD Deficiencies

Isolated long-chain 3-ketoacyl-CoA thiolase (LKAT) deficiency is rare and has only been reported in two patients. Patients with isolated LCHAD deficiency or general MTP deficiency irrespective of the localization of the mutation in the HADHA or HADHB genes present with heterogeneous phenotypes similar to other long-chain FAODs (Spiekerkoetter et al. 2004). Importantly, this is the only FAOD associated with retinopathy and peripheral neuropathy (Tyni et al. 1998). First-line diagnosis is by blood acylcarnitines. However, the acylcarnitine profile may be normal, even during an episode of rhabdomyolysis, especially in patients with primarily neuromyopathic symptoms, therefore enzymatic or molecular testing especially for LCHAD deficiency due to the prevalent 1528G>C mutation is essential in case of clinical suspicion. This common mutation alters the catalytic residue in the LCHAD domain of the MTP alpha subunit. Pregnant women who are heterozygous for LCHAD or MTP deficiencies have an increased risk of HELLP syndrome—Hemolysis, Elevated Liver enzymes and Low Platelets—and acute fatty liver of pregnancy (AFLP) during pregnancies when they are carrying an affected fetus (Wilcken et al. 1993).

### Acyl-CoA Dehydrogenase 9 (ACAD9) Deficiency

ACAD9 is homologous to VLCAD and has dehydrogenase activity toward various long-chain acyl-CoA esters in vitro. Its primary physiological role is in the assembly of the mitochondrial respiratory chain complex I, and it presents predominantly as a respiratory chain deficiency with cardiomyopathy (Repp et al. 2018) and therefore is treated in Table 44.36.

## Medium-Chain Acyl-CoA Dehydrogenase (MCAD) Deficiency

MCAD deficiency (MCADD) has an incidence of approximately 1:10,000 in Europe, Australia, and the USA. Affected patients present clinically primarily if exposed to an appropriate environmental stress such as prolonged fasting or an intercurrent illness. The most common presentations before the era of newborn screening were sudden death or Reye-like symptoms, but many affected individuals identified through family screening were asymptomatic (Pourfarzam et al. 2001; Wilcken et al. 2007). MCADD is readily identifiable by newborn screening and once diagnosed, sudden death is rare as preventive measures can be taken. The risk for hypoglycemia decreases in late childhood and adulthood, but is never zero. Blood octanoylcarnitine (C8) is a highly specific marker, but may be only moderately elevated in mild phenotypes. The excretion of hexanoyl- and phenylpropionylglycine is elevated in urine; however, in milder phenotypes they may not be detectable. Residual enzyme activity correlates with the genotype and the expected clinical phenotype. A common mutation accounts for 75% of the mutations in patients with MCADD. A less common but recurrent c199T>C variant leads to sufficient residual activity to probably be protective from disease in combination with an inactivating mutation on the other allele.

## Short-Chain Acyl-CoA Dehydrogenase (SCAD) Deficiency

There are two polymorphisms in the SCAD gene (c.625G>A and c.511C>T). In northern Europe, 6% of the general population has one of these variants on both alleles. A common inactivating gene variant is present in Ashkenazi Jews. The biochemical diagnosis relies on the finding of increased blood butyrylcarnitine (C4) and/or urine ethylmalonic and methylsuccinic acids. A variety of clinical symptoms has been reported in patients with SCAD mutations, but patients identified through newborn screening have remained well. Thus, SCADD appears to be a biochemical phenotype rather than a clinically relevant disorder (Gallant et al. 2012). Nevertheless, it has been suggested that it may confer susceptibility to neuromuscular disease in combination with other impairments in mitochondrial function (Nochi et al. 2017).

## Short-Chain 3-Hydroxyacyl-CoA Dehydrogenase (SCHAD) Deficiency

SCHAD deficiency is associated with hypoglycemia but due to a different mechanism than the other FAODs. SCHAD has a second role independent of FAO, binding and inhibiting glutamate dehydrogenase (GDH). SCHAD mutations that prevent GDH binding lead to increased GDH activity and insulin secretion and subsequent hypoglycemia, particularly in response to leucine (Li et al. 2010). Increased plasma L-3-hydroxyl-C4-carnitine as well as urine 3-hydroxyglutaric acid are the accepted diagnostic markers.

## Nomenclature

| No | Disease Name | Alternative Disease Name | Abbreviation | Gene Symbol | Chromosomal Localization | Mode of Inheritance | Affected protein | OMIM# |
|---|---|---|---|---|---|---|---|---|
| 48.1 | Carnitine transporter deficiency | Carnitine uptake defect | OCTN2 | SLC22A5 | 5q31.1 | AR | Organic cation carnitine transporter 2 | 212140 |
| 48.2 | Carnitine palmitoyltransferase 1A deficiency | Carnitine palmitoyl-CoA transferase 1 deficiency | CPT1 | CPT1A | 11q22.23 | AR | Carnitine palmitoyltransferase | 255120 |
| 48.3 | Carnitine palmitoyl-transferase IC deficiency | Spastic paraplegia 73 (SPG73) | SPG73 | CPT1C | 19q13.33 | AD | Carnitine palmitoyl-transferase IC | 616282 |
| 48.4 | Carnitine palmitoyltransferase 2 deficiency | Carnitine palmitoyl-CoA transferase 2 deficiency | CPT2 | CPT2 | 1p32 | AR | Carnitine palmitoyltransferase 2 | 255110 |
| 48.5 | Carnitine acylcarnitine translocase deficiency | | CACT | SLC25A20 | 3p21.31 | AR | Carnitine acylcarnitine translocase | 212138 |
| 48.9 | Short-chain acyl CoA dehydrogenase deficiency | Ethylmalonic aciduria | SCAD | ACADS | 12q24.31 | AR | Short-chain acyl CoA dehydrogenase | 201470 |
| 48.10 | Medium-chain acyl CoA dehydrogenase deficiency | | MCAD | ACADM | 1p31 | AR | Medium-chain acyl CoA dehydrogenase | 201450 |
| 48.11 | Very long-chain acyl CoA dehydrogenase deficiency | | VLCAD | ACADVL | 17p13 | AR | Very long-chain acyl CoA dehydrogenase | 201475 |
| 48.12 | Short-chain 3-hydroxyacyl-CoA dehydrogenase deficiency | | SCHAD | HADH | 4q22–q26 | AR | Short-chain 3-hydroxyacyl-CoA dehydrogenase | 231530 |
| 48.13 | Isolated deficiency of long-chain 3-hydroxyacyl-CoA dehydrogenase | | LCHAD | HADHA | 2p23 | AD | Long-chain 3-hydroxyacyl-CoA dehydrogenase | 600890 |
| 48.14 | Isolated deficiency of long-chain 3-ketoacyl CoA thiolase | | LKAT | HADHB | 2p23 | AR | Long-chain 3-ketoacyl CoA thiolase | 143450 |
| 48.15 | Trifunctional protein β subunit deficiency | Long-chain hydroxyacyl-CoA dehydrogenase or complete mitochondrial trifunctional protein deficiency | mTFP, MTP | HADHB | 2p23.3 | AR | Hydroxyacyl-CoA dehydrogenase trifunctional multienzyme complex subunit beta | 609015 |
| 48.16 | Fatty acid transport protein 4 deficiency | Ichthyosis prematurity syndrome | IPS | SLC27A4 | 9q34.11 | AR | Fatty acid transport protein 4 | 608649 |
| 48.17 | Docosahexanoic acid transporter deficiency | Autosomal recessive primary microcephaly type 15 | MCPH15 | MFSD2A | 1p34.2 | AR | Major facilitator superfamily domain-containing protein 2a | 616486 |
| 48.18 | Acyl-CoA dehydrogenase 9 deficiency | Complex I assembly disorder | | ACAD9 | 3q26 | AR | Acyl-CoA dehydrogenase 9 | 611126 |

## Metabolic Pathway

Fatty acids are released from tissue stores or from dietary fat, are transported to cells on carrier proteins, and enter cells in response to hormonal signals including dropping insulin. In the cytoplasm, they are activated to coenzyme A (CoA) esters by acyl-CoA synthases. Long-chain acyl-CoAs must be esterified with carnitine in order to cross the inner mitochondrial membrane, while medium- and short-chain acyl-CoAs appear to enter the mitochondria independent of carnitine. Endogenous synthesis in the liver generally supplies about half of cellular needs and thus the remainder is derived from diet, largely meat. Endogenous production in vegans is enhanced, but in many cases still have clinically insignificant low levels in blood. Carnitine itself is actively transported into cells by the high-affinity organic cation carnitine transporter 2 (OCTN2) carnitine (Fig. 48.1). A low-affinity transporter provides some capacity to transport carnitine into cells in the face of OCTN2 deficiency. At the outer mitochondrial membrane, carnitine palmitoyltransferase I (CPTI) catalyzes the formation of acylcarnitine esters. The carnitine esters are shuttled across the inner membrane by the carnitine acylcarnitine translocase (CACT), and carnitine palmitoyltransferase II (CPTII), which is attached to the inner mitochondrial membrane, catalyzes the release of CoA esters. Within the mitochondria, ß-oxidation is catalyzed by enzymes of different chain length specificities, and each turn of the β-oxidation spiral involves four enzymatic steps, shortening the acyl-CoA by two carbons. The enzymes for the β-oxidation of long-chain substrates (C18-C12 fatty acids) are also membrane-associated, including very long-chain acyl-CoA dehydrogenase (VLCAD) and the mitochondrial trifunctional protein complex (mTFP or MTP) composed of three enzymatic activities on two different subunits. Long-chain enoyl-CoA hydratase (LCEH) and the long-chain 3-hydroxyacyl-CoA dehydrogenase

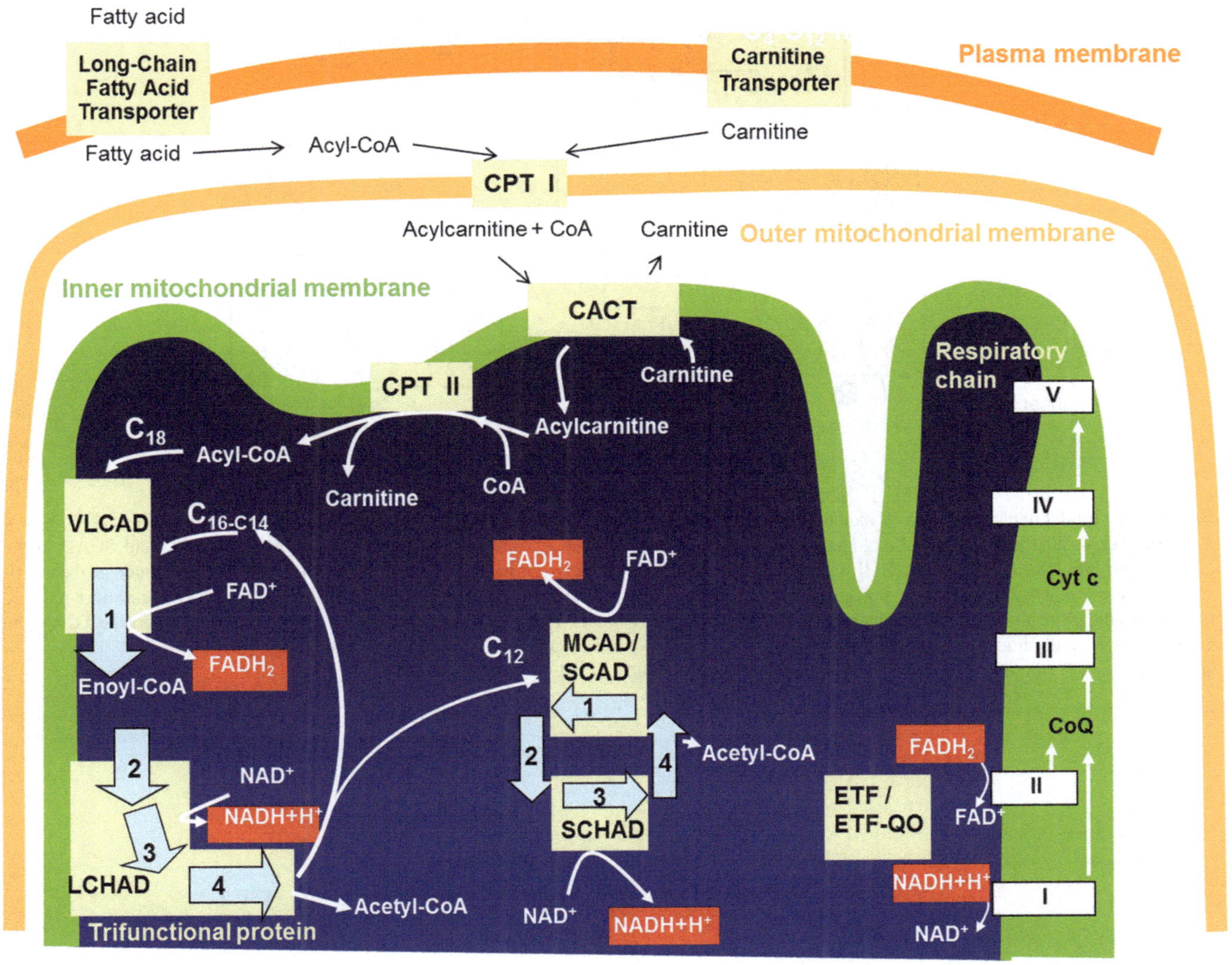


**Fig. 48.1** Transport of fatty acids into the mitochondrion, mitochondrial β-oxidation, and electron transfer. Modified according to Bonnefont et al. (2010)

(LCHAD) both are contained in the α-subunit, while the long-chain 3-ketoacyl-CoA thiolase (LKAT) is localized to the β-subunit. Medium- and short-chain-specific enzymes, including medium-chain acyl-CoA dehydrogenase (MCAD), short-chain acyl-CoA dehydrogenase (SCAD), enoyl-CoA hydratase or crotonase, and short-chain 3-hydroxyacyl-CoA dehydrogenase (SCHAD), are located in the mitochondrial matrix. The acyl-CoA dehydrogenase reaction produces two electrons, which are transferred sequentially to the electron transfer flavoprotein (ETF), ETF-ubiquinone oxidoreductase (ETF:QO), and ultimately to ubiquinone of the mitochondrial electron transfer chain. Flavin adenine dinucleotide (FAD), which is derived from riboflavin, acts as a cofactor in these reactions (see Chap. 32). Acetyl-CoA produced by ß-oxidation can either enter the Krebs cycle or be utilized to synthesize ketone bodies in the liver (Fig. 48.1). The LCHAD reaction utilizes nicotinamide adenine dinucleotide (NAD) as an electron acceptor, which serves as a substrate for complex I of the electron transfer chain. The long-chain fatty acid oxidation enzymes VLCAD and LCHAD, along with electron transfer flavoprotein dehydrogenase (ETFDH), have been shown to interact with respiratory chain supercomplexes in a multiprotein enzyme complex that optimizes catalytic efficiency (Wang et al. 2010; Wang et al. 2019). The LCHAD (alpha) subunit of MTP interacts with the matrix arm of respiratory chain complex I and VLCAD, while ETFDH interacts with the coenzyme Q binding subunit of complex III (Fig. 48.2).

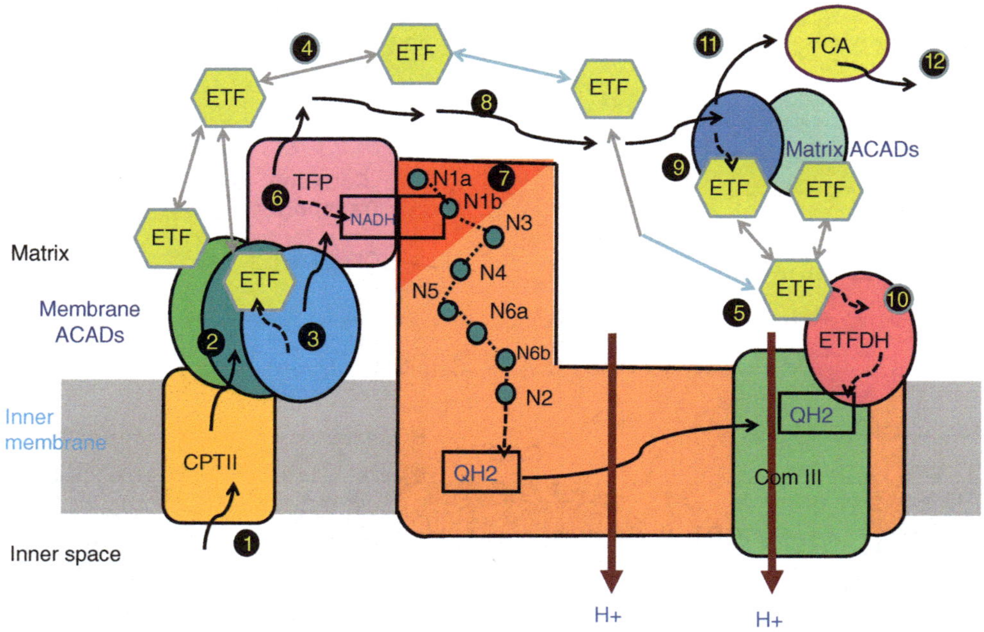


**Fig. 48.2** The model depicts the path of oxidation of long-chain fatty acids (Wang et al. 2019). Steps 1–3: Long-chain acyl-CoA substrates are transferred into VLCAD through CPTII, channeling its product to the MTP (Steps 6–7). Steps 4–5: Reduced ETF is released from VLCAD into the mitochondrial matrix, where it is free to find its redox partner, ETFDH, and shuttle its reducing equivalents ($QH_2$) to ETC complex III. Step 8: In complex I, NADH is oxidized with channeling of electrons to complex III. Medium- and short-chain acyl-CoA substrates produced by TFP are transferred to MCAD and SCAD in the matrix, or in amore weakly associating peripheral domain of the multifunctional FAO-ETC complex (Steps 9–10). ETFDH oxidizes reduced ETF by reducing CoQ to $QH_2$ Finally, acetyl-CoA enters the TCA cycle or is utilized for ketone body production (Steps 12–13)

## Signs and Symptoms

**Table 48.1** Carnitine transporter deficiency

| System | Symptoms and biomarkers | Neonatal (birth–1 month) | Infancy (1–18 months) | childhood (1.5–11 years) | Adolescence (11–16 years) | Adulthood (>16 years) |
|---|---|---|---|---|---|---|
| Cardiovascular | **Cardiomyopathy** | ± | ± | ± | | |
| Digestive | **Liver dysfunction** | ± | ± | ± | | |
| Musculoskeletal | **Hypotonia, muscular-axial** | ± | ± | ± | ± | ± |
| Laboratory findings | **Rhabdomyolysis** | | | ± | ± | ± |
| | **Skeletal myopathy** | ± | ± | ± | ± | ± |
| | Adipic acid (urine) | n-↑ | n-↑ | n-↑ | | |
| | C16:0-Acylcarnitine (dried blood spot) | ↓ | ↓ | ↓ | ↓ | ↓ |
| | C16:0-Acylcarnitine (plasma) | ↓ | ↓ | ↓ | ↓ | ↓ |
| | C18:0-Acylcarnitine (dried blood spot) | ↓ | ↓ | ↓ | ↓ | ↓ |
| | C18:0-Acylcarnitine (plasma) | ↓ | ↓ | ↓ | ↓ | ↓ |
| | C18:1-Acylcarnitine (dried blood spot) | ↓ | ↓ | ↓ | ↓ | ↓ |
| | C18:1-Acylcarnitine (plasma) | ↓ | ↓ | ↓ | ↓ | ↓ |
| | C18:2-Acylcarnitine (dried blood spot) | ↓ | ↓ | ↓ | ↓ | ↓ |
| | C18:2-Acylcarnitine (plasma) | ↓ | ↓ | ↓ | ↓ | ↓ |
| | Carnitine, free (dried blood spot) | ↓↓↓ | ↓↓↓ | ↓↓↓ | ↓↓↓ | ↓↓↓ |
| | Carnitine, free (plasma) | ↓ | ↓ | ↓ | ↓ | ↓ |
| | Carnitine, free (urine) | ↑ | ↑ | ↑ | ↑ | ↑ |
| | Creatine kinase (plasma) | n-↑ | n-↑ | n-↑ | n-↑ | n-↑ |
| | Dicarboxylic acids (urine) | n-↑ | n-↑ | n-↑ | | |
| | Glucose (plasma) | ↓-n | ↓-n | ↓-n | | |
| | Ketones, during hypoglycemia | ↓ | ↓ | ↓ | | |
| | Long-chain acylcarnitine (dried blood spot) | ↓ | ↓ | ↓ | ↓ | ↓ |
| | Long-chain acylcarnitine (plasma) | ↓ | ↓ | ↓ | ↓ | ↓ |
| | Sebacic acid (urine) | n-↑ | n-↑ | n-↑ | | |
| | Suberic acid (urine) | n-↑ | n-↑ | n-↑ | | |
| | Transaminase (plasma) | n-↑ | n-↑ | n-↑ | n-↑ | n-↑ |

**Table 48.2** Carnitine palmitoyltransferase 1A deficiency

| System | Symptoms and biomarkers | Neonatal (birth–1 month) | Infancy (1–18 months) | childhood (1.5–11 years) | Adolescence (11–16 years) | Adulthood (>16 years) |
|---|---|---|---|---|---|---|
| Digestive | **Liver dysfunction** | ± | ± | ± | | |
| Renal | **Renal tubular acidosis** | | ± | ± | ± | ± |
| Laboratory findings | Adipic acid (urine) | n-↑ | n-↑ | n-↑ | n-↑ | n-↑ |
| | C16:0-Acylcarnitine (dried blood spot) | ↓ | ↓ | ↓ | ↓ | ↓ |
| | C16:0-Acylcarnitine (plasma) | ↓ | ↓ | ↓ | ↓ | ↓ |
| | C18:0-Acylcarnitine (dried blood spot) | ↓ | ↓ | ↓ | ↓ | ↓ |
| | C18:0-Acylcarnitine (plasma) | ↓ | ↓ | ↓ | ↓ | ↓ |
| | C18:1-Acylcarnitine (dried blood spot) | ↓ | ↓ | ↓ | ↓ | ↓ |
| | C18:1-Acylcarnitine (plasma) | ↓ | ↓ | ↓ | ↓ | ↓ |
| | C18:2-Acylcarnitine (dried blood spot) | ↓ | ↓ | ↓ | ↓ | ↓ |
| | C18:2-Acylcarnitine (plasma) | ↓ | ↓ | ↓ | ↓ | ↓ |
| | Carnitine, free (dried blood spot) | ↑-↑↑↑ | ↑-↑↑↑ | ↑-↑↑↑ | ↑-↑↑↑ | ↑-↑↑↑ |
| | Carnitine, free (plasma) | n-↑ | n-↑ | n-↑ | n-↑ | n-↑ |
| | Dicarboxylic acids (urine) | n-↑ | n-↑ | n-↑ | n-↑ | n-↑ |
| | Glucose (plasma) | ↓-n | ↓-n | ↓-n | | |
| | Ketones, during hypoglycemia | ↓ | ↓ | ↓ | | |
| | Long-chain acylcarnitine (dried blood spot) | ↓ | ↓ | ↓ | ↓ | ↓ |
| | Long-chain acylcarnitine (plasma) | ↓ | ↓ | ↓ | ↓ | ↓ |
| | Sebacic acid (urine) | n-↑ | n-↑ | n-↑ | n-↑ | n-↑ |
| | Suberic acid (urine) | n-↑ | n-↑ | n-↑ | n-↑ | n-↑ |
| | Transaminase (plasma) | n-↑ | n-↑ | n-↑ | n-↑ | n-↑ |

**Table 48.3** Carnitine palmitoyl-transferase IC deficiency

| System | Symptoms and biomarkers | Neonatal (birth–1 month) | Infancy (1–18 months) | Childhood (1.5–11 years) | Adolescence (11–16 years) | Adulthood (>16 years) |
|---|---|---|---|---|---|---|
| CNS | Evoked potentials +/–, abnormal (EEG) | | | | | + |
| | Hyperreflexia | | | | | + |
| Musculoskeletal | Loss of ambulation | | | | | ± |
| | Muscle atrophy | | | | | + |
| | **Muscle weakness** | | | | | + |
| | Spastic paraparesia/ paraplegia/tetraplegia | | | | | + |
| | **Unable to walk** | | | | | + |

**Table 48.4** Carnitine palmitoyltransferase 2 deficiency

| System | Symptoms and biomarkers | Neonatal (birth–1 month) | Infancy (1–18 months) | childhood (1.5–11 years) | Adolescence (11–16 years) | Adulthood (>16 years) |
|---|---|---|---|---|---|---|
| Cardiovascular | **Cardiomyopathy** | ± | ± | ± | | |
| CNS | **Coma** | ± | ± | ± | | |
| | **Lethargy** | ± | ± | ± | | |
| Digestive | **Liver dysfunction** | ± | ± | ± | | |
| Musculoskeletal | **Hypotonia, muscular-axial** | ± | ± | ± | ± | ± |
| | **Rhabdomyolysis, exercise induced** | | | +++ | +++ | +++ |
| | **Skeletal myopathy** | ± | ± | ± | ± | ± |
| Other | Malformations (brain) | + | | | | |
| | Malformations (kidney) | + | | | | |
| Laboratory findings | Adipic acid (urine) | n-↑ | n-↑ | n-↑ | n-↑ | n-↑ |
| | C14:0-Acylcarnitine (dried blood spot) | n-↑ | n-↑ | n-↑ | n-↑ | n-↑ |
| | C14:0-Acylcarnitine (serum) | n-↑ | n-↑ | n-↑ | n-↑ | n-↑ |
| | C16:0-Acylcarnitine (dried blood spot) | n-↑ | n-↑ | n-↑ | n-↑ | n-↑ |
| | C16:0-Acylcarnitine (plasma) | n-↑ | n-↑ | n-↑ | n-↑ | n-↑ |
| | C16-C18 Acylcarnitine | n-↑ | n-↑ | n-↑ | n-↑ | n-↑ |
| | C18:0-Acylcarnitine (dried blood spot) | n-↑ | n-↑ | n-↑ | n-↑ | n-↑ |
| | C18:0-Acylcarnitine (plasma) | n-↑ | n-↑ | n-↑ | n-↑ | n-↑ |
| | C18:1-Acylcarnitine (dried blood spot) | n-↑ | n-↑ | n-↑ | n-↑ | n-↑ |
| | C18:1-Acylcarnitine (plasma) | n-↑ | n-↑ | n-↑ | n-↑ | n-↑ |
| | C18:2-Acylcarnitine (dried blood spot) | n-↑ | n-↑ | n-↑ | n-↑ | n-↑ |
| | C18:2-Acylcarnitine (plasma) | n-↑ | n-↑ | n-↑ | n-↑ | n-↑ |
| | Carnitine, free (dried blood spot) | ↓-n | ↓-n | ↓-n | ↓-n | ↓-n |
| | Carnitine, free (plasma) | ↓-n | ↓-n | ↓-n | ↓-n | ↓-n |
| | Creatine kinase (plasma) | n-↑ | n-↑ | n-↑↑↑ | n-↑↑↑ | n-↑↑↑ |
| | Dicarboxylic acids (urine) | n-↑ | n-↑ | n-↑ | n-↑ | n-↑ |
| | Glucose (plasma) | ↓-n | ↓-n | ↓-n | | |
| | Ketones, during hypoglycemia | ↓ | ↓ | ↓ | | |
| | Long-chain acylcarnitine | n-↑ | n-↑ | n-↑ | n-↑ | n-↑ |
| | Sebacic acid (urine) | n-↑ | n-↑ | n-↑ | n-↑ | n-↑ |
| | Suberic acid (urine) | n-↑ | n-↑ | n-↑ | n-↑ | n-↑ |
| | Transaminase (plasma) | n-↑ | n-↑ | n-↑↑↑ | n-↑↑↑ | n-↑↑↑ |

**Table 48.5** Carnitine acylcarnitine translocase deficiency (30 patients)

| System | Symptoms and biomarkers | Neonatal (birth–1 month) | Infancy (1–18 months) | childhood (1.5–11 years) | Adolescence (11–16 years) | Adulthood (>16 years) |
|---|---|---|---|---|---|---|
| Cardiovascular | **Cardiac arrhythmias, severe** | +++ | +++ | + | | |
| | **Cardiomyopathy** | +++ | +++ | + | | |
| CNS | **Coma** | ± | ± | ± | | |
| | **Lethargy** | ± | ± | ± | | |
| Digestive | **Liver dysfunction** | ± | ± | ± | | |
| Musculoskeletal | **Hypotonia, muscular-axial** | ± | ± | ± | | |
| | **Skeletal myopathy** | ± | ± | ± | | |
| Other | **Lethality of severe phenotypes, high** | +++ | +++ | + | | |
| | Sudden death | + | + | + | | |
| Laboratory findings | Adipic acid (urine) | n-↑ | n-↑ | n-↑ | n-↑ | n-↑ |
| | C14:0-Acylcarnitine (dried blood spot) | ↑ | ↑ | ↑ | ↑ | ↑ |
| | C14:0-Acylcarnitine (serum) | ↑ | ↑ | ↑ | ↑ | ↑ |
| | C16:0-Acylcarnitine (plasma) | ↑ | ↑ | ↑ | ↑ | ↑ |
| | C16-C18 Acylcarnitine | ↑ | ↑ | ↑ | | |
| | C18:0-Acylcarnitine (dried blood spot) | ↑ | ↑ | ↑ | ↑ | ↑ |
| | C18:0-Acylcarnitine (plasma) | ↑ | ↑ | ↑ | ↑ | ↑ |
| | C18:1-Acylcarnitine (dried blood spot) | ↑ | ↑ | ↑ | ↑ | ↑ |
| | C18:1-Acylcarnitine (plasma) | ↑ | ↑ | ↑ | ↑ | ↑ |
| | C18:2-Acylcarnitine (dried blood spot) | ↑ | ↑ | ↑ | ↑ | ↑ |
| | C18:2-Acylcarnitine (plasma) | ↑ | ↑ | ↑ | ↑ | ↑ |
| | Carnitine, free (dried blood spot) | ↓-n | ↓-n | ↓-n | | |
| | Carnitine, free (plasma) | ↓-n | ↓-n | ↓-n | | |
| | Creatine kinase (plasma) | ↑↑ | ↑↑ | ↑↑↑ | | |
| | Dicarboxylic acids (urine) | n-↑ | n-↑ | n-↑ | | |
| | Glucose (plasma) | ↓-n | ↓-n | ↓-n | | |
| | Ketones, during hypoglycemia | ↓ | ↓ | ↓ | | |
| | Lactate (plasma) | ↑ | ↑ | ↑ | | |
| | Long-chain acylcarnitine | ↑ | ↑ | ↑ | | |
| | Sebacic acid (urine) | n-↑ | n-↑ | n-↑ | n-↑ | n-↑ |
| | Suberic acid (urine) | n-↑ | n-↑ | n-↑ | n-↑ | n-↑ |
| | Transaminase (plasma) | ↑ | ↑ | ↑ | | |

**Table 48.6** ε-N-trimethyllysine hydroxylase deficiency

| System | Symptoms and biomarkers | Neonatal (birth–1 month) | Infancy (1–18 months) | Childhood (1.5–11 years) | Adolescence (11–16 years) | Adulthood (>16 years) |
|---|---|---|---|---|---|---|
| Psychiatric | Autistic spectrum disorder | | | + | + | + |

**Table 48.7** γ-Butyrobetaine hydroxylase deficiency

| System | Symptoms and biomarkers | Neonatal (birth–1 month) | Infancy (1–18 months) | Childhood (1.5–11 years) | Adolescence (11–16 years) | Adulthood (>16 years) |
|---|---|---|---|---|---|---|
| Eye | **Long eye lashes** | | + | | | |
| | **Strabismus** | | + | | | |
| Musculoskeletal | **Facial dysmorphism** | | + | | | |
| | **Growth retardation** | | + | | | |
| | High nasal bridge | | + | | | |
| | Microcephaly | | + | | | |
| Other | **Epicanthal folds** | | + | | | |
| | Epicanthal folds | | + | | | |
| Psychiatric | Behavior, psychotic | | ± | | | |
| | Hyperactivity | | + | + | | |
| Laboratory findings | Carnitine, free (plasma) | | | | | ↓-n |

**Table 48.8** Carnitine acetyltransferase deficiency

| System | Symptoms and biomarkers | Neonatal (birth–1 month) | Infancy (1–18 months) | Childhood (1.5–11 years) | Adolescence (11-16 years) | Adulthood (>16 years) |
|---|---|---|---|---|---|---|
| CNS | Ataxia | | | + | | |
| | Consciousness disturbance | | | + | | |
| | Hypotonia | | | + | | |
| | Intellectual disability | | | + | | |
| | Oculomotor apraxia | | | + | | |

**Table 48.9** Short-chain acyl-CoA dehydrogenase deficiency

| System | Symptoms and biomarkers | Neonatal (birth–1 month) | Infancy (1–18 months) | childhood (1.5–11 years) | Adolescence (11–16 years) | Adulthood (>16 years) |
|---|---|---|---|---|---|---|
| CNS | **Developmental delay** | | ± | ± | ± | ± |
| | **Epilepsy** | | ± | ± | | |
| | **Hypotonia** | ± | ± | ± | | |
| Metabolic | Hypoglycemia | ± | ± | ± | | |
| | Hypoglycemia | | | ± | ± | |
| Musculoskeletal | **Dysmorphic features** | ± | ± | ± | ± | ± |
| | **Exercise intolerance** | | | ± | ± | ± |
| Psychiatric | **Behavioral disorder** | | | ± | ± | ± |
| Other | **Failure to thrive** | | ± | ± | ± | |
| | Predisposition for symptomatic disease | + | + | + | + | + |
| | Second mitochondrial affection | + | + | + | + | + |
| Laboratory findings | Butyrylglycine (urine) | n-↑ | n-↑ | n-↑ | n-↑ | n-↑ |
| | C4 Butyrylcarnitine (blood) | ↑ | ↑ | ↑ | ↑ | ↑ |
| | C4 Butyrylcarnitine (plasma) | ↑ | ↑ | ↑ | ↑ | ↑ |
| | C4-Acylcarnitine (dried blood spot) | ↑ | ↑ | ↑ | ↑ | ↑ |
| | C4-Acylcarnitine (plasma) | ↑ | ↑ | ↑ | ↑ | ↑ |
| | Ethylmalonic acid (urine) | ↑↑ | ↑↑ | ↑↑ | ↑ | n-↑ |
| | Glucose (plasma) | ↓-n | ↓-n | ↓-n | | |
| | Methylsuccinic acid (urine) | ↑ | ↑ | ↑ | ↑ | ↑ |
| | Short-chain acyl-CoA dehydrogenase (fibroblasts) | ↓ | ↓ | ↓ | ↓ | ↓ |

**Table 48.10** Medium-chain acyl-CoA dehydrogenase deficiency

| System | Symptoms and biomarkers | Neonatal (birth–1 month) | Infancy (1–18 months) | childhood (1.5–11 years) | Adolescence (11–16 years) | Adulthood (>16 years) |
|---|---|---|---|---|---|---|
| Digestive | **Liver dysfunction** | ± | ± | ± | | |
| Other | Asymptomatic | ± | ± | ± | ± | ± |
| Laboratory findings | 5-Hydroxyhexanoic acid (urine) | n-↑ | n-↑ | n-↑ | n-↑ | n-↑ |
| | 7-Hydroxyoctanoic acid (urine) | n-↑ | n-↑ | n-↑ | n-↑ | n-↑ |
| | Adipic acid (urine) | n-↑ | n-↑ | n-↑ | n-↑ | n-↑ |
| | C10:0-Acylcarnitine (dried blood spot) | ↑ | ↑ | ↑ | ↑ | ↑ |
| | C10:0-Acylcarnitine (plasma) | ↑ | ↑ | ↑ | ↑ | ↑ |
| | C10:1-Acylcarnitine (dried blood spot) | ↑ | ↑ | ↑ | ↑ | ↑ |
| | C10:1-Acylcarnitine (plasma) | ↑ | ↑ | ↑ | ↑ | ↑ |
| | C6-Acylcarnitine (dried blood spot) | ↑ | ↑ | ↑ | ↑ | ↑ |
| | C6-Acylcarnitine (plasma) | ↑ | ↑ | ↑ | ↑ | ↑ |
| | C6-Acylcarnitine (urine) | ↑ | ↑ | ↑ | ↑ | ↑ |
| | C8/C12 Acylcarnitines ratio | ↑ | ↑ | ↑ | ↑ | ↑ |
| | C8/C2 Acylcarnitines ratio | ↑ | ↑ | ↑ | ↑ | ↑ |
| | C8-Acylcarnitine (dried blood spot) | ↑ | ↑ | ↑ | ↑ | ↑ |
| | C8-Acylcarnitine (plasma) | ↑ | ↑ | ↑ | ↑ | ↑ |
| | C8-Acylcarnitine (urine) | ↑ | ↑ | ↑ | ↑ | ↑ |
| | Carnitine, free (dried blood spot) | ↓-n | ↓-n | ↓-n | ↓-n | ↓-n |
| | Carnitine, free (plasma) | ↓-n | ↓-n | ↓-n | ↓-n | ↓-n |
| | Dicarboxylic acids (urine) | n-↑ | n-↑ | n-↑ | n-↑ | n-↑ |
| | Glucose (plasma) | ↓-n | ↓-n | ↓-n | | |
| | Hexanoylglycine (urine) | n-↑ | n-↑ | n-↑ | n-↑ | n-↑ |
| | Ketones, during hypoglycemia | ↓ | ↓ | ↓ | | |
| | Octanoylglucuronide (urine) | n-↑ | n-↑ | n-↑ | n-↑ | n-↑ |
| | Phenylpropionylglycine (urine) | n-↑ | n-↑ | n-↑ | n-↑ | n-↑ |
| | Phenylpropionylglycine (urine) | n-↑ | n-↑ | n-↑ | n-↑ | n-↑ |
| | Sebacic acid (urine) | n-↑ | n-↑ | n-↑ | n-↑ | n-↑ |
| | Sebacic acid, unsaturated (urine) | n-↑ | n-↑ | n-↑ | n-↑ | n-↑ |
| | Suberic acid (urine) | n-↑ | n-↑ | n-↑ | n-↑ | n-↑ |
| | Suberic acid, unsaturated (urine) | n-↑ | n-↑ | n-↑ | n-↑ | n-↑ |
| | Suberylglycine (urine) | n-↑ | n-↑ | n-↑ | n-↑ | n-↑ |
| | Transaminase (plasma) | n-↑ | n-↑ | n-↑ | n-↑ | n-↑ |

**Table 48.11** Very long-chain acyl-CoA dehydrogenase deficiency

| System | Symptoms and biomarkers | Neonatal (birth–1 month) | Infancy (1–18 months) | childhood (1.5–11 years) | Adolescence (11–16 years) | Adulthood (>16 years) |
|---|---|---|---|---|---|---|
| Cardiovascular | **Cardiomyopathy** | ± | ± | ± | | |
| CNS | **Coma** | ± | ± | ± | | |
| | **Lethargy** | ± | ± | ± | | |
| Digestive | **Liver dysfunction** | ± | ± | ± | ± | ± |
| Musculoskeletal | **Rhabdomyolysis, exercise induced** | | ± | ++ | ++ | ++ |
| Musculoskeletal | **Skeletal myopathy** | ± | ± | ± | ± | ± |
| Musculoskeletal | **Hypotonia, muscular-axial** | ± | ± | ± | ± | ± |
| Laboratory findings | Adipic acid (urine) | n-↑ | n-↑ | n-↑ | n-↑ | n-↑ |
| | C14:0-Acylcarnitine (dried blood spot) | ↑ | ↑ | ↑ | n-↑ | n-↑ |
| | C14:0-Acylcarnitine (serum) | ↑ | ↑ | ↑ | n-↑ | n-↑ |
| | C14:1 Tetradecenoylcarnitine (blood) | n-↑ | n-↑ | n-↑ | n-↑ | n-↑ |
| | C14:1 Tetradecenoylcarnitine (plasma) | n-↑ | n-↑ | n-↑ | n-↑ | n-↑ |
| | C14:1/C12:1 Acylcarnitines ratio | ↑ | ↑ | ↑ | ↑ | ↑ |
| | C14:1/C4 Acylcarnitines ratio | ↑ | ↑ | ↑ | ↑ | ↑ |
| | C14:1-Acylcarnitine (dried blood spot) | ↑ | ↑ | ↑ | n-↑ | n-↑ |
| | C14:1-Acylcarnitine (plasma) | ↑ | ↑ | ↑ | n-↑ | n-↑ |
| | C16:0-Acylcarnitine (dried blood spot) | ↑ | ↑ | ↑ | n-↑ | n-↑ |
| | C16:0-Acylcarnitine (plasma) | ↑ | ↑ | ↑ | n-↑ | ↑n-↑ |
| | C16:1-Acylcarnitine (dried blood spot) | ↑ | ↑ | ↑ | n-↑ | n-↑ |
| | C16:1-Acylcarnitine (plasma) | ↑ | ↑ | ↑ | n-↑ | n-↑ |
| | C18:0-Acylcarnitine (dried blood spot) | ↑ | ↑ | ↑ | n-↑ | n-↑ |
| | C18:0-Acylcarnitine (plasma) | ↑ | ↑ | ↑ | n-↑ | n-↑ |
| | C18:1-Acylcarnitine (dried blood spot) | ↑ | ↑ | ↑ | n-↑ | n-↑ |
| | C18:1-Acylcarnitine (plasma) | ↑ | ↑ | ↑ | n-↑ | n-↑ |
| | C18:2-Acylcarnitine (dried blood spot) | ↑ | ↑ | ↑ | n-↑ | n-↑ |
| | C18:2-Acylcarnitine (plasma) | ↑ | ↑ | ↑ | n-↑ | n-↑ |
| | Carnitine, free (dried blood spot) | ↓-n | ↓-n | ↓-n | ↓-n | ↓-n |
| | Carnitine, free (plasma) | ↓-n | ↓-n | ↓-n | ↓-n | ↓-n |
| | Creatine kinase (plasma) | n-↑ | n-↑ | n-↑↑ | n-↑↑ | n-↑↑ |
| | Dicarboxylic acids (urine) | n-↑ | n-↑ | n-↑ | n-↑ | n-↑ |
| | Glucose (plasma) | ↓-n | ↓-n | ↓-n | | |
| | Ketones, during hypoglycemia | ↓ | ↓ | ↓ | | |
| | Sebacic acid (urine) | n-↑ | n-↑ | n-↑ | n-↑ | n-↑ |
| | Sebacic acid, unsaturated (urine) | n-↑ | n-↑ | n-↑ | n-↑ | n-↑ |
| | Suberic acid (urine) | n-↑ | n-↑ | n-↑ | n-↑ | n-↑ |
| | Suberic acid, unsaturated (urine) | n-↑ | n-↑ | n-↑ | n-↑ | n-↑ |
| | Transaminase (plasma) | n-↑ | n-↑ | n-↑↑ | n-↑↑ | n-↑↑ |

**Table 48.12** Short-chain 3-hydroxyacyl-CoA dehydrogenase deficiency (13 patients)

| System | Symptoms and biomarkers | Neonatal (birth–1 month) | Infancy (1–18 months) | childhood (1.5–11 years) | Adolescence (11–16 years) | Adulthood (>16 years) |
|---|---|---|---|---|---|---|
| Cardiovascular | Cardiomyopathy | ± | | | | |
| CNS | Intellectual disability | ± | ± | ± | ± | ± |
| | Seizures | ± | ± | | | |
| Digestive | Liver failure, Reye-like | | + | + | | |
| Endocrine | **Hyperinsulinism** | + | + | + | | |
| | Protein sensitivity | + | ++ | ++ | ++ | |
| Metabolic | **Hypoglycemia, hypoketotic** | + | + | + | | |
| | 3-Hydroxydicarboxylic acid (urine) | (↑) | (↑) | (↑) | | |
| Laboratory findings | 3-Hydroxyglutarate (urine) | ↑ | ↑ | ↑ | | |
| | Ammonia (blood) | | ↑ | ↑ | ↑ | |
| | C4-OH Hydroxybutyrylcarnitine (dried blood spot) | ↑ | ↑ | ↑ | | |
| | C4-OH Hydroxybutyrylcarnitine (plasma) | ↑ | ↑ | ↑ | | |
| | Glucose (plasma) | ↓ | ↓ | | | |
| | Insulin, durig hypoglycemia | ↑ | ↑ | ↑ | ↑ | ↑ |
| | Ketones (urine) | ↓ | ↓ | | | |
| | Medium chain dicarboxylic acids (urine) | (↑) | (↑) | (↑) | | |

**Table 48.13** Isolated deficiency of long-chain 3-hydroxyacyl-CoA dehydrogenase

| System | Symptoms and biomarkers | Neonatal (birth–1 month) | Infancy (1–18 months) | childhood (1.5–11 years) | Adolescence (11–16 years) | Adulthood (>16 years) |
|---|---|---|---|---|---|---|
| Cardiovascular | **Cardiac arrhythmia** | ± | ± | | | |
| | **Cardiomyopathy** | ± | ± | ± | | |
| CNS | **Coma** | ± | ± | ± | | |
| | **Lethargy** | ± | ± | ± | | |
| | **Neuropathy, peripheral** | | | ± | ± | ± |
| Digestive | **Liver dysfunction** | ± | ± | ± | ± | ± |
| Eye | **Pigmentary retinopathy** | | ± | ± | ± | ± |
| Metabolic | Lactic acidosis | ± | ± | | | |
| Musculoskeletal | **Hypotonia, muscular-axial** | + | + | + | + | + |
| | **Rhabdomyolysis, exercise induced** | | ± | ++ | ++ | ++ |
| | **Skeletal myopathy** | + | + | + | + | + |
| Other | Intrauterine growth retardation | + | | | | |
| | Maternal HELLP syndrome | + | | | | |

**Table 48.13** (continued)

| System | Symptoms and biomarkers | Neonatal (birth–1 month) | Infancy (1–18 months) | childhood (1.5–11 years) | Adolescence (11–16 years) | Adulthood (>16 years) |
|---|---|---|---|---|---|---|
| Laboratory findings | 3-Hydroxydicarboxylic acid (urine) | n-↑ | n-↑ | n-↑ | n-↑ | n |
| | Ammonia (blood) | (↑) | (↑) | (↑) | n | n-↑ |
| | C14-OH 3-Hydroxy tetradecanoylcarnitine (plasma) | n-↑ | n-↑ | n-↑ | n-↑ | n-↑ |
| | C16-C18 Hydroxyacylcarnitine | n-↑ | n-↑ | n-↑ | n-↑ | n-↑ |
| | C16-OH 3-Hydroxy hexadecanoylcarnitine (plasma) | n-↑ | n-↑ | n-↑ | n-↑ | n-↑ |
| | C18:1-OH 3-Hydroxy octadecenoylcarnosine (plasma) | n-↑ | n-↑ | n-↑ | n-↑ | n-↑ |
| | Carnitine, free (dried blood spot) | ↓-n | ↓-n | ↓-n | ↓-n | ↓-n |
| | Carnitine, free (plasma) | ↓-n | ↓-n | ↓-n | ↓-n | ↓-n |
| | Creatine kinase (plasma) | n-↑ | n-↑ | n-↑↑ | n-↑↑ | n-↑↑ |
| | Dicarboxylic acids (urine) | n-↑ | n-↑ | n-↑ | n-↑ | n |
| | Glucose (plasma) | ↓-n | ↓-n | ↓-n | | |
| | Ketones, during hypoglycemia | ↓ | ↓ | ↓ | | |
| | Lactate (plasma) | n-↑ | n-↑ | n | n | n |
| | Transaminase (plasma) | n-↑ | n-↑ | n-↑↑ | n-↑↑ | n-↑↑ |

**Table 48.14** Isolated deficiency of long-chain 3-ketoacyl-CoA thiolase (1 patient)

| System | Symptoms and biomarkers | Neonatal (birth–1 month) | Infancy (1–18 months) | childhood (1.5–11 years) | Adolescence (11–16 years) | Adulthood (>16 years) |
|---|---|---|---|---|---|---|
| Cardiovascular | **Cardiac arrhythmia** | ± | ± | | | |
| | **Cardiomyopathy** | + | + | | | |
| Digestive | **Liver dysfunction** | + | + | | | |
| Musculoskeletal | **Hypotonia, muscular-axial** | + | + | | | |
| | **Skeletal myopathy** | + | + | | | |
| Respiratory | **Pulmonary edema** | + | + | | | |
| Other | **Lethality, high** | + | + | | | |
| Laboratory findings | 3-Hydroxyadipic acid (urine) | ↑ | ↑ | | | |
| | 3-Hydroxyadipic acid lactone (urine) | ↑ | ↑ | | | |
| | 3-Hydroxydicarboxylic acid (urine) | ↑ | ↑ | | | |
| | 3-Hydroxysebacic acid (urine) | ↑ | ↑ | | | |
| | 3-Hydroxysuberic acid (urine) | ↑ | ↑ | | | |
| | Adipic acid (urine) | ↑ | ↑ | | | |
| | C14:0-Hydroxyacylcarnitine (dried blood spot) | ↑ | ↑ | | | |
| | C14:0-Hydroxyacylcarnitine (plasma) | ↑ | ↑ | | | |
| | C14:1-Acylcarnitine (dried blood spot) | ↑ | ↑ | | | |
| | C14:1-Acylcarnitine (plasma) | ↑ | ↑ | | | |

(continued)

**Table 48.14** (continued)

| System | Symptoms and biomarkers | Neonatal (birth–1 month) | Infancy (1–18 months) | childhood (1.5–11 years) | Adolescence (11–16 years) | Adulthood (>16 years) |
|---|---|---|---|---|---|---|
| | C14:1-Hydroxyacylcarnitine (dried blood spot) | ↑ | ↑ | | | |
| | C14:1-Hydroxyacylcarnitine (plasma) | ↑ | ↑ | | | |
| | C16:0-Hydroxyacylcarnitine (dried blood spot) | ↑ | ↑ | | | |
| | C16:0-Hydroxyacylcarnitine (plasma) | ↑ | ↑ | | | |
| | C16:0-Ketoacylcarnitine (dried blood spot) | ↑ | ↑ | | | |
| | C16:0-Ketoacylcarnitine (plasma) | ↑ | ↑ | | | |
| | C16:1-Hydroxyacylcarnitine (dried blood spot) | ↑ | ↑ | | | |
| | C16:1-Hydroxyacylcarnitine (plasma) | ↑ | ↑ | | | |
| | C16-C18 Hydroxyacylcarnitine | ↑ | ↑ | | | |
| | C18:0-Hydroxyacylcarnitine (dried blood spot) | ↑ | ↑ | | | |
| | C18:0-Hydroxyacylcarnitine (plasma) | ↑ | ↑ | | | |
| | C18:1-Hydroxyacylcarnitine (dried blood spot) | ↑ | ↑ | | | |
| | C18:1-Hydroxyacylcarnitine (plasma) | ↑ | ↑ | | | |
| | C18:1-Ketoacylcarnitine (dried blood spot) | ↑ | ↑ | | | |
| | C18:1-Ketoacylcarnitine (plasma) | ↑ | ↑ | | | |
| | C18:2-Hydroxyacylcarnitine (dried blood spot) | ↑ | ↑ | | | |
| | C18:2-Hydroxyacylcarnitine (plasma) | ↑ | ↑ | | | |
| | C18:2-Ketoacylcarnitine (dried blood spot) | ↑ | ↑ | | | |
| | C18:2-Ketoacylcarnitine (plasma) | ↑ | ↑ | | | |
| | Carnitine, free (dried blood spot) | n | n | | | |
| | Carnitine, free (plasma) | n | n | | | |
| | Creatine kinase (plasma) | n | n | | | |
| | Dicarboxylic acids (urine) | ↑ | ↑ | | | |
| | Glucose (plasma) | ± | ± | | | |
| | Ketones, during hypoglycemia | ± | ± | | | |
| | Lactate (plasma) | ↑↑ | ↑ | | | |
| | Sebacic acid (urine) | ↑ | ↑ | | | |
| | Suberic acid (urine) | ↑ | ↑ | | | |
| | Transaminase (plasma) | ↑ | ↑ | | | |

**Table 48.15** Trifunctional protein β subunit deficiency

| System | Symptoms and biomarkers | Neonatal (birth–1 month) | Infancy (1–18 months) | childhood (1.5–11 years) | Adolescence (11–16 years) | Adulthood (>16 years) |
|---|---|---|---|---|---|---|
| Cardiovascular | **Cardiomyopathy** | ± | ± | ± | n | n |
| | **Cardiac arrhythmia** | n - ↑↑↑ | n - ↑↑↑ | | | |
| CNS | **Coma** | ± | ± | ± | n | n |
| | **Lethargy** | ± | ± | ± | n | n |
| | **Neuropathy, peripheral** | n | n | ± | + | ++ |
| Digestive | **Liver dysfunction** | ± | ± | ± | ± | ± |
| Eye | **Pigmentary retinopathy** | n | ± | ± | ± | ± |
| Metabolic | Lactic acidosis | ± | ± | n | n | n |
| Musculoskeletal | **Skeletal myopathy** | + | + | + | + | + |
| Other | Intrauterine growth retardation | + | + | | | |
| | Maternal HELLP syndrome | + | | | | |
| Laboratory findings | 3-Hydroxyadipic acid (urine) | n-↑ | n-↑ | n-↑ | n-↑ | n |
| | 3-Hydroxydicarboxylic acid (urine) | n-↑ | n-↑ | n-↑ | n-↑ | n |
| | 3-Hydroxysebacic acid (urine) | n-↑ | n-↑ | n-↑ | n-↑ | n |
| | 3-Hydroxysuberic acid (urine) | n-↑ | n-↑ | n-↑ | n-↑ | n |
| | Adipic acid (urine) | n-↑ | n-↑ | n-↑ | n-↑ | n |
| | Ammonia (blood) | ↑ | ↑ | ↑ | n | n |
| | C12-OH 3-Hydroxy dodecanoylcarnitine (plasma) | n-↑ | n-↑ | n-↑ | n-↑ | n-↑ |
| | C14:0-Hydroxyacylcarnitine (dried blood spot) | n-↑ | n-↑ | n-↑ | n-↑ | n-↑ |
| | C14:0-Hydroxyacylcarnitine (plasma) | n-↑ | n-↑ | n-↑ | n-↑ | n-↑ |
| | C14:1 Tetradecenoylcarnitine (plasma) | n-↑ | n-↑ | n-↑ | n-↑ | n-↑ |
| | C14:1-Acylcarnitine (dried blood spot) | n-↑ | n-↑ | n-↑ | n-↑ | n-↑ |
| | C14:1-Acylcarnitine (plasma) | n-↑ | n-↑ | n-↑ | n-↑ | n-↑ |
| | C14:1-Hydroxyacylcarnitine (dried blood spot) | n-↑ | n-↑ | n-↑ | n-↑ | n-↑ |
| | C14:1-Hydroxyacylcarnitine (plasma) | n-↑ | n-↑ | n-↑ | n-↑ | n-↑ |
| | C14-OH 3-Hydroxy tetradecanoylcarnitine (plasma) | n-↑ | n-↑ | n-↑ | n-↑ | n-↑ |
| | C16 Palmitoylcarnitine (plasma) | n-↑ | n-↑ | n-↑ | n-↑ | n-↑ |
| | C16:0-Hydroxyacylcarnitine (dried blood spot) | n-↑ | n-↑ | n-↑ | n-↑ | n-↑ |
| | C16:0-Hydroxyacylcarnitine (plasma) | n-↑ | n-↑ | n-↑ | n-↑ | n-↑ |
| | C16:1-Hydroxyacylcarnitine (dried blood spot) | n-↑ | n-↑ | n-↑ | n-↑ | n-↑ |
| | C16:1-Hydroxyacylcarnitine (plasma) | n-↑ | n-↑ | n-↑ | n-↑ | n-↑ |
| | C16-C18 Hydroxyacylcarnitine | n-↑ | n-↑ | n-↑ | n-↑ | n-↑ |
| | C18:0-Hydroxyacylcarnitine (dried blood spot) | n-↑ | n-↑ | n-↑ | n-↑ | n-↑ |

(continued)

**Table 48.15** (continued)

| System | Symptoms and biomarkers | Neonatal (birth–1 month) | Infancy (1–18 months) | childhood (1.5–11 years) | Adolescence (11–16 years) | Adulthood (>16 years) |
|---|---|---|---|---|---|---|
| | C18:0-Hydroxyacylcarnitine (plasma) | n-↑ | n-↑ | n-↑ | n-↑ | n-↑ |
| | C18:1 Octadecenoylcarnitine (plasma) | n-↑ | n-↑ | n-↑ | n-↑ | n-↑ |
| | C18:1-Hydroxyacylcarnitine (dried blood spot) | n-↑ | n-↑ | n-↑ | n-↑ | n-↑ |
| | C18:1-Hydroxyacylcarnitine (plasma) | n-↑ | n-↑ | n-↑ | n-↑ | n-↑ |
| | C18:1-OH 3-Hydroxy octadecenoylcarnosine (plasma) | n-↑ | n-↑ | n-↑ | n-↑ | n-↑ |
| | C18:2 Octadecadienoylcarnitine (plasma) | n-↑ | n-↑ | n-↑ | n-↑ | n-↑ |
| | C18:2-Hydroxyacylcarnitine (dried blood spot) | n-↑ | n-↑ | n-↑ | n-↑ | n-↑ |
| | C18:2-Hydroxyacylcarnitine (plasma) | n-↑ | n-↑ | n-↑ | n-↑ | n-↑ |
| | C18-OH 3-Hydroxy octadecanoylcarnitine (plasma) | n-↑ | n-↑ | n-↑ | n-↑ | n-↑ |
| | Carnitine, free (dried blood spot) | ↓-n | ↓-n | ↓-n | ↓-n | ↓-n |
| | Carnitine, free (plasma) | ↓-n | ↓-n | ↓-n | ↓-n | ↓-n |
| | Creatine kinase (plasma) | n-↑ | n-↑ | n-↑↑ | n-↑↑ | n-↑↑ |
| | Dicarboxylic acids (urine) | n-↑ | n-↑ | n-↑ | n-↑ | n |
| | Glucose (plasma) | ↓-n | ↓-n | ↓-n | | |
| | Ketones, during hypoglycemia | ↓ | ↓ | ↓ | | |
| | Lactate (plasma) | n-↑ | n-↑ | n | n | n |
| | Sebacic acid (urine) | n-↑ | n-↑ | n-↑ | n-↑ | n |
| | Suberic acid (urine) | n-↑ | n-↑ | n-↑ | n-↑ | n |
| | Transaminase (plasma) | n-↑ | n-↑ | n-↑↑ | n-↑↑ | n-↑↑ |

**Table 48.16** Fatty acid transport protein 4 deficiency

| System | Symptoms and biomarkers | Neonatal (birth–1 month) | Infancy (1–18 months) | Childhood (1.5–11 years) | Adolescence (11–16 years) | Adulthood (>16 years) |
|---|---|---|---|---|---|---|
| Hematological | Eosinophilia | ± | ± | | | |
| Dermatological | Hyperkeratosis | + | + | | | |
| | Ichthyosis | + | + | | | |
| | Thick caseous | + | + | | | |

**Table 48.17** Docosahexanoic acid transporter deficiency

| System | Symptoms and biomarkers | Neonatal (birth–1 month) | Infancy (1–18 months) | Childhood (1.5–11 years) | Adolescence (11–16 years) | Adulthood (>16 years) |
|---|---|---|---|---|---|---|
| Autonomic system | **Talipes** | ± | ± | ± | | |
| CNS | Cerebellar hypoplasia | ± | ± | ± | | |
| | **Hyperreflexia** | ± | + | + | | |
| | **Hypotonia** | ± | ± | ± | | |
| | Intellectual disability | | + | + | | |
| | **Loss of speech** | | + | + | | |
| | **Psychomotor delay** | | + | + | | |
| | **Quadriparesis** | | + | + | | |
| | **Seizures** | ± | ± | ± | | |
| | **Thin corpus callosum** | ± | ± | ± | | |
| Eye | Upslanting palpebral fissures | ± | ± | ± | | |
| Musculoskeletal | **Microcephaly** | + | + | + | | |
| Psychiatric | Autistic spectrum disorder | | ± | ± | | |
| Laboratory findings | Lysophosphatidylcholines (plasma) | ↑ | ↑ | ↑ | | |

**Table 48.18** Acyl-CoA Dehydrogenase 9 deficiency

| System | Symptoms and biomarkers | Neonatal (birth–1 month) | Infancy (1–18 months) | childhood (1.5–11 years) | Adolescence (11–16 years) | Adulthood (>16 years) |
|---|---|---|---|---|---|---|
| Cardiovascular | **Cardiomyopathy, dilated** | | + | + | | |
| CNS | **Encephalopathy** | | + | | | |
| | **Neurologic dysfunction** | | + | + | | |
| Digestive | **Liver dysfunction** | | + | + | | |
| | **Liver failure** | | + | + | | |
| | **Liver failure, Reye-like** | | | | + | |
| Ear | **Hearing loss** | | + | + | | |
| Metabolic | Hypoglycemia | | + | + | | |
| | Lactic acidosis | | + | + | | |
| Musculoskeletal | **Exercise intolerance** | | + | + | | |
| | **Hypotonia, muscular-axial** | | + | + | | |
| | **Rhabdomyolysis** | | + | + | | |
| | **Skeletal myopathy** | | + | + | | |
| Other | Complex I assembly disorder | | + | + | | |
| | **Failure to thrive** | | + | + | | |
| Laboratory findings | Transaminase (plasma) | | ↑↑ | ↑↑ | | |
| | Glucose (plasma) | ↓ | ↓ | ↓ | | |
| | Beta-hydroxybutyrate (urine) | | ↑ | | | |
| | Ammonia (blood) | | (↑) | (↑) | (↑) | |
| | Carnitine, free (dried blood spot) | | ↓ | ↓ | | |
| | Carnitine, free (plasma) | | ↓ | ↓ | | |
| | Long-chain acylcarnitine (dried blood spot) | | ↑ | ↑ | | |
| | Long-chain acylcarnitine (plasma) | | ↑ | ↑ | | |
| | Lactate (plasma) | ↑ | ↑ | | | |
| | C14:0-Acylcarnitine (serum) | | ↑ | ↑ | | |
| | C14:0-Acylcarnitine (dried blood spot) | | ↑ | ↑ | | |
| | C16:0-Acylcarnitine (plasma) | | ↑ | ↑ | | |
| | C16:0-Acylcarnitine (dried blood spot) | | ↑ | ↑ | | |
| | C16:1-Acylcarnitine (plasma) | | ↑ | ↑ | | |
| | C16:1-Acylcarnitine (dried blood spot) | | ↑ | ↑ | | |
| | C18:0-Acylcarnitine (plasma) | | ↑ | ↑ | | |
| | C18:0-Acylcarnitine (dried blood spot) | | ↑ | ↑ | | |
| | C18:1-Acylcarnitine (plasma) | | ↑ | ↑ | | |
| | C18:1-Acylcarnitine (dried blood spot) | | ↑ | ↑ | | |
| | C18:2-Acylcarnitine (plasma) | | ↑ | ↑ | | |
| | C18:2-Acylcarnitine (dried blood spot) | | ↑ | ↑ | | |
| | Alanine (plasma) | | ↑ | ↑ | | |
| | Alanine (urine) | | ↑ | ↑ | | |
| | Adipic acid (urine) | | ↑ | ↑ | | |
| | Suberic acid (urine) | | ↑ | ↑ | | |
| | Suberic acid, unsaturated (urine) | | ↑ | ↑ | | |
| | Sebacic acid (urine) | | ↑ | ↑ | | |
| | Sebacic acid, unsaturated (urine) | | ↑ | ↑ | | |
| | Lactate (urine) | ↑ | ↑ | ↑ | | |
| | Lactate/pyruvate ratio | ↑ | ↑ | ↑ | ↑ | |
| | Creatine kinase (plasma) | | ↑ | ↑ | | |

## Reference Values

Measured values of carnitine and acylcarnitines differ in dried blood spots and plasma (de Sain-van der Velden et al. 2013). They also change with age, especially in newborns over the first days of life. Catabolism increases acylcarnitine concentrations in patients and healthy individuals. Reference values are given in Chap. 5. Organic acid analysis in urine reveals a disease-specific profile distinct from healthy individuals; however, organic acids can also be normal in patients during anabolism and in milder phenotypes. Fasting significantly increases the excretion of disease-specific organic acids in patients.

## Pathological Values

An extremely wide variation in blood acylcarnitine values is observed in patients, related both to the specific diagnosis and timing of the most recent meal, and may normalize when the patient is well and not fasting (Smith and Matern 2010). Collecting diagnostic samples immediately prior to a meal or during acute illness maximizes the likelihood of making a diagnosis. In general, patients with milder disease have less dramatic changes in metabolite profiles than those with more severe neonatal/infantile presentations. Normal ketosis increases acylcarnitine levels even in healthy individuals and should not be confused with disease patterns.

Acylcarnitine levels in newborn blood spot samples generally decrease in the first days of life and may normalize, even in patients with FAODs, and therefore late screening can lead to missed diagnoses (Lindner et al. 2010). Importantly, healthy newborns and children may present with abnormal acylcarnitine profiles suggestive of a FAOD during severe catabolism. Pathological reference values taken from a large worldwide cohort have been reported (McHugh et al. 2011). Consideration of the acylcarnitine pattern and calculation of metabolite ratios rather than relying on single metabolite values improve testing accuracy (Marquardt et al. 2012).

## Diagnostic Tools and Flowchart

Laboratory investigation of a suspected FAOD should begin with measurement of the acylcarnitine profile and includes consideration of individual metabolite values as well as the ratios of various acylcarnitines (Fig. 48.3). The acylcarnitine profiles in severe CPTII and CACT are indistinguishable, as are those in LCHAD and MTP deficiencies. In CPTI deficiency, carnitine concentration in dried blood spots is higher than in plasma, and diagnosis may be missed with measurement in plasma.

Clinical circumstances have a major effect on the acylcarnitine profile. Abnormalities are usually more marked during catabolism but, if the plasma-free carnitine concentration is very low, abnormal acylcarnitines may be hard to detect. Abnormalities decrease with intravenous glucose or dietary treatment, and metabolites from medium-chain fat oxidation increase with the use of medium-chain triglycerides (MCTs). An interpretation is especially difficult for terminal or post-mortem samples as they often show multiple raised acylcarnitine species, resembling MAD deficiency (MADD). In cases of very low free carnitine, diagnostic changes may be induced by overnight fasting or carnitine loading, respectively. However, these challenges can be dangerous and should only be considered in the inpatient setting, and the fasting period should be adjusted to the age of the patient. It is probably better to move to functional testing molecular analysis before considering challenge testing.

While acylcarnitine analysis is often consistent with a specific diagnosis, enzyme and/or mutation analyses are required for confirmation. The in vitro assays described below may be useful to reach a diagnosis when metabolite testing is normal in spite of a strong clinical suspicion.

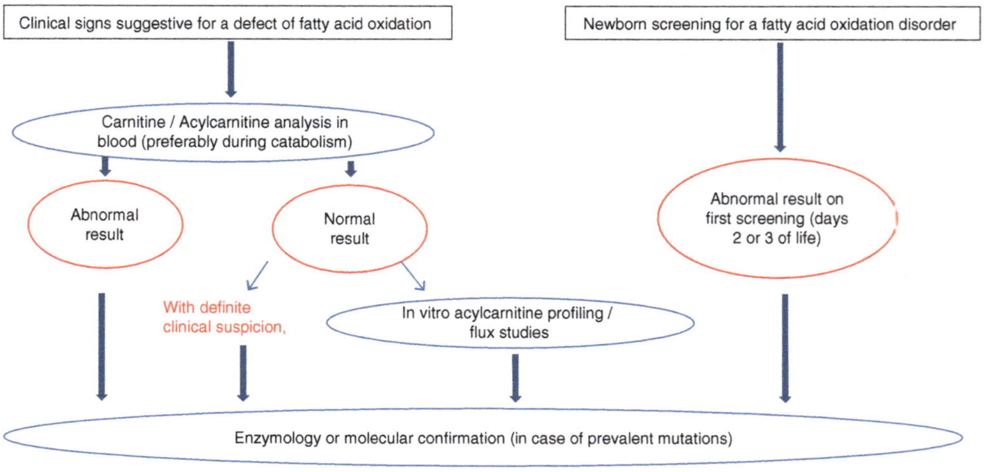


**Fig. 48.3** Diagnostic flow chart

### Enzyme Testing

Enzyme assays are generally performed in cultured fibroblasts or lymphocytes (Wanders et al. 2010) but are available in limited geographic areas. Enzymology in lymphocytes allows a rapid confirmation of diagnosis. Moreover, for VLCAD and MCAD deficiencies, residual activity may allow some predictions with respect to the expected severity of the defect (Hoffmann et al. 2012).

### Fibroblast or Lymphocyte Acylcarnitine Profiling

Fibroblast or lymphocyte acylcarnitine profiling may identify an enzymatic defect if a diagnosis is not clear from blood testing. Here, acylcarnitines are analyzed by tandem mass spectrometry after incubating fibroblasts or lymphocytes with fatty acids' stable isotope-labeled substrates ($^{2}H$ or $^{13}C$) (Ventura et al. 1999; Sim et al. 2002). This technique can identify most FAODs except carnitine transporter and CPTI deficiencies. CACT and severe CPTII deficiencies cannot be distinguished and respiratory chain defects sometimes mimic FAODs (Sim et al. 2002).

### Fatty Acid Oxidation Flux

Fatty acid oxidation flux is measured by incubating cells with radio-labeled fatty acids and collecting the oxidation products (Olpin et al. 1997). This technique identifies a global defect in FAO, is useful in assessing the severity of a disorder, but is not as specific as acylcarnitines in arriving at a diagnosis.

### Urinary Organic Acids and Acylglycines

Urine organic acid analysis is normal in many FAODs when patients are well. Dicarboxylic acids are formed by ß-oxidation in peroxisomes and ω-oxidation in microsomes when plasma-free fatty acid concentrations are increased, but normally they are accompanied by ketonuria. During fasting or illness, however, medium-chain (and sometimes long-chain) dicarboxylic acids are elevated with little or no increase in ketone bodies. Dicarboxylic aciduria without ketonuria can also be seen in some respiratory chain defects. The analysis of acylcarnitines in the urine may identify carnitine esters of dicarboxylic acids that are of additional diagnostic significance. Defects of LCHAD and MTP deficiencies can accumulate unusual 3-hydroxydicarboxylic acids in urine. MCADD is characterized by an abnormal excretion of several acylglycines including hexanoylglycine, suberylglycine, and phenylpropionylglycine. These same acylglycines, in addition to short branched-chain acylcarnitines, are characteristic of MADD and, in general, are accompanied by a variety of dicarboxylic acids including as ethylmalonic acid, glutaric acid, and D-2-hydroxyglutaric acid. Unfortunately, normal organic acids do not exclude an FAO disorder since they can be normal in milder phenotypes and in anabolic situations.

## Specimen Collection

| Test | Material | Handling | Transport | Pitfalls |
|---|---|---|---|---|
| **Acylcarnitines** | Plasma; dried blood spot (DB) | Room temperature (DB); Frozen (plasma) | Normal mail | During anabolism eventually normal values; different profile with MCT diet; long-chain acylcarnitine accumulation also in healthy individuals during catabolism |
| **Carnitine** | Plasma; dried blood spot (DB) | Room temperature (DB); Frozen (plasma) | Normal mail | Blood and tissue concentrations do not correlate; in CPTI deficiency, carnitine is lower in plasma than in DB; it may be missed on analysis in plasma |
| **Dicarboxylic acids** | Spot urine | Frozen for longer storage | Normal mail | MCT diet and glucose infusion change the profile |
| **Free fatty acids** | Plasma | Frozen | Frozen | Determine before the next food intake |
| **Enzyme assays in lymphocytes** | Ethylenediamine tetraacetic acid (EDTA) plasma (2 mL) | Room temperature | Has to reach the laboratory within 48 hours after withdrawal; room temperature | Poor quality of the lymphocytes (due to transport conditions, low temperature, etc.) may result in lower residual enzyme activities |
| **Enzyme assays in fibroblasts** | Skin biopsy | Room temperature, in sterile 0.9% sodium chloride, fibroblast culture | In culture medium | Fibroblast culture must grow 4–8 weeks until enzyme assays can be performed |
| **Molecular analysis** | EDTA blood; dried blood spot | Room temperature | Normal mail | Delineation of only one mutation does not rule out deficiency of the enzyme |

## Prenatal Diagnosis

Prenatal diagnosis is available for all fatty acid oxidation disorders. Mutation analysis is the preferred technique if the molecular defect is known in the index case. Acylcarnitine and acylglycine assays of amniotic fluid have been reported for many FAODs, but are not routinely clinically available. These latter assays do not exclude the disease if metabolites are normal on prenatal diagnosis. All enzymes of fatty acid oxidation are expressed in chorionic villus biopsies and amniocytes and can be used for prenatal diagnosis. Chorionic villus biopsy can be performed at 11 gestational weeks, and amniotic fluid test at 14 + 0 weeks.

| Deficiency of | Prenatal diagnosis suggested | Remarks |
|---|---|---|
| **OCTN2** | – | Very favorable clinical outcome |
| **CPTI** | – | Very favorable outcome |
| **CACT** | + | Majority of patients die in the neonatal period due to severe cardiac arrhythmias |
| **CPTII** | + | Suggested for severe neonatal phenotypes with congenital anomalies |
| | – | Myopathic phenotypes |
| **VLCAD** | – | Very favorable clinical outcome; many asymptomatic "patients"; skeletal myopathy needs to be discussed with the parents |
| **MTP** | + (+) | Suggested for severe phenotypes; neonatal phenotypes generally lethal; irreversible neuropathy/retinopathy needs to be discussed with the parents in milder phenotypes |
| **LCHAD** | ± | Irreversible retinopathy/neuropathy needs to be discussed with the parents |
| **LKAT** | + | Only two patients so far; both died in the neonatal period |
| **ACAD 9** | + | Global mitochondrial dysfunction |
| **MCAD** | – | Very favorable clinical outcome since screening |
| **SCAD** | – | Only predisposition for disease |
| **SCHAD** | ± | Phenotypes of different severity and response to treatment |

## DNA Analysis

All mitochondrial FAODs are inherited in an autosomal recessive pattern. There is molecular heterogeneity in all of the disorders but prevalent mutations have been identified in most. The relationship between genotype and phenotype varies among the different FAODs. In CPTII and VLCAD deficiencies, nonsense mutations on both alleles are generally associated with severe early onset disease, whereas adult onset rhabdomyolysis is associated with conservative missense mutations. A common mutation in VLCAD is found in nearly half of patients identified through newborn screening and is associated with a mild phenotype (c.848T>C). A common mutation accounts for 75% of the mutations in patients with MCADD and leads to complete deficiency, while a recurrent c.199T>C variant is associated with significant residual activity and appears to be benign. A common mutation in the *HADHA* gene alters the catalytic residue in the LCHAD domain and is the predominant cause of isolated LCHAD deficiency.

| Enzyme name | Gene name | Prevalent mutations (Caucasian population) | | Remarks |
|---|---|---|---|---|
| | | Mutation | Amino acid change | |
| **OCTN2** | *SLC22A5* | No prevalent mutation | | |
| **CPTI** | *CPT1* | c.1436C>T (Inuit population) | p.P479L | 70% of babies homozygous for c.1436C>T in the Inuit population (Canada and Greenland) |
| **CACT** | *SLC25A20* | No prevalent mutation | | |
| **CPTII** | *CPT2* | c.338C>T | p.S113L | Allele frequency (60%) |
| **VLCAD** | *ACADVL* | c.848T>C | p.V243A | Suggestive of mild VLCADD |
| **MTP** | *HADHA/HADHB* | No prevalent mutations | | Many deletions and splice site mutations in the HADHA gene;<br>Most compound heterozygotes for c.1528G>C and a second HADHA mutation have MTP deficiency |
| **LCHAD** | *HADHA/HADHB* | c.1528G>C | p.E474Q | Heterogeneous presentations despite one mutation |
| **LKAT** | *HADHA/HADHB* | No prevalent mutation | | Only two patients known |
| **ACAD9** | *ACAD9* | No prevalent mutation | | |
| **MCAD** | *ACADM* | c.985A>G<br>c.199G>C | p.K329E<br>p.Y67H | Classical MCADD; before screening: 80% homozygosity<br>Asymptomatic/(mild) variant; allele frequency: 6% of mutant alleles in screened population; not found in a clinically diagnosed patient before screening |
| **SCAD** | *ACADS* | c.625G>A<br>c.511C>T | p.G209S<br>p.R171W | Polymorphisms with predisposition for disease;<br>625G > A: Allele frequency, 22%;<br>c.511C > T: Allele frequency, 3% |
| **SCHAD** | ***HADH*** | No prevalent mutation | | |

## Treatment

Prolonged fasting should be avoided in all FAODs in order to prevent acute metabolic decompensation. Frequent, regular feeds are recommended, especially during the first year of life, but subsequently overnight fasting (8 h) will be tolerated in most disorders. Prolonged overnight fasting should be postponed until later childhood/adolescence, especially in MTP and LCHAD deficiencies, in order to reduce the risk of retinopathy and neuropathy as a consequence of accumulating toxic metabolites.

Dietary fat restriction is not indicated in MCAD deficiency. In mild long-chain FAODs, the dietary fat intake does not have to be reduced if MCT oil is not prescribed; however, the fat intake should not exceed the dietary recommendation for healthy individuals. If MCT is used in severe long-chain FAODs, some restriction of long-chain fat will be necessary to maintain appropriate nutrient balance. Supplementation with 2–4 gm/kg of body weight per day of MCT oil may be used in young patients (<2 years of age) with a severe phenotype, and may be provided by an MCT-containing formula (Spiekerkoetter et al. 2009). Such high amounts are usually not tolerated in older children or adults, and 1–2 gm/kg/day is more usual. A bolus of MCT before exercise reduces accumulation of long-chain acylcarnitine species and may reduce the risk of rhabdomyolysis in patients with long-chain FAODs (Gillingham et al. 2006). Studies in VLCAD-deficient mice highlight the need to give MCT in accordance to the energy needs, since MCT are otherwise elongated and stored as saturated long-chain fatty acids (Tucci et al. 2015).

Carnitine treatment is undisputedly effective in patients with carnitine transporter deficiency. With a dose of 100–300 mg/kg/day, plasma concentrations may reach the lower normal range but muscle carnitine concentrations remain less than 5% of normal (Stanley et al. 1991). The value of carnitine supplementation in other FAODs is controversial. Plasma-free carnitine concentration is often low, particularly after an acute illness, but tissue concentrations have seldom been measured. In many patients, carnitine concentration in blood reach normal values when well, likely due to induced endogenous carnitine biosynthesis. Carnitine treatment has been hypothesized to be harmful in long-chain FAODs, as it increases the concentrations of potentially arrhythmogenic long-chain acylcarnitines (Primassin et al. 2008). However, this remains unproven and must be balanced against a potential benefit of providing some additional FAO capacity if the free carnitine is exceedingly low.

Bezafibrates (PPARα and PPARδ agonists) may be promising in the treatment of patients with myopathic CPTII or VLCAD deficiencies, though a randomized controlled clinical trial failed to show a clinical effect (Bonnefont et al. 2010). Triheptanoin (C7 odd-chain fatty acid) has been tested anecdotally and in clinical trials as a substitute for MCT (Vockley et al. 2019). It has been presumed that patients with long-chain FAODs have reduced levels of TCA cycle intermediates that is more effectively addressed by supplying both acetyl-CoA and propionyl-CoA from triheptanoin as compared to acetyl-CoA alone from MCT (Vockley et al. 2019). In a double-blind study of the two compounds in patients with long-chain FAODs, patients showed improvement in cardiac function on triheptanoin compared to MCT. A phase-2 open-label trial of triheptanoin in long-chain FAOD patients showed an overall decrease in major clinical events defined as hypoglycemia, development and worsening of cardiomyopathy, and frequency and severity of rhabdomyolysis. A report on compassionate use of triheptanoin with acute onset or exacerbation of cardiomyopathy in long-chain FAOD patients while on MCT, showed rescue of critically ill patients in many cases (Vockley et al. 2016). The drug is being considered for approval in the USA, but has not been extensively tested in Europe. So far it is still considered an experimental treatment and has not been included in general treatment recommendations for FAO defects.

## Emergency Treatment

| Deficiency of | Emergency treatment | Pharmacological emergency treatment |
|---|---|---|
| **OCTN2** | Glucose i.v.; oral glucose monomer (to avoid hypoglycemia)<br>Reach anabolism | L-carnitine i.v.<br>(100–300 mg/kg per day) |
| **CPTI**<br>**CACT**<br>**CPTII**<br>**VLCAD**<br>**MTP**<br>**LCHAD**<br>**LKAT**<br>**ACAD9** | Glucose i.v.; oral glucose monomer<br>(to avoid hypoglycemia)<br>Reach anabolism:<br><3 years: 10–12 mg/kg/min<br>3–10 years: 8–10 mg/kg/min<br>>10 years: 5–8 mg/kg min<br>Oral MCT; i.v. MCT generally not available (only special preparations)<br>When severe decompensation, reach anabolism with use of insulin<br>ACAD 9: Monitor lactate | L-carnitine typically not needed unless free carnitine is very low (<10 mM)<br>D,L-3-hydroxybutyrate with severe cardiomyopathy<br>Pharmacological treatment of arrhythmias |
| **MCAD** | Glucose i.v.; oral glucose monomer<br>(to avoid hypoglycemia)<br>Reach anabolism<br>No MCT | |
| **SCAD** | Glucose i.v. in case of hypoglycemia | |
| **SCHAD** | Glucose i.v. | Glucagon, somatostatin (treatment of hyperinsulinism) |

## Standard Treatment

| Deficiency of | Dietary treatment | Pharmacological treatment |
|---|---|---|
| **OCTN2** | Normal diet; regular meals; avoid catabolism | L-carnitine p.o. (100–300 mg/kg per day) |
| **CPTI** | Normal diet; rarely MCT supplementation in severe phenotypes | L-carnitine supplement only if blood level is very low (<10 mM) |
| **CACT** | MCT modified diet; strictly avoid catabolism (cave arrhythmias!) | |
| **CPTII**<br>**VLCAD** | Severe phenotypes:<br>Carbohydrate-enriched diet (65–75% of total calories); fat restriction (25% of total calories: 10–15% MCT, 4% essential fatty acids, up to 10% long-chain triglyceride [LCT])<br>Regular meals<br>After first year of life: Glucose polymer at night<br>*Myopathic phenotypes*:<br>Fat-reduced or normal diet<br>MCT prior to exercise<br>Regular meals; normal overnight fasting tolerance<br>Asymptomatic patients: No dietary interventions | |
| **MTP**<br>**LCHAD**<br>**LKAT** | Strict long-chain fat reduction<br>MCT supplementation (see CPT2, VLCAD)<br>Docosahexaenoic acid (200–400 mg/kg per day) supplementation to prevent retinopathy is controversial | |
| **ACAD9** | No recommendations available | |
| **MCAD** | No dietary intervention; regular meals | |
| **SCAD** | No dietary intervention; regular meals | |
| **SCHAD** | No dietary intervention; regular meals | Glucagon, somatostatin (treatment of hyperinsulinism) |

## Experimental Treatment

| Treatment | Mechanism of treatment | Current status | Disorders |
|---|---|---|---|
| **Bezafibrate** | PPARα and PPARδ agonists; stimulate residual activity in milder phenotypes | Successful in isolated patients; clinical trials going on | Myopathic CPTII and VLCAD deficiencies |
| **Triheptanoin** | Odd-chain C7 fatty acid; anaplerotic action by provision of propionyl-CoA | Successful clinical trials in the USA | Long-chain FAODs |

## References


Bonnefont JP, Bastin J, Laforet P, Aubey F, Mogenet A, Romano S, Ricquier D, Gobin-Limballe S, Vassault A, Behin A, Eymard B, Bresson JL, Djouadi F. Long-term follow-up of bezafibrate treatment in patients with the myopathic form of carnitine palmitoyltransferase 2 deficiency. Clin Pharmacol Ther. 2010;88(1):101–8.

Bonnet D, Martin D, Pascale L, de Villain E, Jouvet P, Rabier D, Brivet M, Saudubray JM. Arrhythmias and conduction defects as presenting symptoms of fatty acid oxidation disorders in children. Circulation. 1999;100(22):2248–53.

Brunengraber H, Roe CR. Anaplerotic molecules: current and future. J Inherit Metab Dis. 2006;29(2–3):327–31.

Carrasco P, Jacas J, Sahun I, Muley H, Ramirez S, Puisac B, Mezquita P, Pie J, Dierssen M, Casals N. Carnitine palmitoyltransferase 1C deficiency causes motor impairment and hypoactivity. Behav Brain Res. 2013;256:291–7.

de Sain-van der Velden MG, Diekman EF, Jans JJ, van der Ham M, Prinsen BH, Visser G, Verhoeven-Duif NM. Differences between acylcarnitine profiles in plasma and bloodspots. Mol Genet Metab. 2013;110(1–2):116–21.

Gallant NM, Leydiker K, Tang H, Feuchtbaum L, Lorey F, Puckett R, Deignan JL, Neidich J, Dorrani N, Chang E, Barshop BA, Cederbaum SD, Abdenur JE, Wang RY. Biochemical, molecular, and clinical characteristics of children with short chain acyl-CoA dehydrogenase deficiency detected by newborn screening in California. Mol Genet Metab. 2012;106(1):55–61.

Gillingham MB, Scott B, Elliott D, Harding CO. Metabolic control during exercise with and without medium-chain triglycerides (MCT) in children with long-chain 3-hydroxy acyl-CoA dehydrogenase (LCHAD) or trifunctional protein (TFP) deficiency. Mol Genet Metab. 2006;89(1–2):58–63.

Herrema H, Derks TG, van Dijk TH, Bloks VW, Gerding A, Havinga R, Tietge UJ, Muller M, Smit GP, Kuipers F, Reijngoud DJ. Disturbed hepatic carbohydrate management during high metabolic demand in medium-chain acyl-CoA dehydrogenase (MCAD)-deficient mice. Hepatology. 2008;47(6):1894–904.

Hoffmann L, Haussmann U, Mueller M, Spiekerkoetter U. VLCAD enzyme activity determinations in newborns identified by screening: a valuable tool for risk assessment. J Inherit Metab Dis. 2012;35(2):269–77.

Holme E, Jodal U, Linstedt S, Nordin I. Effects of pivalic acid-containing prodrugs on carnitine homeostasis and on response to fasting in children. Scand J Clin Lab Invest. 1992;52(5):361–72.

Li C, Chen P, Palladino A, Narayan S, Russell LK, Sayed S, Xiong G, Chen J, Stokes D, Butt YM, Jones PM, Collins HW, Cohen NA, Cohen AS, Nissim I, Smith TJ, Strauss AW, Matschinsky FM, Bennett MJ, Stanley CA. Mechanism of hyperinsulinism in short-chain 3-hydroxyacyl-CoA dehydrogenase deficiency involves activation of glutamate dehydrogenase. J Biol Chem. 2010;285(41):31806–18.

Lindner M, Hoffmann GF, Matern D. Newborn screening for disorders of fatty-acid oxidation: experience and recommendations from an expert meeting. J Inherit Metab Dis. 2010;33(5):521–6.

Longo N, di San Filippo CA, Pasquali M. Disorders of carnitine transport and the carnitine cycle. Am J Med Genet C Semin Med Genet. 2006;142C(2):77–85.

Makino Y, Sugiura T, Ito T, Sugiyama N, Koyama N. Carnitine-associated encephalopathy caused by long-term treatment with an antibiotic containing pivalic acid. Pediatrics. 2007;120(3):e739–41.

Marquardt G, Currier R, McHugh DM, Gavrilov D, Magera MJ, Matern D, Oglesbee D, Raymond K, Rinaldo P, Smith EH, Tortorelli S, Turgeon CT, Lorey F, Wilcken B, Wiley V, Greed LC, Lewis B, Boemer F, Schoos R, Marie S, Vincent MF, Sica YC, Domingos MT, Al-Thihli K, Sinclair G, Al-Dirbashi OY, Chakraborty P, Dymerski M, Porter C, Manning A, Seashore MR, Quesada J, Reuben A, Chrastina P, Hornik P, Atef Mandour I, Atty Sharaf SA, Bodamer O, Dy B, Torres J, Zori R, Cheillan D, Vianey-Saban C, Ludvigson D, Stembridge A, Bonham J, Downing M, Dotsikas Y, Loukas YL, Papakonstantinou V, Zacharioudakis GS, Barath A, Karg E, Franzson L, Jonsson JJ, Breen NN, Lesko BG, Berberich SL, Turner K, Ruoppolo M, Scolamiero E, Antonozzi I, Carducci C, Caruso U, Cassanello M, la Marca G, Pasquini E, Di Gangi IM, Giordano G, Camilot M, Teofoli F, Manos SM, Peterson CK, Mayfield Gibson SK, Sevier DW, Lee SY, Park HD, Khneisser I, Browning P, Gulamali-Majid F, Watson MS, Eaton RB, Sahai I, Ruiz C, Torres R, Seeterlin MA, Stanley EL, Hietala A, McCann M, Campbell C, Hopkins PV, de Sain-Van der Velden MG, Elvers B, Morrissey MA, Sunny S, Knoll D, Webster D, Frazier DM, McClure JD, Sesser DE, Willis SA, Rocha H, Vilarinho L, John C, Lim J, Caldwell SG, Tomashitis K, Castineiras Ramos DE, Cocho de Juan JA, Rueda Fernandez I, Yahyaoui Macias R, Egea-Mellado JM, Gonzalez-Gallego I, Delgado Pecellin C, Garcia-Valdecasas Bermejo MS, Chien YH, Hwu WL, Childs T, McKeever CD, Tanyalcin T, Abdulrahman M, Queijo C, Lemes A, Davis T, Hoffman W, Baker M, Hoffman GL. Enhanced interpretation of newborn screening results without analyte cutoff values. Genet Med. 2012;14(7):648–55.

McHugh D, Cameron CA, Abdenur JE, Abdulrahman M, Adair O, Al Nuaimi SA, Ahlman H, Allen JJ, Antonozzi I, Archer S, Au S, Auray-Blais C, Baker M, Bamforth F, Beckmann K, Pino GB, Berberich SL, Binard R, Boemer F, Bonham J, Breen NN, Bryant SC, Caggana M, Caldwell SG, Camilot M, Campbell C, Carducci C, Bryant SC, Caggana M, Caldwell SG, Camilot M, Campbell C, Carducci C, Cariappa R, Carlisle C, Caruso U, Cassanello M, Castilla AM, Ramos DE, Chakraborty P, Chandrasekar R, Ramos AC, Cheillan D, Chien YH, Childs TA, Chrastina P, Sica YC, de Juan JA, Colandre ME, Espinoza VC, Corso G, Currier R, Cyr D, Czuczy N, D'Apolito O, Davis T, de Sain-Van der Velden MG, Delgado Pecellin C, Di Gangi IM, Di Stefano CM, Dotsikas Y, Downing M, Downs SM, Dy B, Dymerski M, Rueda I, Elvers B, Eaton R, Eckerd BM, El Mougy F, Eroh S, Espada M, Evans C, Fawbush S, Fijolek KF, Fisher L, Franzson L, Frazier DM, Garcia LR, Bermejo MS, Gavrilov D, Gerace R, Giordano G, Irazabal YG, Greed LC, Grier R, Grycki E, Gu X, Gulamali-Majid F, Hagar AF, Han L, Hannon WH, Haslip C, Hassan FA, He M, Hietala A, Himstedt L, Hoffman GL, Hoffman W, Hoggatt P, Hopkins PV, Hougaard DM, Hughes K, Hunt PR, Hwu WL, Hynes J, Ibarra-Gonzalez I,

Ingham CA, Ivanova M, Jacox WB, John C, Johnson JP, Jonsson JJ, Karg E, Kasper D, Klopper B, Katakouzinos D, Khneisser I, Knoll D, Kobayashi H, Koneski R, Kozich V, Kouapei R, Kohlmueller D, Kremensky I, la Marca G, Lavochkin M, Lee SY, Lehotay DC, Lemes A, Lepage J, Lesko B, Lewis B, Lim C, Linard S, Lindner M, Lloyd-Puryear MA, Lorey F, Loukas YL, Luedtke J, Maffitt N, Magee JF, Manning A, Manos S, Marie S, Hadachi SM, Marquardt G, Martin SJ, Matern D, Mayfield Gibson SK, Mayne P, McCallister TD, McCann M, McClure J, McGill JJ, McKeever CD, McNeilly B, Morrissey MA, Moutsatsou P, Mulcahy EA, Nikoloudis D, Norgaard-Pedersen B, Oglesbee D, Oltarzewski M, Ombrone D, Ojodu J, Papakonstantinou V, Reoyo SP, Park HD, Pasquali M, Pasquini E, Patel P, Pass KA, Peterson C, Pettersen RD, Pitt JJ, Poh S, Pollak A, Porter C, Poston PA, Price RW, Queijo C, Quesada J, Randell E, Ranieri E, Raymond K, Reddic JE, Reuben A, Ricciardi C, Rinaldo P, Rivera JD, Roberts A, Rocha H, Roche G, Greenberg CR, Mellado JM, Juan-Fita MJ, Ruiz C, Ruoppolo M, Rutledge SL, Ryu E, Saban C, Sahai I, Garcia-Blanco MI, Santiago-Borrero P, Schenone A, Schoos R, Schweitzer B, Scott P, Seashore MR, Seeterlin MA, Sesser DE, Sevier DW, Shone SM, Sinclair G, Skrinska VA, Stanley EL, Strovel ET, Jones AL, Sunny S, Takats Z, Tanyalcin T, Teofoli F, Thompson JR, Tomashitis K, Domingos MT, Torres J, Torres R, Tortorelli S, Turi S, Turner K, Tzanakos N, Valiente AG, Vallance H, Vela-Amieva M, Vilarinho L, von Dobeln U, Vincent MF, Vorster BC, Watson MS, Webster D, Weiss S, Wilcken B, Wiley V, Williams SK, Willis SA, Woontner M, Wright K, Yahyaoui R, Yamaguchi S, Yssel M, Zakowicz WM. Clinical validation of cutoff target ranges in newborn screening of metabolic disorders by tandem mass spectrometry: a worldwide collaborative project. Genet Med. 2011;13(3):230–54.

Nakazaki K, Ogawa E, Ishige M, Ishige N, Fuchigami T, Takahashi S. Hypocarnitinemia observed in an infant treated with short-term administration of antibiotic containing pivalic acid. Tohoku J Exp Med. 2018;244(4):279–82.

Nasu T, Suzuki M, Uetake K, Kubota M. Newborn hypocarnitinemia due to long-term transplacental pivalic acid passage. Pediatr Int. 2014;56(5):772–4.

Nochi Z, Olsen RKJ, Gregersen N. Short-chain acyl-CoA dehydrogenase deficiency: from gene to cell pathology and possible disease mechanisms. J Inherit Metab Dis. 2017;40(5):641–55.

North KN, Hoppel CL, De Girolami U, Kozakewich HP, Korson MS. Lethal neonatal deficiency of carnitine palmitoyltransferase II associated with dysgenesis of the brain and kidneys. J Pediatr. 1995;127(3):414–20.

Olpin SE, Bonham JR, Downing M, Manning NJ, Pollitt RJ, Sharrard MJ, Tanner MS. Carnitine-acylcarnitine translocase deficiency—a mild phenotype. J Inherit Metab Dis. 1997;20(5):714–5.

Pena LD, van Calcar SC, Hansen J, Edick MJ, Walsh Vockley C, Leslie N, Cameron C, Mohsen AW, Berry SA, Arnold GL, Vockley J. Outcomes and genotype-phenotype correlations in 52 individuals with VLCAD deficiency diagnosed by NBS and enrolled in the IBEM-IS database. Mol Genet Metab. 2016;118(4):272–81.

Pourfarzam M, Morris A, Appleton M, Craft A, Bartlett K. Neonatal screening for medium-chain acyl-CoA dehydrogenase deficiency. Lancet. 2001;358(9287):1063–4.

Primassin S, Ter Veld F, Mayatepek E, Spiekerkoetter U. Carnitine supplementation induces acylcarnitine production in tissues of very long-chain acyl-CoA dehydrogenase-deficient mice, without replenishing low free carnitine. Pediatr Res. 2008;63(6):632–7.

Rasmussen J, Nielsen OW, Lund AM, Kober L, Djurhuus H. Primary carnitine deficiency and pivalic acid exposure causing encephalopathy and fatal cardiac events. J Inherit Metab Dis. 2013;36(1):35–41.

Repp BM, Mastantuono E, Alston CL, Schiff M, Haack TB, Rotig A, Ardissone A, Lombes A, Catarino CB, Diodato D, Schottmann G, Poulton J, Burlina A, Jonckheere A, Munnich A, Rolinski B, Ghezzi D, Rokicki D, Wellesley D, Martinelli D, Wenhong D, Lamantea E, Ostergaard E, Pronicka E, Pierre G, Smeets HJM, Wittig I, Scurr I, de Coo IFM, Moroni I, Smet J, Mayr JA, Dai L, de Meirleir L, Schuelke M, Zeviani M, Morscher RJ, McFarland R, Seneca S, Klopstock T, Meitinger T, Wieland T, Strom TM, Herberg U, Ahting U, Sperl W, Nassogne MC, Ling H, Fang F, Freisinger P, Van Coster R, Strecker V, Taylor RW, Haberle J, Vockley J, Prokisch H, Wortmann S. Clinical, biochemical and genetic spectrum of 70 patients with ACAD9 deficiency: is riboflavin supplementation effective? Orphanet J Rare Dis. 2018;13(1):120.

Rinaldi C, Schmidt T, Situ AJ, Johnson JO, Lee PR, Chen KL, Bott LC, Fado R, Harmison GH, Parodi S, Grunseich C, Renvoise B, Biesecker LG, De Michele G, Santorelli FM, Filla A, Stevanin G, Durr A, Brice A, Casals N, Traynor BJ, Blackstone C, Ulmer TS, Fischbeck KH. Mutation in CPT1C associated with pure autosomal dominant spastic paraplegia. JAMA Neurol. 2015;72(5):561–70.

Sim KG, Carpenter K, Hammond J, Christodoulou J, Wilcken B. Acylcarnitine profiles in fibroblasts from patients with respiratory chain defects can resemble those from patients with mitochondrial fatty acid beta-oxidation disorders. Metabolism. 2002;51(3):366–71.

Smith EH, Matern D. Acylcarnitine analysis by tandem mass spectrometry. Curr Protoc Hum Genet. 2010; Chapter 17(8): Unit 17 18 11–20.

Spiekerkoetter U, Haussmann U, Mueller M, ter Veld F, Stehn M, Santer R, Lukacs Z. Tandem mass spectrometry screening for very long-chain acyl-CoA dehydrogenase deficiency: the value of second-tier enzyme testing. J Pediatr. 2010;157(4):668–73.

Spiekerkoetter U, Khuchua Z, Yue Z, Bennett MJ, Strauss AW. General mitochondrial trifunctional protein (TFP) deficiency as a result of either alpha- or beta-subunit mutations exhibits similar phenotypes because mutations in either subunit alter TFP complex expression and subunit turnover. Pediatr Res. 2004;55(2):190–6.

Spiekerkoetter U, Lindner M, Santer R, Grotzke M, Baumgartner MR, Boehles H, Das A, Haase C, Hennermann JB, Karall D, de Klerk H, Knerr I, Koch HG, Plecko B, Roschinger W, Schwab KO, Scheible D, Wijburg FA, Zschocke J, Mayatepek E, Wendel U. Treatment recommendations in long-chain fatty acid oxidation defects: consensus from a workshop. J Inherit Metab Dis. 2009;32(4):498–505.

Stanley CA, DeLeeuw S, Coates PM, Vianey-Liaud C, Divry P, Bonnefont JP, Saudubray JM, Haymond M, Trefz FK, Breningstall GN, et al. Chronic cardiomyopathy and weakness or acute coma in children with a defect in carnitine uptake. Ann Neurol. 1991;30(5):709–16.

Tonin AM, Amaral AU, Busanello EN, Gasparotto J, Gelain DP, Gregersen N, Wajner M. Mitochondrial bioenergetics deregulation caused by long-chain 3-hydroxy fatty acids accumulating in LCHAD and MTP deficiencies in rat brain: a possible role of mPTP opening as a pathomechanism in these disorders? Biochim Biophys Acta. 2014;1842(9):1658–67.

Tonin AM, Ferreira GC, Grings M, Viegas CM, Busanello EN, Amaral AU, Zanatta A, Schuck PF, Wajner M. Disturbance of mitochondrial energy homeostasis caused by the metabolites accumulating in LCHAD and MTP deficiencies in rat brain. Life Sci. 2010;86(21–22):825–31.

Tucci S, Behringer S, Spiekerkoetter U. De novo fatty acid biosynthesis and elongation in very long-chain acyl-CoA dehydrogenase-deficient mice supplemented with odd or even medium-chain fatty acids. FEBS J. 2015;282(21):4242–53.

Tyni T, Kivela T, Lappi M, Summanen P, Nikoskelainen E, Pihko H. Ophthalmologic findings in long-chain 3-hydroxyacyl-CoA dehydrogenase deficiency caused by the G1528C mutation: a new type of hereditary metabolic chorioretinopathy. Ophthalmology. 1998;105(5):810–24.

Ventura FV, Costa CG, Struys EA, Ruiter J, Allers P, Ijlst L, de Almeida T, Duran M, Jakobs C, Wanders RJA. Quantitative acylcarnitine profiling in fibroblasts using [U-C-13] palmitic acid: an improved tool for the diagnosis of fatty acid oxidation defects. Clin Chim Acta. 1999;281(1–2):1–17.

Vockley J, Burton B, Berry GT, Longo N, Phillips J, Sanchez-Valle A, Tanpaiboon P, Grunewald S, Murphy E, Bowden A, Chen W, Chen CY, Cataldo J, Marsden D, Kakkis E. Results from a 78-week, single-arm, open-label phase 2 study to evaluate UX007 in pediatric and adult patients with severe long-chain fatty acid oxidation disorders (LC-FAOD). J Inherit Metab Dis. 2019;42(1):169–77.

Vockley J, Charrow J, Ganesh J, Eswara M, Diaz GA, McCracken E, Conway R, Enns GM, Starr J, Wang R, Abdenur JE, Sanchez-de-Toledo J, Marsden DL. Triheptanoin treatment in patients with pediatric cardiomyopathy associated with long chain-fatty acid oxidation disorders. Mol Genet Metab. 2016;119(3):223–31.

Wanders RJ, Ruiter JP, Lodewijk IJ, Waterham HR, Houten SM. The enzymology of mitochondrial fatty acid beta-oxidation and its application to follow-up analysis of positive neonatal screening results. J Inherit Metab Dis. 2010;33(5):479–94.

Wang Y, Mohsen AW, Mihalik SJ, Goetzman ES, Vockley J. Evidence for physical association of mitochondrial fatty acid oxidation and oxidative phosphorylation complexes. J Biol Chem. 2010;285(39):29834–41.

Wang Y, Palmfeldt J, Gregersen N, Makhov AM, Conway JF, Wang M, McCalley SP, Basu S, Alharbi H, Croix CS, Calderon MJ, Watkins S, Vockley J. Mitochondrial fatty acid oxidation and the electron transport chain comprise a multifunctional mitochondrial protein complex. J Biol Chem. 2019;294(33):12380–91.

Wilcken B, Haas M, Joy P, Wiley V, Chaplin M, Black C, Fletcher J, McGill J, Boneh A. Outcome of neonatal screening for medium-chain acyl-CoA dehydrogenase deficiency in Australia: a cohort study. Lancet. 2007;369(9555):37–42.

Wilcken B, Leung KC, Hammond J, Kamath R, Leonard JV. Pregnancy and fetal long-chain 3-hydroxyacyl coenzyme a dehydrogenase deficiency. Lancet. 1993;341(8842):407–8.

# Disorders of Glycerol Metabolism

# 49

Katrina M. Dipple

## Contents



**Summary**

Disorders of glycerol metabolism include glycerol kinase deficiency (GKD: both complex, cGKD, and isolated, iGKD), glycerate kinase deficiency (also known as D-glyceric aciduria), aquaporin 7 deficiency (AQP7, also known as hyperglyceroluria with mild platelet secretion defect), and cytosolic glycerol-3-phosphate dehydrogenase deficiency. GKD is involved in glycerol metabolism while glycerate kinase deficiency is involved in serine and fructose metabolism. Aquaporin 7 is associated with glycerol transport and presents with hyperglyceroluria like GKD. Cytosolic glycerol 3-phosphate dehydrogenase deficiency is a transient infantile hypertriglyceridemia. Disorders of glycerol metabolism vary in severity from asymptomatic to characteristic signs and symptoms. The hallmark of GKD and AQP7 is glyceroluria.

K. M. Dipple (✉)
Division of Genetic Medicine, Department of Pediatrics, University of Washington School of Medicine and Seattle Children's Hospital, Seattle, Washington, USA
e-mail: dipplk@uw.edu



N. Blau et al. (eds.), *Physician's Guide to the Diagnosis, Treatment, and Follow-Up of Inherited Metabolic Diseases*,
https://doi.org/10.1007/978-3-030-67727-5_49

## Introduction

Glycerol kinase deficiency (GKD) has three distinct clinical phenotypes: the complex form and two subtypes of the isolated form—symptomatic (juvenile) and benign (adult) (McCabe 2001a). GKD is due to deletion or mutations within the glycerol kinase (GK) gene on Xp21.2.

The clinical features of a patient with a complex glycerol kinase deficiency will depend on the loci that are involved in this contiguous gene syndrome (McCabe 2001a; McCabe 2001b). Deletion of the adrenal hypoplasia congenita (AHC) locus (*DAX1* gene) results in the cytomegalic form of adrenal hypoplasia (McCabe 2001b). Affected patients exhibit the signs and symptoms of glucocorticoid and mineralocorticoid deficiency, including bronzing of the skin and gums, and inability to respond appropriately to stresses such as intercurrent illnesses, leading to hypoglycemia, hyponatremia, and hyperkalemia. Death may occur during these Addisonian crises. Deletion of *DAX1* also is associated with hypogonadotropic hypogonadism (Zanaria et al. 1994; Muscatelli et al. 1994; Guo et al. 1995; Habiby et al. 1996). Patients with loss of the glycerol kinase (*GK*) gene have episodes of vomiting, acidemia, and stupor that seem to be unrelated to adrenal insufficiency and are similar to those observed in patients with the juvenile form of GKD (see below) (McCabe 2001a). Involvement of the Duchenne muscular dystrophy (DMD) gene may be associated with severe, progressive muscle weakness as in classical Duchenne muscular dystrophy, but also has been associated with milder muscle disease (Guggenheim et al. 1980; McCabe et al. 1989). All patients with involvement of the AHC, GK, and DMD or GK and DMD loci, and many but not all with deletion of the AHC and GK genes, have been mentally retarded (McCabe 2001a). For those with deletions extending telomeric from *DAX1* the mental retardation may be due to loss of a novel interleukin-1 receptor family member, *IL1RAPL1* (Carrié et al. 1999; Jin et al. 2000). Characteristic facies are seen among patients with deletions of all three loci. They have a triangular face with a broad nasal bridge and a bulbous nasal tip, described as an hourglass appearance to the midface (Goubau et al. 2013). The rest of this chapter will focus on isolated GKD (iGKD; Table 49.1).

There are two forms of iGKD: symptomatic (juvenile) and benign (adult) (McCabe 2001a). The symptomatic form of isolated glycerol kinase deficiency presents in early childhood. Affected boys have had hypothermia and lethargy beginning in the first week of life. More commonly, there is episodic vomiting between 2 and 6 years of age variably associated with acidosis and central nervous system depression, which may include lethargy, somnolence, stupor, unconsciousness, and hypoglycemia, interpreted by some as a Reye-like illness (McCabe 2001a).

The benign form of isolated glycerol kinase deficiency is not associated with the episodic metabolic and central nervous system (CNS) deteriorations seen with the other forms. Males with this biochemical phenotype are identified incidentally with pseudo-hypertriglyceridemia when routine laboratory studies incorrectly identify the elevated free glycerol concentration in their blood as triglycerides (McCabe 2001a). These individuals have increased levels of glycerol in blood and urine and may be at an increased risk for insulin resistance and type 2 diabetes mellitus (Basel-Vanagaire et al. 2012). Diagnosis is made by glycerolemia, glyceroluria, and mutations in the *GK* gene.

Glycerate kinase deficiency (GLYCTK-D; Table 49.2) also known as D-glyceric aciduria (DGA) is caused by deficiency of D-glycerate kinase (*GLYCTK*) gene and the glycerate kinase enzyme. It is a rare autosomal recessive inborn error of metabolism of serine and fructose metabolism (Sass et al. 2010). It is characterized by increased D-glyceric acid in the blood and urine. Patients can present with a variety of symptoms ranging from asymptomatic to hypotonia, failure to thrive, encephalopathy, seizures, intellectual disability, microcephaly, metabolic acidosis, to early death. Some consider it a benign disorder. It is distinguished from L-glyceric aciduria, which is primary hyperoxaluria type 2 due to deficiency of glyoxylate reductase/hydroxypyruvate reductase and will not be discussed here (Sass et al. 2020) (see Chap. 67). Diagnosis is made by elevated D-glyceric acid levels in plasma, urine, or cerebrospinal fluid and reduced glycerate kinase activity in the liver.

The aquaglyceroporin family are pore-forming transmembrane proteins that transport glycerol and water (Goubau et al. 2013). Aquaporin 7 (AQP7) is expressed in adipose tissue as well as in the kidney, pancreas, liver, and muscle. AQP7 deficiency (Table 49.3) is an autosomal recessive disorder due to mutations in the aquaporin 7 gene (*AQP7*). Patients with AQP7 deficiency also present with hyperglyceroluria; however, they do not have the hyperglycerolemia seen in GKD. Many patients are asymptomatic, but some patients can have delayed development, autism, epilepsy, hypotonia, and a mild platelet secretion defect. Aquaporin 7 knock out mice are at risk of adult onset diabetes; however, this has not been seen in humans with AQP7 deficiency (Goubau et al. 2013).

Cytosolic glycerol-3-phosphate dehydrogenase is encoded by the *GPD1* gene on 12q13.12 (Basel-Vanagaire et al. 2012). Its deficiency, cytosolic glycerol-3-phosphate dehydrogenase deficiency (HTGT; Table 49.4), is inherited in an autosomal recessive manner and is also known as transient infantile hypertriglyceridemia. Patients may present with elevated triglycerides, cholesterol, and transaminases. In addition, there might be liver steatosis, liver fibrosis, and splenomegaly. The hypertriglyceridemia is transient and normalizes with age (See Tables 49.1, 49.2, 49.3, and 49.4).

## Nomenclature

| No. | Disorder | Alternative name | Abbreviation | Gene symbol | Chromosomal location | Mode of inheritance | Affected protein | OMIM no. |
|---|---|---|---|---|---|---|---|---|
| 49.1 | Glycerol kinase deficiency | Hyperglycerolemia | GKD | *GK* | Xp21.2 | XL | Glycerol kinase | 307030 |
| 49.2 | Glycerate kinase deficiency | D-glyceric acidemia | GLYCTK-D | *GLYCTK* | 3p21.1 | AR | Glycerate kinase | 610516 |
| 49.3 | Aquaporin 7 deficiency | Hyperglyceroluria with mild platelet secretion defect | GLYCQTL | *AQP7* | 9p13.3 | AR | Aquaporin 7 | 614411 |
| 49.4 | Cytosolic glycerol-3-phosphate dehydrogenase deficiency | Transient infantile hypertriglyceridemia | HTGTI | *GPD1* | 12q13.12 | AR | Glycerol-3-phosphate dehydrogenase | 614480 |

Abbreviation: *OMIM* Online Mendelian Inheritance in Man

## Metabolic Pathways

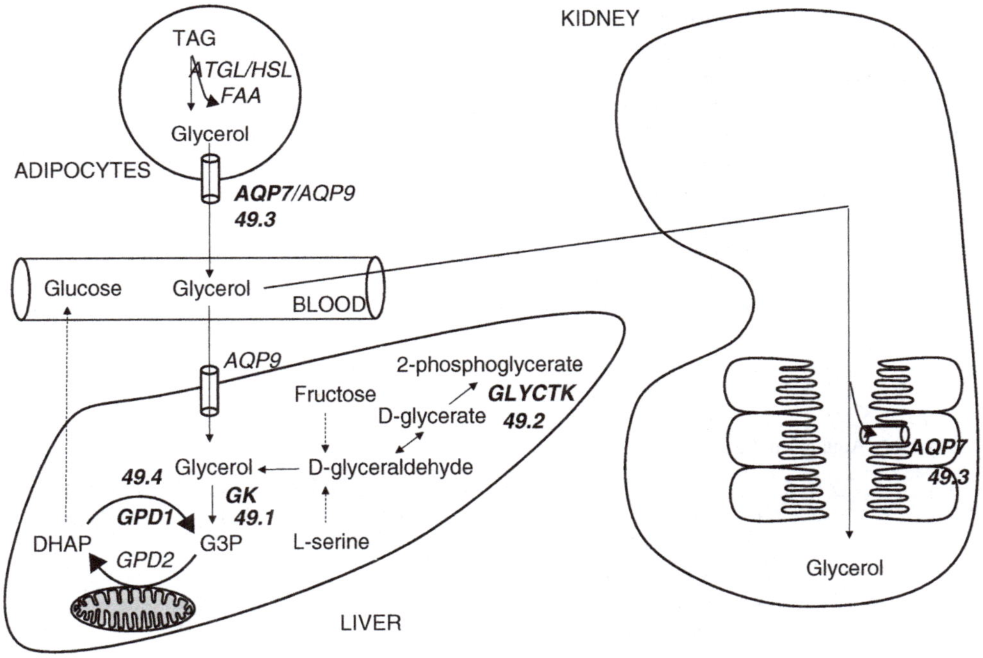


**Fig. 49.1** Metabolic pathway: metabolism of glycerol. *AQP* Aquaglyceroporin, *ATGL* Adipose triglyceride lipase, *DHAP* Dihydroxyacetone phosphate, *G3P* Glycerol-3-phosphate, *GK* Glycerol kinase, *GLYCTK* D-glycerate kinase, *GPD1* Cytosolic glycerol-3-phosphate dehydrogenase, *GPD2* Mitochondrial glycerol-3-phosphate dehydrogenase, *HSL* Hormone-sensitive lipase, *TAG* Triacylglycerol In bold: enzyme deficiencies described in this chapter (GK, GLYCTK, GPD1, AQP7)

## Signs and Symptoms

**Table 49.1** Glycerol kinase deficiency, isolated

| System | Symptoms and biomarkers | Neonatal (birth–1 month) | Infancy (1–18 months) | Childhood (1.5–11 years) | Adolescence (11–16 years) | Adulthood (>16 years) |
|---|---|---|---|---|---|---|
| Other | No clinical significance | + | + | + | + | + |
| Metabolic | Hypoglycemia | ± | ± | ± | ± | ± |
| | Insulin resistance type II diabetes mellitus | | | | | ± |
| Laboratory findings | Glucose (plasma) | ↓-n | ↓-n | ↓-n | ↓-n | ↓-n |
| | Glycerol (plasma) | ↑ | ↑ | ↑ | ↑ | ↑ |
| | Glycerol (urine) | ↑ | ↑ | ↑ | ↑ | ↑ |
| | Triglyceride, pseudo (plasma) | ↑ | ↑ | ↑ | ↑ | ↑ |

**Table 49.2** Glycerate kinase deficiency

| System | Symptoms and biomarkers | Neonatal (birth–1 month) | Infancy (1–18 months) | Childhood (1.5–11 years) | Adolescence (11–16 years) | Adulthood (>16 years) |
|---|---|---|---|---|---|---|
| CNS | **Encephalopathy** | ± | ± | ± | | |
| | **Intellectual disability** | ± | ± | ± | | |
| | **Seizures** | ± | ± | ± | | |
| | **Speech delay** | ± | ± | ± | | |
| Metabolic | Metabolic acidosis | ± | ± | ± | ± | |
| Musculoskeletal | **Hypotonia, muscular-axial** | ± | ± | ± | | |
| | **Microcephaly** | ± | ± | ± | | |
| Other | **Early death** | ± | ± | ± | | |
| | **Failure to thrive** | ± | ± | ± | | |
| Laboratory findings | D-glycerate (cerebrospinal fluid) | ↑ | ↑ | ↑ | ↑ | |
| | D-glycerate (plasma) | ↑ | ↑ | ↑ | ↑ | |
| | D-glycerate (urine) | ↑ | ↑ | ↑ | ↑ | |
| | D-glycerate kinase (liver) | ↓ | ↓ | ↓ | ↓ | |

**Table 49.3** Aquaporin 7 deficiency

| System | Symptoms and biomarkers | Neonatal (birth–1 month) | Infancy (1–18 months) | Childhood (1.5–11 years) | Adolescence (11–16 years) | Adulthood (>16 years) |
|---|---|---|---|---|---|---|
| Other | No clinical significance | | | | | + |
| Laboratory findings | Cholesterol (serum) | | | | | n |
| | Glycerol (plasma) | | | | | ↓-n |
| | Triglyceride (serum) | | | | | n |

**Table 49.4** Cytosolic glycerol-3-phosphate dehydrogenase deficiency

| System | Symptoms and biomarkers | Neonatal (birth–1 month) | Infancy (1–18 months) | Childhood (1.5–11 years) | Adolescence (11–16 years) | Adulthood (>16 years) |
|---|---|---|---|---|---|---|
| Digestive | Hepatomegaly | + | + | + | | |
| | Liver fibrosis | + | + | + | | |
| | Liver steatosis | + | + | + | | |
| | Splenomegaly | ± | ± | ± | | |
| Musculoskeletal | Short stature | + | + | + | | |
| Laboratory findings | ASAT/ALAT (plasma) | ↑ | ↑ | ↑ | | |
| | Cholesterol (serum) | n-↑ | n-↑ | n-↑ | | |
| | Dicarboxylic acids (urine) | ↑ | ↑ | | | |
| | Lipoprotein (a) (plasma) | n-↑ | n-↑ | n-↑ | | |
| | Triglyceride (serum) | ↑ | ↑ | n-↑ | | |

## Reference Values

| Age | Glycerol urine (mmol/L) | Glycerol urine (mmol/mmol creatinine) | Glycerol plasma (mmol/L) |
|---|---|---|---|
| Not specified | ≤0.2 | Not detectable | 0.02–0.27 |

Values taken from McCabe (McCabe 2001a)

## Pathological Values

| No. | Disorder | Glycerol urine | Glycerol plasma | D-glyceric acid: plasma and urine | Triglycerides plasma | Transaminases plasma |
|---|---|---|---|---|---|---|
| 49.1 | Glycerol kinase deficiency | ↑ | ↑ | n | ↑ | n |
| 49.2 | Glycerate kinase deficiency | n | n | ↑ | n | n |
| 49.3 | Aquaporin 7 deficiency | ↑ | n | n | n | n |
| 49.4 | Cytosolic glycerol-3-phosphate deficiency | n | n | n | ↑ | ↑ |

| Disorder | Glycerol urine (mmol/L) | Glycerol urine (mmol/mmol creatinine) | Glycerol plasma (mmol/L) |
|---|---|---|---|
| 49.1 GKD[a] | 41–345 | 90–193 | 1.8–8.3 |

[a]Values taken from McCabe (McCabe 2001a). No differences have been noted with the different phenotypes (McCabe 2001a)

## Diagnostic Flowchart

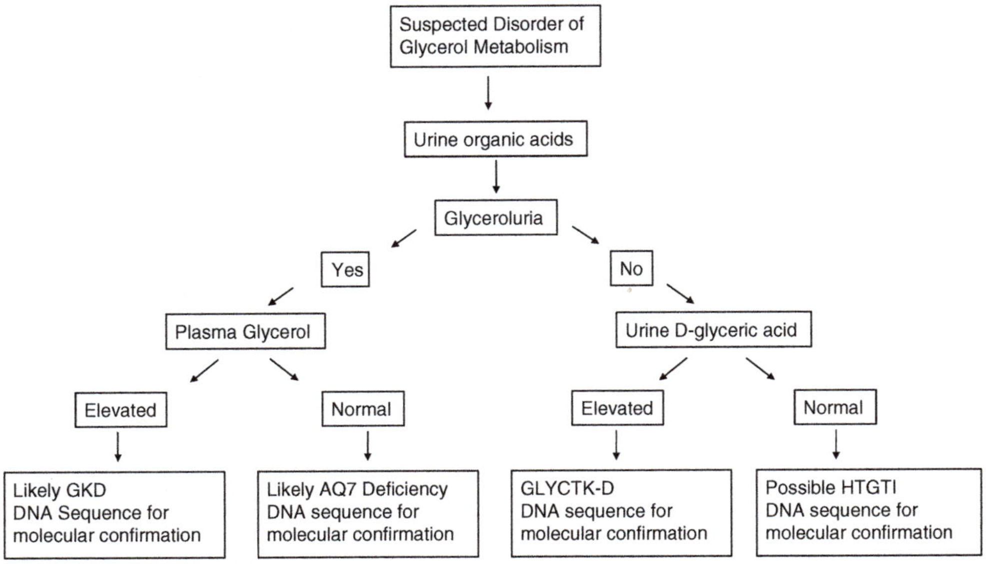


## Specimen Collection

| Test | Preconditions | Material | Handling | Pitfalls |
|---|---|---|---|---|
| Glycerol (U) urine organic acids | None | Random or 24 h | Keep cool or frozen | Contamination by emollients or glycerin suppository |
| Glycerol (S, P) | None | Serum/plasma | Keep cool or frozen | Some rubber stoppers in vacuum tubes use glycerol as lubricant |

## Prenatal Diagnosis

| No. | Disorder | Tests recommended |
|---|---|---|
| 49.1 | Glycerol kinase deficiency | Mutation analysis on DNA from CVS or AF<br>Glycerol level on amniotic fluid |
| 49.2 | Glycerate kinase deficiency | Mutation analysis on DNA from CVS or AF |
| 49.3 | Aquaporin 7 deficiency | Mutation analysis on DNA from CVS or AF |
| 49.4 | Cytosolic glycerol-3-phosphate deficiency | Mutation analysis on DNA from CVS or AF |

Abbreviations: *AF* amniotic fluid, *CVS* chorionic villus, *DNA* deoxyribonucleic acid

## DNA Testing

DNA testing by next-generation sequencing is available for all the disorders in this chapter. DNA can be obtained from peripheral blood leukocytes or buccal swab.

## Treatment

Initial treatment is indicated if the patient is acutely ill, with vomiting and/or CNS depression. Initial treatment for GKD (isolated of complex with metabolic decompensation) includes starting an intravenous (IV) solution containing glucose, evaluating blood pH and serum electrolytes, drawing blood for adrenocorticotropic hormone (ACTH), and, if concerned about adrenal insufficiency (cGKD), considering initiating glucocorticoid and mineralocorticoid treatment. Long-term treatment includes avoiding of fasting in GKD and supportive treatment for the related neuropsychiatric issues with the other disorders.

Emergency treatment

| No. | Disorder | Emergency treatment |
|---|---|---|
| 49.1 | Glycerol kinase deficiency | IV fluids with glucose |
| 49.2 | Glycerate kinase deficiency | IV hydration if metabolic acidosis |
| 49.3 | Aquaporin 7 deficiency | None |
| 49.4 | Cytosolic glycerol-3-phosphate deficiency | Supportive care |

Standard care

| No. | Disorder | Emergency treatment |
|---|---|---|
| 49.1 | Glycerol kinase deficiency | Avoidance of fasting<br>Supportive care |
| 49.2 | Glycerate kinase deficiency | Decreased serine and fructose<br>Supportive care |
| 49.3 | Aquaporin 7 deficiency | Supportive care |
| 49.4 | Cytosolic glycerol-3-phosphate deficiency | Supportive care |

## References


Basel-Vanagaire L, Zevit N, Zadav AH, Guo L, Parathath S, Pasmanik-Chor M, McIntyre AD, Want N, Albin-Kaplanski A, Hartmeah C, Marom D, Zeharia A, Badir A, Shoerman O, Simon AJ, Rechavi G, Shohat M, Hegele RA, Risher EA, Shamir R. Transient infantile hypertriglyceridemia, fatty liver, and hepatic fibrosis caused by mutated GPD1 encoding glycerol-3-phosphate dehydrogenase 1. Am J Hum Genet. 2012;90:49–20.

Carrié A, Jun L, Bienvenu T, Vinet MC, McDonell N, Couvert P, Zemni R, Cardona A, Van Buggenhout G, Frints S, Hamel B, Moraine C, Ropers HH, Strom T, Howell GR, Whittaker A, Ross MT, Kahn A, Fryns JP, Beldjord C, Marynen P, Chelly J. A new member of the IL-1 receptor family highly expressed in hippocampus and involved in X-linked mental retardation. Nat Genet. 1999;23:25–31.

Goubau C, Jaeken J, Levtchenko EN, Thys C, Di Michele M, Martens GA, Gerlo E, De Vos R, Buyse GM, Goemans N, Van Geet C, Freson K. Homozygosity for aquaporin 7 G264V in three unrelated children with hyperglyceroluria and a mild platelet secretion defect. Genet Med. 2013;15(1):55–63.

Guggenheim MA, McCabe ERB, Roig M, Goodman SI, Lum GM, Bullen WW, Ringel SP. Glycerol kinase deficiency with neuromuscular, skeletal and adrenal abnormalities. Ann Neurol. 1980;7:441–9.

Guo W, Mason JS, Stone CG Jr, Morgan SA, Madu SI, Baldini A, Lindsay EA, Biesecker LG, Copeland KC, Horlick MNB, Pettigrew AL, Zanaria E, McCabe ERB. Diagnosis of X-linked adrenal hypoplasia congenita by mutation analysis of the DAX1 gene. JAMA. 1995;274:324–30.

Habiby RL, Boepple P, Nachtigall L, Sluss PM, Crowley WF Jr, Jameson JL. Adrenal hypoplasia congenita with hypogonadotropic hypogonadism: evidence that DAX-1 mutations lead to combined hypothalamic and pituitary defects in gonadotropin production. J Clin Invest. 1996;98:1055–62.

Jin H, Gardner RJ, Viswesvaraiah R, Muntoni F, Roberts RG. Two novel members of the interleukin-1 receptor gene family, one deleted in Xp22.1-Xp21.3 mental retardation. Eur J Hum Genet. 2000;8:87–94.

McCabe ERB. Disorders of glycerol metabolism. In: Scriver CR, Beaudet AL, Sly WS, Valle D, Childs B, Vogelstein B, editors. The metabolic and molecular bases of inherited disease. New York: McGraw-Hill; 2001a. p. 2217–37.

McCabe ERB. Adrenal hypoplasias and aplasias. In: Scriver CR, Beaudet AL, Sly WS, Valle D, Childs B, Vogelstein B, editors. The metabolic and molecular bases of inherited disease. New York: McGraw-Hill; 2001b. p. 4263–74.

McCabe ERB, Towbin J, Chamberlain J, Baumbach L, Witkowski J, van Ommen GJB, Koenig M, Kunkel LM, Seltzer WK. Complementary DNA probes for the Duchenne muscular dystrophy locus demonstrate a previously undetectable deletion in a patient with dystrophic myopathy, glycerol kinase deficiency and congenital adrenal hypoplasia. J Clin Invest. 1989;83:95–9.

Muscatelli F, Strom TM, Walker AP, Zanaria E, Recan D, Meindl A, Bardoni B, Guiolo S, Zehetner G, Rabl W, Schwarz HP, Kaplan JC, Camerino G, Meitinger T, Monaco AP. Mutations in the DAX-1 gene give rise to both X-linked adrenal hypoplasia congenita and hypogonadotropic hypogonadism. Nature. 1994;372:672–6.

Sass JO, Fischer K, Wang R, Christensen E, Scholl-Burgi S, Chang R, Kapelari K, Walter M. D-Glyceric aciduria is caused by genetic deficiency of D-glycerate kinase (GLYCTK). Hum Mutat. 2010;31(12):1280–5.

Sass JO, Behringer S, Fernando M, Cesaroni E, Cusio I, Volpini A, Till C. D-Glycerate kinase deficiency in a neuropediatric patient. Brain Dev. 2020;42:226–30.

Zanaria E, Muscatelli F, Bardoni B, Strom TM, Guioli S, Guo W, Lalli E, Moser C, Walker AP, McCabe ERB, Meitinger T, Monaco AP, Sassone-Corsi P, Camerino G. An unusual member of the nuclear hormone receptor superfamily responsible for X-linked adrenal hypoplasia congenita. Nature. 1994;372:635–41.

# Disorders of Ketone Body Metabolism and Transport

# 50

Jörn Oliver Sass and Sarah C. Grünert

## Contents



**Summary**

Ketone body utilisation is of special importance in times of fasting/starvation or increased energy demand. However, both formation and utilisation of ketone bodies (ketogenesis, ketone body transport and ketolysis) can be impeded by inborn errors of metabolism. In case of genetic deficiency of mitochondrial 3-hydroxy-3-methylglutaryl-coenzyme A synthase (mHMGS) or of 3-hydroxy-3-methylglutaryl-coenzyme A lyase (HMGL), the formation of ketone bodies is impaired. If the monocarboxylate transporter 1 (MCT1, encoded by *SLC16A1*) or one of the enzymes of ketolysis is affected, namely, succinyl-CoA:3-oxoacid CoA transferase (SCOT) or methylacetoacetyl-CoA thiolase (MAT, 'β-ketothiolase'), ketones accumulate and a life-threatening ketoacidosis may result. Since treatment options allow to minimise the risk for metabolic decompensations, awareness of those diseases is important, as is information on how to treat and to prevent clinical manifestations. MCT1 superactivity is clearly different from the other disorders of ketone body metabolism addressed here. While MCT1 is not normally expressed in pancreatic β-cells, gain-of-function mutations in the promoter region of *SLC16A1* enable its expression in those cells, thus causing exercise-induced hyperinsulinism that can result in hypoglycaemia.

J. O. Sass (✉)
Research Group Inborn Errors of Metabolism, Department of Natural Sciences & Institute for Functional Gene Analytics (IFGA), Bonn-Rhein-Sieg University of Applied Sciences, Rheinbach, Germany
e-mail: joern.oliver.oliver.sass@h-brs.de

S. C. Grünert
Zentrum für Kinder- und Jugendmedizin, Universitätsklinikum Freiburg, Freiburg, Germany
e-mail: sarah.gruenert@uniklinik-freiburg.de


N. Blau et al. (eds.), *Physician's Guide to the Diagnosis, Treatment, and Follow-Up of Inherited Metabolic Diseases*, https://doi.org/10.1007/978-3-030-67727-5_50

## Introduction

Ketone bodies acetoacetate and D-3-hydroxy-*n*-butyric acid are mainly formed in the liver. They are derived from fatty acids and ketogenic amino acids (Sass 2012; Sass et al. 2018). In contrast to free fatty acids, acetoacetate and D-3-hydroxy-*n*-butyric acid can be utilised by the brain. After prolonged fasting, they can account for a large proportion of the brain's energy supply.

During ketone body synthesis (ketogenesis), mitochondrial 3-hydroxy-3-methylglutaryl-coenzyme A synthase (mHMGS [EC 4.1.3.5]) catalyses the formation of 3-hydroxy-3-methylglutaryl-coenzyme A (HMG-CoA) from acetyl-CoA and acetoacetyl-CoA (Fig. 50.1). This is the rate-limiting step of ketogenesis. HMG-CoA, which can also result from leucine degradation, is converted by 3-hydroxy-3-methylglutaryl-coenzyme A lyase (HMGL [EC 4.1.3.4]) to acetyl-CoA and acetoacetate.

The interconversion of acetoacetate with D-3-hydroxy-*n*-butyric acid is catalysed by D-3-hydroxy-*n*-butyrate dehydrogenase (EC 1.1.1.30) and essentially reflects the oxidation status of the mitochondrial matrix (Mitchell et al. 1995). So far, genetic deficiency of D-3-hydroxy-*n*-butyrate dehydrogenase has not been identified. Acetone, which may give ketotic patients a typical odour, is formed by nonenzymatic decarboxylation of acetoacetate (Fig. 50.1).

For zebrafish, Hugo et al. reported a transporter of D-3-hydroxy-*n*-butyric acid that is required for hepatocyte secretion of ketone bodies during fasting and to avoid hepatic steatosis (Hugo et al. 2012). However, deficiency in humans of the orthologous human gene *SLC16A6*, encoding MCT7, is not known so far.

Ketone body utilisation (ketolysis) occurs in extrahepatic tissues. Ketone bodies may enter such tissues via monocarboxylate transporter 1 (MCT1, encoded by *SLC16A1*). The first and rate-limiting step of ketolysis requires succinyl-CoA:3-oxoacid CoA transferase (SCOT [EC 2.8.3.5]), which activates acetoacetate to acetoacetyl-CoA (Fig. 50.1). The enzyme methylacetoacetyl-CoA thiolase (MAT [EC 2.3.1.9]) then catalyses the formation of two acetyl-CoA molecules per molecule of acetoacetyl-CoA. Genetic deficiency of mHMGS typically presents as hypoketotic hypoglycaemia, while the lack of HMGL activity not only affects ketone body formation but also results in the accumulation of leucine metabolites (Fig. 50.3). SCOT deficiency is characterised by ketotic episodes or even permanent ketosis, but presents no specific metabolite abnormalities. Since MAT is not only involved in ketone body metabolism but also in the catabolism of the amino acid isoleucine, it may yield a characteristic, isoleucine-derived metabolite pattern in addition to hyperketosis.

Cytosolic acetoacetyl-CoA thiolase (EC 2.3.1.9) also catalyses the thiolytic cleavage of acetoacetyl-CoA. It has been considered the first enzyme of cholesterol synthesis (Fig. 50.2). In two girls, deficiency of cytosolic acetoacetyl-CoA thiolase has been assumed (De Groot et al. 1977; Bennett et al. 1984). One of the patients with developmental delay showed a pronounced metabolic reaction on a ketogenic diet, the other had persistent ketonuria as the only abnormal laboratory finding. However, at that time optimised enzyme assays were not available and the metabolic disorder had never been confirmed on the gene level. Therefore, this supposed metabolic disease will not be addressed further here. However, it may be appropriate to consider detailed studies of cholesterol and ketone body metabolism in future patients with severe neurologic symptoms and persistent ketonuria not explained otherwise. While MCT1 is normally silenced in pancreatic β-cells, certain mutations in the promoter of *SLC16A1* induce expression of MCT1 in this tissue, permitting pyruvate uptake and resulting in pyruvate-stimulated insulin secretion with consecutive hypoglycaemia during anaerobic exercise or following a pyruvate load (Otonkoski et al. 2003, 2007). The majority of the individuals reported with this exercise-induced hyperinsulinism (EIHI) so far is of Finnish origin.

## Nomenclature

| No. | Disorder | Alternative name | Abbreviation | Gene symbol | Chromosomal localisation | Mode of inheritance | Affected protein | OMIM no. |
|---|---|---|---|---|---|---|---|---|
| 50.1 | 3-Hydroxy-3-methylglutaryl-CoA synthase deficiency | Mitochondrial 3-hydroxy-3-methylglutaryl-CoA synthase deficiency | mHMGS deficiency | *HMGCS2* | 1p12 | AR | 3-Hydroxy-3-methylglutaryl-CoA synthase 2 | 605911 |
| 50.2 | 3-Hydroxy-3-methylglutaryl-CoA lyase deficiency | Hydroxymethylglutaryl-CoA lyase deficiency | HMGL deficiency | *HMGCL* | 1p36.11 | AR | 3-Hydroxy-3-methylglutaryl-CoA lyase | 246450 |
| 50.3 | Monocarboxylate transporter 1 deficiency | | MCT1 deficiency | *SLC16A1* | 1p13.2 | AR, AD? | Monocarboxylate transporter 1 | 61095 |

| No. | Disorder | Alternative name | Abbreviation | Gene symbol | Chromosomal localisation | Mode of inheritance | Affected protein | OMIM no. |
|---|---|---|---|---|---|---|---|---|
| 50.4 | Succinyl-CoA: 3-oxoacid CoA transferase deficiency | Succinyl-CoA:3-ketoacid CoA transferase deficiency | SCOT deficiency | *OXCT1* | 5p13.1 | AR, AD? | Succinyl-CoA: 3-oxoacid CoA transferase | 245050 |
| 50.5 | Methylacetoacetyl-CoA thiolase deficiency | Beta-ketothiolase deficiency | MAT deficiency | *ACAT1* | 11q22.3 | AR | Methylacetoacetyl-CoA thiolase | 203750 |
| 50.6 | Cytosolic acetoacetyl-CoA thiolase deficiency | | CT deficiency | *ACAT2* | 6q25.3 | | Cytosolic acetoacetyl-CoA thiolase | 100678 |
| 50.7 | Monocarboxylate transporter 1 superactivity | Hyperinsulinemic hypoglycaemia-7, exercise induced; Monocarboxylate transporter 1 gain-of-function | MCT1 gain-of-function | *SLC16A1* | 1p13.2 | AD | Monocarboxylate transporter 1 | 610021 |

*Abbreviations: IEM* Inborn errors of metabolism, *OMIM* Online Mendelian inheritance in man

## Metabolic Pathways

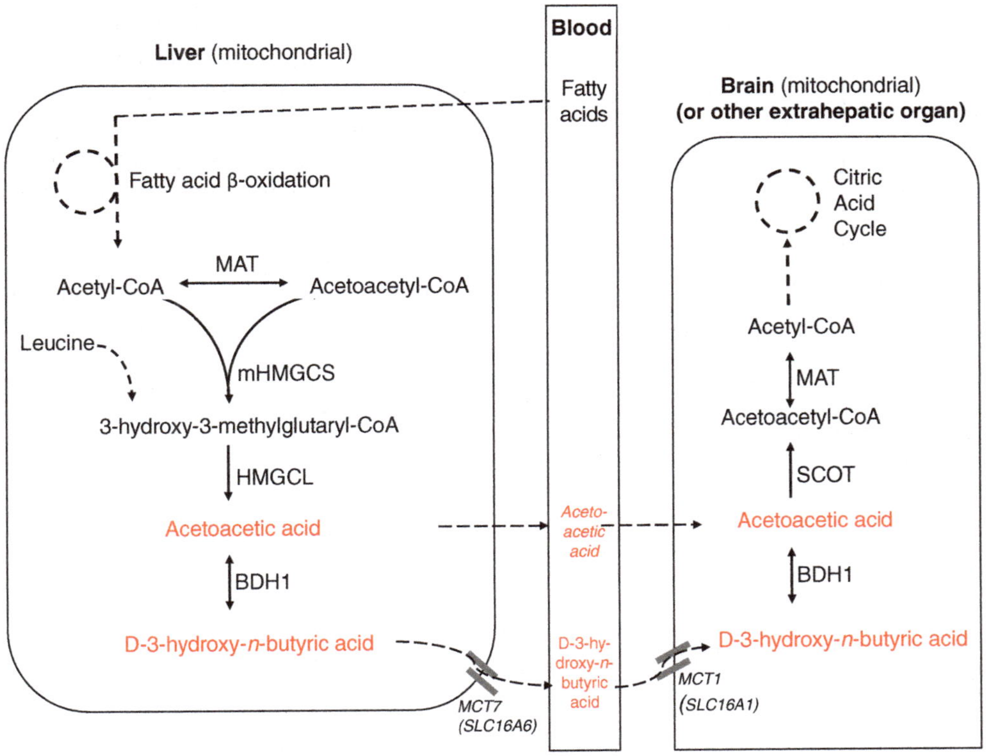


**Fig. 50.1** Ketone body metabolism and transport. Schematic view of the enzymes and transporters of ketone body metabolism that are clearly linked to inborn errors. It is not exhaustive. In particular, additional monocarboxylate transporters (MCT) may be involved in ketone body transfer, and information is very limited regarding the transport of acetoacetic acid. Also, other sites than liver may provide small contributions to ketogenesis, for example, astrocytes and newborn gut. Mitochondrial acetoacetyl-CoA thiolase (MAT) and D-3-hydroxy-*n*-butyrate dehydrogenase (BDH1) participate in both ketogenesis and ketolysis. In liver mitochondria, during ketogenesis, MAT and other thiolases equilibrate the pools of acetoacetyl-CoA and acetyl-CoA. In contrast, in extrahepatic tissues, during ketolysis, MAT is the major mitochondrial thiolase that performs this reaction, and the most critical physiological role of MAT is in ketone body utilisation. Note that up to now the purported role of MCT7 (encoded by *SLC16A6*) has been confirmed in the zebrafish only. Figure and legend taken and slightly modified from the article by Sass et al. (2018), which is distributed under the terms of the Creative Commons Attribution 4.0 License (http://www.creativecommons.org/licenses/by/4.0/) that permits any use, reproduction and distribution of the work without further permission, provided that the original work is attributed as specified on the SAGE and Open Access pages (https://us.sagepub.com/en-us/nam/open-access-at-sage)

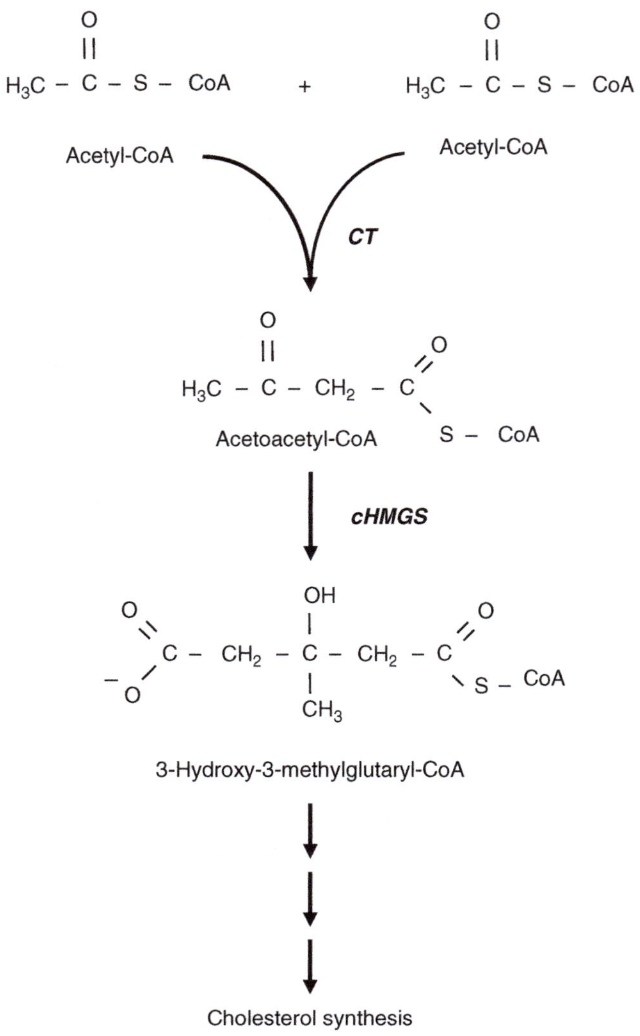


**Fig. 50.2** Cytosolic acetoacetyl-CoA thiolase (*CT*)

## Signs and Symptoms

*Deficiency of mHMGS* (Table 50.1) typically presents with episodes of (mostly) hypoketotic hypoglycaemia, hepatomegaly and acute encephalopathy, much resembling disorders of fatty acid oxidation. During a metabolic crisis, urine organic acids can reveal dicarboxylic aciduria, often—but not always—without ketonuria. Elevated free fatty acids may be found in serum, while levels of lactic acid and ammonia are typically unremarkable. Since leucine enters the pathway at the subsequent step only (Fig. 50.1), mHMGS deficiency affects conversion of fatty acids to ketone bodies, but not amino acid catabolism. Although raised plasma acetylcarnitine (acylcarnitine C2) has been suggested as a marker if associated with hypoketotic hypoglycaemia, hepatomegaly and dicarboxylic aciduria, there are no established specific metabolite markers for this inborn error of metabolism. Crotonylglycine has been suggested as a candidate in this regard based on special investigations in urine of a single patient (Kouremenos et al. 2010). Thompson et al. (1997) reported several novel organic acids in urine of patients with mHMGS deficiency during periods of metabolic decompensation. In particular the pattern of 4-hydroxy-6-methyl-2-pyrone together with high concentrations of adipic acid in urine could be helpful for obtaining a diagnosis of mHMGS deficiency. However, Conboy et al. (2018) have questioned the diagnostic specificity of those biomarkers. All these metabolites warrant confirmation in a higher number of affected individuals and further validation.

*Deficiency of HMGL* (Table 50.2) presents with episodes of hypoketotic hypoglycaemia and metabolic acidosis,

**Fig. 50.3** Accumulation of isoleucine metabolites in deficiency of methylacetoacetyl-CoA thiolase (MAT)

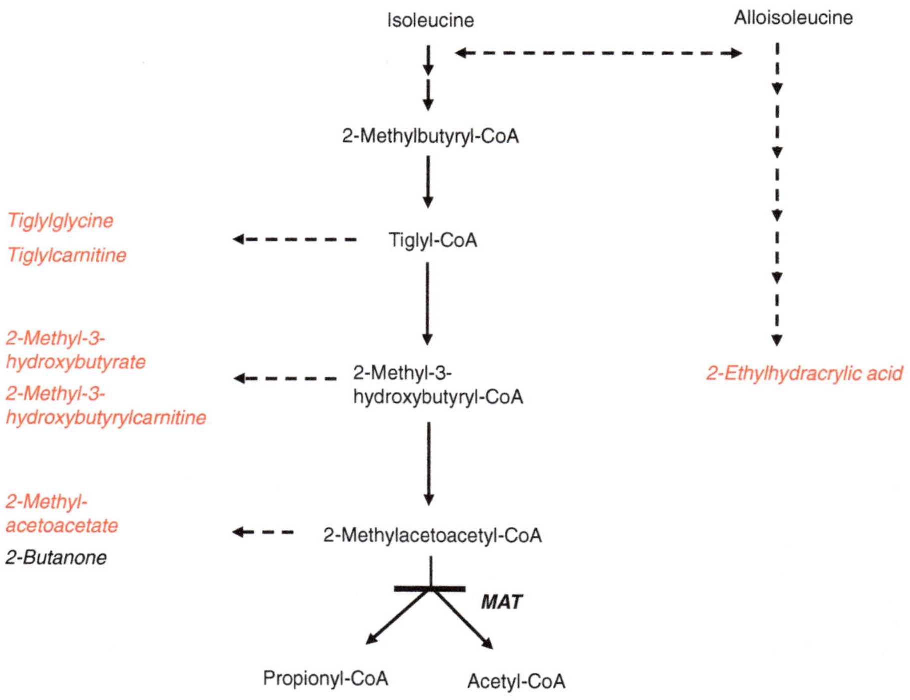

**Table 50.1** 3-Hydroxy-3-methylglutaryl-CoA synthase deficiency

| System | Symptoms and biomarkers | Neonatal (birth–1 month) | Infancy (1–18 months) | Childhood (1.5–11 years) | Adolescence (11–16 years) | Adulthood (>16 years) |
|---|---|---|---|---|---|---|
| CNS | Coma | | ± | ± | | |
| | Coma, during acute episodes | | ± | ± | | |
| | Intellectual development | | n | n | n | n |
| | Lethargy | | ± | ± | | |
| | Lethargy, during acute episodes | | ± | ± | | |
| | Seizures | | | ± | | |
| Digestive | Diarrhea | | ± | ± | | |
| | Liver dysfunction | | ± | ± | | |
| | Vomiting | | ± | ± | | |
| Metabolic | **Acidosis** | | ± | ± | | |
| | **Hypoglycaemia** | | ± | ± | | |
| Laboratory findings | 3-Hydroxy-*n*-butyric acid (plasma, serum) | | ↓-n | ↓ | | |
| | 3-Hydroxy-*n*-butyric acid (urine) | | n-↑ | n-↑ | | |
| | 4-Hydroxy-6-methyl-2-pyrone (urine) | | (↑) | (↑) | | |
| | Acetoacetic acid (plasma) | | ↓-n | ↓-n | | |
| | Acetoacetic acid (urine) | | n-↑ | n-↑ | | |
| | Adipic acid and other dicarboxylic acids (urine) | | n-↑↑ | n-↑↑ | | |
| | ASAT/ALAT (plasma, serum) | | ↑ | ↑ | | |
| | C2 acylcarnitine (acetylcarnitine) (dried blood spot, plasma, serum) | | (↑) | (↑) | | |
| | Carnitine, free (dried blood spot, plasma, serum) | | ↓-n | n | | |
| | Crotonylglycine (urine) | | (↑) | (↑) | | |
| | Free fatty acids (serum) | | ↑ | ↑ | | |
| | Glucose (blood) | | ↓ | ↓ | | |
| | Glucose (plasma) | | ↓ | ↓ | | |
| | Ketones (blood) | | ↓-n | ↓-n | | |
| | Ketones (urine) | | n-↑ | n-↑ | | |
| | Long-chain acylcarnitines | | n | n | | |
| | Medium-chain acylcarnitines | | n | n | | |

usually early in life, although diagnosis may sometimes be delayed until adulthood (Grünert et al. 2017a). Cerebral infarction and pancreatitis are among the reported complications (Muroi et al. 2000).

HMGL deficiency affects not only the synthesis of ketone bodies from fatty acids but also the catabolism of the amino acid leucine. Therefore, both the pattern of urinary organic acids and blood acylcarnitines usually show characteristic abnormalities. Reports on eight pregnancies in five women with HMGCL deficiency suggest that an increased risk of miscarriage is associated with this disease. Pregnancy is a ketogenic state and may make women with this inborn error of metabolism particularly prone to metabolic compensations (Sass et al. 2018).

In nondiabetic patients, repeated or severe ketoacidotic episodes as well as persistent ketonuria without fasting are suggestive of an inborn error of ketone body transport or utilisation. In 2014, MCT1 deficiency (Table 50.3) due to mutations in *SLC16A1* was identified as a cause of ketoacidosis (van Hasselt et al. 2014). Notably, van Hasselt et al. reported clinical symptoms not only in patients who were homozygous or compound-heterozygous for *SLC16A1* mutations but also in some heterozygous individuals with only a single affected allele. This was confirmed by Balasubramaniam et al. who reported symptomatic half-brothers with the same mother but different fathers (Balasubramaniam et al. 2016). Those observations suggest that under some circumstances, heterozygous MCT1 deficiency can lead to ketoacidosis.

**Table 50.2** 3-Hydroxy-3-methylglutaryl-CoA lyase deficiency

| System | Symptoms and biomarkers | Neonatal (birth–1 month) | Infancy (1–18 months) | Childhood (1.5–11 years) | Adolescence (11–16 years) | Adulthood (>16 years) |
|---|---|---|---|---|---|---|
| Cardiovascular | Cardiomyopathy, dilated | | ± | ± | ± | ± |
| CNS | Cerebral infarction | | | ± | | |
| | Lethargy, during acidotic episodes | ± | ± | ± | | |
| | Seizures | ± | ± | ± | ± | ± |
| | Stroke-like encephalopathy | | | ± | | |
| | White matter abnormalities (MRI) | ± | ± | ± | ± | ± |
| Digestive | Hepatomegaly | ± | ± | ± | | |
| | Pancreatitis | | | ± | | |
| Metabolic | **Hypoglycemia, hypoketotic** | ± | ± | ± | ± | ± |
| Other | Coma, during acidotic episodes | ± | ± | ± | | |
| Laboratory findings | 3-Hydroxy-3-methylglutaric acid (urine) | ↑-↑↑↑ | ↑-↑↑↑ | ↑-↑↑↑ | ↑-↑↑↑ | ↑-↑↑↑ |
| | 3-Hydroxy-3-methylglutaryl-CoA lyase activity (fibroblasts, [immortalized] lymphocytes) | ↓-↓↓↓ | ↓-↓↓↓ | ↓-↓↓↓ | ↓-↓↓↓ | ↓-↓↓↓ |
| | 3-Hydroxyisovaleric acid (urine) | ↑-↑↑↑ | ↑-↑↑↑ | ↑-↑↑↑ | ↑-↑↑↑ | ↑-↑↑↑ |
| | 3-Hydroxy-*n*-butyric acid (plasma, serum) | ↓-n | ↓-n | ↓ | | |
| | 3-Hydroxy-n-butyric acid (urine) | n-↑ | n-↑ | n-↑ | | |
| | 3-Methylcrotonylglycine (urine) | n-↑↑ | n-↑↑ | n-↑↑ | n-↑↑ | n-↑↑ |
| | 3-Methylglutaconic acid (urine) | ↑-↑↑↑ | ↑-↑↑↑ | ↑-↑↑↑ | ↑-↑↑↑ | ↑-↑↑↑ |
| | 3-Methylglutaric acid (urine) | ↑-↑↑↑ | ↑-↑↑↑ | ↑-↑↑↑ | ↑-↑↑↑ | ↑-↑↑↑ |
| | Acetoacetic acid (plasma) | ↓-n | ↓-n | ↓-n | | |
| | Acetoacetic acid (urine) | n-↑ | n-↑ | n-↑ | | |
| | Ammonia (blood, plasma) | n-↑↑ | n-↑↑ | n-↑↑ | n-↑↑ | n-↑↑ |
| | ASAT/ALAT (plasma, serum) | n-↑ | n-↑ | n-↑ | n-↑ | n-↑ |
| | C5-OH acylcarnitine (dried blood spot) | ↑-↑↑↑ | ↑-↑↑↑ | ↑-↑↑↑ | ↑-↑↑↑ | ↑-↑↑↑ |
| | C5-OH acylcarnitine (plasma, serum) | ↑-↑↑↑ | ↑-↑↑↑ | ↑-↑↑↑ | ↑-↑↑↑ | ↑-↑↑↑ |
| | C6DC acylcarnitine (blood) | ↑-↑↑↑ | ↑-↑↑↑ | ↑-↑↑↑ | ↑-↑↑↑ | ↑-↑↑↑ |
| | C6DC acylcarnitine (plasma, serum) | ↑-↑↑↑ | ↑-↑↑↑ | ↑-↑↑↑ | ↑-↑↑↑ | ↑-↑↑↑ |
| | Carnitine, free | ↓-n | ↓-n | ↓-n | ↓-n | ↓-n |
| | Dicarboxylic acids (urine) | n-↑↑ | n-↑↑ | n-↑↑ | n-↑↑ | n-↑↑ |
| | Free fatty acids (serum) | n-↑ | n-↑ | n-↑ | n-↑ | n-↑ |
| | Glucose (blood, plasma) | ↓-n | ↓-n | ↓-n | ↓-n | ↓-n |
| | Ketones (blood) | ↓ | ↓ | ↓ | ↓ | ↓ |
| | Ketones (urine) | n-↑ | n-↑ | n-↑ | n-↑ | n-↑ |
| | Lactic acid (plasma) | n-↑↑ | n-↑↑ | n-↑↑ | n-↑↑ | n-↑↑ |

Accumulation of ketone bodies due to insufficient ketolysis because of SCOT deficiency also may result in life-threatening ketoacidosis (Table 50.4). As in MCT1 deficiency, there are no specific metabolite changes pointing to SCOT deficiency. Although permanent/postprandial ketosis/ketonuria may lead to the suspicion of SCOT deficiency, it is not a sensitive marker (Fukao et al. 2011b).

It has been reported that not only homozygous individuals but also heterozygous carriers of *OXCT1* mutations can develop severe ketoacidosis in episodes of ketogenic stress (Sasai et al. 2017).

Differential diagnoses in patients with severe ketonuria include diabetes mellitus type I, endocrine disorders, glycogen storage disease type 0, ketotic types of hepatic glycogen storage diseases and idiopathic ketotic hypoglycaemia. Elevated ketone body levels as a physiological consequence of enhanced ketogenesis (e.g., following heavy physical exercise) will normally not result in a ketoacidotic decompensation, while type I diabetes mellitus may present in such a way, albeit usually associated with polyuria, polydipsia, weight loss and hyperglycaemia. While SCOT deficiency is typically not associated with major abnormalities in

**Table 50.3** Monocarboxylate transporter (MCT1) deficiency

| System | Symptoms and biomarkers | Neonatal (birth–1 month) | Infancy (1–18 months) | Childhood (1.5–11 years) | Adolescence (11–16 years) | Adulthood (>16 years) |
|---|---|---|---|---|---|---|
| CNS | Mild-moderate developmental impairment | | ± | ± | ± | n |
| Metabolic | Hypoglycaemia | ± | ± | ± | | |
| | Ketoacidosis preceded by poor feeding and vomitting | | ± | ± | | |
| Psychiatric | Decreased consciousness, during ketoacidotic episodes | | ± | ± | | |
| Laboratory findings | 3-Hydroxy-*n*-butyric acid (plasma, serum) | | n-↑↑↑ | n-↑↑↑ | | |
| | 3-Hydroxy-*n*-butyric acid (urine) | | n-↑↑↑ | n-↑↑↑ | n-↑↑ | |
| | Acetoacetic acid (plasma) | | n-↑↑↑ | n-↑↑↑ | | |
| | Acetoacetic acid (urine) | | n-↑↑↑ | n-↑↑↑ | n-↑↑ | |
| | Acylcarnitines | | | n | | |
| | Acylglycines (urine) | | n | n | | |
| | Ammonia (blood, plasma) | | n | n | | |
| | Ammonia (plasma, serum) | | n | n | | |
| | Carnitine, free | | n | n | | |
| | Dicarboxylic acids (urine) | | n-↑↑ | n-↑↑ | | |
| | Glucose (blood) | | ↓-n | ↓-n | | |
| | Glucose (plasma, serum) | | ↓-n | ↓-n | | |
| | Ketones (blood) | | n-↑↑↑ | n-↑↑↑ | | |
| | Ketones (urine) | | n-↑↑↑ | n-↑↑↑ | n-↑↑ | n-↑↑ |
| | Lactic acid (plasma) | | n | n | n | |
| | Lactic acid (urine) | | n | n | n | |

blood glucose, ketotic hypoglycaemia may have endocrine causes such as adrenocortical insufficiency, growth hormone deficiency and panhypopituitarism (Mitchell et al. 1995). In contrast to patients with SCOT deficiency, individuals with glycogen storage disease type 0, who also present without hepatomegaly and who suffer from hypoglycaemic-hyperketotic episodes, may show postprandial increase in lactate and alanine (Weinstein et al. 2006). Hyperketotic hypoglycaemia can also be caused by the ketotic forms of glycogen storage diseases affecting the liver (mainly type III, VI and IX). While most patients with these metabolic disorders present with hepatomegaly, some patients may have a normal liver size. Another differential diagnosis of ketoacidosis during the first 8 or 9 years of life is idiopathic ketotic hypoglycaemia. It usually represents an extreme constellation of a high ratio of brain to muscle mass, which can usually be adequately managed by glucose administration, because ketonuria usually precedes hypoglycaemia by hours. Idiopathic ketotic hypoglycaemia essentially represents a diagnosis made by exclusion.

In contrast to SCOT deficiency, MAT deficiency (less precisely called 'β-ketothiolase deficiency') represents not only a disorder of ketolysis but also a defect of isoleucine catabolism (Fig. 50.3; Table 50.5). Consequently, it is more easily identified based on the pattern of urinary organic acids comprising 3-hydroxy-2-methylbutyric acid and usually, but not always, tiglylglycine (Fukao et al. 2011a). If rather labile 2-methylacetoacetate is not detected, this may reflect inadequate preanalytical conditions. However, it may also suggest that a defect of the enzyme catalysing the preceding step in isoleucine catabolism, HSD10 disease (17-β-hydroxysteroid dehydrogenase X [17-β-HSD10], OMIM 300256), needs to be included into the differential diagnosis (Ofman et al. 2003). Although the acylcarnitines C5:1 and C5-OH are sometimes used for newborn screening for MAT deficiency, this is not reliable, as their blood levels can be unremarkable in metabolically stable patients. Although fatal outcomes are documented in some patients with MAT deficiency, a recent study on this inborn error of metabolism suggests that MAT deficiency may be a rather benign metabolic disorder, with a substantial proportion of largely asymptomatic individuals (Grünert et al. 2017b).

Superactivity of MCT1 (Table 50.7) due to gain-of-function mutations in the *SLC16A1* promoter is a cause of exercise-induced hyperinsulinism and underlies familial hyperinsulinemic hypoglycaemia 7 (HHF7).

**Table 50.4** Succinyl-CoA: 3-oxoacid CoA transferase deficiency

| System | Symptoms and biomarkers | Neonatal (birth–1 month) | Infancy (1–18 months) | Childhood (1.5–11 years) | Adolescence (11–16 years) | Adulthood (>16 years) |
|---|---|---|---|---|---|---|
| Cardiovascular | Cardiomyopathy | ± | | | | |
| CNS | Cardiomegaly | ± | | | | |
| | Coma, during ketoacidotic episodes | ± | ± | ± | | |
| | **Lethargy, during ketoacidotic episodes** | ± | ± | ± | | |
| Metabolic | **Acidosis** | ± | ± | ± | | |
| | Hypoglycemia | ↓-n-↑ | ↓-n-↑ | ↓-n-↑ | | |
| Respiratory | **Tachypnea (during ketoacidotic episodes)** | ± | ± | ± | | |
| Laboratory finding | 3-Hydroxy-n-butyric acid (plasma, serum) | n-↑↑↑ | n-↑↑↑ | n-↑↑↑ | n-↑↑ | |
| | 3-Hydroxy-n-butyric acid (urine) | n-↑↑↑ | n-↑↑↑ | n-↑↑↑ | n-↑↑ | |
| | Acetoacetic acid (plasma) | n-↑↑↑ | n-↑↑↑ | n-↑↑↑ | n-↑↑ | |
| | Acetoacetic acid (urine) | n-↑↑↑ | n-↑↑↑ | n-↑↑↑ | n-↑↑ | |
| | Acylcarnitines | | | n | | |
| | Acylglycines (urine) | n | n | n | | |
| | Ammonia (blood, plasma) | n | n | n | | |
| | Ammonia (plasma, serum) | n | n | n | | |
| | Carnitine, free | n | n | n | | |
| | Dicarboxylic acids (urine) | n-↑↑ | n-↑↑ | n-↑↑ | n-↑↑ | |
| | Free fatty acids (serum) | n | n | n | | |
| | Glucose (blood) | ↓-n-↑ | ↓-n-↑ | ↓-n-↑ | | n |
| | Glucose (plasma, serum) | ↓-n-↑ | ↓-n-↑ | ↓-n-↑ | | n |
| | Ketones (blood) | n-↑↑↑ | n-↑↑↑ | n-↑↑↑ | n-↑↑ | |
| | Ketones (urine) | n-↑↑↑ | n-↑↑↑ | n-↑↑↑ | n-↑↑ | |
| | Lactic acid (plasma) | n | n | n | n | n |
| | Lactic acid (urine) | n | n | n | n | n |

It can result in seizures and in loss of consciousness due to hypoglycaemia (Meissner et al. 2001; Otonkoski et al. 2003, 2007).

## Reference Values

In view of the many variables affecting ketone body concentrations physiologically, it is difficult to provide general reference values. The concentrations of ketone bodies fluctuate widely. For details on 3-hydroxy-*n*-butyrate and free fatty acids under fasting conditions, see Bonnefont et al. (1990) and Morris et al. (1996).

Using organic acid analysis according to Lehnert (1994) (applying methylation as the derivatisation procedure), the following reference values have been obtained based on 42 metabolically stable control individuals (mean ± standard deviation): 3-hydroxy-2-methylbutyric acid, 10.7 ± 7.6 mmol/mol creatinine; tiglylglycine, 24.6 ± 14.6 mmol/mol creatinine (Fukao et al. 2011a).

Notably, it is known from quality assessment programs that quantitative organic acid data vary largely between laboratories, and laboratories are encouraged to establish their own reference ranges. However, organic acid analysis is mostly performed on a qualitative/semiquantitative basis based on recognition of diagnostic signal patterns.

## Pathological Values

During metabolic decompensations, levels of diagnostic metabolites may be elevated 100-fold and more. In mHMGCS deficiency, the organic acids of a metabolically decompensated patient may resemble the dicarboxylic aciduria

**Table 50.5** Methylacetoacetyl-CoA thiolase deficiency

| System | Symptoms and biomarkers | Neonatal (birth–1 month) | Infancy (1–18 months) | Childhood (1.5–11 years) | Adolescence (11–16 years) | Adulthood (>16 years) |
|---|---|---|---|---|---|---|
| CNS | Basal ganglia abnormalities (MRI) | | ± | ± | | |
| | Coma, during ketoacidotic episodes | ± | ± | ± | | |
| | **Hyperintensities (T2) of the globus pallidus (MRI)** | ± | ± | ± | ± | |
| | Lethargy, during ketoacidotic episodes | ± | ± | ± | | |
| | Psychomotor impairment | ± | ± | ± | ± | |
| | Seizures | ± | ± | ± | | |
| Digestive | Hepatomegaly | ± | ± | ± | | |
| Metabolic | Acidosis | ± | ± | ± | | |
| | **Ketoacidosis** | ± | ± | ± | | |
| Respiratory | Tachypnea (during ketoacidotic episodes) | + | + | + | | |
| Other | Failure to thrive | ± | ± | ± | ± | |
| Laboratory findings | 2-Ethylhydracrylic acid (urine) | n-↑ | n-↑ | n-↑ | | |
| | 2-Methylacetoacetic acid (urine) | n-↑ | n-↑ | n-↑ | | |
| | 3-hydroxy-2-methylbutyric acid (urine) | ↑-↑↑ | ↑-↑↑ | ↑-↑↑ | ↑-↑↑ | ↑-↑↑ |
| | 3-Hydroxy-n-butyric acid (plasma, serum) | n-↑↑↑ | n-↑↑↑ | n-↑↑↑ | | |
| | 3-Hydroxy-n-butyric acid (urine) | n-↑↑↑ | n-↑↑↑ | n-↑↑↑ | | |
| | Acetoacetic acid (plasma) | n-↑↑↑ | n-↑↑↑ | n-↑↑↑ | | |
| | Acetoacetic acid (urine) | n-↑↑↑ | n-↑↑↑ | n-↑↑↑ | | |
| | Ammonia (blood, plasma) | n-↑ | n-↑ | n-↑ | | |
| | Anion gap | ± | ± | ± | ± | ± |
| | C5:1 acylcarnitine (Tiglylcarnitine) (dried blood spots) | n-↑ | n-↑ | n-↑ | | |
| | C5:1 acylcarnitine (Tiglylcarnitine) (plasma, serum) | n-↑ | n-↑ | n-↑ | | |
| | C5-OH acylcarnitine (3-hydroxy-2-methylbutyrylcarnitine) (dried blood spots) | n-↑ | n-↑ | n-↑ | | |
| | C5-OH acylcarnitine (3-hydroxy-2-methylbutyrylcarnitine) (plasma,serum) | n-↑ | n-↑ | n-↑ | | |
| | Carnitine, free (dried blood spot) | ↓-n | ↓-n | ↓-n | | |
| | Carnitine, free (plasma) | ↓-n | ↓-n | ↓-n | | |
| | Dicarboxylic acids (urine) | n-↑↑ | n-↑↑ | n-↑↑ | | |
| | Free fatty acids (serum) | n | n | n | | |
| | Glucose (blood, plasma, serum) | ± | ± | ± | | |
| | Glycine (plasma, serum) | n-↑ | n-↑ | n-↑ | | |
| | Ketones (blood) | n-↑↑↑ | n-↑↑↑ | n-↑↑↑ | | |
| | Ketones (urine) | n-↑↑↑ | n-↑↑↑ | n-↑↑↑ | | |
| | MAT activity (fibroblasts preferred; lympphocytes of limted use) | ↓↓ | ↓↓ | ↓↓ | ↓↓ | ↓↓ |
| | Tiglylglycine (urine) | n-↑ | n-↑ | n-↑ | | |

**Table 50.7** Monocarboxylate transporter (MCT1) superactivity

| System | Symptoms and biomarkers | Neonatal (birth–1 month) | Infancy (1–18 months) | Childhood (1.5–11 years) | Adolescence (11–16 years) | Adulthood (>16 years) |
|---|---|---|---|---|---|---|
| Cardiovascular | **Syncope** | | | | ± | ± |
| Endocrine | **Hyperinsulinism, exercise induced** | | ± | ± | ± | ± |
| Metabolic | **Hypoglycaemia, exercise induced** | | ± | ± | ± | ± |
| Laboratory findings | Ammonia (plasma) | | | | n | |
| | Free fatty acids (serum) | | | | ↓ | ↓ |
| | Glucose (blood, plasma) | | | | ↓ | ↓ |
| | Ketones (urine) | | | | n-↓ | n-↓ |
| | Ketones, during hypoglycemia (blood) | | | | ↓ | ↓ |
| | Pyruvate- and exercise stimulation of insulin secretion | | | ++ | ++ | ++ |

observed in individuals in ketotic states but without concomitant ketonuria. However, in metabolically stable conditions, defects in ketogenesis or ketolysis may result in unremarkable metabolite profiles, and thus escape detection, which is more easily accomplished in samples obtained during a metabolic decompensation.

### Characteristic abnormalities in laboratory values

| No. | Disorder | Metabolites |
|---|---|---|
| 50.1 | 3-Hydroxy-3-methylglutaryl-CoA synthase deficiency | Ketones ↓ |
| | | Glucose ↓ |
| | | C2 acylcarnitine n-↑↑ |
| 50.2 | 3-Hydroxy-3-methylglutaryl-CoA lyase deficiency | Ketones ↓ |
| | | Glucose n-↓ |
| | | Leucine metabolites ↑-↑↑↑ |
| 50.3 | Monocarboxylate transporter 1 deficiency | Ketones n-↑↑↑ |
| | | Glucose ± |
| | | No specific metabolite abnormalities beyond ketosis |
| 50.4 | Succinyl-CoA:3-oxoacid CoA transferase deficiency | Ketones n-↑↑↑ |
| | | Glucose ± |
| | | No specific metabolite abnormalities beyond ketosis |
| 50.5 | Methylacetoacetyl-CoA thiolase deficiency | Ketones n-↑↑↑ |
| | | Glucose ± |
| | | Isoleucine metabolites ↑↑ |
| 50.7 | Monocarboxylate transporter 1 superactivity | Insulin n-↑↑ |
| | | Glucose n-↓↓ |
| | | Glucagon n-↓ |

## Diagnostic Flowchart

mHMGCS deficiency and HMGCL deficiency are easily distinguished from each other in urinary organic acid profiles and plasma amino acids. MCT1 superactivity is one of many complex differential diagnoses of hypoglycaemia that is beyond the scope of this chapter. However, a flow chart is presented for the disorders of ketone body transport and catabolism (Fig. 50.4).

If characteristic isoleucine metabolites are present, MAT deficiency is the first tentative diagnosis in a ketoacidotic patient. As 2-methylacetoacetic acid is prone to degradation, its absence does not exclude MAT deficiency. If characteristic isoleucine metabolites such as 3-hydroxy-2-methylbutyric acid are not detected, it is useful to start with sequence analysis of *SLC16A1*, which encodes MCT1. If the results are negative, it may be helpful to add a functional test for SCOT deficiency in cells from the same blood sample. Investigations for MAT deficiency would usually follow as last test, if suggestive isoleucine metabolites have not been observed.

## Loading Tests

A leucine load that was performed in one of the first patients with suspected mHMGCS deficiency (Morris et al. 1998), but it is not used anymore today because of the opportunities of genetic testing. Similarly, the intravenous pyruvate test applied in the initial characterisation of several patients with MCT1 superactivity has been replaced by deoxyribonucleic acid (DNA) studies. While an isoleucine loading test was

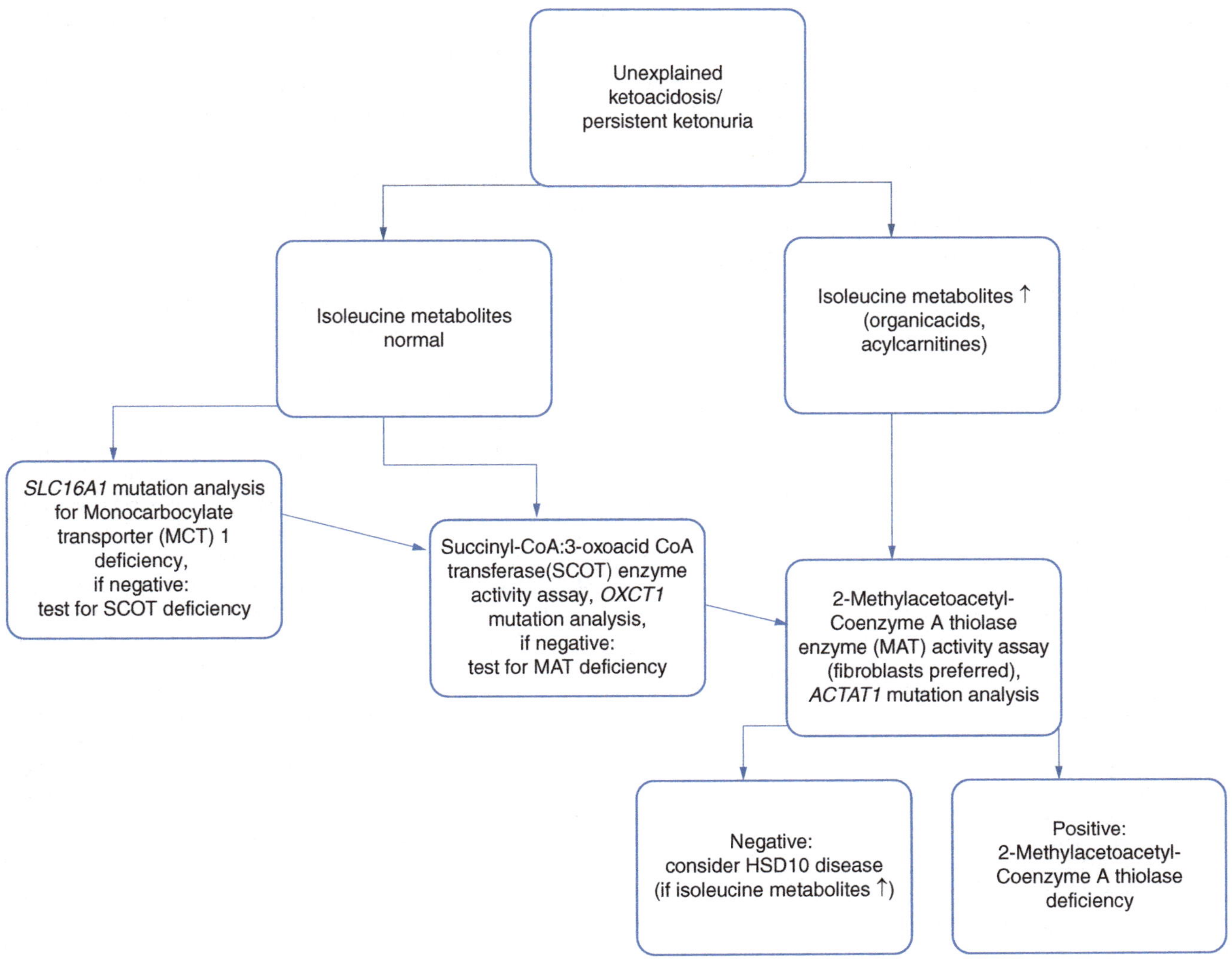


**Fig. 50.4** Diagnostic flowchart for differentiation between inborn errors of ketone body transport and catabolism

important in the discovery of MAT deficiency by Daum et al. in (1971), and was of diagnostic use in subsequent years, it has now been replaced by enzyme activity assays and mutation analysis.

## Specimen Collection

Confirmation of suspected deficiencies of SCOT, MAT and HMGL is usually approached by enzyme activity tests or mutation analyses. In contrast, mutation analysis is the method of choice in suspected deficiencies of mHMGCS or MCT1 (as well as in tentative MCT1 superactivity). If a defect of ketone body transport or catabolism is suspected but no abnormal isoleucine metabolite pattern is found, sequencing of *SLC16A1* (just five exons) can be performed while immortalised lymphocytes from the same blood sample are growing for a SCOT enzyme activity test to be added if the *SLC16A1* testing does not yield a diagnosis.

| No. | Disorder | Metabolites | Enzyme assay | Mutation analysis |
|---|---|---|---|---|
| 50.1 | 3-Hydroxy-3-methylglutaryl-CoA synthase deficiency | U, DBS, P/S | Liver | B |
| 50.2 | 3-Hydroxy-3-methylglutaryl-CoA lyase deficiency | U, DBS, P/S | LYM, FB | B |
| 50.3 | Monocarboxylate transporter 1 deficiency | U | | B |
| 50.4 | Succinyl-CoA:3-oxo-acid CoA transferase deficiency | U | LYM, FB | B |
| 50.5 | Methylacetoacetyl-CoA thiolase deficiency | U[a], DBS, P/S | FB, LYM[b] | B |
| 50.7 | Monocarboxylate transporter 1 superactivity | | | B |

*Abbreviations: U* Urine, *DBS* Dried blood spots, *P/S* Plasma/serum, *LYM* (Immortalised) lymphocytes, *F* Fibroblasts, *B* Blood

[a]Methylacetoacetate, which helps to distinguish MAT deficiency from HSD10 disease, is prone to degradation, thus recommending the shipment of urine in frozen state

[b]Cultured skin fibroblasts preferred, lymphocytes not recommended

## Prenatal Diagnosis

Once the diagnosis is known, disorders of ketone body metabolism are amenable to preventive measures including dietary treatment. However, if prenatal testing is requested, it is technically feasible.

| No. | Disorder | Metabolite | Enzyme assay | Mutation analysis | Source |
|---|---|---|---|---|---|
| 50.1 | 3-Hydroxy-3-methylglutaryl-CoA synthase deficiency | | | X[a] | A, CV |
| 50.2 | 3-Hydroxy-3-methylglutaryl-CoA lyase deficiency | X | X | X | AFC, A, CV |
| 50.3 | Monocarboxylate transporter 1 deficiency | | | X | A, CV[b] |
| 50.4 | Succinyl-CoA: 3-oxoacid CoA transferase deficiency | | X | X[a] | A, CV[b] |
| 50.5 | Methylacetoacetyl-CoA thiolase deficiency | | X | X | A |
| 50.7 | Monocarboxylate transporter 1 superactivity | | | X | A, CV[b] |

*Abbreviations*: *A* Amniocytes, *AFC* Amniotic fluid cells, *CV* Chorionic villi
[a]Not known whether actually done, but can in principle be performed by DNA analysis
[b]For DNA analysis only

## Treatment

The mainstay of therapy in deficiencies of HMG-CoA synthase/lyase, MCT1, SCOT and MAT is a rather preventative measure: ketogenesis has to be obviated to the extent possible.

Therefore, prolonged fasting has to be avoided and increased energy requirements have to be met. During acute decompensations, hypoglycaemia, if present, needs to be corrected immediately followed by constant high-rate intravenous glucose infusion with adequate electrolytes. Carbohydrates have not only antilipolytic effects but may also be useful due to antiproteolytic effects in HMGL, MCT1, SCOT and MAT deficiencies. In the acute phase with ketoacidosis and dehydration, fluid therapy is mandatory. The treatment of metabolic acidosis by bicarbonate is controversial but alkalinisation may be beneficial in severe ketoacidosis (pH < 7.1). Invasive methods such as dialysis have been shown to be effective but are rarely necessary, although haemodiafiltration may play a crucial role in HMG-CoA synthase deficiency. After diagnosis, treatment with frequent carbohydrate-rich meals during mild infections and intercurrent illnesses is advisable to prevent metabolic decompensation. Deficiency of L-carnitine should be compensated, if present. After childhood, metabolic decompensations have hardly been reported in patients with defects in ketone body utilisation or transport.

### Management of acute events

| Nr. | Disorder | Management |
|---|---|---|
| 50.1 | 3-Hydroxy-3-methylglutaryl-CoA synthase deficiency | Immediate correction of hypoglycaemia, if present, followed by constant high-rate glucose infusion |
| | | Consider haemodiafiltration and administration of L-carnitine |
| 50.2 | 3-Hydroxy-3-methylglutaryl-CoA lyase deficiency | Immediate correction of hypoglycaemia, if present, followed by constant high-rate glucose infusion |
| | | Consider administration of L-carnitine |
| 50.3 | Monocarboxylate transporter 1 deficiency | Immediate correction of hypoglycaemia, if present, followed by constant high-rate glucose infusion |
| | | Consider alkalinisation if acidosis is very pronounced (pH < 7.10) |
| 50.4 | Succinyl-CoA:3-oxoacid CoA transferase deficiency | Immediate correction of hypoglycaemia, if present, followed by constant high-rate glucose infusion |
| | | Consider alkalinisation if acidosis is very pronounced (pH < 7.10) |
| 50.5 | Methylacetoacetyl-CoA thiolase deficiency | Immediate correction of hypoglycaemia, if present, followed by constant high-rate glucose infusion |
| | | Consider alkalinisation if acidosis is very pronounced (pH < 7.10) and administration of L-carnitine |
| 50.7 | Monocarboxylate transporter 1 superactivity | Ensure adequate carbohydrate supply (consider glucose infusion) |

In periods of well-being, the avoidance of fasting is considered of crucial importance in all disorders of ketogenesis and ketolysis. This can usually be achieved with a normal meal frequency. In young children, a bedtime snack or the administration of uncooked corn starch at bedtime or midnight might be necessary. A special diet is usually not required; however, extremes of dietary fat intake should be avoided. A ketogenic diet is clearly contraindicated. Protein restriction may be useful in HMGCL and MAT deficiencies and possibly in SCOT deficiencies while a high protein intake may—at least in theory—be beneficial in mHMGS deficiency by compensating for the metabolic block and providing a source of ketone bodies. Most paediatric patients with HMGCL or MAT deficiency are stable on a protein intake of about 1.5 g/kg/day. However, protein intake needs to be individualised (Mitchell et al. 1995) and the expected benefit of protein restriction is based on limited evidence only. In patients with low levels of carnitine, L-carnitine supplementation should be considered and may help to eliminate accumulating tiglyl-CoA. But treatment and outcome studies are still sparse in most of these rare diseases so far.

#### Treatment when metabolically stable (maintenance therapy)

| Nr. | Disorder | Management |
|---|---|---|
| 50.1 | 3-Hydroxy-3-methylglutaryl-CoA synthase deficiency | Avoid fasting and extreme fat intake |
| | | Regular feeding in daytime |
| | | Consider additional bedtime snack in young children and supplementation with L-carnitine |
| 50.2 | 3-Hydroxy-3-methylglutaryl-CoA lyase deficiency | Avoid fasting and extreme fat intake |
| | | Regular feeding in daytime |
| | | Consider additional bedtime snack in young children and mild protein restriction (individualised, about 1.5 g/kg body weight/day) and compensate deficiency of free carnitine, if present |
| 50.3 | Monocarboxylate transporter 1 deficiency | Avoid fasting and extreme fat intake |
| | | Regular feeding in daytime |
| | | Consider additional bedtime snack in young children |
| 50.4 | Succinyl-CoA:3-oxoacid CoA transferase deficiency | Avoid fasting and extreme fat intake |
| | | Regular feeding in daytime |
| | | Consider additional bedtime snack in young children |
| 50.5 | Methylacetoacetyl-CoA thiolase deficiency | Avoid fasting and extreme fat intake |
| | | Regular feeding in daytime |
| | | Consider additional bedtime snack in young children and mild protein restriction (individualised, about 1.5 g/kg body weight/day) and compensate deficiency of free L-Carnitine, if present |
| 50.7 | Monocarboxylate transporter 1 superactivity | Avoid extensive physical exercise |

## References


Balasubramaniam S, Lewis B, Greed L, Meili D, Flier A, Yamamoto R, Bilić K, Till C, Sass JO. Heterozygous monocarboxylate transporter 1 (MCT1, *SLC16A1*) deficiency as a cause of recurrent ketoacidosis. JIMD Rep. 2016;29:33–8.

Bennett MJ, Hosking GP, Smith MF, Gray RGF, Middleton B. Biochemical investigations on a patient with a defect in cytosolic acetoacetyl-CoA thiolase, associated with mental retardation. J Inherit Metab Dis. 1984;7:125–8.

Bonnefont JP, Specola NB, Vassault A, Lombes A, Ogier H, de Klerk JB, Munnich A, Coude M, Paturneau-Jouas M, Saudubray JM. The fasting test in paediatrics: application to the diagnosis of pathological hypo- and hyperketotic states. Eur J Pediatr. 1990;150:80–5.

Conboy E, Vairo F, Schultz M, Agre K, Ridsdale R, Deyle D, Oglesbee D, Gavrilov D, Klee EW, Lanpher B. Mitochondrial 3-hydroxy-3-methylglutaryl-CoA synthase deficiency: unique presenting laboratory values and a review of biochemical and clinical features. JIMD Rep. 2018;40:63–9.

Daum RS, Lamm PH, Mamer OA, Scriver CR. A "new" disorder of isoleucine catabolism. Lancet. 1971;2(7737):1289–90.

De Groot CJ, Luit-De Haan G, Hulstaert CE, Hoomes FA. A patient with severe neurologic symptoms and acetoacetyl-CoA thiolase deficiency. Pediatr Res. 1977;11:1112–6.

Fukao T, Maruyama S, Ohura T, Hasegawa Y, Toyoshima M, Haapalainen AM, Kuwada N, Imamuram I, Yuasa I, Wierenga RK, Yamaguchi S, Kondo N. Three Japanese patients with beta-ketothiolase deficiency who share a mutation, c.431A>C (H144P) in ACAT1. Subtle abnormality in urinary organic acid analysis and blood acylcarnitine analysis using tandem mass spectrometry. JIMD Rep. 2011a;3:107–15.

Fukao T, Sass JO, Kursula P, Thimm E, Wendel U, Ficicioglu C, Monastiri K, Guffon N, Barić I, Zabot MT, Kondo N. Clinical and molecular characterization of five patients with succinyl-CoA:3-ketoacid CoA transferase (SCOT) deficiency. Biochim Biophys Acta. 2011b;1812:619–24.

Grünert SC, Schlatter SM, Schmitt RN, Gemperle-Britschgi C, Mrázová L, Balcı MC, Bischof F, Çoker M, Das AM, Demirkol M, de Vries M, Gökçay G, Häberle J, Uçar SK, Lotz-Havla AS, Lücke T, Roland D, Rutsch F, Santer R, Schlune A, Staufner C, Schwab KO, Mitchell GA, Sass JO. 3-Hydroxy-3-methylglutaryl-coenzyme a lyase deficiency: clinical presentation and outcome in a series of 37 patients. Mol Genet Metab. 2017a;121:206–15.

Grünert SC, Schmitt RN, Schlatter SM, Gemperle-Britschgi C, Balcı MC, Berg V, Çoker M, Das AM, Demirkol M, Derks TGJ, Gökçay G, Uçar SK, Konstantopoulou V, Christoph Korenke G, Lotz-Havla AS, Schlune A, Staufner C, Tran C, Visser G, Schwab KO, Fukao T, Sass JO. Clinical presentation and outcome in a series of 32 patients with 2-methylacetoacetyl-coenzyme A thiolase (MAT) deficiency. Mol Genet Metab. 2017b;122:67–75.

Hugo SE, Cruz-Garcia L, Karanth S, Anderson RM, Stainier DY, Schlegel A. A monocarboxylate transporter required for hepatocyte secretion of ketone bodies during fasting. Genes Dev. 2012;26:282–93.

Kouremenos KA, Pitt J, Marriott PJ. Metabolic profiling of infant urine using comprehensive two-dimensional gas chromatography: application to the diagnosis of organic acidurias and biomarker discovery. J Chromatogr A. 2010;1217:104–11.

Lehnert W. Long-term results of selective screening for inborn errors of metabolism. Eur J Pediatr. 1994;153:S9–S13.

Meissner T, Otonkoski T, Feneberg R, Beinbrech B, Apostolidou S, Sipilä I, Schaefer F, Mayatepek E. Exercise induced hypoglycaemic hyperinsulinism. Arch Dis Child. 2001;84:254–7.

Mitchell GA, Kassovska-Bratinova S, Boukaftane Y, Robert MF, Wang SP, Ashmarina L, Lambert M, Lapierre P, Potier E. Medical aspects of ketone body metabolism. Clin Invest Med. 1995;18:193–216.

Morris AA, Thekekara A, Wilks Z, Clayton PT, Leonard JV, Aynsley-Green A. Evaluation of fasts for investigating hypoglycaemia or suspected metabolic disease. Arch Dis Child. 1996;75:115–9.

Morris AA, Lascelles CV, Olpin SE, Lake BD, Leonard JV, Quant PA. Hepatic mitochondrial 3-hydroxy-3-methylglutaryl-coenzyme a synthase deficiency. Pediatr Res. 1998;44:392–6.

Muroi J, Yorifuji T, Uematsu A, Nakahata T. Cerebral infarction and pancreatitis: possible complications of patients with 3-hydroxy-3-methylglutaryl-CoA lyase deficiency. J Inherit Metab Dis. 2000;23:636–7.

Ofman R, Ruiter JP, Feenstra M, Duran M, Poll-The BT, Zschocke J, Ensenauer R, Lehnert W, Sass JO, Sperl W, Wanders RJ. 2-Methyl-3-hydroxybutyryl-CoA dehydrogenase deficiency is caused by mutations in the HADH2 gene. Am J Hum Genet. 2003;72:1300–7.

Otonkoski T, Kaminen N, Ustinov J, Lapatto R, Meissner T, Mayatepek E, Kere J, Sipilä I. Physical exercise-induced hyperinsulinemic hypoglycemia is anautosomal-dominant trait characterized by abnormal pyruvate-induced insulin release. Diabetes. 2003;52:199–204.

Otonkoski T, Jiao H, Kaminen-Ahola N, Tapia-Paez I, Ullah MS, Parton LE, Schuit F, Quintens R, Sipilä I, Mayatepek E, Meissner T, Halestrap AP, Rutter GA, Kere J. Physical exercise-induced hypoglycemia caused by failed silencing of monocarboxylate transporter 1 in pancreatic beta cells. Am J Hum Genet. 2007;81:467–74.

Sasai H, Aoyama Y, Otsuka H, Abdelkreem E, Naiki Y, Kubota M, Sekine Y, Itoh M, Nakama M, Ohnishi H, Fujiki R, Ohara O, Fukao T. Heterozygous carriers of succinyl-CoA:3-oxoacid CoA transferase deficiency can develop severe ketoacidosis. J Inherit Metab Dis. 2017;40:845–52.

Sass JO. Inborn errors of ketogenesis and ketone body utilization. J Inherit Metab Dis. 2012;35:23–8.

Sass JO, Fukao T, Mitchell GA. Inborn errors of ketone body metabolism and transport: an update for the clinic and for clinical laboratories. J Inborn Errors Metab Screen. 2018; https://doi.org/10.1177/2326409818771101.

Thompson GN, Hsu BY, Pitt JJ, Treacy E, Stanley CA. Fasting hypoketotic coma in a child with deficiency of mitochondrial 3-hydroxy-3-methylglutaryl-CoA synthase. N Engl J Med. 1997;337:1203–7.

van Hasselt PM, Ferdinandusse S, Monroe GR, Ruiter JP, Turkenburg M, Geerlings MJ, Duran K, Harakalova M, van der Zwaag B, Monavari AA, Okur I, Sharrard MJ, Cleary M, O'Connell N, Walker V, Rubio-Gozalbo ME, de Vries MC, Visser G, Houwen RH, van der Smagt JJ, Verhoeven-Duif NM, Wanders RJ, van Haaften G. Monocarboxylate transporter 1 deficiency and ketone utilization. N Engl J Med. 2014;371:1900–7.

Weinstein DA, Correia CE, Saunders AC, Wolfsdorf JI. Hepatic glycogen synthase deficiency: an infrequently recognized cause of ketotic hypoglycemia. Mol Genet Metab. 2006;87:284–8.

# Disorders of Complex Lipids

# 51

Frédéric M. Vaz, Saskia B. Wortmann, and Fanny Mochel

## Contents



## Summary

The advent of exome sequencing has greatly increased the discovery of new disease genes, especially in groups of patients with complex pathology including spastic paraplegias, congenital ichthyosis, and lipodystrophies. Many of these disease-causing genes turned out to be involved in complex lipid metabolism and are dispersed throughout the different branches of the lipid biosynthetic tree. Lipids not only are structural components needed for cell compartmentalization but also are involved in dynamic processes including inter- and intracellular transport and signal transduction. The synthesis, remodeling, and degradation of lipids are tightly coordinated in mammalian cells and involve and affect almost all organelles of the cell. Using simple building blocks including glycerol, amino acids, and radyl units (fatty acids/alcohols), a plethora of lipid species can be produced. The chapter is divided into five parts dealing with disorders in (1) phospholipid and neutral lipid metabolism, (2) fatty acid synthesis and elongation, (3) triglyceride/lipid droplet metabolism, (4) sphingolipid metabolism, and (5) a miscellaneous category. Given the very diverse gene functions and clinical phenotypes, we have chosen a different chapter structure. For each disorder, in addition to the phenotype tables, we have separately listed their function, a brief clinical synopsis, and if known/available specific treatment options, other than supportive care.

F. M. Vaz (✉)
Laboratory Genetic Metabolic Diseases, Amsterdam UMC, location AMC, Amsterdam, The Netherlands
e-mail: f.m.vaz@amsterdamumc.nl

S. B. Wortmann
Paracelsus Medical University, University Children's Hospital, Salzburg, Austria

Radboud Centre for Mitochondrial Medicine, Amalia Children's Hospital, Radboudumc, Nijmegen, The Netherlands
e-mail: s.wortmann@salk.at

F. Mochel
Reference Center for Adult Neurometabolic diseases, La Pitié-Salpêtrière University Hospital, Paris, France
e-mail: fanny.mochel@upmc.fr



N. Blau et al. (eds.), *Physician's Guide to the Diagnosis, Treatment, and Follow-Up of Inherited Metabolic Diseases*,
https://doi.org/10.1007/978-3-030-67727-5_51

## Introduction

Lipids are best known as structural components of biological membranes to form permeability barriers of cells and organelles. In addition, they can function as an energy source, are used to modify proteins, participate in membrane fusion/fission, and can be bioactive messengers that directly or indirectly regulate gene expression. There are many types of lipids, each with different chemical properties that in turn dictate the fluidity and permeability of membranes. By varying the composition of lipids, a huge diversity in membranes can be generated that allows the formation of organelles, cells, and tissues (Harayama and Riezman 2018). Because the chemical properties are crucial to the function of lipids, small changes in lipid structure or composition (a missing double bond or a different fatty acid composition) can have large implications for cells, affecting tissues and therefore the entire human metabolism. The genomics revolution has resulted in the identification of causative genes for many disorders/syndromes, including an increasing number of lipid metabolism genes. Together with considerable advances in lipid analysis, catalyzed by new technological possibilities in mass spectrometry, a new field of inborn errors of lipid metabolism has emerged. Before discussing the clinical, genetic, and functional aspects of these many disorders, it is crucial to first briefly address the metabolism of complex lipids with emphasis on their synthesis.

The synthesis, remodeling, and degradation of lipids are tightly coordinated in mammalian cells, and key organelles involved in this process are the endoplasmic reticulum (ER), mitochondria, lipid droplets (LD), lysosomes, and the Golgi apparatus. At these locations, lipids are assembled from simple building blocks including glycerol, phosphate, fatty acids, fatty alcohols, serine, choline, ethanolamine, and inositol to form a plethora of complex lipids belonging to different major classes. The main categories of lipids discussed in this chapter are fatty acids, glycerophospholipids (from here on called phospholipids), neutral lipids (i.e., sterols and glycerolipids), and sphingolipids. Figure 51.1 shows the molecular structures of the most relevant lipids for this chapter, the three major classes: phospholipids, glycerolipids, and sphingolipids.

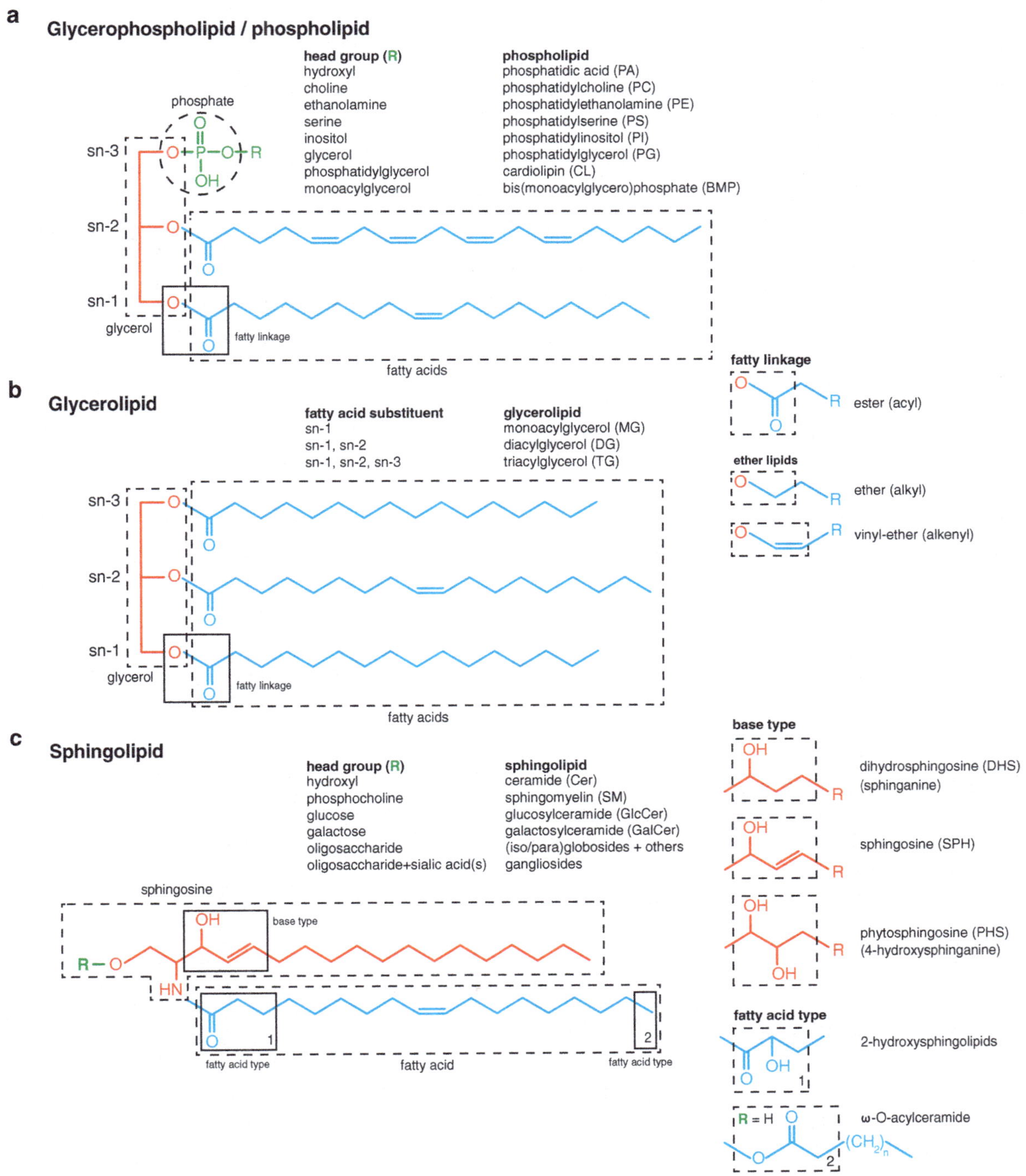


**Fig. 51.1** Molecular structures of different lipid classes. (**a**) Glycerophospholipids or phospholipids contain a glycerol backbone (*red*) attached to one or two fatty acid/fatty alcohol (*blue*) substituents at the *sn*-1 and *sn*-2 position and characteristic phosphate-linked headgroup (*green*) at the *sn*-3 position. Most common headgroups are listed with the name and abbreviation of the corresponding phospholipid. In ether phospholipids, the fatty linkage at the *sn*-1 position is either an ether or a vinyl-ether, and the latter substitution defines the subclass that is known as plasmalogens. (**b**) Glycerolipids contain a glycerol backbone (*red*) attached to one up to three fatty acid/fatty alcohol (*blue*) substituents. In analogy to ether phospholipids, ether variants of glycerolipids also exist with an ether fatty linkage on the *sn*-1 position. (**c**) Sphingolipids consist of a sphingoid base (*red*) coupled to a headgroup (*green*) and an N-linked fatty acid (*blue*). Hydroxylation and (un)saturation define the sphingoid base type. 2-Hydroxylation of the fatty acid (1) or ω-acylation (2) determines the fatty acid type. The headgroup (*green*) defines the type of sphingolipid, common headgroups, and sphingolipids and abbreviations are listed

## Nomenclature

| No. | Disease name | Alternative disease names | Disease abbreviation | Gene symbol | Chromosomal localization | Mode of inheritance | Affected protein | Disease OMIM# |
|---|---|---|---|---|---|---|---|---|
| 51.1 | Acylglycerol kinase deficiency | Sengers syndrome; Autosomal recessive Cataract 38; Mitochondrial DNA depletion syndrome 10 | MTDPS10 | *AGK* | 7q34 | AR | Acylglycerol kinase | 610345 |
| 51.2 | SERAC1 deficiency | 3-methylglutaconic aciduria with deafness, encephalopathy, and Leigh-like syndrome | MEGD(H)EL | *SERAC1* | 6q25.3 | AR | Serine active site-containing protein 1 | 614725 |
| 51.3 | Taffazin deficiency | Barth syndrome | BTHS | *TAZ* | Xq28 | XLR | Tafazzin | 300394 |
| 51.4 | PNPLA8 deficiency | Mitochondrial myopathy with lactic acidosis | MMLA | *PNPLA8* | 7q31.1 | AR | Patatin-like phospholipase domain-containing protein 8 | 612123 |
| 51.5 | Ethanolaminephosphotransferase 1 deficiency | Autosomal recessive spastic paraplegia 81 | SPG81 | *SELENOI* | 2p23.3 | AR | Selenoprotein 1 | 607915 |
| 51.6 | Phosphoethanolamine cytidylyltransferase 2 deficiency | Autosomal recessive spastic paraplegia 82 | SPG82 | *PCYT2* | 17q25.3 | AR | Phosphoethanolamine cytidylyltransferase 2 | 602679 |
| 51.7 | Choline kinase β deficiency | Congenital muscular dystrophy, megaconial type | MDCMC | *CHKB* | 22q13.33 | AR | Choline kinase beta | 612395 |
| 51.8 | Phosphocholine cytidylyltransferase 1α deficiency (retinos keletal type) | Spondylometaphyseal dysplasia with cone-rod dystrophy | SMDCRD | *PCYT1A* | 3q29 | AR | Phosphocholine cytidylyltransferase 1a | 123695 |
| 51.9 | Phosphocholine cytidylyltransferase 1α deficiency (lipody strophy type) | – | | *PCYT1A* | 3q29 | AR | Phosphocholine cytidylyltransferase 1a | 123695 |
| 51.10 | Phosphatidylserine decarboxylase deficiency | – | | *PISD* | 22q12.2 | AR | Phosphatidylserine decarboxylase | 612770 |
| 51.11 | Phosphatidylserine synthase 1 superactivity | Lenz-Majewski syndrome; Lenz-Ma jewski hyperostotic dwarfism | LMHD | *PTDSS1* | 8q22.1 | AD | Phosphatidylserine synthase 1 | 612792 |
| 51.12 | Phospholipase A2 group 6 deficiency | Infantile neuroaxonal dystrophy 1; Neurodegeneration with brain iron accumulation type 2B; Seitelberger disease; Autosomal recessive Parkins on disease 14 | | *PLA2G6* | 22q13.1 | AR | Phospholipase A2 group 6; Patatin-like phospholipase domain-containing protein 9 | 603604 |
| 51.13 | DDHD1 deficiency | Autosomal recessive spastic paraplegia type 28 | SPG28 | *DDHD1* | 14q22.1 | AR | Phosphatidic acid-preferring phospholipase 1 | 614603 |
| 51.14 | DDHD2 deficiency | Autosomal recessive spastic paraplegia type 54 | SPG54 | *DDHD2* | 8p11.23 | AR | Phosphatidic acid-preferring phospholipase 2 | 615003 |
| 51.15 | PNPLA6 deficiency | Autosomal recessive spastic paraplegia type 39; Oliver-McFarlane syndrome; Boucher-Neuhauser syndrome; Laurence-Moon syndrome | SPG39 | *PNPLA6* | 19p13.2 | AR | Patatin-like phospholipase domain-containing protein 6 | 603197 |
| 51.16 | Membrane-bound O-acyltransferase domain-containing 7 deficiency | Autosomal recessive mental retardation type 57 | MRT57 | *MBOAT7* | 19p13.42 | AR | Membrane-bound O-acyltransferase domain-containing 7 | 606048 |
| 51.17 | Diacylglycerol kinase ε deficiency | Nephrotic syndrome type 7; Atypical hemolytic uremic syndrome type 7 | NPHS7 | *DGKE* | 17q22 | AR | Diacylglycerol kinase ε | 601440 |
| 51.18 | Cytosolic acetyl-CoA carboxylase 1 deficiency | – | ACACAD | *ACACA* | 17q12 | AR | Acetyl-CoA carboxylase 1 | 200350 |

| | | | | | | | | |
|---|---|---|---|---|---|---|---|---|
| 51.19 | Mitochondrial acetyl-CoA carboxylase 2 deficiency | ACC1 deficiency | ACACBD | *ACACB* | 12q24.11 | AR | Acetyl-CoA carboxylase 2 | 601557 |
| 51.20 | 3-Hydroxyacyl-CoA dehydratase 1 deficiency | ACC2 deficiency | | *HACD1* | 10p12.33 | AR | 3-Hydroxyacyl-CoA dehydratase 1 | 610467 |
| 51.21 | Trans-2-enoyl-CoA reductase deficiency | Autosomal recessive mental retardation type 14 | MRT14 | *TECR* | 19p13.12 | AR | Trans-2-enoyl-CoA reductase | 610057 |
| 51.22 | Mitochondrial enoyl-CoA reductase deficiency | Mitochondrial enoyl-CoA reductase protein-associated neurodegeneration | MEPAN | *MECR* | 1p35.3 | AR | Mitochondrial enoyl-CoA reductase | 608205 |
| 51.23 | Very long-chain fatty acid elongase 1 deficiency | Ichthyotic keratoderma, spasticity, hypomyelination and dysmorphic features | IKSHD | *ELOVL1* | 1p34.2 | AD | Very long-chain fatty acid elongase 1 | 611813 |
| 51.24 | Very long-chain fatty acid elongase 4 deficiency, neurologic phenotype | Pseudo-Sjögren-Larsson syndrome (recessive); spinocerebellar ataxia type 34 (dominant) | SCA34 | *ELOVL4* | 6q14.1 | AD, AR | Very long-chain fatty acid elongase 4 | 605512 |
| 51.25 | Very long-chain fatty acid elongase 4 deficiency, retinal phenotype | Stargardt disease type 3 | | *ELOVL4* | 6q14.1 | AD | Very long-chain fatty acid elongase 4 | 605512 |
| 51.26 | Very long-chain fatty acid elongase 5 deficiency | Spinocerebellar ataxia type 38 | SCA38 | *ELOVL5* | 6p12.1 | AD | Very long-chain fatty acid elongase 5 | 611805 |
| 51.27 | Long-chain fatty acid-CoA ligase 4 deficiency | X-linked mental retardation 63 | | *ACSL4* | Xq23 | XL | Long-chain fatty acid-CoA ligase 4 | 300157 |
| 51.28 | Lysophosphatidic acid acyltransferase deficiency | Congenital generalized lipodystrophy type 1, Berardinelli-Seip syndrome | BSCL1 | *AGPAT2* | 9q34,3 | AR | Lysophosphatidic acid acyltransferase | 603100 |
| 51.29 | Lipin 1 deficiency | Autosomal recessive acute recurrent myoglobinuria; Familial paroxysmal myoglobinuria; acute recurrent paralytic rhabdomyolysis | | *LPIN1* | 2p25.1 | AR | Lipin 1 | 605518 |
| 51.30 | Lipin 2 deficiency | Majeed syndrome; Congenital chronic recurrent multifocal osteomyelitis; dyserythropoietic anemia and neutrophilic dermatosis | MJDS | *LPIN2* | 18p11.31 | AR | Lipin 2 | 605519 |
| 51.31 | Diacylglycerol acyltransferase deficiency | Congenital diarrhea type 7; Protein-losing enteropathy diarrhea type 7 | DIAR7 | *DGAT1* | 8q24.3 | AR | Diacylglycerol acyltransferase 1 | 604900 |
| 51.32 | CGI-58 deficiency | Chanarin-Dorfman syndrome; Neutral lipid storage disease with ichthyosis | NLSDI | *ABHD5* | 3p21.33 | AR | α/β-hydrolase domain containing 5 | 604780 |
| 51.33 | Adipose triglyceride lipase deficiency | Neutral lipid storage disease with myopathy; Neutral lipid storage without ichthyosis | NLSDM | *PNPLA2* | 11p15.5 | AR | Adipose triglyceride lipase | 609059 |
| 51.34 | Perilipin 1 deficiency | Familial partial lipodystrophy type 4 | FPLD4 | *PLIN1* | 15q26.1 | AD | Perilipin 1 | 170290 |
| 51.35 | Hormone-sensitive lipase deficiency | Familial partial lipodystrophy type 6 | FPLD6 | *LIPE* | 19q13.2 | AR | Hormone-sensitive lipase | 151750 |
| 51.36 | Serine palmitoyltransferase subunit 1 deficiency | Hereditary sensory and autonomic neuropathy type 1A | HSAN1A | *SPTLC1* | 9q22.31 | AD | Serine palmitoyltransferase subunit 1 | 605712 |
| 51.37 | Serine palmitoyltransferase subunit 2 deficiency | Hereditary sensory and autonomic neuropathy type 1C | HSAN1C | *SPTLC2* | 14q24.3 | AD | Serine palmitoyltransferase subunit 2 | 605713 |
| 51.38 | Ceramide synthase 1 deficiency | Progressive myoclonic epilepsy type 8 | EPM8 | *CERS1* | 19p13.11 | AR | Ceramide synthase 1 | 606919 |
| 51.39 | Ceramide synthase 3 deficiency | Autosomal recessive congenital ichthyosis type 9 | ARCI9 | *CERS3* | 15q26.3 | AR | Ceramide synthase 3 | 615276 |

(continued)

| No. | Disease name | Alternative disease name | Disease abbreviation | Gene symbol | Chromosomal localization | Mode of inheritance | Affected protein | Disease OMIM# |
|---|---|---|---|---|---|---|---|---|
| 51.40 | Dihydroceramide desaturase deficiency | Hypomyellinating leukodystrophy 18 | HLD18 | *DEGS1* | 1q42.11 | AR | Δ4-dihydroceramide desaturase | 618404 |
| 51.41 | Alkaline ceramidase 3 deficiency | Early childhood-onset progressive leukodystrophy | PLDECO | *ACER3* | 11q13.5 | AR | Alkaline ceramidase 3 | 617036 |
| 51.42 | CYP4F22 omega hydroxylase deficiency | Autosomal recessive congenital ichthyosis type 5 | ARCI5 | *CYP4F22* | 19p13.12 | AR | cytochrome P450, family 4, subfamily F, polypeptide 22 | 611495 |
| 51.43 | Acylceramide transacylase deficiency | Autosomal recessive congenital ichthyosis type 10 | ARCI10 | *PNPLA1* | 6p21.31 | AR | Acylceramide transacylase; patatin-like phospholipase domain-containing protein 1 | 612121 |
| 51.44 | UDP-glucose ceramide glucosyltransferase deficiency | Autosomal recessive congenital ichthyosis | | *UGCG* | 9q31.3 | AR | UDP-glucose ceramide glucosyltransferase | 602874 |
| 51.45 | Nonlysosomal glucosylceramidase deficiency | Autosomal recessive spastic paraplegia type 46 | SPG46 | *GBA2* | 9p13.3 | AR | Nonlysosomal glucosylceramidase | 609471 |
| 51.46 | Fatty acid 2-hydroxylase deficiency | Autosomal recessive spastic paraplegia type 35; Fatty acid hydroxylaseassociated neurodegeneration | SPG35 | *FA2H* | 16q23.1 | AR | Fatty acid 2-hydroxylase | 611026 |
| 51.47 | Sphingosine-1-phosphate lyase deficiency | Nephrotic syndrome type 14 | NPHS14 | *SGPL1* | 10q22.1 | AR | Sphingosine-1-phosphate lyase | 603729 |
| 51.48 | Ceramide transfer protein superactivity | Autosomal dominant mental retardation type 34 | MRD34 | *COL4A3BP* | 5q13.3 | AD | Ceramide transfer protein | 604677 |
| 51.49 | GM3 synthase deficiency | Amish infantile epilepsy syndrome;salt and pepper developmental regression syndrome; ST3GAL5-CDG | SPDRS | *ST3GAL5* | 2p11.2 | AR | GM3 synthase | 604402 |
| 51.50 | GM2/GD2 synthase deficiency | Autosomal recessive spastic paraplegia type 26 | SPG26 | *B4GALNT1* | 12q13.3 | AR | GM2/GD2 synthase | 601873 |
| 51.51 | GD1a/GT1b synthase deficiency | Autosomal recessive mental retardation 12; ST3GAL3-CDG; Early infantile epileptic encephalopathy 15 | MRT12 | *ST3GAL3* | 1p34.1 | AR | GD1a/GT1b synthase | 606494 |
| 51.52 | GB3 synthase deficiency | NOR polyagglutination syndrome | | *A4GALT* | 22q13.2 | AD | GB3 synthase | 607922 |
| 51.53 | Phospholipid-transporting ATPase IB deficiency | Cerebellar ataxia, mental retardation and dysequilibrium syndrome type 4; Cerebellar ataxia and mental retardation with or without quadrupedal locomotion 4 | CAMRQ4 | *ATP8A2* | 13q12.13 | AR | Phospholipid-transporting ATPase IB | 605870 |
| 51.54 | CYP2U1 deficiency | Autosomal recessive spastic paraplegia type 56 | SPG56 | *CYP2U1* | 4q25 | AR | Cytochrome P450 family 2 subfamily U member 1 | 610670 |
| 51.55 | ABHD12 deficiency | Polyneuropathy, hearing loss, ataxia, retinitis pigmentosa, and cataract syndrome | PHARC | *ABHD12* | 20p11.21 | AR | α/βhydrolase domain—containing protein 12 | 613599 |

## Metabolic Pathways

### Phospholipid and Neutral Lipid Synthesis

Figure 51.2 shows the general metabolic pathways of phospholipid synthesis, fatty acid synthesis, and elongation and triacylglycerol (TG) usage in the lipid droplet. For clarity, only disease genes have been indicated. Briefly, there are two main synthetic pathways with some overlap. The majority of membrane phospholipids are synthesized in the ER and are made from glycerol-3-phosphate that, after two acylations, forms phosphatidic acid (PA). Attachment of a headgroup to this phosphate designates to which major phospholipid class the lipid belongs. Major phospholipid classes include (in order of cellular abundance) phosphatidylcholine (PC), phosphatidylethanolamine (PE), phosphatidylinositol (PI), phosphatidylserine (PS), and phosphatidylglycerol (PG). PG can be further metabolized to cardiolipin (CL) in the mitochondrion, and PG, likely via mitochondria-associated membranes, is the precursor for the late endosomal lipid bis(monoacylglycero)phosphate (BMP). Cytidine triphosphate (CTP) is used to create high-energy molecules of either the headgroup (cytidine diphosphate (CDP)-choline (➔PC) and CDP-ethanolamine (➔PE)) or the acylated glycerol backbone (CDP-diacylglycerol (CDG-DG)) which then condenses with diacylglycerol (DG) or the headgroup (inositol (➔PI), glycerol (➔PG) or phosphatidylglycerol (➔CL)), respectively, to yield the specific lipid. DG is an intermediate metabolite that either is incorporated in phospholipids or that, mainly for energy storage in lipid droplets, is acylated to form TG (Vance 2015). Stepwise hydrolysis of TG at the lipid droplet surface yields three free fatty acids and a glycerol molecule which can be used for energy generation or other metabolism (Fig. 51.2a). Lipid droplet synthesis and degradation plays an important role in cellular lipid homeostasis, storing cholesterol esters and TG that serve as a source of energy substrates or precursors for signaling lipids or membrane (phospho)lipid synthesis (Sztalryd and Brasaemle 2017).

Another important class of lipids is the so-called ether lipids that are characterized by a fatty alcohol on the *sn*-1 position that creates an ether bond with the glycerol backbone (Fig. 51.2b). The precursor is not glycerol-3-phosphate but dihydroxyacetone phosphate, which in a number of steps is converted to 1-alkylglycerol in the peroxisome. The remainder of the synthetic pathway is located at the ER. After acylation of the *sn*-2 position to form 1-alkyl-2-acylglycerol (DG[O]), CDP-choline or CDP-ethanolamine can be used to form the ether phospholipids PC[O] and PE[O]. Desaturation of the ether-linked fatty alcohol on the *sn*-1 position yields a vinyl-ether which is characteristic of plasmalogen species, a subclass of ether phospholipids that are especially important for the brain. Alternatively, DG[O] can be acylated to form 1-alkyl-2,3-diacylglycerol (TG[O]), the ether analog of TG, a relatively uncharacterized ether lipid (Dean and Lodhi 2018; Braverman and Moser 2012).

### Fatty Acid Synthesis and Elongation

Figure 51.2 also shows three relevant auxiliary pathways: the mitochondrial fatty acid synthesis (mFAS), long-chain fatty acid synthesis (FAS) in the cytosol, and very long-chain fatty acid elongation in the ER. mFAS produces mainly octanoate that is subsequently used for synthesis of lipoic acid. Lipoic acid is needed in five mitochondrial reactions including 2-oxoacid dehydrogenases (the pyruvate dehydrogenase, 2-ketoglutarate dehydrogenase, and branched-chain dehydrogenase complexes) and the glycine cleavage system (Kastaniotis et al. 2017). Cytosolic FAS synthesizes mainly palmitate (C16:0) destined for storage in TG, incorporation in other lipids, or further elongation in the ER. Further elongation of saturated or polyunsaturated fatty acids in the ER produces different types of very long-chain fatty acids that can be used for complex lipid synthesis and/or can be used to tune the fatty acid composition of other complex lipids (Kihara 2012). Very and ultra-long-chain fatty acids, for example, are used to synthesize ω-O-acylceramides that are needed for the barrier function of the skin (Kihara 2016a). The three pathways are shown and explained in more detail in Fig. 51.3, including disease genes. mFAS uses acyl carrier protein (ACP) to carry the nascent fatty acid, whereas the cytosolic FAS system and the ER elongation system use coenzyme A. The process of fatty acid synthesis/elongation starts by the generation of malonyl-CoA by carboxylation of acetyl-CoA which condenses with an acyl-CoA or an acyl-unit attached to acyl carrier protein (ACP) to form a 3-ketoacyl-CoA/ACP. Subsequent reduction, dehydrogenation, and another reduction yield an acyl-CoA/ACP with two additional carbon atoms (see Fig. 51.3).

### Sphingolipid Synthesis and Metabolism

Sphingolipids are membrane lipids that not only are structural components but also can participate in membrane microdomain formation, serve as ligands of lectins, and modulate the activity of membrane receptors. They are particularly abundant in the brain and crucial for the development and correct function of the nervous system. Sphingolipid metabolism is shown in Fig. 51.4 and starts by the synthesis of ceramide. The production of ceramide is the backbone of sphingolipid synthesis that branches out into subclasses of complex sphingolipids including phosphocholine-containing sphingomyelins (SM), (oligo)saccharide-containing glycosphingolipids, and

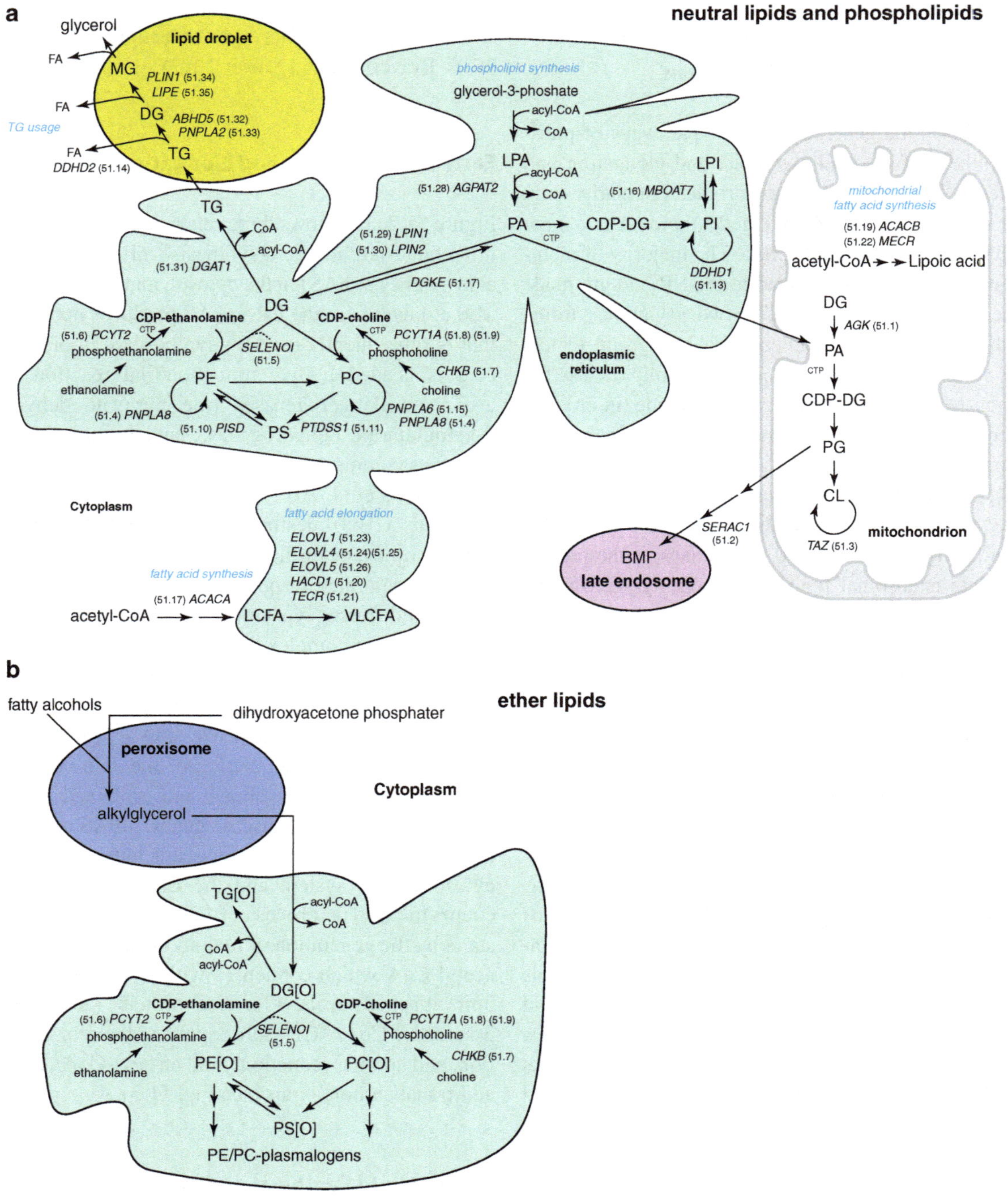


**Fig. 51.2** Phospholipid synthesis, fatty acid synthesis/elongation, and lipid droplet metabolism including disease genes. (**a**) Neutral lipid, fatty acid, and phospholipid synthetic pathways. Glycerol-3-phosphate is acylated on the *sn*-1 position to form lysophosphatidic acid (LPA) followed by a second acylation step on the *sn*-2 position to form phosphatidic acid (PA). At the expense of cytidine triphosphate (CTP), PA can be converted into the high-energy molecule CDP-diacylglycerol (CDP-DG) which can condense with inositol in the endoplasmic reticulum (ER) to form phosphatidylinositol (PI) or in mitochondria with phoshatidylglycerol (PG) to form cardiolipin (CL). PG also is the precursor of the late endosomal lipid bis(monoacylglycero)phosphate (BMP). In the ER, PA can be dephosphorylated to form diacylglycerol (DG) that can condense with activated headgroups CDP-ethanolamine and CDP-choline to form phosphatidylethanolamine (PE) and phosphatidylcholine (PC), respectively. CDP-ethanolamine and CDP-choline are made via phosphorylation and subsequent activation with CTP from ethanolamine and choline, respectively, part of the so-called Kennedy pathway. Phosphatidylserine (PS) can be made by base = headgroup exchange from PE or PC. DG can also be acylated to form triacylglycerol (TG) which can be stored in lipid droplets. Usage of TG is executed by sequential hydrolysis of the fatty acid esters, finally resulting in the formation of glycerol and three fatty acids. Fatty acids can be synthesized from acetyl-CoA in the cytosol to form long-chain fatty acids (LCFA) that can be further elongated in the ER to very long-chain fatty acids. Another fatty acid synthesis system is present in mitochondria, but this is involved in the synthesis of lipoic acid, a special sulfur-containing fatty acid required for three mitochondrial dehydrogenase complexes. (**b**) Ether lipid metabolism. Dihydroxyacetone phosphate and a fatty alcohol is converted to alkylglycerol in the peroxisome after which alkylglycerol is acylated in the ER to form 1-alkyl-2-acylglycerol (DG[O]). Like non-ether lipids, DG[O] can be converted to ether-analogs of PE and PC by condensation with CDP-ethanolamine and CDP-choline, forming plasmanyl-PE and plasmanyl-PC. Creation of a vinyl-ether by desaturation in the ER yields plasmenyl-PE/PC which are collectively called plasmalogens. Like DG, DG[O] can also be acylated which yields 1-alkyl-2,3-diacylglycerol (TG[O]). Remodeling activities are indicated by a circular arrow

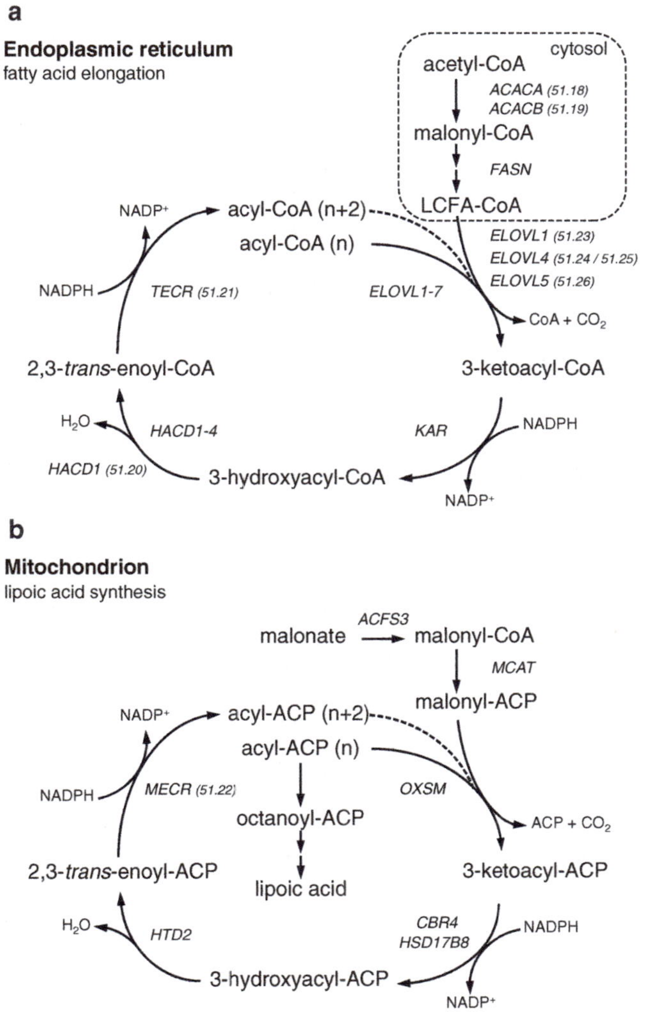


**Fig. 51.3** Fatty acid synthesis and elongation, including disease genes. (**a**) Fatty acids are synthesized in the cytosol from malonyl-CoA by the fatty acid synthase complex (*FASN*) to form a long-chain acyl-CoA (LCFA-CoA). This LCFA-CoA can then be elongated in the ER to yield a variety of very long-chain fatty acids. The first step, the condensation of malonyl-CoA with the LCFA-CoA, is catalyzed by a family of very long-chain 3-oxoacyl-CoA synthases (ELOVLs) with different tissue expression patterns and with variable substrate specificities depending on the fatty acid length and degree of unsaturation. 3-Ketoacyl-CoA-reductase (*KAR*) reduces the keto-group to a hydroxyl-group. The resulting 3-hydroxyacyl-CoA is dehydrated by a family of 3-hydroxyacyl-CoA dehydratases (*HACD1–4*) with different tissue expression patterns to form 2,3-trans-enoyl-CoA. Finally, this double bond is reduced to by trans-2,3-enoyl-CoA reductase (*TECR*) resulting in an acyl-CoA that is two carbon atoms longer. (**b**) The mitochondrial fatty acid synthesis system, also known as mFAS, uses acyl carrier protein (ACP) instead of CoA to carry the growing acyl-unit. After carboxylation of acetyl-CoA to form malonyl-CoA, malonate is transferred by mitochondrial malonyl CoA-acyl carrier protein transacylase to ACP. Malonyl-ACP condenses with acyl-ACP to form 3-ketoacyl-ACP which is catalyzed by 3-oxoacyl-acyl-carrier-protein synthase, encoded by *OXSM*. Carbonyl reductase 4 (*CBR4*) and ketoacyl-ACP reductase (*HSD17B8*) are involved in the NADPH-dependent reduction to form 3-hydroxyacyl-ACP, which is subsequently dehydrated by 3-hydroxyacyl-thioester dehydratase type 2 (*HTD2*) to a 2,3-trans-enoyl-ACP. Mitochondrial trans-2-enoyl-CoA reductase (*MECR*) reduces the double bond to create an acyl-ACP that is two carbon atoms longer. The end product of mitochondrial fatty acid synthesis is octanoyl-ACP. The octanoyl-moiety is then converted into lipoic acid in a number of steps (Mayr et al. 2014)

ω-acylated ceramides. The condensation of L-serine and palmitoyl-CoA leads to the formation of the sphingoid base which is then N-acylated by ceramide synthases resulting in the formation of ceramide. Variation and modification of the molecular structure of either the sphingoid base or the N-acyl group yields many different ceramide species which are precursors of different complex sphingolipids (Figs. 51.1 and 51.4) where the addition of many different headgroups creates an additional multiplication of the amount of subspecies that can be formed. This chapter does not deal with the catabolism of complex sphingolipids (for this metabolism and associated disorders, including sphingolipidoses, see Chap. 60) but does cover ceramide degradation as this not only is the sole exit from the sphingolipid network but also is the way to produce bioactive molecules as sphingosine and sphingosine-1-phosphate (S1P). Ceramide is degraded by first removing the N-acylated fatty acid, followed by phosphorylation to form S1P which is then lysed to phosphoethanolamine and a long-chain aldehyde (Fig. 51.4a). This route controls the levels of ceramide, sphingosine, and S1P which are intra- and intercellular messengers that are involved in cell differentiation, autophagy, and apoptosis (Hannun and Obeid 2018; Jennemann and Gröne 2013).

A particularly important branch of the sphingolipid tree for this chapter is the production of ω-O-acylceramides, shown in Fig. 51.4b, as these ceramide species are required for epithelial permeability and skin barrier function. ω-O-acylceramides are enriched in very long-chain fatty acids, and disturbance of either fatty acid elongation or (ω-O-acyl) ceramide synthesis frequently gives rise to skin phenotypes (Kihara 2016a).

Lastly, ceramide is the precursor for complex sphingolipid synthesis (Fig. 51.4c) which proceeds by the sequential glycosylation of ceramide to form glycosphingolipids or the addition of a phosphocholine headgroup to form sphingomyelins (SM). Glycosphingolipids can contain oligosaccharides with the acidic sugar N-acetylneuraminic acid (gangliosides) or become sulfated (sulfatides) by the action of different biosynthetic enzymes. Deficiency of the corresponding genes gives rise to phenotypes that almost all (severely) affect the central nervous system (Li and Schnaar 2018). As the glycosyltransferases that function in glycosphingolipid metabolism also are involved in protein glycosylation, some of the disorders are also classified as CDG syndromes.

## Remodeling

In addition to the biosynthetic pathways, fatty acid composition of lipids is fine-tuned through a process called remodeling so that the lipid is suited for and supports the function of the cell or organelle. This process is performed by removing a fatty acid side chain from a target lipid by (phospho)lipases, forming a lysolipid, followed by reacylation of the lysolipid by either acyl-CoA-dependent acylases

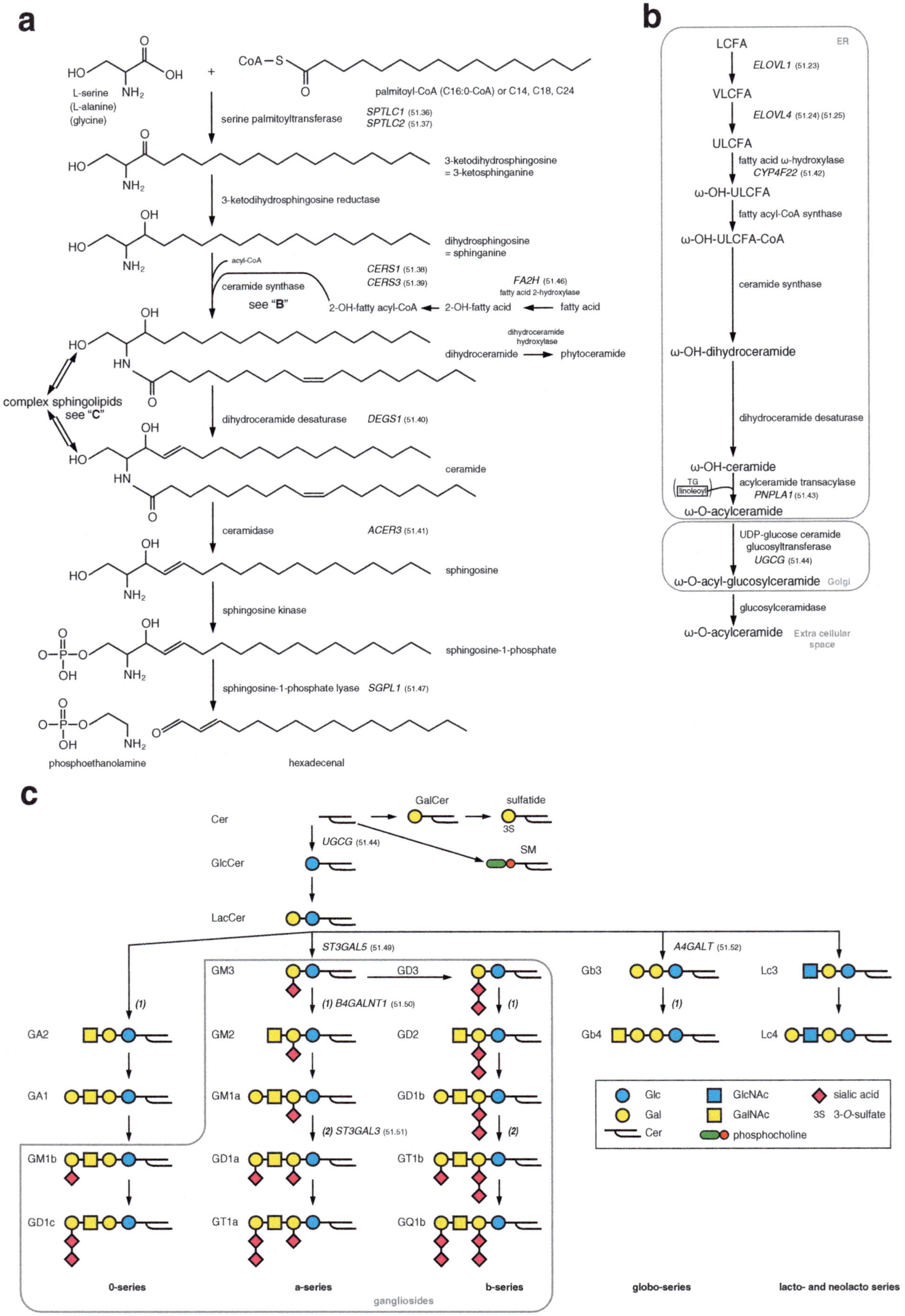
a
L-serine
(L-alanine)
(glycine)
palmitoyl-CoA (C16:0-CoA) or C14, C18, C24
serine palmitoyltransferase
SPTLC1 (51.36)
SPTLC2 (51.37)
3-ketodihydrosphingosine
= 3-ketosphinganine
3-ketodihydrosphingosine reductase
dihydrosphingosine
= sphinganine
acyl-CoA
ceramide synthase
see "B"
CERS1 (51.38)
CERS3 (51.39)
FA2H (51.46)
fatty acid 2-hydroxylase
2-OH-fatty acyl-CoA
2-OH-fatty acid
fatty acid
dihydroceramide hydroxylase
dihydroceramide
phytoceramide
complex sphingolipids
see "C"
dihydroceramide desaturase
DEGS1 (51.40)
ceramide
ceramidase
ACER3 (51.41)
sphingosine
sphingosine kinase
sphingosine-1-phosphate
sphingosine-1-phosphate lyase
SGPL1 (51.47)
phosphoethanolamine
hexadecenal
b
LCFA
ER
ELOVL1 (51.23)
VLCFA
ELOVL4 (51.24) (51.25)
ULCFA
fatty acid ω-hydroxylase
CYP4F22 (51.42)
ω-OH-ULCFA
fatty acyl-CoA synthase
ω-OH-ULCFA-CoA
ceramide synthase
ω-OH-dihydroceramide
dihydroceramide desaturase
ω-OH-ceramide
TG
linoleoyl
acylceramide transacylase
PNPLA1 (51.43)
ω-O-acylceramide
UDP-glucose ceramide
glucosyltransferase
UGCG (51.44)
ω-O-acyl-glucosylceramide
Golgi
glucosylceramidase
ω-O-acylceramide
Extra cellular space
c
Cer
GalCer
sulfatide
3S
UGCG (51.44)
GlcCer
SM
LacCer
ST3GAL5 (51.49)
A4GALT (51.52)
GM3
GD3
Gb3
Lc3
(1)
(1) B4GALNT1 (51.50)
GA2
GM2
GD2
Gb4
Lc4
GA1
GM1a
GD1b
(2) ST3GAL3 (51.51)
(2)
GM1b
GD1a
GT1b
GD1c
GT1a
GQ1b
Glc
Gal
GlcNAc
GalNAc
sialic acid
3S 3-O-sulfate
Cer
phosphocholine
0-series
a-series
b-series
gangliosides
globo-series
lacto- and neolacto series

or by transacylation by so-called transacylases. Transacylases use one of the fatty acids of a donor lipid to reacylate the target lysolipid yielding an acylated lipid (from the target) and a new lysolipid (from the donor). Many of the described disorders are caused by a defect in remodeling of particular lipid species. An overly represented class of genes/proteins in this chapter is the calcium-independent phospholipases of the patatin-like phospholipase domain-containing lipase A (PNPLA) family that has a total of nine members. PNPLAs are active at both *sn*-1 and *sn*-2 positions of phospholipids, depending on its substrate and also can have transacylase activity (Hermansson et al. 2016). Deficiency of the structurally similar PNPLAs 1, 2, 6, 8, and 9 leads to very different disorders as a result of their diverse functions in lipid metabolism (Sects. 51.2.4.8, 51.2.3.6, 51.2.1.15, 51.2.1.4, and 51.2.1.12, respectively).

## Clinical Spectrum of Disorders of Complex Lipid Metabolism in Brief

The clinical spectrum of these disorders is wide and will be presented in more detail in the following sections. Most frequently, the central nervous system is affected which can present with related signs and symptoms (e.g., intellectual disability, developmental delays, (complex) hereditary spastic paraplegia, movement disorder, optic atrophy, hearing loss, etc.). Like other inborn errors of metabolism affecting complex systems such as mitochondrial disorders and congenital disorders of glycosylation, every organ (system) can be affected, which adds to the diversity of symptoms. These include lipodystrophy, insulin resistance, bone abnormalities, recurrent rhabdomyolysis, ichthyosis, anemia, protein-losing enteropathy, and pigmentary retinopathies.

## Chapter Structure

For this chapter, we have divided the metabolism and disorders into five parts: (1) phospholipid and neutral lipid metabolism (Fig. 51.2), (2) fatty acid synthesis and elongation (Figs. 51.2 and 51.3), (3) triglyceride/lipid droplet metabolism (Fig. 51.2), (4) sphingolipid metabolism (Fig. 51.4), and (5) a miscellaneous category. The identification of these disorders mostly has been done by molecular analysis using next-generation sequencing. Given the very wide spectrum of gene functions, if known at all, and the fact that specific diagnostic biomarkers and/or treatments are frequently not available/known, we have chosen a different structure for

**Fig. 51.4** Sphingolipid metabolism, including disease genes. (**a**) Synthesis and degradation of ceramide in the ER. L-Serine condenses with an acyl-CoA (mainly palmitoyl-CoA) to form 3-ketodihydrosphingosine (3-ketosphinganine) by the combined action of serine palmitoyltransferases (SPT) 1, 2, and 3. Alanine or glycine can also be used (instead of serine), yielding 1-deoxysphinganine (from alanine) and 1-deoxymethylsphinganine (from glycine). After reduction of the keto-function to a hydroxyl group by 3-ketodihydrosphingosine reductase, dihydrosphingosine (sphinganine) is produced. Ceramide synthases (*CERS* 1–6) catalyze the condensation of sphinganine with a fatty acyl-CoA on the primary amino group yielding dihydroceramide. Fatty acid 2-hydroxylase (encoded by *FA2H*) can hydroxylate fatty acids at the 2-position, which, after activation to its corresponding 2-OH-acyl-CoA, can be used by ceramide synthases to form 2-OH-ceramides and downstream complex sphingolipids. Dihydroceramide desaturase (encoded by *DEGS1*) creates a trans-double bond at the 4-position that converts the base type from sphinganine to sphingosine and thus yields ceramide. Alternatively, hydroxylation of dihydroceramides by dihydroceramide hydroxylase can lead to the formation of phytoceramides. These different ceramide species can be used to synthesize complex sphingolipids as shown in the remainder of the figure. For the degradation of ceramides, ceramidases (including that encoded by *ACER3*) are responsible for the hydrolysis of the amide bond of ceramide, thereby creating sphingosine and a fatty acid. Sphingosine can be phosphorylated by sphingosine kinases to sphingosine-1-phosphate. Sphingosine-1-phosphate can be cleaved by sphingosine-1-phosphate lyase (encoded by *SGPL1*) yielding a fatty aldehyde (in case of the C18-base shown here; hexadecenal) and phosphoethanolamine. (**b**) ω-O-Acylceramide synthesis. This pathway is especially relevant as ω-O-acylceramides are required for skin permeability barrier formation. Long-chain fatty acids (LCFA) are elongated via very long-chain fatty acids (VLCFA) to ultra-long-chain fatty acids (ULCFA) by *ELOVL1* and *ELOVL4*. The cytochrome P450 enzyme encoded by *CYP4F22* catalyzes the ω-hydroxylation of ULCFA creating ω-OH-ULCFA. After activation to its corresponding CoA-ester, ceramide synthases use ω-OH-ULCFA-CoA to synthesize ω-OH-ceramides. Acylceramide transacylase (encoded by *PNPLA1*) uses a linoleoyl-containing TG to transfer the linoleic acid from TG to the ω-OH group of ω-OH-ceramide yielding ω-O-acylceramide. In the Golgi, UDP-glucose ceramide glucosyltransferase (encoded by *UGCG*) converts ω-O-acylceramide into ω-O-acyl-glucosylceramide, and this molecule is excreted in the extracellular space where glucosylceramidase cleaves off the glucose and thereby regenerates the ω-O-acylceramide to contribute to the lipid lamellae formation of the skin. (**c**) Complex sphingolipid synthesis. Complex sphingolipids are synthesized by the stepwise addition of monosaccharides to ceramide, with the exception of sphingomyelin (SM) where a phosphocholine headgroup is added. Different glycosyltransferases use nucleotide-activated sugars to yield a plethora of glycosphingolipids which takes place mainly in the Golgi. First, glucosylceramide (GlcCer) is produced by UDP-glucose ceramide glucosyltransferase (encoded by *UGCG*) followed by addition of galactose yielding lactosylceramide (LacCer) which is at the main branching point of glycosphingolipids. The action of different glycosyltransferase on LacCer initiates different glycosphingolipid series including ganglio-, globo-, lacto-, and neolacto-series. The presence of N-acetylneuraminic acid = sialic acid makes a glycosphingolipid a "ganglioside"

this chapter. For each disorder, in addition to the signs and symptoms tables, we have separately listed their function, a brief clinical synopsis, and if known/available specific treatment options, other than supportive care.

## Signs, and Symptoms

### Phospholipid and Neutral Lipid Metabolism

#### Acylglycerol Kinase Deficiency AGK, Sengers Syndrome, AGK → See 72.04

**Function:** The mitochondrially located AGK catalyzes the phosphorylation formation of diacylglycerol (DG) and, with lesser affinity, monoacylglycerol (MG) forming phosphatidic acid (PA) and lysophosphatidic acid (LPA), respectively (Fig. 51.2a). In addition to being a lipid kinase at the hinge of neutral lipid and phospholipid metabolism, AGK is believed to be part of the TIM22 import complex that supports the import of a subset of multi-spanning membrane proteins. AGK deficiency causes reduced levels of adenine nucleotide translocator (ANT, SLC25A4) in the heart and muscle, which can lead to multiple respiratory chain complex deficiency. The import function is independent of the lipid kinase activity of AGK, which is required for maintaining mitochondrial cristae integrity (Vukotic et al. 2017; Kang et al. 2017).

**Clinical:** AGK deficiency is characterized by congenital cataracts, hypertrophic cardiomyopathy, skeletal myopathy, and exercise intolerance. The metabolic feature is lactic acidosis (Table 51.1).

#### SERAC1 Deficiency, 3-Methylglutaconic Aciduria with Deafness, Encephalopathy, and Leigh-Like Syndrome (MEGD(H)EL), SERAC1 → See 72.03

**Function:** SERAC1 is localized at the interface of mitochondria and endoplasmic reticulum where it is believed to be involved in phosphatidylglycerol (PG) remodeling (Fig. 51.2a); however, its exact function has not been determined. Additional abnormalities were seen in downstream products of PG, cardiolipin (CL), and bis(monoacylglycero) phosphate (BMP) as well as possible abnormalities of cholesterol trafficking.

**Clinical:** The main features of *SERAC1* deficiency are 3-methylglutaconic aciduria, dystonia-deafness, hepatopathy, encephalopathy, and Leigh-like syndrome, basing the acronym MEGDHEL syndrome. Lactic acidosis and/or respiratory chain complex deficiency in different tissues can be seen (Table 51.2).

#### Tafazzin Deficiency, Barth Syndrome, TAZ → See 72.02

**Function:** The *TAZ* gene encodes a mitochondrial transacylase that is involved in the remodeling of CL. TAZ deficiency causes accumulation of monolysocardiolipins (three instead of four fatty acid side chains) and deficiency of linoleic acid-enriched CL species (Fig. 51.2a).

**Clinical:** Main features of TAZ deficiency are cardiomyopathy, muscle weakness, short stature (when young), and neutropenia. Biochemically, CL metabolism is disturbed which causes monolysocardiolipin accumulation and CL deficiency in addition to impaired oxidative phosphorylation and 3-methylglutaconic aciduria (Table 51.3). A specific blood spot/lymphocyte/fibroblast test based on this biochemical

**Table 51.1** Acylglycerol kinase deficiency

| System | Symptoms and biomarkers | Neonatal (birth–1 month) | Infancy (1–18 months) | Childhood (1.5–11 years) | Adolescence (11–16 years) | Adulthood (>16 years) |
|---|---|---|---|---|---|---|
| Cardiovascular | **Cardiomyopathy, hypertrophic** | + | + | + | + | |
| Eye | **Cataract** | + | + | | | |
| Musculoskeletal | Exercise Intolerance | ± | + | + | + | |
| | Myopathy | + | + | | | |
| | Skeletal myopathy | ± | ± | | | |
| Other | Death | ± | ± | ± | ± | |
| Laboratory findings | 3-Methylglutaconic acid (urine) | ↑ | ↑ | ↑ | ↑ | |
| | Lactate (plasma) | ↑ | ↑ | ↑ | ↑ | |

**Table 51.2** SERAC1 deficiency

| System | Symptoms and biomarkers | Neonatal (birth–1 month) | Infancy (1–18 months) | Childhood (1.5–11 years) | Adolescence (11–16 years) | Adulthood (>16 years) |
|---|---|---|---|---|---|---|
| CNS | **Basal ganglia abnormalities (MRI)** | + | + | + | + | + |
| | **Bilateral hyperintensities of basal ganglia (MRI)** | + | + | + | + | + |
| | **Bilateral sensory hearing loss** | + | + | + | + | + |
| | **Cerebellar atrophy (MRI)** | + | + | + | + | + |
| | **Cerebral atrophy (MRI)** | + | + | + | + | + |
| | **Dystonia** | + | + | + | + | + |
| | **Encephalopathy** | + | + | + | + | + |
| | Epilepsy | ± | ± | ± | ± | ± |
| | **Extrapyramidal signs** | + | + | + | + | + |
| | Leigh syndrome | + | + | + | ± | ± |
| | **Leigh-like lesions (MRI)** | + | + | + | + | + |
| | Metabolic stroke | ± | + | + | + | + |
| | Regression | + | + | + | + | + |
| | Regression, motor | ± | + | + | + | + |
| | Retardation | + | + | + | + | + |
| | **Retardation, psychomotor** | + | + | + | + | + |
| | Spasticity | ± | + | + | + | + |
| Digestive | Feeding difficulties | + | + | + | ± | ± |
| Ear | Deafness, sensorineural | ± | + | + | + | + |
| Hematological | Sepsis | + | + | + | ± | ± |
| Metabolic | Hypoglycemia | ± | ± | ± | ± | ± |
| Other | Failure to thrive | + | + | + | ± | ± |
| Psychiatric | Behavioral disorder | ± | + | + | + | + |
| Laboratory findings | 3-Hydroxyisovaleric acid (urine) | n | n | n | n | n |
| | 3-Methylglutaconic acid (urine) | ↑↑ | ↑↑ | ↑↑ | ↑↑ | ↑↑ |
| | Anion gap | + | ± | + | + | + |
| | Filipin test | + | + | + | + | + |
| | Glucose (plasma) | ↓–n | ↓–n | ↓–n | ↓–n | ↓–n |
| | Lactate (cerebrospinal fluid) | n–↑↑ | n–↑↑ | n–↑↑ | n–↑↑ | n–↑↑ |
| | Lactate (plasma) | n–↑↑↑ | n–↑↑↑ | n–↑↑↑ | n–↑↑↑ | n–↑↑↑ |

abnormality is available for rapid functional diagnostics of this disorder (Houtkooper et al. 2009).

### PNPLA8 Deficiency, Mitochondrial Myopathy with Lactic Acidosis, PNPLA8

**Function:** *PNPLA8* encodes the calcium-independent phospholipase A2γ (iPLA2γ) (Fig. 51.2a) which is a member of the patatin-like phospholipase domain-containing lipase (PNPL) family and is active at both *sn*-1 and *sn*-2 positions of phospholipids, depending on its substrate. Different isoforms are localized to mitochondria, peroxisomes, and possibly also to the ER, where iPLA2γ is believed to be involved (based on mouse models) in the remodeling of phospholipids, in particular plasmalogens containing essential fatty acids as arachidonic acid (AA, C20:4ω6), docosahexaenoic acid (DHA, C22:6ω3), and linoleic acid (LA, C18:2ω6). The activity of iPLA2γ toward arachidonic acid containing PC species is activated by the presence of CL. iPLA2γ also has been shown to deacylate oxidized CL and is suggested to have a role in managing mitochondrial oxidative stress (Liu et al. 2017).

**Clinical:** Only three patients reported from two pedigrees. Patients show progressive muscle weakness, severe global developmental delay, as well as loss of very early milestones, epilepsy, and cardiomyopathy (Saunders et al. 2015; Shukla et al. 2018). Lactic acidosis has been reported. In mice models, CL content was also affected as well as mitochondrial morphology and function (Table 51.4) (Hara et al. 2019).

**Table 51.3** Taffazin deficiency

| System | Symptoms and biomarkers | Neonatal (birth–1 month) | Infancy (1–18 months) | Childhood (1.5–11 years) | Adolescence (11–16 years) | Adulthood (>16 years) |
|---|---|---|---|---|---|---|
| Cardiovascular | Cardiac arrhythmia | ± | ± | ± | ± | ± |
| | **Cardiomyopathy** | + | + | + | + | + |
| | Cardiomyopathy, dilated | ± | + | + | + | + |
| | Clots, stroke | ± | ± | ± | ± | ± |
| | Heart Failure | ± | ± | ± | ± | ± |
| | Left ventricular non-compaction | ± | + | + | + | + |
| CNS | Occasionally cerebral atrophy | ± | ± | ± | ± | ± |
| Dermatological | Chronic aphthous ulceration | ± | ± | ± | ± | ± |
| Digestive | Feeding difficulties | + | + | ± | ± | ± |
| | Vomiting | ± | ± | ± | ± | ± |
| Hematological | **Neutropenia** | + | + | + | + | + |
| | Sepsis | ± | ± | ± | ± | ± |
| Metabolic | Metabolic acidosis | ± | ± | ± | ± | ± |
| | Hypoglycemia | ± | ± | ± | ± | ± |
| Musculoskeletal | Exercise Intolerance | ± | ± | ± | ± | ± |
| | **Growth retardation** | ± | + | + | + | + |
| | Hypotonia, muscular-axial | + | + | + | ± | ± |
| | **Myopathy** | + | + | + | + | + |
| Other | Mild dysmorphic features | ± | ± | ± | ± | ± |
| | Cherubic face | | ± | ± | | |
| Respiratory | Respiratory distress | ± | ± | ± | ± | ± |
| Laboratory findings | 2-Ethylhydracrylic acid (urine) | n–↑ | n–↑ | n–↑ | n–↑ | n–↑ |
| | 3-Methylglutaconic acid (urine) | ↑–↑↑ | ↑–↑↑ | ↑–↑↑ | ↑–↑↑ | ↑–↑↑ |
| | 3-Methylglutaric acid (urine) | ↑ | ↑ | ↑ | ↑ | ↑ |
| | Abnormal cardiolipin profile (blood spot, lymphocytes) | + | + | + | + | + |
| | Ammonia (blood) | n–↑ | n–↑ | n–↑ | n–↑ | n–↑ |
| | Cardiolipin (fibroblasts) | ↓ | ↓ | ↓ | ↓ | ↓ |
| | Cardiolipin (tissue) | ↓ | ↓ | ↓ | ↓ | ↓ |
| | Carnitine, free (dried blood spot) | ↓–n | ↓–n | ↓–n | ↓–n | ↓–n |
| | Carnitine, free (plasma) | ↓–n | ↓–n | ↓–n | ↓–n | ↓–n |
| | Cholesterol (serum) | ↓–n | ↓–n | ↓–n | ↓–n | ↓–n |
| | Creatine kinase (plasma) | n–↑ | n–↑ | n–↑ | n–↑ | n–↑ |
| | Glucose (plasma) | ↓–n | ↓–n | ↓–n | ↓–n | ↓–n |
| | Lactate (plasma) | n–↑ | n–↑ | n–↑ | n–↑ | n–↑ |
| | Uric acid (plasma) | n–↑ | n–↑ | n–↑ | n–↑ | n–↑ |

### Ethanolaminephosphotransferase 1 Deficiency, SELENOI

**Function:** *SELENOI* encodes ethanolaminephosphotransferase 1 and is also known as selenoprotein 1 (Fig. 51.2). It catalyzes the final step in Kennedy pathway that makes ethanolamine glycerophospholipids PE and PE[O] from CDP-ethanolamine and DG or DG[O] (Table 51.5).

**Clinical:** Only five patients from two pedigrees. Severe developmental delay, intellectual disability, demyelinating peripheral neuropathy, pigmentary retinopathy, sensorineural hearing loss, and epilepsy. Lipidomics showed that especially ether lipid metabolism is affected with increases of alkyl-species of PC[O] and decreases of PE[O] plasmalogens in patient fibroblasts (Horibata et al. 2018; Ahmed et al. 2017).

**Table 51.4** PNPLA8 deficiency

| System | Symptoms and biomarkers | Neonatal (birth–1 month) | Infancy (1–18 months) | Childhood (1.5–11 years) | Adolescence (11–16 years) | Adulthood (>16 years) |
|---|---|---|---|---|---|---|
| CNS | Dysarthria | | + | + | | |
| | Dysmetria | + | + | + | | |
| | Dystonia | | + | + | | |
| | Fatigue | | + | + | | |
| | Hypotonia | + | + | + | | |
| | Seizures, complex partial | + | + | + | | |
| | **Spasticity** | + | + | + | | |
| Metabolic | Lactic acidosis | + | + | + | | |
| Musculoskeletal | Gower sign | + | + | + | | |
| | Muscle weakness, proximal | + | + | + | | |
| | **Thin body habitus** | | + | + | | |
| | Toe-walking | | + | + | | |
| Laboratory findings | Lactate (plasma) | ↑ | ↑ | ↑ | | |
| | Pyruvate (plasma) | ↑ | ↑ | ↑ | | |

**Table 51.5** Ethanolaminephosphotransferase 1 deficiency

| System | Symptoms and biomarkers | Neonatal (birth–1 month) | Infancy (1–18 months) | Childhood (1.5–11 years) | Adolescence (11–16 years) | Adulthood (>16 years) |
|---|---|---|---|---|---|---|
| CNS | Developmental delay | | + | + | + | + |
| | Developmental regression | | + | + | + | + |
| | Epileptic seizures | | + | + | + | + |
| | Intellectual disability, mild | | + | + | + | + |
| | Microcephaly | | + | + | + | + |
| | Neuropathy, peripheral, demyelinating | | + | + | + | + |
| | Progressive spastic paraplegia | | + | + | + | + |
| | White matter abnormalities (MRI) | | + | + | + | + |
| Digestive | Bifid uvula | | + | + | + | + |
| Eye | Cone-rod dystrophy | | + | + | + | + |
| | Hyperpigmentation retina | | + | + | + | + |
| Musculoskeletal | Cleft palate | | + | + | + | + |

### Phosphoethanolamine Cytidylyltransferase 2 Deficiency, PCYT2

**Function:** *PCYT2* encodes CTP/phosphoethanolamine cytidylyltransferase (ET) which is the rate-limiting enzyme for PE synthesis via the CDP-ethanolamine pathway (Vaz et al. 2019). ET catalyzes the conversion of CTP and phosphoethanolamine into CDP-ethanolamine. CDP-ethanolamine is then used for the synthesis of PE and PE[O] via condensation with DG or DG[O] (Fig. 51.2).

**Clinical:** One report of four individuals from three families with biallelic *PCYT2* variants with a complex HSP. Patients suffered from global developmental delay with regression, spastic para- or tetraparesis, epilepsy, and progressive cerebral and cerebellar atrophy (Table 51.6) (Vaz et al. 2019).

### Choline Kinase β Deficiency, Congenital Muscular Dystrophy, Megaconial Type, CHKB

**Function:** *CHKB* encodes choline kinase β which catalyzes the phosphorylation of choline to phosphocholine that is used to synthesize PC and PC[O] (Fig. 51.2).

**Clinical:** Congenital muscular dystrophy, cardiomyopathy, developmental delay, intellectual disability, and in the muscle biopsy; peculiar enlarged mitochondria (megaconial) that are prevalent toward the periphery of the fibers but are sparse in the center of the muscle biopsy. Choline kinase activity in muscle tissue was undetectable and decreased PC levels were found (Table 51.7) (Mitsuhashi et al. 2011).

**Phosphocholine Cytidylyltransferase 1α Deficiency, Retinoskeletal Phenotype, PCYT1A**

**Function:** *PCYT1A* encodes the α-form of choline-phosphate cytidylyltransferase that catalyzes the conversion of phosphocholine into CDP-choline (Fig. 51.2). This is the rate-limiting step of PC and PC[O] synthesis (Table 51.8).

**Clinical:** Only two reports, 12 patients from 8 pedigrees. Short stature, spondylometaphyseal dysplasia, progressive lower limb bowing, and cone-rod dystrophy (Hoover-Fong et al. 2014; Yamamoto et al. 2014).

**Phosphocholine Cytidylyltransferase 1α Deficiency, Lipodystrophy Phenotype, PCYT1A**

**Function:** See Sect. Retinoskeletal Phenotype

**Clinical:** Only two patients from two pedigrees. Lipodystrophy, severe insulin resistance, low HDL cholesterol levels, and insulin resistance (Table 51.9) (Payne et al. 2014).

**Phosphatidylserine Decarboxylase Deficiency, PISD**

**Function:** *PISD* encodes phosphatidylserine decarboxylase (PSD) that converts PS to PE in the inner mitochondrial membrane. After production of the PSD enzyme, an autocatalytic processing event generates two subunits (α and β) which is required to form a functional PSD enzyme. In cellular models, severe depletion or complete loss of PSD

**Table 51.6** Phosphoethanolamine cytidylyltransferase 2 deficiency

| System | Symptoms and biomarkers | Neonatal (birth–1 month) | Infancy (1–18 months) | Childhood (1.5–11 years) | Adolescence (11–16 years) | Adulthood (>16 years) |
|---|---|---|---|---|---|---|
| CNS | Ataxia, cerebellar | | + | + | + | + |
| | Cerebellar atrophy (MRI) | | + | + | + | + |
| | Cerebral white matter involvement (MRI) | | + | + | + | + |
| | Developmental delay | | + | + | + | + |
| | Epileptic seizures | | + | + | + | + |
| | Intellectual disability | | + | + | + | + |
| | Intellectual disability | | + | + | + | + |
| | Progressive spastic paraplegia | | + | + | + | + |
| | Regression | | + | + | + | + |
| | Regression | | + | + | + | + |
| Eye | Nystagmus | | + | + | + | + |

**Table 51.7** Choline kinase β deficiency

| System | Symptoms and biomarkers | Neonatal (birth–1 month) | Infancy (1–18 months) | Childhood (1.5–11 years) | Adolescence (11–16 years) | Adulthood (>16 years) |
|---|---|---|---|---|---|---|
| Cardiovascular | Cardiomyopathy | + | + | + | + | + |
| CNS | Developmental delay | + | + | + | + | + |
| | Epileptic seizures | + | + | + | + | + |
| | Hypotonia, generalized | + | + | + | + | + |
| | Intellectual disability | + | + | + | + | + |
| | Microcephaly | + | + | + | + | + |
| Metabolic | Mitochondrial DNA-depletion (muscle) | + | + | + | + | + |
| Musculoskeletal | Muscular dystrophy | + | + | + | + | + |
| | EM, Abnormal mitochondria (muscle) | + | + | + | + | + |
| Laboratory findings | Creatine kinase (plasma) | ↑ | ↑ | ↑ | ↑ | ↑ |
| | Histolochemistry, abnormal fibres (muscle) | + | + | + | + | + |
| | Phosphatidylcholine/ Phosphatidylethanolamine ratio (muscle) | ↓↓↓ | ↓↓↓ | ↓↓↓ | ↓↓↓ | ↓↓↓ |
| | Respiratory chain activity (muscle) | ↓ | ↓ | ↓ | ↓ | ↓ |

**Table 51.8** Phosphocholine cytidylyltransferase 1α deficiency, retinoskeletal phenotype

| System | Symptoms and biomarkers | Neonatal (birth–1 month) | Infancy (1–18 months) | Childhood (1.5–11 years) | Adolescence (11–16 years) | Adulthood (>16 years) |
|---|---|---|---|---|---|---|
| Eye | **Cone-rod dystrophy** | ± | + | + | + | + |
| | Subtype with isolated retinopathy | ± | + | + | + | + |
| Musculoskeletal | Bowing of lower limbs, progressive | ± | + | + | + | + |
| | Short stature | ± | + | + | + | + |
| | **Spondylometaphyseal dysplasia** | ± | + | + | + | + |
| Laboratory findings | Cholesterol (serum) | ↓ | ↓ | ↓ | ↓ | ↓ |
| | HDL cholesterol (plasma) | ↓ | ↓ | ↓ | ↓ | ↓ |
| | Triglyceride (serum) | ↓ | ↓ | ↓ | ↓ | ↓ |

**Table 51.9** Phosphocholine cytidylyltransferase 1α deficiency, lipodystrophy phenotype

| System | Symptoms and biomarkers | Neonatal (birth–1 month) | Infancy (1–18 months) | Childhood (1.5–11 years) | Adolescence (11–16 years) | Adulthood (>16 years) |
|---|---|---|---|---|---|---|
| Digestive | **Liver steatosis** | ± | ± | ± | + | + |
| Endocrine | **Diabetes mellitus** | ± | ± | ± | + | + |
| Other | **Body fat percentage, low** | ± | ± | ± | + | + |
| | **Body mass index, low** | ± | ± | ± | + | + |
| | **Lipodystrophy, partial** | ± | ± | ± | + | + |
| Laboratory findings | HDL cholesterol (plasma) | ↓ | ↓ | ↓ | ↓ | ↓ |
| | Triglyceride (serum) | ↑ | ↑ | ↑ | ↑ | ↑ |

results in decreased mitochondrial oxidative phosphorylation and fragmentation of the mitochondrial network. The complete loss of PSD is embryonically lethal in mice; heterozygote animals show no disease phenotype (Zhao et al. 2019; Girisha et al. 2019).

**Clinical:** Four patients from three families have been reported for this disorder. Two siblings were reported with congenital cataracts in early infancy, progressive sensorineural hearing loss, global developmental delay (mild), short stature with skeletal dysplasia, facial dysmorphism (midface hypoplasia and a depressed nasal ridge), and white matter changes with progressive volume loss and hypomyelination of the corpus callosum (Zhao et al. 2019). Two additional younger individuals were reported with spondyloepimetaphyseal dysplasia with severe platyspondyly (Girisha et al. 2019).

Biochemically, patient-derived fibroblasts showed fragmented mitochondrial morphology and mitochondrial dysfunction which was linked to the (mitochondrial) lack of the fusogenic lipid PE (the product of PSD reaction). Addition of either ethanolamine (Girisha et al. 2019) or lyso-PE (Zhao et al. 2019) appeared to restore the morphological and functional mitochondrial defects. PSD activity was decreased to 50% of control in PSD fibroblasts, and it was shown that the reported point mutation variants of both reports affect the autocatalytic cleavage of PSD needed for functional activity (Table 51.10) (Zhao et al. 2019).

#### Phosphatidylserine Synthase 1 Superactivity, Lenz-Majewski Syndrome, PTDSS1

**Function:** *PTDSS1* encodes phosphatidylserine synthase 1 (PSS1) which is one of the two enzymes that synthesizes PS. PSS1 synthesizes PS through the exchange of serine with the choline moiety of PC (Fig. 51.2a).

**Clinical:** Sclerosing bone dysplasia, developmental delay, intellectual disability, and distinct craniofacial, dental, skin- (cutis laxa), and distal-limb anomalies. All patients harbor de novo heterozygous pathogenic variants that render PSS1 insensitive to feedback inhibition by PS levels leading to enhanced PS synthesis. Recent studies have shown that the pathogenic variants found in Lenz-Majewski syndrome patients also disturb the metabolism of phosphorylated PI species at the Golgi and the plasma membrane (Table 51.11) (Sohn et al. 2016).

**Table 51.10** Phosphatidylserine decarboxylase deficiency

| System | Symptoms and biomarkers | Neonatal (birth–1 month) | Infancy (1–18 months) | Childhood (1.5–11 years) | Adolescence (11–16 years) | Adulthood (>16 years) |
|---|---|---|---|---|---|---|
| CNS | Developmental delay | | ± | ± | ± | ± |
| Ear | Progressive sensorineural hearing loss | | | | | ± |
| Eye | Cataract | | ± | | | |
| Musculoskeletal | Facial dysmorphism | | | + | + | + |
| | Short stature | | + | + | + | + |
| | Skeletal dysplasia | | ± | + | + | + |
| Laboratory findings | PSD activity (fibroblasts) | | ↓–n | | ↓–n | |

**Table 51.11** Phosphatidylserine synthase 1 superactivity

| System | Symptoms and biomarkers | Neonatal (birth–1 month) | Infancy (1–18 months) | Childhood (1.5–11 years) | Adolescence (11–16 years) | Adulthood (>16 years) |
|---|---|---|---|---|---|---|
| CNS | Cervical myelopathy | ± | ± | ± | ± | ± |
| | Hydrocephalus | + | + | + | + | + |
| | Intellectual disability | + | + | + | + | + |
| Dermatological | Cutis laxa | + | + | + | + | + |
| Musculoskeletal | Brachydactyly | + | + | + | + | + |
| | Dwarfism | + | + | + | + | + |
| | **Dysmorphic features** | + | + | + | + | + |
| | **Hyperostosis, generalized** | + | + | + | + | + |
| | Macrocephaly | + | + | + | + | + |
| | **Sclerosing bone dysplasia** | + | + | + | + | + |
| | Short stature | + | + | + | + | + |
| Other | Enamel hypoplasia | + | + | + | + | + |
| | Failure to thrive | + | + | + | + | + |

### Phospholipase A2 Group 6 Deficiency, Infantile Neuroaxonal Dystrophy; Seitelberger Disease; Neurodegeneration with Brain Iron Accumulation Type 2B, PLA2G6

**Function:** *PLA2G6* encodes iPLA2-VI or iPLA$_2$β, a calcium-independent phospholipase from the patatin-like lipase family (also known as *PNPLA9*). It demonstrates no substrate specificity and manifests lipase activity on the *sn*-1 and *sn*-2 position but also lysophospholipase and transacylase activities. Function is unclear. It is likely involved in phospholipid remodeling and has been implicated in nitric oxide-induced or vasopressin-induced arachidonic acid release and in leukotriene and prostaglandin production. Under basal conditions, iPLA$_2$β is predominantly localized in the cytosol, and stimulatory conditions translocate iPLA$_2$β to the Golgi, ER, mitochondria, and nucleus. A role in cardiolipin remodeling was suggested (Table 51.12) (Ramanadham et al. 2015).

**Clinical:** *PLA2G6*-associated neurodegeneration (PLAN). The clinical phenotypes and genotypes of PLAN are closely intertwined and vary widely. Depending on the age of onset and progressive clinical features, there are PLAN subtypes: infantile neuroaxonal dystrophy (INAD), idiopathic neurodegeneration with brain iron accumulation (NBIA), atypical neuroaxonal dystrophy (ANAD), and parkinsonian syndrome which contains adult-onset dystonia-parkinsonism (DP) and autosomal recessive early-onset parkinsonism (AREP) (Guo et al. 2018).

### Phosphatidic Acid-Preferring Phospholipase 1 Deficiency, Autosomal Recessive Spastic Paraplegia Type 28 (SPG28), DDHD1

**Function:** *DDHD1* encodes phosphatidic acid-preferring phospholipase A1. DDHD is the amino acid code sequence, AspAspHisAsp, found in DDHD domain proteins and is involved in the phospholipase activity but also in binding to phosphorylated forms of PI (phosphoinositides) which is believed to be important for specific membrane association to target membranes. *DDHD1* is ubiquitously expressed in human tissues such as the brain and testis, but the physiological role of this enzyme is not clear but is likely involved in remodeling of phospholipids. DDHD1 is mainly localized in cytosol with a partial localization in microsomes and mitochondria. In mouse, DDHD1 was shown to hydrolyze PI/PS to LPI/LPS with *sn*-1 selectivity and to account for a substantial fraction of the PI/PS lipase activity in brain tissue. DDHD1 deletion led to decreased

**Table 51.12** Phospholipase A2 group 6 deficiency

| System | Symptoms and biomarkers | Neonatal (birth–1 month) | Infancy (1–18 months) | Childhood (1.5–11 years) | Adolescence (11–16 years) | Adulthood (>16 years) |
|---|---|---|---|---|---|---|
| CNS | **Adult-onset dystonia parkinson (DP)**[c] | | | | | + |
| | Ataxia | | | ± | ± | ± |
| | **Atypical neuroaxonal dystrophy (ANAD)**[b] | | | | | + |
| | Autism | | | ± | ± | ± |
| | **Autosomal recessive early-onset parkinsonism (AREP)**[d] | | | | | + |
| | Basal ganglia abnormalities (MRI) (iron deposit) | | | ± | ± | ± |
| | Cerebellar atrophy (MRI) | | | ± | ± | ± |
| | Dystrophy, neuroaxonal | | | ± | ± | ± |
| | EEG, abnormal (fast rhythms) | | | ± | ± | ± |
| | Epilepsy | | | ± | ± | ± |
| | Extrapyramidal movement disorder | | | ± | ± | ± |
| | Hypotonia, truncal | | | ± | ± | ± |
| | **Infantile neuroaxonal dystrophy (INAD)**[a] | | | | | + |
| | Interictal nystagmus | | | ± | ± | ± |
| | Nerve conduction velocity, decreased | | | ± | ± | ± |
| | Neurodegeneration with brain iron accumulation (NBIA) | | | ± | ± | ± |
| | Parkinsonism, hypokinetic features | | | ± | ± | ± |
| | Regression, psychomotor | | | ± | ± | ± |
| | Spasticity | | | ± | ± | ± |
| | Tetraparesis | | | ± | ± | ± |
| Eye | Optic atrophy | | | ± | ± | ± |
| | Strabismus | | | ± | ± | ± |
| Musculoskeletal | EMG, abnormal | | | ± | ± | ± |
| Laboratory findings | Iron (brain) | | | ± | ± | ± |

[a]Tetraparesis, truncal hypotonia, dystonia, mental deterioration, cerebellar ataxia, spsticity, optic atrophy, epilepsy
[b]Psychomotor regression, seizure, gait instability, autism, dystonia, dysarthria, eye movement abnormalities, epilepsy, cerebellar ataxia, hypermyotonia
[c]Hypermyotonia, extrapyramidal signs
[d]Bradykinesia, rigidity, tremor

levels of polyunsaturated fatty acids arachidonic acid (AA, C20:4ω6) and docosahexaenoic acid (DHA, C22:6ω3) in lysolipids, particularly lyso-PI (Inloes et al. 2018a) (Fig. 51.2a).

**Clinical:** Autosomal recessive spastic paraplegia type 28 (SPG28): complex HSP with retinal dystrophy and neurodegeneration with brain iron accumulation (NBIA) (Table 51.13).

### Phosphatidic Acid-Preferring Phospholipase 2 Deficiency, Autosomal Recessive Spastic Paraplegia Type 54 (SPG54), DDHD2

**Function:** *DDHD2* encodes phosphatidic acid-preferring phospholipase 2, also known as KIAA0725p, which is ubiquitously expressed and localized to or proximal to ER and Golgi. Functionally (from mouse/rat work), DDHD2 was shown to hydrolyze both DG and TG and is believed to be the principal TG hydrolase of the lipid droplet in the central nervous system (Inloes et al. 2014).

**Clinical:** Autosomal recessive spastic paraplegia type 54 (SPG54), pure or complex with developmental delay, intellectual disability, and abnormal eye movements. An abnormal lipid peak was detected in many patients by brain MR spectroscopy. Genetic deletion in mice leads to ectopic lipid droplet accumulation in neurons throughout the brain, and TG accumulation was established (Inloes et al. 2014; Inloes et al. 2018b) suggesting that disturbed neutral lipid metabolism in CNS is relevant for the pathology in *DDHD2* deficiency (Table 51.14).

**Table 51.13** Phosphatidic acid-preferrin phospholipase 1 deficiency

| System | Symptoms and biomarkers | Neonatal (birth–1 month) | Infancy (1–18 months) | Childhood (1.5–11 years) | Adolescence (11–16 years) | Adulthood (>16 years) |
|---|---|---|---|---|---|---|
| CNS | Ataxia, cerebellar | ± | ± | ± | + | + |
| | Axonal sensory motor polyneuropathy, chronic | ± | ± | ± | + | + |
| | Basal ganglia abnormalities (MRI) (iron deposit) | ± | ± | ± | + | + |
| | Hereditary spastic paraparesis | ± | ± | ± | + | + |
| | Intellectual disability | ± | ± | ± | + | + |
| Eye | Cone-rod dystrophy | ± | ± | ± | + | + |
| | Optic atrophy | ± | ± | ± | + | + |
| | Retinal dystrophy | ± | ± | ± | + | + |
| Laboratory findings | Iron (brain) | ± | ± | ± | + | + |

**Table 51.14** Phosphatidic acid-preferrin phospholipase 2 deficiency

| System | Symptoms and biomarkers | Neonatal (birth–1 month) | Infancy (1–18 months) | Childhood (1.5–11 years) | Adolescence (11–16 years) | Adulthood (>16 years) |
|---|---|---|---|---|---|---|
| CNS | Brainstem atrophy (MRI) | | | + | + | + |
| | Bulbar dysfunction | | | + | + | + |
| | Cerebellar atrophy (MRI) | | | + | + | + |
| | Cerebral white matter involvement (MRI) | | | + | + | + |
| | Developmental delay | | | + | + | + |
| | Hereditary spastic paraparesis, complex or pure | | | + | + | + |
| | Hypoplasia, corpus callosum (MRI) | | | + | + | + |
| | Microcephaly | | | + | + | + |
| | Pyramidal signs | | | + | + | + |
| | Syrinx | | | + | + | + |
| Eye | Eye movements, abnormal | | | + | + | + |
| Psychiatric | Behavioral abnormalities | | | + | + | + |

**PNPLA6 Deficiency, Autosomal Recessive Spastic Paraplegia Type 39; Oliver-McFarlane Syndrome; Boucher-Neuhauser Syndrome; Laurence-Moon Syndrome, PNPLA6**

**Function:** *PNPLA6*, also PLPL6 or NTE (neuropathy target esterase), encodes patatin-like phospholipase domain-containing 6 (PNPLA6) also known as iPLA$_2$δ (Fig. 51.2a). It localizes to ER and Golgi and is expressed primarily in neurons. It liberates fatty acid from phospholipids, monoacylglycerols, and lysophospholipids, with a preference for the latter (van Tienhoven et al. 2002). More recent experiments have shown that PNPLA6 catalyzes the sequential double deacylation of PC to yield glycerophosphocholine and two free fatty acids (Quistad et al. 2003; Zaccheo et al. 2004).

**Clinical:** Main symptoms include ataxia, motor neuron disease, hypogonadism, and chorioretinal dystrophy. Homozygous or compound heterozygous *PNPLA6* variants have been identified in:

- Boucher-Neuhauser syndrome: cerebellar ataxia, chorioretinal dystrophy, and hypogonadotropic hypogonadism (Synofzik et al. 2014).
- Gordon Holmes syndrome: cerebellar ataxia, hypogonadotropic hypogonadism, and pyramidal signs (Synofzik et al. 2014).
- Oliver-McFarlane syndrome: trichomegaly, chorioretinal dystrophy, and congenital or childhood hypopituitarism (Hufnagel et al. 2015).
- Laurence-Moon syndrome: cerebellar ataxia, chorioretinal dystrophy, peripheral neuropathy, spastic paraplegia, and congenital or childhood hypopituitarism (Hufnagel et al. 2015).

Overall, disease onset is usually in the first two decades of life with anterior hypopituitarism, visual impairment, gait alterations, or delayed puberty. Gait alterations may precede visual impairment or anterior hypopituitarism. Conversely, gait disturbance may follow visual impairment or hypopituitarism decades later. Gait disturbances are related to cerebel-

**Table 51.15** PNPLA6 deficiency

| System | Symptoms and biomarkers | Neonatal (birth–1 month) | Infancy (1–18 months) | Childhood (1.5–11 years) | Adolescence (11–16 years) | Adulthood (>16 years) |
|---|---|---|---|---|---|---|
| CNS | Ataxia, cerebellar | | | ± | ± | + |
| | Cerebellar atrophy (MRI) | | | | ± | + |
| | Cognitive dysfunction | | ± | ± | ± | ± |
| | Neuropathy, peripheral | | | | ± | + |
| | Spastic paraplegia | | | | ± | + |
| Endocrine | Growth hormone deficiency | | ± | ± | ± | ± |
| | Hypogonadotropic hypogonadism | | ± | + | + | + |
| | Hypothyroidism | | ± | ± | ± | ± |
| Eye | Chorioretinal degeneration | | ± | ± | ± | + |

lar ataxia more than spasticity or peripheral neuropathy. Rarely, cerebellar ataxia is isolated (Wiethoff et al. 2017). Motor neuron involvement mostly occurs in adults. Congenital hypothyroidism and growth hormone deficiency can cause cognitive dysfunction and short stature. Hypogonadotropic hypogonadism usually becomes manifest during the second decade of life. Hormone deficiencies are responsive to hormone replacement therapy. Cognitive dysfunction may be related to hypothyroidism in some patients (Table 51.15).

#### Membrane-Bound O-Acyltransferase Domain-Containing 7 Deficiency, MBOAT7

**Function:** *MBOAT7* encodes membrane-bound O-acyltransferase domain-containing 7 also known as lyso-phosphatidylinositol (lyso-PI) acyltransferase 1 (LPIAT1) (Fig. 51.2a). LPIAT1 is an ER remodeling enzyme that uses arachidonoyl-CoA to transfer arachidonic acid to lyso-PI yielding an arachidonic acid-containing PI (Johansen et al. 2016). LPIAT1-deficient mice are small and atactic, display atrophy of the cerebral cortex and hippocampus, and have a shorter life span (Lee et al. 2012). There is accumulation of lyso-PI in the brain as well as shortage of arachidonic acid-containing species of PI and selected phosphoinositides in addition to accumulation of other (non-arachidonic acid-containing) PI molecular species (Anderson et al. 2013).
**Clinical:** *MBOAT7* pathogenic variants have been reported in patients with severe intellectual disability, epilepsy (focal and general seizures), and autistic features (Johansen et al. 2016; Jacher et al. 2019). Additional features may include microcephaly, truncal hypotonia (Johansen et al. 2016), ataxic gait, strabismus, and cerebellar cortical dysgenesis on brain MRI (Table 51.16) (Jacher et al. 2019).

#### Diacylglycerol Kinase ε Deficiency, Nephrotic Syndrome Type 7; Atypical Hemolytic Uremic Syndrome Type 7, DGKE

**Function:** *DGKE* encodes diacylglycerol kinase ε (DGKε) that catalyzes the ATP-dependent phosphorylation of DG to form PA. DGKε is associated with ER and plasma membranes. DGKε has been suggested to catalyze one of the steps of the phosphatidylinositol (PI) cycle, the major pathway to regenerate PI and its phosphorylated forms, the phosphoinositides. By its preference for DG species with a fatty acid composition found in PI and phosphoinositide species, DGKε enriches the PA pool with molecular species that are subsequently used for PI and phosphoinositide synthesis (Bozelli and Epand 2019).
**Clinical:** *DGKE* pathogenic variants have been associated with membranoproliferative-like glomerular microangiopathy (MGPN) (Ozaltin et al. 2013) and atypical hemolytic-uremic syndrome (HUS) (Lemaire et al. 2013). It now appears that pathogenic *DGKE* variants cause a heterogeneous glomerular disorder with histopathologic and clinical features ranging from HUS to MPGN. The disease progresses to a chronic nephropathy kidney transplantation which is then indicated with no disease recurrence so far (Table 51.17) (Azukaitis et al. 2017).

### Fatty Acid Synthesis and Elongation

#### Acetyl-CoA carboxylase 1 deficiency, ACACA

**Function:** *ACACA* encodes cytosolic acetyl-CoA carboxylase 1 (ACC1, also known as ACCα) and catalyzes the first committed step of the fatty acid synthesis process which is the biotin-dependent addition of a carboxyl moiety from carbonate to acetyl-CoA producing the malonyl-CoA extender for fatty acyl group elongation (Figs. 51.2a and 51.3a). Its expression is high in the liver, adipose, and other lipogenic tissues (Tong 2013).
**Clinical:** Only one patient was reported in 1981 with a clinical picture clouded by perinatal asphyxia; there was no genetic testing performed. Biochemically, acetyl-CoA carboxylase was measured in the liver of the patient and found to be 2% of control. In fibroblasts of the patient, acetyl-CoA

**Table 51.16** Membrane-bound O-acyltransferase domain-containing 7 deficiency

| System | Symptoms and biomarkers | Neonatal (birth–1 month) | Infancy (1–18 months) | Childhood (1.5–11 years) | Adolescence (11–16 years) | Adulthood (>16 years) |
|---|---|---|---|---|---|---|
| CNS | Ataxia | | ± | ± | ± | ± |
| | Autistic spectrum disorder | | ± | ± | ± | ± |
| | Axial hypotonia | | ± | ± | ± | ± |
| | Cerebellar abnormalities | | ± | ± | ± | ± |
| | Epileptic seizures | ± | + | + | + | + |
| | Microcephaly | | ± | ± | ± | ± |
| | Retardation, psychomotor | + | + | + | + | + |
| | Severe intellectual deficiency | | + | + | + | + |
| Eye | Strabismus | ± | ± | ± | ± | ± |

**Table 51.17** Diacylglycerol kinase ε deficiency

| System | Symptoms and biomarkers | Neonatal (birth–1 month) | Infancy (1–18 months) | Childhood (1.5–11 years) | Adolescence (11–16 years) | Adulthood (>16 years) |
|---|---|---|---|---|---|---|
| Hematological | Hemolytic uremic syndrome (atypical) | ± | + | ± | | |
| Renal | Progressive renal impairment | | ± | ± | ± | |
| | Glomerulopathy | ± | + | + | | |

**Table 51.18** Cytosolic acetyl-CoA carboxylase 1 deficiency

| System | Symptoms and biomarkers | Neonatal (birth–1 month) | Infancy (1–18 months) | Childhood (1.5–11 years) | Adolescence (11–16 years) | Adulthood (>16 years) |
|---|---|---|---|---|---|---|
| CNS | Hypotonia | + | | | | |
| Musculoskeletal | **Growth retardation** | + | | | | |
| | **Myopathy** | + | | | | |
| Laboratory findings | 2-Ethyl-3-hydroxy-hexanoic acid (urine) | ↑ | | | | |
| | 2-Ethyl-3-keto-hexanoic acid (urine) | ↑ | | | | |
| | 2-Ethyl-hexanedioic acid (urine) | ↑ | | | | |

carboxylase activity was 10% of control. Urine organic acid analysis showed presence of 2-ethyl-3-keto-hexanoic acid, 2-ethyl-3-hydroxy-hexanoic acid, and 2-ethyl-hexanedioic acid. The authors explain this as condensation of two butyryl-CoA molecules forming 2-ethyl-3-keto-hexanoyl-CoA (that is converted into the three metabolites mentioned above) and refer to a similar mechanism that has been observed in propionic acidemia where two molecules of propionyl-CoA give rise to 2-methyl-3-keto-valeric acid. The accumulation of butyryl-CoA was suggested to occur because butyryl-CoA is believed to (also) act as a primer for fatty acid synthase which is not used in the absence of malonyl-CoA (Blom et al. 1981). Given the single report and lack of genetic confirmation, this is a candidate gene which needs to be confirmed (Table 51.18).

### Acetyl-CoA Carboxylase 2 Deficiency, ACACB

**Function:** *ACACB* encodes mitochondrial acetyl-CoA carboxylase 2 (ACC2, also known as ACCβ) and like ACC1 catalyzes the biotin-dependent carboxylation of acetyl-CoA to generate malonyl-CoA. ACC2 is located in the outer mitochondrial membrane and is primarily expressed in heart and muscle tissues, as well as the liver (Tong 2013) and is thought to play a role in the production of malonyl-CoA that is used to control the fatty oxidation flux by regulating the activity of carnitine palmitoyltransferase 1 in these tissues.

**Clinical:** Only one patient reported with speech delay and, from 19 months on, recurrent fever-induced and biotin-responsive episodes of lethargy and lactic acidosis with metabolites suggestive of multiple carboxylase deficiency.

Given the single report, this is a candidate gene which needs to be confirmed (Table 51.19) (Tarailo-Graovac et al. 2016).

### 3-Hydroxyacyl-CoA Dehydratase 1 Deficiency, HACD1

**Function:** *HACD1* encodes 3-hydroxyacyl-CoA dehydratase 1 (HACD1) that performs the third of the four reactions of the long-chain fatty acid elongation cycle (Figs. 51.2a and 51.3a). It catalyzes the dehydrogenation of 3-hydroxyacyl-CoA to form 2,3-trans-enoyl-CoA. HACD1 is localized at the ER and forms a complex with the other enzymes of VLCFA synthesis (ELOVL1–7, KAR, and TCER).

**Clinical:** Seven patients from a highly inbred family have been reported with rare, potentially protein disturbing biallelic *HACD1* variants. They showed severe generalized muscular hypotonia with absent deep tendon reflexes that gradually improved, together with a relatively normal cognition (Table 51.20) (Muhammad et al. 2013).

### Trans-2-Enoyl-CoA Reductase Deficiency, Autosomal Recessive Mental Retardation Type 14, TECR

**Function:** *TECR* encodes trans-2,3-enoyl-CoA reductase (TECR) which performs the last step of the four reactions of the long-chain fatty acid elongation cycle (Figs. 51.2a and 51.3a). It is localized at the ER and catalyzes the NADPH-dependent reduction of the trans-2,3-enoyl-CoA to an acyl-CoA.

**Clinical:** Autosomal recessive mental retardation type 14: only five patients were found in one inbred family. Patient displayed nonsyndromic intellectual disability. Functional studies in immortalized B-cells showed that the pathogenic variants lead to decreased trans-2,3-enoyl-CoA reductase activity and decreased level of C24-sphingomyelin and C24-ceramide (Abe et al. 2013; Çalışkan et al. 2011), likely due to shortage of VLCFA due to the elongation defect (Table 51.21).

**Table 51.19** Mitochondrial acetyl-CoA carboxylase 2 deficiency

| System | Symptoms and biomarkers | Neonatal (birth–1 month) | Infancy (1–18 months) | Childhood (1.5–11 years) | Adolescence (11–16 years) | Adulthood (>16 years) |
|---|---|---|---|---|---|---|
| CNS | **Speech delay** | | | + | | |
| | **Lethargy, during crisis** | | | + | | |
| Metabolic | Lactic acidosis | | | + | | |
| Laboratory findings | 2-Methyl-3-hydroxybutyric acid (urine) | | | ↑ | | |
| | 3-Hydroxypropionic acid (urine) | | | ↑ | | |
| | 3-Methylcrotonylglycine (urine) | | | ↑ | | |
| | 3-Methylglutaconic acid (urine) | | | ↑ | | |
| | Glutaric acid (urine) | | | ↑ | | |
| | Lactate (plasma) | | | ↑ | | |
| | Methylcitric acid (urine) | | | ↑ | | |
| | Propionylglycine (urine) | | | ↑ | | |
| | Tiglylglycine (urine) | | | ↑ | | |

**Table 51.20** 3-Hydroxyacyl-CoA dehydratase 1 deficiency

| System | Symptoms and biomarkers | Neonatal (birth–1 month) | Infancy (1–18 months) | Childhood (1.5–11 years) | Adolescence (11–16 years) | Adulthood (>16 years) |
|---|---|---|---|---|---|---|
| CNS | **Hypotonia** | + | + | | | |
| | Regression, motor | | | + | | |
| | **Waddling gait** | | | + | | |
| Digestive | Feeding difficulties | ± | ± | | | |
| Musculoskeletal | Muscle weakness | + | + | | | |
| | **Myopathy** | + | + | + | | |

**Table 51.21** Trans-2-enoyl-CoA reductase deficiency

| System | Symptoms and biomarkers | Neonatal (birth–1 month) | Infancy (1–18 months) | Childhood (1.5–11 years) | Adolescence (11–16 years) | Adulthood (>16 years) |
|---|---|---|---|---|---|---|
| CNS | **Intellectual disability** | | | + | + | + |
| | **Tremor** | ± | ± | + | + | + |

### Enoyl-CoA Reductase Deficiency, Mitochondrial Trans-2-Enoyl-CoA Reductase Protein-Associated Neurodegeneration (MEPAN), MECR

**Function:** *MECR* encodes the mitochondrial trans-2-enoyl-CoA reductase (MECR) and performs the last step of the four reactions of the mitochondrial fatty acid synthesis (mFAS) cycle which is the NADPH-dependent reduction of a trans-2,3-enoyl-ACP to acyl-ACP (Figure 51.3b).

**Clinical:** Only one paper that describes seven individuals from five unrelated families. Patients suffer from developmental delay, intellectual disability, childhood-onset dystonia, optic atrophy, and basal ganglia signal abnormalities on MRI. Fibroblast cell lines from affected individuals displayed reduced levels of both MECR and lipoylated proteins as well as defective mitochondrial respiration (Table 51.22) (Heimer et al. 2016).

### VLCFA Elongase 1 Deficiency, Ichthyotic Keratoderma, Spasticity, Hypomyelination, ELOVL1

**Function:** *ELOVL1* encodes elongation of very long-chain fatty acid protein 1 (ELOVL1) which is localized at the ER and catalyzes the condensation of malonyl-CoA with the growing long-chain fatty acyl-CoA (Figs. 51.2a and 51.3a). ELOVL1 is ubiquitously expressed and prefers saturated and monounsaturated C20–C26 VLCFAs. These VLCFAs are required for the synthesis of ω-O-acylceramides for skin barrier function but also are used for synthesis of complex lipids during myelination of the brain.

**Clinical:** Only two patients (5 and 12 years old) have been reported so far, but surprisingly, they share the same de novo pathogenic variants. They present with an early-onset spastic paraplegia with brain hypomyelination, associated with sensorineural deafness, optic atrophy, ichthyosis, and *acanthosis nigricans*. The pathogenic variants abrogated ELOVL1 enzymatic activity and reduced the levels of ≥C24 ceramides and sphingomyelins in patient cells. Reduced plasma C24:0/C22:0 may be a supportive diagnostic marker (Table 51.23) (Mueller et al. 2019; Kutkowska-Kaźmierczak et al. 2018).

### VLCFA Elongase 4 Deficiency, Neurologic Phenotype, Pseudo-Sjögren-Larsson Syndrome (Recessive); Spinocerebellar Ataxia Type 34 (Dominant), ELOVL4

**Function:** *ELOVL4* encodes elongation of very long-chain fatty acid protein 4 (ELOVL4) which is localized in the ER and catalyzes the condensation of malonyl-CoA with the growing long-chain fatty acyl-CoA (Figs. 51.2a and 51.3a). ELOVL4 is expressed in the retina, brain, testes, and skin

**Table 51.22** Mitochondrial enoyl-CoA reductase deficiency

| System | Symptoms and biomarkers | Neonatal (birth–1 month) | Infancy (1–18 months) | Childhood (1.5–11 years) | Adolescence (11–16 years) | Adulthood (>16 years) |
|---|---|---|---|---|---|---|
| CNS | Abnormalities in the globus pallidus (MRI) | | | + | + | + |
| | Abnormalities in the putamen (MRI) | | | + | + | + |
| | Dystonia | | | + | + | + |
| | Intellectual disability | | | ± | ± | ± |
| Eye | Optic atrophy | | | + | + | + |
| Laboratory findings | Lactate (MRS) | | | + | + | + |

**Table 51.23** Very long-chain fatty acid elongase 1 deficiency

| System | Symptoms and biomarkers | Neonatal (birth–1 month) | Infancy (1–18 months) | Childhood (1.5–11 years) | Adolescence (11–16 years) | Adulthood (>16 years) |
|---|---|---|---|---|---|---|
| CNS | Ataxia, cerebellar | | | ± | ± | |
| | Cerebral hypomyelination | | | + | + | |
| | Spastic paraplegia | | | ++ | ++ | |
| Dermatological | Hyperpigmentation ('acanthosis nigricans') | | | + | + | |
| | Ichthyosis | | | + | + | |
| Ear | Deafness, sensorineural | | | + | + | |
| Eye | Nystagmus | | | + | ± | |
| | Optic atrophy | | | + | + | |
| Laboratory findings | C24:0/C22:0 and C26:0/C22:0 (fibroblasts) | | | ↓–n | ↓–n | |
| | C24:0/C22:0 (plasma) | | | ↓–n | ↓–n | |

and acts on saturated and monounsaturated ≥C26 and elongates up to C38. In addition, ELOVL4 also elongates very long-chain polyunsaturated fatty acids (Cadieux-Dion et al. 2014; Deák et al. 2019).

**Clinical:** Heterozygous inheritance of a different set of autosomal dominant *ELOVL4* pathogenic variants that leads to a full-length protein with single amino acid substitutions causes spinocerebellar ataxia 34 (SCA34). The neurological phenotype is characterized by an adult-onset cerebellar ataxia, but gait ataxia has been reported in adolescence, possibly associated with pyramidal signs and rarely spasticity. Brain MRI shows cerebellar and pons atrophy, called "hot cross bun sign." Often, patients also present with erythrokeratodermia, which may disappear in adulthood. Rarely, patients exhibit a pigmentary retinopathy. Autosomal recessive inheritance of a different set of *ELOVL4* pathogenic variants may cause a severe and early-onset infantile disease characterized by seizures, spasticity, profound psychomotor retardation, ichthyosis, and premature death (Deák et al. 2019). However, biallelic *ELOVL4* pathogenic variants have also been reported with an isolated ichthyosis with dry, erythematous, and hyperkeratotic skin (Table 51.24) (Mir et al. 2014).

### VLCFA Elongase 4 Deficiency, Retinal Phenotype, Stargardt Disease Type 3, ELOVL4

**Function:** See Neurologic Phenotype

**Clinical:** Stargardt disease type 3: heterozygous inheritance of one set of autosomal dominant *ELOVL4* pathogenic variants leads to truncation of the ELOVL4 protein and causes Stargardt-like macular dystrophy (STGD3), a juvenile- or adult-onset retinal degeneration of variable severity (Table 51.25) (Deák et al. 2019).

### VLCFA Elongase 5 Deficiency, Spinocerebellar Ataxia Type 38, ELOVL5

**Function:** *ELOVL5* encodes elongation of very long-chain fatty acid protein 5 (ELOVL5) which is localized at the ER and catalyzes the condensation of malonyl-CoA with the growing long-chain fatty acyl-CoA (Figs. 51.2a and 51.3a). *ELOVL5* is ubiquitously expressed with highest levels in the testis and adrenal gland. ELOVL5 mediates elongation of long-chain polyunsaturated fatty acids (essential fatty acid as linoleic acid (C18:2ω6) and linolenic acid (C18:2ω3)) as well as long-chain straight-chain fatty acids between 18 and 22 carbons in length (Jakobsson et al. 2006).

**Clinical:** Autosomal dominant *ELOVL5* pathogenic variants cause spinocerebellar ataxia type 38. Patients, mostly described in Italy so far, present with a late-onset gait ataxia, nystagmus, and cerebellar atrophy, usually between 30 and 50 years old. The disease is slowly progressive and patients often also present with *pes cavus* and hyposmia and less frequently with hearing loss and peripheral neuropathy (Di Gregorio et al. 2014; Borroni et al. 2016). Low levels of arachidonic acid (AA) and docosahexaenoic acid (DHA) have been measured in patients' plasma.

**Treatment:** Given the decreased plasma levels of AA and DHA, a phase 2 randomized controlled trial was conducted

**Table 51.24** Very long-chain fatty acid elongase 4 deficiency, neurologic phenotype

| System | Symptoms and biomarkers | Neonatal (birth–1 month) | Infancy (1–18 months) | Childhood (1.5–11 years) | Adolescence (11–16 years) | Adulthood (>16 years) |
|---|---|---|---|---|---|---|
| *Autosomal dominant form* | | | | | | |
| CNS | Ataxia, cerebellar | | | | ± | ++ |
| | Nystagmus | | | | | ± |
| | Pyramidal signs | | | | ± | ± |
| Dermatological | Hyperkeratosis | | | + | + | ± |
| | Pigmentary retinopathy | | | | | ± |
| Eye | Cerebellar (and 'pons') atrophy | | | | | ++ |
| | Erythroderma | | | + | + | ± |
| | Ophthalmoplegia | | | | | ± |
| *Autosomal recessive form* | | | | | | |
| CNS | Epilepsy | | ± | ± | | |
| | Retardation, psychomotor | | ± | ± | | |
| | Spastic paraplegia | | ± | ± | | |
| Eye | Ichthyosis | | ++ | ++ | + | + |

**Table 51.25** Very long-chain fatty acid elongase 4 deficiency, retinal phenotype

| System | Symptoms and biomarkers | Neonatal (birth–1 month) | Infancy (1–18 months) | Childhood (1.5–11 years) | Adolescence (11–16 years) | Adulthood (>16 years) |
|---|---|---|---|---|---|---|
| Musculoskeletal | Macular dystrophy | | | ± | ± | + |

using 600 mg of DHA in ten SCA38 patients. After 16 weeks of treatment, the authors observed a mild but significant improvement of cerebellar functions, which was maintained over 40 weeks (Manes et al. 2017) and 104 weeks (Manes et al. 2019) of treatment (open label). Cerebellar glucose metabolism, assessed by PET-FDG, also improved at 40 and 104 weeks of treatment compared to baseline (Table 51.26).

#### LCFA-CoA Ligase 4 Deficiency, X-Linked Mental Retardation 63, FACL4

**Function:** *FACL4* encodes fatty acyl-CoA synthetase 4 (FACL4). It catalyzes the activation of mainly arachidonic acid (C20:4ω6) and eicosapentaenoic acid (C20:5ω3) to their corresponding CoA-ester. FACL4 is expressed in the placenta, brain, testis, ovary, spleen, and adrenal cortex, with low expression in the liver, colon, and small intestine (Cao et al. 1998).

**Clinical:** X-linked mental retardation 63: *FACL4* is deleted—together with the *COL4A5* gene—in X-linked Alport syndrome, elliptocytosis, and mental retardation, a continuous gene deletion syndrome (Piccini et al. 1998). Biallelic point pathogenic variants in *FACL4* were identified as the possible cause for nonspecific X-linked mental retardation in five patients from two families. Males presented with nonsyndromic severe to moderate mental retardation. Heterozygous females showed completely skewed X-inactivation but displayed variable cognition, from mild mental retardation to normal intelligence. Lymphoblast enzyme activity analysis showed low synthetase activity with arachidonic acid as substrate (Meloni et al. 2002). A third family with four affected males carrying a novel *FACL4* mutation was reported in 2003 (Longo et al. 2003) but no more since, only continuous gene deletions encompassing the *FACL4* gene. The *FACL4* gene therefore should be considered a candidate gene (Table 51.27).

### Triglyceride/Lipid Droplet Metabolism

#### Lysophosphatidic Acid Acyltransferase Deficiency, Congenital Generalized Lipodystrophy Type 1, Berardinelli-Seip Syndrome, AGPAT2

**Function:** *AGPAT2* encodes 1-acylglycerol-3-phosphate O-acyltransferase 2 (AGPAT2) which is an acyltransferase involved in the synthesis of TG at the ER (Fig. 51.2a). It catalyzes the acylation of lysophosphatidic acid (LPA) to PA. AGPAT2 is highly expressed in adipose tissues where it is needed for TG synthesis and its storage in adipocytes.

**Clinical:** Congenital generalized lipodystrophy type 1: patients suffer from generalized lipodystrophy, extreme insulin resistance, hypertriglyceridemia, acromegaloid features, hepatic steatosis, and early onset of diabetes (Agarwal et al. 2002; Craveiro Sarmento et al. 2019). One patient was reported with learning disabilities and a non-diabetic polyneuropathy (Oswiecimska et al. 2019). Interestingly,

**Table 51.26** Very long-chain fatty acid elongase 5 deficiency

| System | Symptoms and biomarkers | Neonatal (birth–1 month) | Infancy (1–18 months) | Childhood (1.5–11 years) | Adolescence (11–16 years) | Adulthood (>16 years) |
|---|---|---|---|---|---|---|
| CNS | Anosmia | | | | | + |
| | Ataxia, cerebellar | | | | | ++ |
| | Cerebellar atrophy | | | | | + |
| | Neuropathy, peripheral | | | | | ± |
| | Pyramidal signs | | | | | ± |
| Ear | Hearing loss | | | | | ± |
| Eye | Nystagmus | | | | | ++ |
| Musculoskeletal | Pes cavus | | | | | + |
| Laboratory findings | Arachidonic acid (plasma) | | | | | ↓ |
| | Docosahexaenoic acid (serum) | | | | | ↓ |

**Table 51.27** Long-chain fatty acid-CoA ligase 4 deficiency

| System | Symptoms and biomarkers | Neonatal (birth–1 month) | Infancy (1–18 months) | Childhood (1.5–11 years) | Adolescence (11–16 years) | Adulthood (>16 years) |
|---|---|---|---|---|---|---|
| CNS | Intellectual disability | + | + | + | + | + |
| Laboratory findings | Enzymatic activity (fibroblasts) | | | | | ↓ |
| | Enzymatic activity (leukocytes) | | | | | ↓ |

*AGPAT2* heterozygous pathogenic variant may cause partial lipodystrophy (Broekema et al. 2018).

**Treatment:** Long-term leptin-replacement therapy was shown to be effective and safe in two patients (Table 51.28) (Ebihara et al. 2007).

#### Lipin 1 Deficiency, LPIN1

**Function:** *LPIN1* encodes lipin-1, a phosphatidic acid phosphatase which is a key enzyme in triglyceride and membrane phospholipid biosynthesis (Fig. 51.2a) that catalyzes the removal of the phosphate from PA to form DG. There are three lipins (1, 2, and 3) with different expression tissue patterns (Csaki et al. 2013a). Lipins regulate the levels of both PA and DG and thereby function at the branch point of lipid synthesis channeling it in the direction of neutral lipids, zwitterionic phospholipids (PC and PE), or anionic phospholipids (PG, PS, CL). Lipins may reside in the cytosol and associate with other organellar membranes in a transient manner via a PA-stimulated manner that also depends on the fatty acid composition of the membrane. Lipin-1 is highly expressed in white adipose tissue and skeletal muscle tissue but also, at lower levels, in most other tissues (Csaki et al. 2013a; Zhang and Reue 2017). Lipin 1-can associate with ER and lipid droplets and can translocate to the nucleus in a nutrient-dependent manner, where it has been shown to act as transcriptional co-activator that interacts with PGC1α/PPARα and PPARγ to regulate the expression of genes involved in energy metabolism (Michot et al. 2012). It is this function that is believed to be affected in lipin-1 deficiency leading to inappropriate activation of cell-specific signaling pathways (Lee & Ridgway, 1865).

**Clinical:** Early-onset, recurrent, and acute rhabdomyolysis (Table 51.29).

#### Lipin 2 Deficiency, Majeed Syndrome, LPIN2

**Function:** *LPIN2* encodes lipin-2, a phosphatidic acid phosphatase, and catalyzes the removal of the phosphate from PA to form DG but also, like lipin-1, can act as a transcriptional coregulator (Fig. 51.2a). Lipin-2 is ubiquitously expressed; highest levels are found in the white adipose tissue, liver, intestine, and brain. Although believed to be similar/overlapping with lipin-1, lipin-2 function is unclear. Subcellular localization of lipin-2 is primarily cytosolic (Csaki et al. 2013b).

**Clinical:** Majeed syndrome: early-onset chronic recurrent multifocal osteomyelitis and congenital dyserythropoietic anemia of varying severity.

**Table 51.28** Lysophosphatidic acid acyltransferase deficiency

| System | Symptoms and biomarkers | Neonatal (birth–1 month) | Infancy (1–18 months) | Childhood (1.5–11 years) | Adolescence (11–16 years) | Adulthood (>16 years) |
|---|---|---|---|---|---|---|
| Dermatological | Subcutaneous fat distribution, abnormal | ± | ± | + | + | + |
| Digestive | Hepatomegaly | | ± | ± | ± | ± |
| | Liver steatosis | | ± | ± | ± | ± |
| Endocrine | Diabetes mellitus | ± | ± | + | + | + |
| Laboratory findings | Triglyceride (serum) | ↑↑ | ↑↑ | ↑↑ | ↑↑ | ↑↑ |

**Table 51.29** Lipin 1 deficiency

| System | Symptoms & Biomarkers | Neonatal (birth–1 month) | Infancy (1-18mths) | Childhood (1.5-11yrs) | Adolescence (11-16yrs) | Adulthood (>16yrs) |
|---|---|---|---|---|---|---|
| Musculoskeletal | Muscle cramps, during crisis | | ± | + | + | + |
| | Muscle weakness, during crisis | | ± | + | + | + |
| | Myoglobinuria, during crisis | | ± | + | + | + |
| | Rhabdomyolysis, episodic | | ± | + | + | + |
| | Rhabdomyolysis, precipitated by exercise | | ± | + | + | + |
| | Rhabdomyolysis, precipitated by fever | | | | | |
| Other | Death, during crisis | | ± | ± | ± | ± |
| | Symptome free interval | | ± | + | + | + |
| Renal | Renal failure, acute, during crisis | | ± | + | + | + |
| Laboratory findings | Creatine kinase (plasma), during crisis | | ↑↑↑ | ↑↑↑ | ↑↑↑ | ↑↑↑ |
| | Creatine kinase (plasma), symptom free interval | | n | n | n | n |
| | Myoglobin (urine), during crisis | | ↑↑↑ | ↑↑↑ | ↑↑↑ | ↑↑↑ |

**Table 51.30** Lipin 2 deficiency

| System | Symptoms and biomarkers | Neonatal (birth–1 month) | Infancy (1–18 months) | Childhood (1.5–11 years) | Adolescence (11–16 years) | Adulthood (>16 years) |
|---|---|---|---|---|---|---|
| Dermatological | Dermatitis, psoriasiform | | + | + | + | + |
| Digestive | **Hepatosplenomegaly** | | + | + | + | + |
| | Jaundice, cholestatic | | + | + | + | + |
| | Jaundice, episodic | | + | + | + | + |
| Hematological | **Anemia, dyserythropoietic** | | + | + | + | + |
| | **Anemia, need for blood transfusions** | | + | + | + | + |
| | Anemia, microcytic, hypochromic | | + | + | + | + |
| | Neutropenia | | + | + | + | + |
| Musculoskeletal | **Bone pain** | | + | + | + | + |
| | Bone scan 99Tc radioisotope uptake (bone), enhanced | | + | + | + | + |
| | **CRMO = classic radiographs, multifocal isotope uptake on bone scan, prolonged course, no response to iv antibiotics** | | + | + | + | + |
| | Short stature | | + | + | + | + |
| Other | **Fever, recurrent** | | + | + | + | + |
| Laboratory findings | ASAT/ALAT (plasma) | | ↑ | ↑ | ↑ | ↑ |
| | Blood cultures, sterile | | + | + | + | + |
| | Erythrocyte sedimentation rate | | ↑ | ↑ | ↑ | ↑ |
| | Hemoglobin (blood) | | ↓ | ↓ | ↓ | ↓ |
| | Iron (serum) | n | n | n | n | n |

**Treatment:** TNF-α inhibition was not effective. IL-1 inhibition, however, with either a recombinant IL-1 receptor antagonist (anakinra) or an anti-IL-1β antibody (canakinumab) resulted in clinical and laboratory improvement of bone and systemic inflammation in a sibling pair (Table 51.30) (Herlin et al. 2013).

### Diacylglycerol Acyltransferase Deficiency, Congenital Diarrhea Type 7, DGAT1

**Function:** *DGAT1* encodes diacylglycerol acyltransferase 1 (DGAT1) that acylates DG using acyl-CoA to form TG. DGAT1 is an ER enzyme that diverts DG toward TG and to the lipid droplet, away from phospholipid synthesis (Fig. 51.2a). This is especially relevant for fat absorption in the intestine where absorbed fatty acids are re-esterified into TG and stored in lipid droplets or packaged into chylomicrons before transport into the lymphatic system.

**Clinical:** Congenital diarrhea type 7: early-onset vomiting and/or diarrhea and protein-losing enteropathy with hypoalbuminemia leading to failure to thrive, anemia, and susceptibility to infection.

**Treatment:** Low-free diet with supplementation of essential fatty acids and fat-soluble vitamins is the first line of therapy; often patients depend on total parenteral nutrition (Table 51.31) (van Rijn et al. 2018).

### CGI-58 Deficiency, Chanarin-Dorfman Syndrome; Neutral Lipid Storage Disease with Ichthyosis, ABHD5

**Function:** *ABHD5* encodes α–/β-hydrolase domain-containing 5 (ABHD5) and is also known as CGI-58 (comparative gene identification 58) (Fig. 51.2a). Localized at the lipid droplet, ABHD5 binds to and is a co-activator of ATGL which in turn catalyzes the first step of TG hydrolysis. Independently of ATGL, ABHD5 also is involved in the hydrolysis of TG needed for synthesis of ω-O-acylceramides in the skin (Brown and Mark Brown 2017).

**Clinical:** Neutral lipid storage disease with ichthyosis: ichthyosis and, more variably, liver steatosis with hepatomegaly, short stature, developmental delay, and intellectual disability. Intracellular lipid accumulation is also seen in muscle tissue (mainly TG), and this causes "Jordan's anomaly" of vacuolated polymorphonuclear leukocytes that can be observed in a simple blood smear showing the characteristic lipid droplets in granulocytes. These droplets are also seen in leukocytes of heterozygous carriers (Lefèvre et al. 2001). Skin pathology likely results from the lack of skin ω-O-acylceramides (Table 51.32).

**Table 51.31** Diacylglycerol acyltransferase deficiency

| System | Symptoms and biomarkers | Neonatal (birth–1 month) | Infancy (1–18 months) | Childhood (1.5–11 years) | Adolescence (11–16 years) | Adulthood (>16 years) |
|---|---|---|---|---|---|---|
| CNS | Development, age-adequate | + | + | + | + | + |
| Digestive | Diarrhea, chronic | + | + | + | + | + |
| | Protein-losing enteropathy | + | + | + | + | + |
| | Vomiting | + | + | + | + | + |
| Hematological | Anemia | + | + | + | + | + |
| | Anemia | + | + | + | + | + |
| | Immunodeficiency | + | + | + | + | + |
| Metabolic | Acidosis, recurrent | + | + | + | + | + |
| Other | Diet, low fat | + | + | + | + | + |
| | Failure to thrive | + | + | + | + | + |
| | Infection, suceptibility to | + | + | + | + | + |
| | Total parenteral nutrition | + | + | + | + | + |
| Laboratory findings | Albumin (serum) | ↓ | ↓ | ↓ | ↓ | ↓ |
| | ASAT/ALAT (plasma) | ↑ | ↑ | ↑ | ↑ | ↑ |
| | IgG (serum) | ↓ | ↓ | ↓ | ↓ | ↓ |

**Table 51.32** CGI-58 deficiency

| System | Symptoms and biomarkers | Neonatal (birth–1 month) | Infancy (1–18 months) | Childhood (1.5–11 years) | Adolescence (11–16 years) | Adulthood (>16 years) |
|---|---|---|---|---|---|---|
| CNS | Intellectual disability | + | + | + | + | + |
| Dermatological | **Ichthyosis** | + | + | + | + | + |
| Digestive | **Hepatomegaly** | + | + | + | + | + |
| | Liver steatosis | + | + | + | + | + |
| Hematological | Vacuolated lymphocytes | + | | | | |
| Musculoskeletal | **Short stature** | + | + | + | + | + |

#### Adipose Triglyceride Lipase Deficiency, Neutral Lipid Storage Disease with Myopathy, PNPLA2

**Function:** *PNPLA2* encodes the ubiquitously expressed patatin-like phospholipase domain-containing lipase 2, also known as adipose triglyceride lipase (ATGL) that performs the initial step of TG hydrolysis, converting TG into DG and a fatty acid, at the lipid droplet surface (Fig. 51.2a). ATGL is activated by CGI-58.

**Clinical:** Neutral lipid storage disease with myopathy (calfs, shoulder, and limb girdle), cardiomyopathy elevated creatine kinase levels, and liver steatosis as well as diabetes mellitus. Individuals show Jordan's anomaly, which is diagnostically helpful (see Sect. 51.2.2.3). Heterozygotes can be symptomatic (lipid myopathy, cardiomyopathy, hepatomegaly, insulin resistance, or diabetes) and have lipid accumulation in muscle, leukocytes (also Jordan's anomaly), and basal keratinocytes (Wu et al. 2015).

**Treatment:** Bezafibrate (400 mg/day), a PPARα agonist, was tried and *not* successful in contrast to the promising results in mice models of ATGL deficiency (Table 51.33) (van de Weijer et al. 2013).

#### Perilipin 1 Deficiency, Familial Partial Lipodystrophy Type 4, PLIN1

**Function:** *PLIN1* encodes perilipin 1 (PLIN1) which is a protein that coats lipid droplets, and it is required for optimal lipid incorporation and release from the lipid droplet primarily through the regulation of lipases, including adipose triglyceride lipase (ATGL, 51.33) and hormone-sensitive lipase (HSL, 51.35) which catalyze the hydrolysis of tri- and diacylglycerol, respectively (Fig. 51.2a).

**Clinical:** Familial partial lipodystrophy type 4; autosomal dominant. Patients have partial lipodystrophy, cushingoid appearance, severe dyslipidemia, and insulin-resistant diabetes. Subcutaneous fat from the patients shows smaller adipocytes, suggesting impaired TG storage in lipid droplets. The inability to store TG in adipocytes likely results in the observed ectopic deposition of lipids in tissues such as the

**Table 51.33** Adipose triglyceride lipase deficiency

| System | Symptoms and biomarkers | Neonatal (birth–1 month) | Infancy (1–18 months) | Childhood (1.5–11 years) | Adolescence (11–16 years) | Adulthood (>16 years) |
|---|---|---|---|---|---|---|
| Cardiovascular | Cardiomyopathy | | | ± | ± | + |
| Digestive | Hepatomegaly | | | ± | ± | + |
| | Liver steatosis | | | ± | ± | + |
| Endocrine | Diabetes mellitus | | | ± | ± | + |
| Musculoskeletal | Lipid deposition (muscle) | | | ± | ± | + |
| | Lipid droplets (muscle) | | | + | + | + |
| | Muscle atrophy, calf muscles | | | ± | ± | + |
| | Myopathy, shoulder and limb girdle | | | ± | ± | + |
| | **Vacuolated granulocytes with lipid droplets (Jordans' anomaly)** | | | + | + | + |
| | **Vacuoles, muscle** | | | + | + | + |
| Laboratory findings | Creatine kinase (plasma) | | | + | + | + |

**Table 51.34** Perilipin 1 deficiency

| System | Symptoms and biomarkers | Neonatal (birth–1 month) | Infancy (1–18 months) | Childhood (1.5–11 years) | Adolescence (11–16 years) | Adulthood (>16 years) |
|---|---|---|---|---|---|---|
| Autonomic system | Hypertension | ± | ± | ± | + | + |
| CNS | Stroke | ± | ± | ± | + | + |
| Dermatological | Acanthosis nigricans | ± | ± | ± | + | + |
| Digestive | Liver steatosis | ± | ± | ± | + | + |
| Endocrine | Cushing stigmata | ± | ± | ± | + | + |
| | **Diabetes mellitus** | ± | ± | ± | + | + |
| Genitourinary | Ovarian failure | ± | ± | ± | + | + |
| Musculoskeletal | **Lipodystrophy, partial** | ± | ± | ± | + | + |
| Other | Body fat percentage, low | ± | ± | ± | + | + |
| | Body mass index, low | ± | ± | ± | + | + |
| Laboratory findings | Cholesterol (serum) | ↑↑↑ | ↑↑↑ | ↑↑↑ | ↑↑↑ | ↑↑↑ |
| | Triglyceride (serum) | ↑↑↑ | ↑↑↑ | ↑↑↑ | ↑↑↑ | ↑↑↑ |

skeletal muscle and liver, leading to insulin resistance and hypertriglyceridemia (Gandotra et al. 2011). Interestingly, individuals with a heterozygous *PLIN1* null allele were reported that do not display a partial lipodystrophy phenotype, suggesting that the initially reported heterozygous variants cause a specific disease mechanism leading to the reported partial lipodystrophy phenotype. The authors caution the interpretation of *PLIN1* null allele in diagnostic gene testing for lipodystrophy, insulin resistance, and diabetes (Table 51.34) (Laver et al. 2018).

### Hormone-Sensitive Lipase Deficiency, Familial Partial Lipodystrophy Type 6, LIPE

**Function:** *LIPE* encodes hormone-sensitive lipase (HSL) and is the predominant mediator of the hydrolysis of DG, cholesterol esters, and retinyl esters in human white adipose tissue (Fig. 51.2a). HSL is ubiquitously expressed and involved in lipolysis in adipocytes, steroidogenesis, and spermatogenesis (Albert et al. 2014).

**Clinical:** Familial partial lipodystrophy type 6; heterozygous patients also show symptoms, but symptoms are more prominent in homozygous individuals. Clinically characterized by partial lipodystrophy (reduced lower limb subcutaneous fat), dyslipidemia, hepatic steatosis, and systemic insulin resistance (Table 51.35) (Albert et al. 2014; Zolotov et al. 2017).

## Sphingolipid Metabolism

### Serine Palmitoyltransferase Subunit 1 Deficiency, Hereditary Sensory and Autonomic Neuropathy Type 1A, SPTLC1

**Function:** The de novo biosynthetic pathway is initiated in the ER by the action of serine palmitoyltransferase (SPT) which catalyzes the condensation of L-serine and an acyl-CoA and generates 3-ketodihydrosphingosine (or 3-ketosphinganine). Depending on the tissue/cell requirements, the acyl-CoA is palmitoyl-CoA (C16:0-CoA) or myristoyl- (C14:0), stearyl- (C18:0) or lignoceryl- (C24:0)-CoA. *SPTLC1* encodes serine palmitoyltransferase subunit 1, one of the three SPTLC genes (*SPTLC1–3*) that together with two separately encoded small

**Table 51.35** Hormone-sensitive lipase deficiency

| System | Symptoms and biomarkers | Neonatal (birth–1 month) | Infancy (1–18 months) | Childhood (1.5–11 years) | Adolescence (11–16 years) | Adulthood (>16 years) |
|---|---|---|---|---|---|---|
| Dermatological | Acanthosis nigricans | | | | | + |
| Digestive | Liver steatosis | | | | | + |
| Endocrine | Diabetes mellitus | | | | | + |
| Musculoskeletal | Lipodystrophy, partial | | | | | + |
| Other | Body fat percentage, low | | | | | + |
| | Body mass index, low | | | | | + |
| Laboratory findings | Cholesterol (serum) | ↑↑↑ | ↑↑↑ | ↑↑↑ | ↑↑↑ | ↑↑↑ |
| | Creatine kinase (plasma) | ↑ | ↑ | ↑ | ↑ | ↑ |
| | Triglyceride (serum) | ↑↑↑ | ↑↑↑ | ↑↑↑ | ↑↑↑ | ↑↑↑ |

**Table 51.36** Serine palmitoyltransferase subunit 1 deficiency

| System | Symptoms and biomarkers | Neonatal (birth–1 month) | Infancy (1–18 months) | Childhood (1.5–11 years) | Adolescence (11–16 years) | Adulthood (>16 years) |
|---|---|---|---|---|---|---|
| Autonomic system | Anhidrosis | ± | ± | ± | | |
| CNS | Axonal sensory motor polyneuropathy, chronic | | | | ± | + |
| | Neuropathy, myelinating | | | | | ± |
| | Neuropathy, sensory | | | ± | ± | + |
| Dermatological | Skin ulceration | | | ± | ± | + |
| Eye | Maculopathy | | | | | ± |
| Laboratory findings | 1-Deoxymethylsphiganine (plasma) | | | | ↑ | ↑ |
| | 1-Deoxysphinganine (plasma) | | | | ↑ | ↑ |

subunits, SPTssa and SPTssb, forms different heterotrimeric complexes that have acyl-length specificity and thereby modulate the length of the sphingoid base (Fig. 51.4a). Hereditary sensory and autonomic neuropathy type 1A is caused by (missense) pathogenic variants that induce a shift in the substrate specificity of SPTs, which leads to the formation of the atypical deoxysphingoid bases 1-deoxysphinganine and 1-deoxymethylsphinganine. These deoxysphingoid bases lack the 1-hydroxylgroup required for the coupling of headgroups which abrogates the creation of complex sphingolipids and cannot be degraded. Deoxysphingoid bases, especially deoxysphinganines, are neurotoxic and are elevated in plasma of these patients and can be used as a blood biomarker (Penno et al. 2010).

**Clinical:** Hereditary sensory and autonomic neuropathy type 1A: autosomal and dominantly inherited-axonal neuropathy. Onset is usually in the second or third decade of life, and initial symptoms are sensory loss and pain in the feet and hands followed by distal muscle wasting and weakness caused by motor neuron degeneration. Loss of pain sensation leads to chronic skin ulcers and distal amputations (Dawkins et al. 2001). However, the age of onset can be quite variable (from infancy to late adulthood), disease penetrance is incomplete, and sensory loss may occur without pain (Houlden et al. 2006). In some families, males presented with more severe and earlier onset, with significant motor involvement and demyelinating motor conduction velocities (Houlden et al. 2006). *SPTLC1* variants have also been associated with macular telangiectasia type 2 (Gantner et al. 2019). Most SPTLC1-deficient patients present with both sensory and autonomic neuropathy and macular telangiectasia.

**Treatment:** L-serine has been tested as treatment for SPTLC1 deficiency (400 mg/kg/d L-serine, https://clinicaltrials.gov/ct2/show/NCT01733407) resulting in lower levels of deoxysphingolipids. L-serine treatment in mice and rat has shown positive effects on peripheral nerve function and should be considered a potential treatment in humans (Garofalo et al. 2011). A randomized controlled trial of 16 patients showed a significant improvement on the Charcot-Marie-Tooth neuropathy score of patients treated by 400 mg/kg/d L-serine compared to placebo, with evidence of continued improvement in the second year of treatment (Table 51.36) (Fridman et al. 2019).

### Serine Palmitoyltransferase Subunit 2 Deficiency, Hereditary Sensory and Autonomic Neuropathy Type 1C, SPTLC2

**Function:** *SPTLC2* encodes serine palmitoyltransferase subunit 2 (SPTLC2, Fig. 51.4a).

**Clinical:** *SPTLC2* pathogenic variants are a rarer cause of hereditary sensory and autonomic neuropathy (Rotthier et al. 2010). Age of onset and severity is very variable, from infancy to late adulthood (Suriyanarayanan et al. 2016; Murphy et al. 2013). Patients have elevated plasma levels of deoxysphinganine.

**Treatment:** A small study in one SPTLC2-deficient patient showed that L-serine treatment was well supported and also lowered deoxysphinganine levels in plasma, but there was no change in the Charcot-Marie-Tooth neuropathy score (Auranen et al. 2017). Further studies are warranted in SPTLC2-deficient patients considering the benefit of L-serine supplementation in SPTLC1-deficient patients (Table 51.37).

### Ceramide Synthase 1 Deficiency, Progressive Myoclonic Epilepsy Type 8, CERS1

**Function:** *CERS1* encodes ceramide synthase 1 (CERS1), a transmembrane ER protein that catalyzes the condensation of sphinganine with a fatty acyl-CoA, in case of CERS1 preferably C18-CoA, on the primary amino group yielding dihydroceramides (Fig. 51.4). *CERS1* is highly expressed in the brain, especially in neurons (Kihara 2016b). Mouse models of the disease showed impaired exploration of novel objects, impaired locomotion and motor coordination, neuronal apoptosis in the cerebellum, and dramatic changes in levels of cerebellar sphingolipids (Ginkel et al. 2012).

**Clinical:** Only five patients reported, four from the same family (Ferlazzo et al. 2009; Vanni et al. 2014; Godeiro Junior et al. 2018). Patients presented with action myoclonus with onset in childhood or adolescence, generalized tonic-clonic seizures, and progressive cognitive deterioration up to dementia. Cerebellar ataxia was also present in one patient (Table 51.38) (Godeiro Junior et al. 2018).

### Ceramide Synthase 3 Deficiency, Autosomal Recessive Congenital Ichthyosis Type 9, CERS3

**Function:** *CERS3* encodes ceramide synthase 3 (CERS3), a transmembrane ER protein that catalyzes the condensation of sphinganine with a fatty acyl-CoA to form dihydroceramides (Fig. 51.4). CERS3 has broad substrate specificity, exhibiting activity toward ≥C18-CoAs (Kihara 2016b). CERS3 is also responsible for creating ceramides containing ultra-long-chain fatty acids that are found in the epidermis (saturated and monounsaturated) and testis (polyunsaturated), which corresponds with the expression pattern of *CERS3*.

**Clinical:** Pathogenic variants in *CERS3* cause autosomal recessive congenital ichthyosis (ARCI). Patients are characterized by collodion membranes at birth, generalized scaling of the skin, and mild erythroderma. Ceramides containing ≥C24 fatty acids, including ω-O-acylceramides, are reduced in the epidermis of *Cers3* knockout mice and in *CERS3* patients (Table 51.39) (Eckl et al. 2013).

**Table 51.37** Serine palmitoyltransferase subunit 2 deficiency

| System | Symptoms and biomarkers | Neonatal (birth–1 month) | Infancy (1–18 months) | Childhood (1.5–11 years) | Adolescence (11–16 years) | Adulthood (>16 years) |
|---|---|---|---|---|---|---|
| Autonomic system | Anhidrosis | | | ± | | |
| CNS | Axonal sensory motor polyneuropathy, chronic | | | | ± | + |
| | Neuropathy, myelinating | | | | | ± |
| | Neuropathy, sensory | | | ± | ± | + |
| Dermatological | Skin ulceration | | | ± | ± | + |
| Laboratory findings | 1-Deoxysphinganine (plasma) | | | | ↑ | ↑ |

**Table 51.38** Ceramide synthase 1 deficiency

| System | Symptoms and biomarkers | Neonatal (birth–1 month) | Infancy (1–18 months) | Childhood (1.5–11 years) | Adolescence (11–16 years) | Adulthood (>16 years) |
|---|---|---|---|---|---|---|
| CNS | Ataxia, cerebellar | | ± | ± | ± | ± |
| | Cognitive decline | | | + | + | + |
| | Dementia | | | | ± | ± |
| | Myoclonic epilepsy | | | + | + | + |
| | Seizures, tonic clonic | | | + | ± | ± |

**Table 51.39** Ceramide synthase 3 deficiency

| System | Symptoms and biomarkers | Neonatal (birth–1 month) | Infancy (1–18 months) | Childhood (1.5–11 years) | Adolescence (11–16 years) | Adulthood (>16 years) |
|---|---|---|---|---|---|---|
| Dermatological | Collodion skin, collodion baby | + | | | | |
| | Ichthyosis | | + | + | + | + |

#### Dihydroceramide Desaturase Deficiency, DEGS1

**Function:** *DEGS1* encodes Δ4-dihydroceramide desaturase that converts dihydroceramide to ceramide by creation of a Δ4,5 *trans* double bond into the sphinganine backbone (Karsai et al. 2019) (Fig. 51.4a).

**Clinical:** Nineteen patients from 13 unrelated families were identified with *DEGS1* pathogenic variants (Pant et al. 2019). Most of them presented with very poor psychomotor development, dystonia and severe spasticity, failure to thrive, and frequent seizures. A less severe phenotype was observed in some patients with capacity to sit or walk and to use verbal communication (Pant et al. 2019; Dolgin et al. 2019). Brain MRI was remarkable and showed hypomyelination, sometimes associated with atrophy of the thalami and hypointense T2/FLAIR of the pallidi (Pant et al. 2019). In fibroblasts, dihydroceramide accumulated, and the dihydroceramide/ceramide ratios in patients' plasma, fibroblasts, and muscle were elevated (Karsai et al. 2019; Pant et al. 2019). Lipidomic analyses confirmed elevated levels of dihydroceramides, dihydrosphingosine, dihydro-S1P, and dihydrosphingomyelins in whole blood with concomitant reduced levels of ceramide (mild, still present), sphingosine, S1P, and monohexosylceramides (Table 51.40) (Karsai et al. 2019; Dolgin et al. 2019).

#### Alkaline Ceramidase 3 Deficiency, Early Childhood-Onset Progressive Leukodystrophy, ACER3

**Function:** *ACER3* encodes alkaline ceramidase 3 (ACER3), localized to both the ER and Golgi, and catalyzes the hydrolysis of natural phytoceramide, dihydroceramide, and ceramides carrying an unsaturated fatty acid (C18:1, C20:1, and C20:4) (Fig. 51.4a). Its tissue expression is widespread, but is highly expressed in the placenta (Hu et al. 2010).

**Clinical:** Only one paper reporting two patients (siblings) from Ashkenazi Jewish origin suffering from developmental regression at 6–13 months, truncal hypotonia, appendicular spasticity, dystonia, optic disc pallor, and peripheral neuropathy. The disorder is progressive; both patients (at 11 and 13 years of age) are neurologically severely impaired. Enzyme activity was measured in patients' fibroblasts and lymphoblasts using either C18:1-ceramide or NBD-$C_{12}$-phytoceramide as substrate and was (severely) reduced. Plasma analysis showed increased levels of ACER3 substrates as well as upstream complex sphingolipids (Table 51.41) (Edvardson et al. 2016).

#### CYP4F22 Omega Hydroxylase Deficiency, Autosomal Recessive Congenital Ichthyosis Type 5, CYP4F22

**Function:** *CYP4F22* (cytochrome P450, family 4, subfamily F, polypeptide 22, previously *FLJ39501*) encodes an ER localized ω-hydroxylase that catalyzes the NADPH and $O_2$-dependent ω-hydroxylation of ultra-long-chain fatty acids longer than C26 and is most active toward species with ≥C28 carbon atoms (Ohno et al. 2015) (Fig. 51.4b). These ω-hydroxylated ultra-long-chain fatty acids are used especially in the skin where they are needed for the synthesis of ω-O-acylceramides, which are important for skin permeability barrier formation.

**Clinical:** Autosomal recessive congenital ichthyosis type 5: nonsyndromic autosomal recessive congenital ichthyosis (ARCI), generally mild to moderate ARCI phenotype (Hotz et al. 2018). In rare cases, the skin is minimally involved, the so-called self-healing collodion babies (Noguera-Morel et al. 2016). Pathogenic variants lead to considerably reduced ω-hydroxylase activity, decreased levels of ω-O-acylceramides, and concomitantly increased non-acylated ceramides (Table 51.42) (Ohno et al. 2015).

#### Acylceramide Transacylase Deficiency, Autosomal Recessive Congenital Ichthyosis Type 10, PNPLA1

**Function:** *PNPLA1*, also known as *ARCI10*, encodes patatin-like phospholipase domain-containing 1 (PNPLA1) which is a CoA-independent transacylase (Fig. 51.4b). Linoleate esterified in triglyceride is used as an acyl donor to acylate the ω-hydroxyl group of ω-hydroxyceramide. *PNPLA1* expression is highly restricted to the differentiated, stratified squamous epithelium of the skin but not evident in most other tissues. PNPLA1 is involved in the synthesis of ω-O-acylceramides, which are important for skin permeability barrier formation (Hirabayashi et al. 2018; Ohno et al. 2017).

**Clinical:** Autosomal recessive congenital ichthyosis type 10: Most patients with biallelic *PNPLA1* pathogenic variants are born as collodion babies and show a stable or improving course of the disease with age. Adult patients present with generalized fine lamellar ichthyosis with whitish or brownish scales and mild or moderate erythroderma. Differentiated keratinocytes prepared from a *PNPLA1*-mutated patient showed defective ω-O-acylceramide generation (Table 51.43) (Hirabayashi et al. 2018; Pichery et al. 2017).

**Table 51.40** Dihydroceramide desaturase deficiency

| System | Symptoms and biomarkers | Neonatal (birth–1 month) | Infancy (1–18 months) | Childhood (1.5–11 years) | Adolescence (11–16 years) | Adulthood (>16 years) |
|---|---|---|---|---|---|---|
| CNS | Ataxia, cerebellar | | ± | ± | ± | ± |
| | Basal ganglia abnormalities (MRI) | | ± | ± | ± | ± |
| | Cerebral hypomyelination | | + | + | + | + |
| | Dystonia | | + | + | + | + |
| | Epileptic seizures | | + | + | + | + |
| | Neuropathy, myelinating | | ± | ± | ± | ± |
| | Retardation, psychomotor | + | + | + | + | + |
| | Severe intellectual deficiency | | + | + | + | + |
| | Spasticity | | + | + | + | + |
| Other | Failure to thrive | | + | + | + | + |
| Laboratory findings | Dihydroceramide (plasma, fibroblasts) | | ↑ | ↑ | ↑ | |
| | Dihydroceramide/ceramide ratio (plasma, fibroblasts) | | ↑ | ↑ | ↑ | |

**Table 51.41** Alkaline ceramidase 3 deficiency

| System | Symptoms and biomarkers | Neonatal (birth–1 month) | Infancy (1–18 months) | Childhood (1.5–11 years) | Adolescence (11–16 years) | Adulthood (>16 years) |
|---|---|---|---|---|---|---|
| CNS | Developmental regression | | ± | ± | | |
| | Dystonia | | ± | ± | | |
| | Neuropathy, peripheral | | ± | ± | | |
| | Spasticity | | ± | ± | | |
| Laboratory findings | C(18:1)- and C(20:1)-ceramides (plasma) | | | ↑ | | |
| | C(18:1)- and C(20:1)-dihydroceramides (plasma) | | | ↑ | | |

**Table 51.42** CYP4F22 omega hydroxylase deficiency

| System | Symptoms and biomarkers | Neonatal (birth–1 month) | Infancy (1–18 months) | Childhood (1.5–11 years) | Adolescence (11–16 years) | Adulthood (>16 years) |
|---|---|---|---|---|---|---|
| Dermatological | Collodion skin, collodion baby | + | | | | |
| | Ichthyosis | | + | + | + | + |

**Table 51.43** Acylceramide transacylase deficiency

| System | Symptoms and biomarkers | Neonatal (birth–1 month) | Infancy (1–18 months) | Childhood (1.5–11 years) | Adolescence (11–16 years) | Adulthood (>16 years) |
|---|---|---|---|---|---|---|
| Dermatological | Collodion skin, collodion baby | ± | | | | |
| | Ichthyosis | | + | + | + | + |

## UDP-Glucose Ceramide Glucosyltransferase Deficiency, Autosomal Recessive Congenital Ichthyosis, UGCG

**Function:** *UGCG* encodes UDP-glucose ceramide glucosyltransferase/glucosylceramide synthase (UGCG) that is localized in the ER (Fig. 51.4b). UGCG catalyzes the transfer of glucose to ceramide producing glucosylceramide (GlcCer) which is the precursor for the majority of complex sphingolipids. Production of GlcCer is also important for skin barrier formation as ceramides and acylceramides are transported into the extracellular space of the stratum corneum in glucosylated form and liberated by the action of β-glucosidase 1 (encoded by *GBA1*, defective in Gaucher disease).

**Clinical:** Autosomal recessive congenital ichthyosis: Only two patients from the same family presented with polyhydramnios during pregnancy, collodion membrane, joint contractures, hypernatremic dehydration, and death at 2 months of age. Another molecular event cannot be ruled out with

**Table 51.44** UDP-glucose ceramide glucosyltransferase deficiency

| System | Symptoms and biomarkers | Neonatal (birth–1 month) | Infancy (1–18 months) | Childhood (1.5–11 years) | Adolescence (11–16 years) | Adulthood (>16 years) |
|---|---|---|---|---|---|---|
| Dermatological | Collodion skin, collodion baby | ± | | | | |
| Musculoskeletal | Joint contractures | ± | | | | |
| Other | Dehydration | ± | | | | |

**Table 51.45** Nonlysosomal glucosylceramidase deficiency

| System | Symptoms and biomarkers | Neonatal (birth–1 month) | Infancy (1–18 months) | Childhood (1.5–11 years) | Adolescence (11–16 years) | Adulthood (>16 years) |
|---|---|---|---|---|---|---|
| CNS | Ataxia, cerebellar | | | ± | ± | + |
| | Cerebellar atrophy (MRI) | | | | | ± |
| | Cognitive decline | | | | | ± |
| | Intellectual disability | | ± | ± | ± | ± |
| | Neuropathy, peripheral | | | | | ± |
| | Retardation, psychomotor | ± | ± | | | |
| | Spastic paraplegia | | | ± | ± | + |
| | Thin corpus callosum | | | | | ± |
| Eye | Cataract | | ± | ± | ± | ± |
| Laboratory findings | GBA2 activity in leuckocytes | | | | | ↓ |

respect to the contractures in these patients. In mice, complete UGCG deletion is early embryonic lethal, but the keratinocyte-specific conditional knockout displays a severely impaired skin barrier defect as seen in the two reported patients (Table 51.44) (Monies et al. 2018; Amen et al. 2013).

**Nonlysosomal Glucosylceramidase Deficiency, Autosomal Recessive Spastic Paraplegia Type 46, GBA2**

**Function:** *GBA2* encodes the ubiquitously expressed (highest expression levels found in the liver, brain, and testis) β-glucosidase 2 or nonlysosomal glucosylceramidase 2 (GBA2), an integral membrane protein located at the ER/Golgi and close to the cell surface. The exact function of GBA2 is still under investigation.

**Clinical:** *GBA2* pathogenic variants have been associated predominantly with an early-onset spastic paraplegia, SPG46 (Martin et al. 2013), or cerebellar ataxia (Hammer et al. 2013). Overall, patients usually present with a spastic ataxia in childhood or adolescence, slowly progressive, often associated with intellectual disability and cataract (i.e., Marinesco-Sjögren-like syndrome, (Haugarvoll et al. 2017)). Glucosylceramide levels were elevated in erythrocytes and plasma, in the range of untreated Gaucher patients. Enzyme activity can be measured in leukocytes (not in fibroblasts) by subtraction (with and without GBA2 inhibitor AMP-deoxynojirimycin) to selectively measure GBA2 activity (Table 51.45) (Haugarvoll et al. 2017).

**Fatty Acid 2-Hydroxylase Deficiency, Autosomal Recessive Spastic Paraplegia Type 35 (SPG35); Fatty Acid Hydroxylase-Associated Neurodegeneration (FAHN), FA2H**

**Function:** *FA2H* encodes fatty acid 2-hydroxylase (FA2H) which hydroxylates fatty acids at the 2 (or α)-position (Fig. 51.4a). This can subsequently be activated to its corresponding 2-OH-acyl-CoA and used by ceramide synthases to form 2-OH-ceramides and downstream complex sphingolipids. FA2H is highly expressed in the brain where it is involved in the formation of 2-hydroxy galactosylceramides and 2-hydroxy sulfatides which are critical for normal myelination and myelin function (Alderson et al. 2004).

**Clinical:** Most patients with *FA2H* pathogenic variants present with a rather homogeneous and severe phenotype characterized by an early-onset spastic tetraparesis (SPG35), cerebellar ataxia with dysarthria, dysphagia, truncal hypotonia, and cognitive deficits, frequently accompanied by exotropia and dystonia/rigidity (Edvardson et al. 2008; Kruer et al. 2010; Rattay et al. 2019). Patients may also present with seizures and optic atrophy. Disease onset is usually around 4 years of age, with loss of ambulation within 7 years (Rattay et al. 2019). Rarely, adult-onset forms have been reported (Tonelli et al. 2012). Brain MRI is rather evocative with a combination of periventricular white matter T2 hyperintensities, T2 hypointensity of the globus pallidus as seen in neurodegeneration with brain iron accumulation (NBIA), pontocerebellar atrophy, and thin corpus callosum (Kruer et al. 2010). These four imaging findings have been grouped under the acronym "WHAT"—white

**Table 51.46** Fatty acid 2-hydroxylase deficiency

| System | Symptoms and biomarkers | Neonatal (birth–1 month) | Infancy (1–18 months) | Childhood (1.5–11 years) | Adolescence (11–16 years) | Adulthood (>16 years) |
|---|---|---|---|---|---|---|
| CNS | Abnormalities in the globus pallidus (MRI) | | | ± | + | + |
| | Ataxia, cerebellar | | | ± | + | + |
| | Axial hypotonia | | | ± | ± | ± |
| | Cerebellar hypoplasia | | | ± | + | + |
| | Cognitive dysfunction | | | ± | ± | ± |
| | Dystonia | | | ± | ± | ± |
| | Hypoplasia of pons | | | ± | + | + |
| | Periventricular white matter abnormalities | | | ± | + | + |
| | Seizures | | | ± | ± | ± |
| | Spastic tetraparesis | | ± | ± | + | + |
| | Thin corpus callosum | | | ± | + | + |
| Eye | Exotropia | | ± | ± | ± | ± |
| | Optic atrophy | | | ± | ± | ± |

matter changes, hypointensity of the globus pallidus, pontocerebellar atrophy, and thin corpus callosum (Rattay et al. 2019). The enzyme activity cannot be measured in fibroblasts due to other fatty acid hydroxylation activities (Edvardson et al. 2008). Of note, uniparental disomy seems to be a rather frequent genetic mechanism for homozygous *FA2H* pathogenic variants in non-consanguineous families (Table 51.46) (Soehn et al. 2016).

### Sphingosine-1-Phosphate Lyase Deficiency, SGPL1

**Function:** *SGPL1* encodes the ubiquitously expressed sphingosine-1-phosphate lyase (SGPL1) which cleaves sphingosine-1-phosphate (S1P) yielding a fatty aldehyde and phosphoethanolamine. SGPL1 is an essential enzyme in the sphingolipid catabolic pathway and regulator of S1P levels and other sphingoid bases (Fig. 51.4a). S1P is a bioactive lipid implicated in the regulation of cell survival, apoptosis, proliferation, and migration via both extracellular signaling of G-coupled protein receptors and intracellular signaling (Lovric et al. 2017). Mouse work shows that SGPL1 is also involved in (neuronal) autophagy as the released phosphoethanolamine can be used for synthesis of PE that anchors LC3 to the phagophore membranes.

**Clinical:** *SGPL1* pathogenic variants were identified simultaneously in patients presenting with an atypical form of axonal peripheral neuropathy—characterized by acute or subacute onset and episodes of recurrent mononeuropathy during adolescence (Atkinson et al. 2017)—and children presenting with nephrotic syndrome (NPHS14) and adrenal insufficiency (Lovric et al. 2017; Prasad et al. 2017). Nephrotic syndrome and adrenal insufficiency were variably associated with neurodevelopmental delay, microcephaly, brain malformations, ichthyosis, deafness, and adrenal calcifications (Bamborschke et al. 2018). The levels of SGPL1 substrates, S1P, and sphingosine (latter differentiates best in blood, three- to sixfold elevated) were markedly increased in the patients' blood and fibroblasts. Total serum ceramide levels and C24:0- and C16:0-lactosylceramides were also elevated (Table 51.47) (Lovric et al. 2017).

### Ceramide Transfer Protein Superactivity, Autosomal Dominant Mental Retardation Type 34, COL4A3BP

**Function:** *COL4A3BP* encodes collagen type IV alpha-3-binding protein, also known as ceramide transfer protein (CERT) or StAR-related lipid transfer protein 11 (STARD11). In vitro assays show that this lipid transfer-catalyzing domain specifically extracts ceramide from phospholipid bilayers and is suggested to mediate intracellular trafficking of ceramide in a non-vesicular manner (Hanada et al. 2003).

**Clinical:** Only three patients in large-scale discovery of novel genetic causes of developmental disorders, The Deciphering Developmental Disorders Study: the three identical Ser132Leu pathogenic variants in CERT that remove a serine that when phosphorylated downregulates transporter activity from the ER to the Golgi. Authors suggest that this leads to superactivity of CERT and that this results in intracellular imbalances in ceramide and its downstream metabolic pathways (Deciphering Developmental Disorders Study 2015). As there is no functional proof, it should be considered a candidate gene awaiting confirmation (Table 51.48).

**Table 51.47** Sphingosine-1-phosphate lyase deficiency

| System | Symptoms and biomarkers | Neonatal (birth–1 month) | Infancy (1–18 months) | Childhood (1.5–11 years) | Adolescence (11–16 years) | Adulthood (>16 years) |
|---|---|---|---|---|---|---|
| CNS | Neuropathy, peripheral | | | ± | ± | ± |
| | Retardation, psychomotor | ± | ± | ± | | |
| Dermatological | Ichthyosis | | ± | ± | ± | |
| Ear | Deafness, sensorineural | ± | ± | ± | ± | |
| Endocrine | Adrenal calcification | ± | ± | ± | ± | |
| | Adrenal insufficiency | ± | ± | ± | ± | ± |
| Musculoskeletal | Microcephaly | ± | ± | ± | | |
| Other | Malformations (brain) | ± | ± | | | |
| Renal | Nephrotic syndrome | ± | ± | ± | ± | ± |
| Laboratory findings | C24:0 and C16:0 lactyosylceramides (serum) | | | ↑ | | |
| | Ceramides (serum) | | | ↑ | | |
| | Sphingosine-1-phosphate (plasma) | | | | ↑ | |

**Table 51.48** Ceramide transfer protein superactivity

| System | Symptoms and biomarkers | Neonatal (birth–1 month) | Infancy (1–18 months) | Childhood (1.5–11 years) | Adolescence (11–16 years) | Adulthood (>16 years) |
|---|---|---|---|---|---|---|
| CNS | Intellectual disability | | ± | ± | | |
| | Retardation, psychomotor | | ± | ± | | |

**GM3 Synthase Deficiency, Amish Infantile Epilepsy Syndrome; Salt and Pepper Developmental Regression Syndrome, ST3GAL5 Now Also Called ST3GAL5-CDG**

**Function:** *ST3GAL5* encodes lactosylceramide α-2,3-sialyltransferase, or GM3 synthase, a Golgi enzyme which catalyzes the formation of GM3 ganglioside from lactosylceramide, the first step in the synthesis of complex ganglioside species of the a-, b-, and c-series (Fig. 51.4c).

**Clinical:** Autosomal recessive infantile-onset symptomatic epilepsy syndrome associated with microcephaly, choreoathetosis, blindness, and deafness and failure to thrive (Simpson et al. 2004; Bowser et al. 2019). Pathogenic variants in *ST3GAL5* also have been found in the salt & pepper syndrome, a very similar neurodevelopmental disorder associated with altered "salt & pepper" dermal pigmentation (= freckle-like hyperpigmented and depigmented macules). As *ST3GAL5* deficiency also affects both N-linked and O-linked glycosylation, this disorder is also known as *ST3GAL5*-CDG. Plasma glycosphingolipids of *ST3GAL5*-deficient patients completely lack GM3 and gangliosides derived from GM3 (GM2, GM1a, GD3, GD1a), and its precursor lactosylceramide and its alternative derivatives (LacCer, Gb3, Gb4) are elevated (Simpson et al. 2004). Secondary respiratory chain dysfunction in fibroblasts and the liver was reported (Fragaki et al. 2013) as well as high blood lactate levels (Table 51.49) (Lee et al. 2016).

**GM2_GD2 Synthase Deficiency, Autosomal Recessive Spastic Paraplegia Type 26 (SPG26), B4GALNT1**

**Function:** *B4GALNT1* encodes β-1,4-N-acetyl galactosaminyltransferase 1 (GalNAc-T), or GM2/GD2 synthase, a Golgi enzyme which catalyzes the reaction GM3➔GM2 and GD3➔GD2 in ganglioside synthesis of a-, b-, and c-series, but also lactosylceramide➔GA2 and Gb3➔Gb4 of 0-series and globo-series, respectively (Fig. 51.4c).

**Clinical:** *B4GALNT1* pathogenic variants were identified in patients with an early-onset but slowly progressive spastic paraparesis (SPG26) associated with mild intellectual disability and possibly *pes cavus*, cerebellar ataxia, peripheral neuropathy, dystonia, cataract, and hypogonadism in males (Boukhris et al. 2013). Analysis of patient fibroblasts revealed lack of GM2 production and increased levels of the precursor GM3 (Table 51.50) (Harlalka et al. 2013).

**GD1a_GT1b Synthase Deficiency, ST3GAL3-CDG, ST3GAL3**

**Function:** *ST3GAL3* encodes the Golgi enzyme β-galactoside-α2,3-sialyltransferase-III (ST3Gal-III) that transfers sialic acid (N-acetylneuraminic acid) in α2,3-linkage to galactose and is needed for the synthesis of GD1a and GT1b in ganglioside a-, b-, and c-series but also takes part in the formation of the sialyl-Lewis ($sLe^a$ and $sLe^x$) epitopes on proteins (Edvardson et al. 2013) (Fig. 51.4c).

**Table 51.49** GM3 synthase deficiency

| System | Symptoms and biomarkers | Neonatal (birth–1 month) | Infancy (1–18 months) | Childhood (1.5–11 years) | Adolescence (11–16 years) | Adulthood (>16 years) |
|---|---|---|---|---|---|---|
| CNS | Acquired microcephaly | | + | + | + | |
| | Choreoathetosis | | + | + | + | |
| | Cortical atrophy (MRI) | | | ± | + | |
| | Epilepsy, intractable | | ± | ± | ± | |
| | Regression, psychomotor | | + | + | | |
| | Severe intellectual deficiency | | + | + | + | |
| Dermatological | Pigmentation | | ± | ± | ± | |
| Ear | Deafness, sensorineural | | ± | ± | ± | |
| Eye | Visual impairment | | + | + | + | |
| Other | Failure to thrive | | + | + | + | |
| Laboratory findings | GM3 activity (plasma) | | ↓ | ↓ | ↓ | |
| | GM3 ganglioside (plasma) | | ↓↓ | ↓↓ | ↓↓ | |
| | Lactate (plasma) | | | ↑ | | |
| | Lactosylceramide (plasma) | | ↑ | ↑ | ↑ | |

**Table 51.50** GM2/GD2 synthase deficiency

| System | Symptoms and biomarkers | Neonatal (birth–1 month) | Infancy (1–18 months) | Childhood (1.5–11 years) | Adolescence (11–16 years) | Adulthood (>16 years) |
|---|---|---|---|---|---|---|
| CNS | Ataxia, cerebellar | | ± | ± | ± | ± |
| | Dystonia | | ± | ± | ± | ± |
| | Intellectual disability, mild | | ± | + | + | + |
| | Neuropathy, peripheral | | | ± | ± | ± |
| | Spastic paraparesis | | | ± | + | + |
| Endocrine | Hypogonadism | | | ± | ± | ± |
| Eye | Cataract | | | ± | ± | ± |
| Musculoskeletal | Pes cavus | | ± | ± | ± | ± |
| Laboratory findings | GM2 gangliosides (fibroblasts) | | | ↓↓ | ↓↓ | ↓↓ |
| | GM3 gangliosides (fibroblasts) | | | ↑ | ↑ | ↑ |

**Clinical:** *ST3GAL3* deficiency also affects protein glycosylation, therefore also called *ST3GAL3*-CDG. Few patients have been reported so far with *ST3GAL3* pathogenic variants: two families with nonsyndromic severe intellectual disabilities (Hu et al. 2011) and two families with severe intellectual disability and epileptic encephalopathy (Table 51.51) (Edvardson et al. 2013).

### Gb3 Synthase Deficiency, NOR Polyagglutination Syndrome, A4GALT

**Function:** *A4GALT* encodes α-1,4-galactosyltransferase (A4GALT or Gb3 synthase) that uses UDP-galactose to add a galactose to lactosylceramide forming Gb3 (Fig. 51.4c) as well as reactions more downstream in the globo-series (not shown) that lead to the formation of the human P1PK blood group antigens P1, P(k), and P. The antigen P(k) in fact is Gb3, which is also known as cluster of differentiation 77 (CD77).

**Clinical:** Polyagglutination is the occurrence of red cell agglutination by virtually all human sera, but not by autologous serum or sera from newborns. NOR polyagglutination syndrome was designated "NOR" since the family where this phenomenon was first observed was from Norton, Virginia. The syndrome is transmitted in an autosomal dominant pattern of inheritance and results from a specific mutation in *A4GALT*, c.631C > G, and p. Q211E, which changes the substrate specificity of A4GALT, so it cannot only attach galactose to another galactose but also to N-acetylgalactosamine (GalNac). The latter reaction leads to synthesis of NOR antigens, which are glycosphingolipids with terminal Gal(α1–4)GalNAc sequence, which does not occur in mammals. The NOR-positive individuals do

**Table 51.51** GD1a/GT1b synthase deficiency

| System | Symptoms and biomarkers | Neonatal (birth–1 month) | Infancy (1–18 months) | Childhood (1.5–11 years) | Adolescence (11–16 years) | Adulthood (>16 years) |
|---|---|---|---|---|---|---|
| CNS | Encephalopathy, epileptic | | ± | ± | ± | |
| | Severe intellectual deficiency | + | + | + | + | |

**Table 51.52** GB3 synthase deficiency

| System | Symptoms and biomarkers | Neonatal (birth–1 month) | Infancy (1–18 months) | Childhood (1.5–11 years) | Adolescence (11–16 years) | Adulthood (>16 years) |
|---|---|---|---|---|---|---|
| Other | Polyagglutination syndrome (erythrocytes) | + | + | + | + | + |

not show any morbid symptoms, but their erythrocytes are agglutinated by most human sera, creating a risk of complications during transfusion of NOR erythrocytes. NOR-positive individuals should therefore be disqualified as blood donors (Table 51.52) (Suchanowska et al. 2012; Kaczmarek et al. 2016) (also see https://omim.org/entry/111400).

## Miscellaneous

### Phospholipid-Transporting ATPase IB Deficiency, Cerebellar Ataxia, Mental Retardation, and Dysequilibrium Syndrome Type 4, ATP8A2

**Function:** *ATP8A2* encodes ATPase aminophospholipid transporter type 8A member 2 (ATP8A2) and belongs to the P4-ATPases subfamily of P-type ATPases, which are involved in the transport of aminophospholipids. ATP8A2 is involved in the transport of aminophospholipids (PE and PS) from the outer leaflet of the plasma membrane toward the inner leaflet (PS and to a lesser extent PE) in brain cells, retinal photoreceptors, and the testis. This is important to maintain membrane asymmetry in the plasma membrane (Cacciagli et al. 2010).

**Clinical:** Cerebellar ataxia, mental retardation, and dysequilibrium syndrome type 4 (CAMRQ4): autosomal recessive condition with intellectual disability, developmental delay, ophthalmoplegia, movement disorder, hearing loss, epilepsy, and short stature (Table 51.53) (Guissart et al. 2019).

### CYP2U1 Deficiency, Autosomal Recessive Spastic Paraplegia Type 56, CYP2U1

**Function:** *CYP2U1* encodes cytochrome P450 family 2 subfamily U member 1 (CYP2U1), is localized to both ER and mitochondria, and catalyzes the ω- and (ω-1)-hydroxylation of arachidonic acid (C20:4ω6, AA) as well as hydroxylation of docosahexaenoic acid (C22:6ω3, DHA) and other long-chain fatty acids (saturated/monounsaturated C16-C22). This yields a series of oxygenated products including two bioactive metabolites 19- and 20-hydroxyeicosatetraenoic acid (so-called HETEs). *CYP2U1* is highly expressed in the thymus and cerebellum and has been suggested to modulate the arachidonic acid signaling pathway and play a role in other fatty acid signaling processes (Chuang et al. 2004).

**Clinical:** Autosomal recessive spastic paraplegia type 56. Patients with *CYP2U1* pathogenic variants usually present with an infantile-onset but slowly progressive complicated spastic paraplegia (Tesson et al. 2012). Possible associated symptoms are dystonia, psychomotor retardation or regression, intellectual disability, and/or subclinical sensory motor neuropathy (Tesson et al. 2012; Kariminejad et al. 2016; Iodice et al. 2017). Brain MRI may show delayed myelination, white matter abnormalities, and/or thin corpus callosum (Tesson et al. 2012). CT scan may reveal basal ganglia calcifications (23176821). Adult-onset spastic paraplegia has been reported, associated with a pigmentary maculopathy (Table 51.54) (Leonardi et al. 2016).

### ABHD12 Deficiency, Polyneuropathy, Hearing Loss, Ataxia, Retinitis Pigmentosa, and Cataract (PHARC) Syndrome, ABHD12

**Function:** *ABHD12* encodes α–/β-hydrolase domain-containing protein 12 (ABHD12) which is an integral membrane plasma/ER membrane protein that was shown to hydrolyze the endocannabinoid 2-arachidonoylglycerol (2-AG) into arachidonic acid (C20:4ω6) and monoacylglycerol in vitro. More recently, ABHD12 was shown to be the major lipase acting on VLCFA-containing lysophosphatidylserine (LPS) (Blankman et al. 2013) in the brain and that it also hydrolyzes oxidized PS and LPS species. The oxidation of PS species due to elevated reactive oxygen species is

**Table 51.53** Phospholipid-transporting ATPase IB deficiency

| System | Symptoms and biomarkers | Neonatal (birth–1 month) | Infancy (1–18 months) | Childhood (1.5–11 years) | Adolescence (11–16 years) | Adulthood (>16 years) |
|---|---|---|---|---|---|---|
| CNS | Ataxia, cerebellar | + | + | + | + | + |
| | Bilateral sensory hearing loss | + | + | + | + | + |
| | Dysarthria | + | + | + | + | + |
| | Epileptic seizures | + | + | + | + | + |
| | Extrapyramidal movement disorder | + | + | + | + | + |
| | Gait, atactic | | | + | + | + |
| | Hypotonia, muscular-generalized | + | + | + | + | + |
| | Intellectual disability | ± | ± | + | + | + |
| | Interictal nystagmus | + | + | + | + | + |
| | Sleep disturbances | + | + | + | + | + |
| Digestive | Feeding difficulties | + | + | + | + | + |
| Eye | Ophthalmoplegia | + | + | + | + | + |
| | Optic atrophy | ± | + | + | + | + |
| | Ptosis of eyelid | + | + | + | + | + |
| Musculoskeletal | Microcephaly | + | + | + | + | + |
| | Short stature | + | + | + | + | + |
| Other | Failure to thrive | + | + | + | + | + |

**Table 51.54** CYP2U1 deficiency

| System | Symptoms and biomarkers | Neonatal (birth–1 month) | Infancy (1–18 months) | Childhood (1.5–11 years) | Adolescence (11–16 years) | Adulthood (>16 years) |
|---|---|---|---|---|---|---|
| CNS | Basal ganglia calcifications (CT) | | | ± | ± | ± |
| | Dystonia | | | ± | ± | ± |
| | Intellectual disability | | | ± | ± | ± |
| | Neuropathy, peripheral | | | | ± | ± |
| | Regression, psychomotor | | ± | ± | | |
| | Retardation, psychomotor | ± | ± | ± | | |
| | Spastic paraplegia | ± | ± | ± | ± | + |
| | Thin corpus callosum | | | ± | ± | ± |
| | White matter abnormalities (MRI) | | | ± | ± | ± |
| Eye | Pigmentary maculopathy | | | | | ± |

linked to their transmembrane migration to the exofacial membrane surface which is a pro-apoptotic signal (Kelkar et al. 2019). LPS itself has been recognized as a signaling molecule (Makide et al. 2014), and ABHD12 therefore has been suggested to be involved in the regulation of (L)PS and oxidized (L)PS levels, thereby regulating immunological and neurological processes (Kelkar et al. 2019; Kamat et al. 2015). In *Abhd12−/−* mouse, accumulation of LPS, mainly VLCFA-containing as well as oxidized PS species, has been observed. Lipopolysaccharide challenge of *Abhd12−/−* mice showed a fivefold accumulation of oxidized PS levels in the brain. Reactive oxygen species and oxidative stress may play a role in PHARC pathology where deficient ABHD12 cannot mitigate the excess oxidized PS produced (Blankman et al. 2013; Kelkar et al. 2019).

**Clinical:** *ABHD12* pathogenic variants have been associated with a pseudo-Refsum syndrome called PHARC: polyneuropathy, hearing loss, ataxia, retinitis pigmentosa, and cataract (Fiskerstrand et al. 2010). Disease onset can be in childhood or adolescence, especially hearing loss and gait abnormalities that are related to sensory (i.e., demyelinating neuropathy) and/or cerebellar dysfunction. Visual impairment may occur in adolescence or adulthood due to bilateral cataracts and/or pigmentary retinopathy. *ABHD12* pathogenic variants have also been reported in patients with Usher syndrome (deafness, retinopathy, and sometimes cataract), but neurological examination often revealed cerebellar ataxia or peripheral neuropathy (Eisenberger et al. 2012). Still, some adult patients may present with isolated pigmentary retinopathy (Table 51.55) (Nishiguchi et al. 2014).

**Table 51.55** ABHD12 deficiency

| System | Symptoms and biomarkers | Neonatal (birth–1 month) | Infancy (1–18 months) | Childhood (1.5–11 years) | Adolescence (11–16 years) | Adulthood (>16 years) |
|---|---|---|---|---|---|---|
| CNS | Ataxia, cerebellar | | | ± | ± | ± |
| | Neuropathy, demyelinating | | | ± | ± | + |
| Ear | Deafness, sensorineural | | | | ± | + |
| Eye | Cataract | | | ± | ± | + |
| | Pigmentary retinopathy | | | ± | ± | ± |

## Diagnostic Flowchart

Given the heterogeneity of this group of disorders, no diagnostic flowcharts apply. Depending on the clinical symptoms—if available—specific biomarkers/tests can be measured, but the most common way of diagnosing these disorders is DNA diagnostics by whole-exome/whole-genome sequencing. At this time, lipidomics is not (yet) suited for clinical diagnostics as the measurement is not standardized, the optimal specimen type is variable, and no reference ranges have been established. Still, for disorders where a biomarker profile is known, this measurement can be used for the functional confirmation of the diagnosis. For uncharacterized disorders, however, it should be considered to perform lipidomics to search for new biomarkers that can be developed into targeted tests and/or panels for these types of disorders. To do this, it is crucial that specimens are collected from different cases (or if not available, at least sequential samples from the same patient) and suitable controls to allow comparative lipidomics in search of new biomarkers.

## Specimen Collection

| Test | Preconditions | Material | Handling |
|---|---|---|---|
| DNA analysis | | Whole blood (EDTA) | RT or frozen (−20 °C) |
| Lipidomics (blood) | >4 h after last meal or after overnight fast | Whole blood (EDTA)<br>Plasma (EDTA) | Frozen (−20 °C)<br>Frozen (−20 °C) |
| Lipidomics (fibroblasts) | | Fibroblasts:<br>• Live cells<br>• Cell pellets (from T-175) | RT<br>Frozen (−80 °C) |
| Lipidomics (tissues) | No formalin, rapid transfer to $N_2$ and then freezer | Tissue | Frozen (−80 °C) |

## Prenatal Diagnosis

No specific biochemical tests exist at this time to perform prenatal testing. Like many disorders, if the index patient is known, DNA analysis can be used for prenatal testing if warranted.

## DNA Testing

See Chapter structure.

## References


Abe K, Ohno Y, Sassa T, Taguchi R, Çalışkan M, Ober C, Kihara A. Mutation for nonsyndromic mental retardation in the trans-2-enoyl-CoA reductase TER gene involved in fatty acid elongation impairs the enzyme activity and stability, leading to change in sphingolipid profile. J Biol Chem. 2013;288:36741–9.

Agarwal AK, Arioglu E, De Almeida S, Akkoc N, Taylor SI, Bowcock AM, Barnes RI, Garg A. AGPAT2 is mutated in congenital generalized lipodystrophy linked to chromosome 9q34. Nat Genet. 2002;31:21–3.

Ahmed MY, Al-Khayat A, Al-Murshedi F, et al. A mutation of EPT1 (SELENOI) underlies a new disorder of Kennedy pathway phospholipid biosynthesis. Brain. 2017;140:547–54.

Albert JS, Yerges-Armstrong LM, Horenstein RB, et al. Null mutation in hormone-sensitive lipase gene and risk of type 2 diabetes. N Engl J Med. 2014;370:2307–15.

Alderson NL, Rembiesa BM, Walla MD, Bielawska A, Bielawski J, Hama H. The human FA2H gene encodes a fatty acid 2-hydroxylase. J Biol Chem. 2004;279:48562–8.

Amen N, Mathow D, Rabionet M, Sandhoff R, Langbein L, Gretz N, Jäckel C, Gröne H-J, Jennemann R. Differentiation of epidermal keratinocytes is dependent on glucosylceramide:ceramide processing. Hum Mol Genet. 2013;22:4164–79.

Anderson KE, Kielkowska A, Durrant TN, Juvin V, Clark J, Stephens LR, Hawkins PT. Lysophosphatidylinositol-acyltransferase-1 (LPIAT1) is required to maintain physiological levels of PtdIns and PtdInsP(2) in the mouse. PLoS One. 2013;8:e58425.

Atkinson D, Nikodinovic Glumac J, Asselbergh B, et al. Sphingosine 1-phosphate lyase deficiency causes Charcot-Marie-tooth neuropathy. Neurology. 2017;88:533–42.

Auranen M, Toppila J, Suriyanarayanan S, Lone MA, Paetau A, Tyynismaa H, Hornemann T, Ylikallio E. Clinical and metabolic consequences of L-serine supplementation in hereditary sensory and autonomic neuropathy type 1C. Cold Spring Harb Mol Case Stud. 2017;3:1–9.

Azukaitis K, Simkova E, Majid MA, et al. The phenotypic Spectrum of nephropathies associated with mutations in diacylglycerol kinase ε. J Am Soc Nephrol. 2017;28:3066–75.

Bamborschke D, Pergande M, Becker K, Koerber F, Dötsch J, Vierzig A, Weber LT, Cirak S. A novel mutation in sphingosine-1-phosphate lyase causing congenital brain malformation. Brain and Development. 2018;40:480–3.

Blankman JL, Long JZ, Trauger SA, Siuzdak G, Cravatt BF. ABHD12 controls brain lysophosphatidylserine pathways that are deregulated in a murine model of the neurodegenerative disease PHARC. Proc Natl Acad Sci U S A. 2013;110:1500–5.

Blom W, de Muinck Keizer SM, Scholte HR. Acetyl-CoA carboxylase deficiency: an inborn error of de novo fatty acid synthesis. N Engl J Med. 1981;305:465–6.

Borroni B, Di Gregorio E, Orsi L, et al. Clinical and neuroradiological features of spinocerebellar ataxia 38 (SCA38). Parkinsonism Relat Disord. 2016;28:80–6.

Boukhris A, Schule R, Loureiro JL, et al. Alteration of ganglioside biosynthesis responsible for complex hereditary spastic paraplegia. Am J Hum Genet. 2013;93:118–23.

Bowser LE, Young M, Wenger OK, et al. Recessive GM3 synthase deficiency: natural history, biochemistry, and therapeutic frontier. Mol Genet Metab. 2019;126:475–88.

Bozelli JC, Epand RM. Role of membrane shape in regulating the phosphatidylinositol cycle at contact sites. Chem Phys Lipids. 2019;221:24–9.

Braverman NE, Moser AB. Functions of plasmalogen lipids in health and disease. Biochim Biophys Acta. 2012;1822:1442–52.

Broekema MF, Massink MPG, De Ligt J, Stigter ECA, Monajemi H, De Ridder J, Burgering BMT, van Haaften GW, Kalkhoven E. A single complex Agpat2 allele in a patient with partial lipodystrophy. Front Physiol. 2018;9:1363.

Brown AL, Mark Brown J. Critical roles for α/β hydrolase domain 5 (ABHD5)/comparative gene identification-58 (CGI-58) at the lipid droplet interface and beyond. Biochim Biophys Acta Mol Cell Biol Lipids. 2017;1862:1233–41.

Cacciagli P, Haddad M-R, Mignon-Ravix C, El-Waly B, Moncla A, Missirian C, Chabrol B, Villard L. Disruption of the ATP8A2 gene in a patient with a t(10;13) de novo balanced translocation and a severe neurological phenotype. Eur J Hum Genet. 2010;18:1360–3.

Cadieux-Dion M, Turcotte-Gauthier M, Noreau A, Martin C, Meloche C, Gravel M, Drouin CA, Rouleau GA, Nguyen DK, Cossette P. Expanding the clinical phenotype associated with ELOVL4 mutation: study of a large French-Canadian family with autosomal dominant spinocerebellar ataxia and erythrokeratodermia. JAMA Neurol. 2014;71:470–5.

Çalışkan M, Chong JX, Uricchio L, et al. Exome sequencing reveals a novel mutation for autosomal recessive non-syndromic mental retardation in the TECR gene on chromosome 19p13. Hum Mol Genet. 2011;20:1285–9.

Cao Y, Traer E, Zimmerman GA, McIntyre TM, Prescott SM. Cloning, expression, and chromosomal localization of human long-chain fatty acid-CoA ligase 4 (FACL4). Genomics. 1998;49:327–30.

Chuang SS, Helvig C, Taimi M, Ramshaw HA, Collop AH, Amad M, White JA, Petkovich M, Jones G, Korczak B. CYP2U1, a novel human thymus- and brain-specific cytochrome P450, catalyzes omega- and (omega-1)-hydroxylation of fatty acids. J Biol Chem. 2004;279:6305–14.

Craveiro Sarmento AS, Ferreira LC, Lima JG, de Azevedo Medeiros LB, Barbosa Cunha PT, Agnez-Lima LF, Galvão Ururahy MA, de Melo Campos JTA. The worldwide mutational landscape of Berardinelli-Seip congenital lipodystrophy. Mutat Res. 2019;781:30–52.

Csaki LS, Dwyer JR, Fong LG, Tontonoz P, Young SG, Reue K. Three mammalian lipins act as phosphatidate phosphatases with distinct tissue expression patterns. Prog Lipid Res. 2013a;52:305–16.

Csaki LS, Dwyer JR, Fong LG, Tontonoz P, Young SG, Reue K. Lipins, lipinopathies, and the modulation of cellular lipid storage and signaling. Prog Lipid Res. 2013b;52:305–16.

Dawkins JL, Hulme DJ, Brahmbhatt SB, Auer-Grumbach M, Nicholson GA. Mutations in SPTLC1, encoding serine palmitoyltransferase, long chain base subunit-1, cause hereditary sensory neuropathy type I. Nat Genet. 2001;27:309–12.

Deák F, Anderson RE, Fessler JL, Sherry DM. Novel cellular functions of very long chain-fatty acids: insight from ELOVL4 mutations. Front Cell Neurosci. 2019;13:428.

Dean JM, Lodhi IJ. Structural and functional roles of ether lipids. Protein Cell. 2018;9:196–206.

Deciphering Developmental Disorders Study. Large-scale discovery of novel genetic causes of developmental disorders. Nature. 2015;519:223–8.

Di Gregorio E, Borroni B, Giorgio E, et al. ELOVL5 mutations cause spinocerebellar ataxia 38. Am J Hum Genet. 2014;95:209–17.

Dolgin V, Straussberg R, Xu R, et al. DEGS1 variant causes neurological disorder. Eur J Hum Genet. 2019;27:1668–76.

Ebihara K, Kusakabe T, Hirata M, et al. Efficacy and safety of leptin-replacement therapy and possible mechanisms of leptin actions in patients with generalized lipodystrophy. J Clin Endocrinol Metab. 2007;92:532–41.

Eckl K-M, Tidhar R, Thiele H, et al. Impaired epidermal ceramide synthesis causes autosomal recessive congenital ichthyosis and reveals the importance of ceramide acyl chain length. J Invest Dermatol. 2013;133:2202–11.

Edvardson S, Hama H, Shaag A, Gomori JM, Berger I, Soffer D, Korman SH, Taustein I, Saada A, Elpeleg O. Mutations in the fatty acid 2-hydroxylase gene are associated with leukodystrophy with spastic Paraparesis and dystonia. Am J Hum Genet. 2008;83:643–8.

Edvardson S, Baumann A-M, Mühlenhoff M, et al. West syndrome caused by ST3Gal-III deficiency. Epilepsia. 2013;54:e24–7.

Edvardson S, Yi JK, Jalas C, et al. Deficiency of the alkaline ceramidase ACER3 manifests in early childhood by progressive leukodystrophy. J Med Genet. 2016;53:389–96.

Eisenberger T, Slim R, Mansour A, et al. Targeted next-generation sequencing identifies a homozygous nonsense mutation in ABHD12, the gene underlying PHARC, in a family clinically diagnosed with Usher syndrome type 3. Orphanet J Rare Dis. 2012;7:59.

Ferlazzo E, Italiano D, An I, Calarese T, Laguitton V, Bramanti P, Di Bella P, Genton P. Description of a family with a novel progressive myoclonus epilepsy and cognitive impairment. Mov Disord. 2009;24:1016–22.

Fiskerstrand T, H'Mida-Ben Brahim D, Johansson S, et al. Mutations in ABHD12 cause the neurodegenerative disease PHARC: An inborn error of endocannabinoid metabolism. Am J Hum Genet. 2010;87:410–7.

Fragaki K, Ait-El-Mkadem S, Chaussenot A, et al. Refractory epilepsy and mitochondrial dysfunction due to GM3 synthase deficiency. Eur J Hum Genet. 2013;21:528–34.

Fridman V, Suriyanarayanan S, Novak P, et al. Randomized trial of l-serine in patients with hereditary sensory and autonomic neuropathy type 1. Neurology. 2019;92:e359–70.

Gandotra S, Le Dour C, Bottomley W, et al. Perilipin deficiency and autosomal dominant partial lipodystrophy. N Engl J Med. 2011;364:740–8.

Gantner ML, Eade K, Wallace M, et al. Serine and lipid metabolism in macular disease and peripheral neuropathy. N Engl J Med. 2019;381:1422–33.

Garofalo K, Penno A, Schmidt BP, Lee H-J, Frosch MP, von Eckardstein A, Brown RH, Hornemann T, Eichler FS. Oral L-serine supplementation reduces production of neurotoxic deoxysphingolipids in mice and humans with hereditary sensory autonomic neuropathy type 1. J Clin Invest. 2011;121:4735–45.

Ginkel C, Hartmann D, vom Dorp K, et al. Ablation of neuronal ceramide synthase 1 in mice decreases ganglioside levels and expression of myelin-associated glycoprotein in oligodendrocytes. J Biol Chem. 2012;287:41888–902.

Girisha KM, von Elsner L, Neethukrishna K, Muranjan M, Shukla A, Bhavani GS, Nishimura G, Kutsche K, Mortier G. The homozygous variant c.797G>a/p.(Cys266Tyr) in PISD is associated with a Spondyloepimetaphyseal dysplasia with large epiphyses and disturbed mitochondrial function. Hum Mutat. 2019;40:299–309.

Godeiro Junior CO, Vale TC, Afonso COM, Kok F, Pedroso JL, Barsottini OG. Progressive myoclonic epilepsy type 8 due to CERS1 deficiency: a novel mutation with prominent ataxia. Mov Disord Clin Pract. 2018;5:330–2.

Guissart C, Harrison AN, Benkirane M, et al. ATP8A2-related disorders as recessive cerebellar ataxia. J Neurol. 2019; https://doi.org/10.1007/s00415-019-09579-4.

Guo Y-P, Tang B, Guo J. PLA2G6-associated neurodegeneration (PLAN): review of clinical phenotypes and genotypes. Front Neurol. 2018;9:1100.

Hammer MB, Eleuch-Fayache G, Schottlaender LV, et al. Mutations in GBA2 cause autosomal-recessive cerebellar ataxia with spasticity. Am J Hum Genet. 2013;92:245–51.

Hanada K, Kumagai K, Yasuda S, Miura Y, Kawano M, Fukasawa M, Nishijima M. Molecular machinery for non-vesicular trafficking of ceramide. Nature. 2003;426:803–9.

Hannun YA, Obeid LM. Sphingolipids and their metabolism in physiology and disease. Nat Rev Mol Cell Biol. 2018;19:175–91.

Hara S, Yoda E, Sasaki Y, Nakatani Y, Kuwata H. Calcium-independent phospholipase A2γ (iPLA2γ) and its roles in cellular functions and diseases. Biochim Biophys Acta Mol Cell Biol Lipids. 2019;1864:861–8.

Harayama T, Riezman H. Understanding the diversity of membrane lipid composition. Nat Rev Mol Cell Biol. 2018;19:281–96.

Harlalka GV, Lehman A, Chioza B, et al. Mutations in B4GALNT1 (GM2 synthase) underlie a new disorder of ganglioside biosynthesis. Brain. 2013;136:3618–24.

Haugarvoll K, Johansson S, Rodriguez CE, et al. GBA2 mutations cause a Marinesco-Sjögren-like syndrome: genetic and biochemical studies. PLoS One. 2017;12:e0169309.

Heimer G, Kerätär JM, Riley LG, et al. MECR mutations cause childhood-onset dystonia and optic atrophy, a mitochondrial fatty acid synthesis disorder. Am J Hum Genet. 2016;99:1229–44.

Herlin T, Fiirgaard B, Bjerre M, Kerndrup G, Hasle H, Bing X, Ferguson PJ. Efficacy of anti-IL-1 treatment in Majeed syndrome. Ann Rheum Dis. 2013;72:410–3.

Hermansson M, Hänninen S, Hokynar K, Somerharju P. The PNPLA-family phospholipases involved in glycerophospholipid homeostasis of HeLa cells. Biochim Biophys Acta. 2016;1861:1058–65.

Hirabayashi T, Murakami M, Kihara A. The role of PNPLA1 in ω-O-acylceramide synthesis and skin barrier function. Biochim Biophys Acta Mol Cell Biol Lipids. 2018;1864:869–79.

Hoover-Fong J, Sobreira N, Jurgens J, et al. Mutations in PCYT1A, encoding a key regulator of phosphatidylcholine metabolism, cause spondylometaphyseal dysplasia with cone-rod dystrophy. Am J Hum Genet. 2014;94:105–12.

Horibata Y, Elpeleg O, Eran A, Hirabayashi Y, Savitzki D, Tal G, Mandel H, Sugimoto H. Ethanolamine phosphotransferase 1 (selenoprotein I) is critical for the neural development and maintenance of plasmalogen in human. J Lipid Res. 2018;1:1–47.

Hotz A, Bourrat E, Küsel J, et al. Mutation update for CYP4F22 variants associated with autosomal recessive congenital ichthyosis. Hum Mutat. 2018;39:1305–13.

Houlden H, King R, Blake J, et al. Clinical, pathological and genetic characterization of hereditary sensory and autonomic neuropathy type 1 (HSAN I). Brain. 2006;129:411–25.

Houtkooper RH, Rodenburg RJ, Thiels C, et al. Cardiolipin and monolysocardiolipin analysis in fibroblasts, lymphocytes, and tissues using high-performance liquid chromatography-mass spectrometry as a diagnostic test for Barth syndrome. Anal Biochem. 2009;387:230–7.

Hu W, Xu R, Sun W, Szulc ZM, Bielawski J, Obeid LM, Mao C. Alkaline ceramidase 3 (ACER3) hydrolyzes unsaturated long-chain ceramides, and its down-regulation inhibits both cell proliferation and apoptosis. J Biol Chem. 2010;285:7964–76.

Hu H, Eggers K, Chen W, et al. ST3GAL3 mutations impair the development of higher cognitive functions. Am J Hum Genet. 2011;89:407–14.

Hufnagel RB, Arno G, Hein ND, et al. Neuropathy target esterase impairments cause Oliver-McFarlane and Laurence-Moon syndromes. J Med Genet. 2015;52:85–94.

Inloes JM, Hsu K-L, Dix MM, Viader A, Masuda K, Takei T, Wood MR, Cravatt BF. The hereditary spastic paraplegia-related enzyme DDHD2 is a principal brain triglyceride lipase. Proc Natl Acad Sci U S A. 2014;111:14924–9.

Inloes JM, Jing H, Cravatt BF. The spastic paraplegia-associated phospholipase DDHD1 is a primary brain phosphatidylinositol lipase. Biochemistry. 2018a;57:5759–67.

Inloes JM, Kiosses WB, Wang H, Walther TC, Farese RV, Cravatt BF. Functional contribution of the spastic paraplegia-related triglyceride hydrolase DDHD2 to the formation and content of lipid droplets. Biochemistry. 2018b;57:827–38.

Iodice A, Panteghini C, Spagnoli C, Salerno GG, Frattini D, Russo C, Garavaglia B, Fusco C. Long-term follow-up in spastic paraplegia due to SPG56/CYP2U1: age-dependency rather than genetic variability? J Neurol. 2017;264:586–8.

Jacher JE, Roy N, Ghaziuddin M, Innis JW. Expanding the phenotypic spectrum of MBOAT7-related intellectual disability. Am J Med Genet B Neuropsychiatr Genet. 2019;180:483–7.

Jakobsson A, Westerberg R, Jacobsson A. Fatty acid elongases in mammals: their regulation and roles in metabolism. Prog Lipid Res. 2006;45:237–49.

Jennemann R, Gröne H-J. Cell-specific in vivo functions of glycosphingolipids: lessons from genetic deletions of enzymes involved in glycosphingolipid synthesis. Prog Lipid Res. 2013;52:231–48.

Johansen A, Rosti RO, Musaev D, et al. Mutations in MBOAT7, encoding lysophosphatidylinositol acyltransferase I, lead to intellectual disability accompanied by epilepsy and autistic features. Am J Hum Genet. 2016;99:912–6.

Kaczmarek R, Mikolajewicz K, Szymczak K, Duk M, Majorczyk E, Krop-Watorek A, Buczkowska A, Czerwinski M. Evaluation of an amino acid residue critical for the specificity and activity of human Gb3/CD77 synthase. Glycoconj J. 2016;33:963–73.

Kamat SS, Camara K, Parsons WH, Chen D-H, Dix MM, Bird TD, Howell AR, Cravatt BF. Immunomodulatory lysophosphatidylserines are regulated by ABHD16A and ABHD12 interplay. Nat Chem Biol. 2015;11:164–71.

Kang Y, Stroud DA, Baker MJ, et al. Sengers syndrome-associated mitochondrial acylglycerol kinase is a subunit of the human TIM22 protein import complex. Mol Cell. 2017;67:457–470.e5.

Kariminejad A, Schöls L, Schüle R, Tonekaboni SH, Abolhassani A, Fadaee M, Rosti RO, Gleeson JG. CYP2U1 mutations in two Iranian patients with activity induced dystonia, motor regression and spastic paraplegia. Eur J Paediatr Neurol. 2016;20:782–7.

Karsai G, Kraft F, Haag N, et al. DEGS1-associated aberrant sphingolipid metabolism impairs nervous system function in humans. J Clin Invest. 2019;129:1229–39.

Kastaniotis AJ, Autio KJ, Kerätär JM, Monteuuis G, Mäkelä AM, Nair RR, Pietikäinen LP, Shvetsova A, Chen Z, Hiltunen JK. Mitochondrial fatty acid synthesis, fatty acids and mitochondrial physiology. Biochim Biophys Acta Mol Cell Biol Lipids. 2017;1862:39–48.

Kelkar DS, Ravikumar G, Mehendale N, Singh S, Joshi A, Sharma AK, Mhetre A, Rajendran A, Chakrapani H, Kamat SS. A chemical-genetic screen identifies ABHD12 as an oxidized-phosphatidylserine lipase. Nat Chem Biol. 2019;15:169–78.

Kihara A. Very long-chain fatty acids: elongation, physiology and related disorders. J Biochem. 2012;152:387–95.

Kihara A. Synthesis and degradation pathways, functions, and pathology of ceramides and epidermal acylceramides. Prog Lipid Res. 2016a;63:50–69.

Kihara A. Synthesis and degradation pathways, functions, and pathology of ceramides and epidermal acylceramides. Prog Lipid Res. 2016b;63:50–69.

Kruer MC, Paisán-Ruiz C, Boddaert N, et al. Defective FA2H leads to a novel form of neurodegeneration with brain iron accumulation (NBIA). Ann Neurol. 2010;68:611–8.

Kutkowska-Kaźmierczak A, Rydzanicz M, Chlebowski A, et al. Dominant ELOVL1 mutation causes neurological disorder with ichthyotic keratoderma, spasticity, hypomyelination and dysmorphic features. J Med Genet. 2018;55:408–14.

Laver TW, Patel KA, Colclough K, et al. PLIN1 Haploinsufficiency is not associated with lipodystrophy. J Clin Endocrinol Metab. 2018;103:3225–30.

Lee J, Ridgway ND. Substrate channeling in the glycerol-3-phosphate pathway regulates the synthesis, storage and secretion of glycerolipids. Biochim Biophys Acta Mol Cell Biol Lipids. 2020;1865:158438.

Lee H-C, Inoue T, Sasaki J, et al. LPIAT1 regulates arachidonic acid content in phosphatidylinositol and is required for cortical lamination in mice. Mol Biol Cell. 2012;23:4689–700.

Lee JS, Yoo Y, Lim BC, Kim KJ, Song J, Choi M, Chae J-H. GM3 synthase deficiency due to ST3GAL5 variants in two Korean female siblings: masquerading as Rett syndrome-like phenotype. Am J Med Genet A. 2016;170:2200–5.

Lefèvre C, Jobard F, Caux F, et al. Mutations in CGI-58, the gene encoding a new protein of the esterase/lipase/thioesterase subfamily, in Chanarin-Dorfman syndrome. Am J Hum Genet. 2001;69:1002–12.

Lemaire M, Frémeaux-Bacchi V, Schaefer F, et al. Recessive mutations in DGKE cause atypical hemolytic-uremic syndrome. Nat Genet. 2013;45:531–6.

Leonardi L, Ziccardi L, Marcotulli C, et al. Pigmentary degenerative maculopathy as prominent phenotype in an Italian SPG56/CYP2U1 family. J Neurol. 2016;263:781–3.

Li TA, Schnaar RL. Congenital disorders of ganglioside biosynthesis. Prog Mol Biol Transl Sci. 2018;156:63–82.

Liu G-Y, Moon SH, Jenkins CM, Li M, Sims HF, Guan S, Gross RW. The phospholipase iPLA2γ is a major mediator releasing oxidized aliphatic chains from cardiolipin, integrating mitochondrial bioenergetics and signaling. J Biol Chem. 2017;292:10672–84.

Longo I, Frints SGM, Fryns J-P, et al. A third MRX family (MRX68) is the result of mutation in the long chain fatty acid-CoA ligase 4 (FACL4) gene: proposal of a rapid enzymatic assay for screening mentally retarded patients. J Med Genet. 2003;40:11–7.

Lovric S, Goncalves S, Gee HY, et al. Mutations in sphingosine-1-phosphate lyase cause nephrosis with ichthyosis and adrenal insufficiency. J Clin Invest. 2017;127:912–28.

Makide K, Uwamizu A, Shinjo Y, Ishiguro J, Okutani M, Inoue A, Aoki J. Novel lysophosphoplipid receptors: their structure and function. J Lipid Res. 2014;55:1986–95.

Manes M, Alberici A, Di Gregorio E, et al. Docosahexaenoic acid is a beneficial replacement treatment for spinocerebellar ataxia 38. Ann Neurol. 2017;82:615–21.

Manes M, Alberici A, Di Gregorio E, et al. Long-term efficacy of docosahexaenoic acid (DHA) for spinocerebellar Ataxia 38 (SCA38) treatment: An open label extension study. Parkinsonism Relat Disord. 2019;63:191–4.

Martin E, Schüle R, Smets K, et al. Loss of function of glucocerebrosidase GBA2 is responsible for motor neuron defects in hereditary spastic paraplegia. Am J Hum Genet. 2013;92:238–44.

Mayr JA, Feichtinger RG, Tort F, Ribes A, Sperl W. Lipoic acid biosynthesis defects. J Inherit Metab Dis. 2014;37:553–63.

Meloni I, Muscettola M, Raynaud M, et al. FACL4, encoding fatty acid-CoA ligase 4, is mutated in nonspecific X-linked mental retardation. Nat Genet. 2002;30:436–40.

Michot C, Hubert L, Romero NB, et al. Study of LPIN1, LPIN2 and LPIN3 in rhabdomyolysis and exercise-induced myalgia. J Inherit Metab Dis. 2012;35:1119–28.

Mir H, Raza SI, Touseef M, Memon MM, Khan MN, Jaffar S, Ahmad W. A novel recessive mutation in the gene ELOVL4 causes a neuro-ichthyotic disorder with variable expressivity. BMC Med Genet. 2014;15:25.

Mitsuhashi S, Ohkuma A, Talim B, et al. A congenital muscular dystrophy with mitochondrial structural abnormalities caused by defective de novo phosphatidylcholine biosynthesis. Am J Hum Genet. 2011;88:845–51.

Monies D, Anabrees J, Ibrahim N, Elbardisy H, Abouelhoda M, Meyer BF, Alkuraya FS. Identification of a novel lethal form of autosomal recessive ichthyosis caused by UDP-glucose ceramide glucosyltransferase deficiency. Clin Genet. 2018;93:1252–3.

Mueller N, Sassa T, Morales-Gonzalez S, Schneider J, Salchow DJ, Seelow D, Knierim E, Stenzel W, Kihara A, Schuelke M. De novo mutation in ELOVL1 causes ichthyosis, acanthosis nigricans, hypomyelination, spastic paraplegia, high frequency deafness and optic atrophy. J Med Genet. 2019;56:164–75.

Muhammad E, Reish O, Ohno Y, et al. Congenital myopathy is caused by mutation of HACD1. Hum Mol Genet. 2013;22:5229–36.

Murphy SM, Ernst D, Wei Y, et al. Hereditary sensory and autonomic neuropathy type 1 (HSANI) caused by a novel mutation in SPTLC2. Neurology. 2013;80:2106–11.

Nishiguchi KM, Avila-Fernandez A, van Huet RAC, et al. Exome sequencing extends the phenotypic spectrum for ABHD12 mutations: from syndromic to nonsyndromic retinal degeneration. Ophthalmology. 2014;121:1620–7.

Noguera-Morel L, Feito-Rodríguez M, Maldonado-Cid P, García-Miñáur S, Kamsteeg E-J, González-Sarmiento R, De Lucas-Laguna R, Hernández-Martín A, Torrelo A. Two cases of autosomal recessive congenital ichthyosis due to CYP4F22 mutations: expanding the genotype of self-healing collodion baby. Pediatr Dermatol. 2016;33:e48–51.

Ohno Y, Nakamichi S, Ohkuni A, et al. Essential role of the cytochrome P450 CYP4F22 in the production of acylceramide, the key lipid for skin permeability barrier formation. Proc Natl Acad Sci U S A. 2015;112:7707–12.

Ohno Y, Kamiyama N, Nakamichi S, Kihara A. PNPLA1 is a transacylase essential for the generation of the skin barrier lipid ω-O-acylceramide. Nat Commun. 2017;8:14610.

Oswiecimska J, Dawidziuk M, Gambin T, et al. A patient with Berardinelli-Seip syndrome, novel AGPAT2 Splicesite mutation and concomitant development of non-diabetic polyneuropathy. J Clin Res Pediatr Endocrinol. 2019;11:319–26.

Ozaltin F, Li B, Rauhauser A, et al. DGKE variants cause a glomerular microangiopathy that mimics membranoproliferative GN. J Am Soc Nephrol. 2013;24:377–84.

Pant DC, Dorboz I, Schluter A, et al. Loss of the sphingolipid desaturase DEGS1 causes hypomyelinating leukodystrophy. J Clin Invest. 2019;129:1240–56.

Payne F, Lim K, Girousse A, et al. Mutations disrupting the Kennedy phosphatidylcholine pathway in humans with congenital lipodystrophy and fatty liver disease. Proc Natl Acad Sci. 2014;111:8901–6.

Penno A, Reilly MM, Houlden H, et al. Hereditary sensory neuropathy type 1 is caused by the accumulation of two neurotoxic sphingolipids. J Biol Chem. 2010;285:11178–87.

Piccini M, Vitelli F, Bruttini M, Pober BR, Jonsson JJ, Villanova M, Zollo M, Borsani G, Ballabio A, Renieri A. FACL4, a new gene encoding long-chain acyl-CoA synthetase 4, is deleted in a family with Alport syndrome, elliptocytosis, and mental retardation. Genomics. 1998;47:350–8.

Pichery M, Huchenq A, Sandhoff R, et al. PNPLA1 defects in patients with autosomal recessive congenital ichthyosis and KO mice sustain PNPLA1 irreplaceable function in epidermal omega-O-acylceramide synthesis and skin permeability barrier. Hum Mol Genet. 2017;26:1787–800.

Prasad R, Hadjidemetriou I, Maharaj A, et al. Sphingosine-1-phosphate lyase mutations cause primary adrenal insufficiency and steroid-resistant nephrotic syndrome. J Clin Invest. 2017;127:942–53.

Quistad GB, Barlow C, Winrow CJ, Sparks SE, Casida JE. Evidence that mouse brain neuropathy target esterase is a lysophospholipase. Proc Natl Acad Sci U S A. 2003;100:7983–7.

Ramanadham S, Ali T, Ashley JW, Bone RN, Hancock WD, Lei X. Calcium-independent phospholipases A2 and their roles in biological processes and diseases. J Lipid Res. 2015;56:1643–68.

Rattay TW, Lindig T, Baets J, et al. FAHN/SPG35: a narrow phenotypic spectrum across disease classifications. Brain. 2019;142:1561–72.

Rotthier A, Auer-Grumbach M, Janssens K, et al. Mutations in the SPTLC2 subunit of serine palmitoyltransferase cause hereditary sensory and autonomic neuropathy type I. Am J Hum Genet. 2010;87:513–22.

Saunders CJ, Moon SH, Liu X, et al. Loss of function variants in human PNPLA8 encoding calcium-independent phospholipase A2 $\gamma$ recapitulate the mitochondriopathy of the homologous null mouse. Hum Mutat. 2015;36:301–6.

Shukla A, Saneto RP, Hebbar M, Mirzaa G, Girisha KM. A neurodegenerative mitochondrial disease phenotype due to biallelic loss-of-function variants in PNPLA8 encoding calcium-independent phospholipase A2γ. Am J Med Genet A. 2018;176:1232–7.

Simpson MA, Cross H, Proukakis C, et al. Infantile-onset symptomatic epilepsy syndrome caused by a homozygous loss-of-function mutation of GM3 synthase. Nat Genet. 2004;36:1225–9.

Soehn AS, Rattay TW, Beck-Wödl S, et al. Uniparental disomy of chromosome 16 unmasks recessive mutations of FA2H/SPG35 in 4 families. Neurology. 2016;87:186–91.

Sohn M, Ivanova P, Brown HA, Toth DJ, Varnai P, Kim YJ, Balla T. Lenz-Majewski mutations in PTDSS1 affect phosphatidylinositol 4-phosphate metabolism at ER-PM and ER-Golgi junctions. Proc Natl Acad Sci U S A. 2016;113:4314–9.

Suchanowska A, Kaczmarek R, Duk M, et al. A single point mutation in the gene encoding Gb3/CD77 synthase causes a rare inherited polyagglutination syndrome. J Biol Chem. 2012;287:38220–30.

Suriyanarayanan S, Auranen M, Toppila J, et al. The variant p.(Arg183Trp) in SPTLC2 causes late-onset hereditary sensory neuropathy. NeuroMolecular Med. 2016;18:81–90.

Synofzik M, Gonzalez MA, Lourenco CM, et al. PNPLA6 mutations cause Boucher-Neuhauser and Gordon Holmes syndromes as part of a broad neurodegenerative spectrum. Brain. 2014;137:69–77.

Sztalryd C, Brasaemle DL. The perilipin family of lipid droplet proteins: gatekeepers of intracellular lipolysis. Biochim Biophys Acta Mol Cell Biol Lipids. 2017;1862:1221–32.

Tarailo-Graovac M, Shyr C, Ross CJ, et al. Exome sequencing and the Management of Neurometabolic Disorders. N Engl J Med. 2016;374:2246–55.

Tesson C, Nawara M, Salih MAM, et al. Alteration of fatty-acid-metabolizing enzymes affects mitochondrial form and function in hereditary spastic paraplegia. Am J Hum Genet. 2012;91:1051–64.

Tonelli A, D'Angelo MG, Arrigoni F, Brighina E, Arnoldi A, Citterio A, Bresolin N, Bassi MT. Atypical adult onset complicated spastic paraparesis with thin corpus callosum in two patients carrying a novel FA2H mutation. Eur J Neurol. 2012;19:e127–9.

Tong L. Structure and function of biotin-dependent carboxylases. Cell Mol Life Sci. 2013;70:863–91.

van de Weijer T, Havekes B, Bilet L, et al. Effects of bezafibrate treatment in a patient and a carrier with mutations in the PNPLA2 gene, causing neutral lipid storage disease with myopathy. Circ Res. 2013;112:e51–4.

van Rijn JM, Ardy RC, Kuloğlu Z, et al. Intestinal failure and aberrant lipid metabolism in patients with DGAT1 deficiency. Gastroenterology. 2018;155:130–143.e15.

van Tienhoven M, Atkins J, Li Y, Glynn P. Human neuropathy target esterase catalyzes hydrolysis of membrane lipids. J Biol Chem. 2002;277:20942–8.

Vance JE. Phospholipid synthesis and transport in mammalian cells. Traffic. 2015;16:1–18.

Vanni N, Fruscione F, Ferlazzo E, et al. Impairment of ceramide synthesis causes a novel progressive myoclonus epilepsy. Ann Neurol. 2014;76:206–12.

Vaz FM, McDermott JH, Alders M, et al. Mutations in PCYT2 disrupt etherlipid biosynthesis and cause a complex hereditary spastic paraplegia. Brain. 2019;142:3382–97.

Vukotic M, Nolte H, König T, Saita S, Ananjew M, Krüger M, Tatsuta T, Langer T. Acylglycerol kinase mutated in sengers syndrome is a subunit of the TIM22 protein translocase in mitochondria. Mol Cell. 2017;67:471–483.e7.

Wiethoff S, Bettencourt C, Paudel R, Madon P, Liu YT, Hersheson J, Wadia N, Desai J, Houlden H. Pure cerebellar Ataxia with homozygous mutations in the PNPLA6 gene. Cerebellum. 2017;16:262–7.

Wu JW, Yang H, Wang SP, Soni KG, Brunel-Guitton C, Mitchell GA. Inborn errors of cytoplasmic triglyceride metabolism. J Inherit Metab Dis. 2015;38:85–98.

Yamamoto GL, Baratela WAR, Almeida TF, et al. Mutations in PCYT1A cause spondylometaphyseal dysplasia with cone-rod dystrophy. Am J Hum Genet. 2014;94:113–9.

Zaccheo O, Dinsdale D, Meacock PA, Glynn P. Neuropathy target esterase and its yeast homologue degrade phosphatidylcholine to glycerophosphocholine in living cells. J Biol Chem. 2004;279:24024–33.

Zhang P, Reue K. Lipin proteins and glycerolipid metabolism: roles at the ER membrane and beyond. Biochim Biophys Acta Biomembr. 2017;1859:1583–95.

Zhao T, Goedhart CM, Sam PN, et al. PISD is a mitochondrial disease gene causing skeletal dysplasia, cataracts, and white matter changes. Life Sci Alliance. 2019;2:1–15.

Zolotov S, Xing C, Mahamid R, Shalata A, Sheikh-Ahmad M, Garg A. Homozygous LIPE mutation in siblings with multiple symmetric lipomatosis, partial lipodystrophy, and myopathy. Am J Med Genet A. 2017;173:190–4.

# Disorders of Eicosanoid Metabolism

# 52

Ertan Mayatepek

## Contents



**Summary**

Eicosanoids, including prostaglandins and leukotrienes, are lipid mediators that have been implicated in various pathological processes. They are biologically active metabolites mainly derived from arachidonic acid, a membrane polyunsaturated fatty acid. Prostaglandins (PGs) and thromboxane $A_2$ ($TXA_2$) are formed when arachidonic acid is released from the plasma membrane by phospholipases and metabolized by sequential actions of prostaglandin G/H synthase, cyclooxygenase, or thromboxane synthase (TBXAS1). Leukotrienes (LTs) are synthesized from arachidonic acid by 5-lipoxygnase. This chapter focuses on very rare disorders of eicosanoid metabolism caused by enzymatic defects in the synthesis of $TXA_2$ or of the primary cysteinyl leukotriene $C_4$ ($LTC_4$) as well as defects in the degradation of $PGE_2$.

Thromboxane synthase deficiency (Ghosal hemato-diaphyseal dysplasia (GHDD) syndrome) is caused by mutations in the *TBXAS1* gene. This disorder is characterized by increased bone density (predominantly diaphyseal) and non-regenerative corticosteroid-sensitive anemia.

A defect in the degradation of $PGE_2$, primary hypertrophic osteoarthropathy (PHOAR), is – on the basis of the different pathogenetic genes – categorized into two subtypes. PHOAR type 1 is caused by mutations in the *HPGD* gene encoding for 15-hydroxyprostaglandin dehydroge-

E. Mayatepek (✉)
Department of General Pediatrics, Neonatology and Pediatric Cardiology, University Children's Hospital, Heinrich-Heine University Düsseldorf, Düsseldorf, Germany
e-mail: mayatepek@med.uni-duesseldorf.de


N. Blau et al. (eds.), *Physician's Guide to the Diagnosis, Treatment, and Follow-Up of Inherited Metabolic Diseases*,
https://doi.org/10.1007/978-3-030-67727-5_52

nase whereas PHOAR type 2 is caused by mutations in the *SLCO2A1* gene which encodes for the prostaglandin transporter. Affected patients in both types are mainly characterized by digital clubbing, pachydermia, and periostosis.

In the biosynthesis of leukotrienes, a primary defect has been described in the form of $LTC_4$ synthase deficiency (LTC4SD) leading to decreased levels of cysteinyl leukotrienes in biological fluids. Affected patients seem to be severely affected with symptoms including muscular hypotonia, psychomotor retardation, microcephaly, and failure to thrive. A better understanding of the role of leukotrienes in the brain and their pathophysiological role is a prerequisite for the suggestion of therapeutical approaches. It is possible that this disorder is underdiagnosed since leukotrienes are usually not included in the metabolic workup.

## Introduction

Certain polyunsaturated fatty acids, such as arachidonic acid, are metabolized by oxygenation into a large family of biologically active substances, the eicosanoids. They comprise several compounds including most prominently prostaglandins, thromboxanes, and leukotrienes. Eicosanoids exert their functions through different mechanisms, e.g., by receptor binding and intracellular signaling pathway modulation. Their effects are diverse with a short half-life. A tight regulation on the processes of formation and inactivation is fundamental to prevent exacerbation of their effects. Their actions are primarily linked to inflammatory processes and cellular homeostasis.

Thromboxane synthase deficiency (Ghosal hematodiaphyseal dysplasia (GHDD) syndrome) is an inherited disorder caused by homozygous mutation in the *TBXAS1* gene, which encodes thromboxane synthase (Geneviève et al. 2008). This enzyme catalyzes the conversion of $PGH_2$ to thromboxane $A_2$ ($TXA_2$). Deficiency of thromboxane synthase leads to abnormal bone remodeling and fibrosis of the bone marrow causing non-regenerative severe anemia. Patients, most have been from the Middle East and India, are characterized by sclerosis of long bones with widening of medullary cavities and cortical hyperostosis (Ghosal et al. 1988; Arora et al. 2015). The bone changes specifically affect both diaphysis and metaphysis. Moreover, anemia is a characteristic feature. In addition, defects in arachidonic acid-induced platelet aggregation in vitro have been reported in some patients, although they do not show a clinically significant bleeding diathesis.

Thromboxane synthase seems to be important for bone remodeling. $TXA_2$ modulates the expression of *TNFSF11* and *TNFRSF11B* that encode RANKL and osteoprotegerin in osteoblasts promoting osteosclerosis.

Though mutational analysis is confirmatory, the clinical and radiological picture helps to differentiate from other sclerosing bony disorders. This is important since corticosteroids may lead to considerable improvement, at least with respect to anemia (Mondal et al. 2015; John et al. 2015).

Hypertrophic osteoarthropathy (HO) is a syndrome mainly involving bones and the skin (Martinez-Lavin et al. 1993). It is characterized by a distinct triad: digital clubbing, pachydermia, and periostosis. HO is classified either as primary or secondary. Secondary HO is the most common form and associated with an underlying pulmonary, cardiac, hepatic, or intestinal disease, or it may occur with systemic inflammatory or neoplastic processes (Castori et al. 2005). Primary hypertrophic osteoarthropathy (PHOAR) represents about 3–5% of all cases of HO (Poormoghim et al. 2012). Two causative genes both encoding proteins participating in the degradation of $PGE_2$ were identified. Based on these different pathogenic genes, PHOAR is categorized into two subtypes. Homozygous mutations in the 15-hydroxyprostaglandin dehydrogenase (*HPGD*) gene causes PHOAR type 1 (Uppal et al. 2008). *HPGD* encodes 15-hydroxyprostaglandin dehydrogenase (15-PGDH), which is the main enzyme of prostaglandin degradation. In addition, mutations in the solute carrier organic anion transporter family, member 2A1 (*SLCO2A1*) gene, encoding the prostaglandin transporter (PGT), cause PHOAR type 2 (PGT deficiency) (Zhang et al. 2012). Mutations in the *SLCO2A1* gene are the major cause of PHOAR in the Japanese population, whereas mutations in the *HPGD* gene have not been identified in Japanese patients.

The age of symptom onset has a bimodal distribution, peaking during the first year of life in type 1, with a higher frequency of patent ductus arteriosus and cranial suture defects, and at puberty in PHOAR type 2 (Castori et al. 2005). It has a marked predominance in male, especially in PHOAR type 2. Diagnosis is based on the triad of digital clubbing, pachydermia, and periostosis of the tubular bones. Joint swelling, arthralgia or arthritis, and hyperhidrosis are other common symptoms. Peptic ulcers, chronic gastritis, anemia, and myelofibrosis occur only in patients with PHOAR type 2. Isolated digital clubbing can also be caused by homozygous mutation in the *HPGD* gene.

Both causative genes of PHOAR encode proteins participating in the degradation of $PGE_2$. $PGE_2$ is degraded through two main steps: first, the PGT mediates the uptake of $PGE_2$ across the plasma membrane; then $PGE_2$ is degraded by 15-PGDH in the cell into PGEM. Elevated levels of $PGE_2$ are present in affected patients of both subtypes. In addition, urinary levels of PGEM are elevated in PHOAR type 2 (Hou et al. 2018). Therefore, prostaglandins are considered to be involved in the pathogenesis of PHOAR (Uppal et al. 2008; Zhang et al. 2012). Nonsteroidal anti-inflammatory drugs (NSAIDs) are effective in improving arthralgia or arthritis in majority of affected patients.

Leukotrienes are derived from arachidonic acid via the 5-lipoxygenase pathway. They include the cysteinyl leukotrienes ($LTC_4$, $LTD_4$, $LTE_4$) and $LTB_4$ (Lewis et al. 1990; Mayatepek and Hoffmann 1995). The role of leukotrienes in the CNS is poorly understood, but there is evidence that they are messengers or modulators of CNS activity.

A few disorders have been identified causing secondary disturbances in leukotriene elimination and degradation (Mayatepek et al. 1993; Mayatepek and Lehmann 1996; Willemsen et al. 2000). In the synthesis of leukotrienes, a primary defect has been detected in the enzymatic step in the form of leukotriene $C_4$ synthase deficiency (LTC4SD). So far, this defect has been identified in two independent patients (Mayatepek and Flock 1998; Mayatepek et al. 1999). The clinical picture was mainly characterized by severe muscular hypotonia, psychomotor retardation, failure to thrive, microcephaly, and death in infancy. There was a complete absence of the primary cysteinyl leukotriene, $LTC_4$, and its metabolites in the CSF (Mayatepek et al. 2000). Absence of $LTC_4$, especially in the brain, might at least in part be responsible for the neurological symptoms.

Because of the very limited number of patients identified so far and due to the lack of profound understanding of the role of leukotrienes in the brain and their pathophysiological significance in deficiency states, there exist no therapeutic approaches. It is possible that this disorder is underdiagnosed, suggesting that leukotriene analysis might be included in the metabolic workup in patients with severe neurological symptoms who have no apparently other cause.

## Nomenclature

| No. | Disorder | Alternative name | Abbreviation | Gene symbol | Chromosomal location | Affected protein | OMIM no. |
|---|---|---|---|---|---|---|---|
| 52.1 | Thromboxane synthase deficiency | Ghosal hematodiaphyseal dysplasia syndrome | GHDD | *TBXAS1* | 7q34 | Thromboxane synthase | 231,095 |
| 52.2 | 15-Hydroxyprostaglandin dehydrogenase deficiency | Primary hypertrophic osteoarthropathy type 1 | PHOAR1 | *HPGD* | 4q34.1 | 15-Hydroxyprostaglandin dehydrogenase | 259,100, 119,900 |
| 52.3 | Prostaglandin transporter deficiency | Primary hypertrophic osteoarthropathy type 2 | PHOAR2 | *SLCO2A1* | 3q22.1-q22.2 | Organic anion transporter 2A1 | 259,100; 119,900 |
| 52.4 | Leukotriene $C_4$ synthase deficiency | | LTC4SD | *LTC4S* | 5q35 | Leukotriene $C_4$ synthase | 246,530 |

## Metabolic Pathways

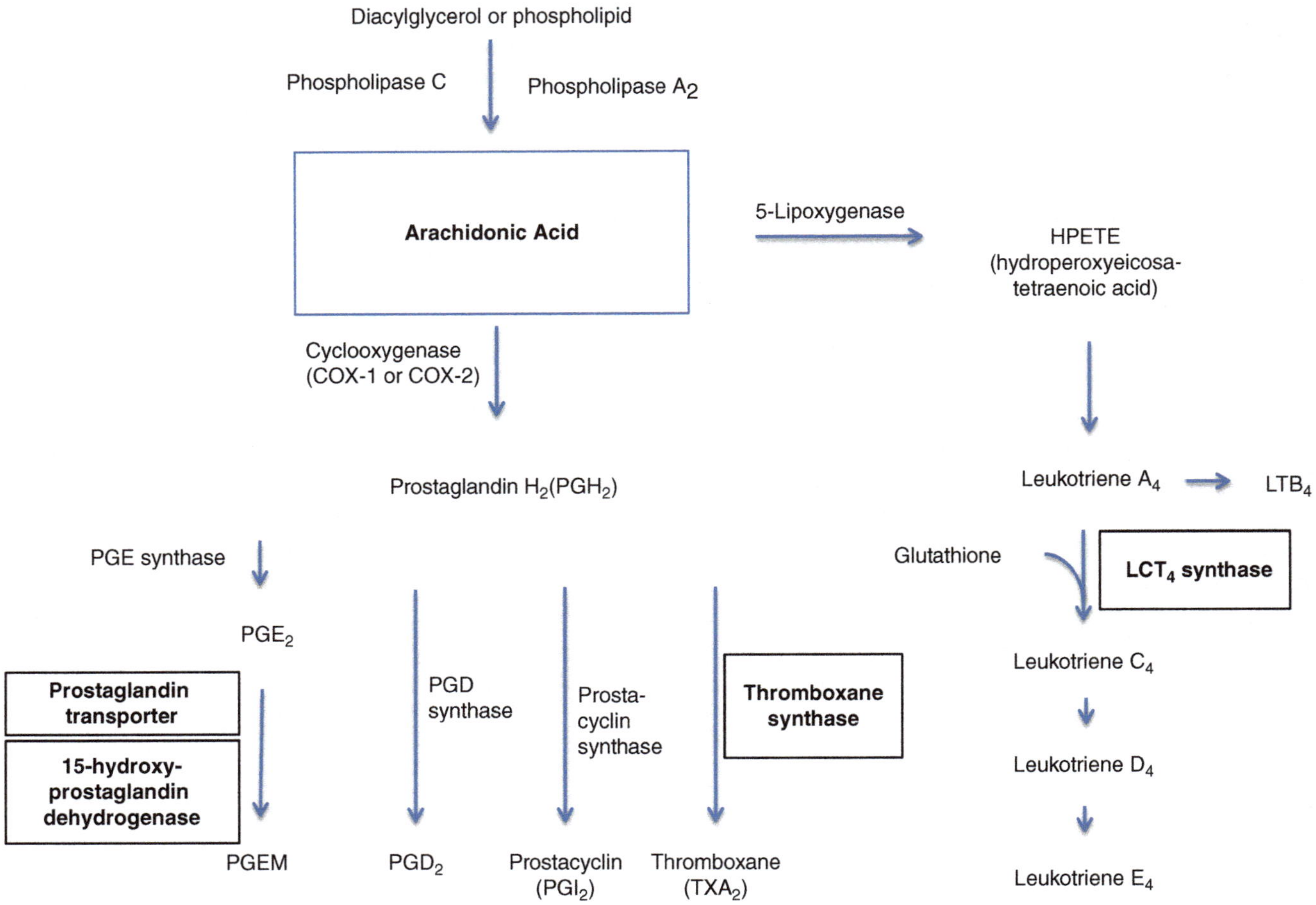


**Fig. 52.1** The arachidonic acid cascade. For simplicity, not all reactions are shown in detail. Prostaglandins (PGs) are derived from enzymatic metabolism of arachidonic acid to $PGG_2$ and subsequently to $PGH_2$ followed by the production of bioactive prostaglandins (e.g., $PGE_2$, $PGI_2$, $PGD_2$) and thromboxane $A_2$ ($TXA_2$) by tissue-specific synthases. Cyclooxygenase (COX-1 or COX-2) is the rate-limiting enzyme responsible for the first two steps in the synthesis of prostaglandins. $TXA_2$ is formed from $PGH_2$ via the enzyme thromboxane synthase. $PGE_2$ is degraded through two main steps: first, the prostaglandin transporter (PGT) mediates the uptake of $PGE_2$ across the plasma membrane. Then $PGE_2$ is degraded by 15-hydroxyprostaglandin dehydrogenase (15-PGDH) in the cell into PGEM. Synthesis of the primary cysteinyl leukotriene (LT), $LTC_4$, results from conjugation of the unstable $LTA_4$ with glutathione and is mediated by $LTC_4$ synthase. Stepwise cleavage of glutamate and glycine from $LTC_4$ by γ-glutamyl transpeptidase membrane-bound dipeptidase yields $LTD_4$ and $LTE_4$, respectively

## Signs and Symptoms

**Table 52.1** Thromboxane synthase deficiency (Ghosal hematodiaphyseal syndrome)

| System | Symptoms and biomarkers | Neonatal (birth–1 month) | Infancy (1–18 months) | Childhood (1.5–11 years) | Adolescence (11–16 years) | Adulthood (>16 years) |
|---|---|---|---|---|---|---|
| Digestive | Splenomegaly | ± | ± | ± | ± | ± |
| Hematological | **Anemia** | ± | + | + | + | + |
| | Leukopenia | ± | ± | ± | ± | ± |
| | Thrombocytopenia | ± | ± | ± | ± | ± |
| Musculoskeletal | Cutis verticis gyrata | | | | + | + |
| | **Diaphyseal thickening** | + | + | + | + | + |
| | **Metaphyseal thickening** | + | + | + | + | + |
| | Swelling or pain of the large bones | ± | ± | + | + | + |

**Table 52.2** 15-Hydroxyprostaglandin dehydrogenase deficiency (primary hypertrophic osteoarthropathy type 1)

| System | Symptoms and biomarkers | Neonatal (birth–1 month) | Infancy (1–18 months) | Childhood (1.5–11 years) | Adolescence (11–16 years) | Adulthood (>16 years) |
|---|---|---|---|---|---|---|
| Autonomic system | Hyperhidrosis | | ± | ± | ± | ± |
| Cardiovascular | Patent ductus arteriosus | ± | ± | | | |
| Dermatological | Thickened skin | ± | ± | ± | ± | ± |
| Musculoskeletal | Arthralgia | ± | ± | + | + | + |
| | Arthritis | ± | ± | + | + | + |
| | Coarse facial features | ± | ± | ± | ± | ± |
| | Cranial suture defects | ± | ± | ± | | |
| | **Digital clubbing** | + | + | + | + | + |
| | Enlargement of hands/feet | ± | ± | ± | ± | ± |
| | **Pachydermia** | + | + | + | + | + |
| | **Periostitis** | + | + | + | + | + |
| | Swollen joints | ± | ± | ± | ± | ± |
| Laboratory findings | Prostaglandin E2 (urine) | ↑ | ↑ | ↑ | ↑ | ↑ |
| | Prostaglandin M (urine) | n | n | n | n | n |

**Table 52.3** Prostaglandin transporter deficiency (primary hypertrophic osteoarthropathy type 2)

| System | Symptoms and Biomarkers | Neonatal (birth–1 month) | Infancy (1-18 months) | childhood (1.5–11 years) | Adolescence (11–16 years) | Adulthood (>16 years) |
|---|---|---|---|---|---|---|
| Autonomic system | Hyperhidrosis | | ± | ± | ± | ± |
| Dermatological | Thickened skin | ± | ± | ± | ± | ± |
| Digestive | Chronic gastritis | | | ± | ± | ± |
| | Peptic ulcer | | | ± | ± | ± |
| Hematological | Anemia | ± | ± | ± | ± | ± |
| | Myelofibrosis | ± | ± | ± | ± | ± |
| Musculoskeletal | Arthralgia | ± | ± | + | + | + |
| | Arthritis | ± | ± | + | + | + |
| | Coarse facial features | ± | ± | ± | ± | ± |
| | **Digital clubbing** | + | + | + | + | + |
| | Enlargement of hands/feet | ± | ± | ± | ± | ± |
| | **Pachydermia** | + | + | + | + | + |
| | **Periostitis** | + | + | + | + | + |
| | Swollen joints | ± | ± | ± | ± | ± |
| Laboratory findings | Prostaglandin E2 (urine) | ↑ | ↑ | ↑ | ↑ | ↑ |
| | Prostaglandin M (urine) | ↑ | ↑ | ↑ | ↑ | ↑ |

**Table 52.4** Leukotriene $C_4$ synthase deficiency

| System | Symptoms and biomarkers | Neonatal (birth–1 month) | Infancy (1–18 months) | childhood (1.5–11 years) | Adolescence (11–16 years) | Adulthood (>16 years) |
|---|---|---|---|---|---|---|
| CNS | Absent head control | + | + | | | |
| | EEG, abnormal | + | + | | | |
| | **Encephalopathy, progressive** | + | + | | | |
| | Hypotonia | ± | + | | | |
| | Lack of facial expression | + | + | | | |
| | Minimal spontaneous movements | + | + | | | |
| | No visual contact | + | + | | | |
| | **Retardation, psychomotor** | + | + | | | |
| | Tendon reflexes, decreased | + | + | | | |
| Musculoskeletal | Dysmorphic features | ± | ± | | | |
| | EMG, abnormal | + | + | | | |
| | Microcephaly | ± | + | | | |
| Other | Death | | + | | | |
| | **Failure to thrive** | + | + | | | |
| | Symmetric extension in the legs | ± | + | | | |
| Laboratory findings | Glutathione (red blood cells) | **n** | **n** | | | |
| | Leukotriene LTC4 (cerebrospinal fluid) | ↓ | ↓ | | | |
| | Leukotriene LTC4 (plasma) | ↓ | ↓ | | | |
| | Leukotriene LTD4 (cerebrospinal fluid) | ↓ | ↓ | | | |
| | Leukotriene LTD4 (plasma) | ↓ | ↓ | | | |
| | Leukotriene LTE4 (cerebrospinal fluid) | ↓ | ↓ | | | |
| | Leukotriene LTE4 (urine) | ↓ | ↓ | | | |
| | Leukotriene LTE4 (plasma) | ↓ | ↓ | | | |
| | Leukotriene LTB4 (cerebrospinal fluid) | n-↑ | n-↑ | | | |
| | Leukotriene LTB4 (plasma) | n-↑ | n-↑ | | | |

## Reference Values

| | |
|---|---|
| **Plasma (nmol/L)** | |
| $LTC_4$ | 14–17 |
| $LTD_4$ | 23–28 |
| $LTE_4$ | 27–33 |
| $LTB_4$ | 27–35 |
| **Urine (nmol/mol creatinine)** | |
| $PGE_2$ | 103–242 |
| PGEM | 70–161 |
| $LTE_4$ | 27–64 |
| **CSF (pmol/L)** | |
| $LTC_4$ | 37–100 |
| $LTD_4$ | 32–70 |
| $LTE_4$ | 46–124 |
| $LTB_4$ | 56–183 |

There exists no significant age dependency in healthy individuals
*LT* leukotriene, *PG* prostaglandin

## Pathological Values

| Disorder | $PGE_2$ (U) | PGEM (U) | $LTC_4$ (CSF) | $LTC_4$ (P) | $LTD_4$ (CSF) | $LTD_4$ (P) | $LTE_4$ (CSF) | $LTE_4$ (P) | $LTE_4$ (U) | $LTB_4$ (CSF) | $LTB_4$ (P) |
|---|---|---|---|---|---|---|---|---|---|---|---|
| PHOAR1 | ↑-↑↑ | N | | | | | | | | | |
| PHOAR2 | ↑-↑↑ | ↑-↑↑↑ | | | | | | | | | |
| LTC4SD | | | ↓ | ↓ | ↓ | ↓ | ↓ | ↓ | ↓ | n-↑ | n-↑ |

## Diagnostic Flowchart

Diagnosis of thromboxane synthase deficiency as well as primary hypertrophic osteoarthropathy is primarily not made on the basis of specific metabolic analyses or profiles but instead based on typically clinical symptoms and especially in the first one on the basis of typical radiological findings. This is completely different in $LTC_4$ synthase deficiency (see Fig. 52.2).

## Specimen Collection

For laboratory measurements of prostaglandins, a thorough drug history is mandatory since nonsteroidal anti-inflammatory drugs or acetylsalicylic acid can affect such analyses.

Leukotrienes are very susceptible to oxidative degradation. Collection of CSF, urine, or plasma (from heparinized blood after centrifugation) and storage should be done preferably in polypropylene tubes (if possible immediately kept in liquid nitrogen) and frozen immediately preferably at −70 °C. Long-term storage may result in lower contents. Bacterial contamination may cause artificial higher contents. Leukotrienes are easily artificially generated and released from leukocytes during blood sampling.

Prostaglandins and leukotrienes are analyzed by liquid chromatography-tandem mass spectrometry (LC-MS/MS).

For mutational analysis, DNA is preferred.

## Prenatal Diagnosis

Prenatal diagnosis has not been performed yet.

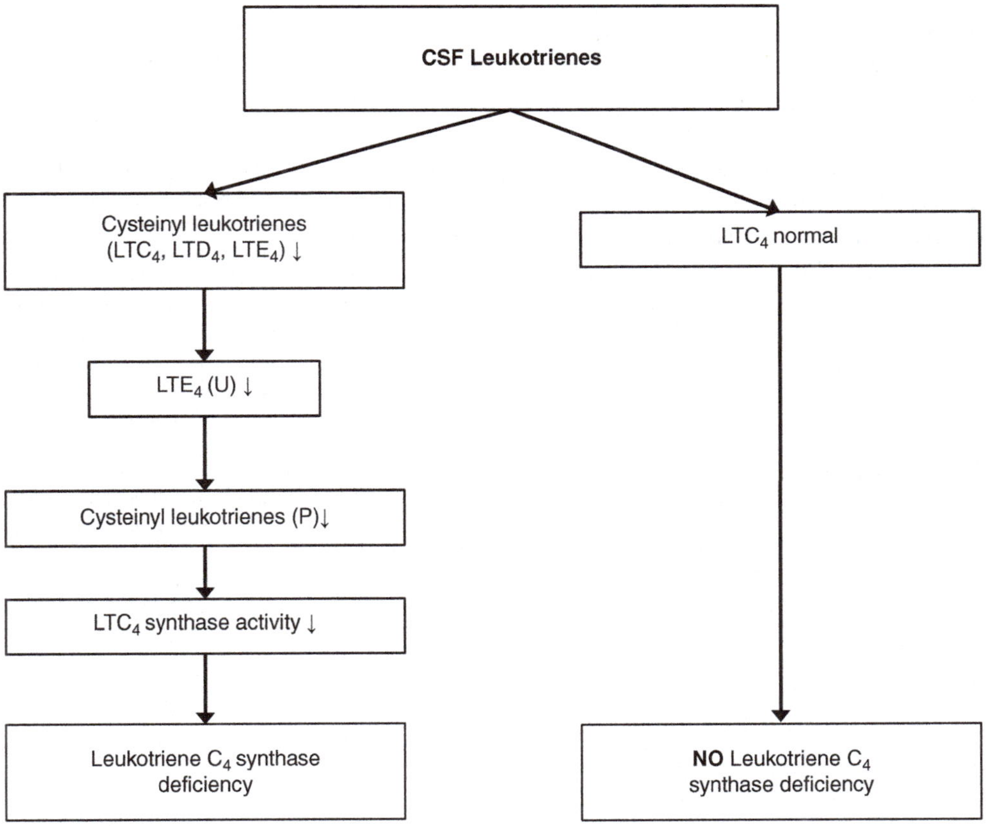


**Fig. 52.2** Diagnostic flow chart for a defect in the primary cysteinyl leukotriene $C_4$ (*LT* leukotriene)

## DNA Testing

Mutational analysis is feasible in GHDD as well as in PHOAR type 1 and type 2. It has not been performed yet in LTC4SD. DNA from peripheral blood leukocytes should be used for PCR and direct sequencing.

## Treatment

### Summary

In GHDD, steroid therapy is the mainstay of treatment especially for hypoplastic anemia negating the need for blood transfusions.

No drug effectively treats PHOAR of both subtypes. NSAID, colchicine, or corticosteroids may be used for symptomatic relief. Bisphosphonates or infliximab has been attempted in patients refractory to these drugs.

There exist no treatment options in LTC4SD.

### Emergency Treatment

No emergency treatment available.

### Standard Treatment

In GHDD, there exists no standard steroid regimen for this steroid-sensitive disorder. Most studies have reported good response to maintenance therapy with low-dose oral prednisolone throughout life.

NSAIDs with their analgesic and anti-inflammatory activities via inhibition of COX activity and prostaglandin synthesis are reasonable in patients with painful osteoarthropathy in both subtypes. Colchicine may be helpful for the pain due to subperiosteal new bone formation. Corticosteroids have been given for rheumatologic symptoms.

No standard treatment available in LTC4SD.

### Experimental Treatment

There exist no experimental treatment options for the disorders discussed here.

## References


Arora R, Aggarwal S, Deme S. Ghosal hematodiaphyseal dysplasia—a concise review including an illustrative patient. Skelet Radiol. 2015;44:447–50.

Castori M, Sinibaldi I, Mingarelli R, et al. Pachydermoperiostosis: an update. Clin Genet. 2005;6:477–86.

Geneviève D, Proulle V, Isidor B, et al. Thromboxane synthase mutations in an increased bone density disorder (Ghosal syndrome). Nat Genet. 2008;40:284–6.

Ghosal SP, Mukherjee AK, Mukherjee D, et al. Diaphyseal dysplasia associated with anemia. J Pediatr. 1988;113:49–57. Erratum in: J Pediatr 113: 410

Hou Y, Lin Y, Qi X, et al. Identification of mutations in the prostaglandin transporter gene SLCO2A1 and phenotypic comparison between two subtypes of primary hypertrophic osteoarthropathy (PHO): a single-center study. Bone. 2018;106:96–102.

John RR, Boddu D, Chaudhary N, et al. Steroid-responsive anemia in patients of Ghosal hematodiaphyseal dysplasia: simple to diagnose and easy to treat. J Pediatr Hematol Oncol. 2015;37:285–9.

Lewis RA, Austen KF, Soberman RJ. Leukotrienes and other products of the 5-lipoxygenase pathway: biochemistry and relation to pathophysiology in human diseases. N Engl J Med. 1990;323:646–55.

Martinez-Lavin M, Matucci-Cerinic M, Jajic I, et al. Hypertrophic osteoarthropathy: consensus on its definition, classification, assessment and diagnostic criteria. J Rheumatol. 1993;20:1386–7.

Mayatepek E, Flock. Leukotriene $C_4$-synthesisis deficiency: a new inborn error of metabolism linked to a fatal developmental syndrome. Lancet. 1998;352:1514–7.

Mayatepek E, Hoffmann GF. Leukotrienes: biosynthesis, metabolism and pathophysiological significance. Pediatr Res. 1995;37:1–9.

Mayatepek E, Lehmann WD. Defective hepatobiliary leukotriene elimination in patients with the Dubin-Johnson syndrome. Clin Chim Acta. 1996;249:37–46.

Mayatepek E, Lehmann WD, Fauler J, et al. Impaired degradation of leukotrienes in patients with peroxisome deficiency disorders. J Clin Invest. 1993;91:881–8.

Mayatepek E, Lindner M, Zelezny R, et al. A severely affected infant with absence of cysteinyl leukotrienes in cerebrospinal fluid: further evidence that leukotriene $C_4$-synthesis deficiency is a new neurometabolic disorder. Neuropediatrics. 1999;30:5–7.

Mayatepek E, Zelezny R, Hoffmann GF. Analysis of leukotrienes in cerebrospinal fluid of a reference population and patients with inborn errors of metabolism: further evidence for a pathognomonic profile in $LTC_4$-synthesis deficiency. Clin Chim Acta. 2000;292:155–62.

Mondal R, Sil A, Nag SS, et al. Ghosal syndrome—ten years follow-up. Indian J Pediatr. 2015;82:568–9.

Poormoghim H, Hosseynian A, Javadi A. Primary hypertrophic osteoarthropathy. Rheumatol Int. 2012;32:607–10.

Uppal S, Diggle CP, Carr IM, et al. Mutations in 15-hydroxyprostaglandin dehydrogenase cause primary hypertrophic osteoarthropathy. Nat Genet. 2008;6:789–93.

Willemsen MAAP, De Jong JGN, Van Domburg PHMF, et al. Defective inactivation of leukotriene $B_4$ in patients with Sjögren-Larsson syndrome. J Pediatr. 2000;136:258–60.

Zhang Z, Xia W, He J, et al. Exome sequencing identifies SLCO2A1 mutations as a cause of primary hypertrophic osteoarthropathy. Am J Hum Genet. 2012;90:125–32.

# Disorders of Lipoprotein Metabolism

# 53

Amanda J. Hooper, Robert A. Hegele, and John R. Burnett

## Contents



A. J. Hooper · J. R. Burnett (✉)
Department of Clinical Biochemistry, Royal Perth Hospital and Fiona Stanley Hospital, PathWest Laboratory Medicine WA, Perth, WA, Australia

School of Medicine, University of Western Australia, Perth, WA, Australia
e-mail: amanda.hooper@health.wa.gov.au; john.burnett@health.wa.gov.au

R. A. Hegele
Schulich School of Medicine and Dentistry, University of Western Ontario, London, ON, Canada
e-mail: hegele@robarts.ca

**Summary**

Disorders of lipoprotein metabolism-dyslipoproteinemias-can be classified based on the primary biochemical disturbance, such as high or low plasma levels of low-density lipoprotein (LDL) cholesterol, high-density lipoprotein (HDL) cholesterol, or triglyceride (TG), or some combination of these. Lipoproteins are physiological transporters of hydrophobic lipids and fat-soluble vitamins through plasma from their site of origin (intestine or liver) to their site of uptake and disposition. Abnormal levels of certain plasma lipids and lipoproteins increase the risk of


N. Blau et al. (eds.), *Physician's Guide to the Diagnosis, Treatment, and Follow-Up of Inherited Metabolic Diseases*,
https://doi.org/10.1007/978-3-030-67727-5_53

cardiovascular disease (CVD) end points, such as myocardial infarction and stroke, and other complications such as pancreatitis. Numerous genetic and environmental factors contribute to inter-individual variation in plasma concentrations of lipids and lipoproteins. Disorders with a monogenic basis typically present earlier in life, while those that present later in life also have genetic, mainly polygenic, determinants, but their expression further depends on interactions with nongenetic environmental or lifestyle factors. Early diagnosis is central to specific dietary, lifestyle, and pharmacological interventions to delay death, disability, and medical complications. For example, to prevent premature CVD in heterozygous familial hypercholesterolemia, it is important to screen subjects at risk, make the appropriate diagnosis (which may include DNA analysis), and initiate treatment, which includes diet, exercise, and lipid-lowering medications. Here we describe the current understanding of genetic determinants, clinical manifestations, and treatment of disorders of lipoprotein metabolism, focusing on defined monogenic disorders that are diagnosed throughout the lifespan.

## Introduction

Disorders of lipoprotein metabolism are usually diagnosed biochemically from a plasma lipid profile. The most important lipids clinically are cholesterol, a key component of cell membranes and a precursor for steroid hormones, and TG, a key energy source comprised of three fatty acids each linked to a glycerol backbone. Due to their hydrophobic nature, lipids are transported in plasma in spheroidal particles called lipoproteins. These consist of a core of cholesterol esters and TG, surrounded by a phospholipid and free cholesterol surface, along with associated proteins called apolipoproteins. Lipoproteins can be distinguished from each other by size, density, composition, and function.

There are three major lipoprotein transport pathways: the exogenous, endogenous, and reverse cholesterol transport. In the exogenous pathway, dietary fats are packaged into large, TG-rich chylomicron particles and secreted from enterocytes via the lymphatic system into plasma. Chylomicrons are rapidly acted upon by lipoprotein lipase (LPL), which hydrolyzes TG to release free fatty acids and to form smaller remnant particles that are cleared by the liver. In the endogenous pathway, the liver produces TG-rich very-low-density lipoproteins (VLDL) that are similarly metabolized by lipase activity to form intermediate-density lipoproteins (IDL) and then low-density lipoproteins (LDL). While the majority of LDL is cleared via the LDL receptor pathway by the liver or peripheral tissues, LDL can become modified, e.g., oxidized, and taken up by foam cells, forming a fatty streak in artery walls that is the early stage of atherosclerosis. This process is a function of atherogenic lipoprotein concentrations over time, with the fatty streak and accompanying inflammation progressing to an atherosclerotic plaque, which may eventually rupture, resulting in CVD end points, such as myocardial infarction or stroke. High-density lipoprotein (HDL) functions to, in part, reverse the process of atherosclerosis, by transporting cholesterol from cells and tissues back to the liver for excretion or reuse.

Apolipoproteins provide lipoproteins with stability and also act as ligands for receptors or activators for enzymes. Apolipoprotein (apo) B forms an integral part of chylomicrons and VLDL and their remnants and, as there is only one molecule of apo B per particle, which stays with the lipoprotein for its circulating life, provides an estimate of atherogenic particle number. The other apolipoproteins are exchangeable between lipoproteins and include apo A-I, the main apolipoprotein of HDL; apo E, a ligand for receptor-mediated clearance particularly for IDL; and apo C-II and apo A-V, cofactors for LPL-mediated hydrolysis of TG.

Plasma lipid and lipoprotein concentrations generally follow a right-skewed Gaussian distribution in the general population. Median levels vary by age and sex, with older age and male sex associated with a less favorable lipid profile. Increased plasma TG concentrations are associated with an increased risk of acute pancreatitis, while plasma concentrations of LDL cholesterol and apo B are directly related to the incidence of coronary events and cardiovascular deaths. Clinical trials using lipid-lowering drugs have unequivocally shown that lowering LDL cholesterol results in significant reductions in both morbidity and mortality in patients with or without established coronary heart disease. While there is an inverse association between HDL cholesterol and CVD, genetic studies suggest that this relationship is not causal; in contrast, increased TG levels appear to have a causative association with CVD.

Important genetic determinants of lipoprotein levels, and therefore targets for novel therapies, have been identified through studies of monogenic lipid disorders. These disorders are generally found at the extremes of the population-specific lipoprotein distribution. While familial hypercholesterolemia (FH) affects ~1 in 250 individuals, other monogenic disorders are classified as rare disorders, affecting less than 1 in 2000 individuals (Ng et al. 2019). Many of these disorders are autosomal recessive, due to homozygous mutations in causative genes. Some affected patients are compound heterozygotes, a category implied whenever the term "homozygous" is used throughout this chapter.

It is important to recognize that common dyslipidemias are often associated with other conditions and therefore are termed secondary. For example, untreated hypothyroidism, nephrotic syndrome, and cholestatic liver disease may cause a marked elevation of LDL cholesterol similar to levels seen in FH. Hypolipidemia may be caused by lipid-lowering therapy, cachexia, hyperthyroidism, or malnutrition/malabsorption. Hypertriglyceridemia is commonly associated with type 2 diabetes, obesity, and alcohol. However, secondary dyslipidemias may have a genetic component that is usually polygenic in nature; subjects who develop secondary dyslipidemia might have inherited one or more subtle metabolic defects that confer susceptibility. It is important to determine whether there is a strong secondary factor underlying the dyslipidemia, since this may guide the preferred means of intervention.

This chapter will focus primarily on genetic disorders that affect the concentrations of the major circulating lipoproteins, indicated biochemically on a lipid profile. Each disorder has specific clinical features, including physical manifestations across a range of tissues and organ systems, a distinctive biochemical profile, and often a discrete molecular genetic basis. The increased availability of DNA sequencing means that this technology is often the most direct and cost-effective path to a diagnosis for monogenic dyslipoproteinemias (Berberich and Hegele 2019; Hegele et al. 2015).

## Nomenclature

| No. | Disorder | Alternative name | Disease abbreviation | Gene symbol | Chromosomal localization | Mode of inheritance | Affected protein | Disease OMIM |
|---|---|---|---|---|---|---|---|---|
| 53.1 | Familial hypercholesterolemia | Autosomal dominant hypercholesterolemia | HeFH | *LDLR* | 19p13.2 | AD | Low-density lipoprotein receptor | 143890 |
| 53.1 | Familial ligand-defective apolipoprotein B-100 | Familial hypercholesterolemia | FDB | *APOB* | 2p24.1 | AD | Apolipoprotein B | 144010 |
| 53.1 | Autosomal dominant hypercholesterolemia | Familial hypercholesterolemia | | *PCSK9* | 1p32.3 | AD | Proprotein convertase subtilisin/kexin type 9 | 603776 |
| 53.2 | Homozygous familial hypercholesterolemia | | HoFH | *LDLR* | 19p13.2 | AR | Low-density lipoprotein receptor | 143890 |
| 53.3 | Autosomal recessive hypercholesterolemia | LDL receptor adaptor protein 1 deficiency | ARH | *LDLRAP1* | 1p36.11 | AR | LDL receptor adaptor protein 1 | 603813 |
| 53.4 | Sitosterolemia | Phytosterolemia | | *ABCG5/ ABCG8* | 2p21 | AR | ATP-binding cassette, subfamily G, members 5 and 8 | 210250 |
| 53.5 | Elevated lipoprotein(a) | | | *LPA* | 6q25-q26 | AD, AR | Apolipoprotein(a) | 152200 |
| 53.6 | Dysbetalipoproteinemia | Hyperlipoproteinemia type 3 | | *APOE* | 19q13.32 | AD, AR | Apolipoprotein E | 617347 |
| 53.7 | Abetalipoproteinemia | Bassen-Kornzweig syndrome | ABL | *MTTP* | 4q23 | AR | Microsomal triglyceride transfer protein | 200100 |
| 53.7 | Homozygous familial hypobetalipoproteinemia | Familial hypobetalipoproteinemia type 1; normotriglyceridemic hypobetalipoproteinemia | HoFHBL | *APOB* | 2p24.1 | AR | Apolipoprotein B | 615558 |
| 53.8 | Familial hypobetalipoproteinemia | Familial hypobetalipoproteinemia type 1 | FHBL | *APOB* | 2p24.1 | AD | Apolipoprotein B | 615558 |
| 53.9 | PCSK9 deficiency | Hypobetalipoproteinemia | | *PCSK9* | 1p32.3 | AD | Proprotein convertase subtilisin/kexin type 9 | 607786 |
| 53.10 | Familial combined hypolipidemia | ANGPTL3 deficiency; familial hypobetalipoproteinemia type 2 | | *ANGPTL3* | 1p31.1 | AR | Angiopoietin-like protein 3 | 605019 |
| 53.11 | Chylomicron retention disease | Anderson disease | | *SAR1B* | 5q31.1 | AR | Secretion-associated Ras related GTPase 1B | 246700 |
| 53.12 | Lipoprotein lipase deficiency | Familial chylomicronemia syndrome; hyperlipoproteinemia type 1 | | *LPL* | 8p21.3 | AR | Lipoprotein lipase | 238600 |
| 53.12 | Apolipoprotein C2 deficiency | Familial chylomicronemia syndrome; hyperlipoproteinemia type 1 | | *APOC2* | 19q13.32 | AR | Apolipoprotein C-II | 207750 |
| 53.12 | Apolipoprotein A5 deficiency | Familial chylomicronemia syndrome; late-onset hyperchylomicronemia; hyperlipoproteinemia type 5 | | *APOA5* | 11q23.3 | AR | Apolipoprotein A-V | 144650 |

| No. | Disorder | Alternative name | Disease abbreviation | Gene symbol | Chromosomal localization | Mode of inheritance | Affected protein | Disease OMIM |
|---|---|---|---|---|---|---|---|---|
| 53.12 | GPIHBP1 deficiency | Familial chylomicronemia syndrome; hyperlipoproteinemia type 1 | | *GPIHBP1* | 8q24.3 | AR | Glycosylphosphatidylinositol-anchored high-density lipoprotein-binding protein 1 | 615947 |
| 53.12 | Lipase maturation factor 1 deficiency | Familial chylomicronemia syndrome; combined lipase deficiency | | *LMF1* | 16p13.3 | AR | Lipase maturation factor 1 | 246650 |
| 53.13 | Hepatic lipase deficiency | | | *LIPC* | 15q21.3 | AR | Hepatic lipase | 614025 |
| 53.14 | Tangier disease | Analphalipoproteinemia | | *ABCA1* | 9q31.1 | AR | ATP-binding membrane cassette transporter A1 | 205400 |
| 53.15 | Apolipoprotein A-I deficiency | Hypoalphalipoproteinemia | | *APOA1* | 11q23.3 | AD | Apolipoprotein A-I | 604091 |
| 53.16 and 53.17 | Lecithin: cholesterol acyltransferase deficiency | Norum disease; fish-eye disease | | *LCAT* | 16q22.1 | AR | Lecithin: cholesterol acyltransferase | 136120, 245900 |
| 53.18 | Cholesteryl ester transfer protein deficiency | Hyperalphalipoproteinemia | | *CETP* | 16q13 | AD | Cholesteryl ester transfer protein | 143470 |

## Metabolic Pathways

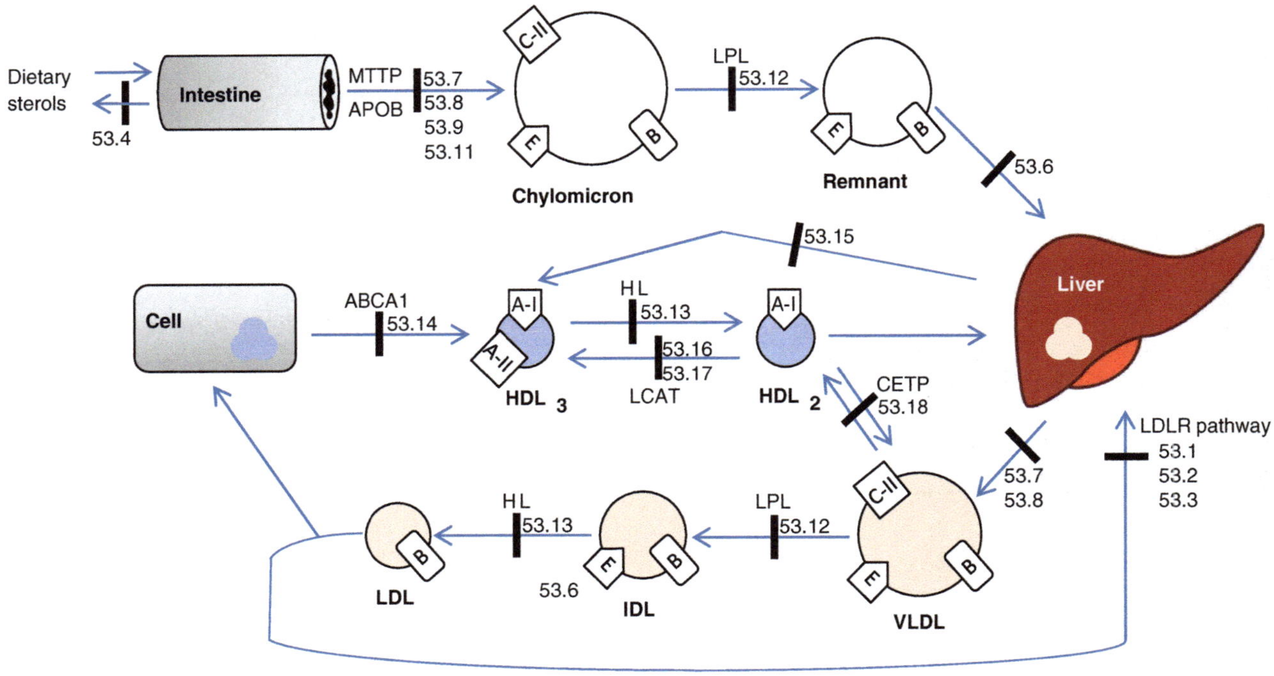


**Fig. 53.1** In enterocytes, dietary fats are loaded onto apoB-48 with the assistance of the microsomal triglyceride transfer protein (MTTP), forming large, triglyceride (TG)-rich chylomicron particles, which enter the plasma via the lymphatic system. Chylomicron TG are hydrolyzed by lipoprotein lipase (LPL) to release free fatty acids and to form smaller remnant particles that are cleared by the liver. Similarly, the liver produces TG-rich very-low-density lipoproteins (VLDL) containing apoB-100 that are metabolized by lipase activity to form intermediate-density lipoproteins (IDL) and then low-density lipoproteins (LDL), which is cleared via the LDL receptor pathway. The ATP-binding cassette transporter A1 (ABCA1) and lecithin: cholesterol acyltransferase (LCAT) facilitate the formation of mature high-density lipoprotein (HDL), while cholesteryl ester transfer protein (CETP) transfers cholesterol from HDL to apoB-containing lipoproteins

## Signs and Symptoms

**Table 53.1** Familial hypercholesterolemia heterozygous (*LDLR*, *APOB*, *PCSK9*)

| System | Symptoms and biomarkers | Neonatal (birth–1 month) | Infancy (1–18 months) | Childhood (1.5–11 years) | Adolescence (11–16 years) | Adulthood (>16 years) |
|---|---|---|---|---|---|---|
| Cardiovascular | Carotid or femoral bruits | | | | | + |
| | Myocardial ischemia | | | | | ++ |
| Dermatological | **Xanthelasmas** | | | | | + |
| | **Xanthomas, tendon** | | | | | ++ |
| Eye | **Arcus cornealis** | | | | | + |
| Laboratory findings | Apo B (plasma) | ↑↑ | ↑↑ | ↑↑ | ↑↑ | ↑↑ |
| | HDL cholesterol (plasma) | ↓-n | ↓-n | ↓-n | ↓-n | ↓-n |
| | LDL cholesterol (plasma) | ↑↑ | ↑↑ | ↑↑ | ↑↑ | ↑↑ |
| | *LDLR, APOB* or *PCSK9* mutation, heterozygous, on DNA sequencing | + | + | + | + | + |
| | TG (plasma) | n | n | n | n | n |

**Table 53.2** Familial hypercholesterolemia homozygous

| System | Symptoms and Biomarkers | Neonatal (birth–1 month) | Infancy (1–18 months) | Childhood (1.5–11 years) | Adolescence (11–16 years) | Adulthood (>16 years) |
|---|---|---|---|---|---|---|
| Cardiovascular | **Aortic valve (AV) disease** | | | + | + | + |
| | **Calcified AV** | | | | + | +++ |
| | Carotid bruits | | | | + | ++ |
| | Carotid stenosis | | | + | + | + |
| | Coronary atherosclerosis | | | + | + | + |
| | Femoral bruits | | | | + | ++ |
| | Myocardial ischemia | | | + | + | +++ |
| Dermatological | **Xanthelasmas** | | | + | ++ | +++ |
| | **Xanthomas, tendon** | | | + | ++ | +++ |
| Eye | **Arcus cornealis** | | | + | ++ | +++ |
| Laboratory findings | Apo B (plasma) | ↑↑↑ | ↑↑↑ | ↑↑↑ | ↑↑↑ | ↑↑↑ |
| | HDL cholesterol (plasma) | n | n | n | n | n |
| | LDL cholesterol (plasma) | ↑↑↑ | ↑↑↑ | ↑↑↑ | ↑↑↑ | ↑↑↑ |
| | *LDLR*, *APOB* or *PCSK9* mutation, homozygous, on DNA sequencing | + | + | + | + | + |
| | TG (plasma) | n | n | n | n | n |

**Table 53.3** Autosomal recessive hypercholesterolemia (ARH)

| System | Symptoms and biomarkers | Neonatal (birth–1 months) | Infancy (1–18 months) | Childhood (1.5–11 years) | Adolescence (11–16 years) | Adulthood (>16 years) |
|---|---|---|---|---|---|---|
| Cardiovascular | Carotid bruits | | | | | ++ |
| | Femoral bruits | | | | | ++ |
| | Myocardial ischemia | | | | + | +++ |
| Dermatological | **Xanthelasmas** | | | + | ++ | +++ |
| | **Xanthomas, tendon** | | | + | ++ | +++ |
| Eye | **Arcus cornealis** | | | | + | +++ |
| Laboratory findings | Apo B (plasma) | ↑↑ | ↑↑ | ↑↑ | ↑↑↑ | ↑↑↑ |
| | HDL cholesterol (plasma) | ↓-n | ↓-n | ↓-n | ↓-n | ↓-n |
| | LDL cholesterol (plasma) | ↑↑ | ↑↑ | ↑↑ | ↑↑↑ | ↑↑↑ |
| | *LDLRAP1* mutation, homozygous, on DNA sequencing | + | + | + | + | + |
| | TG (plasma) | n | n | n | n | n |

**Table 53.4** Sitosterolemia

| System | Symptoms and biomarkers | Neonatal (birth–1 month) | Infancy (1–18 months) | Childhood (1.5–11 years) | Adolescence (11–16 years) | Adulthood (>16 years) |
|---|---|---|---|---|---|---|
| Cardiovascular | Carotid bruits | | | | | + |
| | Femoral bruits | | | | | + |
| | Myocardial ischemia | | | | | ++ |
| Dermatological | **Xanthelasmas** | | | | | + |
| | **Xanthomas** | | | + | + | ++ |
| Laboratory findings | HDL cholesterol (plasma) | n | n | n | n | n |
| | LDL cholesterol (plasma) | ↑↑ | ↑↑↑ | ↑ | ↑ | ↑ |
| | Plant sterols (plasma) | + | + | + | + | + |
| | TG (serum) | n | n | n | n | n |
| | *ABCG5* or *ABCG8* mutation, homozygous, on DNA sequencing | + | + | + | + | + |

**Table 53.5** Elevated lipoprotein(a)

| System | Symptoms and biomarkers | Neonatal (birth–1 month) | Infancy (1–18 months) | childhood (1.5–11 years) | Adolescence (11–16 years) | Adulthood (>16 years) |
|---|---|---|---|---|---|---|
| Cardiovascular | Coronary artery disease | | | | | + |
| | Myocardial ischemia | | | | | + |
| Laboratory findings | Cholesterol (plasma) | n-↑ | n-↑ | n-↑ | n-↑ | n-↑ |
| | HDL cholesterol (plasma) | n | n | n | n | n |
| | Lipoprotein (a) (plasma) | ↑↑ | ↑↑ | ↑↑ | ↑↑ | ↑↑ |
| | Triglyceride (plasma) | n | n | n | n | n |

**Table 53.6** Dysbetalipoproteinemia

| System | Symptoms and biomarkers | Neonatal (birth–1 month) | Infancy (1–18 months) | Childhood (1.5–11 years) | Adolescence (11–16 years) | Adulthood (>16 years) |
|---|---|---|---|---|---|---|
| Cardiovascular | Carotid bruits | | | | | + |
| | Claudication | | | | | ++ |
| | Femoral bruits | | | | | + |
| | Myocardial ischemia | | | | | + |
| Dermatological | **Xanthomas, palmar** | | | | | ++ |
| | **Xanthomas, tuberoeruptive** | | | + | + | +++ |
| Laboratory findings | *APOE* gene ε2/2 or rare mutation on sequencing | | | | | + |
| | Cholesterol (plasma) | n | n | n | n | ↑↑ |
| | HDL cholesterol (plasma) | n | n | n | n | ↓-n |
| | Lipoprotein electrophoresis, broad beta band | n | n | n | n | +++ |
| | TG (plasma) | n | n | n | n | ↑↑ |

**Table 53.7** Abetalipoproteinemia; Homozygous familial hypobetalipoproteinemia

| System | Symptoms and biomarkers | Neonatal (birth–1 month) | Infancy (1–18 months) | Childhood (1.5–11 years) | Adolescence (11–16 years) | Adulthood (>16 years) |
|---|---|---|---|---|---|---|
| CNS | **Ataxia** | | | + | ++ | ++ |
| | Deep tendon reflexes, low | | | + | + | + |
| Digestive | **Malabsorption** | + | + | + | + | + |
| Eye | **Atypical pigmentary retinopathy** | | | + | ++ | ++ |
| Hematological | **Acanthocytosis** | + | + | ++ | ++ | ++ |
| | Bleeding tendency | | | + | + | + |
| Other | **Failure to thrive** | + | + | + | | |
| Laboratory findings | Apo B (plasma) | ↓↓↓ | ↓↓↓ | ↓↓↓ | ↓↓↓ | ↓↓↓ |
| | HDL cholesterol (plasma) | ↓-n | ↓-n | ↓-n | ↓-n | ↓-n |
| | INR | ↑↑ | ↑↑ | ↑↑ | ↑↑ | ↑↑ |
| | LDL cholesterol (plasma) | ↓↓↓ | ↓↓↓ | ↓↓↓ | ↓↓↓ | ↓↓↓ |
| | *MTTP* or *APOB* mutation, homozygous, on DNA sequencing | + | + | + | + | + |
| | Small intestinal biopsy, lipid-laden | ↑ | ↑ | ↑ | ↑ | ↑ |
| | TG (plasma) | ↓↓↓ | ↓↓↓ | ↓↓↓ | ↓↓↓ | ↓↓↓ |
| | Vitamin A (plasma) | ↓↓ | ↓↓ | ↓↓ | ↓↓ | ↓↓ |
| | Vitamin E (plasma) | ↓↓ | ↓↓ | ↓↓↓ | ↓↓↓ | ↓↓↓ |

**Table 53.8** Familial hypobetalipoproteinemia

| System | Symptoms and biomarkers | Neonatal (birth–1 month) | Infancy (1–18 months) | Childhood (1.5–11 years) | Adolescence (11–16 years) | Adulthood (>16 years) |
|---|---|---|---|---|---|---|
| | **No clinical symptoms** | + | + | + | + | + |
| Laboratory findings | Apo B (plasma) | ↓↓ | ↓↓ | ↓↓ | ↓↓ | ↓↓ |
| | *APOB* mutation, heterozygous, on DNA sequencing | + | + | + | + | + |
| | HDL cholesterol (plasma) | n | n | n | n | n |
| | LDL cholesterol (plasma) | ↓↓ | ↓↓ | ↓↓ | ↓↓ | ↓↓ |
| | TG (plasma) | ↓ | ↓ | ↓ | ↓ | ↓ |
| | Vitamin E (plasma) | n-↓ | n-↓ | n-↓ | n-↓ | n-↓ |

**Table 53.9** PCSK9 deficiency with low LDL cholesterol

| System | Symptoms and biomarkers | Neonatal (birth–1 month) | Infancy (1–18 months) | Childhood (1.5–11 years) | Adolescence (11-16 years) | Adulthood (>16 years) |
|---|---|---|---|---|---|---|
| | **No clinical symptoms** | + | + | + | + | + |
| Laboratory findings | Apo B (plasma) | ↓↓ | ↓↓ | ↓↓ | ↓↓ | ↓↓ |
| | HDL cholesterol (plasma) | ↓ | ↓ | ↓ | ↓ | ↓ |
| | LDL cholesterol (plasma) | ↓↓ | ↓↓ | ↓↓ | ↓↓ | ↓↓ |
| | *PCSK9* mutation on DNA sequencing | + | + | + | + | + |
| | TG (plasma) | ↓ | ↓ | ↓ | ↓ | ↓ |

**Table 53.10** Familial combined hypolipidemia

| System | Symptoms and biomarkers | Neonatal (birth–1 month) | Infancy (1–18 months) | Childhood (1.5–11 years) | Adolescence (11–16 years) | Adulthood (>16 years) |
|---|---|---|---|---|---|---|
| | **No clinical symptoms** | + | + | + | + | + |
| Laboratory findings | *ANGPTL3* mutation, homozygous, on DNA sequencing | + | + | + | + | + |
| | Apo B (plasma) | ↓↓ | ↓↓ | ↓↓ | ↓↓ | ↓↓ |
| | HDL cholesterol (plasma) | ↓ | ↓ | ↓ | ↓ | ↓ |
| | LDL cholesterol (plasma) | ↓↓ | ↓↓ | ↓↓ | ↓↓ | ↓↓ |
| | TG (plasma) | ↓↓ | ↓↓ | ↓↓ | ↓↓ | ↓↓ |

**Table 53.11** Chylomicron retention disease

| System | Symptoms and biomarkers | Neonatal (birth–1 month) | Infancy (1–18 months) | Childhood (1.5–11 years) | Adolescence (11–16 years) | Adulthood (>16 years) |
|---|---|---|---|---|---|---|
| Cardiovascular | Cardiomyopathy | | | | | + |
| Digestive | Abdominal distension | + | + | | | |
| | Hepatomegaly | + | + | | | |
| | Malabsorption | + | + | | | |
| Other | Failure to thrive | + | + | | | |
| Laboratory findings | Apo B (plasma) | ↓↓ | ↓↓ | ↓↓ | ↓↓ | ↓↓ |
| | Cholesterol (plasma) | ↓↓ | ↓↓ | ↓↓ | ↓↓ | ↓↓ |
| | HDL cholesterol (plasma) | ↓ | ↓ | ↓ | ↓ | ↓ |
| | *SAR1B* mutation, homozygous, on DNA sequencing | + | + | + | + | + |
| | TG (plasma) | n | n | n | n | n |

**Table 53.12** Lipoprotein lipase deficiency (LPL) and familial chylomicronemia syndrome

| System | Symptoms and biomarkers | Neonatal (birth–1 month) | Infancy (1–18 months) | Childhood (1.5–11 years) | Adolescence (11–16 years) | Adulthood (>16 years) |
|---|---|---|---|---|---|---|
| Dermatological | **Xanthomas, eruptive** | + | + | + | + | + |
| Digestive | Abdominal pain | + | + | + | + | + |
| | **Pancreatitis** | + | + | + | ++ | ++ |
| Eye | **Lipemia retinalis** | + | + | + | + | + |
| Laboratory findings | Cholesterol (plasma) | ↑ | ↑ | ↑ | ↑ | ↑↑ |
| | HDL cholesterol (plasma) | ↓↓ | ↓↓ | ↓↓ | ↓↓ | ↓↓ |
| | LPL activity, post heparin | ↓ | ↓ | ↓ | ↓ | ↓ |
| | *LPL, APOC2, APOA5, LMF1,* or *GPIHBP1* mutation, homozygous, on DNA sequencing | + | + | + | + | + |
| | TG (plasma) | ↑↑↑ | ↑↑↑ | ↑↑↑ | ↑↑↑ | ↑↑↑ |

**Table 53.13** Hepatic lipase deficiency

| System | Symptoms and biomarkers | Neonatal (birth–1 month) | Infancy (1–18 months) | Childhood (1.5–11 years) | Adolescence (11–16 years) | Adulthood (>16 years) |
|---|---|---|---|---|---|---|
| Cardiovascular | Coronary artery disease | | | | | + |
| | Myocardial ischemia | | | | | + |
| Laboratory findings | Cholesterol (plasma) | n | n | n | ↑ | ↑ |
| | HDL cholesterol (plasma) | n | n | n | n | ↑ |
| | Hepatic lipase activity, post heparin | ↓ | ↓ | ↓ | ↓ | ↓ |
| | *LIPC* mutation, homozygous, on DNA sequencing | + | + | + | + | + |
| | Lipoprotein electrophoresis, broad beta band | n | n | n | n | + |
| | TG (plasma) | n | n | n | ↑ | ↑ |

**Table 53.14** Tangier disease

| System | Symptoms and Biomarkers | Neonatal (birth–1 month) | Infancy (1-18 months) | Childhood (1.5–11 years) | Adolescence (11–16 years) | Adulthood (>16 years) |
|---|---|---|---|---|---|---|
| CNS | Neuropathy, peripheral | | | | + | + |
| Digestive | **Hepatosplenomegaly** | | | | + | + |
| Hematological | **Tonsils, enlarged yellow-orange** | + | + | + | + | + |
| Laboratory findings | *ABCA1* mutation, homozygous, on DNA sequencing | + | + | + | + | + |
| | Apo A-I (plasma) | ↓↓↓ | ↓↓↓ | ↓↓↓ | ↓↓↓ | ↓↓↓ |
| | Cholesterol (plasma) | ↓ | ↓ | ↓ | ↓ | ↓ |
| | HDL cholesterol (plasma) | ↓↓↓ | ↓↓↓ | ↓↓↓ | ↓↓↓ | ↓↓↓ |
| | TG (plasma) | n | n | ↑ | ↑ | ↑ |

**Table 53.15** Apolipoprotein A-I deficiency

| System | Symptoms and Biomarkers | Neonatal (birth–1 month) | Infancy (1–18 months) | Childhood (1.5–11 years) | Adolescence (11–16 years) | Adulthood (>16 years) |
|---|---|---|---|---|---|---|
| Cardiovascular | Coronary artery disease | | | | | + |
| Dermatological | Xanthelasmas | | | | | + |
| Laboratory findings | Apo A-I (plasma) | ↓↓ | ↓↓ | ↓↓ | ↓↓ | ↓↓ |
| | *APOA1* mutation, on DNA sequencing | + | + | + | + | + |
| | Cholesterol (plasma) | n | n | n | n | n |
| | HDL cholesterol (plasma) | ↓↓ | ↓↓ | ↓↓ | ↓↓ | ↓↓ |
| | TG (plasma) | n | n | n | n-↑ | n-↑ |

**Table 53.16** Familial LCAT deficiency (complete)

| System | Symptoms and Biomarkers | Neonatal (birth–1 month) | Infancy (1–18 months) | Childhood (1.5–11 years) | Adolescence (11–16 years) | Adulthood (>16 years) |
|---|---|---|---|---|---|---|
| Eye | **Arcus cornealis** | | | | + | + |
| | **Corneal clouding, deposits** | | | | | + |
| Renal | **Kidney disease** | | | | | + |
| | Renal biopsy, abnormal | | | | | + |
| Laboratory findings | Apo A-I (plasma) | ↓↓ | ↓↓ | ↓↓ | ↓↓ | ↓↓ |
| | Cholesterol (plasma) | n | n | n | ↑ | ↑ |
| | Cholesterol esterification rate | ↓↓ | ↓↓ | ↓↓ | ↓↓ | ↓↓ |
| | Cholesterol, unesterified (plasma) | ↑ | ↑ | ↑ | ↑ | ↑ |
| | Creatinine (plasma) | n | n | n | n | ↑ |
| | HDL cholesterol (plasma) | ↓↓ | ↓↓ | ↓↓ | ↓↓ | ↓↓ |
| | LCAT activity (fibroblasts) | ↓↓ | ↓↓ | ↓↓ | ↓↓ | ↓↓ |
| | *LCAT* mutation, homozygous, on DNA sequencing | + | + | + | + | + |
| | Protein, total (urine) | n | n | n | n | ↑ |
| | TG (plasma) | n | n | ↑ | ↑ | ↑ |

**Table 53.17** Familial LCAT deficiency (partial)

| System | Symptoms and Biomarkers | Neonatal (birth–1 month) | Infancy (1–18 months) | Childhood (1.5–11 years) | Adolescence (11–16 years) | Adulthood (>16 years) |
|---|---|---|---|---|---|---|
| Eye | **Arcus cornealis** | | | | + | + |
| Eye | **Corneal clouding, deposits** | | | | | + |
| Laboratory findings | Apo A-I (plasma) | ↓↓ | ↓↓ | ↓↓ | ↓↓ | ↓↓ |
| | Cholesterol (serum) | n | n | n | ↑ | ↑ |
| | Cholesterol esterification rate | n | n | n | n | n |
| | Cholesterol, unesterified (plasma) | n | n | n | n | n |
| | Creatinine (plasma) | n | n | n | n | n |
| | HDL cholesterol (plasma) | ↓↓ | ↓↓ | ↓↓ | ↓↓ | ↓↓ |
| | LCAT activity (fibroblasts) | ↓ | ↓ | ↓ | ↓ | ↓ |
| | *LCAT* mutation, homozygous, on DNA sequencing | + | + | + | + | + |
| | Protein, total (urine) | n | n | n | n | n |
| | TG (plasma) | n-↑ | n-↑ | n-↑ | n-↑ | n-↑ |

**Table 53.18** Cholesteryl ester transfer protein deficiency (CETP)

| System | Symptoms and biomarkers | Neonatal (birth–1 month) | Infancy (1–18 months) | Childhood (1.5–11 years) | Adolescence (11–16 years) | Adulthood (>16 years) |
|---|---|---|---|---|---|---|
| Laboratory findings | *CETP* mutation, on DNA sequencing | + | + | + | + | + |
| | Cholesterol (plasma) | n | n | n | n | ↑ |
| | HDL cholesterol (plasma) | ↑ | ↑ | ↑ | ↑↑ | ↑↑↑ |
| | TG (plasma) | n | n | n | n-↑ | n-↑ |

## Reference Values

| | Infant | Child | Adolescent | Adult | Other comments |
|---|---|---|---|---|---|
| Total cholesterol (mmol/L) | 2.0–3.5 | 2.5–4.0 | 3.0–4.5 | 3.5–5.5 | These are approximate reference intervals/limits across many demographics; there is further variation by age, sex, and ethnic group |
| Triglyceride (mmol/L) | 0.3–1.2 | 0.3–1.5 | 0.3–1.7 | 0.5–1.7 | |
| LDL cholesterol (mmol/L) | 1.0–2.4 | 1.0–3.0 | 1.2–3.5 | 1.4–4.5 | Treatment target for high CVD risk adult is 1.8 mmol/L; there is no specific LDL cholesterol treatment target for children |
| HDL cholesterol (mmol/L) | 0.8–1.6 | 1.0–1.6 | 0.9–1.6 | 0.9–1.8 (men) 1.0–2.4 (women) | |
| Apo B (g/L) | 0.6–1.0 | 0.6–1.0 | 0.6–1.2 | 0.7–1.4 | |
| Apo A-I (g/L) | 1.0–1.5 | 1.0–1.5 | 1.0–1.5 | 1.0–1.6 | |
| Lp(a) (g/L) | <0.50 | <0.50 | <0.50 | <0.50 | Values represent 80th percentile in most populations |

*CVD* cardiovascular disease, *LDL* low-density lipoprotein, *HDL* high-density lipoprotein; *Apo* apolipoprotein, *Lp(a)* lipoprotein(a)

## Pathological Values

| Disorder number | Disorder name | Cholesterol (mmol/L) | LDL-C (mmol/L) | Triglyceride (mmol/L) | HDL-C (mmol/L) | Apo B (g/L) | Other disorder-specific test |
|---|---|---|---|---|---|---|---|
| 53.1 | Familial hypercholesterolemia | >6.0 (child)<br>>7.0 (adult) | >4.0 (child)<br>>5.0 (adult) | n | n | >1.8 | Heterozygous *LDLR*, *APOB*, or *PCSK9* gene mutation |
| 53.2 | Homozygous familial hypercholesterolemia | >10 (child)<br>>13 (adult) | >7.0 (child)<br>>11 (adult) | n | ↓-n | >2.4 | Homozygous *LDLR* gene mutation |
| 53.3 | Autosomal recessive hypercholesterolemia | >10 (child)<br>>13 (adult) | >7.0 (child)<br>>11 (adult) | n | ↓-n | >2.4 | Homozygous *LDLRAP1* gene mutation |
| 53.4 | Sitosterolemia | >6.0 | >4.0 | n | ↓-n | | Increased plasma plant sterols; homozygous *ABCG5/8* mutation |
| 53.5 | Elevated lipoprotein(a) | n | n | n | n | n | Lp(a) >0.5 g/L |
| 53.6 | Dysbetalipoproteinemia | >6.0 | Variable | >3.0 | <1.0 | >1.5 | *APOE* ε2/2 genotype; broad beta band on lipoprotein electrophoresis |
| 53.7 | Abetalipoproteinemia | <1.3 | <0.2 | <0.2 | ↓-n | <0.1 | Homozygous *MTTP* gene mutation, normal lipids in parents |
| 53.7 | Homozygous familial hypobetalipoproteinemia | <1.3 | <0.2 | <0.2 | ↓-n | <0.1 | Homozygous *APOB* gene mutation, half to one-third normal LDL-C and apo B in parents |
| 53.8 | Familial hypobetalipoproteinemia | 2.0–3.0 | 0.5–1.4 | 0.2–0.8 | n | 0.2–0.5 | Heterozygous *APOB* gene mutation |
| 53.9 | PCSK9 deficiency | <2.5 | <0.5 | n | n | <0.2 | Homozygous *PCSK9* gene mutation |
| 53.10 | Familial combined hypolipidemia | 1.3–2.8 | 0.5–1.4 | 0.2–0.8 | 0.3–1.2 | 0.3–0.7 | Homozygous *ANGPTL3* gene mutation |
| 53.11 | Chylomicron retention disease | <1.8 | <1.0 | n | <0.5 | <0.3 | Homozygous *SAR1B* gene mutation |
| 53.12 | Lipoprotein lipase deficiency; familial chylomicronemia syndrome | >6.5 | ↓-n | >10 | <1.0 | <1.0 | Homozygous *LPL, APOC2, APOA5, GPIHBP1 or LMF1* gene mutation; low/absent LPL activity |
| 53.13 | Hepatic lipase deficiency | >6.0 | ↓-n | >3.0 | >2.0 | >1.4 | Homozygous *LIPC* gene mutation |
| 53.14 | Tangier disease | n | ↓-n | Increased | <0.1 | n | Homozygous *ABCA1* gene mutation |
| 53.15 | Apolipoprotein A1 deficiency | n | ↓-n | n | <0.2 | n | *APOA1* gene mutation |
| 53.16 and 53.17 | Lecithin: cholesterol acyltransferase deficiency | n | ↓-n | n-↑ | <0.2 | n | Homozygous *LCAT* gene mutation |
| 53.18 | Cholesteryl ester transfer protein deficiency | n-↑ | n | n | >2.5 | n | *CETP* gene mutation |

*LDL-C* low-density lipoprotein cholesterol, *HDL-C* high-density lipoprotein cholesterol, *Apo B* apolipoprotein B, *Lp(a)* lipoprotein(a)

## Diagnostic Flow Charts

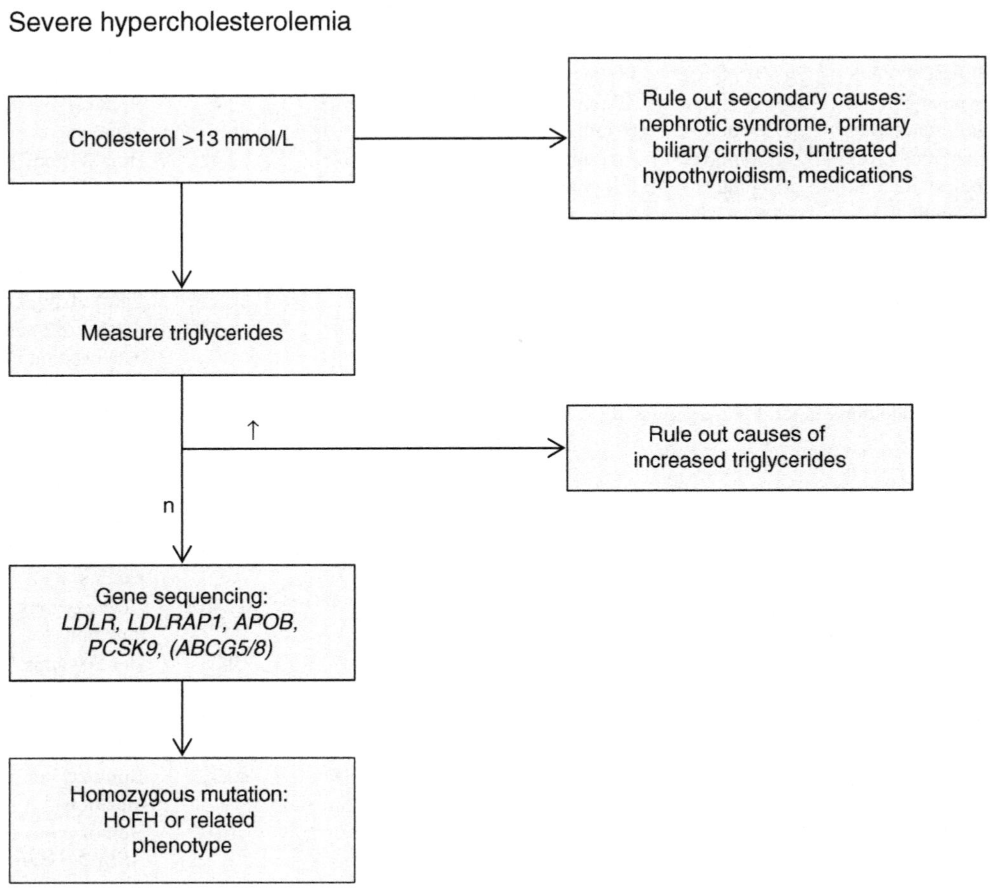

Marked hypercholesterolemia

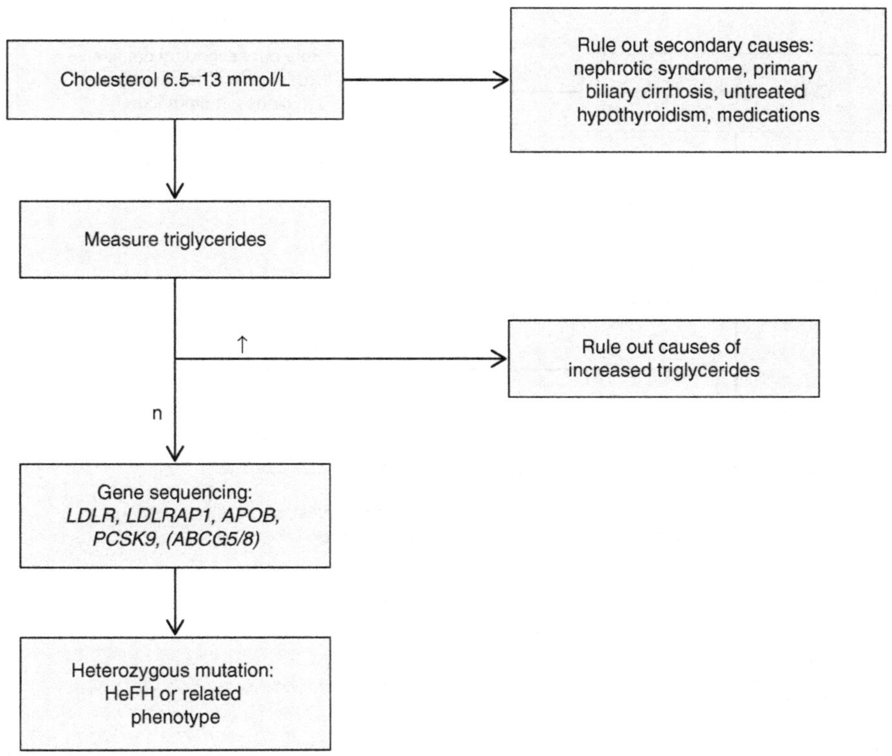


Mixed hyperlipidemia

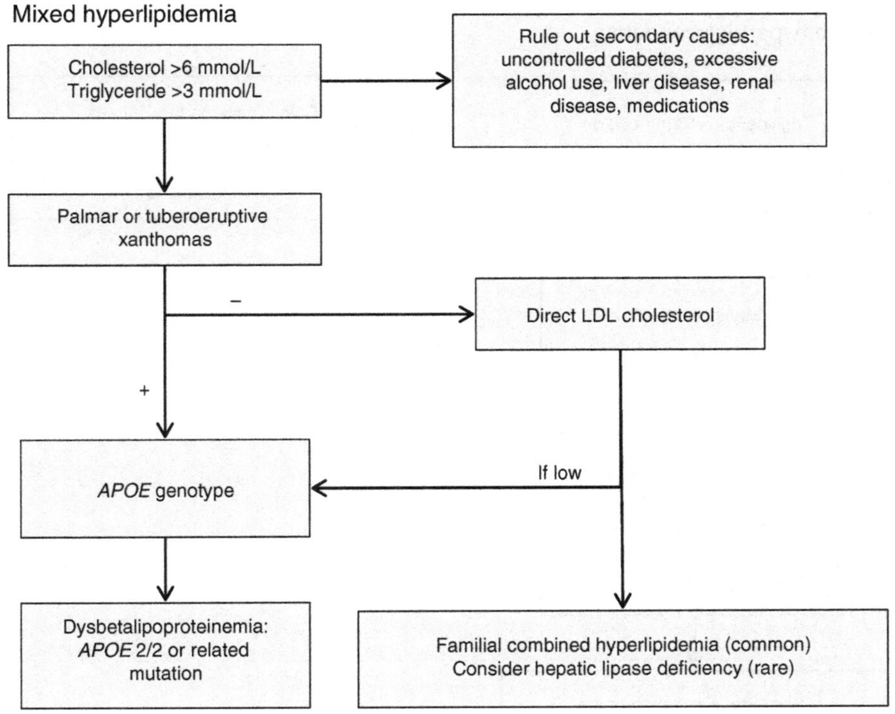

Hypolipidemia

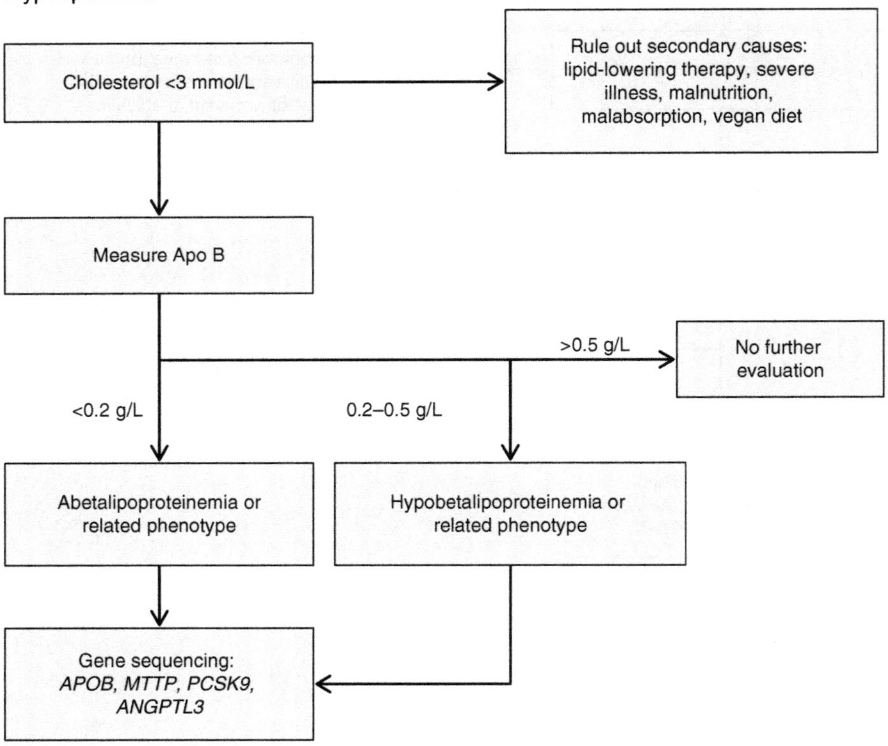


Severe hypertriglyceridemia

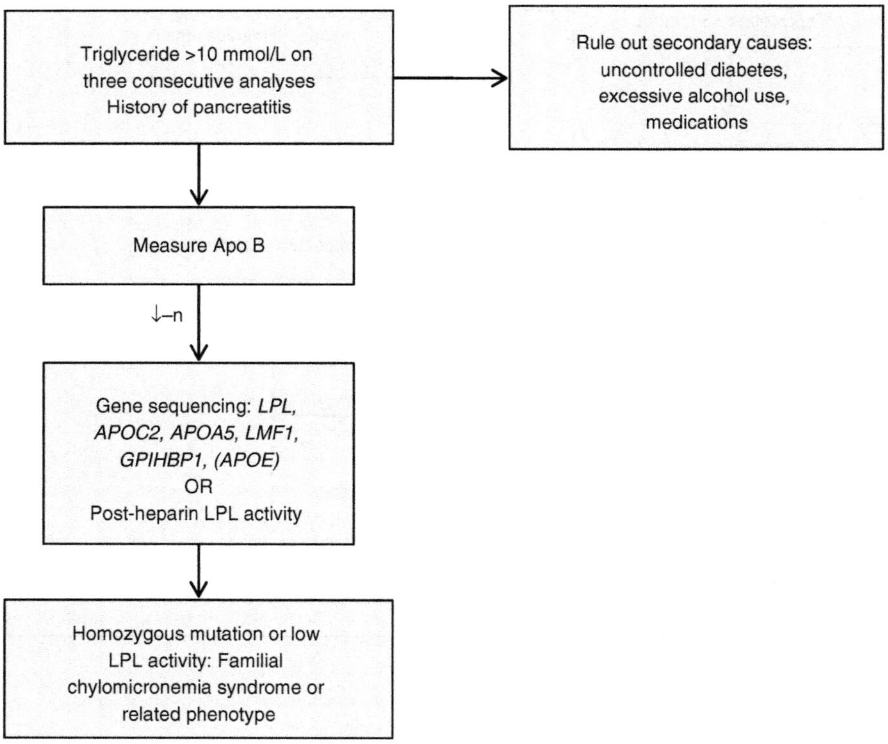

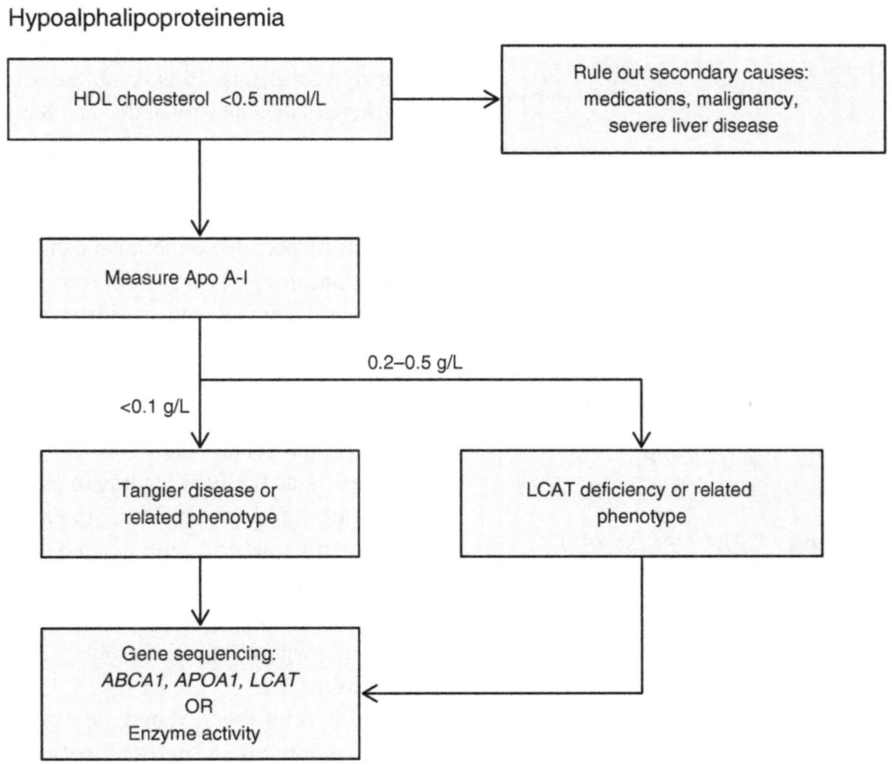


## Specimen Collection

DNA for sequence analysis or genotyping: standard DNA collection procedures from blood, buccal swabs, or saliva.

Skin fibroblasts for LDL receptor activity assay: standard skin biopsy and storage; expertise in performing this test is becoming rare.

Post-heparin plasma for lipase activity: baseline fasting plasma sample, followed by intravenous injection of 50–100 units of normal molecular weight heparin per kg body weight; followed in 30 minutes by a second plasma sample to assay total and fractionated lipase activities; expertise in performing this test is becoming rare.

Other plasma biochemical activities: LCAT activity or cholesterol esterification rate can be measured from plasma, but several available assay kits are research-based and are not standardized for clinical use.

## Prenatal Diagnosis

Prenatal diagnosis for the purpose of pregnancy termination is not usually indicated for monogenic dyslipoproteinemias.

When the index of suspicion for a homozygous illness is high, it is theoretically feasible to sequence genomic DNA sequence of chorionic villus samples for prenatal diagnosis of HoFH for two parents known to have HeFH: vast majority of mutations are found within the *LDLR* gene.

For other severe recessive disorders of lipoprotein metabolism, e.g., LPL deficiency or abetalipoproteinemia, since carrier parents are asymptomatic, diagnosis of the condition within the family follows from diagnosis of an initial offspring. Once the mutation(s) and their segregation within the family are identified, subsequent chorionic villus tissue can be tested with focused genomic DNA analysis.

## DNA Testing

| Clinical suspicion + biochemical disturbance | DNA sequencing of gene(s) |
|---|---|
| HeFH + LDL cholesterol >6.5 mmol/L | *LDLR, APOB, PCSK9,* and possibly *APOE* and *LDLRAP1* |
| HoFH + LDL cholesterol >10 mmol/L | *LDLR, LDLRAP1, APOB,* and possibly *PCSK9* and *ABCG5/G8* |
| Dysbetalipoproteinemia (approximately equimolar total cholesterol and triglyceride elevations) | *APOE* genotype (ε2/2); followed by *APOE* sequencing for rare variants |
| ABL + LDL cholesterol <0.5 mmol/L | *MTTP, APOB,* and possibly *PCSK9* and *ANGPTL3* |
| Hypertriglyceridemia + TG >10 mmol/L | *LPL, APOC2, APOA5, LMF1,* and *GPIHBP1* |
| Hypoalphalipoproteinemia + HDL cholesterol <0.5 mmol/L | *ABCA1, APOA1,* and *LCAT* |
| Hyperalphalipoproteinemia + HDL cholesterol >2.5 mmol/L | *CETP, LIPC, SCARB1* |

## Treatment

National agencies recommend LDL cholesterol as the primary target of therapy to reduce CVD risk (Anderson et al. 2016; Catapano et al. 2016; Grundy et al. 2019). LDL cholesterol goals are recommended for patients stratified into particular risk categories with more stringent goals for patients at high coronary heart disease (CHD) risk. In children, no strong evidence is available to show improvements in end points in regard to achieved LDL cholesterol. Intervention to reduce LDL cholesterol includes lifestyle management and if necessary, pharmacologic therapies. However, certain monogenic disorders are associated with dramatically increased CVD risk, placing these individuals into the highest risk strata (Brunham et al. 2018; Cuchel et al. 2014; Defesche et al. 2017; Raal et al. 2018; Wiegman et al. 2015). Individualized therapies are required for the individual conditions.

General dietary interventions depend on the pattern of dyslipidemia and whether the individual is overweight or obese. *Trans* and saturated fats should be replaced with monounsaturated and polyunsaturated fats and functional foods with beneficial effects on the lipid profile. In overweight or obese individuals, treatment aims to additionally achieve a better balance between energy intake and expenditure. In individuals with high triglycerides, simple sugars and "high glycemic index" foods should be replaced with complex carbohydrates, physical activity increased, and alcohol eliminated in some cases. The intake of animal products should be reduced and fish, seafood, and plant-based foods emphasized. Fish oil supplements may be useful for hypertriglyceridemia. In general, the severity of the dyslipidemia dictates the intensity of the intervention. For severe hyperchylomicronemia, fat intake should be restricted to 10–15% of total calories (Brahm and Hegele 2015; Stroes et al. 2017). For patients with sitosterolemia, elimination of plant sterols is required. A specialized dietician can be very helpful in these circumstances.

Regular exercise and avoiding sedentary behavior are important habits that may be established early. In addition to contributing to energy balance, exercise lowers blood pressure and improves insulin resistance; more directly, it increases the catabolism of TG-rich lipoproteins and increases tissue lipolysis leading to reduced TG and increased HDL cholesterol levels. Recommendations relating to the intensity of regular exercise depend on the health and fitness of the patient; individuals need to engage in the equivalent of 60 minutes of moderately intense physical activity daily. Avoiding cigarettes and other tobacco products is imperative.

Finally, drug therapy may be started together with lifestyle interventions in high-risk patients. The patient's level of risk guides the timing of treatment initiation and also the intensity of the treatment. Moderate- or low-risk patients may be started on medication after a trial period of lifestyle interventions. The main priority of drug therapy is to achieve the identified LDL cholesterol target level. Therefore, once drug therapy has been decided upon for a general patient with high CVD risk and dyslipidemia, an LDL-lowering drug is almost always the first step. Care should be given to choose drugs with documented reductions in cardiovascular disease in adults—no end point trials have been conducted in children.

### Emergency Treatment

| Medical emergency | Treatment |
|---|---|
| Chylomicronemia syndrome (caused by any form of severe hypertriglyceridemia), presenting with sepsis, abdominal pain, pancreatitis | Cessation of oral intake (NPO); intravenous saline to correct or prevent hypovolemia; correction of secondary causes, such as uncontrolled hyperglycemia or alcohol use; with hospitalization, NPO, and hydration, TG will fall with half-life of 2–3 days; there is typically no need for plasmapheresis or heparinization |
| Acute coronary syndromes | As per usual clinical guidelines for the management of acute coronary syndromes |

## Standard Treatment

| Disorder number | Disorder name | Diet | Medications (adult regimens) | Other |
|---|---|---|---|---|
| 53.1 | Familial hypercholesterolemia (HeFH) | Saturated fat <7–10% of energy intake<br>Cholesterol <200 mg/day | Statin as foundation: Simvastatin 10–80 mg/day; atorvastatin 10–80 mg/day; pravastatin 20–80 mg/day; lovastatin 20–40 mg/day; fluvastatin 20–80 mg/day; rosuvastatin 10–40 mg/day<br>Additional agents for combination treatment: Ezetimibe 10 mg/day; cholestyramine 12 g/day or colesevelam 3.75 g/day or colestipol 15 g/day in divided doses; niacin preparations 2–4 g/day; PCSK9 monoclonal antibodies | In children and adolescents, use half-maximal statin dose; half-maximal doses for other medications also |
| 53.2 | Familial hypercholesterolemia homozygous (HoFH) | As above | As above, also lomitapide 5–60 mg/day; mipomersen (where available) or evolocumab (specifically indicated for HoFH with at least one non-null allele) | As above, plus serial plasma exchange, or plasmapheresis or lipoprotein apheresis |
| 53.3 | Autosomal recessive hypercholesterolemia | As above | As above | As above |
| 53.4 | Sitosterolemia | Cessation of plant sterols; reduction of dietary cholesterol | Ezetimibe, bile acid sequestrants, and statins have been shown to have varying effectiveness | Hooper et al. (2017a) |
| 53.5 | Elevated lipoprotein(a) | General prudent diet and lifestyle for CHD prevention | Consider statin therapy as in HeFH if indicated by global cardiovascular risk assessment | |
| 53.6 | Dysbetalipoproteinemia | Balanced diet and physical activity to maintain body weight in relation to growth. Restrict sugars to <10% of energy, saturated fat to <10% of energy | As for HeFH based on clinical assessment of cardiovascular disease risk | |
| 53.7 | Abetalipoproteinemia; homozygous familial hypobetalipoproteinemia | Low-fat diet (<30% total calories) with minimum long-chain FAs; medium-chain TG; essential FA supplements | High doses of oral preparations of vitamins A, D, E, and K | Monitor blood levels of fat-soluble vitamins and titrate therapy (Burnett et al. 2018; Lee and Hegele 2014) |
| 53.8 | Familial hypobetalipoproteinemia | No specific diet | No specific drug therapy | Monitor liver function |
| 53.9 | PCSK9 deficiency with low LDL | No specific diet | No specific drug therapy | Monitor blood levels of fat-soluble vitamins and treat if indicated |
| 53.10 | Familial combined hypolipidemia | No specific diet | No specific drug therapy | As above |
| 53.11 | Chylomicron retention disease | Low-fat diet (<30% total calories) with minimum long-chain FAs; medium-chain TG; essential FA supplements | High doses of oral preparations of vitamins A, D, E, and K | Monitor blood levels of fat-soluble vitamins and titrate therapy (Levy et al. 2019; Peretti et al. 2010) |
| 53.12 | Lipoprotein lipase deficiency; familial chylomicronemia syndrome | Fat <10%–20% of total energy. Medium-chain triglyceride supplements | Try fish oil capsules (EPA mainly) 2–4 g once daily; consider a fibrate (e.g. fenofibrate 145–200 mg/day) | Plasma exchange or plasmapheresis is almost never indicated or definitively helpful in this condition |
| 53.13 | Hepatic lipase deficiency | General prudent diet and lifestyle for CHD prevention | Consider statin therapy as in HeFH if indicated by global cardiovascular risk assessment | |

| Disorder number | Disorder name | Diet | Medications (adult regimens) | Other |
|---|---|---|---|---|
| 53.14 | Tangier disease | As above | As above | Hooper et al. (2017b), Rader and deGoma (2012) |
| 53.15 | Apolipoprotein A-I deficiency | As above | As above | |
| 53.16 and 53.17 | Familial lecithin: cholesterol acyltransferase deficiency | As above | As above | |
| 53.18 | Cholesteryl ester transfer protein deficiency | As above | As above | |

### Experimental Treatment

| Disorder number | Disorder name | Experimental treatment |
|---|---|---|
| 53.1 | Familial hypercholesterolemia (HeFH) | Inclisiran (PCSK9 antisense RNA) |
| 53.2 | Familial hypercholesterolemia homozygous (HoFH) | As for HeFH; also evinacumab (ANGPTL3 monoclonal antibody); LDL receptor gene therapy |
| 53.3 | Autosomal recessive hypercholesterolemia | As for HeFH |
| 53.4 | Sitosterolemia | As for HeFH |
| 53.5 | Elevated lipoprotein(a) | *LPA* antisense RNA |
| 53.6 | Dysbetalipoproteinemia | |
| 53.7 | Abetalipoproteinemia; homozygous familial hypobetalipoproteinemia | |
| 53.8 | Familial hypobetalipoproteinemia | |
| 53.9 | PCSK9 deficiency with low LDL | |
| 53.10 | Familial combined hypolipidemia | |
| 53.11 | Chylomicron retention disease | |
| 53.12 | Lipoprotein lipase deficiency; familial chylomicronemia syndrome | Evinacumab (ANGPTL3 monoclonal antibody), volanesorsen (APOC3 antisense RNA) |
| 53.13 | Hepatic lipase deficiency | |
| 53.14 | Tangier disease | |
| 53.15 | Apolipoprotein A-I deficiency | Apo A-I peptide infusion |
| 53.16 and 53.17 | Familial lecithin: cholesterol acyltransferase deficiency | Recombinant human LCAT enzyme replacement therapy |
| 53.18 | Cholesteryl ester transfer protein deficiency | |

## Follow-Up and Monitoring

| Disorder number | Disorder name | Clinical monitoring | Laboratory investigations |
|---|---|---|---|
| 53.1 | Familial hypercholesterolemia (HeFH) | Cardiovascular examination; coronary atherosclerosis imaging | Lipids, including apolipoproteins |
| 53.2 | Familial hypercholesterolemia homozygous (HoFH) | As above | As above |
| 53.3 | Autosomal recessive hypercholesterolemia | As above | As above |
| 53.4 | Sitosterolemia | As above | As above; plant sterols |
| 53.5 | Elevated lipoprotein(a) | As above | As for HeFH |
| 53.6 | Dysbetalipoproteinemia | As above | As for HeFH |
| 53.7 | Abetalipoproteinemia; homozygous familial hypobetalipoproteinemia | Neurological and ophthalmological examination; hepatic ultrasonography, bone mineral density, echocardiography | Lipids, liver function tests, vitamin A, D, E, INR |
| 53.8 | Familial hypobetalipoproteinemia | Hepatic ultrasonography | Lipids, liver function tests |
| 53.9 | PCSK9 deficiency with low LDL | None | – |
| 53.10 | Familial combined hypolipidemia | None | – |

| Disorder number | Disorder name | Clinical monitoring | Laboratory investigations |
|---|---|---|---|
| 53.11 | Chylomicron retention disease | Neurological and ophthalmological examination; hepatic ultrasonography, bone mineral density, echocardiography | Lipids, liver function tests, vitamin A, D, E, INR |
| 53.12 | Lipoprotein lipase deficiency; familial chylomicronemia syndrome | | Lipids |
| 53.13 | Hepatic lipase deficiency | Cardiovascular examination; coronary atherosclerosis imaging | Lipids |
| 53.14 | Tangier disease | Cardiovascular, gastrointestinal, neurological, and ophthalmological examination; coronary atherosclerosis imaging | Lipids |
| 53.15 | Apolipoprotein A-I deficiency | Cardiovascular, gastrointestinal, neurological, and ophthalmological examination; coronary atherosclerosis imaging | Lipids |
| 53.16 and 53.17 | Familial lecithin: cholesterol acyltransferase deficiency | Renal and ophthalmological examination | Lipids, renal function |
| 53.18 | Cholesteryl ester transfer protein deficiency | None | – |

## Online Resources

Diagnostic Criteria for Familial Hypercholesterolemia https://thefhfoundation.org/diagnostic-criteria-for-familia-hypercholesterolemia.

## References


Anderson TJ, Gregoire J, Pearson GJ, et al. Canadian Cardiovascular Society guidelines for the management of dyslipidemia for the prevention of cardiovascular disease in the adult. Can J Cardiol. 2016;32(11):1263–82.

Berberich AJ, Hegele RA. The role of genetic testing in dyslipidaemia. Pathology. 2019;51(2):184–92.

Brahm AJ, Hegele RA. Chylomicronaemia—current diagnosis and future therapies. Nat Rev Endocrinol. 2015;11(6):352–62.

Brunham LR, Ruel I, Aljenedil S, et al. Canadian Cardiovascular Society position statement on familial hypercholesterolemia: update 2018. Can J Cardiol. 2018;34(12):1553–63.

Burnett JR, Hooper AJ, Hegele RA. Abetalipoproteinemia. In: Adam MP, Ardinger HH, Pagon RA, Wallace SE, Bean LJH, Stephens K, Amemiya A, editors. GeneReviews® [Internet]. Seattle, WA: University of Washington, Seattle; 2018 Oct 25.

Catapano AL, Graham I, De Backer G, et al. ESC/EAS guidelines for the management of dyslipidaemias: the task force for the Management of Dyslipidaemias of the European Society of Cardiology (ESC) and European Atherosclerosis Society (EAS) developed with the special contribution of the European Association for Cardiovascular Prevention & rehabilitation (EACPR). Atherosclerosis. 2016;253: 281–344.

Cuchel M, Bruckert E, Ginsberg HN, et al. Homozygous familial hypercholesterolaemia: new insights and guidance for clinicians to improve detection and clinical management. A position paper from the consensus Panel on Familial Hypercholesterolaemia of the European Atherosclerosis Society. Eur Heart J. 2014;35(32):2146–57.

Defesche JC, Gidding SS, Harada-Shiba M, Hegele RA, Santos RD, Wierzbicki AS. Familial hypercholesterolaemia. Nat Rev Dis Primers. 2017;3:17093.

Grundy SM, Stone NJ, Bailey AL, et al.. AHA/ACC/AACVPR/AAPA/ABC/ACPM/ADA/AGS/APhA/ASPC/NLA/PCNA guideline on the management of blood cholesterol: a report of the American College of Cardiology/American Heart Association Task Force on Clinical Practice Guidelines. Circulation. 2019;139(25):e1082–e1143.

Hegele RA, Ban MR, Cao H, McIntyre AD, Robinson JF, Wang J. Targeted next-generation sequencing in monogenic dyslipidemias. Curr Opin Lipidol. 2015;26(2):103–13.

Hooper AJ, Bell DA, Hegele RA, Burnett JR. Clinical utility gene card for: Sitosterolaemia. Eur J Hum Genet. 2017a;25:4.

Hooper AJ, McCormick SPA, Hegele RA, Burnett JR. Clinical utility gene card for: Tangier disease. Eur J Hum Genet. 2017b;25:7.

Lee J, Hegele RA. Abetalipoproteinemia and homozygous hypobetalipoproteinemia: a framework for diagnosis and management. J Inherit Metab Dis. 2014;37(3):333–9.

Levy E, Poinsot P, Spahis S. Chylomicron retention disease: genetics, biochemistry, and clinical spectrum. Curr Opin Lipidol. 2019;30(2):134–9.

Ng DM, Burnett JR, Bell DA, Hegele RA, Hooper AJ. Update on the diagnosis, treatment and management of rare genetic lipid disorders. Pathology. 2019;51(2):193–201.

Peretti N, Sassolas A, Roy CC, et al. Guidelines for the diagnosis and management of chylomicron retention disease based on a review of the literature and the experience of two centers. Orphanet J Rare Dis. 2010;5:24.

Raal FJ, Hovingh GK, Catapano AL. Familial hypercholesterolemia treatments: guidelines and new therapies. Atherosclerosis. 2018;277:483–92.

Rader DJ, deGoma EM. Approach to the patient with extremely low HDL-cholesterol. J Clin Endocrinol Metab. 2012;97(10):3399–407.

Stroes E, Moulin P, Parhofer KG, Rebours V, Löhr JM, Averna M. Diagnostic algorithm for familial chylomicronemia syndrome. Atheroscler Suppl. 2017;23:1–7.

Wiegman A, Gidding SS, Watts GF, et al. Familial hypercholesterolaemia in children and adolescents: gaining decades of life by optimizing detection and treatment. Eur Heart J. 2015;36(36):2425–37.

# Disorders of Cholesterol Biosynthesis

54

Lisa E. Kratz and Richard I. Kelley

## Contents



**Summary**

Cholesterol has several essential functions in cell physiology. In addition to being a major component of cellular membranes, cholesterol serves as the precursor of bile acids and steroid hormones and plays an important role in embryonic morphogenesis. For many years, mevalonate kinase deficiency (MKD) was the only known genetic disorder of the cholesterol biosynthesis pathway (Hoffmann et al. Pediatrics 91:915–921, 1993). However, the discovery in 1993 of increased levels of 7-dehydrocholesterol (7DHC) and hypocholesterolemia in patients with Smith-Lemli-Opitz syndrome (SLOS) (Irons et al. Lancet 341:1414, 1993) heralded the emergence of a new group of metabolic disorders—inborn errors of cholesterol biosynthesis. The discovery of the biochemical bases of these rare genetic disorders has not only provided biochemical methods for their diagnosis but also allowed the delineation of the broad spectrum of their clinical and biochemical phenotypes.

L. E. Kratz (✉)
Department of Neurogenetics, Kennedy Krieger Institute, Baltimore, MD, USA
e-mail: kratz@kennedykrieger.org

R. I. Kelley
Central Pennsylvania Clinic, Belleville, PA, USA
e-mail: Richard.Kelley@childrens.harvard.edu


N. Blau et al. (eds.), *Physician's Guide to the Diagnosis, Treatment, and Follow-Up of Inherited Metabolic Diseases*,
https://doi.org/10.1007/978-3-030-67727-5_54

## Introduction

***Mevalonate kinase deficiency.*** Mevalonic kinase deficiency (MKD) is a rare, autosomal recessive disorder with principal characteristics of (1) periodic autoinflammatory crises associated with arthralgia, edema, diarrhea, and morbilliform rash; (2) developmental delays, often profound; (3) hepatosplenomegaly secondary to extramedullary hematopoiesis; and (4) marked mevalonic aciduria (Hoffmann et al. 1993). More severely affected patients have dysmorphic facial features, failure to thrive, rhizomelic dwarfism, cataracts, and anemia. Biochemically more mildly affected patients included in the spectrum of MKD may have only minimal psychomotor retardation, hypotonia, myopathy, and cerebellar ataxia. A third group of patients with mild mevalonic kinase deficiency (approximately 5% residual enzyme activity) have recurrent, every 3- to 4-week crises associated with hyperimmunoglobulinemia D (hyper-IgD syndrome), minimally increased urine levels of mevalonic acid and none of the developmental or physical abnormalities associated with classical MKD (Houten et al. 1999). The diagnosis of all forms of MKD is based on finding increased urinary levels of mevalonic acid, deficient activity of mevalonate kinase activity in cultured cells, or disabling mutations in *MVK*.

***Squalene synthase deficiency.*** The condensation of two molecules of farnesyl pyrophosphate to form the 30-carbon molecule, squalene, catalyzed by squalene synthase, FDFT1, is the first committed step in cholesterol synthesis. Squalene synthase deficiency is unique among disorders of cholesterol synthesis in being identifiable by a diagnostic urine organic acid pattern of branched-chain, principally unsaturated dicarboxylic acids produced by the combination of beta- and omega-oxidation of high cytoplasmic levels of farnesol (Coman et al. 2018). Three patients with FDFT1 deficiency, two sibs and an unrelated child, have been described. Clinical characteristics included IUGR, postnatal failure to thrive, neonatal-onset seizures, cerebral defects (agenesis of the corpus callosum, white matter hypoplasia, polymicrogyria), optic atrophy (2/3), SLOS-like facial and skeletal dysmorphisms, and profound developmental delays. All four mutations in the two families were exonic or large intronic deletions but with variable persistence of small amounts of FDFT1 activity. A fourth patient with a deletion/stop-gain mutation and a missense mutation (p. V273G) presented at age 2 days with seizures but had no identifiable physical anomalies (R. Kelley unpublished). Treatment with simvastatin rapidly eliminated the organic aciduria except for minimal residual mevalonic aciduria. At age 6 years, he is developmentally normal except for mild speech delay.

***Lanosterol synthase deficiency.*** Lanosterol synthase (LSS) catalyzes the conversion of (S)-2,3-oxidosqualene to lanosterol, the first sterol in the cholesterol synthesis pathway. Several reports have associated variants in the gene encoding LSS with isolated congenital cataracts (Zhao et al. 2015), hypotrichosis simplex (Romano et al. 2018), or a combination of congenital cataracts and alopecia (Chen and Liu 2017). Identification of an additional 11 individuals from seven unrelated families by Besnard et al. (Besnard et al. 2019) extended the phenotype to include intellectual disability, developmental delays, and seizures. Although plasma sterol levels in these patients are normal, a mildly increased desmosterol level relative to the level of total sterols was observed in cultured lymphoblasts for 2/2 patients tested (L. Kratz unpublished).

***Lanosterol 14α-demethylase deficiency.*** Sterol 14α-demethylase (lanosterol demethylase), encoded by the cytochrome P450 gene, *CYP51A1*, catalyzes an early, rate-limiting step in post-squalene cholesterol biosynthesis. This enzyme, in conjunction with P450 oxidoreductase (POR), removes the 14α-methyl group from lanosterol to form 4,4-dimethylcholesta-8(9),14,24-trien-3ß-ol. Three patients with biochemical evidence and molecular confirmation of lanosterol 14α-demethylase deficiency have been identified [(Gillespie et al. 2014), L. Kratz unpublished, Melissa Crenshaw personal communication]. All cases had congenital cataracts, as did a fourth patient identified by exome sequencing of patients with congenital cataracts (Aldahmesh et al. 2012). Additional features in one patient included microcephaly, short stature, reduced skin pigmentation, developmental delays, and behavioral abnormalities. The second patient had cryptogenic neonatal cirrhosis and spastic diplegia, while the third case had short stature but no other anomalies. Plasma sterol analysis in all three cases and cultured lymphoblasts from case 1 revealed an increased level of lanosterol and dihydrolanosterol. All cases had biallelic mutations in *CYP51A1*.

***Sterol C14-reductase deficiency.*** Hydrops-ectopic calcification-moth-eaten skeletal dysplasia (HEM), or "Greenberg dysplasia," is an especially rare, autosomal recessive, prenatally lethal skeletal dysplasia characterized by fetal hydrops, extreme short-limbed dwarfism, disorganized chondro-osseous mesenchymal proliferation, and abnormal bone mineralization (Konstantinidou et al. 2008). Radiographic findings include marked limb shortening with a "moth-eaten" appearance of the long bones, platyspondyly, ectopic epiphyseal calcifications, and abnormal laryngeal and tracheal calcifications. Sterol analysis in cartilage, cultured fibroblasts, and chondrocytes from affected fetuses revealed small amounts of 14-unsaturated sterols, suggesting a deficiency of sterol C14 reductase. Molecular studies confirmed biallelic pathogenic mutations in the lamin B receptor gene, *LBR* (Waterham et al. 2003), which encodes a fusion protein carrying both sterol C14 reductase enzymatic activity and nuclear lamin B receptor function. Heterozygosity for mutations in *LBR* causes autosomal dominant Pelger-Huët anomaly (PHA) featuring benign, microscopically identifiable, abnormal (reduced) lobation of neutrophils (Hoffmann et al. 2002). A much rarer homozygous form of PHA causes nonlethal skeletal abnormalities of variable severity (Thompson et al. 2019) in addition to abnormally lobated neutrophils. The minimal biochemical abnormality in cells and tissues of a lethal disorder like Greenberg dysplasia presumably indicates the functional importance of a second microsomal enzyme with sterol 14-reductase activity, TM7SF2, for which an associated deficiency in humans remains unknown. However, studies by Clayton et al. (Clayton et al. 2010) indicate that severe skeletal dysplasia is a consequence of the LBR-associated impaired sterol 14α-reductase.

***Sterol C4-methyl oxidase deficiency***. Sterol C4-methyl oxidase, encoded by *SC4MOL*, is one of the three enzymes and one non-enzymatic protein comprising the heteromultimeric enzyme complex, sterol 4α-methyl-4-demethylase. The first patient shown to have SC4MOL deficiency was an adolescent female with congenital cataracts, mild developmental delays, microcephaly, short stature, persistent hypocholesterolemia, and a severe ichthyosiform erythroderma that developed after age 2 years (He et al. 2011). A sibling pair with similar skin manifestations has subsequently been identified (He et al. 2014). However, two additional, unrelated cases of SC4MOL deficiency had no skin involvement, the first presenting with congenital cataracts, microcephaly, hypotonia, and moderate developmental delays (He et al. 2014) and the second with congenital cataracts, growth delay, learning disabilities, behavioral disorders, and short stature (Frisso et al. 2017). While plasma sterol analysis in all reported cases showed increased levels of 4α-methyl and 4,4'α-dimethyl sterols, only the first case had a moderately decreased plasma cholesterol level. The combination of simvastatin treatment and cholesterol supplementation in the first patient was associated with resolution of the ichthyosiform erythroderma and improved growth and development (M. He and J. Vockley personal communication 2011).

***X-linked dominant sterol-4α-carboxylate 3-dehydrogenase deficiency (CHILD syndrome).*** *C*ongenital *h*emidysplasia, *i*chthyosis, and *l*imb *d*efects (CHILD syndrome) is a rare, X-linked dominant disorder defined by unilateral ichthyosiform skin lesions and ipsilateral reduction deformities of the limbs (Happle et al. 1980). Concomitant anomalies on the affected side include punctate epiphyseal calcifications of vertebrae and long bones, abnormal calcification of the laryngeal and tracheal cartilages, and, less frequently, hypoplasia of internal organs, especially the kidney. This syndrome is most often caused by a deficiency of 3ß-hydroxysteroid dehydrogenase, an enzyme encoded by *NSDHL* (NAD(P)H steroid dehydrogenase-like), one of the four proteins constituting the sterol 4α-methyl-4-demethylase complex (König et al. 2000). Patients with NSDHL deficiency CHILD syndrome have abnormal levels of 4α-methylsterols in affected skin and cultured cells, but plasma sterol levels are often normal (Liu et al. 1999). A few patients with unilateral skin and skeletal lesions given an initial diagnosis of CHILD syndrome were later found to have a deficiency of sterol $\Delta^8$-isomerase, the cause of X-linked dominant Conradi-Hünermann syndrome (CDPX2) (Grange et al. 2000). Conversely, one patient with an initial clinical diagnosis of CDPX2 at birth was later found to have a deficiency of NSDHL by biochemical and genetic analysis (R. Kelley unpublished).

***X-linked recessive sterol-4α-carboxylate 3-dehydrogenase deficiency (CK syndrome).*** Although males hemizygous for NSDHL deficiency were assumed to die early in utero, hypomorphic missense mutations in *NSDHL* have recently been reported in three unrelated families with multiple males having an X-linked recessive intellectual disability syndrome (McLarren et al. 2010; Preiksaitiene et al. 2015), now designated "CK syndrome." Plasma sterol levels were normal in these patients.

***X-linked dominant sterol Δ8,Δ7-isomerase deficiency (X-linked dominant Conradi-Hünermann syndrome; CDPX2).*** This is a rare disorder characterized in females by a variable combination of (1) bilateral but asymmetric shortening of long bones; (2) punctate calcifications of the epiphyses, trachea, and larynx; (3) segmental cataracts; and (4) patches of ichthyosiform erythroderma that mostly follow the lines of Blaschko (Silengo et al. 1980). The cause is a deficiency of 3ß-hydroxysteroid-$\Delta^8$,$\Delta^7$-isomerase (sterol-$\Delta^8$,$\Delta^7$-isomerase, emopamil-binding protein, "EBP"), which converts 8(9)-cholestenol into lathosterol (Braverman et al. 1999). The diagnosis of CDPX2 can be made by detection of increased plasma levels of 8(9)-cholestenol and 8-dehydrocholesterol or by mutation analysis. If a mutation in the gene encoding sterol-$\Delta^8$,$\Delta^7$-isomerase (*EBP*) is found, the mother should always be tested, because carrier mothers can have no clinical manifestations of the disorder or only mild short stature. Although rare, there are reports of males with a CDXP2 clinical phenotype and sterol profile who are mosaic for a pathogenic variant in *EBP* (Aughton et al. 2003; Pacault et al. 2018). In one case, paternal transmission of the pathogenic variant resulted in an affected daughter and granddaughter (Pacault et al. 2018).

***X-linked recessive sterol Δ8,Δ7-isomerase deficiency.*** Although *EBP* mutations that cause CDPX2 were once assumed to be uniformly lethal in hemizygous males early in gestation, sterol-$\Delta^8$,$\Delta^7$-isomerase deficiency has been identified in males based on a diagnostic CDPX2 sterol profile and hemizygosity for a damaging mutation in *EBP* (Milunsky et al. 2003; Barboza-Cerda et al. 2014). Males who are hemizygous for mutations in *EBP* have a malformation syndrome distinct from that of heterozygous CDPX2 females, including microcephaly, Dandy-Walker variant, and agenesis of the corpus callosum. Other findings in hemizygous males include seizures, hypotonia, developmental delays, 2/3-toe syndactyly, polydactyly, and heart defects, whereas both chondrodysplasia punctata and other skeletal abnormalities can be absent.

***Sterol Δ5-desaturase deficiency (lathosterolosis).*** Lathosterolosis is caused by a deficiency of lathosterol 5-desaturase (SC5D), which converts lathosterol to 7-dehydrocholesterol (Brunetti-Pierri et al. 2002). Three patients surviving birth had phenotypic findings compatible with the diagnosis of SLOS, but, in contrast to SLOS, two also had progressive hepatosplenomegaly caused by intracellular accumulation of lipids and mucopolysaccharides (Ho et al. 2014). Recently, a lathosterolosis patient with a milder phenotype was ascertained at age 5 years because of bilateral cataracts, developmental delays, and subtle dysmorphic features (Anderson et al. 2019). For all cases, sterol analysis showed a marked increase in the level of lathosterol in plasma and/or cultured fibroblasts but, unlike most individuals with SLOS, a normal plasma cholesterol level. Disabling mutations in *SC5D* were identified in all families. The strong phenotypic resemblance of lathosterolosis to SLOS, a disorder routinely screened in the evaluation of children with dysmorphic features and often just developmental delays, suggests that lathosterolosis is one of the rarest known autosomal recessive enzymopathies, having an estimated incidence substantially less than 1 in a million births.

***24-Dehydrocholesterol reductase deficiency (desmosterolosis).*** Desmosterolosis is a disorder of cholesterol synthesis caused by damaging mutations in *DHCR24*, the gene encoding 3ß-hydroxysteroid-$\Delta^{24}$-reductase (desmosterol reductase) (Waterham et al. 2001) and characterized biochemically by increased plasma and tissue levels of desmosterol [FitzPatrick et al. 1998; Rohanizadegan and Sacharow 2018, L. Kratz unpublished]. All 12 known desmosterolosis patients from eight unrelated families have had structural brain abnormalities, most notably, agenesis of the corpus callosum (12/12) and severe psychomotor delays (10/10). Other variably present abnormalities include arthrogryposis (9/12), microcephaly (7/12), macrocephaly (4/12), cleft palate (5/12), neonatal seizures (5/10), nystagmus, and strabismus (6/10).

***7-Dehydrocholesterol reductase deficiency (Smith-Lemli-Opitz syndrome).*** The most common disorder of cholesterol biosynthesis, with an estimated incidence of 1 in 80,000 births, is Smith-Lemli-Opitz syndrome (SLOS) (Kelley and Hennekam 2000). This well-known, autosomal recessive malformation syndrome is characterized by distinctive facial and oral anomalies, limb and genital malformations, and mild to profound developmental disabilities (Nowaczyk and Irons 2012). In biochemically more severely affected patients, malformations of the kidney, heart, and gastrointestinal tract are common. With the identification in 1993 of diagnostically increased plasma and tissue levels of 7-dehydrocholesterol (7DHC) and later identification of causative mutations in *DHCR7* encoding the last enzyme in the cholesterol biosynthetic pathway, the clinical spectrum for this disorder has broadened to include biochemically minimally affected patients with no discrete malformations and normal intelligence at one extreme and severely affected fetuses dying early in gestation at the other (Nowaczyk and Irons 2012). Although the detection of an increased plasma 7DHC level remains an accurate and efficient screening test for SLOS, rare patients will have normal plasma levels of cholesterol and 7DHC, in which case mutation analysis or sterol analysis in cultured cells must be undertaken. In many patients, treatment with supplemental dietary cholesterol and/or a statin (to upregulate residual DHCR7 activity) leads to clinical and biochemical improvement. A common, nongenetic cause of mildly increased levels of 7DHC is treatment with one of several, mostly psychotropic, medications, which directly inhibit DHCR7 (Hall et al. 2013).

***Porokeratosis.*** Porokeratosis (PK) is a rare dermatologic condition characterized by excessive accumulation of keratin in skin cells, often associated with exposure to ultraviolet light or immunosuppression. Although PK is variable in presentation, with classifications based on number, size, morphology, and distribution of the skin lesions, all variants have cornoid lamellae and a vertical column of parakeratotic cells in the upper epidermis. Recently, certain forms of PK have been associated with heterozygosity for variants in genes responsible for isoprenoid biosynthesis, and autosomal dominant transmission has been demonstrated (Zhang et al. 2015). These genes include *MVK*, *PMVK*, *MVD*, and *FDPS*, encoding the enzymes mevalonate kinase, phosphomevalonate kinase, mevalonate pyrophosphate decarboxylase, and farnesyl diphosphate synthase, respectively. Although there is evidence for genotype-phenotype correlation, no one gene is responsible for all cases of a specific PK variant, suggesting the influence of genetic modifiers of the enzyme deficiencies. No biochemical marker for PK has yet been identified and, thus, evaluation is by molecular testing only.

***Geranylgeranyl pyrophosphate synthase deficiency.*** Although a primary deficiency of geranylgeranyl pyrophosphate synthase has not been described, heterozygous variants in the gene encoding this enzyme (*GGPPS*) have been associated with bisphosphonate-related atypical femoral fractures (Roca-Ayats et al. 2018).

*Note*: The non-metabolic disorders, i.e., those associated with a porokeratosis phenotype and geranylgeranyl pyrophosphate synthase deficiency, will not be described further in this chapter, as they are rare and/or incompletely defined and have no associated clinical biochemical markers at this time.

## Nomenclature

| No. | Disorder[a] | Alternative name | Abbreviation | Gene symbol | Chromosomal localization | Affected protein | OMIM no. |
|---|---|---|---|---|---|---|---|
| 54.1 | Mevalonate kinase deficiency | Mevalonic aciduria | MKD | *MVK* | 12q24.1 | Mevalonate kinase | 610377 |
| 54.2 | Hyper-IgD syndrome | Mevalonic aciduria | HIDS | *MVK* | 12q24.1 | Mevalonate kinase | 260920 |
| 54.3 | Squalene synthase deficiency | Farnesyldiphosphate farnesyltransferase 1 deficiency | | *FDFT1* | 8p23.1 | Farnesyldiphosphate farnesyltransferase (squalene synthase) | 618156 |
| 54.4 | Lanosterol synthase deficiency | | | *LSS* | 21q22.3 | 2,3-Oxidosqualene-lanosterol cyclase (lanosterol synthase) | 618275/616509 |
| 54.5 | Lanosterol 14α-demethylase deficiency | CYP51 deficiency | | *CYP51A1* | 7q21.2 | Lanosterol 14α-demethylase | 601637 |
| 54.6 | Sterol C14-reductase deficiency | Hydrops-ectopic calcification-moth-eaten skeletal dysplasia, Greenberg skeletal dysplasia | HEM dysplasia | *DHCR14* | 1q42.12 | 3β-hydroxysteroid Δ14-reductase | 215140 |
| 54.7 | Sterol C4-methyl oxidase deficiency | SC4MOL deficiency | | *MSMO1* | 4q32.3 | Sterol C4-methyl oxidase | 616834 |
| 54.8 | X-linked dominant sterol 4α-carboxylate 3-dehydrogenase deficiency | Congenital hemidysplasia with ichthyosiform erythroderma and limb defects syndrome | CHILD syndrome | *NSDHL* | Xq28 | 3β-Hydroxysteroid dehydrogenase | 308050 |
| 54.9 | X-linked recessive sterol 4α-carboxylate 3-dehydrogenase deficiency | CK syndrome | | *NSDHL* | Xq28 | 3β-Hydroxysteroid dehydrogenase | 300831 |
| 54.10 | X-linked dominant sterol Δ8,Δ7-isomerase deficiency | X-linked dominant chondrodysplasia punctata type 2; Conradi-Hünermann-Happle syndrome | CDPX2 | *EBP* | Xp11.23 | 3β-Hydroxysteroid Δ8,Δ7-isomerase | 302960 |
| 54.11 | X-linked recessive sterol Δ8,Δ7-isomerase deficiency | Male EBP disorder with neurologic defects | MEND syndrome | *EBP* | Xp11.23 | 3β-Hydroxysteroid Δ8,Δ7-isomerase | 300960 |
| 54.12 | Sterol Δ5-desaturase deficiency | Lathosterolosis | | *SC5D* | 11q23.3 | Sterol Δ5-desaturase | 607330 |
| 54.13 | 24-Dehydrocholesterol reductase deficiency | Desmosterolosis | DHCR24 deficiency | *DHCR24* | 1p32.3 | 3β-Hydroxysteroid 24 reductase | 602398 |
| 54.14 | 7-Dehydrocholesterol reductase deficiency | Smith-Lemli-Opitz syndrome; RSH syndrome | SLOS | *DHCR7* | 11q13.4 | 7-Dehydrocholesterol reductase | 270400 |
| 54.15 | Mevalonate kinase deficiency, Porokeratosis phenotype | Porokeratosis type 3 | | *MVK* | 12q24.1 | Mevalonate kinase | 175900 |
| 54.16 | Phosphomevalonate kinase deficiency | Porokeratosis type 1 | | *PMVK* | 1q21.3 | Phosphomevalonate kinase | 175800 |
| 54.17 | Mevalonate pyrophosphate decarboxylase deficiency | Porokeratosis type 7 | | *MVD* | 16q24.2 | Mevalonate pyrophosphate decarboxylase | 614714 |
| 54.18 | Farnesyl diphosphate synthase deficiency | Porokeratosis type 9 | | *FDPS* | 1q22 | Farnesyl diphosphate synthase | 616631 |
| 54.19 | Geranylgeranyl pyrophosphate synthase deficiency | Atypical femoral fractures with bisphosphonates | | *GGPS1* | 1q42.3 | Geranylgeranyl pyrophosphate synthase | 606982 |

[a]Non-metabolic disorders, including those associated with a porokeratosis phenotype (54.15–54.18) and geranylgeranyl pyrophosphate synthase deficiency (54.19), are not described in detail in this chapter

## Metabolic Pathway

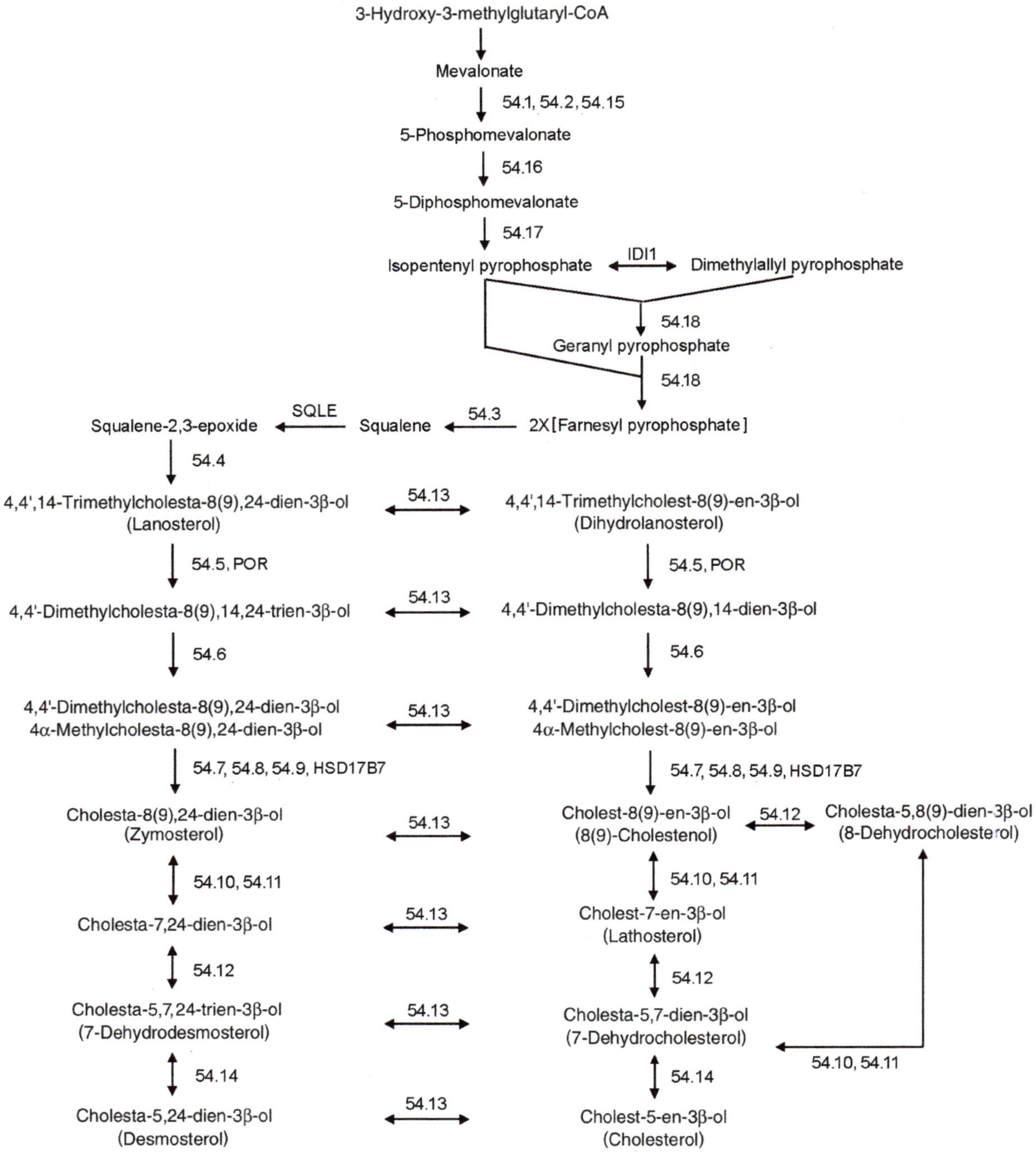


**Fig. 54.1** The pathway of cholesterol biosynthesis. Cholesterol biosynthesis begins with the formation of mevalonate from 3-hydroxy-3-methylglutaryl-CoA by 3-hydroxy-3-methylglutaryl (HMG)-CoA reductase, the major regulatory enzyme of this pathway. From mevalonate are formed the isoprenoids geranyl pyrophosphate and farnesyl pyrophosphate, which are required for the synthesis of squalene, but which also are essential for isoprenylation of proteins and the synthesis of dolichols and coenzyme Q10. Lanosterol is the first sterol in the pathway and is further metabolized to cholesterol by a series of dehydrogenation, reduction, and demethylation steps. In most tissues, the principal route of cholesterol synthesis is through lathosterol and 7-dehydrocholesterol (Kandutsch-Russell pathway). However, an alternative route through desmosterol (Bloch pathway) appears to be important in neuronal cells, given the relative abundance of desmosterol in these tissues. 54.1, 54.2, 54.15 Mevalonate kinase; 54.16 Phosphomevalonate kinase; 54.17 Mevalonate pyrophosphate decarboxylase; *IDI1* Isopentenyl-diphosphate delta isomerase 1; 54.18 Farnesyl diphosphate synthase; 54.3 Farnesyldiphosphate farnesyltransferase 1 (squalene synthase); *SQLE* Squalene epoxidase; 54.4 Lanosterol synthase; 54.5 Lanosterol 14α-demethylase; *POR* Cytochrome P450 oxidoreductase; 54.6 3β-Hydroxysteroid Δ14-reductase (Sterol C14-reductase); 54.7 Sterol C4-methyl oxidase of the sterol 4α-methyl-4-demethylase complex; 54.8, 54.9 3ß-Hydroxysteroid dehydrogenase of the sterol 4α-methyl-4-demethylase complex; *HSD17B7* Hydroxysteroid 17ß-dehydrogenase 7 (3-keto-steroid reductase) of the sterol 4α-methyl-4-demethylase complex; 54.10, 54.11 3ß-Hydroxysteroid $\Delta^8,\Delta^7$-isomerase (sterol $\Delta^8,\Delta^7$-isomerase); 54.12 Sterol $\Delta^5$-desaturase (lathosterol desaturase); 54.13 3ß-Hydroxysteroid $\Delta^{24}$-reductase (desmosterol reductase); 54.14 3ß-Hydroxysteroid $\Delta^7$-reductase (7-dehydrocholesterol reductase)

## Signs and Symptoms

**Table 54.1** Mevalonate kinase deficiency

| System | Symptoms and Biomarkers | Neonatal (birth–1 month) | Infancy (1–18 months) | Childhood (1.5–11 years) | Adolescence (11–16 years) | Adulthood (>16 years) |
|---|---|---|---|---|---|---|
| CNS | Ataxia | | + | + | | |
| | **Cerebellar hypoplasia** | + | + | ++ | | |
| | **Hypotonia** | ++ | + | + | | |
| | **Retardation, psychomotor** | | ++ | ++ | | |
| Digestive | **Hepatosplenomegaly** | ++ | ++ | ++ | | |
| Eye | Cataract | ± | ± | ± | | |
| Hematological | Anemia | ± | ± | ± | | |
| | Leukocytosis | ± | ± | ± | | |
| | Thrombocytopenia | ± | ± | ± | | |
| Musculoskeletal | **Dysmorphic features** | + | + | + | | |
| | **Hypotonia, muscular-axial** | ++ | ++ | ++ | | |
| Respiratory | Respiratory failure | + | + | + | | |
| Laboratory findings | Cholesterol (serum) | ↓-n | ↓-n | ↓-n | | |
| | C-reactive protein (serum) | n-↑ | n-↑ | n-↑ | | |
| | Creatine kinase (plasma) | n-↑ | n-↑ | n-↑ | | |
| | Immunoglobulin D | n-↑ | n-↑ | n-↑ | | |
| | Leukotriene E4 (plasma) | ↑ | ↑ | ↑ | | |
| | Mevalonic acid (urine) | ↑↑↑ | ↑↑↑ | ↑↑↑ | | |
| | Transaminase (plasma) | n-↑ | n-↑ | n-↑ | | |
| | Ubiquinone-50 (plasma) | ↓-n | ↓-n | ↓-n | | |

**Table 54.2** Hyper-IgD syndrome

| System | Symptoms and Biomarkers | Neonatal (birth–1 month) | Infancy (1–18 months) | Childhood (1.5–11 years) | Adolescence (11–16 years) | Adulthood (>16 years) |
|---|---|---|---|---|---|---|
| Digestive | Diarrhea | | ± | ± | ± | ± |
| | Hepatosplenomegaly | ± | ± | ± | ± | ± |
| | Malabsorption | | ± | ± | ± | ± |
| Hematological | **Anemia** | ± | + | + | + | ± |
| | **Leukocytosis** | ± | + | + | + | ± |
| | **Thrombocytopenia** | ± | + | + | + | ± |
| Musculoskeletal | Hypotonia, muscular-axial | n | ± | ± | ± | n |
| Laboratory findings | Cholesterol (serum) | n | n | n | n | n |
| | Erythrocyte sedimentation rate | | n-↑ | n-↑ | n-↑ | n-↑ |
| | Immunoglobulin D | | n-↑ | n-↑ | n-↑ | n-↑ |
| | Leukotriene E4 (plasma) | ↑ | ↑ | ↑ | ↑ | ↑ |
| | Mevalonic acid (urine) | ↑ | ↑ | ↑ | ↑ | ↑ |
| | Ubiquinone-50 (plasma) | ↓-n | ↓-n | ↓-n | ↓-n | ↓-n |

By standard GC/MS urine organic acid quantification, urine mevalonic acid often will be below the limit of detection if not collected during the first 3 days of a febrile episode. Measurement by stable isotope dilution, however, will always be abnormal

**Table 54.3** Squalene synthase deficiency

| System | Symptoms and Biomarkers | Neonatal (birth–1 month) | Infancy (1–18 months) | Childhood (1.5–11 years) | Adolescence (11–16 years) | Adulthood (>16 years) |
|---|---|---|---|---|---|---|
| CNS | Global developmental delay | ± | ± | ± | | |
| | Hypoplastic corpus callosum | ± | ± | ± | | |
| | Irritability | ± | ± | ± | | |
| | **Seizures** | + | + | + | | |
| | White matter loss | ± | ± | ± | | |
| Eye | Optic nerve hypoplasia | ± | ± | ± | | |
| Other | Dysmorphism | ± | ± | ± | | |
| Laboratory findings | Branched-chain dicarboxylic acids (urine) | ↑ | ↑ | ↑ | | |
| | Farnesol (plasma) | ↑ | ↑ | ↑ | | |
| | Mevalonate (urine) | ↑ | ↑ | ↑ | | |

Information provided is based on four known cases

**Table 54.4** Lanosterol synthase deficiency

| System | Symptoms and Biomarkers | Neonatal (birth–1 month) | Infancy (1–18 months) | Childhood (1.5–11 years) | Adolescence (11–16 years) | Adulthood (>16 years) |
|---|---|---|---|---|---|---|
| CNS | Global developmental delay | ± | ± | ± | ± | ± |
| | Hypotonia | ± | ± | ± | ± | ± |
| | **Seizures** | ± | ± | ± | ± | ± |
| Dermatological | **Alopecia** | +++ | +++ | +++ | +++ | +++ |
| | Ichthyosis | ± | ± | ± | ± | ± |
| Eye | **Cataract** | ± | ± | ± | ± | ± |
| Genitourinary | Hypospadias | ± | ± | ± | ± | ± |

**Table 54.5** Lanosterol 14α-demethylase deficiency

| System | Symptoms and Biomarkers | Neonatal (birth–1 month) | Infancy (1–18 months) | Childhood (1.5–11 years) | Adolescence (11–16 years) | Adulthood (>16 years) |
|---|---|---|---|---|---|---|
| CNS | Developmental delay | ± | ± | ± | | |
| | Microcephaly | ± | ± | ± | | |
| | Self-injury | | | ± | | |
| | Spastic diplegia | ± | ± | ± | | |
| Dermatological | Erythema | ± | ± | ± | | |
| | Hypopigmentation | ± | ± | ± | | |
| Digestive | Liver cirrhosis | ± | | | | |
| Eye | **Cataract** | +++ | +++ | +++ | | |
| Musculoskeletal | Short stature | ± | ± | ± | | |
| Laboratory findings | Dihydrolanosterol (lymphoblasts) | ↑ | ↑ | ↑ | ↑ | ↑ |
| | Dihydrolanosterol (plasma) | ↑ | ↑ | ↑ | ↑ | ↑ |
| | Lanosterol (lymphblasts) | ↑ | ↑ | ↑ | ↑ | ↑ |
| | Lanosterol (plasma) | ↑ | ↑ | ↑ | ↑ | ↑ |

Information provided is based on three known unrelated cases where detailed clinical information is available

**Table 54.6** Sterol C14-reductase deficiency

| System | Symptoms and Biomarkers | Neonatal (birth–1 month) | Infancy (1–18 months) | Childhood (1.5–11 years) | Adolescence (11–16 years) | Adulthood (>16 years) |
|---|---|---|---|---|---|---|
| CNS | Cystic hygroma | ± | | | | |
| Digestive | Omphalocele | ± | | | | |
| Musculoskeletal | **Chondrodysplasia punctata** | + | | | | |
| | **Chondro-osseous mineralization** | + | | | | |
| | **Disorganized chondro-osseous proliferation** | + | | | | |
| | Hypoplasia, severe midface | + | | | | |
| | **Platyspondyly** | + | | | | |
| | **Polydactyly, postaxial** | ± | | | | |
| | **Rhizomelic shortness, severe** | + | | | | |
| Other | **Fetal hydrops** | + | | | | |
| | **Intrauterine death** | + | | | | |
| | **Stillbirth** | + | | | | |
| Respiratory | Hypolobated lungs | ± | | | | |
| | Laryngeal calcification | + | | | | |
| | Tracheal calcification | + | | | | |
| | Underdeveloped lungs | ± | | | | |
| Laboratory findings | Cholesta-8,14-dien-3β-ol (fibroblasts) | ↑ | | | | |
| | Cholesta-8,14-dien-3β-ol (tissue) | ↑ | | | | |

**Table 54.7** Sterol C4-methyl oxidase deficiency

| System | Symptoms and Biomarkers | Neonatal (birth–1 month) | Infancy (1–18 months) | Childhood (1.5–11 years) | Adolescence (11–16 years) | Adulthood (>16 years) |
|---|---|---|---|---|---|---|
| CNS | **Developmental delay** | + | + | + | + | + |
| | Hypotonia | ± | ± | ± | ± | ± |
| | **Microcephaly** | ± | ± | ± | ± | ± |
| Dermatological | Dermatitis, psoriasiform | | | ± | ± | ± |
| Eye | **Cataract** | +++ | +++ | +++ | +++ | +++ |
| Musculoskeletal | Arched palate, high | ± | ± | ± | ± | ± |
| | **Short stature** | + | + | + | + | + |
| Other | Failure to thrive | + | + | + | + | + |
| Laboratory findings | 4α-methyl sterols (lymphoblasts) | ↑ | ↑ | ↑ | ↑ | ↑ |
| | 4α-methyl sterols (plasma) | ↑ | ↑ | ↑ | ↑ | ↑ |
| | 4,4-dimethyl sterols (lymphoblasts) | ↑ | ↑ | ↑ | ↑ | ↑ |
| | 4,4-dimethyl sterols (plasma) | ↑ | ↑ | ↑ | ↑ | ↑ |

Information provided is based on four known unrelated cases

**Table 54.8** X-linked dominant sterol 4α-carboxylate 3-dehydrogenase deficiency (CHILD syndrome)

| System | Symptoms and Biomarkers | Neonatal (birth–1 month) | Infancy (1–18 months) | Childhood (1.5–11 years) | Adolescence (11–16 years) | Adulthood (>16 years) |
|---|---|---|---|---|---|---|
| Cardiovascular | Cardiac, anomalies, malformations | ± | ± | ± | ± | ± |
| CNS | Hypoplasia, unilateral | ± | ± | ± | ± | ± |
| Dermatological | Alopecia | ± | ± | ± | ± | ± |
| | Dystrophic nails | ± | ± | ± | ± | ± |
| | Erythema | + | + | + | + | + |
| | **Ichthyosiform skin lesions demarcated at the midline** | + | + | + | + | + |
| Genitourinary | Renal agenesis | ± | ± | ± | ± | ± |
| Musculoskeletal | Absent long bones | ± | ± | ± | ± | ± |
| | Absent phalanges | ± | ± | ± | ± | ± |
| | Hypoplastic long bones | ± | ± | ± | ± | ± |
| | Hypoplastic phalanges | ± | ± | ± | ± | ± |
| | Minor contralateral bone abnormalities | ± | ± | ± | ± | ± |
| | Minor contralateral skin abnormalities | ± | ± | ± | ± | ± |
| | Punctate calcification of nonskeletal cartilage | ± | ± | | | |
| | Punctate calcification of skeletal cartilage | ± | ± | | | |
| | **Unilateral limb defects** | ± | ± | ± | ± | ± |
| | Vertebral anomalies | ± | ± | ± | ± | ± |
| Renal | Renal hypoplasia | ± | ± | ± | ± | ± |
| Laboratory findings | 4-alpha-Carboxymethyl sterol (tissue) | ↑ | ↑ | ↑ | ↑ | ↑ |
| | 4-alpha-Carboxymethyl sterol (lymphoblasts) | ↑ | ↑ | ↑ | ↑ | ↑ |
| | 4-alpha-methyl sterols (tissue) | ↑ | ↑ | ↑ | ↑ | ↑ |
| | 4-alpha-methyl sterols (lymphoblasts) | ↑ | ↑ | ↑ | ↑ | ↑ |

**Table 54.9** X-linked recessive sterol 4α-carboxylate 3-dehydrogenase deficiency (CK syndrome)

| System | Symptoms and Biomarkers | Neonatal (birth–1 month) | Infancy (1–18 months) | Childhood (1.5–11 years) | Adolescence (11–16 years) | Adulthood (>16 years) |
|---|---|---|---|---|---|---|
| CNS | **Cerebral cortical malformations** | + | + | + | + | + |
| | **Cognitive dysfunction** | | ++ | ++ | ++ | ++ |
| | **Microcephaly** | + | + | + | + | + |
| | **Seizures** | + | + | + | + | + |
| Musculoskeletal | Dysmorphic features | ± | ± | ± | ± | ± |
| | Thin body habitus | | | + | + | + |
| Psychiatric | **Behavioral abnormalities** | | + | + | + | + |
| Laboratory findings | 4α-Carboxymethyl sterol (lymphoblasts) | n-↑ | n-↑ | n-↑ | n-↑ | n-↑ |
| | 4α-methyl sterols (lymphoblasts) | n-↑ | n-↑ | n-↑ | n-↑ | n-↑ |

Information provided is based on multiple affected males from two unrelated families

**Table 54.10** X-linked dominant sterol Δ8, Δ7-isomerase deficiency (X-linked dominant Conradi-Hünermann-Happle syndrome) (Chondrodysplasia punctata 2)

| System | Symptoms and Biomarkers | Neonatal (birth–1 month) | Infancy (1–18 months) | Childhood (1.5–11 years) | Adolescence (11–16 years) | Adulthood (>16 years) |
|---|---|---|---|---|---|---|
| Dermatological | **Alopecia** | + | + | + | + | + |
| | **Dystrophic nails** | ± | ± | ± | ± | ± |
| | **Follicular atrophoderma** | ± | + | + | + | + |
| | **Ichthyosiform erythroderma** | + | + | | | |
| Eye | **Cataract** | ± | ± | ± | ± | ± |
| | Microphthalmia | ± | ± | ± | ± | ± |
| Musculoskeletal | Cervical compressive myelopathy | ± | ± | ± | ± | ± |
| | Micrognathia | ± | ± | ± | ± | ± |
| | Midface hypoplasia | ± | ± | ± | ± | ± |
| | Polydactyly | ± | ± | ± | ± | ± |
| | **Punctate calcifications of epiphyses** | + | + | ± | ± | ± |
| | **Punctate calcifications of larynx** | + | + | ± | ± | ± |
| | **Punctate calcifications of trachea** | + | + | ± | ± | ± |
| | Rhizomelia | ± | ± | ± | ± | ± |
| | Scoliosis | ± | ± | ± | ± | ± |
| | Vertebral anomalies | ± | ± | ± | ± | ± |
| Renal | Renal dysgenesis | ± | ± | ± | ± | ± |
| | Renal hypoplasia | ± | ± | ± | ± | ± |
| Laboratory findings | 8(9)-Cholestenol (lymphoblasts) | ↑ | ↑ | ↑ | ↑ | n-↑ |
| | 8(9)-Cholestenol (plasma) | ↑ | ↑ | ↑ | ↑ | n-↑ |
| | 8-Dehydrocholesterol (lymphoblasts) | ↑ | ↑ | ↑ | ↑ | n-↑ |
| | 8-Dehydrocholesterol (plasma) | ↑ | ↑ | ↑ | ↑ | n-↑ |

**Table 54.11** X-linked recessive sterol Δ8, Δ7-isomerase deficiency (MEND syndrome) (Chondrodysplasia punctata 2: male)

| System | Symptoms and Biomarkers | Neonatal (birth–1 month) | Infancy (1–18 months) | Childhood (1.5–11 years) | Adolescence (11–16 years) | Adulthood (>16 years) |
|---|---|---|---|---|---|---|
| Cardiovascular | Cardiac, malformations | ± | ± | ± | | |
| CNS | **Agenesis, corpus callosum (MRI)** | + | + | + | | |
| | **Dandy-Walker variant** | ± | ± | ± | | |
| | **Developmental delay** | + | + | + | | |
| | **Hypogenesis, corpus callosum** | + | + | + | | |
| | Hypotonia | + | + | + | | |
| | **Microcephaly** | + | + | + | | |
| | Seizures | ± | ± | ± | | |
| Dermatological | Hypoplastic nails | ± | ± | ± | | |
| | **Ichthyosis** | ± | ± | ± | | |
| Eye | **Cataract** | ± | ± | ± | | |
| Genitourinary | Cryptorchidism | ± | ± | ± | | |
| | Hypospadias | ± | ± | ± | | |
| Musculoskeletal | Chondrodysplasia punctata | ± | ± | ± | | |
| | Facial dysmorphism | + | + | + | | |
| | Polydactyly | ± | ± | ± | | |
| | Toe syndactyly, 2/3 | ± | ± | ± | | |
| Laboratory findings | 8(9)-Cholestenol (lymphoblasts) | ↑ | ↑ | ↑ | | |
| | 8(9)-Cholestenol (plasma) | ↑ | ↑ | ↑ | | |
| | 8-Dehydrocholesterol (lymphoblasts) | ↑ | ↑ | ↑ | | |
| | 8-Dehydrocholesterol (plasma) | ↑ | ↑ | ↑ | | |

**Table 54.12** Sterol Δ5-desaturase deficiency (Lathosterolosis)

| System | Symptoms and Biomarkers | Neonatal (birth–1 month) | Infancy (1–18 months) | Childhood (1.5–11 years) | Adolescence (11–16 years) | Adulthood (>16 years) |
|---|---|---|---|---|---|---|
| Cardiovascular | Cardiac, anomalies, malformations | ± | ± | ± | | |
| CNS | **Hypotonia** | + | + | ± | | |
| | **Intellectual disability** | | + | + | | |
| | **Microcephaly** | + | + | + | | |
| Eye | **Cataract** | + | + | + | | |
| | Ptosis of eyelid | + | + | + | | |
| Genitourinary | Hypospadias | ± | ± | ± | | |
| Musculoskeletal | Anteverted nares | + | + | + | | |
| | Bitemporal narrowing | ± | ± | ± | | |
| | Cleft palate | ± | ± | ± | | |
| | **Growth retardation** | + | + | + | | |
| | **Micrognathia** | + | + | + | | |
| | Polydactyly, postaxial | + | + | + | | |
| | **Toe syndactyly, 2/3** | + | + | + | | |
| Respiratory | Broad alveolar ridges | + | + | + | | |
| Laboratory findings | Cholesterol (plasma) | n | n | n | | |
| | Lathosterol (fibroblasts) | ↑ | ↑ | ↑ | | |
| | Lathosterol (lymphoblasts) | ↑ | ↑ | ↑ | | |
| | Lathosterol (plasma) | ↑ | ↑ | ↑ | | |

Information provided is based on four known unrelated cases

**Table 54.13** 24-Dehydrocholesterol reductase deficiency (Desmosterolosis)

| System | Symptoms and Biomarkers | Neonatal (birth–1 month) | Infancy (1–18 months) | Childhood (1.5–11 years) | Adolescence (11–16 years) | Adulthood (>16 years) |
|---|---|---|---|---|---|---|
| Cardiovascular | Cardiac, anomalies, malformations | ± | ± | ± | | |
| CNS | **Agenesis, corpus callosum (MRI)** | + | + | + | | |
| | **Cerebral cortical malformations** | ± | ± | ± | | |
| | **Hypogenesis, corpus callosum** | + | + | + | | |
| | **Intellectual disability** | | + | + | | |
| | Microcephaly | ± | ± | ± | | |
| | Seizures | ± | | | | |
| | Ventriculomegaly | + | + | + | | |
| Genitourinary | Renal agenesis | ± | ± | ± | | |
| Musculoskeletal | Arthrogryposis | ± | ± | ± | | |
| | Cleft palate | ± | ± | ± | | |
| | Facial dysmorphism | ± | ± | ± | | |
| | Limb defects | ± | ± | ± | | |
| | Macrocephaly | ± | ± | ± | | |
| | Micrognathia | ± | ± | ± | | |
| Renal | Renal hypoplasia | ± | ± | ± | | |
| Respiratory | Pulmonary hypoplasia | ± | ± | ± | | |
| Laboratory findings | Cholesterol (plasma) | n | n | n | | |
| | Desmosterol (fibroblasts) | ↑ | ↑ | ↑ | | |
| | Desmosterol (lymphoblasts) | ↑ | ↑ | ↑ | | |
| | Desmosterol (plasma) | ↑ | ↑ | ↑ | | |

**Table 54.14** 7-Dehydrocholesterol reductase deficiency (Smith-Lemli-Opitz syndrome)

| System | Symptoms and Biomarkers | Neonatal (birth–1 month) | Infancy (1–18 months) | Childhood (1.5–11 years) | Adolescence (11–16 years) | Adulthood (>16 years) |
|---|---|---|---|---|---|---|
| Cardiovascular | **Cardiac, anomalies, malformations** | ± | ± | ± | ± | ± |
| CNS | Agenesis, corpus callosum (MRI) | ± | ± | ± | ± | ± |
| | **Axial hypotonia** | + | + | ± | | |
| | Cerebellar hypoplasia | ± | ± | ± | ± | ± |
| | **Developmental delay** | + | + | + | + | + |
| | Holoprosencephaly | ± | ± | ± | ± | ± |
| | Hypogenesis, corpus callosum | ± | ± | ± | ± | ± |
| | **Irritability** | + | + | + | + | + |
| | **Microcephaly** | + | + | + | + | + |
| | **Self-injury** | | | ± | ± | ± |
| Dermatological | **Excess digital whorls** | + | + | + | + | + |
| Digestive | Feeding difficulties | + | + | + | ± | ± |
| | Hirschsprung disease | ± | ± | ± | ± | ± |
| | **Intestinal dysmotility** | + | + | ± | ± | ± |
| | Liver dysfunction | ± | ± | | | |
| | **Pyloric stenosis** | ± | ± | | | |
| Ear | Deafness, sensorineural | ± | ± | ± | ± | ± |
| Eye | Cataract | ± | ± | ± | ± | ± |
| | **Ptosis of eyelid** | + | + | + | + | + |
| | Strabismus | ± | ± | ± | ± | ± |
| Genitourinary | Ambiguous genitalia in 46, XY | ± | ± | ± | ± | ± |
| | **Cryptorchidism** | ± | ± | ± | ± | ± |
| | Hypospadias | ± | ± | ± | ± | ± |
| | Renal agenesis | ± | ± | ± | ± | ± |
| Musculoskeletal | **Anteverted nares** | + | + | + | ± | ± |
| | **Cleft palate** | ± | ± | ± | ± | ± |
| | Club foot | ± | ± | ± | ± | ± |
| | **Epicanthal folds** | + | + | + | + | + |
| | **Growth retardation** | + | + | + | + | + |
| | **Micrognathia** | + | + | + | + | + |
| | Polydactyly, postaxial | ± | ± | ± | ± | ± |
| | Rhizomelia | ± | ± | ± | ± | ± |
| | **Toe syndactyly, 2/3** | + | + | + | + | + |
| Psychiatric | **Behavior, aggressive** | | | + | + | + |
| Renal | Renal hypoplasia | ± | ± | ± | ± | ± |
| Respiratory | **Broad alveolar ridges** | + | + | + | + | + |
| | Pulmonary hypoplasia | ± | ± | ± | ± | ± |
| | Pulmonary lobation, abnormal | ± | ± | ± | ± | ± |
| Laboratory findings | 7-Dehydrocholesterol (fibroblasts) | ↑ | ↑ | ↑ | ↑ | ↑ |
| | 7-Dehydrocholesterol (lymphoblasts) | ↑ | ↑ | ↑ | ↑ | ↑ |
| | 7-Dehydrocholesterol (plasma) | ↑ | ↑ | ↑ | ↑ | ↑ |
| | 8-Dehydrocholesterol (fibroblasts) | ↑ | ↑ | ↑ | ↑ | ↑ |
| | 8-Dehydrocholesterol (lymphoblasts) | ↑ | ↑ | ↑ | ↑ | ↑ |
| | 8-Dehydrocholesterol (plasma) | ↑ | ↑ | ↑ | ↑ | ↑ |
| | Cholesterol (serum) | ↓↓↓-n | ↓↓↓-n | ↓↓↓-n | ↓↓-n | ↓↓-n |

## Reference Values

### Organic Acids: Urine (GC/SID GC-MS)

| Age | Mevalonic acid (mmol/mol creat) | **Branched-chain organic acids:** 3-methylhex-2-endioic acid; 2,6-dimethylheptanedioic acid; 3-methylhex-2,4-dienedioic acid; 3,7-dimethyloctanedioic acid; 3,7-dimethyl-2,6-dienedioic acid |
|---|---|---|
| All ages | 0.06–0.21[a] | Below the limit of detection |

[a]Hoffmann et al. (1993)

### Farnesol: Plasma

| Age | Farnesol (μmol/L) |
|---|---|
| All ages | < 0.12[a] |

[a]Coman et al. (2018)

### Sterols: Plasma (GC-MS)

| Age | Cholesterol (mmol/L) |
|---|---|
| <1 week | 1.30–2.59 |
| 1 week–3 months | 1.88–4.79 |
| >3 months | 2.40–5.15 |

| Age | Cholest-8(9)-en-3ß-ol (8(9)-cholestenol) (μmol/L) | Desmosterol (μmol/L) | 4α-Methyl-5α-cholest-8(9)-en-3ß-ol (μmol/L) | 4α-Methyl-5α-cholest-7(8)-en-3ß-ol (μmol/L) |
|---|---|---|---|---|
| <3 months | <1.40 | 0.65–9.06 | <2.48 | <1.50 |
| >3 months | <0.96 | 0.55–7.60 | <1.10 | <0.50 |

| Age | 7-Dehydrocholesterol (μmol/L) | Lathosterol (μmol/L) | 4,4′α-Dimethyl sterols (μmol/L) | Lanosterol (μmol/L) | Dihydrolanosterol (μmol/L) |
|---|---|---|---|---|---|
| All ages | 0.08–1.04 | 0.41–9.90 | <0.02 | <0.35 | <0.23 |

### Sterols: Cells (GC-MS)

| 7-Dehydro-cholesterol | Cholest-8(9)-en-3ß-ol | Desmosterol | Lathosterol | 4α-Methyl sterols | 4,4′α-Dimethyl sterols | Lanosterol | Dihydro-lanosterol | Cholesta-8,14-dien-3ß-ol |
|---|---|---|---|---|---|---|---|---|
| **LYM** | **LYM** | **LYM** | **LYM** | **LYM** | **LYM** | **LYM** | **LYM** | **FB** |
| 0.06–0.35 | <0.01–0.99 | 0.07–0.69 | 0.14–4.30 | <0.1–9.7 | <0.01–3.5 | <0.01–0.67 | <0.01–0.33 | <0.01–0.69 |

Units: % ratio to total sterols. Overall, most sterol levels in fibroblasts (FB) are comparable to levels in lymphoblasts (LYM)

## Pathological Values

| Disorder | Mevalonate urine (mmol/mol creat) |
|---|---|
| 54.1<br>Classic MKD[a] | 3165–51,433 |
| 54.2<br>Hyper-IgD syndrome[b] | Acute: 21–143<br>Well: 4.4–10.3 |

[a]Hoffmann et al. (1993)
[b]Kelley, unpublished data

| Disorder | Cholesterol | Farnesol | Mevalonate | **Branched-chain organic acids:** 3-methylhex-2-enedioic acid; 2,6-dimethylheptanedioic acid; 3-methylhex-2,4-dienedioic acid; 3,7-dimethyloctanedioic acid; 3,7-dimethyl-2,6-dienedioic acid |
|---|---|---|---|---|
| 54.3<br>Squalene synthase deficiency | n-↓ P | ↑ P | ↑ U | ↑ U |

| Disorder | Cholesterol | 7-Dehydro-cholesterol | 8-Dehydro-cholesterol | Desmo-sterol | Lathos-terol | 8(9)-Chole-stenol | 4α-Methyl sterols | 4,4′α-Dimethyl sterols | 4α-Carboxy-methyl-cholest-8(9)-en-3-beta-ol | Cholesta-8,14-dien-3ß-ol | Dihydro-lanosterol | Lanosterol |
|---|---|---|---|---|---|---|---|---|---|---|---|---|
| 54.5 Lanosterol 14α-demethylase deficiency | n P | | | | | | | | | | ↑ P, LYM | ↑ P, LYM |
| 54.6 Greenberg dysplasia | | | | | | | | | | ↑ FB, tis | | |
| 54.7 SC4MOL deficiency | n-↓ P | | | | | | ↑ P, LYM | ↑ P, LYM | n P, LYM | | | |
| 54.8 CHILD syndrome | n P | | | | | | n-↑ P<br>↑ LYM<br>↑ skin flakes | | ↑ LYM<br>↑ skin flakes | | | |
| 54.9 CK syndrome | n P | | | | | | n-↑ LYM | | n-↑ LYM | | | |
| 54.10/54.11 CDPX2/MEND S. | n P | | ↑ P, LYM<br>↑ tis | | | ↑ P, LYM<br>↑ tis | | | | | | |
| 54.12 Lathosterolosis | n P | | | | ↑ P, LYM<br>↑ FIB, tis | | | | | | | |
| 54.13 Desmosterolosis | n P | | | ↑ P, LYM<br>↑ FB, tis | | | | | | | | |
| 54.14 Smith-Lemli-Opitz syndrome | n-↓ P | ↑ P, LYM<br>↑ FB, tis<br>↑ AF, CV | ↑ P, LYM<br>↑ FB, tis<br>↑ AF, CV | | | | | | | | | |

## Diagnostic Flowchart

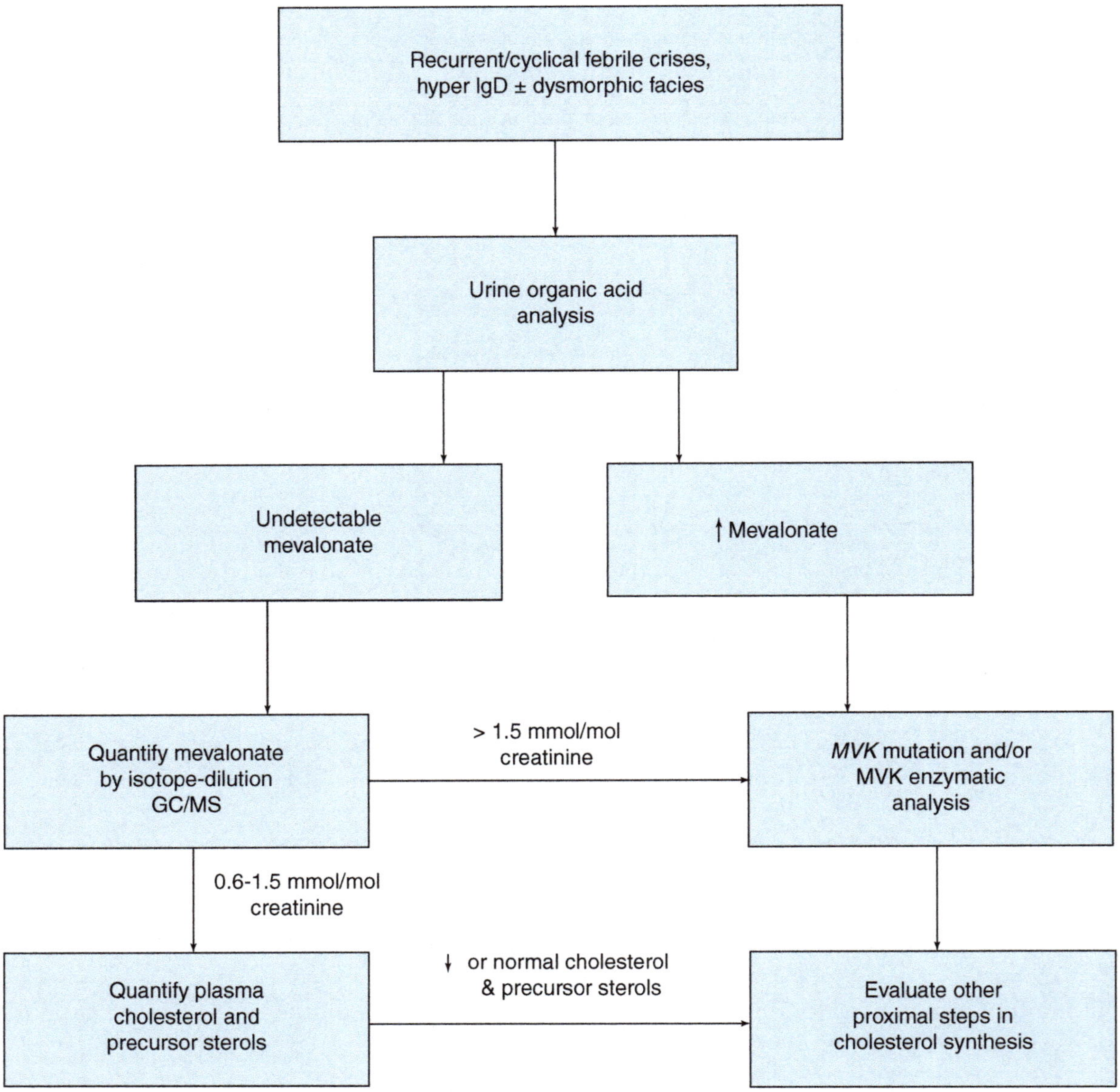


**Fig. 54.2** Diagnostic flow chart for mevalonic aciduria

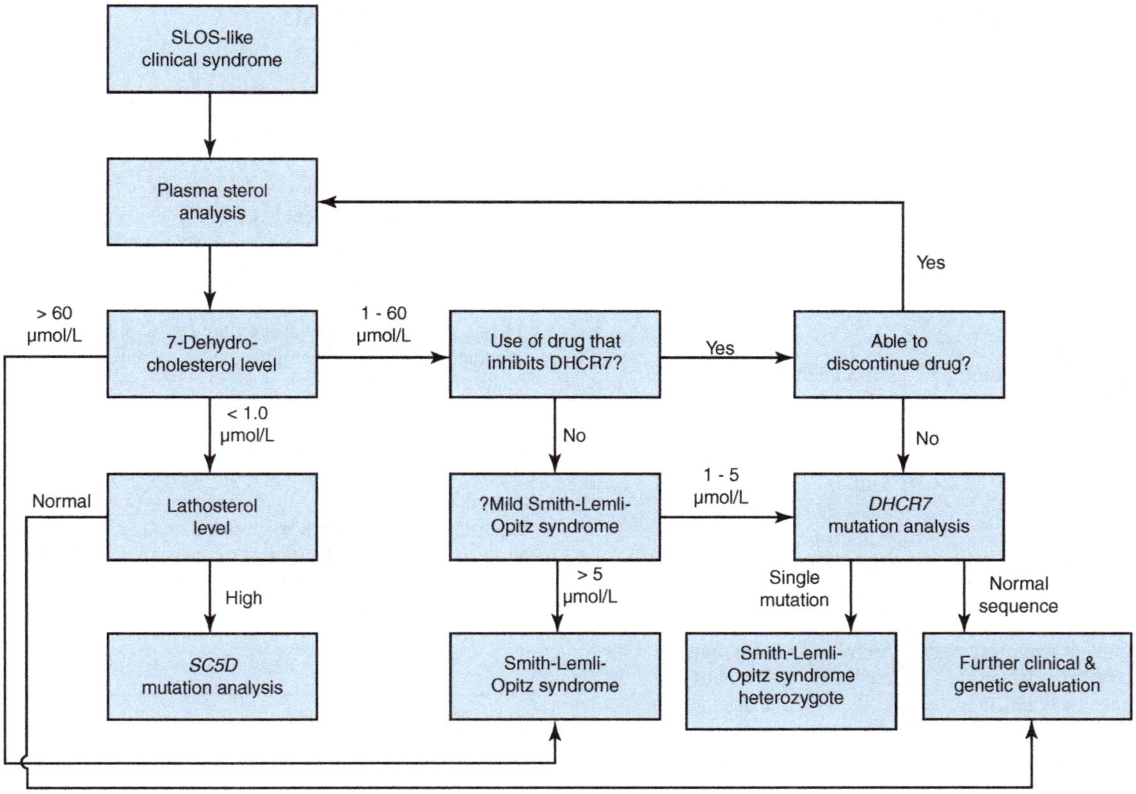


**Fig. 54.3** Diagnostic flowchart for Smith-Lemli-Opitz syndrome and related disorders

**Fig. 54.4** Diagnostic flowchart for chondrodysplasia punctata

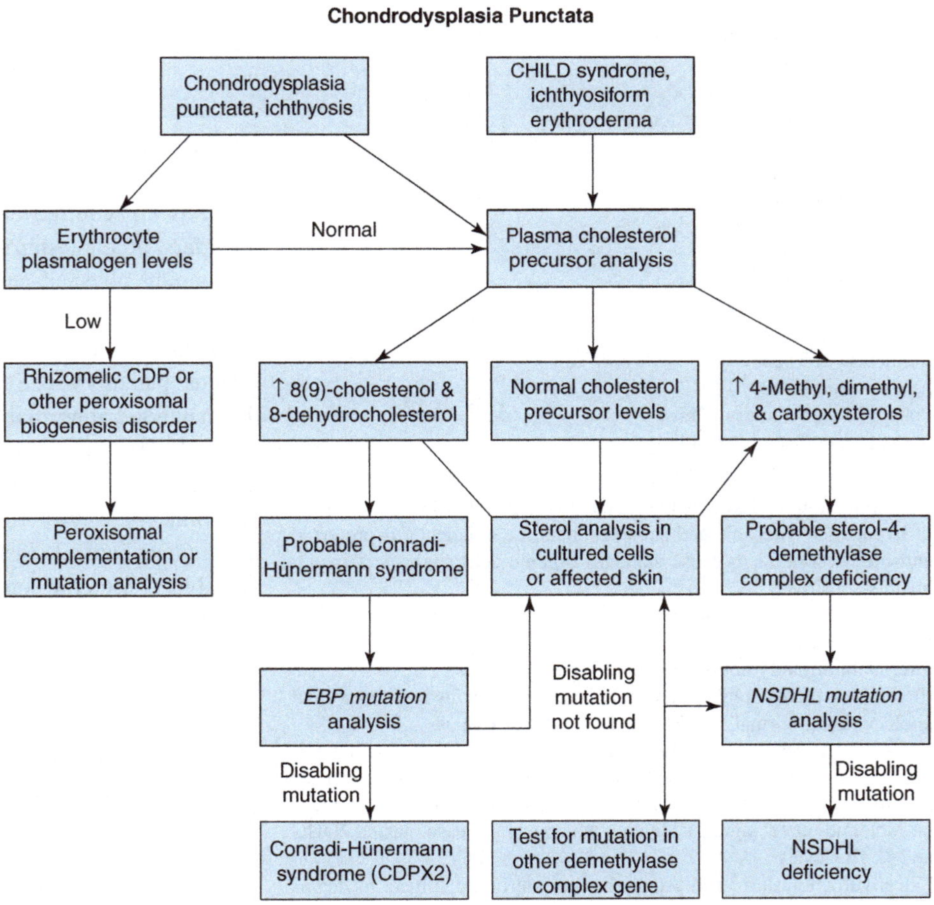

## Specimen Collection

All specimens should be stored frozen at −20 °C.

| Disorder | Test | Sample | Pitfalls |
|---|---|---|---|
| 54.1 Mevalonate kinase deficiency<br>Please insert a box between 54.21 and 54.3 that contains the following information:<br>Test:<br>Sample:<br>Pitfalls: a | Organic acid analysis | Urine (random) | [a] |
| 54.2 Hyper-IgD syndrome | Mevalonate | Urine (acute specimen preferred) | [a] |
| 54.3 Squalene synthase deficiency | Organic acid analysis<br>Farnesol | Urine (random)<br>Plasma | [a] |
| 54.6 Sterol C14-reductase deficiency (Greenberg dysplasia) | Sterol analysis | Tissue, fibroblasts | [b] |
| 54.8 X-linked dominant sterol 4α-carboxylate 3-dehydrogenase deficiency (CHILD syndrome) | Sterol analysis | Skin flakes, lymphoblasts | [c,d] |
| 54.9 X-linked recessive sterol 4α-carboxylate 3-dehydrogenase deficiency (CK syndrome) | Sterol analysis | Lymphoblasts | [b] |
| 54.10 X-linked dominant sterol Δ8,Δ7 isomerase deficiency (CDPX2)<br>54.11 X-linked recessive sterol Δ8,Δ7 isomerase deficiency (MEND syndrome) | Sterol analysis | Plasma, tissue, lymphoblasts, fibroblasts | [d] |
| Autosomal recessive post-squalene inborn errors of cholesterol synthesis:<br>54.5 Lanosterol 14α-demethylase deficiency<br>54.7 Sterol C4-methyl oxidase (SC4MOL) deficiency<br>54.12 Sterol Δ5-desaturase deficiency (Lathosterolosis)<br>54.13 24-Dehydrocholesterol reductase deficiency (Desmosterolosis)<br>54.14 7-Dehydrocholesterol reductase deficiency (Smith-Lemli-Opitz syndrome; SLOS) | Sterol analysis | Plasma, tissue, lymphoblasts, fibroblasts | [e,f] |

[a]Quantification of mevalonate by stable isotope GC-MS for diagnosis of hyper-IgD syndrome and squalene synthase deficiency is preferred and often essential, because standard organic acid analysis is inadequately sensitive

[b]CK syndrome and Greenberg skeletal dysplasia are best diagnosed by targeted mutation analysis

[c]Sterol abnormality not reliably detectable in plasma

[d]In females, there could be skewed X-inactivation in favor of the normal allele, causing normal sterol levels in plasma or tissues

[e]Plasma sterol levels can be mildly increased secondary to certain medications. Most notable are amiodarone and imatinib, which can increase plasma desmosterol levels, and aripiprazole (Abilify), trazodone, haloperidol, and other "sigma-1" ligand, which can increase plasma 7DHC and 8DHC levels

[f]7-Dehydrocholesterol and 8-dehydrocholesterol are subject to degradation (oxidation) over weeks in plasma at room temperature and more slowly (months) when frozen

## Prenatal Diagnosis

| Disorder | Material | Timing, trimester |
|---|---|---|
| 54.1 Mevalonate kinase deficiency | CV, CCV, AF, AFC | I, II |
| 54.10 X-linked dominant sterol-Δ8,Δ7-isomerase deficiency (CDPX2) | CV, AF | II[a] |
| 54.11 X-linked recessive sterol-Δ8,Δ7-isomerase deficiency (MEND syndrome) | AF | II[b] |
| 54.14 7-Dehydrocholesterol reductase deficiency (Smith-Lemli-Opitz syndrome; SLOS) | CV, AF<br>Maternal urine (steroid analysis) | I, II<br>II |

Prenatal diagnosis is possible for all disorders by DNA sequencing

*CV* direct chorionic villi, *CCV* cultured chorionic villi, *AF* amniotic fluid, *AFC* amniocytes

[a]Experience by biochemical prenatal testing limited to four female fetuses with ultrasound anomalies consistent with CDPX2

[b]Experience by biochemical prenatal testing limited to one male fetus originally evaluated for SLOS

## DNA Testing

Molecular testing can be performed for all disorders of cholesterol biosynthesis by direct sequencing and del/dup analysis of DNA isolated from blood or tissue. In addition, some genes may be included on gene panels designed for a specific phenotypic feature, e.g., *CYP51A1* is often included on cataract gene panels.

## Treatment

There is no required emergent metabolic management for disorders of cholesterol biosynthesis, but serious or life-threatening physical anomalies requiring acute medical or surgical intervention are common. For SLOS, cholesterol supplementation has become standard of care, and studies of selected patients with SLOS have also shown amelioration of the metabolic abnormalities with simvastatin treatment (Jira et al. 2000). In addition, when there is an acute life-threatening condition, such as pneumonia or major surgery, and oral cholesterol replacement therapy is not possible, intravenous banked plasma ("fresh-frozen" plasma) can be a valuable parenteral source of cholesterol. Steroid therapy might be required for severely affected patients during periods of stress, usually those with a cholesterol level less than 0.5 mM, because of possible glucocorticoid and/or mineralocorticoid deficiency. Treatment schemes for non-SLOS sterol disorders are limited due, in part, to the rarity of these disorders. Cholesterol supplementation in conjunction with statin therapy has caused improved growth and development in one patient with SC4MOL deficiency, and simvastatin has proved effective in the treatment of squalene synthase deficiency (R. Kelley, unpublished).

For the treatment of periodic severe inflammatory crises, which, among disorders of sterol synthesis, are unique to MKD, especially the HIDS variant, treatment of severe, acute crises with glucocorticoids ("pulse steroids) works rapidly, but overly frequent use of steroids should, of course, be avoided. However, other, often effective, immunosuppressants designed to block cytokines or otherwise blunt the inflammatory response include leukotriene receptors antagonists (e.g., montelukast, zafirlukast), anti-TNF medication (e.g., etanercept), and IL-1 inhibitors (e.g., anakinra), among several others (van der Hilst et al. 2008). Because chronic treatment with these drugs is required, sustained use of these medications risks medically significant immunosuppression, with the exception of the usually mild immunosuppressive effect of montelukast and zafirlukast.

## References


Aldahmesh MA, Khan AO, Mohamed JY, Hijazi H, Al-Owain M, Alswaid A, et al. Genomic analysis of pediatric cataract in Saudi Arabia reveals novel candidate disease genes. Genet Med. 2012;14:955–62.

Anderson R, Rust S, Ashworth J, Clayton-Smith J, Taylor RL, Clayton PT, Morris AAM. Lathosterolosis: a relatively mild case with cataracts and learning difficulties. JIMD Rep. 2019;44:79–84.

Aughton D, Kelley R, Metzenberg A, Pureza V, Pauli R. X-linked dominant chondrodysplasia punctata (CDPX2) caused by single gene mosaicism in a male. Am J Med Genet. 2003;116A:255–60.

Barboza-Cerda MC, Wong LJ, Martínez-de-Villarreal LE, Zhang VW, Déctor MA. A novel EBP c.224T>a mutation supports the existence of a male-specific disorder independent of CDPX2. Am J Med Genet A. 2014;164A:1642–7.

Besnard T, Sloboda N, Goldenberg A, Küry S, Cogné B, Breheret F, et al. Biallelic pathogenic variants in the lanosterol synthase gene LSS involved in the cholesterol biosynthesis cause alopecia with intellectual disability, a rare recessive neuroectodermal syndrome. Genet Med. 2019.

Braverman N, Lin P, Moebius FF, Obie C, Moser A, Glossmann H, et al. Mutations in the gene encoding 3 beta-hydroxysteroid-delta 8, delta 7- isomerase cause X-linked dominant Conradi-Hünermann syndrome. Nat Genet. 1999;22:291–4.

Brunetti-Pierri N, Corso G, Rossi M, Ferrari P, Balli F, Rivasi F, et al. Lathosterolosis, a novel multiple-malformation/mental retardation syndrome due to deficiency of 3b-hydroxysteroid-D5-desaturase. Am J Hum Genet. 2002;71:952–8.

Chen X, Liu L. Congenital cataract with LSS gene mutations: a new case report. J Pediatr Endocrinol Metab. 2017;30:1231–5.

Clayton P, Fischer B, Mann A, Mansour S, Rossier E, Veen M, et al. Mutations causing Greenberg dysplasia but not Pelger anomaly uncouple enzymatic from structural functions of a nuclear membrane protein. Nucleus. 2010;1:354–66.

Coman D, Vissers LELM, Riley LG, Kwint MP, Hauck R, Koster J, et al. Squalene synthase deficiency: clinical, biochemical, and molecular characterization of a defect in cholesterol biosynthesis. Am J Hum Genet. 2018;103:125–30.

FitzPatrick DR, Keeling JW, Evans MJ, Kan AE, Bell JE, Porteous ME, et al. Clinical phenotype of desmosterolosis. Am J Med Genet. 1998;75:145–52.

Frisso G, Gelzo M, Procopio E, Sica C, Lenza MP, Dello Russo A, et al. A rare case of sterol-C4-methyl oxidase deficiency in a young Italian male: biochemical and molecular characterization. Mol Genet Metab. 2017;121:329–35.

Gillespie RL, O'Sullivan J, Ashworth J, Bhaskar S, Williams S, Biswas S, et al. Personalized diagnosis and management of congenital cataract by next-generation sequencing. Ophthalmology. 2014;121:2124–37.

Grange DK, Kratz LE, Braverman NE, Kelley RI. CHILD syndrome caused by deficiency of 3beta-hydroxysteroid-delta8, delta7-isomerase. Am J Med Genet. 2000;90:328–35.

Hall P, Michels V, Gavrilov D, Matern D, Oglesbee D, Raymond K, et al. Aripiprazole and trazodone cause elevations of 7-dehydrocholesterol in the absence of Smith-Lemli-Opitz syndrome. Mol Genet Metab. 2013;110:176–8.

Happle R, Koch H, Lenz W. The CHILD syndrome: congenital hemidysplasia with ichthyosiform erythroderma and limb defects. Eur J Pediatr. 1980;134:27–33.

He M, Kratz LE, Michel JJ, Vallejo AN, Ferris L, Kelley RI, et al. Mutations in the human SC4MOL gene encoding a methyl sterol oxidase cause psoriasiform dermatitis, microcephaly, and developmental delay. J Clin Invest. 2011;121:976–84.

He M, Smith LD, Chang R, Li X, Vockley J. The role of sterol-C4-methyl oxidase in epidermal biology. Biochim Biophys Acta. 2014;1841:331–5.

Ho AC, Fung CW, Siu TS, Ma OC, Lam CW, Tam S, Wong VC. Lathosterolosis: a disorder of cholesterol biosynthesis resembling Smith-Lemli-Opitz syndrome. JIMD Rep. 2014;12:129–34.

Hoffmann GF, Charpentier C, Mayatepek E, Mancini J, Leichsenring M, Gibson KM, et al. Clinical and biochemical phenotype in 11 patients with mevalonic aciduria. Pediatrics. 1993;91:915–21.

Hoffmann K, Dreger CK, Olins AL, Olins DE, Shultz LD, Lucke B, et al. Mutations in the gene encoding the lamin B receptor produce an altered nuclear morphology in granulocytes (Pelger-Huët anomaly). Nat Genet. 2002;31:410–4.

Houten SM, Kuis W, Duran M, de Koning TJ, van Royen-Kerkhof A, Romeijn GJ, et al. Mutations in MVK, encoding mevalonate kinase, cause hyperimmunoglobulinaemia D and periodic fever syndrome. Nat Genet. 1999;22:175–7.

Jira PE, Wevers RA, de Jong J, Rubio-Gozalbo E, Janssen-Zijlstra FS, van Heyst AF, et al. Simvastatin. A new therapeutic approach for Smith-Lemli-Opitz syndrome. J Lipid Res. 2000;41:1339–46.

Kelley RI, Hennekam RC. The Smith-Lemli-Opitz syndrome. J Med Genet. 2000;37:321–35.

König A, Happle R, Bornholdt D, Engel H, Grzeschik KH. Mutations in the NSDHL gene, encoding a 3beta-hydroxysteroid dehydrogenase, cause CHILD syndrome. Am J Med Genet. 2000;90:339–46.

Konstantinidou A, Karadimas C, Waterham HR, Superti-Furga A, Kaminopetros P, Grigoriadou M, et al. Pathologic, radiographic and molecular findings in three fetuses diagnosed with HEM/Greenberg skeletal dysplasia. Prenat Diagn. 2008;28:309–12.

Liu XY, Dangel AW, Kelley RI, Zhao W, Denny P, Botcherby M, et al. The gene mutated in bare patches and striated mice encodes a novel 3beta-hydroxysteroid dehydrogenase. Nat Genet. 1999;22:182–7.

McLarren KW, Severson TM, du Souich C, Stockton DW, Kratz LE, Cunningham D, et al. Hypomorphic temperature-sensitive alleles of NSDHL cause CK syndrome. Am J Hum Genet. 2010;87:905–14.

Milunsky J, Maher T, Metzenberg A. Molecular, biochemical, and phenotypic analysis of a hemizygous male with a severe atypical phenotype for X-linked dominant Conradi-Hunermann-Happle syndrome and a mutation in EBP. Am J Hum Genet. 2003;116A:249–54.

Nowaczyk MJ, Irons MB. Smith-Lemli-Opitz syndrome: phenotype, natural history, and epidemiology. Am J Med Genet C Semin Med Genet. 2012;160C:250–62.

Pacault M, Vincent M, Besnard T, Kannengiesser C, Bénéteau C, Barbarot S, et al. New splicing pathogenic variant in EBP causing extreme familial variability of Conradi-Hünermann-Happle syndrome. Eur J Hum Genet. 2018;26:1784–90.

Preiksaitiene E, Caro A, Benušienė E, Oltra S, Orellana C, Morkūnienė A, et al. A novel missense mutation in the NSDHL gene identified in a Lithuanian family by targeted next-generation sequencing causes CK syndrome. Am J Med Genet A. 2015;167:1342–8.

Roca-Ayats N, Ng PY, Garcia-Giralt N, Falcó-Mascaró M, Cozar M, Abril JF, et al. Functional characterization of a GGPPS variant identified in atypical femoral fracture patients and delineation of the role of GGPPS in bone-relevant cell types. J Bone Miner Res. 2018;33:2091–8.

Rohanizadegan M, Sacharow S. Desmosterolosis presenting with multiple congenital anomalies. Eur J Med Genet. 2018;61:152–6.

Romano MT, Tafazzoli A, Mattern M, Sivalingam S, Wolf S, Rupp A, et al. Bi-allelic mutations in LSS, encoding lanosterol synthase, cause autosomal-recessive hypotrichosis simplex. Am J Hum Genet. 2018;103:777–85.

Silengo MC, Luzzatti L, Silverman FN. Clinical and genetic aspects of Conradi-Hünermann disease. A report of three familial cases and review of the literature. J Pediatr. 1980;97:911–7.

Thompson E, Abdalla E, Superti-Furga A, McAlister W, Kratz L, Unger S, et al. Lamin B receptor-related disorder is associated with a spectrum of skeletal dysplasia phenotypes. Bone. 2019;120:354–63.

van der Hilst JC, Bodar EJ, Barron KS, Frenkel J, Drenth JP, van der Meer JW, Simon A. Long-term follow-up, clinical features, and quality of life in a series of 103 patients with hyperimmunoglobinemia D syndrome. Medicine. 2008;87:301–10.

Waterham H, Koster J, Mooyer P, van Noort G, Kelley R, Wilcox W, et al. Autosomal recessive HEM/Greenberg skeletal dysplasia is caused by 3β-hydroxysterol Δ $^{14}$-reductase deficiency due to mutations in the lamin B receptor gene. Am J Hum Genet. 2003;72:1013–7.

Waterham HR, Koster J, Romeijn GJ, Hennekam RC, Vreken P, Andersson HC, et al. Mutations in the 3beta-hydroxysterol Delta24-reductase gene cause desmosterolosis, an autosomal recessive disorder of cholesterol biosynthesis. Am J Hum Genet. 2001;69:685–94.

Zhang Z, Li C, Wu F, Ma R, Luan J, Yang F, et al. Genomic variations of the mevalonate pathway in porokeratosis. elife. 2015;23(4):e06322.

Zhao L, Chen X, Zhu J, Xi Y, Yang X, Hu L, et al. Lanosterol reverses protein aggregation in cataracts. Nature. 2015;523:607–11.

# Disorders of Adrenals and Gonads

# 55

Anna Biason-Lauber

## Contents



**Summary**

Defects in steroid biosynthesis in adrenals and gonads lead to complex and profound clinical consequences that can be grouped in three categories: (1) defects of saltwater homeostasis and sexual development (DSD), (2) defects of saltwater homeostasis, (3) defects of sexual development, and (4) end-organ steroid hormone resistance. Among the members of the first group, lipoid adrenal hyperplasia is characterized by lack of all steroid hormones, with consequent 46, XY DSD and salt loss in the first weeks of life. 17α-Hydroxylase deficiency leads also to 46, XY DSD associated with hypertension and hypokalemia. 3β-Hydroxysteroid dehydrogenase deficiency causes incomplete virilization in male fetuses, together with salt loss. 21-Hydroxylase deficiency, whose nonclassic form is one of the most common autosomal recessive diseases in humans, is responsible for female ambiguous genitalia at birth and salt loss. 11β-Hydroxylase deficiency differs from 21-hydroxylase deficiency for the absence of salt wasting and later presence of hypertension and hypokalemia. Defects of P450 oxidoreductase, a cofactor common to 21-hydroxylase, 17α-hydroxylase, and aromatase, lead to a complex combined defect of all three enzymes.

Enzymatic defects of the second group cause either salt wasting symptoms in the neonatal period, spontaneously resolving in adulthood, as in the case of corticosterone methyl oxidase II deficiency, or hypertension and hypokalemia as in the cases of glucocorticoid-suppressible hyperaldosteronism and apparent mineralocorticoid excess. The third group of defects includes enzymatic blocks of the last steps of sex hormone biosynthesis. 17,20-Lyase, 17β-hydroxysteroid dehydrogenase, 5α-reductase, and aldo-keto reductase deficiencies determine incomplete virilization of the male fetus. In 17,20-lyase deficiency, there is no spontaneous puberty in males and females; in the lat-

A. Biason-Lauber (✉)
Division of Medicine, University of Fribourg, Fribourg, Switzerland
e-mail: anna.lauber@unifr.ch



N. Blau et al. (eds.), *Physician's Guide to the Diagnosis, Treatment, and Follow-Up of Inherited Metabolic Diseases*,
https://doi.org/10.1007/978-3-030-67727-5_55

ter, two male puberty occurs. Aromatase deficiency is a cause of nonadrenal 46, XX DSD.

The end-organ resistance syndromes, which are still an exclusion diagnosis, represent a further challenge for future diagnostic and therapeutic applications. The treatment of these defects is based on exogenous administration of the deficient hormones and corrective surgery in intersexuality. Given the rarity of most of these diseases, prenatal diagnosis is possible only in a family at risk. In the case of 21-hydroxylase deficiency, however, advances in prenatal diagnosis allowed in utero treatment. Progress in molecular analysis of steroid biosynthesis and action defects will allow a better prenatal diagnosis and treatment of such diseases.

## Introduction

The biosynthesis of steroid hormones is a fascinating process in which the neutral lipid cholesterol, a normal constituent of lipid bilayers, is transformed via a series of hydroxylation, oxidation, and reduction steps into a vast array of biologically active compounds: mineralocorticoids, glucocorticoids, and sex hormones. The majority of these transformations occur in the adrenal, testis, and ovary, although other tissues, such as the liver, kidney, placenta, brain, and skin, are also quite active.

Steroid hormone action is a complex process that is only recently beginning to be understood. Steroid hormones bind to specific intracellular receptors, which upon dimerization interact with the DNA in the nucleus. As a result, gene activity is modulated and a hormone-specific response occurs (Evans 1988). It is logical that abnormalities in any step of this cascade will interfere with the action of a particular hormone. Defects in the receptor or the post-receptor machinery will lead for the most part to abnormalities of action of one specific hormone. Abnormalities of steroid hormone production, however, can result in more profound and complex effects. A block in the pathway of steroid biosynthesis leads to the lack of hormones downstream and accumulation of the upstream compounds that can activate other members of the steroid receptor family. The consequences of such defects can be schematically categorized in three groups: (1) defects leading to abnormalities of sexual differentiation and saltwater balance, (2) defects leading to abnormalities of saltwater balance, and (3) defects leading to abnormalities of sexual differentiation. Abnormalities of end-organ action of steroid hormones, exemplified by the hormone insensitivity syndromes, can be grouped in a fourth category.

The first group of steroid biosynthesis defects include the so-called congenital adrenal hyperplasia (CAH), a collective name given to a group of disorders characterized by inherited inability of the adrenals to secrete cortisol. The consequent compensatory rise of ACTH production causes hyperplastic growth of the adrenal glands. Blocks of the initial steps of the steroidogenic pathway impair the production of all the three types of steroids, causing abnormalities in the saltwater homeostasis and in sexual differentiation. That is the case in *lipoid adrenal hyperplasia*, where no conversion of cholesterol to any steroid takes place. This rare cause of CAH is characterized by salt loss and male pseudohermaphroditism in XY individuals. In XX subjects, internal and external genitalia are female, and the syndrome cannot clinically be separated from congenital adrenal hypoplasia (Prader and Gurtner 1955). The molecular bases of such a defect have been recently clarified as mutations in the steroidogenic acute response protein (StAR) (Lin et al. 1995). *17α-Hydroxylase deficiency* leads to male pseudohermaphroditism, due to the lack of precursors for testosterone. In XX individuals, there is primary amenorrhea and absent development of estrogenic secondary sexual characteristics. Both sexes display hypertension and hypokalemic alkalosis due to accumulation of mineralocorticoid precursors, which do not need 17α-hydroxylation for their synthesis (Biglieri et al. 1966). Adrenal hyperplasia and glucocorticoid deficiency are less marked than in the other types of CAH, because of the ability of corticosterone of suppressing ACTH. Male patients affected by CAH due to *3β-hydroxysteroid dehydrogenase* deficiency display incomplete prenatal masculinization due to the impaired synthesis of bioactive androgens and salt loss due to lack of mineralocorticoid (Bongiovanni 1962). XX subjects have normal female external genitalia or mild virilization due to the action of the weak androgen DHEA. *21-Hydroxylase deficiency* accounts for most cases of CAH (80–90%, depending on the ethnic group). Clinical consequences of 21-hydroxylase deficiency arise from overproduction of androgens. Affected females with the *classical* 21-hydroxylase deficiency are born with ambiguous genitalia. Postnatally, untreated patients of both sexes manifest rapid somatic growth with accelerated skeletal maturation, early closure of the epiphyses, and short adult stature. Other symptoms include excessive pubic and body hair and decreased fertility. Seventy-five per cent of patients with classic 21-hydroxylase deficiency also have reduced synthesis of aldosterone with salt loss. Patients with *nonclassical* disease are born without symptoms of prenatal androgen exposure. Subsequently, they may remain asymptomatic or may develop signs of androgen excess. Deficiency of 21-hydroxylase is inherited as an autosomal recessive trait, closely linked to the HLA major histocompatibility complex on the short arm of chromosome 6. While classic 21-hydroxylase deficiency is found in about 1 in 14.000 births, nonclassical deficiency is far more frequent, occurring in up to 3% of persons amongst certain ethnic groups (New et al. 1989). Steroid *11β-hydroxylase deficiency*, which is responsible for 10–20% of cases of CAH, produces symptoms of androgen excess similar to those in 21-hydroxylase deficiency. The blocked enzymatic step also results in accumulation of 11-deoxycorticosterone which has mineralocorticoid activity, leading in untreated patients to hypertension (New et al. 1989).

The second group of diseases includes rare defects in the final step in the biosynthesis of mineralocorticoid and glucocorticoid that lead to water-sodium disequilibrium. Adrenal *corticosterone methyl oxidase II deficiency* impairs the synthesis of aldosterone with consequent salt loss in the neonatal period. Some patients, however, become completely asymptomatic later in life. *Glucocorticoid-suppressible hyperaldosteronism* is an autosomal dominant disease characterized by mineralocorticoid hypertension due to an abnormal stimulatory action of ACTH on aldosterone synthesis. This is due to unequal crossing over between the *zona glomerulosa* 11β-hydroxylase (angiotensin II regulated) and the *zona fasciculata* 11β-hydroxylase (ACTH regulated) genes (White and Pascoe 1992). Defects in the inactivation of cortisol, such as *11 β-hydroxysteroid dehydrogenase type II deficiency*, can lead to hypertension with hypokalemia in the absence of elevated levels of mineralocorticoids. The mechanism underlying such phenomenon is the prolonged half-life of cortisol that binds to the relatively unselective mineralocorticoid receptor in the kidney and acts like a mineralocorticoid, causing the so-called apparent mineralocorticoid excess syndrome (New 1994). The disorder in which cortisone is overproduced is called *cortisone reductase deficiency* (CRD). CRD (previously known as apparent cortisone reductase deficiency, AERD) is a disorder in which there is a failure to regenerate the active glucocorticoid cortisol (F) from cortisone (E) via the enzyme 11β-hydroxysteroid dehydrogenase (11β-HSD1), encoded by the *HSD11B1* gene. This disease is caused by an increased metabolic rate for cortisol at the expense of ACTH-mediated androgen excess, without any clinical symptoms of hypercortisolism (Biason-Lauber et al. 2000). The cortisol-regenerating reductase activity of 11β-HSD1 is critically dependent upon the provision of reduced nicotinamide adenine dinucleotide phosphate (NADPH) in the endoplasmic reticulum lumen and is provided by the enzyme hexose-6-phosphate dehydrogenase (H6PDH, encoded by the *H6PD* gene). CRD has been shown to demonstrate a triallelic digenic pattern of inheritance involving mutations in the *HSD11B1* and *H6PD* genes (Draper et al. 2003).

The third group is characterized by deficiencies of enzymes responsible for the final steps of sex hormone synthesis, such as *17,20-lyase, 17 β-hydroxysteroid dehydrogenase* (17β-HSD), *5α-reductase, and aromatase*. Deficient activity of 17,20-lyase, 17β-HSD, and 5α-reductase enzymes leads to male pseudohermaphroditism with varying genital ambiguity in XY individuals. In XX individual, the genitalia are generally normal. In 17,20-lyase (or 17,20-desmolase) deficiency, there is no male or female pubertal development. Cortisol is normal, and there is no hypertension. The deficient enzyme is the same as in 17α-hydroxylase deficiency, and it is unknown why the defect manifests itself as 17α-hydroxylase in some and as 17,20-lyase deficiency in other families. Possibly, estrogen replacement induces a conversion to 17α-hydroxylase deficiency (Zachmann et al. 1982). In 17β-HSD deficiency, there is some male pubertal development in XY individuals due to androstenedione and often gynecomastia due to estrone. In XX individuals, there is mild virilization and insufficient development of estrogenic sexual characteristics. In 5α-reductase deficiency, male puberty is present in XY subjects because testosterone is sufficient, and dihydrotestosterone (DHT) is not necessary for expression of male sexual secondary characteristics. In XX individuals, there are no symptoms. Interestingly, at the time of expected puberty, the patients affected by these deficiencies display some degree of virilization. Particularly high is the incidence of 5α-reductase deficiency in the Dominican Republic (Imperato-McGinley et al. 1986). Patients of both sexes affected by *aromatase deficiency* show a delayed somatic development and slower skeletal maturation, with consequent tall adult stature. Female patients affected by aromatase deficiency display various degrees of genital ambiguity, due to the lack of prenatal exposure to estrogens, and signs of hyperandrogenism, such as acne (Conte et al. 1994).

In the fourth class are grouped defects in the action of steroid hormones due to receptor defects. Androgens exert their effects in mediating the development of normal male phenotype via a single receptor protein, the androgen receptor (AR), which is encoded on the X chromosome. Abnormalities that alter the function of this receptor result in a range of abnormalities of male phenotypic development, called *complete and partial androgen insensitivity syndrome* (CAIS and PAIS, respectively). These phenotypes range from normal female (female habitus, normal female breast development, absent pubic and axillary hair, female external genitalia, no internal genital organs, and undescended testes) to those that are characterized by only minor degrees of undervirilization and/or infertility (McPhaul and Griffin 1999).

In patients, loss-of-function mutations in estrogen receptor alpha (or estrogen receptor 1, ESR1) cause *estrogen resistance 1* characterized by osteoporosis, delayed bone age and continuous growth in adulthood, high estrogen levels in both sexes, delayed puberty with no breast development, infantile uteri, primary amenorrhea, and multiple ovarian cysts in women (Smith et al. 1994; Bernard et al. 2017; Quaynor et al. 2013). In addition, the first male patient displayed insulin resistance and glucose intolerance. Genetic abnormalities in the estrogen receptor beta (ESR2, *estrogen resistance 2*) have been reported in genetically male patients (46, XY) with differences of sex development and gonadal dysgenesis, demonstrating an unexpected role for ESR2 in testis formation (Baetens et al. 2018). More recently, we described a female patient (46, XX) with lack of breast development, infantile uterus, primary amenorrhea, and severe osteoporosis but normal bone age and complete primary early-onset ovarian failure (Lang-Muritano et al.

2018). This case suggested that ESR2 is necessary for early human ovarian development and/or maintenance and that ESR1 is not sufficient to support gonadal function.

Although rare, the estrogen resistance was of crucial importance for the understanding of skeletal physiology, since it demonstrated that estrogen is important for bone maturation and mineralization in men as well as in women.

Progesterone prepares the endometrium for blastocyst implantation and allows maintenance of pregnancy. Complete end-organ resistance to progesterone would be incompatible with reproductive competence in females. Males would not be expected to be affected since progesterone has no known function in men. Failure of the uterus to respond to progesterone would lead to the development of a "constantly proliferative" endometrium incompatible with blastocyst implantation. *Partial resistance to progesterone*, on the other hand, would be expected to be associated with various degrees of incomplete maturation of the endometrium, expressed clinically as infertility or early abortions. The syndrome presents with the clinical and histologic picture of a luteal phase defect in which the life span of the corpus luteum and the plasma progesterone concentrations are normal or slightly elevated (Chrousos et al. 1986).

*Glucocorticoid resistance* is characterized by high levels of cortisol (without stigmata of Cushing syndrome), resistance of the hypothalamic-pituitary-adrenal axis to dexamethasone, and an affinity defect of the glucocorticoid receptor. Some of the affected patients presented with hypertension and hypokalemia due to pathological activation of the mineralocorticoid receptor by cortisol (Lipsett et al. 1986).

*Pseudohypoaldosteronism (type I)* is characterized by salt wasting in infancy that is responsive to supplementary sodium but not to mineralocorticoids. Marked aldosterone excess is present in all reported cases and the renin level is increased in most. Salt supplementation often can be discontinued after infancy without adverse effects, even though aldosterone excess is persistent. Sweat and salivary glands and colonic mucosa are unresponsive to mineralocorticoids as is the distal renal tubule. The basic defect in this disease resides in the mineralocorticoid receptor NR3C2 (Geller et al. 1998).

More recently, two new defects in steroid synthesis were identified. An intriguing case is that of *P450 oxidoreductase* (POR) *deficiency*. Cytochrome P450 oxidoreductase is a flavoprotein that donates electrons to all microsomal P450 enzymes, including the steroidogenic enzymes P450c17, P450c21, and CYP51A1 (Miller 1986). In 1985, a clinical report described a patient with genital ambiguity and an abnormal urinary steroid profile suggesting partial combined deficiencies of what was then thought to be three distinct steroidogenic enzymes: 17α-hydroxylase, 17,20-lyase, and 21-hydroxylase (Peterson et al. 1985). Affected girls are born with ambiguous genitalia, indicating intrauterine androgen excess. After birth, however, virilization does not progress, and amounts of circulating androgens are low or normal. Conversely, affected boys are sometimes born undermasculinized. The majority but not all of patients described to date with POR deficiency also had a pattern of skeletal malformations termed Antley-Bixler syndrome (ABS). This disorder is characterized by craniosynostosis (premature fusion of bones of the skull), radio-ulnar or radio-humeral synostosis, bowed femora, and other more variable skeletal disorders (Antley and Bixler 1975; Crisponi et al. 1997). Findings of biochemical investigations of urinary steroid excretion in affected patients have shown accumulation of steroid metabolites, indicating impaired C17 and C21 hydroxylation, suggesting concurrent partial deficiencies of the two steroidogenic enzymes, P450C17 and P450C21. As these steroidogenic enzyme activities were known to be catalyzed by type II cytochrome P450 enzymes, it was suggested that this patient had a disorder in the electron donor for these enzymes, P450 oxidoreductase (Miller 1986). This fascinating idea remained dormant until Fluck first reported four cases of POR deficiency (Fluck et al. 2004). Since that time, about 50 additional patients have been reported (for review, see (Fluck et al. 2008; Scott and Miller 2008).

The other defect concerns the so-called backdoor pathway of fetal androgen synthesis. Following development of the fetal bipotential gonad into a testis, male genital differentiation requires testicular androgens. Fetal Leydig cells produce testosterone that is converted to dihydrotestosterone in genital skin, resulting in labioscrotal fusion. An alternative "backdoor" pathway of dihydrotestosterone synthesis that bypasses testosterone has been described in marsupials, but its relevance to human biology has been uncertain. The classic and backdoor pathways share many enzymes, but a 3α-reductase, AKR1C2, is unique to the backdoor pathway (Fig. 55.1). Human *AKR1C2* mutations cause disordered sexual differentiation, establishing that both pathways are required for normal human male genital development. These observations show that fetal dihydrotestosterone acts both as hormonally and as a paracrine factor, substantially revising the classic paradigm for fetal male sexual development (Fluck et al. 2011).

Defects of the ACTH receptor (M2CR) or of its accessory proteins MRAPs cause *familial glucocorticoid deficiency*. Most of these mutations lead to the production of a MRAP protein that cannot interact with the ACTH receptor and so is unable to transport it out of the ER to the cell membrane. As a result, the ACTH receptor is not at the cell surface where it is needed to bind to ACTH. Without the binding of the ACTH receptor to its hormone, there is no signal to trigger the adrenal glands to produce glucocorticoids. This condition is characterized by potentially life-threatening low blood sugar (hypoglycemia), recurrent infections, and skin coloring darker than that of other family members (hyperpigmentation) (reviewed in Novoselova et al. 2018). These last two conditions will not be discussed in details.

## Nomenclature

| No. | Disorder name | Alternative name | Abbreviation | Gene symbol | Chromosomal localization | Protein | OMIM no. |
|---|---|---|---|---|---|---|---|
| 55.1 | Lipoid congenital adrenal hyperplasia | Steroidogenic acute response protein deficiency | LCAH, StAR def | *STAR* | 8p11.2 | Steroidogenic acute response protein | 600617 |
| 55.2 | Side-chain cleavage deficiency | | SCC def | *CYP11A1* | 15q24.1 | P450scc | 613743 |
| 55.3 | 17α-hydroxylase deficiency | | | *CYP17A1* | 10q24–25 | P450c17 | 609300 |
| 55.4 | 3β-Hydroxysteroid dehydrogenase type II deficiency | | | *HSD3B2* | 1p12 | 3 | 613890 |
| 55.5 | 21-hydroxylase deficiency | Congenital adrenal hyperplasia | CAH/21OHD | *CYP21A2* | 6p21.3 | P450c21 | 613815 |
| 55.6 | 11β-hydroxylase type I deficiency | Congenital adrenal hyperplasia | CAH/11BOHD | *CYP11B1* | 8q24.3 | P450c11 | 610613 |
| 55.7 | Corticosterone methyl oxidase II deficiency | | CMO def | *CYP11B2* | 8q21–22 | CMO | 610600 |
| 55.8 | Glucocorticoid remediable hyperaldosteronism | 11b-hydroxylase 1/2 | GRA | | 8q21–22 | | 610613 |
| 55.9 | Apparent mineralocorticoid excess | 11b-Hydrosteroiddehydrogenase type II deficiency | AME | *HSD11B2* | 16q22 | 11βHSD2 | 614232 |
| 55.10 | Cortisone reductase deficiency | 11b-Hydrosteroiddehydrogenase type I/hexose-6-phosphate dehydrogenase deficiency | CRD | *HSD11B1/H6PD* | 1p36/1q32-q41 | 11βHSD1/H6PD | 600713 |
| 55.11 | 17,20-Lyase deficiency | 17,20-Desmolase deficiency | | | 10q24–25 | P450c17 | 609300 |
| 55.12 | 17β-Hydroxysteroid dehydrogenase type III deficiency | | | *HSD17B3* | 9q22 | 17βHSD3 | 605573 |
| 55.13 | 5α-reductase type II deficiency | Pseudovaginal perineoscrotal hypospadia | | *SRD5A2* | 2p23 | 5α-reductase | 607306 |
| 55.14 | Aromatase deficiency | | | *CYP19A1* | 15q21.1 | P450Aro | 613546 |
| 55.15 | P450 oxidoreductase deficiency | Antley-Bixler syndrome with DSD | POR | *POR* | 7q11.2 | | 613571 |
| 55.16 | Androgen insensitivity syndrome | Testicular feminization | AIS | *AR* | Xq11-q12 | Androgen receptor | 313700 |
| 55.17 | Estrogen resistance 1 | Estrogen receptor alpha defect | | *ESR1* | 6q25.1 | Estrogen receptor 1 | 133430 |
| 55.18 | Estrogen resistance 2 | Estrogen receptor beta defect | | *ESR2* | 14q23.2-q23.3 | Estrogen receptor 2 | 618187 |
| 55.19 | Progesterone resistance | Progesterone receptor defect, pseudocorpus luteum deficiency | | *PGR* | 11q22.1 | Progesterone receptor/NR3C3 | 607311 |
| 55.20 | Glucocorticoid resistance | | | *NR3C1* | 5q31.3 | Glucocorticoid receptor | 138040 |
| 55.21 | Pseudohypoaldosteronism type I | | PHAI | *NR3C2* | 4q31.1 | Mineralocorticoid receptor | 600983 |
| 55.22 | 3α-Hydroxysteroid dehydrogenase deficiency | Aldo-keto reductase 2 deficiency, backdoor pathway defect | AKR1C | *AKR1C2/4* | 10p15.1 | AKR1C2 | 600450 |
| 55.23 | ACTH resistance | Familiar glucocorticoid deficiency | MC2R | *MC2R/MRAP* | 18p11.21/21q22.11 | Melanocortin 2 receptor/Melanocortin 2 receptor accessory protein | 607397/609196 |

## Metabolic Pathways

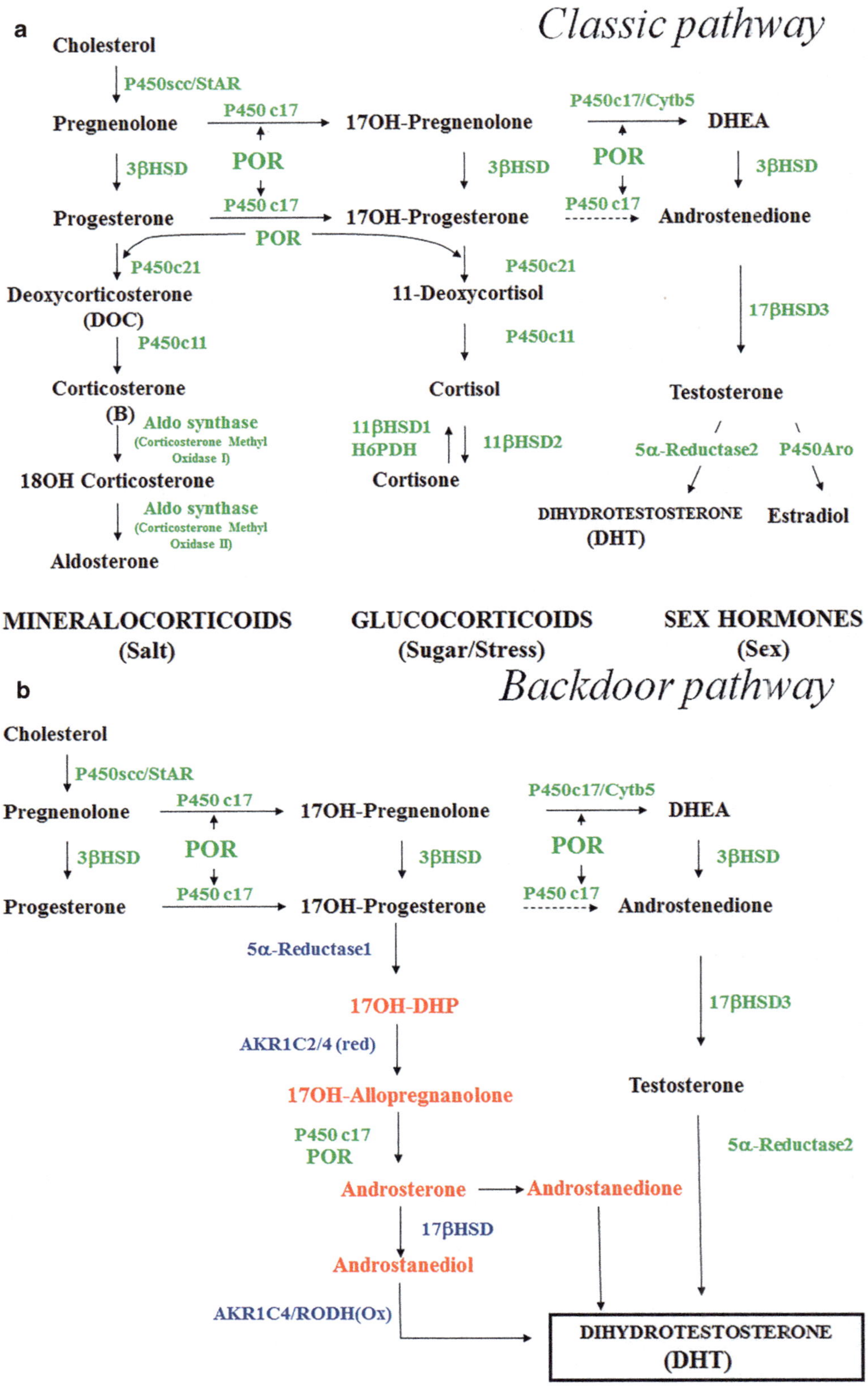


**Fig. 55.1** (**a**) Classic steroidogenesis pathway. (**b**) Backdoor pathway of dihydrotestosterone (DHT) that uses substrates other than testosterone

## Signs and Symptoms

**Table 55.1** Lipoid adrenal hyperplasia (StAR deficiency)

| System | Symptom | Neonatal | Infancy | Childhood | Adolescence | Adulthood |
|---|---|---|---|---|---|---|
| Characteristic clinical findings | Dehydration | +++ | ++ | ++ | + | + |
| | Female external genitalia regardless of genetic sex | +++ | +++ | +++ | +++ | +++ |
| Endocrine | Adrenal hyperplasia | +++ | +++ | +++ | +++ | +++ |
| | Adrenal insufficiency | +++ | +++ | +++ | +++ | ++ |
| | Delayed puberty | n.a. | n.a. | n.a. | +++ | +++ |
| Genitourinary | Ambiguous or female genitalia in 46, XY | +++ | +++ | +++ | +++ | +++ |
| | Cryptorchidism | +++ | +++ | +++ | +++ | +++ |
| Routine laboratory | Alkalosis | ++ | ++ | + | + | + |
| | Potassium (P) | ↑↑↑ | ↑↑↑ | ↑↑ | ↑↑ | ↑↑ |
| | Sodium (P) | ↓↓↓ | ↓↓↓ | ↓↓ | ↓-n | ↓-n |
| Special laboratory | ACTH (P) | ↑↑ | ↑↑↑ | ↑↑↑ | ↑↑ | ↑↑ |
| | Steroids (U, P) | ↓↓↓ | ↓↓↓ | ↓↓ | ↓-n | ↓-n |

**Table 55.2** Cholesterol side-chain cleavage deficiency

| System | Symptom | Neonatal | Infancy | Childhood | Adolescence | Adulthood |
|---|---|---|---|---|---|---|
| Characteristic clinical findings | Ambiguous genitalia in 46, XY | ++ | ++ | ++ | ++ | ++ |
| Endocrine | Adrenal hyperplasia | n | n | n | n | n |
| | Adrenal insufficiency | +++ or +/− | ++ or +/− | ++ or +/− | + or +/− | + or +/− |
| Genitourinary | Cryptorchidism | +++ | +++ | +++ if not corrected | +++ if not corrected | +++ if not corrected |
| Routine laboratory | Sodium (P) | ↓↓ | ↓↓ | ↓ | ↓-n | ↓-n |
| | Potassium (P) | ↑↑ | ↑↑ | ↑ | n-↑ | n-↑ |

**Table 55.3** 17-Alpha-hydroxylase deficiency

| System | Symptom | Neonatal | Infancy | Childhood | Adolescence | Adulthood |
|---|---|---|---|---|---|---|
| Characteristic clinical findings | Episodic vomiting | ± | ± | + | ++ | +++ |
| | Female external genitalia regardless of genetic sex | +++ | +++ | +++ | +++ | +++ |
| | Headache | ± | ± | + | ++ | +++ |
| | Lack of pubertal sex development | n.a. | n.a. | n.a. | +++ | +++ |
| Cardiovascular | Hypertension | - | ± | + | ++ | +++ |
| Endocrine | Adrenal hyperplasia | + | + | + | + | + |
| | Adrenal insufficiency | − | − | − | − | − |
| | Delayed puberty | n.a. | n.a. | n.a. | +++ | +++ |
| Genitourinary | Cryptorchidism | +++ | +++ | +++ | +++ | +++ |
| Reproductive | Ovarian cysts in 46,XX | | | ± | ++ | +++ |
| Routine laboratory | Alkalosis | + | + | + | ++ | ++ |
| | Potassium (P) | ↓ | ↓ | ↓ | ↓↓ | ↓↓ |
| | Sodium (P) | (↑) | (↑) | ↑ | ↑↑ | ↑↑ |
| Special laboratory | ACTH (P) | (↑) | (↑) | (↑) | n | n |
| | Cortisol, sex hormones, aldosterone (P) | ↓↓ | ↓↓ | ↓↓ | ↓↓ | ↓↓ |
| | Deoxycorticosterone, corticosterone (U, P) | ↑↑↑ | ↑↑↑ | ↑↑↑ | ↑↑↑ | ↑↑↑ |
| | Progesterone (P) | ↑↑ | ↑↑ | ↑↑↑ | ↑↑↑ | ↑↑↑ |

**Table 55.4** 3-Beta-hydroxysteroid dehydrogenase type II deficiency

| System | Symptom | Neonatal | Infancy | Childhood | Adolescence | Adulthood |
|---|---|---|---|---|---|---|
| Characteristic clinical findings | Ambiguous genitalia (XY and XX) | +++ | +++ | +++ | +++ | +++ |
| | Dehydration | +++ | ++ | ++ | + | + |
| | Postnatal virilization (XX) | + | ++ | ++ | ++ | ++ |
| Endocrine | Adrenal hyperplasia | ++ | ++ | ++ | + | + |
| | Adrenal insufficiency | +++ | +++ | ++ | ++ | ++ |
| Genitourinary | Clitoromegaly | ++ | ++ | ++ | +++ | +++ |
| | Cryptorchidism | ++ | ++ | ++ | ++ | ++ |
| Routine laboratory | Sodium (P) | ↓↓↓ | ↓↓↓ | ↓↓ | ↓↓ | ↓ |
| | Potassium (P) | ↑↑ | ↑↑ | ↑↑ | ↑↑ | ↑↑ |
| Special laboratory | 17-OH-Pregnenolone (P) | ↑↑ | ↑↑ | ↑↑ | ↑↑↑ | ↑↑↑ |
| | ACTH (P) | ↑↑↑ | ↑↑↑ | ↑↑↑ | ↑↑↑ | ↑↑↑ |
| | Cortisol, aldosterone, sex hormones (P) | ↓↓ | ↓↓ | ↓↓ | ↓↓↓ | ↓↓↓ |
| | DHEA sulfate (P) | ↑↑ | ↑↑ | ↑↑ | ↑↑↑ | ↑↑↑ |

**Table 55.5** 21-Hydroxylase deficiency

| System | Symptom | Neonatal | Infancy | Childhood | Adolescence | Adulthood |
|---|---|---|---|---|---|---|
| Characteristic clinical findings | Advanced somatic development | ± | ± | ++ | +++ | n.a. |
| | Dehydration | +++ | ++ | + | ± | ± |
| | Short stature | n.a. | n.a. | n.a. | ++ | +++ |
| | Various degrees of genital ambiguity (Prader III–V) in XX | +++ | +++ | ++ | ++ | ++ |
| Endocrine | Adrenal hyperplasia | + | ++ | +++ | +++ | +++ |
| | Adrenal insufficiency | +++ | +++ | +++ | ++ | ++ |
| | Virilization (e.g., hirsutism) | n.a. | + | ++ | +++ | +++ |
| Reproductive | Decreased fertility | n.a. | n.a. | n.a. | n.a. | n.a. |
| Other | Accelerated growth | n.a. | n.a. | +++ | + | n.a. |
| | Dehydration | +++ | +++ | ++ | ++ only in stress | ++ only in stress |
| Routine laboratory | Sodium (P) | ↓↓↓ | ↓↓↓ | ↓↓↓ | ↓↓ | ↓↓ |
| | Potassium (P) | ↑↑↑ | ↑↑↑ | ↑↑↑ | ↑↑ | ↑↑ |
| Special laboratory | 17-OH-progesterone (P) | ↑↑↑ | ↑↑↑ | ↑↑↑ | ↑↑↑ | ↑↑↑ |
| | ACTH (P) | ↑↑↑ | ↑↑↑ | ↑↑↑ | ↑↑↑ | ↑↑↑ |
| | Aldosterone (P) | ↓ | ↓↓ | ↓↓ | ↓ | ↓ |
| | Androgens (DHEAS, androstenedione, testosterone) (P) | ↑↑↑ | ↑↑↑ | ↑↑↑ | ↑↑↑ | ↑↑↑ |
| | Cortisol (P) | ↓-n | ↓-n | ↓-n | n | n |
| | Plasma renin activity or renin (P) | ↑↑ | ↑↑ | ↑↑ | ↑↑ | ↑↑ |
| | Progesterone, 17OH-progesterone, and androgen metabolites (U) | ↑↑ | ↑↑↑ | ↑↑↑ | ↑↑↑ | ↑↑↑ |

**Table 55.6** 11-Beta-hydroxylase type I deficiency

| System | Symptom | Neonatal | Infancy | Childhood | Adolescence | Adulthood |
|---|---|---|---|---|---|---|
| Characteristic clinical findings | Short stature | – | – | – | ± | +++ |
| | Advanced somatic development | ± | ± | ++ | +++ | n.a. |
| | Hypertension | ± | ± | + | ++ | +++ |
| | Headache | ± | ± | + | ++ | ++ |
| | Episodic vomiting | ± | ± | + | ++ | ++ |
| | Various degrees of genital ambiguity (Prader III–V) in XX | +++ | +++ | +++ | +++ | +++ |
| Endocrine | Adrenal hyperplasia | ++ | ++ | ++ | ++ | ++ |
| | Adrenal insufficiency | – | – | – | – | – |
| Genitourinary | Various degrees (Prader III–V) of genital ambiguity in 46, XX | ++ | ++ | ++ | ++ | ++ |
| Reproductive | Decreased fertility | n.a. | n.a. | n.a. | + | ++ |
| Other | Short stature | n.a. | n.a. | ± | ++ | ++ |
| | Accelerated growth | – | ± | ++ | ++ | n.a. |
| Routine laboratory | Potassium (P) | ↓↓ | ↓↓ | ↓ | ↓↓ | ↓↓ |
| | Sodium (P) | ↑ | ↑↑ | ↑↑ | ↑↑ | ↑↑ |
| Special laboratory | 17-OH-progesterone (P) | ↑ | ↑ | ↑ | ↑ | ↑ |
| | ACTH (P) | ↑↑ | ↑↑ | ↑↑ | ↑↑ | ↑↑ |
| | Deoxycorticosterone, 11-deoxycortisol (compound S), androgens (P) | ↑↑ | ↑↑ | ↑↑↑ | ↑↑↑ | ↑↑↑ |

**Table 55.7** Corticosterone methyl oxidase deficiency

| System | Symptom | Neonatal | Infancy | Childhood | Adolescence | Adulthood |
|---|---|---|---|---|---|---|
| Characteristic clinical findings | Dehydration | ++ | ++ | ± | – | – |
| | Failure to thrive | ++ | ++ | ± | – | – |
| Routine laboratory | Potassium (P) | ↑↑ | ↑ | n-↑ | n | n |
| | Sodium (P) | ↓↓ | ↓ | ↓-n | n | n |
| Special laboratory | 18-Oxocorticosterone | ↑↑ | ↑↑ | n-↑ | n | n |
| | Aldosterone (P) | ↓↓ | ↓↓ | ↓-n | n | n |

**Table 55.8** Glucocorticoid-suppressible hyperaldosteronism

| System | Symptom | Neonatal | Infancy | Childhood | Adolescence | Adulthood |
|---|---|---|---|---|---|---|
| Characteristic clinical findings | Headache | | ± | ++ | ++ | +++ |
| | Hypertension | ± | ± | + | ++ | +++ |
| Routine laboratory | Potassium (P) | ↓ | ↓↓ | ↓↓ | ↓↓ | ↓↓ |
| Special laboratory | 18-Oxocortisol (U) | | ↑ | ↑↑ | ↑↑ | ↑↑ |
| | Aldosterone (P) | | ↑ | ↑↑ | ↑↑ | ↑↑ |
| | Aldosterone after dexamethasone | | n | n | n | n |

**Table 55.9** Apparent mineralocorticoid excess

| System | Symptom | Neonatal | Infancy | Childhood | Adolescence | Adulthood |
|---|---|---|---|---|---|---|
| Characteristic clinical findings | Headache | | ± | + | ++ | ++ |
| | Hypertension | ± | ± | + | ++ | +++ |
| Routine laboratory | Potassium (P) | ↓ | ↓↓ | ↓↓ | ↓↓ | ↓↓ |
| | Sodium (P) | ↑ | n-↑ | n-↑ | n-↑ | n-↑ |
| Special laboratory | Tetrahydrocortisol/tetrahydrocortisone ratio (U) | ↓↓ | ↓↓ | ↓↓ | ↓↓ | ↓↓ |

**Table 55.10** Cortisone reductase deficiency

| System | Symptom | Neonatal | Infancy | Childhood | Adolescence | Adulthood |
|---|---|---|---|---|---|---|
| Characteristic clinical findings | Signs of androgen excess in women (e.g., hirsutism) | | | | +++ | +++ |
| Endocrine | Adrenal hyperplasia | ± | ± | ± | + | + |
| | Precocious pseudopuberty (46,XY) | n.a | n.a. | + | ++ | n.a. |
| | Virilization (e.g., hirsutism) | | | | ++ | +++ |
| Reproductive | Polycystic ovaries (PCOS) | n.a. | n.a. | n.a. | ++ | +++ |
| Special laboratory | ACTH (P) | | n-↑ | ↑ | ↑↑ | ↑↑ |
| | Adrenal androgens (DHEAS; androstenedione) (P) | n.a. | n.a. | ↑ | ↑↑↑ | ↑↑↑ |
| | Tetrahydrocortisol/tetrahydrocortisone ratio (U) | | ↓ | ↓ | ↓↓ | ↓↓ |

**Table 55.11** 17,20-Lyase deficiency

| System | Symptom | Neonatal | Infancy | Childhood | Adolescence | Adulthood |
|---|---|---|---|---|---|---|
| Characteristic clinical findings | Ambiguous genitalia in 46, XY | +++ | +++ | +++ | +++ | +++ |
| Endocrine | Adrenal hyperplasia | n | n | n | n | n |
| Genitourinary | Cryptorchidism | + | + | + | + | + |
| Special laboratory | Sex hormones | n.a. | n.a. | ↓↓ | ↓↓ | ↓↓↓ |
| | Cortisol, aldosterone (P) | n | n | n | ↓-n under HRT | ↓-n under HRT |
| | 17-OH-progesterone (P) | ↑ | ↑ | ↑ | n-↑ | n-↑ |
| | Progesterone (P) | n | n | n | n | n |

**Table 55.12** 17-Beta-hydroxysteroid dehydrogenase III deficiency

| System | Symptom | Neonatal | Infancy | Childhood | Adolescence | Adulthood |
|---|---|---|---|---|---|---|
| Characteristic clinical findings | Cryptorchidism | +++ | ++ | ++ | ++ | + |
| | Female to ambiguous genitalia in XY | +++ | +++ | +++ | +++ | +++ |
| | Gynecomastia at puberty | | | – | ++ | + |
| Special laboratory | Androstenedione (P) | n-↑ | n-↑ | n-↑ | n-↑ | n-↑ |
| | Androstenedione/testosterone ratio | ↑↑ | ↑↑ | ↑↑ | ↑↑ | ↑↑ |
| | Gonadotropins (FSH, LH) (P) | n-↑ | n-↑ | ↑ | ↑↑ | ↑↑↑ |
| | Testosterone (P) | ↓↓ | ↓↓ | ↓↓ | ↓↓↓ | ↓↓↓ |

**Table 55.13** 5-Alpha-reductase type II deficiency

| System | Symptom | Neonatal | Infancy | Childhood | Adolescence | Adulthood |
|---|---|---|---|---|---|---|
| Characteristic clinical findings | Cryptorchidism | +++ | +++ | +++ | ++ | ++ |
| | Female to ambiguous genitalia in XY | +++ | +++ | +++ | ++ | ++ |
| | Virilization | | | | +++ | +++ |
| Endocrine | Virilization at puberty | n.a. | n.a. | n.a. | +++ | ++ |
| Special laboratory | 5-alpha-/5-beta-reduced metabolites ratio (U) | ↓↓ | ↓↓ | ↓↓ | ↓↓ | ↓↓ |
| | Dihydrotestosterone (DHT) (P) | ↓↓ | Usually not measurable without hCG stimulation | Usually not measurable without hCG stimulation | ↓↓↓ | ↓↓↓ |
| | T/DHT ratio | ↑↑ | n.m. | n.m. | ↑↑ | ↑↑ |
| | Testosterone (P) | n | n | n | n-↑ | n-↑ |

**Table 55.14** Aromatase deficiency

| System | Symptom | Neonatal | Infancy | Childhood | Adolescence | Adulthood |
|---|---|---|---|---|---|---|
| Characteristic clinical findings | Delayed somatic development | | | + | ++ | +++ |
| | Obesity (male) | | | | ++ | +++ |
| | Tall stature | n.a. | n.a. | | ++ | +++ |
| | Various degrees of genital ambiguity (Prader III–V) in XX | +++ | +++ | +++ | +++ | +++ |
| Endocrine | Virilization (e.g., hirsutism) | | | ± | ++ | ++ |
| Reproductive | Ovarian cysts in 46, XX | | | ± | ++ | ++ |
| Other | Maternal virilization during pregnancy | ++ | ++ | ++ | ++ | ++ |
| Special laboratory | Gonadotropins (FSH, LH) (P) | ↑ | n.a. | n.a. | ↑↑ | ↑↑↑ |

**Table 55.15** P450 oxidoreductase deficiency

| System | Symptom | Neonatal | Infancy | Childhood | Adolescence | Adulthood |
|---|---|---|---|---|---|---|
| Characteristic clinical findings | Ambiguous genitalia (XY and XX) | +++ | ++ | ++ | ++ | ++ |
| | Signs of androgen excess | ++ | ± | | | |
| | Skeletal abnormalities | + | + | + | + | + |
| Genitourinary | Ambiguous or female genitalia in 46, XY | +++ | +++ | +++ | +++ | +++ |
| | Various degrees (Prader III–V) of genital ambiguity in 46, XX | +++ | +++ | +++ | +++ | ++ |
| Musculoskeletal | Antley-Bixler syndrome | ++ | ++ | ++ | ++ | ++ |
| Special laboratory | Androgens (DHEAS, androstenedione, testosterone) (P) | ↑↑ | ↓-n | ↓-n | ↓-n | ↓-n |
| | 17-OH-progesterone (P) | ↑↑ | n | n | n | n |

**Table 55.16** Androgen insensitivity syndrome

| System | Symptom | Neonatal | Infancy | Childhood | Adolescence | Adulthood |
|---|---|---|---|---|---|---|
| Characteristic clinical findings | Absent pubic and axillary hair | n.a. | n.a. | +++ | +++ | +++ |
| | Absent uterus | +++ | +++ | +++ | +++ | +++ |
| | Genetic male with female or ambiguous external genitalia | +++ | +++ | +++ | +++ | +++ |
| Genitourinary | Cryptorchidism | +++ | +++ | +++ | +++ | +++ |
| Special laboratory | Androgens (DHEAS, androstenedione, testosterone) (P) | n-↑ | n | n | n for 46, XY | n for 46, XY |
| | Anti-Mullerian hormone (AMH) (P) | n for 46, XY | n for 46, XY | n for 46, XY | n for 46, XY | n for 46, XY |
| | Dihydrotestosterone (DHT) (P) | n | n | n | n | n |
| | Gonadotropins (FSH, LH) (P) | n-↑ | n | n | n-↑ | n-↑ |

**Table 55.17** Estrogen resistance 1

| System | Symptom | Neonatal | Infancy | Childhood | Adolescence | Adulthood |
|---|---|---|---|---|---|---|
| Characteristic clinical findings | Incomplete epiphyseal closure | n.a. | n.a. | n.a. | +++ | +++ |
| | Tall stature | n.a. | n.a. | + | ++ | ++ |
| Endocrine | Glucose tolerance | n | n | n | ↓ | ↓↓ |
| Genitourinary | Genitalia | n | n | n | n | n |
| Other | Delayed somatic development (delayed bone age) | n.a. | n.a. | + | ++ | +++ |
| Special laboratory | Androgens (DHEAS, androstenedione, testosterone) (P) | n | n | n | n | n |
| | Estradiol (P) | (↑) | (↑) | (↑) | ↑↑ | ↑↑ |
| | Gonadotropins (FSH, LH) (P) | (↑) | (↑) | ↑ | ↑↑ | ↑↑↑ |

**Table 55.18** Estrogen resistance 2 (ESR2)

| System | Symptom | Neonatal | Infancy | Childhood | Adolescence | Adulthood |
|---|---|---|---|---|---|---|
| Characteristic clinical findings | Complete epipheseal closure | n.a. | n.a. | n.a. | +++ | +++ |
| | Tall stature | n.a. | n.a. | No | No | No |
| Endocrine | Glucose tolerance | n | n | n | n | n |
| Genitourinary | Genitalia | n | n | n | n | n |
| | Infantile uterus | n.a. | n.a. | n.a. | 0 | |
| Other | Bone age | n | n | n | n | n |
| | Growth and stature | n.a. | n.a. | n | n | n |
| Special laboratory | Androgens (DHEAS, androstenedione, testosterone) (P) | n | n | n | n | n |
| | Estradiol (P) | n.a. | n.a. | n.a. | ↓↓↓ | ↓↓↓ |
| | Gonadotropins (FSH, LH) (P) | (↑) | (↑) | ↑ | ↑-n | Unknown |

**Table 55.19** Progesterone resistance

| System | Symptom | Neonatal | Infancy | Childhood | Adolescence | Adulthood |
|---|---|---|---|---|---|---|
| Characteristic clinical findings | Female infertility | n.a. | n.a. | n.a. | n.a. | +++ |
| Reproductive | Endometrium | n.a. | n.a. | n.a. | Immature | Immature |
| Special laboratory | Progesterone (P) | n.a. | n.a. | n.a. | Inadequately low in luteal phase | Inadequately low in luteal phase |

**Table 55.20** Glucocorticoid resistance

| System | Symptom | Neonatal | Infancy | Childhood | Adolescence | Adulthood |
|---|---|---|---|---|---|---|
| Characteristic clinical findings | Cushing's stigmata | – | – | – | – | – |
| | Hypertension | | | ± | ++ | +++ |
| | Hypokalemic alkalosis | | | ± | ++ | +++ |
| Routine laboratory | Alkalosis | ± | ± | + | ++ | ++ |
| | Potassium (P) | n | n | ↓-n | ↓↓ | ↓↓ |
| Special laboratory | ACTH (P) | | | | n-↑ | n-↑ |
| | Cortisol (P) | n | n | n | ↑ | ↑ |
| | Cortisol (U) | n | n | n | ↑↑ | ↑↑ |
| | Cortisol after dexamethasone suppression | | | | Unresponsive (no suppression) | Unresponsive (no suppression) |

**Table 55.21** Pseudohypoaldosteronism

| System | Symptom | Neonatal | Infancy | Childhood | Adolescence | Adulthood |
|---|---|---|---|---|---|---|
| Characteristic clinical findings | Renal salt loss | ± | ± | + | ++ | ++ |
| Routine laboratory | Potassium (P) | ↑ | ↑ | ↑ | ↑ | ↑ |
| | Sodium (P) | ↓↓ | ↓↓ | ↓ | ↓ | ↓ |
| Special laboratory | Aldosterone (P) | ↑ | ↑↑ | ↑↑ | ↑ | ↑ |
| | Plasma renin activity or renin (P) | ↑ | ↑ | ↑ | ↑ | ↑ |

**Table 55.22** AKR1C2/4 deficiency

| System | Symptom | Neonatal | Infancy | Childhood | Adolescence | Adulthood |
|---|---|---|---|---|---|---|
| Characteristic clinical findings | Cryptorchidism | +++ | +++ | +++ | ++ | ++ |
| | Female to ambiguous genitalia in XY | +++ | +++ | +++ | ++ | ++ |
| | Virilization | | | | +++ | +++ |
| Endocrine | Virilization at puberty (XY) | n.a. | n.a. | n.a. | Probable | n.a. |
| Special laboratory | Androsterone/etiocholanolone ratio (U) | ↓↓ | ↓↓ | | | |
| | Testosterone (P) | n | n | n | n | n |

## Reference Values

**Important note:** Steroid hormone reference values vary enormously depending on the assay and the clinical chemistry laboratory. Therefore, the following values must be considered an example and not used for everyday clinical practice. In the case of the semiquantitative urinary steroid profile using gas chromatography-mass spectrometry (GC-MS), the interpretation of the results is even more complex and should be made by an expert in such assay. For these reasons, only the diagnostic ratios are mentioned in this chapter.

For more information, see also (Wudy and Homoki 2003).

### Plasma

| Age | ACTH pmol/L | FSH/LH mIU/ml | 17OHP nmol/L | DHEA nmol/L | D4A nmol/L | T nmol/L | DHT nmol/L | E2 pmol/L | Aldo pmol/L | DOC pmol/L | B pmol/L | F nmol/L |
|---|---|---|---|---|---|---|---|---|---|---|---|---|
| <6 years | 4.4–22.2 | N/A | 0.3–9.5 | Male: 0.9–4.5 Female: 0.7–4.5 | N/A | Male: 0.28–0.49 Female: 0.17–0.45 | Male: <0.1–04 Female: <0.1–0.3 | Male: <37 Female: <26 | N/A | 1.5–7.5 | 0.6–2.16 | AM 171–536 PM 64–340 |
| 8–10 years | 4.4–22.2 | N/A | 0.3–9.5 | Male: 1.8–4.7 Female: 2.6–6.2 | N/A | Male: 0.28–0.49 Female: 0.17–0.45 | Male: <0.1–04 Female: <0.1–0.3 | Male: <37 Female: 30–65 | m: 83–250 j:11–832[a] | 1.5–7.5 | 0.6–2.16 | AM 171–536 PM 64–340 |
| 10–12 years | 4.4–22.2 | N/A | 0.3–9.5 | Male: 6.3–12.3 Female: 8.1–18.3 | N/A | Male: 0.28–0.49 Female: 0.17–0.45 | Male: <0.1–04 Female: <0.1–0.3 | Male: <37 Female: 30–65 | m: 83–250 j:11–832 | 1.5–7.5 | 0.6–2.16 | AM 171–536 PM 64–340 |
| 14–16 years | 4.4–22.2 | FSH Male: 2–17 Female: 4–20 LH Male: 4–18 Female: 5–25 | 0.3–9.5 | Male: 8.3–18 Female: 7.8–21.2 | 1.4–7.9 | Male: 2.91–6.24 Female: 0.31–0.83 | Male: 1–10.4 Female: 0.2–1.1 | Male: 62–85 Female: 73–250 | m: 83–250 j:11–832 | 1.5–7.5 | 0.6–2.16 | AM 171–536 PM 64–340 |
| Adult | " | " | 0.3–9.5 | Male: 10.6–29 Female: 9.8–27.7 | 1.4–7.9 | Male: 10.4–34.7 Female: 1.04–2.43 | Male: 1–10.4 Female: 0.2–1.1 | Male: 62–184 Female: Follicular 73–367, luteal 367–1836 | m: 83–250 j:11–832 | 1.5–7.5 | 0.6–2.16 | AM 171–536 PM 64–340 |

*ACTH* adrenocorticotropic hormone, *FSH* follicle-stimulating hormone, *LH* luteinizing hormone, *17OHP* 17-hydroxy progesterone, *DHEA* dehydroepiandrosterone, *D4A* androstenedione, *T* testosterone, *DHT* dihydrotestosterone, *E2* estradiol, *Aldo* aldosterone, *DOC* deoxycorticosterone, *B* corticosterone, *F* cortisol, *AM* ante meridiem, *PM post meridiem*

[a]*Sodium intake 100–200 meq/d* recumbent (m) upright:(j); *sodium intake 10 meq/d* recumbent: 333–999 upright: 472–3800

## Pathological Values/Differential Diagnosis

### Plasma

| Disease | ACTH | FSH/LH | 17OHP | DHEA | D4A | T | DHT | E2 | Aldo | DOC | B | F |
|---|---|---|---|---|---|---|---|---|---|---|---|---|
| 55.1 | ↑↑↑ | ↑ | ↓↓ | ↓↓ | ↓↓ | ↓↓ | ↓↓ | ↓↓ | ↓↓ | ↓↓ | ↓↓ | ↓↓ |
| 55.2 | ↑ | ↑-n | ↓ | ↓ | ↓ | ↓ | ↓ | ↓ | ↓ | ↓ | ↓ | ↓-n |
| 55.3 | ↑-n | ↑ | ↓ | ↓ | ↓ | ↓ | ↓ | ↓ | n | ↑↑ | ↑↑ | n |
| 55.4 | ↑↑ | ↑↑ | ↑ | ↑↑ | ↓ | ↓ | ↓ | ↓ | ↓ | ↓ | ↓ | ↓-n |
| 55.5 | ↑↑ | ↑ | ↑↑↑ | ↑↑ | ↑↑↑ | ↑↑ | ↑↑ | n | n | ↓-n | ↓-n | n-↓ |
| 55.6 | ↑ | ↑ | ↑ | ↑↑ | ↑↑↑ | ↑↑ | ↑ | n | n | ↑↑ | ↓ | n |
| 55.7 | n | n | n | n | n | n | n | n | ↓ | ↑ | ↑ | n |
| 55.8 | n | n | n | n | n | n | n | n | ↑ | n-↑ | n-↑ | n |
| 55.9 | n | n | n | n | n | n | n | n | n | n | n | n |
| 55.10 | n-↑ | n | n-↑ | ↑ | ↑ | ↑ | ↑ | n | n | n | n | ↑ |
| 55.11 | n | ↑↑ | ↑ | ↓ | ↓ | ↓ | ↓ | ↓ | n | n | n | n |
| 55.12 | n | ↑↑ | n | n | ↑ | ↓ | ↓ | ↓ | n | n | n | n |
| 55.13 | n | ↑ | n | n | n | n - ↑ | ↓↓ | n | n | n | n | n |
| 55.14 | n | ↑↑ | n | n | n | ↑ | ↑ | ↓↓ | n | n | n | n |
| 55.15 | n-↑ | ↑ | ↑-↓ | ↑ -↓ | ↑-↓ | ↓- | ↓-↑ | ↓ | n | n | n | n |
| 55.16 | n | ↑ | n (XY) | n (XY) | n (XY) | n (XY) | n (XY) | ↑ (XY) | n | n | n | n |
| 55.17 And 55.18 | n | n | n | n | n | n | n | ↑↑ | n | n | n | n |
| 55.19 | n | ↑↑ | n-↑ | n | n | n | n | n | n | n | n | n |
| 55.20 | n-↑ | n | n | n | n | n | n | n | n | n | n | ↑↑ |
| 55.21 | n | n | n | n | n | n | n | n | ↑ | ↑ | n-↑ | n |
| 55.22 | n | n | n | n | n | n | n | n | n | n | n | n |

*ACTH* adrenocorticotropic hormone, *FSH* follicle-stimulating hormone, *LH* luteinizing hormone, *17OHP* 17-hydroxy progesterone, *DHEA* dehydroepiandrosterone, *D4A* androstenedione, *T* testosterone, *DHT* dihydrotestosterone, *E2* estradiol, *Aldo* aldosterone, *DOC* deoxycorticosterone, *B* corticosterone, *F* cortisol

### Special Tests

| Disorder | Test | Procedure | Results |
|---|---|---|---|
| 55.9 | Sodium (P) restriction | 3–5 days of 10 mmol sodium intake. Aldosterone morning plasma levels | Increase two- to threefold over basal levels |
| 55.8<br>55.17 and 55.18 | Dexamethasone suppression test | 1 mg dexamethasone for 2 days p.o. aldosterone morning plasma levels | Decrease of aldosterone<br>Decrease of cortisol |

### Urinary Ratios

| | Pathological |
|---|---|
| **55.2 17α-hydroxylase deficiency** | |
| (THA + THB + 5αTHB)/(THE+THF + 5αTHF) | >10 |
| (THA + THB + 5αTHB)/(AN+ET) | >10 |
| 100*THDOC/(THE+THF + 5αTHF) | >10 |
| **55.5 21-hydroxylase deficiency** | |
| 17HP/(THE+THF + 5αTHF) | >0.25 |
| PT/(THE+THF + 5αTHF) | >0.25 |
| 100*PT'ONE/(THE+THF + 5aTHF) | >10 |
| **55.6 11β-hydroxylase deficiency** | |
| 100*THS/(THE+THF + 5αTHF) | >10 |
| 100*THDOC/(THE+THF + 5αTHF) | >10 |
| **55.7 CMO deficiency** | |
| 18OHTHA/THALDO | >20 |
| (THA + THB + 5αTHB)/(THE+THF + 5αTHF) | >1 |
| **55.9 11ß-HSD2 deficiency** | |
| F/E | >1 |
| (THF + 5αTHF)/THE | >3 |
| (F + E)/(THE+THF + 5αTHF) | >0.1 |
| **55.10 11ß-HSD1 deficiency** | |
| (THF + 5αTHF)/THE | <0.1 |
| **55.13 5α-reductase deficiency** | |
| ET/AN | >5 |
| THF/5αTHF | >10 |
| **55.21 Pseudohypoaldosteronism** | |
| THALDO (μg/24 h) | >90 |
| * 100*THALDO/(THE+THF + 5αTHF) | >5 |

*THA* tetrahydro compound A, *THB* tetrahydrocorticosterone, *THE* tetrahydrocortisone, *THF* tetrahydrocortisol, *AN* androsterone, *ET* etiocholanolone, *THDOC* tetrahydro-deoxycorticosterone, *17HP* metabolites of 17OH-progesterone (pregnanediol; pregnanetriol, 17OH-pregnanolone), *PTONE* pregnanetriolone, *THALDO* terahydroaldosterone, *THS* tetrahydrodeoxycortisol

## Diagnostic Flow Chart

Diagnosis of Disorders of Sex Development (DSD) and Intersexuality.

1. History: family history, pregnancy (hormones, virilization).

Palpation of inguinal region and labioscrotal folds: rectal examination, karyotype.

Initial studies: plasma 17OH-progesterone, DHEA, androstenedione, testosterone, DHT, and estradiol.

Serum electrolytes.

Sonogram of kidneys, ureters, and pelvic content.

2. Provisional diagnosis: "abnormal external genitalia" → proceed as in the following figure.

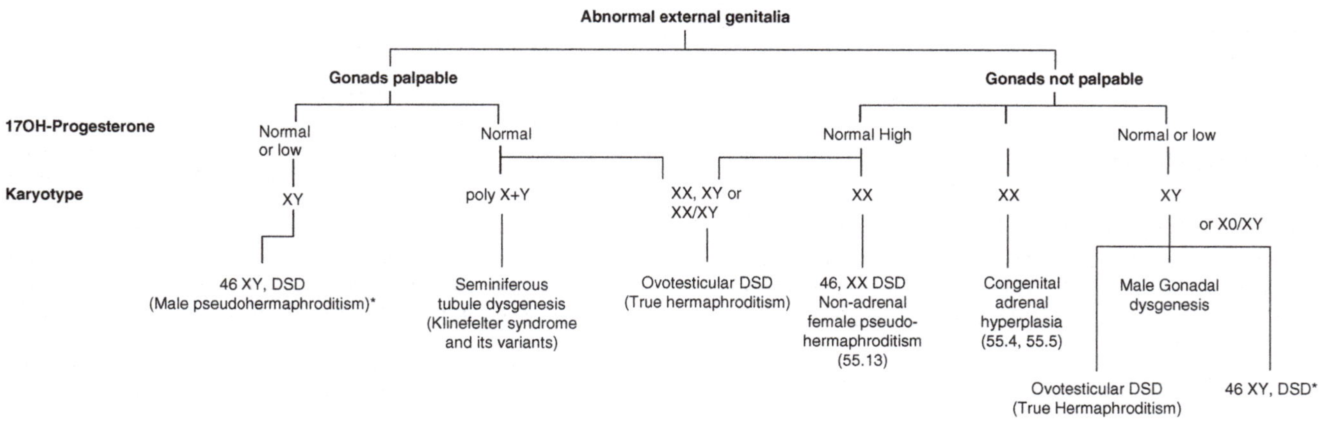


## Specimen Collection

| Test | Preconditions | Material | Handling | Pitfalls |
|---|---|---|---|---|
| Plasma or serum quantitative steroids, ACTH, and gonadotropins | None | Frozen plasma or serum | Keep frozen (−20°C) until analyzed | None, except laboratory error |
| Urine for gas chromatography-mass spectrometry analysis of urinary metabolites | None | Fresh or frozen 24-h urine (discard the morning urine of the first day but collect the morning urine of the second and final day) | Keep frozen (−20 °C) until analyzed | None, except laboratory error |

## Prenatal Diagnosis

| Disorder | Material | Timing, trimester |
|---|---|---|
| All disorders (except 55.9 and 55.15–18 that are adult-onset diseases) | CV, AF | I, II |

## Treatment

The therapeutic management in disorders of steroid synthesis and action can be distinguished in two phases:

1. Management of life-threatening situations (adrenal crisis): emergency.
2. Management of lifelong consequences: no emergency.

Whereas the therapeutic intervention in phase 1 is straightforward, those for phase 2 are complex and different from case to case. It is therefore mandatory to create a multidisciplinary team of experts especially when the patient has a DSD, and not try to manage these complex cases alone.

### Phase 1–Initial Treatment

Disorders 55.1, 55.2, 55.5, 55.7, 55.21 (salt-losing forms)

1. Parenteral isotonic saline.
2. Hydrocortisone (cortisol).

*Note*: salt-loss symptoms do not appear before 6–10 days after birth.

Disorders 55.3, 55.6, 55.8, 55.9 (hypertensive, hypokalemic forms).

1. Restoration of potassium concentrations.
2. Diuretic therapy to reduce blood pressure.

### Phase 2: Disorders 55.1–6, 55.11–16, 55.22 (DSD)

1. Sex assignment.
2. Reconstructive genital surgery.

After the adrenal emergency has been managed, the type and timing of genital surgery and the correspondent sex assignment, necessity, and timing of gonadectomy should be discussed case by case in a multidisciplinary team of experts in DSD.

### Emergency Treatment

All the salt-losing forms (55.1, 55.2, 55.5, 55.7, 55.21) are prone to adrenal crisis in stress situations. Therefore:

| | |
|---|---|
| Initial hydrocortisone i.v. | Infants and preschool children: 25 mg |
| | School-age children: 50 mg |
| | Adults: 100 mg |

Successive i.v. hydrocortisone doses 3–4x the maintenance dose/day, divided in four doses (every 6 h).

### Standard Treatment

Disorders 55.1, 55.2, 55.5, 55.7, 55.21.

| Type of glucocorticoid | Suggested dose (mg/d) | Daily doses |
|---|---|---|
| Hydrocortisone (HC) | 15–25 | 2–3 |
| Prednisone | 5–7.5 | 2 |
| Prednisolone | 4–6 | 2 |
| Dexamethasone | 0.25–0.5 | 1 |
| Fludrocortisone (mineralocorticoid) | 0.05–0.2 | 1 |

Patients affected by the salt-losing forms of steroid synthesis defects should be informed of the necessity of an emergency treatment (55.15).

Disorders: 55.3, 55.6, 55.8, 55.9 (hypertensive, hypokalemic).

DSD (55.3, 55.6, 55.8, 55.9): Induction of puberty according to sex assignment.

## References


Antley R, Bixler D. Trapezoidocephaly, midfacial hypoplasia and cartilage abnormalities with multiple synostoses and skeletal fractures. Birth Defects Orig Artic Ser. 1975;11:397–401.

Baetens D, Guran T, Mendonca BB, Gomes NL, De Cauwer L, Peelman F, Verdin H, Vuylsteke M, Van der Linden M, Esr Study G, Stoop H, Looijenga LH, De Bosscher K, Cools M, De Baere E. Biallelic and monoallelic ESR2 variants associated with 46,XY disorders of sex development. Genet Med. 2018;20:717–27.

Bernard V, Kherra S, Francou B, Fagart J, Viengchareun S, Guechot J, Ladjouze A, Guiochon-Mantel A, Korach KS, Binart N, Lombes M, Christin-Maitre S. Familial multiplicity of Estrogen insensitivity associated with a loss-of-function ESR1 mutation. J Clin Endocrinol Metab. 2017;102:93–9.

Biason-Lauber A, Suter SL, Shackleton CH, Zachmann M. Apparent cortisone reductase deficiency: a rare cause of hyperandrogenemia and hypercortisolism. Horm Res. 2000;53:260–6. 23577

Biglieri EG, Herron MA, Brust N. 17-hydroxylation deficiency in man. J Clin Invest. 1966;45:1946–54.

Bongiovanni AM. The adrenogenital syndrome with deficiency of 3 beta-hydroxysteroid dehydrogenase. J Clin Invest. 1962;41:2086–92.

Chrousos GP, McLusky NJ, Brandon DD, Tomita M, Renquist DM, Loriaux DL, Lipsett MB. Progesterone resistance. In: Chrousos GP, Loriaux DL, Lipsett MB, editors. Steroid hormone resistance: mechanisms and clinical aspects. New York: Plenum Press; 1986.

Conte FA, Grumbach MM, Ito Y, Fisher CR, Simpson ER. A syndrome of female pseudohermaphrodism, hypergonadotropic hypogonadism, and multicystic ovaries associated with missense mutations in the gene encoding aromatase (P450arom). J Clin Endocrinol Metab. 1994;78:1287–92.

Crisponi G, Porcu C, Piu ME. Antley-Bixler syndrome: case report and review of the literature. Clin Dysmorphol. 1997;6:61–8.

Draper N, Walker EA, Bujalska IJ, Tomlinson JW, Chalder SM, Arlt W, et al. Mutations in the genes encoding 11beta-hydroxysteroid dehydrogenase type 1 and hexose-6-phosphate dehydrogenase interact to cause cortisone reductase deficiency. Nat Genet. 2003;34(4):434–9.

Evans RM. The steroid and thyroid hormone receptor superfamily. Science. 1988;240:889–95.

Fluck CE, Meyer-Boni M, Pandey AV, Kempna P, Miller WL, Schoenle EJ, Biason-Lauber A. Why boys will be boys: two pathways of fetal testicular androgen biosynthesis are needed for male sexual differentiation. Am J Hum Genet. 2011;89:201–18.

Fluck CE, Pandey A, Huang N, Agrawal V, Miller WL. P560 oxidoreductase deficiency- a new form of congenital adrenal hyperplasia. Basel: Karger; 2008.

Fluck CE, Tajima T, Pandey AV, Arlt W, Okuhara K, Verge CF, Jabs EW, Mendonca BB, Fujieda K, Miller WL. Mutant P450 oxidoreductase causes disordered steroidogenesis with and without Antley-Bixler syndrome. Nat Genet. 2004;36:228–30.

Geller DS, Rodriguez-Soriano J, Vallo Boado A, Schifter S, Bayer M, Chang SS, Lifton RP. Mutations in the mineralocorticoid receptor gene cause autosomal dominant pseudohypoaldosteronism type I. Nat Genet. 1998;19:279–81.

Imperato-McGinley J, Gautier T, Peterson RE, Shackleton C. The prevalence of 5 alpha-reductase deficiency in children with ambiguous genitalia in the Dominican Republic. J Urol. 1986;136:867–73.

Lang-Muritano M, Sproll P, Wyss S, Kolly A, Hürlimann R, Konrad D, Biason-Lauber A. Estrogen receptor beta is necessary for human ovarian development. J Clin Endocrinol Metab. 2018;103:3748–56.

Lin D, Sugawara T, Strauss JF 3rd, Clark BJ, Stocco DM, Saenger P, Rogol A, Miller WL. Role of steroidogenic acute regulatory protein in adrenal and gonadal steroidogenesis. Science. 1995;267:1828–31.

Lipsett MB, Tomita M, Brandon DD, De Vroede MM. Cortisol resistance in men. In: Chrousos GP, Loriaux MB, editors. Steroid hormone resistance: mechanism and clinical aspects. New York: Plenum Press; 1986.

McPhaul MJ, Griffin JE. Male pseudohermaphroditism caused by mutations of the human androgen receptor. J Clin Endocrinol Metab. 1999;84:3435–41.

Miller WL. Congenital adrenal hyperplasia. N Engl J Med. 1986;314:1321–2.

New MI. The prismatic case of apparent mineralocorticoid excess. J Clin Endocrinol Metab. 1994;79:1–3.

New MI, White PC, Pang SA, Dupont B, Speiser PW. The adrenal hyperplasias. In: Scriver B, editor. The metabolic basis of inherited disease. Valle: Sly; 1989.

Novoselova TV, Chan LF, Clark AJL. Pathophysiology of melanocortin receptors and their accessory proteins. Best Pract Res Clin Endocrinol Metab. 2018;32(2):93–106.

Peterson RE, Imperato-McGinley J, Gautier T, Shackleton C. Male pseudohermaphroditism due to multiple defects in steroid-biosynthetic microsomal mixed-function oxidases. A new variant of congenital adrenal hyperplasia. N Engl J Med. 1985;313:1182–91.

Prader A, Gurtner HP. The syndrome of male pseudohermaphrodism in congenital adrenocortical hyperplasia without overproduction of androgens (adrenal male pseudohermaphrodism). Helv Paediatr Acta. 1955;10:397–412.

Quaynor SD, Stradtman EW Jr, Kim HG, Shen Y, Chorich LP, Schreihofer DA, Layman LC. Delayed puberty and estrogen resistance in a woman with estrogen receptoralpha variant. N Engl J Med. 2013;369:164–71.

Scott RR, Miller WL. Genetic and clinical features of p450 oxidoreductase deficiency. Horm Res. 2008;69:266–75.

Smith EP, Boyd J, Frank GR, Takahashi H, Cohen RM, Specker B, Williams TC, Lubahn DB, Korach KS. Estrogen resistance caused by a mutation in the estrogen-receptor gene in a man. N Engl J Med. 1994;331:1056–61.

Wudy SA and Homoki J. Profiling steroids by gas chromatography-mass spectrometry: clinical applications. In: Ranke MD, editor, Diagnostic of endocrine function in children and adolescents. Basel: Karger; 2003. pp. 427–49.

White PC, Pascoe L. Disorders of steroid 11 beta-hydroxylase isozymes. Trends Endocrinol Metab. 1992;3:229–34.

Zachmann M, Werder EA, Prader A. Two types of male pseudohermaphroditism due to 17, 20-desmolase deficiency. J Clin Endocrinol Metab. 1982;55:487–90.

# Disorders of Bile Acid Synthesis

# 56

Frédéric M. Vaz, David Cassiman,
and Sacha Ferdinandusse

## Contents



**Abstract**

Bile acid synthesis defects often result in a deficiency of the primary bile acids—cholic acid and chenodeoxycholic acid—that are needed for absorption of fats and fat-soluble vitamins. Fat malabsorption leads to steatorrhea and growth retardation, and the fat-soluble vitamin deficiency can lead to coagulation defects and rickets. As bile acids are needed for bile flow, their deficiency can cause cholestasis, jaundice, and liver disease. In addition to the bile acid deficiency, accumulation of bile acid intermediates or their derivatives can cause other symptoms including progressive neurological disease. Bile acid synthesis defects can present from the neonatal period to adulthood. When a bile acid synthesis defect is suspected, bile acid analysis by tandem mass spectrometry in plasma and urine should be performed. As most bile acid synthesis defects have a characteristic bile acid profile, bile acid analysis can readily identify the underlying disorder, but for some disorders genetic analysis is required. Besides supplementation of the fat-soluble vitamins, bile acid replacement therapy can be beneficial in most of the bile acid synthesis disorders. This not only restores the bile acid pool but also strongly reduces the production of toxic bile acid intermediates by feedback inhibition of the bile acid synthesis pathway.

F. M. Vaz (✉) · S. Ferdinandusse
Laboratory Genetic Metabolic Diseases, Amsterdam UMC, Amsterdam, The Netherlands
e-mail: f.m.vaz@amsterdamumc.nl

D. Cassiman
Center for Metabolic Diseases, University of Leuven, Leuven, Belgium

## Introduction

Bile acids are well-known for their role in the absorption of fats and fat-soluble vitamins, but are also important for the maintenance of cholesterol homeostasis, excretion of toxic


N. Blau et al. (eds.), *Physician's Guide to the Diagnosis, Treatment, and Follow-Up of Inherited Metabolic Diseases*,
https://doi.org/10.1007/978-3-030-67727-5_56

substances, induction of bile flow and as signaling molecules that influence glucose homeostasis, lipid metabolism, and energy expenditure (Halilbasic et al. 2013; Russell 2009). The primary bile salts produced in man are the taurine and glycine conjugates of cholic acid (CA) and chenodeoxycholic acid (CDCA). They are synthesized in the liver from cholesterol via numerous modifications of the steroid nucleus and the aliphatic side chain. After synthesis, the (activated = coenzyme A (CoA) esters of the) bile acids (CA-CoA and CDCA-CoA) are converted into bile salts (glycine or taurine conjugates) via a process called amidation. The bile salts are excreted together with other bile components into the canaliculi, and the resulting bile is transported to and stored in the gallbladder. After a meal, the bile is secreted into the duodenum to facilitate fat and fat-soluble vitamin absorption. Gut bacteria modify and/or deconjugate part of the bile salts resulting in secondary bile acids (deoxycholic acid, lithocholic acid, ursodeoxycholic acid (UDCA), hyodeoxycholic acid, and hyocholic acid). Ninety-five percent of the bile acids/salts are recycled in the enterohepatic circulation. The fecal loss is compensated by hepatic bile acid synthesis, thereby maintaining bile acid homeostasis (Heubi et al. 2018).

Many enzymes located in different subcellular compartments including the cytosol, endoplasmic reticulum, mitochondria, and peroxisomes are involved in bile acid biosynthesis (see Figs. 56.1 and 56.2). Bile acid synthesis can roughly be divided into three processes: (1) modifications to the steroid nucleus, (2) modifications to the aliphatic side chain, and (3) amidation. Four main biosynthetic pathways have been delineated, of which the two most commonly described will be briefly discussed: the classic or neutral pathway and the alternative or acidic pathway. The majority of the enzymes are shared between these pathways with the exception of the enzymes involved in 7α-hydroxylation (cholesterol 7α-hydroxylase in the classic pathway and oxysterol-7α-hydroxylase in the acidic pathway) and 12α-hydroxylation, but the order of steps differs. In this respect, it is important to keep in mind that several intermediates are substrates for more than one biosynthetic enzyme. The neutral pathway is considered the most significant in adults, whereas the acidic pathway seems to play a more prominent role early in life. In the classic pathway, which starts with the hydroxylation of cholesterol to 7α-hydroxycholesterol by sterol 7α-hydroxylase (CYP7A1), modifications of the steroid ring structure precede the oxidative chain shortening of the side chain. In the acidic pathway, sterol 27-hydroxylase (CYP27A1) first generates a C27-carboxylic acid, followed by modifications of the steroid nucleus and shortening of the side chain (Fig. 56.1). The side-chain shortening occurs in the peroxisome via β-oxidation and converts C27-bile acid intermediates (cholestanoids) into C24-bile acids (cholanoids). Amidation of the newly synthesized bile acids also occurs in the peroxisome, but amidation of recycled bile acids occurs via cytosolic bile acid-CoA: amino acid *N*-acyltransferase (BAAT), which has a dual localization (Fig. 56.2) (Vaz and Ferdinandusse 2017).

A defect in bile acid biosynthesis results, in most disorders, in a deficiency of the primary bile acids. Because bile acids are crucial for the absorption of fats and fat-soluble vitamins, the characteristic clinical symptoms of a bile acid deficiency are fat malabsorption, leading to steatorrhea and growth retardation and deficiency of fat-soluble vitamins and their sequelae (e.g., coagulation defects and rickets). As bile acids drive bile flow, patients generally present with a failure of bile flow (cholestasis) and a conjugated hyperbilirubinemia (jaundice), but γ-glutamyl transpeptidase (γGT) is characteristically normal as opposed to other causes of cholestasis. Especially in the disorders where transformation of the steroid nucleus is affected (disorders 56.1–56.4), abnormal metabolites are produced which are not proper substrates for excretion into bile and generation of bile flow. Cholesterol 7α-hydroxylase deficiency (56.1) is a notable exception since it does not result in overt bile acid deficiency as the alternative pathway can still produce bile acids via oxysterol 7α-hydroxylase and patients present with statin-resistant hyperlipidemia and gallstones later in life (Pullinger et al. 2002). Oxysterol 7α-hydroxylase deficiency (56.4) not only has been identified in patients with severe neonatal liver disease but also in children or adults with a progressive spastic paraplegia (type SPG5A).

In addition to the bile acid deficiency in the different bile acid biosynthesis defects, there is accumulation of disease-specific bile acid intermediates that can contribute to the clinical presentation. In cerebrotendinous xanthomatosis (CTX), the classic presentation is neonatal cholestasis and intractable diarrhea that is attributed to bile acid deficiency. The progressive deposition of cholestanol and cholesterol, however, can lead to the formation of cataracts, intellectual disability, and developmental delay in the first decade and to tendon xanthomas, premature atherosclerosis, cognitive decline, and motor dysfunction in later life. Especially in disorders that affect the modification of the cholesterol side chain (disorders 56.5–56.8), clinical symptoms appear to be mainly caused by the accumulation of intermediates proximal to the metabolic block. The bile acid deficiency appears to be less important because in these defects, cholestanoids (C27-bile acids) are formed that, to some extent, can still drive bile flow. In peroxisomal disorders, also other metabolic pathways may be affected causing accumulation of different metabolites that may contribute to the clinical presentation. For example, in α-methylacyl-CoA racemase (AMACR) deficiency, not only C27-bile acid intermediates accumulate but also pristanic acid, which causes neurological disease, especially later in life. Still, AMACR deficiency in childhood can present with the bile acid deficiency phenotype characterized by neonatal cholestasis and mild to severe liver disease in addition to fat-soluble vitamin malabsorption and is for that reason discussed in this chapter. Disorders of peroxisome biogenesis (Zellweger spectrum disorders) and defects of peroxisomal β-oxidation (such as D-bifunctional protein deficiency) also affect bile acid synthesis but are considered elsewhere since they clinically do not present as a bile acid deficiency [Ref Chapter Ron Wanders].

In the defects of bile acid amidation (disorders 56.9 and 56.10), 85–95% of the bile acids are unconjugated. They are substrate for active transport into bile and drive bile flow but do not function properly as detergent leading to fat malabsorption and a deficiency of fat-soluble vitamins. In BAAT deficiency, this results in steatorrhea, coagulopathy, rickets, and jaundice, i.e., a classic bile acid deficiency phenotype. The clinical presentation of bile acid-CoA ligase (BACS) deficiency is not entirely clear yet since the only symptomatic patient described also was homozygous for a mutation in the gene encoding the bile salt export pump (BSEP) (Chong et al. 2012).

Overall, most disorders of bile acid biosynthesis present with cholestatic liver disease early in life, but can also cause neurological symptoms (neuropathy, spastic paraplegia, cognitive decline, movement disorder) in juvenile or adult patients. When a bile acid synthesis disorder is considered, both plasma and urine bile acid analysis should be performed. Currently, electrospray ionization-mass spectrometry (ESI-MS) with prior liquid chromatography (LC) separation is the method of choice for analyzing a cholanoid profile (Vaz and Ferdinandusse 2017).

## Nomenclature

| Disease number | Disease name | Alternative disease name 1 | Alternative disease name 2 | Disease abbreviation | Gene symbol | Chromosomal localization | Mode of inheritance | Affected protein | Disease OMIM# |
|---|---|---|---|---|---|---|---|---|---|
| 56.1 | Cholesterol 7α-hydroxylase deficiency | | | CYP7A1 | *CYP7A1* | 8q12.1 | AR | Cholesterol 7α-hydroxylase | 118455 |
| 56.2 | 3β-Hydroxy-Δ5-C27-steroid oxidoreductase deficiency | Congenital bile acid synthesis defect type 1 | | CBAS1 | *HSD3B7* | 16p11.2 | AR | 3β-Hydroxy-Δ5-C27-steroid dehydrogenase | 607764 |
| 56.3 | Δ4–3-Oxosteroid-5β-reductase deficiency | Congenital bile acid synthesis defect type 2 | | CBAS2 | *AKR1D1* | 7q33 | AR | Δ4–3-Oxosteroid-5β-reductase | 604741 |
| 56.4 | Oxysterol 7α-hydroxylase deficiency | Congenital bile acid synthesis defect type 3 | Spastic Paraplegia 5A | CBAS3 | *CYP7B1* | 8q12.3 | AR | Oxysterol 7α-hydroxylase | 603711 |
| 56.5 | Sterol 27-hydroxylase deficiency | Cerebrotendinous xanthomatosis | Cerebral cholesterinosis | CTX | *CYP27A1* | 2q35 | AR | Sterol 27-hydroxylase | 213700 |
| 56.6 | PMP70/ACBD3 deficiency | Congenital bile acid synthesis defect type 5 | | CBAS5 | *ABCD3* | 1p21.3 | AR | ATP-binding cassette protein, subfamily D, member 3 | 616278 |
| 56.7 | α-Methylacyl-CoA racemase deficiency | Congenital bile acid synthesis defect type 4 | | CBAS4 | *AMACR* | 5q13.2 | AR | α-Methylacyl-CoA racemase | 604489 |
| 56.8 | Peroxisomal acyl-CoA oxidase 2 deficiency | Congenital bile acid synthesis defect type 6 | | CBAS6 | *ACOX2* | 3p14.3 | AR | Peroxisomal acyl-CoA oxidase 2 | 617308 |
| 56.9 | Bile acid-CoA:amino acid N-acyltransferase deficiency | Familial hypercholanemia | | FHCA | *BAAT* | 9q31.1 | AR | Bile acid-CoA:amino acid N-acyltransferase | 602938 |
| 56.10 | Bile acid-CoA ligase deficiency | | | SLC27A5 | *SLC27A5* | 19q13.43 | AR | Bile acid-CoA ligase | 603314 |

## Metabolic Pathways

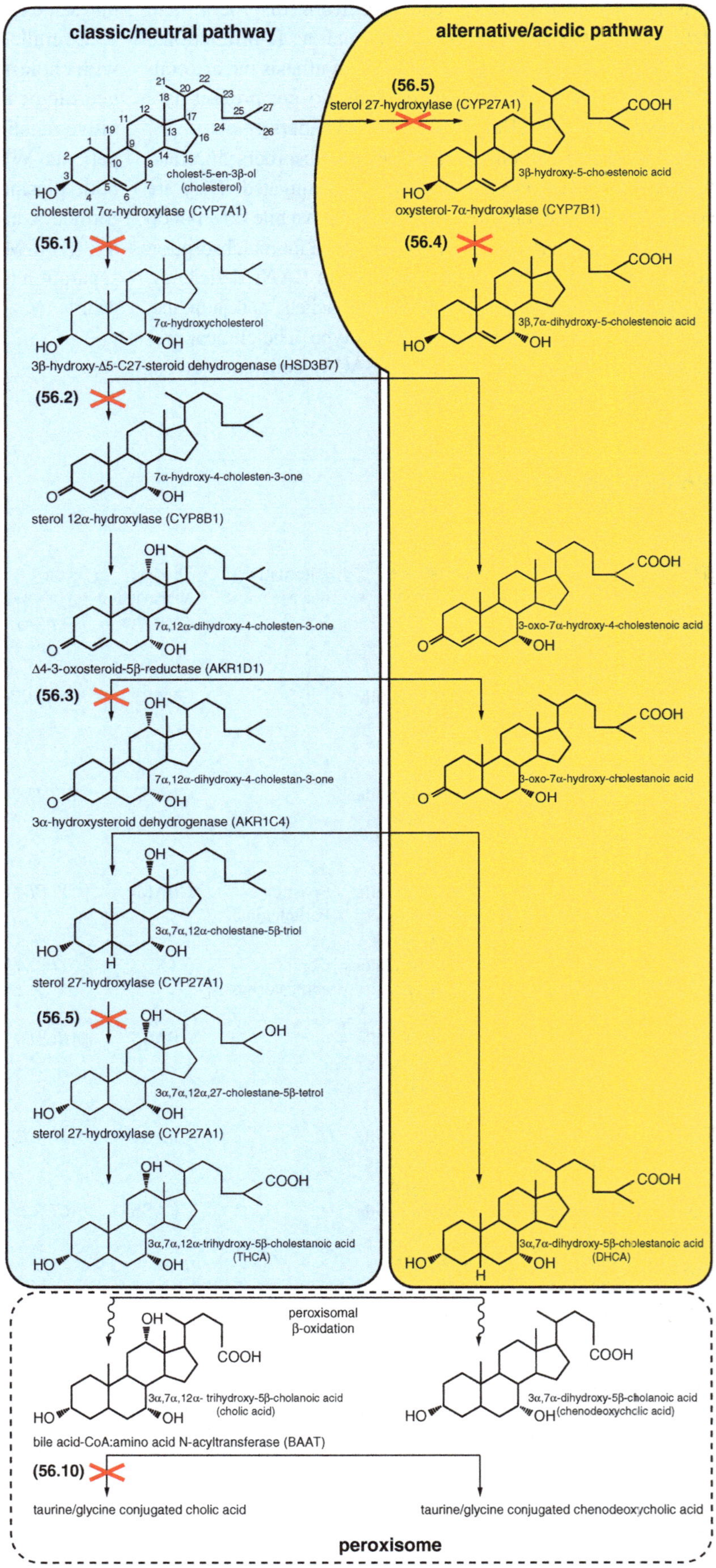


**Fig. 56.1** Schematic representation of the intermediates, enzymes, and corresponding genes of the classic/neutral pathway and the acid/alternative pathway of bile acid synthesis. Known inborn errors discussed in this chapter are indicated by red crosses and the disease number between parentheses. In the neutral pathway, modification of the sterol ring structure precedes the conversion to an acid, whereas in the acidic pathway, an acid = carboxylic group first is formed followed by steroid nucleus modifications. Peroxisomal shortening of the aliphatic side chain of dihydroxy- and trihydroxycholestanoic acid (DHCA and THCA) produces the primary bile acids chenodeoxycholic and cholic acids, respectively. These bile acids can be amidated to form taurine or glycine conjugates, i.e., the bile salts

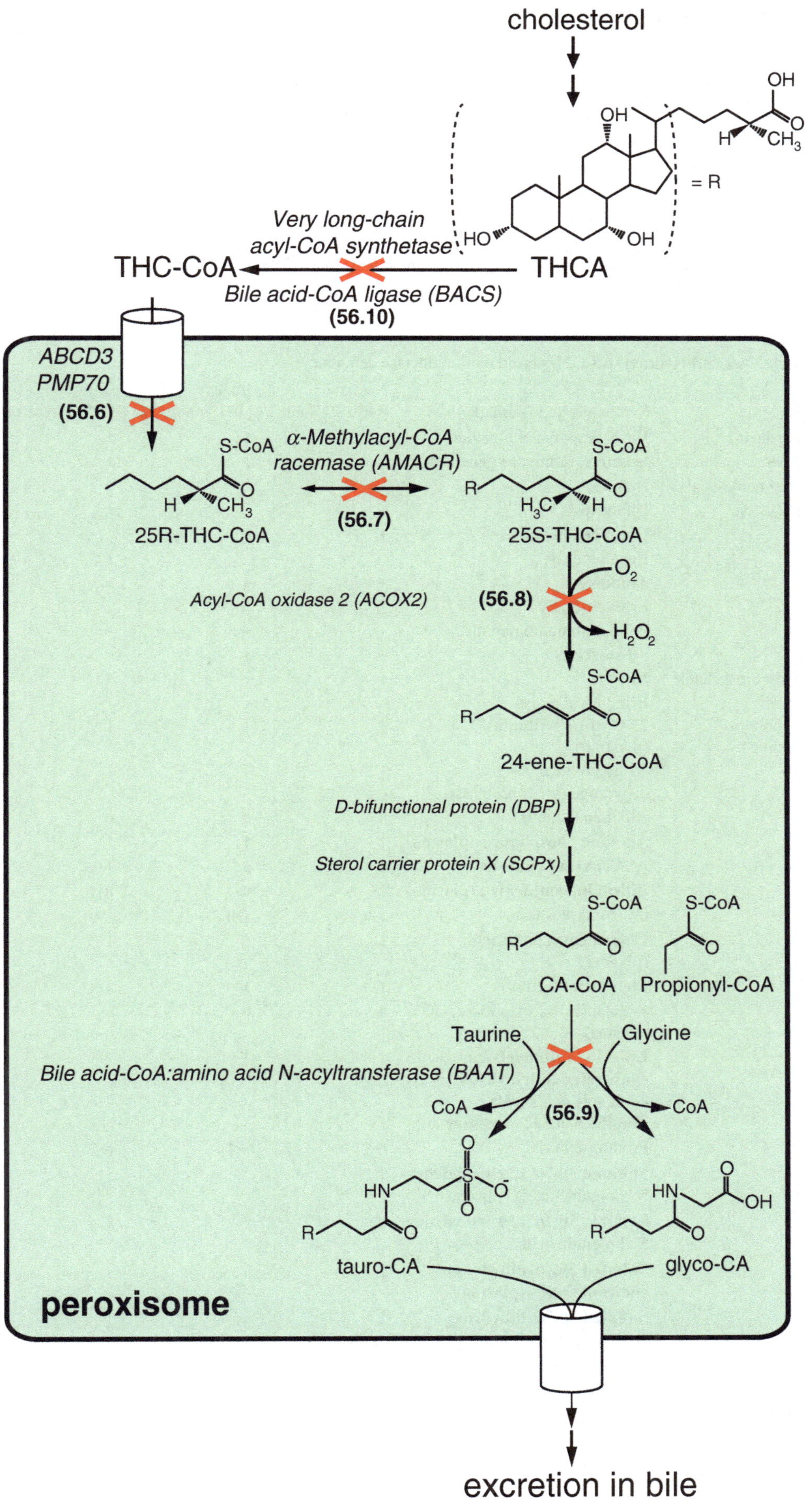


**Fig. 56.2** Schematic representation of the enzymes and bile acid intermediates of the peroxisomal steps in bile acid biosynthesis. Known inborn errors discussed in this chapter are indicated by red crosses and the disease number between parentheses. In short, the C27-bile acid intermediate trihydroxycholestanoic acid (THCA) is formed via several enzymatic steps from cholesterol and then activated to CoA-ester at the endoplasmic reticulum. Subsequently, THC-CoA is transported into the peroxisome via the transporter PMP70/ABCD3 after which the side chain is cleaved via peroxisomal β-oxidation generating choloyl-CoA (CA-CoA) followed by amidation via bile acid-CoA: amino acid *N*-acyltransferase (BAAT)

## Signs and Symptoms

**Table 56.1** Cholesterol 7α-hydroxylase deficiency

| System | Symptoms and Biomarkers | Neonatal (birth–1 month) | Infancy (1–18 months) | Childhood (1.5–11 years) | Adolescence (11–16 years) | Adulthood (>16 years) |
|---|---|---|---|---|---|---|
| Cardiovascular | **Statin resistant hyperlipidemia** | | | | | ± |
| Digestive | Gallstones | | | | | ± |
| DNA testing | *CYP7A1* gene | + | + | + | + | + |

Only three patients (siblings) have been described with a deficiency of cholesterol 7α-hydroxylase (Pullinger et al. 2002)

**Table 56.2** 3β-Hydroxy-Δ5-C27-steroid oxidoreductase deficiency

| System | Symptoms and Biomarkers | Neonatal (birth–1 month) | Infancy (1–18 months) | Childhood (1.5–11 years) | Adolescence (11–16 years) | Adulthood (>16 years) |
|---|---|---|---|---|---|---|
| Cardiovascular | **Vit K responsive bleeding** | ± | ± | ± | | |
| CNS | **Seizures, tetany, hypocalcemic** | | ± | ± | | |
| Dermatological | **Itching** | | ± | ± | | |
| Digestive | **Cholestasis** | + | ± | ± | | ± |
| | **Giant cell hepatitis** | + | + | | | |
| | Hepatomegaly | | | ± | | |
| | **Jaundice** | + | ± | ± | | ± |
| | Liver cirrhosis | | ± | ± | | ± |
| | Periportal inflammation | + | + | + | | |
| | **Steatorrhea** | + | + | + | | |
| Musculoskeletal | **Rickets** | + | + | + | | |
| Other | Bridging fibrosis | | + | + | | |
| Laboratory findings | **25-Hydroxy-vitamin D (plasma)** | ↓ | ↓ | ↓ | | |
| | 7α-hydroxycholesterol dehydrogenase (fibroblasts) | ↑ | ↑ | ↑ | | ↑ |
| | Albumin (serum) | n | n | n | | ↓-n |
| | **Alkaline phosphatase (plasma)** | ↑ | ↑ | ↑ | | **n-↑** |
| | **ASAT/ALAT (plasma)** | ↑ | ↑ | ↑ | | ↑ |
| | **Bilirubin, conjugated (plasma)** | ↑ | **n-↑** | **n-↑** | | |
| | Calcium (plasma) | ↓-n | ↓-n | ↓-n | | |
| | **Chenodeoxycholic acid (plasma)** | ↓ | ↓ | ↓ | | |
| | Cholesterol (serum) | ↓-n | ↓-n | ↓-n | | |
| | γ-glutamyl transpeptidase, GGT (plasma) | n | n | n | | n |
| | **LSI-MS, Sulfate/glycine conjugated di/trihydroxy-5-cholenoic acids (m/z 469,485,526,542)-negative** | ↑ | ↑ | ↑ | | ↑ |
| | Prothrombin ratio | n-↑ | n-↑ | n-↑ | | n-↑ |
| | **Sulfated 3β,7α,12α-trihydroxy-5-cholenoic acids (plasma)** | ↑ | ↑ | ↑ | | |
| | **Sulfated 3β,7α,12α-trihydroxy-5-cholenoic acids (urine)** | ↑ | ↑ | ↑ | | |
| | **Sulfated 3β,7α-dihydroxy--cholenoic acids (plasma)** | ↑ | ↑ | ↑ | | |
| | **Sulfated 3β,7α-dihydroxy--cholenoic acids (urine)** | ↑ | ↑ | ↑ | | |
| | Vitamin A (plasma) | ↓-n | ↓-n | ↓-n | | |
| | **Vitamin E (plasma)** | ↓ | ↓ | ↓ | | |
| DNA testing | ***HSD3B7* gene** | + | + | + | + | + |

**Table 56.3** Δ4–3-Oxosteroid-5β-reductase deficiency

| System | Symptoms and Biomarkers | Neonatal (birth–1 month) | Infancy (1–18 months) | Childhood (1.5–11 years) | Adolescence (11–16 years) | Adulthood (>16 years) |
|---|---|---|---|---|---|---|
| Digestive | **Ascites** | ± | ± | | | |
| | Cholestasis | + | + | | | |
| | Giant cell hepatitis | + | + | | | |
| | **Hepatosplenomegaly** | ± | ± | | | |
| | **Jaundice** | + | ± | | | |
| | Lobular inflammation | ± | ± | | | |
| | Periportal inflammation | ± | ± | | | |
| | Small canaliculi, few microvilli | + | ± | | | |
| Musculoskeletal | **Edema** | ± | ± | | | |
| Other | Pseudoacinar transformation | + | ± | | | |
| Laboratory findings | **7α,12α-dihydroxy-3-oxo--cholenoic acids (urine)** | ↑ | ↑ | | | |
| | 7α-hydroxy-3-oxo-cholenoic acids (urine) | ↑ | ↑ | | | |
| | ***AKR1D1* gene sequencing** | + | + | + | + | + |
| | Albumin (serum) | ↓-n | ↓-n | | | |
| | Alkaline phosphatase (plasma) | n-↑ | n-↑ | | | |
| | **Allochenodeoxycholic acid (plasma)** | ↑ | ↑ | ↑ | | |
| | **Allocholic acid (plasma)** | ↑ | ↑ | ↑ | | |
| | **ASAT/ALAT (plasma)** | ↑ | ↑ | | | |
| | **Bilirubin, conjugated (plasma)** | ↑ | **n-↑** | | | |
| | Cholesterol (serum) | ↓-n | ↓-n | | | |
| | Cortisol metabolites increased 5αH/5βH ratio (urine) | | ↑ | ↑ | ↑ | |
| | γ-glutamyl transpeptidase, GGT (plasma) | n-↑ | n-↑ | | | |
| | Prothrombin ratio | ↑ | n-↑ | | | |

**Table 56.4** Oxysterol 7α-hydroxylase deficiency

| System | Symptoms and Biomarkers | Neonatal (birth–1 month) | Infancy (1–18 months) | Childhood (1.5–11 years) | Adolescence (11–16 years) | Adulthood (>16 years) |
|---|---|---|---|---|---|---|
| Cardiovascular | **Vit K responsive bleeding** | | ± | | | |
| CNS | Ataxia, cerebellar | | | | | ± |
| | **Progressive spastic paraplegia** | | | ± | ± | ± |
| | White matter abnormalities (MRI) | | | | | + |
| Digestive | Bile duct proliferation | | + | | | |
| | Cholestasis | | + | | | |
| | Giant cell hepatitis | | + | | | |
| | **Hepatosplenomegaly** | | + | | | |
| | **Jaundice** | ± | + | | | |
| | **Liver failure** | | + | + | | |
| | Periportal inflammation | | + | | | |
| Eye | Cataract | | | | | ± |
| | Optic atrophy | | | | | ± |
| Metabolic | Hypoglycemia | | + | | | |
| Other | Bridging fibrosis | | + | | | |

(continued)

**Table 56.4** (continued)

| System | Symptoms and Biomarkers | Neonatal (birth–1 month) | Infancy (1–18 months) | Childhood (1.5–11 years) | Adolescence (11–16 years) | Adulthood (>16 years) |
|---|---|---|---|---|---|---|
| Laboratory findings | **27-hydroxycholesterol (plasma)** | | ↑ | ↑ | ↑ | ↑ |
| | **3β-Hydroxy-5-cholenoic acids (urine)** | | ↑ | ↑ | ↑ | ↑ |
| | **3β-Hydroxy-5-cholestenoic acid (plasma)** | | ↑ | ↑ | ↑ | ↑ |
| | **Alkaline phosphatase (plasma)** | | ↑ | | | |
| | **ASAT/ALAT (plasma)** | | ↑ | | | |
| | **Bilirubin, total/direct (plasma)** | | ↑ | | | |
| | Cholesterol (serum) | | n | | | |
| | ***CYP7B1* gene** | + | + | + | + | + |
| | γ-glutamyl transpeptidase, GGT (plasma) | | n | | | |
| | Glucose (plasma) | | ↓ | | | |
| | Prothrombin ratio | | n-↑ | | | |
| | Vitamin E (plasma) | | ↓ | | | |

**Table 56.5** Sterol 27-hydroxylase deficiency

| System | Symptoms and Biomarkers | Neonatal (birth–1 month) | Infancy (1–18 months) | Childhood (1.5–11 years) | Adolescence (11–16 years) | Adulthood (>16 years) |
|---|---|---|---|---|---|---|
| Cardiovascular | Angina | | | | ± | ± |
| | Ischemic heart disease | | | | ± | ± |
| | Myocardial infarction | | | | ± | ± |
| CNS | Ataxia | | | | ± | ± |
| | Dementia | | | | ± | ± |
| | Demyelination | | | | ± | |
| | Developmental delay | | | ± | ± | ± |
| | **Evoked potentials +/–, abnormal (EEG)** | | | ± | ± | ± |
| | Expressive dysphasia | | | | ± | ± |
| | Lipid deposition | | | | ± | |
| | Neuropathy | | | | | ± |
| | Parkinsonism | | | | ± | |
| | Pyramidal signs | | | ± | ± | ± |
| | Regression | | | | ± | ± |
| | Seizures | | | ± | ± | ± |
| | Spastic paresis | | | ± | ± | ± |
| | Spinal cord, myelopathy | | | | | ± |
| Dermatological | **Xanthomas, tendon** | | | | ± | ± |
| Digestive | Diarrhea | | ± | ± | | |
| | Gallstones | | | | | ± |
| | Jaundice | ± | ± | ± | | |
| Endocrine | Adrenal insufficiency | | | | | ± |
| | Hyperthyroidism | | | | | ± |
| | Hypothalamic dysfunction | | | | | ± |
| | Hypothyroidism | | | | | ± |
| | Pituitary dysfunction | | | | | ± |
| Eye | Cataract | | | ± | ± | ± |
| Musculoskeletal | Osteoporosis | | | | | ± |
| | Pes cavus | | | | | ± |
| Respiratory | Respiratory failure | | | | | ± |
| Laboratory findings | 25-Hydroxy-Vitamin D (plasma) | | | | ↓-n | ↓-n |
| | **27-Hydroxylase (fibroblasts)** | ↓ | ↓ | ↓ | ↓ | ↓ |
| | **Cholestane pentol glucuronide (urine)** | ↑ | ↑ | ↑ | ↑ | ↑ |
| | **Cholestanol (plasma)** | **n-↑** | ↑ | ↑ | ↑ | ↑ |
| | Cholesterol (serum) | | | | n-↑ | n-↑ |
| | ***CYP27A1* gene** | + | + | + | + | + |
| | Pigment granules in liver biopsy | | | | | ± |

**Table 56.6** PMP70/ABCD3 deficiency

| System | Symptoms and Biomarkers | Neonatal (birth–1 month) | Infancy (1–18 months) | Childhood (1.5–11 years) | Adolescence (11–16 years) | Adulthood (>16 years) |
|---|---|---|---|---|---|---|
| Digestive | **Hepatosplenomegaly** | | + | + | | |
| | Jaundice | ± | ± | | | |
| | Liver failure | | + | + | | |
| | Liver fibrosis | | + | + | | |
| Hematological | Anemia | | + | + | | |
| Laboratory findings | ***ABCD3* gene** | + | + | + | + | + |
| | ASAT/ALAT (plasma) | | ↑ | ↑ | | |
| | **C27-bile acids (plasma)** | | ↑ | ↑ | | |
| | Iron (serum) | | ↓ | ↓ | | |
| | Phytanic acid (serum) | | n | n | | |
| | Pristanic acid (serum) | | n | n | | |
| | Transaminase (plasma) | | ↑ | ↑ | | |
| | Very-long-chain fatty acids (plasma) | | n | n | | |

Only one patient with a defect of PMP70/ABCD3 has been described in literature so far (Ferdinandusse et al. 2015), who presented with hepatosplenomegaly and severe liver disease

**Table 56.7** α-Methylacyl-CoA racemase deficiency

| System | Symptoms and Biomarkers | Neonatal (birth–1 month) | Infancy (1–18 months) | Childhood (1.5–11 years) | Adolescence (11–16 years) | Adulthood (>16 years) |
|---|---|---|---|---|---|---|
| Cardiovascular | Vit K responsive bleeding | ± | | | | |
| CNS | Ataxia | | | | | ± |
| | Cognitive decline | | | | | ± |
| | Developmental delay | | ± | | | |
| | Dysarthria | | | | | ± |
| | Epilepsy +/– encephalopathy | | | ± | ± | ± |
| | Headache | | | | ± | ± |
| | Hemiparesis | | | | | ± |
| | Neuropathy | | | | | ± |
| | Seizures | | | | ± | ± |
| | Spastic paraparesis | | | | | ± |
| | Tremor | | | | | ± |
| Digestive | Cholestasis | + | | | | |
| | Giant cell hepatitis | + | | | | |
| | Jaundice | ± | ± | | | |
| Endocrine | Hypothyroidism | | | | | ± |
| Eye | Pigmentary retinopathy | | | | ± | ± |
| | Vision, progressive loss | | | | ± | ± |
| Musculoskeletal | Rhabdomyolysis | | | | | ± |
| Laboratory findings | **(25R)-3α,7α,12α-trihydroxy-5β-cholestan-26-oic acid, THCA (plasma)** | ↑ | ↑ | ↑ | ↑ | ↑ |
| | **(25R)-3α,7α-dihydroxy-5β-cholestan-26-oic acid, DHCA (plasma)** | ↑ | ↑ | ↑ | ↑ | ↑ |
| | **25-Hydroxy-vitamin D (plasma)** | ↓ | | | | |
| | ***AMACR* gene** | + | + | + | + | + |
| | ASAT/ALAT (plasma) | | | ↑ | | |
| | **C26:0 fatty acid (plasma)** | | | **n** | **n** | **n** |
| | **C27-bile acid (plasma)** | ↑ | ↑ | ↑ | ↑ | ↑ |

(continued)

**Table 56.7** (continued)

| System | Symptoms and Biomarkers | Neonatal (birth–1 month) | Infancy (1–18 months) | Childhood (1.5–11 years) | Adolescence (11–16 years) | Adulthood (>16 years) |
|---|---|---|---|---|---|---|
| | **LSI-MS, Taurotetra-[tri/penta]-hydroxycholestanoic acids (m/z 556,572,588) (urine)** | ↑ | ↑ | ↑ | ↑ | ↑ |
| | Phosphate (plasma) | | | ↑ | | |
| | Phytanic acid (serum) | | | n-↑ | n-↑ | n-↑ |
| | **Pristanic acid (serum)** | | | ↑ | ↑ | ↑ |
| | **Transaminase (plasma)** | ↑ | | | | |
| | **Vitamin E (plasma)** | ↓ | | | | |
| | **γ-glutamyl transpeptidase, GGT (plasma)** | ↑ | | | | |

**Table 56.8** Peroxisomal acyl-CoA oxidase 2 deficiency

| System | Symptoms and Biomarkers | Neonatal (birth–1 month) | Infancy (1–18 months) | Childhood (1.5–11 years) | Adolescence (11–16 years) | Adulthood (>16 years) |
|---|---|---|---|---|---|---|
| CNS | Ataxia | | | ± | | |
| | Cognitive dysfunction | | | ± | | |
| Digestive | Cholestasis | | | | ± | |
| | Liver fibrosis | | | ± | | |
| | Steatorrhea | | | ± | | |
| Laboratory findings | 25-Hydroxy-Vitamin D (plasma) | | | ↓ | | |
| | ***ACOX2*** **gene** | + | + | + | + | + |
| | ASAT/ALAT (plasma) | | | n-↑ | | |
| | C24-bile acid (plasma) | | | ↓-n | ↓-n | ↓-n |
| | **C27-bile acid (plasma)** | | | ↑ | ↑ | ↑ |
| | C27-bile acid (urine) | | | ↑ | ↑ | ↑ |
| | Cholesterol (serum) | | | ↓ | | |
| | Pristanic acid (plasma) | | | n | n | n |
| | Transaminase (plasma) | | | n-↑ | n-↑ | n-↑ |

Only four patients including two siblings with peroxisomal acyl-CoA oxidase 2 (ACOX2) deficiency have been described so far (Vilarinho et al. 2016; Monte et al. 2017; Ferdinandusse et al. 2018). One patient with a complicated clinical presentation, who died at the age of 5 months, is not included because the patient most likely suffered from another defect underlying the clinical presentation (Ferdinandusse et al. 2018). This patient did have persistently but slightly increased ALAT levels like the other ACOX2 patients

**Table 56.9** Bile acid-CoA: amino acid N-acyltransferase deficiency

| System | Symptoms and Biomarkers | Neonatal (birth–1 month) | Infancy (1–18 months) | Childhood (1.5–11 years) | Adolescence (11–16 years) | Adulthood (>16 years) |
|---|---|---|---|---|---|---|
| Dermatological | **Itching** | | ± | ± | ± | |
| Digestive | **Cholestasis** | ± | ± | ± | ± | |
| | Hepatomegaly | | ± | | | |
| | Hepatosplenomegaly | | ± | | | |
| | **Jaundice** | ± | ± | ± | ± | |
| | Liver cirrhosis | | ± | | | |
| | Steatorrhea | | ± | ± | | |
| Musculoskeletal | **Rickets** | | ± | ± | ± | |
| Other | **Bridging fibrosis** | | ± | | | |
| | **Failure to thrive** | | ± | ± | | |
| Laboratory findings | Alkaline phosphatase (plasma) | | n-↑ | n-↑ | n-↑ | |
| | *BAAT* **gene** | + | + | + | + | + |
| | Bilirubin (plasma) | n-↑ | n-↑ | n-↑ | n-↑ | |
| | **ESI-MS, Unamidated bile acids (m/z 391,407,471,487,567,583)-negative** | | ↑ | ↑ | | |
| | γ-glutamyl transpeptidase, GGT (plasma) | | n | | | |
| | Prothrombin ratio | | n-↑ | | | |
| | Transaminase (plasma) | | n-↑ | n-↑ | n-↑ | |
| | **Vitamin A (plasma)** | | **↓-n** | **↓-n** | **↓-n** | |
| | **Vitamin D (plasma)** | | **↓-n** | **↓-n** | **↓-n** | |
| | **Vitamin E (plasma)** | | **↓-n** | **↓-n** | **↓-n** | |

**Table 56.10** Bile acid-CoA ligase deficiency

| System | Symptoms and Biomarkers | Neonatal (birth–1 month) | Infancy (1–18 months) | Childhood (1.5–11 years) | Adolescence (11–16 years) | Adulthood (>16 years) |
|---|---|---|---|---|---|---|
| Digestive | Cholestasis | ± | | | | |
| | **Jaundice** | ± | | | | |
| Other | **Bridging fibrosis** | ± | | | | |
| Laboratory findings | **Bilirubin, conjugated (plasma)** | **n-↑** | | | | |
| | **Transaminase (plasma)** | **n-↑** | | | | |
| | γ-glutamyl transpeptidase, GGT (plasma) | n | | | | |
| | **ESI-MS, Unamidated bile acids (m/z 391,407,471,487,567,583)-negative** | ↑ | ↑ | | | |
| | *SLC27A5* **gene** | + | + | + | + | + |

Only two siblings with BACS deficiency have been described (Chong et al. 2012). One sibling has remained asymptomatic. The symptomatic sibling also had a homozygous mutation in the gene encoding the bile salt export pump (BSEP)

## Reference Values

Traditionally, urine cholanoid profiles measured by GC-MS were used to investigate a possible bile acid biosynthesis defect. When abnormal metabolites were found, follow-up GC-MS analyses were performed in plasma and/or urine with or without chemical/enzymatic deconjugation to confirm the findings. For details about these procedures, we refer the reader to the previous version of this book, Chapter 34 (Lemonde et al. 2014). Given the established and general use of bile acid analysis by (UPLC)-ESI-MS, we focus on this technique for the diagnosis of bile acid disorders.

As the solubility of the (accumulating) bile acid metabolite greatly determines in which body fluids they are best analyzed, we advise the analysis of cholanoid profiles = bile acid analysis in both plasma (qualitative and quantitative) and urine (qualitative) as this yields the best diagnostic result. Depending on the abnormal metabolites found, MS/MS can be performed to help confirm peak identities by parent/daughter analyses, e.g., m/z 74 for glycine conjugates, m/z 80 for taurine conjugates, m/z 97 for sulfates, and m/z 85 for glucuronides. The advent of high-resolution mass spectrometry with exact mass possibilities, especially with automated fragmentation, will enable better and faster identification of bile acid metabolites, but this equipment is not yet routinely used for diagnostics (Vaz and Ferdinandusse 2017). Anticipating this for the near future, we have included monoisotopic masses in Table below.

Quantitative reference values for bile acid profiles—routine for plasma but less relevant for urine—vary between laboratories as standardization of bile acid measurements is not yet in place and few laboratories offer this service. We therefore chose to concentrate on the presence/absence of metabolites instead of listing quantitative reference and pathological values. For quantitative bile acids/salts in plasma, laboratories generally provide method- and population-specific reference ranges.

Bile acids, bile acid conjugates, and bile alcohols found in urine and plasma of normal and cholestatic[a] individuals by ESI-MS

| Nominal mass | Monoisotopic mass | Compound name | Urine normal | Urine cholestasis | Plasma normal | Plasma cholestasis |
|---|---|---|---|---|---|---|
| 391 | 391,2885 | Dihydroxy-cholanoic acids (e.g., chenodeoxycholic acid) | | ± | | ± |
| 407 | 407,2803 | Trihydroxy-cholanoic acids (e.g., cholic acid) | | ± | | ± |
| 444 | 444,2755 | 7α-Hydroxy-3-oxo-4-cholenoic acid **glycine** | | ± | | |
| 448 | 448,3069 | Dihydroxy-cholanoic acids (e.g., chenodeoxycholic acid, deoxycholic acid) **glycine** | ± | ±/↑ | ± | ↑ |
| 453 | 453,2316 | 3β-Hydroxy-5-cholenoic acid **sulfate** | | ± | | |
| 464 | 464,3018 | Trihydroxy-cholanoic acids **glycine** (e.g., cholic acid) | ± | ±/↑ | ± | ↑ |
| 471 | 471,2422 | Dihydroxy-cholanoic acid **sulfate** | | ± | | |
| 480 | 480,2967 | Tetrahydroxy-cholanoic acids **glycine** | ± | ±/↑ | ± | ±/↑ |
| 494 | 494,2582 | 7α-Hydroxy-3-oxo-4-cholenoic acid **taurine** | | ± | | |
| 498 | 498,2895 | Dihydroxy-cholanoic acids (chenodeoxycholic acid) **taurine** | ± | ±/↑ | ± | ↑ |
| 510 | 510,2531 | 7α,12α-Dihydroxy-3-oxo-4-cholenoic acid **taurine** | ± | ± | | |
| 514 | 514,2844 | Trihydroxy-cholanoic acids (cholic acid) **taurine** | ± | ±/↑ | ± | ↑ |
| 528 | 528,2637 | Dihydroxy-cholanoic acids (e.g., chenodeoxycholic acid) **glycine** and **sulfate** | ± | ±/↑ | | ±/↑ |
| 530 | 530,2793 | Tetrahydroxy-cholanoic acids **taurine** | ± | ±/↑ | | ±/↑ |
| 567 | 567,3175 | Dihydroxy-cholanoic acids **glucuronide** | | ± | | |
| 583 | 583,3124 | Trihydroxy-cholanoic acids **glucuronide** | | ± | | |
| 611 | 611,3801 | 5β-Cholestanetetrol **glucuronide** | ± | ± | | |
| 613 | 613,3593 | 27-nor-5β-Cholestanepentol **glucuronide** | ±/↑ | ± | | |
| 625 | 625,3593 | 5β-Cholestenepentol **glucuronide** | ± | ± | | |
| 627 | 627,3750 | 5β-Cholestanepentol **glucuronide** | ±/↑ | ± | | |
| 643 | 643,3699 | 5β-Cholestanehexol **glucuronide** | ± | ± | | |
| Blank | | Low/not found | | | | |
| ↓ | | Decreased | | | | |
| ± | | (can be) present | | | | |
| ±/↑ | | Moderate/increased | | | | |
| ↑ | | Increased | | | | |

[a]Cholestasis is defined here as hypercholemia (as seen in the laboratory analysis) and can therefore have different clinical etiologies. In cholestatic young children, monohydroxylated species of primary bile acids (m/z 480 and m/z 530) can be more abundant than the primary acids themselves

## Pathological Values

Table 'Bile acids, bile salts, and bile alcohols found in urine and plasma of patients with bile acid synthesis disorders as analyzed by ESI-MS' shows bile acid metabolite changes in both plasma and urine for different bile acid synthesis disorders. In general, most metabolite changes are observed both in urine and plasma where, depending on the solubility and renal excretion of the accumulating metabolites, these can be more predominant in urine or plasma. If relevant, this is indicated. Depending on the disorder, the profile can vary considerably and in some disorders may even be without obvious abnormalities. *CYP7A1* deficiency (56.1), for example, is not in table 'Bile acids, bile salts, and bile alcohols found in urine and plasma of patients with bile acid synthesis disorders as analyzed by ESI-MS' as a normal cholanoid profile is observed, except that possibly relatively more CDCA than CA is present because of upregulation of the CDCA production via the acidic/alternative pathway.

## Diagnostic Flowcharts

Bile acid synthesis defects should be considered, and screened for, in all patients with unexplained jaundice or cholestasis, hepatitis, liver fibrosis or cirrhosis, gallstones, deficiencies in fat-soluble vitamins (e.g., rickets or bleeding problems), hypercholesterolemia, tendon xanthomas, chronic diarrhea or steatorrhea, cataracts, and unexplained neurological disease (e.g., ataxia, spastic paraplegia, neuropathy, cognitive decline, epilepsy). Screening for bile acid synthesis defects should especially, but not exclusively, be considered in patients with cholestasis with low to normal γGT, or low to normal total bile acids. Also patients with genetic variants in the bile acid synthesis pathway genes, detected during, e.g., whole exome and whole genome sequencing, should be screened/confirmed biochemically. Biochemical screening for bile acid synthesis defects is performed in both urine and plasma, preferably using (UPLC-)ESI-MS. For interpretation of the results, see tables 'Plasma cholestanol concentration and % cholestanol', Bile acids, bile acid conjugates, and bile alcohols found in urine and plasma of normal and cholestatica individuals by ESI-MS and 'Bile acids, bile acid conjugates, and bile alcohols found in urine and plasma of normal and cholestatica individuals by ESI-MS'.

Plasma cholestanol concentration and % cholestanol[a]

| | Age < 100 days | Age > 100 days | Cholestatic |
|---|---|---|---|
| Cholestanol (μmol/l) | 2.8–19 | 3.5–10 | Can be elevated |
| % Cholestanol[b] | 0.12–0.72 | 0.1–0.28 | Normal |

[a]Reference values indicative only
[b]Cholestanol concentration/cholesterol concentration * 100%

## Specimen Collection

| Test | Conditions | Material | Handling |
|---|---|---|---|
| Plasma cholanoid profile | No bile acid therapy | Plasma/ serum 0.2–1.0 ml | Ambient temp. 12 h, 4 °C for 48 h, −20 °C for >6 months |
| Urine cholanoid profile | No bile acid therapy | Spot urine ≥0.5 ml | As above |
| Plasma cholestanol | No bile acid therapy | Plasma/ serum 0.2–1.0 ml | As above |

## Prenatal Diagnosis and DNA Testing

Routine specific DNA testing for bile acid biosynthesis defects is not widely available, but the underlying genetic basis can be identified with next-generation sequencing techniques. Now that these NGS techniques become more available, it is likely that the number of patients identified with a bile acid biosynthesis defect will increase. Prenatal diagnosis can be done using genetic analysis.

Bile acids, bile salts, and bile alcohols found in urine and plasma of patients with bile acid synthesis disorders as analyzed by ESI-MS

| Nominal mass | Monoisotopic mass | Compound name | 56.2 *HSD3B7* [a] 3β-HSOR | 56.3 *AKR1D1* [b] 5β-reductase | 56.4 *CYP7B1* [c] Oxysterol-7α-hydroxylase | 56.5 *CYP27A1* [d] Sterol 27-hydroxylase | 56.6 *ABCD3* PMP70 | 56.7 *AMACR* [e] α-Methylacyl-CoA racemase | 56.8 *ACOX2* Acyl-CoA oxidase 2 | 56.9 *BAAT* BA-CoA:amino acid N-acyltransferase | 56.10 *SLC27A5* BA-CoA ligase |
|---|---|---|---|---|---|---|---|---|---|---|---|
| 389 | 389,2697 | Dihydroxy-cholenoic acid | ±/↑ | | | | | | | | |
| 391 | 391,2885 | Dihydroxy-cholanoic acids (e.g., chenodeoxycholic acid) | ↓ | ↓ | | ↓ | | | | ↑ | ↑ |
| 405 | 405,2646 | Trihydroxy-cholenoic acids, 3β,7α,12α-trihydroxy-5-cholenoic acid | ±/↑ | | | | | | | | |
| 407 | 407,2803 | Trihydroxy-cholanoic acids (e.g., cholic acid) | ↓ | ↓ | | ↓ | | | | ↑ | ↑ |
| 430 | 430,2963 | 3β-Hydroxy-5-cholenoic acid **glycine** | | | ±/↑ | | | | | | |
| 431 | 431,3169 | 3β,7α-Dihydroxy-cholestenoic acid | ↑ | | | | | | | | |
| 433 | 433,3323 | Dihydroxy-cholestanoic acid (e.g., DHCA) | | | | | ±/↑ | ±/↑ | ±/↑ | | |
| 444 | 444,2755 | 7α-Hydroxy-3-oxo-4-cholenoic acid **glycine** | | ±/↑ | | | | | | | |
| 446 | 446,2912 | 3β,7α-Dihydroxy-5-cholenoic acid **glycine** | ±/↑ | | | | | | | | |
| 447 | 447,3116 | 3β,7α,12α-Trihydroxy-cholestenoic acid | ± | | | | | | | | |
| 448 | 448,3069 | Dihydroxy-cholanoic acids (e.g., chenodeoxycholic acid, deoxycholic acid) **glycine** | ↓ | ↓ | | ↓ | | | ↓ | ↓ | ↓ |
| 449 | 449,3273 | Trihydroxy-cholestanoic acid (e.g., THCA) | | | | | ±/↑ | ±/↑ | ±/↑ | | |
| 453 | 453,2316 | 3β-Hydroxy-5-cholenoic acid **sulfate** | | | ±/↑ | | | | | | |
| 460 | 460,2705 | 7α,12α-Dihydroxy-3-oxo-4-cholenoic acid **glycine** | | ↑ | | | | | | | |
| 462 | 462,2861 | 3β,7α,12α-Trihydroxy-5-cholenoic acid **glycine** | ↑ | | | | | | | | |
| 464 | 464,3018 | Trihydroxy-cholanoic acids **glycine** (e.g., cholic acid) | ↓ | ↓ | | ↓ | | | ↓ | ↓ | ↓ |
| 465 | 465,3222 | Tetrahydroxy-cholestanoic acid (e.g., OH-THCA, varanic acid) | | | | | ±/↑ | ±/↑ | ±/↑ | | |
| 469 | 469,2265 | 3β,7α-Dihydroxy-5-cholenoic acid **sulfate** | ↑ | | | | | | | | |

| | | | | | | | | | | | |
|---|---|---|---|---|---|---|---|---|---|---|---|
| 471 | 471,2422 | Dihydroxy-cholanoic acid **sulfate** | | | | | | | | ±/↑ | ±/↑ |
| 472 | 472,3432 | 3β-Hydroxy-5-cholestanoic acid **glycine** | | | ±/↑ | | | | | | |
| 480 | 480,2789 | 3β-Hydroxy-5-cholenoic acid **taurine** | | | ±/↑ | | | | | | |
| 485 | 485,2215 | 3β,7α,12α-Trihydroxy-5-cholenoic acid **sulfate** | ±/↑ | | | | | | | | |
| 487 | 487,2371 | Trihydroxy-cholanoic acid **sulfate** | | | | | | | | ±/↑ | ±/↑ |
| 490 | 490,3538 | Dihydroxy-cholestanoic acid (e.g., DHCA) **glycine** | | | | | | ± | | | |
| 494 | 494,2582 | 7α-Hydroxy-3-oxo-4-cholenoic acid **taurine** | | ±/↑ | | | | | | | |
| 498 | 498,2895 | Dihydroxy-cholanoic acids (chenodeoxycholic acid) **taurine** | ↓ | ↓ | | ↓ | | | ↓ | | |
| 506 | 506,3487 | Trihydroxy-cholestanoic acid (e.g., THCA) **glycine** | | | | | | ± | | | |
| 507 | 507,3327 | C29-dicarboxylic acid | | | | | ±/↑ | ±/↑ | ±/↑ | | |
| 510 | 510,2531 | 7α,12α-Dihydroxy-3-oxo-4-cholenoic acid **taurine** | | ↑ | | | | | | | |
| 510 | 510,2531 | 3β-Hydroxy-5-cholenoic acid glycine and **sulfate** | | | ±/↑ | | | | | | |
| 514 | 514,2844 | Trihydroxy-cholanoic acids (cholic acid) **taurine** | ↓ | ↓ | | ↓ | | | ↓ | ↓ | ↓ |
| 522 | 522,3259 | 3β-Hydroxy-5-cholestanoic acid **taurine** | | | ±/↑ | | | | | | |
| 526 | 526,2480 | 3β,7α-Dihydroxy-5-cholenoic acid **glycine** and **sulfate** | ↑ | | | | | | | | |
| 540 | 540,3364 | Dihydroxy-cholestanoic acid (e.g., DHCA) **taurine** | | | | | | ± | | | |
| 542 | 542,2429 | 3β,7α,12α-Trihydroxy-5-cholenoic acid **glycine** and **sulfate** | ↑ | | | | | | | | |
| 552 | 552,3000 | 7α,12α-Dihydroxy-3-oxo-4-cholestenoic acid **taurine** | | ± | | | | | | | |
| 556 | 556,3313 | Trihydroxy-cholestanoic acid (e.g., THCA) **taurine** | | | | | ±/↑ | ±/↑ | ±/↑ | | |
| 567 | 567,3175 | Dihydroxy-cholanoic acids **glucuronide** | | | | | | | | ±/↑ | ±/↑ |

(continued)

(continued)

| Nominal mass | Monoisotopic mass | Compound name | 56.2 *HSD3B7* [a] 3β-HSOR | 56.3 *AKR1D1* [b] 5β-reductase | 56.4 *CYP7B1* [c] Oxysterol-7α-hydroxylase | 56.5 *CYP27A1* [d] Sterol 27-hydroxylase | 56.6 *ABCD3* PMP70 | 56.7 *AMACR* [e] α-Methylacyl-CoA racemase | 56.8 *ACOX2* Acyl-CoA oxidase 2 | 56.9 *BAAT* BA-CoA:amino acid N-acyltransferase | 56.10 *SLC27A5* BA-CoA ligase |
|---|---|---|---|---|---|---|---|---|---|---|---|
| 572 | 572,3263 | Tetrahydroxy-cholestanoic acids (e.g., OH-THCA) **taurine** | | | | | ±/↑ | ±/↑ | ±/↑ | | |
| 583 | 583,3124 | Trihydroxy-cholanoic acids **glucuronide** | | | | | | | | ±/↑ | ±/↑ |
| 609 | 609,3644 | 5β-Cholestenetetrol **glucuronide** | | | | /↑ | | | | | |
| 611 | 611,3801 | 5β-Cholestanetetrol **glucuronide** | | | | ↑ | | | | | |
| 625 | 625,3593 | 5β-Cholestenepentol **glucuronide** | | | | ±/↑ | | | | | |
| 627 | 627,3750 | 5β-Cholestanepentol **glucuronide** | | | | ↑ | | | | | |
| 641 | 641,3543 | 5β-Cholestenehexol **glucuronide** | | | | ±/↑ | | | | | |
| 643 | 643,3699 | 5β-Cholestanehexol **glucuronide** | | | | ±/↑ | | | | | |
| 659 | 659,3648 | 5β-Cholestaneheptol **glucuronide** | | | | ±/↑ | | | | | |
| Blank | | Low/not found | | | | | | | | | |
| ↓ | | Decreased | | | | | | | | | |
| ± | | (can be) present | | | | | | | | | |
| ±/↑ | | Moderate/increased | | | | | | | | | |
| ↑ | | Increased | | | | | | | | | |

[a]56.2 Urine is a better specimen than plasma; biomarker peaks are more pronounced in urine

[b]56.3 Urine is a suitable specimen; plasma less so but corroborates the urine results. Liver disease can mimic a 5β-reductase deficiency profile; however, in these cases, the primary bile acids are usually elevated reflecting cholestasis. Because of the existence of a 5α-reductase, the accumulating C27–3-oxo-Δ4 steroids can be converted to so-called allo-(5α)-bile acids which can account for more than 20% of the total (Setchell et al. 1988). Because the allo-bile acids are isobaric (same molecular mass) to their corresponding natural (5β) bile acids, the diagnosis of 5β-reductase can be missed. When in doubt, perform genetic analysis of the *AKR1D1* gene

[c]56.4 27-Hydroxycholesterol and 25-hydroxycholesterol are additional biomarkers that are grossly elevated (not many laboratories measure these); m/z 453 and m/z 510 are more prominent in urine

[d]56.5 Profile in urine is shifted to more hydroxylated bile alcohol glucuronides (higher m/z). In plasma, m/z 611 (cholestanetetrol glucuronide) is prominent, and m/z 613 is much lower, which in non-CTX liver disease is higher than m/z 611. In urine, m/z 627 (cholestanepentol glucuronide) is the most predominant bile alcohol glucuronide. An additional biomarker for CTX is plasma cholestanol and % cholestanol (from cholesterol). Both are elevated when compared to reference values mentioned. Especially in young children, cholestanol concentration is only slightly elevated, if at all. Bile alcohol glucuronides either in plasma or urine are superior biomarkers for CTX. In addition to these secondary metabolites in CTX, primary metabolites that accumulate are 7α-hydroxycholesterol, 7α-hydroxy-cholest-4-en-3-one, and 7α,12α-dihydroxy-cholest-4-en-3-one

[e]56.7 Sole accumulation of the 25R-isomers of DHCA and THCA. R/S species can usually be separated on UPLC-MS method if appropriate standards are available

## Treatment

In general, standard medical or surgical care is indicated in case of gallstones, cataracts, and epilepsy. Substitution of fat-soluble vitamins A, D, E, and K is indicated in cases of symptomatic, proven deficiency. Patients developing acute liver failure or end-stage liver disease need to be evaluated for liver transplantation.

### Bile Acid Supplementation

Supplementation with CA and/or CDCA has a stabilizing or proven curative effect in several bile acid synthesis defects; in other defects, there are indications of beneficial effects. In general, UDCA supplementation does not have beneficial effects in the bile acid synthesis defects, as it does not exert negative feedback on the first step of the synthesis cascade, at the level of cholesterol 7α-hydroxylase. Therefore, UDCA does not inhibit the formation of bile acid intermediates and derivatives that are considered the source of pathology in these diseases. In addition, combining UDCA with CA or CDCA probably competes for the ileal reuptake and enterohepatic recirculation of CA or CDCA and could thus reduce the effectivity of CA/CDCA supplementation (Heubi et al. 2018). Finally, UDCA appears to be an FXR antagonist and therefore does not suppress bile acid synthesis (Mueller et al. 2015). After initiation of treatment with CDCA or CA, patients should be monitored with liver enzymes and clinical-neurological examination until the bile acid analyses normalize and remain normal. Bile acid therapy is lifelong.

### CTX (56.5) Treatment

Most available data using primary bile acid therapy, accumulated over decades, is for CDCA treatment in the context of CTX. The natural history of CTX is progressive neurodegeneration, most probably due to neurotoxicity of the accumulation of the by-product cholestanol. Long-term treatment with CDCA (10–15 mg/kg/day with a maximum of 750 mg/day in adults) normalizes plasma cholestanol concentrations within months, reduces the urinary excretion of bile alcohols, and stabilizes or improves the neurological symptoms; xanthomas disappear during treatment. Early initiation of therapy improves the outcome (Amador M del et al. 2018; Yahalom et al. 2013; Stelten et al. 2019). In a retrospective Japanese study, the percent decrease of cholestanol by combination therapy of CDCA and statin (59.3%) was not superior to that by CDCA monotherapy (77.6%), and so the efficacy of statin add-on therapy to CDCA remains uncertain (Sekijima et al. 2018). Low-density lipoprotein (LDL) apheresis reduces cholestanol, but the longer-term clinical efficacy is unclear (Berginer and Salen 1994).

Adverse outcomes have been described for the pregnancies and children of untreated CTX mothers, without providing final clarity on the teratogenicity or toxicity of the disease or cholestanol concentrations, nevertheless (Berginer et al. 1988). Developmental toxicity studies in rats, hamsters, and primates showed an absence of teratogenic effects, but CDCA treatment of pregnant rhesus monkeys and baboons (at 5–120 mg/kg/day for rhesus monkey; at 18–38 mg/kg/day for baboons) produced liver pathology in the developing fetus. Pathological effects on adrenals and kidneys were also seen in rhesus monkey fetuses. Maternal effects in the rhesus monkeys, but not baboons, included diarrhea, emesis, weight loss, and reduction in food consumption (Leadiant 2017). According to GeneReviews, it is advised to not interrupt CDCA treatment during pregnancy (Federico et al. 2016). Additional data on the risk of CTX for the fetus, and the risk of CDCA treatment during pregnancy, will be necessary to determine which is preferable.

### Bile Acid Treatment in Other Bile Acid Synthesis Defects

Oral bile acid therapy appears safe; most reported adverse effects are liver toxicity (in some cases attributed to overdosing CDCA) and diarrhea. The success of CDCA and CA for patients with multiple defects in the bile acid biosynthetic pathway is well documented (Clayton 2011). The two most prevalent bile acid synthesis defects, according to a survey in 21 countries, are 3β-hydroxy-Δ5-C27-steroid oxidoreductase (3β-HSOR) deficiency (56.2) ($n$ = 55) and Δ4-3-oxosteroid 5β-reductase deficiency (56.3) ($n$ = 8) (Jahnel et al. 2017). In both these diseases, convincing long-term CA treatment effects at a dose of 15 mg/kg/day have been reported (3β-HSOR, 56.2: $n$ = 13; 5β-reductase, 56.3: $n$ = 2) (Matarazzo et al. 2018). Hepatitis, cholestasis, and even fibrosis/cirrhosis were reversed by CA treatment. Patients grew to adulthood in good health, while the natural history of the disease is an evolution to liver failure and transplantation. Safety of CA treatment during pregnancy seems good, given that ten uneventful pregnancies in five mothers on CA were reported (Matarazzo et al. 2018).

CA treatment failures have been reported in patients with oxysterol 7α-hydroxylase deficiency (CYP7B1) deficiency (SPG5, 56.5), while combination therapy with CDCA and statins appeared beneficial (Marelli et al. 2018).

Very few systematic data are available for the deficiencies of PMP70/ABCD3 (56.6), AMACR (56.7), and ACOX2 (56.8). In AMACR deficiency, primary bile acid therapy with CA is effective in normalizing liver enzymes and preventing the onset of neurologic symptoms in the infant, coupled with dietary restriction of phytanic acid and pristanic acids, which are necessary to prevent neurotoxicity from their accumulation in the brain (Heubi et al. 2018). In view of the rarity of PMP70/ABCD3 ($n = 1$) and ACOX2 ($n = 3$) deficiency, it is hard to make treatment recommendations for these disorders.

A notable exception to the effectivity of CA and CDCA supplementation is the amidation defects (56.9 and 56.10). As conjugation of the primary bile acids CA and CDCA with glycine or taurine is defective in these diseases, they are only responsive to treatment with conjugated bile acids, as was shown for treatment with glycocholic acid (glycine conjugated CA) recently (Heubi et al. 2015).

## References


Amador M del M, Masingue M, Debs R, Lamari F, Perlbarg V, Roze E, Degos B, Mochel F. Treatment with chenodeoxycholic acid in cerebrotendinous xanthomatosis: clinical, neurophysiological, and quantitative brain structural outcomes. J Inherit Metab Dis. 2018;41:799–807.

Berginer VM, Carmi R, Salen G. Pregnancy in women with cerebrotendinous xanthomatosis (CTX): high risk condition for fetus and newborn infant? Am J Med Genet. 1988;31:11–6.

Berginer VM, Salen G. LDL-apheresis cannot be recommended for treatment of cerebrotendinous xanthomatosis. J Neurol Sci. 1994;121:229–32.

Chong CPK, Mills PB, McClean P, Gissen P, Bruce C, Stahlschmidt J, Knisely AS, Clayton PT. Bile acid-CoA ligase deficiency-a new inborn error of bile acid metabolism. J Inherit Metab Dis. 2012;35:521–30.

Clayton PT. Disorders of bile acid synthesis. J Inherit Metab Dis. 2011;34:593–604.

Federico A, Dotti MT, Gallus GN (2016) Cerebrotendinous Xanthomatosis. GeneReviews®.

Ferdinandusse S, Denis S, van Roermund CWTT, Preece MA, Koster J, Ebberink MS, Waterham HR, Wanders RJAA. A novel case of ACOX2 deficiency leads to recognition of a third human peroxisomal acyl-CoA oxidase. Biochim Biophys Acta. 2018;1864:952–8.

Ferdinandusse S, Jimenez-Sanchez G, Koster J, et al. A novel bile acid biosynthesis defect due to a deficiency of peroxisomal ABCD3. Hum Mol Genet. 2015;24:361–70.

Halilbasic E, Claudel T, Trauner M. Bile acid transporters and regulatory nuclear receptors in the liver and beyond. J Hepatol. 2013;58:155–68.

Heubi JE, Setchell KDR, Bove KE. Inborn errors of bile acid metabolism. Clin Liver Dis. 2018;22:671–87.

Heubi JE, Setchell KDR, Jha P, Buckley D, Zhang W, Rosenthal P, Potter C, Horslen S, Suskind D. Treatment of bile acid amidation defects with glycocholic acid. Hepatology. 2015;61:268–74.

Jahnel J, Zöhrer E, Fischler B, et al. Attempt to determine the prevalence of two inborn errors of primary bile acid synthesis: results of a European survey. J Pediatr Gastroenterol Nutr. 2017;64:864–8.

Leadiant (2017) Chenodeoxycholic acid Leadiant : EPAR—Product Information. https://www.ema.europa.eu/documents/product-information/chenodeoxycholic-acid-leadiant-epar-product-information_en.pdf.

Lemonde HA, Gissen P, Clayton PT. Disorders of bile acid synthesis and biliary transport. In: Blau N, Duran M, Gibson KM, Dionisi Vici C, editors. Physician's Guid. To diagnosis, treat. Follow. Inherit. Metab. Dis. Berlin Heidelberg: Springer; 2014. p. 555–75.

Marelli C, Lamari F, Rainteau D, et al. Plasma oxysterols: biomarkers for diagnosis and treatment in spastic paraplegia type 5. Brain. 2018;141:72–84.

Matarazzo L, Myara A, Jacquemin E, et al. Cholic acid for primary bile acid synthesis defects: a life-saving therapy allowing a favorable outcome in adulthood. Orphanet J Rare Dis. 2018;13:1–8.

Monte MJ, Alonso-Peña M, Briz O, Herraez E, Berasain C, Argemi J, Prieto J, Marin JJGG. ACOX2 deficiency: an inborn error of bile acid synthesis identified in an adolescent with persistent hypertransaminasemia. J Hepatol. 2017;66:581–8.

Mueller M, Thorell A, Claudel T, et al. Ursodeoxycholic acid exerts farnesoid X receptor-antagonistic effects on bile acid and lipid metabolism in morbid obesity. J Hepatol. 2015;62:1398–404.

Pullinger CR, Eng C, Salen G, et al. Human cholesterol 7α-hydroxylase (CYP7A1) deficiency has a hypercholesterolemic phenotype. J Clin Invest. 2002;110:109–17.

Russell DW. Fifty years of advances in bile acid synthesis and metabolism. J Lipid Res. 2009;50:S120–5.

Sekijima Y, Koyama S, Yoshinaga T, Koinuma M, Inaba Y. Nationwide survey on cerebrotendinous xanthomatosis in Japan. J Hum Genet. 2018;63:271–80.

Setchell KDR, Suchy FJ, Welsh MB, Zimmer-Nechemias L, Heubi J, Balistreri WF. Δ4-3-oxosteroid 5β-reductase deficiency described in identical twins with neonatal hepatitis. A new inborn error in bile acid synthesis. J Clin Invest. 1988;82:2148–57.

Stelten BML, Huidekoper HH, van de Warrenburg BPC, Brilstra EH, Hollak CEM, Haak HR, Kluijtmans LAJ, Wevers RA, Verrips A. Long-term treatment effect in cerebrotendinous xanthomatosis depends on age at treatment start. Neurology. 2019;92:e83–95.

Vaz FM, Ferdinandusse S. Bile acid analysis in human disorders of bile acid biosynthesis. Mol Asp Med. 2017;56:10–24.

Vilarinho S, Sari S, Mazzacuva F, et al. *ACOX2* deficiency: a disorder of bile acid synthesis with transaminase elevation, liver fibrosis, ataxia, and cognitive impairment. Proc Natl Acad Sci. 2016;113:11289–93.

Yahalom G, Tsabari R, Molshatzki N, Ephraty L, Cohen H, Hassin-Baer S. Neurological outcome in cerebrotendinous xanthomatosis treated with chenodeoxycholic acid: early versus late diagnosis. Clin Neuropharmacol. 2013;36:78–83.

# Part VII

# Disorders of Tetrapyrroles

# Disorders of Heme Metabolism

# 57

Ulrich Stölzel, Ilja Kubisch, Thomas Stauch, and Detlef Schuppan

## Contents




## Summary

Porphyrias are metabolic disorders of the heme biosynthesis. The location of the deficient enzyme within the heme biosynthetic pathway determines the pattern of the accumulated porphyrin precursors and/or porphyrins. Clinically, they can be differentiated into acute and non-acute porphyrias. Acute hepatic porphyrias (AHP) are characterized by overproduction of probably neurotoxic porphyrin precursors and porphyrins. Acute intermittent porphyria (AIP), variegate porphyria (VP), hereditary coproporphyria (HCP), and Doss porphyria (ADP) belong to this group of metabolic disorders. The clinical presentation of acute hepatic porphyrias includes abdominal, psychiatric, neurological, and cardiovascular symptoms. They are diagnosed by an at least fourfold elevated urinary excretion of 5-aminolevulinic acid (ALA) and porphobilinogen (PBG) (except for ADP and lead poisoning (LP)). Besides symptomatic therapy with non-porphyrinogenic drugs, the combination of electrolyte correction, intensive monitoring, intravenous caloric supply (mainly glucose), and heme is established for treatment. Recently, in the Phase 3 ENVISION study in patients with AHP, givosiran, an RNAi therapeutic which targets liver mRNA encoding ALAS1 to reduce 5-ALA/PBG, ameliorates attacks and clinical manifestations.



U. Stölzel (✉) · I. Kubisch
Center of Internal Medicine II, Gastroenterology, Hepatology, Endocrinology, Metabolic Disorders, Oncology, Saxony Porphyria Center, Klinikum Chemnitz gGmbH, Chemnitz, Germany
e-mail: dr.stoelzel@porphyrie.de

T. Stauch
Department of Clinical Chemistry and Toxicology, German Competence Center for Porphyria Diagnosis and Consultation, MVZ Labor PD Dr. Volkmann und Kollegen GbR, Karlsruhe, Germany

D. Schuppan
Institute of Translational Immunology and Research Center for Immune Therapy, University Medical Center, Johannes Gutenberg University, Mainz, Germany

Division of Gastroenterology, Beth Israel Deaconess Medical Center, Harvard Medical School, Boston, MA, USA






N. Blau et al. (eds.), *Physician's Guide to the Diagnosis, Treatment, and Follow-Up of Inherited Metabolic Diseases*,
https://doi.org/10.1007/978-3-030-67727-5_57

Non-acute types are porphyria cutanea tarda (PCT), hepatoerythropoietic porphyria (HEP), erythropoietic protoporphyria (EPP), X-linked protoporphyria (XLP), and congenital erythropoietic porphyria (CEP). Accumulated porphyrins cause photosensitivity of the skin and in some cases severe liver damage. X-linked protoporphyria (XLP) represents a new type of protoporphyria, with 5-aminolevulinic acid synthase 2 gain of function leading to high concentrations of free protoporphyrin IX (PPIX). Treatment of PCT is based on iron depletion, the use of hydroxychloroquine (HCQ), and, in case of chronic hepatitis C virus (HCV) infection, antiviral therapy. Patients with EPP or XLP profit from treatment with an analogue of α-melanocyte-stimulating hormone that reduces sunlight sensitivity and inflammation. Further therapeutic developments directly address dysfunctional steps of the heme biosynthetic pathway.

## Introduction

Porphyrias are a heterogeneous group of metabolic disorders, which are caused by a range enzyme deficiencies or defects due to mutations in genes along the heme synthesis pathway (Puy et al. 2010; Bonkovsky et al. 2013; Bissell et al. 2017; Stölzel et al. 2019) (Fig. 57.1). The majority of patients are carriers of heterozygous mutations. Some patients carry homozygous or compound heterozygous mutations resulting in a reduced enzyme activity. As customary, autosomal dominant disorders porphyrias can vary in penetrance and phenotype; moreover, there are considerable interactions between genetic and environmental factors. Moreover, they can result from combinations of genetic alterations (Lenglet et al. 2018) . In addition, there are considerable interactions between genetic and environmental factors.

PCT is the most common porphyria. Hepatic uroporphyrinogen decarboxylase (UROD) is reduced in all cases with PCT (acquired type 1 or familial type 2). Thus, a cross-sectional registry study comprising 4653 patients showed prevalence ratios of 91/26/9/4/2/1 for PCT/AIP/EPP/VP/HCP/CEP (Stölzel et al. 2019). Among AHPs, AIP is the most frequent type, followed by VP, HCP, and a rare autosomal recessive acute hepatic porphyria ADP (synonym: porphobilinogen synthase defect porphyria, Doss porphyria) which is biochemically very similar to lead poisoning (LP) (Doss et al. 1979) .

Clinically, acute (AIP, VP, HCP, ADP) and non-acute porphyrias (PCT, HEP, EPP, XLP, CEP) can be differentiated, while pathogenetically hepatic (PCT, HEP, AIP, VP, HCP, ALADP) and erythropoietic (EPP, XLP, CEP) porphyrias form two major groups. Dual porphyrias (biochemical findings of two porphyrias) are rare and have been confirmed by mutation analyses. Increased porphyrin precursors and porphyrins are also found in LP.

The clinical presentation of AHP and LP comprises abdominal, neuropsychiatric, and cardiovascular symptoms and hyponatremia, whereas chronic hepatic and erythropoietic porphyrias present with photodermatosis and occasionally severe liver damage. AHP is not just an "acute" disease as its name implies, but also has chronic manifestations that impact patients' lives (Gouya et al. 2020).

All porphyrias are diagnosed and differentiated by specific biochemical patterns of elevated porphyrins and porphyrin precursors in urine, feces, and blood (Bonkovsky et al. 2013; Bissell et al. 2017; Stölzel et al. 2019). AHPs are characterized by excessive accumulation and excretion of the porphyrin precursors 5-ALA (ADP, LP) or 5-ALA and PBG (AIP, VP, HCP) as well as porphyrins. In patients with PCT, but also in patients with HEP, levels of porphyrins are greatly increased in urine and plasma, with uro- and heptacarboxyporphyrins predominating. Increased levels of metal-free protoporphyrin (>4.500 nmol/l, controls <89 nmol/l) in hemolyzed anticoagulated whole blood confirm the diagnosis of EPP or XLP. Here, patients with XLP display a significantly higher proportion of zinc- to metal-free protoporphyrin (>25%) than patients with EPP (<15%).

Erythropoietic and hepatic porphyrias are genetically determined primary porphyrias, whereas clinically asymptomatic secondary porphyrinurias and porphyrinemias are not due to functional mutations of the heme synthetic pathway but caused by a number of different (e.g., metabolic, hepatic, or hematologic) diseases and dysfunctions.

In tyrosinemia type I, the nonfunctional fumarylacetoacetate hydrolase leads to succinylacetone that inhibits the enzyme ALA dehydratase.

## Nomenclature

| No. | Disorder | Alt name | Abbreviation | Gene symbol | Chromosomal localization | Affected protein | OMIM no. | Inheritance |
|---|---|---|---|---|---|---|---|---|
| 57.1 | X-linked sideroblastic anemia | Erythroid 5-aminolevulinate synthase deficiency | XLSA | *ALAS2* | Xp11.21 | 5-Aminolevulinate synthase 2 | 300751 | XL |
| 57.2 | X-linked protoporphyria | Erythroid 5-aminolevulinate synthase gain of function | XLP | *ALAS2* | Xp11.21 | 5-Aminolevulinate synthase 2 | 300752 | XL |
| 57.3 | 5-Aminolevulinate dehydratase deficiency | Doss porphyria | ADP | *ALAD* | 9q32 | Delta-aminolevulinate dehydratase | 612740 | AR |
| 57.4 | Acute intermittent porphyria | Porphobilinogen deaminase deficiency | AIP | *HMBS* | 11q23.3 | Hydroxymethylbilane synthase | 176000 | AD |
| 57.5 | Congenital erythropoietic porphyria | Uroporphyrinogen III synthase deficiency | CEP | *UROS* | 10q25.2–26.3 | Uroporphyrinogen III synthase | 263700 | AR |
| 57.6 | Porphyria cutanea tarda types I, II and hepatoerythropoietic porphyria | Hepatic uroporphyrinogen decarboxylase deficiency | PCT/HEP | *UROD* | 1p34 | Uroporphyrinogen decarboxylase | 176100 | AD, AR |
| 57.7 | Hereditary coproporphyria | Coproporphyrinogen oxidase deficiency | HCP | *CPOX* | 3q12 | Coproporphyrinogen oxidase | 121300 | AD |
| 57.8 | Porphyria variegata | Protoporphyrinogen oxidase deficiency | VP | *PPOX* | 1q22-q23 | Protoporphyrinogen oxidase | 176200 | AD |
| 57.9 | Erythropoietic protoporphyria | Ferrochelatase deficiency | EPP | *FECH* | 18q21.3 | Ferrochelatase | 177000 | AD |

## Metabolic Pathways

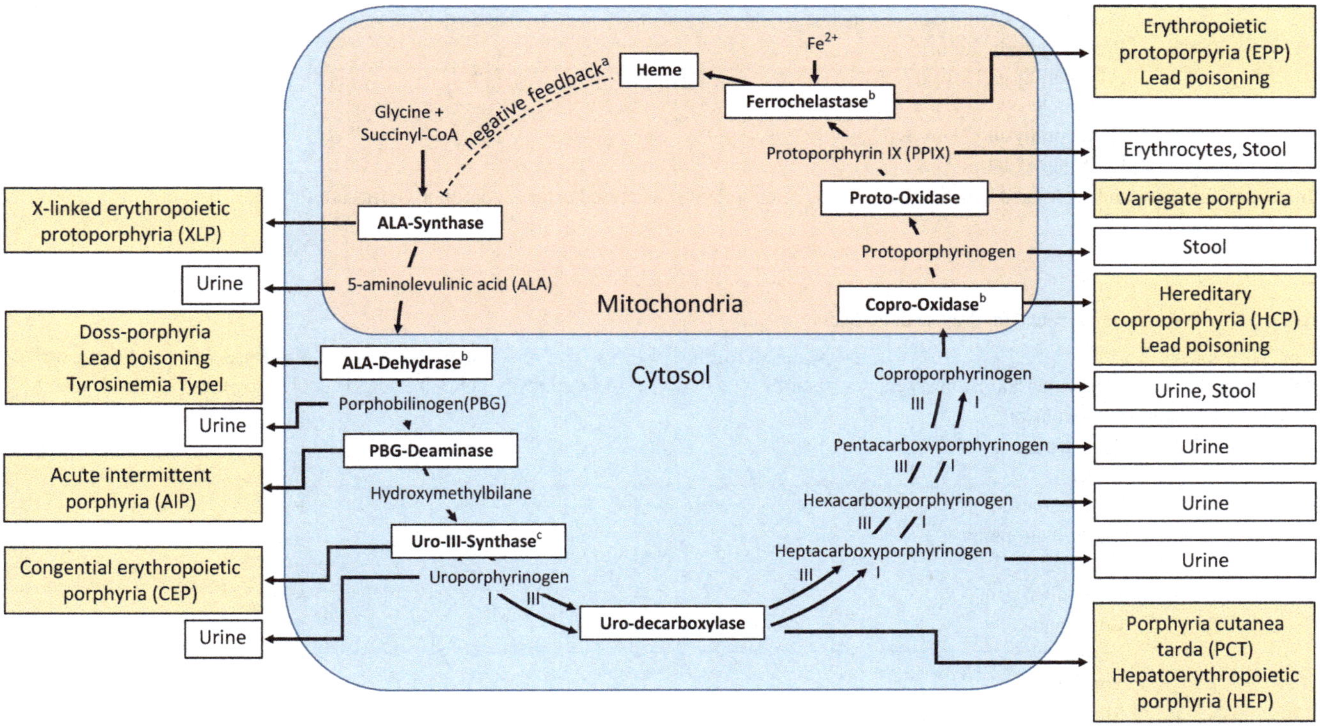


**Fig. 57.1** Localization of characteristic enzyme defects of heme biosynthesis and in porphyrias, lead poisoning, and type I tyrosinemia. The porphyrinogens are excreted after their oxidation to porphyrins. (a) In the liver, the first heme synthetic enzyme ALAS1 is regulated via a negative feedback loop by the end product heme. In contrast, the rate-limiting bone marrow enzyme ALAS2 is regulated by iron and erythropoietin and not by heme. (b) Three enzymes involved in heme biosynthesis are compromised in lead poisoning. (c) The two isomers uroporphyrinogen I and III that are synthesized from hydroxymethylbilane are converted to coproporphyrinogen I and III, respectively. Only isomer III is utilized for heme synthesis. The nonfunctional isomer I is excreted via the hepatobiliary and renal routes in feces and urine, respectively (Modified from Ref. Stölzel et al. 2019)

## Signs and Symptoms

**Table 57.1** X-linked sideroblastic anemia[a]

| System | Symptoms and Biomarkers | Neonatal (birth–1 month) | Infancy (1–18 months) | Childhood (1.5–11 years) | Adolescence (11–16 years) | Adulthood (>16 years) |
|---|---|---|---|---|---|---|
| Hematological | Anemia, microcytic, hypochromic | | | + | + | + |
| | Dimorphism (red blood cells) | | | + | + | + |
| | Sideroblasts (bone marrow) | | | ↑ | ↑ | ↑ |
| Laboratory findings | Delta-ALA synthase (red blood cells) | | | ↓ | ↓ | ↓ |
| | Ferritin (serum) | | | ↑ | ↑ | ↑ |
| | Protoporphyrin-Zn (red blood cells) | | | ↓ | ↓ | ↓ |
| | Transferrin saturation | | | ↑ | ↑ | ↑ |

[a]Note: Other factors and mutations can cause sideroblastic anemias

**Table 57.2** X-linked protoporphyria

| System | Symptoms and Biomarkers | Neonatal (birth–1 month) | Infancy (1–18 months) | Childhood (1.5–11 years) | Adolescence (11–16 years) | Adulthood (>16 years) |
|---|---|---|---|---|---|---|
| Dermatological | Burning sensation after sun exposure | | | + | + | + |
| | Photosensitivity | | | ++ | ++ | ++ |
| Laboratory findings | 5-Aminolevulinic acid (urine) | | | n | n | n |
| | Delta-ALA synthase (red blood cells) | | | ↑ | ↑ | ↑ |
| | Porphyrins, all (urine) | n | n | n[a] | n[a] | n[a] |
| | Protoporphyrin (stool) | | | ± | ± | ± |
| | Protoporphyrin IX (red blood cells) | | | ↑↑↑ | ↑↑↑ | ↑↑↑ |
| | Protoporphyrin IX-Zn (red blood cells) | | | ↑↑ | ↑↑ | ↑↑ |

[a]In case of extensive and prolonged hepatic exposure to protoporphyrin, increased urinary coproporphyrins are found

**Table 57.3** 5-Aminolevulinate dehydratase deficiency

| System | Symptoms and Biomarkers | Neonatal (birth–1 month) | Infancy (1–18 months)[a] | Childhood (1.5–11 years) | Adolescence (11–16 years) | Adulthood (>16 years) |
|---|---|---|---|---|---|---|
| Autonomic system | Hypertension | | | ± | ± | ± |
| Cardiovascular | Tachycardia | | | ± | ± | ± |
| CNS | Coma | | | ± | ± | ± |
| | Hyperesthesia | | | ± | ± | ± |
| | Motor neuropathy | | + | + | + | + |
| | Seizures | | | ± | ± | ± |
| Digestive | Abdominal pain | | + | + | + | + |
| | Constipation | | | ± | ± | ± |
| | Nausea | | + | + | + | + |
| | Vomiting | | + | ± | ± | ± |
| Musculoskeletal | Muscle pain | | | + | + | + |
| Other | Colored red-brown urine | | | + | + | + |

**Table 57.3** (continued)

| System | Symptoms and Biomarkers | Neonatal (birth–1 month) | Infancy (1–18 months)[a] | Childhood (1.5–11 years) | Adolescence (11–16 years) | Adulthood (>16 years) |
|---|---|---|---|---|---|---|
| Laboratory findings | Coproporphyrin III (urine) | | ↑↑↑ | ↑↑↑ | ↑↑↑ | ↑↑↑ |
| | Delta-ALA (urine) | | ↑↑↑ | ↑↑↑ | ↑↑↑ | ↑↑↑ |
| | Delta-ALA dehydratase (red blood cells) | | ↓↓↓ | ↓↓↓ | ↓↓↓ | ↓↓↓ |
| | Fecal porphyrins | | | n-↑ | n-↑ | n-↑ |
| | Free- and zinc protoporphyrin | | ↑ | ↑ | ↑ | ↑ |
| | Porphobilinogen, PBG (urine) | | | n-↑ | n-↑ | n-↑ |
| | Sodium (plasma) | | | ↓-n | ↓-n | ↓-n |
| ALADP deficiency, see also Sect. 21.1 Tyrosinemia type 1 and lead poisoning | | | | | | |

[a]Data not available

**Table 57.4** Acute intermittent porphyria

| System | Symptoms and Biomarkers | Neonatal (birth–1 month) | Infancy (1–18 months) | Childhood (1.5–11 years) | Adolescence (11–16 years) | Adulthood (>16 years) |
|---|---|---|---|---|---|---|
| Autonomic system | Hypertension | | | | + | + |
| Cardiovascular | Tachycardia | | | | + | + |
| CNS | Coma | | | | ± | ± |
| | Hyperesthesia | | | | ± | ± |
| | Motor neuropathy | | | | ± | ± |
| | Seizures | | | | ± | ± |
| Digestive | Abdominal pain | | | | + | + |
| | Constipation | | | | ± | ± |
| | Nausea | | | | ± | ± |
| | Vomiting | | | | ± | ± |
| Musculoskeletal | Muscle pain | | | | + | + |
| Other | Colored red-brown urine | | | | + | + |
| Laboratory findings | Delta-ALA (urine) | | | | ↑↑↑ | ↑↑↑ |
| | Magnesium (plasma) | | | | ↓-n | ↓-n |
| | PBG-deaminase (HMB-synthase) | | | | n-↓ | n-↓ |
| | Porphobilinogen (urine) | | | | ↑↑↑ | ↑↑↑ |
| | Porphyrins, all (urine) | | | | ↑ | ↑ |
| | Sodium (plasma) | | | | ↓-n | ↓-n |

**Table 57.5** Congenital erythropoietic porphyria

| System | Symptoms and Biomarkers | Neonatal (birth–1 month) | Infancy (1–18 months) | Childhood (1.5–11 years) | Adolescence (11–16 years) | Adulthood (>16 years) |
|---|---|---|---|---|---|---|
| Dermatological | Mutilation | | + | + | + | + |
| | Skin blisters | ± | + | + | + | + |
| | Skin fragility | ± | + | + | + | + |
| | Skin scarring | | + | + | + | + |
| Hematological | Anemia, microcytic, hypochromic, hemolytic | ± | + | + | + | + |
| Musculoskeletal | Face disfiguration | | ± | ± | ± | + |
| Other | Colored red-brown urine | + | + | + | + | + |
| Laboratory findings | Porphyrins type I-isomers (plasma) | ↑↑ | ↑↑ | ↑↑ | ↑↑ | ↑↑ |
| | Porphyrins type I-isomers (urine) | ↑↑ | ↑↑ | ↑↑ | ↑↑ | ↑↑ |
| | Porphyrins, all (plasma) | ↑ | ↑↑ | ↑↑ | ↑↑ | ↑↑ |
| | Porphyrins, all (urine) | ↑ | ↑↑ | ↑↑ | ↑↑ | ↑↑ |
| | Uro- and coproporphyrin isomer I (urine/fecal) | ↑↑↑ | ↑↑↑ | ↑↑↑ | ↑↑↑ | ↑↑↑ |

**Table 57.6** Porphyria cutanea tarda type I, II and hepatoerythropoietic porphyria

| System | Symptoms and Biomarkers | Neonatal (birth–1 month) | Infancy (1–18 months) | Childhood (1.5–11 years) | Adolescence (11–16 years) | Adulthood (>15 years) |
|---|---|---|---|---|---|---|
| Dermatological | Skin blisters | | | + | ± | + |
| | Skin fragility | | | + | ± | + |
| Digestive | Liver dysfunction | | | | ± | + |
| Hair | Hypertrichosis | | | ± | ± | ± |
| Other | Colored red-brown urine | | | ± | ± | ± |
| Laboratory findings | Delta-ALA/PBG (urine) | | | n | n | n |
| | Isocoproporphyrin (feces) | | | ↑ | n-↑ | n-↑ |
| | Porphyrins, all (plasma) | | | ↑↑↑ | ↑↑↑ | ↑↑↑ |
| | Porphyrins, all (urine) | | | ↑↑↑ | ↑↑↑ | ↑↑↑ |
| | Porphyrins, heptacarboxy (plasma) | | | ↑↑↑ | ↑↑↑ | ↑↑↑ |
| | Porphyrins, heptacarboxy (urine) | | | ↑↑↑ | ↑↑↑ | ↑↑↑ |
| | Porphyrins, urocarboxy (plasma) | | | ↑↑↑ | ↑↑↑ | ↑↑↑ |
| | Porphyrins, urocarboxy (urine) | | | ↑↑↑ | ↑↑↑ | ↑↑↑ |
| | Uro-decarboxylase | | | ↓-↓↓ | n-↓↓ | n-↓↓ |

**Table 57.7** Hereditary coproporphyria

| System | Symptoms and Biomarkers | Neonatal (birth–1 month) | Infancy (1–18 months) | Childhood (1.5–11 years) | Adolescence (11–16 years) | Adulthood (>16 years) |
|---|---|---|---|---|---|---|
| Autonomic system | Hypertension | | | | + | + |
| Cardiovascular | Tachycardia | | | | + | + |
| CNS | Coma | | | | ± | ± |
| | Hyperesthesia | | | | ± | ± |
| | Motor neuropathy | | | | ± | ± |
| | Seizures | | | | ± | ± |
| Dermatological | Blisters | | | | ± | ± |
| Digestive | Abdominal pain | | | | + | + |
| | Constipation | | | | ± | ± |
| | Nausea | | | | ± | ± |
| | Vomiting | | | | ± | ± |
| Musculoskeletal | Muscle pain | | | | + | + |
| Other | Color red-brown w. pink fluorescence (urine) | | | | + | + |
| Laboratory findings | 5-ALA (urine) | | | | ↑↑ | ↑↑ |
| | Coproporphyrin III (feces) | | | | ↑↑ | ↑↑ |
| | Magnesium (plasma) | | | | ↓-n | ↓-n |
| | Porphobilinogen, PBG (urine) | | | | ↑↑ | ↑↑ |
| | Porphyrins, all (urine) | | | | ↑↑↑ | ↑↑↑ |
| | Sodium (plasma) | | | | ↓-n | ↓-n |

**Table 57.7** (Harderoporphyria)

| System | Symptoms and Biomarkers | Neonatal (birth–1 month) | Infancy (1–18 months) | Childhood (1.5–11 years) | Adolescence (11–16 years) | Adulthood (>16 years) |
|---|---|---|---|---|---|---|
| Autonomic system | Hypertension | | | | | |
| Cardiovascular | Tachycardia | | | | | |
| CNS | Seizures | | | | | |
| | Hyperesthesia | | | | | |
| | Coma | | | | | |
| | Motor neuropathy | | | | | |
| Dermatological | Neonatal Jaundice | + | + | + | + | + |
| Digestive | Abdominal pain | | | | | |
| | Nausea | | | | | |
| | Constipation | | | | | |
| | Vomiting | | | | + | + |
| Musculoskeletal | Muscle pain | | | | + | + |
| Other | Colored red-brown urine | ± | ± | ± | ± | ± |
| Laboratory findings | Hemolytic Anemia | + | + | + | + | + |
| | Delta-ALA (urine) | | | | ↑ | ↑ |
| | Porphobilinogen, PBG (urine) | | | | ↑ | ↑ |
| | Coproporphyrin III (urine) | | | | ↑↑ | ↑↑ |
| | Harderoporpyrin (feces) | | | | ↑↑ | ↑↑ |

**Table 57.8** Porphyria variegata

| System | Symptoms and Biomarkers | Neonatal (birth–1 month) | Infancy (1–18 months) | Childhood (1.5–11 years) | Adolescence (11–16 years) | Adulthood (>16 years) |
|---|---|---|---|---|---|---|
| Autonomic system | Hypertension | | | | + | + |
| Cardiovascular | Tachycardia | | | | + | + |
| CNS | Coma | | | | ± | ± |
| | Hyperesthesia | | | | ± | ± |
| | Motor neuropathy | | | | ± | ± |
| | Seizures | | | | ± | ± |
| Dermatological | Blisters | | | | ± | ± |
| Digestive | Abdominal pain | | | | + | + |
| | Constipation | | | | ± | ± |
| | Nausea | | | | ± | ± |
| | Vomiting | | | | ± | ± |
| Musculoskeletal | Muscle pain | | | | + | + |
| Other | Colored red-brown urine | | | | + | + |
| Laboratory findings | 5-ALA (urine) | | | | ↑↑ | ↑↑ |
| | Coproporphyrin III (feces) | | | | ↑↑↑ | ↑↑↑ |
| | Magnesium (plasma) | | | | ↓-n | ↓-n |
| | Porphobilinogen, PBG (urine) | | | | ↑↑ | ↑↑ |
| | Porphyrins, all (urine) | | | | ↑↑↑ | ↑↑↑ |
| | Protoporphyrin IX (feces) | | | | ↑-↑↑↑ | ↑-↑↑↑ |
| | Sodium (plasma) | | | | ↓ | ↓ |

**Table 57.9** Erythropoietic protoporphyria

| System | Symptoms and Biomarkers | Neonatal (birth–1 month) | Infancy (1–18 months) | Childhood (1.5–11 years) | Adolescence (11–16 years) | Adulthood (>16 years) |
|---|---|---|---|---|---|---|
| Dermatological | Edema in light-exposed areas | | ± | + | + | + |
| | Photosensitivity, acute painful | | ± | + | + | + |
| Digestive | Liver dysfunction | | n | n – ++ | n – ++ | n – ++ |
| Hematological | Anemia | | ± | ± | ± | ± |
| | Microcytosis | | ± | ± | ± | ± |
| Laboratory findings | Ferritin (serum) | | ↓-n | ↓-n | ↓-n | ↓-n |
| | Iron (serum) | | ↓-n | ↓-n | ↓-n | ↓-n |
| | Protoporphyrin IX (feces) | n | n-↑ | n-↑ | n-↑ | n-↑ |
| | Protoporphyrin IX, free (red blood cells) | | ↑↑ | ↑↑ | ↑↑↑ | ↑↑↑ |
| | Protoporphyrin IX, zinc-bound (red blood cells) | | n-↑ | ↑ | ↑ | ↑ |

## Overview on Symptomatology

| Disorder | Leading clinical symptoms | Onset of symptoms | Prevalence |
|---|---|---|---|
| 57.1 X-linked sideroblastic anemia | Anemia | | |
| 57.2 X-linked protoporphyria | Photosensitivity/liver disease/anemia | Childhood | Rare |
| 57.3 ALA-dehydratase deficiency | Abdominal and neurological symptoms | Childhood | Very rare |
| Lead poisoning | Abdominal and neurological symptoms/anemia/lead blue line (Burton's line) | Childhood/adolescence | Rare |
| 21.1 Tyrosinemia type 1 | Failure to thrive, abdominal and neurological symptoms, liver dysfunction | Early childhood | Rare |
| 57.4 Acute intermittent porphyria | Abdominal and neurological symptoms/hyponatremia | After puberty (female>male) | 1: 100,000 |
| 57.5 Congenital erythropoietic porphyria | Photosensitivity: Blisters, erosions, mutilations/ anemia/hemolysis/hepatosplenomegaly/erythrodontia | Neonatal/childhood | Very rare |
| 57.6 Porphyria cutanea tarda I, II, Hepatoerythropoietic porphyria | Liver disease/skin fragility/photosensitivity/ hypertrichosis | Late adolescence | 20: 100,000 Very rare |
| 57.7 Hereditary coproporphyria | Abdominal and neurological symptoms, photosensitivity | After puberty (adolescence And senescence) | 0.1: 100,000 |
| 57.8 Porphyria variegate | Abdominal and neurological symptoms, photosensitivity | After puberty (adolescence And senescence) | 0.3: 100,000 |
| 57.9 Erythropoietic protoporphyria | Photosensitivity, some patients develop liver disease | Infancy/childhood | 1: 100,000 |

## Enzyme Defects along the Heme Biosynthesis in Porphyrias, Regulated Induction of ALAS1, and Major Clinical Manifestation

| | | | Major clinical manifestation | | | |
|---|---|---|---|---|---|---|
| Disorder in heme synthesis | Enzyme | Induction of ALAS1 | Neurovisceral | Cutaneous | Anemia | Liver |
| X-linked sideroblastic anemia (57.1) | ALAS2 | – | | | ++ | |
| XLP (57.2) | ALAS2 | – | – | ++ | –/+ | –/+ |
| ADP (Doss) (57.3) | ALAD | + | + | – | –/+ | – |
| Lead poisoning (57.3) | ALAD | + | + | – | +[a] | +[b] |
| Tyrosinemia type 1[c] (21.1) | ALAD | + | + | | | |
| AIP (57.4) | PBGD | + | + | – | – | –/+ |
| CEP (Günther) (57.5) | UROS | – | – | + | + | –/+ |
| PCT / HEP (57.6) | UROD | – | – | + | – | –/+ |
| HCP (57.7) | CPOX | + | + | –/+ | – | –/+ |
| VP (57.8) | PPOX | + | + | –/+ | – | –/+ |
| EPP (57.9) | FECH | – | – | + | –/+ | –/+ |

[a]Lead inhibits also the enzymes CPOX and FECH
[b]"Lead hepatitis"
[c]Tyrosinemia is not described in detail; the reader is referred to Sect. 21.1

## Reference Ranges

### Urinary Excretion of Porphyrin Precursors and Porphyrins

| | 24-h urine collection | Urine spot sample |
|---|---|---|
| Analyte | Referred to the total excretion volume | Referred to excreted creatinine |
| ALA | <49 µmol/day | <2.6 mmol/mol, BZ 2.6–6.8 |
| PBG | <7.5 µmol/day | <1.0 mmol/mol, BZ 1.0–2.2 |
| Uroporphyrin | <33 nmol/day | <4.5 µmol/mol |
| Coproporphyrin I | <51 nmol/day | <7.0 µmol/mol |
| Coproporphyrin III | <102 nmol/day | <14.0 µmol/mol |
| Total porphyrins | <209 nmol/day | <26.7 µmol/mol |

*BZ* border zone

### Fecal Porphyrin Excretion

| Analyte | Upper limit of reference |
|---|---|
| Coproporphyrin I | <26 nmol/g dry weight |
| Coproporphyrin III | <11 nmol/g dry weight |
| Protoporphyrin | <95 nmol/g dry weight |

### Erythrocytic Porphyrins

| Analyte | Upper limit of reference |
|---|---|
| Zinc protoporphyrin IX | <385 nmol/l or < 40µmol/mol heme |
| Free protoporphyrin IX | <89 nmol/l |

## Pathological Values

### Biochemical Markers in Primary and Secondary Disorders of Heme Biosynthesis

| Sample/metabolite | 57.1 | 57.2 | 57.3 | | 21.1 | 57.4 | 57.5 | 57.6 | 57.7 | 57.8 | 57.9 |
|---|---|---|---|---|---|---|---|---|---|---|---|
| | XLSA | XLP | ADP | LP [a] | TE 1 [b] | AIP | CEP | PCT/ HEP | HCP | VP | EPP |
| *Urine* | | | | | | | | | | | |
| 5-ALA | n | n | ↑↑ | ↑↑ | ↑-↑↑ | ↑↑ | n | n | ↑ | ↑ | n |
| PBG | n | n | n-↑ | n-↑ | n | ↑↑ | n | n | ↑ | ↑ | n |
| Porphyrin I isomers | | | | | | | ↑↑ | | | | |
| Uroporphyrins, total | | n-↑ | n-↑↑ | n-↑↑ | n | ↑↑ | ↑↑ | ↑↑ | n-↓ | n-↓ | n-↑ |
| Uroporphyrins I | | – | – | | | – | ↑↑ | ↑↑ | – | – | |
| Uroporphyrins III | | | | | | ↑ | – | ↑↑ | | | |
| Heptacarboxyporphyrin | | n-↑ | n-↑ | n-↑ | n | ↑ | ↑ | ↑↑ | n-↑ | n-↑ | n-↑ |
| Hexacarboxyporphyrin | | n | n-↑ | n-↑ | n | ↑ | ↑ | ↑ | n-↑ | n-↑ | n |
| Pentacarboxyporphyrin | | n | n-↑ | n-↑ | n-↑ | ↑ | ↑ | ↑ | n-↑ | n-↑ | n |
| Coproporphyrins, total | | n-↑ | ↑↑ | ↑↑ | ↑↑ | ↑↑ | ↑↑ | n-↑ | ↑↑ | ↑↑ | n-↑ |
| Coproporphyrin I > III | | | | | | | +++ | | | | + |
| Coproporphyrin III > I | | | + | + | + | | | | ++ | + | |
| Coproporphyrin III | | | ↑↑ | ↑↑ | ↑↑ | | | | ↑ | ↑ | |
| *Feces* | | | | | | | | | | | |
| Porphyrin I isomers | | | | | | | ↑ | | | | |
| Uroporphyrins | | n | n | n | | | n-↑ | n-↑ | n | n | n |
| Heptacarboxyporphyrin | | n | n | n | | | n-↑ | ↑ | n | n | n |
| Hexacarboxyporphyrin | | n | n | n | | | ↑ | ↑ | n | n | n |
| Pentacarboxyporphyrin | | n | n | n | | | ↑ | ↑ | n | n | n |

| Sample/metabolite | 57.1 | 57.2 | 57.3 | | 21.1 | 57.4 | 57.5 | 57.6 | 57.7 | 57.8 | 57.9 |
|---|---|---|---|---|---|---|---|---|---|---|---|
| | XLSA | XLP | ADP | LP [a] | TE 1 [b] | AIP | CEP | PCT/ HEP | HCP | VP | EPP |
| Isocoproporphyrin | | | | – | | | – | n-↑ | – | – | – |
| Coproporphyrins | | n-↑ | n-↑ | n-↑ | | n-↑ | ↑ | | ↑↑ | ↑ | |
| Coproporphyrin III > I | | | | | | | | | ++ | + | |
| Coproporphyrin I/III | | | | | | | > > 1 | | <1 | <1 | n->1 |
| Protoporphyrin | | n-↑ | n-↑ | n-↑ | | n | n-↑ | | ↑ | ↑↑ | n-↑↑ |
| *Plasma or erythrocytes, resp.* | | | | | | | | | | | |
| Uroporphyrin | | | | | | | ↑ | n | | | |
| Coproporphyrin | | | | | | | ↑ | | | | |
| Zinc protoporphyrin | | ↑↑ | ↑↑ | ↑↑ | | | ↑ | ↑[c] | n | n | ↑↑ |
| Free protoporphyrin | | ↑↑ | ↑ | ↑ | | | ↑ | ↑[c] | n | n | ↑↑ |
| Protoporphyrin free/zinc | ↓ | 2: 1 | < 1 | < 1 | | | | | | | > > 1 |
| *Various* | | | | | | | | | | | |
| PBG deaminase | n | n | n | n | n | ↓↓-n [d] | n-↑ | n-↑ | n | n-↓ | n |
| 5-ALA dehydratase | n | n | ↓↓ | ↓↓ [e] | | n | n | n | n | n | n |
| Uroporphyrinogen-decarboxylase | n | n | n | n | | n | n | n-↓↓ | n | n | n |
| Emission maximum of plasma fluorescence spectrum on excitation with 405 nm (nm) | | 624–635 | 615–620 | 615–620 | | 615–620 | 615–620 | 615–620 | 615–620 | 625–627 | 624–635 |

[a]*LP* lead poisoning
[b]*TE* tyrosinemia type I
[c]Exclusively in HEP
[d]Normal activity only in case of non-erythroid splice site mutation variant
[e]*Reactivated* by *zinc*

## Diagnostic Flowcharts

| | | |
|---|---|---|
| Acute hepatic porphyrias | Porphyria cutanea tarda | Protoporphyrias |
| Patients after puberty | Adult patients<br>Age > 18 years | Children or adolescents |
| • Unexplained gastrointestinal complaints (colic, vomiting, subileus)<br>• Neuropsychiatric symptoms (paresthesia, seizures, paresis, depression, anxiety, hallucination)<br>• Cardiovascular symptoms (tachycardia, hypertension)<br>• Red-colored urine without erythrocytes or hemoglobin<br>• Serum hyponatremia | • Blister-forming dermatosis on light-exposed skin areas<br>• Increased skin vulnerability<br>• Hyper- and hypopigmentation on light-exposed skin<br>• Hypertrichosis of the cheeks, temples, and eyebrows; often associated with:<br>– Iron overload<br>– HCV infection<br>– HIV infection<br>– Alcohol consumption<br>– Hormone (replacement) therapy<br>– Toxic agents, e.g., hexachlorobenzene | • Burning pain<br>• Erythema/redness on light-exposed skin areas<br>• Angioedema-like swelling on the face, on the back of the hands, and on the forearms<br>• Often microcytic anemia |
| Key diagnostic features | | |
| > Fourfold elevated ALA and PBG in urine | ALA and PBG in urine normal, elevated total porphyrins in urine with uroporphyrin > coproporphyrin | ALA and PBG in urine normal, metal-free erythrocyte protoporphyrin increased in blood |

Diagnosis and differential diagnosis of porphyrias rely on biochemical, quantitative determinations of porphyrin precursors and porphyrins in urine, stool, plasma, and heparinized blood. The simplified three scenarios (acute hepatic porphyrias, porphyria cutanea tarda, protoporphyrias) are helpful in clinical practice. Think of porphyria in patients with unexplained abdominal and neuropsychiatric symptoms and/or photosensitivity. Use key diagnostic features. (Modified from Ref. Stölzel et al. 2019)

## Specimen Collection

| Test | Material | Handling |
|---|---|---|
| *First-line diagnostic tests* | | |
| Fluorescence scan | 1 ml serum, plasma (heparin, EDTA) | Light protected and cool |
| 5-Aminolevulinic acid Porphobilinogen (porphyrin precursors) | 5 ml urine (spot sample or 24-h collection) | Light protected and cool |
| Porphyrins | 5 ml urine (spot sample or 24-h collection), 5 g feces | Light protected and cool |
| Free protoporphyrin | 3 ml EDTA blood or | |
| Zinc protoporphyrin | Heparinized blood | Light protected and cool |
| *Second-line diagnostic tests* | | |
| Enzyme activity tests | 5 ml heparinized blood or ACD blood | Cool, not frozen |
| Molecular genetic assays | EDTA blood or | – |
| Genomic DNA | Isolated DNA | |
| cDNA | EDTA blood | Rapid sample transport (<12 h) |

## Treatment

### Acute Porphyrias (ALADP; 57.3, AIP; 57.4, HCP; 57.7, VP; 57.8)

Generally, patients need to be admitted to an intensive care unit, to receive pain treatment and caloric support (mainly glucose infusion) and to have their electrolyte abnormalities corrected. Porphyrinogenic medications and other triggers need to be identified and discontinued (Stölzel et al. 2019). AHP requires specific therapies (see table below).

| | |
|---|---|
| 1. Discontinuation of porphyrinogenic drugs and intensive medical monitoring | www.drugs-porphyria.org and see Fig. 57.2 |
| 2. Caloric support (carbohydrates, protein)<br>And heme treatment: | Intravenous and/or oral carbohydrates as preferred source of energy; beware of dilutional hyponatremia; serum sodium, magnesium, and phosphate must be monitored daily<br>For severe cases, neurologic manifestations and associated hyponatremia: Heme arginate (e.g., Normosang[R]), 3 mg/kg body weight/day in 100 ml human albumin (5%–20%), infused in 15 min, for up to four consecutive days |
| 3. Symptom measures:<br>For pain: | Acetylsalicylic acid, morphine derivatives, gabapentin |
| For tachycardia and hypertension: | Propranolol, metoprolol, valsartan |
| For restlessness or vomiting: | Chlorpromazine, lorazepam, ondansetron |
| For symptoms of ileus: | Neostigmine |
| For respiratory relief: | Assisted or controlled ventilation (possibly tracheotomy) |
| For infections: | Penicillin, cephalosporins, imipenem, gentamicin, amikacin, vancomycin |
| For recurrent attacks and chronic symptoms: | Givosiran (Givlaari[R]) 2.5 mg/kg body weight, s.c., monthly |
| Physiotherapeutic measures from the very beginning | |

Givosiran silences hepatic ALAS1-mRNA, normalizes ALA und PBG overproduction, and significantly reduces pain, the days of administered heme, and annualized rate of porphyria attacks. Givosiran is given once monthly subcutaneously. Modified from Ref. (Stölzel et al. 2019)

Heme therapy is clearly indicated when neurological symptoms occur (Bonkowsky et al. 1971). Usually, these and other symptoms begin to improve within 48 h of early-on intravenous administration of heme (Normosang®, Orphan Europe, Puteaux, France, Europe, and elsewhere; Panhematin®, Recordati Rare Diseases, Lebanon, NJ, United States, Mexico, and elsewhere). Heme is a feedback inhibitor of the rate-limiting hepatic enzyme ALAS1 at the transcriptional level. While being effective in most cases, lack of response can be due to insufficient dosing (<3 mg/kg/day), symptoms that are not caused by porphyria, late start of therapy, or chronified porphyria-related pathology, which includes irreversible neurological damage. Heme therapy is also effective in LP and ALADP. Prophylactic treatment with heme in fixed intervals, e.g., up to weekly in severe cases, is justified for patients with recurrent attacks (defined as more than three per year). However, regular heme infusions over prolonged periods have significant side effects, especially iron overload and venous damage and obliteration caused by heme degradation products that bind to clotting factors, platelets, and endothelial cells. These patients require an intravenous port for blood sampling and intravenous heme therapy. Administration of heme bound to albumin is an easy measure to reduce intravenous heme toxicity (see table above). We dilute the heme arginate in 100 ml of human albumin (5–20%). After infusion into a large vein or the port, physiological saline is infused for 15 min to reduce local toxicity. In rare cases that require highly frequent heme infusions, because of severe clinical manifestations, the accumulating heme can activate heme oxygenase 1, which results in accelerated heme degradation and loss of feedback inhibition of ALAS1. This can explain the more than fourfold increase of reported AIP patients that experience recurrent attacks since the introduction of heme therapy in 1985

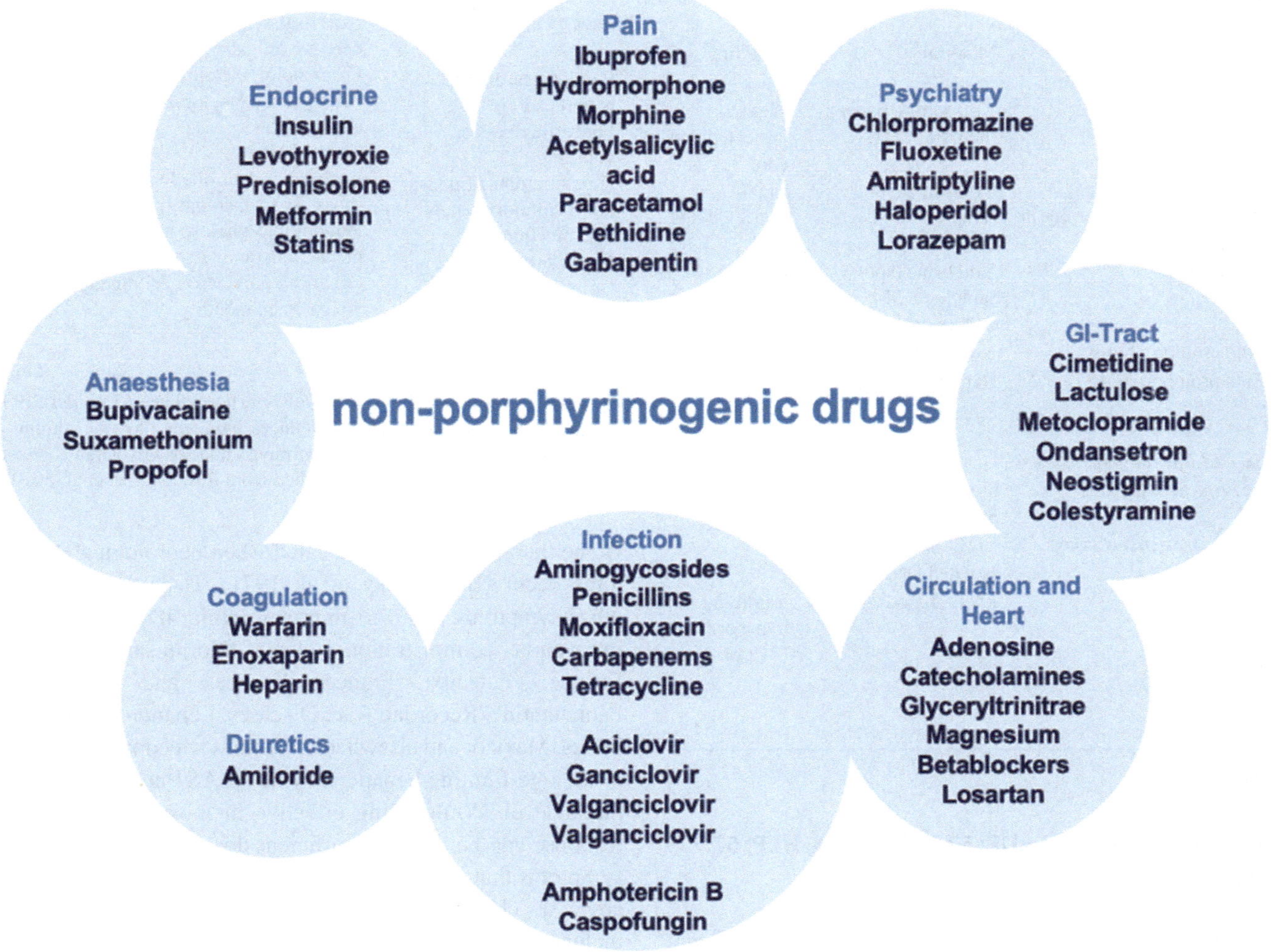


**Fig. 57.2** Non-porphyrinogenic drugs

(from 4/230 in 1985 to 40/536 in 2008), but improved survival with heme therapy may also have contributed (Schmitt et al. 2018). Taken together, if feasible, high-frequency heme therapy should be avoided.

Sufficient caloric support (especially with carbohydrates and protein) is a central basic therapy for AHP. Attacks are often induced by low caloric intake and worsened by nausea and vomiting (Doss et al. 1985). The infused glucose inhibits the peroxisome proliferator-activated receptor-$\gamma$ (PPAR-$\gamma$) coactivator-1$\alpha$ that otherwise upregulates transcription of ALAS1 (Handschin et al. 2005). Glucose combined with insulin may be more effective than glucose alone, but controlled studies are lacking. A too rapid glucose infusion may lead to a dangerous refeeding syndrome, promoting, e.g., hyponatremia. Therefore, patients with hyponatremia should first receive heme therapy followed by careful glucose infusion.

Pain, another component of the vicious cycle, needs to be treated immediately and rigorously prevented. Well-tolerated drugs used by us are opiates and gabapentin. They do not induce hepatic ALAS1 and are excreted via the kidneys. Mild acute hepatic porphyria cases should be treated with pain medication and caloric support alone. Figure 57.2 lists safe drugs, based on numerous experimental studies, pharmacological data, and clinical reports (Stölzel et al. 2009). We recommend to consult the International Guidelines (www.drugs-porphyria.org, www.porphyria-europe.com).

In women with acute porphyria, pregnancy is in general not at risk, although progesterone potently induces liver heme production. However, pregnancy-associated vomiting and subsequent caloric deficiency should be normalized promptly by caloric supply with parenteral nutrition. For those women suffering from frequent attacks related to menstrual cycle, gonadotropin-releasing hormone analogues, combined subsequently with low-dose estrogen patch to suppress menopausal symptoms, can be helpful.

Ultimately, in severe and complicated disease, liver transplantation was shown to cure the disease (Seth et al. 2007). Complete normalization of porphyrin metabolism after liver transplantation proves that acute porphyrias are diseases of the liver.

Small interfering RNA (givosiran, Givlaari®, Alnylam, USA) silences hepatic ALAS1-mRNA, normalizes ALA und PBG overproduction (Tschudy et al. 1965), and significantly reduces the annualized rate of porphyria attacks (Balwani et al. 2020). After 12 months of follow-up, 62% of patients on givosiran were attack-free. Safety profile was acceptable. However, 10 (11%) and 16 (17%) of the treated patients had renal and/or hepatic adverse events, respectively.

Overall, the rigorous elimination of precipitating factors in daily life remains the mainstay of prevention and therapy. Avoiding porphyrinogenic medication, including alcohol, smoking, and physical stress, is of major importance, as well as a balanced diet with a high percentage of carbohydrates. Patients with acute porphyria should take special care to avoid infections and other diseases, and the porphyrin precursors ALA and PBG should be monitored. We recommend liberal vaccination.

**Porphyria Cutanea Tarda/Hepatoerythropoietic Porphyria (PCT I, II/HEP; 57.6)**

Vitamin D supplementation and adequate sun protection is indispensable. The skin should not be exposed to intensive artificial light sources. Patients are advised to avoid known precipitating factors, especially alcohol and smoking, that upregulate CyP450 enzymes and thus the heme synthetic machinery. Alcohol further contributes by downregulating hepcidin, which increases iron resorption and enhances oxidative stress. Women must discontinue hormonal contraception or replacement therapy. Photoprotection, phlebotomy, and treatment with hydroxychloroquine (HCQ) (100 mg twice per week, respectively) are effective first-line therapies (Kordac and Semrádová 1973). Phlebotomy is employed to remove excess iron. Initially, a biweekly phlebotomy up to 500 ml is performed and monitored by serum ferritin concentrations (target value near the lower limit of normal) to avoid iron deficiency. When phlebotomy is not possible, such as in severe anemia, oral iron chelators or low-dose HCQ can be given. Phlebotomy and low-dose HCQ are also effective baseline therapies for the majority of patients with PCT, with comparable efficacy. HCQ can mobilize cellular porphyrin aggregates with subsequent elimination mainly via the urine. With HCQ, urinary porphyrin excretion usually increases at least twofold, and skin photosensitivity can worsen during the first 3 months, but then starts to decrease, followed by clinical remission which is accompanied by normalization of elevated liver enzyme activities in 95% of patients. Long-term HCQ therapy can lead to retinopathy, requiring (baseline and annual) regular ophthalmologic monitoring. Patients with PCT and iron overload related to HFE mutations should preferentially undergo phlebotomy (Stölzel et al. 2003). In general, in patients with increased serum ferritin, the combination of phlebotomy with low-dose HCQ shortens the time of remission. Even advanced liver damage and siderosis, such as in patients that are homozygous for the HFE C282Y mutation, can regress after combined phlebotomy and HCQ therapy.

In patients with chronic HCV infection, treatment with iron depletion combined with highly effective antiviral therapy induces rapid clinical and biochemical remission (Combalia et al. 2017).

Treatment should be discontinued once urinary porphyrin levels stabilize around 400 nmol/day (normal <209 nmol/day). Such mild porphyrinuria usually persists during clinical remission. Still, biochemical and clinical relapse occurred in 36% and 20% of patients in the first year after discontinuation of HCQ or phlebotomy, respectively (Salameh et al. 2018).

**Erythropoietic Protoporphyrias (EPP/XLP 57.1/57.9)**

EPP and XLP require effective sun protection, including protection from intensive artificial light sources. Conventional sunscreens are insufficient, since photosensitivity is mainly due to visible blue light (Soret band: near 400 nm). Appropriate skin protectants contain zinc oxide or titanium oxide. Since sunlight exposure triggers pain, patients quickly learn and adopt light protection measures. Vitamin D substitution (1000–2000 U of D3 daily) is necessary. Afamelanotide (Scenesse®, Clinuvel Pharmaceuticals, Melbourne, VIC, Australia), an α-melanocyte-stimulating hormone analogue, promotes skin pigmentation independent of sunlight via the activation of the melanocyte melanocortin-1 receptor and improves sunlight protection and tolerance (Langendonk et al. 2015).

In uncontrolled observational studies, ursodeoxycholic acid appears to increase hepatic clearance, and cholestyramine may bind excess protoporphyrin IX (PPIX) in the gut to interrupt its enterohepatic circulation. Excess metal-free PPIX has also been removed by plasma exchange in the treatment of liver failure or for prevention of hepatic decompensation. Erythrocytapheresis may be useful, since patients' red blood cells contain high amount of toxic PPIX. Moreover, iron depletion should be beneficial, since iron stimulates ALAS2. Patients with advanced cholestasis or cirrhosis should receive liver transplants. Before liver transplantation, excess circulating PPIX must be removed. During transplantation, but also during other abdominal surgeries, the use of special yellow filters prevents light-induced damage of visceral organs. Unfortunately, and in contrast to patients with AHP, liver transplantation does not cure patients with EPP or XLP, where the excessively elevated PPIX originates from the bone marrow. Consequently, allogeneic hematopoietic stem cell transplantation has led to a PPIX reduction of up to 85% and a resolution of inflammatory liver damage, regardless of prior liver transplantation.

Patients with EPP or XLP are not sensitive to numerous drugs, as are patients with AHP. Paradoxical on a first glance, iron substitution can decrease PPIX concentrations and improve symptoms in patients with XLP, which can be explained by iron serving as secondary substrate to promote conversion of toxic PPIX to heme by FECH (Landefeld et al. 2016). In contrast, EPP is exacerbated by iron substitution, since iron induces the bone marrow enzyme ALAS2 (Barman-Aksoezen et al. 2017). In this line, mild iron deficiency may rather protect patients with EPP. Should iron substitution in patients with EPP be necessary, as in cases of severe anemia, it should be done during the darker seasons with low-intensity sunlight. There is some hope for gene therapeutic approaches to EPP.

#### Congenital Erythropoietic Porphyria (CEP; 57.5)

As in EPP and XLP, baseline treatment and prevention for CEP are light protection and vitamin D supplementation. Some patients with anemia have benefited from splenectomy. The indication for splenectomy must be personalized, since clinical presentation is highly variant, with different degrees of splenomegaly, anemia, and thrombocytopenia. Allogeneic hematopoietic stem cell transplantation is curative and should be performed at younger age. A single case was reported, where iron depletion with deferasirox improved photosensitivity, likely by reducing the activity of ALAS2. This mechanism is supported by another case, where an ALAS2 gain-of-function mutation increased the severity of CEP. Furthermore, proteasome inhibitors or chemical chaperones could stabilize the otherwise dysfunctional UROS variants to increase their activity, reduce porphyrin accumulation, and ameliorate skin photosensitivity in CEP patients.

## References


Balwani M, Sardh E, Ventura P, et al. Phase 3 trial of RNAi therapeutic givosiran for acute intermittent porphyria. N Engl J Med. 2020;382:2289–301.

Barman-Aksoezen J, Girelli D, Aurizi C, Schneider-Yin X, Campostrini N, Barbieri L, Minder EI, Biolcati G. Disturbed iron metabolism in erythropoietic protoporphyria and association of GDF15 and gender with disease severity. J Inherit Metab Dis. 2017;40:433–41.

Bissell DM, Anderson KE, Bonkovsky HL. Porphyria. N Engl J Med. 2017;377:2101.

Bonkovsky HL, Guo J-T, Hou W, Li T, Narang T, Thapar M. Porphyrin and heme metabolism and the porphyrias. In: Compr. Physiol: American Cancer Society; 2013. p. 365–401.

Bonkowsky HL, Tschudy DP, Collins A, Doherty J, Bossenmaier I, Cardinal R, Watson CJ. Repression of the overproduction of porphyrin precursors in acute intermittent porphyria by intravenous infusions of hematin. Proc Natl Acad Sci U S A. 1971;68:2725–9.

Combalia A, To-Figueras J, Laguno M, Martínez-Rebollar M, Aguilera P. Direct-acting antivirals for hepatitis C virus induce a rapid clinical and biochemical remission of porphyria cutanea tarda. Br J Dermatol. 2017;177:e183–4.

Doss M, Sixel-Dietrich F, Verspohl F. "Glucose effect" and rate limiting function of uroporphyrinogen synthase on porphyrin metabolism in hepatocyte culture: relationship with human acute hepatic porphyrias. J Clin Chem Clin Biochem. 1985;23:505–13.

Doss M, von Tiepermann R, Schneider J, Schmid H. New type of hepatic porphyria with porphobilinogen synthase defect and intermittent acute clinical manifestation. Klin Wochenschr. 1979;57:1123–7.

Gouya L, Ventura P, Balwani M, et al. EXPLORE: a prospective, multinational, natural history study of patients with acute hepatic porphyria with recurrent attacks. Hepatology. 2020;71:1546–58.

Handschin C, Lin J, Rhee J, Peyer A-K, Chin S, Wu P-H, Meyer UA, Spiegelman BM. Nutritional regulation of hepatic heme biosynthesis and porphyria through PGC-1alpha. Cell. 2005;122:505–15.

Kordac V, Semrádová M. Therapy of patients with porphyria cutanea tarda with antimalarials. Cas Lek Cesk. 1973;112:762–5.

Landefeld C, Kentouche K, Gruhn B, Stauch T, Rößler S, Schuppan D, Whatley SD, Beck JF, Stölzel U. X-linked protoporphyria: iron supplementation improves protoporphyrin overload, liver damage and anaemia. Br J Haematol. 2016;173:482–4.

Langendonk JG, Balwani M, Anderson KE, et al. Afamelanotide for Erythropoietic Protoporphyria. N Engl J Med. 2015;373:48–59.

Lenglet H, Schmitt C, Grange T, et al. From a dominant to an oligogenic model of inheritance with environmental modifiers in acute intermittent porphyria. Hum Mol Genet. 2018;27:1164–73.

Puy H, Gouya L, Deybach J-C. Porphyrias. Lancet. 2010;375:924–37.

Salameh H, Sarairah H, Rizwan M, Kuo Y-F, Anderson KE, Singal AK. Relapse of porphyria cutanea tarda after treatment with phlebotomy or 4-aminoquinoline antimalarials: a meta-analysis. Br J Dermatol. 2018;179:1351–7.

Schmitt C, Lenglet H, Yu A, et al. Recurrent attacks of acute hepatic porphyria: major role of the chronic inflammatory response in the liver. J Intern Med. 2018;284:78–91.

Seth AK, Badminton MN, Mirza D, Russell S, Elias E. Liver transplantation for porphyria: who, when, and how? Liver Transpl. 2007;13:1219–27.

Stölzel U, Brosche C, Koszka C, Stauch T, Teubner A, Doss MO. Safe and probably safe drugs in acute hepatic porphyria. Cell Mol Biol (Noisy-le-Grand). 2009;55:147–51.

Stölzel U, Doss MO, Schuppan D. Clinical guide and update on Porphyrias. Gastroenterology. 2019;157:365–81.e4

Stölzel U, Köstler E, Schuppan D, Richter M, Wollina U, Doss MO, Wittekind C, Tannapfel A. Hemochromatosis (HFE) gene mutations and response to chloroquine in porphyria cutanea tarda. Arch Dermatol. 2003;139:309–13.

Tschudy DP, Perlroth MG, Marver HS, Collins A, Hunter G, Rechcigl M. Acute intermittent porphyria: the first "overproduction disease" localized to a specific enzyme. Proc Natl Acad Sci U S A. 1965;53:841–7.

# Inherited Disorders of Bilirubin Metabolism

# 58

Namita Roy-Chowdhury, Chandan Guha,
and Jayanta Roy-Chowdhury

## Contents



### Summary

Bilirubin is the breakdown product of heme, which is the iron-containing tetrapyrrole moiety of hemoglobin, myoglobin, and several enzymes. Heme cleavage, catalyzed by microsomal heme oxygenases, gives rise to biliverdin, which is reduced to bilirubin by biliverdin reductase. As an antioxidant, bilirubin provides health benefits at low concentrations, but at very high concentrations, it can cause bilirubin-induced neurological damage (BIND). Binding to plasma albumin, rapid uptake by hepatocytes, UGT1A1-mediated conjugation with glucuronide, and ATP-dependent pumping into bile canaliculi maintain low plasma concentrations of bilirubin, preventing its tissue toxicity. A fraction of bilirubin glucuronides formed in periportal hepatocytes is pumped out into sinusoidal blood and undergoes reuptake by hepatocytes located downstream to sinusoidal blood flow. Inherited disorders causing excessive bilirubin production, reduced glucuronidation, defective canalicular excretion, or abnormal reuptake can cause hyperbilirubinemia. Newborns have transient hyperbilirubinemia that normally resolves in 1–2 weeks, but can be prolonged or exacerbated by breast-feeding, delayed UGT1A1 maturation, or several inherited disorders of bilirubin metabolism. Mutations of *UGT1A1* gene that cause complete or partial loss of the

N. Roy-Chowdhury · J. Roy-Chowdhury (✉)
Depatments of Medicine and Genetics, Albert Einstein College of Medicine, Bronx, NY, USA

Marion Bessin Liver Research Center, Albert Einstein College of Medicine, Bronx, NY, USA
e-mail: namita.roychowdhury@einsteinmed.org; jayanta.roy-chowdhury@einsteinmed.org

C. Guha
Marion Bessin Liver Research Center, Albert Einstein College of Medicine, Bronx, NY, USA

Departments of Radiation Oncology and Pathology, Albert Einstein College of Medicine, Bronx, NY, USA
e-mail: cguha@Montefiore.org


N. Blau et al. (eds.), *Physician's Guide to the Diagnosis, Treatment, and Follow-Up of Inherited Metabolic Diseases*,
https://doi.org/10.1007/978-3-030-67727-5_58

enzyme activity (Crigler-Najjar syndromes, types 1 and 2, respectively) increase specifically the unconjugated fraction of plasma bilirubin. A common polymorphism of *UGT1A1* promoter causes mild and harmless increase of plasma bilirubin (Gilbert syndrome). Both conjugated and unconjugated bilirubin fractions are increased in disorders of canalicular organic anion excretion (Dubin-Johnson syndrome) or reuptake of bilirubin glucuronides (Rotor syndrome). A group of monogenic disorders, termed progressive familial intrahepatic cholestasis, cause hyperbilirubinemia not by specifically perturbing the bilirubin excretory pathway, but through extensive liver injury.

## Introduction

Bilirubin is the breakdown product of the heme (ferroprotoporphyrin IX) moiety of hemoproteins. Hemoglobin, derived from senescent erythrocytes, contributes 80% of the daily bilirubin production of approximately 4 mg/kg body weight in normal adults. Reticuloendothelial cells in the spleen and bone marrow are major sites of bilirubin production. The remainder comes from rapidly turning over hepatic hemoproteins, such as cytochrome P450s, catalase, peroxidase, and tryptophan pyrrolase, a small free hemoglobin pool, and the slowly turning over myoglobin. Heme degradation begins with the oxidation of the α-methene bridge carbon by microsomal heme oxygenase isoforms 1 and 2 (HO-1 and HO-2) by a reaction requiring oxygen and a reducing agent, such as NADPH. HO inhibition by non-metabolized "dead-end" inhibitors, such as tin-protoporphyrin or tin-mesoporphyrin, reduces serum bilirubin levels in neonates (Kappas and Drummond 1995). Oxidation of the α-methene bridge carbon of the ferroprotoporphyrin ring converts it to the linear tetrapyrrole, biliverdin, releasing 1 mol each of CO and iron. Heme breakdown can be quantified from CO exhaled in breath. CO regulates vascular tone in the liver and other organs, such as the heart under stressful conditions. The iron molecule is reutilized.

HO-1, encoded by the *HMOX1* gene, is ubiquitous and inducible by protoheme IX and oxidative/electrophilic stress signals. HO-1 is cytoprotective against oxygen radicals both directly and through its products, biliverdin and bilirubin. Induction of intestinal HO-1 protects against ischemia-reperfusion injury and bacterial lipopolysaccharides, as well as injury caused by indomethacin, trinitrobenzene sulfonic acid, and dextran sulfate. The physiological importance of HO-1 is highlighted by extensive endothelial injury, causing consumption coagulopathy, microangiopathic hemolytic anemia, low serum bilirubin, hyperlipidemia, and growth retardation observed in a patient with inherited frameshift mutation of *HMOX1* (Yachie et al. 1999). HO-2 is expressed mainly in the brain, and its induction in response to anoxia may be protective during ischemic attacks.

Two biliverdin reductase isozymes, BVRA and BVRB, reduce biliverdin to bilirubin. The *BVRB* gene, located at chromosome 19.q13, is expressed during early embryogenesis and primarily reduces biliverdin IXβ, the product of fetal heme-IXβ. *BVRA*, located on chromosome 7 (pter>q22), is expressed later and mediates the reduction of biliverdin IXα, the product of adult heme-IXα (O'Brien et al. 2015). The N-terminal domains of both isozymes contain catalytic sites for biliverdin reduction. The C-terminal region of BVRA (but not BVRB) contains a basic leucine zipper (bZiP) domain, which functions as a transcription factor that binds the antioxidant response element (ARE) and hypoxia response elements (HRE), and recruits the transcription factor, Nrf2. Nrf2 induces HO-1, thereby protecting against oxidative injury. Additionally, BVRA is an insulin receptor substrate and interacts with both major arms of insulin signalling, namely, the PI3-kinase/Akt and the IRK/IRS/PI3-kinase/MAPK pathways (Choi et al. 2013).

The antioxidant activity of bilirubin may be particularly important during the neonatal period, when intracellular availability of other antioxidants is low. Also there is accumulating evidence for the physiological benefit of bilirubin in adults. At relatively low serum bilirubin concentrations, an inverse relationship has been reported between bilirubin levels and the incidence of ischemic heart disease (Breimer et al. 1995), colon cancer (Zucker et al. 2004), abdominal visceral obesity, and metabolic syndrome (Choi et al. 2013). On the other hand, clinicians are more concerned with abnormal elevation of serum bilirubin, as an indicator of acquired hepatobiliary diseases, hemolysis, or a number of inherited disorders, which are the focus of this chapter. Bilirubin toxicity manifests primarily as bilirubin-induced neurological damage (BIND), caused by unconjugated bilirubin. BIND most commonly occurs when there is exaggerated neonatal jaundice. It can also occur in adults with severe inherited UGT1A1 deficiency, as seen in Crigler-Najjar syndrome type 1.

*Bilirubin chemistry:* Bilirubin IXα is a linear tetrapyrrole, the two dipyrrolic halves of which are joined by a central methene bridge. The propionic acid side chain of each dipyrrolic half is internally hydrogen-bonded to the pyrrolic and lactam sites on the opposite dipyrrolic half (Bonnet et al. 1976), thereby engaging all polar groups. This renders bilirubin water-insoluble. Bilirubin remains in solution by binding to plasma albumin. In clinical laboratories, bilirubin is measured using the van den Bergh reaction (Van den Bergh and Muller 1916), in which diazo reagents attack the central methane bridge, generating two moles of azodipyrrole. Unconjugated bilirubin reacts slowly because of the inaccessibility of the central methene bridge due to hydrogen bonding. Disruption of hydrogen bonds by adding chemical accelerators makes the reaction rapid and complete ("total" bilirubin). In conjugated bilirubin, glucuronidation of the propionic acid carboxyls disrupts the hydrogen bonds, allowing the diazo reagents to react rapidly without accelerators ("direct-reacting" bilirubin).

*Hepatic metabolism and elimination*: Non-covalent binding to plasma albumin keeps unconjugated bilirubin in solution, preventing its tissue toxicity and renal excretion. Normally, albumin is in ~3-fold molar excess to bilirubin. As some metabolites and drugs can interfere with albumin binding, measurement of reserve bilirubin binding capacity may be needed for assessing BIND risk, particularly in premature infants. Peroxidase treatment, gel chromatography, electrophoretic analysis, and direct fluorimetry can be used for unbound bilirubin determination (Ahlfors et al. 2007). Conjugated bilirubin binds less tightly to albumin, and the unbound fraction is excreted in urine. Prolonged conjugated hyperbilirubinemia results in covalent binding of bilirubin to albumin (delta-bilirubin), delaying its clearance from plasma.

In liver sinusoids, bilirubin dissociates from albumin and undergoes facilitated diffusion into hepatocytes, where it is retained by binding to cytosolic glutathione S-transferases. Microsomal uridinediphosphoglucuronate glucuronosyltransferase type 1 (UGT1A1) catalyzes the transfer of glucuronic acid from UDP-glucuronate to bilirubin, forming mono- and diglucuronides. Glucuronidation makes bilirubin water-soluble, reduces its toxicity, and enables its secretion into bile canaliculi by the ATP-consuming pump, ABCC2 (also termed MRP2) (Fig. 58.1). A fraction of the bilirubin glucuronides is secreted into sinusoidal blood by ABCC3 and undergoes reuptake by hepatocytes located downstream to the blood flow via organic anion transporting polypeptides OATP1B1 (SLC01B1) and OATP1B3 (SLC01B3). This process increases bilirubin excreting capacity of the liver by recruiting additional hepatocytes to this process (see under Rotor syndrome).

Bilirubin glucuronides secreted into bile are degraded by intestinal bacteria into urobilinogen, stercobilinogen, and related products. Urobilinogen is partly reabsorbed from the intestine and undergoes enterohepatic circulation, but a small fraction is excreted in urine. Urobilinogen is colorless; but its yellow oxidation product, urobilin, contributes to the normal color of urine and stool.

To adapt to the demand for increased bilirubin clearance, such as during elevated bilirubin production due to hemolysis, bilirubin uptake, conjugation, and excretion need to be coordinately upregulated. Several nuclear receptors, including CAR and PXR, mediate coordinated regulation of these processes (Roy-Chowdhury et al. 2003).

Measurement of serum bilirubin has been used as a test for liver function and disease for many decades. In clinical laboratories, the fraction of bilirubin that reacts with diazo reagents rapidly without addition of a chemical "accelerator" is termed "direct"-reacting bilirubin. Total bilirubin is determined in the presence of an accelerator. The "indirect" bilirubin fraction is determined by subtracting the direct fraction from total bilirubin (Van den Bergh and Muller 1916). Direct bilirubin slightly overestimates the conjugated bilirubin fraction. More accurate measurements are possible using high-pressure liquid chromatography (HPLC) or thin-layer chromatography (TLC). By chromatographic analysis, approximately 4% of serum bilirubin is conjugated. When necessary, it is also possible to analyze bile pigments excreted in duodenal bile by HPLC. Inherited disorders of bilirubin metabolism can be classified into hyperbilirubinemia (a) due to exclusive increase in the unconjugated serum bilirubin fraction and (b) those associated with both conjugated and unconjugated bilirubin fractions (Nomenclature Table).

## Nomenclature

| No. | Disorder | Abbreviation | Gene symbol | Chromosomal localization | Affected protein | OMIM no. |
|---|---|---|---|---|---|---|
| 58.1.1 | Crigler-Najjar syndrome type 1 | UGT1A1 deficiency (complete); CN-1 | *UGT1A1* | 2q37.1 | Uridine diphosphoglucuronate-glucuronosyl transferase 1A1 | 218800 |
| 58.1.2 | Crigler-Najjar syndrome type 2 | UGT1A1 deficiency (incomplete) CN-2; Arias syndrome | *UGT1A1* | 2q37.1 | Uridine diphosphoglucuronate-glucuronosyl transferase 1A1 | 606785 |
| 58.1.3 | Gilbert syndrome | UGT1A1 deficiency (partial) | *UGT1A1* | 2q37.1 | Uridine diphosphoglucuronate-glucuronosyl transferase 1A1 | 143500 |
| 58.2 | Dubin-Johnson syndrome | ABCC2 deficiency; DJS | *ABCC2* | 10q24.2 | Multidrug resistance-associated protein 2 | 237500 |
| 58.3 | Rotor syndrome | OATP1B1 and OATP1B3 disease | *SLCO1B1; SLCO1B3* (digenic) | 12p12.2-p12.1; 12p12.2 | Organic anion transporter proteins OATP1B1 and OATP1B3 | 605495604843 |
| 58.4 | Progressive familial intrahepatic cholestasis type 1 (and benign recurrent intrahepatic cholestasis type 1) | Byler's disease; PFIC-1 (and BRIC-1) | *ATP8B1* | 18q21.31 | ATP8B1 (type-4 P-type ATPase) | 211600 |
| 58.5 | Progressive familial intrahepatic cholestasis type 2 (and benign recurrent intrahepatic cholestasis type 2) | PFIC-2; BSEP deficiency (and BRIC-2) | *ABCB11* | 2q31.1 | ATP binding cassette subfamily B member 11 (canalicular bile salt export pump) | 601847 |
| 58.6 | Progressive familial intrahepatic cholestasis type 3 (and benign recurrent intrahepatic cholestasis type 3) | PFIC-3 (ABCB4 deficiency) (and BRIC-3) | *ABCB4* | 7q21.12 | ABCB4 (MDR3) | 602347 |
| 58.7 | Progressive familial intrahepatic cholestasis type 4 | PFIC-4 | *TJP2* | 9q21.11 | Tight junction protein ZO-2 | 615878 |
| 58.8 | Progressive familial intrahepatic cholestasis type 5 | PFIC-5; NR1H4 deficiency | *NR1H4* | 12q23.1 | Farnesoid X receptor (FXR) | 617049 |

## Metabolic Pathways

Effective biliary excretion of unconjugated bilirubin internalized into hepatocytes requires its conversion to polar conjugates by conjugation of one or both of its carboxyl groups with the glucuronic acid moiety transferred from UDP-glucuronic acid by the microsomal enzyme UDP-glucuronosyltransferase isoform 1A1 (UGT1A1). Absence or reduction of UGT1A1-mediated glucuronidation results in accumulation of unconjugated bilirubin in hepatocytes, which diffuses out into the sinusoidal blood. This results in an increase in the unconjugated fraction of serum bilirubin, along with reduction of the conjugated bilirubin fraction. Thus, the hyperbilirubinemia is contributed solely by unconjugated bilirubin, which is measured by subtracting the direct-reacting fraction from total bilirubin.

Following glucuronidation, conjugated bilirubin is pumped into bile across the biliary canaliculus by ABCC2, while a smaller component secreted into liver sinusoidal blood undergoes reuptake via sinusoidal organic anion transporters OATPB1 and OATPB3. Inherited disorders of canalicular secretion or sinusoidal reuptake cause Dubin-Johnson syndrome or Rotor syndrome, respectively. These disorders cause conjugated hyperbilirubinemia, without significant liver injury. Several other inherited disorders, termed progressive familial intrahepatic cholestasis, cause hyperbilirubinemia as a part of severe liver injury and cholestasis.

## Signs, Symptoms, and Treatment

### Inherited Disorders of Bilirubin Metabolism Associated with Increase of Exclusively Unconjugated Serum Bilirubin

UGT1A1-mediated glucuronidation is essential for effective excretion of bilirubin into the bile. Three inherited disorders

**Table 58.1** Signs and symptoms of Crigler-Najjar syndrome type 1

| System | Symptoms and signs | Neonatal | Infancy | Childhood | Adolescence | Adulthood |
|---|---|---|---|---|---|---|
| Conjunctiva, mucous membranes, skin | Yellow discoloration (jaundice) | ++ | +++ | +++ | +++ | +++ |
| Central nervous system | Abnormal eye movements | ++ | ± | ± | ± | ± |
| | Convulsions | ± | ++ | ++ | +++ | ++ |
| | Drowsiness, high-pitched crying | ++ | ± | | | |
| | Inability to gaze upward | ± | ++ | ++ | ++ | + |
| | Reduced muscle tone or muscle stiffness, choreoathetoid movements | + | ++ | ++ | +++ | ++ |
| | Temperature instability | + | ± | | | |
| Hearing | Loss of hearing | ± | ± | ± | + | + |
| Routine laboratory tests | ALT, AST, alkaline phosphatase | n | n | n | n | n |
| | Serum bilirubin (all unconjugated) | 425–500 µmol/L at 96 h | 340–510 µmol/L | 340–510 µmol/L | 340–600 µmol/L | 340–600 µmol/L |
| Special laboratory tests | Chromatographic analysis of pigments in duodenal bile | | | | Only unconjugated bilirubin | Only unconjugated bilirubin |
| Pharmacological tests | Phenobarbital administration for 1 week | | | Total bilirubin reduced by <25% | Total bilirubin reduced by <25% | |

result in various degrees of unconjugated hyperbilirubinemia from absence or reduction of UGT1A1 activity (Tables 58.1 and 58.2). The UGT1A locus, located at chromosome 2q37, consists of 4 exons (e2–e5) located at the 3′ end and a series of 12 additional exons (e1A1–e1A12) upstream (5′) to these exons. The bilirubin-conjugating enzyme, UGT1A1 is encoded by the UGT1A1 mRNA, which consists of five exons (exon e1A1 and e2-5). Notably, e2-5 also participate in mRNAs for several other UGT1A isoforms. Complete absence of UGT1A1 activity due to nonsense or missense coding region mutations of the UGT1A1 or splice site mutations leading to aberrant splicing of the RNA transcript results in Crigler-Najjar syndrome type 1 (DNA Testing Table). Lack of UGT1A1-mediated glucuronidation of bilirubin results in failure of biliary excretion and accumlation of unconjugated bilirubin in blood (Fig. 58.1). Crigler-Najjar syndrome type II is a milder disorder caused by missense coding region mutations that results in amino acid substitutions that markedly reduce the catalytic activity of UGT1A1 (DNA Testing Table). Finally, Gilbert syndrome is caused by reduced expression of catalytically normal UGT1A1 due to a common promoter variation consisting of insertion of TA dinucleotide in the TATAA box upstream to the UGT1A1 translation initiation site. Gilbert syndrome is associated with mild and/or intermittent unconjugated hyperbilirubinemia.

Comparison of inherited unconjugated hyperbilirubinemia syndromes

| Features | Crigler-Najjar syndrome type 1 (CN1) | Crigler-Najjar syndrome type 2 (CN2) | Gilbert syndrome (GS) |
|---|---|---|---|
| Serum alanine aminotransferase (ALT), aspartate aminotransferase (AST), alkaline phosphatase | Normal | Normal | Normal |
| Pigments excreted in bile | Small amounts of unconjugated bilirubin | Increased proportion of bilirubin monoglucuronide (>10%) | Increased proportion of bilirubin monoglucuronide (>10%) |
| Hepatic bilirubin-UGT1A1 activity | Undetectable | Detectable but markedly reduced | Approximately 30% of normal |
| Effect of phenobarbital administration | No significant reduction of serum bilirubin | Reduction of serum bilirubin by <25% (with rare exceptions) | Normalization of serum bilirubin |
| Prevalence | Rare: <1 in 1,000,000 | Rare: <1 in 1,000,000 | Clinically in 3–5% of most populations. Genotypically ~9% in most populations |
| Prognosis | BIND unless vigorously treated. Cured by liver transplantation | BIND is uncommon, but occurs rarely | Innocuous, but may increase the toxicity of certain drugs. |

*BIND* bilirubin-induced neurologic dysfunction

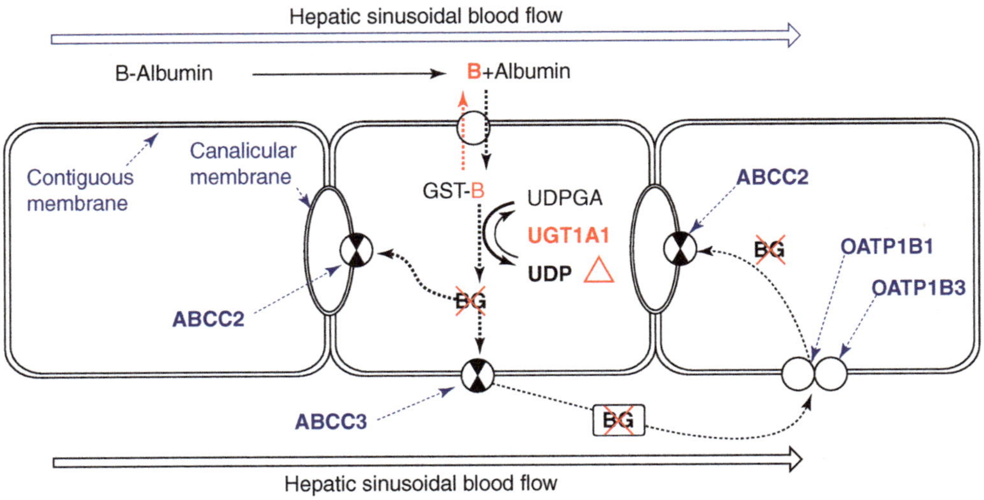


**Fig. 58.1** Metabolic pathway of bilirubin disposal: Unconjugated bilirubin [B] enters hepatic sinusoids bound to serum albumin. At the sinusoidal surface of hepatocytes, bilirubin dissociates from albumin and is internalized by facilitated diffusion. In hepatocyte cytosol, bilirubin remains in solution bound to glutathione S-transferases [GSTs]. In the endoplasmic reticulum, UGT1A1 catalyzes the transfer of glucuronic acid from UDP-glucuronic acid (UDPGA) to bilirubin, forming bilirubin mono- and diglucuronides [BGs]. BGs are pumped out into the bile canaliculus by the ATP-consuming pump ABCC2, as well as by electrogenic mechanisms. A fraction of the BGs is pumped out into hepatic sinusoidal blood by ABCC3 and undergoes reuptake by hepatocytes located downstream to the blood flow via OATP1B1 and OATP1B3 and is subsequently excreted into the bile canaliculus by ABCC2

## Crigler-Najjar Syndrome Type 1 (CN1)

**Signs and Symptoms**: This rare autosomal recessive disorder was originally described by Crigler and Najjar in six infants from three families (Crigler and Najjar 1952). The patients exhibited lifelong severe unconjugated hyperbilirubinemia resulting in bilirubin-induced neurological damage (BIND). Five of the 6 original cases died by 15 months of age, and the remaining patient lived for 15 years. Since then, several hundred CN1 patients have been reported in all races. With routine early implementation of phototherapy and plasmapheresis during acute hyperbilirubinemic crisis, many CN1 patients now survive beyond adolescence, but they remain at the risk of developing BIND around puberty or early adulthood (Wolkoff et al. 1979).

CN1 babies have normal serum bilirubin at birth, because during fetal life, bilirubin is cleared by the placenta. Serum bilirubin levels change from hour to hour after birth, and BIND risk depends on both the rate of rise and peak concentrations of bilirubin. Age-related curves have been constructed to correlate BIND risk to age-related bilirubin levels in newborns (Maisels 2015). In nearly all babies, serum bilirubin increases to above normal adult levels between 24 and 96 h of age. In healthy full-term newborns in Europe and North America, the 50th percentile for total serum bilirubin is 137–154 μmol/L (8–9 mg/dL), and the 95th percentile is about 257–300 μmol/L (15–17.5 mg/dL). In newborns with CN1 not treated with phototherapy or exchange transfusion, bilirubin levels at 96 h of age can exceed 425–510 μmol/L (25–30 mg/dL), at which levels penetration of the blood-brain barrier by bilirubin can lead to kernicterus with acute, and subsequently chronic, BIND, characteristically manifesting as choreoathetoid cerebral palsy and auditory neuropathy causing dyssynchrony with or without hearing loss. Normally, after 96 h, serum bilirubin declines rapidly. CN1 is suspected when serum bilirubin levels fail to normalize in 1 week despite phototherapy with or without plasmapheresis. Jaundice is usually the only initial presenting feature, although some patients may already exhibit signs of BIND. In older children maintained on phototherapy, a small amount of unconjugated bilirubin is excreted in bile, increasing the incidence of pigment gallstones and the risk of biliary obstruction.

Serum bilirubin levels usually range from 340 to 425 μmol/L, but may reach 850 μmol/L (Crigler and Najjar 1952) during intercurrent illness or if phototherapy is missed. Serum bilirubin is all unconjugated and tightly bound to albumin; therefore, bilirubinuria is absent. Bile samples obtained by duodenal intubation or endoscopy show the presence of small amounts of unconjugated bilirubin (Wolkoff et al. 1979). Fecal urobilinogen excretion is reduced, but the stool color remains normal (Crigler and Najjar 1952). As the bile canalicular transport mechanism remains normal, the biliary tree is visualized normally by cholecystographic agents, and bromosulfophthalein and indocyanine green are cleared normally from plasma after intravenous injection (Crigler and Najjar 1952) (See Table 58.1).

Liver biopsy is not usually required for the diagnosis. In infants, liver histology is normal, except for bilirubin plugs in bile canaliculi and bile ducts (Crigler and Najjar 1952; Maisels 2015). Older children may develop hepatic fibrosis. A recent study of 22 CN1 patients undergoing liver transplantation showed various degrees of liver fibrosis in 41% of the explanted livers (Mitchell et al. 2018). The fibrosis was not correlated with the presence of gallstones, and there was no evidence of portal hypertension.

*Abnormalities of Hepatic UGT1A1.* Hepatic UGT1A1 activity toward bilirubin is virtually absent in CN1. Depending on the site of mutation, additional UGT1A isoforms may be catalytically inactive, so that glucuronidation of phenolic substrates may also be reduced (Bosma et al. 1992).

**Treatment**: Goal of the treatment of CN1 is to maintain serum bilirubin concentrations below neurotoxic levels. Liver transplantation is curative, but commits the patient to prolonged immunosuppressive therapy. Following is a brief discussion of the treatment modalities.

*Phototherapy*. Daily phototherapy is the standard maintenance therapy for reducing plasma unconjugated bilirubin (Maisels 2015). Banks of fluorescent lamps or more light-emitting diode (LED) lamps are used along with shielding the eyes. Exposure of the skin to light converts bilirubin $IX_{\alpha}$-ZZ to its photoisomers that are excreted in bile. In newborns, use of phototherapy is based on age-related serum bilirubin concentrations: 260 μM at age 24–48 h, 310 μM at 49–72 h, and 340 μM at 72 h. If intensive phototherapy does not reduce serum bilirubin by at least 1–2 mg/dL within 4–6 h, plasmapheresis is considered (see below). By the age of 3 or 4 years, efficiency of phototherapy declines because of the thickening of skin, pigmentation, and reduction of surface area relative to body mass, requiring readjustment of the intensity and duration of phototherapy.

*Plasmapheresis.* If despite intensive phototherapy, serum bilirubin levels exceed the target levels described above by 85 μM, plasmapheresis is added to continued intensive phototherapy (Maisels 2015). Intensive phototherapy needs to be continued for several days because removal of albumin-bound bilirubin from blood mobilizes bilirubin from tissue stores to plasma, leading to secondary increase of bilirubin levels.

*Orthotopic Liver Transplantation.* Presently, the transplantation of whole liver or a liver lobe is the only available curative therapy for CN1 (Mazariegos et al. 2014). Liver transplantation has dramatically improved the prognosis of CN1 patients, although it commits the patient to prolonged immunosuppression.

## Experimental Therapies

*Heme oxygenase inhibition:* Non-iron metalloporphyrins are dead-end heme oxygenase inhibitors (Kappas and Drummond 1995). Serum bilirubin concentrations were modestly reduced after tin-mesoporphyrin injection (0.5 μmol/kg, three times a week for 13–23 weeks) in two 17-year-old male CN1 patients. However, the duration of effect and safety of this treatment have not been established.

*Hepatocyte transplantation:* Hepatocytes have a high reserve UGT1A1 activity. Therefore, partial restitution of the enzyme activity in livers of CN1 patients should enable therapeutically significant reduction of serum bilirubin. After evaluation of the efficiency of hepatocyte transplantation in UGT1A1-deficient Gunn rats (Polgar et al. 2017), isolated allogeneic human hepatocytes were transplanted into the liver of an adolescent CN1 patient. Transplantation of $7.5 \times 10^9$ hepatocytes by infusion into the portal vein via a percutaneously placed catheter reduced serum bilirubin levels by about 50% and permitted reduction of the duration of phototherapy (Fox et al. 1998). Bilirubin glucuronides were detectable in duodenal bile samples for up to two and a half years, but after 2 years, serum bilirubin gradually increased to pretransplantation levels, requiring auxiliary liver transplantation, which normalized serum bilirubin levels (J. Roy-Chowdhury, personal communication). These results in this study and experience derived from a number of hepatocyte transplantations for CN1 performed by several investigators indicated that the number of hepatocytes that can be transplanted at a time, without causing prolonged portal hypertension, is insufficient for fully obviating the requirement for continued phototherapy (Iansante et al. 2018). Therefore, novel strategies are being explored to expand the mass of the engrafted hepatocytes. As the liver to body weight ratio is regulated tightly by physiological mechanisms, the engrafted hepatocytes can proliferate significantly only by replacing the mutant host hepatocytes by cell competition. Liver repopulation has been achieved in Gunn rats by preparative regional irradiation of the liver, combined with a variety of mitotic stimuli (Zhou et al. 2012). Partial hepatic irradiation enhanced both initial hepatocyte engraftment and subsequent proliferation of the donor hepatocytes, resulting in complete normalization of serum bilirubin levels (Zhou et al. 2012). Preparative irradiation for hepatocyte transplantation has been evaluated in non-human primates and in a patient with phenylketonuria (Soltys et al. 2016).

*Gene Therapy.* To reconstitute the missing hepatic UGT1A1 activity, gene therapy is being evaluated through (a) ex vivo gene therapy, consisting of transduction of primary hepatocytes using viral vectors, followed by transplantation into the liver, and (b) systemic administration of viral or non-viral vectors to express wild-type UGT1A1 in host hepatocytes in vivo. After initial validation in animal experiments, a clinical trial using recombinant adeno-associated viral vectors has been initiated for CN1 patients and (c) targeted gene editing by homologous recombination (Asp et al. 2019).

Targeted gene editing by homologous recombination is being explored using three different strategies (Asp et al. 2019): (a) gene repair to correct mutations, insertions, or deletions or (b) insertion of a UGT1A1 transcription unit at a genomic "safe haven" (such as the AAV-S1 site on human chromosome 19) or (c) insertion of a promoterless UGT1A1 open reading frame (orf) downstream to a highly expressed gene (e.g., albumin) to take advantage of the strong endogenous promoter. Homologous recombination is augmented by generating a nuclease-mediated DNA break which recruits DNA repair proteins at the break site. This can be achieved by expressing a peptide-nuclease fusion protein, e.g., zinc-finger nuclease (ZFN) or transcription activator-like effector nuclease (TALEN). Alternatively, site-directed DNA break can be generated using the CRISPR system, in which a nuclease, such as Cas9, can be guided to the site of interest and activated using a guide strand RNA. In in vivo experiments, usually recombinant adeno-associated viral vectors are used to express the transgenes for inducing targeted DNA breaks, as well as for delivering the DNA strand for homologous recombination. Interestingly, expression from the albumin promoter is so efficient that a low level of homology-directed insertion of the UGT1A1 open reading orf 3′ to the albumin coding sequences is sufficient to reduce serum bilirubin levels in *Ugt1A1* gene-deleted jaundiced mice.

#### Crigler-Najjar Syndrome Type 2 (CN2, Also Termed Arias Syndrome)

**Signs and Symptoms**: Arias described a milder variant of Crigler-Najjar syndrome (Arias 1962) in which serum bilirubin usually ranges from 136 to 306 μmol/L (see Table 58.1), but can increase to 500 μmol/L during intercurrent illness, general anesthesia, or prolonged fasting. Kernicterus is unusual, but can occur during episodes of exacerbated hyperbilirubinemia (Arias 1962). As in CN1, the inheritance shows autosomal recessive pattern, and jaundice due to increased plasma unconjugated bilirubin is the main presenting feature. As there is some residual UGT1A1 activity, CN2 can be usually differentiated from CN1 by induction of UGT1A1 by phenobarbital administration. Also in contrast to CN1, bile contains a significant amount of bilirubin glucuronides. Whereas normal human bile contains predominantly bilirubin diglucuronide, in CN2 and Gilbert syndrome (see below), bilirubin monoglucuronide exceeds 30% of total bilirubin in duodenal bile (normal, ~10%). Liver biopsy is not necessary for diagnosis, but when performed shows normal histology. Hepatic UGT1A1 activity toward bilirubin is usually reduced to 10% normal.

**Treatment**: The baseline level of hyperbilirubinemia in CN2 patients does not increase the BIND risk sufficiently to require routine phototherapy. However, highly stressful situations, such as severe infections, major surgery, or prolonged fasting, can increase bilirubin concentrations to dangerous levels. In these cases, the patients can be treated on a short-term basis with phototherapy or, rarely, plasmapheresis. In special situations, phenobarbital may be used to reduce serum bilirubin levels.

#### Gilbert Syndrome

**Signs and Symptoms**: This very common disorder associated with mild, fluctuating, and occasionally intermittent unconjugated hyperbilirubinemia was described by Gilbert and Lereboullet in 1901 (Gilbert and Lereboullet 1901). More than a century later, Bosma and colleagues showed that Gilbert syndrome is caused by the insertion of a TA dinucleotide into the TATAA element in the proximal promoter of *UGT1A1* (Bosma et al. 1995). Gilbert syndrome is usually diagnosed incidentally in young adults from routine blood tests or during investigation of unrelated illnesses. Mild icterus is the only positive physical finding, and serum bilirubin is predominantly unconjugated. Bilirubin levels can be within normal limits, and are only elevated intermittently. In the absence of coexisting hemolytic conditions, e.g., glucose-6-phosphate dehydrogenase deficiency, or stressful situations, serum bilirubin usually remains below 51 μmol/L. Hyperbilirubinemia is exacerbated during intercurrent illness, stress, fasting, or menstruation. Not uncommonly, patients with known diagnosis of Gilbert syndrome erroneously ascribe fatigue and abdominal discomfort caused by other conditions to Gilbert syndrome. Incidence of pigment gallstones is higher in subjects with Gilbert syndrome than in general population. Liver biopsy is not necessary for diagnosis, but, when performed, shows normal histology.

Gilbert syndrome is one of the most common inherited disorders (Roy-Chowdhury et al. 2019). Clinical diagnosis of Gilbert syndrome has been reported in 3–7% of most populations, although prevalence of homozygous promoter variance (~9%) indicates that all cases are clinically diagnosed. Gilbert syndrome is diagnosed more frequently in males (Roy-Chowdhury et al. 2019), who have a higher baseline bilirubin levels. Increased erythrocyte mass during puberty with consequent increase in bilirubin production and inhibition of bilirubin glucuronidation by endogenous steroid hormones may make the diagnosis clinically apparent at adolescence.

Gilbert syndrome is diagnosed in individuals with mild unconjugated hyperbilirubinemia, but otherwise normal liver serology and no evidence of hemolysis. However, coexistent hemolytic disorders can make jaundice clinically obvious, bringing the patient to medical attention. Liver biopsy is not indicated for the diagnosis, but, when performed, shows reduced hepatic UGT1A1 activity (approximately 30% of normal) (Arias and London 1957). Where the diagnosis is in question, genetic analysis can be performed from a small amount of whole blood sample, usually submitted as a filter paper blot. Homozygosity for a TA dinucleotide insertion into the TATAA element within the proximal promoter region of UGT1A1 establishes the diagnosis. Chromatographic analysis of bile collected by duodenal aspiration via endoscopy shows an increased proportion of bilirubin monoglucuronide (>10%), reflecting reduced hepatic UGT1A1 activity. Reduction of caloric intake to 400 kcal/day for 2 days or nicotinic acid administration may make jaundice clinically detectable in Gilbert syndrome, but since these "challenges" also increase serum bilirubin in normal subjects, they do not provide definitive diagnosis.

Gilbert syndrome is not only innocuous; mild serum bilirubin elevation may have significant health benefits as suggested by reduced incidence of obesity and metabolic syndrome (Choi et al. 2013), ischemic coronary artery disease (Breimer et al. 1995), and colon cancer (Zucker et al. 2004). However, reduced UGT1A1 expression can affect glucuronidation and excretion of certain drugs (Roy-Chowdhury et al. 2019). Gilbert syndrome is associated with a high incidence of diarrhea in patients treated with the anticancer drug, irinotecan (Iyer et al. 1998). Oxidative intermediates of acetaminophen are associated with its drug toxicity. There is conflicting evidence in literature for reduced glucuronidation of these oxidative metabolites in subjects with the UGT1A1*28 allele.

**Treatment**. No treatment is necessary for Gilbert syndrome.

## Inherited Disorders of Bilirubin Metabolism Associated with Predominantly Conjugated Hyperbilirubinemia

By chromatographic measurement, about 4% of serum biliru bin is conjugated, although diazo-based measurements in clinical laboratories overestimate the proportion to some extent (Roy-Chowdhury et al. 2019). Proportion of conjugated bilirubin increases in conditions where bilirubin glucuronides formed in hepatocytes are pumped out to plasma because of bile duct obstruction, inflammatory or ischemic liver injury, as well as inherited disorders of bile canalicular transport or failure of reuptake of bilirubin glucuronides transported out of the hepatocytes into sinusoidal blood. In addition, a number of cholestatic disorders termed progressive familial intrahepatic cholestasis can lead to various degrees of liver injury. In this chapter we will describe in brief two inherited disorders of bilirubin metabolism that cause accumulation of both conjugated and unconjugated bilirubin in plasma, without causing significant liver injury, Dubin-Johnson syndrome (Table 58.2) and Rotor syndrome (Table 58.3), and five inherited types of progressive familial intrahepatic cholestasis that cause hyperbilirubinemia in the context of significant liver injury.

### Dubin-Johnson Syndrome (Table 58.2)

**Signs and Symptoms**: Dubin-Johnson syndrome is characterized by chronic or intermittent conjugated hyperbilirubinemia and grossly pigmented, but otherwise histologically normal liver. Mild jaundice is the only consistent presenting feature. Usually, the patients are otherwise asymptomatic, but vague abdominal pain and hepatosplenomegaly occur in some cases (Dubin 1958; Shani et al. 1970). Serum bile acid levels are nearly normal (Dubin 1958), and in contrast to chronic cholestatic disorders, pruritus is absent. Serum bilirubin levels increase during intercurrent illness, intake of oral contraceptives, and pregnancy (Iyer et al. 1998). Diagnosis is usually made in young adults. In some cases, the condition is identified during pregnancy or contraceptive use (Dubin 1958; Shani et al. 1970). Dubin-Johnson syndrome is innocuous, but the diagnosis is important, because increased serum conjugated bilirubin levels suggest inflammatory or cholestatic hepatobiliary diseases.

Serum bilirubin levels usually range from 34 to 85 μmol/L, but levels as high as 340–425 μmol/L have been reported in rare situations. More than half of serum bilirubin is direct-reacting, and bilirubin is excreted in urine. Liver serology, including ALT, AST, and alkaline phosphatase, is normal. In contrast to other cholestatic conditions, serum bile acid levels are normal in adult patients with Dubin-Johnson syndrome (Shani et al. 1970). As the functional defect involves hepatocellular canalicular excretion for multiple organic anions, other than most bile acids, oral cholecystography does not visualize the gallbladder even using the contrast material at "double dose." Intravenous administration of meglumine iodipamide (Biligrafin) may enable visualization of the gallbladder after 4–6 h (Roy-Chowdhury et al. 2019).

*Organic Anion Transport.* A large variety of organic anions, including bilirubin glucuronides, but not most bile acids are pumped out into the bile canaliculus from the hepatocyte against a concentration gradient by an energy-consuming ATP-dependent protein ABCC2 or MRP2 (Fig. 58.2) (Roy-Chowdhury et al. 2019; Shani et al. 1970). Much of the information on the function of Abcc2 has come from studies in the jaundiced $TR^-$ rat strain (Paulusma et al. 1996). In this rat strain, biliary excretion of sulfated or glucuronidated bile acids was found to be deficient. Consistent with this, in a subsequent multicenter study, neonates with Dubin-Johnson syndrome were found to have significantly increased serum total

**Table 58.2** Signs and symptoms of Dubin-Johnson syndrome

| System | Symptoms and signs | Neonatal | Infancy | Childhood | Adolescence | Adulthood |
|---|---|---|---|---|---|---|
| Conjunctiva, mucous membranes, skin | Yellow discoloration (jaundice) | ± | ± | + | ++ | ++ |
| | Increased jaundice during pregnancy and contraceptive use | | | | | + |
| Abdominal pain | Vague upper abdominal pain | | | | ± | ± |
| Routine laboratory tests | ALT, AST, alkaline phosphatase, γ-glutamyl transpeptidase | + | | | | |
| | Elevated serum bilirubin (predominantly conjugated) | + | ± | + | ++ | ++ |
| | Plasma bile salt elevation | + | ± | | | |
| Special laboratory tests | Urinary coproporphyrinogen chromatography: Increased proportion of isoform I | + | + | ++ | +++ | +++ |
| Oral cholecystography | Non-visualization even with double dose of contrast | | | + | + | + |
| Liver biopsy | Macroscopic: Black liver | | | + | ++ | +++ |
| | Microscopic: Dark brown pigments | | | + | ++ | +++ |
| Pharmacological tests | Plasma bromosulfophthalein clearance: Normal at 45 min, secondary rise at 90 min | | | + | ++ | ++ |

**Table 58.3** Signs and symptoms of Rotor syndrome

| System | Symptoms and signs | Neonatal | Infancy | Childhood | Adolescence | Adulthood |
|---|---|---|---|---|---|---|
| Conjunctiva, mucous membranes, skin | Yellow discoloration (jaundice) | ± | ± | + | ++ | ++ + |
| Routine laboratory tests | ALT, AST, alkaline phosphatase, γ-glutamyl transpeptidase | | | | | |
| | Elevated serum bilirubin (predominantly conjugated) | ± | ± | + | ++ | ++ |
| Special laboratory tests | Urinary coproporphyrin chromatography: Increased total coproporphyrins. Both isomers I and II are increased | + | + | ++ | +++ | +++ |
| Oral cholecystography | Gallbladder visualized normally | | | + | + | + |
| Liver biopsy | No pigmentation | n | n | n | n | n |
| Pharmacological tests | Plasma bromosulfophthalein retention at 45 min, no secondary rise | | | + | ++ | ++ |

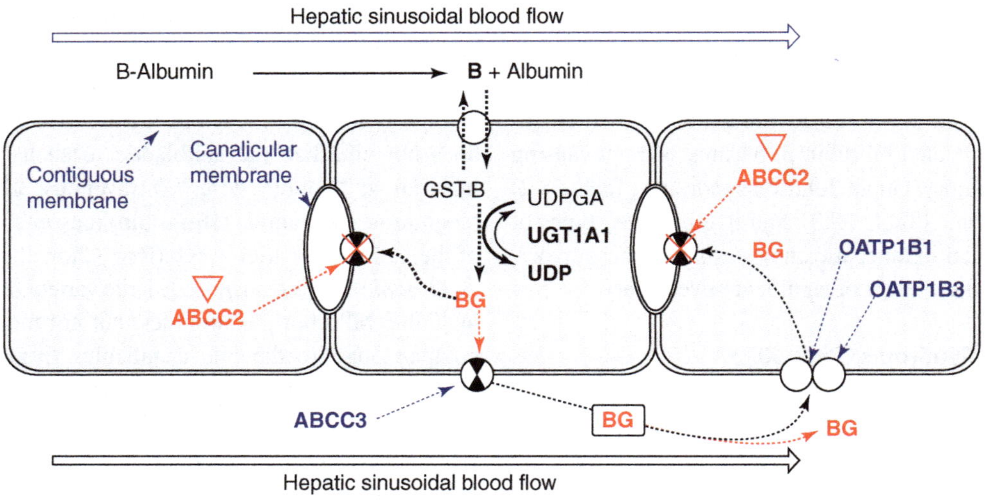


**Fig. 58.2** Dubin-Johnson syndrome is caused by mutations of the bile canalicular ATP-utilizing pump, ABCC2. This protein is involved in pumping a large number of organic anions into the bile canaliculus, including bilirubin glucuronides (BGs), but not including most bile salts. Conjugated bilirubin retained in the hepatocytes is pumped out across the sinusoidal surface membrane of hepatocytes by alternative pumps, such as ABCC3, resulting in an increase in the conjugated fraction of serum bilirubin

bile acid levels (Togawa et al. 2018). Despite the lack of ABCC2, serum bilirubin is only mildly elevated, suggesting additional pathways of excretion of bilirubin conjugates in bile. In addition, accumulated organic anions within the hepatocytes upregulate the expression of ABCC11 and ABCC3 at the basolateral surface of the hepatocytes. These and possibly additional ATP-consuming pumps may transport both unconjugated and conjugated bilirubin from the hepatocyte to plasma (Roy-Chowdhury et al. 2019).

*Urinary Coproporphyrin Excretion.* In normal adults approximately 75% of the urinary coproporphyrin is isomer III, the precursor of heme. The remaining is coproporphyrin I. In Dubin-Johnson syndrome, over 80% of total urinary coproporphyrin is isomer I, but total urinary coproporphyrin excretion is normal (Kaplowitz et al. 1972). In neonates, the proportion of urinary coproporphyrin I is higher than in adults, but not as high as in Dubin-Johnson syndrome. The relationship of the abnormal urinary porphyrin excretion pattern to defective organic anion transport is not known. Together with consistent clinical presentation, the urinary coproporphyrin excretion pattern is diagnostic of Dubin-Johnson syndrome.

As indicated in Fig. 58.2, the uptake mechanism at the sinusoidal surface of hepatocytes is unaffected in Dubin-Johnson syndrome. Consistent with this, after intravenous injection of the organic anion BSP (bromosulfophthalein), initial decline of plasma BSP concentration is nearly normal for 45 min, but, in most patients, there is a secondary increase in plasma BSP concentration at 90 min because of the reflux of glutathione-conjugated BSP from hepatocytes into the circulation (Roy-Chowdhury et al. 2019). However, such secondary rise of plasma BSP can also occur in other cholestatic disorders (Roy-Chowdhury et al. 2019). Therefore, the BSP clearance pattern is not pathognomonic of Dubin-Johnson syndrome.

*Liver Histology:* The liver is black in color, which is a distinguishing characteristic of Dubin-Johnson syndrome. Light microscopy reveals a dense brown pigment (Fig. 58.3). After intravenous infusion of $^{3}$H-epinephrine into mutant Corriedale sheep (an animal model for Dubin-Johnson syndrome), radioactivity is incorporated into the pigment, which may consist of polymers of epinephrine metabolites (Roy-Chowdhury et al. 2019). Following liver regeneration after massive hepatocellular death, the pigment is cleared from the liver, but reaccumulates slowly after recovery.

**Treatment***:* No treatment is required for Dubin-Johnson syndrome.

**Rotor Syndrome** (Table 58.3)

**Signs and Symptoms**: Rotor syndrome is characterized by lifelong mild hyperbilirubinemia without evidence of hemolysis (Rotor et al. 1948). Elevation of serum bilirubin levels is predominantly due to increase in the conjugated bilirubin fraction. Serum ALT, AST, alkaline phosphatase, and other routine blood biochemistries are normal (Table 58.3). In these respects, the clinical phenotype resembles that of Dubin-Johnson syndrome. However, in contrast to Dubin-Johnson syndrome, there is no pigmentation accumulation in the liver. Liver histology is normal. Rotor syndrome is harmless (Kaplowitz et al. 1972), but the diagnosis is important because, as in Dubin-Johnson syndrome, increased serum conjugated bilirubin fraction may suggest inflammatory or cholestatic hepatobiliary diseases. Rotor syndrome is rare, but has been reported in several races.

*Organic Anion Excretion.* In contrast to Dubin-Johnson syndrome, canalicular secretion of organic anions is normal in Rotor syndrome, but the reuptake of bilirubin glucuronides and several other conjugated substances by hepatocyte sinusoidal membranes is defective as result of complete deficiency of two organic anion transport proteins, OATP1B1 and OATP1B3 (Fig. 58.4) (Roy-Chowdhury et al. 2019; van de Steeg et al. 2012). As in many acquired liver diseases, and in contrast with Dubin-Johnson syndrome, over 25% of injected BSP is retained in serum at 45 min, and there is no secondary rise of plasma BSP level (Roy-Chowdhury et al. 2019). Plasma clearance of intravenously administrated unconjugated bilirubin and ICG is also delayed. In contrast to the findings in Dubin-Johnson syndrome, bile canalicular export pumps are normal in Rotor syndrome; therefore, the gallbladder is visualized by oral cholecystography (Fig. 58.4).

*Urinary Coproporphyrin Excretion.* Total urinary coproporphyrin excretion in Rotor syndrome is increased two- to fivefold over normal. Approximately 65% of the urinary cop-

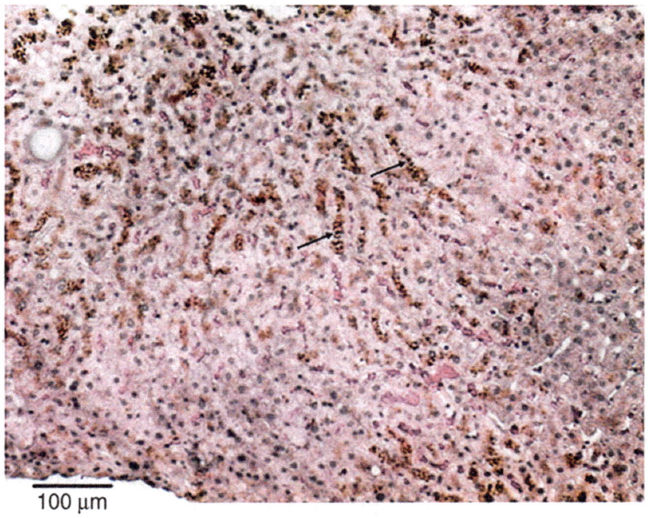


**Fig. 58.3** Hematoxylin/eosin staining of liver section in a patient with Dubin-Johnson syndrome. The liver architecture and histology are normal, except for dark brown pigments (arrows) predominantly in centrizonal (Zone 3) hepatocytes

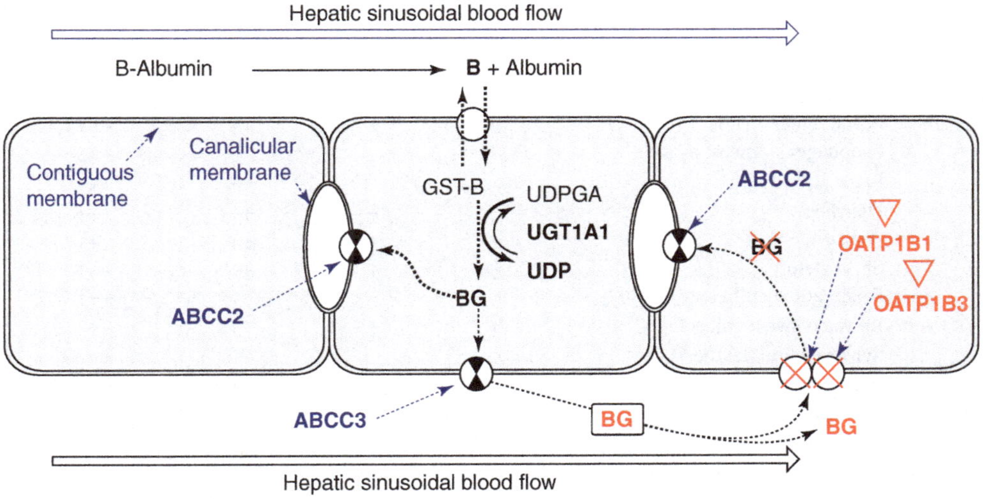


**Fig. 58.4** Rotor syndrome is caused by simultaneous deficiency of the organic anion transporters OATP1B1 and OATP1B3 at the sinusoidal membrane of hepatocytes. While the majority of bilirubin glucuronides (BGs) formed by the action of UGT1A1 is normally secreted into the bile canaliculus, a fraction is pumped out into the hepatic sinusoidal blood by ABCC3. This fraction of bilirubin glucuronides undergoes reuptake by hepatocytes located downstream to the blood flow via OATP1B1 and OATP1B3 (encoded by the *SLCO1B1* and *SLCO1B3* genes, respectively). Lack of bilirubin glucuronide reuptake results in mild conjugated hyperbilirubinemia

roporphyrin has been reported to be isomer I (Roy-Chowdhury et al. 2019). This pattern is similar to that found in many other hepatobiliary disorders, but is distinct from that seen in Dubin-Johnson syndrome (see above). However, in two brothers with characteristic clinical features of Rotor syndrome, over 80% of urinary coproporphyrins was isomer I (Roy-Chowdhury et al. 2019), raising doubts about the utility of urinary coproporphyrin analysis in distinguishing Rotor from Dubin-Johnson syndrome.

**Treatment**: No treatment is required for Rotor syndrome.

***Progressive Familial Intrahepatic Cholestasis.*** These conditions do not affect the bilirubin throughput pathway directly, but result in elevation of both serum unconjugated and conjugated bilirubin levels as a result of hepatocellular injury. Five life-threatening monogenic disorders, collectively termed progressive familial intrahepatic cholestasis (PFIC-1, PFIC-2, PFIC-3, PFIC-4, PFIC-5), can cause cholestasis, associated with severe liver injury, affecting the secretion of bile acids or other components of bile into the bile canaliculi. It is likely that additional gene mutations causing PFIC will be discovered. Some mutations of the genes associated with the PFIC syndromes cause only partial loss of function, resulting in a milder phenotype of the diseases, namely, benign recurrent intrahepatic cholestasis (BRIC) or mild chronic liver disease, resulting in delayed liver fibrosis or cirrhosis. Inherited cholestatic diseases including the PFIC syndromes have been reviewed recently (Henkel et al. 2019), and a brief discussion follows.

#### Progressive Familial Intrahepatic Cholestasis Type 1 (Table 58.4)

**Signs and Symptoms**: Progressive familial intrahepatic cholestasis type 1 (PFIC 1) was originally described in an Amish Mennonite family and was named Byler's disease, after the family name of the first patient (Roy-Chowdhury et al. 2019; Henkel et al. 2019). It has been also termed Greenland-Eskimo familial cholestasis. PFIC-1 is associated with severe life-threatening cholestatic liver disease along with extrahepatic manifestations. Abnormality of aminophospholipid transfer from the outer leaflet of plasma membrane to the inner leaflet results in hyperbilirubinemia and accumulation of bile salts in plasma. Infants often present with jaundice, pruritus, and hepatosplenomegaly. When the disease is severe, cholestasis is persistent and progressive resulting in development of portal hypertension in early childhood. Although serum ALT and AST are elevated, γ-glutamyl transpeptidase (GGT) level remains normal. Severe extrahepatic manifestations, such as profound diarrhea, poor growth, short stature, pancreatic insufficiency, elevated sweat chloride, and sensorineural deafness (Henkel et al. 2019; Clayton et al. 1969), distinguish this disease from other inherited cholestatic disorders. The liver shows canalicular cholestasis with biliary plugs, giant cell transformation, paucity of bile ducts, and lobular disarray. The bile has a granular appearance.

**Treatment**: As with all forms of PFIC, no definitive medical therapies are available. Supportive measures include improving nutritional deficiencies by caloric, fat (mainly

**Table 58.4** Signs and symptoms of progressive familial intrahepatic cholestasis type 1

| System | Symptoms and signs | Neonatal | Infancy | Childhood | Adolescence | Adulthood |
|---|---|---|---|---|---|---|
| Hepatic | | | | | | |
| Skin and conjunctiva | Jaundice | | ++ | +++ | +++ | +++ |
| | Pruritus | ± | ++ | +++ | +++ | +++ |
| Liver and spleen size | Liver and spleen are enlarged | | + | ++ | +++ | +++ |
| End-stage liver disease | Portal hypertension<br>Esophageal varices, ascites | n | ± | ++ | +++ | +++ |
| | Liver failure | | | ++ | +++ | +++ |
| Digestive system | Diarrhea | ± | ++ | +++ | +++ | +++ |
| | Poor growth | ± | + | ++ | +++ | +++ |
| | Short stature | | + | ++ | +++ | +++ |
| | Pancreatic insufficiency | | | | ++ | |
| Skin | Elevated sweat chloride | ± | ++ | ++ | ++ | ++ |
| Neurological | Sensorineural deafness | | | + | + | ++ |
| Routine laboratory tests | ALT, AST | | ± | ++ | ++ | ++ |
| | Elevated serum bilirubin (predominantly conjugated) | ± | + | ++ | ++ | ++ |
| | γ-Glutamyl transpeptidase | | | | | |
| Special laboratory tests | Biliary primary bile acids (low) | | + | + | + | + |
| | Electron microscopy shows granular bile | | + | + | + | + |
| | Serum bile acids (increased) | | ++ | ++ | ++ | ++ |
| Liver histology | Bland cholestasis<br>Mild lobular fibrosis | | + | ++ | ++ | ++ |

medium chain triglycerides), and vitamin supplementation. Ursodeoxycholic acid (UDCA) is administered to replace the hydrophobic bile salt pool, as well as to induce bile salt excretory protein (BSEP) and MDR3 expression. UDCA administration usually improves pruritus (Roy-Chowdhury et al. 2019; Henkel et al. 2019).

*Surgical Interruption of Bile Salt Reabsorption*: When medical therapy is insufficient, surgical procedures aimed at interruption of enterohepatic recycling of bile acids have been used for the treatment of PFIC. Partial external biliary diversion (cholecysto-jejunal cutaneous fistula) or ileal bypass can reduce pruritus and improve growth rate in many cases. More recently, partial internal biliary diversion (PIBD) has been utilized by creating a neo-conduit between the gallbladder and the colon to prevent reabsorption of bile acids in the terminal ileum (Clayton et al. 1969). In addition to relieving pruritus, these procedures have been reported to reduce plasma bile acid and bilirubin levels.

*Liver Transplantation*: Patients with a refractory course and those who have developed end-stage liver disease require liver transplantation. It should be noted that diarrhea associated with PFIC-1 may persist or even worsen after liver transplantation. Furthermore, the allograft may develop steatosis and fibrosis, and in some cases ileal diversion has been performed at the time of liver transplantation to prevent hepatic steatosis. (Gunaydin et al. 2016).

#### Progressive Familial Intrahepatic Cholestasis Type 2 (PFIC-2) (Table 58.5)

This condition results from defective transport of bile acids from hepatocytes into the bile canaliculi, leading to hepatotoxicity from accumulated bile salts. Deficiency of bile salts in the intestinal lumen results in fat indigestion and malabsorption.

**Signs and Symptoms***:* Affected infants initially present with jaundice. Pruritus develops at 4–5 months of age. Hepatomegaly and growth retardation due to malabsorption of fat and fat-soluble vitamins may also be apparent. Extrahepatic symptoms are less pronounced than in FIC1 deficiency, but the disease often progresses to portal hypertension within the first year of life (Henkel et al. 2019). Typically, serum aminotransferase levels are over twice the upper limit, and both conjugated and unconjugated bilirubin are elevated. But serum GGT levels remain normal (Henkel et al. 2019).

Liver biopsy typically shows evidence of canalicular cholestasis, hepatocellular disarray, and lobular and portal fibrosis (Roy-Chowdhury et al. 2019; Henkel et al. 2019). Up to 15% of PFIC-2 patients develop liver malignancy (hepatocellular carcinoma and cholangiocarcinoma), which can occur in children as early as at 13 months of age (Knisely et al. 2006). Therefore, PFIC-2 patients need to be screened for liver cancer by serum α-fetoprotein (AFP) level and abdominal ultrasonography every 6–12 months.

**Treatment**: Medical treatment is primarily supportive and includes nutritional supplementation and antipruritic agents. Enhancers of the residual cell surface BSEP such as 4-phenylbutyrate have been promising. Surgical interruption of the enterohepatic circulation ameliorates pruritus but not progression of liver injury (Wang et al. 2017). In general, patients with some residual BSEP function have better prognosis than those with severely dysfunctional or absent BSEP (Roy-Chowdhury et al. 2019; Henkel et al. 2019).

Liver transplantation: Liver transplantation has been performed in PFIC-2 patients with a severe course and in those who develop tumor. However, some recipients develop alloreactive antibodies specific to the extracellular loop of the BSEP protein, which may cause an immune-mediated recur-

**Table 58.5** Signs and symptoms of progressive familial intrahepatic cholestasis type 2

| System | Symptoms and signs | Neonatal | Infancy | Childhood | Adolescence | Adulthood |
|---|---|---|---|---|---|---|
| Hepatic | | | | | | |
| Skin and conjunctiva | Jaundice | | ++ | +++ | +++ | +++ |
| | Pruritus | ± | ++ | +++ | +++ | +++<br>+++ |
| Liver and spleen size | Liver and spleen are enlarged | | + | ++ | +++ | |
| End-stage liver disease | Portal hypertension with esophageal varices and ascites | n | + | +++ | +++ | +++ |
| | Risk of hepatocellular carcinoma | n | n | + | ++ | +++ |
| Gallbladder | Cholesterol gallstones | n | ± | ++ | +++ | +++ |
| Routine laboratory tests | AFP | | ± | + | +++ | +++ |
| | ALT, AST | | + | ++ | ++ | ++ |
| | Elevated serum bilirubin (predominantly conjugated) | ± | + | ++ | ++ | ++ |
| | γ-Glutamyl transpeptidase | | | | | |
| Special laboratory tests | Biliary primary bile acids (low) | | +++ | +++ | +++ | +++ |
| | Electron microscopy shows amorphous bile | | | + | + | + |
| | Serum bile acids (high) | + | +++ | +++ | +++ | +++ |
| Liver histology | Cholestasis, giant cell hepatitis, hepatocellular necrosis, portal fibrosis | | ± | ++ | +++ | +++ |

rence of BSEP disease in the allograft, which may respond to standard immunosuppression, although refractory disease recurrence may require B-cell-depleting antibody therapy and allogeneic hematopoietic stem cell transplantation (Krebs-Schmitt et al. 2019). Some patients have required repeat liver transplantation (Krebs-Schmitt et al. 2019).

### Progressive Familial Intrahepatic Cholestasis Type 3 (PFIC-3) (Table 58.6)

PFIC-3 results from defects of energy-consuming transport of phosphatidylcholine from the inner lipid leaflet of the bile canaliculus to the outer leaflet. This process normally replenishes the phospholipid in the outer leaflet, which is continuously removed by high concentrations of bile acid in the bile canaliculi. Failure of phosphatidylcholine replenishment results in chronic bile salt-mediated injury of the canalicular membrane and small bile ducts (Roy-Chowdhury et al. 2019; Henkel et al. 2019).

**Signs and Symptoms***:* PFIC-3 has been diagnosed in some cases in the first months of life or in children, but patients usually present in late adolescence or even adulthood (Schatz et al. 2018). Those diagnosed in childhood present with pruritus at about 1 year of age, and most have hepatosplenomegaly, portal hypertension, and jaundice at presentation. Children and adolescents may initially present with variceal bleeding, without significant prior symptoms. Many patients in the pediatric age group also have growth restriction, reduced bone density, and learning disability (Schatz et al. 2018). Adult patients can present with slowly progressive disease, cholelithiasis, drug-induced cholestasis, or benign recurrent intrahepatic cholestasis (also see below under BRIC).

In contrast to other PFICs, GGT is typically elevated at presentation, despite relatively milder elevation of serum bilirubin and transaminases.

Portal fibrosis and bile duct proliferation with mild giant cell hepatitis are usually seen early in the course of the disease with occasional intraductal cholelithiasis (Roy-Chowdhury et al. 2019; Henkel et al. 2019). MDR3 is often absent by immunohistochemical staining, but may be visualized when there are functional protein defects. Both hepatoma and cholangiocarcinomas may be found.

**Treatment**: Supportive management includes nutritional supplements and antipruritic agents. Liver transplantation offers the only definitive therapy.

***Benign Recurrent Intrahepatic Cholestasis (BRIC)*** presents with recurrent episodes of cholestasis in adolescence or early adulthood, characterized by both conjugated and unconjugated hyperbilirubinemia, malaise, anorexia, pruritus, weight loss, and malabsorption. During the attacks that last weeks to months, laboratory tests are typical of cholestasis without severe hepatocellular injury (Biempica et al. 1967). The cholestatic episodes are followed by a complete clinical, biochemical, and histological resolution. In individual patients, the clinical features and duration of the episodes resemble those in previous attacks. Liver biopsy shows noninflammatory intrahepatic cholestasis without fibrosis, even after multiple episodes. During remission, the liver appears normal by light and electron microscopy (Roy-Chowdhury et al. 2019; Biempica et al. 1967). Interestingly, this relatively benign disorder is also caused by certain missense mutations of the *ATP8B1, ABCB11*, or *ABCB4* genes (BRIC-1, BRIC-2, and BRIC-3, respectively).

**Table 58.6** Signs and symptoms of progressive familial intrahepatic cholestasis type 3

| System | Symptoms and signs | Neonatal | Infancy | Childhood | Adolescence | Adulthood |
|---|---|---|---|---|---|---|
| Hepatic | | | | | | |
| Skin and conjunctiva | Jaundice | + | ± | ++ | +++ | +++ |
| | Pruritus | + | ± | + | ++ | ++<br>+++ |
| Liver and spleen size | Liver and spleen are enlarged | | + | ++ | +++ | |
| End-stage liver disease | Portal hypertension with esophageal varices and ascites | n | n | + | ++ | +++ |
| | Risk of hepatocellular carcinoma | n | n | + | + | ++ |
| Gallbladder | Cholesterol gallstones | n | ± | ++ | +++ | +++ |
| Routine laboratory tests | Elevated serum bilirubin (predominantly conjugated) | ± | + | ++ | ++ | ++ |
| | ALT, AST | n | + | ++ | ++ | ++ |
| | γ-Glutamyl transpeptidase high | | ++ | +++ | +++ | +++ |
| Special laboratory tests | Biliary phospholipids (low) | | +++ | +++ | +++ | +++ |
| | Biliary primary bile acids (low) | n | n | n | n | n |
| | Serum bile acids (high) | n | ± | + | + | ++ |
| Liver histology | Inflammatory infiltrates<br>Bile ductular proliferation<br>Biliary fibrosis | | ± | ++ | +++ | +++ |

### Progressive Familial Intrahepatic Cholestasis Type 4 (PFIC-4)

In a multi-institution collaborative study, 33 children with severe chronic cholestatic liver disease but with low GGT for the degree of cholestasis were found to have no mutations of either *ABCB11* or *ATP8B1*, which cause PFIC-1 or PFIC-2, respectively. Therefore, these patients were designated as having PFIC-4. Subsequently, histological analysis showed deficiency of the tight junction protein 2 (TJP2) (Henkel et al. 2019; Sambrotta et al. 2014).

**Signs and Symptoms**: Infants present with severe liver disease during the first few months of life. Although only a small number of patients have been reported so far, retrospective re-classification suggests that TJP2 deficiency may be more common than previously thought.

Increased serum bilirubin and transaminase levels indicate severe liver injury, but as in PFIC-1 and PFIC-2, serum GGT levels are normal or low for the degree of cholestasis. Histological examination of the liver shows evidence of intracellular cholestasis and giant cell transformation. Immunohistochemical staining reveals absence of TJP2. Hepatocellular carcinoma was found at presentation in several infants (Zhou et al. 2015).

***Treatment***: As the liver injury and cholestasis are severe from the onset, 9 of the 12 initially reported patients have undergone liver transplantation. Two others who did not receive liver transplantation have survived, but have developed portal hypertension (Henkel et al. 2019; Zhou et al. 2015).

### Progressive Familial Intrahepatic Cholestasis Type 5 (PFIC-5) (Table 58.7)

This is a rare disease caused by abnormality of the nuclear receptor FXR, which in turn regulates BSEP. So far five patients have been reported in literature (Henkel et al. 2019; Gomez-Ospina et al. 2016).

**Signs and Symptoms**: All reported patients with this defect presented in the neonatal period and rapidly progressed to end-stage liver disease with coagulopathy and hyperammonemia.

Serum ALT and AST are initially normal, and as in PFIC 1, 2, and 4, GGT remains normal. Serum bile acid levels are elevated and AFP levels can be very high. With the onset of end-stage liver disease, coagulopathy that is not reversed by vitamin K and hyperammonemia occur (Henkel et al. 2019).

Histologically, the liver shows evidence of intralobular cholestasis with ductular reaction, hepatocellular ballooning, giant cell transformation, and fibrosis with progression to micronodular cirrhosis.

**Treatment**: Of the five patients reported in literature, three underwent liver transplantation. However two of the transplant recipients showed steatosis in the graft organ on follow-up.

**Table 58.7** Signs and symptoms of progressive familial intrahepatic cholestasis type 5

| System | Symptoms and signs | Neonatal | Infancy | Childhood | Adolescence | Adulthood |
|---|---|---|---|---|---|---|
| Hepatic | | | | | | |
| Skin and conjunctiva | Jaundice | | ++ | +++ | +++ | +++ |
| | Pruritus | ± | ++ | +++ | +++ | +++<br>+++ |
| Liver and spleen size | Liver and spleen are enlarged | | + | ++ | +++ | |
| End-stage liver disease | Portal hypertension with esophageal varices and ascites | n | + | +++ | +++ | +++ |
| | Risk of hepatocellular carcinoma | n | n | + | ++ | +++ |
| Gallbladder | Cholesterol gallstones | n | ± | ++ | +++ | +++ |
| Routine laboratory tests | AFP | n | + | ++ | +++ | +++ |
| | ALT, AST | n | + | ++ | ++ | ++ |
| | Elevated serum bilirubin (predominantly conjugated) | ± | + | ++ | ++ | ++ |
| | Hyperammonemia | | ± | ++ | +++ | +++ |
| | Increased prothrombin time (INR) | n | + | ++ | +++ | +++ |
| | γ-Glutamyl transpeptidase | n | n | n | n | n |
| Special laboratory tests | Serum bile acids (high) | + | +++ | +++ | +++ | +++ |
| | Biliary primary bile acids (low) | | +++ | +++ | +++ | +++ |
| Liver histology | Intralobular cholestasis, ductular reaction, hepatocellular ballooning, Giant cell transformation, fibrosis progressing to micronodular cirrhosis | | ± | ++ | +++ | +++ |

## Reference Values

| Age | Serum total bilirubin (μmol/L) | Serum unconjugated bilirubin (μmol/L)[a] | Serum conjugated bilirubin (μmol/L)[a] | Total plasma bile acids (μmol/L) |
|---|---|---|---|---|
| **Newborn** | | | | |
| At birth | 1.71–25 | 1.2–17.5 | 0.51–7.5[a] | 3.85–6.32 (isomer I: 25%) |
| *At 96 hr* | | | | |
| 50th percentile | 137–154 | 124–139[a] | 13–15[a] | |
| 96th percentile | 257–300 | 251–270 | 26–30[a] | |
| **Infant** | 1.71–17 | 1.21–12[a] | 0.5–5.1[a] | 6.61–9.43 (isomer I 25%) |
| **Adult** | 1.71–20.5 | 1.21–14.5[a] | 0.5–6.0[a] | 0.28–6.50 (isomer I 25%) |

[a]By methods using diazo reagents, which overestimate conjugated bilirubin. By chromatographic measurements, approximately 4% of total serum bilirubin in normal adults is conjugated

## Pathological Values

| Disorder | Serum unconjugated bilirubin (μmol/L) | Serum conjugated bilirubin (μmol/L)[a] | Plasma bile acids (μmol/L) | Total urine coproporphyrin (μmol/L) (% isomer-I) |
|---|---|---|---|---|
| Crigler-Najjar type 1 | 340–600 | 0[a] | | |
| Crigler-Najjar type 2 | 136–306 | >4% of total[a] | | |
| Gilbert syndrome | 15–51 | >4% of total[a] | | |
| Dubin-Johnson syndrome | 9–35 | 25–50 | 0.28–6.50[b] | 0.28–6.50 (isomer I: 80%) |
| Rotor syndrome | | | 20–33 | 16–33 (isomer I: ~50%) |

[a]Conjugated bilirubin values obtained by chromatographic analysis. Diazo reagent-based assays show artifactually higher proportions of conjugated ("direct-reacting") bilirubin

[b]Neonates with Dubin-Johnson syndrome may have abnormally high serum bile acid levels

## Diagnostic Flowchart

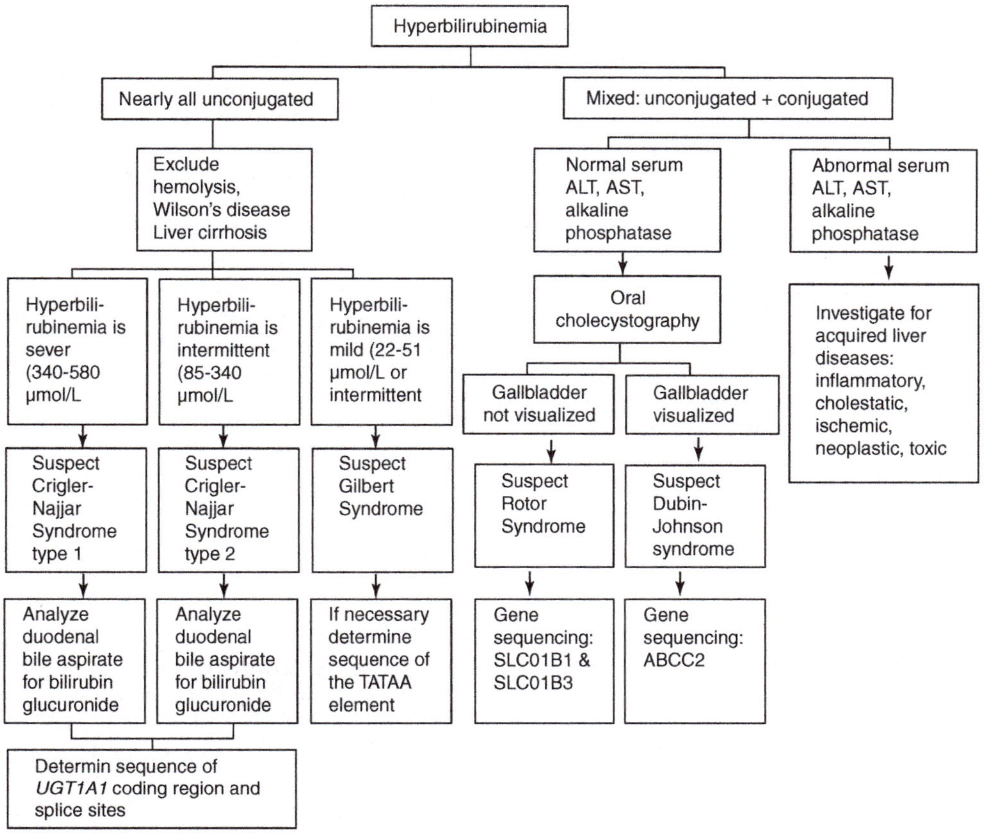


## Specimen Collection

| Test | Sample requirement | Special handling/storage |
|---|---|---|
| **Bilirubin:**<br>• Total<br>• conjugated<br>• unconjugated | Serum sample, at least 0.5 ml | Protect from bright light<br>Analysis to be completed by:<br>• room temperature: 2 days<br>• 0–4.0 °C: 3 days<br>• frozen (−20 °C): 14 days |
| **Plasma bile acid** | Anticoagulated blood (EDTA or heparin)<br>At least 0.2 ml | Analysis to be completed by:<br>• Room temperature: 1 day<br>• 0–4.0 °C: 3 days<br>• Frozen (−20 °C): 7 days |

## Prenatal Diagnosis

| Disorder | Material | Timing (post-conception) |
|---|---|---|
| Crigler-Najjar syndrome type 1 | • Amniotic fluid (30 ml) collected by amniocentesis<br>• Chorionic villus sampling | 16–20 weeks (or later)<br>11–14 weeks |
| Crigler-Najjar syndrome type 2 | • Amniotic fluid (30 ml) collected by amniocentesis<br>• Chorionic villus sampling | 16–20 weeks (or later)<br>11–14 weeks |
| Progressive familial intrahepatic cholestasis type 1 (PFIC-1) | • Amniotic fluid (30 ml) collected by amniocentesis<br>• Chorionic villus sampling | 16–20 weeks (or later)<br>11–14 weeks |
| PFIC-2 | • Amniotic fluid (30 ml) collected by amniocentesis<br>• Chorionic villus sampling | 16–20 weeks (or later)<br>11–14 weeks |
| PFIC-3 | • Amniotic fluid (30 ml) collected by amniocentesis<br>• Chorionic villus sampling | 16–20 weeks (or later)<br>11–14 weeks |
| PFIC-4 | • Amniotic fluid (30 ml) collected by amniocentesis<br>• Chorionic villus sampling | 16–20 weeks (or later)<br>11–14 weeks |
| PFIC-5 | • Amniotic fluid (30 ml) collected by amniocentesis<br>• Chorionic villus sampling | 16–20 weeks (or later)<br>11–14 weeks |

## DNA testing

| Disorder | Gene | Comments |
|---|---|---|
| Crigler-Najjar syndrome type 1 (CN1) | *UGT1A1* | Insertions, deletions, or single nucleotide mutations (nonsense or missense) within any of the five exons comprising the coding region of UGT1A1 can result in complete or near-complete loss of UGT1A1 activity. Genetic lesions within exon 1 affect only UGT1A1, but lesions within exons 2–5 affect all UGT isoforms expressed from the UGT1A locus. Intronic lesions leading to splicing abnormalities can also cause CN1 |
| Crigler-Najjar syndrome type 2 (CN2) | *UGT1A1* | CN2 is caused by nonsynonymous missense mutations within coding region of UGT1A1 that lead to a single amino acid substitution, causing reduction of UGT1A1 catalytic activity to ~10% of normal |
| Gilbert syndrome (GS) | *UGT1A1*28* | GS is caused by homozygosity for the insertion of a TA dinucleotide within the TATAA element 29 nt 5′ of the translation initiation site of UGT1A1. The GS-type promoter reduces UGT1A1 expression to ~30% of normal. Because of the high frequency of the GS promoter in general population, it may coexist with other genetic disorders. In heterozygote carriers of CN1 or CN2, presence of a GS promoter in the allele with normal coding region reduces UGT1A1 expression, resulting in an intermediate level of jaundice |
| Dubin-Johnson syndrome (DJS) | *ABCC2* | Genetic lesions within the coding region include insertions, deletions (in-frame or frameshift), non-sense mutations, or nonsynonymous single nucleotide transitions. In addition, splice site mutations within introns may result in exon skipping |
| Rotor syndrome | *SLCO1B1; SLCO1B3* (digenic) | The Rotor syndrome phenotype requires simultaneous genetic lesions within the coding regions of both *SLCO1B1*and *SLCO1B3*. In addition, inversion of exon 4 of *SLCO1B3* has been reported |
| Progressive familial intrahepatic cholestasis type 1 (PFIC-1) and benign recurrent intrahepatic cholestasis (BRIC-1) | *ATP8B1* | Nonsense mutations, nonsynonymous nucleotide transitions, small (three-base) or large deletions, a seven-base duplication, and intronic mutations leading to splicing abnormality of ATP8B1 pre-mRNA have been reported to cause PFIC1. Patients are homozygotes or compound heterozygotes<br>In BRIC-1, *ATP8B1* point mutations are nonsynonymous |
| PFIC-2 and BRIC-2 | *ABCB11* | Nonsense mutations, small insertions, or deletions leading to truncated protein, and single nonsynonymous mutations within the ABCB11 coding region can cause PFIC-2. In addition, intronic mutations and a synonymous mutation predicted to affect splicing have been reported<br>In BRIC-2, *ABCB11* point mutations are nonsynonymous. |
| PFIC-3 and BRIC-3 | *ABCB4* | A large number of nonsynonymous, nonsense, or frameshift mutations and short insertions within the coding region of the ABCB4 gene have been reported to affect the function of various domains of ABCB4 (bile canalicular "flopase")<br>In BRIC3, the point mutations are nonsynonymous. |
| PFIC-4 | *TJP2* | Patients are homozygotes or compound heterozygotes for a variety of genetic lesions of *TJP2*. Small deletions (1–4 bases) within exons, causing frameshift, and a nonsense mutation have been described. Intronic mutations can result in deletions ranging from 2-nt to 11 entire exons |
| PFIC-5 | *NR1H4* | Patients are homozygotes or compound heterozygotes for nonsense mutations, in-frame insertions, or large deletions (37.2 kb) spanning exons 1 and in the *NR1H4* gene |

## References


Ahlfors CE, Vreman HJ, Wong RJ, Bender GJ, Oh W, Morris BH, Stevenson DK. Effects of sample dilution, peroxidase concentration, and chloride ion on the measurement of unbound bilirubin in premature newborns. Clin Biochem. 2007;40:261–7.

Arias IM. Chronic unconjugated hyperbilirubinemia without overt signs of hemolysis in adolescents and adults. J Clin Invest. 1962;41:2233.

Arias IM, London IM. Bilirubin glucuronide formation in vitro: demonstration of a defect in Gilbert's disease. Science. 1957;126:563.

Asp P, Guha C, Roy Chowdhury N, Roy Chowdhury J. Chapter 73. Liver-directed gene therapy. In The liver: biology and pathobiology, 6th edition, Arias, IM, editor in chief. Wiley-Blackwell, Oxford 2019.

Biempica L, Gutstein S, Arias IM. Morphological and biochemical studies of benign recurrent cholestasis. Gastroenterology. 1967;52:521.

Bonnet RJ, Davis E, Hursthouse MB. Structure of bilirubin. Nature. 1976;262:326.

Bosma PJ, Roy Chowdhury J, Bakker C, et al. A sequence abnormality in the promoter region results in reduced expression of bilirubin-UDP-glucuronosyltransferase-1 in Gilbert syndrome. N Engl J Med. 1995;333:1171.

Bosma PJ, Roy Chowdhury N, Goldhoorn BG, et al. Sequence of exons and the flanking regions of human bilirubin-UDP-glucuronosyltransferase gene complex and identification of a genetic mutation in a patient with Crigler-Najjar syndrome, type I. Hepatology. 1992;15:941.

Breimer LH, Wannamethee G, Ebrahim S, Shaper AG. Serum bilirubin and risk of ischemic heart disease in middle-aged British men. Clin Chem. 1995;41:1504.

Choi SH, Yun KE, Choi HJ. Relationships between serum total bilirubin levels and metabolic syndrome in Korean adults. Nutr Metab Cardiovasc Dis. 2013;23:31.

Clayton RJ, Iber FL, Ruebner BH, et al. Byler disease: fatal familial intrahepatic cholestasis in an Amish kindred. Am J Dis Child. 1969;117:112.

Crigler JF, Najjar VA. Congenital familial non-hemolytic jaundice with kernicterus. Pediatrics. 1952;10:169.

Dubin IN. Chronic idiopathic jaundice: a review of fifty cases. Am J Med. 1958;23:268.

Fox IJ, Roy Chowdhury J, Kaufman SS, et al. Treatment of Crigler-Najjar syndrome type I with hepatocyte transplantation. N Engl J Med. 1998;333:1422.

Gilbert A, Lereboullet P. La cholamae simple familiale. Semin Med. 1901;21:241.

Gomez-Ospina N, Potter CJ, Xiao R, et al. Mutations in the nuclear bile acid receptor FXR cause progressive familial intrahepatic cholestasis. Nat Commun. 2016;7:10713. [PMID: 123]

Gunaydin M, Tander B, Demirel D, Caltepe G, Kalayci AG, Eren E, Bicakcı U, Rizalar R, Ariturk E, Bernay F. Different techniques for biliary diversion in progressive familial intrahepatic cholestasis. J Pediatr Surg. 2016;51:386–9.

Henkel SAF, Squires JH, Ayers M, Ganoza A, Mckiernan P, Squires JE. Expanding etiology of progressive familial intrahepatic cholestasis. World J Hepatol. 2019;11:450–63.

Iansante V, Mitry RR, Filippi C, Fitzpatrick E, Dhawan A. Human hepatocyte transplantation for liver disease: current status and future perspectives. Pediatr Res. 2018;83:232–40.

Iyer L, King CD, Whittington PF, et al. Genetic predisposition to the metabolism of irinotecan (CPT-11): role of uridine diphosphate glucuronosyltransferase isoform 1A1in the glucuronidation of its active metabolite (SN-38) in human liver microsomes. J Clin Invest. 1998;101:847.

Kaplowitz N, Javitt N, Kappas A. Coproporphyrin I and III excretion in bile and urine. J Clin Invest. 1972;51:2895.

Kappas A, Drummond GS. Direct comparison of Sn-mesoporphyrin, an inhibitor of bilirubin production, and phototherapy in controlling hyperbilirubinemia in term and near-term newborns. Pediatrics. 1995;95:468.

Knisely AS, Strautnieks SS, Meier Y, Stieger B, Byrne JA, et al. Hepatocellular carcinoma in ten children under five years of age with bile salt export pump deficiency. Hepatology. 2006;44:478–86.

Krebs-Schmitt D, Briem-Richter A, Brinkert F, et al. Alloimmunity and cholestasis after liver transplantation in children with progressive familial intrahepatic cholestasis. J Pediatr Gastroenterol Nutr. 2019;68:169–74.

Maisels MJ. Managing the jaundiced newborn: a persistent challenge. Can Med Assoc J. 2015;187:335–43.

Mazariegos G, Benjamin Shneider B, Barbara Burton B, Fox IJ, Hadzic N, Kishnani P, Morton H, Mcintire S, Sokol RJ, Summar l M, White D, Chavanon V, Vockley J. Liver transplantation for pediatric metabolic disease. Mol Genet Metab. 2014;111:418–27.

Mitchell E, Ranganathan S, McKiernan P, Squires RH, Strauss K, Soltys K, Mazariegos G, Squires JE. Hepatic parenchymal injury in Crigler-Najjar type I. J Pediatr Gastroenterol Nutr. 2018;66:588–94.

O'Brien L, Hosick PA, John K, Stec DE, Hinds TD Jr. Biliverdin reductase isozymes in metabolism. Trends Endocrinol Metab. 2015;26:212–20.

Paulusma CC, Bosma PJ, Zaman GJR, et al. Congenital jaundice in rats with a mutation in a multidrug resistance-associated protein gene. Science. 1996;271:1126.

Polgar Z, Li Y, Li Wang X, Guha C, Roy-Chowdhury N, Roy-Chowdhury J. Gunn rats as a surrogate model for evaluation of hepatocyte transplantation-based therapies of Crigler-Najjar syndrome type 1. Methods Mol Biol. 2017;1506:131–47.

Rotor AB, Manahan L, Florentin A. Familial nonhemolytic jaundice with direct van den Bergh reaction. Acta Med Philos. 1948;5:37.

Roy-Chowdhury J, Locker J, Roy-Chowdhury N. Nuclear receptors orchestrate detoxification pathways. Dev Cell. 2003;4:607.

Roy-Chowdhury N, Wang X, Roy-Chowdhury J. In: Rimoin DL, Connor JM, Pyeritz RE, Korf BR, editors. Chapter 19. Bile pigment metabolism and its disorders. Emery and Rimoin's principle and practice of medical genetics. 7th ed. Philadelphia, PA: Churchill-Livingstone-Elsevier; 2019. p. 507–53.

Sambrotta M, Strautnieks S, Papouli E, et al. Mutations in TJP2 cause progressive cholestatic liver disease. Nat Genet. 2014;46:326–8.

Schatz SB, Jüngst C, Keitel-Anselmo V, et al. Phenotypic spectrum and diagnostic pitfalls of ABCB4 deficiency depending on age of onset. Hepatol Commun. 2018;2:504–14.

Shani M, Seligshon U, Gilon E, et al. Dubin-Johnson syndrome in Israel: clinical, laboratory, and genetic aspects of 101 cases. West J Med. 1970;39:549.

Soltys KA, Setoyama K, Tafaleng EN, et al. Host conditioning and rejection monitoring in hepatocyte transplantation in humans. J Hepatol. 2016;66:987–1000.

Togawa T, Mizuochi T, Sugiura T, et al. Clinical, pathologic, and genetic features of neonatal Dubin-Johnson syndrome: a Multicenter study in Japan. J Pediatr. 2018;196:161.

van de Steeg E, Stranecky V, Hartmannova H, et al. Complete OATP1B1 and OATP1B3 deficiency causes human Rotor syndrome by interrupting conjugated bilirubin uptake into the liver. J Clin Invest. 2012;122:519.

Van den Bergh AAH, Muller P. Uber eine direkte und eine indirekte Diazoreaktion auf Bilirubin. Biochem Z. 1916;77:90.

Wang KS, Tiao G, Bass LM, et al. Childhood liver disease research network (ChiLDReN). Analysis of surgical interruption of the enterohepatic circulation as a treatment for pediatric cholestasis. Hepatology. 2017;65:1645–54.

Wolkoff AW, Roy Chowdhury J, Gartner LA, et al. Crigler-Najjar syndrome (type I) in an adult male. Gastroenterology. 1979;76:338023.

Yachie A, Niida Y, Wada T, Igarashi N, Kaneda H, Toma T, et al. Oxidative stress causes enhanced endothelial cell injury in human heme oxygenase-1 deficiency. J Clin Invest. 1999;103:129–35.

Zhou H, Dong X, Kabarriti R, Chen Y, Avsar A, Wang X, Ding J, Liu L, Fox IJ, Roy-Chowdhury J, Roy-Chowdhury N, Guha C. Single liver lobe repopulation with wildtype hepatocytes using regional hepatic irradiation cures jaundice in Gunn rats. PLoS One. 2012;7:e46775.

Zhou S, Hertel PM, Finegold MJ, Wang L, Kerkar N. Hepatocellular carcinoma associated with tight-junction protein 2 deficiency. Hepatology. 2015;62:1914.

Zucker SD, Horn PS, Sherman KE. Serum bilirubin levels in the US population: gender effect and inverse correlation with colorectal cancer. Hepatology. 2004;40:827.

# Part VIII

# Storage Disorders

# Disorders of Autophagy

# 59

Carlo Dionisi Vici, Heinz Jungbluth, Rita Carsetti, and Clara D. M. van Karnebeek

## Contents



**Summary**

The term autophagy derives from the Greek word autóphagos, which means "self-eating" or "self-digestion." Autophagy is a fundamental and highly conserved intracellular pathway that in its most basic sense involves the delivery of cytoplasmic cargo to the lysosome for degradation. The Nobel Laureate in Physiology and Medicine in 1974, Christian de Duve, introduced this term to describe the self-eating function of lysosomes in degrading intracellular debris, including damaged organelles (mitochondria, endoplasmic reticulum membranes, ribosomes), and other cellular components such as larger protein aggregates (Harnett et al. 2017). Based on different modes of cargo delivery to lysosomes, three subtypes of autophagy have been defined: macro-autophagy, micro-autophagy, and chaperone-mediated autophagy. In macro-autophagy, cargo is transported inside double-membrane vesicles (or autophagosomes) which are delivered to and fused with lysosomes to form the autolysosome. In micro-autophagy, the cytosolic cargo is trapped in small vesicles formed by invagination of the lysosomal membrane. In chaperone-mediated autophagy, substrates are selectively targeted by hsp70 to the microvesicles and delivered by the receptor protein LAMP2 for lysosomal degradation.

C. Dionisi Vici (✉)
Division of Metabolic Disease, Bambino Gesù Children's Hospital IRCCS, Rome, Italy
e-mail: carlo.dionisivici@opbg.net

H. Jungbluth
Department of Paediatric Neurology, Evelina Children's Hospital, Guy's and St Thomas' Hospital NHS Foundation Trust, London, UK

R. Carsetti
Diagnostic Immunology Clinical Unit, Bambino Gesù Children's Hospital IRCCS, Rome, Italy

C. D. M. van Karnebeek
Department of Pediatrics, Emma Children's Hospital, Amsterdam University Medical Centres, Amsterdam, The Netherlands


N. Blau et al. (eds.), *Physician's Guide to the Diagnosis, Treatment, and Follow-Up of Inherited Metabolic Diseases*, https://doi.org/10.1007/978-3-030-67727-5_59

## Introduction

The term autophagy derives from the Greek word autóphagos, which means "self-eating" or "self-digestion." Autophagy is a fundamental and highly conserved intracellular pathway that in its most basic sense involves the delivery of cytoplasmic cargo to the lysosome for degradation. The Nobel Laureate in Physiology and Medicine in 1974, Christian de Duve, introduced this term to describe the self-eating function of lysosomes in degrading intracellular debris, including damaged organelles (mitochondria, endoplasmic reticulum membranes, ribosomes), and other cellular components such as larger protein aggregates (Harnett et al. 2017). Based on different modes of cargo delivery to lysosomes, three subtypes of autophagy have been defined: macro-autophagy, micro-autophagy, and chaperone-mediated autophagy. In macro-autophagy, cargo is transported inside double-membrane vesicles (or autophagosomes) which are delivered to and fused with lysosomes to form the autolysosome. In micro-autophagy, the cytosolic cargo is trapped in small vesicles formed by invagination of the lysosomal membrane. In chaperone-mediated autophagy, substrates are selectively targeted by hsp70 to the microvesicles and delivered by the receptor protein LAMP2 for lysosomal degradation.

Besides its key function in degradative pathways, autophagy contributes to biosynthetic and secretory processes and is associated with a wide range of physiological processes including embryogenesis, adaptation to changed metabolic requirements and stress, cellular remodeling and quality control of organelles, tumor suppression, pathogen elimination, immune and inflammatory responses, and aging. Macro-autophagy plays a major role and as a pathway can be divided into six consecutives steps—initiation, nucleation, elongation, closure, maturation, and fusion—closely related to the cascade activation of the AuTophaGy-related (or ATG) genes. The whole process is under the tight control of pathways crucial for cellular metabolic control such as the mTOR and AMPK pathways and requires tight regulation of each step, fine-tuning at the substrate level, and crosstalk with other vesicular and cellular trafficking machineries. The term "selective autophagy" refers to the specificity of autophagy for certain cargos that in mammalian cells include peroxisomes ("pexophagy"), mitochondria ("mitophagy"), the endoplasmic reticulum ("reticulophagy"), lysosomes ("lysophagy"), pathogens ("xenophagy"), lipid droplets ("lipophagy"), ferritin ("ferritinophagy"), and glycogen ("glycophagy") (Gatica et al. 2018).

Given its crucial role in many essential cellular processes, the involvement of autophagy has been implicated in a wide range of human diseases, manifesting as organ-specific or as systemic disorders, including infections; cancer; neurodegenerative, cardiovascular, autoimmune, and inflammatory disorders; chronic liver disease; myopathies; obesity and metabolic syndrome; diabetes; and even aging. In the specific field of metabolic diseases, a secondary involvement of autophagy has been reported in lysosomal storage disorders and, more recently, also in urea cycle defects and organic acidurias (Luciani et al. 2020; Settembre et al. 2013; Soria and Brunetti-Pierri 2019).

The advent of next-generation sequencing has allowed the discovery of several disorders primarily affecting the genes of the autophagy machinery, and these single gene disorders, recently named congenital disorders of autophagy, represent an emerging category of inborn errors of metabolism (Ferreira et al. 2021; García-Cazorla and Saudubray 2018; Teinert et al. 2020).

Despite a growing interest over the last years in congenital disorders of autophagy, a consensus in the classification of autophagy-related diseases is still missing (Fig. 59.1) (Ferreira et al. 2021; García-Cazorla and Saudubray 2018; Levine and Kroemer 2019; Stamatakou et al. 2020; Teinert et al. 2020; Zatyka et al. 2020).

## Nomenclature

In this chapter, we propose a new classification of congenital disorders of autophagy, which includes 25 genetic disorders responsible for over 30 different OMIM phenotypes, the number of which will likely increase with genomic disease discovery. These genetic defects that primarily involve the different steps of the autophagy machinery are clinically heterogeneous yet invariably present with a characteristic involvement of the CNS and the peripheral nervous system. Given their post-mitotic nature, neurons are highly sensitive to the accumulation of toxic proteins and damaged organelles and are therefore highly dependent on the autophagy machinery to maintain their homeostasis even already from early embryonic and perinatal stages (Fassio et al. 2020). This dependency makes autophagy a key player for early neurogenesis and central nervous system development, neuronal polarity, and synaptic function. Neurological signs include developmental delay, intellectual disability, ataxia, epilepsy, myopathies, psychiatric manifestations, pyramidal dysfunction, neuropathy, sensorineural deafness, and various manifestations of neurodegeneration, including parkinsonism. Neuroimaging often reveals corpus callosum agenesis or hypoplasia, cerebral and cerebellar atrophy, and, in some cases, a characteristic brain iron accumulation. Non-neurological manifestations include ocular, skeletal, respiratory, renal, hepatic, gastrointestinal, cardiac, cutaneous, and immunological abnormalities and dysmorphic, i.e., storage-like, features in certain conditions.

| No. | Disease name | Alternative name | Abbreviation | Gene symbol | Chromosomal localization | Inheritance | Affected protein | OMIM phenotype | OMIM genotype |
|---|---|---|---|---|---|---|---|---|---|
| 59.1 | Vici syndrome | EPG5 deficiency | VICIS | *EPG5* | 18q12.3-q21.1 | AR | Ectopic P-granules autophagy protein 5 | 242840 | 615068 |
| 59.2 | Neurodegeneration with brain iron accumulation 5 | Static encephalopathy of childhood with neurodegeneration in adulthood (SENDA) | NBIA5 | *WDR45* | Xp11.23 | XLD | WD40 repeat protein | 300894 | 300526 |
| 59.3 | Spinocerebellar ataxia 20 | SNX14 deficiency | SCAR20 | *SNX14* | 6q14.3 | AR | Sorting nexin 14 | 616354 | 616105 |
| 59.4 | Spastic paraplegia 11 | SPG11 deficiency type 1 | SPG11 | *SPG11* | 15q21.1 | AR | SPATACSIN | 604360 | 610844 |
| 59.5 | Charcot-Marie-tooth disease 2X | SPG11 deficiency type 2 | CMT2X | *SPG11* | 15q21.1 | AR | SPATACSIN | 616668 | 610844 |
| 59.6 | Amyotrophic lateral sclerosis 5 | SPG11 deficiency type 3 | ALS5 | *SPG11* | 15q21.1 | AR | SPATACSIN | 602099 | 610844 |
| 59.7 | Spastic paraplegia 15 | Kjellin syndrome | SPG15 | *ZFYVE26* | 14q24.1 | AR | Zinc finger FYVE domain-containing protein 26 | 270700 | 612012 |
| 59.8 | Spastic paraplegia 48 | Adaptor-related protein complex 5 ζ-1 subunit deficiency | SPG48 | *AP5Z1* | 7p22.1 | AR | Adaptor-related protein complex 5, ZETA-1 subunit | 613647 | 613653 |
| 59.9 | Spastic paraplegia 49 | TECPR2 deficiency | SPG49 | *TECPR2* | 14q32.31 | AR | Tectonin beta-propeller repeat-containing protein 2 | 615031 | 615000 |
| 59.10 | Frontotemporal dementia and/or amyotrophic lateral sclerosis 4 | TBK1 deficiency | FTDALS4 | *TBK1* | 17q21.32 | AD | Serine/threonine-protein kinase | 616439 | 604834 |
| 59.11 | Charcot-Marie-tooth disease 2B | RAB7 deficiency | CMT2B | *RAB7A* | 3q21.3 | AD | RAS-associated protein RAB7 | 600882 | 602298 |
| 59.12 | Spinocerebellar ataxia 25 | ATG5 deficiency | SCAR25 | *ATG5* | 6q21 | AR | Autophagy-related 5 | 617584 | 604261 |
| 59.13 | Parkinson disease 2 | Parkin deficiency | PARK2 | *PRKN* | 6q26 | AR | Parkin | 600116 | 602544 |
| 59.14 | Parkinson disease 6 | PINK1 deficiency | PARK6 | *PINK1* | 1p36.12 | AR | PTEN-induced putative kinase 1 | 605909 | 608309 |
| 59.15 | Frontotemporal dementia and/or amyotrophic lateral sclerosis 3 | SQSTM1 deficiency type 1 | FTDALS3 | *SQSTM1* | 5q35.3 | AD | Sequestosome 1 | 616437 | 601530 |
| 59.16 | Myopathy distal with rimmed vacuoles | SQSTM1 deficiency type 2 | DMRV | *SQSTM1* | 5q35.3 | AD | Sequestosome 1 | 617158 | 601530 |
| 59.17 | Neurodegeneration with ataxia, dystonia, and gaze palsy | SQSTM1 deficiency type 3 | NADGP | *SQSTM1* | 5q35.3 | AR | Sequestosome 1 | 617145 | 601530 |
| 59.18 | Paget disease of bone 3 | SQSTM1 deficiency type 4 | PDB3 | *SQSTM1* | 5q35.3 | AD | Sequestosome 1 | 167250 | 601530 |
| 59.19 | Spastic paraplegia 52 | AP4S1 deficiency | SPG52 | *AP4S1* | 14q12 | AR | Adaptor-related protein complex 4, Sigma-1 subunit | 614067 | 607243 |
| 59.20 | Spastic paraplegia 47 | AP4B1 deficiency | SPG47 | *AP4B1* | 1p13.2 | AR | Adaptor-related protein complex 4, Beta-1 subunit | 614066 | 607245 |
| 59.21 | Spastic paraplegia 50 | AP4M1 deficiency | SPG50 | *AP4M1* | 7q22.1 | AR | Adaptor-related protein complex 4, MU-1 subunit | 612936 | 602296 |

(continued)

| No. | Disease name | Alternative name | Abbreviation | Gene symbol | Chromosomal localization | Inheritance | Affected protein | OMIM phenotype | OMIM genotype |
|---|---|---|---|---|---|---|---|---|---|
| 59.22 | Spastic paraplegia 51 | AP4E1 deficiency | SPG51 | *AP4E1* | 15q21.2 | AR | Adaptor-related protein complex 4, Epsilon-1 subunit | 613744 | 607244 |
| 59.23 | Hypotonia, infantile, with psychomotor retardation and characteristic facies 3 | TBCK deficiency | IHPRF3 | *TBCK* | 4q24 | AR | TBC1 domain-containing kinase | 616900 | 616899 |
| 59.24 | Amyotrophic lateral sclerosis 2 | ALS2 deficiency type 1 | ALS2 | *ALS2* | 2q33.1 | AR | ALSIN | 205100 | 606352 |
| 59.25 | Primary lateral sclerosis juvenile | ALS2 deficiency type 2 | PLSJ | *ALS2* | 2q33.1 | AR | ALSIN | 606353 | 606352 |
| 59.26 | Spastic paralysis, infantile onset ascending | ALS2 deficiency type 3 | IAHSP | *ALS2* | 2q33.1 | AR | ALSIN | 607225 | 606352 |
| 59.27 | Neuropathy, distal hereditary motor, type VIIB | DCTN1 deficiency type 1 | HMN7B | *DCTN1* | 2p13.1 | AD | DYNACTIN 1 | 607641 | 601143 |
| 59.28 | Perry syndrome | DCTN1 deficiency type 2 | PERRYS | *DCTN1* | 2p13.1 | AD | DYNACTIN 1 | 168605 | 601143 |
| 59.29 | Polymicrogyria bilateral temporo-occipital | FIG4 deficiency type 1 | BTOP | *FIG4* | 6q21 | AR | SAC domain-containing inositol phosphatase 3 | 612691 | 609390 |
| 59.30 | Amyotrophic lateral sclerosis 11 | FIG4 deficiency type 2 | ALS11 | *FIG4* | 6q21 | AD | Sac domain-containing inositol phosphatase 3 | 612577 | 609390 |
| 59.31 | Charcot-Marie-tooth disease 4 J | FIG4 deficiency type 3 | CMT4J | *FIG4* | 6q21 | AR | SAC domain-containing inositol phosphatase 3 | 611228 | 609390 |
| 59.32 | Yunis-Varon syndrome | FIG4 deficiency type 4 | YVS | *FIG4* | 6q21 | AR | SAC domain-containing inositol phosphatase 3 | 216340 | 609390 |
| 59.33 | Yunis-Varon syndrome | VAC14 deficiency type 1 | YVS | *VAC14* | 16q22 | AR | VAC14 component of PIKFYVE complex | 216340 | 604632 |
| 59.34 | Striatonigral degeneration, childhood-onset | VAC14 deficiency type 2 | SDCO | *VAC14* | 16q22 | AR | VAC14 component of PIKFYVE complex | 617054 | 604632 |
| 59.35 | Centronuclear myopathy 1 | MTMR14 deficiency | CNM1 | *MTMR14* | 3p25.3 | AD | Myotubularin-related protein 14 | 160150 | 611089 |
| 59.36 | Centronuclear myopathy 1 | DNM2 deficiency type 1 | CNM1 | *DNM2* | 19p13.2 | AD | Dynamin 2 | 160150 | 602378 |
| 59.37 | Charcot-Marie-tooth disease 2 M | DNM2 deficiency type 2 | CMT2M | *DNM2* | 19p13.2 | AD | Dynamin 2 | 606482 | 602378 |
| 59.38 | Amyotrophic lateral sclerosis 17 | CHMP2B deficiency type 1 | ALS17 | *CHMP2B* | 3p11.2 | AD | Charged multivesicular body protein 2B | 614696 | 609512 |
| 59.39 | Frontotemporal dementia chromosome 3 linked | CHMP2B deficiency type 2 | FTD3 | *CHMP2B* | 3p11.2 | AD | Charged multivesicular body protein 2B | 600795 | 609512 |

## Metabolic Pathway

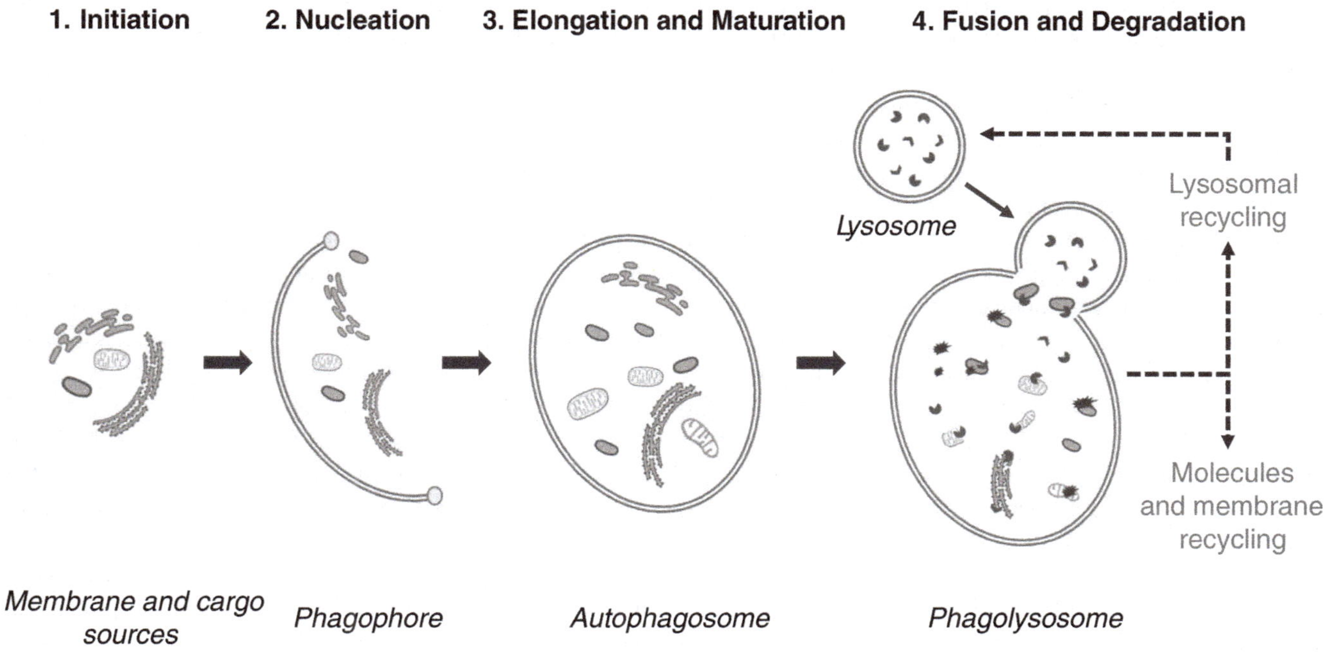


**Fig. 59.1** Schematic illustration of the main steps of Macroautophagy

## Signs and Symptoms

Based on the main clinical presentation, congenital or monogenic disorders of autophagy can be grouped into different subtypes: multisystem diseases, hereditary spastic paraplegia, amyotrophic lateral sclerosis, Parkinson disease, neurodegeneration with brain iron accumulation, Charcot-Marie-Tooth disease, and other complex neurodegenerative diseases.

### Multisystem Disease

Four diseases, Vici syndrome, Yunis-Varon syndrome, spinocerebellar ataxia 20 (SCARS20), and TBCK deficiency, present with multisystemic clinical storage-like pictures, affecting the central nervous system and other organs and systems.

Vici syndrome (59.1, AR, MIM 615068), caused by autosomal recessive mutations in *EPG5*, was initially described as a new syndrome characterized by agenesis of the corpus callosum, skin and hair hypopigmentation, cataracts, cleft lip and palate, cardio/myopathy, and immunodeficiency. After this first report, numerous other cases were described, and the genetic cause, mutations in *EPG5*, a gene encoding ectopic P granules protein 5 (EPG5) playing a key role in the autophagy machinery, was reported in 2013 (Cullup et al. 2013). EPG5 deficiency causes impaired fusion of autophagosomes with lysosomes and subsequent accumulation of autophagosomes. The disease has a pan-ethnic distribution and over 60 patients are known (Byrne et al. 2016). In addition to a wide range of other multisystem features, EPG5 deficiency causes a complex immunological dysfunction, with selective involvement of memory B cells, whose pathophysiology implicates a perturbation of the cell signaling cascade mediated by toll-like receptor 7 and 9 affecting both innate and adaptive immunity (Piano Mortari et al. 2018).

Yunis-Varon syndrome (59.32, AR, MIM 609390; and 59.33, AR, MIM 604632) has been reported in association with two different genetic defects of autophagy, *FIG4* and *VAC14*, coding for two proteins involved in the conversion of phosphoinositide PI(3)P to PI(3,5)P and causing a perturbation in the homeostasis of cellular vacuoles containing LAMP1 and LAMP2 proteins (Campeau et al. 2013; Lines et al. 2017). This syndrome shares some similarities with Vici syndrome such as corpus callosum agenesis/hypoplasia, cardio/myopathy, cataract, cleft lip and palate, and tissue lysosomal storage. An abnormal urine oligosaccharide profile has been reported in Yunis-Varon syndrome. Mutations in *FIG4* and *VAC14* have also been associated with additional clinical manifestations. For *FIG4*, other associated phenotypes include bilateral temporo-occipital polymicrogyria (59.29, AR, MIM 609390) (Baulac et al. 2014), amyotrophic lateral sclerosis type 11 (59.30, AD, MIM 609390) (Nguyen et al. 2019), and Charcot-Marie-Tooth disease type 4 J (59.31, AR, MIM 609390) (Nicholson et al. 2011), while mutations in *VAC14* have been reported in a Leigh-like disease with childhood-onset striato-nigral degeneration (59.34, AR, MIM 604632) (Lenk et al. 2016).

Spinocerebellar ataxia 20 (59.3, AR, 616105) is an autosomal recessive disorder due to mutations in *SNX14*, encoding a protein involved in phosphatidylinositol (3,5)-bisphosphate metabolism and maturation of the autophagy pathway, resulting in a dysfunction of lysosome-autophagosome fusion (Akizu et al. 2015). Patients present between birth and 1 year of age with developmental delay and hypotonia, with development of age-dependent cerebellar atrophy. Coarse facial features similar to those of mucopolysaccharidosis and other lysosomal storage disorders, seizures, hepatosplenomegaly, skeletal abnormalities, hypertrichosis, nystagmus, and hearing loss represent additional clinical signs. An abnormal pattern of urine oligosaccharides and elevated excretion of glycosaminoglycans have been observed in some patients.

Mutations in *TBCK*, encoding for TBC1-domain-containing kinase, a protein implicated in the mTOR pathway, cause a complex storage-like disease with autophagosomal-lysosomal dysfunction (59.23, AR, MIM 616899) (Bhoj et al. 2016; Beck-Wödl et al. 2018). The main phenotypic features described in over 30 patients reported to date include distinctive facial features with bitemporal narrowing, macroglossia, severe motor and cognitive delay, seizures, hypo/areflexia, generalized hypotonia, endocrinological abnormalities, dysgenesis of the corpus callosum, and cerebellar atrophy. Autopsy where performed revealed lipofuscin-like storage material in CNS neurons; storage deposits in astrocytes and microglia; PAS-positive deposits in the pons, cerebellum, spleen, and liver in two sibs; and GM2-ganglioside storage in spinal motor neurons in another patient (Strømme et al. 1997), all showing normal total glycosaminoglycans and oligosaccharide profiles in urine.

## Hereditary Spastic Paraplegia

Hereditary spastic paraplegias (HSPs) are a heterogeneous group of neurodegenerative diseases, inherited in an autosomal dominant, autosomal recessive, or X-linked manner, characterized by retrograde degeneration of the long corticospinal motor neuron axons, resulting in progressive lower limb spasticity, weakness, reduced vibration sense, and urinary incontinence. To date, HSPs encompass more than 80 loci and over 60 genes, with some labeled complex HSPs, presenting additional phenotypic features, in particular cerebellar signs and cognitive impairment. Spastic gait genes (SPG) are involved in several cellular pathways, including ER and vesicle trafficking, mitochondrial regulation, myelination, lipid metabolism, and autophagy. Thus far, eight different inherited defects of autophagy have been implicated in hereditary spastic paraplegia. These include SPG11 (59.4, AR, MIM 610844), SPG15 (59.7, AR, MIM 612012), and SPG47 (59.20, AR, MIM 607245), SPG48 (59.8, AR, MIM 613653), SPG49 (59.9, AR, MIM 615000), SPG50 (59.21, AR, MIM 602296), SPG51 (59.22, AR, MIM 607244), and SPG52 (59.19, AR, MIM 607243) (Ebrahimi-Fakhari et al. 2018; Hirst et al. 2015; Oz-Levi et al. 2012; Vantaggiato et al. 2019). All these disorders can be classified as complex HSPs and are clinically characterized by lower limb spasticity, developmental delay/mental retardation, and, frequently, corpus callosum and white matter abnormalities. Additional findings often include cerebellar atrophy, seizures, ataxia, neuropathy, dysmorphic features, psychiatric manifestations, retinopathy, and deafness. SPG11 and SPG15, which are clinically indistinguishable, are the most frequent form of complex HSPs. *SPG11* encodes spatacsin, a protein involved in autophagosome maturation, and mutations in *SPG11* have been associated also with Charcot-Marie-Tooth disease type 2X (59.5, AR, MIM 610844) and to amyotrophic lateral sclerosis type 5 (59.6, AR, MIM 610844) (Montecchiani et al. 2016; Orlacchio et al. 2010). SPG15 is due to mutation in the *ZFYVE26* gene, coding for spastizin, also involved in autophagosome maturation (Vantaggiato et al. 2019). SPG49 is caused by mutations in the *TECPR2* gene, encoding tectonin beta-propeller repeat-containing protein 2, which interacts with ATG8 in phagophore membrane elongation (Oz-Levi et al. 2012). SPG47, SPG50, SPG51, and SPG52 are caused by mutations in genes that encode the subunits of adaptor-protein 4, involved in autophagosome turnover and resulting in impaired autophagic degradation of protein aggregates (Ebrahimi-Fakhari et al. 2018). These "adaptinopathies," together with SPG48, caused by mutation in a gene encoding a subunit of adaptor protein 5 (Hirst et al. 2015), represent a specific subtype of complex HSPs. Interestingly, spastizin and spatacsin physically interact and have similar subcellular distributions and co-localize with adaptor protein 5 in a multiprotein complex expressed in endosomes and lysosomes and are involved in autophagosome-endosome fusion.

## Amyotrophic Lateral Sclerosis

Amyotrophic lateral sclerosis (ALS) is an invariably fatal neurodegenerative disease involving neurons controlling voluntary muscles. ALS is characterized by the progressive degeneration of motor neurons in the spinal cord and brain, which leads to neuromuscular denervation, atrophy, and paralysis of voluntary skeletal muscles and ultimately to death. ALS is most commonly a sporadic disease, but approximately 5%–10% of cases are familial. Six genetic defects affecting the autophagy pathway cause different forms of amyotrophic lateral sclerosis often associated with frontotemporal dementia (Nguyen et al. 2019): ALS 2, ALS 2 deficiency (59.24, AR, 606352); ALS 3, SQSTM1 deficiency (59.15, AD, MIM 601530); ALS 4, TBK1 deficiency (59.10, AD, MIM 604834); ALS 5, spatacsin deficiency (59.6, AR, MIM 610844), involved in autophagosome maturation; ALS 11, FIG4 deficiency (59.30, AD, MIM 609390); and ALS 17, CHMP2B deficiency (59.38, AD, MIM 609512). Besides ALS, other phenotypic manifestations have been reported in association with these genetic defects: distal myopathy with rimmed vacuoles (59.16, AD, MIM 601530) (Bucelli et al. 2015), neurodegeneration, ataxia, dystonia, and gaze palsy (59.17, AR, MIM 601530) (Haack et al. 2016), and Paget disease of bone 3 (59.18, AD, MIM 601530) (Laurin et al. 2002) with mutations in *SQSTM1*; spastic paraplegia (59.4, AR, MIM 610844) (Vantaggiato et al. 2019) with mutations in *SPG11*; primary lateral sclerosis juvenile (59.25, AR, MIM 606352) and infantile-onset ascending spastic paralysis (59.26, AR, MIM 606352) with mutations in *ALS2* (Eymard-Pierre et al. 2002); bilateral temporo-occipital polymicrogyria (59.29, AR, 609390) (Baulac et al. 2014), Charcot-Marie-Tooth disease type 4 (59.31, AR, MIM 609390) (Nicholson et al. 2011), and Yunis-Varon syndrome (59.32, AR, 609390) (Campeau et al. 2013), with mutations in *FIG4*; and frontotemporal dementia without ALS (59.39, AS, MIM 609512) with mutations in *CHMP2B* (Skibinski et al. 2005).

### Parkinson Disease

Three genes of the autophagy machinery, *PARK2* (59.13, AR, MIM 602544) (Kitada et al. 1998), *PINK1* (59.14, AR, MIM 608309) (Valente et al. 2004), selectively affecting mitochondria target cargos (mitophagy), and *DCTN1* (59.27, AD, MIM 601143) (Konno et al. 2017), cause autosomal recessive and dominant forms of Parkinson disease. *PINK1* encodes a mitochondrially located serine/threonine kinase which phosphorylates parkin, encoded by *PARK2*, and ubiquitin to regulate mitophagy. *DCTN1* gene encodes the subunit p150$^{\mathrm{Glued}}$ of the protein complex dynactin, which participates with dynein in autophagosome-lysosome fusion, playing a key role in retrograde axonal transport. *DCTN1* mutations, which cause pathological protein accumulation and aggregation in neurons, were identified in patients with Perry syndrome (59.28, AD, MIM 601143), a rare hereditary neurodegenerative disease characterized by dominantly inherited parkinsonism, psychiatric symptoms, weight loss, and central hypoventilation (Konno et al. 2017). *DCTN1* variants have also been found in patients with distal hereditary motor neuropathy type VIIB (59.27, AD, MIM 601143) and other neurodegenerative phenotypes, such as amyotrophic lateral sclerosis, with or without frontotemporal dementia, and a progressive supranuclear palsy (PSP)-like syndrome (Konno et al. 2017).

### Neurodegeneration with Brain Iron Accumulation

Neurodegeneration with brain iron accumulation (NBIA) comprises a group of disorders characterized by abnormal accumulation of iron in the basal ganglia, most often in the globus pallidus and/or substantia nigra. NBIA 5 (59.2, XLD, MIM 300526), also known as beta-propeller protein-associated neurodegeneration (BPAN), is due to X-linked dominant mutations in *WDR45*, a gene involved in autophagosome formation and elongation by binding phosphatidylinositol 3-phosphate (Haack et al. 2012). The characteristic features of the disease include childhood-onset developmental delay with slow motor and cognitive gains; little to no expressive language; seizures of various types, prominent in childhood but may resolve in adolescence; autistic-like behavioral abnormalities; motor dysfunction; and ataxia, hypotonia, and spasticity, progressing into dystonia-parkinsonism and dementia, with a biphasic disease course. MRI can feature hypomyelination and a thin corpus callosum.

### Charcot-Marie-Tooth Disease

Charcot-Marie-Tooth (CMT) disease comprises a heterogeneous group of progressive hereditary sensory and motor neuropathy with onset between the 5th and the 15th year of age. Patients present with muscle weakness, walking difficulties, abnormal gait, pes cavus, and progressive distal-muscle wasting of lower and upper limbs. Charcot-Marie-Tooth disease has been associated with some genetic defects linked to autophagy, including *SPG11* (CMT 2x, 59.5, AR 610844) (Montecchiani et al. 2016), involved in autophagosome maturation, *RAB7A* (CMT 2b, 59.11, AD, MIM 602298) (Verhoeven et al. 2003), *FIG4* (CMT 4 J, 59.31, AR, MIM 609390) (Nicholson et al. 2011), and *DNM2* which has also been implicated in a form of centronuclear myopathy (CNM) (59.36, AD, MIM 602378) (Bitoun et al. 2005). Remarkably, the extremely rare form of CNM due to mutations in *MTMR14* (59.35, AD, MIM 611089) (Tosch et al. 2006), encoding myotubularin-related protein 14, also causes a dysregulation of autophagy in relation to an abnormal metabolism of phosphoinositides, a group of phospholipids that play a critical role in the control of organelle and membrane traffic. Interestingly, also myotubularin, the gene implicated in X-linked myotubular myopathy, the X-linked form of CNM, plays a crucial role in the regulation of PI3P levels.

### Other Complex Neurodegenerative Diseases

Mutations in *ATG5*, coding for ATG protein 5 which plays a key role in the elongation process of phagophore, cause spinocerebellar ataxia 25 (59.12, AR, MIM 604261), a childhood-onset disorder with walking difficulties, ataxia, nystagmus, variable degrees of intellectual disability, pyramidal signs, and cerebellar hypoplasia, with evidence of a reduced autophagic flux (Kim et al. 2016).

**Table 59.1** Vici syndrome (EPG5)

| System | Symptoms and biomarkers | Neonatal (birth–1 month) | Infancy (1–18 months) | Childhood (1.5–11 years) | Adolescence (11–16 years) | Adulthood (>16 years) |
|---|---|---|---|---|---|---|
| Cardiovascular | Cardiomyopathy, dilated | + | + | + | | |
| | Heart failure | | + | + | | |
| | Left ventricular hypertrophy | + | + | + | | |
| CNS | Agenesis, corpus callosum (MRI) | + | + | + | | |
| | Bilateral schizencephaly | + | + | + | | |
| | Cerebellar vermis agenesis, hypoplasia | + | + | + | | |
| | Hypotonia | + | + | + | | |
| | Retardation, psychomotor | | + | + | | |
| | Seizures | + | + | + | | |
| Dermatological | Chronic mucocutaneous candidiasis | | + | + | | |
| | Cutaneous albinism | + | + | + | | |
| Ear | Hearing loss, sensorineural | + | + | + | | |
| | Low-set ears | + | + | + | | |
| Eye | **Cataract** | + | + | + | | |
| | Hypopigmentation, retinal | + | + | + | | |
| | **Nystagmus** | + | + | + | | |
| | Ocular albinism | + | + | + | | |
| Genitourinary | Hypospadias | + | + | + | | |
| Musculoskeletal | Cleft lip | + | + | + | | |
| | Cleft palate | + | + | + | | |
| | **Growth retardation** | | + | + | | |
| | **Hypertelorism** | + | + | + | | |
| | Microcephaly | + | + | + | | |
| | Micrognathia | + | + | + | | |
| Other | **Failure to thrive** | + | + | + | | |
| | Frequent infections | + | + | + | | |
| | **Immunodeficiency** | + | + | + | | |
| | Recurrent bacterial infections | + | + | + | | |
| Renal | Renal tubular acidosis | ± | ± | ± | | |
| Laboratory findings | IgA (serum) | n | n | n | | |
| | IgG (serum) | ↓ | ↓ | ↓ | | |
| | IgM (serum) | n | n | n | | |

**Table 59.2** Neurodegeneration with brain iron accumulation 5

| System | Symptoms and biomarkers | Neonatal (birth–1 month) | Infancy (1–18 months) | Childhood (1.5–11 years) | Adolescence (11–16 years) | Adulthood (>16 years) |
|---|---|---|---|---|---|---|
| CNS | Ataxia | | | + | + | + |
| | Cerebral atrophy (MRI) | | | | + | + |
| | Dementia | | | | | + |
| | **Dystonia** | | | | + | + |
| | **Extrapyramidal signs** | | | + | + | + |
| | **Seizures** | | | + | + | + |
| Laboratory findings | Iron (brain) | | | ↑ | ↑ | ↑ |

**Table 59.3** Spinocerebellar ataxia 20 – SNX14 deficiency

| System | Symptoms and biomarkers | Neonatal (birth–1 month) | Infancy (1–18 months) | Childhood (1.5–11 years) | Adolescence (11–16 years) | Adulthood (>16 years) |
|---|---|---|---|---|---|---|
| CNS | **Ataxia** | | | | + | + |
| | **Cerebral atrophy (MRI)** | | | | + | + |
| | Deep tendon reflexes | | | | ± | ± |
| | Gait disturbance | | | | + | + |
| | Hyporeflexia | | | | ± | ± |
| | Hypotonia | | | | ± | ± |
| | **Loss of speech** | | | | + | + |
| | Oculomotor apraxia | | | | ± | ± |
| | **Retardation, psychomotor** | | | | + | + |
| Musculoskeletal | **Coarse facial features** | | | | + | + |
| | Facial dysmorphism | | | | ± | ± |
| | Macrocephaly | | | | ± | |

**Table 59.4** Spastic paraplegia 11 (SPG11)

| System | Symptoms and biomarkers | Neonatal (birth–1 month) | Infancy (1–18 months) | Childhood (1.5–11 years) | Adolescence (11–16 years) | Adulthood (>16 years) |
|---|---|---|---|---|---|---|
| CNS | Areflexia | + | + | + | | |
| | Gait disturbance | | + | + | + | |
| | Neuropathy, axonal motor | + | + | + | | |
| | Thin corpus callosum | ± | | | | |
| | Tremor | | | ± | ± | |
| Genitourinary | Urinary incontinence | | ± | ± | ± | |
| Musculoskeletal | Contractures | ± | ± | ± | ± | |
| | Hand and feet anomalies | ± | ± | ± | ± | |
| | Kyphoscoliosis | ± | ± | ± | ± | |
| | Muscle weakness, distal | + | + | + | + | |

**Table 59.5** Charcot–Marie–Tooth disease 2X (SPG11)

| System | Symptoms and biomarkers | Neonatal (birth–1 month) | Infancy (1–18 months) | Childhood (1.5–11 years) | Adolescence (11–16 years) | Adulthood (>16 years) |
|---|---|---|---|---|---|---|
| CNS | Agenesis, corpus callosum (MRI) | + | + | + | + | |
| | Ataxia | + | + | + | + | |
| | Cortical atrophy (MRI) | + | + | + | + | |
| | Dysarthria | + | + | + | + | |
| | Hyperreflexia | + | + | + | + | |
| | Intellectual disability | | + | + | + | + |
| | Neuropathy, sensory | | + | + | + | + |
| | Pyramidal signs | + | + | + | + | |
| | Spasticity | + | + | + | + | |
| | Sphincter control problems | | + | + | + | + |
| | Thin corpus callosum | + | + | + | + | |
| | Walking on tiptoes | | + | + | + | |
| Digestive | Dysphagia | + | + | + | + | |
| | Obesity | | + | + | + | |
| Eye | Macular dystrophy | | | | | + |
| | Nystagmus | + | + | + | + | |
| | Poor visual fixation | | | | | + |
| | Retinal dystrophy | | | | | + |
| Genitourinary | Urinary incontinence | | + | + | + | + |
| Musculoskeletal | Amyotrophy | + | + | + | + | + |
| | Muscle atrophy | | + | + | + | + |
| | Pes cavus | + | + | + | + | |
| Psychiatric | Learning disabilities | | + | + | + | |

**Table 59.6** Amyotrophic lateral sclerosis 5 (SPG11)

| System | Symptoms and biomarkers | Neonatal (birth–1 month) | Infancy (1–18 months) | Childhood (1.5–11 years) | Adolescence (11–16 years) | Adulthood (>16 years) |
|---|---|---|---|---|---|---|
| CNS | Bulbar dysfunction | | | + | + | |
| | Dysarthria | | | + | + | |
| | Extensor plantar responses | | | + | + | |
| | Hyperreflexia | | | + | | |
| | Pyramidal signs | | | + | + | |
| | **Spasticity** | | | + | + | |
| Musculoskeletal | Fasciculations | | | + | + | |
| | Fibrillations | | | + | + | |
| | **Muscle weakness, distal** | | | + | + | |
| Respiratory | Respiratory failure | | | + | + | |

**Table 59.7** Spastic paraplegia 15 (ZFYVE26)

| System | Symptoms and biomarkers | Neonatal (birth–1 month) | Infancy (1–18 months) | Childhood (1.5–11 years) | Adolescence (11–16 years) | Adulthood (>16 years) |
|---|---|---|---|---|---|---|
| CNS | **Ataxia** | | | + | + | + |
| | Brain atrophy (MRI) | | | + | + | + |
| | Dysarthria | | | + | + | + |
| | **Extensor plantar responses** | | | + | + | + |
| | Gait disturbance | | | + | + | + |
| | Hyperreflexia | | | + | + | + |
| | **Intellectual disability** | | | + | + | + |
| | Myoclonus | | | + | + | + |
| | Neuropathy, axonal motor | | | + | + | + |
| | Spasticity | | | + | + | + |
| | Thin corpus callosum | | | + | + | + |
| | White matter abnormalities (MRI) | | | + | + | + |
| Genitourinary | **Urinary incontinence** | | | + | + | + |
| Musculoskeletal | Amyotrophy | | | + | + | + |
| | Pes cavus | | | + | + | + |
| Psychiatric | Mood swings | | | + | + | + |
| | Psychosis | | | + | + | + |

**Table 59.8** Spastic paraplegia 48 (AP5Z1)

| System | Symptoms and biomarkers | Neonatal (birth–1 month) | Infancy (1–18 months) | Childhood (1.5–11 years) | Adolescence (11–16 years) | Adulthood (>16 years) |
|---|---|---|---|---|---|---|
| CNS | Ataxia | | | | | + |
| | Cognitive decline | | | | | + |
| | Dysmetria | | | | | + |
| | Gait disturbance | | | | | + |
| | Intellectual disability, mild | | | | | + |
| | Neuropathy | | | | | + |
| | Parkinsonism | | | | | + |
| | Retardation, psychomotor | | | | | + |
| | Spasticity, limbs | | | | | + |
| | Thin corpus callosum | | | | | + |
| | White matter abnormalities (MRI) | | | | | + |
| Eye | Retinopathy | | | | | ± |
| Genitourinary | **Urinary incontinence** | | | | | + |

**Table 59.9** Spastic paraplegia 49 (TECPR2)

| System | Symptoms and biomarkers | Neonatal (birth–1 month) | Infancy (1–18 months) | Childhood (1.5–11 years) | Adolescence (11–16 years) | Adulthood (>16 years) |
|---|---|---|---|---|---|---|
| CNS | Areflexia | | + | + | | |
| | Cerebral atrophy (MRI) | | + | + | | |
| | Dysarthria | | + | + | | |
| | Dysmetria | | + | + | | |
| | Gait ataxia | | + | + | | |
| | Hypomimia | | + | + | | |
| | Hypotonia | | + | + | | |
| | Regression, psychomotor | | + | + | | |
| | Seizures | | ± | ± | | |
| | Thin corpus callosum | | + | + | | |
| Digestive | Gastroesophageal reflux | | + | + | | |
| Hair | Low anterior hairline | | + | + | | |
| Musculoskeletal | **Short stature** | | + | + | | |
| | **Microcephaly** | | + | + | | |
| | Brachycephaly | | + | + | | |
| | Round face | | + | + | | |
| | Dental crowding | | + | + | | |
| Respiratory | Apnea | | ± | ± | | |

**Table 59.10** Frontotemporal dementia and/or amyotrophic lateral sclerosis 4 (TBK1)

| System | Symptoms and biomarkers | Neonatal (birth–1 month) | Infancy (1–18 months) | Childhood (1.5–11 years) | Adolescence (11–16 years) | Adulthood (>16 years) |
|---|---|---|---|---|---|---|
| CNS | Amyotrophic lateral sclerosis | | | | | + |
| | Bulbar dysfunction | | | | | + |
| | Cortical atrophy (MRI) | | | | | + |
| | Dysarthria | | | | | + |
| | **Frontotemporal dementia** | | | | | + |
| | Hyperreflexia | | | | | + |
| | Hyporeflexia | | | | | + |
| | Mutism | | | | | + |
| | Swallowing difficulties | | | | | + |
| Digestive | **Dysphagia** | | | | | + |
| Musculoskeletal | Amyotrophy | | | | | + |
| | Fasciculations | | | | | + |
| | Fibrillations | | | | | + |
| | **Muscle weakness** | | | | | + |
| Psychiatric | Apathy | | | | | + |
| | Behavioral disorder | | | | | + |
| | Disinhibition | | | | | + |
| | Personality changes | | | | | + |

**Table 59.11** Charcot–Marie–Tooth disease 2B (RAB7A)

| System | Symptoms and biomarkers | Neonatal (birth–1 month) | Infancy (1–18 months) | Childhood (1.5–11 years) | Adolescence (11–16 years) | Adulthood (>16 years) |
|---|---|---|---|---|---|---|
| CNS | Areflexia | | | | + | + |
| | Hyporeflexia | | | | + | + |
| Dermatological | Dystrophic toenail changes | | | | + | + |
| | Ulcers, distal | | | | + | + |
| Musculoskeletal | Autoamputation | | | | + | + |
| | Foot deformities | | | | + | + |
| | Hammer toes | | | | + | + |
| | Muscle weakness, distal | | | | + | + |
| | **Pes cavus** | | | | + | + |
| | Pes planus | | | | + | + |

**Table 59.12** Spinocerebellar ataxia 25 (ATG5)

| System | Symptoms and biomarkers | Neonatal (birth–1 month) | Infancy (1–18 months) | Childhood (1.5–11 years) | Adolescence (11–16 years) | Adulthood (>16 years) |
|---|---|---|---|---|---|---|
| CNS | **Cerebellar hypoplasia** | | | | + | |
| | **Dysmetria** | | | | + | |
| | **Truncal ataxia** | | | | + | |
| Eye | **Nystagmus** | | | | + | |

**Table 59.13** Parkinson disease 2 (PRKN)

| System | Symptoms and biomarkers | Neonatal (birth–1 month) | Infancy (1–18 months) | Childhood (1.5–11 years) | Adolescence (11–16 years) | Adulthood (>16 years) |
|---|---|---|---|---|---|---|
| CNS | Bradykinesia | | | | | + |
| | Dystonia | | | | + | + |
| | **Hyperreflexia** | | | | + | + |
| | **Parkinsonism, hypokinetic features** | | | | + | + |
| | **Retropulsion** | | | | + | + |
| | Tremor | | | | ± | ++ |
| Musculoskeletal | Postural instability | | | | | ± |
| | Rigidity | | | | | ± |

**Table 59.14** Parkinson disease 6 early onset (PINK1)

| System | Symptoms and biomarkers | Neonatal (birth–1 month) | Infancy (1–18 months) | Childhood (1.5–11 years) | Adolescence (11–16 years) | Adulthood (>16 years) |
|---|---|---|---|---|---|---|
| CNS | Anxiety | | | | ± | = |
| | Asymmetry | | | | ± | + |
| | Autonomic instability | | | | ± | ± |
| | **Bradykinesia** | | | | ± | + |
| | Dementia | | | | ± | ± |
| | Depression | | | | ± | ± |
| | Dystonia | | | | ± | ± |
| | Gait impairment | | | | ± | + |
| | **Hyperreflexia** | | | | ± | + |
| | **Parkinsonism** | | | | ± | + |
| | Psychiatric disturbances | | | | ± | ± |
| | Sleep benefit | | | | ± | ± |
| | Tremor | | | | ± | + |
| Musculoskeletal | Postural instability | | | | ± | ± |
| | **Rigidity** | | | | ± | + |
| Genitourinary | Urinary urgency | | | | ± | ± |

**Table 59.15** Frontotemporal dementia and/or amyotrophic lateral sclerosis 3 (SQSTM1)

| System | Symptoms and biomarkers | Neonatal (birth–1 month) | Infancy (1–18 months) | Childhood (1.5–11 years) | Adolescence (11–16 years) | Adulthood (>16 years) |
|---|---|---|---|---|---|---|
| CNS | Amyotrophic lateral sclerosis | | | | | + |
| | Bulbar dysfunction | | | | | + |
| | Dysarthria | | | | | + |
| | **Frontotemporal dementia** | | | | | + |
| | Hyperreflexia | | | | | + |
| | Hyporeflexia | | | | | + |
| | Language difficulties | | | | | + |
| | Mutism | | | | | + |
| | **Orofacial apraxia** | | | | | + |
| | **Swallowing difficulties** | | | | | + |
| Digestive | **Dysphagia** | | | | | + |
| Musculoskeletal | **Amyotrophy** | | | | | + |
| | Fasciculations | | | | | + |
| | Fibrillations | | | | | + |
| | **Muscle weakness** | | | | | + |
| Psychiatric | Apathy | | | | | + |
| | Behavioral disorder | | | | | + |
| | **Disinhibition** | | | | | + |
| | Personality changes | | | | | + |

**Table 59.16** Myopathy distal with rimmed vacuoles (SQSTM1)

| System | Symptoms and biomarkers | Neonatal (birth–1 month) | Infancy (1–18 months) | Childhood (1.5–11 years) | Adolescence (11–16 years) | Adulthood (>16 years) |
|---|---|---|---|---|---|---|
| CNS | Gait disturbance | | | | | + |
| Musculoskeletal | **Foot drop** | | | | | + |
| | **Muscle atrophy** | | | | | + |
| | **Muscle weakness, distal** | | | | | + |
| Laboratory findings | Creatine kinase (plasma) | | | | | ↑ |

**Table 59.17** Neurodegeneration with ataxia, dystonia, and gaze palsy (SQSTM1)

| System | Symptoms and biomarkers | Neonatal (birth–1 month) | Infancy (1–18 months) | Childhood (1.5–11 years) | Adolescence (11–16 years) | Adulthood (>16 years) |
|---|---|---|---|---|---|---|
| CNS | Cerebellar atrophy (MRI) | | | ± | ± | |
| | Cognitive decline | | | + | + | |
| | Dysarthria | | | + | + | |
| | Dysdiadochokinesis | | | + | + | |
| | Dysmetria | | | + | + | |
| | Dystonia | | | + | + | |
| | **Gait ataxia** | | | + | + | |
| | **Gait disturbance** | | | + | + | |
| | Hyperreflexia | | | + | + | |
| | **Iron deposition in the basal ganglia** | | | + | + | |
| | **Oculomotor apraxia** | | | + | + | |
| | Pyramidal signs | | | + | + | |
| | Tremor | | | + | + | |
| Ear | Hearing loss | | | ± | ± | |
| Eye | Nystagmus | | | + | + | |
| Genitourinary | Urinary incontinence | | | ± | ± | |

**Table 59.18** Paget disease of bone 3 (SQSTM1)

| System | Symptoms and biomarkers | Neonatal (birth–1 month) | Infancy (1–18 months) | Childhood (1.5–11 years) | Adolescence (11–16 years) | Adulthood (>16 years) |
|---|---|---|---|---|---|---|
| Ear | Deafness | | | | | ± |
| Musculoskeletal | Bone fractures | | | | | ± |
| | **Bone pain** | | | | | + |
| | Osteoarthrosis | | | | | + |
| | **Osteosclerosis** | | | | | + |
| Laboratory findings | Alkaline phosphatase (plasma) | | | | | ↑ |

**Table 59.19** Spastic paraplegia 52 (AP4S1)

| System | Symptoms and biomarkers | Neonatal (birth–1 month) | Infancy (1–18 months) | Childhood (1.5–11 years) | Adolescence (11–16 years) | Adulthood (>16 years) |
|---|---|---|---|---|---|---|
| CNS | Axial hypotonia | + | + | + | + | |
| | Extensor plantar responses | + | + | + | + | |
| | Hyperreflexia | + | + | + | + | |
| | Hypertonia | + | + | + | + | |
| | Intellectual disability | | + | + | + | |
| | Loss of speech | | + | + | + | |
| | Retardation, psychomotor | | + | + | + | |
| | Seizures | + | + | + | | |
| | Spasticity | + | + | + | + | |
| Digestive | Big open mouth | + | + | + | | |
| Musculoskeletal | Broad nasal bridge | + | + | + | + | |
| | Bulbous nose | + | + | + | + | |
| | Coarse facial features | + | + | + | + | |
| | Hypertelorism | + | + | + | + | |
| | Inability to walk | | ± | + | + | |
| | Joint contractures | | + | + | + | |
| | Microcephaly | + | + | + | + | |
| | Short philtrum | + | + | + | + | |
| | **Short stature** | | + | + | + | |
| | Talipes equinovarus | + | + | + | + | |
| Psychiatric | Amicable character | | + | + | + | |
| | Shy character | | + | + | + | |
| | Stereotypic behaviors | | + | + | + | |

**Table 59.20** Spastic paraplegia 47 (AP4B1)

| System | Symptoms and biomarkers | Neonatal (birth–1 month) | Infancy (1–18 months) | Childhood (1.5–11 years) | Adolescence (11–16 years) | Adulthood (>16 years) |
|---|---|---|---|---|---|---|
| CNS | Dysarthria | | + | + | + | |
| | Dystonia | | + | + | | |
| | Extensor plantar responses | + | + | + | + | |
| | Hyperreflexia | + | + | + | + | |
| | Hypertonia | | + | + | + | |
| | Hypotonia | + | | | | |
| | Intellectual disability | | + | + | + | |
| | Retardation, psychomotor | | + | + | + | |
| | Seizures | + | + | + | + | |
| | Spasticity | + | + | + | | |
| | Speech delay | | + | + | + | |
| | Thin corpus callosum | + | + | + | + | |
| | Ventriculomegaly | + | + | + | | |
| | Waddling gait | | + | + | + | |
| Musculoskeletal | Bitemporal narrowing | + | + | + | + | |
| | Bulbous nose | + | + | + | | |
| | Club foot | ± | ± | ± | ± | |
| | Coarse face | + | + | + | + | |
| | Contractures | + | + | + | + | |
| | Joint hypermobility | ± | ± | ± | ± | |
| | Microcephaly | + | + | + | + | |
| | Pes planus | ± | ± | ± | ± | |
| | Short philtrum | + | + | + | + | |
| | Short stature | | + | + | + | |
| | Wide mouth | + | + | + | | |
| | Wide nasal bridge | + | + | + | + | |
| Psychiatric | Shy character | | + | + | + | |
| | Stereotypic behaviors | | + | + | + | |

**Table 59.21** Spastic paraplegia 50 (AP4M1)

| System | Symptoms and biomarkers | Neonatal (birth–1 month) | Infancy (1–18 months) | Childhood (1.5–11 years) | Adolescence (11–16 years) | Adulthood (>16 years) |
|---|---|---|---|---|---|---|
| CNS | Cerebellar atrophy (MRI) | + | + | + | + | |
| | Extensor plantar responses | + | + | + | + | |
| | Gliosis | + | + | + | + | |
| | Hyperreflexia | + | + | + | + | |
| | Hypertonia | | + | + | + | |
| | Hypotonia | + | | | | |
| | Intellectual disability | | + | + | + | |
| | Retardation, psychomotor | | + | + | + | |
| | Spastic quadriplegia | | + | + | + | |
| | Speech delay | | + | + | + | |
| | Thin corpus callosum | + | + | + | + | |
| | Ventriculomegaly | + | + | + | + | |
| | White matter abnormalities (MRI) | + | + | + | + | |
| Eye | **Strabismus** | + | + | + | + | |
| Musculoskeletal | Arched palate, high | + | + | + | + | |
| | Bitemporal narrowing | + | + | + | + | |
| | Broad nasal bridge | + | + | + | + | |
| | Bulbous nose | + | + | + | + | |
| | Club foot | + | + | + | + | |
| | Coarse face | + | + | + | + | |
| | Facial dysmorphism | ± | ± | ± | + | |
| | **Microcephaly** | + | + | + | + | |
| | Short philtrum | + | + | + | + | |
| | Wide mouth | + | + | + | | |

**Table 59.22** Spastic paraplegia 51 (AP4E1)

| System | Symptoms and biomarkers | Neonatal (birth–1 month) | Infancy (1–18 months) | Childhood (1.5–11 years) | Adolescence (11–16 years) | Adulthood (>16 years) |
|---|---|---|---|---|---|---|
| CNS | Cerebellar atrophy (MRI) | + | + | + | + | |
| | Cortical atrophy (MRI) | + | + | + | + | |
| | Extensor plantar responses | + | + | + | + | |
| | Hyperreflexia | + | + | + | + | |
| | Hypotonia | + | + | + | + | |
| | Intellectual disability | | + | + | + | |
| | Retardation, psychomotor | | + | + | + | |
| | Seizures | + | + | + | + | |
| | Spastic quadriplegia | + | + | + | + | |
| | Speech delay | | + | + | + | |
| | White matter abnormalities (MRI) | + | + | + | + | |
| Digestive | Drooling | + | + | + | | |
| Ear | Prominent antihelix | + | + | + | | |
| Eye | Downslanting palpebral fissures | + | + | + | | |
| | Nystagmus | + | + | + | + | |
| Musculoskeletal | Bitemporal narrowing | + | + | + | + | |
| | Bulbous nose | + | + | + | | |
| | Coarse facial features | + | + | + | + | |
| | Joint contractures | | + | + | + | |
| | Microcephaly | + | + | + | | |
| | Narrow, elongated face | + | + | + | + | |
| | Short philtrum | + | + | + | | |
| | Short stature | + | + | + | + | |
| | Talipes equinovarus | | + | + | + | |
| | Wide mouth | + | + | + | | |
| | Wide nasal bridge | + | + | + | | |
| Psychiatric | Amicable character | | + | + | + | |
| | Shy character | | + | + | + | |
| | Stereotypic behaviors | | + | + | + | |

**Table 59.23** Hypotonia, infantile, with psychomotor retardation and characteristic facies 3 (TBCK)

| System | Symptoms and biomarkers | Neonatal (birth–1 month) | Infancy (1–18 months) | Childhood (1.5–11 years) | Adolescence (11–16 years) | Adulthood (>16 years) |
|---|---|---|---|---|---|---|
| CNS | Cerebellar hypoplasia | + | + | + | | |
| | Cerebral atrophy (MRI) | + | + | + | | |
| | Developmental delay | + | + | + | | |
| | Hyporeflexia | + | + | + | | |
| | Hypotonia | ++ | ++ | ++ | | |
| | Retardation, psychomotor | | + | + | | |
| | Seizures | + | + | + | | |
| | Small basal ganglia | + | + | + | | |
| | Speech delay | | + | + | | |
| | Thin corpus callosum | + | + | + | | |
| Digestive | Feeding difficulties | + | + | + | | |
| | Macroglossia | + | + | + | | |
| Eye | Deeply set eyes | + | + | + | | |
| | Visual loss | + | + | + | | |
| Hair | Arched eyebrows | + | + | + | | |
| Musculoskeletal | Anteverted nares | + | + | + | | |
| | Bitemporal narrowing | + | + | + | | |
| | Bulbous nose | + | + | + | | |
| | Coarse face | + | + | + | | |
| | Gingival hyperplasia | + | + | + | | |
| | High nasal bridge | + | + | + | | |
| | Microcephaly | ± | ± | ± | | |
| | Thick lips | + | + | + | | |
| Respiratory | Respiratory insufficiency | + | + | + | | |

**Table 59.24** Amyotrophic lateral sclerosis 2 (ALS2)

| System | Symptoms and biomarkers | Neonatal (birth–1 month) | Infancy (1–18 months) | Childhood (1.5–11 years) | Adolescence (11–16 years) | Adulthood (>16 years) |
|---|---|---|---|---|---|---|
| CNS | Anarthria | | + | + | + | |
| | Dysarthria | | + | + | + | |
| | Extensor plantar responses | + | + | + | + | |
| | Hyperreflexia | | + | + | + | |
| | Sialorrhea | + | + | + | + | |
| | Spastic tetraparesis | | + | + | + | |
| | **Spasticity** | | + | + | + | |
| Digestive | **Dysphagia** | + | + | + | + | |
| Musculoskeletal | **Amyotrophy** | + | + | + | + | |

**Table 59.25** Primary lateral sclerosis juvenile (PLSJ)

| System | Symptoms and biomarkers | Neonatal (birth–1 month) | Infancy (1–18 months) | Childhood (1.5–11 years) | Adolescence (11–16 years) | Adulthood (>16 years) |
|---|---|---|---|---|---|---|
| CNS | **Cortical atrophy (MRI)** | + | + | + | | |
| | Extensor plantar responses | + | + | + | | |
| | Hyperreflexia | | + | + | | |
| | **Spastic tetraparesis** | + | + | + | | |
| | **Spasticity** | + | + | + | | |
| Digestive | Dysphagia | + | + | + | | |

**Table 59.26** Spastic paralysis, infantile onset ascending (IAHSP)

| System | Symptoms and biomarkers | Neonatal (birth–1 month) | Infancy (1–18 months) | Childhood (1.5–11 years) | Adolescence (11–16 years) | Adulthood (>16 years) |
|---|---|---|---|---|---|---|
| CNS | Anarthria | | + | + | + | |
| | Bulbar dysfunction | | + | + | | |
| | Dysarthria | | + | + | + | |
| | Extensor plantar responses | | + | + | + | |
| | Hyperreflexia | | + | + | | |
| | Motor developmental delay | | + | + | + | |
| | Spastic paraplegia | | + | + | | |
| | **Spasticity** | | + | + | + | |
| | Stiffness | | + | + | | |
| Digestive | **Dysphagia** | | | + | + | |
| Eye | Eyes opening, delayed | | | + | + | |
| | **Ocular abnormalities** | | | + | + | |
| Genitourinary | **Urinary incontinence** | | + | + | + | |
| Musculoskeletal | Muscle weakness | | + | + | + | |
| | **Muscle weakness, facial** | | + | + | + | |
| | Pes cavus | | + | + | | |

**Table 59.27** Neuropathy, distal hereditary motor, type VIIB (DCTN1)

| System | Symptoms and biomarkers | Neonatal (birth–1 month) | Infancy (1–18 months) | Childhood (1.5–11 years) | Adolescence (11–16 years) | Adulthood (>16 years) |
|---|---|---|---|---|---|---|
| Musculoskeletal | **Muscle atrophy** | | | | | + |
| | **Muscle weakness** | | | | | + |
| | **Muscle weakness, facial** | | | | + | + |
| Respiratory | Breathing difficulty | | | | + | + |

**Table 59.28** Perry syndrome (DCTN1)

| System | Symptoms and biomarkers | Neonatal (birth–1 month) | Infancy (1–18 months) | Childhood (1.5–11 years) | Adolescence (11–16 years) | Adulthood (>16 years) |
|---|---|---|---|---|---|---|
| CNS | Axonal spheroids | | | | | + |
| | Brain, abnormal (MRI) | | | | | + |
| | **Frontal lobe atrophy** | | | | | + |
| | Frontotemporal dementia | | | | | + |
| | Insomnia | | | | | + |
| | **Parkinsonism** | | | | | + |
| | Vertical gaze palsy | | | | | + |
| Other | **Weight loss** | | | | | + |
| Psychiatric | **Behavioral disorder** | | | | | + |
| | **Depression** | | | | | + |
| Respiratory | **Hypoventilation, central** | | | | | + |
| | **Respiratory insufficiency** | | | | | + |

**Table 59.29** Polymicrogyria bilateral temporo-occipital (FIG4)

| System | Symptoms and biomarkers | Neonatal (birth–1 month) | Infancy (1–18 months) | Childhood (1.5–11 years) | Adolescence (11–16 years) | Adulthood (>16 years) |
|---|---|---|---|---|---|---|
| CNS | Polymicrogyria | | | + | + | |
| | Psychiatric symptoms | | | + | + | |
| | Seizures | | | + | + | |
| | Ventriculomegaly | | | + | + | |
| Eye | Visual hallucinations | | | + | + | |
| Psychiatric | Behavior, aggressive | | | + | + | |

**Table 59.30** Amyotrophic lateral sclerosis 11 (FIG4)

| System | Symptoms and biomarkers | Neonatal (birth–1 month) | Infancy (1–18 months) | Childhood (1.5–11 years) | Adolescence (11–16 years) | Adulthood (>16 years) |
|---|---|---|---|---|---|---|
| CNS | Bulbar dysfunction | | | | | + |
| | Corticospinal tract abnormalities | | | | | + |
| | EEG, abnormal | | | | | + |

**Table 59.31** Charcot-Marie-Tooth disease 4 J (FIG4)

| System | Symptoms and biomarkers | Neonatal (birth–1 month) | Infancy (1–18 months) | Childhood (1.5–11 years) | Adolescence (11–16 years) | Adulthood (>16 years) |
|---|---|---|---|---|---|---|
| CNS | Areflexia | | + | + | | |
| | Delayed myelination | | + | + | | |
| | Distal sensory loss | | + | + | | |
| | Gait disturbance | | + | + | | |
| | Motor developmental delay | | ± | ± | | |
| Musculoskeletal | Amyotrophy | | + | + | | |
| | Contractures | | + | + | | |
| | Muscle weakness, proximal | | + | + | | |

**Table 59.32** Yunis-Varon syndrome (FIG4)

| System | Symptoms and biomarkers | Neonatal (birth–1 month) | Infancy (1–18 months) | Childhood (1.5–11 years) | Adolescence (11–16 years) | Adulthood (>16 years) |
|---|---|---|---|---|---|---|
| Cardiovascular | **Cardiomyopathy** | + | + | + | | |
| | Congenital heart defects | + | + | + | | |
| | Pulmonary hypertension | + | + | + | + | |
| | **Tetralogy of Fallot** | + | + | + | + | |
| | Ventricular septal defect | + | + | + | + | |
| CNS | Agenesis, corpus callosum (MRI) | + | + | + | | |
| | Developmental delay | | + | + | + | |
| | Hypotonia | + | + | + | | |
| Dermatological | Single transverse palmar crease | + | + | + | | |
| Digestive | Pyloric stenosis | + | + | | | |
| Ear | Hearing loss | + | + | + | + | |
| | Low-set ears | + | + | + | + | |
| Eye | Cataract | + | + | + | + | |
| | Pachygyria | + | + | + | | |
| | Protruding eyes | + | + | + | + | |
| | Sclerocornea | + | + | + | + | |
| Genitourinary | Cryptorchidism | + | + | | | |
| | Hypospadias | + | + | + | | |
| | Micropenis | + | + | + | | |
| Hair | Sparse eyebrows and eyelashes | + | + | + | | |
| | Sparse hair | | + | + | | |
| Musculoskeletal | Absent clavicle | + | + | + | + | |
| | **Absent nipples** | + | + | | | |
| | Anteverted nares | + | + | + | + | |
| | Dolichocephaly | + | + | + | + | |
| | Hip dislocation | | + | + | + | |
| | **Hypertelorism** | + | + | + | + | |
| | Microcephaly | + | + | + | + | |
| | Micrognathia | + | + | + | + | |
| | Narrow palate | + | + | + | + | |
| | Premature loss of teeth | | + | + | | |
| | Short philtrum | + | + | + | + | |
| | Syndactyly | + | + | + | | |
| | Tin upper lips | + | + | + | + | |
| Other | Death | ± | ± | | | |
| | **Failure to thrive** | +++ | | | | |
| | **Intrauterine growth retardation** | + | | | | |

**Table 59.33** Yunis-Varon syndrome (VAC14)

| System | Symptoms and biomarkers | Neonatal (birth–1 month) | Infancy (1–18 months) | Childhood (1.5–11 years) | Adolescence (11–16 years) | Adulthood (>16 years) |
|---|---|---|---|---|---|---|
| CNS | Basal ganglia abnormalities (MRI) | + | | | | |
| | Developmental delay | + | | | | |
| | Hydrocephalus | + | | | | |
| | Hypotonia | + | | | | |
| | Irritability | + | + | | | |
| | Leukodystrophy, progressive | + | | | | |
| Digestive | Feeding difficulties | + | + | | | |
| Eye | Eye movements, roving | + | + | | | |
| Musculoskeletal | Dysmorphic features | + | | | | |
| | Skeletal abnormalities | + | | | | |
| Other | Intracytoplasmic vacuolation | + | | | | |

**Table 59.34** Striatonigral degeneration, childhood-onset (VAC14)

| System | Symptoms and biomarkers | Neonatal (birth–1 month) | Infancy (1–18 months) | Childhood (1.5–11 years) | Adolescence (11–16 years) | Adulthood (>16 years) |
|---|---|---|---|---|---|---|
| CNS | Developmental regression | | + | + | | |
| | Dystonia | | + | + | | |
| | Facial dystonia | + | + | + | | |
| | Hyperreflexia | + | + | + | | |
| | Hypersalivation | + | + | + | | |
| | Involuntary movements | + | + | + | | |
| | Speech disturbances | | + | + | | |
| Digestive | Drooling | + | + | + | | |
| | Dysphagia | + | + | + | | |
| Musculoskeletal | Inability to walk | | + | + | | |

**Table 59.35** Centronuclear myopathy 1 (MTMR14)

| System | Symptoms and biomarkers | Neonatal (birth–1 month) | Infancy (1–18 months) | Childhood (1.5–11 years) | Adolescence (11–16 years) | Adulthood (>16 years) |
|---|---|---|---|---|---|---|
| CNS | Areflexia | | | + | + | + |
| | Motor developmental delay | | | + | + | + |
| Eye | **Ophthalmoparesis** | | | + | + | + |
| | Ptosis of eyelid | | | + | + | + |
| Musculoskeletal | **Muscle weakness, facial** | | | + | + | + |
| | Walking difficulty | | | + | + | + |

**Table 59.36** Centronuclear myopathy 1 (DNM2)

| System | Symptoms and biomarkers | Neonatal (birth–1 month) | Infancy (1–18 months) | Childhood (1.5–11 years) | Adolescence (11–16 years) | Adulthood (>16 years) |
|---|---|---|---|---|---|---|
| CNS | Areflexia | + | + | + | + | + |
| Eye | Ophthalmoparesis | + | + | + | + | + |
| | Ptosis of eyelid | + | + | + | + | + |
| Musculoskeletal | Contractures | | + | + | + | + |
| | Muscle weakness | + | + | + | + | + |
| | Walking difficulty | | + | + | + | + |

**Table 59.37** Charcot-Marie-Tooth disease 2 M (DNM2)

| System | Symptoms and biomarkers | Neonatal (birth–1 month) | Infancy (1–18 months) | Childhood (1.5–11 years) | Adolescence (11–16 years) | Adulthood (>16 years) |
|---|---|---|---|---|---|---|
| CNS | Areflexia | | + | + | + | |
| | Distal sensory loss | | + | + | + | |
| | Hyperreflexia | | + | + | + | |
| Musculoskeletal | Muscle weakness | | + | + | + | |
| | Pes cavus | | + | + | + | |

**Table 59.38** Amyotrophic lateral sclerosis 17 (CHMP2B)

| System | Symptoms and biomarkers | Neonatal (birth–1 month) | Infancy (1–18 months) | Childhood (1.5–11 years) | Adolescence (11–16 years) | Adulthood (>16 years) |
|---|---|---|---|---|---|---|
| CNS | Areflexia | | | | | + |
| | Bulbar dysfunction | | | | | + |
| | Dysarthria | | | | | + |
| | Extensor plantar responses | | | | | ± |
| | Hyporeflexia | | | | | + |
| Digestive | Dysphagia | | | | | + |
| Musculoskeletal | Fasciculations | | | | | + |
| | **Muscle atrophy** | | | | | + |
| | **Muscle weakness** | | | | | + |
| Respiratory | **Respiratory insufficiency** | | | | | + |

**Table 59.39** Frontotemporal dementia chromosome 3 linked (CHMP2B)

| System | Symptoms and biomarkers | Neonatal (birth–1 month) | Infancy (1–18 months) | Childhood (1.5–11 years) | Adolescence (11–16 years) | Adulthood (>16 years) |
|---|---|---|---|---|---|---|
| CNS | Astrocytosis | | | | | + |
| | **Cortical atrophy (MRI)** | | | | | + |
| | Dyscalculia | | | | | + |
| | Dystonia | | | | | + |
| | Extensor plantar responses | | | | | + |
| | **Frontotemporal dementia** | | | | | + |
| | **Hyperreflexia** | | | | | + |
| | Loss of speech | | | | | + |
| | Memory problems | | | | | + |
| | Mutism | | | | | + |
| | Myoclonus | | | | | + |
| | Orofacial dyskinesia | | | | | + |
| | **Pyramidal signs** | | | | | + |
| | **White matter abnormalities (MRI)** | | | | | + |
| Genitourinary | **Urinary incontinence** | | | | | + |
| Musculoskeletal | Rigidity | | | | | + |
| Psychiatric | Apathy | | | | | + |
| | Behavior, aggressive | | | | | + |
| | Disinhibition | | | | | + |
| | Personality changes | | | | | + |
| | Stereotypic behaviors | | | | | + |

## Diagnosis

The diagnosis of an autophagy-related disorder should be prompted by a characteristic combination of features as outlined above. Mutation analysis via targeted Sanger or exome analysis is the only reliable method of diagnosis of an autophagy-related disorder. Non-specific laboratory changes, such as abnormalities of urinary oligosaccharides profile or increased GAG, have been reported in a few disorders presenting with a multisystem storage-like disease, such as Yunis-Varon syndrome (59.32; 59.33) and spinocerebellar ataxia 20 (59.3) (Akizu et al. 2015; Dworzak et al. 1995).

## Treatment

There are currently no approved therapies available for inherited disorders of autophagy; therefore, current treatment is limited to symptomatic and supportive management. However, there are several therapeutic modalities under investigation (Morel et al. 2017; Maiuri and Kroemer 2019; Yang et al. 2013).

## References


Akizu N, Cantagrel V, Zaki MS, et al. Biallelic mutations in SNX14 cause a syndromic form of cerebellar atrophy and lysosome-autophagosome dysfunction. Nat Genet. 2015;47:528–34.

Baulac S, Lenk GM, Dufresnois B, et al. Role of the phosphoinositide phosphatase FIG4 gene in familial epilepsy with polymicrogyria. Neurology. 2014;82:1068–75.

Beck-Wödl S, Harzer K, Sturm M, et al. Homozygous TBC1 domain-containing kinase (TBCK) mutation causes a novel lysosomal storage disease—a new type of neuronal ceroid lipofuscinosis (CLN15)? Acta Neuropathol Commun. 2018;6:145.

Bhoj EJ, Li D, Harr M, et al. Mutations in TBCK, encoding TBC1-domain-containing kinase, Lead to a recognizable syndrome of intellectual disability and Hypotonia. Am J Hum Genet. 2016;98:782–8.

Bitoun M, Maugenre S, Jeannet, et al. Mutations in dynamin 2 cause dominant centronuclear myopathy. Nat Genet. 2005;37:1207–9.

Bucelli RC, Arhzaouy K, Pestronk A, et al. SQSTM1 splice site mutation in distal myopathy with rimmed vacuoles. Neurology. 2015;85:665–74.

Byrne S, Jansen L, U-King-Im JM, et al. EPG5-related Vici syndrome: a paradigm of neurodevelopmental disorders with defective autophagy. Brain. 2016;139:765–81.

Campeau PM, Lenk GM, Lu JT, et al. Yunis-Varón syndrome is caused by mutations in FIG4, encoding a phosphoinositide phosphatase. Am J Hum Genet. 2013;92:781–91.

Cullup T, Kho AL, Dionisi-Vici C, et al. Recessive mutations in EPG5 cause Vici syndrome, a multisystem disorder with defective autophagy. Nat Genet. 2013;45:83–7.

Dworzak F, Mora M, Borroni C, et al. Generalized lysosomal storage in Yunis Varón syndrome. Neuromuscul Disord. 1995;5:423–8.

Ebrahimi-Fakhari D, Behne R, Davies AK, et al. AP-4-associated hereditary spastic paraplegia. In: Adam MP, Ardinger HH, Pagon RA, et al., editors. GeneReviews® [Internet]. Seattle, WA: University of Washington, Seattle; 2018. 1993-2020. Bookshelf URL: https://www.ncbi.nlm.nih.gov/books/.

Eymard-Pierre E, Lesca G, Dollet S, et al. Infantile-onset ascending hereditary spastic paralysis is associated with mutations in the alsin gene. Am J Hum Genet. 2002;71:518–27.

Fassio A, Falace A, Esposito A, Aprile D, Guerrini R, Benfenati F. Emerging role of the autophagy/lysosomal degradative pathway in neurodevelopmental disorders with epilepsy. Front Cell Neurosci. 2020;14:39.

Ferreira CR, Rahman S, Keller M, Zschocke J, ICIMD Advisory Group. An international classification of inherited metabolic disorders (ICIMD). J Inherit Metab Dis. 2021;44:164–77.

García-Cazorla À, Saudubray JM. Cellular neurometabolism: a tentative to connect cell biology and metabolism in neurology. J Inherit Metab Dis. 2018;41:1043–54.

Gatica D, Lahiri V, Klionsky DJ. Cargo recognition and degradation by selective autophagy. Nat Cell Biol. 2018;20:233–42.

Haack TB, Hogarth P, Kruer MC, et al. Exome sequencing reveals de novo WDR45 mutations causing phenotypically distinct, X-linked dominant form of NBIA. Am J Hum Genet. 2012;91:1144–9.

Haack TB, Ignatius E, Calvo-Garrido J, et al. Absence of the autophagy adaptor SQSTM1/p62 causes childhood-onset neurodegeneration with ataxia, dystonia, and gaze palsy. Am J Hum Genet. 2016;99:735–43.

Harnett MM, Pineda MA, Latré de Laté P, et al. From Christian de Duve to Yoshinori Ohsumi: more to autophagy than just dining at home. Biom J. 2017;40:9–22.

Hirst J, Edgar JR, Esteves T, et al. Loss of AP-5 results in accumulation of aberrant endolysosomes: defining a new type of lysosomal storage disease. Hum Mol Genet. 2015;24:4984–96.

Kim M, Sandford E, Gatica D, et al. Mutation in ATG5 reduces autophagy and leads to ataxia with developmental delay. elife. 2016;5:e12245.

Kitada T, Asakawa S, Hattori N, et al. Mutations in the parkin gene cause autosomal recessive juvenile parkinsonism. Nature. 1998;392:605–8.

Konno T, Ross OA, Teive HAG, Sławek J, Dickson DW, Wszolek ZK. DCTN1-related neurodegeneration: Perry syndrome and beyond. Parkinsonism Relat Disord. 2017;41:14–24.

Laurin N, Brown JP, Morissette J, Raymond V. Recurrent mutation of the gene encoding sequestosome 1 (SQSTM1/p62) in Paget disease of bone. Am J Hum Genet. 2002;70:1582–8.

Lenk GM, Szymanska K, Debska-Vielhaber G, et al. Biallelic mutations of VAC14 in pediatric-onset neurological disease. Am J Hum Genet. 2016;99:188–94.

Levine B, Kroemer G. Biological functions of autophagy genes: a disease perspective. Cell. 2019;176:11–42.

Lines MA, Ito Y, Kernohan KD, et al. Yunis-Varón syndrome caused by biallelic VAC14 mutations. Eur J Hum Genet. 2017;25:1049–54.

Luciani A, Schumann A, Berquez M, et al. Impaired mitophagy links mitochondrial disease to epithelial stress in methylmalonyl-CoA mutase deficiency. Nat Commun. 2020;11:970.

Maiuri MC, Kroemer G. Therapeutic modulation of autophagy: which disease comes first? Cell Death Differ. 2019;26:680–9.

Montecchiani C, Pedace L, Lo Giudice T, et al. ALS5/SPG11/KIAA1840 mutations cause autosomal recessive axonal Charcot-Marie-tooth disease. Brain. 2016;139:73–85.

Morel E, Mehrpour M, Botti J, et al. Autophagy: a druggable process. Annu Rev Pharmacol Toxicol. 2017;57:375–98.

Nguyen DKH, Thombre R, Wang J. Autophagy as a common pathway in amyotrophic lateral sclerosis. Neurosci Lett. 2019;697:34–48.

Nicholson G, Lenk GM, Reddel SW, et al. Distinctive genetic and clinical features of CMT4J: a severe neuropathy caused by mutations in the PI(3,5)$P_2$ phosphatase FIG4. Brain. 2011;134:1959–71.

Orlacchio A, Babalini C, Borreca A, et al. SPATACSIN mutations cause autosomal recessive juvenile amyotrophic lateral sclerosis. Brain. 2010;133:591–8.

Oz-Levi D, Ben-Zeev B, Ruzzo EK, et al. Mutation in TECPR2 reveals a role for autophagy in hereditary spastic paraparesis. Am J Hum Genet. 2012;91:1065–72.

Piano Mortari E, Folgiero V, Marcellini V, et al. The Vici syndrome protein EPG5 regulates intracellular nucleic acid trafficking linking autophagy to innate and adaptive immunity. Autophagy. 2018;14:22–37.

Settembre C, Fraldi A, Medina DL, Ballabio A. Signals from the lysosome: a control Centre for cellular clearance and energy metabolism. Nat Rev Mol Cell Biol. 2013;14:283–96.

Skibinski G, Parkinson NJ, Brown JM, et al. Mutations in the endosomal ESCRTIII-complex subunit CHMP2B in frontotemporal dementia. Nat Genet. 2005;37:806–8.

Soria LR, Brunetti-Pierri N. Ammonia and autophagy: an emerging relationship with implications for disorders with hyperammonemia. J Inherit Metab Dis. 2019;42:1097–104.

Stamatakou E, Wróbel L, Hill SM, et al. Mendelian neurodegenerative disease genes involved in autophagy. Cell Discov. 2020;6:24.

Strømme P, Månsson JE, Scott H, Skullerud K, Hovig T. Encephaloneuropathy with lysosomal zebra bodies and GM2 ganglioside storage. Pediatr Neurol. 1997;16:141–4.

Teinert J, Behne R, Wimmer M, Ebrahimi-Fakhari D. Novel insights into the clinical and molecular spectrum of congenital disorders of autophagy. J Inherit Metab Dis. 2020;43:51–62.

Tosch V, Rohde HM, Tronchere H, et al. A novel PtdIns3P and PtdIns(3,5)P2 phosphatase with an inactivating variant in centronuclear myopathy. Hum Mol Genet. 2006;15:3098–106.

Valente EM, Abou-Sleiman PM, Caputo V, et al. Hereditary early-onset Parkinson's disease caused by mutations in PINK1. Science. 2004;304:1158–60.

Vantaggiato C, Panzeri E, Castelli M, et al. ZFYVE26/SPASTIZIN and SPG11/SPATACSIN mutations in hereditary spastic paraplegia types AR-SPG15 and AR-SPG11 have different effects on autophagy and endocytosis. Autophagy. 2019;15:34–57.

Verhoeven K, De Jonghe P, Coen K, et al. Mutations in the small GTPase late endosomal protein RAB7 cause Charcot-Marie-tooth type 2B neuropathy. Am J Hum Genet. 2003;72:722–7.

Yang YP, Hu LF, Zheng HF, et al. Application and interpretation of current autophagy inhibitors and activators. Acta Pharmacol Sin. 2013;34:625–35.

Zatyka M, Sarkar S, Barrett T. Autophagy in rare (nonlysosomal) neurodegenerative diseases. J Mol Biol. 2020;432:2735–53.

# Lipidoses: The Sphingolipidoses, Lysosomal Acid Lipase Deficiency, and Niemann-Pick Type C

60

Carla Hollak

## Contents



**Abstract**

Metabolic disorders that affect the lysosomal degradation of complex carbohydrates, lipids, and proteins are associated with a wide variety of clinical symptoms. The lipidoses are the most common of the lysosomal storage disorders and are increasingly recognized in adults with a more attenuated phenotype. At the severe end of the clinical spectrum, neurological symptoms are frequently seen and go along with significant brain pathology. The high abundance of sphingolipids in the brain partially explains the major neurodegenerative effect of disturbed sphingolipid breakdown. For most of the sphingolipidoses, new treatments have emerged, which provides hope for the future of patients, in particular for those with non-neurological disease, such as renal and cardiac disease in Fabry disease and hepatosplenomegaly with bone symptoms in Gaucher disease. Neurological disease has so far been very difficult to manage, although hematopoietic stem cell transplantation in metachromatic leukodystrophy and gene therapy approaches hold promise for the future as well.

C. Hollak (✉)
Division of Endocrinology and Metabolism, Department of Internal Medicine, F5-170, Academic Medical Center, University of Amsterdam, 22700, Amsterdam, The Netherlands
e-mail: c.e.hollak@amsterdamumc.nl

## Introduction

This chapter deals with lysosomal lipid storage disorders, in particular the sphingolipidoses, Niemann-Pick type C disease, and lysosomal acid lipase deficiency. The mucolipidoses




N. Blau et al. (eds.), *Physician's Guide to the Diagnosis, Treatment, and Follow-Up of Inherited Metabolic Diseases*,
https://doi.org/10.1007/978-3-030-67727-5_60

and the neuronal ceroid lipofuscinoses are described elsewhere (cross refs).

Sphingolipids are catabolized by hydrolases in lysosomes, followed by sequential removal of the degraded components. The various enzymes participating in this degradative pathway include galactosidases, hexosaminidases, neuraminidase (sialidase), glucosidases, sphingomyelinase (a phosphodiesterase), sulfatase, and ceramidase (an amidase). Specific activator proteins, saposins, or sphingolipid activator proteins (SAPs) are needed for sphingolipid degradation. These small, nonenzymatic glycoproteins bind the respective hydrolases and can support connection of lipids accessible to the hydrolases. Apart from deficient activities of lysosomal enzymes, defects in saposins can also give rise to sphingolipid storage disorders. Lysosomal cholesterol accumulation occurs as the main feature of lysosomal acid lipase deficiency and Niemann-Pick disease type C. Lysosomal acid lipase normally hydrolyzes cholesteryl esters and triglycerides to generate free fatty acids and cholesterol, while in Niemann-Pick disease type C, a defect in NPC1 or NPC2 proteins hampers transport of cholesterol out of the lysosomal/endosomal compartment, which in addition leads to secondary accumulation of sphingolipids.

Depending on the defect, different cells can be the target of lysosomal storage: macrophages are a frequent target, but neuronal cells, endothelial cells, cardiomyocytes, etc. can be affected. This results in a wide variety of symptoms: from neuronal damage to visceral enlargement or renal insufficiency. In addition, the type of mutation will lead to different residual enzyme activities, which importantly determines the age of onset of symptoms. However, genotype-phenotype relationships are generally poor especially for the late-onset disorders resulting in a wide variety of signs and symptoms, even within families. Clearly modifier genes or epigenetic or environmental factors influence the clinical manifestations in the majority of disorders. Many of these factors have so far not been identified, which may hamper family counseling and interpret results of screening. Treatment options have rapidly evolved over the last two decades, with more success to target visceral symptoms than neurological features. Intravenous enzyme replacement therapy is now available for several disorders, and oral substrate reduction therapy is authorized for Gaucher disease and under investigation for Fabry disease, while a first chaperone treatment is now available for the latter. In addition, hematopoietic stem cell transplantation has a place for metachromatic leukodystrophy, and several gene therapy options are currently explored. The different disorders, their characteristic features, guidelines for follow-up, and treatments are discussed separately below.

## Gangliosidoses: GM1, GM2 (Sandhoff and Tay-Sachs Diseases), and Galactosialidosis

### The Gangliosidoses

The general clinical hallmark of the gangliosidoses is neurodegeneration, due to accumulation of substrates in the central nervous system. GM1 gangliosidosis is caused by deficiency of β-galactosidase due to a mutation in *GLB1*. This gene is also mutated in Morquio type B, with a completely different phenotype, indicating different substrate binding sites, protein folding-relevant sites, or subdomains in the enzyme (Sandhoff and Harzer 2013). GM1 gangliosidosis encompasses a spectrum of clinical phenotypes, depending on the age of onset: a rapidly progressive infantile form (most common) with early developmental delay followed by severely progressive neurological disease with blindness, deafness, and death by 1–2 years of age. These children have visceral disease as well with hepatosplenomegaly, coarse features, and corneal clouding; the late infantile or juvenile form is characterized by a slower course with loss of developmental milestones; in adults a variant is described mainly with extrapyramidal manifestations (Brunetti-Pierri and Scaglia 2008). GM2 gangliosidosis is caused by deficiency of β-hexosaminidase or in very exceptional cases due to a defect in the GM2 activator protein. The enzyme has two isoforms, A and B: HEXA, encoded by *HEXA*, has α and β subunits, and isoenzyme HEXB consists of two β subunits encoded by *HEXB*. Tay-Sachs disease is caused by *HEXA* mutations, while Sandhoff disease is caused by HEXB mutations (Bley et al. 2011). Similar to GM1 disease, GM2 gangliosidosis has different phenotypes: infantile, juvenile, and adult forms. The infantile form is characterized by hyperacusis and visual impairment, developmental regression, and seizures. The juvenile form has a slower progressive course with psychomotor retardation. The adult form presents mostly with either cerebellar or anterior motor neuron involvement. Affected individuals may also develop psychotic episodes (Neudorfer et al. 2005).

Galactosialidosis clinically resembles GM1 gangliosidosis. In this disorder, a secondary deficiency of acid β-galactosidase is present, together with deficiency in sialidase and a specific sulfatase, all caused by mutations in *CTSA* encoding the protective protein/cathepsin A (PPCA). A defect in this protein hampers the stabilization of the enzymes, resulting in deficiency of their activities. For an appropriate diagnosis of GM1 gangliosidosis, a differentiation with galactosialidosis needs to be made on the basis of enzyme activities or molecular analysis.

## Krabbe Disease

Krabbe disease (globoid cell leukodystrophy) is a rare, autosomal recessively inherited sphingolipid storage disorder with a neurological phenotype. As a result of deficiency of galactocerebrosidase, galactolipids including galactocerebroside and psychosine (the lyso compound, i.e., galactosylsphingosine) accumulate in the brain. In particular galactosylsphingosine is toxic for oligodendrocytes and leads to severe white matter involvement of the peripheral and central nervous system. Mutations in the gene for the lysosomal enzyme galactocerebrosidase (GALC) result in different residual activity with accordingly variable clinical disease manifestations, although phenotype-genotype correlations are imperfect. The most severe cases of early infantile disease manifest with ataxia, spasticity, rapid psychomotor decline, and early death, usually before the age of 2 years. This form is associated in a high percentage of European and Mexican patients with one specific mutation (Rafi et al. 1995). Juvenile and adult patients have a more variable and attenuated course with differences in onset and progression of ataxia, spasticity, peripheral neuropathy, and sometimes loss of vision and dementia. Imaging of the brain may be normal for a long time in attenuated cases (Bajaj et al. 2002).

For counseling purposes and selection of infantile cases for hematopoietic stem cell transplantation, neonatal screening programs have been set up (Kwon et al. 2018).

## Metachromatic Leukodystrophy

Metachromatic leukodystrophy (MLD) is an autosomal recessive disease caused by mutations in the arylsulfatase A (ARSA) leading to a deficiency of the enzyme, which is involved in the breakdown of sulfatide. Accumulation of sulfatide and related compounds affects the central and peripheral nervous system, which leads to demyelination. MLD is clinically characterized by progressive neurological decay: based on the age of onset three sybtypes can roughly be distinguished (Gomez-Ospina [Internet], n.d.). A late infantile form manifests before the age of 2,5 years and has a rapidly progressive course with loss of motor function and early death. The juvenile form starts between 2,5 and 16 years and the adult form beyond 16 years of age. This group has variable progression of disease, with adults remaining mildly symptomatic for years. In the latter group, psychiatric symptoms may be a first manifestation of the disorder. In those less severe phenotypes, hematopoietic cell transplantation (HCT) can arrest progression of disease, especially when patients are pre-symptomatic or very early symptomatic. Characteristic white matter lesions on MRI may even improve after transplantation, although peripheral neuropathy will persist. Recently, visceral symptoms have been described as well, mainly in relation to the gastrointestinal tract, specifically the occurrence of gallbladder polyps (van Rappard et al. 2016a, b). Atypical presentations have been described in relation to saposin B deficiency with flaccid paralysis and gallbladder abnormalities as well (Madaan et al. 2019).

## Gaucher Disease, Saposin C Deficiency, and Limp2 Deficiency

The lysosomal enzyme β-glucocerebrosidase (β-GCase) is involved in the degradation of the natural glycosphingolipid glucocerebroside (or glucosylceramide; GC) into glucose and ceramide (Brady et al. 1966). Deficient activity of this enzyme causes Gaucher disease. The enzyme β-GCase is activated by saposin C, which is derived from proteolytic cleavage of prosaposin. Deficiency of saposin C results in a decrease in β-GCase and gives rise to a clinical variant of Gaucher disease with neuronopathic features (Christomanou et al. 1986). More recently, another disease subtype associated with deficiency of β-GCase in skin fibroblasts, but not in leukocytes, has been described. In this disorder, lysosomal integral membrane protein type 2 (LIMP-2) is deficient. This protein has been shown to be the mannose-6-phosphate-independent trafficking receptor for β-GCase (Reczek et al. 2007), which may result in tissue-dependent decreases in intralysosomal β-GCase activities (Berkovic et al. 2008; Balreira et al. 2008). Clinically this disorder was previously described as action myoclonus renal failure syndrome.

### Gaucher Disease

Gaucher disease has first been described by Philippe Gaucher in 1882 and is now recognized as one of the most prevalent lysosomal storage disorders. Its inheritance is autosomal recessive and the disease is panethnic, but there are some ethnic predilections. In Western countries, type I Gaucher disease or the non-neuronopathic variant is most common and has a high prevalence in the Ashkenazi Jewish population of 1 in 850 (Zimran and Elstein 2010). In general, the prevalence is believed to be around 1 in 75,000 (Meikle et al. 1999; Poorthuis et al. 1999), but it is likely that this is an underestimation since milder variants remain undiagnosed. The neuronopathic variants are extremely rare, with variable ethnic background, although clusters of these patients have been described in Norrbotten (Sweden), in Poland, and in the Jenin Arab population (Vellodi et al. 2009).

Type 1 Gaucher disease has a wide phenotypic variability. In general, the buildup of undegraded GC in macrophages results in hepatosplenomegaly, bone marrow involvement, cytopenia, and skeletal disease (Grabowski 2008). Most patients with this disorder present with unexplained thrombocytopenia and splenomegaly. More exceptionally, the first symptoms can be related to skeletal involvement, such as painful bone crises or avascular necrosis. Although the majority is diagnosed during adolescence/adulthood, severe manifestations may already be present during early childhood. Spleens can become massively enlarged, which necessitated splenectomy before enzyme replacement therapy was available (Beutler 1988). After splenectomy, these patients are vulnerable to septicaemia and progressive skeletal, liver, and pulmonary disease. Once extreme bone marrow infiltration has occurred, the risk for bone complications increases (Hollak et al. 2001). This can be shown by a reduction in fat signal in the bone marrow on MRI. Skeletal complications include avascular necrosis, specifically of the femoral head but also in other joints, pathological fractures, and bone crises. These crises resemble the acute bone pain seen in sickle cell disease and can only be managed by supportive measures such as morphinomimetics. Imaging of the skeleton shows characteristic, although not pathognomonic, features including osteopenia, sclerosis, Erlenmeyer flask deformities of the femurs, lytic lesions, and fractures (Maas et al. 2002). On MRI, decrease in fat signal and sometimes areas with high water signal can be seen. This last feature does not always indicate acute disease. Early AVN and infarcts can also be recognized on MRI. While severe, progressive disease in children and young adults has been described, on the other end of the clinical spectrum, a diagnosis of Gaucher disease can be made as a coincidental finding in an otherwise healthy person. The very mild patients have usually little disease progression (Beutler et al. 1995). Gaucher disease type 1 is also associated with other conditions, including a higher risk for malignancies, specifically multiple myeloma. As a large proportion (up to 20%) of adult Gaucher disease patients have a monoclonal protein, it is clear that there is an increased risk and patients should be monitored for this (De Fost et al. 2008). In addition, several cases of hepatocellular carcinoma have been reported, presumably associated with advanced liver involvement. Pulmonary hypertension and renal and cardiac involvement have all been reported. The increased risk for these conditions should be kept in mind during clinical follow-up. Individual factors that put patients at risk for these complications are currently under investigation. Another intriguing association is that of Parkinson's disease, not only in patients but also in carriers of a *GBA1* mutation: in fact, recent research indicates that *GBA1* mutations are the most common known genetic risk factor for Parkinson's disease and dementia with Lewy bodies. The clinical phenotype of carriers and patients with Gaucher disease and Parkinson's disease resembles sporadic Parkinson's disease, but with an earlier onset and more severe course (Ryan et al. 2019.)

Type 2 and 3 Gaucher disease are the neuronopathic Gaucher disease forms which are traditionally distinguished based upon the onset of neurological disease and the rate of deterioration. Type 2 patients always present with very early developmental delay and a rapidly fatal course. However, an early diagnosis can also be made in a type 3 patient, and considerable overlap of disease manifestations between type 2 and 3 disease exists. Therefore, neuropathic forms are increasingly regarded as a phenotypic continuum (Hruska et al. 2008). Since management decisions will be made primarily based upon the course of progression, Vellodi and coworkers have suggested using the terms "acute" and "chronic" (Vellodi et al. 2009) instead of type 2 and type 3. Acute neuropathic disease then refers to onset at <1 year of age with progressive neurological features including bulbar and pyramidal signs and cognitive impairment. Chronic neuropathic disease encompasses all patients with neurological disease manifestations in the context of Gaucher disease, who do not have the acute form (Vellodi et al. 2009). The chronic neuropathic disease group harbors several variants: the subtype living in Northern Sweden (Norrbotten) with relatively mild neurological features but extensive visceral disease is sometimes referred to as type 3a, to distinguish these from patients with more prominent neurological features, including myoclonic epilepsy (type 3b). Another atypical variant of chronic neuropathic disease is referred to as type 3c and has first been reported in a group of Jenin Arab patients (Abrahamov et al. 1995). Homozygosity for the D409H mutation in these patients is associated with valvular heart disease with cardiovascular calcifications in addition to oculomotor apraxia and mild visceromegaly.

#### Saposin C Deficiency or Prosaposin Deficiency

Patients with saposin C deficiency or prosaposin deficiency have been described with clinical features of neuronopathic Gaucher disease, including the characteristic horizontal ophthalmoplegia, epilepsy, and pyramidal and cerebellar signs (Pampols et al. 1999), but also non-neuronopathic variants with extensive visceral involvement have been described (Tylki-Szymanska et al. 2007). Diagnosis can be difficult as β-GCase activity is normal. The clinical presentation, presence of Gaucher cells, high levels of chitotriosidase, and storage of glucosylceramide will point to the direction of saposin C deficiency. Molecular analysis of *PSAP* can confirm the diagnosis. Treatment with substrate reduction therapy (miglustat, Zavesca ™) has been attempted but did not have any effect (Tylki-Szymańska et al. 2011).

#### LIMP2 Deficiency

Patients diagnosed with action myoclonus-renal failure syndrome have been identified as carrying a mutation in *SCARB2/LIMP2*. Several non-sense mutations in this gene have been shown to impair trafficking of β-GCase to the lysosome. Deficiency of active β-GCase that differs between tissues can hamper a diagnosis, as only fibroblasts and not leukocytes have low activity. Molecular analysis needs to be performed for a final diagnosis. The diversity in β-GCase deficiency throughout the body gives a totally different clinical picture, although some of the neurological features resemble those found in neuronopathic Gaucher disease. In addition to myoclonus epilepsy, demyelinating peripheral neuropathy, hearing loss, and dementia can occur in the presence or absence of renal failure (Dibbens et al. 2016). However, no visceromegaly is present, and no evidence of systemic storage of glucosylceramide is established in bone marrow and kidney biopsies, which is in agreement with the presence of normal chitotriosidase activities (Chaves et al. 2011).

### Combined Saposin Deficiency

Prosaposin (PSAP) deficiency is caused by mutations in *PSAP* that codes for the 65–70 kDa prosaposin protein, which is the precursor for four sphingolipid activator proteins, saposins A–D. This ultra-rare disorder can have features of severe Gaucher disease or metachromatic leukodystrophy and has a rapidly fatal course. Lysolipid analysis has revealed elevated levels of globotriaosylsphingosine (LysoGb3) and glucosylsphingosine (GlSph) in some cases (Motta et al. 2016).

## Fabry Disease

The enzyme $\alpha$-galactosidase A (aGalA) is deficient in Fabry disease, which results in storage of glycosphingolipids, mainly globotriaosylceramide (ceramide trihexoside, CTH, Gb3), in multiple cell types (Schiffmann 2015). Most involved are cells of the vascular system, including endothelial and smooth muscle cells. Storage can also be found in podocytes in the kidney, cardiomyocytes, sweat glands, and peripheral nerves. Fabry disease is X-linked, with severe manifestations in male patients without any residual aGalA activity. In carrier females and in non-classical male patients, the disease is much more variable. Variants in males have been described in which only the heart or kidney is involved. It is important to discriminate between classical and non-classical disease as well as in males and females, as for each of these subgroups, the natural disease course is different (Arends et al. 2017). In classically affected males, severe pain in hands and feet caused by acroparesthesia is one of the earliest symptoms starting in the first or second decade of life. Some children may have severe abdominal pain as well or unexplained periods of fever. Angiokeratoma may start to appear at the same age, located primarily in the genital area and around the umbilicus (Germain 2010). Gradually, further storage in the kidney, heart, and brain results in end-organ damage: proteinuria is one of the first signs of kidney involvement and is associated with further deterioration in both kidney and heart (Wanner et al. 2010). The heart may become extremely hypertrophic, with areas of fibrosis. Already at an early stage, most patients have bradycardia or other rhythm disturbances, and many need to receive a pacemaker or ICD later in life (Germain 2010). White matter lesions in the brain are believed to represent small vessel involvement, and there is an increased risk of stroke/TIA. Hearing loss, both acute and chronic, is probably also related to ischemia in the brain and has frequently been reported in Fabry disease. Classically affected males usually develop kidney disease, while this is more exceptional in non-classical males and classical females. In general, the life expectation of classically affected males is reduced with around 20 years (Schiffmann et al. 2009). In non-classical males and classical females, cardiac manifestations and brain white matter lesions are the most prominent features. These symptoms usually develop very gradually but may lead to a reduced life expectation of around 10 years (MacDermot et al. 2001), although there is probably some bias in studies reporting on this, since many asymptomatic females may remain undiagnosed or are not regularly followed in the clinic.

The disease is panethnic, with an estimated birth prevalence of classically affected patients of ~1:40,000 (Desnick 2003). However, awareness for the disease after the introduction of enzyme replacement therapy has resulted in the identification of large groups of individual carrying a *GLA*-mutation. For example, neonatal screening and screening in "high-risk" populations have shown an abundance of *GLA* variant of unknown significance (van der Tol et al. 2014; Spada et al. 2006; Hwu et al. 2009). To avoid anxiety and unnecessary treatment or inappropriate counseling, a diagnosis should only be made based on solid criteria, which may need additional testing, for example histology (Smid et al. 2014). The European Fabry Working Group recently launched an independent database which is freely accessible and provides guidance on genetics, biochemical parameters, and diagnostic criteria (http://www.fabrygenphen.com/).

## Farber Disease

Farber disease is an autosomal recessive disorder caused by mutations in the acid ceramidase gene (*ASAH1*) leading to a deficiency of the lysosomal enzyme acid ceramidase (AC). The disorder is extremely rare with less than 100 patients described in the world. Ceramide accumulation can be found in the central nervous system as well as in the skin, kidney, liver, and lungs, leading to a complex and often difficult-to-diagnose phenotype. Main clinical manifestations are neurological and rheumatological. A triad of subcutaneous nodules, joint swellings/arthritis, and a hoarse or weak voice impairment is suggestive of the disease, but this is not present in all cases (Levade et al. 2017).

Onset is usually in infancy with a progressive and lethal course. Most patients die during childhood, at a median age of 3 years (Zielonka M, Garbade SF, Kölker S, Hoffmann GF, Ries M. A cross-sectional quantitative analysis of the natural history of Farber disease: an ultra-orphan condition with rheumatologic and neurological cardinal disease features. Genet Med. 2018 Apr;20(5):524–530).

## Niemann-Pick Diseases

The Niemann-Pick disease group encompasses two distinct entities: acid sphingomyelinase-deficient Niemann-Pick disease (ASMD) resulting from mutations in *SMPD1* and Niemann-Pick disease type C (NP-C) including also type D, resulting from mutations in either *NPC1* or *NPC2* (Vanier 2013). These rare autosomal recessively inherited disorders have a wide spectrum of phenotypical manifestations with mainly neurovisceral characteristics.

Traditionally, ASMD has been classified as Niemann-Pick disease (NPD) types A (NPD A) and B (NPD B). NPD A has mainly neurological features starting in infancy followed by a rapidly progressive course, usually lethal before the age of 3 years. Patients with NPDB may have an intermediate phenotype (or variant NPDB) with both visceral and neurological symptoms starting and progressing during childhood. These patients frequently die early, usually from respiratory failure or liver failure. Older patients typically lack neurological symptoms and may have variable degrees of hepatosplenomegaly, thrombocytopenia, interstitial lung disease, and an abnormal, atherogenic, lipid profile. In these attenuated patients, the disease may remain stable during adult life (Hollak et al. 2012a, b). Studies are performed for a better understanding of symptom diversity and the natural history across the disease spectrum, which is needed to improve disease recognition, timely diagnosis, and appropriate disease management (McGovern et al. 2017).

NP-C usually presents with both visceral and neurological manifestations at a wide range of ages. Due to the variability in symptoms, which may be subtle and aspecific, a diagnosis of NP-C is often delayed. A neonatal form with severe jaundice and hepatosplenomegaly can be the first sign of the disease, but since this is often temporary and not immediately followed by systemic or neurological manifestations, the diagnosis may be missed. At a later age, subtle or more prominent hepatosplenomegaly can be present, but the neurological symptoms are more prominent and devastating, including vertical supranuclear gaze palsy, cerebellar ataxia, seizures, and progressive dementia.

## Lysosomal Acid Lipase Deficiency

Lysosomal acid lipase deficiency (LAL-D) is an extremely rare, autosomal recessive disorder caused by lysosomal acid lipase deficiency as a result of mutations in *LIPA*. LAL hydrolyzes cholesteryl esters and triglycerides to generate free fatty acids and cholesterol in lysosomes. As a consequence of the deficiency, storage of cholesteryl esters in macrophages and hepatocytes occurs, giving rise to hepatosplenomegaly and liver dysfunction. Residual enzyme activity determines the clinical severity: in Wolman's disease no residual activity is present leading to a severe disorder that presents during infancy with failure to thrive, diarrhea, malabsorption, hepatomegaly, and hepatic failure and involvement of the adrenal glands. These infants have a rapidly devastating course with death occurring in the first year of life. On the other end of the phenotypic spectrum is cholesteryl ester storage disease, ranging from early dyslipidemia, hepatomegaly, and cirrhosis to minimal symptoms without progression in adults (Pericleous et al. 2017).

While misdiagnosis as non-alcoholic fatty liver disease (NAFLD), non-alcoholic steatohepatitis (NASH), or other causes of dyslipidemia and cirrhosis may occur, recent screening studies have shown that the extreme rarity of LALD of around 1 in 175,000 does not justify screening in dyslipidemia cohorts or only as second tier in non-obese patients with fatty liver (Carter et al. 2019).

## Nomenclature

| No. | Disorder | Alternative name | Abbreviation | Gene symbol | Chromosomal localization | Affected protein | OMIM No. |
|---|---|---|---|---|---|---|---|
| 60.1 | GM1 gangliosidosis | Beta-galactosidase-1 deficiency | | *GLB1* | 3p22.3 | Beta-galactosidase | 230500 |
| 60.2 | Sandhoff disease | GM2 gangliosidosis O-variant | | *HEXB* | 5q13.3 | Beta-subunit of hexosaminidase | 268800 |
| 60.3 | Tay-Sachs disease | GM2 gangliosidosis B-variant | TSD | *HEXA* | 15q23 | Alpha-subunit of hexosaminidase | 272800 |
| 60.4 | GM2 gangliosidosis AB variant | GM2 activator deficiency | | *GM2A* | 5q33.1 | GM2 activator | 272750 |
| 60.5 | Galactosialidosis | Protective protein/cathepsin A deficiency | GSL | *CTSA* | 20q13.12 | Protective protein/cathepsin A | 256540 |
| 60.6 | Krabbe disease | Globoid cell leukodystrophy | GLD | *GALC* | 14q31.3 | Galactocerebrosidase | 245200 |
| 60.6 | Krabbe disease-like disorder due to saposin A deficiency | Saposin A deficiency | | *PSAP* | 10q22.1 | Saposin A | 611722 |
| 60.7 | Metachromatic leukodystrophy | Arylsulfatase A deficiency | MLD | *ARSA* | 22q13.33 | Arylsulfatase A | 250100 |
| 60.7 | Metachromatic leukodystrophy-like disorder due to saposin B deficiency | Saposin B deficiency | | *PSAP* | 10q22.1 | Saposin B, cerebroside sulfatase activator | 249900 |
| 60.8 | Gaucher disease | Glucocerebrosidase deficiency | | *GBA* | 1q22 | Glucocerebrosidase | 230800 |
| 60.9 | Gaucher disease-like disorder due to saposin C deficiency | Saposin C deficiency | | *PSAP* | 10q22.1 | Saposin C | 610539 |
| 60.10 | Action myoclonus-renal failure syndrome | Myoclonus-neuropathy syndrome progressive myoclonic epilepsy type 4 | AMRF, EPM4 | *SCARB2/ LIMP-2* | 4q21.1 | Scavenger receptor class B, member 2/ lysosomal integral membrane protein 2 | 254900 |
| 60.11 | Combined saposin deficiency | Prosaposin deficiency | PSAPD | *PSAP* | 10q22.1 | Saposins A–D | 611721 |
| 60.12 | Fabry disease | Alpha-galactosidase A deficiency | | *GLA* | Xq22.1 | Alpha-galactosidase | 301500 |
| 60.13 | Farber disease | Farber lipogranulomatosis | | *ASAH1* | 8p22 | Acid ceramidase | 228000 |
| 60.14 | Niemann-pick disease type A or B | Sphingomyelinase deficiency | NPD | *SMPD1* | 11p15.4 | Acid sphingomyelinase (ASM) | 257200 607616 |
| 60.15 | Niemann-pick disease type C1 | | NPC1 | *NPC1* | 18q11.2 | NPC1 protein | 257220 |
| 60.15 | Niemann-pick disease type C2 | | NPC2 | *NPC2* | 14q24.3 | NPC2 protein | 607625 |
| 60.16 | Lysosomal acid lipase deficiency | Wolman disease, cholesteryl ester storage disease | CESD | *LIPA* | 10q23.31 | Acid lipase | 278000 |

## Metabolic Pathway

Glycosphingolipids and sphingolipids are components of cell membranes. They are formed of ceramide, a molecule formed of sphingosine and long-chain fatty acids. After synthesis in the ER, glucose and carbohydrates are added to ceramide in a series of modification steps in the Golgi apparatus before the newly synthesized glycosphingolipids reach membrane compartments by vesicular membrane transport. Glycosphingolipids comprise gangliosides, and cerebrosides, named according to the composition of their sugar chain, and sulfatides in case of sulfation of cerebrosides. Sphingomyelin is a sphingolipid composed of ceramide and phosphocholine or phosphoethanolamine instead. The degradation of glycosphingolipids and sphingolipids is driven by a stepwise degradation through a series of specific hydrolases in the lysosome after their transport via the endosomal pathway. Hydrolase defects result in accumulation and lysosomal storage of substrates, thereby leading to cell pathology. Membrane-rich tissues or tissues with a high membrane turnover, e.g., myelin in the central and peripheral nervous system or cells of the reticuloendothelial system like macrophages with a high amount of glycosphingolipids and sphingolipids, are prone to an early cellular dysfunction in case of a hydrolase defect. This primarily affects the CNS, liver, and spleen to a variable extent in every disease due to the different content of defined glycosphingolipids and sphingolipids in cell membranes. A detailed pathway of the lysosomal degradation of sphingolipids is given in Fig. 60.1 (Schulze et al. 2009; Kolter and Sandhoff 2006; Kolter et al. 2002).

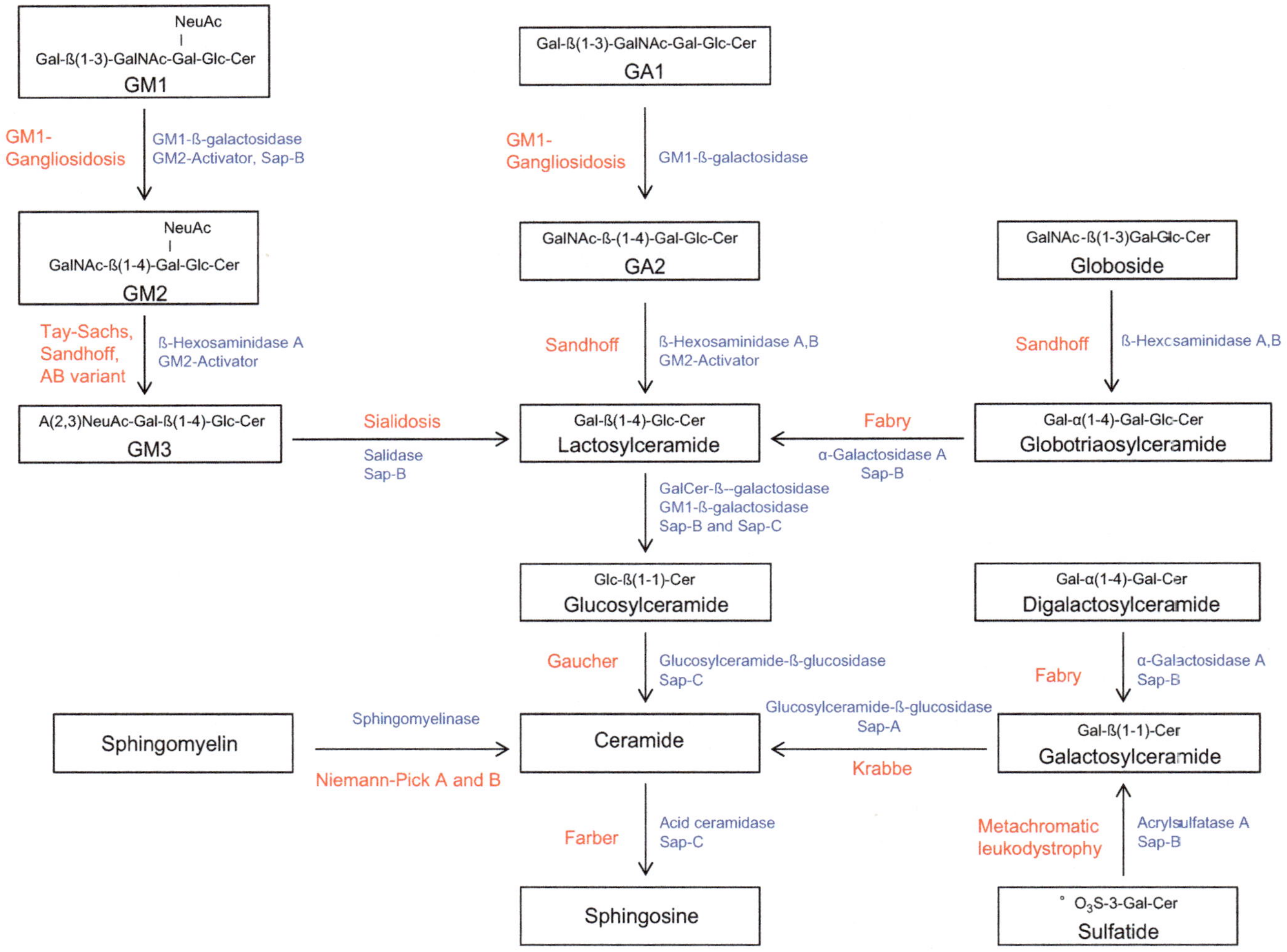


**Fig. 60.1** Degradation pathway of sphingolipids. The major metabolites are framed, the enzymes and activator proteins that catalyze the degradation step are colored *blue*, and the disorders resulting from the corresponding enzyme defect are highlighted in *red*

Single lysosomal hydrolase deficiencies comprise disorders like gangliosidosis, galactosialidosis, Krabbe disease, metachromatic leukodystrophy, Gaucher disease, Fabry disease, Farber disease, lysosomal acid lipase deficiency, and Niemann-Pick disease types A and B or acid sphingomyelinase deficiency (ASMD).

In gangliosidosis the deficiency of β-galactosidase leads to the disease pattern of GM1 gangliosidosis (Wenger et al. 1978; D'Azzo et al. 1982; Galjart et al. 1988), and the deficiency of hexosaminidase subunit alpha and beta as well as the deficiency of GM2 activator leads to the phenotype of Tay-Sachs disease (B variant), Sandhoff disease (0 variant), and AB variant of GM2 gangliosidosis (Adams and Green 1986; Beck et al. 1998; Hendriksz et al. 2004). Galactosialidosis is characterized by combined deficiency of β-galactosidase and neuraminidase (sialidase) activity due to a defect in the protective protein/cathepsin A (PPCA). PPCA stabilized and routed the β-galactosidase/neuraminidase complex on their way from endoplasmic reticulum to lysosome and protected them against rapid proteolysis (Abaroa et al. 2011). While β-galactosidase cleaves β-galactosyl residues from GM1-gangliosides, glycoproteins, and glycosaminoglycans, neuraminidase (sialidase) cleaves sialic acid mainly *N*-acetylneuraminic acid from glycoproteins. PPCA itself has a catalytic deaminase/esterase activity on neuropeptides, but this activity is presumably irrelevant for the pathophysiology of galactosialidosis disease.

In mammalian neuronal tissue, there are two isoenzymes of β-hexosaminidase, and each isoenzyme consists of two polypeptide chains. β-Hexosaminidase A is a heterodimer (α/β), whereas β-hexosaminidase B is a homodimer (β/β). Only the β-hexosaminidase A is able to cleave *N*-acetyl-d-glucosamine and *N*-acetyl-d-galactosamine from GM2 gangliosides in presence of GM2 activator, a substrate-specific cofactor. Due to this fact, there are three genes that can lead to impaired GM2 ganglioside hydrolysis: *HEXA* which encodes β-hexosaminidase A subunit-α, *HEXB* which encodes β-hexosaminidase A/B subunit-β, and *GM2A* which encodes the GM2 activator. Mutations of HEXA lead to impaired β-hexosaminidase A activity with normal β-hexosaminidase B activity in Tay-Sachs disease (B variant). Mutations of HEXB lead to impaired β-hexosaminidase A and B activity in Sandhoff disease (0 variant). And at last mutations in *GM2A* lead to failure of GM2 activator in GM2 gangliosidosis AB variant.

In Krabbe disease cerebroside beta-galactosidase catabolizes galactosylceramide to ceramide and galactosylsphingosine to sphingosine. The degradation step further requires the saposin A protein that presents the substrate to the enzyme. Mutations in *GALC* encoding cerebroside beta-galactosidase lead to impaired enzymatic function with storage of galactosylceramide in the pathognomonic "globoid cells," macrophages with storage material, in the CNS as well as toxic galactosylsphingosine in oligodendrocytes and Schwann cells (Wenger et al. 2000).

Arylsulfatase A (ASA) conducts the desulfation of 3-O-sulfogalactosyl-containing glycolipids. 3-O-sulfogalactosyl-containing glycolipids are mainly present in the myelin sheaths of central and peripheral nervous system. The desulfation requires the combined action of ASA and saposin B, a nonenzymatic protein, supposed to present the substrate to ASA, similar to the action of saposin A and cerebroside beta-galactosidase (see above). Deficiency of either ASA activity, which is much more common, or saposin B causes metachromatic leukodystrophy (Gieselmann and Krageloh-Mann 2010; Grossi et al. 2008).

Farber disease is a rare disorder due to the deficiency of the lysosomal hydrolase acid ceramidase with accumulation of undegraded ceramide. An accumulation of macrophages and histiocytes in different tissues as well as ceramide accumulation in brain cells defines the histopathology.

Wolman disease and the milder phenotype cholesteryl ester storage disease are due to the deficiency of lysosomal acid lipase, which is needed to cleave cholesteryl esters in various tissues. The deficiency results in a massive accumulation of cholesteryl esters and triglycerides in lysosomes of most body tissues (Scriver 2002).

Deficiency of lysosomal acid sphingomyelinase in Niemann-Pick type A and B that catalyzes the degradation of sphingomyelin to ceramide and phosphocholine results in the accumulation of sphingomyelin and other lipids in the monocyte-macrophage system. Residual enzymatic activity of sphingomyelinase is much more reduced in patients presenting with the severe form type A compared to milder activities in patients with type B, displaying a more attenuated course of disease.

Besides single lysosomal hydrolase deficiencies leading to glycosphingolipid and sphingolipid storage in lysosomes, the group of sphingolipidoses comprises diseases due to deficiencies of activator proteins, defects of posttranslational modification of lysosomal hydrolases, and lipid trafficking, primarily displaying the clinical picture of sphingolipidosis or in combination with clinical signs of mucopolysaccharidosis (Klima et al. 1993; Vielhaber et al. 1996; Dierks et al. 2009). For the function of different lysosomal hydrolases in the degradation of cerebrosides and gangliosides, the so-called saposins, a group of intralysosomal activator proteins, are a prerequisite. Defective saposin proteins lead to lysosomal hydrolase dysfunction and substrate accumulation resulting in a nearly identical clinical phenotype (Spiegel et al. 2005; Christomanou et al. 1986).

In case of mucolipidosis, a defect in the posttranslational glycosylation of lysosomal hydrolases results in a missorting of lysosomal hydrolases to the extracellular space (Tiede et al. 2005). This is further discussed in the chapter on mucopolysaccharidoses (cross ref).

Niemann-Pick type C (NPC) is caused by mutations in *NPC1* or *NPC2*. The disease is caused by a defect in the very complex coordinated action of *NPC1* or *NPC2* with regard to intralysosomal transport and efflux of cholesterol (Wheeler et al. 2019).

Combined saposin deficiency is characterized by the absence of all four types of saposin (saposins A–D) and already manifests in the newborn period with hypotonia, myoclonus, and hepatosplenomegaly. Patients usually develop generalized brain atrophy and epileptic seizures and die during infancy. As in the case of the isolated saposin deficiencies, the enzymatic activities of lysosomal enzymes (e.g., glycosylceramidase, galactosylceramidase, and ceramidase) may be normal in leukocytes but are reduced in cultured fibroblasts. In addition, increased urinary excretion of glycosphingolipids, such as globotriaosylceramide, is found. The diagnosis is confirmed by detection of (often truncating) mutations in *PSAP*.

## Signs and Symptoms

**Table 60.1** GM1-gangliosidosis

| System | Symptoms and biomarkers | Neonatal (birth–1 month) | Infancy (1–18 months) | Childhood (1.5–11 years) | Adolescence (11–16 years) | Adulthood (>16 years) |
|---|---|---|---|---|---|---|
| Cardiovascular | Cardiomyopathy | ± | ± | ± | | |
| CNS | Brain atrophy (MRI) | ++ | ++ | + | | |
| | Dystonia | ± | ± | ++ | ++ | ++ |
| | Gait disturbance | | | ± | ++ | ++ |
| | Hypotonia | +++ | +++ | + | | |
| | Intellectual disability | +++ | +++ | ++ | ± | ± |
| | Leukodystrophy (MRI) | ++ | ++ | + | + | + |
| | Seizures | ++ | ++ | ++ | | |
| | Spasticity | +++ | +++ | ++ | ± | ± |
| | Speech disturbances | | | ± | ++ | ++ |
| | Startle response, exaggerated | ++ | ++ | + | | |
| Digestive | Ascites, edema | ± | | | | |
| | Hepatosplenomegaly | ++ | ++ | ± | | |
| Eye | Cherry-red spot | ++ | ++ | ± | | |
| | Corneal clouding | + | + | ± | ± | ± |
| | Optic atrophy | ++ | ++ | ± | ± | ± |
| Hematological | Vacuolated lymphocytes | + | + | + | + | + |
| Musculoskeletal | Coarse facial features | ++ | ++ | + | | |
| | Dysostosis multiplex | ++ | ++ | ± | | |
| | Gingival hypertrophy, macroglossia | ++ | + | ± | | |
| Laboratory findings | LysoGM1 | ↑ | ↑ | n-↑ | | |
| | Molecular analysis | + | + | + | + | + |
| | Mucopolysaccharides (unsaturated keratan sulfate) | ↑ | ↑ | ↑ | | |
| | Oligosaccharides (U) | ↑↑↑ | ↑↑↑ | ↑↑ | ↑ | ↑ |

There is no involvement of peripheral nerve system.

**Table 60.2** Sandhoff disease

| System | Symptoms and biomarkers | Neonatal (birth–1 month) | Infancy (1–18 months) | Childhood (1.5–11 years) | Adolescence (11–16 years) | Adulthood (>16 years) |
|---|---|---|---|---|---|---|
| CNS | Ataxia | | ± | ± | ++ | ++ |
| | Brain atrophy (MRI) | | ++ | ++ | + | + |
| | Choreoathetosis | | | | ++ | ++ |
| | Dementia | | +++ | ++ | + | + |
| | Dystonia | | | | ++ | ++ |
| | Hypotonia | | +++ | ++ | + | + |
| | Leukodystrophy (MRI) | | ++ | ++ | ± | ± |
| | Mental deterioration | | +++ | ++ | ± | ± |
| | Seizures | | ± | ± | + | + |
| | Spasticity | | +++ | +++ | + | + |
| | Speech disturbances | | +++ | ++ | ++ | ++ |
| | Startle response, exaggerated | | +++ | ++ | + | + |
| | Visual evoked potential | | ↓↓↓ | ↓↓↓ | | |
| Digestive | Hepatosplenomegaly | | ± | ± | ± | ± |
| Eye | Cherry-red spot | | ++ | ++ | ± | ± |
| | Vision, impaired | | ++ | ++ | + | + |
| Genitourinary | Urinary incontinence | | ++ | ++ | + | + |
| Hematological | Vacuolated lymphocytes | | + | + | + | + |
| Musculoskeletal | Doll-like face | | ++ | ++ | | |
| | Macrocephaly | | | ++ | + | + |
| | Muscle weakness | | +++ | +++ | ++ | ++ |
| Laboratory findings | Beta-hexosaminidase activity A + B[a] | ↓↓↓ | ↓↓↓ | ↓↓↓ | ↓↓ | ↓ |
| | Beta-hexosaminidase activity A[a] | ↓↓↓ | ↓↓↓ | ↓↓↓ | ↓↓ | ↓ |
| | LysoGM2 | ↑ | ↑ | n-↑ | | |
| | Molecular analysis | + | + | + | + | + |
| | Oligosaccharides (U) | | ↑↑↑ | ↑↑↑ | ↑↑↑ | ↑↑↑ |

[a]Enzyme activity is measured with synthetic substrates without need of GM2-activator

**Table 60.3** Tay-Sachs disease

| System | Symptoms and biomarkers | Neonatal (birth–1 month) | Infancy (1–18 months) | Childhood (1.5–11 years) | Adolescence (11–16 years) | Adulthood (>16 years) |
|---|---|---|---|---|---|---|
| CNS | Ataxia | | ± | ± | ++ | ++ |
| | Dementia | | +++ | ++ | ± | ± |
| | Dystonia | | | | ++ | ++ |
| | Hypotonia | | +++ | ++ | ++ | ++ |
| | Megalencephaly | | ++ | + | | |
| | Mental deterioration | | +++ | ++ | ± | ± |
| | Psychiatric symptoms | | | +++ | ± | ± |
| | Psychosis | | | | ++ | ++ |
| | Seizures[a] | | ++ | ++ | ± | ± |
| | Spasticity | | +++ | +++ | + | + |
| | Speech disturbances | | +++ | ++ | ± | ± |
| | Startle response, exaggerated | | +++ | ++ | ± | ± |
| Digestive | Hepatosplenomegaly | | ± | ± | ± | ± |
| Eye | Cherry-red spot | | ++ | ++ | ± | ± |
| | Vision, impaired | | ++ | ++ | ± | ± |
| Genitourinary | Urinary incontinence | | ++ | ++ | | |
| Musculoskeletal | Macrocephaly | | | ++ | | |
| | Muscle weakness | | +++ | +++ | ++ | ++ |

(continued)

**Table 60.3** (continued)

| System | Symptoms and biomarkers | Neonatal (birth–1 month) | Infancy (1–18 months) | Childhood (1.5–11 years) | Adolescence (11–16 years) | Adulthood (>16 years) |
|---|---|---|---|---|---|---|
| Laboratory findings | Beta-hexosaminidase activity A + B[b] | n-↑ | n-↑ | n-↑ | n-↑ | n-↑ |
| | Beta-hexosaminidase activity A[b] | ↓↓↓ | ↓↓↓ | ↓↓↓ | ↓↓ | ↓↓ |
| | LysoGM2 | ↑ | ↑ | n-↑ | | |
| | Molecular analysis | + | + | + | + | + |
| | Oligosaccharides (U) | ↑↑ | ↑↑↑ | ↑↑↑ | ↑↑↑ | ↑↑↑ |

There is no neonatal form of Tay-Sachs disease
Chronic/adult form is clinical related to an atypical Friedreich's ataxia (spinoqcerebellar ataxia); juvenile form is clinical related to juvenile spinal muscular atrophy (Kugelberg-Welander syndrome)
[a]Seizures develop in infancy with disease duration time
[b]Enzyme activity is measured with synthetic substrates without need of GM2-activator

**Table 60.4** GM2-gangliosidosis AB variant

| System | Symptoms and biomarkers | Neonatal (birth–1 month) | Infancy (1–18 months) | Childhood (1.5–11 years) | Adolescence (11–16 years) | Adulthood (>16 years) |
|---|---|---|---|---|---|---|
| CNS | Megalencephaly | | ++ | + | | |
| | Mental deterioration | | +++ | ++ | | |
| | Muscular hypotonia | | ++ | ++ | | |
| | Psychiatric symptoms | | | +++ | | |
| | Spasticity | | ++ | ++ | | |
| | Speech disturbances | | +++ | ++ | | |
| | Startle response, exaggerated | | +++ | + | | |
| Eye | Cherry-red spot | | ++ | ++ | | |
| | Vision, impaired | | ++ | ++ | | |
| Genitourinary | Urinary incontinence | | ++ | ++ | | |
| Laboratory findings | Beta-hexosaminidase activity A | n-↑ | n-↑ | n-↑ | | |
| | Molecular analysis | + | + | + | | |
| | Oligosaccharides (U) | n-↑ | n-↑ | n-↑ | | |
| | Oligosaccharides (U) | ↑↑ | ↑↑↑ | ↑↑↑ | | |

All forms of GM2-gangliosidosis AB variant are infantile; no chronic forms described
There is no possibility to measure the functionality of GM2-activator, so in clinical suspicion of GM2-gangliosidosis with normal activity of β-hexosaminidases, Molecular analysis of GM2A should be done

**Table 60.5** Galactosialidosis

| System | Symptoms and biomarkers | Neonatal (birth–1 month) | Infancy (1–18 months) | Childhood (1.5–11 years) | Adolescence (11–16 years) | Adulthood (>16 years) |
|---|---|---|---|---|---|---|
| Cardiovascular | Cardiomyopathy | +++ | ± | + | + | + |
| | Valvular thickening | ± | +++ | | | |
| CNS | Ataxia | | | + | ++ | ++ |
| | Intellectual disability | +++ | ± | + | + | + |
| | Myoclonus | | | ++ | ++ | ++ |
| | Seizures | ± | ± | + | + | + |
| | Spasticity | | | + | + | + |
| Dermatological | Angiokeratoma | ± | ± | + | ++ | ++ |
| | Telangiectasia | +++ | ± | ± | ± | ± |
| Digestive | Hepatosplenomegaly | +++ | +++ | ++ | | |
| Eye | Cherry-red spot | + | + | +++ | ++ | ++ |
| | Corneal clouding | + | + | + | + | + |
| | Vision, impaired | ± | ± | +++ | +++ | +++ |
| Hematological | Foam cells | +++ | +++ | +++ | +++ | +++ |
| | Vacuolated lymphocytes | +++ | +++ | +++ | +++ | +++ |

**Table 60.5** (continued)

| System | Symptoms and biomarkers | Neonatal (birth–1 month) | Infancy (1–18 months) | Childhood (1.5–11 years) | Adolescence (11–16 years) | Adulthood (>16 years) |
|---|---|---|---|---|---|---|
| Musculoskeletal | Coarse facial features | + | + | + | + | + |
| | Dysostosis multiplex | ++ | +++ | +++ | + | + |
| | Edema | ++ | | | | |
| | Growth retardation | + | +++ | ++ | ++ | ++ |
| | Hernias | + | | | | |
| Renal | Renal failure, proteinuria | +++ | ++ | | | |
| Other | **Fetal hydrops** | ++ | | | | |
| Laboratory findings | Alpha-neuraminidase activity | ↓↓↓ | ↓↓↓ | ↓↓ | ↓ | ↓ |
| | Beta-galactosidase activity | ↓↓↓ | ↓↓↓ | ↓↓ | ↓ | ↓ |
| | Cathepsin A—activity[a] | ↓-n | ↓-n | ↓-n | ↓-n | ↓-n |
| | Molecular analysis | + | + | + | + | + |
| | Sialic acid-rich oligosaccharides (U)[b] | ↑↑↑ | ↑↑↑ | ↑↑↑ | ↑↑ | ↑↑ |

[a]Catalytic activity of PPCA is an indication for galactosialidosis but is not needed for diagnosis of galactosialidosis, because not all mutations that avoid the interaction of the multienzyme complex lead to poor or absent catalytic activity of PPCA
[b]Atypical forms with absence of sialyloligosacchariduria are described (Darin et al. 2009)

**Table 60.6** Krabbe disease and Krabbe disease-like disorder due to saposin A deficiency

| System | Symptoms and biomarkers | Neonatal (birth–1 month) | Infancy (1–18 months) | Childhood (1.5–11 years) | Adolescence (11–16 years) | Adulthood (>16 years) |
|---|---|---|---|---|---|---|
| CNS | Ataxia | | | | ++ | ++ |
| | Irritability | | +++ | ++ | | |
| | **Leukodystrophy** | | +++ | +++ | ++ | ++ |
| | Nerve conductive velocity | | ↓↓↓ | ↓↓↓ | ↓ | ↓-n |
| | Neurological deterioration | | +++ | +++ | | |
| | Neuropathy | | +++ | +++ | | |
| | Seizures | | +++ | +++ | | |
| | Spasticity | | +++ | +++ | | |
| Digestive | Feeding difficulties | | +++ | +++ | | |
| Ear | Deafness | | ++ | | | |
| Eye | Blindness | | +++ | +++ | | |
| Other | Fever | | +++ | +++ | | |
| Laboratory findings | Lysogalactosylceramide[a] | ↑ | ↑ | ↑ | ↑ | ↑ |
| | Protein (CSF) | | ↑↑↑ | (↑) | (↑) | (↑) |

[a]Lysoglucosylceramide (glucosylsphingosine) are measured as lysohexosylceramide

**Table 60.7** Metachromatic leukodystrophy and Metachromatic leukodystrophy-like disorder due to saposin B deficiency

| System | Symptoms and biomarkers | Neonatal (birth–1 month) | Infancy (1–18 months) | Childhood (1.5–11 years) | Adolescence (11–16 years) | Adulthood (>16 years) |
|---|---|---|---|---|---|---|
| CNS | Ataxia | | | +++ | ++ | ++ |
| | Dysarthria | | | +++ | ++ | ++ |
| | Emotion ability | | | + | ++ | +++ |
| | Gait disturbance | | | | ++ | ++ |
| | Irritability | | +++ | ++ | | |
| | Leukodystrophy | | +++ | +++ | ++ | ++ |
| | Nerve conductive velocity | | ↓↓↓ | ↓↓↓ | ↓↓↓ | ↓↓↓ |
| | Neurological deterioration | | +++ | +++ | | |
| | Neuropathy | | +++ | +++ | | |
| | Psychosis | | – | – | + | +++ |
| | Seizures | | +++ | +++ | ± | ± |
| | Spasticity | | +++ | +++ | ± | ± |
| Musculoskeletal | Muscle weakness | | +++ | +++ | | |
| Laboratory findings | Protein (CSF) | | ↑↑↑ | ↑↑↑ | ↑↑↑ | n |
| | Sulfatide (U) | | ↑↑↑ | ↑↑↑ | ↑↑↑ | ↑↑↑ |

(continued)

**Table 60.8** Gaucher disease

| System | Symptoms and biomarkers | Neonatal (birth–1 month) | Infancy (1–18 months) | Childhood (1.5–11 years) | Adolescence (11–16 years) | Adulthood (>16 years) |
|---|---|---|---|---|---|---|
| CNS | Developmental delay | | +++ | ++ | ± | |
| | Seizures | | +++ | ++ | ± | |
| Dermatological | Collodion skin, collodion baby | +++ | | | | |
| Digestive | Hepatosplenomegaly | ++ | +++ | +++ | +++ | +++ |
| | Liver cirrhosis | | | | | ± |
| Eye | Eye movements, abnormal | | +++ | ++ | ± | |
| Hematological | Anemia | | + | +++ | ++ | + |
| | Foam cells | ++ | +++ | +++ | +++ | +++ |
| | Pancytopenia | | + | + | + | + |
| | Thrombocytopenia | | + | +++ | +++ | ++ |
| Musculoskeletal | Bone pain | | | + | +++ | ++ |
| | Kyphosis | | | ± | ++ | ± |
| | Osteoporosis | | | ± | ++ | + |
| | Pathological fractures | | | ± | + | ++ |
| Respiratory | Restrictive lung disease | | ++ | ++ | + | ± |
| Other | Early death | +++ | +++ | ± | | |
| Laboratory findings | Beta-d-glucosidase | ↓↓↓ | ↓↓ | ↓↓ | ↓↓ | ↓↓ |
| | Chitotriosidase | ↑↑ | ↑↑ | ↑↑↑ | ↑↑↑ | ↑↑ |
| | Glucosylsphingosine[a] | ↑↑ | ↑↑ | ↑↑↑ | ↑↑↑ | ↑↑ |

[a]Lysogalactosylceramide and lysoglucosylceramide (glucosylsphingosine) are measured as lysohexosylceramide

**Table 60.9** Gaucher disease-like disorder due to saposin C deficiency

| System | Symptoms and biomarkers | Neonatal (birth–1 month) | Infancy (1–18 months) | Childhood (1.5–11 years) | Adolescence (11–16 years) | Adulthood (>16 years) |
|---|---|---|---|---|---|---|
| CNS | Developmental delay | | ++ | ++ | ± | |
| | Seizures, myoclonic | | ++ | ++ | ± | |
| Digestive | Hepatosplenomegaly | | | ++ | +++ | +++ |
| Eye | Eye movements, abnormal | | +++ | ++ | ± | |
| Hematological | Anemia | | + | ++ | ++ | +++ |
| | Foam cells | ++ | +++ | +++ | +++ | +++ |
| | Thrombocytopenia | | + | ++ | +++ | +++ |
| Musculoskeletal | Bone pain | | | ± | + | ++ |
| | Pathological fractures | | | ± | + | ++ |
| Special laboratory | Beta-δ-glucosidase | n | n | n | n | n |
| | Chitotriosidase | ↑↑ | ↑↑ | ↑↑↑ | ↑↑↑ | ↑↑↑ |
| | Glucosylsphingosine[a] | ↑↑ | ↑↑ | ↑↑↑ | ↑↑↑ | ↑↑ |

[a]Lysogalactosylceramide and lysoglucosylceramide (glucosylsphingosine) are measured as lysohexosylceramide

**Table 60.10** Action myoclonus-renal failure syndrome

| System | Symptoms and biomarkers | Neonatal (birth–1 month) | Infancy (1–18 months) | Childhood (1.5–11 years) | Adolescence (11–16 years) | Adulthood (>16 years) |
|---|---|---|---|---|---|---|
| CNS | Dementia | | | | ± | ++ |
| | Polyneuropathy | | | + | ++ | +++ |
| | Seizures, myoclonic | | | + | ++ | +++ |
| Heart | Dilated cardiomyopathy | | | | ± | ± |
| Renal | Renal failure | | | + | ++ | +++ |
| Laboratory findings | Beta-δ-glucosidase | | | n in leukocytes, decreased in fibroblasts | n in leukocytes, decreased in fibroblasts | n in leukocytes, decreased in fibroblasts |

**Table 60.11** Combined saposin deficiency

| System | Symptoms and biomarkers | Neonatal (birth–1 month) | Infancy (1–18 months) | Childhood (1.5–11 years) | Adolescence (11–16 years) | Adulthood (>16 years) |
|---|---|---|---|---|---|---|
| CNS | Cerebral and cerebellar atrophy | + | +++ | | | |
| | Developmental delay | ++ | +++ | | | |
| | Hyperkinesia | ++ | +++ | | | |
| | Hypotonia | ± | ++ | | | |
| | Myoclonus | ++ | +++ | | | |
| | Seizures, myoclonic | + | ++ | | | |
| Digestive | Hepatosplenomegaly | ++ | +++ | | | |
| Hematological | Foam cells | ++ | +++ | | | |
| Laboratory findings | Ceramidase (fibroblasts) | ↓↓ | ↓↓↓ | | | |
| | Chitotriosidase—Glucosylsphingosine | ↑↑ | ↑↑ | | | |
| | Galactosylceramidase (fibroblasts) | ↓↓ | ↓↓ | | | |
| | Glycosylceramidase (fibroblasts) | ↓↓ | ↓↓↓ | | | |

**Table 60.12** Fabry disease

| System | Symptoms and biomarkers | Neonatal (birth–1 month) | Infancy (1–18 months) | Childhood (1.5–11 years) | Adolescence (11–16 years) | Adulthood (>16 years) |
|---|---|---|---|---|---|---|
| Cardiovascular | Cardiomyopathy, hypertrophic | | | | | ++ |
| CNS | Cerebral infarction/stroke-like encephalopathy | | | | ± | ++ |
| | Neuropathic pain | | | ± | ++ | + |
| Dermatological | Angiokeratoma | | | ± | ++ | ++ |
| Digestive | Abdominal pain | | | + | + | + |
| Ear | Hearing loss, sensorineural | | | | ± | + |
| Eye | Cornea verticillata | | | + | + | + |
| Renal | Proteinuria | | | ± | ± | ++ |
| | Renal failure, chronic | | | | | ++ |
| Laboratory findings | Globotriaosylceramide | (↑) | ↑ | ↑ | ↑ | ↑ |
| | Globotriaosylsphingosine | ↑ | ↑ | ↑↑ | ↑↑ | ↑↑ |

**Table 60.13** Farber disease

| System | Symptoms and biomarkers | Neonatal (birth–1 month) | Infancy (1–18 months) | Childhood (1.5–11 years) | Adolescence (11–16 years) | Adulthood (>16 years) |
|---|---|---|---|---|---|---|
| CNS | Deep tendon reflexes | | ↓↓ | ↓ | | |
| | Developmental delay | | ++ | ± | | |
| | Hypotonia | ± | ++ | | | |
| | Intellectual diasability | | ++ | ± | | |
| | Seizures | | ++ | + | | |
| Dermatological | Subcutaneous nodules | +++ | +++ | +++ | | |
| Digestive | Hepatosplenomegaly | ++ | + | + | | |
| Eye | Cherry-red spot | | + | | | |
| Hematological | Foam cells | ± | ± | ± | | |
| | Lymphadenopathy | | + | | | |
| Musculoskeletal | Arthritis | +++ | +++ | +++ | | |
| Respiratory | Hoarseness | +++ | +++ | +++ | | |
| | Lung infiltrates | | ++ | + | | |
| Other | Failure to thrive | | ++ | | | |
| Laboratory findings | Acid ceramidase activity (LC) | ↓↓↓ | ↓↓↓ | ↓↓↓ | | |
| | C26-ceramide | ↑ | ↑ | ↑ | ↑ | ↑ |
| | Protein (CSF) | | n-↑ | n-↑ | | |

**Table 60.14** Niemann-Pick disease type A or B

| System | Symptoms and biomarkers | Neonatal (birth–1 month) | Infancy (1–18 months) | Childhood (1.5–11 years) | Adolescence (11–16 years) | Adulthood (>16 years) |
|---|---|---|---|---|---|---|
| CNS | Developmental delay | +++ | | | | |
| | Hypotonia | +++ | | | | |
| | Seizures | ± | | | | |
| Digestive | Feeding difficulties | +++ | | | | |
| | Hepatosplenomegaly | +++ | +++ | +++ | +++ | +++ |
| | Jaundice | ↑↑ | | | | |
| | Liver cirrhosis | | +++ | +++ | +++ | +++ |
| Ear | Deafness | +++ | | | | |
| Eye | Cherry-red spot | +++ | ± | ± | ± | ± |
| | Vision loss | +++ | | | | |
| Hematological | Foam cells | +++ | +++ | +++ | +++ | +++ |
| | Lymphadenopathy | +++ | | | | |
| | Pancytopenia | | + | + | + | + |
| | **Thrombocytopenia** | +++ | | | | |
| Respiratory | Hypoxia | | +++ | +++ | +++ | +++ |
| | Pulmonary interstitial changes | | +++ | +++ | +++ | +++ |
| Other | Failure to thrive | +++ | | | | |
| Laboratory findings | Lysosphingomyelin | ↑ | ↑ | ↑↑ | ↑↑ | ↑↑ |
| | Sphingomyelinase | ↓↓↓ | ↓↓ | ↓↓ | ↓↓ | ↓↓ |

**Table 60.15** Niemann-Pick disease type C1 and Niemann-Pick disease type C2

| System | Symptoms and biomarkers | Neonatal (birth–1 month) | Infancy (1–18 months) | Childhood (1.5–11 years) | Adolescence (11–16 years) | Adulthood (>16 years) |
|---|---|---|---|---|---|---|
| CNS | Action dystonia | | + | + | + | |
| | Ataxia | | | +++ | +++ | ± |
| | Behavioral disorder | | | | + | + |
| | Clumsiness | | +++ | +++ | +++ | |
| | Cognitive dysfunction | | +++ | +++ | | |
| | Dysarthria | | + | + | + | ± |
| | Dystonia | | + | + | + | ± |
| | Gait disturbance | | +++ | +++ | | |
| | Gelastic cataplexy | | + | + | + | |
| | Language difficulties | | +++ | +++ | | |
| | Psychosis | | | | + | + |
| | School problems (difficulties in writing, attention) | | +++ | +++ | | |
| | Seizures | | ± | ± | ± | |
| | Vertical gaze palsy | | + | + | + | |
| Digestive | Hepatosplenomegaly | +++ | +++ | ± | ± | |
| | Jaundice, cholestatic | +++ | | | | |
| Hematological | Foam cells | + | + | + | + | + |
| Laboratory findings | Blue histiocytes | + | + | + | + | + |
| | Chitotriosidase | ↑↑↑ | ↑↑↑ | ↑↑↑ | ↑↑↑ | ↑↑↑ |
| | Filipin test | ↓↓↓ | ↓↓↓ | ↓↓↓ | ↓↓↓ | ↓↓↓ |
| | Oxysteroles, LysoSM-509/LysoSM Chitotriosidase | ↑ | ↑ | ↑↑ | ↑↑ | ↑↑ |

**Table 60.16** Lysosomal acid lipase deficiency

| System | Symptoms and biomarkers | Neonatal (birth–1 month) | Infancy (1–18 months) | Childhood (1.5–11 years) | Adolescence (11–16 years) | Adulthood (>16 years) |
|---|---|---|---|---|---|---|
| Cardiovascular | Atherosclerosis, severe | | | + | ++ | +++ |
| CNS | Developmental delay | + | + | | | |
| Digestive | Abdominal distension | + | + | | | |
| | Failure to thrive | ++ | ++ | | | |
| | Hepatosplenomegaly | +++ | +++ | + | + | + |
| | Steatorrhea | + | + | | | |
| | Vomiting | + | + | | | |
| Endocrine | Adrenal calcification | + | + | | | |
| Routine laboratory | Cholesterol (S) | n-↑ | n-↑ | n-↑ | n-↑ | n-↑ |
| | Triglycerides (S) | n-↑ | n-↑ | n-↑ | n-↑ | n-↑ |
| Special laboratory | Acid lipase activity | ↓↓↓ | ↓↓↓ | ↓ | ↓ | ↓ |
| | Molecular analysis | + | + | + | + | + |

## Reference Values

Reference values for fluorometric enzyme assays given as ratio enzyme/beta-galactosidase activity (normal ranges depend on assays and detection devices)

| No. | Disorder | Enzyme | Enzyme/beta-galactosidase (%) | Material |
|---|---|---|---|---|
| 60.1 | GM1 gangliosidosis | Beta-galactosidase | 54–146 | Leukocytes |
| 60.2 | Sandhoff disease | Beta-hexosaminidase A + B | 284–1345 | Leukocytes |
| 60.3 | Tay-Sachs disease | Beta-hexosaminidase A | 46–171 | Leukocytes |
| 60.6 | Krabbe disease | Galactocerebrosidase | 0.2–3.2 | Leukocytes |
| 60.8 | Gaucher disease | Beta-d-glucosidase | 2,2–22 | Leukocytes |
| 60.12 | Fabry disease | Alpha-galactosidase[a] | 5,9–59 | Leukocytes |
| 60.14 | Niemann-Pick disease type A or B | Sphingomyelinase | 0.2–0.8 | Leukocytes |

[a]In females activities can be decreased or normal; family, clinical, biochemical, and genetic and sometimes histological studies are needed for confirmation

Reference values for spectrophotometric enzyme assays given as ratio enzyme/beta-hexosaminidase activity (normal ranges depend on assays and detection devices)

| No. | Disorder | Enzyme | Enzyme/beta-hexosaminidase (%) | Material |
|---|---|---|---|---|
| 60.1 | GM1 gangliosidosis | Beta-galactosidase | 6.6–33 | Leukocytes |
| 60.2 | Sandhoff disease | Beta-hexosaminidase A + B | 53–147 | Leukocytes |
| 60.7 | Metachromatic leukodystrophy | Arylsulfatase A | 1.7–8.5 | Leukocytes |

## Laboratory Investigations

Specific laboratory investigations for the diagnostic work-up of sphingolipidoses

| No. | Disorder | Metabolite analysis diagnostic feature | Enzyme assay | Molecular analysis | Prenatal diagnosis |
|---|---|---|---|---|---|
| 60.1 | GM1 gangliosidosis | LysoGM1 (S); GAGs (U); oligosaccharides (U) | L, FB | L, FB | A, CV |
| 60.2 | Sandhoff disease | LysoGM2 (S); oligosaccharides (U) | L, S, FB | L, FB | A, CV |
| 60.3 | Tay-Sachs disease | LysoGM2 (S); oligosaccharides (U) | L, S, FB | L, FB | A, CV |
| 60.4 | GM2 gangliosidosis AB variant | lysoGM2 (S); oligosaccharides (U) | – | L, FB | A, CV |
| 60.5 | Galactosialidosis | Oligosaccharides (U), vacuolated lymphos | FB | L, FB | A, CV, oligo[a] |
| 60.6 | Krabbe disease | Lysogalactosylceramide[b] | L, FB | L, FB | A, CV |
| 60.6 | Krabbe disease-like disorder due to saposin A deficiency | Low galactocerebrosidase activity in L | L | L, FB | A, CV |
| 60.7 | Metachromatic leukodystrophy | Sulfatides (U) | L, FB | L, FB | A, CV |
| 60.7 | Metachromatic leukodystrophy-like disorder due to saposin B deficiency | Sulfatides (U) | – | L, FB | A, CV |
| 60.8 | Gaucher disease | Glucosylsphingosine[b], chitotriosidase (S) | L, FB | L, FB | A, CV |
| 60.9 | Gaucher disease-like disorder due to saposin C deficiency | Chitotriosidase (S) | – | L, FB | A, CV |
| 60.10 | Action myoclonus-renal failure syndrome | – | L, FB | L, FB | A, CV |
| 60.11 | Combined saposin deficiency | – | L, FB | L, FB | A, CV |
| 60.12 | Fabry disease | Globotriaosylsphingosine (lysoGb3) | L, S FB | L, FB | A, CV |
| 60.13 | Farber disease | C26-ceramide | FB | L, FB | A, CV |
| 60.14 | Niemann-Pick disease types A or B | Lysosphingomyelin (lysoSM) | L, FB | L, FB | A, CV |
| 60.15 | Niemann-Pick disease type C1 | Oxysteroles, LysoSM-509/LysoSM Chitotriosidase (S), vacuolated lymphos | – | L, FB | A, CV |
| 60.15 | Niemann-Pick disease type C2 | Oxysteroles, LysoSM-509/LysoSM Chitotriosidase (S), vacuolated lymphos | – | L, FB | A, CV |
| 60.16 | Lysosomal acid lipase deficiency | High LDL cholesterol, low HDL cholesterol; vacuolated lymphos | L | L, FB | A, CV |

*GAGs* Glycosaminoglycans, *L* Leukocytes, *S* Serum/plasma, *FB* Fibroblasts, *A* Amniotic fluid cells, *CV* Chorionic villi, *EM* Electron microscopy, *lymphos* lymphocytes

[a]Sialyloligosaccharides in amniotic fluid supernatant

[b]Lysogalactosylceramide and lysoglucosylceramide (glucosylsphingosine) are measured as lysohexosylceramide

## Diagnosis and Reference Values

The diagnostic work-up of the sphingolipidoses should begin with the clinical assessment of the patients and should consider the general classification. The characteristic combination of symptoms determines the further diagnostic investigations as outlined in the diagnostic flowcharts (see Fig. 60.2). Depending on the disorder and signs as shown in the tables, these may comprise full blood count and smear, fundoscopy, cardiac assessment (ECG/ECHO), skeletal status (X-ray), cranial MRI, and electrophysiology (VEP, SEP, ERG).

Specific tests for sphingolipidoses, LAL deficiency, and NPC should be performed in specialized laboratories. Diagnostic procedures include specific enzyme assays of lysosomal hydrolases in plasma, leukocytes, or fibroblasts as well as quantitative analysis of metabolites, mostly in plasma, serum, urine, or CSF. In case the disorder is not associated with an enzyme deficiency or in order to confirm the diagnosis, DNA mutational analysis in the affected gene should be performed. DNA testing is also important in cases where enzymatic diagnosis is already made for counseling purposes, which may include prediction of phenotypes. For further details on specific investigations, see Table 'Specific laboratory investigations for the diagnostic work-up of sphingolipidoses'. For reference values see corresponding lysosomal Tables.

## Diagnostic Flowchart

Figure 60.2 shows a diagnostic follow-up of patients presenting with visceral symptoms, mainly hepatosplenomegaly, and with or without neurological presentation. In the case of a multisystem disease with one or more of the specific symptoms in the figure, a further work-up can be performed with screening panels followed by specific enzyme and molecular analysis.

## Pathological Values

Specific laboratory investigations for the diagnostic work-up of sphingolipidoses are given below. Of note, dried blood spots (DBS) are increasingly used for screening purposes. However, enzyme assays based upon DBS alone are not always reliable and should be confirmed with other specific tests including enzyme analysis in plasma, leukocytes, or fibroblasts and molecular analysis. Studies have shown that many of the biomarkers can also be determined from blood spots. Again, confirmation by state-of-the-art enzymatic and genetic studies is always necessary to avoid misdiagnosis resulting in erroneous treatment and counseling decisions.

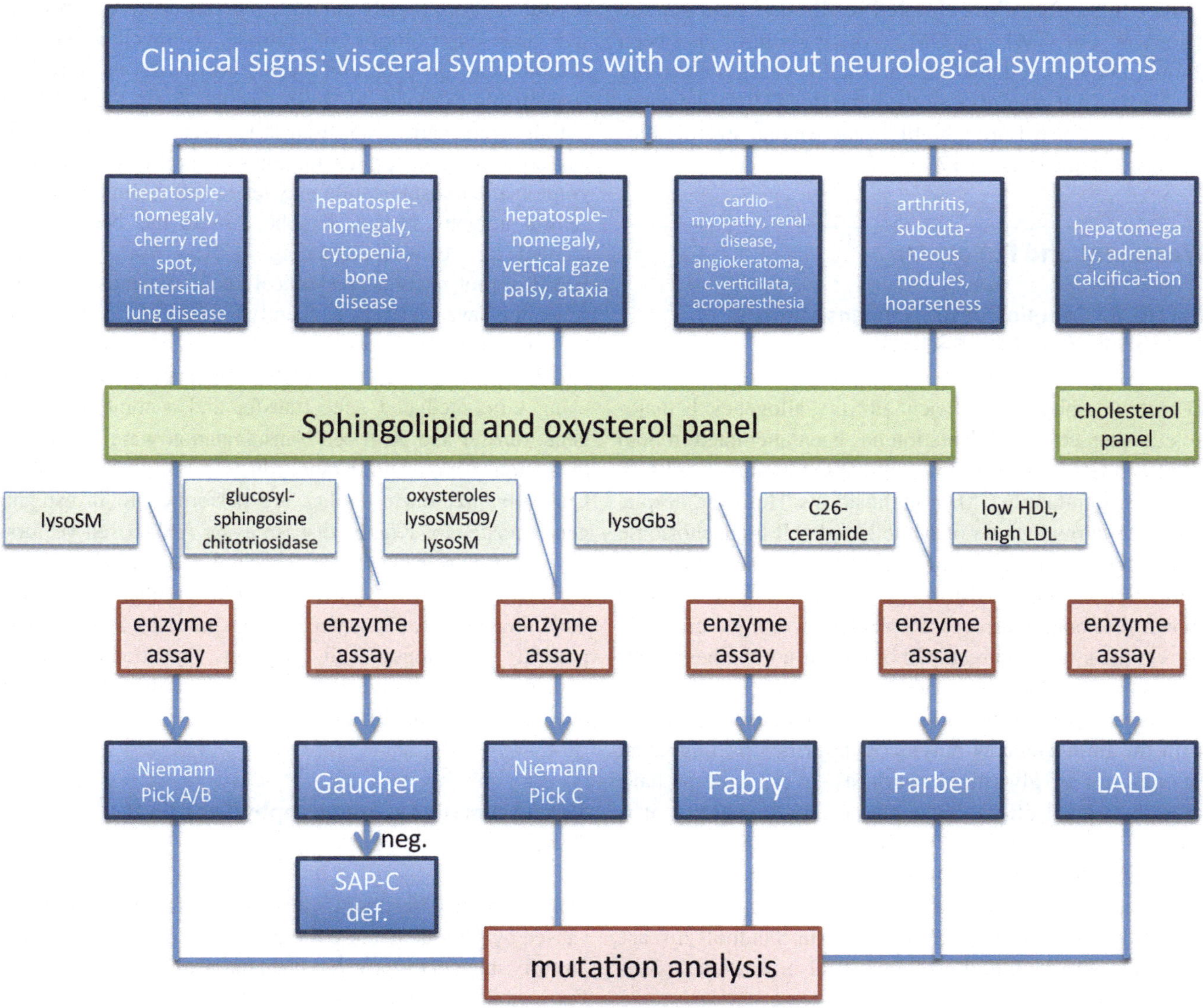


**Fig. 60.2** Diagnostic follow-up based upon presenting symptoms

A screening panel consisting of the lysosphingolipids lysoglobotriaosylceramide (LysoGb3), lysohexosylceramide (LysoHexCer: both lysoglucosylceramide and lysogalactosylceramide), lysosphingomyelin (LysoSM), and its carboxylated analogue lysosphingomyelin-509 (LysoSM-509) and oxysterols cholestane-3β,5α,6β-triol and 7-ketocholesterol by UPLC-MS/MS and chitotriosidase activity can be used for a rapid screening to identify lipid storage disorders (Voorink-Moret et al. 2018). Specific elevations, i.e., without overlap between controls and other lipid storage disorders, can be used: LysoSM levels in acid sphingomyelinase deficiency (Niemann-Pick disease type A/B), LysoGb3 levels in males with classical phenotype Fabry disease, and LysoHexCer (i.e., lysoglucosylceramide/lysogalactosylceramide) in Gaucher and Krabbe diseases. In Niemann-Pick diseases, oxysterols were elevated, but LysoSM-509/LysoSM ratio was specifically abnormal in Niemann-Pick disease type C. In Gaucher disease type I, chitotriosidase was grossly elevated while only mildly elevated in all other lipid storage disorders. For GM1 and GM2, lysolipids have also been found to be elevated but only in infantile cases (Pettazzoni et al. n,d). In Farber disease the ceramide C26:0 and especially its isoform 1 are a highly sensitive and specific biomarker (Cozma et al. 2017).

## Treatment and Follow-Up

### GM1/GM2 Gangliosidosis, Galactosialidosis, and Sandhoff and Tay-Sachs Diseases

In order to replace the deficient enzyme, allogeneic hematopoietic stem cell transplantation has been attempted in both GM1 and GM2 gangliosidoses with disappointing results: in a child with infantile GM1 gangliosidosis. However, despite complete normalization of white blood cell β-galactosidase levels, the patient continued to deteriorate neurologically (Shield et al. 2005). Also for galactosialidosis it has been shown that bone marrow transplantation in mice can fully correct the systemic organ pathology but not the neurological phenotype (Zhou et al. 1995).

In some patients with GM1 gangliosidosis, treatment with the iminosugar N-butyldeoxynojirimycin, miglustat, an inhibitor of glycolipid synthesis, is reported to have some beneficial effect, but without a control group, it is difficult to ascertain its value (Deodato et al. 2017). Based upon its ability to reduce the generation of complex glycolipids, miglustat was also tried in GM2 gangliosidosis. However, no clear effect of miglustat in Sandhoff disease has been observed, and a clinical trial of late-onset Tay-Sachs patients failed.

The most promising therapeutic intervention at this moment is gene therapy: adeno-associated viruses (AAV) seem to have the greatest potential to treat the nervous system because most serotypes preferentially transduce neurons after intraparenchymal injection. Currently intravenous gene transfer with an AAV9 vector is studied for GM1 gangliosidosis, and gene therapy trials for Tay-Sachs and Sandhoff disease are underway. Similar gene transfer therapies are currently being studied for galactosialidosis.

For late-onset patients with relatively milder mutations, pharmacological chaperones, such as pyrimethamine for GM2 gangliosidosis, which enhance residual enzyme activity may be an option. So far no clinical successes have been established (Clarke et al. 2011).

### Krabbe Disease

Hematopoietic stem cell transplantation appeared to be successful in asymptomatic infantile patients or slowly progressive later-onset forms of disease. Demyelination and neurological deterioration were prevented or arrested, respectively (Krivit et al. 1998; Escolar et al. 2005). While initially bone marrow was used as a source, nowadays umbilical cord blood is applied for transplants. Since only presymptomatic transplantation may lead to remyelination of the central nervous system, Krabbe disease has been implemented for newborn screening in New York. However, HSCT is not a cure, and ethical issues towards newborn screening have been raised recently because of the identification of uncertain phenotypes based upon GALC enzyme levels (Ehmann and Lantos 2019). Therapeutic approaches using virus-mediated gene transfer and a combination of gene transfer and stem cell transplantation were performed in a mouse model of Krabbe disease (Biffi et al. 2012). Currently preclinical studies are performed to investigate gene transfer for Krabbe disease using AAV-based vectors. No treatment is available for saposin A deficiency.

Supportive care requires a multidisciplinary approach, including measures to manage pain, spasticity, and seizures, prevent infections, and support nutrition. Disease management recommendations are provided by Escolar et al. (Escolar et al. 2016).

### Metachromatic Leukodystrophy/Saposin B Deficiency

Only supportive treatment is available for late-infantile MLD caused by ASA deficiency. Stem cell transplantation, even at an early stage of disease, has been mainly proven ineffective. For juvenile and adult forms of MLD caused by ASA deficiency, hematopoietic stem cell transplantation is able to stabilize cerebral demyelination and arrests or slows disease progression, but without influence on the peripheral nervous system. ERT trials are taking place in animal models (Batzios and Zafeiriou 2012; Matthes et al. 2012; Biffi et al. 2008). Gene therapy trials using a lentiviral vector to transfer a functional *ARSA* into hematopoietic stem cells are currently conducted with promising preliminary results (Sessa et al. 2016). Additional gene therapy trials using AAV-based vectors are under investigation. Enzyme replacement therapy through intrathecal administration of the recombinant ARSA is piloted in a phase ½ study that was completed in 2017. Further results are awaited.

There is no treatment available for MLD due to saposin B deficiency (Landrieu et al. 1998).

As for Krabbe disease, supportive care managing pain and spasms as well as nutrition is the cornerstone of treatment of these patients, especially when they are not eligible for transplantation. A specific concern is the risk for gallbladder polyps that may evolve to carcinoma, even in transplanted patients, requiring follow-up and surgical intervention in some cases (van Rappard et al. 2016a, b).

## Gaucher Disease

Before enzyme replacement therapy became available, the treatment of a Gaucher disease patient has been symptomatic (Beutler 1988). Splenectomy was performed usually in case of grossly enlarged spleens, leading to infarcts, abdominal discomfort, or severe cytopenia secondary to hypersplenism. After splenectomy, cytopenia is usually immediately resolved. However, the patient is at risk for further liver involvement, hepatopulmonary syndrome, and pulmonary hypertension. In addition, splenectomized patients more frequently develop bone crises and pathological fractures (Mikosch and Hughes 2010). Also, absence of the spleen puts them at a higher risk of septicemia from pneumococci and other encapsulated bacteria. Thus, splenectomy should be avoided whenever possible. Bone crises usually present as acute, circumscript, severe, persistent pain in a long bone, pelvis, or spine, often with signs of inflammation. No other treatment than supportive care with bed rest and nonsteroidal anti-inflammatory drugs or morphine is available. Orthopedic procedures such as joint replacement in case of avascular necrosis are sometimes necessary. Bleeding has been a major problem related to thrombocytopenia, thrombocytopathy, and decreased clotting factors (Hollak et al. 1997). Coagulation studies, including PT and aPTT, need to be performed around every surgical procedure or pregnancy. Supplementation with coagulation factors or plasma may be indicated. For patients with severe skeletal disease, especially those with fractures and osteoporosis, bisphosphonates have been used. While they lead to an increase in bone density, the clinical relevance of this treatment is unclear. Also, new evidence points towards decreased osteoblast activity rather than increased bone loss, and prolonged bisphosphonate therapy may further impair bone remodelling (Van Dussen et al. 2011).

### Hematopoietic Stem Cell Transplantation (HSCT)

Allogeneic bone marrow transplantation or HSCT has been used specifically in the past to treat neuronopathic Gaucher disease (Ringdén et al. 1995). The aim of this approach is to replace hematopoietic stem cells with healthy donor cells secreting normal enzyme. Since enzyme replacement therapy does not reach the central nervous system, HSCT may still be an option for patients with chronic neuronopathic disease. However, this procedure is rarely performed nowadays considering the high risk and the beneficial effects of ERT. Updated outcomes of patients transplanted in the past showed that HSCT had no potential to completely prevent the development of neurological damage since patients developed epilepsy over time (Machaczka 2013).

### Enzyme Replacement Therapy (ERT)

The prospects of patients with type 1 Gaucher disease have improved dramatically with the advent of ERT. Intravenous administration, usually once every 2 weeks, of recombinant β-GCase (Cerezyme, Genzyme Corp., MA) has proven to result in reversal of most disease manifestations (Barton et al. 1991). In patients with advanced liver, lung, or bone disease, the effectiveness is more limited. But in those initiating therapy before irreversible damage has occurred, the responses are very good. Many dosing regimens have been explored, with higher doses generally leading to more robust responses (Grabowski et al. 2009). However, individualization of dosing has become standard practice, since doses between 15 and 60 U/kg eow may all produce sustained responses. It needs to be emphasized that many patients do not need to be treated as they have very mild, nonprogressive disease manifestations (Beutler et al. 1995). The precise criteria to start ERT in type 1 Gaucher disease are not unequivocal. Some believe that most patients need ERT, while others tend to be more conservative. In general, children with symptoms are always treated, while adults with stable disease and mild splenomegaly without severe platelet count (e.g., below 60 × 109/L) and without severe bone marrow infiltration may remain untreated. Currently, the risk factors for late complications, such as multiple myeloma, osteoporosis, or liver/lung disease, are unknown. Whether early initiation of ERT can prevent this is unclear and needs to be investigated. Patients with the acute neuronopathic form of Gaucher disease do not benefit from ERT, and it is now generally accepted that these should not be treated (Vellodi et al. 2009). In a very young patient with neurological symptoms, it may be difficult to decide whether this represents an acute or a chronic form. In such a case, it may be an option to discuss temporary treatment with the option to stop when the course of disease is rapidly progressive (Vellodi et al. 2009). In patients with the chronic neuronopathic form, ERT may certainly alleviate the symptoms related to hepatosplenomegaly and partially also skeletal disease. However, there is no evidence that ERT has reversed, stabilized, or slowed the progression of neurological involvement. Detailed recommendations for treatment are provided in the consensus paper by Vellodi et al. (2009). In type 3c, ERT is usually not indicated, as these patients do not have extensive visceral disease. Over the last years, new ERTs have been developed. Currently, velaglucerase (VPRIV, Shire HGT) has also received marketing authorization in the EU and the USA, whereas taliglucerase (Uplyso, Protalix/Pfizer) has been approved by the FDA only (Zimran et al. 2010, 2011). All these enzymes have shown effectiveness, and choices for treatment will probably depend on whether there are any potential differences in effectiveness or safety, as well as reimbursement strategies and costs.

**Substrate Reduction Therapy (SRT) and Gene Therapy**
An alternative approach is based on small molecules that inhibit substrate synthesis. The authorized treatment is miglustat (*N*-butyl deoxynojirimycin, Zavesca, Actelion/Janssen). As mentioned before, this compound is an iminosugar, which inhibits the glucosyltransferase involved in the first step in the formation of complex glycosphingolipids. The rationale is that the reduction in substrate is balanced against the residual β-GCase activity, which ultimately results in degradation of stored glycolipids. Indeed, miglustat results in reductions in liver and spleen size and gradual improvements in hemoglobin and platelet counts (Cox et al. 2000). The limitations of miglustat are the inferior effects in relation to ERT and unpleasant, mainly gastrointestinal, side effects. With the authorization of a second-generation substrate inhibitor, eliglustat (Lukina et al. 2010), with a more favorable safety and efficacy profile, miglustat is rarely used for type 1 Gaucher disease. While miglustat failed in type 3 Gaucher disease (Schiffmann et al. 2008), newer SRTs such as venglustat (Sanofi/Genzyme) are currently under development that have the ability to cross the blood-brain barrier and can be used in neuropathic Gaucher disease. Preclinical data on gene therapy for type 1 Gaucher disease with lentiviral or liver-directed AAV-based vectors have been promising, and clinical trial programs are about to start.

**Follow-Up and Monitoring of Gaucher Disease**
Follow-up should in principle be individualized, as the heterogeneity of the disease and a number of associated conditions precludes strict protocolized follow-up. However, recommendations for follow-up of patients with Gaucher disease have been previously published (Charrow et al. 2004; Baldellou et al. 2004; Grabowski 2004; Zimran 2011). For neuronopathic disease, a helpful scheme for follow-up of neurological symptoms has been published (Vellodi et al. 2009). Some of the recommendations for follow-up in non-neuronopathic Gaucher disease refer to earlier-defined therapeutic goals (Pastores et al. 2004). It should be kept in mind that these goals are in fact mean responses in blood counts, liver and spleen volumes, and skeletal parameters, rather than clinically meaningful endpoints. Dose adjustment should be made on an individual basis rather than on achievement of these goals. For example, in patients with very large spleens, platelet responses will initially be very slow, and in the absence of clinically relevant bleeding episodes, there is no justification for a dose increase (Hollak et al. 2012a, b). In general, bleeding, severe anemia, and symptomatic organomegaly are alleviated within 12–24 months. Of importance is that good clinical responses are always accompanied by substantial decreases in chitotriosidase (Aerts et al. 2005) or in deficient patients, in CCL18/PARC, ACE, or ferritin levels. Absence of a response in these parameters indicates failure of treatment. Table 'Follow-up and monitoring of non-neuronopathic (type 1) Gaucher disease' shows the minimal recommended follow-up procedures. Because of the increased risk for multiple myeloma, pulmonary hypertension, Parkinson's disease, and perhaps other conditions such as diabetes, it may be wise to include relevant physical, laboratory, or imaging parameters in the follow-up (Zimran 2011). Skeletal imaging should preferably be performed with MRI, as this allows the assessment of the degree of bone marrow involvement. Serial follow-up with skeletal X-rays is unnecessary and exposes patients at high levels of radiation (Poll et al. 2002). DEXA scanning has difficulties in interpreting results in pediatric patients and in adults with sclerotic lesions may also give false outcomes. However, in those with milder disease, regular follow-up to detect early osteopenia or osteoporosis is of importance (Hughes et al. 2019).

## Fabry Disease

Multidisciplinary care for a Fabry disease patient is usually required because of the complexity of the manifestations (Desnick et al. 2003). Since the natural disease course differs between man and women and classically and non-classically affected patients (Arends et al. 2017), management needs to be tailored to the patients' needs. Adequate pain management and early treatment with ACE inhibitors or angiotensin receptor blockers may be needed in case of proteinuria or cardiac symptoms (Jain and Warnock 2011). The use of aspirin is mostly recommended, certainly after TIA or stroke, but whether use of antiplatelet therapy prevents new white matter lesions is unknown. Cardiovascular risk factors independent of Fabry disease are likely to influence the disease course and deserve adequate identification and strict treatment, including hypertension, diabetes, and hypercholesterolemia. Those with rhythm disturbances, frequently bradycardia and AV blocks with ventricular escape tachycardias, may experience syncope. Those patients carry a risk for acute cardiac death and need cardiological monitoring (Pierre-Louis et al. 2009). Patients with end-stage renal failure may benefit greatly from kidney transplantation. The graft survival is not different compared with other patients with renal failure (Ojo et al. 2000).

#### Enzyme Replacement Therapy

In 2001, two recombinant enzymes were approved for use in Fabry disease: agalsidase alpha (Replagal®) and agalsidase beta (Fabrazyme®), referred to as enzyme replacement therapy (ERT). While these enzymes are produced in different cell systems, their biochemical properties are very similar. They have been investigated in different doses: agalsidase beta at 1.0 mg/kg eow and agalsidase alpha at 0.2 mg/kg eow. The first placebo-controlled trials showed some beneficial effect on reduction of storage in endothelial cells and improvement in pain, with stable parameters of renal and cardiac disease (Eng et al. 2001; Schiffmann et al. 2001; Hughes et al. 2008). In a phase IV placebo-controlled trial, treatment with agalsidase beta resulted in a reduction of Fabry-related complications in patients with advanced disease at baseline (Banikazemi et al. 2007). However, complications can still occur during treatment, specifically in patients with advanced disease (Schiffmann et al. 2006; Germain et al. 2007; Weidemann et al. 2009). The occurrence of antibodies may also influence the clinical outcome, as has been recently shown (Lenders et al. 2018; van der Veen et al. 2019). Antibodies almost exclusively emerge in male patients, in particular those without any residual enzyme activity. Their presence is frequently associated with infusion-associated reactions such as chills and fever. This can usually be managed by premedication with corticosteroids and/or slowing down of the infusion rate. Benefits of ERT have also been reported in children, but whether early treatment can prevent the occurrence of late complications is still unknown. There is increasing consensus that not all patients will benefit, and therefore start and stop criteria have been developed and should be regularly evaluated (Biegstraaten et al. 2015).

More recently migalastat and oral chaperone treatment has been authorized for treatment of Fabry disease patients with amenable mutations (Germain et al. 2016). Only a subset of patients, mainly non-classical, have amenable mutations. For which patients this oral alternative is an effective option needs further study, including the reliability of the amenability assay, as some switch patients may show biochemical evidence of disease progression (Lenders et al. 2019). Many questions are thus still unanswered regarding the appropriate use of Fabry treatments. A major concern in this respect is that screening initiatives (neonatal or screening in high-risk groups) may reveal many individuals with variants of unknown significance that may be misdiagnosed as Fabry cases. A diagnosis should be carefully considered before costly and burdensome treatments are recommended.

#### Alternative or Investigational Treatments for Fabry Disease

New enzyme replacement therapies are being developed that hopefully will have less immunological side effects and a better biodistribution. Of these, pegunigalsidase, a pegylated dimer of aGal-A, is a promising agent as shown in a phase 1/2 study (Schiffmann et al. 2019.) A moss-derived enzyme with a different glycosylation and therefore biodistribution, perhaps better targeting kidney cells, is also investigated in Fabry disease patients (Hennermann et al. 2019).

Other small molecules, specifically substrate inhibitors (see Gaucher disease), are under investigation. Currently lucerastat (*N*-butyl deoxygalactonojirimycin, Idorsia) is investigated in Fabry disease and has shown to be safe (Guérard et al. 2018). Its effectiveness is now studied in a phase 3 trial. In addition, a new oral substrate inhibitor is developed by Sanofi/Genzyme, venglustat, for treatment of Fabry disease but also for neuropathic Gaucher disease and Parkinson's disease. Gene therapy has been successfully used in animal models of Fabry disease. As for Gaucher disease, lentiviral or liver-directed AAV-based vectors are currently explored in clinical trials of adult Fabry disease patients. All these developments hold great promise for the future, but results of safety and efficacy studies have to be awaited.

#### Follow-Up and Monitoring of Fabry Disease

As discussed before, Fabry disease is extremely variable. Hence an individualized approach is the cornerstone of management and follow-up. ERT is usually initiated in symptomatic patients, but those who are asymptomatic should receive follow-up as well. Early recognition of organ failure and adequate and timely initiation of appropriate therapy are important. ERT is probably of limited effectiveness in advanced cases, and benefits should be outweighed against the burden of frequent intravenous administration and costs (Biegstraaten et al. 2015). In advanced cases, follow-up schedules need to be extended based on the most severe end-organ damage, following general practice guidelines for patients with renal or cardiac failure. A proposal for follow-up measures is shown in Table 'Follow-up and monitoring of Fabry disease'.

## Farber Disease

There is no effective treatment for Farber disease at this moment. Hematopoietic stem cell transplantation (HSCT) has been explored in Farber disease showing some improvement in peripheral manifestations but without effect on the central nervous system (Ehlert et al. 2018). Enzyme replacement therapy with recombinant human ACDase (rhACDase) is not yet in clinical phase of development, but is currently being investigated as potential treatment. Finally, gene therapy strategies hold promise for the treatment of ACDase deficiency. Gene therapy was performed in mouse models showing long-term expression of ACDase for up to 13 weeks (Ramsubir et al. 2008). An ex vivo strategy with transduction of hematopoietic stem cells seems an attractive approach as well. No clinical trials have so far started in Farber disease.

## Niemann-Pick Type a or B

For patients with Niemann-Pick A and B, supportive therapy to treat the pulmonary manifestations or liver disease is still the mainstay of treatment. Splenectomy is rarely done as it aggravates the liver and lung disease, but may be required in case of extensive enlargement and infarcts or rupture. Standard lipid-lowering agents are indicated for the treatment of ASMD-associated lipid abnormalities in adult patients. Bronchoalveolar lavage has been tried in some cases of extreme pulmonary involvement to relieve symptoms, but its effect is unclear.

Hematopoietic stem cell transplantation (HSCT) has not been very successful, with several patients succumbing due to peritransplant complications (Schuchman and Wasserstein et al. 2015).

Enzyme replacement therapy (ERT) with recombinant human ASM (Sanofi/Genzyme) is currently explored in a phase 3 clinical study. In a 26-week phase 1 study, decreases in spleen and liver volumes and sphingomyelin accumulation in liver biopsies have been observed (Wasserstein et al. 2015).

## Niemann-Pick Disease Type C

Treatment of NPC should involve symptom management, employing disease-modifying agent(s) when available. Several supportive therapies for neurological symptoms are listed in an extensive review from the International Niemann-Pick Disease Registry (INPDR) (Geberhiwot et al. 2018). Bone marrow transplantation in a child with NPC did not improve neurological deterioration (Hsu et al. 1999), whereas trials with hematopoietic stem cell transplantation are in progress in an animal model of NPC (Seo et al. 2011). In infantile-onset NPC presenting with jaundice and hepatosplenomegaly, liver transplantation can be a temporary life-saving measure, but the outcome is poor due to neurological deterioration, despite miglustat therapy (Yamada et al. 2019).

Substrate reduction therapy with miglustat is the only authorized treatment for NPC so far. A randomized controlled trial of 12-month duration reported improvements or stabilization of saccadic eye movements, and in later cohort studies, neurological symptoms including swallowing have been reported to improve or stabilize (Pineda et al. 2018). In a retrospective study in France, patients with less severe neurological disability had a better outcome while using miglustat. Since the disease course is very variable, and with the lack of an untreated comparator, it remains unclear whether this is due to a milder disease course or a neuroprotective effect of miglustat (Nadjar et al. 2018). Current consensus states that only patients with milder phenotypes and early neurological disease should receive treatment (Geberhiwot et al. 2018).

New treatments are arimoclomol, a small-molecule co-inducer of heatshock proteins, which is currently in phase 2/3 trial, and cyclodextrins. The latter compounds are small oligosaccharide rings that can capture cholesterol, a specific mixture of which was piloted in a phase 1/2a clinical trial with intrathecal administration followed by a phase 2/3 clinical trial. In addition, phase 1 clinical studies utilizing high-dose intravenous administration of different cyclodextrins are currently executed. N-Acetyl-L-leucine, which is an amino acid used traditionally for vertigo as well as several causes of ataxia, is also evaluated in NPC.

The INPDR has proposed a schedule for follow-up on a regular basis including neurocognitive, ophthalmological, audiological, and swallowing assessments (Geberhiwot et al. 2018).

## Lysosomal Acid Lipase Deficiency

HMG-CoA reductase inhibitors are given in cholesteryl ester storage disease to prevent early complications of atherosclerosis. HSCT and liver transplantation have been employed with successes in some patients but also with disease recurrence and complications in others (Bernstein et al. 2018).

Currently, ERT with recombinant human acid lipase (Alexion) is authorized to treat patients of all ages, including infants with Wolman disease, where it has shown to improve survival and growth (Jones et al. 2017). In attenuated phenotypes with significant and progressive disease, ERT can improve cholesterol profiles and liver enzymes and volume and hopefully prevent liver failure. Older patients with very mild phenotypes and minimal symptoms may remain stable and probably do not require treatment (Burton et al. 2015).

## Follow-up and Monitoring

Follow-up and monitoring of non-neuronopathic (type 1) Gaucher disease

| Assessment | | Untreated | Treated | |
|---|---|---|---|---|
| Schedule | | Every 12–24 months | Every 3 months during the first year, every 6 months thereafter | Every 12 months during the first 2–4 years, on an individual basis thereafter |
| Physical examination | | X | X | X |
| Laboratory | Ab testing[b] | | | X |
| | ACE | X | | X |
| | CBC | X | X | X |
| | Chitotriosidase or CCL18/PARC[a] | X | X | X |
| | Ferritin | X | | X |
| | Glucosylsphingosine | X | X | X |
| | Liver enzymes | X | | X |
| | M-protein | X | | X |
| Imaging | DEXA scan[d] | X | | X |
| | Liver and spleen volume (MRI, US) | | | |
| | Skeletal MRI | X | | X |
| | Skeletal X-rays[c] | X | | X |
| QoL scores | | X | | X |

[a]CCL18/PARC is recommended in case of chitotriosidase deficiency
[b]Testing for antibodies should be done at baseline and after 12 months. If negative, this should only be repeated in case of infusion-associated reactions or lack of response
[c]Skeletal X-rays are recommended to be made only once, to serve as baseline; follow-up X-rays should only be made upon clinical indication (Maas et al. 2002)
[d]DEXA scans should be performed at baseline and on an individual basis thereafter

Follow-up and monitoring of Fabry disease

| Assessment | | At first visit | Untreated | Treated | |
|---|---|---|---|---|---|
| | | | Every 12–24 months | Every 3 months during the first year, every 6 months thereafter | Every 12 months during the first 2–4 years, on an individual basis thereafter |
| Physical examination | General Neurological[a] | X | X | X | X |
| Laboratory | 24 h urinary protein | X | X | X | |
| | Ab testing | | | | X[c] |
| | Cholesterol profile[b] | X | | | |
| | Creatinine/eGFR | X | X | X | |
| | Electrolytes | X | | | X |
| | Gb3/lysoGb3 | | | X | |
| Imaging | Brain MRI[d] | X | | | X |
| | Cardiac MRI or | X | X | | |
| | US[d] | | X | | X |
| Others | Audiogram | X | X | | X |
| | EKG | X | X | | X |
| | Ocular examination | X | | | |
| | Qol scores | X | X | | X |

[a]At first visit, the presence of angiokeratoma and small fiber neuropathy should be investigated
[b]Cholesterol profile and other cardiovascular risk factors should be recorded carefully at first visit and followed on an individual basis
[c]Testing for antibodies should be done at baseline and after 12 months. If negative, this should only be repeated in case of infusion-associated reactions or lack of response
[d]MRI or US of the heart and MRI of the brain in adults only or upon clinical indication in children

## References

Abaroa L, Garretto NS, et al. Myoclonus and angiokeratomas in adult galactosialidosis. Mov Disord. 2011;26(4):756–7.

Abrahamov A, Elstein D, Horowitz M, et al. A new Gaucher disease variant characterized by progressive calcification of heart valves and unique genotype. Lancet. 1995;346(8981):1000–3.

Adams C, Green S. Late-onset hexosaminidase a and hexosaminidase a and B deficiency: family study and review. Dev Med Child Neurol. 1986;28(2):236–43.

Aerts JM, Hollak CE, van Breemen M, Maas M, Groener JE, Boot RG. Identification and use of biomarkers in Gaucher disease and other lysosomal storage diseases. Acta Paediatr Suppl. 2005;94(447):43–6; discussion 37–8.

Arends M, Wanner C, Hughes D, Mehta A, Oder D, Watkinson OT, Elliott PM, Linthorst GE, Wijburg FA, Biegstraaten M, Hollak CE. Characterization of classical and nonclassical fabry disease: a multicenter study. J Am Soc Nephrol. 2017;28(5):1631–41.

Bajaj NP, Waldman A, Orrell R, Wood NW, Bhatia KP. Familial adult onset of Krabbe's disease resembling hereditary spastic paraplegia with normal neuroimaging. J Neurol Neurosurg Psychiatry. 2002;72(5):635–8.

Baldellou A, Andria G, Campbell PE, Charrow J, Cohen I, Grabowski GA, Harris CH, Kaplan P, McHugh K, Mengel E, Vellodi A. Paediatric non-neuronopathic Gaucher disease: recommendations for treatment and monitoring. Eur J Pediatr. 2004;16:67–75.

Balreira A, Gaspar P, Caiola D, Chaves J, Beirao I, Lopes Lima J, Azevedo JE, Sa Miranda MC. A nonsense mutation in the LIMP-2 gene associated with progressive myoclonic epilepsy and nephrotic syndrome. Hum Mol Genet. 2008;17:2238–43.

Banikazemi M, Bultas J, Waldek S, et al. Agalsidase-beta therapy for advanced Fabry disease: a randomized trial. Ann Intern Med. 2007;146(2):77–86.

Barton NW, Brady RO, Dambrosia JM, et al. Replacement therapy for inherited enzyme deficiency–macrophage-targeted glucocerebrosidase for Gaucher's disease. NEngl J Med. 1991;324:1464–70.

Batzios SP, Zafeiriou DI. Developing treatment options for metachromatic leukodystrophy. Mol Genet Metab. 2012;105(1):56–63.

Beck M, Sieber N, et al. Progressive cerebellar ataxia in juvenile GM2-gangliosidosis type Sandhoff. Eur J Pediatr. 1998;157(10):866–7.

Berkovic SF, Dibbens LM, Oshlack A, Silver JD, Katerelos M, Vears DF, Lullmann-Rauch R, Blanz J, Zhang KW, Stankovich J, Kalnins RM, Dowling JP, et al. Array-based gene discovery with three unrelated subjects shows SCARB2/LIMP-2 deficiency causes myoclonus epilepsy and glomerulosclerosis. Am J Hum Genet. 2008;82:673–84.

Bernstein DL, Lobritto S, Iuga A, Remotti H, Schiano T, Fiel MI, Balwani M. Lysosomal acid lipase deficiency allograft recurrence and liver failure- clinical outcomes of 18 liver transplantation patients. Mol Genet Metab. 2018;124(1):11–9.

Beutler E. Gaucher disease. Blood Rev. 1988;2(1):59–70. Review

Beutler E, Demina A, Laubscher K, Garver P, Gelbart T, Balicki D, Vaughan L. The clinical course of treated and untreated Gaucher disease. A study of 45 patients. Blood Cells Mol Dis. 1995;21(2):86–108.

Biegstraaten M, Arngrímsson R, Barbey F, Boks L, Cecchi F, Deegan PB, Feldt-Rasmussen U, Geberhiwot T, Germain DP, Hendriksz C, Hughes DA, Kantola I, Karabul N, Lavery C, Linthorst GE, Mehta A, van de Mheen E, Oliveira JP, Parini R, Ramaswami U, Rudnicki M, Serra A, Sommer C, Sunder-Plassmann G, Svarstad E, Sweeb A, Terryn W, Tylki-Szymanska A, Tøndel C, Vujkovac B, Weidemann F, Wijburg FA, Woolfson P, Hollak CE. Recommendations for initiation and cessation of enzyme replacement therapy in patients with Fabry disease: the European Fabry Working Group consensus document. Orphanet J Rare Dis. 2015;10:36.

Biffi A, Lucchini G, et al. Metachromatic leukodystrophy: an overview of current and prospective treatments. Bone Marrow Transplant. 2008;42(Suppl 2):S2–6.

Biffi A, Aubourg P, et al. Gene therapy for leukodystrophies. Hum Mol Genet. 2012;20(R1):R42–53.

Bley AE, Giannikopoulos OA, et al. Natural history of infantile G(M2) gangliosidosis. Pediatrics. 2011;128(5):e1233–41

Brady RO, Kanfer JN, Bradley RM, Shapiro D. Demonstration of a deficiency of glucocerebroside-cleaving enzyme in Gaucher's disease. J Clin Invest. 1966;45(7):1112–5.

Brunetti-Pierri N, Scaglia F. GM1 gangliosidosis: review of clinical, molecular, and therapeutic aspects. Mol Genet Metab. 2008;94(4):391–6.

Burton BK, Balwani M, Feillet F, Barić I, Burrow TA, Camarena Grande C, Coker M, Consuelo-Sánchez A, Deegan P, Di Rocco M, Enns GM, Erbe R, Ezgu F, Ficicioglu C, Furuya KN, Kane J, Laukaitis C, Mengel E, Neilan EG, Nightingale S, Peters H, Scarpa M, Schwab KO, Smolka V, Valayannopoulos V, Wood M, Goodman Z, Yang Y, Eckert S, Rojas-Caro S, Quinn AG. A phase 3 trial of Sebelipase alfa in lysosomal acid lipase deficiency. N Engl J Med. 2015;373:1010–20.

Carter A, Brackley SM, Gao J, Mann JP. The global prevalence and genetic spectrum of lysosomal acid lipase deficiency: a rare condition that mimics NAFLD. J Hepatol. 2019;70(1):142–50.

Charrow J, Andersson HC, Kaplan P, Kolodny EH, Mistry P, Pastores G, Prakash-Cheng A, Rosenbloom BE, Scott CR, Wappner RS, Weinreb NJ. Enzyme replacement therapy and monitoring for children with type 1 Gaucher disease: consensus recommendations. J Pediatr. 2004;144:112–20.

Chaves J, Beirão I, Balreira A, Gaspar P, Caiola D, Sá-Miranda MC, Lima JL. Progressive myoclonus epilepsy with nephropathy C1q due to SCARB2/LIMP-2 deficiency: clinical report of two siblings. Seizure. 2011;20(9):738–40.

Christomanou H, Aignesberger A, Linke RP. Immunochemical characterization of two activator proteins stimulating enzymic sphingomyelin degradation in vitro: absence of one of them in a human Gaucher disease variant. Biol Chem Hoppe Seyler. 1986;367:879–90.

Clarke JT, Mahuran DJ, et al. An open-label phase I/II clinical trial of pyrimethamine for the treatment of patients affected with chronic GM2 gangliosidosis (Tay-Sachs or Sandhoff variants). Mol Genet Metab. 2011;102(1):6–12.

Cozma C, Iurașcu MI, Eichler S, Hovakimyan M, Brandau O, Zielke S, Böttcher T, Giese AK, Lukas J, Rolfs A. C26-ceramide as highly sensitive biomarker for the diagnosis of Farber disease. Sci Rep. 2017;7(1):6149.

Cox T, Lachmann R, Hollak C, Aerts J, van Weely S, Hrebicek M, Platt F, Butters T, Dwek R, Moyses C, Gow I, Elstein D, Zimran A. Novel oral treatment of Gaucher's disease with *N*-butyldeoxynojirimycin (OGT 918) to decrease substrate biosynthesis. Lancet. 2000;355:1481–5.

D'Azzo A, Hoogeveen A, et al. Molecular defect in combined beta-galactosidase and neuraminidase deficiency in man. Proc Natl Acad Sci U S A. 1982;79(15):4535–9.

Darin N, Kyllerman M, et al. Juvenile galactosialidosis with attacks of neuropathic pain and absence of sialyloligosacchariduria. Eur J Paediatr Neurol. 2009;13(6):553–5.

De Fost M, Out TA, de Wilde FA, et al. Immunoglobulin and free light chain abnormalities in Gaucher disease type I: data from an adult cohort of 63 patients and review of the literature. Ann Hematol. 2008;87(6):439–49.

Deodato F, Procopio E, Rampazzo A, Taurisano R, Donati MA, Dionisi-Vici C, Caciotti A, Morrone A, Scarpa M. The treatment of juvenile/adult GM1-gangliosidosis with Miglustat, the iminosugar may reverse disease progression. Metab Brain Dis. 2017;32(5):1529–36.

Desnick RJ, Brady R, et al. Fabry disease, an under-recognized multisystemic disorder: expert recommendations for diagnosis, management, and enzyme replacement therapy. Ann Intern Med. 2003;138(4):338–46

Dibbens L, Schwake M, Saftig P, Rubboli G. SCARB2/LIMP2 deficiency in action myoclonus-renal failure syndrome. Epileptic Disord. 2016;18(S2):63–72.

Dierks T, Schlotawa L, et al. Molecular basis of multiple sulfatase deficiency, mucolipidosis II/III and Niemann-pick C1 disease—lysosomal storage disorders caused by defects of non-lysosomal proteins. Biochim Biophys Acta. 2009;1793(4):710–25.

Ehmann P, Lantos JD. Ethical issues with testing and treatment for Krabbe disease. Dev Med Child Neurol. 2019; [Epub ahead of print].

Ehlert K, Levade T, Di Rocco M, Lanino E, Albert MH, Führer M, Jarisch A, Güngör T, Ayuk F, Vormoor J. Allogeneic hematopoietic cell transplantation in Farber disease. J Inherit Metab Dis. 2018:1–8.

Eng CM, Guffon N, Wilcox WR, et al. Safety and efficacy of recombinant human alpha-galactosidase a – replacement therapy in Fabry's disease. N Engl J Med. 2001;345(1):9–16.

Escolar ML, Poe MD, et al. Transplantation of umbilical-cord blood in babies with infantile Krabbe's disease. N Engl J Med. 2005;352(20):2069–81.

Escolar ML, West T, Dallavecchia A, Poe MD, LaPoint K. Clinical management of Krabbe disease. J Neurosci Res. 2016;94(11):1118–25.

Galjart NJ, Gillemans N, et al. Expression of cDNA encoding the human "protective protein" associated with lysosomal beta-galactosidase and neuraminidase: homology to yeast proteases. Cell. 1988;54(6):755–64.

Geberhiwot T, Moro A, Dardis A, Ramaswami U, Sirrs S, Marfa MP, Vanier MT, Walterfang M, Bolton S, Dawson C, Héron B, Stampfer M, Imrie J, Hendriksz C, Gissen P, Crushell E, Coll MJ, Nadjar Y, Klünemann H, Mengel E, Hrebicek M, Jones SA, Ory D, Bembi B, Patterson M, International Niemann-Pick Disease Registry (INPDR). Consensus clinical management guidelines for Niemann-Pick disease type C. Orphanet J Rare Dis. 2018; 13(1):50.

Germain DP. Fabry disease. Orphanet J Rare Dis. 2010;5:30.

Germain DP, Waldek S, Banikazemi M, et al. Sustained, long-term renal stabilization after 54 months of agalsidase beta therapy in patients with Fabry disease. J Am Soc Nephrol. 2007;18(5):1547–57.

Germain DP, Hughes DA, Nicholls K, Bichet DG, Giugliani R, Wilcox WR, Feliciani C, Shankar SP, Ezgu F, Amartino H, Bratkovic D, Feldt-Rasmussen U, Nedd K, Sharaf El Din U, Lourenco CM, Banikazemi M, Charrow J, Dasouki M, Finegold D, Giraldo P, Goker-Alpan O, Longo N, Scott CR, Torra R, Tuffaha A, Jovanovic A, Waldek S, Packman S, Ludington E, Viereck C, Kirk J, Yu J, Benjamin ER, Johnson F, Lockhart DJ, Skuban N, Castelli J, Barth J, Barlow C, Schiffmann R. Treatment of Fabry's disease with the pharmacologic chaperone migalastat. N Engl J Med. 2016;375(6):545–55.

Gieselmann V, Krageloh-Mann I. Metachromatic leukodystrophy–an update. Neuropediatrics. 2010;41(1):1–6.

Gomez-Ospina N. In: Adam MP, Ardinger HH, Pagon RA, Wallace SE, Bean LJH, Stephens K, Amemiya A, editors. SourceGeneReviews® [Internet]; n.d.

Grabowski GA, Andria G, et al. Pediatric non-neuronopathic Gaucher disease: presentation, diagnosis and assessment. Consensus statements. Eur J Pediatr. 2004;163(2):58–66.

Grabowski GA. Phenotype, diagnosis, and treatment of Gaucher's disease. Lancet. 2008;372(9645):1263–71.

Grabowski GA, Kacena K, Cole JA, et al. Dose-response relationships for enzyme replacement therapy with imiglucerase/alglucerase in patients with Gaucher disease type 1. Genet Med. 2009;11(2):92–100.

Grossi S, Regis S, et al. Molecular analysis of ARSA and PSAP genes in twenty-one Italian patients with metachromatic leukodystrophy: identification and functional characterization of 11 novel ARSA alleles. Hum Mutat. 2008;29(11):E220–30.

Guérard N, Oder D, Nordbeck P, Zwingelstein C, Morand O, Welford RWD, Dingemanse J, Wanner C. Lucerastat, an Iminosugar for substrate reduction therapy: tolerability, pharmacodynamics, and pharmacokinetics in patients with Fabry disease on enzyme replacement. Clin Pharmacol Ther. 2018;103(4):703–11.

Hendriksz CJ, Corry PC, et al. Juvenile Sandhoff disease—nine new cases and a review of the literature. J Inherit Metab Dis. 2004;27(2):241–9.

Hennermann JB, Arash-Kaps L, Fekete G, Schaaf A, Busch A, Frischmuth T. Pharmacokinetics, pharmacodynamics, and safety of moss-aGalactosidase a in patients with Fabry disease. J Inherit Metab Dis. 2019;42(3):527–33.

Hollak CE, Levi M, Berends F, Aerts JM, van Oers MH. Coagulation abnormalities in type 1 Gaucher disease are due to low-grade activation and can be partly restored by enzyme supplementation therapy. Br J Haematol. 1997;96(3):470–6.

Hollak C, Maas M, Akkerman E, den Heeten A, Aerts H. Dixon quantitative chemical shift imaging is a sensitive tool for the evaluation of bone marrow responses to individualized doses of enzyme supplementation therapy in type 1 Gaucher disease. Blood Cells Mol Dis. 2001;27(6):1005–12.

Hollak CE, Belmatoug N, Cole JA, Vom Dahl S, Deegan PB, Goldblatt J, Rosenbloom B, van Dussen L, Tylki-Szymańska A, Weinreb NJ, Zimran A, Cappellini MD. Characteristics of type I Gaucher disease associated with persistent thrombocytopenia after treatment with imiglucerase for 4-5 years. Br J Haematol. 2012a;158(4):528–38.

Hollak CE, de Sonnaville ES, Cassiman D, Linthorst GE, Groener JE, Morava E, Wevers RA, Mannens M, Aerts JM, Meersseman W, Akkerman E, Niezen-Koning KE, Mulder MF, Visser G, Wijburg FA, Lefeber D, Poorthuis BJ. Acid sphingomyelinase (Asm) deficiency patients in the Netherlands and Belgium: disease spectrum and natural course in attenuated patients. Mol Genet Metab. 2012b;107(3):526–33.

Hruska KS, LaMarca ME, Scott CR, Sidransky E. Gaucher disease: mutation and polymorphism spectrum in the glucocerebrosidase gene (GBA). Hum Mutat. 2008;29(5):567–83, Review.

Hsu YS, Hwu WL, et al. Niemann-pick disease type C (a cellular cholesterol lipidosis) treated by bone marrow transplantation. Bone Marrow Transplant. 1999;24(1):103–7.

Hughes DA, Elliott PM, et al. Effects of enzyme replacement therapy on the cardiomyopathy of Anderson-Fabry disease: a randomised, double-blind, placebo-controlled clinical trial of agalsidase alfa. Heart. 2008;94:153–8.

Hughes D, Mikosch P, Belmatoug N, Carubbi F, Cox T, Goker-Alpan O, Kindmark A, Mistry P, Poll L, Weinreb N, Deegan P. Gaucher disease in bone: from pathophysiology to practice. J Bone Miner Res. 2019;34(6):996–1013.

Hwu WL, Chien YH, Lee NC, et al. Newborn screening for Fabry disease in Taiwan reveals a high incidence of the later-onset GLA mutation c.936+919G>A (IVS4+919G>A). Hum Mutat. 2009;30(10):1397–405.

Jain G, Warnock DG. Blood pressure, proteinuria and nephropathy in Fabry disease. Nephron Clin Pract. 2011;118(1):c43–8, [Epub 2010 Nov 11].

Jones SA, Rojas-Caro S, Quinn AG, Friedman M, Marulkar S, Ezgu F, Zaki O, Gargus JJ, Hughes J, Plantaz D, Vara R, Eckert S, Arnoux JB, Brassier A, Le Quan Sang KH, Valayannopoulos V. Survival in infants treated with sebelipase alfa for lysosomal acid lipase deficiency: an open-label, multicenter, dose-escalation study. Orphanet J Rare Dis. 2017;12(1):25.

Klima H, Klein A, et al. Over-expression of a functionally active human GM2-activator protein in Escherichia coli. Biochem J. 1993;292(Pt 2):571–6.

Kolter T, Sandhoff K. Sphingolipid metabolism diseases. Biochim Biophys Acta. 2006;1758(12):2057–79.

Kolter T, Proia RL, et al. Combinatorial ganglioside biosynthesis. J Biol Chem. 2002;277(29):25,859–62.

Krivit W, Shapiro EG, et al. Hematopoietic stem-cell transplantation in globoid-cell leukodystrophy. N Engl J Med. 1998;338(16):1119–26.

Kwon JM, Matern D, Kurtzberg J, Wrabetz L, Gelb MH, Wenger DA, Ficicioglu C, Waldman AT, Burton BK, Hopkins PV, Orsini JJ. Consensus guidelines for newborn screening, diagnosis and treatment of infantile Krabbe disease. Orphanet J Rare Dis. 2018;13(1):30.

Landrieu P, Blanche S, et al. Bone marrow transplantation in metachromatic leukodystrophy caused by saposin-B deficiency: a case report with a 3-year follow-up period. J Pediatr. 1998;133(1):129–32.

Lenders M, Neußer LP, Rudnicki M, Nordbeck P, Canaan-Kühl S, Nowak A, Cybulla M, Schmitz B, Lukas J, Wanner C, Brand SM, Brand E. Dose-dependent effect of enzyme replacement therapy on neutralizing antidrug antibody titers and clinical outcome in patients with Fabry disease. J Am Soc Nephrol. 2018;29(12): 2879–89.

Lenders M, Stappers F, Niemietz C, Schmitz B, Boutin M, Ballmaier PJ, Zibert A, Schmidt H, Brand SM, Auray-Blais C, Brand E. Mutation-specific Fabry disease patient-derived cell model to evaluate the amenability to chaperone therapy. J Med Genet. 2019;56(8):548–56.

Levade T, Sandhoff K, Schulze H, Medin JA. 143: Acid ceramidase deficiency: Farber lipogranulomatosis. In: Valle D, editor. The online metabolic and molecular bases of inherited disease. McGraw-Hill, USA. 2017. http://ommbid.mhmedical.com/content.aspx?bookid=971&sectionid=62643272.

Lukina E, Watman N, Avila Arreguin E, et al. Improvement in hematological, visceral, and skeletal manifestations of Gaucher disease type 1 with oral eliglustat tartrate (Genz-112638) treatment: two-year results of a phase 2 study. Blood. 2010;116(20):4095–8.

Maas M, Poll LW, Terk MR. Imaging and quantifying skeletal involvement in Gaucher disease. Br J Radiol. 2002;75(Suppl 1):A13–24.

Machaczka M. Allogeneic hematopoietic stem cell transplantation for treatment of Gaucher disease. Pediatr Hematol Oncol. 2013;30(5):459–61.

MacDermot KD, Holmes A, Miners AH. Anderson-Fabry disease: clinical manifestations and impact of disease in a cohort of 60 obligate carrier females. J Med Genet. 2001;38:769–75.

Madaan P, Jauhari P, Chakrabarty B, Kumar A, Gulati S. Saposin B-deficient metachromatic leukodystrophy mimicking acute flaccid paralysis. Neuropediatrics. 2019;

Matthes F, Stroobants S, et al. Efficacy of enzyme replacement therapy in an aggravated mouse model of metachromatic leukodystrophy declines with age. Hum Mol Genet. 2012;21(11):2599–609.

McGovern MM, Avetisyan R, Sanson BJ, Lidove O. Disease manifestations and burden of illness in patients with acid sphingomyelinase deficiency (ASMD). Orphanet J Rare Dis. 2017;12(1):41.

Meikle PJ, Hopwood JJ, Clague AE, Carey WF. Prevalence of lysosomal storage disorders. JAMA. 1999;281:249–54.

Mikosch P, Hughes D. An overview on bone manifestations in Gaucher disease. Wien Med Wochenschr. 2010;160(23–24): 609–24.

Motta M, Tatti M, Furlan F, Celato A, Di Fruscio G, Polo G, Manara R, Nigro V, Tartaglia M, Burlina A, Salvioli R. Clinical, biochemical and molecular characterization of prosaposin deficiency. Clinically the disorder. Clin Genet. 2016;90(3):220–9.

Nadjar Y, Hütter-Moncada AL, Latour P, Ayrignac X, Kaphan E, Tranchant C, Cintas P, Degardin A, Goizet C, Laurencin C, Martzolff L, Tilikete C, Anheim M, Audoin B, Deramecourt V, De Gaillarbois TD, Roze E, Lamari F, Vanier MT, Héron B. Adult Niemann-pick disease type C in France: clinical phenotypes and long-term miglustat treatment effect. Orphanet J Rare Dis. 2018;13(1):175.

Neudorfer O, Pastores GM, Zeng BJ, Gianutsos J, Zaroff CM, Kolodny EH. Late-onset Tay-Sachs disease: phenotypic characterization and genotypic correlations in 21 affected patients. Genet Med. 2005;7(2):119–23.

Ojo A, Meier-Kriesche HU, Friedman G, Hanson J, Cibrik D, Leichtman A, Kaplan B. Excellent outcome of renal transplantation in patients with Fabry's disease. Transplantation. 2000;69(11):2337–9.

Pampols T, Pineda M, Giros ML, Ferrer I, Cusi V, Chabas A, Sanmarti FX, Vanier MT, Christomanou H. Neuronopathic juvenile glucosylceramidosis due to sap-C deficiency: clinical course, neuropathology and brain lipid composition in this Gaucher disease variant. Acta Neuropathol. 1999;97:91–7.

Pastores GM, Weinreb NJ, Aerts H, et al. Therapeutic goals in the treatment of Gaucher disease. Semin Hematol. 2004;41(4 Suppl 5):4–14.

Pericleous M, Kelly C, Wang T, Livingstone C, Ala A. Wolman's disease and cholesteryl ester storage disorder: the phenotypic spectrum of lysosomal acid lipase deficiency. Lancet Gastroenterol Hepatol. 2017;2(9):670–9.

Pettazzoni M, Froissart R, Pagan C, Vanier MT, Ruet S, Latour P, Guffon N, Fouilhoux A, Germain DP, Levade T, Vianey-Saban C, Piraud M, Cheillan D. LC-MS/MS multiplex analysis of lysosphingolipids in plasma and amniotic fluid: A novel tool for the screening of sphingolipidoses and Niemann-Pick type C disease. n.d.

Pierre-Louis B, Kumar A, Frishman WH. Fabry disease: cardiac manifestations and therapeutic options. Cardiol Rev. 2009;17(1):31–5.

Pineda M, Walterfang M, Patterson MC. Miglustat in Niemann-pick disease type C patients: a review. Orphanet J Rare Dis. 2018; 13(1):140.

Poll LW, Maas M, Terk MR, Roca-Espiau M, Bembi B, Ciana G, Weinreb NJ. Response of Gaucher bone disease to enzyme replacement therapy. Br J Radiol. 2002;75(Suppl 1):A25–36.

Poorthuis BJ, Wevers RA, Kleijer WJ, Groener JE, de Jong JG, van Weely S, Niezen-Koning KE, van Diggelen OP. The frequency of lysosomal storage diseases in the Netherlands. Hum Genet. 1999;105:151–6.

Rafi MA, Luzi P, Chen YQ, et al. A large deletion together with a point mutation in the GALC gene is a common mutant allele in patients with infantile Krabbe disease. Hum Mol Genet. 1995;4:1285–9.

Ramsubir S, Nonaka T, et al. In vivo delivery of human acid ceramidase via cord blood transplantation and direct injection of lentivirus as novel treatment approaches for Farber disease. Mol Genet Metab. 2008;95(3):133–41.

van Rappard DF, Bugiani M, Boelens JJ, van der Steeg AF, Daams F, de Meij TG, van Doorn MM, van Hasselt PM, Gouma DJ, Verbeke JI, Hollak CE, van Hecke W, Salomons GS, van der Knaap MS, Wolf NI. Gallbladder and the risk of polyps and carcinoma in metachromatic leukodystrophy. Neurology. 2016a;87(1):103–11.

van Rappard DF, Bugiani M, Boelens JJ, van der Steeg AF, Daams F, de Meij TG, van Doorn MM, van Hasselt PM, Gouma DJ, Verbeke JI, Hollak CE, van Hecke W, Salomons GS, van der Knaap MS, Wolf NI. Gallbladder and the risk of polyps and carcinoma in metachromatic leukodystrophy. Neurology. 2016b;87(1):103–11.

Reczek D, Schwake M, Schröder J, Hughes H, Blanz J, Jin X, Brondyk W, Van Patten S, Edmunds T, Saftig P. LIMP-2 is a receptor for lysosomal mannose-6-phosphate-independent targeting of beta-glucocerebrosidase. Cell. 2007;131(4):770–83.

Ringdén O, Groth CG, Erikson A, Granqvist S, Månsson JE, Sparrelid E. Ten years' experience of bone marrow transplantation for Gaucher disease. Transplantation. 1995;59(6):864–70.

Ryan E, Seehra G, Sharma P, Sidransky E. GBA1-associated parkinsonism: new insights and therapeutic opportunities. Curr Opin Neurol. 2019;32(4):589–96.

Sandhoff K, Harzer K. Gangliosides and gangliosidoses: principles of molecular and metabolic pathogenesis konrad. J Neurosci. 2013;33(25):10,195–208.

Schiffmann R, Kopp JB, Austin HA III, et al. Enzyme replacement therapy in Fabry disease: a randomized controlled trial. JAMA. 2001;285(21):2743–9.

Schiffmann R, Ries M, Timmons M, Flaherty JT, Brady RO. Long-term therapy with agalsidase alfa for Fabry disease: safety and effects on renal function in a home infusion setting. Nephrol Dial Transplant. 2006;21(2):345–54.

Schiffmann R, Fitzgibbon EJ, Harris C, et al. Randomized, controlled trial of miglustat in Gaucher's disease type 3. Ann Neurol. 2008;64(5):514–22.

Schiffmann R, Warnock DG, Banikazemi M, Bultas J, Linthorst GE, Packman S, Sorensen SA, Wilcox WR, Desnick RJ. Fabry disease: progression of nephropathy, and prevalence of cardiac and cerebrovascular events before enzyme replacement therapy. Nephrol Dial Transplant. 2009;24:2102–11.

Schiffmann R. Fabry disease. Handb Clin Neurol. 2015;132:231–48.

Schiffmann R, Goker-Alpan O, Holida M, Giraldo P, Barisoni L, Colvin RB, Jennette CJ, Maegawa G, Boyadjiev SA, Gonzalez D, Nicholls K, Tuffaha A, Atta MG, Rup B, Charney MR, Paz A, Szlaifer M, Alon S, Brill-Almon E, Chertkoff R, Hughes D. Pegunigalsidase alfa, a novel PEGylated enzyme replacement therapy for Fabry disease, provides sustained plasma concentrations and favorable pharmacodynamics: a 1-year phase 1/2 clinical trial. J Inherit Metab Dis. 2019;42(3):534–44.

Schuchman EH. The pathogenesis and treatment of acid sphingomyelinase-deficient Niemann-pick disease. J Inherit Metab Dis. 2007;30(5):654–63.

Schulze H, Kolter T, et al. Principles of lysosomal membrane degradation: cellular topology and biochemistry of lysosomal lipid degradation. Biochim Biophys Acta. 2009;1793(4):674–83.

Scriver CR. The metabolic and molecular bases of inherited diseases. New York/London: McGraw-Hill; 2002.

Seo Y, Yang SR, et al. Human umbilical cord blood-derived mesenchymal stem cells protect against neuronal cell death and ameliorate motor deficits in Niemann pick type C1 mice. Cell Transplant. 2011;20(7):1033–47.

Sessa M, Lorioli L, Fumagalli F, Acquati S, Redaelli D, Baldoli C, Canale S, Lopez ID, Morena F, Calabria A, Fiori R, Silvani P, Rancoita PM, Gabaldo M, Benedicenti F, Antonioli G, Assanelli A, Cicalese MP, Del Carro U, Sora MG, Martino S, Quattrini A, Montini E, Di Serio C, Ciceri F, Roncarolo MG, Aiuti A, Naldini L, Biffi A. Lentiviral haemopoietic stem-cell gene therapy in early-onset metachromatic leukodystrophy: an ad-hoc analysis of a non-randomised, open-label, phase 1/2 trial. Lancet. 2016;388(10043):476–87.

Shield JP, Stone J, et al. Bone marrow transplantation correcting beta-galactosidase activity does not influence neurological outcome in juvenile GM1-gangliosidosis. J Inherit Metab Dis. 2005;28(5):797–8.

Smid BE, van der Tol L, et al. Uncertain diagnosis of Fabry disease: consensus recommendation on diagnosis in adults with left ventricular hypertrophy and genetic variants of unknown significance. Int J Cardiol. 2014;177(2):400–8.

Spada M, Pagliardini S, Yasuda M, et al. High incidence of later-onset fabry disease revealed by newborn screening. Am J Hum Genet. 2006;79(1):31–40.

Spiegel R, Bach G, et al. A mutation in the saposin a coding region of the prosaposin gene in an infant presenting as Krabbe disease: first report of saposin a deficiency in humans. Mol Genet Metab. 2005;84(2):160–6.

Tiede S, Storch S, et al. Mucolipidosis II is caused by mutations in GNPTA encoding the alpha/beta GlcNAc-1-phosphotransferase. Nat Med. 2005;11(10):1109–12.

Tylki-Szymanska A, Czartoryska B, Vanier M-T, Poorthuis BJMH, Groener JAE, Lugowska A, Millat G, Vaccaro AM, Jurkiewicz E. Non-neuronopathic Gaucher disease due to saposin C deficiency. Clin Genet. 2007;72:538–42.

Tylki-Szymańska A, Groener JE, Kamiński ML, Ługowska A, Jurkiewicz E, Czartoryska B. Gaucher disease due to saposin C deficiency, previously described as non-neuronopathic form--no positive effects after 2-years of miglustat therapy. Mol Genet Metab. 2011;104(4):627–30.

Van Dussen L, Lips P, Everts VE, Bravenboer N, Jansen ID, Groener JE, Maas M, Blokland JA, Aerts JM, Hollak CE. Markers of bone turnover in Gaucher disease: modeling the evolution of bone disease. J Clin Endocrinol Metab. 2011;96(7):2194–205.

Vanier MT. Niemann-pick diseases. Handb Clin Neurol. 2013;113:1717–21.

van der Tol L, Smid BE, Poorthuis BJ, Biegstraaten M, Deprez RH, Linthorst GE, Hollak CE. A systematic review on screening for Fabry disease: prevalence of individuals with genetic variants of unknown significance. J Med Genet. 2014;51(1):1–9.

van der Veen SJ, van Kuilenburg ABP, Hollak CEM, Kaijen PHP, Voorberg J, Langeveld M. Antibodies against recombinant alpha-galactosidase A in Fabry disease: subclass analysis and impact on response to treatment. Mol Genet Metab. 2019;126(2):162–8.

Vellodi A, Tylki-Szymanska A, Davies EH, Kolodny E, Bembi B, Collin-Histed T, Mengel E, Erikson A, Schiffmann R, European Working Group on Gaucher Disease. Management of neuronopathic Gaucher disease: revised recommendations. J Inherit Metab Dis. 2009;32(5):660–4.

Vielhaber G, Hurwitz R, et al. Biosynthesis, processing, and targeting of sphingolipid activator protein (SAP) precursor in cultured human fibroblasts. Mannose 6-phosphate receptor-independent endocytosis of SAP precursor. J Biol Chem. 1996;271(50):32,438–46.

Voorink-Moret M, Goorden SMI, van Kuilenburg ABP, Wijburg FA, der Vlugt JMM G-v, Beers-Stet FS, Zoetekouw A, Kulik W, Hollak CEM, Vaz FM. Rapid screening for lipid storage disorders using biochemical markers. Expert center data and review of the literature. Mol Genet Metab. 2018;123(2):76–84.

Wanner C, Oliveira JP, Ortiz A, Mauer M, Germain DP, Linthorst GE, Serra AL, Marodi L, Mignani R, Cianciaruso B, Vujkovac B, Lemay R, Beitner-Johnson D, Waldek S, Warnock DG. Prognostic indicators of renal disease progression in adults with Fabry disease: natural history data from the Fabry registry. Clin J Am Soc Nephrol. 2010;5(12):2220–8.

Wasserstein MP, Jones SA, Soran H, Diaz GA, Lippa N, Thurberg BL, et al. Successful within-patient dose escalation of olipudase alfa in acid sphingomyelinase deficiency. Mol Genet Metab. 2015;116:88–97.

Weidemann F, Niemann M, Breunig F, et al. Long-term effects of enzyme replacement therapy on fabry cardiomyopathy: evidence for a better outcome with early treatment. Circulation. 2009;119(4):524–9.

Wenger DA, Tarby TJ, et al. Macular cherry-red spots and myoclonus with dementia: coexistent neuraminidase and beta-galactosidase deficiencies. Biochem Biophys Res Commun. 1978;82(2):589–95.

Wenger DA, Rafi MA, et al. Krabbe disease: genetic aspects and progress toward therapy. Mol Genet Metab. 2000;70(1):1–9.

Wheeler S, Schmid R, Sillence DJ. Lipid–protein interactions in Niemann–pick type C disease: insights from molecular modeling. Int J Mol Sci. 2019;20:717.

Yamada N, Inui A, Sanada Y, Ihara Y, Urahashi T, Fukuda A, Sakamoto S, Kasahara M, Yoshizawa A, Okamoto S, Okajima H, Fujisawa T, Mizuta K. Pediatric liver transplantation for neonatal-onset Niemann-Pick disease type C: Japanese multicenter experience. Pediatr Transplant. 2019;23(5):e13462.

Zhou XY, Morreau H, et al. Mouse model for the lysosomal disorder galactosialidosis and correction of the phenotype with overexpressing erythroid precursor cells. Genes Dev. 1995;9(21):2623–34.

Zimran A. How I, treat Gaucher disease. Rev Blood. 2011;118(6):1463–71.

Zimran A, Elstein D. Lipid storage diseases. In: Lichtman MA, Kipps T, Seligsohn U, Kaushansky K, Prchal JT, editors. Williams hematology. 8th ed. New York: McGraw-Hill; 2010. p. 1065–71.

Zimran A, Altarescu G, Philips M, et al. Phase 1/2 and extension study of velaglucerase alfa replacement therapy in adults with type 1 Gaucher disease: 48-month experience. Blood. 2010;115(23):4651–6.

Zimran A, Brill-Almon E, Chertkoff R, Petakov M, Blanco-Favela F, Muñoz ET, Solorio-Meza SE, Amato D, Duran G, Giona F, Heitner R, Rosenbaum H, Giraldo P, Mehta A, Park G, Phillips M, Elstein D, Altarescu G, Szleifer M, Hashmueli S, Aviezer D. Pivotal trial with plant cell-expressed recombinant glucocerebrosidase, taliglucerase alfa, a novel enzyme replacement therapy for Gaucher disease. Blood. 2011;118(22):5767–73.

# 61 The Neuronal Ceroid Lipofuscinoses

Maurizio Scarpa, Cinzia Maria Bellettato, and Annalisa Sechi

## Contents




M. Scarpa (✉) · C. M. Bellettato
Regional Coordinating Center for Rare Diseases, Udine University Hospital, Udine, Italy
e-mail: maurizio.scarpa@hsk-wiesbaden.de

A. Sechi
Regional Coordinating Center for Rare Diseases, Udine University Hospital, Udine, Italy





N. Blau et al. (eds.), *Physician's Guide to the Diagnosis, Treatment, and Follow-Up of Inherited Metabolic Diseases*,
https://doi.org/10.1007/978-3-030-67727-5_61

## Introduction

Neuronal ceroid lipofuscinoses (NCLs) are a heterogeneous group of inherited neurodegenerative diseases characterized by the lysosomal accumulation of autofluorescent material, revealed upon electron microscopy of neurons and many other cell types. The autofluorescent storage material is most commonly represented by subunit c of mitochondrial ATP synthase and sphingolipid activator proteins A and C. Nearly all of the NCL diseases can be subdivided in different clinical forms by age of onset and severity due to residual activity of the corresponding enzyme.

The overall incidence of the NCL is estimated to be 1:20.000. The disorders primarily affect the cerebral gray matter. Signs and symptoms vary widely between the forms, but generally the major clinical symptoms include psychomotor regression, movement disorder, myoclonic epilepsy, progressive loss of vision, behavioral disturbance, and cognitive decline leading to dementia. The early-onset forms of NCL are characterized by severe brain atrophy, decerebration, and premature death. Five clinical groups—congenital, infantile, late infantile, juvenile, and adult—refer to the age of disease onset and are caused by mutations in at least 13 different genes (see Table 61.1). Three enzymes have been recognized as responsible, when deficient, of NCL cases: palmitoyl-protein thioesterase 1 (*PPT1*), tripeptidyl-peptidase 1 (*TPP1*), and cathepsin D (CTSD).

CLN9 is not genetically defined yet. *SGSH* gene mutations usually cause mucopolysaccharidosis type IIIA. SGSH mutations that are associated with high residual sulfamidase activity may also cause adult onset of NCL.

Most NCL diseases are inherited in an autosomal recessive manner. As by current knowledge, only the CLN4B follows an autosomal dominant inheritance. There is a rough genotype-phenotype correlation in the sense that several missense mutations with minor residual enzymatic activity in the palmitoyl protein thioesterase 1 (CLN1), the tripeptidyl peptidase 1 (CLN2), and cathepsin D (CLN10) are correlated with protracted clinical courses (Das et al. 2001; Steinfeld et al. 2004, 2006).

## Nomenclature

| No. | Disorder | Alternative names | Abbreviation | Gene symbol | Chromosomal localization | Affected protein | Protein (type) | OMIN | Subtypes | Typical NCL disease | Atypical NCL disease |
|---|---|---|---|---|---|---|---|---|---|---|---|
| 61.1 | Ceroid lipofuscinosis, neuronal, 1 | Santavuori-Haltia disease | CLN1 | PPT1 | 1p34.2 | Lysosomal palmitoyl protein thioesterase-1 | Palmitoyl protein thioesterase 1 (lysosomal enzyme) | 256730 | All forms | Infantile | Late infantile, juvenile, adult |
| 61.2 | Ceroid lipofuscinosis, neuronal, 2 | Jansky-Bielschowsky disease | CLN2 | TPP1 | 11p15.4 | Lysosomal tripeptidyl-peptidase-1 | Tripeptidyl peptidase 1 (lysosomal enzyme) | 204500 | All forms | Late infantile | Juvenile |
| 61.3 | Ceroid lipofuscinosis, neuronal, 3 | Batten-Spielmeyer-Vogt disease | CLN3 | CLN3 | 16p11.2 | Lysosomal transmembrane CLN3 protein | CLN3 (Golgi lysosome transmembrane protein) | 204200 | All forms | Juvenile | |
| 61.4 | Ceroid lipofuscinosis, neuronal, 4A | Kufs disease recessive type A | CLN4A | CLN6 | 15q23 | CLN6 | CLN6 (ER transmembrane protein) | 204300 | | | |
| 61.5 | Ceroid lipofuscinosis, neuronal, 4B | Kufs disease dominant type A | CLN4B | DNAJC5 | 20q13.33 | DNAJC5 Cysteine string protein alpha | Soluble cysteine string protein alpha (synaptic vesicle protein) | 162350 | Adult form | Adult | |
| 61.6 | Ceroid lipofuscinosis, neuronal, 5 | Lysosomal CLN5 protein deficiency | CLN5 | CLN5 | 13q22.3 | Lysosomal CLN5 protein | CLN5 (soluble lysosomal protein) | 256731 | All forms | Late infantile | Juvenile, adult |
| 61.7 | Ceroid lipofuscinosis, neuronal, 6 | CLN6 late infantile variant | CLN6 | CLN6 | 15q23 | CLN6 | CLN6 (ER transmembrane protein) | 601780 | All forms | Late infantile | Adult |
| 61.8 | Ceroid lipofuscinosis, neuronal, 7 | CLN7 Turkish variant | CLN7 | MFSD8 | 4q28.2 | Major facilitator superfamily domain-containing protein-8 (MFSD8) | MFSD8 (lysosomal transporter) | 610951 | All forms | Late infantile | Juvenile |
| 61.9 | Ceroid lipofuscinosis, neuronal, 8 | CLN8 disease, late infantile variant | CLN8 | CLN8 | 8p23.3 | CLN8 | CLN8 (ER-Golgi transmembrane protein) | 600143 | | Late infantile | Juvenile (EPMR) |
| 61.10 | Ceroid lipofuscinosis, neuronal, 8, Northern epilepsy variant | CLN8 disease, progressive epilepsy with mental retardation | CLN8 | CLN8 | 8p23.3 | CLN8 | CLN8 (ER-Golgi transmembrane protein) | 610003 | All forms | | |

(continued)

| No. | Disorder | Alternative names | Abbreviation | Gene symbol | Chromosomal localization | Affected protein | Protein (type) | OMIN | Subtypes | Typical NCL disease | Atypical NCL disease |
|---|---|---|---|---|---|---|---|---|---|---|---|
| 61.11 | Ceroid lipofuscinosis, neuronal, 10 | Ceroid lipofuscinosis, neuronal, cathepsin D-deficient | CLN10 | CTSD | 11p15.5 | Cathepsin D | Cathepsin D (lysosomal enzyme) | 610127 | Late infantile form | Congenital | Late infantile, juvenile, adult |
| 61.12 | Ceroid lipofuscinosis, neuronal, 11 | Progranulin deficiency | CLN11 | GRN | 17q21.31 | Progranulin | Progranulin (autocrine growth factor) | 614706 | Juvenile form | Adult | |
| 61.13 | Ceroid lipofuscinosis, neuronal, 12 | Kufor-Rakeb syndrome, Parkinson's disease 9 | CLN12/ PARK9 | ATP13A2 | 1p36.13 | Lysosomal type 5 P-type ATPase | ATP13A2 (P-type ATPase, lysosomal cation transporter) | 606693 | All forms | Juvenile | |
| 61.14 | Ceroid lipofuscinosis, neuronal, 13 | Kufs disease recessive type B | CLN13 | CTSF | 11q13 | Cathepsin F | KCTD7 (potassium channel) | 615362 | Adult form | Adult | |
| 61.15 | Ceroid lipofuscinosis, neuronal, 14 | Progressive myoclonic epilepsy type 3 | CLN14/ EPM3 | KCTD7 | 7q11.22 | Potassium channel tetramerization domain-containing protein 7 | Cathepsin F (lysosomal enzyme) | 611726 | Juvenile form | Infantile | |

## NCL Phenotypes Classified by Age at Onset

The *congenital NCL* (CLN10) begins in utero and is associated with intrauterine growth retardation and fetal microcephaly. At birth, affected infants show intractable seizures, spasticity, and central apnea. These newborns usually survive only days, seldom weeks.

The *infantile NCL* is a rapidly progressive form and presents between 6 and 18 months with hyperexcitability, muscular hypotonia, psychomotor retardation, myoclonic seizures, visual failure, and microcephaly. Later, by the age of 3 years, loss of motor abilities, increasing spasticity, and lack of environmental contact comprise the clinical picture.

The *classical late infantile NCL* is characterized by normal development to the age of 2 years, followed by developmental delay, motor regression, myoclonic seizures, and visual failure. After the onset of symptoms, the disease progresses in a program-like manner over 2–3 years leading to chair boundness, spasticity, blindness, and dementia (Steinfeld et al. 2002).

The *juvenile NCL* is characterized by progressive visual failure beginning at the age of 4–9 years, followed by developmental delay, motor regression, myoclonic seizures, and visual failure. Cognitive decline and motor deterioration follow and finally lead to death in the third or fourth decades. Seizures are a variable feature. Atypical juvenile forms (CLN2 and CLN5) initially present with motor symptoms and behavioral problems before they develop visual disturbance.

The *variant forms of late infantile NCL* have clinical presentations intermediate between the classical late infantile and juvenile forms.

The *adult* NCL is distinguished from the other NCL types by the absence of visual failure and an onset at 20–30 years of age with mild progression (Mole et al. 2005, Mole and Williams 2010).

The diagnostic work-up of the NCL should begin with the clinical assessment of the patients and should mainly consider the presence of major neurodegeneration (Mole and Williams 2001). The assessment of the specific combination of symptoms is important to determine the further diagnostic investigations that commonly comprise full blood count and smear, fundoscopy, cardiac assessment (ECG/ECHO), skeletal status (X-ray), brain MRI, and electrophysiology (VEP, SEP, ERG). Specific tests should be performed in specialized laboratories. Diagnostic procedures include quantitative analysis of metabolites in body fluids (urine, serum, CSF) and fibroblasts as well as specific assays of lysosomal hydrolases. DNA mutation analysis in the affected gene should be performed to confirm the diagnosis. DNA testing is particularly important for prenatal diagnosis. More specific information are available in the following specific sessions.

## Tripeptidyl-Peptidase 1 Deficiency (NCL2)

### Physiopathology

The lipopigment pattern seen most often in CLN2 consists of "curvilinear" profiles. Patients with CLN2 are deficient in a pepstatin-insensitive lysosomal peptidase called tripeptidyl peptidase 1 (TTP1). TTP1 removes tripeptides from the N-terminal of polypeptides. The mechanism by which failure to cleave these N-terminal peptides leads to neuronal degeneration of the hippocampus, cortical interneurons, cerebellum, and thalamocortical neurons with consequent neuronal death is still poorly understood.

**Table 61.1** Ceroid lipofuscinosis, neuronal, 2

| System | Symptoms and biomarkers | Neonatal (birth–1 month) | Infancy (1–18 months) | Childhood (1.5–11 years) | Adolescence (11–16 years) | Adulthood (>16 years) |
|---|---|---|---|---|---|---|
| CNS | Ataxia | | ± | +++ | +++ | +++ |
| | Cerebellar atrophy (MRI) | | ± | +++ | +++ | +++ |
| | **Cerebral atrophy (MRI)** | | ± | +++ | +++ | +++ |
| | **Developmental regression** | | | +++ | +++ | +++ |
| | Developmental regression | | ± | +++ | +++ | +++ |
| | Dystonia | | ± | +++ | +++ | +++ |
| | EEG, abnormal | | ± | +++ | +++ | +++ |
| | ERG, abnormal | | | +++ | +++ | +++ |
| | **Movement disorder** | | | +++ | +++ | +++ |
| | Myoclonic epilepsy | | ± | +++ | +++ | +++ |
| | Myoclonus | | ± | +++ | +++ | +++ |
| | Neurodegenerative disease | | | +++ | +++ | +++ |
| | **Seizures** | | | +++ | +++ | +++ |
| | **Seizures, myoclonic** | | | +++ | +++ | +++ |
| | Seizures, tonic clonic | | | +++ | +++ | +++ |
| | Spasticity | | | +++ | +++ | +++ |
| | Speech delay | | + | +++ | +++ | +++ |
| | SSEP, abnormal | | ± | +++ | +++ | +++ |
| | VEP, abnormal | | n | +++ | +++ | +++ |
| | White matter abnormalities (MRI) | | ± | + | ± | ± |

(continued)

**Table 61.1** (continued)

| System | Symptoms and biomarkers | Neonatal (birth–1 month) | Infancy (1–18 months) | Childhood (1.5–11 years) | Adolescence (11–16 years) | Adulthood (>16 years) |
|---|---|---|---|---|---|---|
| Eye | **Optic atrophy** | | | +++ | +++ | +++ |
| | **Pigmentary retinopathy** | | | +++ | +++ | +++ |
| | **Retinal dystrophy** | | | +++ | +++ | +++ |
| | **Vision loss** | | | +++ | +++ | +++ |
| Metabolic | EM, Storage material | ++ | +++ | +++ | +++ | +++ |
| Musculoskeletal | Muscular atrophy | n | + | +++ | +++ | +++ |
| | Spinal muscular atrophy | n | + | +++ | +++ | +++ |
| Laboratory findings | Lysosomal tripeptidyl-peptidase-1 (dried blood spot) | ↓↓↓ | ↓↓↓ | ↓↓↓ | ↓↓↓ | ↓↓↓ |
| | Lysosomal tripeptidyl-peptidase-1 (fibroblasts) | ↓↓↓ | ↓↓↓ | ↓↓↓ | ↓↓↓ | ↓↓↓ |
| | Lysosomal tripeptidyl-peptidase-1 (leukocytes) | ↓↓↓ | ↓↓↓ | ↓↓↓ | ↓↓↓ | ↓↓↓ |

Laboratory and instrumental examinations (NCL2)

| | |
|---|---|
| Histologic findings (electron microscopic findings) | Electron microscopy ultrastructural studies in peripheral blood lymphocytes or other tissues (conjunctiva, skin. or other tissues) show the presence of the curvilinear profiles (CVB). Histologic findings include neuronal loss and the presence of distended neurons with granular PAS-positive material |
| Enzyme activity | Tripeptidyl peptidase 1 (TPP1) levels can be measured in leukocytes, cultured fibroblasts, dried blood spots, and saliva. Fibroblast TPP1 activity is approximately 17,000 micromoles of amino acids produced per hour per mg of protein<br>The TPP1 activity in CLN2 is less than 4% of normal |
| Molecular genetic testing | Molecular genetic testing of TPP1 gene. More than 90 mutations of TPP1 are known. The common mutations are p. Arg208Ter and c.509-1G>C; the others are uncommon or private mutations |
| Instrumental tests | *Electroencephalography:* Abnormal EEG with spikes in the occipital region in response to photic stimulation at 1–2 Hz<br>*Electroretinography:* Electroretinogram (ERG) is usually abnormal at presentation and becomes undetectable soon thereafter. On occasion, the ERG may be normal at presentation<br>*Visual evoked potential:* Abnormally enhanced for a long period and diminish in the final stage of the disease<br>*Somatosensory evoked potential:* Progressive attenuation in all NCLs is seen in somatosensory evoked potential studies<br>*MRI and MR spectroscopy:* Progressive cerebellar and cerebral atrophy with normal basal ganglia and thalami. In a study, Dyke et al. elaborate a multiparametric disease severity score, correlating with the patient's age and disease duration; it is obtained from the combination of the whole-brain apparent diffusion coefficient (ADC), the volume percentage of CSF, and N-acetylaspartate-to-creatine metabolite ratios and const. They determined that children in the study with CLN2 began to differ from controls at age 5 years<br>*Positron emission tomography:* a severe, generalized hypometabolism is seen |
| Other tests | *Neurologic examination*<br>*Developmental/cognitive and educational assessment*<br>*Ophthalmic examination:* Ophthalmic scale may serve as an objective marker of LINCL (late infantile neuronal ceroid lipofuscinosis) severity and disease progression<br>*A total disability score* is derived by summing up the single scores for motor, visual, and verbal functions<br>*A Weill Cornell LINCL (late infantile neuronal ceroid lipofuscinosis) scale,* based on neurologic, ophthalmologic, and CNS imaging, has been developed, which correlate with age and time since the onset of initial clinical manifestations |

### Prevention

Prenatal diagnosis is an option in patients with family history of CLN2 or known carriers. It can be done through electron microscopic examination of uncultured amniocytes for typical curvilinear bodies and through mutation analysis.

Genetic counseling should be offered to family members, and the risk of CLN2 should be assessed for subsequent pregnancies.

## Neuronal Ceroid Lipofuscinosis Type 3

### Physiopathology

In CLN3 NCL, mutations in CLN3 gene, coding for a protein involved in lysosomal function, in particular in microtubule-dependent, anterograde transport of late endosomes and lysosomes, have been found. These mutations result in a substantial decrease in mRNA expression and stability. Consequently, several cellular processes are affected, such as

**Table 61.2** Ceroid lipofuscinosis, neuronal, 3

| System | Symptoms and biomarkers | Neonatal (birth–1 month) | Infancy (1–18 months) | Childhood (1.5–11 years) | Adolescence (11–16 years) | Adulthood (>16 years) |
|---|---|---|---|---|---|---|
| Cardiovascular | Cardiac arrhythmia | | | | + | ++ |
| | Cardiomyopathy | | | | + | ++ |
| CNS | Cerebellar atrophy (MRI) | | | n | + | ++ |
| | **Cerebral atrophy (MRI)** | | | n | + | ++ |
| | Cognitive dysfunction | | | + | ++ | +++ |
| | Developmental regression | | | + | ++ | +++ |
| | Dysarthria | | | + | ++ | +++ |
| | EEG, abnormal | | | + | ++ | +++ |
| | ERG, abnormal | | | ++ | +++ | +++ |
| | Extrapyramidal movement disorder | | | | ++ | +++ |
| | Gait disturbance | | | | ++ | +++ |
| | Hallucinations | | | | ++ | ++ |
| | Hypokinesia | | | | ++ | +++ |
| | **Movement disorder** | | | + | ++ | +++ |
| | Neurodegenerative disease | | | + | ++ | +++ |
| | Psychiatric symptoms | | | | ++ | +++ |
| | **Seizures** | | | | + | ++ |
| | Seizures, complex partial | | | | + | ++ |
| | Seizures, tonic clonic | | | | + | ++ |
| | SSEP, abnormal | | | + | ++ | +++ |
| | VEP, abnormal | | | ++ | +++ | +++ |
| | White matter abnormalities (MRI) | | | + | + | + |
| Eye | Optic atrophy | | | + | ++ | +++ |
| | **Pigmentary retinopathy** | | | ++ | +++ | +++ |
| | **Retinal dystrophy** | | | ++ | +++ | +++ |
| | **Vision loss** | | | +++ | +++ | +++ |
| Hematological | Vacuolated lymphocytes | | ++ | ++ | ++ | ++ |
| Metabolic | EM, Storage material | | ++ | +++ | +++ | +++ |
| Musculoskeletal | Muscular atrophy | | | ± | + | ++ |
| | Rigidity | | | | ++ | +++ |
| | Spinal muscular atrophy | | | ± | + | ++ |
| Psychiatric | Anxiety | | | | ++ | ++ |
| | Behavior, aggressive | | | | ++ | ++ |
| | **Behavioral disorder** | | | ++ | +++ | +++ |
| | Depression | | | | ++ | ++ |

Laboratory and instrumental examinations (CLN3)

| | |
|---|---|
| Histologic findings (electron microscopic findings) and laboratory tests | The analysis of *blood smears* through light microscopy reveals the presence of lymphocyte vacuoles<br>*Electron microscopy ultrastructural studies* in peripheral blood lymphocytes or other tissues (conjunctiva, skin, or other tissues) show the presence of vacuoles and the storage of lipopigment with a "fingerprint" profile. The fingerprint profile can have three different appearances: pure within a lysosomal residual body; in conjunction with curvilinear or rectilinear profiles; and as a small component within large membrane-bound lysosomal vacuoles. The combination of fingerprint profiles within lysosomal vacuoles is a regular feature of blood lymphocytes from patients with CLN3<br>*Histological studies* reveal severe widespread neuronal degeneration resulting in retinal atrophy and in massive loss of brain substance, the selective necrosis of stellate cells in layers II and III and loss of pyramidal cells in layer V, and the accumulation of lipofuscin in neuronal perikaryon and in the thyroid<br>*Muscle biopsy:* In muscle tissue, autophagic vacuoles and intermyofibrillar and subsarcolemmal accumulation of electrodense material are seen on biopsy (in some patients)<br>*Biochemical abnormalities* include the accumulation of subunit C of the ATP synthase complex (SCMAS) in the lysosomes of patients<br>*Lymphoblast cell analysis:* Enhanced levels of α-synuclein oligomers and gangliosides GM1, GM2, and GM3 and reduced levels of sphingomyelin and autophagy in CLN3 disease lymphoblast cells compared with normal cells<br>CLN3-deficient cells display defects in the ARF1-Cdc42 pathway and actin-dependent events |
| Enzyme activity | Not applicable |
| Molecular genetic testing | *Molecular genetic testing* of CLN3 gene |

| | |
|---|---|
| Instrumental tests | *Electroencephalography:* The EEG shows nonspecific disorganization and spike-and-slow-wave complexes<br>*Electroretinography:* Abnormal early ERG shows loss of photoreceptor function<br>*Visual evoked potential:* Abnormal early with delayed latency<br>*Somatosensory evoked potential:* Progressive attenuation<br>*Magnetic resonance imaging (MRI) and MR spectroscopy:* Cerebral atrophy and cerebellar atrophy are seen usually after age 15 years. Progressive hippocampal atrophy is one of the characteristic features of brain atrophy in CLN3 in adolescence<br>*Longitudinal MRI* shows that the annual rate of the gray matter loss in adolescent CLN3 patients is as high as 2.4%<br>*In voxel-based morphometric study,* marked reduction in the gray matter volume of the dorsomedial thalami in particular and decreased white matter volume of the corona radiata are seen<br>*Positron emission tomography (PET):* Hypometabolism, earliest in the calcarine area |
| Other tests | *Neurologic examination*<br>*Ophthalmologic examination* (early in the course of disease may reveal macular changes only; gradually, typical signs of pan-retinal degeneration develop, such as pigmentary changes in the retinal periphery, vascular attenuation, and optic nerve pallor)<br>*Developmental/cognitive and educational assessment*<br>*Use of the multimodal clinical rating instrument, the Unified Batten Disease Rating Scale (UBDRS),* to assess motor, behavioral, and functional capabilities of patients with juvenile onset |

lysosomal pH, endocytosis, autophagy, transport of proteins from the TGN, cell proliferation, apoptosis, and synaptic transmission. Nevertheless, it is still not clear what precise biological function(s) CLN3 regulates and what is the mechanism of such regulation (Anil B. Mukherjee et al. 2019).

### Prevention

Prenatal testing for pregnancies at increased risk is possible if the disease-causing mutation(s) have been identified in the family.

## Neuronal Ceroid Lipofuscinosis Type 4 (Parry Type) (CLN4B)

### Physiopathology

In CLN4B NCL, the DNAJ homolog subfamily C member 5 (DNAJC5) is deficient. DNAJC5 functions in many cellular processes by regulating the ATPase activity of 70-kd heat-shock proteins. In particular cysteine string protein alpha (CSP$\alpha$) encoded by the DNAJC5 gene plays critical acting as a chaperone to facilitate correct folding of proteins.

### Prevention

Prenatal testing for pregnancies at increased risk is possible if the disease-causing mutation(s) have been identified in the family.

## Neuronal Ceroid Lipofuscinosis Type 5

### Physiopathology

The lipopigment patterns observed most often in CLN5 comprise mixed combinations of "granular," "curvilinear," and "fingerprint" profiles. The functions of these soluble lysosomal glycoproteins are still unknown, but it seems to play a role in endosomal sorting.

### Prevention

Prenatal testing for pregnancies at increased risk is possible if the disease-causing mutation(s) have been identified in the family.

**Table 61.3** Ceroid lipofuscinosis, neuronal, 4B

| System | Symptoms and biomarkers | Neonatal (birth–1 month) | Infancy (1–18 months) | Childhood (1.5–11 years) | Adolescence (11–16 years) | Adulthood (>16 years) |
|---|---|---|---|---|---|---|
| CNS | Ataxia | | | | | ++ |
| | Cerebellar atrophy (MRI) | | | | | + |
| | Cerebral atrophy (MRI) | | | | | + |
| | **Cognitive decline** | | | | | +− |
| | EEG, abnormal | | | | | +− |
| | Extrapyramidal movement disorder | | | | | ++ |
| | **Movement disorder** | | | | | ++ |
| | Myoclonus | | | | | ++ |
| | Neurodegenerative disease | | | | | +++ |
| | Psychiatric symptoms | | | | | ++ |
| | **Seizures** | | | | | ++ |
| | **Seizures, tonic clonic** | | | | | +++ |
| | Spasticity | | | | | ++ |
| Metabolic | EM, Storage material | | | | | + |
| Psychiatric | Behavioral disorder | | | | | ++ |

Laboratory and instrumental examinations (CLN4B)

| | |
|---|---|
| Histologic findings and laboratory tests (electron microscopic findings) and laboratory tests | *Histologic analysis:* Electron microscopy ultrastructural studies in peripheral blood lymphocytes or other tissues (conjunctiva, skin, or other tissues) show the presence of mixed-type inclusions (curvilinear bodies, rectilinear complex, and granular osmiophilic deposits)<br>In neural tissues, histopathologic features included neuronal loss, accumulation of lipopigment in remaining neurons, and PAS-positive intraneuronal storage material<br>*Biochemical tests:* Abnormalities include the accumulation of subunit C of the ATP synthase complex (SCMAS) in the lysosomes of patients |
| Enzyme activity | Not applicable |
| Molecular genetic testing | *Molecular genetic testing* in DNAJC5 gene |
| Instrumental tests | *Electroencephalogram:* Abnormal with recurrent burst of 4- to 6-Hz slow waves<br>*Somatosensory evoked potential:* Progressive attenuation |
| Other tests | *Neurologic examination*<br>*Ophthalmologic examination*<br>*Developmental/cognitive and educational assessment* |

**Table 61.4** Ceroid lipofuscinosis, neuronal, 5

| System | Symptoms and biomarkers | Neonatal (birth–1 month) | Infancy (1–18 months) | Childhood (1.5–11 years) | Adolescence (11–16 years) | Adulthood (>16 years) |
|---|---|---|---|---|---|---|
| CNS | Ataxia | | ± | +++ | +++ | +++ |
| | **Cerebellar atrophy (MRI)** | | ± | +++ | +++ | +++ |
| | **Cerebral atrophy (MRI)** | | ± | +++ | +++ | +++ |
| | Developmental regression | | ± | +++ | +++ | +++ |
| | Dystonia | | ± | +++ | +++ | +++ |
| | EEG, abnormal | | ± | +++ | +++ | +++ |
| | ERG, abnormal | | | +++ | +++ | +++ |
| | **Movement disorder** | | | +++ | +++ | +++ |
| | Myoclonic epilepsy | | ± | +++ | +++ | +++ |
| | Myoclonus | | ± | +++ | +++ | +++ |
| | Neurodegenerative disease | | | +++ | +++ | +++ |
| | **Seizures** | | | +++ | +++ | +++ |
| | **Seizures, myoclonic** | | | +++ | +++ | +++ |
| | Seizures, tonic clonic | | | +++ | +++ | +++ |
| | Spasticity | | | + | ++ | +++ |
| | **Speech delay** | | | + | ++ | +++ |
| | SSEP, abnormal | | ± | +++ | +++ | +++ |
| | VEP, abnormal | | | +++ | +++ | +++ |
| | White matter abnormalities (MRI) | | ± | + | ± | ± |
| Eye | Macular dystrophy | | | +++ | +++ | +++ |
| | **Optic atrophy** | | | ++ | +++ | +++ |
| | **Retinal dystrophy** | | | ++ | +++ | +++ |
| | **Vision loss** | | | +++ | +++ | +++ |
| Metabolic | **EM, Storage material** | ++ | +++ | +++ | ++ | ++ |
| Musculoskeletal | **Muscular atrophy** | | + | +++ | +++ | +++ |
| | Spinal muscular atrophy | | + | +++ | +++ | +++ |

Laboratory and instrumental examinations (CLN5)

| | |
|---|---|
| Histologic findings and laboratory tests (electron microscopic findings) and laboratory tests | *Histologic analysis.* Electron microscopy ultrastructural studies in peripheral blood lymphocytes or other tissues (conjunctiva, skin, or other tissues) show the presence of "fingerprint," curvilinear," and "rectilinear" profiles. No storage material is seen in lymphocytes. Histologic findings also include neuronal loss in the neocortex and cerebellum, laminar pattern of neuronal loss (most severe in layers III and V), meganeurites in layer III, extensive gliosis, and an almost complete loss of Purkinje and granule cells<br>Accumulation of subunit C of the mitochondrial adenosine triphosphate (ATP) synthase complex in lysosomes |
| Enzyme activity | Not applicable |
| Molecular genetic testing | *Molecular genetic testing* on CLN5 gene |
| Instrumental tests | *Neurophysiologic inspection:* Neurophysiologic abnormalities in electroencephalography and visual evoked potential<br>*MRI*: Cerebral and cerebellar atrophy<br>*Somatosensory evoked potential*: Enlarged SI (primary somatosensory cortex) and SII (secondary somatosensory cortex) somatosensory evoked responses |
| Other tests | *Neurologic examination*<br>*Ophthalmologic examination*<br>*Developmental/cognitive and educational assessment* |

## Neuronal Ceroid Lipofuscinosis Type 6

### Physiopathology

CLN6 encodes a protein of unknown function with seven transmembrane domains localizing to the endoplasmic reticulum (ER). It has been reported that CLN6 has a role in the regulation of cellular acidification, endocytosis, and autophagy, but how the altered function of this gene leads to the accumulation of biometals and how this defect leads to CLN6 disease pathogenesis must still be clarified.

### Prevention

Prenatal testing for pregnancies at increased risk is possible if the disease-causing mutation(s) have been identified in the family.

## Neuronal Ceroid Lipofuscinosis Type 7

### Physiopathology

In NCL 7, the major facilitator superfamily domain of the CLN7 gene containing protein-8 (MFSD8), an acid membrane protein that belongs to the major facilitator superfamily of transporter proteins (active permeases), is deficient. The precise role of this protein is still not well understood, but active permeases function as transporters of sugars, sugar phosphates, drugs, inorganic and organic cations, amino acids, and neurotransmitters across membranes, so mutations in gene cause depletion of soluble proteins in the lysosomes that in turn impairs the reactivation of mTOR signalling, thus being responsible for impaired anabolic regulator of cell growth and metabolism. The protein likely localizes to lysosomal membranes. MFSD8 is ubiquitously expressed at a very low level; only in the liver, heart, and pancreas its expression is consistently higher.

### Prevention

Prenatal testing for pregnancies at increased risk is possible if the disease-causing mutation(s) have been identified in the family.

## Neuronal Ceroid Lipofuscinosis Type 8

### Physiopathology

The CLN8 gene encodes a transmembrane protein belonging to a family of proteins containing TLC domains, which are postulated to function in lipid synthesis, transport, or sensing. The protein localizes to the endoplasmic reticulum (ER) and may recycle between the ER and ER-Golgi intermediate compartment. The exact function is still not clear, but it is known that CLN8 protein belongs to the TRAM-

**Table 61.5** Ceroid lipofuscinosis, neuronal, 6

| System | Symptoms and biomarkers | Neonatal (birth–1 month) | Infancy (1–18 months) | Childhood (1.5–11 years) | Adolescence (11–16 years) | Adulthood (>16 years) |
|---|---|---|---|---|---|---|
| CNS | Ataxia | | ± | +++ | +++ | +++ |
| | **Cerebellar atrophy (MRI)** | | ± | +++ | +++ | +++ |
| | **Cerebral atrophy (MRI)** | | ± | +++ | +++ | +++ |
| | Developmental regression | | ± | +++ | +++ | +++ |
| | Dystonia | | ± | +++ | +++ | +++ |
| | EEG, abnormal | | ± | +++ | +++ | +++ |
| | ERG, abnormal | | | +++ | +++ | +++ |
| | **Movement disorder** | | | +++ | +++ | +++ |
| | Myoclonic epilepsy | | ± | +++ | +++ | +++ |
| | Myoclonus | | ± | +++ | +++ | +++ |
| | Neurodegenerative disease | | | +++ | +++ | +++ |
| | **Seizures** | | | +++ | +++ | +++ |
| | **Seizures, myoclonic** | | | +++ | +++ | +++ |
| | Seizures, tonic clonic | | | +++ | +++ | +++ |
| | Spasticity | | | +++ | +++ | +++ |
| | **Speech delay** | | | ++ | ++ | +++ |
| | SSEP, abnormal | | ± | +++ | +++ | +++ |
| | VEP, abnormal | | n | +++ | +++ | +++ |
| | White matter abnormalities (MRI) | | ± | + | ± | ± |
| Eye | **Optic atrophy** | | | ++ | +++ | +++ |
| | **Pigmentary retinopathy** | | | ++ | +++ | +++ |
| | **Retinal dystrophy** | | | ++ | +++ | +++ |
| | **Vision loss** | | | +++ | +++ | +++ |
| Musculoskeletal | **Muscular atrophy** | | + | +++ | +++ | +++ |
| | **Spinal muscular atrophy** | | + | +++ | +++ | +++ |

Laboratory and instrumental examinations (CLN6)

| | |
|---|---|
| Histologic findings and laboratory tests (electron microscopic findings) and laboratory tests | *Histologic analysis:* Electron microscopy ultrastructural studies in peripheral blood lymphocytes or other tissues (conjunctiva, skin, or other tissues) show the presence of mixed-type inclusions (curvilinear bodies, fingerprint profiles, rectilinear complex, and granular osmiophilic deposits). In neural tissues, histologic findings also include the presence of autofluorescent lipopigment in neurons; neuronal loss, especially layer V; and loss of granule cells, with relative preservation of Purkinje cells<br>Subunit C of the mitochondrial adenosine triphosphate (ATP) synthase complex accumulates in the lysosomes of patients |
| Enzyme activity | Not applicable |
| Molecular genetic testing | *Genetic variants* in CLN6 gene associated with CLN6 disease, late infantile |
| Instrumental tests | *Electroencephalogram*: Abnormal patterns of electrical activity<br>*MRI and MR spectroscopy*: Severe cerebral and cerebellar atrophy<br>*Somatosensory evoked potential*: Progressive attenuation |
| Other tests | *Neurologic examination*<br>*Ophthalmologic examination*<br>*Developmental/cognitive and educational assessment* |

Lag1p-CLN8 (TLC) family. Members of this family are involved in the biosynthesis, metabolisms, transport, and sensing of lipids. However, the specific function of the CLN8 is not known.

## Prevention

Prenatal testing for pregnancies at increased risk is possible if the disease-causing mutation(s) have been identified in the family.

**Table 61.6** Ceroid lipofuscinosis, neuronal, 7

| System | Symptoms and biomarkers | Neonatal (birth–1 month) | Infancy (1–18 months) | Childhood (1.5–11 years) | Adolescence (11–16 years) | Adulthood (>16 years) |
|---|---|---|---|---|---|---|
| CNS | Ataxia | | ± | +++ | +++ | +++ |
| | **Cerebellar atrophy (MRI)** | | ± | +++ | +++ | +++ |
| | **Cerebral atrophy (MRI)** | | ± | +++ | +++ | +++ |
| | Developmental regression | | ± | +++ | +++ | +++ |
| | Dystonia | | ± | +++ | +++ | +++ |
| | EEG, abnormal | | ± | +++ | +++ | +++ |
| | ERG, abnormal | | n | +++ | +++ | +++ |
| | **Movement disorder** | | | +++ | +++ | +++ |
| | Myoclonic epilepsy | | ± | +++ | +++ | +++ |
| | Myoclonus | | ± | +++ | +++ | +++ |
| | Neurodegenerative disease | | | +++ | +++ | +++ |
| | **Seizures** | | | +++ | +++ | +++ |
| | Seizures, myoclonic | | | +++ | +++ | +++ |
| | Seizures, tonic clonic | | | +++ | +++ | +++ |
| | Spasticity | | | +++ | +++ | +++ |
| | Speech delay | | | ++ | ++ | +++ |
| | SSEP, abnormal | | ± | +++ | +++ | +++ |
| | VEP, abnormal | | | +++ | +++ | +++ |
| | White matter abnormalities (MRI) | | ± | + | ± | ± |
| Eye | Optic atrophy | | | ++ | +++ | +++ |
| | Pigmentary retinopathy | | | ++ | +++ | +++ |
| | Retinal dystrophy | | | ++ | +++ | +++ |
| | **Vision loss** | | | +++ | +++ | +++ |
| Musculoskeletal | **Muscular atrophy** | | + | +++ | +++ | +++ |
| | **Spinal muscular atrophy** | | + | +++ | +++ | +++ |
| Psychiatric | **Behavioral disorder** | | | + | ++ | +++ |

Laboratory and instrumental examinations (CLN7)

| | |
|---|---|
| Histologic findings and laboratory tests (electron microscopic findings) and laboratory tests | *Histologic analysis*: Electron microscopy ultrastructural studies in peripheral blood lymphocytes or other tissues (conjunctiva, skin, or other tissues) show the presence of "curvilinear profiles," "fingerprint profiles" (FP), and "rectilinear complex." Intracellular accumulation of material can occur in neuronal and nonneuronal cells and may not always be apparent<br>Histologic findings also include neurodegeneration<br>Storage of subunit C of the mitochondrial adenosine triphosphate (ATP) synthase complex in lysosomes |
| Enzyme activity | Not applicable |
| Molecular genetic testing | *Molecular genetic testing* of MFSD8 gene |
| Instrumental tests | *Electroencephalography:* Shows EEG abnormalities with diffuse slowing and frequent, multifocal sharp waves<br>*Brain magnetic resonance imaging (MRI)*<br>shows atrophic changes which are more in the occipital lobe |
| Other tests | *Neurologic examination*<br>*Ophthalmologic examination*<br>*Developmental/cognitive and educational assessment* |

**Table 61.7** Ceroid lipofuscinosis, neuronal, 8

| System | Symptoms and biomarkers | Neonatal (birth–1 month) | Infancy (1–18 months) | Childhood (1.5–11 years) | Adolescence (11–16 years) | Adulthood (>16 years) |
|---|---|---|---|---|---|---|
| CNS | Ataxia | | ± | +++ | +++ | +++ |
| | **Cerebellar atrophy (MRI)** | | ± | +++ | +++ | +++ |
| | **Cerebral atrophy (MRI)** | | ± | +++ | +++ | +++ |
| | Developmental regression | | ± | +++ | +++ | +++ |
| | Dystonia | | ± | +++ | +++ | +++ |
| | EEG, abnormal | | ± | +++ | +++ | +++ |
| | ERG, abnormal | | | +++ | +++ | +++ |
| | **Movement disorder** | | | +++ | +++ | +++ |
| | Myoclonic epilepsy | | ± | +++ | +++ | +++ |
| | Myoclonus | | ± | +++ | +++ | +++ |
| | Neurodegenerative disease | | | +++ | +++ | +++ |
| | **Seizures** | | | +++ | +++ | +++ |
| | Seizures, complex partial | | | +++ | +++ | +++ |
| | Seizures, tonic clonic | | | +++ | +++ | +++ |
| | Spasticity | | | +++ | +++ | +++ |
| | Speech delay | | | ++ | ++ | +++ |
| | SSEP, abnormal | | ± | +++ | +++ | +++ |
| | VEP, abnormal | | | +++ | +++ | +++ |
| | White matter abnormalities (MRI) | | ± | + | ± | ± |
| Eye | **Optic atrophy** | | | ++ | +++ | +++ |
| | **Pigmentary retinopathy** | | | ++ | +++ | +++ |
| | **Retinal dystrophy** | | | ++ | +++ | +++ |
| | **Vision loss** | | | ++ | +++ | +++ |
| Musculoskeletal | **Muscular atrophy** | | + | +++ | +++ | +++ |
| | **Spinal muscular atrophy** | | + | +++ | +++ | +++ |
| Psychiatric | Behavioral disorder | | | + | ++ | +++ |

**Table 61.8** Ceroid lipofuscinosis, neuronal, 8, Northern Epilepsy variant (CLN8)

| System | Symptoms and biomarkers | Neonatal (birth–1 month) | Infancy (1–18 months) | Childhood (1.5–11 years) | Adolescence (11–16 years) | Adulthood (>16 years) |
|---|---|---|---|---|---|---|
| CNS | Ataxia | | | + | ++ | ++ |
| | Cerebellar atrophy (MRI) | | | | ± | + |
| | Cerebral atrophy (MRI) | | | | ± | + |
| | **Cognitive decline** | | | + | ++ | ++ |
| | EEG, abnormal | | | | +++ | +++ |
| | **Movement disorder** | | | + | ++ | ++ |
| | Myoclonus | | ± | ++ | ++ | ++ |
| | Neurodegenerative disease | | | ++ | + | + |
| | **Seizures** | | | +++ | +++ | +++ |
| | **Seizures, complex partial** | | | +++ | +++ | +++ |
| | **Seizures, tonic clonic** | | | +++ | +++ | +++ |
| | Speech delay | | | ++ | ++ | +++ |
| Metabolic | EM, Storage material | ++ | ++ | ++ | ++ | ++ |
| Psychiatric | **Behavioral disorder** | | | + | ++ | ++ |

Laboratory and instrumental examinations (CLN8)

| | |
|---|---|
| Histologic findings and laboratory tests (electron microscopic findings) and laboratory tests | *Electron microscopy studies of tissue specimens* (5–10 mL of heparinized whole blood (lymphocytes)) or tissue biopsies (now usually of skin, but previously of conjunctiva or other tissues) show intracellular accumulation of granular storage material and autofluorescent lipopigment in neurons<br>Intracellular curvilinear profiles on ultrastructural analysis<br>Lymphocytes are not usually vacuolated |
| Enzyme activity | Not applicable |
| Molecular genetic testing | Molecular analysis to confirm the diagnosis |
| Instrumental tests | *Neurologic examination with developmental/cognitive and educational assessment*<br>*EEG* shows abnormalities<br>*MRI* shows cerebral and cerebellar atrophy, progressive<br>*Somatosensory evoked magnetic field (SEF) studies* within normal limits<br>*Magnetic resonance imaging* shows slight to moderate cerebellar atrophy and might reveal slightly enlarged cerebral sulci |
| Other tests | *Clinical examination*<br>*Family history* |

## Cathepsin D Deficiency (NCL Type 10)

### Physiopathology

The CLN10 gene encodes cathepsin D, a lysosomal aspartic protease belonging to the pepsin superfamily. Cathepsin D is important for neuronal stability and maintenance of the extracellular environment. It is associated with several physiological processes such as protein degradation, autophagy, and apoptosis since it hydrolyzes a wide variety of substrates including the extracellular matrix proteins fibronectin and laminin. So far, the in vivo substrates of this enzyme have not been clearly identified although it has been reported that CTSD catalyzes the cleavage of α-synuclein, a protein associated with Parkinson's disease.

Alterations in a macroautophagy-lysosomal degradation pathway appear to mediate neurodegeneration in this disease.

### Prevention

Prenatal testing is possible in pregnancies at increased risk if biochemical studies in the proband have revealed deficient activity of the enzyme CTSD, or if the disease-causing mutation(s) have been identified in the proband and parents. In these instances, testing is performed on fetal cells obtained by chorionic villus sampling (CVS) at about 10–12 weeks' gestation or amniocentesis usually performed at about 15–18 weeks' gestation. (Gestational age is expressed as menstrual weeks calculated either from the first day of the last normal menstrual period or by ultrasound measurements.)

Preimplantation genetic diagnosis (PGD) may be an option for some families in which the disease-causing mutations have been identified.

## Progranulin Deficiency (NCL Type 11 Recessive)

### Physiopathology

The CLN11 gene encodes progranulin (PGRN), originally described as a growth factor that regulates wound healing, vasculogenesis, and tumor growth. Within the central nervous system, GRN-mRNA is expressed in a variety of cell types including neuron, microglia, astrocytes, and endothelial cells. It has been suggested that signaling pathways downstream of Akt may also be activated by progranulin. In macrophages, granulins, cleaved from PGRN, bind to CpG oligodeoxynucleotides in lysosomes, enabling Toll-like receptor-9 signaling. Mutations in the PGRN gene are responsible for frontotemporal lobar degeneration with distinct neuropathological features consisting of ubiquitin-positive protein aggregates in the nucleus and cytoplasm of cortical neurons related to the lysosomal dysfunction. The role of PGRN in this disease is anyway still not clear, and more research is needed to advance our understanding of the induced pathogenesis.

### Prevention

Prenatal testing for pregnancies at increased risk is possible if the disease-causing mutation(s) have been identified in the family.

**Table 61.9** Ceroid lipofuscinosis, neuronal, 10

| System | Symptoms and biomarkers | Neonatal (birth–1 month) | Infancy (1–18 months) | Childhood (1.5–11 years) | Adolescence (11–16 years) | Adulthood (>16 years) |
|---|---|---|---|---|---|---|
| CNS | Ataxia | | + | +++ | +++ | +++ |
| | **Cerebellar atrophy (MRI)** | +++ | +++ | + | ++ | + |
| | **Cerebral atrophy (MRI)** | +++ | +++ | + | ++ | + |
| | **Congenital encephalopathy** | +++ | +++ | | | |
| | Developmental regression | | | + | ++ | ++ |
| | **EEG, abnormal** | +++ | +++ | + | + | + |
| | **Epilepsy** | +++ | +++ | + | + | + |
| | ERG, abnormal | | | +++ | +++ | +++ |
| | Language difficulties | | | ++ | +++ | +++ |
| | **Movement disorder** | +++ | +++ | + | ++ | ++ |
| | Myoclonus | | | + | + | + |
| | Neurodegenerative disease | +++ | +++ | ++ | ++ | ++ |
| | Seizures | +++ | +++ | + | + | + |
| | **Spasticity** | +++ | +++ | + | + | + |
| | SSEP, abnormal | | | ++ | ++ | + |
| | VEP, abnormal | | | +++ | +++ | +++ |
| Eye | Optic atrophy | | | + | ++ | ++ |
| | Pigmentary retinopathy | | | +++ | +++ | +++ |
| | Retinal dystrophy | | | ++ | +++ | ++ |
| | Vision loss | | | ++ | +++ | +++ |
| Metabolic | EM, Storage material | +++ | +++ | +++ | +++ | +++ |
| Musculoskeletal | **Microcephaly** | +++ | +++ | | | |
| | Microcephaly | +++ | +++ | | | |
| | **Muscular atrophy** | +++ | +++ | + | ++ | + |
| | Spinal muscular atrophy | +++ | +++ | + | ++ | + |
| Laboratory findings | Cathepsin D (dried blood spot) | ↓↓↓ | ↓↓↓ | ↓↓↓ | ↓↓↓ | ↓↓↓ |
| | Cathepsin D (fibroblasts) | ↓↓↓ | ↓↓↓ | ↓↓↓ | ↓↓↓ | ↓↓↓ |
| | Cathepsin D (leukocytes) | ↓↓↓ | ↓↓↓ | ↓↓↓ | ↓↓↓ | ↓↓↓ |

Laboratory and instrumental examinations (CLN10)

| | |
|---|---|
| Histologic findings and laboratory tests (electron microscopic findings) and laboratory tests | *Electron microscopy ultrastructural studies* in peripheral blood lymphocytes or other tissues (conjunctiva, skin, or other tissues) show the presence of autofluorescent granular osmiophilic deposits (GRODs). This granular lipopigment material can be identified in astrocytes, macrophages, and residual neurons. Similar material can be observed in cells from the liver, spleen, thymus, and lung. Histologic findings also include severe neuronal loss in the cerebrum and cerebellum, extensive gliosis, and white matter almost devoid of axons and myelin<br>*Neuropathologic examination* showed severe cerebral atrophy and diffuse ballooning of neurons with autofluorescent lipid accumulation<br>Decrease or absence of cathepsin D (CTSD) protein immunostaining in brain tissue<br>Presence of non-vacuolated lymphocytes |
| Enzyme activity | *Measurement of enzymatic activity of cathepsin D* (CTSD) in leukocytes and cultured skin fibroblast cells |
| Molecular genetic testing | *Molecular genetic testing* of CTSD gene |
| Instrumental tests | *Magnetic resonance imaging (MRI)* shows cerebral and cerebellar atrophy |
| Other tests | |

**Table 61.10** Ceroid lipofuscinosis, neuronal, 11

| System | Symptoms and biomarkers | Neonatal (birth–1 month) | Infancy (1–18 months) | Childhood (1.5–11 years) | Adolescence (11–16 years) | Adulthood (>16 years) |
|---|---|---|---|---|---|---|
| CNS | **Ataxia** | | | | | + |
| | **Cerebellar atrophy (MRI)** | | | | | + |
| | EEG, abnormal | | | | | + |
| | ERG, abnormal | | | | | ++ |
| | Language difficulties | | | | | + |
| | Movement disorder | | | | | + |
| | Seizures | | | | | + |
| Eye | **Retinal dystrophy** | | | | | ++ |
| | **Vision loss** | | | | | ++ |
| Metabolic | EM, Storage material | | | | | +++ |
| Musculoskeletal | **Muscular atrophy** | | | | | + |
| | **Spinal muscular atrophy** | | | | | + |

Laboratory and instrumental examinations (CLN11)

| | |
|---|---|
| Histologic findings and laboratory tests (electron microscopic findings) and laboratory tests | *Electron microscopy ultrastructural studies* in peripheral blood lymphocytes or other tissues (conjunctiva, skin, or other tissues) show the presence of numerous "fingerprint profiles"<br>*Measurement of plasma progranulin levels*: undetectable in the homozygous patients and about 50% decreased in the heterozygous parents<br>Presence of non-vacuolated lymphocytes |
| Enzyme activity | Not applicable |
| Molecular genetic testing | *Molecular genetic testing* of GRN gene |
| Instrumental tests | *Electroencephalography* showed generalized polyspike wave discharges<br>*Electroretinography* showed severe attenuation of both rod and cone responses<br>*Magnetic resonance imaging (MRI)* showed cerebellar atrophy<br>Visual evoked potential (VEP): polyphasic VEP waveform suggesting hyperexcitability of the occipital cortex<br>*Somatosensory evoked potential*: progressive attenuation in all NCLs<br>*Visual evoked potential (VEP):* polyphasic VEP waveform suggesting hyperexcitability of the occipital cortex |
| Other tests | *Neurologic examination*<br>*Ophthalmologic examination*<br>*Developmental/cognitive and educational assessment* |

## ATP13A2 Deficiency (NCL Type 12)

### Physiopathology

The ATP13A2 gene encodes a member of the P5 subfamily of ATPases which transports inorganic cations as well as other substrates. In most human tissues, ATP13A2-mRNA is detectable, but it is expressed at a high level in the ventral midbrain, including substantia nigra, and to a lesser extent in the kidney and skeletal muscle. Interestingly, oxidative stress is found to increase the expression of the CLN12/ATP13A2-mRNA. This protein is highly expressed in neurons and is predicted to function as a cation pump, playing a role as a cation transporter regulating Mn2+, Zn2+, and Mg2+ homeostasis with H+ ion concentration in the cell. Being cation regulation and homeostasis vital for neuronal function including intra- and intercellular signaling, dysfunction of the ATP13A2 may be responsible for the dysregulated neurotransmission and eventual dementia characteristic of this disease. Indeed, accumulation of zinc and mitochondrial dysfunction are established etiological factors that contribute to Parkinson's disease; however, their underlying molecular mechanisms are largely unknown.

Mitochondrial dysfunction and autophagy are centrally implicated in Parkinson's disease (PD). It has been suggested that ATP13A2 helps maintain optimal pH in lysosomes where ceramide is also metabolized. The apoptosis that appears to cause NCLs is associated with increased levels of ceramide, which might have also been linked to α-synuclein deposition, contributing to PD pathogenesis. It may be that ATP13A2 helps regulate ceramide metabolism, such that significant changes inATP13A2 activity may contribute to the pathogenesis of both PD and NCLs.

**Table 61.11** Ceroid lipofuscinosis, neuronal, 12

| System | Symptoms and biomarkers | Neonatal (birth–1 month) | Infancy (1–18 months) | Childhood (1.5–11 years) | Adolescence (11–16 years) | Adulthood (>16 years) |
|---|---|---|---|---|---|---|
| CNS | **Akinesia** | | | | ++ | +++ |
| | Cognitive dysfunction | | | + | ++ | +++ |
| | Dysarthria | | | | + | ++ |
| | Extrapyramidal movement disorder | | | | + | ++ |
| | Gait disturbance | | | | ++ | +++ |
| | **Movement disorder** | | | | + | ++ |
| | **Myoclonus** | | | | + | +++ |
| | Neurodegenerative disease | | | | + | ++ |
| Metabolic | EM, Storage material | | | | +++ | +++ |
| Musculoskeletal | **Rigidity** | | | | ++ | +++ |
| Psychiatric | **Behavioral disorder** | | | | + | ++ |

Laboratory and instrumental examinations (CLN12/PARK9)

| | |
|---|---|
| Histologic findings and laboratory tests (electron microscopic findings) and laboratory tests | *Light and electron microscopy ultrastructural studies:* Light and electron microscopic investigations of intracellular storage that, when performed in the logical order shown, lead straight and economically to adequate molecular genetic confirmation<br>Presence of non-vacuolated lymphocytes |
| Enzyme activity | Not applicable |
| Molecular genetic testing | *Sequences analysis* ATP13A2 |
| Instrumental tests | *EEG* shows nonspecific disorganization and spike-and-slow-wave complexes<br>*Computed tomography and MRI* reveal cerebral and, to a lesser degree, cerebellar atrophy in the later stages (age > 15 years)<br>*Ophthalmologic examination* may reveal macular changes only; gradually, typical signs of pan-retinal degeneration develop: pigmentary changes in the retinal periphery, vascular attenuation, and optic nerve pallor<br>*ERG* shows loss of photoreceptor function early on<br>*Developmental/cognitive and educational assessment*: Speech disturbances (festinating stuttering, often mislabelled as echolalia) and slow decline in cognition occur around the time of onset of seizures. Behavioral problems, extrapyramidal signs, and sleep disturbance occur in the second decade<br>*Cardiological assessment*: Cardiac involvement late in the disease, progressive cardiac involvement with repolarization disturbances, ventricular hypertrophy, and sinus node dysfunction |
| Other tests | *Medical genetics consultation*<br>*Psychiatric examination*: Psychiatric problems including disturbed thoughts, attention problems, somatic complaints, and aggressive behavior |

### Prevention

Prenatal testing is possible in pregnancies at increased risk if the disease-causing mutation(s) have been identified in the proband and parents. In these instances, testing is performed on fetal cells obtained by chorionic villus sampling (CVS) at about 10–12 weeks' gestation or amniocentesis usually performed at about 15–18 weeks' gestation.

## Cathepsin F Deficiency (NCL Type 13)

### Physiopathology

Kufs disease type B can be due to variants to the *DNAJC5* and cathepsin F (CTSF) genes with *CTSF* mutations accounting for a minority of cases of type B Kufs. Mutations in cathepsin F as the causative gene for autosomal recessive Kufs disease type B have been only recently identified. When the *CTSF* gene is mutated, it cannot produce cathepsin F, an enzyme that cuts proteins in the lysozyme. CTSF is a cysteine protease synthesized in the ER. CTSF is tagged with mannose 6-phosphate residues in the cis-Golgi and transported by CI-M6PR to the late endosomal/lysosomal compartment. CTSF is highly expressed in cerebrocortical, hippocampal, and cerebellar neurons. By cutting proteins, cathepsin F can modify the function of the proteins as well as help break them down. Dysfunction leads to incomplete breakdown of proteins. Once again, lipopigments build up, and brain function is decreased as the neuron cells.

### Prevention

Prenatal testing for pregnancies at increased risk is possible if the disease-causing mutation(s) have been identified in the family.

**Table 61.12** Ceroid lipofuscinosis, neuronal, 13

| System | Symptoms and biomarkers | Neonatal (birth–1 month) | Infancy (1–18 months) | Childhood (1.5–11 years) | Adolescence (11–16 years) | Adulthood (>16 years) |
|---|---|---|---|---|---|---|
| CNS | Ataxia | | | | | + |
| | **Cerebellar atrophy (MRI)** | | | | | + |
| | **Cerebral atrophy (MRI)** | | | | | + |
| | **Cognitive decline** | | | | | ++ |
| | Dysarthria | | | | | + |
| | **Extrapyramidal movement disorder** | | | | | ++ |
| | Movement disorder | | | | | + |
| | **Neurodegenerative disease** | | | | | ++ |
| | Seizures | | | | | + |
| | Seizures, tonic clonic | | | | | + |
| Metabolic | EM, Storage material | | | | | ± |
| Musculoskeletal | Muscular atrophy | | | | | + |
| | Spinal muscular atrophy | | | | | + |
| Psychiatric | **Behavioral disorder** | | | | | + |

Laboratory and instrumental examinations (CLN13)

| | |
|---|---|
| Histologic findings and laboratory tests (electron microscopic findings) and laboratory tests | *Histologic findings:* Electron microscopy ultrastructural studies in peripheral blood lymphocytes or other tissues (conjunctiva, skin, or other tissues) often show the presence of fingerprint profiles<br>Abundant autofluorescent material is found in the cytoplasm of neurons of the cerebral cortex, thalamus, striatum, brainstem nuclei, and Purkinje cells. This storage material is immunoreactive for ubiquitin and contained fingerprint profiles |
| Enzyme activity | *Measurement of enzymatic activity of cathepsin F (CTSF)* in leukocytes and cultured skin fibroblast cells |
| Molecular genetic testing | *Molecular genetic testing* on CTSF gene |
| Instrumental tests | *Brain MRI* showed diffuse cerebral atrophy |
| Other tests | |

## Neuronal Ceroid Lipofuscinosis Type 14

### Physiopathology

KCTD7 gene (potassium channel tetramerization domain containing 7) encodes a member of the potassium channel tetramerization domain-containing protein family. Family members are identified on a structural basis and contain an amino-terminal domain similar to the T1 domain present in the voltage-gated potassium channel. Mutations in this gene have been associated with progressive myoclonic epilepsy-3, a clinically defined epileptic syndrome that manifests as myoclonic seizures and progressive neurological dysfunction before age 2 years and accompanied by developmental regression. Alternative splicing results in multiple transcript variants. KCTD7 encoded protein is a highly conserved soluble cytosolic protein localized in various organs indicating that it plays a role in the hyperpolarization of the cell membrane via interaction with a component of the ubiquitin ligase complex. It also directly interacts with Cullin-3, a component of E3 ubiquitin-protein ligases, for degradation by ubiquitin proteasome system. Missense mutations in the KCTD gene found in CLN14 disease disrupt KCTD7-Cullin-3 interactions, suggesting a role in the impairment of the cellular degradative process.

### Prevention

No data.

## Ceroid Lipofuscinosis, Neuronal, 1

### Physiopathology

The neuronal ceroid lipofuscinoses (NCLs; CLNs) are a clinically and genetically heterogeneous group of neurodegenerative disorders characterized by the intracellular accumulation of autofluorescent lipopigment storage material in different patterns.

The lipopigment pattern seen most often in CLN1 is referred to as granular osmiophilic deposits (GROD), with characteristic accumulation of saposins A and D.

In CLN1 NCL, a lysosomal enzyme, palmitoyl protein thioesterase 1 (PPT1), is deficient. PPT1, which removes fatty acyl groups from cysteine residues on fatty acid-modified proteins, remains in the endoplasmic reticulum, where it is inactive, causing saposins A and D to accumulate in the lysosomes.

**Table 61.13** Ceroid lipofuscinosis, neuronal, 14

| System | Symptoms and biomarkers | Neonatal (birth–1 month) | Infancy (1–18 months) | Childhood (1.5–11 years) | Adolescence (11–16 years) | Adulthood (>16 years) |
|---|---|---|---|---|---|---|
| CNS | Ataxia | | | ++ | +++ | +++ |
| | **Cerebellar atrophy (MRI)** | | + | ++ | +++ | +++ |
| | **Cerebral atrophy (MRI)** | | + | ++ | +++ | +++ |
| | Developmental regression | | | +++ | +++ | +++ |
| | EEG, abnormal | | + | +++ | +++ | +++ |
| | **Epilepsy** | | + | +++ | +++ | +++ |
| | Hypokinesia | | | ++ | +++ | +++ |
| | **Language difficulties** | | | +++ | +++ | +++ |
| | **Movement disorder** | | | +++ | +++ | +++ |
| | Myoclonic epilepsy | | + | +++ | +++ | +++ |
| | Neurodegenerative disease | | | +++ | +++ | +++ |
| | Seizures, myoclonic | | + | +++ | +++ | +++ |
| | Speech delay | | | +++ | +++ | +++ |
| Eye | **Optic atrophy** | | | +++ | +++ | +++ |
| | **Vision loss** | | | +++ | +++ | +++ |
| Metabolic | EM, Storage material | | | | +++ | +++ |
| Musculoskeletal | Microcephaly | | | +++ | +++ | +++ |
| | **Muscular atrophy** | ± | ++ | +++ | +++ | +++ |
| | **Spinal muscular atrophy** | ± | ++ | +++ | +++ | +++ |

Laboratory and instrumental examinations (CLN14/EPM3)

| | |
|---|---|
| Histologic findings and laboratory tests (electron microscopic findings) and laboratory tests | Electron microscopy ultrastructural studies: Presence of granular osmiophilic deposits with fingerprint profiles<br>Lymphocytes' vacuolation is absent |
| Enzyme activity | Not applicable |
| Molecular genetic testing | KCTD7 mutation screening should be considered in progressive myoclonus epilepsies (PME) patients with onset around 2 years of age followed by rapid mental and motor deterioration<br>Metabolic screening and normal routine blood test including lactate, chromatography of amino acids in plasma and urine, organic acids in urine<br>Genetic variations associated with progressive myoclonic epilepsy type 3 |
| Instrumental tests | EEG shows slowed dysrhythmia and multifocal discharges<br>EEG with photic stimulation to provoke frequency-dependent spike-wave activity with increase of myoclonic seizures raising<br>Cerebral morphological magnetic resonance imaging can show cerebral and cerebellar atrophy, thinning of the corpus callosum<br>Evoked potential of nervus tibialis and medianus on both sides might present a slightly delayed cortical answer to stimulation with normal amplitude (no giant potentials)<br>Fundoscopy<br>Abdominal ultrasonography |
| Other tests | Family pedigree |

## Prevention

Prenatal testing is possible in pregnancies at increased risk if biochemical studies in the proband have revealed deficient activity of the enzyme PPT-1, or if the disease-causing mutation(s) have been identified in the proband and parents. In these instances, testing is performed on fetal cells obtained by chorionic villus sampling (CVS) at about 10–12 weeks' gestation or amniocentesis usually performed at about 15 to 18 weeks' gestation. (Gestational age is expressed as menstrual weeks calculated either from the first day of the last normal menstrual period or by ultrasound measurements.)

Preimplantation genetic diagnosis (PGD) may be an option for some families in which the disease-causing mutations have been identified.

**Table 61.14** Ceroid lipofuscinosis, neuronal, 1

| System | Symptoms and biomarkers | Neonatal (birth–1 month) | Infancy (1–18 months) | Childhood (1.5–11 years) | Adolescence (11–16 years) | Adulthood (>16 years) |
|---|---|---|---|---|---|---|
| CNS | Ataxia | | + | +++ | +++ | +++ |
| | Cerebellar atrophy (MRI) | ± | ++ | +++ | +++ | +++ |
| | **Cerebral atrophy (MRI)** | ± | ++ | +++ | +++ | +++ |
| | **Developmental regression** | | ++ | +++ | +++ | +++ |
| | Dystonia | | + | +++ | +++ | +++ |
| | EEG, abnormal | | + | +++ | +++ | +−+ |
| | **Epilepsy** | | ± | +++ | +++ | +++ |
| | ERG, abnormal | | + | +++ | +++ | +++ |
| | Language difficulties | | + | +++ | +++ | +++ |
| | **Movement disorder** | | + | +++ | +++ | +++ |
| | Myoclonic epilepsy | | ± | +++ | +++ | +++ |
| | Myoclonus | | + | +++ | +++ | +++ |
| | Neurodegenerative disease | | ++ | +++ | +++ | +++ |
| | **Seizures, myoclonic** | | ± | +++ | +++ | +++ |
| | Seizures, tonic clonic | | ± | +++ | +++ | +++ |
| | Spasticity | | ± | +++ | +++ | +++ |
| | Speech delay | | + | +++ | +++ | +++ |
| | SSEP, abnormal | | ± | +++ | +++ | +++ |
| | VEP, abnormal | | ± | +++ | +++ | +++ |
| | White matter abnormalities (MRI) | | ++ | ++ | ± | ± |
| Eye | **Maculopathy** | | ± | +++ | +++ | +++ |
| | Optic atrophy | | + | +++ | +++ | +++ |
| | **Retinopathy** | | ± | +++ | +++ | +++ |
| | **Vision loss** | ± | + | +++ | +++ | +++ |
| Metabolic | EM, Storage material | ++ | +++ | +++ | +++ | ++− |
| Musculoskeletal | Microcephaly | ± | ++ | +++ | +++ | +++ |
| | Muscular atrophy | ± | ++ | +++ | +++ | +++ |
| | Spinal muscular atrophy | ± | ++ | +++ | +++ | +++ |
| Laboratory findings | Lysosomal palmitoyl protein thioesterase-1 (dried blood spot) | ↓↓↓ | ↓↓↓ | ↓↓↓ | ↓↓↓ | ↓↓↓ |
| | Lysosomal palmitoyl protein thioesterase-1 (fibroblasts) | ↓↓↓ | ↓↓↓ | ↓↓↓ | ↓↓↓ | ↓↓↓ |
| | Lysosomal palmitoyl protein thioesterase-1 (leukocytes) | ↓↓↓ | ↓↓↓ | ↓↓↓ | ↓↓↓ | ↓↓↓ |

Laboratory and instrumental examinations (CLN1)

| | |
|---|---|
| Histologic findings (electron microscopic findings) | Electron microscopy ultrastructural studies in peripheral blood lymphocytes or other tissues (conjunctiva, skin, or other tissues) show the presence of autofluorescent granular osmiophilic deposits (GROD) with characteristic accumulation of saposins A and D<br>Not vacuolated lymphocytes<br>Almost complete loss of cortical neurons |
| Enzyme activity | Deficient activity of palmitoyl-protein thioesterase 1 (PPT-1) encoded by PPT1 evidenced by fluorimetric assay based on the fluorochrome 4-methylumbelliferone in leukocytes, dry blood samples, cultured skin fibroblast cells, amniotic fluid cells, or chorionic villi |
| Molecular genetic testing | Targeted analysis for pathogenic variants<br>Sequence analysis for assessment of sequence variants<br>Deletion/duplication analysis |
| Instrumental tests | *Electroencephalography:* Electroencephalographic characteristics seen in CLN1 NCL include lack of attenuation of posterior dominant rhythm to eye opening, loss of sleep spindles, progressive background abnormality, and attenuation with the background flat by age 3 years<br>*Electroretinography*: Unrecordable at age 3 years<br>*Visual evoked potential*: Unrecordable at age 4 years<br>*Somatosensory evoked potential*: Progressive attenuation in all NCLs<br>*Magnetic resonance imaging (MRI):* Mild cerebral atrophy that progresses after 4 years, decreased T2 signal intensity in the thalami, callosal thinning, periventricular rims of hyperintensity that progress to diffuse white matter hyperintensity on T2, and cerebellar atrophy after age 3 years<br>*Magnetic resonance (MR) spectroscopy:* Almost complete loss of N-acetylaspartate (metabolite present only in neurons), reduction in creatine- and choline-containing compounds (i.e., markers for glial membrane turnover), elevation of myoinositol (i.e., a glial marker), elevation of lactate in gray and white matter |

## Current Treatment Strategies

Being the NCL inherited metabolic disorders, any therapeutic approach will need to be strictly connected to the primary metabolic defect. For the majority of NCLs, so far, there is no specific treatment, and current disease management is mainly aimed at controlling the symptoms rather than "curing" the disease.

**The only specific treatment available for NCL is cerliponase alfa for neuronal ceroid lipofuscinosis type 2 (CLN2, also known as tripeptidyl peptidase 1 [TPP1] deficiency).** Cerliponase alfa is an enzyme replacement therapy (ERT) approved by the FDA in April 2017 and by the CE in June 2017, to slow the loss of ambulation in symptomatic pediatric patients aged 3 years or older with late infantile neuronal CLN2. Recent studies confirm that the decline in motor and language functions is decreased in patients treated with alfa cerliponase compared to their historical controls (Schulz et al. 2018).

The drug requires weekly intraventricular administration via a reservoir surgically implanted under the scalp. The recommended dosage for cerliponase alfa is 300 mg (10 mL solution) administered every other week by intraventricular infusion.

**Standard anticonvulsant drugs to control seizures in NCLs** to terminate clinical and electrical seizure activity as rapidly as possible and to prevent seizure recurrence (from Goldenberg 2010)

| Drug | Chemical name | Molecular weight | Brand and other names | Indication | Action | Mechanism of action |
|---|---|---|---|---|---|---|
| Carbamazepine | 5H-Dibenz[b, f] azepine-5-carboxamide | 236.27 | (Tegretol, Carbatrol, Epitol, Equetro) | Treatment of complex partial seizures (To control generalized tonic-clonic (grand mal) and complex partial (psychomotor, temporal lobe) seizures and for preventing and treating seizures occurring during or following neurosurgery) | May reduce polysynaptic responses and block post-tetanic potentiation | Reduction of sustained, high-frequency, repetitive neural firing |
| Oxcarbazepine | 10,11-Dihydro-10-oxo-5H-dibenz[b,f] aze-pine-5-carboxamide | 252.27 | (Trileptal) | Anticonvulsant Monotherapy for adults and in children 4 to 16 years of age with partial seizures and as adjunctive therapy for children 2 years of age and older and for adults and children 2 to 16 years of age with partial seizures | May block voltage-sensitive sodium channels, inhibit repetitive neuronal firing, and impair synaptic impulse propagation | Increased potassium conductance and modulation of high-voltage activated calcium channels |

| Drug | Chemical name | Molecular weight | Brand and other names | Indication | Action | Mechanism of action |
|---|---|---|---|---|---|---|
| Valproic | -N-propyl acetic acid | 144 | Acid (Depakote, Depakene, Depacon, Stavzor) | Status epilepticus: primary generalized tonic-clonic seizures Partial and generalized seizures and is indicated as monotherapy and adjunctive therapy for complex partial seizures, which begin in a limited area of the brain. These seizures may occur either in isolation or in association with other types of seizures | Increase brain concentrations of GABA.1 | Not established |
| Gabapentin | 1-(Aminomethyl) cyclohexaneacetic acid | 171.24 | (Neurontin) | Status epilepticus: Adjunctive therapy for patients older than 12 years of age with partial seizures with and without secondary generalization Adjunctive therapy for pediatric patients 3–12 years of age with partial seizures Nerve pain | Mimic the neurotransmitter GABA | Not established |
| Topiramate | 2,3:4,5-Di-O-isopropylidene-β-d-fructopyranose sulfamate | 339.36 | (Topamax) | Primary generalized tonic-clonic seizures Adjunctive therapy for adult and pediatric patients 2 to 16 years of age with partial-onset seizures Initial monotherapy in patients 10 years of age and older with partial-onset or primary generalized tonic-clonic seizures | Potentiate the inhibitory activity of the neurotransmitter GABA. In addition, topiramate may block glutamate activity | Not well established: Probable inhibition of voltage-dependent sodium channels; may increase activity of the neurotransmitter GABA at some subtypes of the GABAA receptor, and antagonize the AMPA/kainate subtype of the glutamate receptor, and inhibit the carbonic anhydrase enzyme, particularly isozymes II and IV |
| Tiagabine | (−)-(R)-1-[4,4-Bis(3-methyl-2-thienyl)-3-butenyl]nipecotic acid HCl | 412.0 | (Gabitril) | Adjunctive therapy in adults and children 12 years of age and older with partial seizures | Enhanced activity of GABA | Not well established: It is believed to be related to recognition sites associated with the GABA uptake carrier, therefore blocking GABA uptake into presynaptic neurons and thus increasing the quantity of GABA available for receptor binding on the surfaces of postsynaptic cells |

| Drug | Chemical name | Molecular weight | Brand and other names | Indication | Action | Mechanism of action |
|---|---|---|---|---|---|---|
| Felbamate | 2-Phenyl-1,3-propanediol dicarbamate | 238.24 | (Felbatol) | | Weak inhibitory effects on GABA receptor binding and benzodiazepine receptor binding | Antagonist at the strychnine-insensitive glycine recognition site of the N-methyl-D-aspartate (NMDA) receptor-ionophore complex |
| Midazolam | 8-Chloro-6-(2-fluorophenyl)-1-methyl-4H-imidazo[1,5-a][1,4] benzodiazepine | 325.8 | (Versed) | Emergency management of seizures<br>Sleep problems | Anxiolytic, amnestic, hypnotic, anticonvulsant, and sedative action | Binding to the benzodiazepine receptor at the GABA receptor-chloride ionophore complex in the central nervous system (CNS). It induces an increase in the opening of chloride channels and membrane hyperpolarization and increases the inhibitory effect of GABA in the CNS. Midazolam may also interfere with the reuptake of GABA, thereby causing accumulation of GABA in the synaptic cleft |
| Phenobarbital | 5-Ethyl-5-phenylpyrimidine-2,4,6(1H,3H,5H)-trione | 232.24 | (Solfoton, Luminal) | Seizures that occur in neonates and in the first year of life<br>Both generalized tonic-clonic seizures and partial seizures in patients of all ages<br>Phenobarbital is used to treat status epilepticus (continuous seizures with impaired consciousness between episodes) | Potentiated inhibitory neurotransmission | Increased duration of time that GABA-mediated chloride channels remain open and reduced neurotransmitter release from nerve terminals, probably due to effect on calcium channels<br>Decreased excitatory neurotransmission due to a reduced effect of glutamate |
| Valproate | 2-Propylpentanoic acid | 144.21 | (Convulex, Depakote, Epilim, Stavzor, and others) | Tonic-clonic seizures<br>Mioclonus | Anticonvulsant effect | Not well established: It seems to be due to the blockade of voltage-gated sodium channels and increased brain levels of gamma-aminobutyric acid (GABA) |
| Zonisamide | 1,2-Benzisoxazole-3-methanesulfonamide | 212.23 | (Zonegran) | Adjunctive therapy for treating partial seizures in adults | Reduces sustained high-frequency repetitive firing of action potentials and prevents the spread of seizure discharge across cells | Not well established, probable inactivation of voltage-sensitive sodium channels and inhibition of low-threshold T-type calcium channels in neurons |

| Drug | Chemical name | Molecular weight | Brand and other names | Indication | Action | Mechanism of action |
|---|---|---|---|---|---|---|
| Levetiracetam | (−)-(S)-α-Ethyl-2-oxo-1-pyrrolidine acetamide | 170.21 | (Keppra, Keppra XR, Spritam) | Adjunctive therapy for partial-onset seizures and epilepsy in adults and children 4 years of age and older<br>Myoclonic seizures in adults and adolescents 12 years of age and older with juvenile myoclonic epilepsy<br>And primary generalized tonic-clonic seizures in adults and children 6 years of age and older with idiopathic generalized epilepsy | May selectively prevent hypersynchronization of epileptiform burst firing and propagation of seizure activity | Modulation of synaptic neurotransmitter release through binding to the synaptic vesicle protein SV2A in the brain |

Drugs used to control myoclonia and spasticity

| Drug | Chemical name | Molecular weight | Brand and other names | Indication | Action | Mechanism of action |
|---|---|---|---|---|---|---|
| Baclofen | 4-Amino-3-(4-chlorophenyl) butyric acid | 213.661 | Lioresal | Myoclonia and spasticity | GABA agonist used as a skeletal muscle relaxant | Reduces the release of excitatory neurotransmitters and substance P by binding to the GABA-B receptor |
| Tizanidine | 5-Chloro-4-(2-imidazolin-2-yl-amino)-2,1,3-benzothiadiazole monohydrochloride | 253.71 | Zanaflex | Myoclonia and spasticity | Central alpha-2-adrenergic receptor agonist | Reduces spasticity by increasing presynaptic inhibition of motor neurons |
| Piracetam | 2-(2-Oxopyrrolidin-1-yl) acetamide | 142.156 | Nootropil | Adult patients suffering from myoclonus of cortical origin | Neuroprotective and anticonvulsant | Piracetam's mode of action in cortical myoclonus is as yet unknown |

Other helping supportive means of utmost importance in these chronic diseases characterized by a multiplicity of symptoms and affected systems include chest physiotherapy, nasogastric or gastric tube feeding in the later stages of the disease, orthopedic treatment, speech therapy, and psychological and transition (Kohlschütter et al. 2019). In particular physical and occupational therapies are routinely used to aid in the retention of physical abilities (Neverman et al. 2015).

Some antiepileptic drugs like carbamazepine, phenytoin, and vigabatrin can exacerbate myoclonia. These drugs should therefore be avoided especially in the late infantile NCL types that commonly manifest a high prevalence of myoclonic seizures, although they can improve control of tonic-clonic seizures when these are refractory to other medications. Clinical distinction among NCL forms is therefore important for the therapeutic choice (Augustine et al. 2015).

Drug to be avoided

| Drug | Chemical name | Molecular weight | Brand and other names | Indication | Action | Mechanism of action |
|---|---|---|---|---|---|---|
| Carbamazepine | 5H-Dibenz[b, f] azepine-5-carboxamide | 236.27 | (Tegretol, Carbatrol, Epitol, Equetro) | Treatment of complex partial seizures (To control generalized tonic-clonic (grand mal) and complex partial (psychomotor, temporal lobe) seizures and for preventing and treating seizures occurring during or following neurosurgery) | May reduce polysynaptic responses and block post-tetanic potentiation | Reduction of sustained, high-frequency, repetitive neural firing |
| Phenytoin | Sodium 5,5-diphenyl-2, 4-imidazolidinedione | 274.3 | (Dilantin, Phenytek) | Status epilepticus: For controlling generalized tonic-clonic (grand mal) and complex partial (psychomotor, temporal lobe) seizures and for preventing and treating seizures occurring during or following neurosurgery | Selective block of high-frequency neuronal activity | Suppression of the sodium action potential through a voltage-dependent blockade of membrane sodium channels (Yaari et al. 1986) |
| Vigabatrin | 4-Amino-5-hexenoic acid | 129.16 | (Sabril, Vigadrone) | It is used in patients who have already been treated with other medicines that did not work well. For treating complex partial seizures in adults and children 10 years of age and older and infantile spasms in children | Increased concentrations of GABA in the CNS | The precise mechanism of the antiseizure effect is unknown, but it is believed to result from its action as an irreversible inhibitor of GABA transaminase (GABA-T), the enzyme responsible for the metabolism of the inhibitory neurotransmitter GABA |

Recently also the use and effectiveness of Lamotrigine have been debated since it may worsen myoclonus in the early stages of CLN2 disease, late infantile (Shorvon, et al. 2019).

| | | | | | | |
|---|---|---|---|---|---|---|
| Lamotrigine | 3,5-Diamino-6-(2,3-dichlorophenyl)-as-triazine | 256.09 | (Lamictal) | Adjunctive therapy for partial seizures, and primary generalized tonic-clonic seizures Neuralgic pain | Diminished neuronal activity | Inhibition of the release of glutamate and also inactivation of voltage-sensitive sodium channels, with stabilization of the neuronal membrane |

## Emerging Causal Treatment

Several major therapeutic options are under investigations: The majority - enzyme replacement therapy; gene therapy; bone marrow transplantation; neural stem cell therapy; and molecular or pharmacological chaperone therapy—are aimed at reducing the levels of the compounds that accumulate in the lysosomes.

- **Enzyme replacement therapy (ERT):** It usually consists in the regular intravenous infusions of a recombinant form of the defective enzyme which is then scavenged by affected cells, endocytosed, and incorporated into lysosomes restoring functional activity. Unfortunately, ERT does not cross the blood-brain barrier, thus hindering effective treatment of CLNs with CNS involvement. Therefore, it is necessary to inject the enzyme to the cerebrospinal fluid, either directly into the lateral ventricles or by intrathecal injection (needle in the back). ERT is currently available for CLN2 and under study for CLN1.
- **Gene therapy** is currently only utilized in animal models. Multiple viral vectors have been used to accomplish in vivo gene transfer, such as herpesviruses, lentiviruses, adeno-associated viruses (AAV), adenoviruses (Ad), and others. Gene therapy approaches have shown promising results in animal models of various NCLs with improvements already made in vectors used for delivery of the genes. Importantly recent findings indicate that early ther-

apy (i.e., presymptomatic) provides best results (Kohlschütter et al. 2019).

- **Bone marrow transplant (BMT):** It consists in using donor bone marrow-derived cells as a source of enzyme. Studies in animal models as well as in a few infants have so far not showed satisfactory results. Nevertheless, BMT in combination with gene therapy provides an unprecedented increase in lifespan as well as dramatic improvement on functional and histological parameters (Macauley et al. 2012).
- **Molecular or pharmacological chaperone therapy (protein chaperone therapy, PCT):** It consists in the use of small molecule compounds to assist the folding of mutated enzymes, therefore restoring their catalytic activity. This type of therapy is still highly experimental, but testing in cell culture models has shown promising results. Currently, no pharmacological chaperones have been tested in NCL cell lines or animal models except one study in lymphoblast lines from patients with CLN1where increase in PPT1 activity was showed (Dawson et al. 2010). Currently, no other pharmacological chaperones have been tested in NCL cell lines or animal models.
- **Stem cell transplant (SCT):** It is useful for the enzymatic deficiencies and it can intravenous transplantation of different types of donor cells. Generally it consists of healthy hematopoietic stem cells (usually from bone marrow, sometimes from cord blood) or neural stem cells (nerve cells). The newly produced enzymes can be taken up by the enzyme-deficient cells (cross-correction), or in certain cases stem cells can also have the capacity to differentiate and replace the person's own (diseased) cells. Both types have been used in animal models and clinical trials. Unfortunately, this therapy showed to have minimal effects on disease progression and to be largely ineffective against LINCL and JNCL. Nevertheless, this is not an approach to be eliminated since more promising outcomes have been obtained using HSC, specifically bone marrow treatment, in combination with gene therapy in Ppt1 −/− mice where neurodegeneration in the brain was attenuated, even if not in the retina (Arrant et al. 2018).
- **Substrate reduction therapy (SRT):** It consists in the oral administration of a drug capable of inhibiting/reducing the rate of production of the substrate reducing the metabolic load on the lysosome. Clinical trials that studied the effect of combining cysteamine bitartrate and N-acetylcysteine to treat INCL have been performed, but no effect on the progression of the disease was shown even if the treatment succeeded in reducing the amount of storage material in peripheral leucocytes and parents reported less irritability and increased concentration.

Nowadays CLN1, CLN2, CLN3, and CLN6 are the diseases for which the current therapeutic approaches have reached preclinical or clinical trials (see Table below). Both small and large animal models of various forms of NCLs are being developed. These animal models are likely to be very useful for the preclinical evaluation of novel therapeutic strategies.

## Moving Towards Effective Therapeutic Strategies

For ongoing trial for NCL see ClinicalTrials.gov.

**Acknowledgments** We thank Carla E Hollak for her help in the preparation of the paper.

**Funding** This work was generated within the European Reference Network for Rare Hereditary Metabolic Disorders (MetabERN), co-funded by the European Union within the framework of the Third Health Programme ERN-2016 - Framework Partnership Agreement 2017–2021, Project ID No. 739543.

## References

Arrant AE, et al. Progranulin gene therapy improves lysosomal dysfunction and microglial pathology associated with frontotemporal dementia and neuronal ceroid lipofuscinosis. J Neurosci. 2018;38:2341e.

Augustine EF, Adams HR, Beck CA, et al. Standardized assessment of seizures in patients with juvenile neuronal ceroid lipofuscinosis. Dev Med Child Neurol. 2015;57(4):366–71.

Das AK, Lu JY, et al. Biochemical analysis of mutations in palmitoyl-protein thioesterase causing infantile and late-onset forms of neuronal ceroid neuronal ceroid lipofuscinosis. Hum Mol Genet. 2001;10(13):1431–9.

Dawson G, Schroeder C, Dawson PE. Palmitoyl:protein thioesterase (PPT1) inhibitors can act as pharmacological chaperones in infantile Batten disease. Biochem Biophys Res Commun. 2010;395:66–9.

Goldenberg MM. Overview of drugs used for epilepsy and seizures: etiology, diagnosis, and treatment. P T. 2010;35(7):392–415.

Kohlschütter A, et al. Current and Emerging Treatment Strategies for Neuronal Ceroid Lipofuscinoses. CNS drugs vol. 2019;33(4):315–25.

Macauley SL, Roberts MS, Wong AM, McSloy F, Reddy AS, Cooper JD, Sands MS. Synergistic effects of central nervous system-directed gene therapy and bone marrow transplantation in the murine model of infantile neuronal ceroid lipofuscinosis. Ann Neurol. 2012;71(6):797–804.

Mole SE, Williams RE. Neuronal ceroid-lipofuscinoses. In: Adam MP, Ardinger HH, Pagon RA, et al., editors. GeneReviews® [Internet]. Seattle, WA: University of Washington, Seattle; 1993-2019; 2001. [Updated 2013 Aug 1].

Mole SE, Williams RE, Goebel HH. Correlations between genotype, ultrastructural morphology and clinical phenotype in the neuronal ceroid lipofuscinoses. Neurogenetics. 2005;6:107–26.

Mole SE, Williams RE. Neuronal Ceroid-Lipofuscinoses. Gene Reviews; 2010.

Mukherjee AB, Appu AP, Sadhukhan T, Casey S, Mondal A, Zhang Z, Bagh MB. Emerging new roles of the lysosome and neuronal ceroid lipofuscinoses. Mol Neurodegener. 2019;14(1):4.

Neverman NJ, Best HL, et al. Experimental therapies in the neuronal ceroid lipofuscinoses. Biochim Biophys Acta. 2015;1852(10 Pt B):2292–300.

Schulz A, Ajayi T, et al. CLN2 study group. Study of intraventricular cerliponase alfa for CLN2 disease. N Engl J Med. 2018;378(20):1898–907.

Shorvon S, Guerrini R, Trinka E, Schachter S. The causes of epilepsy: diagnosis and investigation. Cambridge: Cambridge University Press; 2019.

Steinfeld R, Heim P, et al. Late infantile neuronal ceroid lipofuscinosis: quantitative description of the clinical course in patients with CLN2 mutations. Am J Med Genet. 2002;112:347–54.

Steinfeld R, Steinke HB, et al. Mutations in classical late infantile neuronal ceroid lipofuscinosis disrupt transport of tripeptidyl-peptidase I to lysosomes. Hum Mol Genet. 2004;13(20):2483.

Steinfeld R, Reinhardt K, et al. Cathepsin D deficiency is associated with a human neurodegenerative disorder. Am J Hum Genet. 2006;78(6):988–98.

Yaari Y, Selzer ME, Pincus JH. Phenytoin: mechanisms of its anticonvulsant action. Ann Neurol. 1986;20(2):171–84.

# Mucolipidoses, Multiple Sulfatase Deficiency, and Cathepsin K and C Deficiency

# 62

Hidde H. Huidekoper and Esmee Oussoren

## Contents




## Summary

Mucolipidosis type II/III (ML II/III) and multiple sulfatase deficiency (MSD) share clinical features with the mucopolysaccharidoses. Both ML II/III and MSD result from enzymatic defects that affect the post-translational modification of lysosomal enzymes. In ML II/III the mannose-6-phosphate marker, essential for routing lysosomal enzymes towards the lysosomes, is lacking. This leads to the excretion of lysosomal enzymes in plasma where they are unable to execute their function. In MSD lysosomal sulfatases, as well as sulfatases from the endoplasmic reticulum and Golgi complex, cannot be activated due to the inability to modify a conserved cysteine residue at the active site. In mucolipidosis type IV (ML IV), lysosomal dysfunction is caused by the deficiency of transient receptor potential channel mucolipin-1 (TRPML1), a nonselective cation channel present in late endosomal and lysosomal membranes necessary for autophagy, vesicular trafficking, and mTOR and TFEB signaling. Neurological dysfunction and visual impairment are the most predominant clinical features; skeletal abnormalities are not seen in ML IV. Deficiency of the lysosomal enzymes cathepsin K (pycnodysostosis) and C (Papillon–Lefèvre or Haim–Munk syndrome) presents both with a very distinct clinical picture. Cathepsin K is important for bone resorption and extracellular matrix remodeling. Its deficiency results in stunted growth, facial dysmorphism, osteopetrosis, and dental abnormalities. In cathepsin C deficiency, premature loss of both deciduous and permanent teeth due to periodontitis in combination with palmoplantar keratosis is the main clinical feature.

All disorders are ultra-rare and have autosomal recessive inheritance. Their clinical spectrum is not yet fully



H. H. Huidekoper (✉) · E. Oussoren (✉)
Center for Lysosomal and Metabolic diseases, Department of Pediatrics, Erasmus MC University Medical Center, Rotterdam, The Netherlands
e-mail: h.huidekoper@erasmusmc.nl; e.oussoren@erasmusmc.nl







N. Blau et al. (eds.), *Physician's Guide to the Diagnosis, Treatment, and Follow-Up of Inherited Metabolic Diseases*,
https://doi.org/10.1007/978-3-030-67727-5_62

known, and patients are likely still underdiagnosed. No specific biomarkers are available that can lead to the diagnosis. All disorders have in common that no curative treatments are available and specialized multidisciplinary supportive care is needed to minimize the disease burden and provide an adequate quality of life.

## Introduction

In this chapter different lysosomal storage disorders are described that do not necessarily share a mutual pathophysiological mechanism, but do cause lysosomal dysfunction and have overlap in clinical presentation. In both mucolipidosis type II and III (ML II/III) and in multiple sulfatase deficiency (MSD), the deficiency of an extra-lysosomal enzyme results in the deficiency of lysosomal enzymes. In mucolipidosis type IV, lysosomal dysfunction is caused by a defect in a cation channel in the membrane of lysosomes, and both cathepsin K and C deficiency are lysosomal proteases whose deficiency results in a distinct clinical picture. We will briefly introduce all disorders separately.

*Mucolipidoses:* **mucolipidosis type II** (ML II; **I-cell disease** OMIM#252500) and **mucolipidosis type III α/β** or **γ** (**pseudo-Hurler dystrophy**, ML III α/β; OMIM#252600, ML III γ; OMIM#252605) are rare autosomal recessive lysosomal storage disorders (Maroteaux and Lamy 1966; Leroy and Martin 1975). The birth prevalence in the Netherlands is less than 1 per 100.000. In ML II and ML III, there is absent or reduced activity of the membrane-bound enzyme **UDP-*N*-acetyl glucosamine-1-phosphotransferase** (GlcNAc-1-phosphotransferase), a hexameric complex, with three subunits; α2, β2 (*GNPTAB*), and γ2 (*GNPTG*). **GlcNAc-1-phosphotransferase** is responsible for the first step in the phosphorylation of enzyme-conjugated mannose residues to form mannose-6-phosphate (Reitman and Kornfeld 1981). Mannose-6-phosphate serves as the recognition marker for the targeting of more than 70 newly synthesized soluble lysosomal enzymes to the lysosome. Absence or reduced presence of this marker results in secretion of lysosomal enzymes in the plasma, where they are unable to execute their function and substrates, such as glycosaminoglycans (GAGs) and (glyco)sphingolipids, accumulate in the lysosome. The clinical picture of ML II and ML III mostly resembles that of the mucopolysaccharidoses and much less that of the sphingolipidoses and other lysosomal storage disorders. There is a clinical spectrum with severely affected patients (MLII) at one end of the spectrum and milder patients at the other end (ML III). There is also an "intermediate" phenotype with features of both ML II and ML III patients (Cathey et al. 2010). The patients with the most severe form of ML II are already severely affected at birth and develop rapidly progressive airway, cardiac, skeletal, and nervous system disease, resulting in death in early childhood. The ML III α/β patients present with a broader clinical phenotype ranging from severely affected patients that die in childhood to milder affected patients displaying primarily skeletal symptoms, who survive into adulthood (Cathey et al. 2010). ML III γ patients have a milder phenotype with onset in early school age, but are phenotypically not distinguishable from the ML III α/β patients (Nampoothiri et al. 2019).

In **mucolipidosis type IV** (ML VI; OMIM#252650), another ultra-rare autosomal recessive disorder predominantly present among Ashkenazi Jews (Bargal et al. 2001), mutations in *MCOLN1*, which encodes for the transient receptor potential cation channel, mucolipin-1 subfamily member 1 (**TRPML1**), lead to lysosomal dysfunction (Clapham et al. 2001). This channel is distributed in the membranes of late endosomes and lysosomes in all tissues, with the highest expression in the brain, kidney, liver, spleen, and heart (Cheng et al. 2010). It is nonselective permeable to several cations. Abnormal flux of calcium probably is the most important in the lysosomal dysfunction in ML IV, resulting in dysregulation of autophagy, vesicular trafficking, and mammalian target of rapamycin (mTOR) and transcription factor EB (TFEB) signaling (Boudewyn and Walkley 2019). Patients with ML IV do not have the typical dysmorphic features, as seen in ML II/III. Patients can have severe psychomotor delay (slowly progressive over time) due to neuronal dysmyelination, hypotonia which gradually progresses to spasticity during childhood, speech deficits, retinal degeneration, and optic atrophy causing visual impairment. Other symptoms are cornea clouding, achlorhydria with increased gastrin secretion and iron deficiency anemia, and kidney disease and failure, which finally leads to a shortened life span in the patients (Boudewyn and Walkley 2019). Most of them are still alive at least in the first two to three decades; thereafter, it is still unknown. From the patients that died in the second decade, the cause of death was not exactly known (Bargal et al. 2001).

*Multiple sulfatase deficiency:* **multiple sulfatase deficiency** (MSD; OMIM #272200), an ultra-rare disorder with autosomal recessive inheritance, was first described in 1964 by Austin et al. (Austin et al. 1964) and results from the deficiency of **formylglycine-generating enzyme (FGE)** due to mutations in *SUMF1* (sulfatase-modifying factor 1). Only approximately 100 cases have been described to date, but MSD is most likely still underdiagnosed due to the broad clinical spectrum seen in patients. FGE plays a crucial role in the post-translational activation of sulfatases by modifying a conserved cysteine residue into formylglycine at the active site, necessary for the catalytic activity of sulfatases. Its deficiency therefore affects the activity of all known 17 sulfatases, including 8 lysosomal sulfatases, of which 6 are associated with well-characterized lysosomal storage disorders (i.e., **metachromatic leukodystrophy** (OMIM #250100), **mucopolysaccharidoses types II** (OMIM #309900), **III A** (OMIM #252900) **and D** (OMIM #252940), **IV A** (OMIM #253000), **and VI** (OMIM #253200)), 1 in the endoplasmatic reticulum associated with **X-linked ichthyosis** (OMIM #308100), and 1 in the Golgi complex associated with **chondrodysplasia punctata type I** (OMIM #302950). The clinical phenotype of MSD can be very heterogeneous and is dependent on FGE protein stability and residual enzyme activity and the degree the different sulfatases are affected. Four clinical subtypes can be distinguished based on the main presenting symptoms and age of symptom onset: a neonatal, severe late infantile, mild late infantile, and juvenile form of MSD (Ahrens-Nicklas et al. 2018).

*Cathepsin K deficiency (pycnodysostosis):* **pycnodysostosis** (OMIM #265800) is an ultra-rare, prevalence is estimated at one to three per million, **osteochondrodysplasia** with autosomal recessive inheritance (Bizaoui et al. 2019). It was first described in 1962 (Maroteaux and Lamy 1962), and since a few hundred cases have been published, the most well-known being the French painter Henri de Toulouse-Lautrec (Markatos et al. 2018). Pycnodysostosis is caused by the deficiency of lysosomal **cathepsin K** encoded by *CTSK*. Cathepsin K belongs to the papain-like cysteine protease family and is mainly expressed in osteoclasts where it plays a central role in bone resorption by degrading collagen type I. Cathepsin K is also expressed in other tissues where it is involved in extracellular matrix remodeling, adipogenesis, thyroxine liberation, and peptide hormone regulation (Novinec and Lenarcic 2013). Its deficiency causes a distinct clinical phenotype characterized by short stature and the formation of hard and dense bones with thick cortices (osteopetrosis), resulting in frequent fractures and skeletal problems including dysplasia of the cranium, mandible, clavicle, and distal phalanges. In addition, dental abnormalities are frequently seen including dental crowding, delayed eruption of permanent teeth, enamel hypoplasia, and hypercementosis (Xue et al. 2011; Wen et al. 2016).

*Cathepsin C deficiency:* **cathepsin C deficiency** is best known as **Papillon–Lefèvre syndrome** (PLS; OMIM #245000) characterized by a severe early-onset periodontitis, resulting in the premature loss of both deciduous and permanent teeth, and palmoplantar keratosis. It is also associated with **Haim–Munk syndrome** (HMS; OMIM #245010), which resembles PLS but in addition also exhibits arachnodactyly, acro-osteolysis, and onychogryphosis (Hart TC et al. 2000). PLS is an ultra-rare disorder with an estimated prevalence of approximately one to four per million and autosomal recessive inheritance (Machado et al. 2019). Cathepsin C, encoded by *CTSC* and also known as **dipeptidyl peptidase 1**, also belongs to the papain-like cysteine protease family and is ubiquitously expressed. By removing dipeptides from the N-terminus of its substrates, it has a major role in the activation of pro-inflammatory granule-associated serine proteases, which degrade various extracellular matrix compounds causing tissue damage and chronic inflammation. It also has been suggested to play an important role in epithelial differentiation and desquamation, which could explain the palmoplantar keratosis seen in patients (Korkmaz et al. 2018). Besides the characteristic severe periodontitis and palmoplantar keratosis, patients have a higher susceptibility to infections, especially skin, respiratory, and urinary tract infections, and may exhibit a delay in somatic development, keratosis pilaris, and hyperhidrosis.

## Nomenclature

| No. | Disorder | Alternative name | Abbreviation | Gene symbol | Chromosomal localization | Inheritance | Affected protein | OMIM no. |
|---|---|---|---|---|---|---|---|---|
| 62.1 | Mucolipidosis type II | I-cell disease | ML II | *GNPTAB* | 12q23.3 | AR | UDP-*N*-acetyl glucosamine-1-phosphotransferase (GlcNAc-PTase) | 252500 |
| 62.2 | Mucolipidosis type III alpha, beta | Pseudo-hurler | ML III α, β | *GNPTAB* | 12q23.3 | AR | UDP-*N*-acetyl glucosamine-1-phosphotransferase (GlcNAc-PTase) | 252600 |
| 62.2 | Mucolipidosis type III, gamma | Pseudo-hurler | ML III γ | *GNPTG* | 16p13.3 | AR | UDP-*N*-acetyl glucosamine-1-phosphotransferase (GlcNAc-PTase) | 252605 |
| 62.3 | Mucolipidosis type IV | | ML IV | *MCOLN1* | 19p13.2 | AR | Transient receptor potential channel mucolipin-1 (TRPML1) | 252650 |
| 62.4 | Multiple sulfatase deficiency | Mucosulfatidosis<br>Austin disease | MSD | *SUMF1* | 3p26.1 | AR | Formylglycine-generating enzyme (FGE) | 272200 |
| 62.5 | Cathepsin K deficiency | Pycnodysostosis | | *CTSK* | 1q21.3 | AR | Cathepsin K | 265800 |
| 62.6 | Cathepsin C deficiency | Papillon–Lefèvre syndrome<br>Haim–Munk syndrome | PLS/HMS | *CTSC* | 11q14.2 | AR | Cathepsin C | 245000/245010 |

## Metabolic Pathways

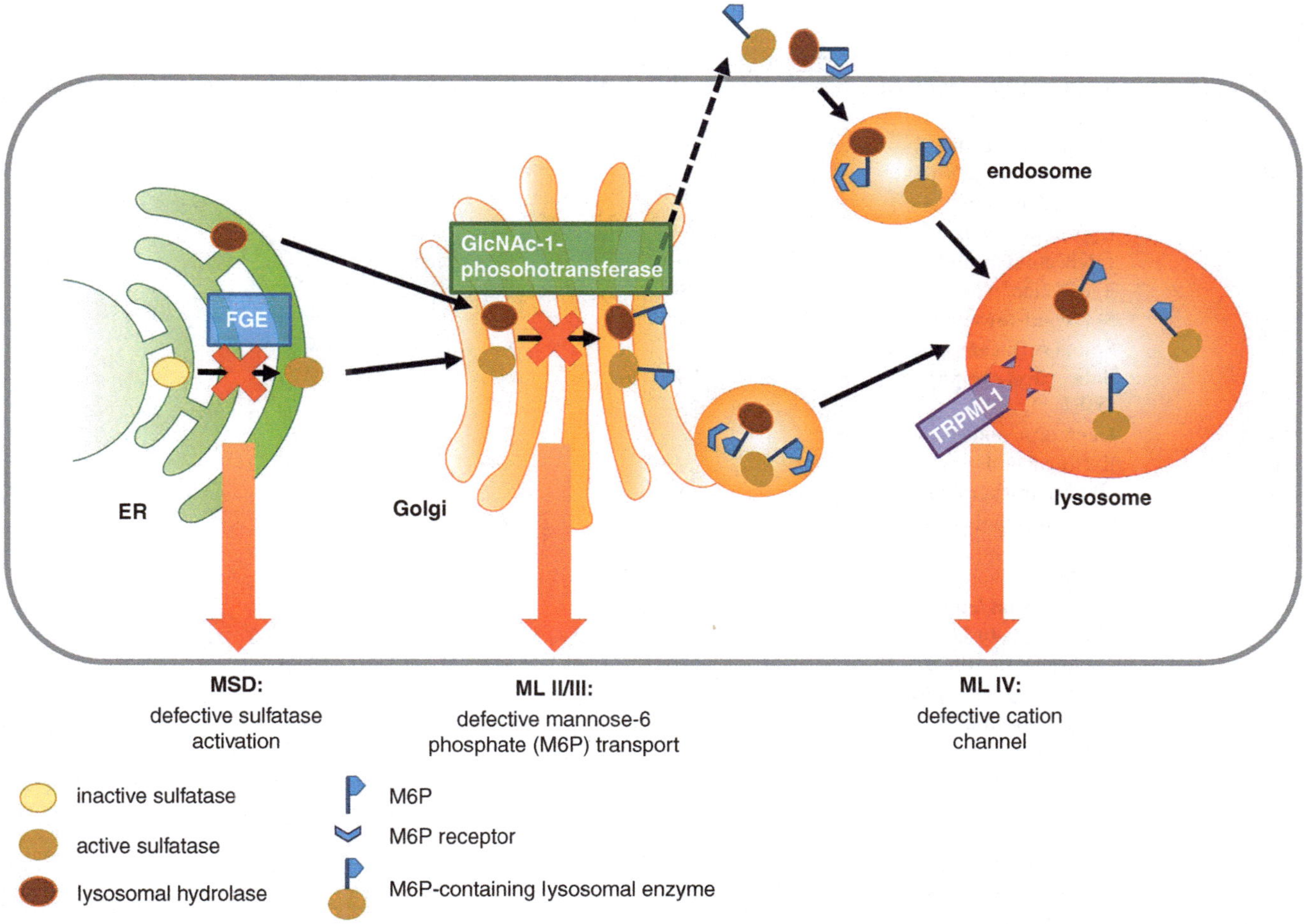


**Fig. 62.1** Intracellular lysosomal enzyme processing and trafficking. After production more than 70 lysosomal enzymes are transported from the ER to the Golgi complex where a mannose-6-phosphate residue is added by UDP-*N*-acetyl glucosamine-1-phosphotransferase (GlcNAc-1-phosphotransferase), defective in mucolipidosis type II/III (ML II/III), which serves as a key targeting signal for the intracellular routing of enzymes towards lysosomes. In addition, lysosomal sulfatases need to be activated by formylglycine-generating enzyme (FGE), defective in multiple sulfatase deficiency (MSD), in the ER before transportation to the Golgi complex. The TRPML1 cation channel present in the membranes of late endosomes and lysosomes, defective in mucolipidosis type IV, is essential for the nonselective flux of cations, necessary for regulation of lysosomal autophagy and vesicular trafficking and mammalian target of rapamycin (mTOR) and transcription factor EB (TFEB) signaling

## Signs and Symptoms

**Table 62.1** Mucolipidosis II alpha-beta

| System | Symptoms and biomarkers | Neonatal (birth–1 month) | Infancy (1–18 months) | Childhood (1.5–11 years) | Adolescence (11–16 years) | Adulthood (>16 years) |
|---|---|---|---|---|---|---|
| Cardiovascular | Cardiomyopathy | ± | ± | + | + | |
| | **Valvular thickening** | ± | + | ++ | ++ | |
| CNS | Cortical atrophy (MRI) | + | + | ++ | + | |
| | **Cortical atrophy (MRI)** | ± | + | ++ | + | |
| | Hypomyelination, CNS | + | ++ | +++ | ± | |
| | **Intellectual disability** | + | ++ | +++ | ± | |
| | Retardation, motor | + | ++ | +++ | ++ | |
| | **Speech disturbances** | | + | ++ | | |
| | **Spinal cord compression** | | + | ++ | ++ | |
| | **Subcortical atrophy (MRI)** | ± | + | ++ | + | |
| Digestive | **Hepatosplenomegaly** | ± | + | ++ | ++ | |
| Ear | Recurrent otitis media | + | ++ | +++ | ± | |
| Endocrine | **Hyperparathyroidism** | ± | ± | n | n | |
| Eye | **Corneal clouding** | + | ++ | ++ | ++ | |
| Musculoskeletal | **Carpal and tarsal syndrome** | n | ± | + | ++ | |
| | **Coarse facial features** | + | ++ | +++ | ++ | |
| | **Craniosynostosis** | + | + | + | ± | |
| | **Dysostosis multiplex** | + | ++ | +++ | +++ | |
| | **Gingival hypertrophy** | + | ++ | +++ | ++ | |
| | **Hernias (umbilical, inguinalis)** | + | + | + | + | |
| | **Hip dislocation** | ± | + | ++ | +++ | |
| | **Hypotonia, muscular-axial** | + | + | ± | ± | |
| | **Joint contractures** | + | ++ | ++ | ++ | |
| Laboratory findings | Glycosaminoglycans | n-↑ | n-↑ | n-↑ | | |
| | Lysosomal enzyme activities (fibroblast) | ↓↓↓ | ↓↓↓ | ↓↓↓ | | |
| | Lysosomal enzyme activities (serum) | ↑↑↑ | ↑↑↑ | ↑↑↑ | | |
| | Oligosaccharide (urine) | ↑↑ | ↑↑ | ↑↑ | | |

**Table 62.2** Mucolipidosis III alpha-beta-gamma

| System | Symptoms and biomarkers | Neonatal (birth–1 month) | Infancy (1–18 months) | Childhood (1.5–11 years) | Adolescence (11–16 years) | Adulthood (>16 years) |
|---|---|---|---|---|---|---|
| CNS | Intellectual disability | | ± | + | + | ± |
| | Spinal cord compression | | | ± | ± | + |
| Ear | Recurrent otitis media | | + | ++ | ++ | ++ |
| Musculoskeletal | **Carpal tunnel syndrome** | | | ± | + | + |
| | Coarse facial features (puffy cheeks) | | | ± | ± | ± |
| | **Dysostosis multiplex** | | ± | + | + | + |
| | **Joint contractures** | | ± | ++ | ++ | ++ |
| | **Osteoarthritis (all joints can be involved)** | | | | + | ++ |
| Laboratory findings | Glycosaminoglycans | | | n-↑ | n-↑ | n-↑ |
| | Lysosomal enzymes (fibroblasts) | | | ↓↓ | ↓↓ | ↓↓ |
| | Lysosomal enzymes (serum) | | | ↑↑ | ↑↑ | ↑↑ |
| | Oligosaccharide (urine) | | | n-↑ | n-↑ | n-↑ |

**Table 62.3** Mucolipin 1 deficiency

| System | Symptoms and biomarkers | Neonatal (birth–1 month) | Infancy (1–18 months) | Childhood (1.5–11 years) | Adolescence (11–16 years) | Adulthood (>16 years) |
|---|---|---|---|---|---|---|
| CNS | Bilateral tract pyramidal tract signs | | ± | ± | ± | |
| | Cerebellar atrophy | ± | + | + | ++ | ++ |
| | Epilepsy | | ± | ± | ± | ± |
| | **Hypotonia** | ± | + | + | | |
| | **Intellectual disability** | ± | + | ++ | ++ | ++ |
| | **Motor delay** | ± | + | ++ | ++ | +++ |
| | **Reduced size of corpus callosum** | ± | + | + | + | + |
| | **Spasticity** | | + | ++ | +++ | +++ |
| | **Speech delay** | | | + | ++ | ++ |
| Eye | Cornea clouding | ± | ± | ± | ± | ± |
| | Myopia | | ± | ± | ± | ± |
| | **Optic nerve atrophy** | ± | ± | + | ++ | +++ |
| | Photophobia | | | ± | | |
| | **Retinal degeneration** | ± | ± | + | ++ | +++ |
| | Strabismus | + | + | + | + | + |
| | **Visual impairment** | + | ++ | +++ | +++ | +++ |
| Digestive | **Achlorhydria** | + | + | + | + | + |
| Hematological | Iron deficiency anemia | ± | ± | ± | ± | ± |
| Renal | Kidney disease (failure) | | | ± | + | ++ |
| Musculoskeletal | Growth retardation | | ± | + | ± | ± |
| Laboratory findings | Blood gastrin | ↑ | ↑ | ↑ | ↑ | |
| | Blood Iron (iron deficiency anemia) | ↓-n | ↓-n | ↓-n | ↓-n | |

**Table 62.4** Multiple sulfatase deficiency

| System | Symptoms and biomarkers | Neonatal (birth-1 month) | Infancy (1–18 months) | Childhood (1.5–11 years) | Adolescence (11–16 years) | Adulthood (>16 years) |
|---|---|---|---|---|---|---|
| CNS | **Gait disturbance** | | +++ | +++ | | |
| | **Hypomyelination, CNS** | +++ | + | + | | |
| | **Intellectual disability** | | +++ | ++ | + | |
| | **Leukodystrophy** | | +++ | + | | |
| | **Slow nerve conductive velocity** | | + | + | | |
| | Cortical atrophy (MRI) | | + | + | | |
| | Hydrocephalus | ± | ± | ± | | |
| | Neurologic deterioration | +++ | ++ | ++ | | |
| | Retardation, psychomotor | | +++ | ++ | | |
| | Seizures | ± | ± | ± | | |
| | Spasticity | | +++ | +++ | | |
| | Speech disturbances | | +++ | +++ | | |
| Dermatological | Ichthyosis | ++ | + | + | + | |
| Digestive | Hepatosplenomegaly | +++ | ± | ± | ++ | |
| Eye | Ophthalmological anomalies | + | ± | ± | | |
| Musculoskeletal | **Coarse facial features** | +++ | + | + | + | |
| | Dysostosis multiplex | +++ | ± | ± | | |
| | Growth retardation | +++ | + | ± | | |
| | Hypotonia, muscular-axial | +++ | ± | ± | | |
| Respiratory | Cardiopulmonary involvement | ++ | ± | ± | | |

**Table 62.5** Cathepsin K deficiency

| System | Symptoms and biomarkers | Neonatal (birth to 1 month) | Infancy (1–18 months) | Childhood (1.5–11 years) | Adolescence (11–16 years) | Adulthood (>16 years) |
|---|---|---|---|---|---|---|
| Digestive | Dental crowding/displacement | | | ± | ± | ± |
| | Delayed eruption of permanent teeth | | ± | ± | ± | ± |
| | Enamel hypoplasia | – | ± | ± | ± | ± |
| | Hypercementosis | | | ± | ± | ± |
| | Obliteration of pulp chambers | | | ± | ± | ± |
| | Periodontitis | | | ± | ± | ± |
| | Persistant desiduous teeth | | ± | ± | ± | ± |
| Eye | Blue sclera | – | ± | ± | ± | ± |
| Musculoskeletal | **Abnormal cranial suture closure** | | + | + | + | + |
| | **Acro-osteolysis** | ± | + | ++ | ++ | ++ |
| | **Aquiline nose** | ± | ± | ± | ± | ± |
| | **Growth retardation** | ± | ++ | +++ | +++ | +++ |
| | **Increased bone density (osteopetrosis)** | + | ++ | +++ | +++ | +++ |
| | **Mandibular and/or maxillary hypoplasia** | + | ++ | ++ | ++ | ++ |
| | **Short stature** | ± | ++ | +++ | +++ | +++ |
| | **Skull deformity** | | + | + | + | + |
| Respiratory | Upper airway obstruction | ± | ± | ± | ± | ± |

**Table 62.6** Cathepsin C deficiency

| System | Symptoms and biomarkers | Neonatal (birth–1 month) | Infancy (1–18 months) | Childhood (1.5–11 years) | Adolescence (11–16 years) | Adulthood (>16 years) |
|---|---|---|---|---|---|---|
| Autonomic system | Hyperhidrosis | | | ± | ± | ± |
| Dermatological | Keratosis pilaris | | | ± | ± | ± |
| | **Onychogryphosis*** | | | ± | ++ | ++ |
| | **Palmoplantar hyperkeratosis** | ± | + | + | ++ | ++ |
| Digestive | **Periodontitis** | | + | +++ | +++ | + |
| | **Loss of deciduous teeth** | | ± | +++ | | |
| | **Loss of permanent teeth** | | | ± | +++ | + |
| Musculoskeletal | **Acro-osteolysis*** | | | ± | ++ | ++ |
| | **Arachnodactyly*** | | ± | ± | ++ | ++ |
| Other | Delay in somatic development | | | ± | ± | ± |
| | Increased susceptibility to infections | | ± | ± | ± | ± |

* Characteristic for Haim-Munk syndrome (HMS)

## Reference Values

For the diagnosis of mucolipidosis type II/III and cathepsin C deficiency, the following enzymatic assays are used (normal ranges may vary between laboratories). Please see Chaps. 60 "Lipidoses" and 64 "Mucopolysaccharidoses" for details on the different sulfatase assays which can be used for the diagnosis of multiple sulfatase deficiency.

| No. | Disorder | Enzyme(s) | Material | Normal range | Reference |
|---|---|---|---|---|---|
| 62.1 | Mucolipidosis type II | β-Hexosaminidase A<br>β-Hexosaminidase A+B<br>α-L-Fucosidase<br>β-D-Glucuronidase<br>α-D-Mannosidase<br>β-D-Galactosidase | Plasma/fibroblasts | In nmol/h/mg:<br>22–63/292–1,200<br>620–3,700/4,000–23,900<br>80–800/35–160<br>12–160/78–270<br>20–120/39–180<br>N.A./320–1,900 | Erasmus MC[a] |
| 62.2 | Mucolipidosis type III alpha, beta | See 62.1 | See 62.1 | See 62.1 | See 62.1 |
| 62.2 | Mucolipidosis type III, gamma | See 62.1 | See 62.1 | See 62.1 | See 62.1 |
| 62.4 | Multiple sulfatase deficiency | See Chaps. 60 and 64 | See Chaps. 60 and 64 | See Chaps. 60 and 64 | See Chaps. 60 and 64 |
| 62.6 | Cathepsin C deficiency | Cathepsin C | Leucocytes<br>Fibroblasts | 685–1,200 μmol/min/mg<br>4030–11,700 nmol/h/mg<br>1,180–9,610 nmol/h/mg | Hart PS et al. (2000)<br>Erasmus MC[a]<br>Erasmus MC[a] |

*N.A.* Not applicable
[a]Control values obtained in the laboratory of Clinical Genetics at the Erasmus MC University Medical Center, Rotterdam, The Netherlands

## Pathological Values

The diagnosis of mucolipidoses (ML), multiple sulfatase deficiency (MSD), and cathepsin K and C deficiency is based on enzymatic analysis and/or molecular analysis. No specific diagnostic biomarkers are known for these disorders, although biochemical abnormalities are seen: urinary **glycosaminoglycans** (GAGs) excretion can be increased in ML II and III as well as in MSD. Urinary **sulfatides** may be increased in MSD, in ML II, bound **sialic acid** is elevated in urine. As these can also be normal in ML and MSD, they cannot be used to exclude these disorders. In ML and MSD, as well as in attenuated forms of cathepsin K and C deficiency, the clinical phenotype may be less distinct. These forms are more likely to be diagnosed through untargeted molecular analysis, especially with exome sequencing since this is now more widely used in patients with an unexplained clinical phenotype.

*Mucolipidoses:* for ML II/III first-level diagnostic procedures include measurement of the activity of several lysosomal enzymes including β-hexosaminidase A, β-hexosaminidase A+B, α-L-fucosidase, β-D-glucuronidase, α-D-mannosidase, and β-D-galactosidase in plasma and/or fibroblasts, where these enzymes are elevated in plasma and decreased in fibroblasts. In addition, GlcNAc-1-phophotransferase activity can be measured in fibroblasts. Finally, molecular analysis of *GNPTAB* (ML II and III α, β) or *GNPTG* (ML III γ) can be performed. Genotype-phenotype correlations in the MLII/III are difficult to establish due to the high proportion of individual mutations and the variable expressivity in patients carrying the same mutation (Velho et al. 2019).

ML IV can only be diagnosed by molecular analysis of *MCOLN1*. Increased **gastrin** secretion and **iron deficiency anemia** are indicative for ML IV and can support the diagnosis.

*Multiple sulfatase deficiency:* the diagnosis of MSD is based on demonstrating reduced activity of at least two sulfatases in leucocytes or fibroblasts as patients can be missed if only one sulfatase is assayed (Schlotawa et al. 2011). Hereafter, the diagnosis should be confirmed with molecular analysis by demonstrating a pathogenic alteration on both alleles of *SUMF1*. Several specific genotype–phenotype correlations have been established, where mutations strongly affecting protein stability and residual enzyme activity are associated with a more severe clinical phenotype (Sabourdy et al. 2015).

*Cathepsin K deficiency (pycnodysostosis):* the distinct clinical and radiographic features of pycnodysostosis are the most important clues towards diagnosis. Detecting acro-osteolysis in combination with increased bone density upon radiological evaluation is almost pathognomonic of the disorder. The diagnosis can only be confirmed by molecular analysis of *CTSK* demonstrating pathologic alterations on both alleles. Until now genotype–phenotype relations have not been established (Bizaoui et al. 2019). *CTSK* mutations have also been detected in patients with a more attenuated osteopetrosis phenotype without the distinct clinical features of pycnodysostosis and should therefore be considered in all patients with unexplained osteopetrosis (Schlotawa et al.

2011). Differentiating pycnodysostosis from other forms of osteopetrosis is important as the latter may benefit from early hematopoietic stem cell transplantation whereas this has no proven benefit in pycnodysostosis (Bizaoui et al. 2019).

*Cathepsin C deficiency:* as with cathepsin K deficiency, the distinct clinical features of palmoplantar hyperkeratosis and periodontitis seen in Papillon–Lefèvre syndrome offer the most important clues for cathepsin C deficiency. An enzymatic assay for cathepsin C has been described (Hart PS et al. 2000), but is not widely available. Diagnosis should be confirmed with molecular analysis of *CTSC*. To date 89 disease-causing mutations have been described, all affecting the heavy chain of cathepsin C which is essential for its tetramer formation and protein function. No consistent genotype–phenotype relations have been established (Machado et al. 2019).

## Diagnostic Flowchart

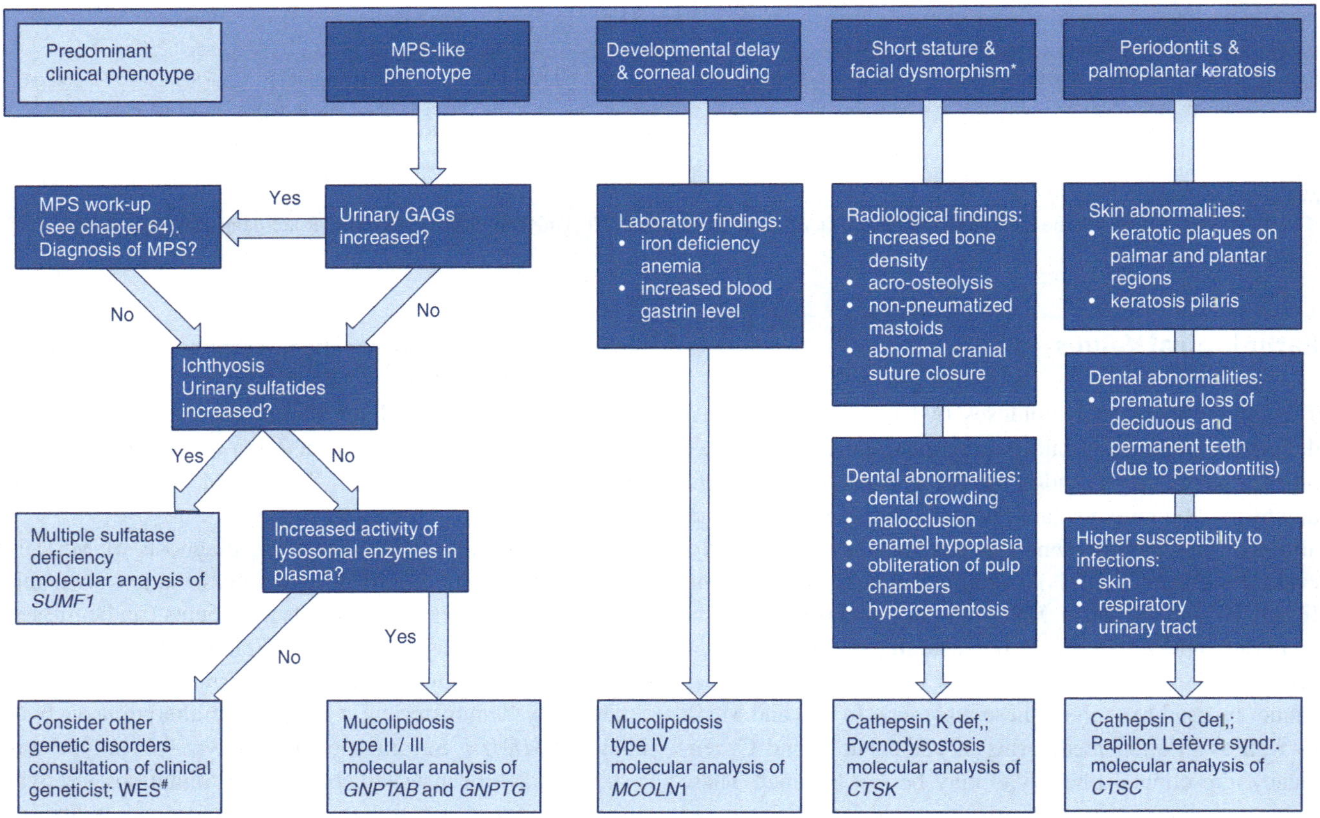


**Fig. 62.2** Diagnostic flowchart based on predominant clinical features
*Frontal bossing, mandibular and/or maxillary hypoplasia, aquiline nose, proptosis, blue sclera
#Whole exome sequencing

## Treatment and Follow-Up

All lysosomal disorders discussed in this chapter are multisystem diseases for which no curative treatments are available. Multidisciplinary supportive treatment is therefore essential, as well as palliative care for the patients with a shortened life span. Supportive treatment and developments in innovative treatment approaches are discussed below.

### Supportive Treatment

*Mucolipidoses:* as the clinical phenotype of ML II/III patients is similar to the patients with mucopolysaccharidosis (MPS), the multidisciplinary supportive care described for MPS patients in Chap. 64 can also be used for patients with ML II/III. Patients with ML II are poor feeders with stunted growth and are often overfed. Most children need nasogastric tube feeding and dietary support. Patients with ML III have skeletal problems and often develop secondary osteoarthritis (more severe than observed in MPS patients), necessitating **surgical orthopedic interventions** relatively early in life.

Orthopedic follow-up is necessary, with involvement of the care of a rehabilitation specialist and occupational therapist. ML III patients experience bone pain due to secondary osteoarthritis and osteopenia causing microfractures. Adequate pain management is important in this patient group, which may require an expert in **pain management**. **Bisphosphonates** have been given to ML III patients (Robinson et al. 2002; Zolkipli et al. 2005; Kerr et al. 2011; Kobayashi et al. 2011). Their effect on bone pain remains unclear. Since long-term use of these drugs suppresses bone turnover and consequently may have a negative effect on final height, they may be of limited use in ML III.

For patients with ML IV, neurological and pediatric follow-up is important. There is a psychomotor delay in all the patients, and in infancy patients are hypotonic, which gradually progresses to spasticity during childhood. All patients develop visual impairment due to corneal clouding, strabismus, myopia, retinal degeneration, and/or optic atrophy, for which they need ophthalmologic follow-up. It has been noted that many patients in the second to third decades of life suffer from kidney disease and kidney failure, which needs follow-up by a nephrologist (Boudewyn and Walkley 2019). Patient with ML IV can have iron deficiency anemia for which they need iron supplementation, which must be monitored over time by measuring iron and hemoglobin levels in the blood.

*Multiple sulfatase deficiency:* the clinical spectrum in MSD is highly variable. Therefore, a tailor-made multidisciplinary approach is required in each patient in order to support motor function, prevent secondary complications, and maintain an adequate quality of life. Most patients have musculoskeletal problems, including dysostosis multiplex, contractures, and muscle tone dysregulation and/or muscle weakness, requiring the involvement of a physiotherapist and rehabilitation specialist as well as pharmacological management of tone abnormalities. A specialized dermatologist is needed to treat ichthyosis. Other potential clinical issues requiring specialized care include symptoms related to GAG accumulation in different tissues as seen in MPS; see details in Chap. 64. Patients should be seen at regular time intervals (every 3–6 months is suggested depending on the disease burden) to monitor the progression of the disease and its complications, preferably using standardized outcome measures in order to obtain more knowledge about the natural course of MSD. For more details and a comprehensive guideline on treatment and follow-up in MSD, see Ahrens-Nicklas et al. 2018 (Ahrens-Nicklas et al. 2018).

*Cathepsin K deficiency (pycnodysostosis):* as pycnodysostosis is primarily a bone disease and patients are prone to fractures, (parents of) patients should be instructed to avoid activities that increase the risk of fractures. Nevertheless, most patients require at least one surgical intervention in their life span (Bizaoui et al. 2019). As bone remodeling is impaired due to the osteoclastic dysfunction, open reduction with internal fixation (direct bone healing) is advised over external fixation with casting (indirect bone healing) in fracture management (Grewal et al. 2019). It should be noted there is an increased risk of developing osteomyelitis with all surgical procedures as bone blood supply in pycnodysostosis is decreased. An important aspect of the disease is upper airway obstruction due to the mandibular and/or maxillary hypoplasia, the long soft palate, and possible laryngomalacia. This can lead to severe obstructive apnea requiring a nasopharyngeal tube and/or noninvasive ventilation and possibly surgical interventions, during childhood. Patients can be very difficult to intubate, and airway management should be carefully evaluated before any procedure requiring general anesthesia is scheduled. Dental hygiene and management are essential as patients are prone to develop severe caries with the dental abnormalities seen in pycnodysostosis; patients should be seen by a (specialized) dentist at least once a year. Patients may exhibit a Chiari malformation related to the cranial dysplasia; it is therefore advised to do a cerebral MRI in all patients after diagnosis. Finally, as stunted growth is important in pycnodysostosis, supplementation of **growth hormone** can be considered and was reported to be effective in 40% of the patients (Bizaoui et al. 2019).

*Cathepsin C deficiency:* management in Papillon–Lefèvre syndrome focuses on the preservation of permanent teeth in young patient by controlling factors that contribute to the destruction of the periodontium. This requires frequent (every 3 months) specialized dentist care aimed at prevention and early treatment of periodontitis with oral hygiene instructions using **chlorhexidine gluconate** 0.2% mouth rinses and antibiotic treatment when necessary. Development of pyogenic liver and skin abscesses due to bacteremia is a complication of periodontitis seen in PLS because of impairment of the immune system. Renal and cerebral abscesses have also been described. Deciduous teeth should be extracted when they have a poor prognosis and cause a potential problem for the eruption of permanent teeth. Extraction of permanent teeth with advanced periodontal disease is also required. In order to preserve chewing function, dental prostheses are needed involving fabrication of partial or complete dentures with an age-specific approach. Management of the dermatological manifestations seen in PLS requires the involvement of a specialized dermatologist. The mainstay of treatment is anti-inflammatory emollients; keratolytics, such as **salicylic acid** and **topical steroids**; and **oral retinoids**, which have been shown to improve both dental and cutaneous lesions of PLS. Retinoids decrease the total keratin content of keratinocytes, are involved in the regulation of growth and differentiation of epithelial cells, and may have a positive effect on inflammation by stimulating both humoral and cellular immunity. Prescribers should be aware of adverse effects which include dryness of lips, mild pruritus, transient hair loss, and elevated serum triglycerides and liver enzymes due to liver toxicity and teratogenicity. Long-term use of retinoids can cause bone toxicity with growth disturbances due to premature epiphyseal closure and traumatic fractures (Sreeramulu et al. 2015; Korkmaz et al. 2018).

### Innovative Treatments

*Mucolipidoses:* in ML II patients, hematopoietic stem cell transplantation (HSCT) has been explored but was proven ineffective (Lund et al. 2014). As in both ML II/III and ML IV, a transmembrane protein is involved, it is highly unlikely that this approach would be effective (Boudewyn and Walkley 2019). In patients with lysosomal storage diseases, an inflammatory component, arising from the accumulation of lysosomal storage products, contributes to the pathophysiology. Reducing this inflammatory response could be a possible target of treatment. This may be achieved by drugs such as pentosan polysulfate (PPS), as this drug has shown to improve range of motion and reduce pain in MPS I patients in a short-term study (Hennermann et al. 2016). Recently, a proof of concept for the development of an anti-sense oligonucleotide to induce exon skipping of exon 19 in *GNPTAB*, in order to overcome the deleterious effect of the most common c.3503_3504del mutation in ML II, was reported (Matos et al. 2020). Some clinical aspects, like bone disease, in ML II are less likely to be treated with this approach, as they have their origin in fetal development.

*Multiple sulfatase deficiency:* combined rAAV9 gene therapy, where a single injection of this vector was given both systemic and in the cerebral ventricles, was shown to result in a widespread transduction of tissues, leading to the activation of sulfatases, a near complete clearance of glycosaminoglycans (GAGs), a decrease in inflammation in both the central nervous system and visceral organs, and an improvement in behavior and survival of *SUMF1* knockout mice (Spampanato et al. 2011). Further work on the development of gene therapy for MSD has not been reported. Currently, there is no evidence to support the use of HSCT in MSD (Tan et al. 2019).

*Cathepsin K deficiency (pycnodysostosis):* to our knowledge no innovative treatment approaches for pycnodysostosis are under development. This may be related to the fact that enzyme replacement treatment strategies are known to be less effective for skeletal disease manifestations. Hematopoietic stem cell transplantation has been proven effective in several genetic forms of osteopetrosis, but its therapeutic potential in pycnodysostosis remains yet to be shown (Bizaoui et al. 2019).

*Cathepsin C deficiency:* autophagic flux has been shown to be impaired in Papillon–Lefèvre syndrome and is suggested to play an important role in PLS pathophysiology. Providing recombinant cathepsin C to fibroblasts of PLS patients partially restored autophagic flux, reduced lysosomal membrane permeability, and improved the fibroblast growth rate (Bullon et al. 2018). This suggests that enzyme replacement therapy and gene therapy approaches may be of interest in PLS.

## References

Ahrens-Nicklas R, Schlotawa L, Ballabio A, et al. Complex care of individuals with multiple sulfatase deficiency: clinical cases and consensus statement. Mol Genet Metab. 2018;123:337–46.

Austin J, McAfee D, Armstrong D, O'Rourke M, Shearer L, Bachhawat B. Abnormal sulphatase activities in two human diseases (metachromatic leucodystrophy and gargoylism). Biochem J. 1964;93:15C–7C.

Bargal R, Avidan N, Olender T, et al. Mucolipidosis type IV: novel MCOLN1 mutations in Jewish and non-Jewish patients and the frequency of the disease in the Ashkenazi Jewish population. Hum Mutat. 2001;17:397–402.

Bizaoui V, Michot C, Baujat G, et al. Pycnodysostosis: natural history and management guidelines from 27 French cases and a literature review. Clin Genet. 2019;96:309–16.

Boudewyn LC, Walkley SU. Current concepts in the neuropathogenesis of mucolipidosis type IV. J Neurochem. 2019;148:669–89.

Bullon P, Castejon-Vega B, Roman-Malo L, et al. Autophagic dysfunction in patients with Papillon-Lefevre syndrome is restored by recombinant cathepsin C treatment. J Allergy Clin Immunol. 2018;142:1131–1143.e1137.

Cathey SS, Leroy JG, Wood T, et al. Phenotype and genotype in mucolipidoses II and III alpha/beta: a study of 61 probands. J Med Genet. 2010;47:38–48.

Cheng X, Shen D, Samie M, Xu H. Mucolipins: intracellular TRPML1-3 channels. FEBS Lett. 2010;584:2013–21.

Clapham DE, Runnels LW, Strubing C. The TRP ion channel family. Nat Rev Neurosci. 2001;2:387–96.

Grewal S, Kilic O, Savci-Heijink CD, Kloen P. Disturbed remodeling and delayed fracture healing in pediatric pycnodysostosis patients. J Orthop. 2019;16:373–7.

Hart PS, Zhang Y, Firatli E, et al. Identification of cathepsin C mutations in ethnically diverse papillon-Lefevre syndrome patients. J Med Genet. 2000;37:927–32.

Hennermann JB, Gokce S, Solyom A, Mengel E, Schuchman EH, Simonaro CM. Treatment with pentosan polysulphate in patients with MPS I: results from an open label, randomized, monocentric phase II study. J Inherit Metab Dis. 2016;39:831–7.

Kerr DA, Memoli VA, Cathey SS, Harris BT. Mucolipidosis type III alpha/beta: the first characterization of this rare disease by autopsy. Arch Pathol Lab Med. 2011;135:503–10.

Kobayashi H, Takahashi-Fujigasaki J, Fukuda T, et al. Pathology of the first autopsy case diagnosed as mucolipidosis type III alpha/beta suggesting autophagic dysfunction. Mol Genet Metab. 2011;102:170–5.

Korkmaz B, Caughey GH, Chapple I, et al. Therapeutic targeting of cathepsin C: from pathophysiology to treatment. Pharmacol Ther. 2018;190:202–36.

Leroy JG, Martin JJ. Mucolipidosis II (I-cell disease): present status of knowledge. Birth Defects Orig Artic Ser. 1975;11:283–93.

Lund TC, Cathey SS, Miller WP, et al. Outcomes after hematopoietic stem cell transplantation for children with I-cell disease. Biol Blood Marrow Transplant. 2014;20:1847–51.

Machado RA, Cuadra-Zelaya FJM, Martelli-Junior H, et al. Clinical and molecular analysis in Papillon-Lefevre syndrome. Am J Med Genet A. 2019;179:2124–31.

Markatos K, Mavrogenis AF, Karamanou M, Androutsos G. Pycnodysostosis: the disease of Henri de Toulouse-Lautrec. Eur J Orthop Surg Traumatol. 2018;28:1569–72.

Maroteaux P, Lamy M. Pyknodysostosis. Presse Med. 1962;70:999–1002.

Maroteaux P, Lamy M. [Hurler's pseudo-polydystrophy] La pseudo-polydystrophie de Hurler. Presse Med. 1966;74:2889–92.

Matos L, Vilela R, Rocha M, et al. Development of an antisense oligonucleotide-mediated exon skipping therapeutic strategy for mucolipidosis II: validation at RNA level. Hum Gene Ther. 2020;31:775–83.

Nampoothiri S, Elcioglu NH, Koca SS, et al. Does the clinical phenotype of mucolipidosis-IIIgamma differ from its alphabeta counterpart?: Supporting facts in a cohort of 18 patients. Clin Dysmorphol. 2019;28:7–16.

Novinec M, Lenarcic B. Cathepsin K: a unique collagenolytic cysteine peptidase. Biol Chem. 2013;394:1163–79.

Reitman ML, Kornfeld S. UDP-N-acetylglucosamine:glycoprotein N-acetylglucosamine-1-phosphotransferase. Proposed enzyme for the phosphorylation of the high mannose oligosaccharide units of lysosomal enzymes. J Biol Chem. 1981;256:4275–81.

Robinson C, Baker N, Noble J, et al. The osteodystrophy of mucolipidosis type III and the effects of intravenous pamidronate treatment. J Inherit Metab Dis. 2002;25:681–93.

Sabourdy F, Mourey L, Le Trionnaire E, et al. Natural disease history and characterisation of SUMF1 molecular defects in ten unrelated patients with multiple sulfatase deficiency. Orphanet J Rare Dis. 2015;10:31.

Schlotawa L, Ennemann EC, Radhakrishnan K, et al. SUMF1 mutations affecting stability and activity of formylglycine generating enzyme predict clinical outcome in multiple sulfatase deficiency. Eur J Hum Genet. 2011;19:253–61.

Spampanato C, De Leonibus E, Dama P, et al. Efficacy of a combined intracerebral and systemic gene delivery approach for the treatment of a severe lysosomal storage disorder. Mol Ther. 2011;19:860–9.

Sreeramulu B, Shyam ND, Ajay P, Suman P. Papillon-Lefevre syndrome: clinical presentation and management options. Clin Cosmet Investig Dent. 2015;7:75–81.

Tan EY, Boelens JJ, Jones SA, Wynn RF. Hematopoietic stem cell transplantation in inborn errors of metabolism. Front Pediatr. 2019;7:433.

Velho RV, Harms FL, Danyukova T, et al. The lysosomal storage disorders mucolipidosis type II, type III alpha/beta, and type III gamma: update on GNPTAB and GNPTG mutations. Hum Mutat. 2019;40:842–64.

Wen X, Yi LZ, Liu F, Wei JH, Xue Y. The role of cathepsin K in oral and maxillofacial disorders. Oral Dis. 2016;22:109–15.

Xue Y, Cai T, Shi S, et al. Clinical and animal research findings in pycnodysostosis and gene mutations of cathepsin K from 1996 to 2011. Orphanet J Rare Dis. 2011;6:20.

Zolkipli Z, Noimark L, Cleary MA, Owens C, Vellodi A. Temporomandibular joint destruction in mucolipidosis type III necessitating gastrostomy insertion. Eur J Pediatr. 2005;164:772–4.

# Oligosaccharidoses and Sialic Acid Disorders

# 63

Michael Beck and Zoltan Lukacs

## Contents



**Zoltan Lukacs** was deceased on 13. August 2020.

M. Beck (✉)
SphinCS GmbH–Clinical Science for LSD, Hochheim, Germany
e-mail: michael.beck@sphincs.de

Z. Lukacs
Newborn Screening and Metabolic Diagnostics Unit, Hamburg University Medical Center, Hamburg, Germany

**Summary**

Oligosaccharidoses comprise a group of disorders which show glycoprotein excretion in urine and diminished activity of lysosomal enzymes that are involved in the degradation of sugar side chains (Tables 63.1–63.14). Among those are glycosylasparaginase deficiency (aspartylglucosaminuria), α-L-fucosidase deficiency (fucosidosis), α- and β-mannosidase deficiency (α- and β-mannosidosis), α-*N*-acetylgalactosaminidase deficiency (Kanzaki and Schindler disease), and neuraminidase deficiency (siali-



N. Blau et al. (eds.), *Physician's Guide to the Diagnosis, Treatment, and Follow-Up of Inherited Metabolic Diseases*,
https://doi.org/10.1007/978-3-030-67727-5_63

dosis) (Fig. 63.1). In contrast to the latter, where the degradation of glycosides is impaired, disorders of sialic acid (= N-acetyl neuraminic acid, Neu5Ac) metabolism are based on different mechanisms: A defect of sialin, a transporter protein of the lysosomal membrane, leads to accumulation of sialic acid within the lysosomes and clinical consequences, namely to Salla disease and the more severe form, free sialic acid storage disorder (Fig. 63.2). Sialuria, inclusion body myopathy and a defect of N-acetylneuraminic acid synthase (NANS) are due to a disturbance of sialic acid biosynthesis. In patients with a deficiency of N-acetylneuraminate pyruvate lyase (NPL) the degradation of sialic acid is impaired. Oligosaccharidoses and sialic acid disorders are rare and present a wide phenotypic spectrum. Detection of oligosaccharides in urine and enzyme activity measurements in leukocytes or fibroblasts is usually diagnostic. Free sialic acid has to be assessed by HPLC. For final confirmation a molecular genetic test should be carried out. To date mainly palliative therapies can be provided.

## Introduction

The term oligosaccharidoses comprises a group of disorders that are caused by defective degradation of protein-bound sugar side chains as a result of deficiency in certain lysosomal enzymes. Hurler-like symptoms, skeletal abnormalities, hearing impairment, and neurological symptoms are common features of most of these conditions. As it is common to all lysosomal storage disorders, a broad phenotypic heterogeneity is observed within each of the oligosaccharidoses, ranging from a severe neonatal to a milder adult form, making the clinical diagnosis often difficult.

In sialidosis the enzyme neuraminidase is deficient. In vivo this enzyme is found within a multienzyme complex consisting of protective protein/cathepsin A (PPCA), neuraminidase and β-galactosidase. Cathepsin A stabilizes this structure, and a defect of that protein leads to the disease galactosialidosis in which both neuraminidase and ß-galactosidase are deficient. Clinically galactosialidosis resembles sialidosis.

The diseases named after Schindler and Kanzaki represent different phenotypic expressions of α-*N*-acetylgalactosaminidase (α-NAGA) deficiency. However, it seems that α-NAGA deficiency alone cannot explain the phenotypic variation among patients with the same mutation. The first two brothers described by Schindler et al. (Schindler et al. 1989) had clinical signs of neuroaxonal dystrophy, a neurodegenerative disorder that is now known to be caused by mutations of the *PLA2G6* gene. Therefore it must be suggested that mutations in this gene have caused neuroaxonal dystrophy in the original patients with Schindler disease (Westaway et al. 2007). And also in other patients with α-NAGA deficiency, no clear correlation between residual enzyme activity and the severity of symptoms exists. Therefore, most likely other factors or genes contribute to this clinical heterogeneity (Bakker et al. 2001).

In contrast to oligosaccharidoses, where the degradation of sugar side chains is impaired, other pathogenetic mechanisms are responsible for sialic acid disorders. A defect of sialin, a specific carrier protein of the lysosomal membrane that transports sialic acid out of the lysosomes, leads to progressive accumulation of this compound in the cell, resulting in the allelic disorders free sialic acid storage disease and Salla disease. Free sialic acid storage disease represents the severe infantile form, characterized by global developmental delay, hepatosplenomegaly, cardiomegaly, and early death. The less severe adult form is named Salla disease after a geographic region in Finland where the patients' families have lived. Patients with Salla disease show a broad phenotypic spectrum ranging from mild cognitive dysfunction and ataxia to an intermediate severe form characterized by coarse facial features, intellectual disability, hypotonia, and hepatosplenomegaly (Barmherzig et al. 2017).

The biosynthesis of sialic acid is a complex process in which the enzyme UDP-GlcNac 2-epimerase/ManNAc kinase (GNE) plays an essential role as the master regulator. This enzyme consists of two independent functional domains, an N-terminal domain covering the epimerase activity and a C-terminal domain responsible for ManNAc kinase activity. In the initial step of sialic acid synthesis, the active site of UDP-GlcNac 2-epimerase converts UDP-GlcNAc into ManNAc. The activity of UDP-GlcNac 2-epimerase is regulated by allosteric feedback inhibition by CMP-sialic acid, the final product of the synthetic pathway.

Two disorders are known in GNE deficiency: hereditary inclusion body myopathy (or Nonaka myopathy; autosomal recessive) and sialuria (autosomal dominant). Sialuria is a genetic defect of the feedback inhibition of UDP-GlcNac 2-epimerase resulting in cytoplasmic accumulation and urinary excretion of large amounts of free sialic acid. Characteristic clinical signs of sialuria include developmental delay, mildly coarse features, hepatomegaly, and prolonged neonatal jaundice (Ferreira et al. 2018). Until now, only nine patients with sialuria have been described (Martinez et al. 2018).

The C-terminal domain of UDP-GlcNac 2-epimerase/ManNAc kinase converts ManNAc into ManNAc-6-phosphate. Mutations of this domain, but in some cases also of the epimerase domain, lead to the autosomal recessive adult-onset hereditary inclusion body myopathy (HIBM), also called distal myopathy with rimmed vacuoles or Nonaka myopathy. In affected patients progressive muscle weakness and limb atrophy are the leading clinical signs. This is associated with muscle hyposialylation. A unique feature of hereditary inclusion body myopathy is the sparing of the quadriceps muscles, even in advanced stages of the disease.

Since both disorders hereditary inclusion body myopathy and sialuria represent defects in the biosynthesis of sialic acid, an important component of the glycosylation machinery, they are also classified as congenital disorders of glycosylation (CDG) (Ferreira et al. 2018).

As the next step in the sialic acid biosynthetic pathway, ManNAc-6-phosphate is converted to N-acetylneuraminic acid (Neu5Ac) by N-acetylneuraminic acid synthase (NANS) and N-acetylneuraminic acid phosphatase (NANP), respectively. Finally, Neu5Ac is transported to the nucleus and there activated to CMP-sialic acid by the enzyme cytidine monophosphate N-acetylneuraminic acid synthase (CMAS). CMP-sialic acid is transferred to the Golgi apparatus by the specific transporter SLC35A1 for sialylation of gangliosides and glycoproteins (Willems et al. 2016).

A genetic defect of the enzyme N-acetylneuraminic acid synthase (NANS) leads to a disorder characterized by severe developmental delay, intellectual disability, skeletal dysplasia, and coarse facial features (van Karnebeek et al. 2016; van Karnebeek et al. 2017). In the affected patients, the urine concentration of N-acetylmannosamine is increased, but not of sialic acid.

Wen et al. have detected a defect not in the biosynthesis, but in the degradation of sialic acid in two siblings who presented with dilated cardiomyopathy, proximal myopathy, and sensorineural hearing loss. In these patients compound heterozygous mutations in the gene *NPL* have been found that codes for the enzyme N-acetylneuraminate pyruvate lyase NPL (Wen et al. 2018). And a defect of this enzyme that is responsible for the degradation of sialic acid to N-acetylmannosamine and pyruvate leads to significant sialic aciduria, but not to accumulation of sialic acid in fibroblasts.

For the diagnosis of oligosaccharidoses and sialic acid disorders usually thin-layer chromatography (TLC) combined with enzyme measurement and/or mutation analysis is employed. Free sialic acid will not prominently show on thin-layer chromatography, and therefore a dedicated high-performance-liquid-chromatography method is necessary to assess the concentration of sialic acid in urine and possibly fibroblasts. More recently, tandem-mass spectrometry (TMS) has been applied for the determination of oligosaccharides and sialic acid. However, as the differentiation of sugar moieties by TMS is difficult, TLC will probably remain the screening method of choice for the time being. N-Acetylmannosamine has been measured by NMR-spectroscopy.

Finally, molecular genetic testing by using modern methods such as next-generation sequencing will become more important for the diagnosis of these rare disorders.

Unfortunately, despite progress in therapies for many lysosomal storage diseases, the oligosaccharidoses and sialic acid disorders still lack an effective treatment; only for patients affected by alpha-mannosidosis enzyme replacement therapy has become available. However, further understanding of disease mechanism and phenotypic differences between patients with the same mutation may help to pave the way to novel therapies and better care for the patients.

## Nomenclature

| No. | Disorder name | Alternative name 1 | Alternative name 2 | Abbreviation | Gene | Chromosomal localization | Mode of inheritance | Affected protein | OMIM no. | Phenotype |
|---|---|---|---|---|---|---|---|---|---|---|
| 63.1 | Sialidosis | Mucolipidosis type I | Neuraminidase deficiency | NEU | *NEU1* | 6p21.3 | AR | Neuraminidase | 256550 | All forms |
| 63.2 | Galactosialidosis | Protective protein/ cathepsin A deficiency | Goldberg syndrome | GSL | *CTSA* | 20q13.12 | AR | Protective protein/ cathepsin A | 256540 | All forms |
| 63.3 | α-Mannosidosis | α-mannosidase B deficiency | ∅ | LAMAN | *MAN2B1* | 19p13.13 | AR | α-mannosidase B | 248500 | All forms |
| 63.4 | ß-Mannosidosis | ß-mannosidase deficiency | ∅ | LBMAN | *MANBA* | 4q24 | AR | ß-mannosidase | 248510 | All forms |
| 63.5 | Kanzaki disease | α-N-Acetylgalactosaminidase deficiency II | Schindler disease type II | NAGA | *NAGA* | 22q13.2 | AR | α-N-Acetylgalactosaminidase | 609242 | Adult form |
| 63.6 | Schindler disease type III | α-N-Acetylgalactosaminidase deficiency III | ∅ | NAGA | *NAGA* | 22q13.2 | AR | α-N-Acetylgalactosaminidase | 609241 | Juvenile form |
| 63.7 | Fucosidosis | α-Fucosidase deficiency | ∅ | FUCO | *FUCA1* | 1p36.11 | AR | α-Fucosidase | 230000 | All forms |
| 63.8 | Aspartylglucosaminuria | Glycosylasparaginase deficiency | Aspartylglucosaminidase deficiency | AGU | *AGA* | 4q34.3 | AR | Glycosylasparaginase | 208400 | All forms |
| 63.9 | Infantile sialic acid storage disease | ISSD | Solute carrier family 17 member 5 (SLC17A5) deficiency | SLC17A5 | *SLC17A5* | 6q13 | AR | Sialin | 269920 | Infantile form |
| 63.10 | Salla disease | Sialuria, Finnish type | Solute carrier family 17 member 5 (SLC17A5) deficiency | SLC17A5 | *SLC17A5* | 6q13 | AR | Sialin | 604369 | Juvenile/ adult form |
| 63.11 | GNE myopathy | Nonaka myopathy | Hereditary inclusion body myopathy 2 | HIBM | *GNE* | 9p13.3 | AR | UDP-GlcNAc 2-epimerase/ManNac kinase | 605820 | Adult form |
| 63.12 | Sialuria | Sialuria, French type | UDP-GlcNAc 2-epimerase/ManNac kinase superactivity | ∅ | *GNE* | 9p13.3 | AD | UDP-GlcNAc 2-epimerase/ManNac kinase | 269921 | Infantile form |
| 63.13 | Neuraminic acid pyruvate-lyase deficiency | NPL deficiency | ∅ | ∅ | *NPL* | 1q25.3 | AR | N-Acetylneuraminate pyruvate lyase | 611412 | Infantile/ adult form |
| 63.14 | N-Acetylneuraminic acid synthase deficiency | Sialic acid synthase deficiency | Spondyloepimetaphyseal dysplasia Geneviève type | ∅ | *NANS* | 9q22.33 | AR | N-Acetylneuraminic acid synthase | 605202 | Infantile/ adult form |

## Signs and Symptoms

**Table 63.1** Sialidosis

| System | Symptoms and biomarkers | Neonatal (birth–1 month) | Infancy (1–18 months) | Childhood (1.5–11 years) | Adolescence (11–16 years) | Adulthood (>16 years) |
|---|---|---|---|---|---|---|
| CNS | Ataxia | | | ± | ++ | ++ |
| | Developmental delay | | +++ | +++ | + | + |
| | Intellectual disability | | ++ | ++ | + | + |
| | Myoclonic epilepsy | | ± | ± | ++ | +++ |
| | Seizures | ++ | + | + | ± | ± |
| | Spasticity | | + | ++ | + | + |
| | Startle response, exaggerated | | | + | | |
| Dermatological | Angiokeratoma | | | ± | ± | ± |
| Digestive | Hepatosplenomegaly | +++ | ++ | ++ | ± | ± |
| Ear | Hearing loss | | | + | | |
| Eye | Cherry red spot | | ++ | ++ | ++ | ++ |
| | Corneal clouding | ± | + | ± | ± | ± |
| Hematological | Vacuolated lymphocytes | | + | ++ | ± | ± |
| Musculoskeletal | Coarse facial features | ++ | ++ | ++ | | |
| | Dysostosis multiplex | | ++ | ++ | | + |
| | Hernias | + | + | + | ± | ± |
| | Macrocephaly | ± | ± | ± | | |
| | Short stature | | ± | ++ | | |
| Other | Fetal hydrops | +++ | | | | |
| Renal | Renal failure, chronic | | ± | ± | ± | ± |
| Laboratory findings | Alpha-neuraminidase activity | ↓ | ↓ | ↓ | ↓ | ↓ |
| | Sialic acid-rich oligosaccharide (urine) | ↑ | ↑ | ↑ | ↑ | ↑ |

**Table 63.2** Galactosialidosis

| System | Symptoms and biomarkers | Neonatal (birth–1 month) | Infancy (1–18 months) | Childhood (1.5–11 years) | Adolescence (11–16 years) | Adulthood (>16 years) |
|---|---|---|---|---|---|---|
| Cardiovascular | Cardiomyopathy | +++ | ± | + | + | + |
| | Valvular thickening | ± | +++ | – | – | – |
| CNS | Ataxia | | | + | ++ | ++ |
| | Intellectual deterioration | +++ | ± | + | + | + |
| | Myoclonus | | | ++ | ++ | ++ |
| | Seizures | ± | ± | + | + | + |
| | Spasticity | | | + | + | + |
| Dermatological | Angiokeratoma | ± | ± | + | ++ | ++ |
| | Telangiectasia | +++ | ± | ± | ± | ± |
| Digestive | Hepatosplenomegaly | +++ | +++ | ++ | | |
| Eye | Cherry red spot | + | + | +++ | ++ | ++ |
| | Corneal clouding | + | + | + | + | + |
| | Vision, impaired | ± | ± | +++ | +++ | +++ |
| Hematological | Foam cells | +++ | +++ | +++ | +++ | +++ |
| | Vacuolated lymphocytes | +++ | +++ | +++ | +++ | +++ |
| Musculoskeletal | Coarse facial features | + | + | + | + | + |
| | Dysostosis multiplex | ++ | +++ | +++ | + | + |
| | Edema | ++ | ± | – | | |
| | Growth retardation | + | +++ | ++ | ++ | ++ |
| | Hernias | + | – | – | – | – |
| Other | Fetal hydrops | ++ | ± | | | |
| Renal | Proteinuria | +++ | ++ | ± | ± | ± |
| | Renal failure | +++ | ++ | ± | ± | ± |
| Laboratory findings | Alpha-neuraminidase activity | ↓↓↓ | ↓↓↓ | ↓↓ | ↓ | ↓ |
| | Beta-galactosidase | ↓↓↓ | ↓↓↓ | ↓↓ | ↓ | ↓ |
| | Cathepsin A activity | ↓-n | ↓-n | ↓-n | ↓-n | ↓-n |
| | Sialic acid-rich oligosaccharide (urine) | ↑↑↑ | ↑↑↑ | ↑↑↑ | ↑↑ | ↑↑ |

**Table 63.3** Alpha-mannosidosis

| System | Symptoms and biomarkers | Neonatal (birth–1 month) | Infancy (1–18 months) | Childhood (1.5–11 years) | Adolescence (11–16 years) | Adulthood (>16 years) |
|---|---|---|---|---|---|---|
| CNS | Ataxia | | | + | ++ | +++ |
| | Intellectual disability | | ± | + | ++ | +++ |
| | Spasticity | | | ± | ± | ± |
| Digestive | Hepatomegaly | ++ | | | | |
| Ear | Deafness, sensorineural | | ++ | +++ | +++ | +++ |
| Eye | Corneal clouding | | | ± | ± | ± |
| | Corneal deposits | | | ± | ± | ± |
| Hematological | Vacuolated lymphocytes | ± | + | + | + | + |
| Musculoskeletal | Coarse facial features | | ++ | ++ | + | + |
| | Dysostosis multiplex | | + | + | ± | ± |
| | Hernias | ± | + | + | + | ± |
| | Macrocephaly | | + | + | + | ± |
| Other | Immunodeficiency | | ++ | ++ | ++ | + |
| Psychiatric | Psychosis | | | | + | + |
| Laboratory findings | Alpha-mannosidase B (fibroblasts) | ↓ | ↓ | ↓ | ↓ | ↓ |
| | Alpha-mannosidase B (white blood cells) | ↓ | ↓ | ↓ | ↓ | ↓ |
| | Mannose-oligosaccharides (urine) | ↑ | ↑ | ↑ | ↑ | ↑ |

**Table 63.4** β-Mannosidase deficiency

| System | Symptoms and biomarkers | Neonatal (birth–1 month) | Infancy (1–18 months) | Childhood (1.5–11 years) | Adolescence (11–16 years) | Adulthood (>16 years) |
|---|---|---|---|---|---|---|
| CNS | Ataxia | | | | ± | ± |
| | Intellectual disability | | + | + | + | ++ |
| | Polyneuropathy | | | | ± | ± |
| | Spasticity | | ± | ± | ± | ± |
| Dermatological | Angiokeratoma | | ± | ± | ± | ± |
| Ear | Hearing loss | | + | ++ | +++ | +++ |
| Musculoskeletal | Coarse facial features | | | + | + | |
| | Dysostosis multiplex | | ± | ± | ± | ± |
| | Short stature | | ± | ± | ± | ± |
| Laboratory findings | Beta-mannosidase (fibroblasts) | ↓ | ↓ | ↓ | ↓ | ↓ |
| | Beta-mannosidase (white blood cells) | ↓ | ↓ | ↓ | ↓ | ↓ |

**Table 63.5** Kanzaki disease

| System | Symptoms and biomarkers | Neonatal (birth–1 month) | Infancy (1–18 months) | Childhood (1.5–11 years) | Adolescence (11–16 years) | Adulthood (>16 years) |
|---|---|---|---|---|---|---|
| Cardiovascular | Cardiomyopathy, hypertrophic | | | | | + |
| CNS | Intellectual disability, mild | | | | | ± |
| | Neuropathy, sensory | | | | | ± |
| Dermatological | Angiokeratoma | | | | | ++ |
| | Lymphedema | | | | ± | ± |
| Eye | Corneal clouding | | | | | |
| Musculoskeletal | Coarse facial features | | | | | ± |
| Laboratory findings | Alpha-N-acetylgalactosaminidase (fibroblasts) | ↓ | ↓ | ↓ | ↓ | ↓ |
| | Alpha-N-acetylgalactosaminidase (white blood cells) | ↓ | ↓ | ↓ | ↓ | ↓ |

**Table 63.6** Schindler disease

| System | Symptoms and biomarkers | Neonatal (birth–1 month) | Infancy (1–18 months) | Childhood (1.5–11 years) | Adolescence (11–16 years) | Adulthood (>16 years) |
|---|---|---|---|---|---|---|
| CNS | Autism | | | ± | | |
| | Developmental delay | | ± | ± | | |
| | Intellectual disability | | + | | | |
| | Seizures | | ± | ± | | |
| Eye | Cataract | | ± | | | |
| Cardiovascular | Cardiomyopathy | | ± | | | |
| Digestive | Hepatomegaly | | ± | | | |
| Laboratory findings | Alpha-N-acetylgalactosaminidase (fibroblasts) | ↓ | ↓ | ↓ | ↓ | ↓ |
| | Alpha-N-acetylgalactosaminidase (white blood cells) | ↓ | ↓ | ↓ | ↓ | ↓ |

**Table 63.7** Fucosidosis

| System | Symptoms and biomarkers | Neonatal (birth–1 month) | Infancy (1–18 months) | Childhood (1.5–11 years) | Adolescence (11–16 years) | Adulthood (>16 years) |
|---|---|---|---|---|---|---|
| Autonomic system | Sweating | | | ± | ± | ± |
| CNS | Epileptic seizures | | ± | + | + | ± |
| | Intellectual disability | | ± | ++ | ++ | + |
| | Spasticity | | ± | ++ | ++ | +++ |
| Dermatological | Angiokeratoma | | ± | + | + | + |
| Digestive | Hepatosplenomegaly | | ± | ± | ± | ± |
| Ear | Hearing loss | | | ± | ± | ± |
| Eye | Corneal clouding | | ± | ± | ± | ± |
| Hematological | Vacuolated lymphocytes | | ± | ± | ± | ± |
| Musculoskeletal | Coarse facial features | | ± | + | + | + |
| | Dysostosis multiplex | | ± | + | + | ± |
| | Hernias | ± | ± | ± | ± | ± |
| | Short stature | | | + | + | ± |
| Laboratory findings | Alpha-L-fucosidase (fibroblasts) | ↓ | ↓ | ↓ | ↓ | ↓ |
| | Alpha-L-fucosidase (white blood cells) | ↓ | ↓ | ↓ | ↓ | ↓ |
| | Fucose (urine) | ↑ | ↑ | ↑ | ↑ | ↑ |

**Table 63.8** Aspartylglucosaminuria

| System | Symptoms and biomarkers | Neonatal (birth–1 month) | Infancy (1–18 months) | Childhood (1.5–11 years) | Adolescence (11–16 years) | Adulthood (>16 years) |
|---|---|---|---|---|---|---|
| Cardiovascular | Cardiomyopathy, hypertrophic | | – | ± | ± | ± |
| CNS | Epileptic seizures | | ± | ± | ± | ± |
| | Intellectual disability | | | + | ++ | ++ |
| | Spasticity | | – | ± | + | + |
| Dermatological | Angiokeratoma | ± | ± | ± | ± | ± |
| Digestive | Hepatosplenomegaly | ± | ± | ± | ± | ± |
| Hematological | Vacuolated lymphocytes | + | + | ± | ± | ± |
| Musculoskeletal | Club foot | ± | | | | |
| | Coarse facial features | – | – | ± | + | + |
| | Dysostosis multiplex | ± | ± | + | + | + |
| | Hernias | ± | ± | ± | ± | ± |
| | Hypotonia, muscular-axial | ++ | ± | | | |
| | Macrocephaly | ± | ± | ± | ± | |
| | Short stature | | | | ± | ± |
| Other | Accelerated growth | ++ | + | | | |
| Laboratory findings | Aspartylglucosamine (urine) | ↑ | ↑ | ↑ | ↑ | ↑ |
| | Aspartylglucosaminidase (fibroblasts) | ↓ | ↓ | ↓ | ↓ | ↓ |
| | Aspartylglucosaminidase (lymphocytes) | ↓ | ↓ | ↓ | ↓ | ↓ |
| | Aspartylglucosaminidase (white blood cells) | ↓ | ↓ | ↓ | ↓ | ↓ |

**Table 63.9** Free sialic acid storage disease

| System | Symptoms and biomarkers | Neonatal (birth–1 month) | Infancy (1–18 months) | Childhood (1.5–11 years) | Adolescence (11–16 years) | Adulthood (>16 years) |
|---|---|---|---|---|---|---|
| CNS | Ataxia | | | ± | | |
| | Developmental delay | ± | +++ | +++ | | |
| | Hypotonia | ± | ± | + | | |
| | Spasticity | | + | + | | |
| Digestive | Hepatosplenomegaly | + | ++ | ++ | | |
| Eye | Nystagmus | | | + | | |
| Musculoskeletal | Coarse facial features | ± | ± | ± | | |
| | Growth retardation | | + | ++ | | |
| | Hernias | ± | ± | ± | | |
| Other | Fetal hydrops | ± | | | | |
| Laboratory findings | N-Acetylneuraminic acid (urine) | ↑ | ↑ | ↑ | ↑ | ↑ |
| | Sialic acid, free (urine) | ↑ | ↑ | ↑ | ↑ | ↑ |

**Table 63.10** Salla disease

| System | Symptoms and biomarkers | Neonatal (birth–1 month) | Infancy (1–18 months) | Childhood (1.5–11 years) | Adolescence (11–16 years) | Adulthood (>16 years) |
|---|---|---|---|---|---|---|
| CNS | Ataxia | | | ± | +++ | +++ |
| | Developmental delay | | + | + | + | + |
| | Hypotonia | | | + | ± | ± |
| | Intellectual disability | | | ++ | ++ | +++ |
| | Seizures | | | + | + | + |
| | Spasticity | | + | + | ++ | +++ |
| Digestive | Hepatosplenomegaly | | ± | ± | ± | ± |
| Eye | Nystagmus | | | + | + | + |
| | Optic atrophy | | | ± | ± | ± |
| Musculoskeletal | Coarse facial features | | ± | ± | ± | ± |
| | Growth retardation | | | + | + | + |
| | Hernias | | ± | | | |
| Laboratory findings | N-Acetylneuraminic acid (urine) | ↑ | ↑ | ↑ | ↑ | ↑ |
| | Sialic acid, free (urine) | ↑ | ↑ | ↑ | ↑ | ↑ |

**Table 63.11** UDP-GlcNAc epimerase-kinase deficiency

| System | Symptoms and biomarkers | Neonatal (birth–1 month) | Infancy (1–18 months) | Childhood (1.5–11 years) | Adolescence (11–16 years) | Adulthood (>16 years) |
|---|---|---|---|---|---|---|
| Cardiovascular | Cardiomyopathy | | | | | ± |
| Musculoskeletal | Foot drop | | | | ± | ± |
| | Muscle dystrophy, progressive | | | | ± | ++ |
| | Muscle histopathology, rimmed vacuoles | | | | ± | + |
| | Muscle histopathology, tubulofilaments | | | | ± | + |
| | Muscle wasting of limbs with sparing of quadriceps muscles | | | | ± | +++ |
| Respiratory | Respiratory dysfunction | | | | | + |
| Laboratory findings | Creatine kinase (plasma) | n | n | n | n-↑ | n-↑ |
| | Sialotransferrins (serum) | n | n | n | n | n |

**Table 63.12** UDP-GlcNAc epimerase-kinase superactivity

| System | Symptoms and biomarkers | Neonatal (birth–1 month) | Infancy (1–18 months) | Childhood (1.5–11 years) | Adolescence (11–16 years) | Adulthood (>16 years) |
|---|---|---|---|---|---|---|
| CNS | Cognitive decline | | ++ | + | ± | |
| | Intellectual disability, mild | | | | ± | |
| | Jaundice, prolonged neonatal | ± | | | | |
| | Motor developmental delay | | ++ | + | ± | |
| Digestive | Hepatomegaly | | + | + | + | |
| Musculoskeletal | Coarse facial features | | + | + | ± | |
| Laboratory findings | N-Acetylneuraminic acid (urine) | ↑↑↑ | ↑↑↑ | ↑↑↑ | ↑↑↑ | ↑↑↑ |
| | Sialic acid, free (urine) | ↑↑↑ | ↑↑↑ | ↑↑↑ | ↑↑↑ | ↑↑↑ |

**Table 63.13** Neuraminic acid pyruvate-lyase deficiency[a]

| System | Symptoms and biomarkers | Neonatal (birth–1 month) | Infancy (1–18 months) | Childhood (1.5–11 years) | Adolescence (11–16 years) | Adulthood (>16 years) |
|---|---|---|---|---|---|---|
| Cardiovascular | Cardiomyopathy, dilated | | | | | + |
| | Fetal arrhythmia | ± | | | | |
| Ear | Hearing loss, sensorineural | | | | | + |
| Musculoskeletal | Proximal myopathy | | | | | + |
| Other | Fetal hydrops | ± | | | | |
| Laboratory findings | N-Acetylneuraminic acid (urine) | ↑ | ↑ | ↑ | ↑ | ↑ |
| | Sialic acid, free (urine) | ↑ | ↑ | ↑ | ↑ | ↑ |

[a]Wen et al. (2018)

**Table 63.14** N-acetylneuraminic acid synthase deficiency[a]

| System | Symptoms and biomarkers | Neonatal (birth–1 month) | Infancy (1–18 months) | Childhood (1.5–11 years) | Adolescence (11–16 years) | Adulthood (>16 years) |
|---|---|---|---|---|---|---|
| CNS | Developmental delay | | +++ | +++ | | |
| | Epileptic seizures | | | | ± | ± |
| | Hydrocephalus | ± | | | | |
| | Intellectual disability | | | | +++ | +++ |
| | Muscle hypotonia | | + | + | | |
| Musculoskeletal | Coarse facial features | | | | +++ | +++ |
| | Short limbs | + | + | + | +++ | +++ |
| | Short stature | | | | +++ | +++ |
| Laboratory findings | N-acetylmannosamine (urine) | Not known | Not known | ↑↑ | ↑↑ | ↑↑ |
| | Sialic acid, free (urine) | n | n | n | n | n |

[a]van Karnebeek et al. (2017)

## Metabolic Pathways

Lysosomal enzymes that cleave sugar residues from glycoproteins are deficient in oligosaccharidoses (Fig. 63.1). In aspartylglucosaminuria, glycosylasparaginase shows diminished activity (Fig. 63.1, step 2). This enzyme requires prior hydrolysis of both peptide bonds joined to the asparagine (Asn). This is achieved by lysosomal cathepsins. In addition, the enzyme is inhibited by fucose that is bound to the core reducing end of N-acetylglucosamine (Fig. 63.1, step 1). This special property explains why most of fragments that accumulate in fucosidosis are glycopeptides that retain the Asn residue (Aronson Jr. 1999). In α-mannosidosis oligosaccharides containing α-1–3 and α-1–6 linkages accumulate, while in β-mannosidosis the disaccharide Man-β1-4GlcNAc is the major storage material (Fig. 63.1, step 4α/β). For α-NAGA deficiency the major compounds are sialylglycopeptides of the O-linked type. However, they seem not to be the primary lysosomal storage product (Keulemans et al. 1996). Sialidosis is characterized by increased amounts of sialylated oligosaccharides and glycoproteins (Fig. 63.1, step 3).

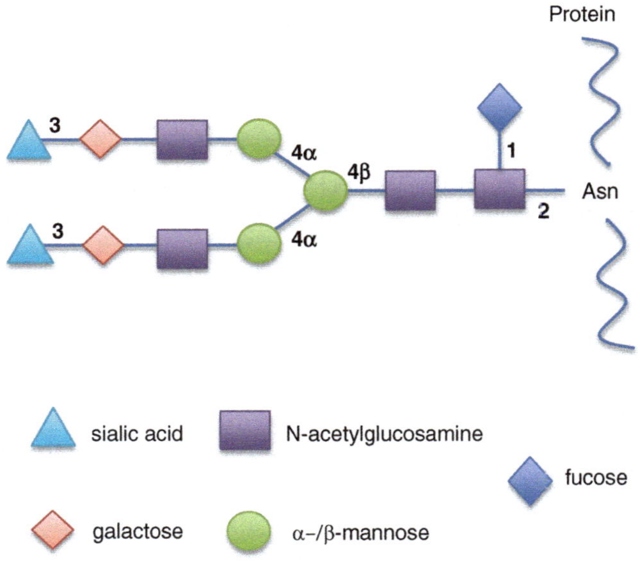


**Fig. 63.1** Degradation of complex oligosaccharides. Liberation of the glycoside from the protein by lysosomal cathepsins is followed by a sequential degradation of the sugar moieties (steps 1–4). Galactose and N-acetylglucosamine are cleaved by β-galactosidase and hexosaminidase, respectively, between steps 3 and 4

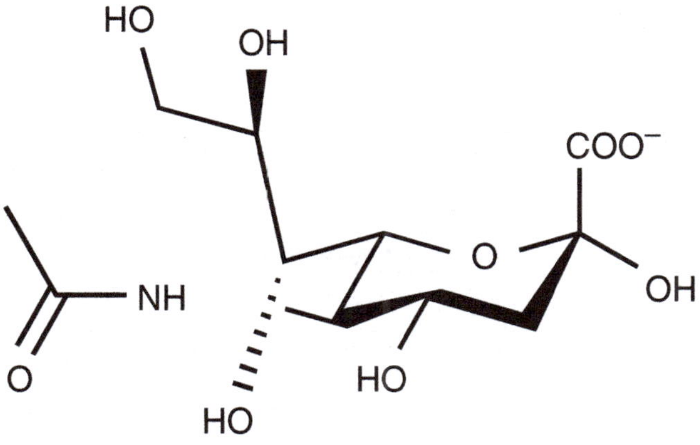


**Fig. 63.2** Sialic acid (N-acetyl neuraminic acid, Neu5Ac)

In Salla disease, a defect in the membrane transporter protein, sialin, impairs efflux of sialic acid (Fig. 63.2) from the lysosomes, so that this compound accumulates in the cell.

## Reference Values

Reference values for analysis of the specific enzymes deficient in the respective disorders and free sialic acid. Activities are usually independent of age and gender. Ranges are listed according to methods and materials used.

| Entry | Protein | Method | Material | Range (unit) |
|---|---|---|---|---|
| 1 | AGU | 2-AADG[a] | Fibroblasts | 45–333 (nmol/min*g) |
| 2 | AGU | 2-AADG[a] | Lymphocytes | 91–243 (nmol/min*g) |
| 3 | AGU | 2-AADG[a] | Leukocytes | 22–132 (nmol/min*g) |
| 4 | AGU | 2-AADG[a] | Plasma | 45–170 (nmol/min*mL) |
| 5 | AGU | AspAMC[b] | Lymphocytes | 87–493 (μU/mg) |
| 6 | AGU | AspAMC[b] | Serum | 10.6–28.2 (mU/L) |
| 7 | AGU | AspAMC[b] | Plasma | 10.2–26.0 (mU/L) |
| 8 | FUCO | NitroF[c] | Fibroblasts | 2.3–41.9 (nmol/mg*h) |
| 9 | FUCO | MUF[d] | DBS | 0.2–2.1 (nmol/spot*21 h) |
| 10 | FUCO | MUF[d] | Leukocytes | 0.05–0.4 (nmol/mg*min) |
| 11 | FUCO | MUF[d] | Fibroblasts | 0.05–0.33 (nmol/mg*min) |
| 12 | FUCO | MUF[d] | Plasma | 2.4–7.3 (nmol/min*mL) |
| 13 | LAMAN | MUAM[e] | DBS | 0.3–1.3 (nmol/spot*21 h) |
| 14 | LAMAN | MUAM[e] | Leukocytes | 0.09–0.7 (nmol/min*mg) |
| 15 | LBMAN | MUBM[f] | Plasma | 240–800 (μM/h*L) |
| 16 | LBMAN | MUBM[f] | Leukocytes | 245–467 (μM/h*g) |
| 17 | LBMAN | MUBM[f] | Fibroblasts | 58–389 (μM/h*g) |
| 18 | LBMAN | MUBM[f] | DBS | 0.92–2.89 (nmol/spot*21 h) |
| 18 | NAGA | MUNAC[g] | Fibroblasts | 40–130 (nmol/h*mg) |
| 19 | NAGA | MUNAC[g] | Plasma | 4–8.33 (nmol/s*L) |
| 20 | NAGA | MUNAC[g] | Lymphoblasts | 10.5–27.2 (nmol/s*g) |
| 21 | NEU | MUNEU[h] | Fibroblasts | 17.6–189 (nmol/h*mg) |
| 22 | Sialin[i] | HPLC | Fibroblasts | < 1.3 (nmol/mg protein) |
| 23 | Sialin[i] | HPLC | Urine | <1 y < 58<br>1–4 y < 40<br>4–15 y < 30<br>> 15 y < 21<br>(mmol/Mol Crea) |
| 24 | N-Acetyl-man-nosamine[j] | NMR spectros-copy | Urine | < 10 (μmol/mmol Crea) |

[a]2-Acetamido-*N*-(L-aspart-4′-oyl)-2-deoxy-β-glucopyranosylamine
[b]*L*-Aspartic acid β-(7-amido-4-methylcoumarin)
[c]p-Nitrophenyl-α-L-fucopyranoside
[d]4-Methylumbelliferyl-α-L-fucoside
[e]4-Methylumbelliferyl-α-D-mannopyranoside
[f]4-Methylumbelliferyl-β-D-mannopyranoside
[g]4-Methylumbelliferyl-α-*N*-acetylgalactosaminide
[h]4-Methylumbelliferyl-α-neuraminide
[i]Free sialic acid has been determined by HPLC
[j]N-Acetylmannosamine has been determined by NMR spectroscopy (van Karnebeek et al. 2016; 2017)

## Pathological Values

Pathological values for the analysis of the specific enzymes deficient in the listed disorders and free sialic acid. Activities are usually independent of age and gender. Pathological values are restricted to those methods and analytical materials that either have been used at the Hamburg University Medical Center or have been published in peer-reviewed journals.

| Entry | Protein | Method | Material | Range (unit) |
|---|---|---|---|---|
| 1 | AGU | 2-AADG[a] | Fibroblasts | 0–9 (nmol/min*g) |
| 2 | AGU | 2-AADG[a] | Lympho-cytes | 0–5 (nmol/min*g) |
| 3 | AGU | 2-AADG[a] | Leukocytes | 0 (nmol/min*g) |
| 4 | AGU | 2-AADG[a] | Plasma | 0–2 (nmol/min*mL) |
| 5 | AGU | AspAMC[b] | Lympho-cytes | 1.2–11.4 (μU/mg) |
| 6 | AGU | AspAMC[b] | Serum | 0–1.2 (mU/L) |
| 7 | AGU | AspAMC[b] | Plasma | 0–0.9 (mU/L) |

| Entry | Protein | Method | Material | Range (unit) |
|---|---|---|---|---|
| 8 | FUCO | NitroP[c] | Fibroblasts | 0–0.08 (nmol/mg*h) |
| 9 | FUCO | MUF[d] | Plasma[e] | 0 (nmol/mL*min) |
| 10 | LAMAN | MUAM[f] | Leukocytes | <0.05[g] (nmol/mg*min) |
| 11 | LBMAN | MUBM[h] | Plasma | 0–10 (μM/h*L) |
| 12 | LBMAN | MUBM[h] | Leukocytes | < 1 (μM/h*g) |
| 13 | LBMAN | MUBM[h] | Fibroblasts | 4 ($n$ = 1) (μM/h*g) |
| 14 | NAGA | MUNAC[i] | Fibroblasts | 0.2–3.2 (nmol/h*mg) |
| 15 | NAGA | MUNAC[i] | Plasma | 0.05 ($n$ = 1) (nmol/s*L) |
| 16 | NAGA | MUNAC[i] | Lymphoblasts | 0.05 ($n$ = 1) (nmol/s*g) |
| 17 | NEU | MUNEU[j] | Fibroblasts[k] | 0–5.3 (sialidosis) 0.8–17.0 (galactosialidosis) (nmol/h*mg) |
| 18 | Sialin[l] | HPLC | Fibroblasts | 2.6–23.5 (nmol/mg protein) |
| 19 | Sialin[l] | HPLC | Urine | 48–402 (mmol/Mol Crea) |
| 20 | N-Acetyl-mannosamine[m] | NMR spectroscopy | Urine | 41–295 (μmol/mmol Crea) |

[a]2-Acetamido-*N*-(L-aspart-4′-oyl)-2-deoxy-β-glucopyranosylamine
[b]*L*-Aspartic acid β-(7-amido-4-methylcoumarin)
[c]p-Nitrophenyl-α-L-fucopyranoside
[d]4-Methylumbelliferyl-α-L-fucoside
[e]A polymorphism is responsible for enzyme activities of approx. 25% of the control mean in ca. 10% of the population. This affects only measurements in fibroblasts and plasma. Activity in leukocytes remains unaffected (Willems et al. 1999)
[f]4-Methylumbelliferyl-α-D-mannopyranoside
[g]In affected individuals the residual activity is found to be between 5 and 15% of normal activity. This may be due to the fact that other mannosidases are present and can contribute some activity. Following immunoprecipitation, only 0.1–1.3% of the normal activity has been detected (Malm and Nilssen 2008)
[h]4-Methylumbelliferyl-β-D-mannopyranoside
[i]4-Methylumbelliferyl-α-*N*-acetylgalactosaminide
[j]4-Methylumbelliferyl-α-neuraminide
[k]Enzyme is labile to sonication and freezing. Activity in leukocytes is approx. Tenfold lower than in fibroblasts. For this reason, leukocyte activity measurement is not recommended for diagnosis in sialidosis
[l]Free sialic acid has been determined by HPLC
[m]N-Acetylmannosamine has been determined by NMR spectroscopy (van Karnebeek et al. 2016; 2017)

## Diagnostic Flowcharts (Figs. 63.3, 63.4 and 63.5)

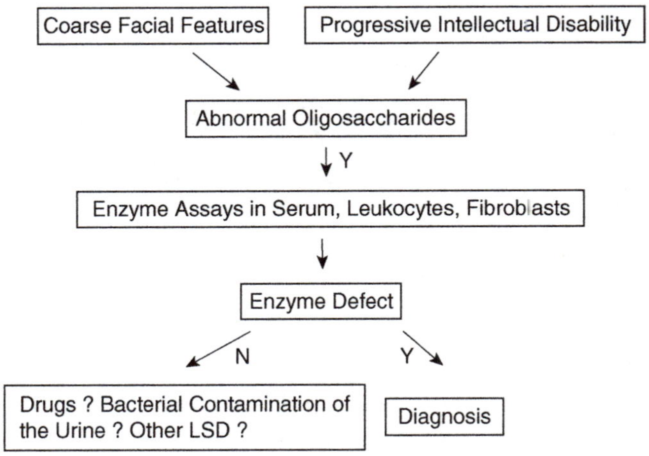


**Fig. 63.3** Flowchart for the diagnosis of oligosaccharide storage disorders

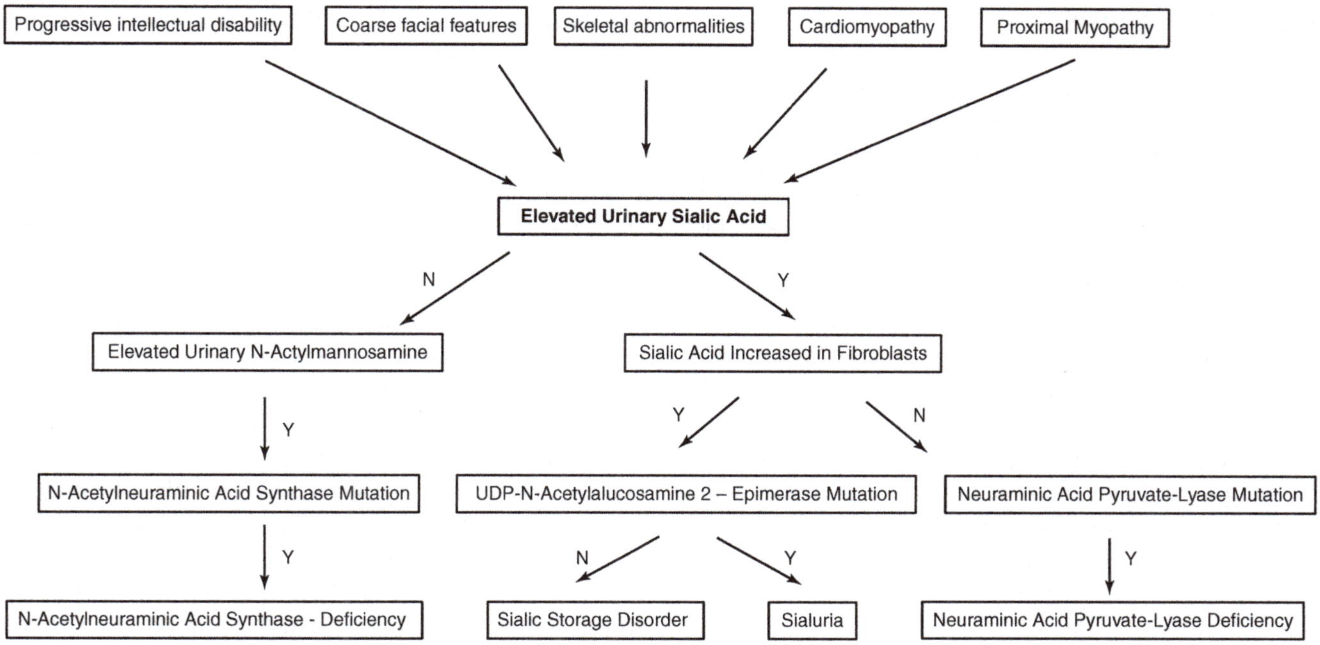


**Fig. 63.4** Flowchart for the diagnosis of sialic acid disorder and sialuria

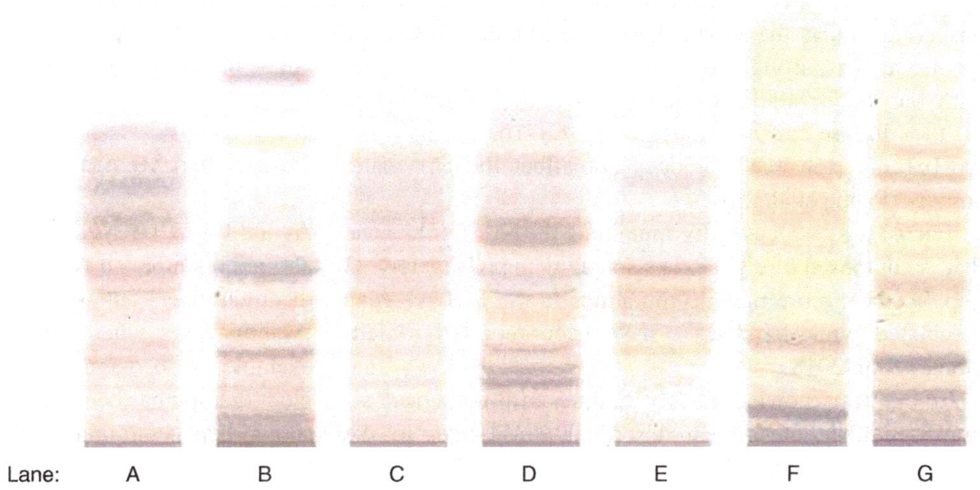


**Fig. 63.5** Oligosaccharides in urine analyzed by thin-layer chromatography provide a simple tool for a primary biochemical diagnosis. This figure shows examples of certain oligosaccharidosis (urines kindly provided by Prof. Beck, Mainz, Germany). Urines from patients with the following disorders have been analyzed: GM2-gangliosidosis, Sandhoff type (lane *A*), fucosidosis (lane *B*), GM1-gangliosidosis, patient 1 (lane *C*), aspartylglucosaminuria (lane *D*), mannosidosis (lane *E*), sialidosis (lane *F*), GM1-gangliosidoses, patient 2 (lane *G*)

## Specimen Collection

For enzyme analysis either fibroblasts, leukocytes/lymphocytes, plasma or dried blood spots can be used, depending on the enzyme that should be determined. Fibroblasts should be taken by specialized staff in a hospital environment. They can be shipped in sterile growth medium or, if shipping time does not exceed 1–2 days, in physiological NaCl solution (also sterile). For leukocytes and lymphocytes whole blood is required (usually approx. 5 mL). Shipping time should be kept to a minimum (less than 3 days). Nevertheless, the likelihood of hemolysis increases with prolonged shipping time. Plasma samples should be shipped after centrifugation and removal of any cell pellet to avoid contamination with hemolyzed cells during shipment. Dried blood specimens can be prepared either from tubes of whole blood or directly from venous/capillary blood. In the case of newborns, the usual procedures for taking newborn screening samples can also be followed. It is especially important that samples are prepared swiftly after the blood has been taken. In addition, they should be dried at room temperature (ca. 20°C) over night before shipment. The stability of enzymes varies widely in dried condition, so that timely shipping and analysis are always preferable.

Oligosaccharides and sialic acid are analyzed from urine. Spontaneous urine samples (ca. 3–5 mL) can be shipped without additives at room temperature, provided no bacterial contamination is present. Otherwise, samples should be shipped on dry ice.

## Prenatal Diagnosis

Preferably, prenatal diagnosis should be performed by molecular genetic testing, especially if mutations from an index patient in the family are already known. Enzyme testing of amniotic cells is also possible. However, it has to be checked whether maternal cells are present and thus may contribute to enzyme activity. In addition, interpretation of low enzyme activity becomes problematic in cases of heterozygote carriers, especially as only a few laboratories have a significant number of normal controls to determine a statistically reliable reference range. In any case, requirements and the possibility of prenatal enzyme testing should be checked with the specialized laboratory before shipment of samples. As in all autosomal-recessive disorders with a known disease-causing mutation, also in lysosomal storage disorders, a preimplantation diagnosis can be performed.

## DNA Testing

In aspartylglucosaminuria the *AGA* gene is comprised of nine exons. About 30 different *AGA* mutations have been observed around the world. Due to a founder effect, the incidence of aspartylglucosaminuria is very high in Finland, with one major allele, named $AGU_{FIN}$, that is composed of the disease-causing substitution Cys163Ser and the Arg161Gln exchange that does not affect the enzymatic activity (Pande et al. 2018).

Fucosidosis is caused by mutations in the *FUCA1* gene that is composed of eight exons spanning approximately 23 kbp. To date, more than 30 mutations in the FUCA1 gene associated with the disease have been reported (Saleh-Gohari et al. 2018).

To our best knowledge, only 22 cases of β-mannosidosis in 18 families have been described worldwide. In the ß-mannosidosis gene *MANBA* that consists of 17 exons, so far 18 disease-causing variants have been reported including both null and missense mutations (Blomqvist et al. 2019).

The α-*N*-acetylgalactosaminidase gene *NAGA* consists of 9 exons coding for 411 amino acids. An overview of mutations is given by Bakker et al. (Bakker et al. 2001).

Sialidosis is caused by mutations in the *NEU1* gene that consists of 6 exons and codes for a protein of 368 amino acid moieties. So far, more than 40 mutations within the *NEU1* gene have been identified in patients with sialidosis type I and II (Khan and Sergi 2018).

Salla disease is caused by mutations in the *SLC17A5* gene that codes for a lysosomal membrane transporter (sialin). The disease is mainly found in Finland, where the missense mutation Arg39Cys is responsible for 95% of cases. An overview of mutations is given by Barmherzig et al. (Barmherzig et al. 2017).

Mutations in the *CTSA* gene lead to the lysosomal storage disorder galactosialidosis that is characterized by the combined deficiency of ß-galactosidase and neuraminidase. More than 30 *CTSA* mutations are known until now (Aldamiz-Echevarria et al. 2018).

The enzyme UDP-GlcNac 2-epimerase/ManNAc kinase (GNE) that plays an essential role in the biosynthesis of sialic acid is encoded by the *GNE* gene on chromosome 9p13.3. Mutations of the *GNE* gene are responsible for two different disorders (See Introduction): Heterozygous missense variants at the allosteric site, specifically at Arginine 294 and Arginine 297, result in sialuria. A new heterozygous pathogenic variant (Asp84His) has been detected in a 2-year-old boy who was diagnosed with sialuria (Martinez et al. 2018).

Mutations elsewhere in the *GNE* gene, which lead to decreased sialylation, are responsible for the hereditary inclusion body myopathy, also called distal myopathy with rimmed vacuoles or Nonaka myopathy. In a study performed by Mori-Yoshimura et al. in order to examine the correlation between genotype and phenotype in 71 patients with genetically confirmed GNE myopathy, it was found that patients with a homozygous mutation in the N-acetylmannosamine kinase domain had an earlier disease onset and exhibited a more severe phenotype compared to compound heterozygous individuals with mutations in the uridine diphosphate-N-acetylglucosamine (UDP-GlcNAc) 2-epimerase and N-acetylmannosamine kinase domains (Mori-Yoshimura et al. 2012).

## Treatment Summary

As until now no specific treatment is available for almost all patients affected by an oligosaccharidosis or sialic acid disorder, they will require significant supportive therapy even in cases where specific therapies are effective, for example, in α-mannosidosis for which enzyme replacement therapy has been approved. The supportive care given should be custom tailored to each disease and each patient, based on the organs affected and the degree of severity of this involvement.

## Standard Treatment

As oligosaccharidoses and sialic acid disorders are multisystemic diseases, the affected individuals often need surgical procedures. The anesthetic management of these patients, however, is often complicated by airway problems such as difficult laryngoscopy secondary to dysmorphic facial features, thoracic deformities, and impaired visualization of the vocal cords (Hallas et al. 2011). In those cases, intubation by fiber-optic laryngoscopy is strongly recommended in order to prevent the necessity of performing a tracheostomy. Preoperative examination should be carefully performed to rule out the presence of cardiomyopathy and hepatosplenomegaly. Epileptic seizures are not uncommon in oligosaccharidoses; they should be treated according to general therapeutic guidelines; in aspartylglucosaminuria patients carbamazepine has been shown to be very effective (Arvio and Mononen 2016). In a 15-year-old sialidosis patient, severe myoclonic seizures could be successfully treated with perampanel, a non-competitive, selective glutamate receptor antagonist (Hu et al. 2018). In fucosidosis, the occurrence of dystonic symptoms has been observed that did not respond to drugs that are commonly used for the treatment of dystonia such as carbamazepine, L-dopa, anticholinergics, or baclofen (Gordon et al. 1995).

Enzyme replacement therapy is now available for α-mannosidosis. In patients treated with the recombinant human α-mannosidase enzyme velmanase alfa, biochemical and functional improvements were seen for up to 4 years (Lund et al. 2018).

## Experimental Treatment

### Substrate Supplementation

Several mouse models of GNE myopathy have been developed that recapitulate the pathological changes of the human disease. To elucidate whether inclusion body myopathy can be treated by sialic acid supplementation, 6′-sialyllactose or free sialic acid was orally given to GNE myopathy mice. After several weeks of treatment in 6′-sialyllactose-treated mice, spontaneous locomotion activity improved, while in sialic acid-treated mice, just a slowing down of disease progression could be observed (Yonekawa et al. 2014). As this and other animal studies provided a proof of concept of substrate replacement, clinical trials with substrate supplementation in GNE myopathy patients have been initiated.

In a human placebo-controlled, double-blind, single-ascending dose study, 22 subjects suffering from GNE myopathy received N-acetyl-D-mannosamine (ManNAc), the first committed precursor in the sialic acid biosynthetic pathway, at single doses of 3 g, 6 g, or 10 g or placebo. The administration of a single dose of ManNAc resulted in a significant and sustained increase in plasma free sialic acid. In subjects who received a dose of 6 g or 10 g, the sialic acid levels remained above baseline 2 days post-dose (Xu et al. 2017).

Free sialic acid was considered as a therapeutic agent in GNE myopathy and other disorders of sialic acid metabolism. However, as orally administered sialic acid is rapidly cleared from the circulation via the kidney, an extended release formulation of sialic acid (aceneuramic acid extended release; Ace-ER) was developed to achieve a continuous elevated substrate concentration in serum and thereby to attain sufficient muscle uptake (Argov et al. 2016). To investigate the efficacy and safety of Ace-ER, a phase 3, double-blind, placebo-controlled study was performed in 89 patients with GNE myopathy. Clinical endpoints were changes in muscle strength of upper and lower extremity and knee extensor strength. After 48 weeks of treatment with 6 g/day Ace-ER, muscle strength did not differ between the Ace-ER and the placebo group (Lochmüller et al. 2019). The authors come to the conclusion that in future studies the clinical heterogeneity and the rate of progression of the disease need more attention when planning clinical trials in patients with GNE myopathy.

Substrate supplementation may be effective also in other disorders of sialic acid metabolism: A knockdown of *NPL* (N-acetylneuraminate pyruvate lyase deficiency) in zebra fish resulted in skeletal myopathy and cardiac edema, and these abnormalities could be rescued by treatment of embryos with N-acetylglucosamine or N-acetylmannosamine, the catabolic products of NPL (Wen et al. 2018). Knockdown of *NANS* (N-acetylneuraminic acid synthase deficiency) in zebra fish embryos leads to an abnormal skeletal phenotype that can be rescued by exogenously added sialic acid (van Karnebeek et al. 2016; van Karnebeek et al. 2017).

### Enzyme Replacement Therapy

Enzyme replacement therapy has been studied in several animal models of oligosaccharide storage disorders: Dunder and co-workers have given mice affected by aspartylglucosaminuria different dosages of recombinant glycosylasparaginase at the age of 1 week. In the mice who have received the highest amount of enzyme, a reduction of the storage material aspartylglucosamine was observed not only in the visceral organs but also in the brain tissue (Dunder et al. 2010).

Kondagari et al. evaluated the effect of intracisternal infusions of recombinant α-fucosidase on neuropathological findings in the naturally occurring dog model of fucosidosis (Kondagari et al. 2015). The procedure resulted in improvement in almost all measures of neurodegeneration and inflammation in several brain regions. These animal studies may pave the way for clinical trials using recombinant fucosidase.

### Chaperones

An efficient mechanism exists in each cell that controls correct folding of newly synthesized enzymes. As misfolded enzymes are degraded by proteasomes, they cannot reach the Golgi apparatus for further maturation. Specific molecules, named *chaperones*, help the proteins to be folded into the appropriate confirmation. Missense mutations that affect accurate folding of lysosomal enzymes prevent them from reaching the lysosome, so that they cannot fulfill their function. Small pharmacological molecules are able to correct the folding of mutant enzymes and increase their enzymatic activities.

O'Leary et al. used fibroblasts from sialidosis patients in order to examine the efficacy of the immunosuppressant (Celastrol) and a proteosomal inhibitor (MG132) to rescue mutant enzymes with altered conformation. In their study they demonstrated that MG132 could reduce the accumulation of gangliosides, but Celastrol diminished sialidase activity. The combination of both, MG132 and Celastrol, however, resulted in a significant increase in specific sialidase activity beyond that of the enzyme activity measured in normal fibroblasts (O'Leary and Igdoura 2012). This study points to a potential therapeutic strategy for the treatment of sialidosis.

### Hematopoietic Stem Cell Transplantation (HSCT)

Hematopoietic stem cell transplantation (HSCT) was the first approach for the treatment of lysosomal storage disorders. Previously, bone marrow has been traditionally the graft source for this procedure. However, in the last years, more and more patients have been treated with unrelated donor umbilical cord blood transplant, allowing rapid and increased access to transplantation. Krivit et al. analyzed the clinical results of HSCT in over 500 patients with a peroxisomal or lysosomal storage disorder. This study included also individuals with α-mannosidosis, fucosidosis, and aspartylglucosaminuria (Krivit 2004). In those disorders HSCT did not lead to a significant clinical improvement, most probably as the patients were older and had already irreversible organ damage. Arvio et al. reported five patients with aspartylglucosaminuria in whom HSCT was not successful; therefore the authors do not recommend this treatment of patients with this lysosomal storage disorder (Arvio et al. 2001). Some positive were seen in fucosidosis patients who underwent bone marrow transplantation; however, considering the transplantation-related risk, this therapeutic option should be recommended for patients only at an early stage of disease (Jiang et al. 2017).

### Gene Therapy

As lysosomal storage disorders in general represent well-characterized single gene disorders and in addition are not subject to complex regulation mechanisms, they are excellent candidates for therapy by gene transfer. In addition, an enzyme activity of only 15%–20% of the normal level is sufficient for clinical efficacy (Sands and Davidson 2006). A gene can be delivered to the organism by two ways, the ex vivo and the in vivo technique. For ex vivo therapy, stem cells of the patient are transfected with the gene and thereafter returned to the body. This technique was used in a study with a mouse model of galactosialidosis, in which the animals received hematopoietic progenitor cells transduced with a retroviral vector overexpressing the protein protective/cathepsin A (PPCA) that is deficient in galactosialidosis. The procedure resulted in a complete correction of systemic organ damage and in an improvement of CNS pathology (Leimig et al. 2002). The results support the use of this approach for the treatment of patients affected by a galactosialidosis.

The in vivo technique was studied in α-mannosidosis cats that received an intracisternal infusion of adeno-associated virus type 1 (AAV1) expressing the feline α-mannosidase gene. The lifespan of the treated animals was significantly prolonged, the α-mannosidase activity was increased, and the neuropathology showed a reduction of storage material within the whole brain (Yoon et al. 2016).

### Gene Editing

The elegant and easy-to-manage gene editing system CRISPR/Cas9 (clustered regularly interspaced short palindromic repeats/CRISPR-associated protein 9) seems to represent a conceivable therapeutic option for patients affected by a lysosomal storage disorder. This sophisticated technique that is able to selectively target genes containing deleterious mutations and correct the disease-causing mutations is currently used in human pluripotent stem cells taken from patients to correct several genetic diseases and will be probably soon applied in clinical studies in patients with a lysosomal storage disorder (Christensen and Choy 2017).

Besides the CRISPR/Cas9 system, two other gene editing techniques have been developed, namely, zinc finger nucleases (ZFNs) and transcription activator-like effector nucleases (TALENs) (Schneller et al. 2017). These alternative gene editing tools, however, have some disadvantages in comparison with the CRISPR/Cas9 technique.

When and how the results of the experiments with pluripotent stem cells can be transferred to clinical trials cannot be answered now, as this transformation requires the development of quality assays, demonstration of safety and efficacy of new gene therapy protocols, and, last but not least, the approval and consensus of the scientific and biomedical communities (Giugliani et al. 2017).

## References

Aldamiz-Echevarria L, Couce ML, Villate O, Fernandez-Marmiesse A, Pinan MA. New CTSA mutation in early infantile galactosialidosis. Pediatr Int. 2018;60(8):761–2.

Argov Z, Caraco Y, Lau H, Pestronk A, Shieh PB, Skrinar A, et al. Aceneuramic acid extended release administration maintains upper limb muscle strength in a 48-week study of subjects with GNE myopathy: results from a phase 2, randomized, controlled study. J Neuromuscul Dis. 2016;3(1):49–66.

Aronson NN Jr. Aspartylglycosaminuria: biochemistry and molecular biology. Biochim Biophys Acta. 1999;1455(2–3):139–54.

Arvio M, Mononen I. Aspartylglycosaminuria: a review. Orphanet J Rare Dis. 2016;11(1):162.

Arvio M, Sauna-Aho O, Peippo M. Bone marrow transplantation for aspartylglucosaminuria: follow-up study of transplanted and non-transplanted patients. J Pediatr. 2001;138(2):288–90.

Bakker HD, de Sonnaville ML, Vreken P, Abeling NG, Groener JE, Keulemans JL, et al. Human alpha-N-acetylgalactosaminidase (alpha-NAGA) deficiency: no association with neuroaxonal dystrophy? Eur J Hum Genet. 2001;9(2):91–6.

Barmherzig R, Bullivant G, Cordeiro D, Sinasac DS, Blaser S, Mercimek-Mahmutoglu S. A new patient with intermediate severe Salla disease with hypomyelination: a literature review for Salla disease. Pediatr Neurol. 2017;74:87–91.

Blomqvist M, Smeland MF, Lindgren J, Sikora P, Riise Stensland HMF. Asin-Cayuela J. beta-Mannosidosis caused by a novel homozygous intragenic inverted duplication in MANBA. Cold Spring Harb Mol Case Stud. 2019;5:3.

Christensen CL, Choy FYMA. Prospective treatment option for lysosomal storage diseases: CRISPR/Cas9 gene editing technology for mutation correction in induced pluripotent stem cells. Diseases. 2017;5:1.

Dunder U, Valtonen P, Kelo E, Mononen I. Early initiation of enzyme replacement therapy improves metabolic correction in the brain tissue of aspartylglycosaminuria mice. J Inherit Metab Dis. 2010;33(5):611–7.

Ferreira CR, Altassan R, Marques-Da-Silva D, Francisco R, Jaeken J, Morava E. Recognizable phenotypes in CDG. J Inherit Metab Dis. 2018;41(3):541–53.

Giugliani R, Federhen A, Michelin-Tirelli K, Riegel M, Burin M. Relative frequency and estimated minimal frequency of lysosomal storage diseases in Brazil: report from a reference laboratory. Genet Mol Biol. 2017;40(1):31–9.

Gordon BA, Gordon KE, Seo HC, Yang M, DiCioccio RA, O'Brien JS. Fucosidosis with dystonia. Neuropediatrics. 1995;26(6): 325–7.

Hallas P, Borgwardt LG, Roed J, Lauritsen T, Dali CI, Lund AM. Anesthesia for patients with alpha-mannosidosis—a case series of 10 patients. Paediatr Anaesth. 2011;21(12):1269–70.

Hu SC, Hung KL, Chen HJ, Lee WT. Seizure remission and improvement of neurological function in sialidosis with perampanel therapy. Epilepsy Behav Case Rep. 2018;10:32–4.

Jiang M, Liu S, Jiang H, Lin Y, Shao Y, Hu H, et al. Brain abnormalities in fucosidosis: transplantation or supportive therapy? Metab Brain Dis. 2017;32(2):317–20.

Keulemans JL, Reuser AJ, Kroos MA, Willemsen R, Hermans MM, van den Ouweland AM, et al. Human alpha-N-acetylgalactosaminidase (alpha-NAGA) deficiency: new mutations and the paradox between genotype and phenotype. J Med Genet. 1996;33(6):458–64.

Khan A, Sergi C. Sialidosis: a review of morphology and molecular biology of a rare pediatric disorder. Diagnostics (Basel). 2018;8(2):29.

Kondagari GS, Fletcher JL, Cruz R, Williamson P, Hopwood JJ, Taylor RM. The effects of intracisternal enzyme replacement versus sham treatment on central neuropathology in preclinical canine fucosidosis. Orphanet J Rare Dis. 2015;10(1):143.

Krivit W. Allogeneic stem cell transplantation for the treatment of lysosomal and peroxisomal metabolic diseases. Springer Semin Immunopathol. 2004;26(1–2):119–32.

Leimig T, Mann L, Martin Mdel P, Bonten E, Persons D, Knowles J, et al. Functional amelioration of murine galactosialidosis by genetically modified bone marrow hematopoietic progenitor cells. Blood. 2002;99(9):3169–78.

Lochmüller H, Behin A, Caraco Y, Lau H, Mirabella M, Tournev I, et al. A phase 3 randomized study evaluating sialic acid extended-release for GNE myopathy. Neurology. 2019;92(18):e2109–e17.

Lund AM, Borgwardt L, Cattaneo F, Ardigo D, Geraci S, Gil-Campos M, et al. Comprehensive long-term efficacy and safety of recombinant human alpha-mannosidase (velmanase alfa) treatment in patients with alpha-mannosidosis. J Inherit Metab Dis. 2018;41(6):1225–33.

Malm D, Nilssen O. Alpha-mannosidosis. Orphanet J Rare Dis. 2008;3:21.

Martinez NN, Lipke M, Robinson J, Sialuria WB. Ninth patient described has a novel mutation in GNE. JIMD Rep. 2018;44:17–21.

Mori-Yoshimura M, Monma K, Suzuki N, Aoki M, Kumamoto T, Tanaka K, et al. Heterozygous UDP-GlcNAc 2-epimerase and N-acetylmannosamine kinase domain mutations in the GNE gene result in a less severe GNE myopathy phenotype compared to homozygous N-acetylmannosamine kinase domain mutations. J Neurol Sci. 2012;318(1–2):100–5.

O'Leary EM, Igdoura SA. The therapeutic potential of pharmacological chaperones and proteosomal inhibitors, Celastrol and MG132 in the treatment of sialidosis. Mol Genet Metab. 2012;107(1–2):173–85.

Pande S, Bizilj W, Guo HC. Biochemical and structural insights into an allelic variant causing the lysosomal storage disorder—aspartylglucosaminuria. FEBS Lett. 2018;592(15):2550–61.

Saleh-Gohari N, Saeidi K, Zeighaminejad R. A novel homozygous frameshift mutation in the FUCA1 gene causes both severe and mild fucosidosis. J Clin Pathol. 2018;71(9):821–4.

Sands MS, Davidson BL. Gene therapy for lysosomal storage diseases. Mol Ther. 2006;13(5):839–49.

Schindler D, Bishop DF, Wolfe DE, Wang AM, Egge H, Lemieux RU, et al. Neuroaxonal dystrophy due to lysosomal alpha-N-acetylgalactosaminidase deficiency. N Engl J Med. 1989;320(26): 1735–40.

Schneller JL, Lee CM, Bao G, Venditti CP. Genome editing for inborn errors of metabolism: advancing towards the clinic. BMC Med. 2017;15(1):43.

van Karnebeek CDM, Bonafe L, Wen XY, Tarailo-Graovac M, Balzano S, Royer-Bertrand B, et al. Corrigendum: NANS-mediated synthesis of sialic acid is required for brain and skeletal development. Nat Genet. 2017;49(6):969.

van Karnebeek CDM, Bonafé L, Wen X-Y, Tarailo-Graovac M, Balzano S, Royer-Bertrand B, et al. NANS-mediated synthesis of sialic acid is required for brain and skeletal development. Nat Genet. 2016;48:777.

Wen XY, Tarailo-Graovac M, Brand-Arzamendi K, Willems A, Rakic B, Huijben K, et al. Sialic acid catabolism by N-acetylneuraminate pyruvate lyase is essential for muscle function. JCI Insight. 2018;3:24.

Westaway SK, Gregory A, Hayflick SJ. Mutations in PLA2G6 and the riddle of Schindler disease. J Med Genet. 2007;44(1):e64.

Willems AP, van Engelen BG, Lefeber DJ. Genetic defects in the hexosamine and sialic acid biosynthesis pathway. Biochim Biophys Acta. 2016;1860(8):1640–54.

Willems PJ, Seo HC, Coucke P, Tonlorenzi R, O'Brien JS. Spectrum of mutations in fucosidosis. Eur J Hum Genet. 1999;7(1):60–7.

Xu X, Wang AQ, Latham LL, Celeste F, Ciccone C, Malicdan MC, et al. Safety, pharmacokinetics and sialic acid production after oral administration of N-acetylmannosamine (ManNAc) to subjects with GNE myopathy. Mol Genet Metab. 2017;122(1–2): 126–34.

Yonekawa T, Malicdan MC, Cho A, Hayashi YK, Nonaka I, Mine T, et al. Sialyllactose ameliorates myopathic phenotypes in symptomatic GNE myopathy model mice. Brain. 2014;137(Pt 10): 2670–9.

Yoon SY, Bagel JH, O'Donnell PA, Vite CH, Wolfe JH. Clinical improvement of alpha-mannosidosis cat following a single cisterna magna infusion of AAV1. Mol Ther. 2016;24(1):26–33.

# The Mucopolysaccharidoses

# 64

Giancarlo Parenti and Roberto Giugliani

## Contents




**Summary**

The mucopolysaccharidoses (MPS) are a group of inborn errors of metabolism caused by the deficiency of lysosomal hydrolases that degrade glycosaminoglycans (GAGs). These disorders are associated with a progressive accumulation of different types of GAGs within the cells of various organs and are characterized by somatic manifestations (facial dysmorphisms, hepatosplenomegaly, cardiac, respiratory, and skeletal involvement) and neurological, hematologic, and ocular symptoms. These manifestations are variably associated in each disorder. In most cases the disease phenotypes encompass a spectrum ranging from severe to attenuated clinical forms. Initial clinical assessment should include the evaluation of different organs and systems. Biochemical and genetic investigations are an important part of the diagnostic process and include the analysis of GAGs, the demonstration of a specific enzyme defect, and the identification of mutations in the relevant gene. Neonatal screening programs for selected MPS types have been implemented in some countries. Carrier detection and prenatal diagnosis are possible. Management of any MPS requires supportive care and multidisciplinary treatment. Specific treatment is available for several MPS, based on different approaches. Hematopoietic stem cell transplantation is indicated for MPS IH patients under the age of 2 years who have normal or near-normal developmental scores, but is not standard practice in other MPS types. Enzyme replacement therapy (ERT) is currently available for MPS I, MPS II, MPS IVA, MPS VI, and MPS



G. Parenti (✉)
Department of Translational Medical Sciences, Federico II University, Naples, Italy

Telethon Institute of Genetics and Medicine, Pozzuoli, Italy
e-mail: parenti@unina.it

R. Giugliani
Department of Genetics, Federal University of Rio Grande do Sul, Porto Alegre, RS, Brazil

Medical Genetics Service, Hospital de Clinicas de Porto Alegre, Porto Alegre, RS, Brazil
e-mail: rgiugliani@hcpa.edu.br






N. Blau et al. (eds.), *Physician's Guide to the Diagnosis, Treatment, and Follow-Up of Inherited Metabolic Diseases*,
https://doi.org/10.1007/978-3-030-67727-5_64

VII. ERT results in improvement of somatic manifestations and of motor performance and in reduced urinary GAG excretion. However, other clinical features, particularly those related to central nervous system involvement, respond to a lesser extent to therapy. Newer therapeutic approaches involving the use of small molecules, ERT with enzymes that bypass the blood-brain barrier, intrathecal or intracerebroventricular enzyme delivery, and gene therapy/gene editing approaches are still in preclinical or clinical development.

## Introduction

The mucopolysaccharidoses (MPS) are a broad group of lysosomal storage diseases, classically caused by the deficiency of lysosomal hydrolases that degrade the glycosaminoglycans (GAGs). These disorders are associated with a progressive accumulation of different types of GAGs within the cells of various organs, ultimately compromising their function. The cumulative incidence of these disorders varies between approximately 1.5 and 4.5 in 100,000 live births/year, depending on ethnicity (Kobayashi 2019).

The pathophysiology of MPS is complex. Recent studies suggest that the clinical manifestations of these disorders not only are the direct effects of GAG storage but also derive from a cascade of secondary events, triggered by storage, that ultimately lead to dysfunction or inappropriate activation of different cellular processes and pathways (Parenti and Fraldi 2018). These events include secondary storage of substrates unrelated to the defective enzyme; abnormal composition of membranes, impaired vesicle fusion and trafficking; impairment or block of autophagy; oxidative stress; dysregulation or activation of signaling pathways; and abnormalities of calcium homeostasis. These abnormalities are emerging as key factors in the pathophysiology of the MPS and may represent potential new targets of therapies. Particular attention has been paid to the impairment of autophagy, a catabolic pathway that mediates the degradation of macromolecules and organelles in lysosomes. The autophagic pathway was shown to be affected in the MPS (Pshezhetsky 2016; Shapiro et al. 2014; Settembre et al. 2008), with a block or reduction of the autophagic flux and consequent autophagosome accumulation. Both the impairment of the autophagic flux and activation of inflammation have been recognized as important pathogenic factors for neurodegeneration, one of the most debilitating manifestations of MPS (Martins et al. 2015).

The major manifestations of disease differ depending on the specific deficiency and on the turnover of substrates. Therefore, the clinical presentation and approach to therapy is different across the various disease types. The clinical presentation of the MPS is broad. They are characterized by somatic manifestations (facial dysmorphisms, hepatosplenomegaly, cardiac, respiratory, and skeletal involvement) and neurological, hematologic, and ocular symptoms. These manifestations are variably associated in each disorder. In most cases the disease phenotypes encompass a spectrum ranging from severe to attenuated clinical forms.

Because of the multisystem involvement in these patients, initial clinical assessment should rely on the evaluation of different organs and systems, and the involvement of a multidisciplinary team, including neurologist, ophthalmologist, ENT specialist, cardiologist, orthopedic surgeon, hematologist, and pulmonologist, is recommended. Imaging and functional studies are also valuable.

Biochemical investigations are needed to confirm the specific diagnosis, and genetic analyses, which are important for phenotype prediction, carrier detection, and prenatal diagnosis, may be required for diagnosis confirmation. These include the analysis of GAGs, the demonstration of a specific enzyme defect, and the identification of mutations in the relevant gene.

The evidence that earlier introduction of therapy improves the disease outcome supports the expansion of neonatal screening for selected MPS, which has already been introduced in some countries. Carrier detection, aiming to genetic counseling and/or family planning, is especially important in the X-linked recessive MPS II. This requires identification of the family mutation to investigate potential carriers, although in some cases this could be made by pedigree analysis. Prenatal diagnosis is possible either by assay of enzyme activity or by molecular analysis. As for other genetic conditions, preimplantation genetic diagnosis is also possible in the MPS.

Management of all MPS requires both supportive care and specific treatment. Supportive care should be based on multidisciplinary treatment of a variety of systemic complications and personalized in individual patients. Specific treatment is based on different approaches, depending on the MPS subtype. Hematopoietic stem cell transplantation (HSCT) has been performed in several MPS types, with variable results, being its most consistent indication MPS IH patients under the age of 2–3 years who have normal or near-normal developmental scores. Data of HSCT in MPS VI are also encouraging (Turbeville et al. 2011). Mortality and morbidity risks associated to HSCT are not negligible and should be taken into account.

Enzyme replacement therapy (ERT) with recombinant human enzymes has been approved for MPS I, MPS II, MPS IVA, MPS VI, and MPS VII. ERT reduces urinary GAG excretion and results in improvement of somatic manifestations and functional performance. However, some disease features (as heart valves pathology) respond to a lesser extent to therapy, and the inability of the recombinant enzymes to cross the blood-brain barrier limits its effect on the CNS. Strategies to address these important limitations and to facilitate recombinant enzyme delivery to the central nervous system are currently under development.

Other therapeutic approaches for the treatment of the MPS include substrate reduction, modulation of inflammation, gene therapy, and genome editing, among others, and are still under preclinical and clinical evaluation.

## Nomenclature

| No. | Disorder | Alternative name | Abbreviation | Gene symbol | Chromosomal localization | Affected protein | OMIM no. |
|---|---|---|---|---|---|---|---|
| 64.1 | Hurler-Scheie disease | Alpha-Iduronidase deficiency | MPS I | *IDUA* | 4p16.3 | Alpha-Iduronidase | 607014, 607015, 607016 |
| 64.2 | Hunter disease | Iduronate 2-sulfatase deficiency | MPS II | *IDS* | Xq28 | Iduronate 2-sulfatase | 309900 |
| 64.3 | Sanfilippo A disease | Heparan-N-sulfatase deficiency | MPS IIIA | *SGSH* | 17q25.3 | Heparan-N-sulfatase | 252900 |
| 64.4 | Sanfilippo B disease | N-acetyl-alpha-D-glucosaminidase deficiency | MPS IIIB | *NAGU* | 17q21 | N-acetyl-alpha-D-glucosaminidase | 252920 |
| 64.5 | Sanfilippo C disease | Acetyl-CoA alpha-glucosaminide acetyltransferase deficiency | MPS IIIC | *MPS3C* | 8p11.1 | Acetyl-CoA alpha-glucosaminide acetyltransferase | 252930 |
| 64.6 | Sanfilippo D disease | N-Acetylglucosamine-6-sulfatase deficiency | MPS IIID | *GNS* | 12q14 | N-Acetylglucosamine-6-sulfatase | 252940 |
| 64.7 | Morquio A disease | N-Acetylgalactosamine-6-sulfatase deficiency | MPS IVA | *GALNS* | 16q24.3 | N-Acetylgalactosamine-6-sulfatase | 253000 |
| 64.8 | Morquio B disease | Beta-galactosidase deficiency | MPS IVB | *GLB1* | 3p21.33 | Beta-galactosidase | 253010 |
| 64.9 | Maroteaux-Lamy disease | N-Acetylgalactosamine-4-sulfatase deficiency | MPS VI | *ARSB* | 5q11-q13 | N-Acetylgalactosamine-4-sulfatase | 253200 |
| 64.10 | Sly disease | Beta-Glucuronidase deficiency | MPS VII | *GUSB* | 7q21.11 | Beta-Glucuronidase | 253220 |
| 64.11 | Natowicz disease | Hyaluronidase deficiency | MPS IX | *HYAL1* | 3p21.31 | Hyaluronidase | 601492 |
| 64.12 | MPS plus | – | MPSPS | *VPS33A* | 12q24.3 | Vacuolar protein sorting-associated protein 33A | 61730 |

## Metabolic Pathway

The degradation of GAGs is performed through the sequential action of lysosomal hydrolases. As the majority of these enzymes are either exoglycosidases (they cleave the sugar moiety at the end of the oligosaccharide chains) or sulfatases, a deficiency of one of these activities results in a block of further degradation of GAGs. The degradation pathways of HS, KS, and DS are shown in Fig. 64.1.

## Signs and Symptoms

The major and evocative clinical features of MPS include somatic manifestations (facial dysmorphism, hepatosplenomegaly, cardiac, respiratory, and skeletal involvement) and neurological, hematologic, and ocular symptoms. These disease manifestations are variably associated in each disorder. The combination of the clinical features may be an important clue for the differential diagnosis in a patient in whom a MPS is suspected.

In most cases the disease phenotypes encompass a spectrum ranging from early-onset (severe) to late-onset (attenuated) clinical forms. The clinical presentation of each disease is reported in Tables 64.1, 64.2, 64.3, 64.4, 64.5, 64.6, 64.7, 64.8, 64.9, 64.10, 64.11, and 64.12 (signs and symptoms).

Patients with the severe form of MPS I (Hurler disease, MPS IH), MPS II (Hunter disease), and MPS VI (Maroteaux-Lamy disease) generally present with facial dysmorphism and persistent respiratory disease in the early years of life. Many patients will have undergone surgical procedures for recurrent otitis media, removal of tonsils and/or adenoids, and hernia repair before the diagnosis is established. Infants with MPS III (Sanfilippo A, B, C, or D disease) present with cognitive difficulties and then develop a profound behavioral disturbance. The behavior disorder is characteristic and often leads to the diagnosis. Somatic features are less pronounced in these patients. Children with MPS IVA (Morquio disease, type A) have normal cognitive functions but are affected by severe spondyloepiphyseal dysplasia, which in most patients leads to extreme short stature, deformity of the chest, marked shortening and instability of the neck, and joint laxity. MPS IVB (Morquio disease, type B) has similar features of the skeletal dysplasia of MPS IVA but is much more variable in its effects; MPS VII (Sly disease) often presents as nonimmune hydrops fetalis. Those patients who survive or who present later resemble patients

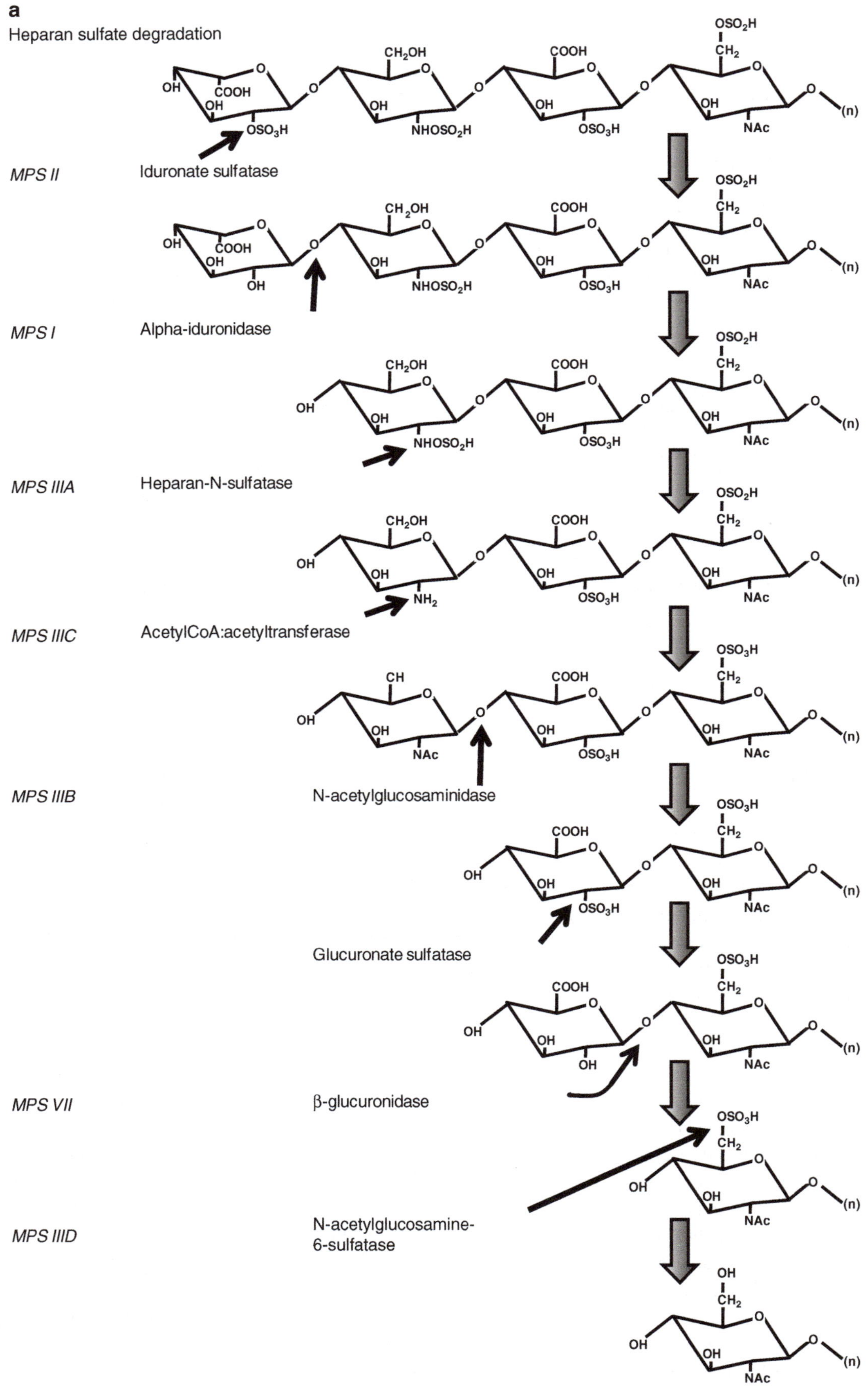


**Fig. 64.1** Metabolic pathways of (**a**) heparan sulfate, (**b**) keratan sulfate, and (**c**) dermatan sulfate degradation. The diseases associated with each specific enzyme deficiency are indicated

**Fig. 64.1** (continued)

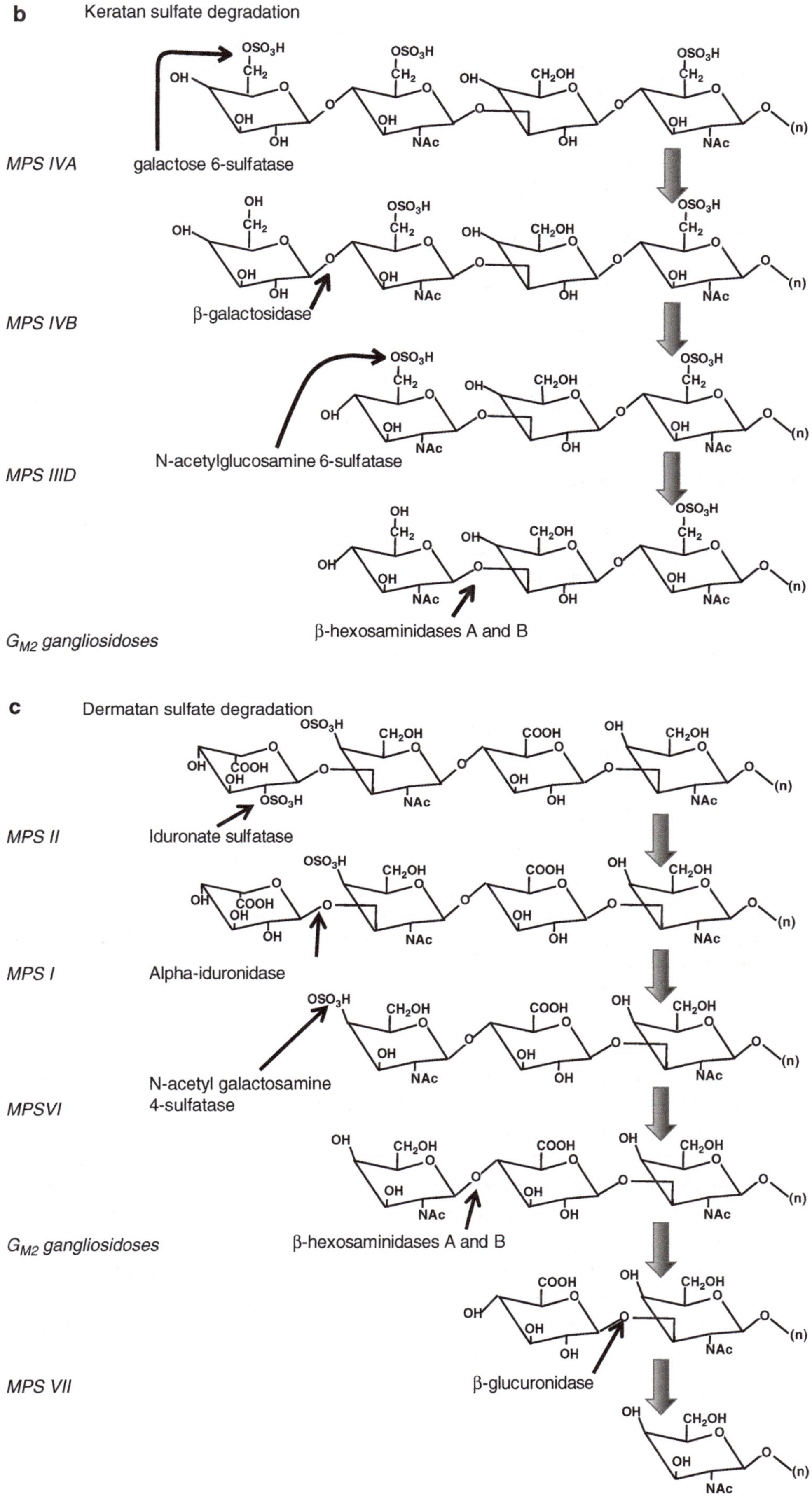

**Table 64.1** Hurler–Scheie disease (MPS I)[a]

| System | Symptoms and biomarkers | Neonatal (birth–1 month) | Infancy (1–18 months) | Childhood (1.5–11 years) | Adolescence (11–16 years) | Adulthood (>16 years) |
|---|---|---|---|---|---|---|
| Cardiovascular | Cardiomyopathy | | + | + | + | + |
| | Coronary artery disease | | + | + | + | + |
| | Valvular thickening | | ++ | +++ | +++ | +++ |
| CNS | Behavioral disorder | | | ± | | |
| | Cervical myelopathy | | | ++ | ++ | ± |
| | Hydrocephalus | | ++ | ++ | ++ | |
| | **Retardation and regression** | | ++ | +++ | ± | |
| | Seizures | | ± | ± | | |
| | Swallowing difficulties | | + | + | + | |
| Digestive | Diarrhea | | + | + | + | |
| | Hepatosplenomegaly | | ++ | +++ | +++ | + |
| Ear | Hearing loss | | ± | + | + | + |
| | Recurrent otitis media | | ++ | ++ | ++ | – |
| Eye | Corneal clouding | | + | +++ | +++ | +++ |
| | Glaucoma | | ± | + | | |
| | Retinal dystrophy | | ± | ± | ++ | ++ |
| Musculoskeletal | Atlantoaxial instability | | ± | + | + | |
| | Carpal tunnel syndrome | | ± | ++ | ++ | ++ |
| | **Coarse facial features** | | ++ | +++ | ++ | ++ |
| | Degenerative hip dysplasia | | + | ++ | ++ | ++ |
| | Dysostosis multiplex | | +++ | +++ | ++ | ++ |
| | Genu valgum | | ± | ± | ± | ± |
| | Hernias | | ++ | ++ | ++ | + |
| | Joint contractures | | ++ | +++ | +++ | ++ |
| | Kyphosis | | + | ++ | + | |
| | **Macrocephaly** | | +++ | +++ | ++ | + |
| Respiratory | Obstructive sleep apnea | | ++ | +++ | +++ | ++ |
| | Restrictive lung disease | | ± | + | + | ± |
| | Upper airway obstruction | | ++ | +++ | +++ | ++ |
| Laboratory findings | Alpha-Iduronidase activity | ↓↓↓ | ↓↓↓ | ↓↓↓ | ↓↓↓ | ↓↓↓ |
| | Dermatan sulfate (U) | ↑↑ | ↑↑ | ↑↑ | ↑↑ | ↑↑ |
| | Heparan sulfate (U) | ↑↑ | ↑↑ | ↑↑ | ↑↑ | ↑↑ |
| | Total GAGs (U) | ↑↑ | ↑↑ | ↑↑ | ↑↑ | ↑↑ |

[a]MPS I presents with wide variability. Traditionally, phenotypes were described as Hurler (severe, MPS IH) and Scheie (attenuated, MPS IS), with an intermediate, Hurler-Scheie (MPS IH/S) in between. From the clinical perspective, the classification in severe and attenuated types makes more sense. The severe phenotype is quite well defined and corresponds to the Hurler syndrome. The attenuated phenotype is a spectrum of presentations that range from the severe end of the Hurler-Scheie phenotype, which could have some cognitive involvement, to the mild end of the Scheie phenotype that has limited clinical impact

with MPS I with respect to clinical phenotype and supportive management. Potentially life-threatening manifestations, such as tracheal compression and aortic dilatation, have been reported in some MPS. Cognitive impairment is a feature of MPS III and of the severe forms of MPS I, MPS II, and MPS VII. Patients with the rare MPS IX (Natowicz disease) show a clinical picture limited to joint involvement and proliferative synovitis (Imundo et al. 2011). The recently described MPSPS (MPS Plus) has an early presentation with coarse face, dysostosis multiplex, respiratory difficulty, visceromegaly, neurological involvement, and other severe manifestations (Kondo et al. 2017).

The phenotype of patients with attenuated forms of MPS I (MPS IH/S and MPS IS, Hurler-Scheie or Scheie disease, respectively), MPS II, and MPS VI is much more difficult to predict, and treatment needs in this group of patients may be very variable. The MPS disorders in general present as a continuum of clinical involvement, and even patients with the most attenuated forms of Scheie syndrome may have severe disabilities, requiring major medical and surgical interventions.

**Table 64.2** Hunter disease (MPS II)[a]

| System | Symptoms and biomarkers | Neonatal (birth–1 month) | Infancy (1–18 months) | Childhood (1.5–11 years) | Adolescence (11–16 years) | Adulthood (>16 years) |
|---|---|---|---|---|---|---|
| Cardiovascular | Cardiomyopathy | | + | + | + | + |
| | Valvular thickening | | ++ | +++ | +++ | +++ |
| CNS | Behavioral disorder | | | ++ | ++ | |
| | Cervical myelopathy | | | ++ | ++ | |
| | Hydrocephalus | | ++ | ++ | ++ | |
| | Retardation and regression | | ++ | +++ | ++ | |
| | Seizures | | + | + | ++ | |
| | Swallowing difficulties | | ± | + | ± | |
| Digestive | Diarrhea | | ± | + | ± | |
| | Hepatosplenomegaly | | ++ | +++ | +++ | ++ |
| Ear | Hearing loss | | ++ | ++ | ++ | ++ |
| | Recurrent otitis media | | ++ | ++ | ++ | ++ |
| Eye | Retinal dystrophy | | | ± | ± | ± |
| Musculoskeletal | Atlantoaxial instability | | ± | + | + | ± |
| | Carpal tunnel syndrome | | ± | ++ | ++ | ++ |
| | Coarse facial features | | ++ | +++ | ++ | ++ |
| | Degenerative hip dysplasia | | + | ++ | ++ | + |
| | Dysostosis multiplex | | + | + | + | + |
| | Hernias | | +++ | +++ | ++ | + |
| | Joint contractures | | +++ | +++ | +++ | ++ |
| | Kyphosis | | + | ++ | + | ± |
| | Macrocephaly | | +++ | +++ | ++ | + |
| Respiratory | Obstructive sleep apnea | | ++ | +++ | +++ | ++ |
| | Restrictive lung disease | | ± | + | + | ± |
| | Upper airway obstruction | | ++ | +++ | +++ | ++ |
| Laboratory findings | Dermatan sulfate (U) | ↑↑ | ↑↑ | ↑↑ | ↑↑ | ↑↑ |
| | Heparan sulfate (U) | ↑↑ | ↑↑ | ↑↑ | ↑↑ | ↑↑ |
| | Iduronate-2-sulfatase (LC) | ↓↓↓ | ↓↓↓ | ↓↓↓ | ↓↓↓ | ↓↓↓ |
| | Total GAGs (U) | ↑↑ | ↑↑ | ↑↑ | ↑↑ | ↑↑ |

[a]Hunter disease phenotype is variable. The adolescence and adult phenotypes refer to the attenuated form of the disease

**Table 64.3** Sanfilippo A disease (MPS IIIA)

| System | Symptoms and biomarkers | Neonatal (birth–1 month) | Infancy (1–18 months) | Childhood (1.5–11 years) | Adolescence (11–16 years) | Adulthood (>16 years) |
|---|---|---|---|---|---|---|
| CNS | Behavior, aggressive | | ± | +++ | ++ | + |
| | Hyperactivity | | ± | +++ | ++ | + |
| | Retardation and regression | | ± | +++ | +++ | +++ |
| | Seizures | | | ± | ++ | ++ |
| | Sleep disturbances | | ++ | +++ | ++ | + |
| | Swallowing difficulties | | ± | + | +++ | +++ |
| Digestive | Diarrhea | | ++ | ++ | + | − |
| | Liver dysfunction | | ± | ± | + | + |
| Ear | Hearing loss | | ± | ± | ± | ± |
| Musculoskeletal | Coarse facial features | | ± | + | + | + |
| | Dysostosis multiplex | | ± | ± | ± | ± |
| Laboratory findings | Heparan sulfate (U) | ↑↑ | ↑↑ | ↑↑ | ↑↑ | ↑↑ |
| | Heparan-N-sulfatase (LC) | ↓↓↓ | ↓↓↓ | ↓↓↓ | ↓↓↓ | ↓↓↓ |
| | Total GAGs (U) | ↑↑ | ↑↑ | ↑↑ | ↑↑ | ↑↑ |

**Table 64.4** Sanfilippo B disease (MPS IIIB)

| System | Symptom | Neonatal (birth–1 month) | Infancy (1–18 months) | Childhood (1.5–11 years) | Adolescence (11–16 years) | Adulthood (>16 years) |
|---|---|---|---|---|---|---|
| CNS | Behavior, aggressive | | ± | +++ | ++ | + |
| | Hyperactivity | | ± | +++ | ++ | + |
| | Retardation and regression | | ± | +++ | +++ | +++ |
| | Seizures | | | ± | ++ | ++ |
| | Sleep disturbances | | ++ | +++ | ++ | + |
| | Swallowing difficulties | | ± | + | +++ | +++ |
| Digestive | Diarrhea | | ++ | ++ | + | ± |
| | Liver dysfunction | | ± | ± | + | + |
| Ear | Hearing loss | | ± | ± | ± | ± |
| Musculoskeletal | Coarse facial features | | ± | + | + | + |
| | Dysostosis multiplex | | ± | ± | ± | ± |
| Laboratory findings | Alpha-N-acetylglucosaminidase | ↓↓↓ | ↓↓↓ | ↓↓↓ | ↓↓↓ | ↓↓↓ |
| | Heparan sulfate (U) | ↑↑ | ↑↑ | ↑↑ | ↑↑ | ↑↑ |
| | Total GAGs (U) | ↑↑ | ↑↑ | ↑↑ | ↑↑ | ↑↑ |

**Table 64.5** Sanfilippo C disease (MPS IIIC)

| System | Symptoms and biomarkers | Neonatal (birth–1 month) | Infancy (1–18 months) | Childhood (1.5–11 years) | Adolescence (11–16 years) | Adulthood (>16 years) |
|---|---|---|---|---|---|---|
| CNS | Behavior, aggressive | | ± | +++ | ++ | + |
| | Hyperactivity | | ± | +++ | ++ | + |
| | Retardation and regression | | ± | +++ | +++ | +++ |
| | Seizures | | | ± | ++ | ++ |
| | Sleep disturbances | | ± | ++ | ++ | + |
| | Swallowing difficulties | | ± | + | +++ | +++ |
| Digestive | Diarrhea | | ++ | ++ | + | ± |
| | Liver dysfunction | | ± | ± | + | + |
| Ear | Hearing loss | | ± | ± | ± | ± |
| Musculoskeletal | Coarse facial features | | ± | + | + | + |
| | Dysostosis multiplex | | ± | ± | ± | ± |
| Laboratory findings | Acetyl-CoA:Alpha-N-glucosaminide-N-acetyl transferase (LC) | ↓↓↓ | ↓↓↓ | ↓↓↓ | ↓↓↓ | ↓↓↓ |
| | Heparan sulfate (U) | ↑↑ | ↑↑ | ↑↑ | ↑↑ | ↑↑ |
| | Total GAGs (U) | ↑↑ | ↑↑ | ↑↑ | ↑↑ | ↑↑ |

**Table 64.6** Sanfilippo D disease (MPS IIID)

| System | Symptom | Neonatal (birth–1 month) | Infancy (1–18 months) | Childhood (1.5–11 years) | Adolescence (11–16 years) | Adulthood (>16 years) |
|---|---|---|---|---|---|---|
| CNS | Behavior, aggressive | | | +++ | ++ | + |
| | Hyperactivity | | | +++ | ++ | + |
| | Retardation and regression | | | +++ | +++ | +++ |
| | Seizures | | | | ++ | ++ |
| | Swallowing difficulties | | ± | + | +++ | +++ |
| Digestive | Diarrhea | | ++ | ++ | + | ± |
| | Liver dysfunction | | | ± | + | + |
| Ear | Hearing loss | | | ± | ± | ± |
| Musculoskeletal | Coarse facial features | | | + | + | + |
| | Dysostosis multiplex | | | ± | ± | ± |
| Laboratory findings | Heparan sulfate (U) | ↑↑ | ↑↑ | ↑↑ | ↑↑ | ↑↑ |
| | N-Acetylglucosamine-6-sulfatase (LC) | ↓↓↓ | ↓↓↓ | ↓↓↓ | ↓↓↓ | ↓↓↓ |
| | Total GAGs (U) | ↑↑ | ↑↑ | ↑↑ | ↑↑ | ↑↑ |

**Table 64.7** Morquio A disease (MPS IVA)

| System | Symptoms and biomarkers | Neonatal (birth–1 month) | Infancy (1–18 months) | Childhood (1.5–11 years) | Adolescence (11–16 years) | Adulthood (>16 years) |
|---|---|---|---|---|---|---|
| Cardiovascular | Valvular thickening | | | + | + | + |
| CNS | Cervical myelopathy | | | + | ++ | ++ |
| Digestive | Liver dysfunction | | | + | + | + |
| Ear | Hearing loss | | | + | + | + |
| Eye | Corneal clouding | | | + | ++ | ++ |
| Musculoskeletal | Atlantoaxial instability | | +++ | +++ | +++ | +++ |
| | Coarse facial features | | | ± | ± | ± |
| | Degenerative hip dysplasia | | | ++ | ++ | ++ |
| | Dysostosis multiplex | | | + | + | + |
| | Genu valgum | | | +++ | +++ | +++ |
| | Joint laxity | | | + | + | + |
| | Kyphosis | | ++ | ++ | ++ | ++ |
| | Odontoid hypoplasia | | | ++ | ++ | ++ |
| | Short stature | | + | +++ | +++ | +++ |
| | Sternal bulging | | + | ++ | ++ | ++ |
| Respiratory | Restrictive lung disease | | | + | + | + |
| Laboratory findings | Chondroitin sulfate (U) | n- ↑ | ↑ | ↑ | n- ↑ | n- ↑ |
| | Keratan sulfate (U) | n- ↑ | n- ↑ | n- ↑ | n | n |
| | N-Acetylgalactosamine-6-sulfatase (LC) | ↓↓↓ | ↓↓↓ | ↓↓↓ | ↓↓↓ | ↓↓↓ |
| | Total GAGs (U) | – | n- ↑ | n- ↑ | n | n |

**Table 64.8** Morquio B disease (MPS IVB)

| System | Symptom | Neonatal (birth–1 month) | Infancy (1–18 months) | Childhood (1.5–11 years) | Adolescence (11–16 years) | Adulthood (>16 years) |
|---|---|---|---|---|---|---|
| Cardiovascular | Valvular thickening | | | + | + | + |
| CNS | Cervical myelopathy | | | + | ++ | ++ |
| Digestive | Liver dysfunction | | | + | + | + |
| Ear | Hearing loss | | | ± | ± | ± |
| Eye | Corneal clouding | | | + | ++ | ++ |
| Musculoskeletal | Atlantoaxial instability | | | ++ | ++ | ++ |
| | Coarse facial features | | | ± | ± | ± |
| | Degenerative hip dysplasia | | | ++ | ++ | ++ |
| | Dysostosis multiplex | | | + | + | + |
| | Genu valgum | | | ++ | ++ | ++ |
| | Joint laxity | | | + | + | + |
| | Kyphosis | | | ++ | ++ | ++ |
| | Odontoid hypoplasia | | | + | + | + |
| | Short stature | | | +++ | +++ | +++ |
| | Sternal bulging | | | + | + | + |
| Respiratory | Restrictive lung disease | | | + | + | + |
| Laboratory findings | Beta-galactosidase | ↓↓↓ | ↓↓↓ | ↓↓↓ | ↓↓↓ | ↓↓↓ |
| | Keratan sulfate (U) | n- ↑ | n- ↑ | n- ↑ | n- ↑ | n- ↑ |
| | Total GAGs (U) | n- ↑ | n- ↑ | n- ↑ | n | n |

**Table 64.9** Maroteaux-Lamy disease (MPS VI)

| System | Symptoms and biomarkers | Neonatal (birth–1 month) | Infancy (1–18 months) | Childhood (1.5–11 years) | Adolescence (11–16 years) | Adulthood (>16 years) |
|---|---|---|---|---|---|---|
| Cardiovascular | Cardiomyopathy | | ± | + | + | + |
| | Valvular thickening | | | +++ | +++ | +++ |
| CNS | Spinal cord, compression | | – | ++ | ++ | ++ |
| Digestive | Hepatosplenomegaly | | ++ | +++ | +++ | ++ |
| Ear | Hearing loss | | | + | + | + |
| | Recurrent otitis media | | + | ++ | ++ | + |
| Eye | Corneal clouding | | + | +++ | +++ | +++ |
| | Glaucoma | | | + | + | + |
| Musculoskeletal | Carpal tunnel syndrome | | ± | ++ | ++ | ++ |
| | Coarse facial features | | | ++ | ++ | ++ |
| | Degenerative hip dysplasia | | | ++ | ++ | ++ |
| | Dysostosis multiplex | | + | +++ | +++ | +++ |
| | Hernias | | + | + | + | + |
| | Joint contractures | | + | +++ | +++ | +++ |
| | Kyphosis | | + | ++ | ++ | ++ |
| | Short stature | | + | ++ | ++ | ++ |
| | Sternal bulging | | | + | + | + |
| Respiratory | Obstructive sleep apnea | | + | ++ | ++ | ++ |
| | Upper airway obstruction | | + | ++ | ++ | ++ |
| Laboratory findings | Dermatan sulfate (U) | ↑↑ | ↑↑ | ↑↑ | ↑↑ | ↑↑ |
| | N-Acetylgalactosamine-4-sulfatase | ↓↓↓ | ↓↓↓ | ↓↓↓ | ↓↓↓ | ↓↓↓ |
| | Total GAGs (U) | ↑↑ | ↑↑ | ↑↑ | ↑↑ | ↑↑ |

**Table 64.10** Sly disease (MPS VII)

| System | Symptoms and biomarkers | Neonatal (birth–1 month) | Infancy (1–18 months) | Childhood (1.5–11 years) | Adolescence (11–16 years) | Adulthood (>16 years) |
|---|---|---|---|---|---|---|
| Cardiovascular | Valvular thickening | | ++ | ++ | | |
| CNS | Retardation and regression | | +++ | +++ | ± | ± |
| Digestive | Hepatosplenomegaly | + | ++ | ++ | ++ | ++ |
| Eye | Corneal clouding | | ± | ± | ± | ± |
| Musculoskeletal | Coarse facial features | | ++ | ++ | ++ | ++ |
| | Dysostosis multiplex | | + | + | + | + |
| | Hernias | | + | + | | |
| | Joint contractures | | ++ | ++ | ++ | ++ |
| | Macrocephaly | + | + | | | |
| | Short stature | + | + | + | + | + |
| Others | Fetal hydrops | ++ | | | | |
| Laboratory findings | Beta-Glucuronidase | ↓↓↓ | ↓↓↓ | ↓↓↓ | ↓↓↓ | ↓↓↓ |
| | Chondroitin sulfate (U) | ↑↑ | ↑↑ | ↑↑ | ↑↑ | ↑↑ |
| | Dermatan sulfate (U) | ↑↑ | ↑↑ | ↑↑ | ↑↑ | ↑↑ |
| | Heparan sulfate (U) | ↑↑ | ↑↑ | ↑↑ | ↑↑ | ↑↑ |
| | Total GAGs (U) | ↑↑ | ↑↑ | ↑↑ | ↑↑ | ↑↑ |

**Table 64.11** Hyaluronidase deficiency (MPS IX)

| System | Symptoms and biomarkers | Neonatal (birth–1 month) | Infancy (1–18 months) | Childhood (1.5–11 years) | Adolescence (11–16 years) | Adulthood (>16 years) |
|---|---|---|---|---|---|---|
| Dermatological | Cutaneous nodules and swelling | | | ++ | ++ | ++ |
| Musculoskeletal | Degenerative hip dysplasia | | | + | + | + |
| | Joint contractures | | | ++ | ++ | + |
| | Scoliosis | | | + | + | + |
| Laboratory findings | Hyaluronan (U) | ↑↑ | ↑↑ | ↑↑ | ↑↑ | ↑↑ |
| | Hyaluronidase (P) | ↓↓↓ | ↓↓↓ | ↓↓↓ | ↓↓↓ | ↓↓↓ |
| | Total GAGs (U) | n | n | n | n | n |

**Table 64.12** Mucopolysaccharidosis Plus (MPSPS)

| System | Symptoms and biomarkers | Neonatal (birth–1 month) | Infancy (1–18 months) | Childhood (1.5–11 years) | Adolescence (11–16 years) | Adulthood (>16 years) |
|---|---|---|---|---|---|---|
| Cardiovascular | Congenital heart defect | + | + | + | | |
| | Heart failure | + | + | + | | |
| | Hypertrophic cardiomyopathy | + | + | + | | |
| CNS | Developmental delay | + | + | + | | |
| | Pyramidal signs | | + | + | | |
| Digestive | Hepatosplenomegaly | + | ++ | ++ | | |
| Pulmonary | Respiratory disturbance | ++ | ++ | ++ | | |
| | Respiratory infections | ++ | ++ | ++ | | |
| Renal | Foamy cells | + | + | + | | |
| Eye | Optic atrophy | | + | + | | |
| Musculoskeletal | Coarse facial features | | ++ | ++ | | |
| | Dysostosis multiplex | + | ++ | ++ | | |
| | Hernias | | | | | |
| | Hirsutism | | + | + | | |
| | Joint contractures | + | + | + | | |
| | Macrocephaly | | | | | |
| | Macroglossia | | + | + | | |
| | Short stature | | + | + | | |
| Others | Anemia | ++ | ++ | ++ | | |
| | Bone marrow hypoplasia | + | + | + | | |
| | Granulation in lymphocytes | + | + | + | | |
| | Proteinuria | ++ | ++ | ++ | | |
| | Thrombocytopenia | + | + | + | | |
| Laboratory findings | Dermatan sulfate (U) | | ↑ | ↑ | | |
| | Heparan sulfate (U/P) | ↑↑↑ | ↑↑↑ | ↑↑↑ | | |
| | Oligosaccharides | | ↑ | ↑ | | |
| | Sialic acid | | ↑ | ↑ | | |
| | Total GAGs (U) | ↑↑↑ | ↑↑↑ | ↑↑↑ | | |

## Diagnostic Flowcharts

The diagnosis workup for MPS is complex and relies on clinical evaluation and multiple laboratory tests.

The first step in the diagnostic workup of MPS is the clinical evaluation of patients and first-level diagnostic procedures (x-ray, blood smear, eye examination, ECG, cardiac ECHO, etc.; see Fig. 64.2).

Laboratory tests to complete the diagnosis should be performed in laboratories with specific expertise. These procedures usually start by the search for metabolites (quantitative and qualitative analysis of urinary GAGs; Fig. 64.3) using colorimetric methods and/or tandem mass spectrometry procedures; the assay of GAGs in blood is being developed and may play a role in MPS screening and diagnosis; enzyme assay of specific hydrolases in dried blood spots, plasma, leucocytes, or fibroblasts; and molecular analysis of the relevant gene (usually in DNA samples from peripheral blood, but DNA can be obtained also from other sources). Molecular analysis may be based on next-generation sequencing of multiple genes, including the ones involved in other lysosomal processes (Di Fruscio et al. 2015).

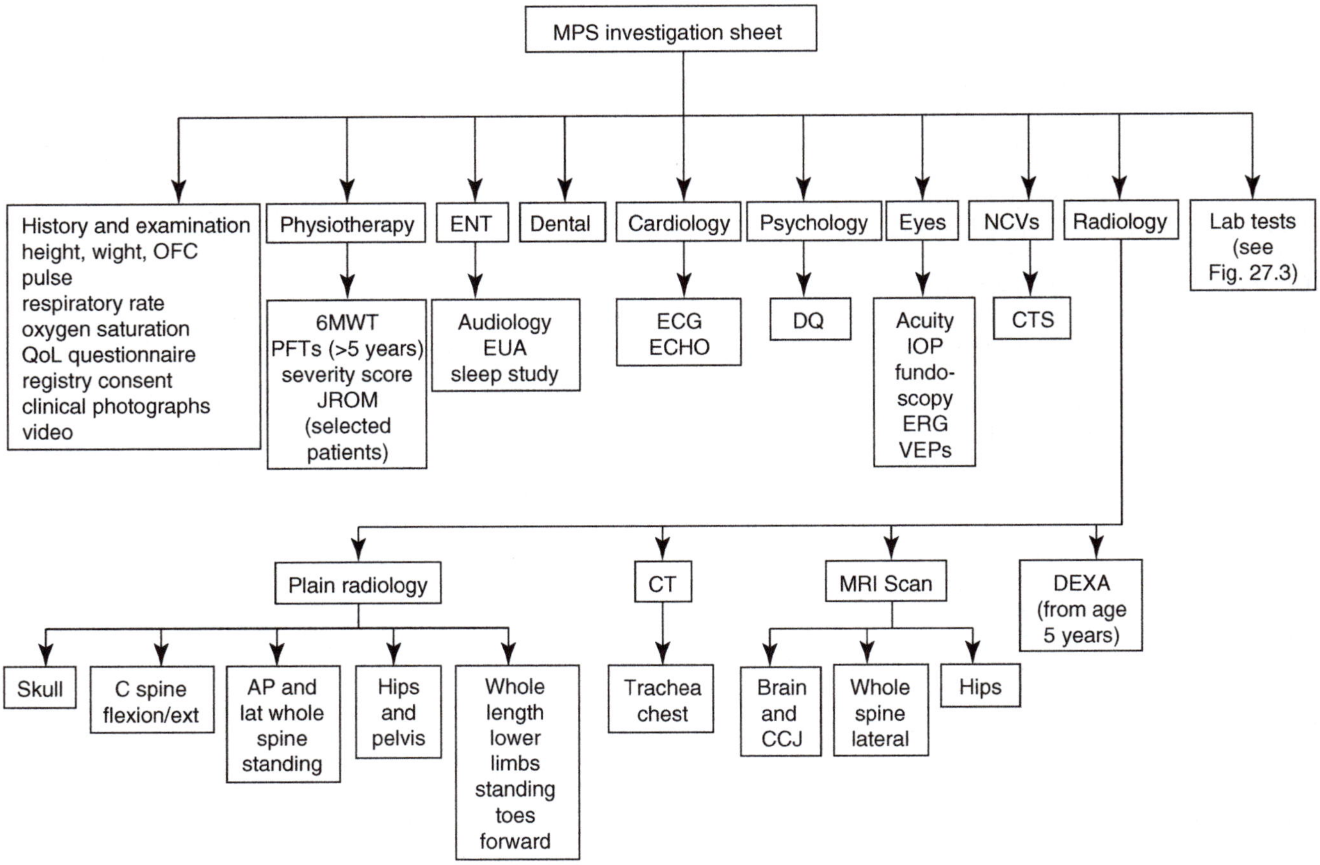


**Fig. 64.2** The MPS investigation sheet. History, clinical examination, and imaging studies are associated with evaluation of multisystem involvement and laboratory tests to confirm the diagnosis

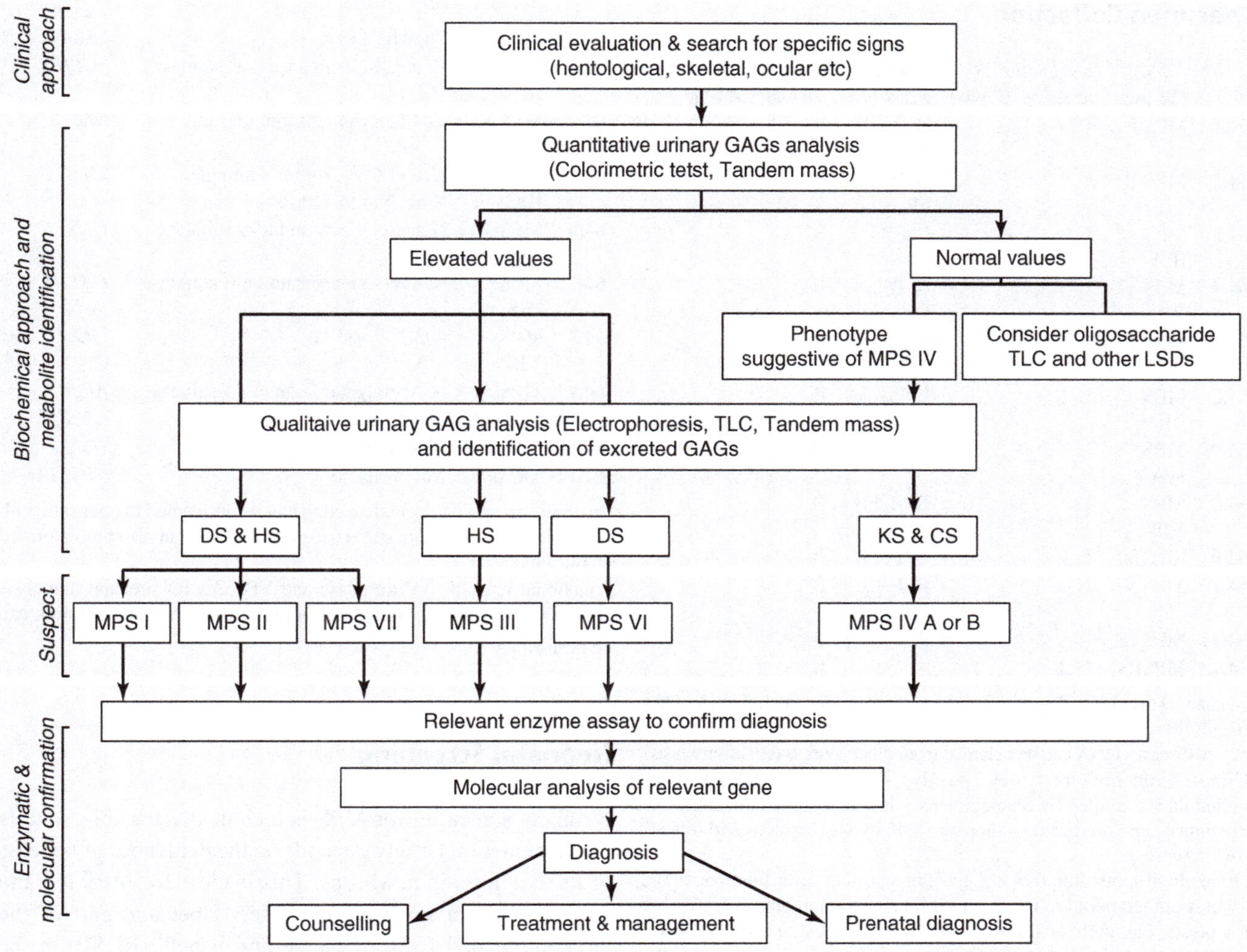


**Fig. 64.3** The assay of urinary GAGs and the identification of specific excretion patterns, performed by thin-layer chromatography (TLC), electrophoretic separation, or tandem mass spectrometry (depending on the availability of these techniques in the laboratory), help to select the specific enzyme(s) to be tested in the appropriate sample. Enzyme assays in dried blood spots or plasma are considered screening methods that should be validated by the enzyme assay in leucocytes or fibroblasts and/or by genetic analysis. The diagnosis should be confirmed by molecular analysis of the relevant gene. *LSDs* Lysosomal storage diseases

## Specimen Collection

| No. | Disorder | Metabolite analysis (GAGs) | Enzyme assay | Molecular characterization[a] |
|---|---|---|---|---|
| 64.1 | MPS I | U[b] | D[c], P[d], L[e], FB[f] | B |
| 64.2 | MPS II | U | D, P, L, FB | B |
| 64.3 | MPS IIIA | U | L, FB | B |
| 64.4 | MPS IIIB | U | D, P, L, FB | B |
| 64.5 | MPS IIIC | U | L, FB | B |
| 64.6 | MPS IIID | U | L, FB | B |
| 64.7 | MPS IVA | U | D, L, FB | B |
| 64.8 | MPS VIB | U | D, L, FB | B |
| 64.9 | MPS VI | U | D, L, FB | B |
| 64.10 | MPS VII | U | D, P, L, FB | B |
| 64.11 | MPS IX | – | P | B |
| 64.12 | MPSPS | U, P | – | B |

*U* Urine, *D* dried blood spots, *P* plasma, *S* serum, *B* blood, *L* leucocytes, *FB* fibroblast

[a]For all diseases DNA can be obtained from other sources (e.g., fibroblasts)

[b]Urine should be kept frozen (positive screening for MPS may be missed due to diluted urine specimens – low creatinine concentration, proteinuria, and medications; heparan sulfate may be increased in non-MPS diseases)

[c]Dried blood spots should be collected in a protein saver filter paper and dry at room temperature for at least 4 hours and then placed preferably in a plastic bag with desiccant; could be transported at room temperature; and should be stored at refrigerator until analysis, noting that the activity of some enzymes, as GALNS, is time-sensitive

[d]Fibroblasts are obtained by skin biopsy, obtained under sterile conditions, and kept in culture medium or saline solution at room temperature until the culture is started; after harvested, fibroblasts could be stored frozen

[e]Plasma could be obtained preferably by collection of blood with EDTA, so the material could be used for the measurement of GAGs, when available; transport the blood at room temperature or refrigerated until plasma is obtained; the plasma sample could be stored frozen (−20°C)

[f]Leucocytes and lymphocytes could be obtained from blood collected with EDTA, as it could allow assay of GAGs; blood should be kept at room temperature or refrigerated (do not freeze) until isolation of leucocytes or lymphocytes, which should be performed no more than 48–72 h after collection; after isolation, leucocytes and lymphocytes could be stored frozen

## Prenatal Diagnosis

| No. | Disorder | Enzyme assay | Genetic testing |
|---|---|---|---|
| **64.1** | MPS I | α-Iduronidase | *IDUA* |
| **64.2** | MPS II | Iduronate-2-sulfatase | *IDS* |
| **64.3** | MPS IIIA | Heparan-N-sulfatase (sulfamidase) | *SGSH* |
| **64.4** | MPS IIIB | α-N-acetylglucosaminidase | *NAGU* |
| **64.5** | MPS IIIC | Acetyl-CoA:α-glucosaminide N-acetyltransferase | *MPS3C* |
| **64.6** | MPS IIID | N-acetyl glucosamine-6-sulfatase | *GNS* |
| **64.7** | MPS IVA | N-Acetylgalactosamine-6-sulfatase | *GALNS* |
| **64.8** | MPS VIB | β-Galactosidase | *GLB1* |
| **64.9** | MPS VI | N-Acetylgalactosamine-4-sulfatase | *ARSB* |
| **64.10** | MPS VII | β-Glucuronidase | *GUSB* |
| **64.11** | MPS IX | Hyaluronidase | *HYAL1* |
| **64.12** | MPSPS | Not available | *VPS33A* |

Enzyme analysis and genetic testing can be performed in chorionic villi or amniocytes. Iduronate sulfatase enzyme assay can also be performed in amniotic fluid

Functional tests of hyaluronidase and VPS33A for prenatal diagnosis are not reported in the literature. For both disorders genetic testing can be performed

## Neonatal Screening

Neonatal screening for MPS is technically feasible, and its implementation largely depends on the evidences of benefits of its diagnosis in newborns. This is clear for MPS IH, and so the newborn screening for MPS I became part of the "Recommended Uniform Screening Panel" (RUSP) in the United States (http://www.hrsa.gov/advisorycommittees/mchbadvisory/heritabledisorders/recommendedpanel/index.html) in 2016 and is now routine in several US states (https://www.newsteps.org/), in Taiwan (Chan et al. 2019; Chuang et al. 2018), and in a growing number of regions, including regular schemes and pilot programs (Taylor et al. 2019a, b; Bronstein et al. 2019; Burlina et al. 2018; Bravo et al. 2017; Navarrete-Martínez et al. 2017; Burton et al. 2017).

Screening for MPS II is in place in Taiwan since 2015 (Chuang et al. 2018) and the US state of Illinois since 2017 and will probably expand to other states and countries in the short term (Joseph et al. 2018).

Screening for other MPS, which is technically possible, is under consideration for MPS IVA, MPS VI, and MPS VII, which have specific therapy available (Donati et al. 2018; Liu et al. 2017). Screening for MPS III still needs that specific therapies become available in order to move to practice (Yi et al. 2018; Kuiper et al. 2018).

The present newborn screening techniques are based on the measurement of specific enzymes, by tandem mass spectrometry (Gelb 2018; Schielen et al. 2017; Gelb et al. 2017) or digital microfluidics (Sista et al. 2011; Millington et al. 2010). Postanalytical tools can help to reduce false-positive rates regardless of the methodology chosen for the enzyme assay (Minter Baerg et al. 2018; Gelb 2018).

However, the possibility of measuring GAGs in dried blood spots is being tested (Maccari et al. 2018; Kubaski et al. 2017) and if approved may bring the possibility of detecting almost all MPS cases with just one assay (Saville et al. 2019).

Newborn screening with genetic analyses is also being developed and may become an alternative technology for the detection of not only MPS but also of a large number of other treatable diseases; however currently major concerns with this type of analyses are due to new variants or variants of unknown significance (VUS) (Donati et al. 2018).

## Treatment

Because of the multisystem involvement in these patients, treatment is multidisciplinary and encompasses both the specific and general management elements.

### Supportive Treatment

Irrespective of the type, the management of all MPS requires supportive care and multidisciplinary treatment of a variety of systemic complications.

Regular evaluation at a major center with special interest and expertise in the management of the diseases is important in the coordination of interdisciplinary input and to coordinate multispecialty treatment strategies. In addition to the neurological complications experienced by many, distortion and narrowing of the upper airway and deformities of the chest present potential fatal anesthetic risks for most patients with MPS. Even the most trivial procedures requiring general anesthesia should be done at centers with anesthetists who are experienced with MPS disorders (Moretto et al. 2018; Madoff et al. 2019).

Because of the progressive nature of the diseases, individuals with MPS need to be evaluated regularly in order to identify potential problems early at a time when intervention would decrease morbidity, prevent premature mortality, and enhance the quality of life of affected patients. Every patient with MPS is unique; therefore, treatment options need to be individually based.

The table summarizes the types of problems experienced by patients with MPS disorders and strategies for their management.

Supportive treatment of mucopolysaccharidoses

| System | Problem | Intervention |
|---|---|---|
| Cardiovascular | Cardiomyopathy | Anti-heart failure medication |
| | Valve lesions | Anti-heart failure medication; valve replacement |
| | Coronary artery disease | None |
| CNS | Hydrocephalus | Ventriculoperitoneal shunt |
| | Atlantoaxial instability | Surgical decompression or fusion of cervical spine |
| | Cervical myelopathy | Surgical decompression or fusion |
| | Seizures | Anticonvulsant medication |
| | Behavior problems | Behavior management, medication |
| | Sleep disturbance | Medication |
| | Mental retardation | Appropriate educational support and interventions |
| Digestive | Hepatosplenomegaly | None |
| | Umbilical and inguinal hernias | Surgical repair |
| | Swallowing problems | Pureed diet; small, frequent meals; gastrostomy |
| | Drooling | Hyoscine glycopyrrolate, Botox injections |
| | Diarrhea | Antimotility medication |
| Ear | Recurrent otitis media | Antibiotic therapy; ENT surgery [a] |
| | Sensorineural deafness | Hearing aids |
| Eye | Corneal clouding | Avoid direct sunlight; corneal transplantation |
| | Glaucoma | Topical beta-blockers; trabecular surgery |
| | Retinal dystrophy | None |
| Musculoskeletal | Degenerative hip dysplasia | Analgesics; orthopedic surgical correction |
| | Kyphosis or kyphoscoliosis | Bracing or orthopedic surgical correction |
| | Joint contractures | Physiotherapy and orthoses |
| | Genu valgum deformities | Osteotomies |
| Respiratory | Upper airway obstruction | ENT surgery [a] |
| | Obstructive sleep apnea | Oxygen therapy, CPAP, or BiPAP |
| | Restrictive lung disease | Oxygen therapy, CPAP, or BiPAP |
| Dental | Caries, dental abscess | Oral hygiene; dental extraction |
| Peripheral nerve | Carpal tunnel syndrome | Surgical decompression |

*ENT* Ears, nose, throat, *CPAP* continuous positive airway pressure
[a]Including various combinations of tonsillectomy, adenoidectomy, myringotomy, the insertion of ventilation tubes, and tracheostomy

## Specific Treatment

### Hematopoietic Stem Cell Transplantation (HSCT)

In patients with MPS IH under the age of 2–3 years who have normal or near-normal developmental scores (DQ > 70), HSCT should be considered, using either HLA-matched bone marrow or umbilical cord blood cells as the donor cells (Taylor et al. 2019a, b). The best results are achieved with HLA-matched sibling donors, although using heterozygous carriers as donors should be avoided. Successful engraftment is associated with resolution of hepatosplenomegaly and upper airway obstruction. Corneal clouding usually resolves slowly, but never completely. Intraocular pressures may decrease. Cardiac manifestations attributable to muscle involvement are corrected, but valvular abnormalities are resistant to HSCT and often progress. Improvements in joint mobility are routinely experienced, and growth may approach normal rates for children of the same age. However, some skeletal abnormalities, especially abnormalities of the spine, do not respond to HSCT, and most severely affected children still require major orthopedic interventions. HSCT has been used occasionally to treat other MPS types, with controversial findings. The most consistent results, other than in young MPS IH patients, is in MPS VI (Turbeville et al. 2011), although it has been not routinely used where ERT is available due to the mortality and morbidity risks associated to the transplantation, which also limits its use in attenuated forms of MPS I. Limited data are available on HSCT in other MPS (Kubaski et al. 2017; Selvanathan et al. 2018; Taylor et al. 2019a, b).

### Enzyme Replacement Therapy

ERT has been demonstrated in randomized, double-blind, placebo-controlled studies to produce improvements in general performance, joint mobility, pulmonary function, and exercise tolerance in patients with MPS I (laronidase), MPS II (idursulfase), MPS IVA (elosulfase alfa), MPS VI (galsulfase), and MPS VII (vestronidase alfa). These enzymes are licensed in the European Union, United States, and several other countries to treat the non-neurological aspects of the specific MPS.

As there is no evidence that any of the replacement proteins cross the blood-brain barrier in significant amounts, an approach based on repeated intrathecal ERT has been used in MPS I (Muñoz-Rojas et al. 2008) and MPS VI patients (Muñoz-Rojas et al. 2010) and later further tested in clinical trials on MPS I (ClinicalTrials.gov Identifier: NCT02232477), MPS II (ClinicalTrials.gov Identifier: NCT00920647), and MPS IIIA (ClinicalTrials.gov Identifier: NCT01299727), but so far is not an approved therapeutic approach. Intracerebroventricular ERT is presently in development for MPS II and for MPS III B.

Another approach to provide enzyme to the CNS is the use of fusion proteins that could bypass the blood-brain barrier. A fusion protein combining laronidase and the antibody for the insulin receptor was tested in MPS I patients (Giugliani et al. 2018), and a similar product with idursulfase is in clinical trial for MPS II. Another fusion protein, combining idursulfase with the antibody for the transferrin receptor, was developed to treat MPS II (ClinicalTrials.gov Identifier: NCT02262338) and is presently in clinical development, with a similar approach being planned also for MPS I (ClinicalTrials.gov Identifier: NCT02371226).

### Other Therapeutic Approaches

The treatment of MPS is rapidly evolving and other therapeutic approaches are currently under evaluation.

Small molecules have been considered in the treatment of MPS I. Genistein was proposed as a substrate reduction therapy that could bring benefit to neuronopathic MPS as MPS III and the severe forms of MPS I and MPS II (de Ruijter et al. 2012; Marucha et al. 2011; Kloska et al. 2011). Despite good results in preclinical studies and safety demonstrated in clinical trials (Kim et al. 2013), no benefits to MPS patients were clearly demonstrated so far. Rhodamine B was also proposed as drug that could lead to substrate inhibition (Roberts et al. 2007). Ataluren was proposed as a stop-codon read-through strategy which could improve the outcome on severe MPS I patients (Hein et al. 2004), but no successful clinical use was reported so far. Odiparcil, a drug that makes GAGs (especially dermatan sulfate) more soluble and could reduce its storage (Myers et al. 2008), is under evaluation in a clinical trial (ClinicalTrials.gov Identifier: NCT03370653). Pentosan polysulfate was proposed to reduce inflammation (Hennermann et al. 2016; Simonaro et al. 2016), suspected to be one of the major players in MPS pathology.

Gene therapy is in clinical development for several types of MPS (MPS I, MPS II, MPS IIIA, MPS IIIB, and MPS VI), using different vectors (adeno-associated virus, lentivirus) and different administration routes (intravenous, intrathecal, intraparenchymal).

The results of clinical trials of gene therapy for MPS IIIA and IIIB have been published (Tardieu et al. 2014; Tardieu et al. 2017). Adeno-associated virus-mediated intraparenchymal gene therapy resulted in stabilized or delayed disease progression, particularly in patients treated at earlier ages.

Genome editing, which is also in clinical trials (MPS I and MPS II), may become another therapeutic alternative in the future (Ho et al. 2018).

Different therapeutic options may be available for the same disorder, and the appropriate treatment should be considered in individual patients.

Patients with severe central nervous system involvement (MPS III, Sanfilippo disease) or severe bone dysplasia (MPS IVA, Morquio disease) present particular challenges to management, as current therapies are poor in correcting the effects of the genetic lesion in the brain and bone, respectively.

Treatment of mucopolysaccharidoses by ERT

| No. | Disorder | Age | Medication | Dosage | Route and frequency |
|---|---|---|---|---|---|
| 64.1 | MPS I | All | Laronidase | 100 U/kg | IV weekly |
| 64.2 | MPS II | All | Idursulfase | 0.5 mg/kg | IV weekly |
| 64.7 | MPS IVA | All | Elosulfase alfa | 2 mg/kg | IV weekly |
| 64.9 | MPS VI | All | Galsulfase | 1 mg/kg | IV weekly |
| 64.10 | MPS VII | All | Vestronidase alfa | 4 mg/kg | IV every two weeks |

Therapeutic options for mucopolysaccharidoses

| No. | Disorder | HSCT | ERT | Small molecules | Gene therapy |
|---|---|---|---|---|---|
| 64.1 | MPS I | + | + | Preclinical studies | Clinical development |
| 64.2 | MPS II | (+) | + | Preclinical studies | Clinical development |
| 64.3 | MPS IIIA | | | | Clinical development |
| 64.4 | MPS IIIB | | Clinical development | | Clinical development |
| 64.5 | MPS IIIC | | | | Preclinical studies |
| 64.6 | MPS IIID | | Preclinical studies | | |
| 64.7 | MPS IVA | (+) | + | | Preclinical studies |
| 64.8 | MPS IVB | | | | Preclinical studies |
| 64.9 | MPS VI | + | + | Clinical development | Clinical development |
| 64.10 | MPS VII | (+) | + | | Preclinical studies |
| 64.11 | MPS IX | | | | |
| 64.12 | MPSPS | | | | |

## Follow-Up and Monitoring

The objectives of monitoring patients with MPS disorders are:

1. To provide ongoing support for the patient and family.
2. To anticipate complications, identify them early when they occur, and treat them in order to decrease morbidity.
3. To monitor specific therapies, such as HSCT and ERT, to assess their effectiveness, and, in the case of ERT, to manage infusion reactions which may occur.

Recommended follow-up and monitoring of MPS disorders

| | | Initial | Every 6 months | Every 12 months | Every 2 years |
|---|---|---|---|---|---|
| General | Medical history and physical examination[a] | * | * | | |
| Neurological | Neurological examination | * | * | | |
| | Developmental assessment | * | | * | |
| | MRI of brain | * | | | * |
| | MRI of spine | * | | | * |
| Ophthalmologic[b] | Visual acuity | * | | * | |
| | Retinal examination | * | | * | |
| | Corneal examination | * | | * | |
| Auditory | ENT consultation | * | | * | |
| | Audiometry | * | | * | |

| | | Initial | Every 6 months | Every 12 months | Every 2 years |
|---|---|---|---|---|---|
| Cardiac | Chest radiograph (for heart size) | * | | * | |
| | ECG | * | | | * |
| | Echocardiogram | * | | | * |
| Respiratory | Pulmonary function tests[c] | * | * | | |
| | Sleep study | * | | * | |
| Gastrointestinal | Spleen and liver volumes[d] | * | | | * |
| Musculoskeletal | Skeletal radiographs[e] | * | | | * |
| Laboratory studies[f] | Enzyme assay[g] | * | | | |
| | Urinary GAG level | * | * | | |
| | Urine analysis | * | * | | |
| | Antibody testing | *[h] | * | | |

[a]Including measurement of height, weight, head circumference, and blood pressure

[b]Including measurement of intraocular pressures

[c]Forced vital capacity (FVC) and 1-s forced expiratory volume ($FEV_1$)

[d]Best measured by MRI or CT scan

[e]AP and lateral views of the skull, PA view of the chest, lateral views of the spine (including the cervical spine), AP view of the hips and pelvis, single AP view of both hands together. In the case of MPS IV, include lateral views of the neck in flexion and extension to assess stability of the atlantoaxial joint and a single AP view of the upper cervical spine through the open mouth to assess the integrity of the odontoid process. These studies are primarily for the assessment of disease in children; the menu and schedule for radiographic studies in adults would be more limited, emphasizing the assessment of osteoarthritis

[f]In patients who have undergone hematopoietic stem cell transplantation (HSCT), leucocytes alpha-l-iduronidase assays and VNTR analyses on DNA extracted from peripheral blood should be done monthly from the time of transplantation and then every 6 months to assess engraftment

[g]For assessment of response to enzyme replacement therapy or HSCT

[h]To be performed initially 3 months after the start of ERT

## References


Bravo H, Neto EC, Schulte J, Pereira J, Filho CS, Bittencourt F, Sebastião F, Bender F, de Magalhães APS, Guidobono R, Trapp FB, Michelin-Tirelli K, Souza CFM, Rojas Málaga D, Pasqualim G, Brusius-Facchin AC, Giugliani R. Investigation of newborns with abnormal results in a newborn screening program for four lysosomal storage diseases in Brazil. Mol Genet Metab Rep. 2017;12:92–7.

Bronstein MG, Pan RJ, Dant M, Lubin B. Leveraging evidence-based public policy and advocacy to advance newborn screening in California. Pediatrics. 2019;143:2).

Burlina AB, Polo G, Salviati L, Duro G, Zizzo C, Dardis A, Bembi B, Cazzorla C, Rubert L, Zordan R, Desnick RJ, Burlina AP. Newborn screening for lysosomal storage disorders by tandem mass spectrometry in North East Italy. J Inherit Metab Dis. 2018;41(2):209–19.

Burton BK, Charrow J, Hoganson GE, Waggoner D, Tinkle B, Braddock SR, Schneider M, Grange DK, Nash C, Shryock H, Barnett R, Shao R, Basheeruddin K, Dizikes G. Newborn screening for lysosomal storage disorders in Illinois: the initial 15-month experience. J Pediatr. 2017;190:130–5.

Chan MJ, Liao HC, Gelb MH, Chuang CK, Liu MY, Chen HJ, Kao SM, Lin HY, Huang YH, Kumar AB, Chennamaneni NK, Pendem N, Lin SP, Chiang CC. Taiwan National Newborn Screening Program by tandem mass spectrometry for mucopolysaccharidoses types I, II, and VI. J Pediatr. 2019;205:176–82.

Chuang CK, Lin HY, Wang TJ, Huang YH, Chan MJ, Liao HC, Lo YT, Wang LY, Tu RY, Fang YY, Chen TL, Ho HC, Chiang CC, Lin SP. Status of newborn screening and follow up investigations for Mucopolysaccharidoses I and II in Taiwan. Orphanet J Rare Dis. 2018;13(1):84.

de Ruijter J, Valstar MJ, Narajczyk M, Wegrzyn G, Kulik W, Ijlst L, Wagemans T, van der Wal WM, Wijburg FA. Genistein in Sanfilippo disease: a randomized controlled crossover trial. Ann Neurol. 2012;71(1):110–20.

Di Fruscio G, Schulz A, De Cegli R, Savarese M, Mutarelli M, Parenti G, Banfi S, Braulke T, Nigro V, Ballabio A. Lysoplex: an efficient toolkit to detect DNA sequence variations in the autophagy-lysosomal pathway. Autophagy. 2015;11(6):928–38.

Donati MA, Pasquini E, Spada M, Polo G, Burlina A. Newborn screening in mucopolysaccharidoses. Ital J Pediatr. 2018;44(Suppl 2):126.

Gelb MH. Newborn screening for lysosomal storage diseases: methodologies, screen positive rates, normalization of datasets, second-tier tests, and post-analysis tools. Int J Neonatal Screen. 2018;4(3):23.

Gelb MH, Ronald Scott C, Turecek F, Liao HC. Comparison of tandem mass spectrometry to fluorimetry for newborn screening of LSDs. Mol Genet Metab Rep. 2017;12:80–1.

Giugliani R, Giugliani L, de Oliveira Poswar F, Donis KC, Corte AD, Schmidt M, Boado RJ, Nestrasil I, Nguyen C, Chen S, Pardridge WM. Neurocognitive and somatic stabilization in pediatric patients with severe mucopolysaccharidosis type I after 52 weeks of intravenous brain-penetrating insulin receptor antibody-iduronidase fusion protein (valanafusp alpha): an open label phase 1-2 trial. Orphanet J Rare Dis. 2018;13(1):110.

Hein LK, Bawden M, Muller VJ, Sillence D, Hopwood JJ, Brooks DA. Alpha-L-iduronidase premature stop codons and potential read-through in mucopolysaccharidosis type I patients. J Mol Biol. 2004;338(3):453–62.

Hennermann JB, Gökce S, Solyom A, Mengel E, Schuchman EH, Simonaro CM. Treatment with pentosan polysulphate in patients with MPS I: results from an open label, randomized, monocentric phase II study. J Inherit Metab Dis. 2016;39(6):831–7.

Ho BX, Loh SJH, Chan WK, Soh BS. In vivo genome editing as a therapeutic approach. Int J Mol Sci. 2018;19(9):E2721.

Imundo L, Leduc CA, Guha S, Brown M, Perino G, Gushulak L, Triggs-Raine B, Chung WK. A complete deficiency of Hyaluronoglucosaminidase 1 (HYAL1) presenting as familial juvenile idiopathic arthritis. J Inherit Metab Dis. 2011;34(5):1013–22.

Joseph R, DiCesare EB, Miller A. Hunter syndrome: is it time to make it part of newborn screening? Adv Neonatal Care. 2018;18(6):480–7.

Kim KH, Dodsworth C, Paras A, Burton BK. High dose genistein aglycone therapy is safe in patients with mucopolysaccharidoses involving the central nervous system. Mol Genet Metab. 2013;109(4):382–5.

Kloska A, Jakóbkiewicz-Banecka J, Narajczyk M, Banecka-Majkutewicz Z, Węgrzyn G. Effects of flavonoids on glycosaminoglycan synthesis: implications for substrate reduction therapy in Sanfilippo disease and other mucopolysaccharidoses. Metab Brain Dis. 2011;26(1):1–8.

Kobayashi H. Recent trends in mucopolysaccharidosis research. J Hum Genet. 2019;64(2):127–37.

Kondo H, Maksimova N, Otomo T, Kato H, Imai A, Asano Y, Kobayashi K, Nojima S, Nakaya A, Hamada Y, Irahara K, Gurinova E, Sukhomyasova A, Nogovicina A, Savvina M, Yoshimori T, Ozono K, Sakai N. Mutation in VPS33A affects metabolism of glycosaminoglycans: a new type of mucopolysaccharidosis with severe systemic symptoms. Hum Mol Genet. 2017;26(1):173–83.

Kubaski F, Mason RW, Nakatomi A, Shintaku H, Xie L, van Vlies NN, Church H, Giugliani R, Kobayashi H, Yamaguchi S, Suzuki Y, Orii T, Fukao T, Montaño AM, Tomatsu S. Newborn screening for mucopolysaccharidoses: a pilot study of measurement of glycosaminoglycans by tandem mass spectrometry. J Inherit Metab Dis. 2017;40(1):151–8.

Kuiper GA, Meijer OLM, Langereis EJ, Wijburg FA. Failure to shorten the diagnostic delay in two ultra-orphan diseases (mucopolysaccharidosis types I and III): potential causes and implications. Orphanet J Rare Dis. 2018;13(1):2.

Liu Y, Yi F, Kumar AB, Kumar Chennamaneni N, Hong X, Scott CR, Gelb MH, Turecek F. Multiplex tandem mass spectrometry enzymatic activity assay for Newborn screening of the Mucopolysaccharidoses and type 2 neuronal ceroid Lipofuscinosis. Clin Chem. 2017;63(6):1118–26.

Maccari F, Galeotti F, Mantovani V, Zampini L, Padella L, Rigon L, Concolino D, Fiumara A, Pascale E, Pittalà A, Galeazzi T, Monachesi C, Marchesiello RL, Coppa G, Gabrielli O, Volpi N. Composition and structure of glycosaminoglycans in DBS from 2-3-day-old newborns for the diagnosis of mucopolysaccharidosis. Anal Biochem. 2018;557:34–41.

Madoff LU, Kordun A, Cravero JP. Airway management in patients with mucopolysaccharidoses: the progression toward difficult intubation. Paediatr Anaesth. 2019;29:620.

Martins C, Hůlková H, Dridi L, Dormoy-Raclet V, Grigoryeva L, Choi Y, Langford-Smith A, Wilkinson FL, Ohmi K, DiCristo G, Hamel E, Ausseil J, Cheillan D, Moreau A, Svobodová E, Hájková Z, Tesařová M, Hansíková H, Bigger BW, Hrebícek M, Pshezhetsky AV. Neuroinflammation, mitochondrial defects and neurodegeneration in mucopolysaccharidosis III type C mouse model. Brain. 2015;138(Pt 2):336–55.

Marucha J, Tylki-Szymańska A, Jakóbkiewicz-Banecka J, Piotrowska E, Kloska A, Czartoryska B, Węgrzyn G. Improvement in the range of joint motion in seven patients with mucopolysaccharidosis type II during experimental gene expression-targeted isoflavone therapy (GET IT). Am J Med Genet A. 2011;155A(9):2257–62.

Millington DS, Sista R, Eckhardt A, Rouse J, Bali D, Goldberg R, Cotten M, Buckley R, Pamula V. Digital microfluidics: a future technology in the newborn screening laboratory? Semin Perinatol. 2010;34(2):163–9.

Minter Baerg MM, Stoway SD, Hart J, Mott L, Peck DS, Nett SL, Eckerman JS, Lacey JM, Turgeon CT, Gavrilov D, Oglesbee D, Raymond K, Tortorelli S, Matern D, Mørkrid L, Rinaldo P. Precision newborn screening for lysosomal disorders. Genet Med. 2018;20(8):847–54.

Moretto A, Bosatra MG, Marchesini L, Tesoro S. Anesthesiological risks in mucopolysaccharidoses. Ital J Pediatr. 2018;44(Suppl 2):116.

Muñoz-Rojas MV, Horovitz DD, Jardim LB, Raymundo M, Llerena JC Jr, de Magalhães Tde S, Vieira TA, Costa R, Kakkis E, Giugliani R. Intrathecal administration of recombinant human N-acetylgalactosamine 4-sulfatase to a MPS VI patient with pachymeningitis cervicalis. Mol Genet Metab. 2010;99(4):346–50.

Muñoz-Rojas MV, Vieira T, Costa R, Fagondes S, John A, Jardim LB, Vedolin LM, Raymundo M, Dickson PI, Kakkis E, Giugliani R. Intrathecal enzyme replacement therapy in a patient with mucopolysaccharidosis type I and symptomatic spinal cord compression. Am J Med Genet A. 2008;146A(19):2538–44.

Myers AL, Upreti VV, Khurana M, Eddington ND. Characterization of total plasma glycosaminoglycan levels in healthy volunteers following oral administration of a novel antithrombotic odiparcil with aspirin or enoxaparin. J Clin Pharmacol. 2008;48(10):1158–70.

Navarrete-Martínez JI, Limón-Rojas AE, Gaytán-García MJ, Reyna-Figueroa J, Wakida-Kusunoki G, Delgado-Calvillo MDR, Cantú-Reyna C, Cruz-Camino H, Cervantes-Barragán DE. Newborn screening for six lysosomal storage disorders in a cohort of Mexican patients: three-year findings from a screening program in a closed Mexican health system. Mol Genet Metab. 2017;121(1):16–21.

Parenti G, Fraldi A. Pathogenesis of mucopolysaccharidoses. In: Tomatsu S, Lavery C, Giugliani R, Harmatz P, Scarpa M, Wegrzyn G, Orii T, editors. Mucopolysaccharidoses update: Nova Science Publisher; 2018. Chapter 5.

Pshezhetsky AV. Lysosomal storage of heparan sulfate causes mitochondrial defects, altered autophagy, and neuronal death in the mouse model of mucopolysaccharidosis III type C. Autophagy. 2016;12(6):1059–60.

Roberts AL, Rees MH, Klebe S, Fletcher JM, Byers S. Improvement in behaviour after substrate deprivation therapy with rhodamine B in a mouse model of MPS IIIA. Mol Genet Metab. 2007;92(1–2):115–21.

Saville JT, McDermott BK, Fletcher JM, Fuller M. Disease and subtype specific signatures enable precise diagnosis of the mucopolysaccharidoses. Genet Med. 2019;21(3):753–7.

Schielen PCJI, Kemper EA, Gelb MH. Newborn screening for lysosomal storage diseases: a concise review of the literature on screening methods, therapeutic possibilities and regional programs. Int J Neonatal Screen. 2017;3(2):6.

Selvanathan A, Ellaway C, Wilson C, Owens P, Shaw PJ, Bhattacharya K. Effectiveness of early hematopoietic stem cell transplantation in preventing neurocognitive decline in Mucopolysaccharidosis type II: a case series. JIMD Rep. 2018;41:81–9.

Settembre C, Fraldi A, Jahreiss L, Spampanato C, Venturi C, Medina D, de Pablo R, Tacchetti C, Rubinsztein DC, Ballabio A. A block of autophagy in lysosomal storage disorders. Hum Mol Genet. 2008;17(1):119–29.

Shapiro IM, Layfield R, Lotz M, Settembre C, Whitehouse C. Boning up on autophagy: the role of autophagy in skeletal biology. Autophagy. 2014;10(1):7–19.

Simonaro CM, Tomatsu S, Sikora T, Kubaski F, Frohbergh M, Guevara JM, Wang RY, Vera M, Kang JL, Smith LJ, Schuchman EH, Pentosan Polysulfate HME. Oral versus subcutaneous injection in mucopolysaccharidosis type I dogs. PLoS One. 2016;11(4):e0153136.

Sista RS, Eckhardt AE, Wang T, Graham C, Rouse JL, Norton SM, Srinivasan V, Pollack MG, Tolun AA, Bali D, Millington DS, Pamula VK. Digital microfluidic platform for multiplexing enzyme assays: implications for lysosomal storage disease screening in newborns. Clin Chem. 2011;57(10):1444–51.

Tardieu M, Zérah M, Gougeon ML, Ausseil J, de Bournonville S, Husson B, Zafeiriou D, Parenti G, Bourget P, Poirier B, Furlan V, Artaud C, Baugnon T, Roujeau T, Crystal RG, Meyer C, Deiva K. Heard JM. Intracerebral gene therapy in children with mucopolysaccharidosis type IIIB syndrome: an uncontrolled phase 1/2 clinical trial. Lancet Neurol. 2017;16(9):712–20.

Tardieu M, Zérah M, Husson B, de Bournonville S, Deiva K, Adamsbaum C, Vincent F, Hocquemiller M, Broissand C, Furlan V, Ballabio A, Fraldi A, Crystal RG, Baugnon T, Roujeau T, Heard JM, Danos O. Intracerebral administration of adeno-associated viral vector serotype rh.10 carrying human SGSH and SUMF1 cDNAs in children with mucopolysaccharidosis type IIIA disease: results of a phase I/II trial. Hum Gene Ther. 2014;25(6):506–16.

Taylor JL, Clinard K, Powell CM, Rehder C, Young SP, Bali D, Beckloff SE, Gehtland LM, Kemper AR, Lee S, Millington D, Patel HS, Shone SM, Woodell C, Zimmerman SJ, Bailey DB Jr, Muenzer J. The North Carolina experience with mucopolysaccharidosis type I newborn screening. J Pediatr. 2019a; pii: S0022-3476(19)30509-8

Taylor M, Khan S, Stapleton M, Wang J, Chen J, Wynn R, Yabe H, Chinen Y, Boelens JJ, Mason RW, Kubaski F, Horovitz DDG, Barth AL, Serafini M, Bernardo ME, Kobayashi H, Orii KE, Suzuki Y, Orii T, Tomatsu S. Hematopoietic stem cell transplantation for mucopolysaccharidoses: past, present, and future. Biol Blood Marrow Transplant. 2019b; pii: S1083-8791(19)30137-5

Turbeville S, Nicely H, Rizzo JD, Pedersen TL, Orchard PJ, Horwitz ME, Horwitz EM, Veys P, Bonfim C, Al-Seraihy A. Clinical outcomes following hematopoietic stem cell transplantation for the treatment of mucopolysaccharidosis VI. Mol Genet Metab. 2011;102(2):111–5.

Yi F, Hong X, Kumar AB, Zong C, Boons GJ, Scott CR, Turecek F, Robinson BH, Gelb MH. Detection of mucopolysaccharidosis III-A (Sanfilippo syndrome-a) in dried blood spots (DBS) by tandem mass spectrometry. Mol Genet Metab. 2018;125(1–2):59–63.

# Cystinosis

# 65

Elena Levtchenko and Francesco Emma

## Contents



E. Levtchenko
Department of Pediatric Nephrology, University Hospitals Leuven, Catholic University of Leuven, Leuven, Belgium
e-mail: elena.levtchenko@uzleuven.be

F. Emma (✉)
Department of Pediatric Subspecialties, Division of Nephrology and Dialysis, Bambino Gesù Children's Hospital, IRCCS, Rome, Italy
e-mail: francesco.emma@opbg.net

## Summary

Infantile nephropathic cystinosis is an autosomal recessive disorder caused by mutations in the *CTNS* gene that encodes for cystinosin, a lysosomal cystine/$H^+$ symporter. With time, cystine accumulation leads to cell dysfunction in various tissues. The kidneys are initially more involved. Most patients are asymptomatic at birth but present in the first or second



N. Blau et al. (eds.), *Physician's Guide to the Diagnosis, Treatment, and Follow-Up of Inherited Metabolic Diseases*,
https://doi.org/10.1007/978-3-030-67727-5_65

year of life with failure to thrive, polyuria, dehydration, and/or rickets, which are secondary to the renal Fanconi syndrome. With very few exceptions, all patients have corneal cystine crystals by 18 months of age that can help in recognizing the disease. The diagnosis of cystinosis is based on the detection of increased leukocyte cystine levels and demonstration of mutations in the *CTNS* gene (detection rate > 95%). In Northern Europe, 75% of mutated alleles carry a 57-kb deletion; all other types of mutations, generally resulting in a complete or severe loss of function of the cystinosin protein, have been described.

Introduction of cysteamine treatment in the late 1980s and improvements in dialysis and renal transplantation have considerably improved the prognosis of cystinosis. Cysteamine significantly delays progression to end-stage renal kidney disease, but cannot prevent it in most cases. The majority of patients live well into adulthood but, if not appropriately treated with cysteamine, develop other symptoms related to cystine accumulation in various tissues. These include retinal degeneration, hypothyroidism, diabetes mellitus, exocrine pancreatic insufficiency, pubertal retardation and gonadal dysfunction, restrictive pulmonary disease, myopathy, neurological deterioration, and liver involvement. Two milder forms of the disease, namely, juvenile cystinosis and ocular cystinosis, caused by mutations that allow residual function of the cystinosin protein, have also been reported. These patients present with milder symptoms later in childhood or with isolated corneal cystine depositions.

## Introduction

Cystinosis is an inherited autosomal recessive disease caused by mutations in the *CTNS* gene, which encodes for cystinosin, a cystine/$H^+$ symporter that is primarily expressed at the lysosomal membrane (Kalatzis et al. 2001). The *CTNS* gene is located on chromosome 17p13 and was cloned in 1998 (Town et al. 1998). To date, more than 140 different mutations have been identified with a detection rate that exceeds 95% (David et al. 2019).

The *CTNS* gene is composed of 12 exons and spans 23 kb. Cystinosin is composed of 367 amino acids that form a 7-transmembrane domain cotransporter with 2 lysosomal targeting motifs (Cherqui et al. 2001). The most common mutation, accounting for 75% of the affected alleles in Northern Europe, is a 57-kb deletion that removes the first nine exons and part of exon 10 of the *CTNS* gene, the upstream 5′ region of the *CARKL* gene, and the first two non-coding exons of the *TRPV1* gene (Nesterova and Gahl 2017). The function of the *CARKL* gene has been identified in the phosphorylation of sedoheptulose, an intermediate metabolite of the pentose phosphate pathway. The transient receptor potential channel vanilloid subfamily member 1 (*TRPV1*) encodes for an ion channel that is primarily expressed in sensory nerves and is activated by a wide range of chemical stimuli. Patients with a homozygous 57-kb deletion have elevated blood and urinary levels of sedoheptulose. The contribution of the *CARKL* and *TRPV1* genes to the pathogenesis of the disease in patients with homozygous 57-kb deletion has not been fully studied. No major differences in the clinical evolution, however, have been reported when comparing these patients to patients carrying other *CTNS* gene mutations (Wilmer et al. 2010). These include smaller deletions, insertions, nonsense mutations, missense mutations, mutations within the promoter region, and splice site mutations. Intronic mutations affecting normal splicing have also been reported in families whose standard genetic testing failed to identify mutations in one or both alleles, indicating that cystinosis is a monogenic disorder and that intronic regions should be analyzed when no mutations are found in the *CTNS* coding sequence (Taranta et al. 2010; David et al. 2019).

A transcript variant originating from an alternative splicing of exon 12 has been reported and was shown to be expressed also in other cell compartments, including the plasma membrane (Taranta et al. 2008). The contribution of this isoform to the physiopathology of the disease is not known yet (Wilmer et al. 2010).

The incidence of cystinosis varies among countries between 0.5 and 1.0/100,000 live births; several founder mutations have been observed in different geographic regions, such as the 57-kb deletion that originated in Germany around A.D. 500 (Nesterova and Gahl 2017). In its most frequent form, termed infantile nephropathic cystinosis (MIM 219800), children are usually asymptomatic at birth and develop normally during the first 2–3 months of life. They generally present around the age of 6 months with failure to thrive, vomiting, constipation, polyuria, excessive thirst, dehydration, and sometimes rickets (Nesterova and Gahl 2017; Elmonem et al. 2016). These symptoms are the consequence of the renal Fanconi syndrome, which is characterized by excessive urinary losses of water, amino acids, phosphate, uric acid, bicarbonate, glucose, sodium, potassium, low-molecular-weight proteins, and other solutes. Untreated children develop chronic renal failure during early childhood that progresses to end-stage kidney disease in the first decade of life. Patients with cystinosis have a characteristic facial appearance. Typically, Caucasian children have blond hair, although children from other ethnic groups may retain normal or near-normal pigmentation. With time, cystine crystals deposit in the cornea and are nearly always observed by 18 months of age (Tsilou et al. 2002). They may cause photophobia and chronic inflammatory changes of the anterior chamber, if not treated.

The diagnosis of cystinosis is based on the measurement of leukocyte cystine levels by tandem mass spectrometry or HPLC. Abnormal results need to be confirmed by molecular analysis of the *CTNS* gene. Leukocyte cystine levels are increased up to 100-fold in affected individuals compared with control subjects; levels in heterozygous carriers are only slightly increased.

Since the late 1980s, improvements in dialysis and renal transplantation and the introduction of treatment with the cystine-depleting agent cysteamine have considerably prolonged the life expectancy of patients with cystinosis (Markello et al. 1993; Van Stralen et al. 2011). However, they have also revealed hitherto long-term complications resulting from cystine accumulation in other tissues. These include retinal degeneration, hypothyroidism, diabetes mellitus, exocrine pancreatic insufficiency, pubertal retardation and gonadal dysfunction, restrictive pulmonary disease, myopathy, neurological deterioration, and liver involvement (Gahl et al. 2007; Nesterova and Gahl 2013; Brodin-Sartorius et al. 2012). A few female patients have given birth to normal healthy children, but nearly all tested male patients with infantile cystinosis are infertile. Most late-onset complications improve or are prevented by cysteamine (Gahl et al. 2007; Nesterova and Gahl 2013; Brodin-Sartorius et al. 2012). Corneal cystine crystals do not respond to oral cysteamine and require topical administration. Cysteamine treatment should be optimized by regular measurements of leukocyte cystine levels that allow adapting the dose to target levels (Levtchenko et al. 2004).

Renal transplantation is a well-established treatment for patients reaching end-stage renal disease. Transplanted cystinotic patients have longer renal survival, probably because they have a lower risk of rejection (Van Stralen et al. 2011). They require, nonetheless, standard immunosuppression. Although cysteamine has considerably improved the outcome, progression to end-stage kidney diseases usually cannot be prevented beyond the second or third decade of life (Van Stralen et al. 2011; Nesterova and Gahl 2013).

Early recognition of complications, optimization of nutritional intake, early treatment of Fanconi syndrome and rickets, and growth hormone therapy have also considerably improved the clinical outcome.

In addition to the infantile form, two other milder variants have been identified (Nesterova and Gahl 2017). These include the "juvenile" or "intermediate" form (MIM 219900), which is usually diagnosed during childhood or adolescence and is characterized by less severe renal symptoms, and a third form that has been reported primarily in adults and is characterized by isolated ocular symptoms and is termed "ocular" or "non-nephropathic" cystinosis (MIM 219750).

The severity of the disease co-segregates within family members with very few exceptions. *In vitro* studies of residual cystine transport activity have shown that infantile cystinosis generally results from severe mutations leading to complete loss of function of cystinosin (David et al. 2019).

To date, the physiopathology of cell damage in cystinosis has not been fully elucidated. *In vitro* and *in vivo* studies have shown that cystinotic cells are more prone to apoptosis; abnormalities in glutathione and ATP metabolism, as well as defects in intracellular trafficking and mTOR signaling and impaired autophagy, have been reported (Wilmer et al. 2010; Cherqui and Courtoy 2017; Festa et al. 2018).

## Nomenclature

| No. | Disorder name | Alternative disorder names | Disorder abbreviation | Gene symbol | Chromosomal localization | Affected protein | OMIM # |
|---|---|---|---|---|---|---|---|
| 65.1 | Infantile nephropathic cystinosis | | – | *CTNS* | 17p13 | Cystinosin | 219800 |
| 65.2 | Juvenile cystinosis | Intermediate form | – | *CTNS* | 17p13 | Cystinosin | 219900 |
| 65.3 | Non-nephropathic cystinosis | Ocular form | – | *CTNS* | 17p13 | Cystinosin | 219750 |

## Metabolic Pathways

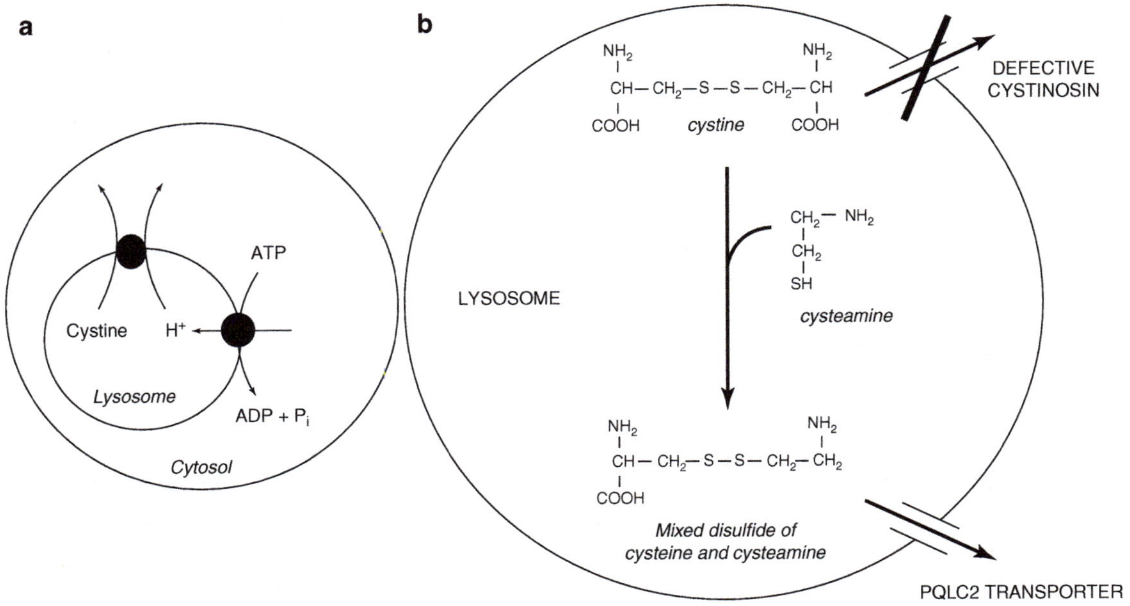


**Fig. 65.1** *Panel* (**a**). Cystinosin is a lysosomal cystine carrier. Cystine efflux from lysosomes is dependent on the proton gradient generated by the vacuolar $H^+$ ATPase. *Panel* (**b**). Mechanism of action of cysteamine. In the presence of cystine, cysteamine forms a mixed disulfide molecule resembling lysine, which is more soluble than cystine and exits the lysosome through a PQLC2 transporter

## Signs and Symptoms

**Tables 65.1 and 65.2** Nephropathic cystinosis (infantile)

| System | Symptom | Neonatal (birth–1 month) | Infancy (1–18 months) | Childhood (1.5–11 years) | Adolescence (11–16 years) | Adulthood (>16 years)[a] |
|---|---|---|---|---|---|---|
| CNS | Cognitive dysfunction | | | ± | ± | ± |
| | Peripheral neuropathy | | | | | ± |
| | Pyramidal signs | | | | | ± |
| | Stroke-like episodes | | | | ± | ± |
| | Swallowing difficulties | | | | | ± |
| Digestive | Hepatomegaly | | | | ± | ± |
| | Liver fibrosis | | | | | ± |
| | Splenomegaly | | | | | ± |
| Endocrine | Diabetes mellitus | | | | ± | ± |
| | Hypogonadism | | | | ± | + |
| | Hypothyroidism | | | ± | ± | ± |
| | Infertility (men) | | | | + | + |
| | Pancreatic dysfunction, endocrine | | | | ± | ± |
| | Puberty, delayed | | | | + | |
| Eye | Photophobia | | | ± | + | + |
| | Retinopathy | ± | ± | ± | + | + |
| | Vision, impaired | | | | ± | ± |

**Tables 65.1 and 65.2** (continued)

| System | Symptom | Neonatal (birth–1 month) | Infancy (1–18 months) | Childhood (1.5–11 years) | Adolescence (11–16 years) | Adulthood (>16 years)[a] |
|---|---|---|---|---|---|---|
| Musculoskeletal | Dental defects | | | + | + | + |
| | Diaphragm dysfunction | | | | | ± |
| | Genu valgum | | ± | ± | ± | ± |
| | Muscle weakness | | | | | ± |
| | Myopathy, peripheral | | | | | ± |
| | Osteopenia | | | ± | ± | ± |
| | Osteoporosis | | | ± | ± | ± |
| | Pes planus | | | ± | ± | ± |
| | Renal osteodystrophy | | | ± | ± | ± |
| | Rickets | | ± | ± | ± | ± |
| | Scoliosis | | | ± | ± | ± |
| Renal | Nephrocalcinosis | | ± | ± | ± | ± |
| | Nephrolithiasis | | | ± | ± | ± |
| | Polyuria | | + | + | + | ± |
| | Renal failure, chronic | | | ± | ± | + |
| | Renal Fanconi syndrome | | + | + | ± | ± |
| Other | Corneal cystine crystals | | ± | + | + | + |
| | Failure to thrive | | + | + | | |
| Routine laboratory | Albumin (U) | | ↑ | ↑ | ↑ | |
| | Bicarbonate (P) | | ↓ | ↓ | ↓-n[b] | |
| | Calcium (U) | | ↑ | ↑ | ↑[b] | |
| | Creatinine (P) | n | n | n-↑ | n-↑ | |
| | Glucose (U) | | ↑ | ↑ | ↑[b] | |
| | Phosphate (P) | n | ↓ | ↓-n | ↓-n[b] | |
| | Phosphate (U) | ↑ | ↑ | ↑ | ↑[b] | |
| | Potassium (P) | n | ↓ | ↓ | ↓-n[b] | |
| | Potassium (U) | | ↑ | ↑ | n-↑[b] | |
| | Sodium (U) | | ↑ | ↑ | ↑[b] | |
| | Uric acid (P) | n | ↓ | ↓-n | n-↑[b] | |
| | Uric acid (U) | | ↑ | ↑ | ↑[b] | |
| Special laboratory | Amino acids (P) | n | n | n | n | |
| | Amino acids (U) | ↑ | ↑ | ↑ | n-↑[b] | |
| | Carnitine, total and free (P) | n | ↓ | ↓-n | n | |
| | Cystine (P) | n | n | n | n | |
| | Cystine (WBC, FB)[c] | ↑ | ↑ | ↑ | ↑ | |
| | T4 | n | n | ↓-n | ↓-n | |
| | TSH (S) | | n-↑ | n-↑ | n-↑ | |

Patients with juvenile cystinosis present with symptoms similar to the infantile form, but usually at older age. Renal Fanconi syndrome is usually less pronounced. Non-nephropathic cystinosis 65.3 are exceptional patients that only have corneal cystine crystals.

Patients with ocular cystinosis present only with ocular complaints related to corneal cystine crystals, but not with systemic symptoms

[a]Patients have usually a kidney transplant at that age; symptoms and routine biochemical parameters depend on the graft function

[b]Biochemical features of renal Fanconi syndrome decrease during the decline of the GFR. Urinary features of renal Fanconi syndrome mostly persist even at advanced stages of renal failure and after renal transplantation if the diuresis of the native kidneys is still present

[c]Cystine measurements in cultured fi broblasts (FB) are not recommended routinely. The diagnosis of cystinosis should be confi rmed by molecular diagnosis of the *CTNS* gene

## Reference Values

Reference values for leukocyte cystine

| | |
|---|---|
| Cystine (WBC) | <0.1–0.2 nmol cystine/mg protein[a] |
| Cystine (PMN) | <0.1–0.2 nmol cystine/mg protein[a] |

Conversion factor ½ cystine/mg protein = 2× cystine/mg protein
[a]Cystine is sometimes expressed as nmol ½ cystine/mg protein

## Pathological Values

Pathological values for leukocyte cystine

| | | |
|---|---|---|
| Cystine (PMN) | Heterozygotes | 0.09–0.65 nmol cystine/mg protein |
| | Patients at diagnosis | >2 nmol cystine/mg protein |
| | Patients under cysteamine therapy | <0.6 nmol cystine/mg protein |
| Cystine (WBC) | Heterozygotes | 0.05–0.5 nmol cystine/mg protein |
| | Patients at diagnosis | >2 nmol cystine/mg protein |
| | Patients under cysteamine therapy | <0.5 nmol cystine/mg protein |

## Diagnostic Flowchart

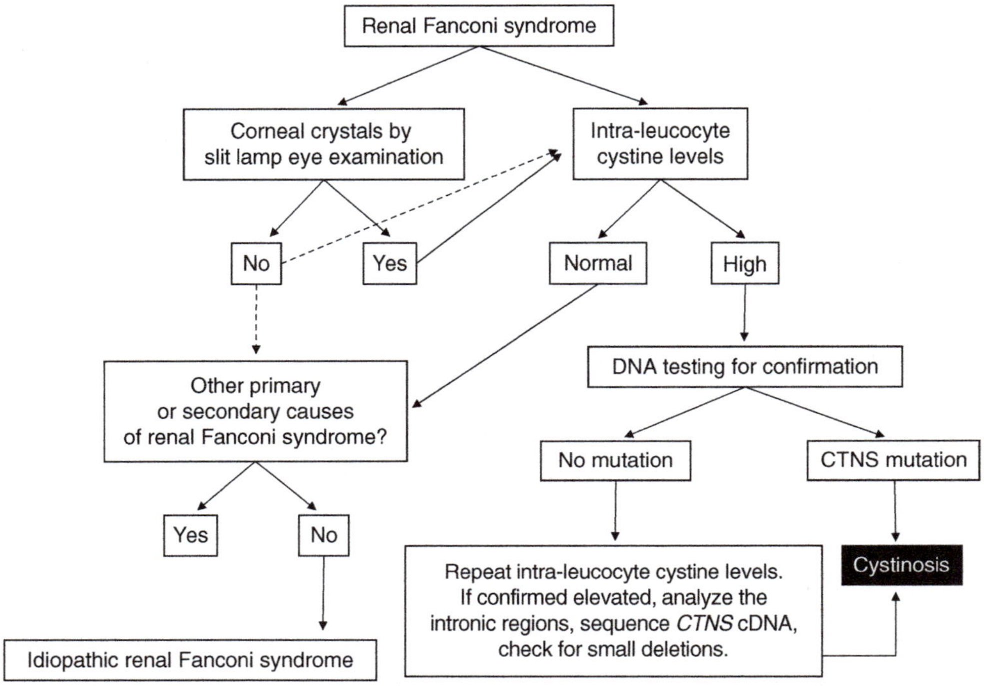


## Specimen Collection

Leukocyte cystine measurement is a particularly sensitive test that should be performed in certified laboratories. Each laboratory should produce its own reference values for healthy subjects, heterozygotes carriers, patients at diagnosis, and patients under cysteamine treatment.

Blood is usually collected in heparin or citrate tubes according to the laboratory recommendation; results are significantly influenced by the type of anticoagulant. After collecting blood samples, specimens should be processed as soon possible. The pre-analytic phase is the most delicate part of the analysis. Cystine is currently measured by tandem mass spectrometry (MS-MS) and, less frequently, by high-performance liquid chromatography (HPLC). Results are usually normalized per mg of proteins. Sample contamination with other non-leukocyte proteins (e.g., erythrocyte ghosts) may result in falsely low values. Measurements performed on the granulocyte fraction after Ficoll fractionation are more reliable than measurements on the entire leukocyte population, because granulocytes contain significantly more lysosomes than lymphocytes.

## Prenatal Diagnosis

Fetal DNA sequencing allows accurate prenatal diagnosis. In the past, cystine measurements were performed on cultured amniotic cells, but this approach has been abandoned.

## Treatment Summary

Oral cysteamine bitartrate efficiently depletes lysosomes from cystine (Fig. 65.1) at a recommended dose of 1.3–1.9 g/m$^2$/day given at 6-hour intervals (Markello et al. 1993; Elmonem et al. 2016; Gahl et al. 2007). A delayed release preparation is also available in some countries, allowing treatment every 12 hours at a dose that is usually 80% of the regular cysteamine bitartrate dose (Langman et al. 2016). Treatment should be started as soon as the diagnosis is made and continued lifelong. Trough levels should be used to monitor leukocyte cystine levels (Levtchenko et al. 2004). Side effects of cysteamine are mostly restricted to gastrointestinal discomfort, bad breath, and sweat odor. Gastric tolerance can be improved by proton pump inhibitors. Noncompliance because of foul odor and strict administration schedules (especially for standard cysteamine bitartrate) occur frequently, particularly in adolescents, and often correspond to worsening clinical symptoms and prognosis.

Symptomatic therapy includes prescription of appropriate fluid and electrolyte intake, adequate nutrition, and prevention of rickets. Patients with cystinosis should always have free access to water; prolonged heat exposure should be avoided. Young children frequently require tube feeding. Renal tubular waste is significantly reduced by indomethacin (1–3 mg/kg/day in 2–3 separate doses), but this therapy can be nephrotoxic; it can be, however, particularly useful in the first years of life. The doses of potassium, sodium, bicarbonate, and phosphate supplements should be regularly adapted; 1,25-dihydroxycholecalciferol should be prescribed very early to prevent rickets. Carnitine supplementation is recommended in some centers (Veys et al. 2017).

Treatment with recombinant growth hormone improves growth of children that are growth retarded despite cysteamine therapy and adequate metabolic control. Other complications such as hypothyroidism, diabetes, or hypogonadism are treated with L-thyroxin, insulin, or testosterone, respectively. ACE inhibitors can decrease albuminuria and may delay progression of renal failure; however, they may also cause hypotension and impair renal function in patients that are fluid and salt depleted. They should be used therefore with caution, preferably not in conjunction with indomethacin; the dose should be reduced or stopped during the hot weather season (Veys et al. 2017).

## Experimental Treatment

The FDA has approved in 2019 a clinical trial in humans for the use of autologous hematopoietic stem cells after gene repair (https://clinicaltrials.gov, trial no. NCT03897361), based on encouraging results obtained in a cystinosis mouse model (Rocca and Cherqui 2018). Up to six subjects will undergo in this phase I/II trial autologous hematopoietic stem cell transplantation after ex vivo gene modification with a pCCL-CTNS lentiviral vector to express CTNS gene.

## Online Resources

https://www.cystinosisresearch.org/
https://cystinosis.org/
http://cystinosis-europe.eu/network/
http://www.cystinosisfoundation.org/

## References


Brodin-Sartorius A, Tête MJ, Niaudet P, Antignac C, Guest G, Ottolenghi C, Charbit M, Moyse D, Legendre C, Lesavre P, Cochat P, Servais A. Cysteamine therapy delays the progression of nephropathic cystinosis in late adolescents and adults. Kidney Int. 2012;81(2):179–89.

Cherqui S, Courtoy PJ. The renal Fanconi syndrome in cystinosis: pathogenic insights and therapeutic perspectives. Nat Rev Nephrol. 2017;13(2):115–31.

Cherqui S, Kalatzis V, Trugnan G, et al. The targeting of cystinosin to the lysosomal membrane requires a tyrosine-based signal and a novel sorting motif. J Biol Chem. 2001;276:13314–21.

David D, Princiero Berlingerio S, Elmonem MA, Oliveira Arcolino F, Soliman N, van den Heuvel B, Gijsbers R, Levtchenko E. Molecular basis of cystinosis: geographic distribution, functional consequences of mutations in the CTNS gene, and potential for repair. Nephron. 2019;141(2):133–46.

Elmonem MA, Veys KR, Soliman NA, van Dyck M, van den Heuvel LP, Levtchenko E. Cystinosis: a review. Orphanet J Rare Dis. 2016;11:47.

Festa BP, Chen Z, Berquez M, Debaix H, Tokonami N, Prange JA, Hoek GV, Alessio C, Raimondi A, Nevo N, Giles RH, Devuyst O, Luciani A. Impaired autophagy bridges lysosomal storage disease and epithelial dysfunction in the kidney. Nat Commun. 2018;9(1):161.

Gahl WA, Balog JZ, Kleta R. Nephropathic cystinosis in adults: natural history and effects of oral cysteamine therapy. Ann Intern Med. 2007;147:242–50.

Kalatzis V, Cherqui S, Antignac C, et al. Cystinosin, the protein defective in cystinosis, is a H(+)-driven lysosomal cystine transporter. EMBO J. 2001;20:5940–9.

Langman CB, Barshop BA, Deschênes G, Emma F, Goodyer P, Lipkin G, Midgley JP, Ottolenghi C, Servais A, Soliman NA, Thoene JG, Levtchenko EN, Conference Participants. Controversies and research agenda in nephropathic cystinosis: conclusions from a "kidney disease: improving global outcomes" (KDIGO) controversies conference. Kidney Int. 2016;89(6):1192–203.

Levtchenko E, de Graaf-Hess A, Wilmer M, et al. Comparison of cystine determination in mixed leukocytes vs polymorphonuclear leukocytes for diagnosis of cystinosis and monitoring of cysteamine therapy. Clin Chem. 2004;50:1686–8.

Markello TC, Bernardini IM, Gahl WA. Improved renal function in children with cystinosis treated with cysteamine. N Engl J Med. 1993;328:1157–62.

Nesterova G, Gahl WA. Cystinosis: the evolution of a treatable disease. Pediatr Nephrol. 2013;28(1):51–9.

Nesterova G, Gahl WA. Cystinosis. Updated Dec 7. In: Adam MP, Ardinger HH, Pagon RA, et al., editors. GeneReviews® [internet]. Seattle (WA). Seattle: University of Washington; 2017. p. 1993–2019.

Rocca CJ, Cherqui S. Potential use of stem cells as a therapy for cystinosis. Pediatr Nephrol. 2018; https://doi.org/10.1007/s00467-018-3974-7. [Epub ahead of print]

Taranta A, Petrini S, Palma A, et al. Identification and sub-cellular localization of a new cystinosin isoform. Am J Physiol Renal Physiol. 2008;294:F1101–8.

Taranta A, Wilmer MJ, van den Heuvel LP, et al. Analysis of CTNS gene transcripts in nephropathic cystinosis. Pediatr Nephrol. 2010;25(7):1263–7.

Town M, Jean G, Cherqui S, et al. A novel gene encoding an integral membrane protein is mutated in nephropathic cystinosis. Nat Genet. 1998;18:319–24.

Tsilou ET, Rubin BI, Reed GF, et al. Age-related prevalence of anterior segment complications in patients with infantile nephropathic cystinosis. Cornea. 2002;21:173–6.

Van Stralen KJ, Emma F, Jager KJ, Verrina E, Schaefer F, Laube GF, Lewis MA, Levtchenko EN. Improvement in the renal prognosis in nephropathic cystinosis. Clin J Am Soc Nephrol. 2011;6(10):2485–91.

Veys KR, Elmonem MA, Arcolino FO, van den Heuvel L. Levtchenko E. Nephropathic cystinosis: an update. Curr Opin Pediatr. 2017;29(2):168–78.

Wilmer MJ, Emma F, Levtchenko EN. The pathogenesis of cystinosis: mechanisms beyond cystine accumulation. Am J Physiol Renal Physiol. 2010;299:F905–16.

# Part IX

# Disorders of Peroxisomes and Oxalate

# Peroxisomal Disorders

# 66

Ronald J. A. Wanders, Femke C. C. Klouwer, Marc Engelen, and Hans R. Waterham

## Contents



R. J. A. Wanders (✉) · H. R. Waterham (✉)
Departments of Pediatrics, Emma Children's Hospital, and Laboratory Medicine, Amsterdam University Medical Centers, Academic Medical Center, Amsterdam, The Netherlands
e-mail: r.j.wanders@amsterdamumc.nl; h.r.waterham@amsterdamumc.nl

F. C. C. Klouwer
Departments of Neurology and Pediatric Neurology, Emma Children's Hospital, Amsterdam University Medical Centers, Academic Medical Center, Amsterdam, The Netherlands
e-mail: f.c.klouwer@amsterdamumc.nl

M. Engelen
Departments of Pediatric Neurology, Emma Children's Hospital, Amsterdam University Medical Centers, Academic Medical Center, Amsterdam, The Netherlands
e-mail: m.engelen@amsterdamumc.nl


N. Blau et al. (eds.), *Physician's Guide to the Diagnosis, Treatment, and Follow-Up of Inherited Metabolic Diseases*, https://doi.org/10.1007/978-3-030-67727-5_66

## Summary

The peroxisomal disorders comprise a heterogeneous group of genetic diseases either caused by a defect in peroxisome biogenesis or in one of the metabolic functions of peroxisomes. Diagnosis of patients affected by a certain peroxisomal disorder can be simple if the clinical signs and symptoms of the patient involved are suggestive as in Zellweger syndrome. Through the years, however, we have seen a tremendous increase in the phenotypic variability among patients with a peroxisomal disorder which makes diagnosis on clinical grounds increasingly difficult. The availability of a set of highly sensitive metabolite biomarkers, which can be measured in a small blood sample, followed by enzyme studies and flux analysis of the different peroxisomal pathways in fibroblasts has been of great importance in this respect. Moreover, these biochemical markers and assays remain instrumental for the confirmation of the pathogenicity of DNA variants of uncertain significance identified through whole exome and whole genome sequencing, which have taken over as first-line diagnostic test, at least in several centers around the world. Despite the progress in the clinical and laboratory diagnosis of peroxisomal patients, much less progress has been made with respect to the treatment options. For some disorders there is curative treatment for some aspects of the disease. For instance, the leukodystrophy of XALD responds to hematopoietic cell transplantation (HCT), either heterologous from a matched donor or autologous employing lentiviral gene therapy. Another peroxisomal disorder for which therapeutic options are truly on the horizon is hyperoxaluria Type 1 for which different therapeutic trials are underway.


## Introduction

The peroxisomal disorders (PDs) represent a heterogeneous group of genetic diseases in man caused either by a defect in the biogenesis of peroxisomes or an impairment in one of its metabolic functions. Zellweger syndrome (ZS) is generally considered to be the prototype of the group of peroxisomal disorders, and studies on ZS in the early 1980s have laid the basis for our current knowledge about peroxisomes, at least to a significant extent. This applies to the resolution of the basic principles of peroxisome biogenesis as well as the identification of the various metabolic pathways in peroxisomes which often started with some metabolic abnormality first identified in ZS patients. Indeed, it was the finding of elevated very-long-chain fatty acids, the bile acid intermediates di- and trihydroxycholestanoic acid and phytanic acid which led to the discovery of the pathways of fatty acid beta-oxidation, bile acid synthesis, and alpha-oxidation in peroxisomes. The same is true for the discovery of the role of peroxisomes in ether phospholipid biosynthesis. Studies on ZS have also set the stage for the discovery of the various biomarkers we now have for the proper laboratory diagnosis of patients with a PD. Moreover, these biomarkers have been very instrumental in identifying all the different PDs and the recognition of their tremendous clinical heterogeneity. In this chapter we will describe our current state of knowledge about PDs as listed in Table below.

## Nomenclature

| No. | Disorder | Alternative name 1 | Alternative name 2 | Disease abbreviation | Gene symbol | Chromosomal localization | Mode of inheritance | Affected protein | OMIM no |
|---|---|---|---|---|---|---|---|---|---|
| 66.1.1 | Zellweger spectrum disorder | Peroxisome biogenesis disorder | Zellweger syndrome<br>Neonatal adrenoleukodystrophy<br>Infantile Refsum disease | ZSD | *PEX1* | 7q21.2 | AR | PEX1 | 602136 |
| 66.1.2 | Zellweger spectrum disorder | Peroxisome biogenesis disorder | Zellweger syndrome<br>Neonatal adrenoleukodystrophy<br>Infantile Refsum disease | ZSD | *PEX2* | 8q21.1 | AR | PEX2 | 170993 |
| 66.1.3 | Zellweger spectrum disorder | Peroxisome biogenesis disorder | Zellweger syndrome<br>Neonatal adrenoleukodystrophy<br>Infantile Refsum disease | ZSD | *PEX3* | 6q23–24 | AR | PEX3 | 603164 |
| 66.1.4 | Zellweger spectrum disorder | Peroxisome biogenesis disorder | Zellweger syndrome<br>Neonatal adrenoleukodystrophy<br>Infantile Refsum disease | ZSD | *PEX5* | 12p13.3 | AR | PEX5 | 600414 |
| 66.1.5 | Zellweger spectrum disorder | Peroxisome biogenesis disorder | Zellweger syndrome<br>Neonatal adrenoleukodystrophy<br>Infantile Refsum disease | ZSD | *PEX6* | 6q21.1 | AR | PEX6 | 601498 |
| 66.1.6 | Zellweger spectrum disorder | Peroxisome biogenesis disorder | Zellweger syndrome<br>Neonatal adrenoleukodystrophy<br>Infantile Refsum disease | ZSD | *PEX10* | 1q36.32 | AR | PEX10 | 602859 |
| 66.1.7 | Zellweger spectrum disorder | Peroxisome biogenesis disorder | Zellweger syndrome<br>Neonatal adrenoleukodystrophy<br>Infantile Refsum disease | ZSD | *PEX12* | 17q12 | AR | PEX12 | 601758 |
| 66.1.8 | Zellweger spectrum disorder | Peroxisome biogenesis disorder | Zellweger syndrome<br>Neonatal adrenoleukodystrophy<br>Infantile Refsum disease | ZSD | *PEX13* | 2p14-p16 | AR | PEX13 | 601789 |
| 66.1.9 | Zellweger spectrum disorder | Peroxisome biogenesis disorder | Zellweger syndrome<br>Neonatal adrenoleukodystrophy<br>Infantile Refsum disease | ZSD | *PEX14* | 1p36.2 | AR | PEX14 | 601791 |
| 66.1.10 | Zellweger spectrum disorder | Peroxisome biogenesis disorder | Zellweger syndrome<br>Neonatal adrenoleukodystrophy<br>Infantile Refsum disease | ZSD | *PEX16* | 11p11.2 | AR | PEX16 | 603360 |
| 66.1.11 | Zellweger spectrum disorder | Peroxisome biogenesis disorder | Zellweger syndrome<br>Neonatal adrenoleukodystrophy<br>Infantile Refsum disease | ZSD | *PEX19* | 1q23.2 | AR | PEX19 | 600279 |
| 66.1.12 | Zellweger spectrum disorder | Peroxisome biogenesis disorder | Zellweger syndrome<br>Neonatal adrenoleukodystrophy<br>Infantile Refsum disease | ZSD | *PE26* | 22q11.21 | AR | PEX26 | 608666 |
| 66.2.1 | Rhizomelic chondrodysplasia punctata type 1 | RCDP type 1 | | RCDP1 | *PEX7* | 6q23.3 | AR | PEX7 | 215100 |

(continued)

| No. | Disorder | Alternative name 1 | Alternative name 2 | Disease abbreviation | Gene symbol | Chromosomal localization | Mode of inheritance | Affected protein | OMIM no |
|---|---|---|---|---|---|---|---|---|---|
| 66.2.2 | Rhizomelic chondrodysplasia punctata type 2 | RCDP type 2 | | RCDP2 | *GNPAT* | 1q42.1–42.3 | AR | Glycerone-3-phosphate acyltransferase | 222765 |
| 66.2.3 | Rhizomelic chondrodysplasia punctata type 3 | RCDP type 3 | | RCDP3 | *AGPS* | 2q31.2 | AR | Alkyl-glycerone-3-synthase | 600121 |
| 66.2.4 | Rhizomelic chondrodysplasia punctata type 4 | RCDP type 4 | Peroxisomal fatty acyl-CoA reductase 1 disorder | RCDP4 | *FAR1* | 11p15.3 | AR | Fatty acyl-CoA reductase 1 | 616154 |
| 66.2.5 | Rhizomelic chondrodysplasia punctata type 5 | RCDP type 5 | | RCDP5 | *PEX5L* | 12p13.3 | AR | PEX5L | 616716 |
| 66.3 | X-linked adrenoleukodystrophy | X-linked adrenomyeloneuropathy | | XALD | *ABCD1* | Xq28 | X-linked | ALD protein | 300100 |
| 66.4 | Peroxisomal acyl-CoA oxidase 1 deficiency | Straight-chain acyl-CoA oxidase deficiency | | ACOX1 deficiency SCOX deficiency | *ACOX1* | 17q25 | AR | Peroxisomal straight-chain acyl-CoA oxidase | 264470 |
| 66.5 | Peroxisomal acyl-CoA oxidase 2 deficiency | Branched-chain acyl-CoA oxidase deficiency | | ACOX2 deficiency | *ACOX2* | 3p14.3 | AR | Peroxisomal branched-chain acyl-CoA oxidase | 601641 |
| 66.6 | D-bifunctional protein deficiency | DBP deficiency | | DBP deficiency | *HSD17B4* | 5q2 | AR | D-bifunctional protein | 261515 |
| 66.7 | ACBD5 deficiency | | | ACBD5 deficiency | *ACBD5* | 10p12.1 | AR | Acyl-CoA-binding domain-containing protein 5 | 616618 |
| 66.8.1 | Refsum disease | Adult Refsum disease | | ARD, RD | *PHYH* | 10p13 | AR | Phytanoyl-CoA hydroxylase | 266500 |
| 66.8.2 | Refsum disease | Adult Refsum disease | | ARD, RD | *PEX7* | 6q23.3 | AR | PEX7 | 614879 |
| 66.9 | Alpha-methylacyl-CoA racemase deficiency | AMACR deficiency | | Racemase deficiency | *AMACR* | 5p13.2 | AR | AMACR | 604489 |
| 66.10 | Bile acid-CoA: Amino acid N-acyltransferase deficiency | BAAT deficiency | | BAAT deficiency | *BAAT* | 9q31.1 | AR | Peroxisomal bile acid-CoA: Amino acid N-acyl transferase | 602938 |
| 66.11 | ABCD3 deficiency | PMP70 deficiency | | ABCD3 deficiency | *ABCD3* | 1p21.3 | AR | ABCD3 | 170995 |
| 66.12 | Primary hyperoxaluria type 1 | | | PH1 | *AGXT* | 2q36-q37 | AR | Alanine-glyoxylate and serine-pyruvate aminotransferase | 259900 |

| No. | Disorder | Alternative name 1 | Alternative name 2 | Disease abbreviation | Gene symbol | Chromosomal localization | Mode of inheritance | Affected protein | OMIM no |
|---|---|---|---|---|---|---|---|---|---|
| 66.13 | PEX11 beta deficiency | | | PEX11B deficiency | *PEX11B* | 1q21.1 | AR | PEX11 beta | 603867 |
| 66.14 | Dynamin-like protein 1 deficiency | DLP1 deficiency | | DLP1 deficiency | *DNM1L* | 12p11.21 | AR & AD | Dynamin-like protein 1 | 603850 |
| 66.15 | MFF deficiency | | | MFF deficiency | *MFF* | 2q36.3 | AR | Mitochondrial fission factor | 614785 |
| 66.16 | FIS1 deficiency | | | FIS1 deficiency | *FIS1* | 7q22.1 | AR | Mitochondrial fission 1 | 609003 |
| 66.17 | Charcot-Marie-tooth disease 4A | GDAP1 deficiency | | GDAP1 deficiency | *GDAP1* | 8q21.11 | AR | Ganglioside-induced differentiation-associated protein 1 | 606598 |

## Metabolic Pathways

### Peroxisome Biogenesis

Peroxisomes were long thought to be solely derived from pre-existing peroxisomes through a mechanism of growth and division and would therefore belong to the group of non-autonomous cell organelles just like mitochondria. However, it is now clear that peroxisomes are in fact semi-autonomous organelles which may form de novo from a special subcompartment of the endoplasmic reticulum or by growth and division of pre-existing peroxisomes. Importantly, all peroxisomal proteins albeit matrix or membrane proteins are synthesized on free polyribosomes and are directed to the peroxisome through specific targeting signals which are an integral part of each peroxisomal protein. Peroxisomal matrix proteins for instance are targeted to peroxisomes via one of the two different targeting signals (see Legend to Fig. 66.1) named peroxisome targeting signal (PTS) 1 and 2. These two PTS sequences are recognized by their cognate receptors PEX5 and PEX7, respectively, and the cargo-loaded receptors are subsequently recognized by the peroxisomal protein import machinery followed by transfer of the matrix proteins across the peroxisomal membrane and recycling of the unloaded receptors back into the cytosol (Fig. 66.1). The complexity of peroxisome biogenesis as briefly outlined above immediately explains why so many different proteins collectively named PEX proteins are required to maintain peroxisome biosynthesis and also explains why the disorders of peroxisome biogenesis are so genetically heterogeneous as discussed later. For a review on peroxisome biogenesis, see Waterham et al. (2016).

### Metabolic Functions of Peroxisomes

Peroxisomes in humans catalyze a great number of different metabolic functions (for reviews see Wanders et al. (2016) and Van Veldhoven (2010)), but so far defects in only a few of these metabolic pathways have been identified, which is why we have chosen to limit our discussion to the pathways described below:

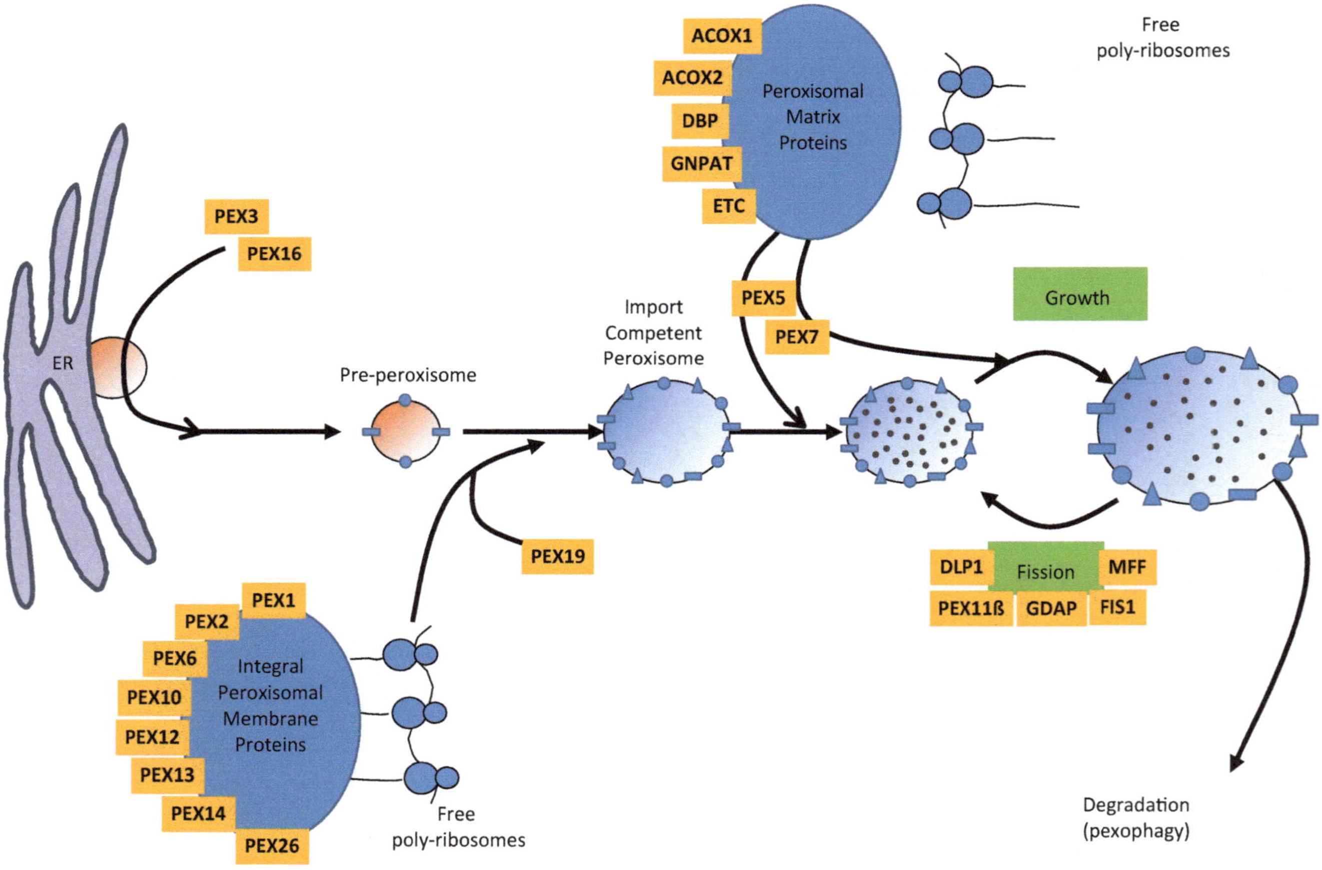


**Fig. 66.1** Schematic diagram showing the essential features of peroxisome biogenesis in humans. In short, peroxisomes may be formed by one of the two different pathways, which include a de novo pathway whereby a pre-peroxisome is formed from a special subcompartment of the endoplasmic reticulum as mediated by PEX3 and PEX16. Hereafter the peroxisomal membrane proteins that are all synthesized on free polyribosomes are inserted into the pre-peroxisomal membrane so that an import-competent peroxisome arises able to accept the peroxisomal matrix proteins, which are also all synthesized on free polyribosomes. In the second pathway, peroxisomes are formed by growth and division of pre-existing peroxisomes. Abbreviations used: *ACOX1* acyl-CoA oxidase 1, *ACOX2* acyl-CoA oxidase 2, *DBP* D-bifunctional protein, *GNPAT* glycerone-3-phosphate acyltransferase, *DLP1* dynamin-like protein 1, *MFF* mitochondrial fission factor, *FIS1* fission 1, *GDAP1* ganglioside-induced differentiation-associated protein 1

## Fatty Acid Oxidation

The majority of dietary fatty acids (FAs) is oxidized by mitochondria with only a minor role for peroxisomes. Nevertheless, peroxisomes do play an indispensable role in cellular fatty acid homeostasis since they catalyze the oxidation of a range of different FAs which cannot be degraded by mitochondria. These include:

(a) Very-long-chain FAs, notably hexacosanoic acid (C26:0), which are derived from dietary sources but mostly from chain elongation of shorter-chain saturated FAs.
(b) Pristanic acid (2,6,10,14-tetramethylpentadecanoic acid), which is to some extent derived from dietary sources but mostly originates from phytanic acid (3,7,11,15-tetramethylhexadecanoic acid) which upon alpha-oxidation produces pristanic acid.
(c) Di- and trihydroxycholestanoic acid (DHCA and THCA) which are intermediates in the biosynthesis of the primary bile acids cholic acid and chenodeoxycholic acid.
(d) Tetracosahexaenoic acid (C24:6w3), which upon beta-oxidation in peroxisomes yields docosahexaenoic acid (C22:6w3).
(e) Other FAs including long-chain dicarboxylic fatty acids, etc. (Fig. 66.2).

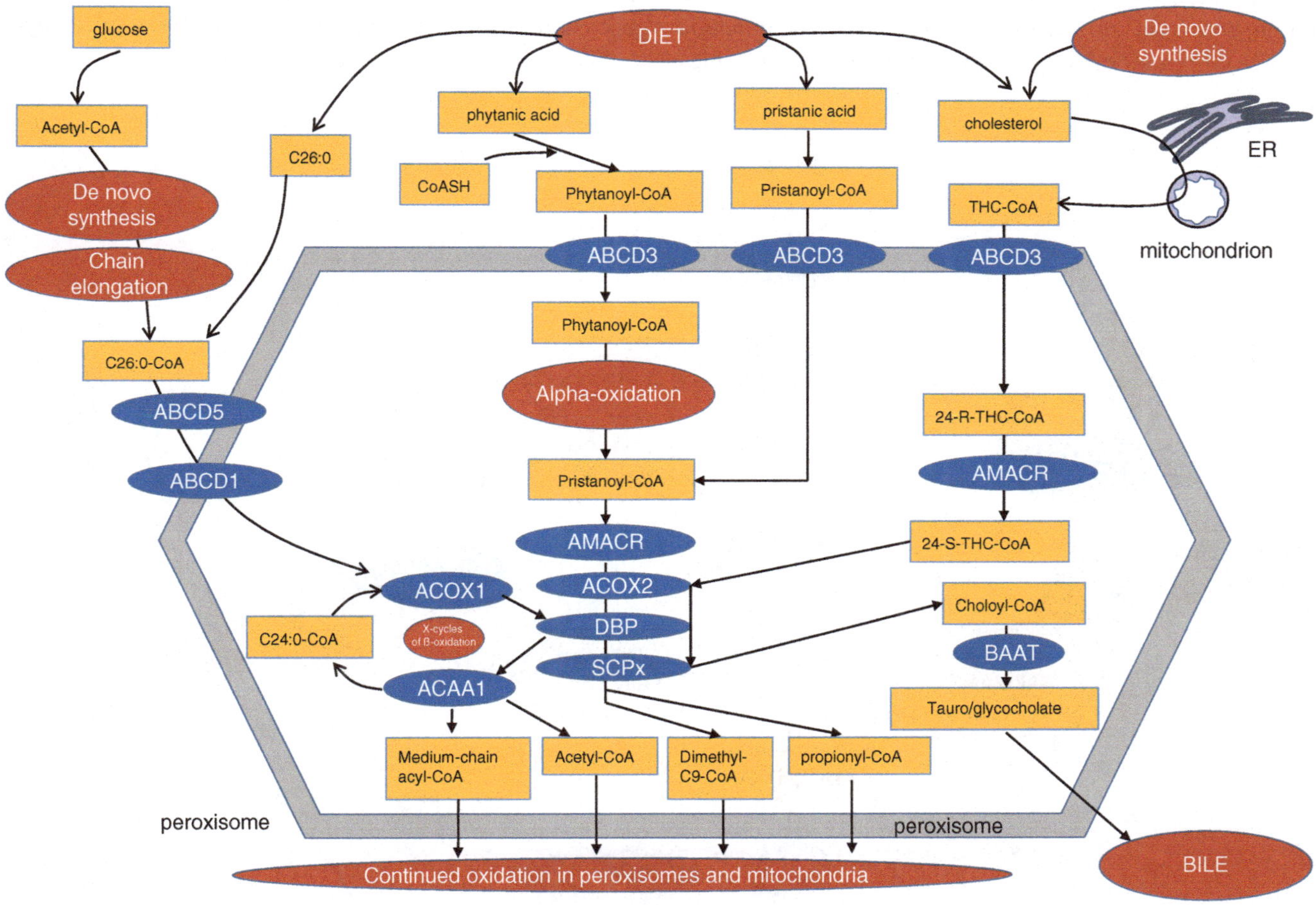


**Fig. 66.2** Schematic diagram showing the essential features of the peroxisomal fatty acid beta-oxidation machinery. The main substrates oxidized in peroxisomes include (1) very-long-chain FAs with C26:0 as typical example which is either derived from exogenous, dietary sources or synthesized de novo from acetyl-CoA via the FAS complex followed by chain elongation; (2) pristanic acid which cannot be synthesized endogenously but is only derived from exogenous, dietary sources either directly or indirectly via alpha-oxidation of phytanic acid which also comes from dietary sources only; and (3) di- and trihydroxycholestanoic acid as derived from cholesterol via a series of enzymes localized in different subcellular compartments including the mitochondrion, cytosol, and endoplasmic reticulum. The actual beta-oxidation machinery is different for each of the three substrates as indicated in Fig. 66.2 except that the enzyme DBP (D-bifunctional protein) is involved in the beta-oxidation of all three substrates. The end products of the beta-oxidation of C26:0 and pristanic acid are acetyl-CoA, propionyl-CoA, and several medium-chain acyl-CoAs, which are then shuttled to the mitochondrion for full oxidation to CO2 and H2O via one of the two different routes including a free-acid route and a carnitine-mediated pathway. In case of di- and trihydroxycholestanoic acid, the end products are choloyl-CoA and chenodeoxycholoyl-CoA which then undergo transamination via the peroxisomal enzyme BAAT (bile acid-CoA: amino acid N-acyltransferase) to give rise to tauro/glycocholic acid and tauro/glycochenodeoxycholic acid, which are then transported out of the peroxisome to end up in the bile

## Ether Phospholipid Biosynthesis

Ether phospholipids (EPLs) are a special class of phospholipids which differ from their more well-known sister molecules the diacylphospholipids in one major aspect, which is the presence of an ether bond rather than an ester bond at the sn-1 position of the glycerol backbone (see Fig. 66.3). Furthermore, EPLs catalyze a number of unique functions in human physiology different from diacylphospholipids. Importantly, peroxisomes play an indispensable role in the synthesis of EPLs since the characteristic ether bond is generated by a unique peroxisomal enzyme named alkylglycerone-3-phosphate synthase (AGPS, formerly called alkylDHAP synthase (ADHAPS)), which, if deficient, causes one of the different forms of rhizomelic chondrodysplasia punctata (RCDP). Figure 66.3 depicts the ether phospholipid biosynthesis pathway and the enzymes plus the deficiencies involved (see Braverman and Moser 2012).

## Fatty Acid Alpha-Oxidation

Fatty acids with a methyl group at the 3-position, like in phytanic acid 3,7,11,15-tetramethylhexadecanoic acid, cannot undergo beta-oxidation because of the location of the methyl group at the 3-position and first require one round of alpha-oxidation to turn the 3-methyl FA into the corresponding 2-methyl FA which in case of phytanic acid is pristanic acid.

Figure 66.4 shows the alpha-oxidation pathway. Refsum disease is so far the only peroxisomal disorder in which the alpha-oxidation pathway is affected due to mutations in the gene coding for the first enzyme of the pathway phytanoyl-CoA hydroxylase (see Wanders et al. 2011).

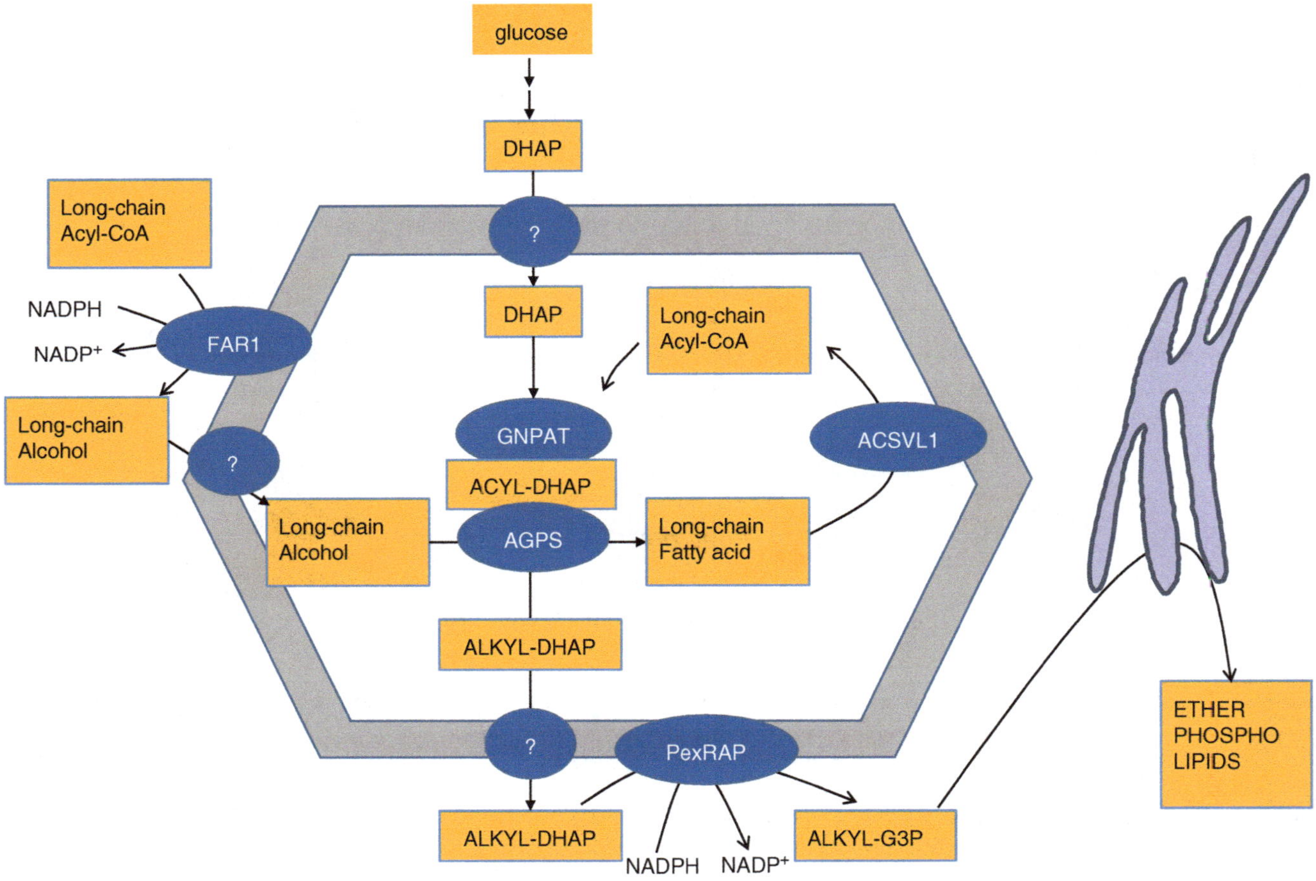


**Fig. 66.3** Schematic diagram showing the essential features of the ether phospholipid biosynthesis pathway. Peroxisomes play a key role in the synthesis of ether phospholipids by virtue of the fact that the enzyme responsible for the introduction of the characteristic ether bond (AGPS, alkyl glycerone 3-phosphate synthase) is strictly peroxisomal. The long-chain alcohol required in the AGPS reaction is provided by the enzyme fatty acyl-CoA reductase of which there are two isoforms, FAR1 and FAR2. Furthermore, the enzyme GNPAT (glycerone-3-phosphate acyltransferase) provides the other substrate for the AGPS reaction, which is acylglycerone 3-phosphate. The end product of the peroxisomal part of the ether phospholipid biosynthetic machinery is alkyl-DHAP, which is converted into alkyl-G3P via the enzyme PexRAP and then transported to the ER where the subsequent steps take place. The importance of each of the individual steps involved in ether phospholipid synthesis is exemplified by the fact that deficiencies of GNPAT, AGPS, and FAR1 give rise to (rhizomelic) chondrodysplasia punctata

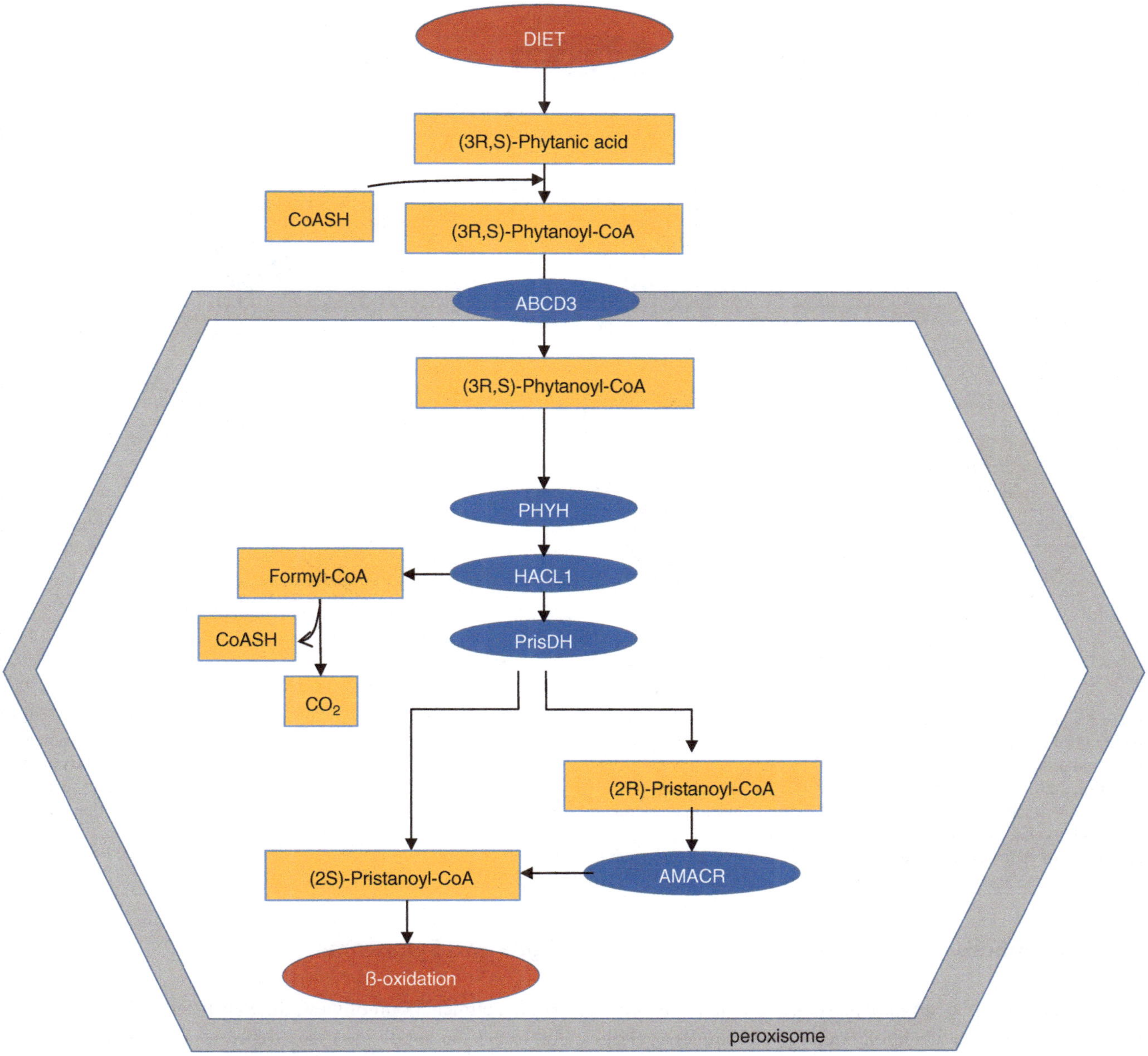


**Fig. 66.4** Schematic diagram showing the essential features of the fatty acid alpha-oxidation pathway in humans. Phytanic acid cannot be synthesized endogenously but is derived from dietary sources only. Phytanic acid first undergoes activation to the corresponding coenzyme A ester, i.e., phytanoyl-CoA, which then enters the peroxisome via the half-ABC transporter ABCD3. Once inside, phytanoyl-CoA is converted into 2-hydroxyphytanoyl-CoA by the enzyme phytanoyl-CoA hydroxylase (PHYH) after which the enzyme hydroxyacyl-CoA lyase 1 (HACL1) splits the molecule into two parts including formyl-CoA plus pristanal, followed by dehydrogenation of pristanal to pristanic acid which then undergoes activation to the corresponding coenzyme-A ester to yield pristanoyl-CoA which can then enter the beta-oxidation machinery. In vivo, phytanic acid occurs as a racemic mixture of two different stereoisomers including (3R,7R,11R,15)-tetramethylhexadecanoic acid and (3S,7R,11R,15)-tetramethylhexadecanoic acid which are both substrates for the alpha-oxidation system, thus yielding (2S,6R,10R,14)-pristanoyl-CoA and (2R,6R,10R,14)-pristanoyl-CoA. The latter pristanoyl-CoA requires the enzyme AMACR to convert the (2R)-form into the (2S)-form because the beta-oxidation machinery only accepts (2S)-acyl-CoAs as substrate

## Glyoxylate Metabolism

Peroxisomes play a key role in the metabolism of glyoxylate: the ultimate detoxification of glyoxylate is catalyzed by the peroxisomal enzyme alanine glyoxylate aminotransferase (AGXT), which, if deficient, causes hyperoxaluria Type 1. Glyoxylate is generated from different precursors including hydroxyproline and glycolate, and its toxicity is due to the fact that, if not immediately detoxified by AGXT, glyoxylate is converted into oxalate which precipitates into calcium oxalate in multiple tissues including the kidneys (Fig. 66.5).

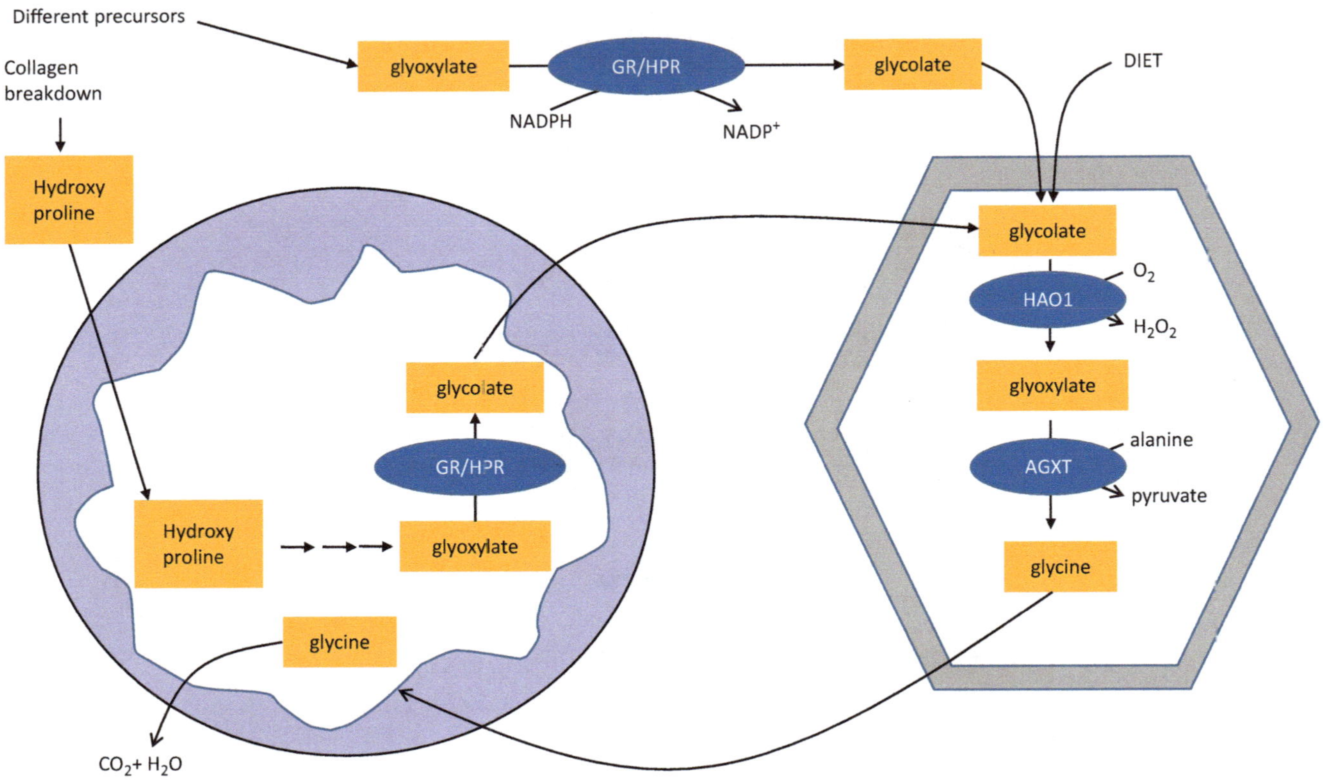


**Fig. 66.5** Essential features of the glyoxylate detoxification pathway in humans. Glyoxylate is a highly toxic molecule since it readily undergoes oxidation to oxalate as mediated by the ubiquitous enzyme lactate dehydrogenase followed by precipitation of oxalate as calcium oxalate in different tissues including the kidneys. Peroxisomes play a crucial role in glyoxylate detoxification by virtue of the fact that the enzyme alanine glyoxylate aminotransferase (AGXT) is strictly peroxisomal. Two of the primary precursors of glyoxylate in humans are hydroxyproline, which is generated in lysosomes upon breakdown of collagen, and glycolate, derived from plant-derived foodstuffs. Shown is the complicated crosstalk between different subcellular compartments with the peroxisome as ultimate site of final glyoxylate detoxification by converting glyoxylate into glycine

### Bile Acid Synthesis

Peroxisomes also play an indispensable role in the synthesis of the primary bile acids cholic acid and chenodeoxycholic acid from cholesterol in the liver (Vaz and Ferdinandusse 2017). The final steps in the formation of bile acids from di- and trihydroxycholestanoic acid to chenodeoxycholic acid and cholic acid, respectively, occur exclusively in peroxisomes. Furthermore, the formation of the taurine and glycine derivatives of cholic acid and chenodeoxycholic acid also takes place solely in peroxisomes.

### Additional Peroxisomal Pathways

Peroxisomes are involved in various additional metabolic pathways including the oxidation of L-pipecolic acid, hydrogen peroxide metabolism, and other pathways not detailed here.

## Signs and Symptoms

From a clinical point of view, the PDs listed in Nomenclature Table can be subdivided into different subgroups based on the similarity in clinical signs and symptoms including:

A. The Zellweger spectrum disorders (PD66.1.1–66.1.12), acyl-CoA oxidase 1 deficiency (PD66.4), and D-bifunctional protein deficiency (PD66.6).
B. The rhizomelic chondrodysplasia punctata spectrum (PD:66.2.1–66.2.5).
C. X-linked adrenoleukodystrophy (PD66.3).
D. Refsum disease (PD66.8.1 and PD66.8.2).
E. Hyperoxaluria Type 1 (PD66.11).
F. The disorders of bile acid biosynthesis including acyl-CoA oxidase 2 deficiency (PD66.5), BAAT deficiency (PD66.10), PMP70 deficiency (PD66.11), and racemase deficiency (PD66.9).

G. The peroxisomal fission defects including PEX11 beta deficiency (PD66.13), DLP1 deficiency (PD66.14), MFF deficiency (PD66.15), FIS1 deficiency (PD66.16), and GDAP1 deficiency (PD66.17).
H. The separate disorder, ACBD5 deficiency (PD66.7).

We will restrict discussion of the signs and symptoms to the main groups of peroxisomal disorders including the ZSDs, RCDPs, XALD, Refsum disease, and AMACR deficiency (see Table below).

## Zellweger Spectrum Disorders (PD66.1, PD66.4, PD66.6, PD66.7, and PD 66.13)

The prototype of the Zellweger spectrum disorders (ZSDs) is Zellweger syndrome (ZS), which is a multisystem disorder dominated by (1) typical craniofacial dysmorphic features including a high forehead, a large anterior fontanelle, hypoplastic supraorbital ridges, and epicanthic folds; (2) profound developmental delay and neurological abnormalities including severe hypotonia and seizures; and (3) liver dysfunction

Possible symptoms related to age in peroxisomal disorders

| | System | Symptoms | ZSD[a] | RCDP | ALD | RD | AMACR |
|---|---|---|---|---|---|---|---|
| Neonatal period | Neurological | Hypotonia | + | | | | |
| | | Seizures | + | | | | |
| | | Spastic paresis | | + | | | |
| | Vision | Cataract | + | + | | | |
| | | Glaucoma, retinitis pigmentosa | + | | | | |
| | Hearing | Sensorineural hearing loss | + | | | | |
| | Musculoskeletal | Enlarged fontanel | + | | | | |
| | | Contractures, rhizomelia | | + | | | |
| | | Dysmorphic features | + | + | | | |
| | Cardiopulmonal | Congenital heart defects | | + | | | |
| | Endocrinological | Adrenal insufficiency | + | | | | |
| | Gastrointestinal | Cholestasis | + | | | | + |
| | | Hepatomegaly, jaundice | + | | | | |
| | Other | Coagulopathy | + | | | | + |
| | | Failure to thrive | + | | | | |
| Early childhood | Neurological | Developmental regression | + | | | | |
| | | Developmental delay | + | + | | | |
| | | Hypotonia | + | | | | |
| | | Intellectual disability | + | + | | | |
| | | Seizures | + | + | | | |
| | | Spastic paresis | | + | | | |
| | Vision | Cataract | + | + | | | |
| | | Glaucoma, retinitis pigmentosa | + | | | | |
| | Hearing | Sensorineural hearing loss | + | | | | |
| | Musculoskeletal | Enlarged fontanel | + | | | | |
| | | Contractures, rhizomelia, growth retardation | | + | | | |
| | | Dysmorphic features | + | + | | | |
| | Cardiopulmonal | Congenital heart defects | | + | | | |
| | | Increased rate of infections (pneumonia, otitis) | | + | | | |
| | Dermatological | Ichthyosis | | + | | | |
| | Endocrinological | Adrenal insufficiency | + | | | | |
| | Gastrointestinal | Diarrhea | + | | | | |
| | | Hepatomegaly, liver dysfunction | + | | | | |
| | Others | Coagulopathy | + | | | | |

Possible symptoms related to age in peroxisomal disorders (continued)

| | System | Symptoms | ZSD[a] | RCDP | ALD | RD | AMACR |
|---|---|---|---|---|---|---|---|
| Late childhood | Neurological | Developmental delay | + | + | | | + |
| | | Developmental regression | + | | + | | |
| | | Behavioral changes | | | + | | |
| | | Ataxia | + | | + | + | |
| | | Neuropathy | + | | | + | |
| | | Intellectual disability | + | + | | | |
| | | Seizures | + | + | + | | + |
| | | Spastic paresis | + | + | + | | |
| | Vision | Cataract | + | + | | + | |
| | | Retinitis pigmentosa | + | | | + | |
| | | Glaucoma | + | | | | |
| | Hearing | Sensorineural hearing loss | + | | | + | |
| | Olfaction | Anosmia | | | | + | |
| | Musculoskeletal | Dysmorphic features | + | + | | | |
| | | Osteopenia | + | | | | |
| | | Contractures, rhizomelia, growth retardation | | + | | | |
| | Cardiopulmonal | Congenital heart defects | | + | | | |
| | | Increased rate of infections (pneumonia, otitis) | | + | | | |
| | | Cardiac conduction abnormalities | | | | + | |
| | Dermatological | Ichthyosis | | + | | + | |
| | Endocrinological | Adrenal insufficiency | + | | + | | |
| | Gastrointestinal | Diarrhea | + | | | | |
| | | Hepatomegaly, liver dysfunction | + | | | | |
| | | Liver cirrhosis, hepatocellular carcinoma | + | | | | + |
| | Others | Coagulopathy | + | | | | |
| Adulthood | Neurological | Developmental delay | + | + | | | + |
| | | Behavioral changes, cognitive deterioration | | | + | | |
| | | Intermittent encephalopathy | | | | | + |
| | | Ataxia | + | | + | + | |
| | | Neuropathy | + | | + | + | + |
| | | Intellectual disability | + | + | | | + |
| | | Seizures | | + | + | | + |
| | | Spastic paresis | + | + | + | | + |
| | Vision | Cataract | + | + | | + | + |
| | | Retinitis pigmentosa | + | | | + | + |
| | | Glaucoma | + | | | | |
| | Hearing | Sensorineural hearing loss | + | | | + | |
| | Olfaction | Anosmia | | | | + | |
| | Musculoskeletal | Dysmorphic features | + | + | | | |
| | | Osteopenia | + | | | | |
| | | Rhabdomyolysis | | | | | + |
| | | Contractures, rhizomelia, growth retardation | | + | | | |
| | Cardiopulmonal | Congenital heart defects | | + | | | |
| | | Increased rate of infections (pneumonia, otitis) | | + | | | |
| | | Cardiac conduction abnormalities | | | | + | |
| | Dermatological | Ichthyosis | | + | | + | |
| | Endocrinological | Adrenal insufficiency | + | | + | | |
| | Gastrointestinal | Diarrhea | + | | | | |
| | | Hepatomegaly, liver dysfunction | + | | | | |
| | | Liver cirrhosis, hepatocellular carcinoma | + | | | | + |

*AMACR*, α-Methylacyl-CoA racemase deficiency, *RCDP* rhizomelic chondrodysplasia punctata, *RD* Refsum disease (classic), *ALD* adrenoleukodystrophy

[a]Includes Zellweger spectrum disorders (ZSDs), peroxisomal acyl-CoA oxidase type 1 (ACOX1) deficiency, and D-bifunctional protein (DBP) deficiency

along with additional aberrations in multiple organs. Apart from ZS with its neonatal onset and early fatal course, milder variants have been identified originally labeled under the names neonatal adrenoleukodystrophy and infantile Refsum disease. Since the realization that we are dealing with a disease spectrum rather than distinct, well-defined phenotypes, the collective term Zellweger spectrum disorders (ZSDs) has been coined. Roughly three main phenotypic groups can be discerned based on age of presentation: (1) the neonatal-infantile presentation, essentially resembling the classic Zellweger syndrome with severe hypotonia, seizures, failure to thrive, liver dysfunction, and craniofacial dysmorphism; (2) the childhood presentation characterized by failure to thrive, developmental delay, liver dysfunction, adrenal insufficiency, and less profound hypotonia and craniofacial dysmorphism; and (3) the adolescent-adult presentation with visual and hearing impairment as most consistent symptoms, developmental delay, and in some cases cerebellar ataxia and neuropathy at the time of presentation (see Table above).

Importantly, the group of Zellweger spectrum disorders also includes the single peroxisomal enzyme deficiencies acyl-CoA oxidase 1 deficiency (PD66.4) and D-bifunctional protein deficiency (PD66.6) because of the marked similarity in the clinical signs and symptoms (Ferdinandusse et al. 2006; Ferdinandusse et al. 2007). Patients with the single peroxisomal enzyme deficiency ACBD5 deficiency (PD66.7) and the peroxisomal fission defect PEX11 beta deficiency (PD66.13) which have been described in only a few patients so far, are also showing symptoms resembling the Zellweger spectrum (Ferdinandusse et al. 2017; Ebberink et al., 2012). This has major implications for the laboratory diagnosis of patients as discussed later (for reviews see Argyriou et al. (2016) and Klouwer et al. (2015, 2017)).

## Rhizomelic Chondrodysplasia Punctata (RCDP) Spectrum (PD66.2.1–5)

The RCDP spectrum is a clinically heterogeneous group with, at the severe end of the spectrum, patients showing severe growth retardation, proximal shortening of the extremities, contractures, spasticity, severe developmental delay, and cataracts. Life expectancy is considerably reduced. At the other end of the spectrum are patients with mild to moderate developmental delay, cataracts, and bone dysplasia but no rhizomelic shortening. It is important to note that many patients with the mild phenotype reach adulthood and that progression of disease is common (with progressive deterioration of joint and spinal cord compression at the craniocervical junction) (Poll-The, personal observation). The characteristic biochemical abnormality in RCDP patients is the deficiency of plasmalogens, which can either be caused by a (partial) deficiency in peroxisome biogenesis (PEX7 and PEX5) or by a deficiency of one of the enzymes involved in the synthesis of plasmalogens (GNPAT, AGPS, and FAR1) (see Braverman and Moser 2012).

## X-Linked Adrenoleukodystrophy (PD66.3)

Patients with XALD are normal at birth. Although patients are traditionally classified in distinct "phenotypes", XALD should be considered as a progressive neurodegenerative disease. In male patients, adrenal failure is often the first symptom and can occur in (early) childhood but also in adulthood (lifetime prevalence is about 80%) (Huffnagel et al. 2019a). A progressive gait disorder and incontinence due to spinal cord disease (with involvement of predominantly the pyramidal tracts and the dorsal columns) develop on average in the third decade in males (Engelen et al. 2012; Huffnagel et al. 2019b) and the fifth decade in females (Huffnagel et al. 2019c; Engelen et al. 2014). About 60% of males will develop a progressive leukodystrophy (about 40% in childhood) (de Beer et al. 2014). Hematopoietic cell transplantation (HCT) (either heterologous or, more recently, autologous after ex vivo lentiviral gene therapy) is available as treatment for the leukodystrophy in an early stage (preferably with few lesions on MRI of the brain and without symptoms) (Miller et al. 2011; Eichler et al. 2017).

## Refsum Disease (PD66.8)

Refsum disease is due to a deficiency of the peroxisomal enzyme phytanoyl-CoA hydroxylase (Fig. 66.4) and is characterized by anosmia and early-onset retinitis pigmentosa in virtually all patients with variable combinations of cerebellar ataxia, polyneuropathy, sensorineural hearing loss, ichthyosis, skeletal abnormalities, and cardiac arrhythmias. The clinical picture of Refsum disease is usually that of a slowly developing retinopathy and progressive neuropathy with severe motor weakness and muscular wasting especially of the lower extremities (see Wierzbicki et al. 2002 and Wanders et al. 2011).

## Hyperoxaluria Type 1 (PD66.11)

Hyperoxaluria Type 1 is caused by a deficiency of the peroxisomal enzyme alanine glyoxylate aminotransferase (AGXT). This leads to the accumulation of glyoxylate which is then converted to oxalate by the enzyme lactate dehydrogenase. Oxalate precipitates as calcium oxalate in all tissues including the kidneys with all the consequences involved as discussed elsewhere in detail in Chap. 67.

## Disorders of Peroxisomal Bile Acid Biosynthesis (PD66.5, PD66.9, PD66.10, and PD66.11)

The disorders of peroxisomal bile acid biosynthesis include PMP70 deficiency (PD66.11), acyl-CoA oxidase 2 deficiency (PD66.5), 2-methylacyl-CoA racemase deficiency (PD66.9), and bile acid-CoA: amino acid N-acyltransferase (BAAT) deficiency (PD66.10) in increasing order of incidence. The first two disorders have only been described in only a few patients (1 and 3, respectively) with divergent clinical signs and symptoms not detailed here. AMACR deficiency has been described in about ten patients, again with various symptoms. The childhood form of AMACR deficiency presents with the typical features reminiscent of the bile acid deficiency phenotype (see Chap. 40) dominated by variable liver abnormalities which may progress into liver failure if untreated, fat malabsorption with steatorrhea and growth retardation, and fat-soluble vitamin deficiency leading to coagulation defects and rickets. Apart from this severe childhood form, we have recently identified several patients with AMACR deficiency, who showed a much more slowly developing phenotype characterized by developmental delay, neuropathy, intellectual disability, seizures, spastic paresis, as well as cataract, retinitis pigmentosa, and rhabdomyolysis (see Table above). Furthermore, based on a previously reported specific MRI pattern of the brain suggestive for AMACR deficiency (Haugarvoll et al. 2013), our clinic recently identified five adult patients, who all had an unremarkable childhood, developed retinitis pigmentosa in early adulthood and peripheral neuropathy after the fourth decade (M. Engelen, personal observation). All five patients had increased transaminases and one patient developed hepatocellular carcinoma. We also follow three children that were identified because of increased transaminases but are otherwise asymptomatic (Poll-The and Engelen, personal observation). It is possible this is the typical disease course of AMACR; however, more observations are needed.

Since AMACR plays a key role in the degradation of both pristanic acid and the bile acid intermediates di- and trihydroxycholestanoic acid, there is accumulation of all these metabolites in plasma from AMACR-deficient patients. BAAT deficiency has been described more frequently and is caused by a deficiency of the peroxisomal enzyme bile acid-CoA: amino acid N-acyltransferase (BAAT) deficiency, which leaves di- and trihydroxycholestanoic acid unconjugated and leads to a deficiency of the conjugated forms of the primary bile acids cholic acid and chenodeoxycholic acid which results in steatorrhea, coagulopathy, rickets, and jaundice, which are all features observed in patients affected by one of the classic bile acid synthesis deficiencies (see Heubi et al. 2018). These disorders are dealt with in more detail in Chap. 40 by Vaz et al. (see also Vaz and Ferdinandusse 2017).

## Reference Values

The laboratory diagnosis of peroxisomal disorders involves the analysis of only a limited set of biomarkers including the analysis of very-long-chain fatty acids or rather C26:0-lysoPC, phytanic acid, pristanic acid, and di- and trihydroxycholestanoic acid in plasma, pipecolic acid in urine, and plasmalogens in erythrocytes. In literature many different methods have been described for these metabolites either measured individually or in combination. Indeed, we analyze the very-long-chain fatty acid, phytanic acid, and pristanic acid levels in a single assay essentially as described in Vreken et al. (Vreken et al. 1998) although we now prefer to analyze C26:0-lysoPC because of its superior sensitivity (see Klouwer et al. 2017). The analysis of di- and trihydroxycholestanoic acid is part of a much more elaborate analysis which involves the analysis of all bile acids, bile acid conjugates, and bile alcohols as discussed in detail in Chap. 40 by Vaz et al. The best diagnostic markers next to di- and trihydroxycholestanoic acid coming out of this analysis include tetrahydroxycholestanoic acid, C29-dicarboxylic cholestanoic acid, tauro-trihydroxycholestanoic acid, and tauro-tetrahydroxycholestanoic acid.

Plasmalogen analysis in erythrocytes can best be done using the method originally described by Bjorkhem et al. (Bjorkhem et al. 1986) as modified by Dacremont and Vincent (Dacremont and Vincent 1995) although plasmalogen analysis can also be done using lipidomics technology (see Herzog et al. 2018).

Table below lists the reference values for the various metabolites described above.

Reference values of peroxisomal biomarker metabolites

| Biomarker | Reference level |
|---|---|
| *Plasma (P), erythrocyte (E), dried blood spot (D)* | |
| C26:0-lysoPC (D) | <72 nmol/L |
| C26:0 (P) | 0.45–1.32 µmol/L |
| C26:0/C22:0 (P) | 0.0–0.02 |
| Phytanic acid (P) | 0.5–9.9 µmol/L |
| Pristanic acid (P) | 0.1–3.0 µmol/L |
| Pipecolic acid (P) | 0.1–7.0 µmol/L |
| Dihydroxycholestanoic acid (P) | 0.0–0.0 µmol/L |
| Tetrahydroxycholestanoic acid (P) | 0.0–0.1 µmol/L |
| *Plasmalogens (E)* | |
| C16:0-dimethylacetal | 6.8–11.9% |
| C18:0-dimethylacetal | 10.6–24.9% |

## Pathological Values

Table below lists the different peroxisomal biomarker metabolites and their levels in blood from patients affected by one of the peroxisomal disorders illustrated in Nomenclature Table.

Peroxisomal biomarker metabolites and their levels in blood, urine, or erythrocytes from patients affected by one of the peroxisomal disorders shown in Nomenclature Table

| Peroxisomal biomarker | Type of peroxisomal disorder | | | | | | | | | | |
|---|---|---|---|---|---|---|---|---|---|---|---|
| | Zellweger spectrum disorders | | | Rhizomelic chondrodysplasia punctata types 1–5 | | | | | Single enzyme deficiencies | | |
| Plasma (P), erythrocyte (E), dried blood spot (D), and urine (U) | PBD | ACOX1D | DBPD | 1 (PEX7) | 2 (GNPAT) | 3 (AGPS) | 4 (FAR1) | 5 (PEX5L) | XALD | RD | AMACR def |
| C26:0-lysoPC (D) | N - ↑ | N - ↑ | N - ↑ | N | N | N | N | N | ↑ | N | N |
| C26:0-lysoPC (P) | N - ↑ | N - ↑ | N - ↑ | N | N | N | N | N | ↑ | N | N |
| VLCFA (C26:0; C26:0/C22:0) (P) | N - ↑ | N - ↑ | N - ↑ | N | N | N | N | N | N - ↑ | N | N |
| Phytanic acid (P) | N - ↑ | N | N - ↑ | N - ↑ | N | N | N | N - ↑ | N | ↑ | N - ↑ |
| Pristanic acid (P) | N - ↑ | N | N - ↑ | N | N | N | N | N - ↑ | N | N | N - ↑ |
| Pipecolic acid (PU) | N - ↑ | N | N | N | N | N | N | N | N | N | N |
| Dihydroxycholestanoic acid (P) | N - ↑ | N | N - ↑ | N | N | N | N | N | N | N | N - ↑ |
| Trihydroxycholestanoic acid (P) | N - ↑ | N | N - ↑ | N | N | N | N | N | N | N | N - ↑ |
| Tetrahydroxycholestanoic acid (P) | N - ↑ | N | N - ↑ | N | N | N | N | N | N | N | N - ↑ |
| Tauro-tetrahydroxycholestanoic acid (P) | N - ↑ | N | N - ↑ | N | N | N | N | N | N | N | N - ↑ |
| Plasmalogens (E) | N - ↓ | N | N | ↓ | ↓ | ↓ | ↓ | ↓ | N | N | N |

## Diagnostic Flowcharts

The flowcharts for the Zellweger spectrum disorders (Fig. 66.6), rhizomelic chondrodysplasia punctata (Fig. 66.7), X-linked adrenoleukodystrophy/adrenomyeloneuropathy in males and females (Fig. 66.8), and Refsum disease (Fig. 66.9) are shown below. Metabolite analysis is the first essential step in the laboratory diagnosis of the different peroxisomal disorders, and, when abnormal, the results obtained immediately guide the way to the identification of the enzyme defect and subsequent molecular analysis to pinpoint the molecular defect in the gene involved. In recent years there has been a shift in the laboratory diagnosis of patients away from metabolite analysis as first-line diagnostic method thanks to the revolutionary developments of different sequencing methods. As a consequence whole exome and/or whole genome sequencing has gained popularity as first-line test in patients suspected to suffer from an inborn error of metabolism, which includes the peroxisomal disorders. It should be stressed that functional studies, including metabolite analyses, enzymatic assays, and/or metabolic pathway flux analysis, remain of key importance for the interpretation of whole exome/whole genome data especially when the mutations identified are novel and have not been

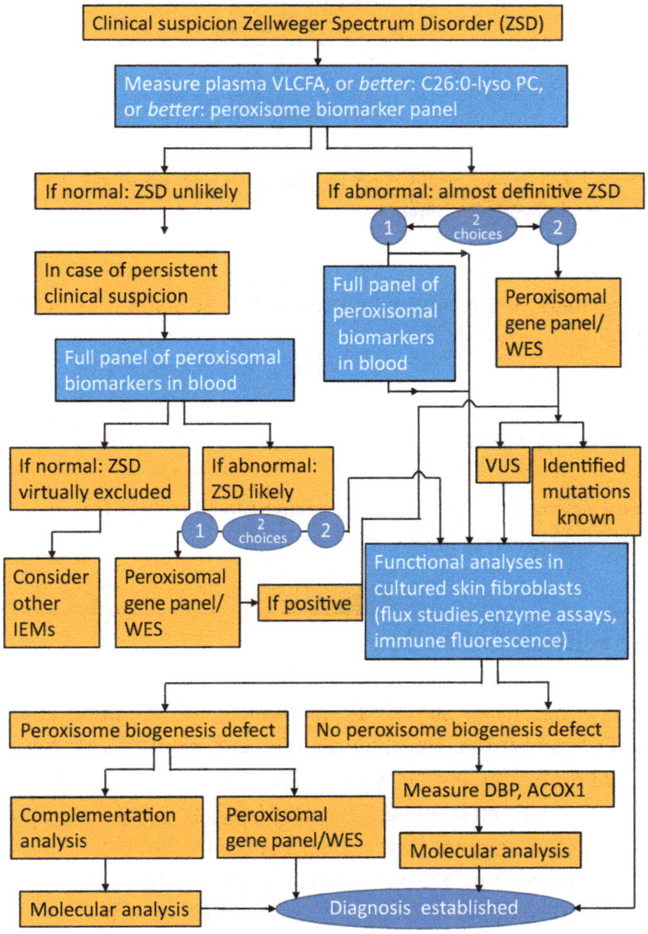


**Fig. 66.6** Diagnostic flowchart for patients suspected to suffer from a Zellweger spectrum disorder (ZSD)

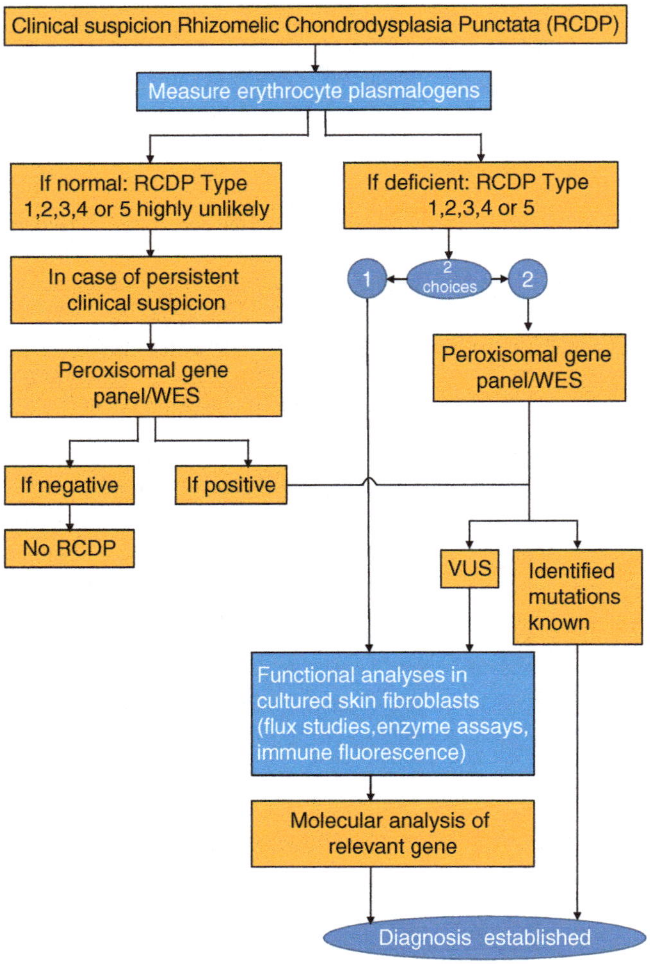


Fig. 66.7 Diagnostic flowchart for patients suspected to suffer from (rhizomelic) chondrodysplasia punctate

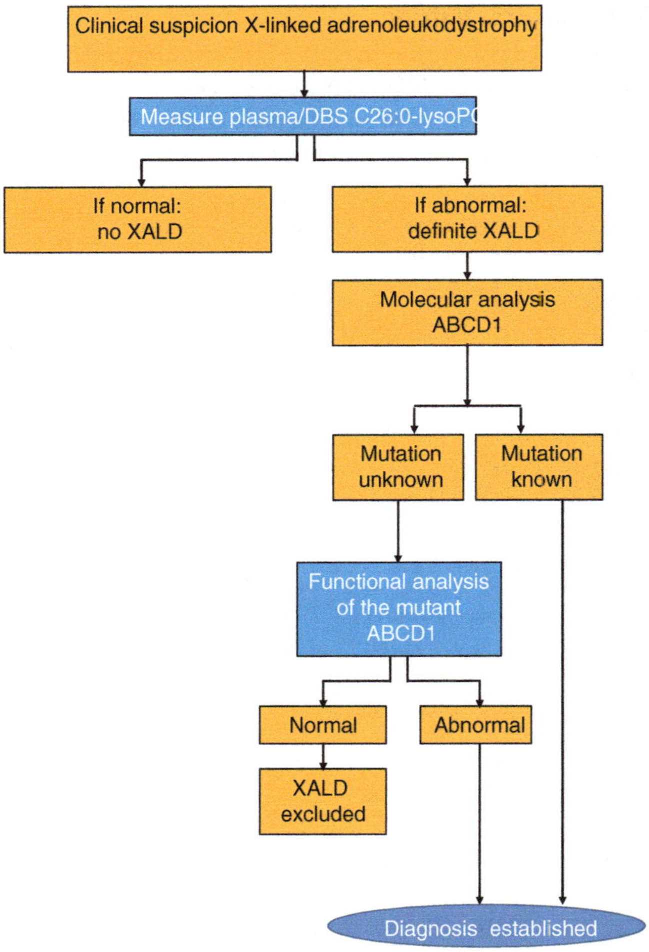


Fig. 66.8 Diagnostic flowchart for patients suspected to suffer from X-linked adrenoleukodystrophy/adrenomyeloneuropathy

described in literature before (see Ferdinandusse et al. 2016).

## Loading Tests

No loading tests have been described in literature for any of the PDs shown in Nomenclature Table.

## Specimen Collection

Very-long-chain fatty acids, phytanic acid, pristanic acid, and di- and trihydroxycholestanoic acid should all be measured preferably in EDTA plasma (or serum) and, if possible, in samples taken from patients after 1-night fasting. From the same blood sample, erythrocytes can be prepared for subsequent analysis of plasmalogens and DHA. Although glycolate and oxalate are mostly measured in urine, these metabolites can also be measured in plasma samples, which is especially relevant for some hyperoxaluria Type 1 patients (see Chap. 67 on hyperoxaluria).

## Prenatal Diagnosis

In the past, prenatal diagnostic methods have been developed for all PDs using biochemical methods including the analysis of specific metabolites, enzyme activity measurements, and immunoblot analysis, but these methods have become relatively obsolete thanks to the progress in molecular techniques. Indeed, molecular analysis of the gene involved is now the method of choice for the prenatal diagnosis of all PDs except in rare cases in which the molecular defect has not been established with certainty. In few patients with a clear-cut peroxisomal defect on biochemical grounds, the gene involved has remained unidentified, whereas in few other cases, molecular analysis has only identified one heterozygous mutation in the index patient.

## DNA Testing

Because it is not possible to predict from the biochemical and clinical phenotype of a patient with ZSD which of the known 13 *PEX* genes is defective, different approaches have

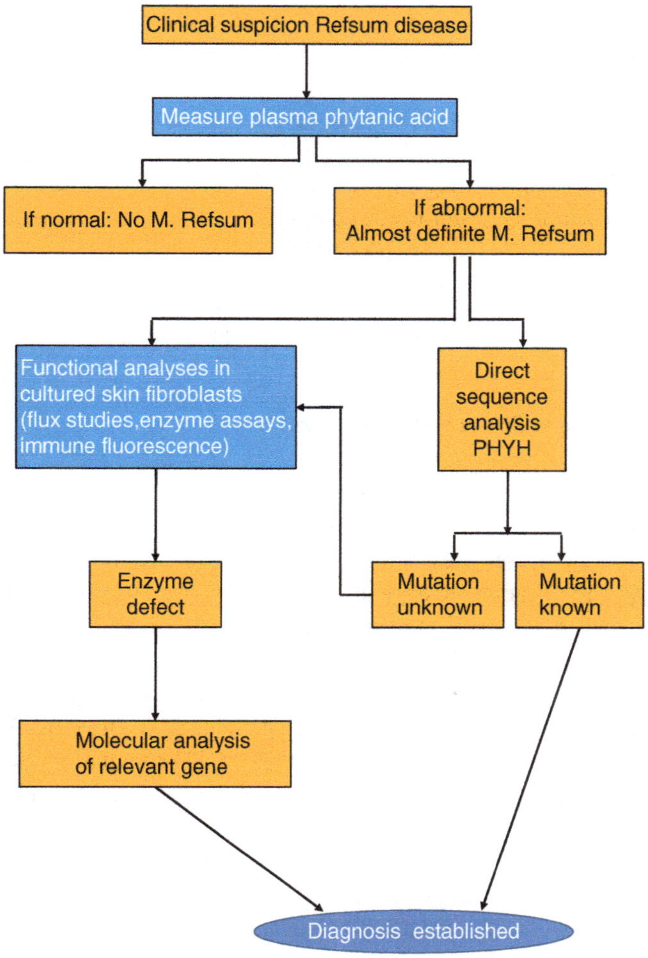


**Fig. 66.9** Diagnostic flowchart for patients suspected to suffer from Refsum disease

been developed to rapidly identify the affected gene. This includes *PEX* cDNA transfection complementation assays followed by sequencing of the implicated *PEX* gene and parallel sequencing of multiple genes involved in peroxisome biogenesis and maintenance, either by means of diagnostic peroxisomal gene panels or by exome sequencing (Waterham et al. 2016).

Genetic confirmation of patients suspected from any of the single enzyme defects (based on clinical presentation and/or biochemical parameters) is performed by sequencing of the encoding genes.

Genetic confirmation of patients suspected from a peroxisomal fission defect (usually after observing abnormal peroxisomal morphology upon microscopy) is performed by sequencing of the candidate genes, including DLP1, MFF, FIS1, GDAP1, and the PEX11B genes.

The identification of mutations causing a peroxisomal disorder enables carrier testing in relatives of patients and allows early prenatal testing or preimplantation genetic diagnosis in families with a recurrence risk for such disorders.

## Treatment Summary

For many of the PDs, no curative treatment has been described so far, which implies that treatment options are restricted to symptomatic and supportive care only (see Tables below).

Supportive treatment of ZSD, DBP, acyl-CoA oxidase 1 deficiency

| System | Problem | Intervention |
|---|---|---|
| Nervous system | Seizures | Anti-epileptic drugs |
| | Behavioral problems | Antipsychotics, behavioral management |
| | Intellectual disability | Educational support and intervention |
| | Drooling | Anti-cholinergic medication, botulinum toxin injection in salivary glands, surgical removal of submandibular salivary |
| | Neuropathy | Management of complications, referral to rehabilitation physician if severe |
| | Ataxia | Physical therapy, referral to rehabilitation physician |
| Eye | Retinopathy | Glasses |
| | Cataract | Lens replacement |
| Ear | Hearing impairment | Hearing aids |
| Dental | Enamel hypoplasia, caries | Oral hygiene, dental referral |
| Digestive | Dysphagia | Speech therapist; gastrostomy tube placement |
| | Steatorrhea | Surveillance of malabsorption; elemental formulas may be better tolerated |

Therapeutic options for Zellweger spectrum disorders

| Defect/deficiency | Medication/diet | Dosage |
|---|---|---|
| Low levels of fat-soluble Vitamins (A, D, E) | Vitamin A, D, E | Depending on plasma levels |
| Vitamin K-dependent coagulopathy | Vitamin K (phytomenadione) | Up to 1 mg/day or more |
| Accumulation of bile acid intermediates (di- and trihydroxycholestanoic acids) | Cholic acid | 10–20 mg/kg/day |
| Phytanic acid accumulation | Dietary restriction of phytanic acid with adequate caloric intake | Reduce following products: Dairy products, fish |
| Hyperoxaluria and/or kidney stones | Sufficient fluid intake and citrate therapy | |
| Adrenal insufficiency | Adrenal hormone replacement | |

Supportive treatment of rhizomelic chondrodysplasia punctata spectrum

| System | Problem | Intervention |
|---|---|---|
| Nervous system | Seizures | Anti-epileptic drugs |
| | Intellectual impairment | Educational support and intervention |
| | Spastic paresis | Spasmolytics, referral to rehabilitation physician |
| Eye | Cataract | Lens replacement |
| Digestive | Dysphagia | Gastrostomy tube placement |
| Cardiovascular | Congenital heart defects | Appropriate support and intervention |
| Musculoskeletal | Contractures | Physical therapy |
| Respiratory | Respiratory tract infections | Prophylactic antibiotics |
| Skin | Ichthyosis | Hydrating creams |

Therapeutic options for rhizomelic chondrodysplasia punctata spectrum

| Defect/deficiency | Medication/diet | Dosage |
|---|---|---|
| Phytanic acid accumulation | Dietary restriction of phytanic acid intake | Reduce following products: Dairy products, fish |

Supportive treatment of XALD males

| System | Problem | Intervention |
|---|---|---|
| Nervous system | Behavioral problems | Behavioral management, psychiatric consultation |
| | Myeloneuropathy (adult man), myelopathy with spastic paraparesis, incontinence, and sexual dysfunction | Supportive care by rehabilitation medicine and urologist, physical therapy, treatment of spasticity, neuropathic pain, and bladder issues |

Therapeutic options for XALD males

| Defect/deficiency | Medication/diet |
|---|---|
| Adrenal insufficiency | Adrenal hormone replacement |
| Neurologic dysfunction | Hematopoietic stem cell or bone marrow transplants |
| | Autologous hematopoietic stem cell gene therapy (phase IV study) |

Supportive treatment of Refsum disease

| System | Problem | Intervention |
|---|---|---|
| Nervous system | Ataxia | Physical therapy, referral to rehabilitation physician |
| | Neuropathy | Management of complications, referral to rehabilitation physician if severe |
| Eye | Retinitis pigmentosa | Glasses |
| | Cataract | Lens replacement |
| Ear | Hearing impairment | Hearing aids |
| Smell | Anosmia | None |
| Cardiovascular | Arrhythmia, cardiomyopathy | Antiarrhythmic drugs and other cardiac medication |
| Skin | Ichthyosis | Hydrating creams |

Therapeutic options for Refsum disease

| Defect/deficiency | Medication/diet | Dosage |
|---|---|---|
| Phytanic acid accumulation | Dietary restriction of phytanic acid intake | |
| | Plasmapheresis, lipopheresis | |
| | Avoidance of sudden weight loss | Appropriate caloric intake |

## Zellweger Spectrum Disorders

The symptomatic and supportive care options for ZSD patients include treatment of adrenal insufficiency (Berendse et al. 2014); seizures; low levels of fat-soluble vitamins A, D, and E; vitamin K-dependent coagulopathy; hearing and visual impairment; kidney stones due to hyperoxaluria; and dental abnormalities. Because supplementation of cortisone may be associated with severe side effects such as growth suppression and osteoporosis, only patients with a true insufficiency as established by means of an ACTH stimulation test qualify for this therapy. For hearing and visual impairments, ophthalmologists and ENT specialists can sometimes provide symptomatic treatment. In exceptional cases, cataract removal in infancy is advised.

Patients with renal calcium oxalate stones due to hyperoxaluria should be treated with citrate to prevent the formation of these stones. No evidence that ZSD patients benefit from a phytanic acid low diet is available at this point; therefore a phytanic acid-restricted diet is not advised when patients have only slightly increased phytanic acid levels. Some patients will need a gastrostomy tube to provide adequate intake of calories. On top of the symptomatic measures described above, several therapeutic options have been tried in the past. This includes a dietary therapy based on docosahexaenoic acid supplementation to patients to correct the deficiency of DHA in ZSD patients. Despite initial claims of a beneficial effect of DHA, a randomized, double-blind placebo-controlled trial in ZSD patients failed to show improvements of visual function and growth despite the increased DHA levels in plasma (Paker et al. 2010). Cholic acid therapy has also been advocated to be beneficial for ZSD patients, although recent clinical studies were unable to support this claim.

## Rhizomelic Chondrodysplasia Punctata

Also for the different RCDPs, treatment is only supportive and symptomatic. This may include cataract extraction in order to restore some vision, physical therapy to prevent contractures, and anti-epileptic drugs. Dietary restriction of phytanic acid as described for Refsum disease may be beneficial for RCDP patients especially in the milder forms dominated by ataxia and bone dysplasia (Smeitink et al. 1992) when phytanic acid levels are high. Inspired by the work of Brites and coworkers in a mouse model for RCDP Type 1 (Brites et al. 2011), alkylglycerol supplementation therapy has been tried in several RCDP patients with inconclusive results, which warrant additional work (Poll-The, personal communication).

### XALD

Corticosteroid replacement therapy is of crucial importance in every XALD patient with adrenal insufficiency. Indeed, if untreated, patients may succumb to adrenal crises. HLA-matched hematopoietic stem cell transplantation using HLA-matched donor or cord blood can stabilize or even reverse the cerebral demyelination at least to some extent when the procedure is performed at an early stage of the disease (Miller et al. 2011). More recently, following the initial encouraging work by Cartier and Aubourg (Cartier et al. 2009), Eichler and coworkers have shown that autologous hematopoietic stem cell gene therapy using a lentiviral vector may well be the treatment of choice especially when a matching HLA donor is missing (Eichler et al. 2017). These new developments are especially important since XALD has been included in several neonatal screening programs around the world.

#### Refsum Disease

Owing to the pathogenic role of excessive phytanic acid accumulation and its strict dietary source, therapeutic measures are aimed at lowering phytanic acid levels. Serial plasmapheresis or lipid apheresis should be initiated promptly if levels are excessively high as in some patients with levels >1000 micromol/L (normal levels = <15 micromol/L). Lipid apheresis can be done serially over a long period of time and usually is well tolerated. The mainstay of therapy in Refsum patients, however, is dietary restriction of phytanic acid which implies elimination of dairy products as well as certain fish and other ingredients from the diet (Baldwin et al. 2010). With long-term treatment and depending on the dietary compliance, patients do show stabilization or even improvement of the neuropathy, ataxia, and cardiac arrhythmias, whereas the retinitis pigmentosa, deafness, and anosmia seem more refractory.

#### **Hyperoxaluria Type 1** (See Chap. 67)

#### Disorders of Peroxisomal Bile Acid Synthesis Including ACOX2 Deficiency, PMP70 Deficiency, AMACR Deficiency, and BAAT Deficiency

So far only few patients have been described with deficiencies at the level of PMP70/ABCD3 (PD66.7), ACOX2 (PD66.5), and AMACR deficiency (PD66.12). Like all disorders of bile acid biosynthesis, the peroxisomal defects in bile acid synthesis also qualify for oral bile acid therapy, although evidence of clinical benefit is very limited in this subgroup. As discussed in more detail by Vaz et al. in Chap. 40, the mainstay of the treatment of BAAT-deficient patients involves supplementation of conjugated bile acids like glycocholic acid rather than unconjugated cholic acid or chenodeoxycholic acid as in the other bile acid synthesis defects.

## Standard Treatment Tables

Tables above show the supportive and therapeutic options for the main peroxisomal disorders including the Zellweger spectrum disorders, rhizomelic chondrodysplasia punctata, XALD, and Refsum disease.

## Experimental Treatment

There are no experimental treatment options studied at present, but retinal gene therapy for mildly affected ZSD patients is considered based on successful preliminary work in a mouse model for Zellweger syndrome (Argyriou et al., unpublished) and gene therapy and substrate deprivation therapy in hyperoxaluria Type 1, which is discussed in Chap. 67.

## Follow-Up and Monitoring

### Zellweger Spectrum Disorders

Follow-up should be aimed at screening for treatable complications as described in paragraph 66.11. This includes periodic blood withdrawal to assess adrenal function, fat-soluble vitamin levels, phytanic acid level, liver enzymes, and coagulation parameters. Screening for kidney stones should be done by performing abdominal ultrasound in combination with measuring urine oxalate levels to detect hyperoxaluria. Additional recommendations for follow-up and monitoring include regular assessment of growth and nutritional status and periodic ophthalmologic, audiological, neurological, and dental evaluation. Depending on the specific symptoms an individual patient is experiencing, additional follow-up may be indicated.

### Rhizomelic Chondrodysplasia Punctate

Recommendations for follow-up include regular assessment of growth and nutritional status and periodic ophthalmologic, cardiac, dental, orthopedic, and neurological evaluation including seizure frequency. Periodic blood withdrawal to assess phytanic acid levels is advised.

### XALD

Follow-up for male patients is recommended every 6 months from the age of 2–12 years and yearly from that age to monitor for complications and initiate timely treatment. Visits are preferably organized in a specialized clinic with a (pediatric) neurologist and endocrinologist. Aside from clinical evaluation, an MRI of the brain is done and an ACTH stimulation test (in those patients that have not developed adrenal failure) (Engelen et al. 2012). When lesions with gadolinium enhancement develop on the MRI, HCT treatment is advised. HCT is not recommended for patients with a symptomatic leukodystrophy or extensive lesions on MRI of the brain (Loes score of 9 or higher) (Miller et al. 2011). For the myelopathy of adulthood (that also occurs in those patients who received HSCT for cerebral ALD), there is currently no disease modifying or curative treatment, and only supportive care is available. Women with ALD do not develop adrenal failure or cerebral ALD and yearly follow-up is therefore not necessary.

#### Refsum Disease

The following evaluations are recommended to be performed on a regular basis: ophthalmologic, audiological, cardiac, and neurological assessment and testing for anosmia. Weight and plasma phytanic acid levels should be evaluated at least on a yearly basis in order to adapt the diet and perform plasmapheresis and/or lipid apheresis.

**Hyperoxaluria Type 1** (See Chap. 67)

**Disorders of Bile Acid Biosynthesis** (See Chap. 40).

## Online Resources

**GeneReviews Series:**

- Steinberg SJ, Raymond GV, Braverman NE, et al. Zellweger spectrum disorder. 2003 Dec 12 [Updated 2017 Dec 21] In: Adam MP, Ardinger HH, Pagon RA, et al., editors. GeneReviews® [Internet]. Seattle, WA: University of Washington, Seattle; 1993–2020.
- Newman WG, Friedman TB, Conway GS, et al. Perrault syndrome. 2014 Sep 25 [Updated 2018 Sep 6] In: Adam MP, Ardinger HH, Pagon RA, et al., editors. GeneReviews® [Internet]. Seattle, WA: University of Washington, Seattle; 1993–2020.
- Braverman NE, Steinberg SJ, Fallatah W, et al. Rhizomelic chondrodysplasia punctata type 1. 2001 Nov 16 [Updated 2020 Jan 30] In: Adam MP, Ardinger HH, Pagon RA, et al., editors. GeneReviews® [Internet]. Seattle, WA: University of Washington, Seattle; 1993–2020.
- Wanders RJA, Waterham HR, Leroy BP. Refsum Disease. 2006 Mar 20 [Updated 2015 Jun 11] In: Adam MP, Ardinger HH, Pagon RA, et al., editors. GeneReviews® [Internet]. Seattle, WA: University of Washington, Seattle; 1993–2020.
- Raymond GV, Moser AB, Fatemi A. X-Linked Adrenoleukodystrophy. 1999 Mar 26 [Updated 2018 Feb 15] In: Adam MP, Ardinger HH, Pagon RA, et al., editors. GeneReviews® [Internet]. Seattle, WA: University of Washington, Seattle; 1993–2020.
- Milliner DS, Harris PC, Cogal AG, et al. Primary Hyperoxaluria Type 1. 2002 Jun 19 [Updated 2017 Nov 30] In: Adam MP, Ardinger HH, Pagon RA, et al., editors. GeneReviews® [Internet]. Seattle (WA): University of Washington, Seattle; 1993–2020.

## References


Argyriou C, D'Agostino MD, Braverman N. Peroxisome biogenesis disorders. Transl Sci Rare Dis. 2016;1(2):111–44.

Baldwin EJ, Gibberd FB, Harley C, Sidey MC, Feher MD, Wierzbicki AS. The effectiveness of long-term dietary therapy in the treatment of adult Refsum disease. J Neurol Neurosurg Psychiatry. 2010;81(9):954–7.

Berendse K, Engelen M, Linthorst GE, van Trotsenburg ASP, Poll-The BT. High prevalence of primary adrenal insufficiency in Zellweger spectrum disorders. Orphanet J Rare Dis. 2014;9:133.

Bjorkhem I, Sisfontes L, Bostrom B, Kase BF, Blomstrand R. Simple diagnosis of the Zellweger syndrome by gas-liquid chromatography of dimethylacetals. J Lipid Res. 1986;27:786–91.

Braverman NE, Moser AB. Functions of plasmalogen lipids in health and disease. Biochim Biophys Acta. 2012;1822(9):1442–52.

Brites P, Ferreira AS, da Silva TF, Sousa VF, Malheiro AR, Duran M, Waterham HR, Baes M, Wanders RJ. Alkyl-glycerol rescues plasmalogen levels and pathology of ether-phospholipid deficient mice. PLoS One. 2011;6(12):e28539.

Cartier N, Hacein-Bey-Abina S, Bartholomae CC, Veres G, Schmidt M, Kutschera I, Vidaud M, Abel U, Dal-Cortivo L, Caccavelli L, Mahlaoui N, Kiermer V, Mittelstaedt D, Bellesme C, Lahlou N, Lefrère F, Blanche S, Audit M, Payen E, Leboulch P, l'Homme B, Bougnères P, Von Kalle C, Fischer A, Cavazzana-Calvo M, Aubourg P. Hematopoietic stem cell gene therapy with a lentiviral vector in X-linked adrenoleukodystrophy. Science. 2009;326(5954):818–23.

Dacremont G, Vincent G. Assay of plasmalogens and polyunsaturated fatty acids (PUFA) in erythrocytes and fibroblasts. J Inherit Metab Dis. 1995;18:84–9.

de Beer M, Engelen M, van Geel BM. Frequent occurrence of cerebral demyelination in adrenomyeloneuropathy. Neurology 2014;83:2227–31.

Ebberink MS, Koster J, Visser G, van Spronsen FJ, Stolte-Dijkstra I, Smit GPA, Fock JM, Wanders RJA, Waterham HR. A novel defect of peroxisome division due to a homozygous non-sense mutation in the PEX11B gene. J Med Genet. 2012;49:307–13.

Eichler F, Duncan C, Musolino PL, Orchard PJ, De Oliveira S, Thrasher AJ, Armant M, Dansereau C, Lund TC, Miller WP, Raymond GV, Sankar R, Shah AJ, Sevin C, Gaspar HB, Gissen P, Amartino H, Bratkovic D, Smith NJC, Paker AM, Shamir E, O'Meara T, Davidson D, Aubourg P, Williams DA. Hematopoietic stem-cell gene therapy for cerebral Adrenoleukodystrophy. N Engl J Med. 2017;377(17):1630–8.

Engelen M, Barbier M, Dijkstra IM, Schür R, de Bie RM, Verhamme C, Dijkgraaf MG, Aubourg PA, Wanders RJ, van Geel BM, de Visser M, Poll-The BT, Kemp S. X-linked adrenoleukodystrophy in women: a cross-sectional cohort study. Brain 2014;137(Pt 3):693–706.

Engelen M, Kemp S, de Visser M, van Geel BM, Wanders RJ, Aubourg P, Poll-The BT. X-linked adrenoleukodystrophy (X-ALD): clinical presentation and guidelines for diagnosis, follow-up and management. Orphanet J Rare Dis. 2012;7:51.

Ferdinandusse S, Denis S, Hogenhout EM, Koster J, van Roermund CW, IJlst L, Moser AB, Wanders RJ, Waterham HR. Clinical, biochemical, and mutational spectrum of peroxisomal acyl-coenzyme A oxidase deficiency. Hum Mutat. 2007;28(9):904–12.

Ferdinandusse S, Denis S, Mooyer PA, Dekker C, Duran M, Soorani-Lunsing RJ, Boltshauser E, Macaya A, Gärtner J, Majoie CB, Barth PG, Wanders RJ, Poll-The BT. Clinical and biochemical spectrum of D-bifunctional protein deficiency. Ann Neurol. 2006;59(1):92–104.

Ferdinandusse S, Ebberink MS, Vaz FM, Waterham HR, Wanders RJA. The important role of biochemical and functional studies in the diagnosis of peroxisomal disorders. J Inherit Metab Dis. 2016;39:531–43.

Ferdinandusse S, Falkenberg KD, Koster J, Mooyer PA, Jones R, van Roermund CWT, Pizzino A, Schrader M, Wanders RJA, Vanderver A, Waterham HR. ACBD5 deficiency causes a defect in peroxisomal very long-chain fatty acid metabolism. J Med Genet. 2017;54(5):330–7.

Haugarvoll K, Johansson S, Tzoulis C, Haukanes BI, Bredrup C, Neckelmann G, Boman H, Knappskog PM, Bindoff LA. MRI characterisation of adult onset alpha-methylacyl-coA racemase deficiency diagnosed by exome sequencing. Orphanet J Rare Dis. 2013;8:1.

Herzog K, Pras-Raves ML, Ferdinandusse S, Vervaart MAT, Luyf ACM, van Kampen AHC, Wanders RJA, Waterham HR, Vaz FM. Plasma lipidomics as a diagnostic tool for peroxisomal disorders. J Inherit Metab Dis. 2018;41(3):489–98.

Heubi JE, Bove KE, Setchell KDR. Oral cholic acid is efficacious and well tolerated in patients with bile acid synthesis and Zellweger spectrum disorders. J Pediatr Gastroenterol Nutr. 2018;66(2): e57–9.

Huffnagel IC, Laheji FK, Aziz-Bose R, Tritos NA, Marino R, Linthorst GE, Kemp S, Engelen M, Eichler F. The natural history of adrenal insufficiency:and international collaboration. J Clin Endocrinol Metab 2019a;104:118–26.

Huffnagel IC, van Ballegoij WJC, van Geel BM, Vos JMBW, Kemp S, Engelen M. Progression of myelopathy in males with adrenoleukodystrophy: towards clinical trail readiness. Brain 2019b;142:334–43.

Huffnagel IC, Dijkgraaf MGW, Janssens GW, van Weeghel M, van Geel BM, Poll-the BT, Kemp s, Engelen M. Disease progression in women with X-linked adrenoleukodystrophy is slow. Orphanet J rare Dis. 2019c;14:30.

Klouwer FC, Berendse K, Ferdinandusse S, Wanders RJ, Engelen M, Poll-The BT. Zellweger spectrum disorders: clinical overview and management approach. Orphanet J Rare Dis. 2015;10:151.

Klouwer FCC, Ferdinandusse S, van Lenthe H, Kulik W, Wanders RJA, Poll-The BT, Waterham HR, Vaz FM. Evaluation of C26:0-lysophosphatidylcholine and C26:0-carnitine as diagnostic markers for Zellweger spectrum disorders. J Inherit Metab Dis. 2017;40(6):875–81.

Miller WP, Rothman SM, Nascene D, Kivisto T, DeFor TE, Ziegler RS, Eisengart J, Leiser K, Raymond G, Lund TC, Tolar J, Orchard PJ. Outcomes after allogeneic hematopoietic cell transplantation for childhood cerebral adrenoleukodystrophy: the largest single-institution cohort report. Blood 2011;118(7):1971–1978.

Paker AM, Sunness JS, Brereton NH, Speedie LJ, Albanna L, Dharmaraj S, Moser AB, Jones RO, Raymond GV. Docosahexaenoic acid therapy in peroxisomal diseases: results of a double-blind, randomized trial. Neurology. 2010;75(9):826–30.

Smeitink JA, Beemer FA, Espeel M, Donckerwolcke RA, Jakobs C, Wanders RJ, Schutgens RB, Roels F, Duran M, Dorland L, et al. Bone dysplasia associated with phytanic acid accumulation and deficient plasmalogen synthesis: a peroxisomal entity amenable to plasmapheresis. J Inherit Metab Dis. 1992;15(3):377–80.

Van Veldhoven PP. Biochemistry and genetics of inherited disorders of peroxisomal fatty acid metabolism. J Lipid Res. 2010;51(10):2863–95.

Vaz FM, Ferdinandusse S. Bile acid analysis in human disorders of bile acid biosynthesis. Mol Asp Med. 2017;56:10–24.

Vreken P, van Lint AE, Bootsma AH, Overmars H, Wanders RJ, van Gennip AH. Rapid stable isotope dilution analysis of very-long-chain fatty acids, pristanic acid, and phytanic acid using gas chromatography-electron impact mass spectrometry. J Chromatogr B Biomed Sci Appl 1998;25:281–7.

Wanders RJ, Komen J, Ferdinandusse S. Phytanic acid metabolism in health and disease. Biochim Biophys Acta. 2011;1811(9):498–507.

Wanders RJ, Waterham HR, Ferdinandusse S. Metabolic interplay between peroxisomes and other subcellular organelles including mitochondria and the endoplasmic reticulum. Front Cell Dev Biol. 2016;3:83.

Waterham HR, Ferdinandusse S, Wanders RJ. Human disorders of peroxisome metabolism and biogenesis. Biochim Biophys Acta. 2016;1863(5):922–33.

Wierzbicki AS, Lloyd MD, Schofield CJ, Feher MD, Gibberd FB. Refsum's disease: a peroxisomal disorder affecting phytanic acid alpha-oxidation. J Neurochem. 2002;80(5):727–35.

# 67 Disorders of Oxalate Metabolism

Bernd Hoppe, Bodo B. Beck,
and Cristina Martin-Higueras

## Contents




B. Hoppe (✉)
Hyperoxaluria Center, German Hyperoxaluria Center, Bonn, Germany
e-mail: bernd.hoppe@knz-bonn.de

B. B. Beck
Department of Human Genetics, University Hospital Cologne, Cologne, Germany

C. Martin-Higueras
Department of Pediatrics, Division of Pediatric Nephrology, University Hospital Bonn, Bonn, Germany

Department of Basic Medical Science, Fac. of Medicine, University of La Laguna, La Laguna, Spain



## Summary

Hyperoxaluria is one of the most important promoters of crystallization, which might induce a chronic inflammatory process if crystals are internalized in the tubular system, leading later to early end-stage renal failure (Kurts 2013; Beck et al. 2016). Urinary oxalate is mostly of endogenous origin, and only ~10% derive from the daily nutritional intake (Whittamore et al. 2019). Primary causes are distinguished from secondary ones: The autosomal recessive inherited primary hyperoxaluria (PH) types I, II, and III are defects of the glyoxylate metabolism leading to endogenous (primary) overproduction of oxalate (Hoppe





N. Blau et al. (eds.), *Physician's Guide to the Diagnosis, Treatment, and Follow-Up of Inherited Metabolic Diseases*,
https://doi.org/10.1007/978-3-030-67727-5_67

2012; Belostotsky et al. 2010). A significant number of hyperoxaluric patients, who would classify for PH, have yet unknown genetic basis of disease; thus, further types of PH are likely to exist (unclassified PH). Urinary excretion of oxalate is strongly elevated (>1 mmol/1.73 m$^2$ BSA/day, normal <0.5) in all forms of PH, resulting in recurrent stone formation and/or nephrocalcinosis and in progressive kidney damage leading to systemic calcium oxalate deposition (systemic oxalosis), primarily in PH type I (100%), but also in PH II (50%). Systemic oxalosis in PH I is a catastrophic situation that must be prevented by all means. Yet, diagnosis is all too often missed or delayed until end-stage renal failure occurs (in more than one third of adult patients). This is particularly unfortunate because progressive renal damage can be delayed or even prevented by early intervention (Garrelfs et al. 2021; Weigert et al. 2018). Secondary hyperoxaluria is due either to excessive oxalate or vitamin C intake (dietary hyperoxaluria), the latter being metabolized to oxalate, or to increased intestinal oxalate absorption (enteric, mostly based on chronic inflammatory bowel syndromes, Hoppe et al. 2003). Although the urinary oxalate excretion is usually <1 mmol/1.73 m$^2$ BSA/24 h, it may nevertheless lead to significant morbidity, i.e., to recurrent urolithiasis or progressive nephrocalcinosis with renal failure, especially in patients with Crohn's disease and ileocecal valve resections.

## Introduction

### Glyoxylate Reductase/Hydroxypyruvate Reductase (GRHPR) Deficiency

All currently known types of primary hyperoxaluria (PH I–III) are rare, autosomal recessive disorders of the glyoxylate metabolism (Hoppe 2012; Belostotsky et al. 2010). Primary hyperoxaluria type II (PH II) seems to be even more rare (under one tenth of the PH fraction) or remains markedly underdiagnosed. It is characterized by increased urinary excretion of oxalate and L-glyceric acid due to a defect in glyoxylate reductase/hydroxypyruvate reductase (GRHPR) activity (Cregeen et al. 2003). *GRHPR*, located on chromosome 9p11, is composed of 9 exons with >30 known causative mutations (Garrelfs et al. 2019). The clinical course of PH II is comparable, but generally more benign as compared to PH I, but symptoms may be clinically indistinguishable from PH I. CKD/ESRF occurs less frequently, has not been reported in childhood, but still affects about 50% of adults (Garrelfs et al. 2019).

### 4-Hydroxy-2-Oxoglutarate Aldolase 1 (HOGA1) Deficiency

Mutations in the seven exons spanning gene on chromosome 10 (*HOGA1*) were found to cause PH III (Belostotsky et al. 2010; Monico et al. 2011). *HOGA1* encodes for a mitochondrial 4-hydroxy-2-oxoglutarate aldolase. The findings of nonsense mutations in *HOGA1* suggested that a loss of function may lead to glyoxylate accumulation and hence the production of oxalate (Beck et al. 2013) by lactate dehydrogenase A. PH III patients also show increased urinary 4-hydroxy-2-oxoglutarate (HOG), which serves as a diagnostic biomarker together with urinary oxalate (PMID: 22771891). Also, dihydroxyglutarate and 4-hydroxy-glutamate excretion is elevated. What may be extrapolated from the limited data available is the fact that this subtype is about to become the second most frequent form. Also adults presenting with recurrent kidney stones and CKD stages 2 or higher are observed in more than 20 % of patients. Although PH III so far has only two documented cases of ESRF, long term follow up data is still missing, but it is already clear that it is not as benign as it was initially reported (Monico et al. 2011, Ventzke et al. 2017).

### Oxalate Transporter Deficiencies

In the intestine, oxalate is secreted by the soluble intestinal oxalate transporter (SLC26A6), and in the kidney, next to the fact that it is freely filtered, tubular secretion and reabsorption processes are regulated via SLC26A1 and SLC26A6, finally resulting in a net secretion (Knauf et al. 2011; Knauf et al. 2019). A reduced secretion of oxalate via SLC24A6 may therefore lead way to increased plasma oxalate levels and hence to elevated urinary oxalate excretion. This was reported in mice with a defect in SLC26A6, showing a defective interplay of net absorption of oxalate and net secretion, thus inducing hyperoxalemia and hyperoxaluria (Knauf et al. 2011). Next to that, mice who lack the sulfate anion transporter-1 (Sat1 or SLC26A1), which mediates intestinal oxalate transport, also have a phenotype of hyperoxalemia, hyperoxaluria, and calcium oxalate stones (Ko et al. 2012). Also, in obese mice, a reduced active transcellular intestinal oxalate secretion was recently found, which induces sometimes severe hyperoxalemia and hyperoxaluria (Amin et al. 2018). Here, however, it has to be considered that data of mice studies are not always applicable to the human situation and that there are also conflicting results even for mice data using an equivalent research approach (here *SLC26A1* knockout mice with/without hyperoxalemia and hyperoxaluria) (Dawson et al. 2010; Whittamore et al. 2019).

## Alanine-Glyoxylate Aminotransferase (AGT) Deficiency

In PH I, mistargeting or low/absent activity of liver-specific peroxisomal alanine-glyoxylate aminotransferase (AGT) causes massive hyperoxaluria (Danpure et al. 1989). PH I is the most frequent and most severe subtype. The underlying defective *AGXT* comprises 11 exons, located on chromosome 2q36–37 (Purdue et al. 1991). Diagnosis is mostly based on complete *AGXT* sequencing, with >200 mutations identified nowadays throughout the gene. Genetic testing in patients with suspected disease is now considered the gold standard for diagnosis. The disease prevalence is approximately two patients per million populations (van Woerden et al. 2003), but newer genomic data let us suspect that the prevalence is even higher (1:58,000, Hopp et al. 2015). The highly elevated urinary excretion of oxalate and glycolate (>1 mmol/1.73 $m^2$ body surface area/day, normal <0.5) causes renal calculi (medullary), nephrocalcinosis (NC), or both (Hoppe 2012). While the disease progresses and renal function declines, calcium oxalate crystals systemically deposit (Cochat and Rumsby 2013, Hoppe 2012), when plasma oxalate (Pox) and plasma calcium oxalate saturation (ßPCaOx) increase dramatically, both being inversely correlated with glomerular filtration rate (GFR) in patients with severely impaired renal function (Hoppe et al. 1999). CaOx supersaturation then leads to systemic CaOx crystal deposition and hence a multisystemic disorder with extreme morbidity. PH I patients show a substantial genetic, biochemical, and phenotypic heterogeneity ranging from end-stage renal failure (ESRF) already in infancy (infantile oxalosis) to a late onset or oligosymptomatic course in advanced adulthood. Unfortunately, most patients will develop ESRF over time, if no measures are taken. Systemic oxalosis in PH I is a catastrophic situation that must be prevented by all means. Yet, diagnosis is all too often missed or delayed until ESRF had occurred (in approx. a third of adult patients) (Zhao et al. 2016, Hopp et al. 2015, Mandrile et al. 2014). Early intervention can delay or even prevent progressive renal damage, though.

## Secondary Hyperoxaluria

Distinction between PH and secondary hyperoxalurias may be difficult (Robijn et al. 2011). The latter is due either to excessive dietary oxalate intake (dietary hyperoxaluria); to massive vitamin C intake, which is metabolized to oxalate; or to increased intestinal oxalate absorption (enteric). Patients with intestinal disease have an increased risk of hyperoxaluria, particularly after bowel resection (short bowel syndrome), after bypass surgery, in chronic inflammatory bowel disease or cystic fibrosis, and in other malabsorption syndromes. Although the urinary oxalate excretion is usually <1 mmol/1.73 $m^2$ BSA/24 h, it may nevertheless lead to significant morbidity, i.e., to recurrent urolithiasis or progressive nephrocalcinosis with renal failure and also to systemic oxalosis subsuming multisystemic disorder like in PH I (Hoppe 2012). Therapy is primarily directed toward the underlying disease, but additional measures are still very important.

## Hydroxyacid Oxidase 1 (HAO1) Deficiency

Up to now, there are only two reports presenting patients with HAO1 deficiency leading to either only elevated urinary glycolate excretion in two brothers (Frishberg et al. 2014) or an (unexplained) hyperoxaluria in another young patient (Clifford-Mobley et al. 2017, Frishberg et al. 2014). The first report of Frishberg et al. pointed out that GO (glycolate oxidase) inhibition by RNA interference treatment (see below) would be safe, as no hyperoxaluria would be expected after that blockage. We are now aware of three other families with homozygous HAO1 mutations leading to extremely elevated uinary glycolate, but also to some amount of hyperoxaluria!

## Nomenclature

| No. | Disorder | Alternative name | Abbreviation | Gene symbol | Chromosomal localization | Affected protein | OMIM no. |
|---|---|---|---|---|---|---|---|
| 67.1 | Primary hyperoxaluria type II | Glyoxylate reductase deficiency | PH 2 | *GRHPR* | 9p13.2 | D-Glycerate dehydrogenase | 260000 |
| 67.2 | Primary hyperoxaluria type III | 4-Hydroxy-2-oxoglutarate aldolase deficiency (mitochondrial) | PH 3 | *HOGA1* | 10q24.2 | 4-Hydroxy-2-oxoglutarate aldolase | 613616 |
| 67.3 | Oxalate transporter deficiency | Solute carrier transporter deficiencies | SLC | *SLC26A6* *SLC26A1* | 3p21.31 4p16.3 | SLC26A6 SAT1 | 610068 610130 |
| 67.4 | Primary hyperoxaluria type I | Alanine-glyoxylate aminotransferase deficiency (peroxisomal) | PH 1 | *AGXT* | 2q36–37 | Alanine-glyoxylate aminotransferase | 259900 |
| 67.5 | Hydroxyacid oxidase 1 deficiency | Glycolate oxidase deficiency; isolated glycolic aciduria | HAO | *HAO1* | 20p12.3 | Glycolate oxidase deficiency | 605023 |

### Secondary Hyperoxalurias

| Disorder | Definition/comment |
|---|---|
| Dietary hyperoxaluria (normalized on low-oxalate diet) | Oxalate (U) > 0.5 mmol/1.73 m²/day Elevated urinary oxalate/ creatinine ratios (age specific) |
| Enteric, absorptive hyperoxaluria (inflammatory bowel diseases, malabsorption syndromes, post bowel resection; lack of intestinal oxalate-degrading bacteria like *Oxalobacter formigenes*) | Oxalate (U) > 0.5 mmol/1.73 m²/day Elevated urinary oxalate/ creatinine ratios (age specific) |

## Metabolic Pathways

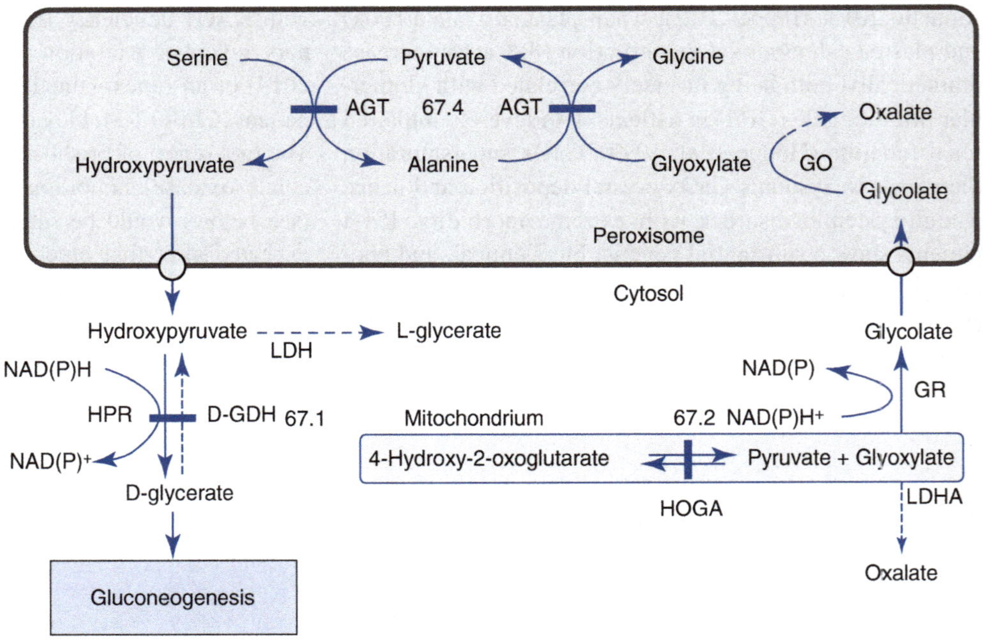


**Fig. 67.1** Hepatic glyoxylate metabolism

## Signs and Symptoms

**Table 67.1** Primary hyperoxaluria type II

| System | Symptoms and biomarkers | Neonatal (birth–1 month) | Infancy (1–18 months) | Childhood (1.5–11 years) | Adolescence (11–16 years) | Adulthood (>16 years) |
|---|---|---|---|---|---|---|
| Cardiovascular | Cardiomyopathy | ± | ± | ± | ± | ± |
| | Cardiac oxalate deposition | ± | ± | ± | ± | ± |
| Dermatological | Calcinosis cutis | ± | ± | ± | ± | ± |
| | Livedo reticularis | ± | ± | ± | ± | ± |
| Eye | Optic atrophy | ± | ± | ± | ± | ± |
| | Pigmentary retinopathy | ± | ± | ± | ± | ± |
| Hematological | Pancytopenia | ± | ± | ± | ± | ± |
| Musculoskeletal | Bone pain | ± | ± | ± | ± | ± |
| | Derangement of trabecular structure | ± | ± | ± | ± | + |
| | Growth retardation | ± | ± | ± | ± | |
| | Pathological fractures | ± | ± | ± | ± | ± |
| | Radiolucent metaphyseal bands | ± | ± | ± | ± | + |
| Renal | Nephrocalcinosis | + | + | + | + | + |
| | Nephrolithiasis | + | + | + | ++ | ++ |
| | Renal colic | + | + | + | ++ | ++ |
| | Renal failure, chronic | ± | ± | ± | + | + |
| | Urinary infections | ± | ± | ± | ± | ± |
| Other | Failure to thrive | ± | ± | ± | ± | |
| Laboratory findings | Creatinine (S) | n-↑ | n-↑ | n-↑ | n-↑ | n-↑↑ |
| | Glyceric acid (P) | n-↑ | n-↑ | n-↑ | n-↑ | n-↑ |
| | Glyceric acid (U) | ↑↑ | ↑↑ | ↑↑ | ↑↑ | ↑↑ |
| | Hematuria | ± | ± | ± | ± | ± |
| | Oxalic acid (P) | n-↑ | n-↑ | n-↑ | n-↑ | n-↑↑ |
| | Oxalic acid (U) | ↑↑ | ↑↑ | ↑↑ | ↑↑ | ↑↑ |
| | Urea (S) | n-↑ | n-↑ | n-↑ | n-↑ | n-↑ |

**Table 67.2** Primary hyperoxaluria type III

| System | Symptoms and biomarkers | Neonatal (birth–1 month) | Infancy (1–18 months) | Childhood (1.5–11 years) | Adolescence (11–16 years) | Adulthood (>16 years) |
|---|---|---|---|---|---|---|
| Cardiovascular | Cardiomyopathy | ± | ± | ± | ± | ± |
| | Cardiac oxalate deposition | ± | ± | ± | ± | ± |
| Dermatologica | Calcinosis cutis | ± | ± | ± | ± | ± |
| | Livedo reticularis | ± | ± | ± | ± | ± |
| Eye | Optic atrophy | ± | ± | ± | ± | ± |
| | Pigmentary retinopathy | ± | ± | ± | ± | ± |
| Hematological | Pancytopenia | ± | ± | ± | ± | ± |
| Musculoskeletal | Bone pain | ± | ± | ± | ± | ± |
| | Derangement of trabecular structure | ± | ± | ± | ± | ± |
| | Growth retardation | ± | ± | ± | ± | |
| | Pathological fractures | ± | ± | ± | ± | ± |
| | Radiolucent metaphyseal bands | ± | ± | ± | ± | ± |
| Renal | Nephrocalcinosis | + | + | + | + | + |
| | Nephrolithiasis | ++ | ++ | ++ | + | + |
| | Renal colic | ++ | ++ | ++ | + | + |
| | Renal failure, chronic | ± | ± | ± | + | + |
| | Urinary infections | ± | ± | ± | ± | ± |
| Other | Failure to thrive | ± | ± | ± | ± | |
| Laboratory findings | Creatinine (S) | n-↑ | n-↑ | n-↑ | n-↑ | n-↑ |
| | Calcium (U) | n-↑ | n-↑ | n-↑ | n-↑ | n-↑ |
| | HOG (U) | ↑ | ↑ | ↑ | ↑ | ↑ |
| | Hematuria | ± | ± | ± | ± | ± |
| | Oxalic acid (P) | ± | ± | ± | ± | ± |
| | Oxalic acid (U) | ↑↑ | ↑↑ | ↑↑ | ↑↑ | ↑↑ |
| | Urea (S) | n-↑ | n-↑ | n-↑ | n-↑ | n-↑ |

**Table 67.3** Secondary hyperoxaluria incl. SLC26A1 and SLC26A6

| System | Symptom | Neonatal (birth–1 month) | Infancy (1–18 months) | Childhood (1.5–11 years) | Adolescence (11–16 years) | Adulthood (>16 years) |
|---|---|---|---|---|---|---|
| Cardiovascular | Cardiomyopathy | | | | | ± |
| | Cardiac oxalate deposition | | | | | ± |
| Dermatological | Calcinosis cutis | | | | | ± |
| | Livedo reticularis | | | | | ± |
| | Pigmentary retinopathy | | | | | |
| Hematological | Pancytopenia | | | | | ± |
| Musculoskeletal | Bone pain | | | | | ± |
| | Derangement of trabecular structure | | | | | ± |
| | Pathological fractures | | | | | ± |
| | Radiolucent metaphyseal bands | | | | | ± |
| Renal | Nephrocalcinosis | ± | ± | ± | ± | ± |
| | Nephrolithiasis | + | + | + | + | + |
| | Renal colic | + | + | + | + | + |
| | Renal failure, chronic | | | | ± | + |
| | Urinary infections | ± | ± | ± | ± | ± |
| Other | Failure to thrive | ± | ± | ± | ± | |
| Laboratory findings | Creatinine (serum) | n-↑ | n-↑ | n-↑ | n-↑ | n-↑ |
| | Citrate (urine) | n-↓ | n-↓ | n-↓ | n-↓ | n-↓ |
| | Hematuria | ± | ± | ± | ± | ± |
| | Oxalic acid (serum) | n-↑ | n-↑ | n-↑ | n-↑ | n-↑ |
| | Oxalic acid (urine) | ↑–↑↑ | ↑–↑↑ | ↑–↑↑ | ↑–↑↑ | ↑–↑↑ |
| | Urea (serum) | n-↑ | n-↑ | n-↑ | n-↑ | n-↑ |

**Table 67.4** Primary hyperoxaluria Type I

| System | Symptoms and biomarkers | Neonatal (birth–1 month) | Infancy (1–18 months) | Childhood (1.5–11 years) | Adolescence (11–16 years) | Adulthood (>16 years) |
|---|---|---|---|---|---|---|
| Cardiovascular | Cardiomyopathy | ± | ± | ± | ± | ± |
| | Cardiac oxalate deposition | ± | ± | ± | ± | ± |
| Dermatological | Calcinosis cutis | ± | ± | ± | ± | ± |
| | Livedo reticularis | ± | ± | ± | ± | ± |
| Eye | Optic atrophy | ± | ± | ± | ± | ± |
| | Pigmentary retinopathy | ± | ± | ± | ± | ± |
| Hematological | Pancytopenia | ± | ± | ± | ± | ± |
| Musculoskeletal | Bone pain | ± | ± | ± | ± | ± |
| | Derangement of trabecular structure | ++ | ± | ± | + | + |
| | Growth retardation | ++ | ++ | ++ | ++ | |
| | Pathological fractures | ± | ± | ± | ± | ± |
| | Radiolucent metaphyseal bands | + | + | + | + | + |
| Renal | Nephrocalcinosis | ++ | ++ | ++ | + | + |
| | Nephrolithiasis | ± | ± | ± | + | ++ |
| | Renal colic | ± | ± | + | ++ | ++ |
| | Renal failure, chronic | +++ | ++ | ++ | + | + |
| | Urinary infections | ± | ± | ± | ± | ± |
| Other | Failure to thrive | +++ | +++ | +++ | +++ | |
| Laboratory findings | Creatinine (S) | n-↑ | n-↑ | n-↑ | n-↑ | n-↑ |
| | Hematuria | ± | ± | ± | ± | ± |
| | Glycolic acid (P) | n-↑ | n-↑ | n-↑ | n-↑ | n-↑ |
| | Glycolic acid (U) | n-↑ | n-↑ | n-↑ | n-↑ | n-↑ |
| | Oxalic acid (P) | ↑↑ | ↑↑ | ↑↑ | ↑↑ | ↑↑ |
| | Oxalic acid (U) | ↑↑ | ↑↑ | ↑↑ | ↑↑ | ↑↑ |
| | Urea (S) | n-↑ | n-↑ | n-↑ | n-↑ | n-↑ |

**Table 67.5** Glycolate oxidase 1 deficiency

| System | Symptoms and biomarkers | Neonatal (birth–1 month) | Infancy (1–18 months) | Childhood (1.5–11 years) | Adolescence (11–16 years) | Adulthood (>16 years) |
|---|---|---|---|---|---|---|
| CNS | Retardation, psychomotor | ± | ± | ± | ± | ± |
| Eye | **Anisocoria** | ± | ± | ± | ± | ± |
| | **Alacrima** | ± | ± | ± | ± | ± |
| Musculoskeletal | Achalasia | ± | ± | ± | ± | ± |
| Renal | Kidney stones | ± | ± | ± | ± | ± |
| Laboratory findings | Citric acid (urine) | n | n | n | n | n |
| | Glycolic acid (urine) | ↑↑↑ | ↑↑↑ | ↑↑↑ | ↑↑↑ | ↑↑↑ |
| | Glyceric acid (urine) | n | n | n | n | n |
| | Oxalic acid (urine) | n-↑(↑) | n-↑(↑) | n-↑(↑) | n-↑(↑) | n-↑(↑) |

**Table 67.6** Secondary hyperoxaluria

| System | Symptoms and biomarkers | Neonatal (birth–1 month) | Infancy (1–18 months) | Childhood (1.5–11 years) | Adolescence (11–16 years) | Adulthood (>16 years) |
|---|---|---|---|---|---|---|
| Cardiovascular | Cardiomyopathy | | | | | ± |
| | Cardiac oxalate deposition | | | | | ± |
| Dermatological | Calcinosis cutis | | | | | ± |
| | Livedo reticularis | | | | | ± |
| | Pigmentary retinopathy | | | | | |
| Hematological | Pancytopenia | | | | | ± |
| Musculoskeletal | Bone pain | | | | | ± |
| | Derangement of trabecular structure | | | | | ± |
| | Pathological fractures | | | | | ± |
| | Radiolucent metaphyseal bands | | | | | ± |
| Renal | Nephrocalcinosis | ± | ± | ± | ± | ± |
| | Nephrolithiasis | + | + | + | + | + |
| | Renal colic | + | + | + | + | + |
| | Renal failure, chronic | | | | ± | + |
| | Urinary infections | ± | ± | ± | ± | ± |
| Other | Failure to thrive | ± | ± | ± | ± | |
| Laboratory findings | Creatinine (serum) | n-↑ | n-↑ | n-↑ | n-↑ | n-↑ |
| | Citrate (urine) | n-↓ | n-↓ | n-↓ | n-↓ | n-↓ |
| | Hematuria | ± | ± | ± | ± | ± |
| | Oxalic acid (serum) | n-↑ | n-↑ | n-↑ | n-↑ | n-↑ |
| | Oxalic acid (urine) | ↑–↑↑ | ↑–↑↑ | ↑–↑↑ | ↑–↑↑ | ↑–↑↑ |
| | Urea (serum) | n-↑ | n-↑ | n-↑ | n-↑ | n-↑ |

## Reference Values

| Metabolite | Age | Normal value |
|---|---|---|
| Oxalate (U)<br>Glycolate (U)<br>L-Glycerate (U) | All ages | <0.5 mmol<br>(45 mg)/1.73 m²/day<br><0.5 mmol<br>(45 mg)/1.73 m²/day<br><5 µmol/l |
| Oxalate (U, molar creatinine ratio, mmol/mol) | <6 months<br>7 months–2 years<br>2–5 years<br>5–15 years<br>>16 years | <325–360<br><132–174<br><98–101<br><70–82<br><40 |
| Oxalate (P) | | 6.3 ± 1.4 µmol/l |
| Glycolate (U, molar creatinine ratio, mmol/Mol) | <6 months<br>7 months–2 years<br>2–5 years<br>5–15 years<br>>16 years | <363–425<br><245–293<br><191–229<br><166–186<br><99–125 |
| Glycolate (P) | | 7.9 ± 2.4 µmol/l |
| L-Glycerate (U, molar creatinine ratio, mmol/mol) | <6 months<br>7 months–2 years<br>2–5 years<br>5–15 years<br>>16 years | 14–205<br>14–205<br>14–205<br>23–138<br><138 |
| Hydroxy-oxoglutarate (HOG) (U, molar creatinine ratio, µmol/mg) | All age groups | <2.5 |
| Calcium (U) | All age groups | <0.1 mmol/kg body weight/24 h |

## Pathological Values

| Disorder | Oxalate (U) | Oxalate (P) | Glycolate (U) | Glycolate (P) | L-Glycerate (U) | HOG (U) |
|---|---|---|---|---|---|---|
| 67.1 | ↑ | ↑ | ↑ | ↑ | n | n |
| 67.2 | ↑ | ↑ | n | n | ↑ | n |
| 67.3 | ↑ | ↑ | n | n | n | ↑ |

## Diagnostic Flowchart(s)

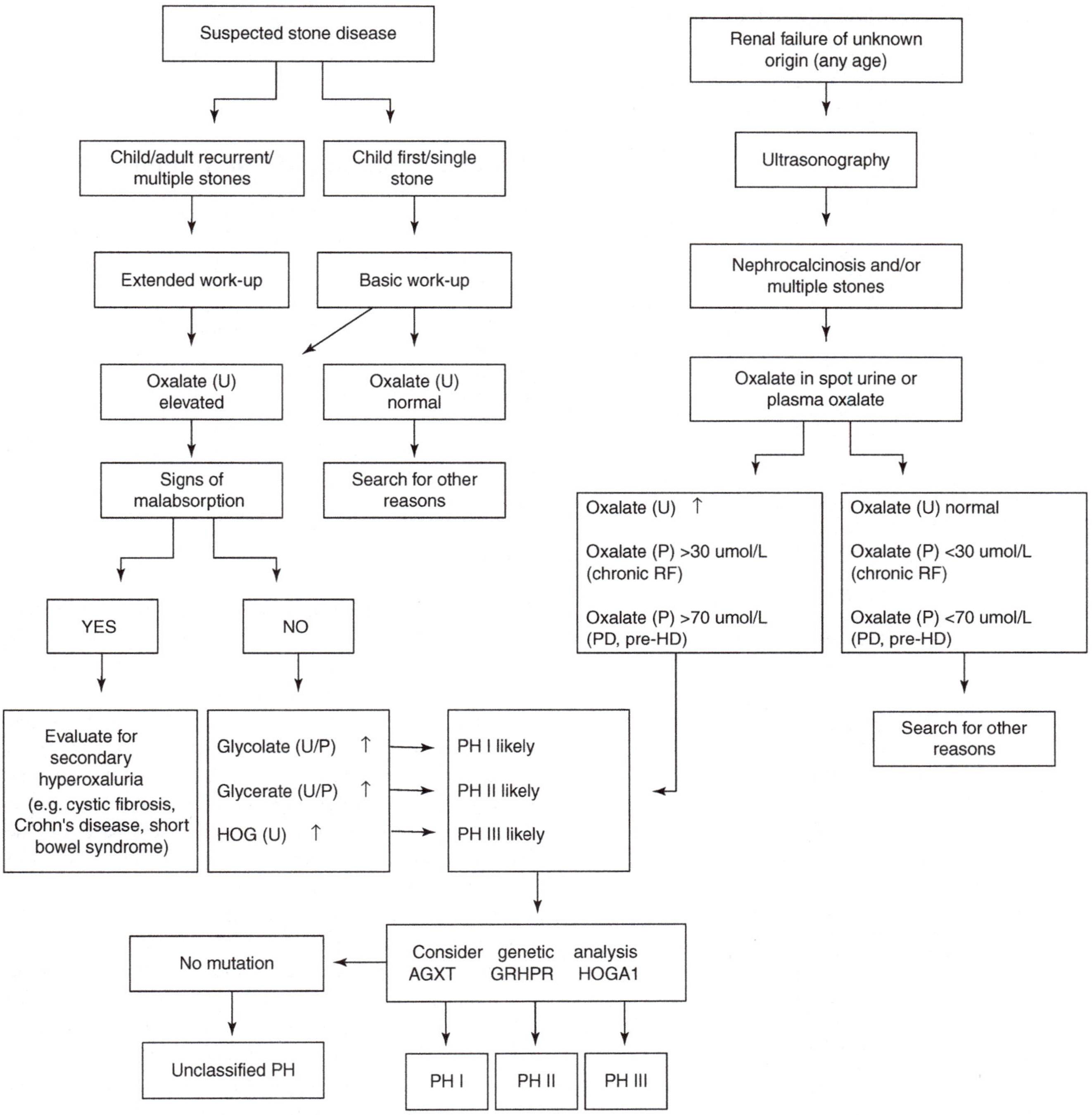


**Fig. 67.2** Flowchart of diagnostic evaluation of hyperoxaluria

## Specimen Collection

| Metabolite | Material | Handling | Pitfalls |
|---|---|---|---|
| Oxalate | Urine | Immediately acidify with 0.02 ml, 6 mol/l HCl/ml to pH < 3. Dilute 20-fold with 0.3 mol/l boric acid | 1. Excess alimentary oxalate or precursors (increased enteral uptake)<br>2. Vitamin B6 deficiency<br>3. Chronic renal failure<br>4. Parenteral nutrition in prematures<br>5. Alkaline pH aids spontaneous formation of oxalate from ascorbate<br>6. Precipitation of oxalate from urine sample before analysis |
| | Blood, heparinized | Keep ice-cold after collection<br>Separate red cells and ultrafilter (cutoff 10,000 Da) 2 ml plasma onto 0.06 ml, 1 mol/l hydrochloric acid/ml. Dilute ultrafiltrate 1:1 with 0.3 mol/l boric acid. All steps at 4 °C. Store at −20 °C until analysis | |
| Glycolate | Urine | Immediately acidify with 0.02 ml, 6 mol/l HCl/ml to pH < 3. Dilute 20-fold with 0.3 mol/l boric acid | |
| | Blood, heparinized | Keep ice-cold after collection<br>Separate red cells and ultrafilter (cutoff 10,000 Da) 2 ml plasma onto 0.06 ml, 1 mol/l hydrochloric acid/ml. Dilute ultrafiltrate 1:1 with boric acid. All steps at 4 °C. Store at −20 °C until analysis | |
| Glycerate | Urine | Immediately acidify with 0.02 ml, 6 mol/l HCl/ml to pH < 3. Dilute 20-fold with 0.3 mol/l boric acid | |
| HOG | Urine | Immediately acidify with 0.02 ml, 6 mol/l HCl/ml to pH < 3. Dilute 20-fold with 0.3 mol/l boric acid | |

## Prenatal Diagnosis and DNA Testing

| | Amniotic fluid metabolites | Fetal liver biopsy (enzyme activity) | CV (enzyme activity) | DNA testing[a] (from CV or biopsy) |
|---|---|---|---|---|
| PH 1 | Non-diagnostic | 2 trimester | 1 and 2 trimester | + |
| PH 2 | Non-diagnostic | | | + |
| PH 3 | Non-diagnostic | | | + |

[a]In PH patients, genomic DNA sequencing or linkage analysis (if an index patient exist)

## Treatment

The management greatly depends on the degree of renal function, especially in PH type I. About one third of patients with PH I respond to pharmacological doses of pyridoxine (Milliner et al. 1994), but the majority of patients only show a decline in urinary oxalate excretion of 30–50% (Hoyer-Kuhn et al. 2014). Normalization of urinary oxalate excretion is only achieved in some patients. In case of renal failure, the waiting time until transplantation must be kept as short as possible, as no form of dialysis is able to keep pace with the extreme amounts of endogenous oxalate production (Hoppe et al. 2008). Thus, systemic oxalosis develops, which greatly reduces the success of transplantation (Jamieson 2005). Isolated kidney transplantation in PH I is only a reasonable option in fully pyridoxine-responsive patients or, perhaps, in older patients. The transplantation treatment of choice in all other patients with PH I is combined liver-kidney transplantation or kidney after liver transplantation in those with a massive burden of systemic oxalate deposition. Preemptive liver transplantation as enzyme replacement therapy may be considered in patients with remaining stable kidney function (GFR >50 ml/min, Nolkemper et al. 2000); however, the timing of the transplantation is considered to be difficult. In PH type II, isolated kidney transplantation is the treatment of choice, as the underlying enzyme defect is not only located within the liver. However, combined liver-kidney transplantation was now also reported in PH II patients with problematic disease courses or after failed isolated kidney transplantation. A report in one adult patient showed that normal urinary oxalate and glycerate levels were achieved after 1-year follow-up (Dhondup et al. 2018). Currently, only two patients with PH III have reached end-stage renal failure (Hopp et al. 2015; Richard et al. 2017), although, to our knowledge, no transplantation has been considered for them to date.

Conservative and palliative measures are mandatory for patients diagnosed with PH. High fluid intake and crystallization inhibitors (sodium-potassium citrate) must be advised as soon as PH (of any type) is diagnosed or even suspected. In the last decade, many innovative therapeutic approaches have emerged aiming to tackle the disease from different perspectives: targeting the hepatic metabolism, the oxalate absorption in the gut, or the renal consequences of CaOx deposition. Currently, four drugs are being evaluated in human clinical trials or has already been licenced:

1. Oxabact® (OxThera AB, Stockholm, Sweden), phase III (NCT03116685): composed of *Oxalobacter formigenes*, a commensal anaerobic bacterium of the human intestinal tract that uses oxalate as its carbon source. Oral administration of Oxabact® reduces oxalate absorption, hence Uox, by activating the intestinal oxalate transporter SLC26A6, thus shifting the blood-lumen gradient concentration of oxalate toward its elimination through the feces (Hoppe et al. 2006; Hoppe et al. 2017). Therefore, Oxabact® would be applicable for all types of PH and secondary hyperoxaluria.
2. Oxlumo® (Lumasiran, Alnylam Pharmaceuticals, Boston, MA, USA), was recently approved from FDA and EMA for treatment of PH I. It is a small interference RNA (siRNA) against the *HAO1* gene, encoding for the liver-specific protein glycolate oxidase (GO). Blockade of GO reduces the formation of glyoxylate, upstream of the metabolic blockade by AGT deficiency, thus reducing the burden of oxalate produced in the liver and excreted through the kidneys (Liebow et al. 2017, Dutta et al. 2016, Martin-Higueras et al. 2016). In principle, this substrate reduction therapy is only useful for PH I patients. In the recently published paper a decline of 65.4% in urinary oxalate excretion was reported and most of the patients reached near-normal urinary oxalate values (Garrelfs et al. 2021).
3. DCR-PHXC/Nedosiran® (Dicerna Pharmaceuticals, Boston, MA, USA), phase II (NCT03847909): hepatic lactate dehydrogenase type V (LDH-A) inhibition by siRNA, which blocks the ultimate conversion of glyoxylate into oxalate, thus being suitable for treating at least PH I and PH II patients (Lai et al. 2018). In the recent PHYOX1 study, the safety and efficacy of medication were shown. A mean maximum reduction of 72% of urinary oxalate excretion was achieved in patients with PH I and of 49% in patients with PH II after a single dose of Nedosiran® (Hoppe et al. 2020). The pivotal trial (PHYOX2) is ongoing, but open label data from a long term follow up study (PHYOX3) of the patients being included in PHYOX1 shows normalization of urinary oxalate excretion in all patients (Coenen et al. 2020).
4. ALLN-177 (Allena Pharmaceuticals, Newton, MA, USA), phase II (NCT03391804): a recombinant oxalate decarboxylase that enzymatically degrades oxalate in the intestinal lumen. Because of an oxalate gradient toward the intestinal lumen, but without any intestinal transporter activation, it may help to secrete blood oxalate, which can then be further metabolized (Langman et al. 2016; Leumann et al. 2016). This medication is currently being evaluated in patients with secondary hyperoxaluria and also PH II and PH III. A recent study showed a 22.6% mean reduction of urinary oxalate excretion in patients with enteric hyperoxaluria (Lieske et al. 2019).

Many other drugs are still under evaluation at preclinical stage using animal models of disease (AAV vectors, CRISPR/Cas9, CRID3, R-7050, stiripentol, huAGT-RHEAM mRNA) (Salido et al. 2011; Le Dudal et al. 2019; Kukreja et al. 2019). Although some drugs may reach the market soon, no curative options are available nowadays beyond combined liver-kidney transplantation.

### PH Type I (AGT Deficiency)

- New RNAi medication available (Oxluma, Alnylam Pharmaceuticals).
- Systematic evaluation of pyridoxine (vitamin B6) treatment, starting with 5 mg/kg body weight/day, increasing every 6 weeks by 5 mg until 20 mg/kg body weight/day, is necessary in all patients (Cochat et al. 2012). Reliable and repeated baseline values for Uox (in normal renal function) or Pox in chronic renal failure are essential. If reduction of Uox or Pox is >30%, continue with dose of best response in B6 trial. If no effect, discontinue pyridoxine. Beware of side effects (e.g., neuropathy).
- Reduce intake of vitamin C, vitamin D, and eventually dietary oxalate.

### PH Type II (GRHPR Deficiency)

- No effect of pyridoxine to be expected.
- Possible benefit of liver transplantation in renal failure.
- Other measures as for PH I.

### PH Type III (HOGA1 Deficiency)

- No benefit of pyridoxine to be expected.
- Only two patients with ESRD reported, but transplant option not yet determined.
- Other measures as for PH I.
- Dietary (low-hydroxyproline, low-oxalate) diet recommendable.

### Oxalate Transporter Deficiencies and Secondary Hyperoxaluria

- Dietary intervention, low-oxalate diet.
- Avoid vitamin C intake.

**Beware: Pitfalls in Hyperoxaluria**

1. Urinary oxalate excretion and oxalate/creatinine ratios are falsely low in renal insufficiency because of oxalate retention.
2. Ascorbic acid is a precursor of oxalate and may interfere with oxalate determination. Vitamin C intake should be avoided.
3. Poor compliance is a serious problem in patients with hyperoxaluria who require long-term therapy.
4. Calcium restriction is contraindicated because it leads to enhanced intestinal oxalate absorption.
5. Renal replacement therapy by dialysis (hemo, peritoneal) should be avoided by all means or, at least, not be extended beyond 6 months in patients with primary hyperoxaluria. No form of dialysis is able to eliminate all oxalate generated; thus ongoing systemic deposition of calcium oxalate is inevitable.

### Standard Protocol for Intercurrent Illness

Make sure patients get a high fluid intake at all times. Early intravenous fluid administration is indicated in case of severe diarrhea, vomiting, infection, and high fever. A medical emergency card with appropriate instructions is recommended for patients going abroad.

## References

Amin R, Asplin J, Jung D, Bashir M, Alshaikh A, Ratakonda S, Sharma S, Jeon S, Granja I, Matern D, Hassan H. Reduced active transcellular intestinal oxalate secretion contributes to the pathogenesis of obesity-associated hyperoxaluria. Kidney Int. 2018;93(5):1098–107.

Beck et al. Pediatric kidney disease. New York: Elsevier/WB Saunders; 2016. pp. 1037–58.

Belostotsky R, Seboun E, Idelson GH, Milliner DS, Becker-Cohen R, Rinat C, Monico CG, Feinstein S, Ben-Shalom E, Magen D, Weissman I, Charon C, Frishberg Y. Mutations in DHDPSL are responsible for primary hyperoxaluria type III. Am J Hum Genet. 2010;87(3):392–9.

Clifford-Mobley O, Rumsby G, Kanodia S, Didi M, Holt R, Senniappan S. Glycolate oxidase deficiency in a patient with congenital hyperinsulinism and unexplained hyperoxaluria. Pediatr Nephrol. 2017;32(11):2159–63.

Cochat P, Hulton SA, Acquaviva C, Danpure CJ, Daudon M, De Marchi M, Fargue S, Groothoff J, Harambat J, Hoppe B, Jamieson NV, Kemper MJ, Mandrile G, Marangella M, Picca S, Rumsby G, Salido E, Straub M, van Woerden CS, OxalEurope. Primary hyperoxaluria Type 1: indications for screening and guidance for diagnosis and treatment. Nephrol Dial Transplant. 2012;27(5):1729–36.

Coenen M, Schalk G, Cochat P, et al. PHYOX3: A long term, open-label extension trial of nedosiran in patients with primary hyperoxaluria type 1, 2, or 3 (abstract). J Am Soc Nephrol 31. 2020;515.

Cregeen DP, Williams EL, Hulton S, Rumsby G. Molecular analysis of the glyoxylate reductase (GRHPR) gene and description of mutations underlying primary hyperoxaluria type 2. Hum Mutat. 2003;22(6):497.

Danpure CJ, Cooper PJ, Wise PJ, Jennings PR. An enzyme trafficking defect in two patients with primary hyperoxaluria type 1: peroxisomal alanine/glyoxylate aminotransferase rerouted to mitochondria. J Cell Biol. 1989;108(4):1345–52.

Dawson PA, et al. Urolithiasis and hepatotoxicity are linked to the anion transporter Sat1 in mice. J Clin Invest. 2010;120(3):706–12.

Dhondup T, Lorenz EC, Milliner DS, Lieske JC. Combined liver-kidney transplantation for primary hyperoxaluria type 2: a case report. Am J Transplant. 2018;18(1):253–7.

Dutta C, Avitahl-Curtis N, Pursell N, Larsson Cohen M, Holmes B, Diwanji R, Zhou W, Apponi L, Koser M, Ying B, Chen D, Shui X, Saxena U, Cyr WA, Shah A, Nazef N, Wang W, Abrams M, Dudek H, Salido E, Brown BD, Lai C. Inhibition of glycolate oxidase with dicer-substrate siRNA reduces calcium oxalate deposition in a mouse model of primary hyperoxaluria type 1. Mol Ther. 2016;24(4):770–8.

Frishberg Y, Zeharia A, Lyakhovetsky R, Bargal R, Belostotsky R. Mutations in HAO1 encoding glycolate oxidase cause isolated glycolic aciduria. J Med Genet. 2014;51(8):526–9.

Garrelfs SF, Frishberg Y, Hulton SA, Koren MJ, O'Riordan WD, Cochat P, Deschênes G, Shasha-Lavsky H, Saland JM, Van't Hoff WG, Fuster DG, Magen D, Moochhala SH, Schalk G, Simkova E, Groothoff JW, Sas DJ, Meliambro KA, Lu J, Sweetser MT, Garg PP, Vaishnaw AK, Gansner JM, McGregor TL, Lieske JC. ILLUMINATE-A Collaborators. Lumasiran, an RNAi Therapeutic for Primary Hyperoxaluria Type 1. N Engl J Med. 2021;384(13):1216–26.

Garrelfs SF, Rumsby G, Peters-Sengers H, Erger F, Groothoff JW, Beck BB, Oosterveld MJS, Pelle A, Neuhaus T, Adams B, Cochat P, Salido E, Lipkin GW, Hoppe B, Hulton SA, OxalEurope Consortium. Patients with primary hyperoxaluria type 2 have significant morbidity and require careful follow-up. Kidney Int. 2019;96(6):1389–99.

Hueppelshaeuser R, von Unruh GE, Habbig S, Beck BB, Buderus S, Hesse A, Hoppe B. Enteric hyperoxaluria, recurrent urolithiasis, and systemic oxalosis in patients with Crohn's disease. Pediatr Nephrol. 2012;27(7):1103–9.

Hopp K, Cogal AG, Bergstralh EJ, Seide BM, Olson JB, Meek AM, Lieske JC, Milliner DS, Harris PC. Rare kidney stone consortium. Phenotype-genotype correlations and estimated carrier frequencies of primary hyperoxaluria. J Am Soc Nephrol. 2015;26(10):2559-70. 2

Hoppe B. An update on primary hyperoxaluria. Nat Rev Nephrol. 2012;8(8):467–75.

Hoppe B, Beck B, Gatter N, von Unruh G, Tischer A, Hesse A, Laube N, Kaul P, Sidhu H. Oxalobacter formigenes: a potential tool for the treatment of primary hyperoxaluria type 1. Kidney Int. 2006;70(7):1305–11.

Hoppe B, Cochat P, Lemoine S, Lipkin G, Gentile AM, Brown BD, Rosskamp R, Hulton S, Groothoff JW, Baum MA. PHYOX: A Safety and Tolerability Study of DCR-PHXC in Primary Hyperoxaluria Types 1 and 2 and outlook of future studies. Abstract GPN 2020.

Hoppe B, Kemper MJ, Bökenkamp A, Portale AA, Cohn RA, Langman CB. Plasma calcium-oxalate supersaturation in children with primary hyperoxaluria and end-stage renal failure. Kidney Int. 1999;56(1):268–74.

Hoppe B, Leumann E, von Unruh G, Laube N, Hesse A. Diagnostic and therapeutic approaches in patients with secondary hyperoxaluria. Front Biosci. 2003;8:e437–43.

Hoppe B, Leumann E, Milliner D. Urolithiasis in childhood. In: Geary D, Schäfer F, editors. Comprehensive Pediatric nephrology. New York: Elsevier/WB Saunders; 2008. p. 499–525.

Hoppe B, Niaudet P, Salomon R, Harambat J, Hulton SA, Van't Hoff W, Moochhala SH, Deschênes G, Lindner E, Sjögren A, Cochat P. A randomised phase I/II trial to evaluate the efficacy and safety of orally administered Oxalobacter formigenes to treat primary hyperoxaluria. Pediatr Nephrol. 2017;32(5):781–90.

Hoyer-Kuhn H, Kohbrok S, Volland R, Franklin J, Hero B, Beck BB, Hoppe B. Vitamin B6 in primary hyperoxaluria I: first prospective trial after 40 years of practice. Clin J Am Soc Nephrol. 2014;9(3):468–77.

Jamieson NV. A 20-year experience of combined liver/kidney transplantation for primary hyperoxaluria (PH1): the European PH1 transplant registry experience 1984-2004. Am J Nephrol. 2005;25(3):282–9. European PHI Transplantation Study Group; Epub 2005 Jun 15

Knauf F, Ko N, Jiang Z, Robertson WG, Van Itallie CM, Anderson JM, Aronson PS. Net intestinal transport of oxalate reflects passive absorption and SLC26A6-mediated secretion. J Am Soc Nephrol. 2011;22(12):2247–55.

Knauf F, Velazquez H, Pfann V, Jiang Z, Aronson PS. Characterization of renal NaCl and oxalate transport in Slc26a6. Am J Physiol Renal Physiol. 2019;316(1):F128–33.

Ko N, Knauf F, Jiang Z, Markovich D, Aronson PS. Sat1 is dispensable for active oxalate secretion in mouse duodenum. Am J Physiol Cell Physiol. 2012;303(1):C52–7.

Kukreja A, Lasaro M, Cobaugh C, Forbes C, Tang JP, Gao X, Martin-Higueras C, Pey AL, Salido E, Sobolov S, Subramanian RR. Systemic alanine Glyoxylate aminotransferase mRNA improves Glyoxylate metabolism in a mouse model of primary Hyperoxaluria type 1. Nucleic Acid Ther. 2019;29(2):104–13.

Kurts C. A crystal-clear mechanism of chronic kidney disease. Kidney Int. 2013;84(5):859–61.

Lai C, Pursell N, Gierut J, Saxena U, Zhou W, Dills M, Diwanji R, Dutta C, Koser M, Nazef N, Storr R, Kim B, Martin-Higueras C, Salido E, Wang W, Abrams M, Dudek H, Brown BD. Specific inhibition of hepatic lactate dehydrogenase reduces oxalate production in mouse models of primary hyperoxaluria. Mol Ther. 2018;26(8):1983–95.

Langman CB, Grujic D, Pease RM, Easter L, Nezzer J, Margolin A, Brettman L. A double-blind, placebo controlled, randomized phase 1 cross-over study with ALLN-177, an orally administered oxalate degrading enzyme. Am J Nephrol. 2016;44(2):150–8.

Le Dudal M, Huguet L, Perez J, Vandermeersch S, Bouderlique E, Tang E, Martori C, Chemaly N, Nabbout R, Haymann JP, Frochot V, Baud L, Deschênes G, Daudon M, Letavernier E. Stiripentol protects against calcium oxalate nephrolithiasis and ethylene glycol poisoning. J Clin Invest. 2019;129(6):2571–7.

Leumann EP, Dietl A, Matasovic A. Urinary oxalate and glycolate excretion in healthy infants and children. Pediatr Nephrol. 2016;4:493–7.

Liebow A, Li X, Racie T, Hettinger J, Bettencourt BR, Najafian N, Haslett P, Fitzgerald K, Holmes RP, Erbe D, Querbes W, Knight J. An investigational RNAi therapeutic targeting glycolate oxidase reduces oxalate production in models of primary hyperoxaluria. J Am Soc Nephrol. 2017;28(2):494–503.

Lieske JC, Lingeman JE, Ferraro PM, Zhang Z,Kausz AT. A phase 3, randomized, placebo-controlled trial of reloxaliase in enteric hyperoxaluria (URIROX-1): clinical characteristics and burden of illness. ASN abstract 2019.

Mandrile G, van Woerden CS, Berchialla P, Beck BB, Acquaviva Bourdain C, Hulton SA, Rumsby G, OxalEurope Consortium. Data from a large European study indicate that the outcome of primary hyperoxaluria type 1 correlates with the AGXT mutation type. Kidney Int. 2014;86(6):1197–204.

Marangella M, Petrarulo M, Vitale C, Cosseddu D, Linari F. Plasma and urine glycolate assays for differentiating the hyperoxaluria syndromes. J Urol. 1992;148:986–9.

Martin-Higueras C, Luis-Lima S, Salido E. Glycolate oxidase is a safe and efficient target for substrate reduction therapy in a mouse model of primary hyperoxaluria type I. Mol Ther. 2016;24(4):719–25.

Milliner DS, Eickholt JT, Bergstralh EJ, Wilson DM, Smith LH. Results of long-term treatment with orthophosphate and pyridoxine in patients with primary hyperoxaluria. N Engl J Med. 1994;331(23):1553-8.

Monico CG, Rossetti S, Belostotsky R, Cogal AG, Herges RM, Seide BM, Olson JB, Bergstrahl EJ, Williams HJ, Haley WE, Frishberg Y, Milliner DS. Primary hyperoxaluria type III gene HOGA1 (formerly DHDPSL) as a possible risk factor for idiopathic calcium oxalate urolithiasis. Clin J Am Soc Nephrol. 2011;6(9):2289–95.

Nolkemper D, Kemper MJ, Burdelski M, Vaismann I, Rogiers X, Broelsch CE, Ganschow R, Müller-Wiefel DE. Long-term results of pre-emptive liver transplantation in primary hyperoxaluria type 1. Pediatr Transplant. 2000;4(3):177–81.

Purdue PE, Allsop J, Isaya G, Rosenberg LE, Danpure CJ. Mistargeting of peroxisomal L-alanine:glyoxylate aminotransferase to mitochondria in primary hyperoxaluria patients depends upon activation of a cryptic mitochondrial targeting sequence by a point mutation. Proc Natl Acad Sci U S A. 1991;88(23):10900–4.

Richard E, Blouin JM, Harambat J, Llanas B, Bouchet S, Acquaviva C, de la Faille R. Late diagnosis of primary hyperoxaluria type III. Ann Clin Biochem. 2017;54(3):406–11.

Robijn S, Hoppe B, Vervaet BA, D'Haese PC, Verhulst A. Hyperoxaluria: a gut-kidney axis? Kidney Int. 2011;80(11):1146–58.

Salido E, Rodriguez-Pena M, Santana A, Beattie SG, Petry H, Torres A. Phenotypic correction of a mouse model for primary hyperoxaluria with adeno-associated virus gene transfer. Mol Ther. 2011;19(5):870–5.

Shrikant RM, Jonathan NE, Jyaysi D, Julian AM, Santhosh VRK, Marc W, Melissa G, Maciej L, Nuru E, Lisa M, Wolfgang H, Martin H de Angelis, Volker V, Hoppe B, Asplin J, Burzlaff N, Herrmann M, Evan A, Anders H.-J. Hyperoxaluria requires TNF receptors to initiate crystal adhesion and kidney stone disease. J Am Soc Nephrol. 2017;28(3):761–68.

van Woerden CS, Groothoff JW, Wanders RJ, Davin JC, Wijburg FA. Primary hyperoxaluria type 1 in The Netherlands: prevalence and outcome. Nephrol Dial Transplant. 2003;18(2):273–9.

Ventzke A, Feldkötter M, Wei A, Becker J, Beck BB, Hoppe B. Systematic assessment of urinary hydroxy-oxo-glutarate for diagnosis and follow-up of primary hyperoxaluria type III. Pediatr Nephrol. 2017;32(12):2263–71. (2018)

Weigert A, Martin-Higueras C, Hoppe B. Novel therapeutic approaches in primary hyperoxaluria. Expert Opin Emerg Drugs. 2018;23(4):349–57.

Whittamore JM, Stephens CE, Hatch M. Absence of the sulfate transporter SAT-1 has no impact on oxalate handling by mouse intestine and does not cause hyperoxaluria or hyperoxalemia. Am J Physiol Gastrointest Liver Physiol. 2019;316(1):G82–94.

Zhao F, Bergstralh EJ, Mehta RA, Vaughan LE, Olson JB, Seide BM, Meek AM, Cogal AG, Lieske JC, Milliner DS. Investigators of Rare Kidney Stone Consortium. Predictors of Incident ESRD among patients with primary hyperoxaluria presenting prior to kidney failure. Clin J Am Soc Nephrol. 2016;11(1):119–26.

# Part X

# Congenital Disorders of Glycosylation

# Congenital Disorders of Glycosylation

# 68

Jaak Jaeken and Lambert van den Heuvel

## Contents




**Summary**

Congenital defects of glycosylation (CDG) are genetic diseases due to deficient glycosylation of glycoconjugates (glycoproteins, glycolipids) and to deficient synthesis of glycosylphosphatidylinositol anchors. Since the first clinical description, in 1980, of patients with a CDG, this disease family has shown an exponential expansion. At least 145 CDG have been reported. They can be divided into five groups: (1) defects in protein N-glycosylation, (2) defects in protein O-glycosylation, (3) defects in lipid glycosylation, (4) defects in multiple glycosylation pathways, and (5) defects in glycosylphosphatidylinositol anchor biosynthesis. In 2009, a novel, transparent CDG nomenclature was introduced that covers all (known and still to be discovered) CDG. It consists of the official gene symbol (unitalicized) followed by "-CDG." The majority of CDG patients show neurological disease associated with variable involvement of nearly all other organs. Only a few CDG are mono-organ diseases (e.g., ALG2-CDG, ALG14-CDG, GFPT1-CDG



J. Jaeken (✉)
Center for Metabolic Disease, University Hospital Gasthuisberg, Leuven, Belgium
e-mail: jaak.jaeken@kuleuven.be

L. van den Heuvel
Institute for Genetic and Metabolic Disease, Nijmegen Medical Centre, Radboud University, Nijmegen, The Netherlands
e-mail: bert.vandenheuvel@uzleuven.be







N. Blau et al. (eds.), *Physician's Guide to the Diagnosis, Treatment, and Follow-Up of Inherited Metabolic Diseases*,
https://doi.org/10.1007/978-3-030-67727-5_68

(retina), EXT1/EXT2-CDG (cartilage), GNE-CDG (skeletal muscles), POFUT1-CDG (skin), POGLUT1-CDG (skin or skeletal muscles), SEC23B-CDG (erythrocytes), ST3GAL3-CDG (brain), TMEM199-CDG (liver), TUSC3-CDG (brain)). The known CDG present autosomal recessive inheritance except for ALG13-CDG, ATP6AP1-CDG, MAGT1-CDG, PIGA-CDG, SLC35A2-CDG, and SSR4-CDG (X-linked) and EXT1/EXT2-CDG, GANAB-CDG, POFUT1-CDG, POGLUT1-CDG, and PRKCSH-CDG (autosomal dominant). Some CDG can be diagnosed clinically such as EXT1/EXT2-CDG and the typical PMM2-CDG presentation. Two screening techniques are available: serum transferrin isoelectrofocusing (or similar techniques such as capillary zone electrophoresis) for the diagnosis of protein N-glycosylation disorders associated with sialic acid deficiency and serum apolipoprotein C-III isoelectrofocusing for the diagnosis of core 1 mucin-type O-glycans. Treatment possibilities are still frustratingly limited. An efficient therapy is available for only two CDG, namely, oral mannose for MPI-CDG and oral uridine for CAD-CDG. Since about 1–2% of the human genome is involved in glycosylation, it appears that a substantial number of CDG have still to be discovered. Elucidation of the basic defects of these CDG will increasingly require next-generation sequencing techniques such as whole exome and whole genome sequencing. Metabolomics and glycomics technology will reveal novel insights into the molecular basis of CDG.

## Introduction

Congenital disorders of glycosylation (CDG) are genetic diseases caused by defective glycosylation of glycoproteins and glycolipids and defective synthesis of glycosylphosphatidylinositol anchors (reviews in Abu Bakar et al. (2018), Ferreira et al. (2018), Jaeken and Péanne (2017), Ng and Freeze (2018); reviews on specific aspects of CDG in Coman et al. (2008) (skeleton), Francisco et al. (2018b), Morava et al. (2009) (eyes), Marques-da-Silva et al. (2017b) (heart), Marques-da-Silva et al. (2017a) (liver), Monticelli et al. (2016) (immune system)). A novel CDG nomenclature was recently introduced that covers all (known and still to be discovered) CDG. It consists of the official gene symbol (unitalicized) followed by "-CDG" (Jaeken et al. 2009). Among the 145 known CDG, 118 are disorders of glycoprotein glycosylation. This CDG group comprises disorders of N-glycosylation, disorders of O-glycosylation, and disorders with a combined N- and O-glycosylation defect. C-Glycosylation defects have not yet been reported. The N-glycosylation pathway encompasses three cellular compartments: the cytosol, the endoplasmic reticulum (ER), and the Golgi. It starts in the cytosol with the formation of the mannose donor GDP-mannose from fructose 6-phosphate, an intermediate of the glycolytic pathway. In the ER, the dolichol-linked oligosaccharide $GlcNAc_2Man_9Glc_3$ is assembled and subsequently transferred from dolichol to selected asparagines of nascent proteins. Still in the ER, this glycan starts to be processed by trimming off the three glucoses. This processing is continued in the Golgi by trimming off six mannoses and replacing them by two residues each of N-acetylglucosamine, galactose and finally sialic acid. O-Glycosylation is usually limited to the Golgi and has no processing pathway. The O-glycans are linked to the hydroxyl group of selected threonine and serine residues.

The first report on CDG was on patients who were subsequently shown to have an N-glycosylation disorder, phosphomannomutase 2 deficiency (PMM2-CDG) (Jaeken et al. 1980; Van Schaftingen and Jaeken 1995; Matthijs et al. 1997). It is a cytosolic assembly defect and turned out to be, by far, the most frequent N-glycosylation disorder with around 900 patients known worldwide. They show mild to severe neurological disease and variable involvement of many other organs. Dysmorphism ranges from mild and aspecific to a characteristic abnormal subcutaneous adipose tissue distribution with fat pads and nipple retraction. Mortality is about 20% in the first years of life (review in Grünewald 2009). The second most frequent N-glycosylation disorder is an ER assembly defect, glucosyltransferase 1 deficiency (ALG6-CDG). It is mainly a neurological disorder but usually milder than that of PMM2-CDG, with limb anomalies in some 10% of these patients (92 patients reported) (review in Morava et al. 2016). The third most reported N-glycosylation disorder is ALG1-CDG with 58 patients, also a predominant neurological disease (review in Ng et al. 2016). The fourth place is occupied by two CDG, on the one hand MAN1B1-CDG and on the other mannose phosphate isomerase deficiency (MPI-CDG), each with around 40 reported patients. MPI-CDG (review in Jaeken et al. 2014) is a remarkable disorder not only because of its pure hepatic-intestinal presentation but particularly because it is one of only two, more or less efficiently, treatable CDG (with oral mannose). The other is CAD-CDG, a defect in pyrimidine biosynthesis causing a deficiency in uridine diphosphate (UDP) (Koch et al. 2017). UDP monosaccharides are necessary for the transport of monosaccharides into the Golgi.

The protein N-glycosylation disorders can be divided into three groups: (1) defects in nucleotide-sugar biosynthesis (e.g., PMM2-CDG, MPI-CDG), (2) defects in lipid-linked oligosaccharide biosynthesis (e.g., DPAGT1-CDG, ALG1-CDG), and (3) defects in protein-linked oligosaccharide biosynthesis (e.g., MAN1B1-CDG, MGAT2-CDG).

A number of protein N-glycosylation disorders are associated with a protein O-glycosylation defect. These comprise defects in dolichol phosphate biosynthesis (e.g., DK1-CDG, SRD5A3-CDG), in dolichol phosphomannose synthesis (e.g., DPM1-CDG, DPM3-CDG), in dolichol phosphomannose utilization (MPDU1-CDG), in galactosylation (B4GALT1-CDG), in sialylation (SLC35A1-CDG), in fucosylation (SLC35C1-CDG), in ER-Golgi intermediate compartment proteins (SEC23B-CDG), and in other vesicular transport proteins (e.g., COG-CDG, ATP6V0A2-CDG). The latter two groups comprise defects in proteins that are not only involved in glycosylation but also in other functions (such as Golgi pH regulation). It has been proposed to name them "CDG-plus."

The protein O-glycosylation disorders can be divided on the basis of the monosaccharide which links the glycan to the protein. Seven groups have been described: (1) defects in O-xylosylglycan synthesis (e.g., XYLT1-CDG, B4GALT7-CDG, EXT1/EXT2-CDG, CHSY1-CDG); (2) defect in O-*N*-acetylglucosaminylglycan synthesis (EOGT-CDG); (3) defect in O-*N*-acetylgalactosaminylglycan synthesis (GALNT3-CDG); (4) defect in O-xylosyl/*N*-acetylgalactosaminylglycan synthesis (SLC35D1-CDG); (5) defects in O-mannosylglycan synthesis (e.g., POMT1/POMT2-CDG, POMGNT1-CDG, B3GALNT2-CDG, LARGE-CDG); (6) defects in O-fucosylglycan synthesis (POFUT1-CDG, B3GALTL-CDG, LFNG-CDG); and (7) defect in O-glucosylglycan synthesis (POGLUT1-CDG). Several of these diseases have also a descriptive name, based on their typical clinical presentation: multiple cartilaginous exostoses (EXT1/EXT2-CDG), familial tumoral calcinosis (GALNT3-CDG), Schneckenbecken dysplasia (SLC35D1-CDG), muscle-eye-brain disease (POMGNT1-CDG, POMT1/POMT2-CDG), and spondylocostal dysostosis type 3 (LFNG-CDG).

Most CDG present an autosomal recessive inheritance. ALG13-CDG, ATP6AP1-CDG, MAGT1-CDG, PIGA-CDG, SLC35A2-CDG, and SSR4-CDG are X-linked, and EXT1/EXT2-CDG, GANAB-CDG, POFUT1-CDG, POGLUT1-CDG, and PRKCSH-CDG display an autosomal dominant inheritance.

Essentially two techniques are available for CDG screening: serum transferrin isoelectrofocusing (IEF) detects protein N-glycosylation disorders associated with sialic acid deficiency (Jaeken et al. 1984), and serum apolipoprotein C-III IEF detects core 1 mucin-type O-glycosylation defects (Wopereis et al. 2003). Serum transferrin IEF can be replaced by other techniques such as capillary zone electrophoresis (Carchon et al. 2004). Serum transferrin IEF detects only about 50% of the known CDG. It does not pick up the O-glycosylation disorders that are not associated with an N-glycosylation defect, the lipid glycosylation defects, and the glycosylphosphatidylinositol (GPI) anchor synthesis defects, as well as defects in the N-glycosylation pathway that do not show a deficiency of sialic acid (PMM2-CDG due to a promotor defect, GMPPA-CDG, GMPPB-CDG, TUSC3-CDG, MOGS-CDG, GANAB-CDG, PRKCSH-CDG, FUT8-CDG, GNE-CDG, NANS-CDG, DHDDS-CDG, SLC35A1-CDG, SLC35A3-CDG, SLC35C1-CDG, SEC23B-CDG, PGM3-CDG). In case of an abnormal transferrin IEF profile, first an artifact, a protein polymorphism, and a secondary CDG (fructosemia, galactosemia, alcohol abuse, bacterial sialidase) should be excluded. Two types of abnormal transferrin IEF profiles can be distinguished: a type 1 pattern, characterized by an increase of di- and/or asialoprotein (CDG-I), and a type 2 pattern, characterized by an increase of tri-, di-, mono-, and/or asialoprotein (CDG-II). A type 1 pattern points to an assembly or transfer defect of the dolichol-linked glycan (in the cytosol or the ER). When there is a typical PMM2-CDG or MPI-CDG phenotype, measurement of the phosphomannomutase or mannose phosphate isomerase activity in fibroblasts or leukocytes is the next step, or direct mutation analysis of the involved genes. If there is no typical phenotype, next-generation sequencing (CDG gene panel analysis, WES, or WGS) is indicated. A type 2 pattern indicates a glycan processing defect (in the ER or the Golgi). If this is associated with a typical MAN1B1-CDG, MGAT2-CDG, or PGM1-CDG phenotype, mutation analysis is indicated, preceded or not by structural analysis of serum transferrin glycans. In the absence of a typical phenotype, CDG gene panel analysis, WES, or WGS should be performed. In order to know whether there is an associated O-glycosylation defect, apolipoprotein C-III IEF can be performed. When there is a normal serum transferrin IEF pattern but a strong clinical and/or biochemical suspicion (e.g., fat pads, cerebellar hypoplasia, and decreased coagulation factor XI (PMM2-CDG); intellectual disability with increased serum alkaline phosphatases (GPI anchor synthesis defect)), mutation analysis of the suspected gene or next-generation sequencing (using gene panels, WES, and/or WGS) should be performed (Francisco et al. 2018a).

The nomenclature and signs and symptoms tables are limited in this article to 124 CDG, namely, 30 disorders of N-linked glycosylation, 16 disorders of O-mannosylglycan synthesis, 1 disorder of O-*N*-acetylgalactosaminylglycan synthesis, 2 disorders of O-*N*-acetylglucosaminylglycan synthesis, 1 disorder of O-glucosylglycan synthesis, 2 disorders of O-fucosylglycan synthesis, 1 disorder of a galactosyltransferase-specific chaperone, 8 disorders of dolichol metabolism, 4 disorders of monosaccharide synthesis and interconversion, 1 disorders of nucleotide-sugar synthesis, 6 disorders of Golgi transport, 1 disorder of plasma membrane transport, 8 disorders of Golgi homeostasis, 24 disorders of glycosaminoglycan synthesis, and 19 GPI anchor synthesis disorders. N-Glycanase 1 deficiency (68.125) is not a CDG but a congenital disorder of deglycosylation (CDDG).

## Nomenclature

| No. | Disorder | Alternative names | Gene symbol | Chromosomal localization | Mode of inheritance | Affected protein | OMIM |
|---|---|---|---|---|---|---|---|
| 68.1 | PMM2-CDG | Phosphomannomutase 2 deficiency | *PMM2* | 16p13.2 | AR | Phosphomannomutase 2 | 601785 |
| 68.2 | MPI-CDG | Phosphomannose isomerase deficiency | *MPI* | 15q24.1 | AR | Phosphomannose isomerase | 602579 |
| 68.3 | DPAGT1-CDG | UDP-GlcNAc:Dol-P-GlcNac-P transferase deficiency | *DPAGT1* | 11q23.3 | AR | UDP-GlcNAc:dolichol-phosphate-N-Acetylglucosamine-1-phosphotransferase | 608093 |
| 68.4 | ALG13-CDG | X-linked recessive UDP-N-acetylglucosamine transferase catalytic subunit deficiency | *ALG13* | Xq23 | XLR | UDP-GlcNAc:dolichol pyrophosphate N-acetylglucosamine transferase (cytosolic) | 300884 |
| 68.5 | ALG13-CDG | X-linked dominant UDP-N-acetylglucosamine transferase catalytic subunit deficiency | *ALG13* | Xq23 | XLD | UDP-GlcNAc:dolichol pyrophosphate N-acetylglucosamine transferase (cytosolic) | 300884 |
| 68.6 | ALG14-CDG | UDP-N-acetylglucosamine transferase anchoring subunit deficiency | *ALG14* | 1p21.3 | AR | UDP-GlcNAc:dolichol pyrophosphate N-acetylglucosamine transferase (membrane-bound) | 616227, 612866 |
| 68.7 | ALG1-CDG | Mannosyltransferase 1 deficiency | *ALG1* | 16p13.3 | AR | GDP-Man:GlcNAc2-PP-dolichol mannosyltransferase | 608540 |
| 68.8 | ALG2-CDG | Mannosyltransferase 2 deficiency | *ALG2* | 9q22.33 | AR | GDP-mannose:Man1GlcNAc2-PP-dolichol mannosyltransferase | 607906 |
| 68.9 | ALG11-CDG | Mannosyltransferase 4–5 deficiency | *ALG11* | 13q14.3 | AR | GDP-Man:Man3-4GlcNAc2-PP-dolichol mannosyltransferase | 613661 |
| 68.10 | RFT1-CDG | Flippase of Man5GlcNAc2-PP-Dol deficiency | *RFT1* | 3p21.1 | AR | Flippase of Man5GlcNAc2-PP-Dol | 612015 |
| 68.11 | ALG3-CDG | Mannosyltransferase 6 deficiency | *ALG3* | 3q27.1 | AR | Dolichol-P-mannose: Man5GlcNAc2-PP-dolichol mannosyltransferase | 601110 |
| 68.12 | ALG9-CDG | Mannosyltransferase 7–9 deficiency | *ALG9* | 11q23.1 | AR | Dolichol-P-mannose:α1,2 mannosyltransferase | 608776 |
| 68.13 | ALG12-CDG | Mannosyltransferase 8 deficiency | *ALG12* | 22q13.33 | AR | Dolichol-P-mannose: Man7GlcNAc2-PP-dolichol mannosyltransferase | 607143 |
| 68.14 | ALG6-CDG | Glucosyltransferase 1 deficiency | *ALG6* | 1p22.3 | AR | Dolichol-P-glucose:Man9GlcNAc2-PP-dolichol glucosyltransferase | 603147 |
| 68.15 | ALG8-CDG | Glucosyltransferase 2 deficiency | *ALG8* | 11q14.1 | AR | Dolichol-P-glucose: Glc1Man9GlcNAc2-PP-dolichol- α1,3-glucosyltransferase | 608104 |
| 68.16 | TUSC3-CDG | Oligosaccharyltransferase subunit TUSC3 deficiency | *TUSC3* | TUSC3 | AR | Subunit N33-TUSC3 of the OST complex | 611093 |
| 68.17 | DDOST-CDG | Oligosaccharyltransferase subunit DDOST deficiency | *DDOST* | 1p36.12 | AR | Subunit DDOST of the OST complex | 614507, 602202 |
| 68.18 | STT3A-CDG | Oligosaccharyltransferase subunit STT3A deficiency | *STT3A* | 11q24.2 | AR | Subunit STT3A of the OST complex | 615596, 601134 |
| 68.19 | STT3B-CDG | Oligosaccharyltransferase subunit STT3B deficiency | *STT3B* | 3p23 | AR | Subunit STT3B of the OST complex | 615597 |

| No. | Disorder | Alternative names | Gene symbol | Chromosomal localization | Mode of inheritance | Affected protein | OMIM |
|---|---|---|---|---|---|---|---|
| 68.20 | MAGT1-CDG | Magnesium transporter 1 deficiency | *MAGT1* | Xq21.1 | XL | Magnesium transporter 1 | 300716, 300853 |
| 68.21 | SSR4-CDG | Translocon-associated protein δ subunit deficiency | *SSR4* | Xq28 | XL | Signal sequence receptor 4 protein of the TRAP complex | 300934 |
| 68.22 | MOGS-CDG | Glucosidase 1 deficiency | *MOGS* | 2p13.1 | AR | Endoplasmic reticulum glucosidase I | 606056 |
| 68.23 | GANAB-CDG | Polycyctic kidney disease 3 | *GANAB* | 11q12.3 | AD | Alpha subunit of glucosidase II | 600666 |
| 68.24 | PRKCSH-CDG | α-1,3-glucosidase II subunit β deficiency | PRKCSH | 19p13.2 | AD | Protein kinase C substrate, 80-KD, heavy chain | 174050 |
| 68.25 | MAN1B1-CDG | Mental retardation, autosomal recessive 15 | *MAN1B1* | 9q34.3 | AR | Endoplasmic reticulum 1,2-α-mannosidase | 614202, 604346 |
| 68.26 | MGAT2-CDG | N-acetylglucosaminyl-transferase 2 deficiency | *MGAT2* | 14q21.3 | AR | Golgi N-acetyl-glucosaminyltransferase II | 212066 |
| 68.27 | B4GALT1-CDG | Beta-1,4-galactosyltransferase 1 deficiency | *B4GALT1* | 9p21.1 | AR | Beta-1,4-galactosyltransferase 1 | 607091 |
| 68.28 | FUT8-CDG | α-1,6-fucosyltransferase deficiency | *FUT8* | 14q23.3 | AR | Fucosyltransferase 8 | 602589 |
| 68.29 | POMT1-CDG | Protein O-mannosyltransferase 1 deficiency | *POMT1* | 9q34.13 | AR | O-mannosyltransferase 1 | 236670, 613555, 609308 |
| 68.30 | POMT2-CDG | Protein O-mannosyltransferase 2 deficiency | *POMT2* | 14q24.3 | AR | O-mannosyltransferase 2 | 613150, 613156, 613158 |
| 68.31 | POMGNT1-CDG | O-mannose beta-1,2-N-acetyglucosaminyltrans-ferase deficiency | *POMGNT1* | 1p34.1 | AR | O-Mannose beta-1,2-N-acetyglucosaminyltrans-ferase | 253280, 613151, 613157 |
| 68.32 | POMGNT2-CDG | O-mannose β-1,4-N-acetylglucosaminyltrans-ferase deficiency | *POMGNT2* | 3p22.1 | AR | Protein O-mannose beta-1,4-N-acetylglucosaminyl-transferase 2 | 614830 |
| 68.33 | B3GALNT2-CDG | β-1,3-galactosaminyltransferase 2 deficiency | *B3GALNT2* | 1q42.3 | AR | Beta-1,3-N-acetylgalactos-aminyltransferase 2 | 615181 |
| 68.34 | POMK-CDG | O-mannose kinase deficiency | *POMK* | 8p11.21 | AR | Protein-O-mannose kinase | 616094; 615249 |
| 68.35 | CRPPA-CDG | Methylerythritol 4-phosphate cytidylyltransferase deficiency | *CRPPA* | 7p21.2 | AR | 2-C-methyl-D-erythritol 4-phosphate cytidylyltransferase | |
| 68.36 | FKTN-CDG A | Fukutin type A deficiency | *FKTN* | 9q31.2 | AR | Fukutin | 253800 |
| 68.37 | FKTN-CDG B | Fukutin type B deficiency | *FKTN* | 9q31.3 | AR | Fukutin | 613152 |
| 68.38 | FKTN-CDG C | Fukutin limb-girdle type C deficiency | *FKTN* | 9q31.4 | AR | Fukutin | 611588 |
| 68.39 | FKRP-CDG A | FKRP type A deficiency | *FKRP* | 19q13.32 | AR | Fukutin-related protein | 613153 |
| 68.40 | FKRP-CDG B | FKRP type B deficiency | *FKRP* | 19q13.33 | AR | Fukutin-related protein | 606612 |
| 68.41 | FKRP-CDG C | FKRP limb-girdle type C deficiency | *FKRP* | 19q13.34 | AR | Fukutin-related protein | 606596 |
| 68.42 | RXYLT1-CDG | Ribitol β1,4-xylosyltransferase deficiency | *RXYLT1* | 12q14.2 | AR | Ribitol β1,4-xylosyltransferase | 615041 |
| 68.43 | B4GAT1-CDG | β-1,4-glucuronyltransferase 1 deficiency | *B4GAT1* | 11q13.2 | AR | Beta-1,4-glucuronyltransferase 1 | 615287 |
| 68.44 | LARGE1-CDG | β-1,3-glucuronyltransferase/α-1,3-xylosytransferase deficiency | *LARGE1* | 22q12.3 | AR | Acetylglucosaminyltransfer-ase-like protein | 613154; 608840 |

(continued)

| No. | Disorder | Alternative names | Gene symbol | Chromosomal localization | Mode of inheritance | Affected protein | OMIM |
|---|---|---|---|---|---|---|---|
| 68.45 | XYLT1-CDG | Xylosyltransferase 1 deficiency | *XYLT1* | 16p12.3 | AR | Xylosyltransferase 1 | 615777 |
| 68.46 | XYLT2-CDG | Xylosyltransferase 2 deficiency | *XYLT2* | 17q21.33 | AR | Xylosyltransferase 2 | 605822 |
| 68.47 | B4GALT7-CDG | β-1,4-galactosyltransferase 7 deficiency | *B4GALT7* | 5q35.3 | AR | Golgi UDP-galactose:N-acetylglucosamine β-1,4-galactosyltransferase | 130070 |
| 68.48 | B3GALT6-CDG | β-1,3-galactosyltransferase 6 deficiency | *B3GALT6* | 1p36.33 | AR | Beta-1,3-galactosyltransferase 6 | 271640; 615349 |
| 68.49 | B3GAT3-CDG | β-1,3-glucuronyltransferase 3 deficiency | *B3GAT3* | 11q12.3 | AR | Beta-1,3-glucuronyltransferase 3 | 245600 |
| 68.50 | EXT1-CDG | Exostosin 1 deficiency | *EXT1* | 8q24.11 | AD | Exostosin glycosyltransferase 1 | 133700 |
| 68.51 | EXT2-CDG | Exostosin 2 deficiency | *EXT2* | 11p11.2 | AD | Exostosin glycosyltransferase 2 | 133701 |
| 68.52 | EXT2-CDG | Autosomal recessive exostosin 2 deficiency | *EXT2* | 11p11.2 | AR | Exostosin glycosyltransferase 2 | 616682 |
| 68.53 | EXTL3-CDG | Exostosin-like glycosyltransferase 3 deficiency | *EXTL3* | 8p21.1 | AR | Exostosin-like glycosyltransferase 3 | 617425 |
| 68.54 | CHSY1-CDG | Chondroitin sulfate synthase 1 deficiency | *CHSY1* | 15q26.3 | AR | Chondroitin sulfate synthase 1 | 605282 |
| 68.55 | CHST11-CDG | Chondroitin 4-sulfotransferase 1 deficiency | *CHST11* | 12q23.3 | AR | Carbohydrate sulfotransferase 11 | 610128 |
| 68.56 | CHST3-CDG | Chondroitin 6-sulfotransferase deficiency | *CHST3* | 10q22.1 | AR | Chondroitin 6-sulfotransferase 3 | 143095 |
| 68.57 | CHST14-CDG | Dermatan 4-sulfotransferase 1 deficiency | *CHST14* | 15q15.1 | AR | Carbohydrate sulfotransferase 14 | 601776 |
| 68.58 | DSE-CDG | Dermatan sulfate epimerase deficiency | *DSE* | 6q22.1 | AR | Dermatan sulfate epimerase | 615539 |
| 68.59 | CSGALNACT1-CDG | Chondroitin sulfate N-acetylgalactosaminyl-transferase 1 deficiency | *CSGALN-ACT1* | 8p21.3 | AR | Chondroitin sulfate N-acetylgalactosaminyl-transferase 1 | 616615 |
| 68.60 | CHST6-CDG | Corneal N-acetylglucosamine 6-O-sulfotransferase deficiency | *CHST6* | 16q23.1 | AR | N-Acetylglucosamine 6-O-sulfotransferase | 217800 |
| 68.61 | NDST1-CDG | Heparan sulfate N-deacetylase/N-sulfotransferase 1 deficiency | *NDST1* | 5q33.1 | AR | N-deacetylase/N-sulfotransferase 1 | 616116 |
| 68.62 | HS6ST1-CDG | Heparan sulfate 6-O-sulfate transferase 1 deficiency | *HS6ST1* | 2q14.3 | AD | Heparan sulfate 6-O-sulfotransferase 1 | 614880 |
| 68.63 | CANT1-CDG | Calcium-activated nucleotidase 1 deficiency | *CANT1* | 17q25.3 | AR | Calcium-activated nucleotidase 1 | 251450; 617719 |
| 68.64 | SLC26A2-CDG | Sulfate transporter deficiency | *SLC26A2* | 5q32 | AR | Solute carrier family 26 (sulfate transporter), member 2 | 226900; 222600; 256050; 600972 |

| No. | Disorder | Alternative names | Gene symbol | Chromosomal localization | Mode of inheritance | Affected protein | OMIM |
|---|---|---|---|---|---|---|---|
| 68.65 | PAPSS2-CDG | Phosphoadenosine 5′-phosphosulfate synthetase 2 deficiency | *PAPSS2* | 10q23.2-q23.3 | AR | 3-Prime-phosphoadenosine 5-prime-phosphosulfate synthase 2 | 612847 |
| 68.66 | IMPAD1-CDG | Inositol monophosphate domain-containing protein 1 deficiency | *IMPAD1* | 8q12.1 | AR | Inositol monophosphatase domain-containing protein 1 | 614078 |
| 68.67 | TGDS-CDG | TDP-D-glucose 4,6-dehydrogenase deficiency | *TGDS* | 13q32.1 | AR | TDP-D-glucose 4,6-dehydrogenase | 616145 |
| 68.68 | GALTNT3-CDG | Polypeptide N-acetyl-galactosaminyltransferase 3 deficiency | *GALNT3* | 2q24.3 | AR | Polypeptide N-acetylgalactosaminyltransferase 3 | 211900 |
| 68.69 | C1GATLT1C1-CDG | Core 1 β-1,3-galactosyltransferase chaperone deficiency | *C1GALT1C1* | Xq24 | XL | C1GALT1-specific chaperone 1 | 300622 |
| 68.70 | OGT-CDG | O-linked N-acetylglucosamine transferase deficiency | *OGT* | Xq13.1 | XL | O-linked N-acetylglucosamine transferase | 300997 |
| 68.71 | EOGT-CDG | Adams-Oliver syndrome type 4 | *EOGT* | 3p14.1 | AR | EGF domain-specific O-linked N-acetylglucosamine transferase | 615297 |
| 68.72 | POGLUT1-CDG | Muscular dystrophy, limb-girdle, type 2Z | *POGLUT1* | 3q13.33 | AR | Endoplasmic reticulum O-glucosyltransferase | 617232 |
| 68.73 | POGLUT2-CDG | Dowling-Degos disease 4 | *POGLUT2* | 3q13.34 | AR | Endoplasmic reticulum O-glucosyltransferase | 615696 |
| 68.74 | POFUT1-CDG | Protein O-fucosyltransferase deficiency | *POFUT1* | 20q11.21 | AD | Protein o-fucosyltransferase 1 | 615327 |
| 68.75 | LFNG-CDG | O-fucose-specific beta-1,3-N-acetylglucosaminyltransferase deficiency | *LFNG* | 7p22.3 | AR | O-Fucose-specific beta-1,3-N-acetylglucosaminyl-transferase | 609813 |
| 68.76 | B3GLCT-CDG | O-fucose-specific beta-1,3-N-glucosyltransferase deficiency | *B3GLCT* | 13q12.3 | AR | O-Fucose-specific beta-1,3-N-glucosyltransferase | 261540 |
| 68.77 | PIGA-CDG | PIGA deficiency | *PIGA* | Xp22.2 | XL | Phosphatidylinositol glycan anchor biosynthesis class A protein | 300868; 300818 |
| 68.78 | PIGC-CDG | PIGC deficiency | *PIGC* | 1q24.3 | AR | Phosphatidylinositol glycan anchor biosynthesis class C protein | 617816 |
| 68.79 | PIGQ-CDG | PIGQ deficiency | *PIGQ* | 16p13.3 | AR | Phosphatidylinositol glycan anchor biosynthesis class Q protein | 618548 |
| 68.80 | PIGP-CDG | PIGP deficiency | *PIGP* | 21q22.13 | AR | Phosphatidylinositol glycan anchor biosynthesis class P protein | 617599 |
| 68.81 | PIGY-CDG | PIGY deficiency | *PIGY* | 1p36.11 | AR | Phosphatidylinositol glycan anchor biosynthesis class Y protein | 239300 |
| 68.82 | PIGH-CDG | PIGH deficiency | *PIGH* | 14q24.1 | AR | Phosphatidylinositol glycan anchor biosynthesis class H protein | 618010 |

(continued)

| No. | Disorder | Alternative names | Gene symbol | Chromosomal localization | Mode of inheritance | Affected protein | OMIM |
|---|---|---|---|---|---|---|---|
| 68.83 | PIGL-CDG | PIGL deficiency | *PIGL* | 17p11.2 | AR | Phosphatidylinositol glycan anchor biosynthesis class L protein | 280000 |
| 68.84 | PIGW-CDG | PIGW deficiency | *PIGW* | 17q12 | AR | Phosphatidylinositol glycan anchor biosynthesis class W protein | 616025 |
| 68.85 | PIGM-CDG | PIGM deficiency | *PIGM* | 1q23.2 | AR | Phosphatidylinositol glycan anchor biosynthesis class M protein | 610293 |
| 68.86 | PIGV-CDG | PIGV deficiency | *PIGV* | 1p36.11 | AR | Phosphatidylinositol glycan anchor biosynthesis class V protein | 239300 |
| 68.87 | PIGN-CDG | PIGN deficiency | *PIGN* | 18q21.33 | AR | Phosphatidylinositol glycan anchor biosynthesis class N protein | 614080 |
| 68.88 | PIGO-CDG | PIGO deficiency | *PIGO* | 9p13.3 | AR | Phosphatidylinositol glycan anchor biosynthesis class O protein | 614749 |
| 68.89 | PIGG-CDG | PIGG deficiency | *PIGG* | 4p16.3 | AR | Glycosylphosphatidylinositol glycan anchor biosynthesis G protein | 616917 |
| 68.90 | PIGT-CDG | PIGT deficiency | *PIGT* | 20q13.12 | AR | Phosphatidylinositol glycan anchor biosynthesis class T protein | 615398 |
| 68.91 | GPAA1-CDG | GPAA1 deficiency | *GPAA1* | 8q24.3 | AR | Glycosylphosphatidylinositol anchor attachment protein 1 | 617810 |
| 68.92 | PGAP1-CDG | PGAP1 deficiency | *PGAP1* | 2q33.1 | AR | GPI deacylase | 615802 |
| 68.93 | PGAP3-CDG | PGAP3 deficiency | *PGAP3* | 17q12 | AR | PER1-like domain-containing protein 1 | 615716 |
| 68.94 | PGAP2-CDG | PGAP2 deficiency | *PGAP2* | 11p15.4 | AR | Post-gpi attachment to proteins 2 | 614207 |
| 68.95 | PIGS-CDG | PIGS deficiency | *PIGS* | 17q11.2 | AR | Phosphatidylinositol glycan anchor biosynthesis class S protein | 618143 |
| 68.96 | DHDDS-CDG | Dehydrodolichyl diphosphate synthase deficiency | *DHDDS* | 1p36.11 | AR | Dehydrodolichyl diphosphate synthase | 613861, 608172 |
| 68.97 | NgBR-CDG | Nogo-B receptor deficiency | *NUS1* | 6q22.1 | AR | Subunit of cis-prenyltransferase (cis-PTase) | 617082 |
| 68.98 | SRD5A3-CDG | Steroid 5 alpha-reductase 3 deficiency | *SRD5A3* | 4q12 | AR | Steroid 5 alpha-reductase 3 | 612379 |
| 68.99 | DK1-CDG | Dolichol kinase deficiency | *DOLK* | 9q34.11 | AR | Dolichol kinase | 610768 |
| 68.100 | DPM1-CDG | GDP-Man:Dol-P mannosyltransferase subunit 1 deficiency | *DPM1* | 20q13.13 | AR | GDP-Man:Dol-P mannosyltransferase subunit 1 | 608799 |
| 68.101 | DPM2-CDG | Dolichol-P-mannose synthase-2 deficiency | *DPM2* | 9q34.11 | AR | Dolichol-P-mannose synthase-2 | 615042 |
| 68.102 | DPM3-CDG | GDP-Man:Dol-P mannosyltransferase 3 deficiency | *DPM3* | 1q22 | AR | Dolichol-P-mannose synthase 3 | 612937 |
| 68.103 | MPDU1-CDG | Dol-P-Man utilization 1 deficiency | *MPDU1* | 17p13.1 | AR | Dol-P-Man utilization 1 | 609180 |
| 68.104 | GFPT1-CDG | Glutamine:fructose-6-phosphate transaminase deficiency | *GFPT1* | 2p13.3 | AR | Glutamine:fructose-6-phosphate transaminase 1 | 610542 |

| No. | Disorder | Alternative names | Gene symbol | Chromosomal localization | Mode of inheritance | Affected protein | OMIM |
|---|---|---|---|---|---|---|---|
| 68.105 | PGM1-CDG | Phosphoglucomutase 1 deficiency | *PGM1* | 1p31.3 | AR | Phosphoglucomutase 1 | 614921 |
| 68.106 | PGM3-CDG | Phosphoglucomutase 3 deficiency | *PGM3* | 6q14.1 | AR | Phosphoglucomutase 3 | 615816, 172100 |
| 68.107 | G6PC3-CDG | Glucose-6-phosphatase catalytic subunit 3 deficiency | *G6PC3* | 17q21.31 | AR | Glucose-6-phosphatase catalytic subunit 3 | 612541 |
| 68.108 | GMPPA-CDG | GDP-mannose pyrophosphorylase α subunit deficiency | *GMPPA* | 2q35 | AR | GDP-mannose pyrophosphorylase subunit A | 615510 |
| 68.109 | GMPPB-CDG | GDP-mannose pyrophosphorylase β subunit deficiency | *GMPPB* | 3p21.31 | AR | GDP-mannose pyrophosphorylase subunit B | 615350, 615351, 615352 |
| 68.110 | CAD-CDG | Epileptic encephalopathy, early infantile, 50 | *CAD* | 2p23.3 | AR | Carbamoyl phosphate synthetase, aspartate transcarbamoylase, and dihydroorotase trifuntional protein (CPSase/ATCase/ DHOase) | 616457 |
| 68.111 | SLC35A1-CDG | CMP-sialic acid transporter deficiency | *SLC35A1* | 6q15 | AR | CMP-sialic acid transporter | 603585 |
| 68.112 | SLC35A2-CDG | UDP-galactose transporter deficiency | *SLC35A2* | Xp11.23 | XL | Golgi UDP-galactose transporter | 314375 |
| 68.113 | SLC35A3-CDG | UDP-N-acetylglucosamine transporter deficiency | *SLC35A3* | 1p21.2 | AR | Solute carrier family 35 (udp-n-acetylglucosamine transporter), member 3 | 615553 |
| 68.114 | SLC35C1-CDG | GDP-fucose transporter deficiency | *SLC35C1* | 11p11.2 | AR | GDP-fucose transporter | 266265 |
| 68.115 | SLC35D1-CDG | UDP-glucuronic acid/ UDP-N-acetylgalactosamine dual transporter deficiency | *SLC35D1* | 1p31.3 | AR | UDP-glucuronic acid-UDP-N-acetylgalactosamine dual transporter | 269250 |
| 68.116 | SLC39A8-CDG | Solute carrier family 39 (Zn transporter) deficiency | *SLC39A8* | 4q24 | AR | SLC39A8 transporter of divalent cations, including manganese (Mn), zinc (Zn), cadmium (Cd), and iron (Fe) | 616721 |
| 68.117 | ATP6V0A2-CDG | V0 subunit a2 of vesicular H(+)-ATPase deficiency | *ATP6V0A2* | 12q24.31 | AR | The multisubunit vacuolar-type proton pump (H(+)-ATPase or V-ATPase) | 219200, 278250 |
| 68.118 | ATP6V1A-CDG | Cutis laxa, autosomal recessive, type IID | *ATP6V1A* | 3q13.31 | AR | V-ATPase A subunit 1 | 617403 |
| 68.119 | ATP6V1E1-CDG | Cutis laxa, autosomal recessive, type IIC | *ATP6V1E1* | 22q11.21 | AR | ATPase subunit E, ATP6E | 617402 |
| 68.120 | ATP6AP1-CDG | Immunodeficiency 47 | *ATP6AP1* | Xq28 | XL | Accessory subunit 1 of the vacuolar-ATPase protein | 300972 |
| 68.121 | ATP6AP2-CDG | X-linked mental retardation, Hedera type | *ATP6AP2* | Xp11.4 | XL | ATPase, h + transporting, lysosomal, accessory protein 2 | 300423 |
| 68.122 | TMEM199-CDG | TMEM199 deficiency | *TMEM199* | 17q11.2 | AR | Transmembrane protein 199 | 616829 |
| 68.123 | CCDC115-CDG | CCDC115 deficiency | *CCDC115* | 2q21.1 | AR | Coiled-coil domain-containing protein 115 | 616828 |
| 68.124 | TMEM165-CDG | TMEM165 deficiency | *TMEM165* | 4q12 | AR | TMEM165 (TPARL) protein | 614727, 614726 |
| 68.125 | NGLY1-CDDG | N-glycanase 1 deficiency | *NGLY1* | 3p24.2 | AR | N-glycanase 1 | 615273 |

## Metabolic Pathway

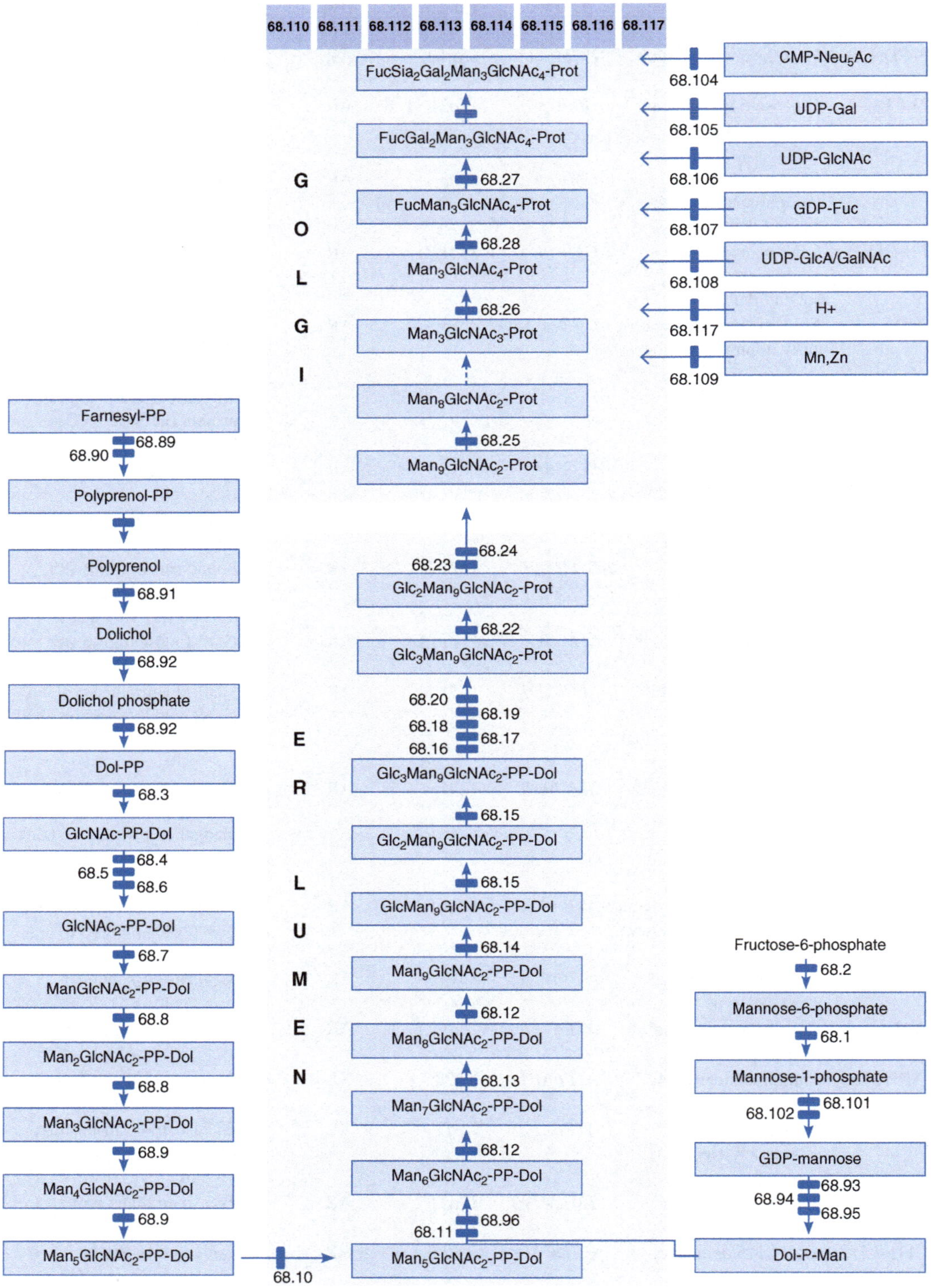


**Fig. 68.1** Abbreviated scheme of the synthesis of a biantennary N-glycan linked to dolichol pyrophosphate (Dol-PP) and subsequently, in the Golgi apparatus, to proteins (Prot). *68.1*, PMM2-CDG; *68.2*, MPI-CDG; *68.3*, DPAGT1-CDG; *68.4*, ALG13-CDG; *68.5*, ALG13-CDG; *68.6*, ALG14-CDG; *68.7*, ALG1-CDG; *68.8*, ALG2-CDG; *68.9*, ALG11-CDG; *68.10*, RFT1-CDG; *68.11*, ALG3-CDG; *68.12*, ALG9-CDG; *68.13*, ALG12-CDG; *68.14*, ALG6-CDG; *68.15*, ALG8-CDG; *68.16*, TUSC3-CDG; *68.17*, DDOST-CDG; *68.18*, STT3A-CDG; *68.19*, STT3B-CDG; *68.20*, MAGT1-CDG; *68.22*, MOGS-CDG; *68.23*, GANAB-CDG; *68.24*, PRKCSH-CDG; *68.25*, MAN1B1-CDG; *68.26*, MGAT2-CDG; *68.27*, B4GALT1-CDG; *68.28*, FUT8-CDG; *68.96*, DHDDS-CDG; *68.97*, NgBR-CDG; *68.98*, SRD5A3-CDG; *68.99*, DK1-CDG; *68.100*, DPM1-CDG; *68.101*, DPM2-CDG; *68.102*, DPM3-CDG; *68.108*, GMPPA-CDG; *68.109*, GMPPB-CDG; *68.111*, SLC35A1-CDG; *68.112*, SLC35A2-CDG; *68.113*, SLC35A3-CDG; *68.114*, SLC35C1-CDG; *68.115*, SLC35D1-CDG; *68.116*, SLC39A8-CDG; *68.117*, ATP6V0A2-CDG; *68.118*, ATP6V1A-CDG; *68.119*, ATP6V1E1-CDG; *68.120*, ATP6AP1-CDG; *68.121*, ATP6AP2-CDG; *68.122*, TMEM199-CDG; *68.123*, CCDC115-CDG; *68.124*, TMEM165-CDG. *GDP* guanosine diphosphate, *Man* mannose, *GlcNAc* N-acetylglucosamine, *Dol* dolichol, *P* phosphate, *Glc* glucose, *Gal* galactose, *Sia* sialic acid. Dotted arrow indicates multiple steps

## Signs and Symptoms

**Table 68.1** Phosphomannomutase 2 deficiency PMM2-CDG

| System | Symptoms and biomarkers | Neonatal (birth–1 month) | Infancy (1–18 months) | Childhood (1.5–11 years) | Adolescence (11–16 years) | Adulthood (>16 years) |
|---|---|---|---|---|---|---|
| Cardiovascular | Cardiomyopathy | ± | ± | ± | ± | ± |
| | **Pericardial effusion** | ± | ± | ± | ± | ± |
| CNS | **Cerebellar hypoplasia** | + | ++ | ++ | ++ | ++ |
| | Demyelination | + | + | + | + | + |
| | Epilepsy | ± | ± | + | ± | ± |
| | **Hypotonia** | ++ | ++ | + | + | + |
| | **Retardation, psychomotor** | ++ | ++ | ++ | ++ | ++ |
| | **Stroke-like episodes** | ± | ± | ± | ± | ± |
| | **Tendon reflexes, decreased** | ± | + | + | + | + |
| Dermatological | **Inverted nipples** | + | + | + | | |
| | **Subcutaneous fat distribution, abnormal** | ± | ± | ± | ± | ± |
| Digestive | **Anorexia** | ± | ± | ± | ± | ± |
| | Ascites | ± | ± | ± | ± | ± |
| | Diarrhea | ± | ± | ± | ± | ± |
| | **Liver dysfunction** | + | + | + | ± | ± |
| | Vomiting | ± | ± | ± | – | – |
| Endocrine | **Hypergonadotropic hypogonadism, female** | – | – | – | + | + |
| Eye | **Pigmentary retinopathy** | ± | + | + | + | + |
| | **Strabismus** | ± | ± | ± | ± | ± |
| Musculoskeletal | Cervical compressive myelopathy | – | – | ± | ± | ± |
| | **Dysmorphic features** | ± | ± | ± | ± | ± |
| | Dysostosis multiplex | ± | ± | ± | ± | ± |
| | **Joint contractures** | – | – | ± | ± | ± |
| | **Osteopenia** | – | ± | + | + | + |
| | Vertebral anomalies | ± | ± | ± | ± | ± |
| Other | **Failure to thrive** | ± | ± | ± | ± | ± |
| | Fetal hydrops | ± | – | – | – | – |
| Renal | **Proteinuria** | ± | ± | ± | ± | ± |
| | Renal enlargement | ± | ± | ± | ± | ± |
| Laboratory findings | Albumin (serum) | ↓ | ↓ | ↓ | ↓ | ↓ |

**Table 68.2** Phosphomannose isomerase deficiency MPI-CDG

| System | Symptoms and biomarkers | Neonatal (birth–1 month) | Infancy (1–18 months) | Childhood (1.5–11 years) | Adolescence (11–16 years) | Adulthood (>16 years) |
|---|---|---|---|---|---|---|
| CNS | Hypotonia | ± | ± | ± | ± | ± |
| | Retardation, psychomotor | ± | ± | ± | ± | ± |
| Digestive | Diarrhea | | +/++ | +/++ | ± | ± |
| | **Liver fibrosis** | | + | + | + | + |
| | **Protein-losing enteropathy** | | +/++ | +/++ | ± | ± |
| Endocrine | **Hyperinsulinism** | ± | ± | ± | | |
| Hematological | Thrombosis | | ± | ± | ± | ± |
| Metabolic | **Hypoglycemia, hypoketotic** | ± | ± | ± | | |
| Laboratory findings | Albumin (serum) | ↓ | ↓ | ↓ | ↓ | ↓ |
| | Antithrombin III (plasma) | ↓ | ↓ | ↓ | | |
| | Arylsulfatase A (serum) | ↑ | ↑ | ↑ | n-↑ | n-↑ |
| | Asialotransferrin (serum) | ↑ | ↑ | ↑ | | |
| | Cholesterol (serum) | ↓ | ↓ | ↓ | ↓ | ↓ |
| | Cholesterol (serum) | ↓ | ↓ | ↓ | | |
| | Cholinesterase (plasma) | ↓ | ↓ | ↓ | | |
| | Disialotransferrin (serum) | ↑ | ↑ | ↑ | | |
| | Factor XI (blood) | ↓ | ↓ | ↓ | ↓ | ↓ |
| | Free fatty acids (serum), during hypoglycemia | ↓↓↓ | ↓↓↓ | ↓↓ | | |
| | Glucose (plasma) | ↓ | ↓ | ↓ | | |
| | Insulin, during hypoglycemia | ↑ | ↑ | ↑ | ↑ | ↑ |
| | Ketones, during hypoglycemia | ↓↓↓ | ↓↓↓ | ↓↓ | | |
| | Protein C (serum) | ↓ | ↓ | ↓ | | |
| | Sialotransferrins, type 1 pattern (serum) | ++ | ++ | ++ | + | –/+ |
| | Tetrasialotransferrin (serum) | ↓ | ↓ | ↓ | | |
| | Thyroxin-binding globulin (serum) | ↓ | ↓ | ↓ | ↓-n | ↓-n |
| | Transaminase (plasma) | ↑ | ↑ | ↑ | n-↑ | n-↑ |

**Table 68.3** UDP–GlcNAc:Dol-P-GlcNac-P transferase deficiency DPAGT1-CDG

| System | Symptoms and biomarkers | Neonatal (birth–1 month) | Infancy (1–18 months) | Childhood (1.5–11 years) | Adolescence (11–16 years) | Adulthood (>16 years) |
|---|---|---|---|---|---|---|
| CNS | **Congenital myasthenic syndrome** | | | ± | ± | ± |
| | **Epilepsy** | ± | ± | ± | ± | ± |
| | Fetal hypokinesia phenotype | ± | ± | | | |
| | Hypertonia | ± | ± | ± | ± | ± |
| | **Hypotonia** | ± | ± | ± | ± | ± |
| | Intellectual disability | ± | ± | ± | ± | ± |
| | Retardation, motor | + | + | + | + | + |
| Digestive | Feeding difficulties | ± | ± | ± | ± | |
| Eye | Cataract | ± | ± | | | |
| | Exotropia | ± | | | | |
| | Nystagmus | ± | ± | ± | | |
| | Strabismus | ± | ± | ± | ± | ± |
| Musculoskeletal | Arched palate, high | ± | | | | |
| | Contractures | ± | ± | ± | | |
| | EM, type 2 fiber tubular aggregates (muscle) | | | ± | ± | |
| | Microcephaly | – | ± | ± | ± | ± |
| | Micrognathia | ± | | | | |

**Table 68.3** (continued)

| System | Symptoms and biomarkers | Neonatal (birth–1 month) | Infancy (1–18 months) | Childhood (1.5–11 years) | Adolescence (11–16 years) | Adulthood (>16 years) |
|---|---|---|---|---|---|---|
| Other | Dysmorphism | ± | ± | ± | ± | ± |
| | Fatal outcome | ± | ± | ± | | |
| Laboratory findings | Antithrombin III (plasma) | ↓ | ↓ | ↓ | | |
| | Asialotransferrin (serum) | n-↑ | n-↑ | n-↑ | | |
| | Creatine kinase (plasma) | n-↑ | n-↑ | n-↑ | n-↑ | n-↑ |
| | Disialotransferrin (serum) | n-↑ | n-↑ | n-↑ | | |
| | Lipid-linked Man9GlcNAc2 (fibroblasts) | ↓-n | ↓-n | ↓-n | ↓-n | |
| | Sialotransferrins, type 1 pattern (serum) | ± | ± | ± | ± | |
| | Tetrasialotransferrin (serum) | ↓-n | ↓-n | ↓-n | | |
| | Transaminase (plasma) | n-↑ | n-↑ | n-↑ | n-↑ | n-↑ |

**Table 68.4** X-linked recessive UDP-N-acetylglucosamine transferase catalytic subunit deficiency X-linked recessive ALG13-CDG

| System | Symptoms and biomarkers | Neonatal (birth–1 month) | Infancy (1–18 months) | Childhood (1.5–11 years) | Adolescence (11–16 years) | Adulthood (>16 years) |
|---|---|---|---|---|---|---|
| CNS | Developmental regression | – | ± | ± | | |
| | **Epilepsy, refractory** | – | + | + | | |
| | Extrapyramidal signs | – | ± | ± | | |
| | Intellectual disability | – | + | + | | |
| | Pyramidal signs | – | ± | ± | | |
| Digestive | Feeding difficulties | ± | ± | ± | | |
| | **Hepatomegaly** | – | ± | ± | | |
| Eye | **Delayed visual maturation** | ± | ± | ± | | |
| Musculoskeletal | Dysmorphic features | + | + | + | | |
| | **Microcephaly** | ± | ± | ± | | |
| Laboratory findings | Asialotransferrin (serum) | n-↑ | n-↑ | n-↑ | | |
| | Disialotransferrin (serum) | n-↑ | n-↑ | n-↑ | | |
| | Tetrasialotransferrin (serum) | ↓-n | ↓-n | ↓-n | | |
| | Thromboplastin time (blood) | n-↑ | n-↑ | n-↑ | | |

**Table 68.5** X-linked dominant UDP-N-acetylglucosamine transferase catalytic subunit deficiency X-linked dominant ALG13-CDG

| System | Symptoms and biomarkers | Neonatal (birth–1 month) | Infancy (1–18 months) | Childhood (1.5–11 years) | Adolescence (11–16 years) | Adulthood (>16 years) |
|---|---|---|---|---|---|---|
| CNS | Developmental regression | – | ± | ± | | |
| | **Epilepsy, refractory** | – | + | + | | |
| | Extrapyramidal signs | – | ± | ± | | |
| | Intellectual disability | – | + | + | | |
| | Pyramidal signs | – | ± | ± | | |
| Digestive | Feeding difficulties | ± | ± | ± | | |
| | **Hepatomegaly** | – | ± | ± | | |
| Eye | **Delayed visual maturation** | ± | ± | ± | | |
| Musculoskeletal | **Microcephaly** | ± | ± | ± | | |
| Other | **Dysmorphism** | + | + | + | | |
| Laboratory findings | Asialotransferrin (serum) | n-↑ | n-↑ | n-↑ | | |
| | Disialotransferrin (serum) | n-↑ | n-↑ | n-↑ | | |
| | Tetrasialotransferrin (serum) | ↓-n | ↓-n | ↓-n | | |
| | Thromboplastin time (blood) | n-↑ | n-↑ | n-↑ | | |

**Table 68.6** Congenital myasthenic syndrome, without tubular aggregates-15 ALG14-CDG

| System | Symptoms and biomarkers | Neonatal (birth–1 month) | Infancy (1–18 months) | Childhood (1.5–11 years) | Adolescence (11–16 years) | Adulthood (>16 years) |
|---|---|---|---|---|---|---|
| CNS | **Congenital myasthenic syndrome** | ± | ± | ± | ± | ± |
| | Developmental delay | | ± | ± | ± | |
| | Epilepsy | ± | ± | ± | ± | ± |
| | Hypotonia | ± | ± | ± | ± | ± |
| Musculoskeletal | Contractures | ± | ± | ± | ± | ± |
| Other | Fetal hydrops | ± | | | | |
| Psychiatric | Behavioral abnormalities | | | ± | ± | ± |
| Laboratory findings | Creatine kinase (plasma) | n | n | n | n | n |
| | Sialotransferrin type 1 (serum) | ± | ± | ± | ± | ± |

**Table 68.7** Mannosyltransferase 1 deficiency ALG1-CDG

| System | Symptoms and biomarkers | Neonatal (birth–1 month) | Infancy (1–18 months) | Childhood (1.5–11 years) | Adolescence (11–16 years) | Adulthood (>16 years) |
|---|---|---|---|---|---|---|
| Cardiovascular | Cardiomyopathy | ± | ± | ± | | |
| CNS | Axial hypotonia | ± | ± | ± | | |
| | Cerebellar hypoplasia (MRI) | ± | ± | ± | | |
| | Cortical atrophy (MRI) | ± | ± | ± | | |
| | **Epilepsy** | + | + | + | | |
| | Retardation, psychomotor | + | + | + | | |
| Digestive | Diarrhea, chronic | ± | ± | ± | | |
| | Feeding difficulties | ± | ± | ± | | |
| Eye | **Poor visual fixation** | ± | ± | ± | | |
| | Strabismus | ± | ± | ± | | |
| Hematological | Thrombocytopenia | ± | ± | ± | | |
| Musculoskeletal | Contractures | ± | ± | ± | | |
| | **Facial dysmorphism** | ± | ± | ± | | |
| | Microcephaly | ± | ± | + | | |
| | Scoliosis | ± | ± | ± | | |
| Other | **Fatal outcome** | ± | ± | ± | | |
| Renal | **Nephrotic syndrome** | ± | ± | ± | | |
| Laboratory findings | Albumin (serum) | ↓-n | ↓-n | ↓-n | | |
| | Asialotransferrin (serum) | ↑ | ↑ | ↑ | | |
| | Disialotransferrin (serum) | ↑ | ↑ | ↑ | | |
| | Dolichol-linked GlcNAc2 (serum) | ↑ | ↑ | ↑ | | |
| | Lipid-linked GlcNAc2 (fibroblasts) | ↑ | ↑ | ↑ | | |
| | Protein C (plasma) | ↓-n | ↓-n | ↓-n | | |
| | Sialotransferrins, type 1 pattern (serum) | + | + | + | | |
| | Tetrasialotransferrin (serum) | ↓ | ↓ | ↓ | | |
| | Transaminase (plasma) | n-↑ | n-↑ | n-↑ | | |
| | Xeno-tetrasaccharide (serum, fibroblasts) | ± | ± | | | |

**Table 68.8** Mannosyltransferase 2 deficiency ALG2-CDG

| System | Symptoms and biomarkers | Neonatal (birth–1 month) | Infancy (1–18 months) | Childhood (1.5–11 years) | Adolescence (11–16 years) | Adulthood (>16 years) |
|---|---|---|---|---|---|---|
| CNS | **Abnormal jitter** | | | | + | + |
| | **Bulbar dysfunction** | | | | ± | ± |
| | **Congenital myasthenic syndrome** | ± | ± | ± | | |
| | **Demyelination** | + | + | + | | |
| | Epilepsy | + | + | + | | |
| | **Facial weakness, mild** | ± | ± | ± | ± | ± |
| | Hyperreflexia | + | + | + | | |
| | Hypotonia | + | + | + | | |
| | Motor developmental delay | + | + | + | + | + |
| Eye | **Cataract** | + | + | + | | |
| | **Coloboma** | + | + | + | ± | ± |
| Laboratory findings | Asialotransferrin (serum) | ↑ | ↑ | ↑ | | |
| | Creatine kinase (plasma) | n-↑ | n-↑ | n-↑ | n-↑ | n-↑ |
| | Disialotransferrin (serum) | ↑ | ↑ | ↑ | | |
| | Dolichol-linked Man1GlcNAc2 (serum) | ↑ | ↑ | ↑ | | |
| | Dolichol-linked Man2GlcNAc2 (serum) | ↑ | ↑ | ↑ | | |
| | Factor XI (blood) | ↓ | ↓ | ↓ | | |
| | Lipid-linked Man1GlcNAc2 (fibroblasts) | ↑ | ↑ | ↑ | | |
| | Lipid-linked Man2GlcNAc2 (fibroblasts) | ↑ | ↑ | ↑ | | |
| | Sialotransferrins, type 1 pattern (serum) | + | + | + | | |
| | Tetrasialotransferrin (serum) | ↓ | ↓ | ↓ | | |
| | Thromboplastin time | ↑ | ↑ | ↑ | | |

**Table 68.9** Mannosyltransferase 4–5 deficiency ALG11-CDG

| System | Symptoms and biomarkers | Neonatal (birth–1 month) | Infancy (1–18 months) | Childhood (1.5–11 years) | Adolescence (11–16 years) | Adulthood (>16 years) |
|---|---|---|---|---|---|---|
| CNS | **Axial hypotonia** | + | + | + | | |
| | **Cerebral atrophy (MRI)** | ± | ± | ± | | |
| | Demyelination | ± | ± | ± | | |
| | **Epilepsy** | ± | + | + | | |
| | **Hearing, impaired** | ± | ± | ± | | |
| | Hyperreflexia | ± | ± | ± | | |
| | Hypertonia, extremities | ± | ± | ± | | |
| | **Retardation, psychomotor** | + | + | + | | |
| Dermatological | Fat pads | ± | ± | ± | | |
| | **Inverted nipples** | ± | ± | ± | | |
| Digestive | Feeding difficulties | ± | ± | ± | | |
| | Vomiting, episodic | ± | ± | ± | | |
| Eye | **Optic atrophy** | ± | ± | ± | | |
| | **Retinal dystrophy** | ± | ± | ± | | |
| | **Strabismus** | + | + | + | | |
| Hematological | Leukocytosis | + | + | + | | |
| Musculoskeletal | **Facial dysmorphism** | ± | ± | ± | | |
| | Microcephaly | ± | ± | ± | | |
| Other | **Early death** | ± | ± | ± | – | – |
| Respiratory | Stridor, inspiratory | ± | ± | ± | | |

(continued)

**Table 68.9** (continued)

| System | Symptoms and biomarkers | Neonatal (birth–1 month) | Infancy (1–18 months) | Childhood (1.5–11 years) | Adolescence (11–16 years) | Adulthood (>16 years) |
|---|---|---|---|---|---|---|
| Laboratory findings | Albumin (serum) | ↓-n | ↓-n | ↓-n | | |
| | Antithrombin III (plasma) | ↓ | ↓ | ↓ | | |
| | APTT | ↑ | ↑ | ↑ | | |
| | Asialotransferrin (serum) | ↑ | ↑ | ↑ | | |
| | Disialotransferrin (serum) | ↑ | ↑ | ↑ | | |
| | Dolichol-linked Man3GlcNAc2 (serum) | ↑ | ↑ | ↑ | | |
| | Dolichol-linked Man4GlcNAc2 (serum) | ↑ | ↑ | ↑ | | |
| | Factor XI (blood) | ↓-n | ↓-n | ↓-n | | |
| | Lactate (plasma) | n-↑ | n-↑ | n-↑ | | |
| | Lipid-linked Man3GlcNAc2 (fibroblasts) | ↑ | ↑ | ↑ | | |
| | Lipid-linked Man4GlcNAc2 (fibroblasts) | ↑ | ↑ | ↑ | | |
| | Prolactin (plasma) | ↑ | ↑ | ↑ | | |
| | Sialotransferrins, type 1 pattern (serum) | + | + | + | | |
| | Tetrasialotransferrin (serum) | ↓ | ↓ | ↓ | | |

**Table 68.10** Flippase of Man5GlcNAc2-PP-Dol deficiency RFT1-CDG

| System | Symptoms and biomarkers | Neonatal (birth–1 month) | Infancy (1–18 months) | Childhood (1.5–11 years) | Adolescence (11–16 years) | Adulthood (>16 years) |
|---|---|---|---|---|---|---|
| CNS | Ataxia | ± | ± | ± | ± | ± |
| | Cerebral atrophy (MRI) | ± | ± | ± | ± | – |
| | Epilepsy | ± | ± | ± | ± | ± |
| | **Hearing, impaired** | ± | ± | ± | ± | ± |
| | **Hypotonia** | + | + | + | + | + |
| | **Retardation, psychomotor** | + | + | + | + | + |
| Dermatological | Inverted nipples | ± | ± | ± | ± | – |
| Digestive | Feeding difficulties | ± | ± | ± | ± | – |
| | Hepatomegaly | ± | ± | ± | ± | ± |
| Eye | Vision, impaired | ± | ± | ± | ± | – |
| Hematological | Thrombosis | ± | ± | ± | ± | – |
| Musculoskeletal | Microcephaly | ± | ± | ± | – | – |
| Other | Dysmorphism | ± | ± | ± | ± | ± |
| | Failure to thrive | ± | ± | ± | – | – |
| Laboratory findings | Antithrombin III (plasma) | ↓ | ↓ | ↓ | ↓ | ↓ |
| | Asialotransferrin (serum) | ↑ | ↑ | ↑ | ↑ | ↑ |
| | Creatine kinase (plasma) | n | n | n | n | n |
| | Disialotransferrin (serum) | ↑ | ↑ | ↑ | ↑ | ↑ |
| | Dolichol-linked Man5GlcNAc2 (serum) | ↑ | ↑ | ↑ | ↑ | |
| | Factor XI (blood) | ↓ | ↓ | ↓ | ↓ | ↓ |
| | Lipid-linked Man5GlcNAc2 (fibroblasts) | ↑ | ↑ | ↑ | ↑ | |
| | Protein C (serum) | ↓ | ↓ | ↓ | ↓ | ↓ |
| | Sialotransferrins, type 1 pattern (serum) | ↑ | ↑ | ↑ | ↑ | ↑ |
| | Tetrasialotransferrin (serum) | ↓ | ↓ | ↓ | ↓ | ↓ |
| | Transaminase (plasma) | n | n | n | n | n |

**Table 68.11** Mannosyltransferase 6 deficiency ALG3-CDG

| System | Symptoms and biomarkers | Neonatal (birth–1 month) | Infancy (1–18 months) | Childhood (1.5–11 years) | Adolescence (11–16 years) | Adulthood (>16 years) |
|---|---|---|---|---|---|---|
| Cardiovascular | **Congenital heart defects** | ± | ± | ± | ± | ± |
| CNS | **Axial hypotonia** | + | ++ | ++ | + | + |
| | Cerebral atrophy (MRI) | ± | ± | ± | + | + |
| | **Epilepsy** | ++ | ++ | ++ | ++ | ++ |
| | **Hypertonia, extremities** | + | + | + | + | + |
| | **Retardation, psychomotor** | +++ | +++ | +++ | +++ | +++ |
| | **Hypsarrhythmia (EEG)** | + | + | + | + | + |
| | **Microcephaly** | + | + | + | + | + |
| Digestive | Feeding difficulties | ± | ± | ± | ± | ± |
| Eye | Optic atrophy | ± | ± | ± | ± | |
| | Strabismus | ± | ± | ± | ± | ± |
| Musculoskeletal | **Arachnodactyly** | ± | ± | ± | ± | ± |
| | **Club foot** | ± | ± | ± | ± | ± |
| | **Facial dysmorphism** | ± | + | + | + | + |
| | Microcephaly | ± | + | ++ | + | |
| | Micrognathia | ± | ± | ± | ± | ± |
| | **Skeletal dysplasia** | ± | ± | ± | ± | ± |
| Laboratory findings | Antithrombin III (plasma) | ↓ | ↓ | ↓ | | |
| | Apolipoprotein B (serum) | ↓ | ↓ | ↓ | | |
| | Asialotransferrin (serum) | ↑ | ↑ | ↑ | ↑ | ↑ |
| | Disialotransferrin (serum) | ↑ | ↑ | ↑ | ↑ | ↑ |
| | Lipid-linked Man5GlcNAc2 (fibroblasts) | ↑↑ | ↑↑ | ↑↑ | ↑↑ | ↑↑ |
| | Protein S (serum) | ↓ | ↓ | ↓ | | |
| | Sialotransferrins, type 1 pattern (serum) | + | + | + | + | + |
| | Tetrasialotransferrin (serum) | ↓ | ↓ | ↓ | ↓ | ↓ |
| | Glucose (plasma) | ↓ | ↓ | | | |
| | Free fatty acids (serum), during hypoglycemia | ↓↓↓ | ↓↓↓ | | | |
| | Ketones, during hypoglycemia | ↓↓↓ | ↓↓↓ | | | |
| | Insulin, durig hypoglycemia | ↑ | ↑ | | | |

**Table 68.12** Mannosyltransferase 7–9 deficiency ALG9-CDG

| System | Symptoms and biomarkers | Neonatal (birth–1 month) | Infancy (1–18 months) | Childhood (1.5–11 years) | Adolescence (11–16 years) | Adulthood (>16 years) |
|---|---|---|---|---|---|---|
| Cardiovascular | Pericardial effusion | ± | ± | ± | ± | |
| CNS | Brain atrophy (MRI) | ± | ± | ± | ± | |
| | Demyelination | ± | ± | ± | ± | |
| | **Epilepsy** | + | + | + | ± | |
| | **Hypotonia** | + | + | + | ± | |
| | **Retardation, psychomotor** | + | + | + | + | |
| Dermatological | Inverted nipples | ± | ± | ± | ± | |
| Digestive | Hepatomegaly | ± | ± | ± | ± | |
| | Splenomegaly | ± | ± | ± | ± | |
| Eye | Strabismus | ± | ± | ± | ± | |
| Musculoskeletal | **Facial dysmorphism** | ± | ± | ± | ± | |
| | Microcephaly | ± | ± | ± | ± | |
| | **Skeletal dysplasia** | + | + | ± | ± | |
| Other | Failure to thrive | ± | ± | ± | + | |

(continued)

**Table 68.12** (continued)

| System | Symptoms and biomarkers | Neonatal (birth–1 month) | Infancy (1–18 months) | Childhood (1.5–11 years) | Adolescence (11–16 years) | Adulthood (>16 years) |
|---|---|---|---|---|---|---|
| Renal | Renal cysts | ± | ± | ± | ± | |
| Laboratory findings | Albumin (serum) | ↓-n | ↓-n | ↓-n | | |
| | Asialotransferrin (serum) | ↑ | ↑ | ↑ | ↑ | |
| | Cholesterol (serum) | ↓-n | ↓-n | ↓-n | | |
| | Disialotransferrin (serum) | ↑ | ↑ | ↑ | ↑ | |
| | Dolichol-linked Man6GlcNAc2 (serum) | ↑ | ↑ | ↑ | | |
| | Dolichol-linked Man8GlcNAc2 (serum) | ↑ | ↑ | ↑ | | |
| | Factor XI (blood) | ↓-n | ↓-n | ↓-n | | |
| | Lipid-linked Man6GlcNA2 | ↑ | ↑ | ↑ | | |
| | Lipid-linked Man8GlcNA2 | ↑ | ↑ | + | | |
| | Sialotransferrins, type 1 pattern (serum) | + | + | + | + | |
| | Tetrasialotransferrin (serum) | ↓ | ↓ | ↓ | ↓ | |

**Table 68.13** Mannosyltransferase 8 deficiency ALG12-CDG

| System | Symptoms and biomarkers | Neonatal (birth–1 month) | Infancy (1–18 months) | Childhood (1.5–11 years) | Adolescence (11–16 years) | Adulthood (>16 years) |
|---|---|---|---|---|---|---|
| Cardiovascular | Cardiomyopathy, hypertrophic | ± | ± | ± | | |
| | Ventricular septal defect | ± | ± | ± | | |
| CNS | Agenesis, corpus callosum (MRI) | ± | ± | ± | | |
| | Cerebellar hypoplasia | ± | ± | ± | | |
| | **Hearing, impaired** | ± | ± | ± | | |
| | Hypotonia | ± | ± | ± | | |
| | **Retardation, psychomotor** | ++ | ++ | ++ | | |
| | Temporal hypoplasia, dilated external CSF spaces | ± | ± | ± | | |
| Dermatological | Hypoplastic nails | ± | ± | ± | | |
| | Inverted nipples | ± | ± | ± | | |
| Digestive | Feeding difficulties | ± | ± | ± | | |
| | Gastric tube feeding | ± | ± | ± | | |
| | Gastrointestinal dysmotility | ± | ± | ± | | |
| | Malrotation | ± | ± | ± | | |
| Eye | **Retinal detachment** | ± | ± | ± | | |
| | Strabismus | ± | ± | ± | | |
| Genitourinary | Hypospadias | ± | ± | ± | | |
| | **Male genital hypoplasia** | ± | ± | ± | | |
| | **Micropenis** | ± | ± | ± | | |
| Hematological | Thrombocytopenia | ± | ± | ± | | |
| Metabolic | Hypoglycemia | ± | ± | – | | |
| Musculoskeletal | Club foot | ± | ± | ± | | |
| | Dwarfism | ± | ± | ± | | |
| | Edema | ± | – | – | | |
| | Facial dysmorphism | ± | ± | ± | | |
| | Microcephaly | ± | ± | ± | | |
| | **Skeletal dysplasia** | ± | ± | ± | | |
| Other | Early death | ± | ± | ± | | |
| | Failure to thrive | ± | ± | ± | | |
| | Maternal HELLP syndrome | ± | | | | |
| | Prematurity | ± | | | | |

**Table 68.13** (continued)

| System | Symptoms and biomarkers | Neonatal (birth–1 month) | Infancy (1–18 months) | Childhood (1.5–11 years) | Adolescence (11–16 years) | Adulthood (>16 years) |
|---|---|---|---|---|---|---|
| Laboratory findings | Antithrombin III (plasma) | ↓ | ↓ | ↓ | | |
| | Asialotransferrin (serum) | ↑ | ↑ | ↑ | | |
| | Cholesterol (serum) | ↓-n | ↓-n | ↓-n | | |
| | Disialotransferrin (serum) | ↑ | ↑ | ↑ | | |
| | Dolichol-linked Man7GlcNAc2 (serum) | ↑ | ↑ | | | |
| | Glucose (plasma) | ↓-n | ↓-n | | | |
| | IGF BP3 | ↓-n | ↓-n | ↓-n | | |
| | IGF1 | ↓-n | ↓-n | ↓-n | | |
| | Immunoglobulins (serum) | ↓-n | ↓-n | ↓-n | | |
| | Lipid-linked Man7GlcNA2 (fibroblasts) | ↑ | ↑ | ↑ | | |
| | Sialotransferrins, type 1 pattern (serum) | + | + | + | | |
| | Tetrasialotransferrin (serum) | ↓ | ↓ | ↓ | | |
| | Transaminase (plasma) | n-↑ | n-↑ | n-↑ | | |

**Table 68.14** Glucosyltransferase 1 deficiency ALG6-CDG

| System | Symptoms and biomarkers | Neonatal (birth–1 month) | Infancy (1–18 months) | Childhood (1.5–11 years) | Adolescence (11–16 years) | Adulthood (>16 years) |
|---|---|---|---|---|---|---|
| CNS | **Ataxia** | ± | ± | ± | ± | ± |
| | **Axial hypotonia** | ++ | ++ | + | ± | – |
| | **Epileptic seizures** | + | ++ | + | ± | ± |
| | **Retardation, psychomotor** | ++ | ++ | ++ | ++ | ++ |
| Eye | **Nystagmus** | ± | ± | ± | ± | ± |
| | **Strabismus** | ++ | ++ | ++ | ++ | ++ |
| Musculoskeletal | **Skeletal abnormalities** | ± | ± | ± | ± | ± |
| Psychiatric | **Behaviour difficulties** | ± | ± | ± | ± | ± |
| Laboratory findings | Antithrombin III (plasma) | ↓ | ↓ | ↓ | | |
| | Arylsulfatase A (serum) | ↑ | ↑ | ↑ | n-↑ | n-↑ |
| | Asialotransferrin (serum) | ↑ | ↑ | ↑ | | |
| | Cholesterol (serum) | ↓↓ | ↓↓ | ↓↓ | ↓↓ | ↓↓ |
| | Disialotransferrin (serum) | ↑ | ↑ | ↑ | | |
| | Dolichol-linked Man9GlcNAc2 (serum) | ↑ | ↑ | ↑ | | |
| | Factor XI (blood) | ↓ | ↓ | ↓ | ↓ | ↓ |
| | Factor XI (blood) | ↓ | ↓ | ↓ | | |
| | Free fatty acids (serum), during hypoglycemia | ↓↓↓ | ↓↓↓ | ↓↓ | ↓↓ | ↓↓ |
| | Glucose (plasma) | ↓ | ↓ | ↓ | ↓ | ↓ |
| | Insulin, during hypoglycemia | ↑ | ↑ | ↑ | ↑ | ↑ |
| | Ketones, during hypoglycemia | ↓↓↓ | ↓↓↓ | ↓↓ | ↓↓ | ↓↓ |
| | Lipid-linked Man9GlcNAc2 (fibroblasts) | ↑ | ↑ | ↑ | ↑ | ↑ |
| | Sialotransferrins, type 1 pattern (serum) | + | + | + | + | –/+ |
| | Tetrasialotransferrin (serum) | ↓ | ↓ | ↓ | | |
| | Thyroxin-binding globulin (serum) | ↓ | ↓ | ↓ | ↓-n | ↓-n |
| | Transaminase (plasma) | ↑ | ↑ | ↑ | n-↑ | n-↑ |

**Table 68.15** Glucosyltransferase 2 deficiency ALG8-CDG

| System | Symptoms and biomarkers | Neonatal (birth–1 month) | Infancy (1–18 months) | Childhood (1.5–11 years) | Adolescence (11–16 years) | Adulthood (>16 years) |
|---|---|---|---|---|---|---|
| Cardiovascular | Ventricular septal defect | ± | ± | ± | | |
| CNS | Cerebellar hypoplasia | ± | ± | ± | | |
| | Cerebral atrophy (MRI) | ± | ± | ± | | |
| | **Hypotonia** | + | + | + | | |
| | **Retardation, psychomotor** | ++ | ++ | ++ | | + |
| | Seizures | ± | ± | ± | ± | |
| Dermatological | **Edema, generalized** | ± | ± | ± | | |
| | Excess skin | ± | ± | ± | | |
| | Inverted nipples | ± | ± | ± | | |
| Digestive | Cholestasis | ± | ± | ± | | |
| | Feeding difficulties | ± | ± | ± | ± | |
| | Hepatomegaly | ± | ± | ± | ± | + |
| | **Protein-losing enteropathy** | ± | ± | ± | ± | + |
| Endocrine | Hypothyroidism | ± | ± | ± | | |
| Eye | Cataract | ± | ± | ± | | |
| | Optic atrophy | ± | ± | ± | | |
| Genitourinary | Cryptorchidism | ± | ± | ± | | |
| Hematological | Anemia | ± | ± | ± | | |
| | Coagulopathy | ± | ± | ± | | |
| | Thrombocytopenia | ± | ± | ± | | |
| Musculoskeletal | Camptodactyly | ± | ± | ± | | |
| | Closure of fontanels, delayed | ± | ± | – | | |
| | Facial dysmorphism | ± | ± | ± | | |
| | Macrocephaly | ± | ± | ± | | |
| | Microcephaly | ± | ± | ± | | |
| | Osteopenia | ± | ± | ± | | |
| Other | **Early death** | ± | ± | | | |
| Renal | Renal cysts | ± | ± | ± | | |
| | Renal tubulopathy | ± | ± | ± | | |
| Laboratory findings | Albumin (serum) | ↓↓ | ↓↓ | ↓↓ | | ↓ |
| | Antithrombin III (plasma) | ↓ | ↓ | ↓ | | ↓ |
| | Asialotransferrin (serum) | ↑ | ↑ | ↑ | | ↑ |
| | Disialotransferrin (serum) | ↑ | ↑ | ↑ | | ↑ |
| | Dolichol-linked Glc1Man9GlcNAc2 (serum) | ↑ | ↑ | ↑ | | |
| | Factor XI (blood) | ↓ | ↓ | ↓ | | ↓ |
| | Lipid-linked Glc1Man9GlcNAc2 (fibroblasts) | ↑ | ↑ | ↑ | | |
| | Protein C (serum) | ↓ | ↓ | ↓ | | ↓ |
| | Sialotransferrins, type 1 pattern (serum) | + | + | + | | + |
| | Tetrasialotransferrin (serum) | ↓ | ↓ | ↓ | | ↓ |

**Table 68.16** Oligosaccharyltransferase subunit tusc3 deficiency TUSC3-CDG

| System | Symptoms and biomarkers | Neonatal (birth–1 month) | Infancy (1–18 months) | Childhood (1.5–11 years) | Adolescence (11–16 years) | Adulthood (>16 years) |
|---|---|---|---|---|---|---|
| CNS | **Retardation, psychomotor** | | ++ | ++ | ++ | ++ |
| Musculoskeletal | Facial dysmorphism | ± | ± | ± | ± | ± |
| | Short stature | ± | ± | ± | ± | ± |
| Laboratory findings | Sialotransferrins (serum) | n | n | n | n | n |

**Table 68.17** Congenital disorder of glycosylation DDOST-CDG

| System | Symptoms and biomarkers | Neonatal (birth–1 month) | Infancy (1–18 months) | Childhood (1.5–11 years) | Adolescence (11–16 years) | Adulthood (>16 years) |
|---|---|---|---|---|---|---|
| CNS | Delayed myelination | | + | + | | |
| | Developmental delay | + | | | | |
| | Hypotonia | + | | | | |
| | **Intellectual disability** | | + | + | | |
| | **Oromotor dysfunction** | + | | | | |
| Digestive | **Constipation** | | + | + | | |
| | Gastroesophageal reflux | + | | | | |
| | **Liver dysfunction, mild to moderate** | + | | | | |
| Ear | Ear infections | | + | + | | |
| | **Strabismus** | + | | | | |
| Musculoskeletal | Osteopenia | | ± | ± | | |
| Other | Failure to thrive | + | | | | |
| Laboratory findings | Antithrombin (blood) | ↓ | | | | |
| | Asialotransferrin (serum) | ↑ | | | | |
| | Disialotransferrin (serum) | ↑ | | | | |
| | Factor XI (blood) | ↓ | | | | |
| | Monosialotransferrin (serum) | ↑ | | | | |
| | Protein C (serum) | ↓ | | | | |
| | Protein S (serum) | ↓ | | | | |
| | Tetrasialotransferrin (serum) | ↓ | | | | |

**Table 68.18** Congenital disorder of glycosylation STT3A-CDG

| System | Symptoms and biomarkers | Neonatal (birth–1 month) | Infancy (1–18 months) | Childhood (1.5–11 years) | Adolescence (11–16 years) | Adulthood (>16 years) |
|---|---|---|---|---|---|---|
| CNS | **Cerebellar atrophy (MRI)** | | ± | ± | ± | |
| | **Developmental delay** | | + | + | + | + |
| | Hypotonia | | + | + | + | − |
| | **Intellectual disability** | | + | + | + | + |
| | **Seizures** | | + | + | + | + |
| Digestive | Gastrointestinal dysmotility | | + | + | | |
| Musculoskeletal | **Microcephaly** | | ± | ± | ± | ± |
| Other | Failure to thrive | | ± | ± | ± | − |
| Laboratory findings | Asialotransferrin (serum) | | n-↑ | n-↑ | n-↑ | n-↑ |
| | Disialotransferrin (serum) | | n-↑ | n-↑ | n-↑ | n-↑ |
| | Factor VIII (plasma) | | ↓-n | ↓-n | ↓-n | ↓-n |
| | Tetrasialotransferrin (serum) | | ↓-n | ↓-n | ↓-n | ↓-n |
| | von Willebrand factor (plasma) | | ↓-n | ↓-n | ↓-n | ↓-n |

**Table 68.19** Congenital disorder of glycosylation STT3B-CDG

| System | Symptoms and biomarkers | Neonatal (birth–1 month) | Infancy (1–18 months) | Childhood (1.5–11 years) | Adolescence (11–16 years) | Adulthood (>16 years) |
|---|---|---|---|---|---|---|
| CNS | **Intellectual disability** | + | | | | |
| | **Cerebral atrophy (MRI)** | + | | | | |
| | **Seizures** | + | | | | |
| | Hypotonia | + | | | | |
| | Developmental delay | + | | | | |
| Digestive | Gastrointestinal dysmotility | + | | | | |
| | **Hepatopathy** | + | | | | |
| Eye | **Optic atrophy** | + | | | | |
| Genitourinary | **External genitalia abnormality** | + | | | | |
| | **Scrotum, hypoplastic** | + | | | | |
| | Testes, undescended | + | | | | |
| Hematological | **Thrombocytopenia** | + | | | | |
| Musculoskeletal | **Microcephaly** | + | | | | |
| Other | Failure to thrive | + | | | | |
| Respiratory | Respiratory failure | + | | | | |
| Laboratory findings | Disialotransferrin (serum) | ↑ | | | | |
| | Asialotransferrin (serum) | ↑ | | | | |
| | Tetrasialotransferrin (serum) | ↓ | | | | |

**Table 68.20** Magnesium transporter 1 deficiency MAGT1-CDG

| System | Symptoms and biomarkers | Neonatal (birth–1 month) | Infancy (1–18 months) | Childhood (1.5–11 years) | Adolescence (11–16 years) | Adulthood (>16 years) |
|---|---|---|---|---|---|---|
| CNS | Sialotransferrin type 1 pattern (serum) | ± | ± | ± | ± | ± |
| Hematological | **Epstein-Barr virus infection** | ± | ± | ± | ± | ± |
| | **Neoplasm** | ± | ± | ± | ± | ± |
| Other | **Immunodeficiency, T-cell** | ± | ± | ± | ± | ± |
| | **Magnesium transport defect** | ± | ± | ± | ± | ± |
| | **Retardation, psychomotor** | ± | ± | ± | ± | ± |

**Table 68.21** Congenital disorder of glycosylation SSR4-CDG

| System | Symptoms and biomarkers | Neonatal (birth–1 month) | Infancy (1–18 months) | Childhood (1.5–11 years) | Adolescence (11–16 years) | Adulthood (>16 years) |
|---|---|---|---|---|---|---|
| CNS | Developmental delay | + | + | + | | |
| | Failure to thrive | + | + | + | | |
| | Hypotonia | + | | | | |
| | **Microcephaly** | + | + | + | | |
| Dermatological | Hypospadias | ± | | | | |
| | Subcutaneous fat distribution, abnormal | + | | | | |
| Eye | Skeletal malformations | ± | ± | ± | | |
| Genitourinary | **Clinodactyly** | + | | | | |
| Musculoskeletal | **Facial dysmorphism** | + | + | + | | |
| | Intellectual disability | + | + | + | | |
| | Micrognathia | + | | | | |
| | Seizures | | ± | ± | | |
| | Subcutaneous fat distribution, abnormal | + | | | | |
| Other | Strabismus | + | + | + | | |
| Laboratory findings | Disialotransferrin (serum) | ↑ | | | | |
| | Tetrasialotransferrin (serum) | ↓ | | | | |

**Table 68.22** Glucosidase 1 deficiency GCS1-CDG

| System | Symptoms and biomarkers | Neonatal (birth–1 month) | Infancy (1–18 months) | Childhood (1.5–11 years) | Adolescence (11–16 years) | Adulthood (>16 years) |
|---|---|---|---|---|---|---|
| CNS | Apnea | ++ | ++ | | | |
| | **BAER, abnormal** | + | + | + | | |
| | **Burst-suppression (EEG)** | + | + | | | |
| | Developmental delay | | + | + | | |
| | **Epilepsy** | + | + | + | | |
| | **Hypokinesia** | + | + | | | |
| | **Hypotonia** | + | + | + | | |
| | **Neuropathy, myelinating** | + | + | | | |
| | **VEP, abnormal** | +++ | +++ | | | |
| Digestive | Gastric tube feeding | + | + | | | |
| | **Hepatomegaly** | + | + | | | |
| Eye | **Long eye lashes** | + | + | | | |
| | **Short palpebral fissures** | + | + | | | |
| Genitourinary | **Hypoplastic labia majora** | + | + | + | | |
| Hair | **Alopecia areata** | | ± | | | |
| Musculoskeletal | **Arched palate, high** | ± | ± | | | |
| | **Facial dysmorphism** | + | + | + | | |
| | **Fingers, overlapping** | + | + | | | |
| Respiratory | **Respiratory failure** | + | + | | | |
| Laboratory findings | Immunoglobulins (serum) | ↓ | ↓ | ↓ | | |
| | Sialotransferrin abnormal pattern (serum) | ± | ± | ± | | |
| | Tetrasaccharide (urine) | ↑ | ↑ | | | |

**Table 68.23** Polycyctic kidney disease 3 GANAB-CDG

| System | Symptoms and biomarkers | Neonatal (birth–1 month) | Infancy (1–18 months) | Childhood (1.5–11 years) | Adolescence (11–16 years) | Adulthood (>16 years) |
|---|---|---|---|---|---|---|
| Renal | **Polycystic kidney** | | | | | + |
| Digestive | **Polycystic liver disease** | | | | | ± |
| Laboratory findings | Sialotransferrins (serum) | | | | | n |

**Table 68.24** α-1,3-glucosidase II subunit β deficiency

| System | Symptoms and biomarkers | Neonatal (birth–1 month) | Infancy (1–18 months) | Childhood (1.5–11 years) | Adolescence (11–16 years) | Adulthood (>16 years) |
|---|---|---|---|---|---|---|
| Digestive | **Polycystic liver disease 1** | | | | | + |
| Renal | **Kidney cysts** | | | | | ± |
| Laboratory findings | Sialotransferrins (serum) | | | | | n |

**Table 68.25** Mental retardation, autosomal recessive 15 MAN1B1-CDG

| System | Symptoms and biomarkers | Neonatal (birth–1 month) | Infancy (1–18 months) | Childhood (1.5–11 years) | Adolescence (11–16 years) | Adulthood (>16 years) |
|---|---|---|---|---|---|---|
| CNS | **Hypotonia** | + | + | + | ± | ± |
| | **Intellectual disability** | | + | + | + | + |
| | Seizures | | | | ± | ± |
| | **Speech delay** | | + | + | + | + |
| Dermatological | **Inverted nipples** | ± | ± | ± | | |
| Digestive | **Obesity** | ± | ± | ± | ± | + |
| Eye | Strabismus | ± | ± | ± | ± | ± |
| Musculoskeletal | **Bulbous nose** | ± | ± | ± | ± | ± |
| | **Flat oval face** | + | + | + | + | + |
| | **Macrocephaly** | ± | ± | ± | ± | ± |
| | **Tin upper lips** | ± | ± | + | ± | ± |
| Psychiatric | **Behaviour difficulties** | | | ± | ± | ± |
| Laboratory findings | Tetrasialotransferrin (serum) | ↓ | ↓ | ↓ | ↓ | ↓ |
| | Transaminase (plasma) | n-↑ | n-↑ | n-↑ | n-↑ | n |
| | Trisialotransferrin (serum) | ↑ | ↑ | ↑ | ↑ | ↑ |

**Table 68.26** N-acetylglucosaminyltransferase 2 deficiency MGAT2-CDG

| System | Symptoms and biomarkers | Neonatal (birth–1 month) | Infancy (1–18 months) | Childhood (1.5–11 years) | Adolescence (11–16 years) | Adulthood (>16 years) |
|---|---|---|---|---|---|---|
| Cardiovascular | Ventricular septal defect | ± | ± | ± | ± | ± |
| CNS | Cortical atrophy (MRI) | ± | ± | ± | ± | ± |
| | **Epilepsy, intractable** | ± | ± | ± | ± | ± |
| | **Hypotonia** | + | + | + | + | + |
| | Movement, abnormal | ± | ± | ± | ± | ± |
| | **Retardation, psychomotor** | ++ | ++ | ++ | ++ | ++ |
| Digestive | **Big open mouth** | + | + | + | + | + |
| | Diarrhea, chronic | ± | ± | ± | | |
| | Everted lower lip | ± | ± | ± | ± | ± |
| | Feeding difficulties | ± | ± | ± | ± | ± |
| | Gastroesophageal reflux | ± | ± | ± | | |
| | Gastrointestinal bleeding | ± | ± | ± | | |
| | Volvulus of the stomach | ± | ± | ± | | |
| Ear | **Dysplastic ears** | + | + | + | + | + |
| | **Hearing loss** | ± | ± | ± | ± | ± |
| Endocrine | Absent puberty | | | | ± | ± |
| | Decreased body height | ± | + | + | + | + |
| Eye | Delayed visual maturation | | ± | ± | | |
| | Myopia | ± | ± | ± | ± | ± |
| Genitourinary | **Male genital hypoplasia** | ± | ± | ± | ± | ± |
| Hematological | Bleeding tendency | ± | ± | ± | ± | ± |
| | Problematic lymphocyte growth | ± | ± | ± | ± | ± |
| Musculoskeletal | **Facial dysmorphism** | + | + | + | + | + |
| | Foot deformity | ± | ± | ± | ± | ± |
| | **Kyphosis** | ± | ± | ± | ± | ± |
| | Microcephaly | ± | ± | ± | ± | ± |
| | Muscular dystrophy | | ± | ± | ± | ± |
| | Osteoporosis | | ± | ± | ± | ± |
| | Pectus excavatum | ± | ± | ± | ± | ± |
| | **Radius dislocation** | ± | ± | ± | ± | ± |
| | Scoliosis | ± | ± | ± | ± | ± |
| | Vertebral anomalies | ± | ± | ± | ± | ± |
| Respiratory | Respiratory insufficiency | | | | ± | ± |
| Other | Beaked nose | ± | ± | ± | ± | ± |
| | Drug reactions | ± | ± | ± | ± | ± |
| | Fatal evolution before 1 year | ± | ± | | | |
| | Gum hypertrophy | | ± | ± | ± | ± |
| | Recurrent infections | ± | ± | ± | ± | ± |
| | **Teeth malposition** | | ± | ± | ± | ± |
| Laboratory findings | Antithrombin III (plasma) | ↓ | ↓ | ↓ | | |
| | Arylsulfatase A (serum) | n | n | n | n | n |
| | ASAT (plasma) | ↑ | ↑ | ↑ | ↑ | ↑ |
| | Factor IX (blood) | ↓ | ↓ | ↓ | | |
| | Factor XI (blood) | ↓ | ↓ | ↓ | | |
| | Haptoglobin (serum) | ↓ | ↓ | ↓ | ↓ | ↓ |
| | Immunoglobulin G (serum) | ↓ | ↓ | ↓ | n | n |
| | Sialotransferrins, type 2 pattern (serum) | + | + | + | + | + |
| | Thyroxin-binding globulin (serum) | ↓ | ↓ | ↓ | ↓ | ↓ |

**Table 68.27** Beta-1,4-galactosyltransferase 1 deficiency B4GALT1-CDG

| System | Symptoms and biomarkers | Neonatal (birth–1 month) | Infancy (1–18 months) | Childhood (1.5–11 years) | Adolescence (11–16 years) | Adulthood (>16 years) |
|---|---|---|---|---|---|---|
| CNS | **Axial hypotonia** | + | + | | | |
| Eye | **Myopia** | + | + | + | | |
| Digestive | Diarrhea, recurrent episodes | ± | ± | | | |
| Hematological | Perinatal bleeding diathesis | ± | | | | |
| Musculoskeletal | **Facial dysmorphism** | + | + | + | | |
| Laboratory findings | Antithrombin (blood) | ↓ | ↓ | ↓ | | |
| | Antithrombin III (plasma) | ↓ | ↓ | ↓ | | |
| | APTT | ↑ | ↑ | ↑ | | |
| | ASAT (plasma) | ↑↑ | ↑↑ | ↑↑ | ↑↑ | |
| | Asialotransferrin (serum) | ↑ | ↑ | ↑ | | |
| | Cholinesterase (plasma) | ↓ | ↓ | ↓ | | |
| | Creatine kinase (plasma) | ↑ | ↑ | ↑ | | |
| | Disialotransferrin (serum) | ↑ | ↑ | ↑ | | |
| | Factor XI (blood) | ↓ | ↓ | ↓ | | |
| | Fibrinogen | ↓ | ↓ | ↓ | | |
| | Hypogalactosylation Tf glycans | + | + | + | | |
| | Monosialotransferrin (serum) | ↑ | ↑ | ↑ | | |
| | Sialotransferrins, type 2 pattern (serum) | + | + | + | | |
| | Tetrasialotransferrin (serum) | ↓ | ↓ | ↓ | | |
| | Trisialotransferrin (serum) | ↑ | ↑ | ↑ | | |

**Table 68.28** α-1,6-fucosyltransferase deficiency FUT8-CDG

| System | Symptoms and biomarkers | Neonatal (birth–1 month) | Infancy (1–18 months) | Childhood (1.5–11 years) | Adolescence (11–16 years) | Adulthood (>16 years) |
|---|---|---|---|---|---|---|
| CNS | **Developmental delay** | | ++ | ++ | | |
| | **Epilepsy** | + | + | + | | |
| | **Hypotonia** | + | + | + | | |
| | **Intellectual disability** | | + | + | | |
| Digestive | **Feeding difficulties** | + | + | + | | |
| Endocrine | Hypothyroidism | ± | ± | ± | | |
| Eye | **Buphthalmos** | ± | ± | ± | | |
| | **Glaucoma** | ± | ± | ± | | |
| Musculoskeletal | **Contractures** | ± | ± | ± | | |
| | **Facial dysmorphism** | + | + | + | | |
| | **Microcephaly** | + | + | + | | |
| | **Short stature** | + | + | + | | |
| Renal | **Nephrocalcinosis** | ± | ± | ± | | |
| Respiratory | Recurrent bronchopneumonia | ± | ± | ± | | |
| | Tracheostomy | ± | ± | ± | | |
| Other | **Failure to thrive** | ++ | ++ | ++ | | |
| Laboratory findings | Sialotransferrins (serum) | n | n | n | | |

**Table 68.29** O-Mannosyltransferase 1 deficiency POMT1-CDG

| System | Symptoms and biomarkers | Neonatal (birth–1 month) | Infancy (1–18 months) | Childhood (1.5–11 years) | Adolescence (11–16 years) | Adulthood (>16 years) |
|---|---|---|---|---|---|---|
| CNS | **Agenesis, corpus callosum (MRI)** | ± | ± | ± | ± | ± |
| | **Cerebellar abnormalities** | ± | ± | ± | ± | ± |
| | **Cerebral cortical malformations** | ± | ± | ± | ± | ± |
| | **Cobblestone lissencephaly** | ± | ± | ± | ± | ± |
| | **Encephalocele** | ± | ± | ± | ± | ± |
| | Epilepsy | ± | ± | ± | ± | ± |
| | Hydrocephalus | ± | ± | ± | ± | ± |
| | **Retardation, psychomotor** | +++ | +++ | +++ | +++ | +++ |
| Eye | **Buphthalmos** | ± | ± | ± | ± | ± |
| | **Cataract** | ± | ± | ± | ± | ± |
| | Exophthalmia | ± | ± | ± | ± | ± |
| | **Glaucoma** | ± | ± | ± | ± | ± |
| | **Megalocornea** | ± | ± | ± | ± | ± |
| | **Microphthalmia** | ± | ± | ± | ± | ± |
| | **Pigmentary retinopathy** | ± | ± | ± | ± | ± |
| Musculoskeletal | **Dysmorphic features** | ± | ± | ± | ± | ± |
| | **Muscular dystrophy** | + | + | + | + | + |
| Other | Fatal evolution before 1 year | ± | ± | – | – | – |
| | **Walker-Warburg syndrome** | ± | ± | ± | ± | ± |
| Laboratory findings | Creatine kinase (plasma) | ↑↑ | ↑↑ | ↑↑ | ↑↑ | ↑↑ |
| | Sialotransferrins (serum) | n | n | n | n | n |

**Table 68.30** O-Mannosyltransferase 2 deficiency POMT2-CDG

| System | Symptoms and biomarkers | Neonatal (birth–1 month) | Infancy (1–18 months) | Childhood (1.5–11 years) | Adolescence (11–16 years) | Adulthood (>16 years) |
|---|---|---|---|---|---|---|
| CNS | **Agenesis, corpus callosum (MRI)** | ± | ± | ± | ± | ± |
| | Cerebellar abnormalities | ± | ± | ± | ± | ± |
| | **Cerebral cortical malformations** | ± | ± | ± | ± | ± |
| | **Cobblestone lissencephaly** | ± | ± | ± | ± | ± |
| | **Encephalocele** | ± | ± | ± | ± | ± |
| | Epilepsy | ± | ± | ± | ± | ± |
| | **Hydrocephalus** | ± | ± | ± | ± | ± |
| | **Retardation, psychomotor** | +++ | +++ | +++ | +++ | +++ |
| Eye | **Buphthalmos** | ± | ± | ± | ± | ± |
| | **Cataract** | ± | ± | ± | ± | ± |
| | Exophthalmia | ± | ± | ± | ± | ± |
| | **Glaucoma** | ± | ± | ± | ± | ± |
| | **Megalocornea** | ± | ± | ± | ± | ± |
| | **Microphthalmia** | ± | ± | ± | ± | ± |
| | **Pigmentary retinopathy** | ± | ± | ± | ± | ± |
| Musculoskeletal | **Dysmorphic features** | ± | ± | ± | ± | ± |
| | **Muscular dystrophy** | + | + | + | + | + |
| Other | Fatal evolution before 1 year | ± | ± | – | – | – |
| | **Walker-Warburg syndrome** | ± | ± | ± | ± | ± |
| Laboratory findings | Creatine kinase (plasma) | ↑↑ | ↑↑ | ↑↑ | ↑↑ | ↑↑ |
| | Sialotransferrins (serum) | n | n | n | n | n |

**Table 68.31** O-Mannose beta-1,2-N-acetyglucosaminyltransferase deficiency POMGNT1-CDG

| System | Symptoms and biomarkers | Neonatal (birth–1 month) | Infancy (1–18 months) | Childhood (1.5–11 years) | Adolescence (11–16 years) | Adulthood (>16 years) |
|---|---|---|---|---|---|---|
| CNS | **Agenesis, corpus callosum (MRI)** | ± | ± | ± | ± | ± |
| | **Cerebellar abnormalities** | ± | ± | ± | ± | ± |
| | **Cerebral cortical malformations** | ± | ± | ± | ± | ± |
| | **Cobblestone lissencephaly** | ± | ± | ± | ± | ± |
| | **Encephalocele** | ± | ± | ± | ± | ± |
| | **Epilepsy** | ± | ± | ± | ± | ± |
| | Hydrocephalus | ± | ± | ± | ± | ± |
| | **Retardation, psychomotor** | +++ | +++ | +++ | +++ | +++ |
| Eye | **Buphthalmos** | ± | ± | ± | ± | ± |
| | **Cataract** | ± | ± | ± | ± | ± |
| | Exophthalmia | ± | ± | ± | ± | ± |
| | **Glaucoma** | ± | ± | ± | ± | ± |
| | **Megalocornea** | ± | ± | ± | ± | ± |
| | **Microphthalmia** | ± | ± | ± | ± | ± |
| | Myopia | ± | ± | ± | ± | ± |
| | **Pigmentary retinopathy** | ± | ± | ± | ± | ± |
| Musculoskeletal | **Dysmorphic features** | ± | ± | ± | ± | ± |
| | **Muscle-eye-brain disease** | ± | ± | ± | ± | ± |
| | **Muscular dystrophy** | + | + | + | + | + |
| Laboratory findings | Creatine kinase (plasma) | ↑↑ | ↑↑ | ↑↑ | ↑↑ | ↑↑ |
| | Sialotransferrins (serum) | n | n | n | n | n |

**Table 68.32** Protein O-mannose β-1,4-N-acetylglucosaminyltransferase deficiency POMGNT2-CDG

| System | Symptoms and biomarkers | Neonatal (birth-1 month) | Infancy (1–18 months) | Childhood (1.5–11 years) | Adolescence (11–16 years) | Adulthood (>16 years) |
|---|---|---|---|---|---|---|
| CNS | **Cerebellar hypoplasia** | ± | ± | ± | ± | ± |
| | **Cobblestone lissencephaly** | ± | ± | ± | ± | ± |
| | Hydrocephalus | ± | ± | ± | ± | ± |
| | **Hypotonia** | ± | ± | ± | ± | ± |
| | **Retardation, psychomotor** | ± | ± | ± | ± | ± |
| Eye | **Macrophthalmia** | ± | ± | ± | ± | ± |
| | **Microphthalmia** | ± | ± | ± | ± | ± |
| | **Retinal dysplasia** | ± | ± | ± | ± | ± |
| Musculoskeletal | **Limb-girdl muscular dystrophy** | ± | ± | ± | ± | ± |
| Other | **Death** | ± | ± | | | |
| | **Walker-Warburg syndrome** | ± | ± | ± | ± | ± |
| Laboratory findings | Creatine kinase (plasma) | ↑↑ | ↑↑ | ↑↑ | ↑↑ | ↑↑ |
| | Sialotransferrins (serum) | n | n | n | n | n |

**Table 68.33** β-1,3-galactosaminyltransferase 2 deficiency B3GALNT2-CDG

| System | Symptoms and biomarkers | Neonatal (birth–1 month) | Infancy (1–18 months) | Childhood (1.5–11 years) | Adolescence (11–16 years) | Adulthood (>16 years) |
|---|---|---|---|---|---|---|
| CNS | **Cortical malformation/ dysplasia** | ± | ± | ± | ± | ± |
| | **Epilepsy** | ± | ± | ± | ± | ± |
| | **Hydrocephalus** | ± | ± | ± | ± | ± |
| | **Hypotonia** | ± | ± | ± | ± | ± |
| | **Intellectual disability** | ± | ± | ± | ± | ± |
| | **Pontocerebellar abnormalities** | ± | ± | ± | ± | ± |
| | **Retardation, psychomotor** | ± | ± | ± | ± | ± |
| | **Speech disorder** | ± | ± | ± | ± | ± |
| Eye | **Cataract** | ± | ± | ± | ± | ± |
| | **Glaucoma** | ± | ± | ± | ± | ± |
| | **Microphthalmia** | ± | ± | ± | ± | ± |
| | **Optic nerve hypoplasia** | ± | ± | ± | ± | ± |
| Musculoskeletal | **Muscular dystrophy** | ± | ± | ± | ± | ± |
| Psychiatric | Behaviour difficulties | ± | ± | ± | ± | ± |
| Other | **Walker-Warburg syndrome/ muscle-eye-brain disease** | ± | ± | ± | ± | ± |
| Laboratory findings | Creatine kinase (plasma) | ↑↑ | ↑↑ | ↑↑ | ↑↑ | ↑↑ |
| | Sialotransferrins (serum) | n | n | n | n | n |

**Table 68.34** Protein O-mannose kinase deficiency POMK-CDG

| System | Symptoms and biomarkers | Neonatal (birth–1 month) | Infancy (1–18 months) | Childhood (1.5–11 years) | Adolescence (11–16 years) | Adulthood (>16 years) |
|---|---|---|---|---|---|---|
| CNS | **Cerebellar hypoplasia** | ± | ± | ± | ± | ± |
| | **Cobblestone lissencephaly** | ± | ± | ± | ± | ± |
| | **Cognitive disability** | ± | ± | ± | ± | ± |
| | **Hydrocephalus** | ± | ± | ± | ± | ± |
| | **Hyporeflexia** | ± | ± | ± | ± | ± |
| | **Hypotonia** | ± | ± | ± | ± | ± |
| | Mirror movements, upper limbs | ± | ± | ± | ± | ± |
| | **Retardation, motor** | | ± | ± | ± | ± |
| Ear | Hearing loss, sensorineural | ± | ± | ± | ± | ± |
| Eye | **Glaucoma** | ± | ± | ± | ± | ± |
| | **Retinal dystrophy** | ± | ± | ± | ± | ± |
| Musculoskeletal | **Calf pseudohypertrophy** | ± | ± | ± | ± | ± |
| | **Limb-girdle congenital muscular dystrophy** | ± | ± | ± | ± | ± |
| | **Macrocephaly** | ± | ± | ± | ± | ± |
| | **Muscle cramps** | ± | ± | ± | ± | ± |
| | **Muscle weakness, proximal** | ± | ± | ± | ± | ± |
| Other | **Walker Warburg syndrome/ muscle-eye-brain disease** | ± | ± | ± | ± | ± |
| Laboratory findings | Creatine kinase (plasma) | ↑↑ | ↑↑ | ↑↑ | ↑↑ | ↑↑ |
| | Sialotransferrins (serum) | n | n | n | n | n |

**Table 68.35** Muscular dystrophy-dystroglycanopathy type A7 and C7 CRPPA-CDG

| System | Symptoms and biomarkers | Neonatal (birth–1 month) | Infancy (1–18 months) | Childhood (1.5–11 years) | Adolescence (11–16 years) | Adulthood (>16 years) |
|---|---|---|---|---|---|---|
| Cardiovascular | Cardiac dysfunction | ± | ± | ± | ± | ± |
| CNS | **Agenesis, corpus callosum (MRI)** | ± | ± | ± | ± | ± |
| | Anterior chamber abnormalities | ± | ± | ± | ± | ± |
| | **Brain stem hypoplasia** | + | ± | ± | ± | ± |
| | Brain vascular anomalies | ± | ± | ± | ± | ± |
| | **Cerebellar dys/hypoplasia** | + | ± | ± | ± | ± |
| | **Cobblestone lissencephaly** | + | ± | ± | ± | ± |
| | **Hydrocephalus** | ± | ± | ± | ± | ± |
| | **Hypotonia** | ± | ± | ± | ± | ± |
| | **Neural tube defects** | ± | ± | ± | ± | ± |
| Endocrine | Gonadal dysgenesis | | | | ± | ± |
| Eye | Agyria | ± | ± | ± | ± | ± |
| | **Cataract** | + | ± | ± | ± | ± |
| | **Chorioretinal degeneration** | ± | ± | ± | ± | ± |
| | Corneal clouding | ± | ± | ± | ± | ± |
| | **Microphthalmia** | ± | ± | ± | ± | ± |
| | **Optic nerve hypoplasia** | ± | ± | ± | ± | ± |
| | Pachygyria | ± | ± | ± | ± | ± |
| | Vitreous, persistent hyperplastic primary | ± | ± | ± | ± | ± |
| Musculoskeletal | **Calf pseudohypertrophy** | ± | ± | ± | ± | ± |
| | **Limb deformities** | ± | ± | ± | ± | ± |
| | **Muscular dystrophy** | ± | ± | ± | ± | ± |
| Other | **Walker-Warburg syndrome/ muscle-eye-brain disease** | ± | ± | ± | ± | ± |
| Laboratory findings | Creatine kinase (plasma) | n-↑ | n-↑ | n-↑ | n-↑ | n-↑ |
| | Sialotransferrins (serum) | n | n | n | n | n |

**Table 68.36** Muscular dystrophy-dystroglycanopathy (congenital with brain and eye anomalies), type A, 4 FKTN-CDG A

| System | Symptoms and biomarkers | Neonatal (birth–1 month) | Infancy (1–18 months) | Childhood (1.5–11 years) | Adolescence (11–16 years) | Adulthood (>16 years) |
|---|---|---|---|---|---|---|
| Cardiovascular | **Cardiomyopathy, dilated** | ± | ± | ± | ± | ± |
| CNS | **Brainstem hypoplasia** | ± | ± | ± | ± | ± |
| | **Cerebellar abnormalities** | ± | ± | ± | ± | ± |
| | **Cobblestone lissencephaly** | ± | ± | ± | ± | ± |
| | **Corpus callosum abnormalities** | ± | ± | ± | ± | ± |
| | **Epilepsy** | ± | ± | ± | ± | ± |
| | **Hydrocephalus** | ± | ± | ± | ± | ± |
| | **Hypotonia** | ± | ± | ± | ± | ± |
| | **Polymicrogyria** | ± | ± | ± | ± | ± |
| | **Regression, psychomotor** | | ± | ± | ± | ± |
| Eye | Agyria | ± | ± | ± | ± | ± |
| | **Cataract** | ± | ± | ± | ± | ± |
| | **Chorioretinal degeneration** | ± | ± | ± | ± | ± |
| | **Microphthalmia** | ± | ± | ± | ± | ± |
| | **Optic atrophy** | ± | ± | ± | ± | ± |
| | Pachygyria | ± | ± | ± | ± | ± |
| Musculoskeletal | **Calf muscle hypertrophy** | ± | ± | ± | ± | ± |
| | Contractures, progressive | ± | ± | ± | ± | ± |
| | **Muscular dystrophy** | + | + | + | + | + |
| | **Scoliosis** | | ± | ± | ± | ± |
| Respiratory | **Respiratory insufficiency** | | ± | ± | ± | ± |
| Other | **Walker-Warburg syndrome/ muscle-eye-brain disease** | ± | ± | ± | ± | ± |
| Laboratory findings | Creatine kinase (plasma) | ↑↑ | ↑↑ | ↑↑ | ↑↑ | ↑↑ |
| | Sialotransferrins (serum) | n | n | n | n | n |

**Table 68.37** Muscular dystrophy-dystroglycanopathy (congenital without mental retardation), type B, 4 FKTN-CDG B

| System | Symptoms and biomarkers | Neonatal (birth–1 month) | Infancy (1–18 months) | Childhood (1.5–11 years) | Adolescence (11–16 years) | Adulthood (>16 years) |
|---|---|---|---|---|---|---|
| CNS | **Hypotonia** | + | + | + | | |
| Musculoskeletal | **Muscular dystrophy** | + | + | + | | |
| Laboratory findings | Creatine kinase (plasma) | ↑↑ | ↑↑ | ↑↑ | | |
| Laboratory findings | Sialotransferrins (serum) | n | n | n | | |

**Table 68.38** Muscular dystrophy-dystroglycanopathy (limb-girdle), type C, 4 FKTN-CDG C

| System | Symptoms and biomarkers | Neonatal (birth–1 month) | Infancy (1–18 months) | Childhood (1.5–11 years) | Adolescence (11–16 years) | Adulthood (>16 years) |
|---|---|---|---|---|---|---|
| Cardiovascular | **Cardiomyopathy** | ± | ± | ± | ± | ± |
| CNS | **Hypotonia** | ± | ± | ± | ± | ± |
| Musculoskeletal | **Limb-girdle muscular dystrophy** | + | + | + | + | + |
| | Rigid spine | | | ± | ± | ± |
| Laboratory findings | Creatine kinase (plasma) | ↑↑ | ↑↑ | ↑↑ | ↑↑ | ↑↑ |
| | Sialotransferrins (serum) | n | n | n | n | n |

**Table 68.39** Muscular dystrophy-dystroglycanopathy (congenital with brain and eye anomalies), type A, 5 FKRP-CDG A

| System | Symptoms and biomarkers | Neonatal (birth–1 month) | Infancy (1–18 months) | Childhood (1.5–11 years) | Adolescence (11–16 years) | Adulthood (>16 years) |
|---|---|---|---|---|---|---|
| Cardiovascular | Cardiomyopathy | ± | ± | ± | | |
| CNS | **Brainstem hypoplasia** | ± | ± | ± | | |
| | **Cerebellar abnormalities** | + | + | + | | |
| | **Cobblestone lissencephaly** | + | + | + | | |
| | **Corpus callosum abnormalities** | + | + | + | | |
| | Dandy-Walker malformation | ± | ± | ± | | |
| | **Hydrocephalus** | ± | ± | ± | | |
| | **Hypotonia** | + | + | + | | |
| | **Regression, psychomotor** | | ++ | ++ | | |
| Eye | Agyria | ± | ± | ± | | |
| | Cataract | ± | ± | ± | | |
| | Coloboma | ± | ± | ± | | |
| | Corneal clouding | ± | ± | ± | | |
| | **Eye movements, roving** | ± | ± | ± | | |
| | **Microphthalmos** | ± | ± | ± | | |
| | Pachygyria | ± | ± | ± | | |
| | **Retinal abnormalities** | + | + | + | | |
| Musculoskeletal | **Calf pseudohypertrophy** | ± | ± | ± | | |
| | **Muscular dystrophy** | + | + | + | | |
| Other | **Walker-Warburg syndrome/ muscle-eye-brain disease** | + | + | + | | |
| Laboratory findings | Creatine kinase (plasma) | ↑↑ | ↑↑ | ↑↑ | | |
| | Sialotransferrins (serum) | n | n | n | | |

**Table 68.40** Muscular dystrophy-dystroglycanopathy (congenital with or without mental retardation), type B, 5 FKRP-CDG B

| System | Symptoms and biomarkers | Neonatal (birth–1 month) | Infancy (1–18 months) | Childhood (1.5–11 years) | Adolescence (11–16 years) | Adulthood (>16 years) |
|---|---|---|---|---|---|---|
| CNS | Cerebellar abnormalities | ± | ± | ± | ± | ± |
| | **Hypotonia** | + | + | + | + | + |
| | Intellectual disability | | ± | ± | ± | ± |
| | Nodular heterotopia | ± | ± | ± | ± | ± |
| | Spinal abnormalities | ± | ± | ± | ± | ± |
| | White matter abnormalities | ± | ± | ± | ± | ± |
| Digestive | Feeding difficulties | ± | ± | ± | ± | ± |
| Eye | Pachygyria | ± | ± | ± | ± | ± |
| Musculoskeletal | Microcephaly | ± | ± | ± | ± | ± |
| | **Muscular dystrophy** | + | + | + | + | + |
| Laboratory findings | Creatine kinase (plasma) | ↑↑ | ↑↑ | ↑↑ | ↑↑ | ↑↑ |
| | Sialotransferrins (serum) | n | n | n | n | n |

**Table 68.41** Muscular dystrophy-dystroglycanopathy (limb-girdle), type C, 5 FKRP-CDG C

| System | Symptoms and biomarkers | Neonatal (birth–1 month) | Infancy (1–18 months) | Childhood (1.5–11 years) | Adolescence (11–16 years) | Adulthood (>16 years) |
|---|---|---|---|---|---|---|
| Cardiovascular | Cardiomyopathy | ± | ± | ± | ± | ± |
| CNS | **Spinal abnormalities** | | ± | ± | ± | ± |
| Musculoskeletal | **Calf muscle hypertrophy** | | ± | ± | + | + |
| | **Limb-girdle muscular dystrophy** | + | + | + | + | + |
| | Myoglobinuria | ± | ± | ± | ± | ± |
| | Tongue hypertrophy | | ± | ± | ± | ± |
| Respiratory | Respiratory failure | | ± | ± | ± | ± |
| Laboratory findings | Creatine kinase (plasma) | ↑↑ | ↑↑ | ↑↑ | ↑↑ | ↑↑ |
| | Sialotransferrins (serum) | n | n | n | n | n |

**Table 68.42** Muscular dystrophy-dystroglycanopathy (congenital with brain and eye anomalies), type A, 10 TMEM5-CDG

| System | Symptoms and biomarkers | Neonatal (birth–1 month) | Infancy (1–18 months) | Childhood (1.5–11 years) | Adolescence (11–16 years) | Adulthood (>16 years) |
|---|---|---|---|---|---|---|
| CNS | Cerebellar dysplasia | ± | ± | ± | ± | |
| | Cobblestone lissencephaly | ± | ± | ± | ± | |
| | **Hypotonia** | + | + | + | + | |
| | Intellectual disability | | ± | ± | ± | |
| | Neural tube defect | ± | | | | |
| Endocrine | Gonadal dysgenesis | ± | ± | ± | ± | |
| Eye | Retinal dysplasia | ± | ± | ± | ± | |
| Musculoskeletal | **Muscular dystrophy** | + | + | + | + | |
| Laboratory findings | Creatine kinase (plasma) | ↑↑ | ↑↑ | ↑↑ | ↑↑ | |
| | Sialotransferrins (serum) | n | n | n | n | |

**Table 68.43** β-1,4-glucuronyltransferase 1 deficiency B4GAT1-CDG

| System | Symptoms and biomarkers | Neonatal (birth–1 month) | Infancy (1–18 months) | Childhood (1.5–11 years) | Adolescence (11–16 years) | Adulthood (>16 years) |
|---|---|---|---|---|---|---|
| CNS | **Brainstem hypoplasia** | + | + | | | |
| | **Cerebellar hypoplasia** | + | + | | | |
| | **Cobblestone lissencephaly** | + | + | | | |
| | **Corpus callosum hypogenesis** | + | + | | | |
| | **Cortical dysplasia** | + | + | | | |
| | **Epilepsy** | ± | ± | | | |
| | **Hydrocephalus** | + | + | | | |
| | **Hypotonia** | + | + | | | |
| | Nodular heterotopia | ± | ± | | | |
| | **Psychomotor development, absent** | + | + | | | |
| Eye | Corneal clouding | ± | ± | | | |
| | **Optic nerve dysplasia** | + | + | | | |
| | **Retinal dysplasia** | + | + | | | |
| Genitourinary | **Micropenis** | ± | ± | | | |
| | **Testicular hypoplasia** | ± | ± | | | |
| Musculoskeletal | Anencephaly | ± | | | | |
| | Encephalocoele, occipital | ± | ± | | | |
| | **Muscular dystrophy** | + | + | | | |
| Renal | Hydronephrosis | ± | ± | | | |
| | **Kidney dysplasia** | ± | ± | | | |
| | **Renal cysts** | ± | ± | | | |
| Other | Dandy-Walker malformation | ± | ± | | | |
| Laboratory findings | Creatine kinase (plasma) | ↑↑ | ↑↑ | | | |
| | Sialotransferrins (serum) | n | n | | | |

**Table 68.44** β-1,3-glucuronyltransferase/α-1,3-xylosyltransferase deficiency LARGE1-CDG

| System | Symptoms and biomarkers | Neonatal (birth–1 month) | Infancy (1–18 months) | Childhood (1.5–11 years) | Adolescence (11–16 years) | Adulthood (>16 years) |
|---|---|---|---|---|---|---|
| CNS | **Brainstem hypoplasia** | ± | ± | ± | ± | |
| | **Cerebellar hypoplasia** | + | + | + | + | |
| | **Developmental regression** | | + | + | + | |
| | **Hypotonia** | + | + | + | + | |
| | **Neuronal migration abnormalities** | + | + | + | + | |
| | Nystagmus, horizontal | ± | ± | ± | ± | |
| | Pachygyria, frontoparietal | ± | ± | ± | ± | |
| | White matter changes (MRI) | ± | ± | ± | ± | |
| Musculoskeletal | Camptodactyly | ± | ± | ± | ± | |
| | **Muscle dystrophy, progressive** | + | + | + | + | |
| | Muscle hypertrophy | ± | + | + | + | |
| Laboratory findings | Creatine kinase (plasma) | ↑↑ | ↑↑ | ↑↑ | ↑↑ | |
| | Sialotransferrins (serum) | n | n | n | n | |

**Table 68.45** XYLT1 deficiency XYLT1-CDG

| System | Symptoms and biomarkers | Neonatal (birth–1 month) | Infancy (1–18 months) | Childhood (1.5–11 years) | Adolescence (11–16 years) | Adulthood (>16 years) |
|---|---|---|---|---|---|---|
| CNS | **Intellectual disability** | | + | + | + | + |
| Digestive | Obesity | | ± | ± | ± | |
| Eye | Myopia | | ± | ± | | |
| Musculoskeletal | **Brachydactyly** | + | + | + | + | + |
| | Cleft palate | ± | ± | ± | | |
| | Clubfoot | ± | | | | |
| | **Depressed nasal bridge** | + | | | | |
| | **Flat midface** | + | + | + | + | + |
| | **Joint laxity** | + | + | + | | |
| | **Patellar dislocation** | | | + | + | + |
| | **Short stature** | + | + | + | + | + |
| | Synophrys | ± | ± | ± | ± | ± |
| Radiographic findings | Advanced bone age | + | + | + | | |
| | Coronal clefts | + | | | | |
| | Monkey wrench appearance of femora | + | + | + | | |
| | Short femoral necks | + | + | + | | |
| | Short metacarpals | + | + | + | + | + |
| | Short phalanges | + | + | + | + | + |

**Table 68.46** XYLT2 deficiency XYLT2-CDG

| System | Symptoms and biomarkers | Neonatal (birth–1 month) | Infancy (1–18 months) | Childhood (1.5–11 years) | Adolescence (11–16 years) | Adulthood (>16 years) |
|---|---|---|---|---|---|---|
| Cardiovascular | Atrial septal defect | ± | ± | | | |
| CNS | Intellectual disability | | | ± | | |
| Ear | **Hearing loss** | + | + | + | | |
| Eye | **Cataract** | + | + | + | | |
| | **Retinal detachment** | | | + | + | |
| Musculoskeletal | Kyphosis | | | ± | ± | ± |
| | **Long bone fractures** | + | + | + | | |
| | **Short stature** | | | ± | ± | ± |
| Radiographic findings | **Low bone mineral density** | | + | + | + | + |
| | **Vertebral compression fractures** | | + | + | + | + |

**Table 68.47** Beta-1,4-galactosyltransferase 7 deficiency B4GALT7-CDG

| System | Symptoms and biomarkers | Neonatal (birth–1 month) | Infancy (1–18 months) | Childhood (1.5–11 years) | Adolescence (11–16 years) | Adulthood (>16 years) |
|---|---|---|---|---|---|---|
| CNS | Developmental delay | ± | ± | ± | | |
| Dermatological | **Atrophic scars** | | + | + | + | + |
| | **Hyperelastic, loose skin** | + | + | + | + | + |
| Eye | Cataracts | ± | ± | ± | | |
| | **Proptosis** | + | + | + | + | + |
| Musculoskeletal | **Arachnodactyly** | + | + | + | + | + |
| | Dental defects | | + | + | + | + |
| | **Flat midface** | + | + | + | + | + |
| | **Frontal bossing** | + | + | + | + | + |
| | **Joint laxity** | ++ | ++ | ++ | ++ | ++ |
| | **Overlapping fingers** | + | + | + | + | + |
| | **Scoliosis** | | + | + | + | + |
| | **Short stature** | + | + | + | + | + |
| | Talipes equinovarus | + | + | + | + | + |
| Laboratory findings | Sialotransferrins (serum) | n | n | n | n | n |
| Radiographic findings | Advanced bone age | ± | ± | ± | | |
| | **Large joint dislocations** | + | + | + | + | + |
| | Low bone mineral density | | | + | + | + |
| | **Radioulnar synostosis** | + | + | + | + | + |

**Table 68.48** Beta-1,3-galactosyltransferase 6 deficiency B3GALT6-CDG

| System | Symptoms and biomarkers | Neonatal (birth–1 month) | Infancy (1–18 months) | Childhood (1.5–11 years) | Adolescence (11–16 years) | Adulthood (>16 years) |
|---|---|---|---|---|---|---|
| Cardiovascular | Congenital heart defects | ± | ± | | | |
| CNS | Hypotonia | ± | ± | ± | | |
| Dermatological | Hyperelastic skin | ± | ± | ± | | |
| Eye | Corneal clouding | ± | ± | ± | ± | ± |
| Musculoskeletal | Cleft palate | ± | ± | ± | | |
| | Flat midface | + | + | + | | |
| | **Joint laxity** | ++ | ++ | ++ | ++ | ++ |
| | **Kyphoscoliosis** | + | + | ++ | ++ | ++ |
| | Short stature | + | + | + | + | + |
| | Spatulate distal phalanges | + | + | + | | |
| | Talipes equinovarus | + | + | + | | |
| Other | Pectus carinatum | ± | ± | ± | | |
| Radiographic findings | Epiphyseal dysplasia | + | + | + | + | |
| | Hip dislocation | + | + | + | | |
| | Long bone fractures | ± | ± | ± | ± | ± |
| | Platyspondyly | + | + | | | |
| | **Radial head dislocation** | + | + | + | + | + |

**Table 68.49** Beta-1,3-glucuronyltransferase 3 deficiency B3GAT3-CDG

| System | Symptoms and biomarkers | Neonatal (birth–1 month) | Infancy (1–18 months) | Childhood (1.5–11 years) | Adolescence (11–16 years) | Adulthood (>16 years) |
|---|---|---|---|---|---|---|
| Cardiovascular | Congenital heart defects | ± | ± | | | |
| CNS | Hypotonia | ± | ± | ± | | |
| Eye | Proptosis | ± | ± | ± | | |
| Musculoskeletal | Cleft palate | ± | ± | ± | | |
| | Clubfoot | ± | ± | ± | | |
| | Flat midface | + | + | + | | |
| | **Joint laxity** | + | + | + | + | + |
| | **Kyphoscoliosis** | + | + | + | | |
| | **Overlapping, long fingers** | ± | ± | ± | | |
| | Pectus carinatum | ± | ± | ± | | |
| | **Scoliosis** | + | + | + | | |
| | Short stature | + | + | + | + | + |
| Radiographic findings | Bowing of long bones | ± | ± | | | |
| | Craniosynostosis | ± | ± | | | |
| | Joint dislocations | + | + | + | + | + |
| | Long bone fractures | ± | ± | ± | ± | ± |
| | Radioulnar synostosis | + | + | + | + | + |

**Table 68.50** Exostosin 1 deficiency EXT1-CDG

| System | Symptoms and biomarkers | Neonatal (birth–1 month) | Infancy (1–18 months) | Childhood (1.5–11 years) | Adolescence (11–16 years) | Adulthood (>16 years) |
|---|---|---|---|---|---|---|
| Musculoskeletal | **Bone deformity** | | | ± | ± | ± |
| | **Chondrosarcoma** | | | ± | ± | ± |
| | **Functional joint impairment** | | | ± | ± | ± |
| | **Osteochondroma** | | + | ++ | ++ | ++ |
| Laboratory findings | Sialotransferrins (serum) | n | n | n | n | n |

**Table 68.51** Exostosin 2 deficiency EXT2-CDG

| System | Symptoms and biomarkers | Neonatal (birth–1 month) | Infancy (1–18 months) | Childhood (1.5–11 years) | Adolescence (11–16 years) | Adulthood (>16 years) |
|---|---|---|---|---|---|---|
| Musculoskeletal | **Bone deformity** | | | ± | ± | ± |
| | **Chondrosarcoma** | | | ± | ± | ± |
| | **Functional joint impairment** | | | ± | ± | ± |
| | **Osteochondroma** | | + | ++ | ++ | ++ |
| Laboratory findings | Sialotransferrins (serum) | n | n | n | n | n |

**Table 68.52** Autosomal recessive exostosin 2 deficiency autosomal recessive EXT2-CDG

| System | Symptoms and biomarkers | Neonatal (birth–1 month) | Infancy (1–18 months) | Childhood (1.5–11 years) | Adolescence (11–16 years) | Adulthood (>16 years) |
|---|---|---|---|---|---|---|
| CNS | Hypotonia | + | + | + | + | + |
| | **Intellectual disability** | | + | + | + | + |
| | **Seizures** | | + | + | + | + |
| Musculoskeletal | **Hypertelorism** | + | + | + | + | + |
| | **Kyphoscoliosis** | | | | + | + |
| | **Macrocephaly** | | | + | + | + |
| Radiographic findings | Low bone mineral density | | | ± | ± | ± |

**Table 68.53** Exostosin-like glycosyltransferase 3 deficiency EXTL3-CDG

| System | Symptoms and biomarkers | Neonatal (birth–1 month) | Infancy (1–18 months) | Childhood (1.5–11 years) | Adolescence (11–16 years) | Adulthood (>16 years) |
|---|---|---|---|---|---|---|
| CNS | Developmental delay | + | + | | | |
| | **Intellectual disability** | + | + | + | + | |
| | Opisthotonus | ± | ± | | | |
| | Hyperreflexia | ± | ± | | | |
| | Seizures | ± | ± | | | |
| | Spinal cord compression | + | + | + | + | |
| Digestive | **Liver cysts** | + | + | + | + | |
| Hematological | Hypogammaglobulinemia | ± | ± | | | |
| | **Immunodeficiency, T-cell** | + | + | + | | |
| Musculoskeletal | **Kyphosis** | + | + | + | + | + |
| | **Short stature** | + | + | + | + | + |
| Radiographic findings | **Brachydactyly** | + | + | + | + | + |
| | Craniosynostosis | ± | ± | | | |
| | Dislocated radial heads | | | + | + | + |
| | **Platyspondyly** | + | + | + | + | + |
| | Small capital femoral epiphyses | | + | + | + | |

**Table 68.54** Chondroitin sulfate synthase 1 deficiency CHSY1-CDG

| System | Symptoms and biomarkers | Neonatal (birth–1 month) | Infancy (1–18 months) | Childhood (1.5–11 years) | Adolescence (11–16 years) | Adulthood (>16 years) |
|---|---|---|---|---|---|---|
| CNS | Cerebellar vermis hypoplasia | ± | ± | ± | ± | ± |
| | Developmental delay | ± | ± | ± | ± | |
| Ear | Sensorineural hearing loss | ± | ± | ± | ± | ± |
| Eye | Optic atrophy | ± | ± | ± | ± | ± |
| Musculoskeletal | **Abducted thumbs** | + | + | + | + | + |
| | **Clinodactyly** | + | + | + | + | + |
| | Kyphoscoliosis | ± | ± | ± | ± | ± |
| | **Medial deviations of fingers** | + | + | + | + | + |
| | **Medial deviations of toes** | + | + | + | + | + |
| | Pectus excavatum | ± | ± | ± | ± | ± |
| | **Preaxial brachydactyly** | + | + | + | + | + |
| | **Syndactyly** | + | + | + | + | + |
| Radiographic findings | **Carpal/tarsal fusion** | | | + | + | + |
| | **Delta-shaped phalanges** | + | + | + | + | + |
| | **Hyperphalangism** | + | + | + | + | + |
| | Radioulnar synostosis | ± | ± | ± | ± | ± |
| | **Symphalangism** | + | + | + | + | + |

**Table 68.55** Chondroitin 4-sulfotransferase 1 deficiency CHST11-CDG

| System | Symptoms and biomarkers | Neonatal (birth–1 month) | Infancy (1–18 months) | Childhood (1.5–11 years) | Adolescence (11–16 years) | Adulthood (>16 years) |
|---|---|---|---|---|---|---|
| Musculoskeletal | **Clinodactyly** | + | + | + | + | + |
| | Kyphoscoliosis | | | | + | + |
| | **Medial deviations of fingers** | + | + | + | + | + |
| | **Medial deviations of toes** | + | + | + | + | + |
| | Pectus excavatum | | | | | ± |
| | **Preaxial brachydactyly** | + | + | + | + | + |
| | **Syndactyly** | + | + | + | + | + |
| `Radiographic findings | **Delta-shaped phalanges** | + | + | + | + | + |
| | **Dislocated patellae** | | | | + | + |
| | **Hyperphalangism** | + | + | + | + | + |
| | **Symphalangism** | + | + | + | + | + |

**Table 68.56** Chondroitin 6-sulfotransferase deficiency CHST3-CDG

| System | Symptoms and biomarkers | Neonatal (birth–1 month) | Infancy (1–18 months) | Childhood (1.5–11 years) | Adolescence (11–16 years) | Adulthood (>16 years) |
|---|---|---|---|---|---|---|
| Cardiovascular | Heart valve dysplasia | ± | ± | ± | | |
| Ear | Hearing loss | ± | ± | ± | | |
| Musculoskeletal | Clubfoot | + | + | + | | |
| | **Joint dislocations** | + | + | + | | |
| | **Kyphoscoliosis** | | + | + | + | + |
| | **Short stature** | + | + | + | + | + |
| Radiographic findings | **Bifid distal humerus** | ± | ± | | | |
| | **Coronal clefts** | + | | | | |
| | Small epiphyses | | ± | ± | ± | |

**Table 68.57** Dermatan 4-sulfotransferase 1 deficiency CHST14-CDG

| System | Symptoms and biomarkers | Neonatal (birth–1 month) | Infancy (1–18 months) | Childhood (1.5–11 years) | Adolescence (11–16 years) | Adulthood (>16 years) |
|---|---|---|---|---|---|---|
| Hematological | **Large subcutaneous hematomas** | + | + | + | + | + |
| Dermatological | Atrophic scars | | + | + | + | + |
| | **Excessively wrinkled palms** | + | + | + | + | + |
| | **Hyperextensible skin** | + | + | + | + | + |
| Eye | Glaucoma | | | | | + |
| Musculoskeletal | **Adducted thumbs** | ± | ± | | | |
| | **Downslanted palpebral fissures** | + | + | + | + | + |
| | **Joint laxity** | + | + | + | + | + |
| | **Long tapered fingers and toes** | + | + | + | + | + |
| | **Myopathy** | + | + | + | + | + |
| | **Scoliosis** | | | + | + | + |
| | **Short stature** | | | + | + | + |
| | **Talipes equinovarus** | + | + | | | |

**Table 68.58** Dermatan sulfate epimerase deficiency DSE-CDG

| System | Symptoms and biomarkers | Neonatal (birth–1 month) | Infancy (1–18 months) | Childhood (1.5–11 years) | Adolescence (11–16 years) | Adulthood (>16 years) |
|---|---|---|---|---|---|---|
| Hematological | **Large subcutaneous hematomas** | + | + | + | + | + |
| Dermatological | Atrophic scars | | + | + | + | + |
| | **Excessively wrinkled palms** | + | + | + | + | + |
| | **Hyperextensible skin** | + | + | + | + | + |
| CNS | Hypotonia | + | + | + | | + |
| Musculoskeletal | Adducted thumbs | ± | ± | | | |
| | **Downslanted palpebral fissures** | + | + | + | + | + |
| | **Joint laxity** | + | + | + | + | + |
| | **Long tapered fingers and toes** | + | + | + | + | + |
| | **Scoliosis** | | | + | + | + |
| | **Short stature** | | | + | + | + |
| | **Talipes equinovarus** | + | + | | | |

**Table 68.59** Chondroitin sulfate N-acetylgalactosaminyltransferase 1 deficiency CSGALNACT1-CDG

| System | Symptoms and biomarkers | Neonatal (birth–1 month) | Infancy (1–18 months) | Childhood (1.5–11 years) | Adolescence (11–16 years) | Adulthood (>16 years) |
|---|---|---|---|---|---|---|
| Cardiovascular | Congenital heart defect | ± | | | | |
| CNS | Hypotonia | ± | | | | |
| Musculoskeletal | Flat midface | + | + | | | |
| | Genu valgum | | | + | + | |
| | Joint laxity | | + | + | + | |
| | Short stature | + | + | + | + | |
| Radiographic findings | Advanced bone age | + | + | + | | |
| | Coronal clefts | + | | | | |
| | Enlarged lesser trochanter | + | + | | | |
| | Mild tibial bowing | | | + | + | |

**Table 68.60** Corneal N-acetylglucosamine 6-O-sulfotransferase deficiency CHST6-CDG

| System | Symptoms and biomarkers | Neonatal (birth–1 month) | Infancy (1–18 months) | Childhood (1.5–11 years) | Adolescence (11–16 years) | Adulthood (>16 years) |
|---|---|---|---|---|---|---|
| Eye | Corneal erosion | | | + | + | + |
| | **Corneal opacities** | | | + | + | + |
| | **Macular corneal dystrophy** | | | + | + | + |
| | **Photophobia** | | | + | + | + |

**Table 68.61** Heparan sulfate N-deacetylase N-sulfotransferase 1 deficiency NDST1-CDG

| System | Symptoms and biomarkers | Neonatal (birth–1 month) | Infancy (1–18 months) | Childhood (1.5–11 years) | Adolescence (11–16 years) | Adulthood (>16 years) |
|---|---|---|---|---|---|---|
| Respiratory | Apnea | ± | | | | |
| CNS | Ataxia | | | ± | ± | ± |
| | Cranial nerve dysfunction | ± | | | | |
| | **Epilepsy** | + | + | + | + | + |
| | **Hypotonia** | + | + | + | + | + |
| | **Intellectual disability** | | + | + | + | + |
| | Sleep disturbances | | ± | ± | ± | |
| Psychiatric | Aggressive behavior | | ± | ± | ± | ± |
| | Self-injury | | ± | ± | ± | ± |

**Table 68.62** Heparan sulfate 6-O-sulfate transferase 1 deficiency HS6ST1-CDG

| System | Symptoms and biomarkers | Neonatal (birth–1 month) | Infancy (1–18 months) | Childhood (1.5–11 years) | Adolescence (11–16 years) | Adulthood (>16 years) |
|---|---|---|---|---|---|---|
| CNS | **Anosmia** | | | ± | ± | |
| Ear | Sensorineural hearing loss | | | ± | ± | |
| Endocrine | **Hypogonadotropic hypogonadism** | | | + | + | + |
| | **Self-limited delayed puberty** | | | | + | |
| Musculoskeletal | Cleft palate | | | ± | ± | |
| Laboratory findings | Gonadotropins (plasma) | | | ↓ | ↓ | |
| | Testosterone (plasma) | | | ↓ | ↓ | |

**Table 68.63** Calcium-activated nucleotidase 1 deficiency CANT1-CDG

| System | Symptoms and biomarkers | Neonatal (birth–1 month) | Infancy (1–18 months) | Childhood (1.5–11 years) | Adolescence (11–16 years) | Adulthood (>16 years) |
|---|---|---|---|---|---|---|
| CNS | Motor developmental delay | | ± | ± | | |
| Eye | **Glaucoma** | ± | ± | ± | ± | |
| | Myopia | | + | + | + | |
| | Prominent eyes | + | + | + | + | |
| Musculoskeletal | Clubfoot | + | + | + | | |
| | Finger deviation | + | + | | | |
| | **Joint laxity** | + | + | + | + | |
| | Microretrognathia | + | + | + | + | |
| | Midface hypoplasia | + | + | + | + | |
| | Round face | + | + | + | + | |
| | **Short stature** | + | + | + | + | + |
| Radiographic findings | **Advanced bone age** | + | + | + | + | |
| | Coronal clefts | + | + | | | |
| | **Hyperphalangy** | ± | ± | ± | ± | |
| | Joint dislocations | ± | ± | | | |
| | Prominent lesser trochanters | + | + | + | | |
| | Short metacarpals | ± | ± | ± | ± | |
| | Small epiphyses | | | + | + | |

**Table 68.64** Sulfate transporter deficiency SLC26A2-CDG

| System | Symptoms and biomarkers | Neonatal (birth–1 month) | Infancy (1–18 months) | Childhood (1.5–11 years) | Adolescence (11–16 years) | Adulthood (>16 years) |
|---|---|---|---|---|---|---|
| Ear | **Cauliflower ear** | | | ± | ± | ± |
| | **Cystic ear** | ± | ± | | | |
| Musculoskeletal | **Abducted ("hitchhiker") thumbs** | + | + | + | + | + |
| | Cleft palate | ± | ± | | | |
| | Joint contractures | + | + | + | + | + |
| | **Kyphoscoliosis** | | + | + | + | + |
| | **Short stature** | + | + | + | + | + |
| | Talipes equinovarus | + | + | + | + | + |
| Radiographic findings | **Advanced carpal bone age** | + | + | + | + | |
| | Bowing of radius and ulna | ± | | | | |
| | **Delta-shaped phalanges** | + | + | + | + | |
| | **Flat epiphyses** | + | + | + | + | |
| | **Multilayered patellae** | | | ± | ± | ± |
| | **Short long bones** | + | + | + | + | + |
| Other | Fetal hydrops | ± | | | | |
| | Intrauterine death | ± | | | | |
| Respiratory | Respiratory insufficiency | ± | | | | |

**Table 68.65** Phosphoadenosine 5′-phosphosulfate synthetase 2 deficiency PAPSS2-CDG

| System | Symptoms and biomarkers | Neonatal (birth–1 month) | Infancy (1–18 months) | Childhood (1.5–11 years) | Adolescence (11–16 years) | Adulthood (>16 years) |
|---|---|---|---|---|---|---|
| Dermatological | Acne, severe | | | + | + | |
| | Hirsutism | | | + | + | |
| Endocrine | **Premature pubarche** | | | ± | ± | |
| | Secondary amenorrhea | | | | + | + |
| Musculoskeletal | **Bowed limbs** | | + | + | + | + |
| | Brachydactyly | ± | ± | ± | ± | ± |
| | Enlarged knee joints | | + | + | + | + |
| | **Kyphosis** | | | + | + | + |
| | **Short stature** | | + | + | + | + |
| Radiographic findings | Advanced bone age | | | + | + | |
| | Delayed epiphyseal ossification | ± | ± | ± | ± | ± |
| | **Platyspondyly** | + | + | + | + | + |
| | Precocious osteoarthropathy | | | | + | + |
| | Short metacarpals | ± | ± | ± | ± | ± |
| Laboratory findings | Androstenedione (plasma) | | | ↑ | ↑ | ↑ |
| | Dehydroepiandrosterone DHEA (plasma) | | | n-↑ | n-↑ | n-↑ |
| | **Dehydroepiandrosterone sulfate DHEAS (plasma)** | | | ↓ | ↓ | ↓ |
| | Testosterone (plasma) | | | ↑ | ↑ | ↑ |

**Table 68.66** Inositol monophosphate domain-containing protein 1 deficiency IMPAD1-CDG

| System | Symptoms and biomarkers | Neonatal (birth–1 month) | Infancy (1–18 months) | Childhood (1.5–11 years) | Adolescence (11–16 years) | Adulthood (>16 years) |
|---|---|---|---|---|---|---|
| Ear | Brachydactyly | + | + | | | |
| | **Cleft palate** | + | + | | | |
| | Hearing loss | | | | ± | ± |
| | **Joint dislocations** | + | + | + | + | + |
| | **Joint laxity** | + | + | + | + | + |
| | **Lateral deviation of the fifth toe** | + | + | + | + | + |
| | **Micrognathia** | + | + | | | |
| Musculoskeletal | **Short stature** | + | + | + | + | + |
| Radiographic findings | Accesory ossification centers of hands and feet | ± | ± | | | |
| | Advanced carpal bone age | ± | ± | ± | | |
| | Carpal fusion | | + | + | + | + |
| | Dislocated patellae | + | + | | | |
| | **Short metacarpals** | + | + | | | |

**Table 68.67** TDP-D-glucose 4,6-dehydrogenase deficiency—Catel–Manzke syndrome TGDS-CDG

| System | Symptoms and biomarkers | Neonatal (birth–1 month) | Infancy (1–18 months) | Childhood (1.5–11 years) | Adolescence (11–16 years) | Adulthood (>16 years) |
|---|---|---|---|---|---|---|
| Cardiovascular | Ventricular septal defect | ± | ± | | | |
| Musculoskeletal | Cleft palate | + | + | + | + | + |
| | Hyperphalangy of index finger | + | + | + | + | |
| | Joint laxity | ± | ± | ± | | |
| | Micrognathia | + | + | + | + | + |
| | Radial deviation of the index finger | + | + | + | + | + |
| | Short stature | ± | ± | ± | | |

**Table 68.68** Polypeptide N-acetylgalactosaminyltransferase 3 deficiency GALTNT3-CDG

| System | Symptoms and biomarkers | Neonatal (birth–1 month) | Infancy (1–18 months) | Childhood (1.5–11 years) | Adolescence (11–16 years) | Adulthood (>16 years) |
|---|---|---|---|---|---|---|
| Dermatological | **Cutaneous calcifications** | ++ | ++ | ++ | ++ | ++ |
| | **Subcutaneous calcifications** | ++ | ++ | ++ | ++ | ++ |
| Digestive | Visceral calcifications | ± | ± | ± | ± | ± |
| Musculoskeletal | Bone pain | ± | ± | ± | ± | ± |
| | **Ectopic calcifications** | + | + | + | + | + |
| | Hyperostosis | ± | ± | ± | ± | ± |
| Laboratory findings | Phosphate (plasma) | ↑↑ | ↑↑ | ↑↑ | ↑↑ | ↑↑ |
| | Sialotransferrins (serum) | n | n | n | n | n |

**Table 68.69** Core 1 β-1,3-galactosyltransferase chaperone deficiency C1GALT1C1-CDG

| System | Symptoms and biomarkers | Neonatal (birth–1 month) | Infancy (1–18 months) | Childhood (1.5–11 years) | Adolescence (11–16 years) | Adulthood (>16 years) |
|---|---|---|---|---|---|---|
| Hematological | Leukemia | ± | ± | ± | ± | ± |
| | Myelodysplasia | ± | ± | ± | ± | ± |
| | **Polyagglutination syndrome** | + | + | + | + | + |
| Laboratory findings | Hemoglobin (blood) | ↓ | ↓ | ↓ | ↓ | ↓ |
| | Neutrophils (blood) | ↓ | ↓ | ↓ | ↓ | ↓ |
| | Platelets (blood) | ↓ | ↓ | ↓ | ↓ | ↓ |

**Table 68.70** O-linked N-acetylglucosamine transferase deficiency OGT-CDG

| System | Symptoms and biomarkers | Neonatal (birth–1 month) | Infancy (1–18 months) | Childhood (1.5–11 years) | Adolescence (11–16 years) | Adulthood (>16 years) |
|---|---|---|---|---|---|---|
| CNS | **Intellectual disability** | | + | + | + | + |
| | **Psychomotor disability** | | + | + | + | + |
| Eye | Amblyopia | ± | ± | ± | ± | ± |
| | Hypermetropia | ± | ± | ± | ± | ± |
| | Nystagmus | ± | ± | ± | ± | ± |
| Genitourinary | Hypogenitalism | ± | ± | ± | ± | ± |
| | Hypospadias | ± | ± | ± | ± | ± |
| Musculoskeletal | Facial dysmorphism, minor | + | + | + | + | + |
| Laboratory findings | Sialotransferrins (serum) | n | n | n | n | n |

**Table 68.71** EGF domain-specific O-linked N-acetylglucosamine transferase deficiency EOGT-CDG

| System | Symptoms and biomarkers | Neonatal (birth-1 month) | Infancy (1–18 months) | Childhood (1.5–11 years) | Adolescence (11–16 years) | Adulthood (>16 years) |
|---|---|---|---|---|---|---|
| Cardiovascular | Heart defects | ± | ± | ± | ± | |
| CNS | Epilepsy | ± | ± | ± | ± | |
| | Periventricular calcifications | ± | ± | ± | ± | |
| Dermatological | **Nail abnormalities** | + | + | + | + | |
| | **Scalp skin defects** | + | + | + | + | |
| Musculoskeletal | **Distal phalanges hypoplasia** | + | + | + | + | |
| | **Facial dysmorphism** | + | + | + | + | |
| | **Skull defects** | ± | ± | ± | ± | |
| | Syndactyly | ± | ± | ± | ± | |
| Laboratory findings | Sialotransferrins (serum) | n | n | n | n | |

**Table 68.72** Muscular dystrophy, limb-girdle, type 2Z autosomal recessive POGLUT1-CDG

| System | Symptoms and biomarkers | Neonatal (birth–1 month) | Infancy (1–18 months) | Childhood (1.5–11 years) | Adolescence (11–16 years) | Adulthood (>16 years) |
|---|---|---|---|---|---|---|
| Musculoskeletal | **Muscular dystrophy** | | | | | + |
| | **Muscle weakness, proximal** | | | | | + |
| | **Scapular winging** | | | | | + |
| Laboratory findings | Sialotransferrins (serum) | | | | | n |

**Table 68.73** Dowling–Degos disease 4 autosomal dominant POGLUT1-CDG

| System | Symptoms and biomarkers | Neonatal (birth–1 month) | Infancy (1–18 months) | Childhood (1.5–11 years) | Adolescence (11–16 years) | Adulthood (>16 years) |
|---|---|---|---|---|---|---|
| Dermatological | **Hyperkeratotic dark-brown papules** | | | + | + | |
| | **Hyperpigmentation** | | | + | + | |
| | Pruritus | | | ± | ± | |
| Laboratory findings | Sialotransferrins (serum) | | | n | n | |

**Table 68.74** Protein O-fucosyltransferase deficiency POFUT1-CDG

| System | Symptoms and biomarkers | Neonatal (birth–1 month) | Infancy (1–18 months) | Childhood (1.5–11 years) | Adolescence (11–16 years) | Adulthood (>16 years) |
|---|---|---|---|---|---|---|
| Dermatological | **Hyperkeratotic papules** | | | | + | + |
| | **Hyperpigmentation** | | | | + | + |
| | **Hypopigmented macules** | | | | + | + |
| Eye | **Hypopigmentation, reticular** | | | | + | + |
| Laboratory findings | Sialotransferrins (serum) | | | | n | n |

**Table 68.75** O-Fucose-specific beta-1,3-N-acetylglucosaminyltransferase deficiency LFNG-CDG

| System | Symptoms and biomarkers | Neonatal (birth–1 month) | Infancy (1–18 months) | Childhood (1.5–11 years) | Adolescence (11–16 years) | Adulthood (>16 years) |
|---|---|---|---|---|---|---|
| Endocrine | **Decreased body height** | + | + | + | + | + |
| Musculoskeletal | **Long, slender fingers** | + | + | + | + | + |
| | **Scoliosis** | + | + | + | + | + |
| | **Vertebral anomalies of the whole spine** | + | + | + | + | + |
| Laboratory findings | Sialotransferrins (serum) | n | n | n | n | n |

**Table 68.76** O-Fucose-specific beta-1,3-N-glucosyltransferase deficiency B3GALTL-CDG

| System | Symptoms and biomarkers | Neonatal (birth-1 month) | Infancy (1–18 months) | Childhood (1.5–11 years) | Adolescence (11–16 years) | Adulthood (>16 years) |
|---|---|---|---|---|---|---|
| Cardiovascular | **Cardiac, anomalies, malformations** | ± | ± | ± | ± | ± |
| CNS | **Hydrocephalus** | ± | ± | ± | ± | ± |
| | Retardation, psychomotor | ± | ± | ± | ± | ± |
| Digestive | Anteriorly placed anus | ± | ± | ± | ± | ± |
| | Gastroesophageal reflux | ± | ± | ± | ± | ± |
| | Malrotation | ± | ± | ± | ± | ± |
| Ear | **Anterior eye chamber anomalies** | + | + | + | + | + |
| | **Hearing loss** | ± | ± | ± | ± | ± |
| Genitourinary | **Cryptorchidism** | ± | ± | ± | ± | ± |
| | Hydroureter | ± | ± | ± | ± | ± |
| Musculoskeletal | Brachydactyly | ± | ± | ± | ± | ± |
| | **Facial dysmorphism** | + | + | + | + | + |
| | Growth retardation | ± | ± | ± | ± | ± |
| Renal | Hydronephrosis | ± | ± | ± | ± | ± |
| Laboratory findings | Sialotransferrins (serum) | n | n | n | n | n |

**Table 68.77** PIGA-CDG

| System | Symptoms and biomarkers | Neonatal (birth–1 month) | Infancy (1–18 months) | Childhood (1.5–11 years) | Adolescence (11–16 years) | Adulthood (>16 years) |
|---|---|---|---|---|---|---|
| CNS | **Hypotonia** | + | + | + | | |
| | **Intellectual disability** | + | + | + | | |
| | **Seizures** | + | + | + | | |
| Musculoskeletal | **Broad nasal bridge** | ± | ± | ± | | |
| | **Coarse face** | ± | ± | ± | | |
| Gastrointestinal | Feeding difficulty | + | + | | | |
| Laboratory findings | Alkaline phosphatase (plasma) | ± | ± | ± | | |
| | Flow cytometry of GPI markers (granulocytes) | ↓ | ↓ | ↓ | | |

**Table 68.78** Developmental disability, severe intellectual disability, and drug-responsive epilepsy PIGC-CDG

| System | Symptoms and biomarkers | Neonatal (birth–1 month) | Infancy (1–18 months) | Childhood (1.5–11 years) | Adolescence (11–16 years) | Adulthood (>16 years) |
|---|---|---|---|---|---|---|
| CNS | **Developmental delay** | + | + | + | | |
| | **Epilepsy** | + | + | + | | |
| | **Intellectual disability** | | + | + | | |
| Laboratory findings | Flow cytometry of GPI markers (granulocytes) | ↓ | ↓ | ↓ | | |

**Table 68.79** PIGQ-CDG

| System | Symptoms and biomarkers | Neonatal (birth–1 month) | Infancy (1–18 months) | Childhood (1.5–11 years) | Adolescence (11–16 years) | Adulthood (>16 years) |
|---|---|---|---|---|---|---|
| CNS | Delayed myelination | ± | ± | | | |
| | Developmental delay | + | + | | | |
| | Encephalopathy, epileptic | + | + | | | |
| | Hypotonia | + | + | | | |
| | Seizures, refractory | + | + | | | |
| Eye | Alacrima | ± | ± | | | |
| | Optic atrophy | ± | ± | | | |
| Laboratory findings | Alkaline phosphatase (plasma) . | ↑ | ↑ | | | |

**Table 68.80** PIGP-CDG

| System | Symptoms and biomarkers | Neonatal (birth–1 month) | Infancy (1–18 months) | Childhood (1.5–11 years) | Adolescence (11–16 years) | Adulthood (>16 years) |
|---|---|---|---|---|---|---|
| CNS | **Dyskinesias** | + | + | + | | |
| | **Epileptic seizures** | + | + | + | | |
| | Hypotonia | + | + | + | | |
| | **Intellectual disability** | + | + | + | | |
| | Microcephaly | ± | ± | ± | | |
| Laboratory findings | Flow cytometry of GPI markers (granulocytes) | ↓ | ↓ | ↓ | | |

**Table 68.81** PIGY-CDG

| System | Symptoms and biomarkers | Neonatal (birth–1 month) | Infancy (1–18 months) | Childhood (1.5–11 years) | Adolescence (11–16 years) | Adulthood (>16 years) |
|---|---|---|---|---|---|---|
| CNS | Epilepsy | ± | ± | ± | | |
| | **Intellectual disability** | | + | + | | |
| Musculoskeletal | Brachytelephalangy | ± | ± | ± | | |
| | **Large, fleshy earlobes** | + | + | + | | |
| Laboratory findings | **Alkaline phosphatase (plasma)** | ↑-↑↑ | ↑-↑↑ | ↑-↑↑ | | |
| | Flow cytometry of GPI markers (fibroblasts) | ↓ | ↓ | ↓ | | |

**Table 68.82** PIGH-CDG

| System | Symptoms and biomarkers | Neonatal (birth–1 month) | Infancy (1–18 months) | Childhood (1.5–11 years) | Adolescence (11–16 years) | Adulthood (>16 years) |
|---|---|---|---|---|---|---|
| CNS | **Developmental delay** | | + | + | | |
| | Hypotonia | | ± | ± | | |
| | Seizures | | ± | ± | | |
| Psychiatric | **Autism** | | + | + | | |
| | **Behavior, aggressive** | | + | + | | |
| Laboratory findings | Flow cytometry of GPI markers (granulocytes) | ↓ | ↓ | ↓ | | |

**Table 68.83** PIGL-CDG

| System | Symptoms and biomarkers | Neonatal (birth–1 month) | Infancy (1–18 months) | Childhood (1.5–11 years) | Adolescence (11–16 years) | Adulthood (>16 years) |
|---|---|---|---|---|---|---|
| Cardiovascular | **Congenital heart defects** | + | + | | | |
| CNS | **Intellectual disability** | | + | + | | |
| Dermatological | **Ichthyosis** | + | + | + | | |
| Ear | **Hearing loss** | + | + | + | | |
| Eye | **Coloboma** | + | + | + | | |
| Laboratory findings | Alkaline phosphatase (plasma) | ± | ± | ± | | |
| | Flow cytometry of GPI markers (granulocytes) | ↓ | ↓ | ↓ | | |

**Table 68.84** PIGW-CDG

| System | Symptoms and biomarkers | Neonatal (birth–1 month) | Infancy (1–18 months) | Childhood (1.5–11 years) | Adolescence (11–16 years) | Adulthood (>16 years) |
|---|---|---|---|---|---|---|
| CNS | **Developmental delay** | + | + | + | | |
| | Epilepsy | + | + | + | | |
| | **Hypotonia** | ± | ± | ± | | |
| Laboratory findings | Alkaline phosphatase (plasma) | n-↑ | n-↑ | n-↑ | | |
| | Flow cytometry of GPI markers (granulocytes) | ↓ | ↓ | ↓ | | |

**Table 68.85** PIGM-CDG

| System | Symptoms and biomarkers | Neonatal (birth-1 month) | Infancy (1–18 months) | Childhood (1.5–11 years) | Adolescence (11–16 years) | Adulthood (>16 years) |
|---|---|---|---|---|---|---|
| CNS | **Absence seizures** | | | + | + | |
| | Developmental delay | | ± | ± | | |
| Hematological | **Cerebral vein thrombosis** | | ± | ± | | |
| | **Hepatic vein thrombosis** | | + | + | + | |
| | **Portal vein thrombosis** | | + | + | + | |
| Dermatologic | Prominent superficial veins | ± | ± | ± | | |
| Laboratory findings | Flow cytometry of GPI markers (granulocytes) | ↓ | ↓ | ↓ | | |

**Table 68.86** PIGV-CDG

| System | Symptoms and biomarkers | Neonatal (birth–1 month) | Infancy (1–18 months) | Childhood (1.5–11 years) | Adolescence (11–16 years) | Adulthood (>16 years) |
|---|---|---|---|---|---|---|
| CNS | Hearing, impaired | | + | + | + | |
| | Hypotonia | + | + | + | | |
| | **Intellectual disability** | | ++ | ++ | ++ | |
| | Seizures | + | + | + | + | |
| Dermatological | **Hypoplastic nails** | ± | ± | ± | | |
| Digestive | Anorectal anomalies | ± | ± | | | |
| | Feeding difficulties | + | + | + | | |
| | Megacolon | ± | ± | ± | | |
| Eye | Upslanted palpebral fissures | + | + | + | + | |
| Musculoskeletal | **Brachytelephalangy** | + | + | + | + | |
| | Broad nasal bridge | + | + | + | + | |
| | Hypertelorism | + | + | + | + | |
| Laboratory findings | **Alkaline phosphatase (plasma)** | ↑ | ↑ | ↑ | ↑ | |
| | Flow cytometry of GPI markers (granulocytes) | ↓ | ↓ | ↓ | ↑ | |

**Table 68.87** PIGN-CDG

| System | Symptoms and biomarkers | Neonatal (birth–1 month) | Infancy (1–18 months) | Childhood (1.5–11 years) | Adolescence (11–16 years) | Adulthood (>16 years) |
|---|---|---|---|---|---|---|
| Cardiovascular | **Cardiac anomalies** | ± | ± | ± | | |
| Gastrointestinal | **Diaphragmatic defect** | ± | ± | ± | | |
| CNS | Hypotonia | + | + | + | | |
| | **Seizures** | + | + | + | | |
| Musculoskeletal | **Brachytelephalangy** | ± | ± | ± | | |
| | **Dysmorphic features** | + | + | + | | |
| Laboratory findings | Flow cytometry of GPI markers (granulocytes) | ↑ | ↑ | ↑ | | |

**Table 68.88** PIGO-CDG

| System | Symptoms and biomarkers | Neonatal (birth–1 month) | Infancy (1–18 months) | Childhood (1.5–11 years) | Adolescence (11–16 years) | Adulthood (>16 years) |
|---|---|---|---|---|---|---|
| Cardiovascular | Cardiac anomalies | ± | ± | | | |
| CNS | **Hypotonia** | + | + | + | | |
| | **Intellectual disability** | | + | + | | |
| | **Seizures** | | + | + | | |
| Dermatological | **Hypoplastic nails** | + | + | + | | |
| Musculoskeletal | **Brachytelephalangy** | + | + | + | | |
| | **Facial dysmorphism** | + | + | + | | |
| Gastrointestinal | **Anal stenosis** | ± | ± | | | |
| Laboratory findings | Alkaline phosphatase (plasma) | ↑ | ↑ | ↑ | | |
| | Flow cytometry of GPI markers (granulocytes) | ↓ | ↓ | ↓ | | |

**Table 68.89** PIGG-CDG

| System | Symptoms and biomarkers | Neonatal (birth–1 month) | Infancy (1–18 months) | Childhood (1.5–11 years) | Adolescence (11–16 years) | Adulthood (>16 years) |
|---|---|---|---|---|---|---|
| CNS | Ataxia | | ± | ± | | |
| | Cerebellar hypoplasia | | ± | ± | | |
| | **Epilepsy** | | + | + | | |
| | Hypotonia | | + | + | | |
| | **Intellectual disability** | | + | + | | |
| Laboratory findings | Flow cytometry of GPI markers (fibroblasts) | | ↓ | ↓ | | |
| | Flow cytometry of GPI markers (granulocytes) | | n | n | | |

**Table 68.90** PIGT-CDG

| System | Symptoms and biomarkers | Neonatal (birth–1 month) | Infancy (1–18 months) | Childhood (1.5–11 years) | Adolescence (11–16 years) | Adulthood (>16 years) |
|---|---|---|---|---|---|---|
| CNS | **Hypotonia** | + | + | + | | |
| | **Intellectual disability** | | + | + | | |
| | **Seizures** | + | + | + | | |
| Musculoskeletal | **Dysmorphic features** | ± | ± | ± | | |
| Hematologic | **Intravascular hemolysis** | | | | | ± |
| Immunologic | **Autoinflammation** | | | | | ± |
| Laboratory findings | Alkaline phosphatase (plasma) | ↓ | ↓ | | | |
| | Flow cytometry of GPI markers (granulocytes) | ↓ | ↓ | ↓ | | |

**Table 68.91** GPAA1-CDG

| System | Symptoms and biomarkers | Neonatal (birth–1 month) | Infancy (1–18 months) | Childhood (1.5–11 years) | Adolescence (11–16 years) | Adulthood (>16 years) |
|---|---|---|---|---|---|---|
| CNS | **Ataxia** | | | + | + | + |
| | **Cerebellar atrophy (MRI)** | | | + | + | + |
| | Developmental delay | | | + | + | + |
| | Hypotonia | | | + | + | + |
| | **Intellectual disability** | | | + | + | + |
| | **Seizures** | | | ± | ± | ± |
| Eye | **Nystagmus** | | | + | + | + |
| Musculoskeletal | Osteopenia | | | ± | ± | ± |
| Laboratory findings | Flow cytometry of GPI markers (granulocytes) | | | ↓ | ↓ | ↓ |

**Table 68.92** PGAP1-CDG

| System | Symptoms and biomarkers | Neonatal (birth-1 month) | Infancy (1–18 months) | Childhood (1.5–11 years) | Adolescence (11–16 years) | Adulthood (>16 years) |
|---|---|---|---|---|---|---|
| CNS | Brain atrophy (MRI) | | + | + | | |
| | Delayed myelination | | + | + | | |
| | **Epilepsy** | | + | + | | |
| | Hypotonia | | + | + | | |
| | **Intellectual disability** | | + | + | | |
| | Movement disorder | | + | + | | |
| Musculoskeletal | Facial dysmorphism | | + | + | | |
| Respiratory | Apnea | | ± | ± | | |

**Table 68.93** PGAP3–CDG

| System | Symptoms and biomarkers | Neonatal (birth–1 month) | Infancy (1–18 months) | Childhood (1.5–11 years) | Adolescence (11–16 years) | Adulthood (>16 years) |
|---|---|---|---|---|---|---|
| CNS | **Ataxia** | | ± | ± | | |
| | **Epilepsy** | | + | + | | |
| | Hypotonia | + | + | + | | |
| | **Intellectual disability** | | + | + | | |
| Musculoskeletal | **Micrognathia** | ± | ± | ± | | |
| Respiratory | **Cleft palate** | ± | ± | ± | | |
| Laboratory findings | Alkaline phosphatase (plasma) | | ↑ | ↑ | | |
| | Flow cytometry of GPI markers (granulocytes) | | ↓ | ↓ | | |

**Table 68.94** PGAP2-CDG

| System | Symptoms and biomarkers | Neonatal (birth–1 month) | Infancy (1–18 months) | Childhood (1.5–11 years) | Adolescence (11–16 years) | Adulthood (>16 years) |
|---|---|---|---|---|---|---|
| CNS | **Developmental delay** | | + | + | | |
| | Hypotonia | ± | ± | ± | + | + |
| | **Intellectual disability** | | + | + | + | + |
| | Seizures | ± | ± | ± | | |
| Ear | Hearing loss, sensorineural | ± | ± | ± | | |
| Musculoskeletal | Microcephaly | ± | ± | ± | | |
| Laboratory findings | Alkaline phosphatase (plasma) | | ↑-↑↑ | ↑-↑↑ | | |

**Table 68.95** PIGS-CDG

| System | Symptoms and biomarkers | Neonatal (birth–1 month) | Infancy (1–18 months) | Childhood (1.5–11 years) | Adolescence (11–16 years) | Adulthood (>16 years) |
|---|---|---|---|---|---|---|
| CNS | **Ataxia** | | + | + | | |
| | **Cerebellar atrophy (MRI)** | ± | ± | ± | | |
| | **Hypotonia** | + | + | + | | |
| | **Intellectual disability** | | + | + | | |
| | **Seizures, intractable** | + | + | + | | |
| Musculoskeletal | Coarse facial features | + | + | + | | |
| Laboratory findings | Flow cytometry of GPI markers (granulocytes) | ↓ | ↓ | ↓ | | |

**Table 68.96** Dehydrodolichyl diphosphate synthase deficiency DHDDS-CDG

| System | Symptoms and biomarkers | Neonatal (birth–1 month) | Infancy (1–18 months) | Childhood (1.5–11 years) | Adolescence (11–16 years) | Adulthood (>16 years) |
|---|---|---|---|---|---|---|
| CNS | Ataxia | ± | ± | ± | ± | ± |
| | Dystonia | ± | ± | ± | ± | ± |
| | Epilepsy | ± | ± | ± | ± | ± |
| | Hypotonia | ± | ± | ± | ± | ± |
| | Intellectual disability | | ± | ± | ± | ± |
| | **Retinitis pigmentosa** | | ± | ± | ± | ± |
| Genitourinary | Micropenis | ± | ± | ± | ± | ± |
| Renal | Renal failure, acute | ± | ± | ± | ± | ± |
| Laboratory findings | Sialotransferrins (serum) | n | n | n | n | n |

**Table 68.97** Nogo-B receptor deficiency NgBR-CDG

| System | Symptoms and biomarkers | Neonatal (birth–1 month) | Infancy (1–18 months) | Childhood (1.5–11 years) | Adolescence (11–16 years) | Adulthood (>16 years) |
|---|---|---|---|---|---|---|
| CNS | **Cortical atrophy (MRI)** | + | | | | |
| | **Developmental delay** | | + | | | |
| | **Epilepsy** | + | | | | |
| | Hypotonia, axial | + | | | | |
| | **Spasticity, acral** | + | | | | |
| Eye | **Retinitis pigmentosa** | + | | | | |
| Musculoskeletal | **Microcephaly** | + | | | | |
| | **Scoliosis** | + | | | | |
| Other | **Failure to thrive** | + | | | | |
| Laboratory findings | Cholesterol (fibroblasts) | ↑ | | | | |
| | Dolichols (fibroblasts) | ↓ | | | | |

**Table 68.98** Steroid 5 alpha-reductase 3 deficiency SRD5A3-CDG

| System | Symptoms and biomarkers | Neonatal (birth–1 month) | Infancy (1–18 months) | Childhood (1.5–11 years) | Adolescence (11–16 years) | Adulthood (>16 years) |
|---|---|---|---|---|---|---|
| CNS | Cerebellar abnormalities | ± | ± | ± | ± | ± |
| | Hypotonia | ± | ± | ± | ± | ± |
| | **Midline brain malformations** | ± | ± | ± | ± | ± |
| Dermatological | Dry skin | ± | ± | ± | ± | ± |
| | **Erythroderma** | ± | ± | ± | ± | ± |
| | Ichthyosis | ± | ± | ± | ± | ± |
| Endocrine | Growth hormone deficiency | ± | ± | ± | ± | ± |
| Eye | **Cataract** | ± | ± | ± | ± | ± |
| | **Coloboma** | ± | ± | ± | ± | ± |
| | Microphthalmia | ± | ± | ± | ± | ± |
| | Nystagmus | ± | ± | ± | ± | ± |
| | Optic atrophy | ± | ± | ± | ± | ± |
| Musculoskeletal | **Facial dysmorphism** | + | + | + | + | + |
| | **Hypotonia, muscular-axial** | + | + | + | + | + |
| | Kyphosis | | | | ± | ± |
| Other | Failure to thrive | ± | ± | ± | ± | ± |
| Laboratory findings | Antithrombin III (plasma) | ↓ | ↓ | ↓ | | |
| | Dolichol-linked Glc3Man9GlcNAc2 (serum) | ↓ | ↓ | ↓ | | |
| | Dolichol-phosphate (serum) | ↓ | ↓ | ↓ | | |
| | Partial thromboplastin time (PTT) | ↑ | ↑ | ↑ | | |
| | Protein C (serum) | ↓ | ↓ | ↓ | | |
| | Protein S (serum) | ↓ | ↓ | ↓ | | |
| | Sialotransferrins, type 1 pattern (serum) | ± | ± | ± | ± | ± |
| | Transaminase (plasma) | ↑ | ↑ | ↑ | | |

**Table 68.99** Dolichol kinase deficiency DK1-CDG

| System | Symptoms and biomarkers | Neonatal (birth–1 month) | Infancy (1–18 months) | Childhood (1.5–11 years) | Adolescence (11–16 years) | Adulthood (>16 years) |
|---|---|---|---|---|---|---|
| Cardiovascular | Cardiomyopathy, dilated | ± | ± | ± | ± | ± |
| CNS | Epilepsy | ± | ± | ± | ± | |
| | Hypotonia | ± | ± | ± | ± | |
| Dermatological | Hair abnormality | ± | ± | ± | ± | |
| | Ichthyosiform erythroderma | ± | ± | ± | ± | ± |
| Endocrine | Puberty, delayed | | | | | ± |
| Eye | Nystagmus | ± | ± | ± | | |
| Musculoskeletal | Digital necrosis (distal phalanges) | ± | | | | |
| | **Facial dysmorphism** | – | – | – | – | – |
| | Microcephaly | | ± | ± | ± | ± |
| Other | **Early death** | | ± | | | |
| | Failure to thrive | ± | ± | ± | ± | |
| Laboratory findings | Lipid-linked oligosaccharides (fibroblasts) | ↓ | ↓ | ↓ | ↓ | |
| | Sialotransferrins, type 1 pattern (serum) | + | + | + | + | |
| | Transaminase (plasma) | n-↑ | n-↑ | n-↑ | n-↑ | |

**Table 68.100** GDP-Man:Dol-P mannosyltransferase subunit 1 deficiency DPM1-CDG

| System | Symptoms and biomarkers | Neonatal (birth–1 month) | Infancy (1–18 months) | Childhood (1.5–11 years) | Adolescence (11–16 years) | Adulthood (>16 years) |
|---|---|---|---|---|---|---|
| CNS | Ataxia | ± | ± | ± | ± | |
| | Cerebral atrophy (MRI) | | ± | ± | ± | ± |
| | Dentate nucleus lesions (MRI) | | ± | ± | | |
| | Epilepsy | ± | ± | ± | ± | |
| | **Hypotonia** | + | + | + | + | |
| | **Intellectual disability** | ++ | ++ | ++ | ++ | |
| | Neuropathy, peripheral | | ± | ± | ± | ± |
| | Tremor | ± | ± | ± | ± | |
| Digestive | Feeding difficulties | ± | ± | ± | | |
| | **Hepatosplenomegaly** | ± | ± | ± | | |
| Eye | **Nystagmus** | ± | ± | ± | | |
| | **Retinal dystrophy** | ± | ± | ± | | |
| | **Strabismus** | + | + | + | | |
| Musculoskeletal | **Microcephaly** | − | + | + | + | + |
| Laboratory findings | Creatine kinase (plasma) | | ↑ | ↑ | | |
| | Dolichol-linked Man5GlcNAc2 (serum) | ↑ | ↑ | ↑ | | |
| | Factor XI (blood) | ↑ | ↑ | ↑ | | |
| | Sialotransferrins, type 1 pattern (serum) | + | + | + | | |
| | Transaminase (plasma) | | ↑ | ↑ | | |

**Table 68.101** Dolichol-P-mannose synthase-2 deficiency DPM2-CDG

| System | Symptoms and biomarkers | Neonatal (birth–1 month) | Infancy (1–18 months) | Childhood (1.5–11 years) | Adolescence (11–16 years) | Adulthood (>16 years) |
|---|---|---|---|---|---|---|
| CNS | **Cerebral atrophy (MRI)** | + | + | | | |
| | Epilepsy | + | + | | | |
| | Hypotonia | +++ | +++ | | | |
| Digestive | **Hepatomegaly** | + | + | | | |
| Musculoskeletal | **Dysmorphic features** | + | + | | | |
| | **Joint contractures** | + | + | | | |
| | **Microcephaly** | + | + | | | |
| | **Muscular dystrophy** | + | + | | | |
| | **Scoliosis** | + | + | | | |
| Respiratory | Respiratory infections/distress | + | + | | | |
| Laboratory findings | Creatine kinase (plasma) | ↑ | ↑ | | | |
| | Dolichol-linked Man5GlcNAc2 (fibroblasts) | ↑ | ↑ | | | |
| | Sialotransferrin type 1 pattern (serum) | + | + | | | |
| | Transaminases (serum) | ↑ | ↑ | | | |

**Table 68.102** GDP-Man:Dol-P mannosyltransferase 3 deficiency DPM3-CDG

| System | Symptoms and biomarkers | Neonatal (birth–1 month) | Infancy (1–18 months) | Childhood (1.5–11 years) | Adolescence (11–16 years) | Adulthood (>16 years) |
|---|---|---|---|---|---|---|
| Cardiovascular | **Cardiomyopathy, dilated** | | | | | ± |
| CNS | **Gait disturbance** | | | | + | + |
| | Retardation, psychomotor | n | n | n | n | n |
| | Stroke-like episode | – | – | – | – | + |
| Musculoskeletal | Dysmorphic features | n | n | n | n | n |
| | **Limb girdle muscular dystrophy** | | | + | + | + |
| | **Muscle weakness, proximal** | | | + | + | + |
| | **Pes planus** | | | | + | + |
| Laboratory findings | Creatine kinase (plasma) | | | | | ↑↑ |
| | Dolichol-linked Man5GlcNAc2 (serum) | | | ↑ | ↑ | ↑ |
| | Dolichol-P-mannose (serum) | | | ↓ | ↓ | ↓ |
| | Factor XI (blood) | n | n | n | n | n |
| | Sialotransferrins, type 1 pattern (serum) | | | | | ± |
| | Transaminase (plasma) | | | | | ↑ |

**Table 68.103** Dol-P-Man utilization 1 deficiency MPDU1-CDG

| System | Symptoms and biomarkers | Neonatal (birth–1 month) | Infancy (1–18 months) | Childhood (1.5–11 years) | Adolescence (11–16 years) | Adulthood (>16 years) |
|---|---|---|---|---|---|---|
| CNS | Cerebral atrophy (MRI) | ± | ± | ± | ± | ± |
| | Hypotonia | ± | ± | ± | ± | ± |
| | **Retardation, psychomotor** | | ++ | ++ | ++ | ++ |
| | Seizures | ± | ± | ± | ± | ± |
| | **Tendon reflexes** | n | n | n | n | n |
| Dermatological | **Erythroderma** | ± | ± | ± | ± | ± |
| | **Hyperkeratosis** | ± | ± | ± | ± | ± |
| | **Ichthyosis** | ± | ± | ± | ± | ± |
| Digestive | Feeding difficulties | ± | ± | ± | ± | ± |
| Endocrine | Growth hormone deficiency | | | ± | ± | ± |
| Eye | Optic atrophy | ± | ± | ± | ± | ± |
| | Strabismus | ± | ± | ± | ± | ± |
| | Vision, impaired | | ± | ± | ± | ± |
| Musculoskeletal | Dysmorphic features | ± | ± | ± | ± | ± |
| Laboratory findings | Antithrombin III (plasma) | ↓ | ↓ | ↓ | ↓ | ↓ |
| | Creatine kinase (plasma) | n-↑ | n-↑ | n-↑ | n-↑ | n-↑ |
| | Dolichol-linked Man5GlcNAc2 (serum) | ↑ | ↑ | ↑ | ↑ | ↑ |
| | Dolichol-linked Man9GlcNAc2 (serum) | ↑ | ↑ | ↑ | ↑ | ↑ |
| | Lipid-linked Man5GlcNAc2 (fibroblasts) | ↑ | ↑ | ↑ | ↑ | ↑ |
| | Lipid-linked Man9GlcNAc2 (fibroblasts) | ↑ | ↑ | ↑ | ↑ | ↑ |
| | Sialotransferrins, type 1 pattern (serum) | + | + | + | + | + |
| | Transaminase (plasma) | n | n | n | n | n |

**Table 68.104** Glutamine:fructose-6-phosphate transaminase deficiency GFPT1-CDG

| System | Symptoms and biomarkers | Neonatal (birth–1 month) | Infancy (1–18 months) | Childhood (1.5–11 years) | Adolescence (11–16 years) | Adulthood (>16 years) |
|---|---|---|---|---|---|---|
| CNS | Cerebral white matter involvement (MRI) | ± | ± | ± | ± | ± |
| | **Congenital myasthenic syndrome** | + | + | + | + | + |
| Eye | **Ophthalmoparesis** | – | – | – | – | – |
| | Retinoschizis | ± | ± | ± | ± | ± |
| Other | **Response to anticholinesterase therapy** | + | + | + | + | + |
| Laboratory findings | Creatine kinase (plasma) | ± | ± | ± | ± | ± |
| | Sialotransferrin, type 1 pattern (serum) | + | + | + | + | + |

**Table 68.105** Phosphoglucomutase 1 deficiency PGM1-CDG

| System | Symptoms and biomarkers | Neonatal (birth–1 month) | Infancy (1–18 months) | Childhood (1.5–11 years) | Adolescence (11–16 years) | Adulthood (>16 years) |
|---|---|---|---|---|---|---|
| Cardiovascular | Cardiomyopathy, dilated | ± | ± | ± | ± | ± |
| CNS | Fatigue | | ± | ± | ± | ± |
| | **Thrombosis, cerebral** | ± | ± | ± | ± | ± |
| Digestive | **Bifid uvula** | ± | ± | ± | ± | ± |
| | Hepatopathy | + | + | + | + | + |
| Endocrine | **Growth hormone deficiency** | ± | ± | ± | ± | ± |
| | Hyperinsulinism | ± | ± | | | |
| | Hypogonadotropic hypogonadism | ± | ± | ± | ± | ± |
| Musculoskeletal | **Cleft palate** | ± | ± | ± | ± | ± |
| | **First arch syndrome** | ± | ± | ± | ± | ± |
| | Muscle weakness | ± | ± | ± | ± | ± |
| | Rhabdomyolysis | ± | ± | ± | ± | ± |
| | **Short stature** | ± | ± | ± | ± | ± |
| Metabolic | Hypoglycemia (episodic) | ± | ± | | | |
| Other | Increased susceptibility to malignant hyperthermia | ± | ± | ± | ± | ± |
| Laboratory findings | Ammonia (blood) | ↑ | ↑ | ↑ | ↑ | ↑ |
| | Antithrombin (plasma) | ↓ | ↓ | ↓ | ↓ | ↓ |
| | Asialotransferrin (serum) | ↑ | ↑ | ↑ | ↑ | ↑ |
| | Creatine kinase (plasma) | ↑ | ↑ | ↑ | ↑ | ↑ |
| | Disialotransferrin (serum) | ↑ | ↑ | ↑ | ↑ | ↑ |
| | Free fatty acids (serum), during hypoglycemia | ↓↓↓ | ↓↓↓ | | | |
| | Glucose (plasma) | ↓ | ↓ | | | |
| | Insulin, durig hypoglycemia | ↑ | ↑ | ↑ | ↑ | ↑ |
| | Ketones, during hypoglycemia | ↓↓↓ | ↓↓↓ | | | |
| | Monosialotransferrin (serum) | ↑ | ↑ | ↑ | ↑ | ↑ |
| | Tetrasialotransferrin (serum) | ↓ | ↓ | ↓ | ↓ | ↓ |
| | Transaminase (plasma) | ↑ | ↑ | ↑ | ↑ | ↑ |
| | Trisialotransferrin (serum) | ↑ | ↑ | ↑ | ↑ | ↑ |

**Table 68.106** Immunodeficiency-23 PGM3-CDG

| System | Symptoms and biomarkers | Neonatal (birth–1 month) | Infancy (1–18 months) | Childhood (1.5–11 years) | Adolescence (11–16 years) | Adulthood (>16 years) |
|---|---|---|---|---|---|---|
| CNS | Intellectual disability | | ± | ± | ± | ± |
| Hematological | **Immunodeficiency, T-cell** | + | + | + | + | + |
| | **Neutropenia** | + | + | + | + | + |
| Musculoskeletal | Brachydactyly | ± | ± | ± | ± | ± |
| | Facial dysmorphism | ± | ± | ± | ± | ± |
| | **Short stature** | | ± | ± | ± | ± |
| | **Skeletal dysplasia** | ± | ± | ± | ± | ± |
| Other | Atopy | + | + | + | + | + |
| | **Recurrent infections** | + | + | + | + | + |
| Laboratory findings | B-cells | ↓ | ↓ | ↓ | ↓ | ↓ |
| | IgE (serum) | n-↑ | n-↑ | n-↑ | n-↑ | n-↑ |
| | Sialotransferrins (serum) | n | n | n | n | n |

**Table 68.107** Glucose-6-phosphatase catalytic subunit 3 deficiency G6PC3-CDG

| System | Symptoms and biomarkers | Neonatal (birth–1 month) | Infancy (1–18 months) | Childhood (1.5–11 years) | Adolescence (11–16 years) | Adulthood (>16 years) |
|---|---|---|---|---|---|---|
| Cardiovascular | Atrial septal defect | ± | ± | ± | ± | ± |
| | Patent ductus arteriosus | ± | ± | ± | ± | ± |
| | Pulmonary arterial hypertension | ± | ± | ± | ± | ± |
| | Skin veins, prominent | + | + | + | + | + |
| CNS | Intellectual disability | ± | ± | ± | ± | ± |
| Digestive | Inflammatory bowel disease | ± | ± | ± | ± | ± |
| Genitourinary | Urogenital abnormalities | ± | ± | ± | ± | ± |
| Hematological | Anemia, mild | ± | ± | ± | ± | ± |
| | Neutropenia | ++ | ++ | ++ | ++ | ++ |
| | Neutrophil hypoglycosylation | + | + | + | + | + |
| | Thrombocytopenia | ± | ± | ± | ± | ± |
| Musculoskeletal | Facial dysmorphism | ± | ± | ± | ± | ± |
| Other | Respiratory infections, recurrent | ± | ± | ± | ± | ± |

**Table 68.108** GDP–mannose pyrophosphorylase B deficiency GMPPA-CDG

| System | Symptoms and biomarkers | Neonatal (birth–1 month) | Infancy (1–18 months) | Childhood (1.5–11 years) | Adolescence (11–16 years) | Adulthood (>16 years) |
|---|---|---|---|---|---|---|
| Cardiovascular | Hypotension, postural | | | ± | ± | ± |
| CNS | **Developmental delay** | | + | + | | |
| | **Gait disturbance** | | ± | ± | ± | ± |
| | Hearing, impaired | ± | ± | ± | ± | ± |
| | Hypotonia | ± | ± | ± | ± | ± |
| | **Intellectual disability** | | + | + | + | + |
| Digestive | **Dysphagia** | + | + | + | | |
| | **Regurgitation** | + | + | + | | |
| Eye | **Alacrima** | + | + | + | + | + |
| | **Ocular abnormalities** | | ± | ± | ± | ± |
| Musculoskeletal | **Achalasia** | + | + | + | + | + |
| | Facial dysmorphism | ± | ± | ± | ± | ± |
| | Growth retardation | ± | ± | ± | ± | ± |
| Laboratory findings | Sialotransferrins (serum) | n | n | n | n | n |

**Table 68.109** Muscular dystrophy-dystroglycanopathy GMPPB-CDG

| System | Symptoms and biomarkers | Neonatal (birth–1 month) | Infancy (1–18 months) | Childhood (1.5–11 years) | Adolescence (11–16 years) | Adulthood (>16 years) |
|---|---|---|---|---|---|---|
| CNS | **Cerebellar hypoplasia (MRI)** | ± | ± | ± | ± | ± |
| | **Congenital myasthenic syndrome** | ± | ± | ± | ± | ± |
| | Epilepsy | ± | ± | ± | ± | ± |
| | Hypotonia | + | + | + | + | + |
| | Intellectual disability | | ± | ± | ± | ± |
| Eye | **Cataract** | ± | ± | ± | ± | ± |
| Musculoskeletal | Microcephaly | ± | ± | ± | ± | ± |
| | **Muscle weakness** | + | + | + | + | + |
| | **Muscular dystrophy, limb-girdle** | | ± | ± | ± | ± |
| | Myoglobinuria | | | ± | ± | ± |
| Laboratory findings | Creatine kinase (plasma) | ↑ | ↑ | ↑ | ↑ | ↑ |
| | Hypoglycosylation of α-dystroglycan (muscle) | + | + | + | + | + |

**Table 68.110** Epileptic encephalopathy, early infantile, 50 CAD-CDG

| System | Symptoms and biomarkers | Neonatal (birth-1 month) | Infancy (1–18 months) | Childhood (1.5–11 years) | Adolescence (11–16 years) | Adulthood (>16 years) |
|---|---|---|---|---|---|---|
| CNS | **Developmental regression** | | + | + | | |
| | **Epilepsy** | | + | + | | |
| | Swallowing difficulties | | ± | ± | | |
| Hematological | **Anemia (dyserythropoietic)** | | + | + | | |
| | **Anisocytosis** | | + | + | | |
| | **Poikilocytosis** | | + | + | | |
| Laboratory findings | Orotic acid (urine) | | n | n | | |
| | Pyrimidines (urine) | | n | n | | |
| | Sialotransferrins (serum) | | n | n | | |

**Table 68.111** CMP–sialic acid transporter deficiency SLC35A1-CDG

| System | Symptoms and biomarkers | Neonatal (birth–1 month) | Infancy (1–18 months) | Childhood (1.5–11 years) | Adolescence (11–16 years) | Adulthood (>16 years) |
|---|---|---|---|---|---|---|
| CNS | Ataxia | + | + | + | + | + |
| | Epilepsy | | + | + | + | + |
| | Hypotonia | ± | ± | ± | ± | ± |
| | Intellectual disability | | + | + | + | + |
| Hematological | Bleeding, easy | ± | ± | ± | ± | ± |
| | Macrothrombocytopenia | + | + | + | + | + |
| Musculoskeletal | Microcephaly | ± | ± | ± | ± | ± |
| Psychiatric | Behaviour difficulties | | ± | ± | ± | ± |
| Laboratory findings | Sialotransferrins, type 2 pattern (serum) | + | + | + | + | + |
| | Sialylation of platelet glycoproteins | ↓ | ↓ | ↓ | ↓ | ↓ |

**Table 68.112** Congenital disorder of glycosylation SLC35A2-CDG

| System | Symptoms and biomarkers | Neonatal (birth–1 month) | Infancy (1–18 months) | Childhood (1.5–11 years) | Adolescence (11–16 years) | Adulthood (>16 years) |
|---|---|---|---|---|---|---|
| CNS | **Cerebellar abnormalities** | ± | ± | ± | ± | ± |
| | **Cerebral abnormalities** | ± | ± | ± | ± | ± |
| | **Corpus callosum abnormalities** | ± | ± | ± | ± | ± |
| | **Developmental disability** | | + | + | | |
| | Epilepsy | + | + | + | + | + |
| | Hypotonia | + | + | + | | |
| | **Intellectual disability** | | + | + | + | + |
| Digestive | Feeding difficulties | ± | ± | ± | ± | ± |
| Eye | Cortical visual impairment | | ± | ± | ± | ± |
| | Nystagmus | | ± | ± | ± | ± |
| | Retinitis pigmentosa | | ± | ± | ± | ± |
| Musculoskeletal | **Dysmorphic features** | + | + | + | + | + |
| | **Hand/finger abnormalities** | ± | ± | ± | ± | ± |
| | **Microcephaly** | ± | ± | ± | ± | ± |
| | **Shortened limbs** | ± | ± | ± | ± | ± |
| Other | Frequent infections | ± | ± | ± | ± | ± |
| Laboratory findings | Sialotransferrins, type 2 pattern (serum) | ± | ± | ± | ± | ± |

**Table 68.113** UDP-N-acetylglucosamine transporter deficiency SLC35A3-CDG

| System | Symptoms and biomarkers | Neonatal (birth–1 month) | Infancy (1–18 months) | Childhood (1.5–11 years) | Adolescence (11–16 years) | Adulthood (>16 years) |
|---|---|---|---|---|---|---|
| CNS | **Autistic spectrum disorder** | | ± | ± | | |
| | **Epilepsy** | | ± | ± | | |
| | Hypotonia | ± | + | + | | |
| | **Intellectual disability** | | + | + | | |
| Musculoskeletal | **Arthrogryposis** | + | + | + | | |
| | **Facial dysmorphism** | + | + | + | | |
| | **Skeletal abnormalities** | + | + | + | | |
| | **Vertebral abnormalities** | + | + | + | | |
| Laboratory findings | Sialotransferrins (serum) | ? | ? | ? | | |

**Table 68.114** GDP-fucose transporter deficiency SLC35C1-CDG

| System | Symptoms and biomarkers | Neonatal (birth–1 month) | Infancy (1–18 months) | Childhood (1.5–11 years) | Adolescence (11–16 years) | Adulthood (>16 years) |
|---|---|---|---|---|---|---|
| CNS | **Retardation, psychomotor** | | +++ | +++ | +++ | +++ |
| Digestive | **Periodontitis** | | ++ | ++ | ++ | ++ |
| Endocrine | **Decreased body height** | + | + | + | + | + |
| Hematological | **Bombay blood group phenotype** | + | + | + | + | + |
| | Delayed separation umbilical cord | – | – | – | – | – |
| | **Neutrophilia** | ++ | ++ | ++ | ++ | ++ |
| Musculoskeletal | Facial dysmorphism | ++ | ++ | ++ | ++ | ++ |
| | **Pus formation, inability to** | + | + | + | + | + |
| Other | **Recurrent infections** | + | + | + | + | + |
| Laboratory findings | B-cell function | n | n | n | n | n |
| | Neutrophil motility | ↓↓↓ | ↓↓↓ | ↓↓↓ | ↓↓↓ | ↓↓↓ |
| | Neutrophil rolling | ↓↓↓ | ↓↓↓ | ↓↓↓ | ↓↓↓ | ↓↓↓ |
| | Sialotransferrins (serum) | n | n | n | n | n |
| | Sialyl-Lewis on neutrophils | ↓ | ↓ | ↓ | | |
| | T-cell function | n | n | n | n | n |

**Table 68.115** UDP–glucuronic acid/UDP-N-acetylgalactosamine dual transporter deficiency SLC35D1-CDG

| System | Symptoms and biomarkers | Neonatal (birth–1 month) | Infancy (1–18 months) | Childhood (1.5–11 years) | Adolescence (11–16 years) | Adulthood (>16 years) |
|---|---|---|---|---|---|---|
| Digestive | **Abdominal distension** | ++ | | | | |
| Musculoskeletal | **Advanced ossification** | + | | | | |
| | **Club foot** | + | | | | |
| | **Dwarfism** | ++ | | | | |
| | **Nasal hypoplasia** | + | | | | |
| | **Platyspondyly** | ++ | | | | |
| | **Shortening of long bones** | +++ | | | | |
| | **Small ilia with snail-like appearance** | ++ | | | | |
| | **Thoracic hypoplasia** | +++ | | | | |
| Other | **Hydrops** | ++ | | | | |
| | **Perinatal lethality** | + | | | | |
| Laboratory findings | Sialotransferrins (serum) | n | | | | |

**Table 68.116** Solute carrier family 39 (Zn transporter) deficiency SLC39A8-CDG

| System | Symptoms and biomarkers | Neonatal (birth–1 month) | Infancy (1–18 months) | Childhood (1.5–11 years) | Adolescence (11–16 years) | Adulthood (>16 years) |
|---|---|---|---|---|---|---|
| CNS | **Cerebellar atrophy (MRI)** | | ± | ± | ± | ± |
| | **Cerebral atrophy (MRI)** | | ± | ± | ± | ± |
| | Hyperreflexia | | | ± | ± | |
| | Hypotonia | + | + | + | + | + |
| | Intellectual disability | | ++ | ++ | ++ | ++ |
| | Seizures | | ± | ± | ± | ± |
| Eye | **Strabismus** | | + | + | + | + |
| Musculoskeletal | Osteopenia | | | ± | ± | ± |
| | **Scoliosis** | | ± | ± | ± | ± |
| | **Short stature** | | ± | ± | ± | ± |
| Other | Recurent infections | | | ± | ± | |
| Laboratory findings | Manganese (blood) | | ↓↓ | ↓↓ | ↓↓ | |
| | Manganese (urine) | | n-↑ | n-↑ | n-↑ | |
| | Sialotransferrins, type 2 pattern (serum) | + | + | + | + | |
| | Zinc (serum) | | ↓ | ↓ | ↓ | |
| | Zinc (urine) | | n | n | n | |

**Table 68.117** V0 subunit a2 of vesicular H(+)-ATPase deficiency ATP6V0A2-CDG

| System | Symptoms and biomarkers | Neonatal (birth–1 month) | Infancy (1–18 months) | Childhood (1.5–11 years) | Adolescence (11–16 years) | Adulthood (>16 years) |
|---|---|---|---|---|---|---|
| CNS | Cerebral cortical malformations | ± | ± | ± | ± | ± |
| | Intellectual disability | ± | ± | ± | ± | ± |
| Dermatological | **Cutis laxa** | + | + | ± | ± | ± |
| | **Skin histology, abnormal elastin fibers** | + | + | ± | ± | ± |
| Eye | Amblyopia | ± | ± | ± | ± | ± |
| | Myopia | ± | ± | ± | ± | ± |
| | Strabismus | ± | ± | ± | ± | ± |
| Musculoskeletal | **Closure of fontanels, delayed** | – | – | ± | – | – |
| | Facial dysmorphism | + | + | + | + | + |
| | **Fat distribution, subcutaneous, abnormal** | ± | ± | ± | ± | ± |
| | Growth retardation | ± | ± | ± | ± | ± |
| | **Joint laxity** | + | + | + | + | + |
| | **Microcephaly** | ± | ± | ± | ± | ± |
| | **Osteoporosis** | ± | ± | ± | ± | ± |
| Other | **Aged appearance** | + | + | + | + | + |
| Laboratory findings | Apolipoproteine C-III isoelectrofocusing, abnormal (serum) | + | + | + | + | + |
| | Sialotransferrins, type 2 pattern (serum) | n-↑ | n-↑ | n-↑ | n-↑ | n-↑ |

**Table 68.118** Cutis laxa, autosomal recessive, type IID ATP6V1A-CDG

| System | Symptoms and biomarkers | Neonatal (birth–1 month) | Infancy (1–18mths) | Childhood (1.5–11 years) | Adolescence (11–16 years) | Adulthood (>16 years) |
|---|---|---|---|---|---|---|
| Cardiovascular | **Cardiovascular abnormalities** | | ± | ± | ± | |
| CNS | **Brain, abnormal (MRI)** | | ± | ± | ± | |
| | **Hypotonia** | | + | + | + | |
| | Intellectual disability | | ± | ± | ± | |
| | **Seizures** | | + | + | + | |
| Dermatological | **Cutis laxa** | | ± | ± | ± | |
| Musculoskeletal | Contractures | | ± | ± | | |
| | **Facial dysmorphism** | | ± | ± | ± | |
| | Kyphoscoliosis | | ± | ± | | |
| | Marfanoid features | | ± | ± | | |
| Laboratory findings | Sialotransferrins, type 2 pattern | | ± | ± | | |

**Table 68.119** Cutis laxa, autosomal recessive, type IIC ATP6V1E1-CDG

| System | Symptoms and biomarkers | Neonatal (birth–1 month) | Infancy (1–18 months) | Childhood (1.5–11 years) | Adolescence (11–16 years) | Adulthood (>16 years) |
|---|---|---|---|---|---|---|
| Cardiovascular | **Cardiovascular abnormalities** | | + | + | | |
| CNS | **Hypotonia** | | + | + | | |
| Dermatological | **Cutis laxa** | | + | + | | |
| Eye | Entropion | | ± | ± | | |
| Musculoskeletal | Contractures | | ± | ± | | |
| | **Facial dysmorphism** | | + | + | | |
| | Hip dysplasia | | ± | ± | | |
| | Kyphoscoliosis | | ± | ± | | |
| | Marfanoid habitus | | ± | ± | | |
| Laboratory findings | Sialotransferrins, type 2 pattern (serum) | | + | + | | |

**Table 68.120** Immunodeficiency 47 ATP6AP1-CDG

| System | Symptoms and biomarkers | Neonatal (birth–1 month) | Infancy (1–18 months) | Childhood (1.5–11 years) | Adolescence (11–16 years) | Adulthood (>16 years) |
|---|---|---|---|---|---|---|
| CNS | Neurological symptoms | | ± | ± | ± | ± |
| Dermatological | Cutis laxa, improving with age | ± | ± | ± | ± | – |
| Digestive | **Hepatosplenomegaly** | | + | + | + | + |
| | Pancreatic insufficiency, exocrine | | ± | ± | ± | ± |
| Hematological | Leukopenia | | | ± | ± | ± |
| Other | **Recurrent infections** | | + | + | + | + |
| Laboratory findings | Alkaline phosphatase (plasma) | | | n-↑ | n-↑ | n-↑ |
| | Apolipoprotein C-III, abnormal IEF (serum) | | ± | ± | ± | ± |
| | Ceruloplasmin (serum) | | | ↓ | ↓ | ↓ |
| | Copper (serum) | | | ↓ | ↓ | ↓ |
| | IgA (serum) | | | ↓-n | ↓-n | ↓-n |
| | IgG (serum) | | | ↓ | ↓ | ↓ |
| | IgM (serum) | | | ↓-n | ↓-n | ↓-n |
| | Sialotransferrins, type 2 pattern (serum) | | + | + | + | + |
| | Transaminase (plasma) | | | n-↑ | n-↑ | n-↑ |

**Table 68.121** ATP6AP2-CDG

| System | Symptoms and biomarkers | Neonatal (birth–1 month) | Infancy (1–18 months) | Childhood (1.5–11 years) | Adolescence (11–16 years) | Adulthood (>16 years) |
|---|---|---|---|---|---|---|
| CNS | Cognitive impairment, mild | | ± | ± | ± | ± |
| Dermatological | **Cutis laxa** | + | + | + | + | + |
| Digestive | **Liver involvement** | + | + | + | + | + |
| Other | Dysmorphism | ± | ± | ± | ± | ± |
| | **Recurrent infections** | | + | + | + | + |
| Laboratory findings | Factor IX (blood) | ↓ | ↓ | ↓ | ↓ | ↓ |
| | Gammaglobulins (serum) | ↓ | ↓ | ↓ | ↓ | ↓ |
| | Sialotransferrins, type 2 pattern (serum) | + | + | + | + | + |
| | Transaminase (plasma) | ↑ | ↑ | ↑ | ↑ | ↑ |

**Table 68.122** Congenital disorder of glycosylation, type IIp TMEM199-CDG

| System | Symptoms and biomarkers | Neonatal (birth–1 month) | Infancy (1–18 months) | Childhood (1.5–11 years) | Adolescence (11–16 years) | Adulthood (>16 years) |
|---|---|---|---|---|---|---|
| Digestive | Hepatomegaly | | | ± | | |
| Laboratory findings | Alkaline phosphatase (plasma) | ↑↑ | ↑↑ | ↑↑ | ↑↑ | n-↑ |
| | Ceruloplasmin (serum) | ↓ | ↓ | ↓ | ↓ | ↓ |
| | Hypoglycosylation of apolipoprotein CIII (serum) | ± | ± | ± | ± | ± |
| | Sialotransferrins, type 2 pattern (serum) | + | + | + | + | + |
| | Transaminase (plasma) | ↑ | ↑ | ↑ | ↑ | n |

**Table 68.123** CCDC115 deficiency CCDC115-CDG

| System | Symptoms and biomarkers | Neonatal (birth–1 month) | Infancy (1–18 months) | Childhood (1.5–11 years) | Adolescence (11–16 years) | Adulthood (>16 years) |
|---|---|---|---|---|---|---|
| CNS | Hypotonia | | ± | ± | | |
| | **Retardation, psychomotor** | | + | + | + | + |
| | Seizures | | ± | ± | ± | ± |
| Digestive | Cholestasis | ± | ± | ± | ± | ± |
| | **Hepatosplenomegaly** | ± | ± | ± | ± | ± |
| | Liver failure | ± | ± | ± | ± | ± |
| Musculoskeletal | Facial dysmorphism | ± | ± | ± | ± | ± |
| Psychiatric | Behaviour difficulties | | | | ± | ± |
| Laboratory findings | Alkaline phosphatase (plasma) | | ↑↑ | ↑↑ | ↑↑ | ↑↑ |
| | Apolipoprotein CIII hypoglycosylation (serum) | | + | + | + | + |
| | Ceruloplasmin (serum) | | ↓ | ↓ | ↓ | ↓ |
| | Cholesterol (serum) | | ↑ | ↑ | ↑ | ↑ |
| | LDL cholesterol (serum) | | ↑ | ↑ | ↑ | ↑ |
| | Sialotransferrins, type 2 pattern (serum) | | + | + | + | + |
| | Transaminase (plasma) | | ↑ | ↑ | ↑ | ↑ |

**Table 68.124** Congenital disorder of glycosylation TMEM165-CDG

| System | Symptoms and biomarkers | Neonatal (birth–1 month) | Infancy (1–18 months) | Childhood (1.5–11 years) | Adolescence (11–16 years) | Adulthood (>16 years) |
|---|---|---|---|---|---|---|
| CNS | Retardation, psychomotor | | + | + | + | + |
| Digestive | **Hepatomegaly** | + | + | + | | |
| | Obesity | + | + | + | + | + |
| Endocrine | **Growth hormone deficiency** | | + | + | + | |
| Musculoskeletal | **Dysmorphic features** | + | + | + | + | + |
| | **Growth retardation** | ++ | ++ | ++ | ++ | ++ |
| | **Joint laxity** | + | + | + | | |
| | **Midface hypoplasia** | + | + | + | + | + |
| | Muscle weakness | + | + | + | | |
| | **Skeletal abnormalities** | ++ | ++ | ++ | ++ | ++ |
| Other | Failure to thrive | | + | + | | |
| | Fever of unknown origin | ± | ± | ± | ± | ± |
| Laboratory findings | ASAT:ALAT ratio (plasma) | ↑ | ↑ | ↑ | ↑ | ↑ |
| | Creatine kinase (plasma) | ↑ | ↑ | ↑ | ↑ | ↑ |
| | Sialotransferrins, type 2 pattern (serum) | + | + | + | + | + |

**Table 68.125** N-glycanase 1 deficiency

| System | Symptoms and biomarkers | Neonatal (birth–1 month) | Infancy (1–18 months) | Childhood (1.5–11 years) | Adolescence (11–16 years) | Adulthood (>16 years) |
|---|---|---|---|---|---|---|
| CNS | **Developmental/intellectual disability** | | ++ | ++ | ++ | ++ |
| | **Epilepsy** | | ± | ± | ± | – |
| | **Hyporeflexia** | + | + | + | + | + |
| | **Hypotonia** | | + | + | + | + |
| | **Microcephaly, acquired** | | ± | ± | ± | + |
| | **Movement abnormalities** | ± | ± | ± | ± | ± |
| | **Peripheral neuropathy** | | ± | ± | ± | ± |
| Digestive | **Feeding difficulties** | ± | ± | ± | | |
| | **Liver storage** | | + | + | + | + |
| Endocrine | Adrenal insufficiency | | ± | ± | ± | |
| Eye | **Alacrima, hypolacrima** | + | + | + | + | + |
| | **Corneal ulceration, scarring** | ± | ± | ± | ± | – |
| | **Ocular apraxia** | | | ± | ± | ± |
| | Strabismus | ± | ± | ± | ± | ± |
| Musculoskeletal | **Hands/feet, small** | ± | ± | ± | ± | |
| | **Scoliosis** | | ± | ± | ± | ± |
| Other | Anhydrosis | | | ± | | |
| | Dysmorphism | ± | ± | ± | ± | |
| | **Mortality increased** | | + | + | + | |
| | Pain sensation diminished | | ± | ± | ± | |
| Laboratory findings | Sialotransferrins (serum) | n | n | n | n | n |
| | Transaminase (plasma) | ↑ | ↑ | n-↑ | n-↑ | n-↑ |

## Reference Values

| *Serum sialotransferrins (isoelectrofocusing) (P3–P97 centiles, $n = 96$, all ages) | |
|---|---|
| Monosialotransferrins | 0.0–3.7 |
| Disialotransferrins | 2.0–6.1 |
| Trisialotransferrins | 5.5–15.1 |
| Tetrasialotransferrins | 48.5–65.3 |
| Pentasialotransferrins | 14.9–28.7 |
| Hexasialotransferrins | 2.3–8.1 |

| *Enzyme analyses | |
|---|---|
| *Phosphomannose mutase (mU/mg protein)* | |
| Leukocytes | 1.8–3.2 (range); 2.2 (median) |
| Fibroblasts | 3.8 ± 0.9 (mean ± 1 SD) |
| *Phosphomannose isomerase (mU/mg protein)* | |
| Leukocytes | 860–1800 (nmol/h/mg protein, range) |
| Fibroblasts | 6.8 ± 1.0 (mean ± 1 SD) |

## Pathological Values

| Disease | Sialotransferrin IEF pattern (S) |
|---|---|
| 68.1–68.15 | Type 1 pattern[a] |
| 68.17–68.21 | |
| 68.96–68.104 | |
| 68.25–68.27 | Type 2 pattern° |
| 68.105, 68.111, 68.112 | |
| 68.116–68.124 | |
| All other CDG | Normal pattern |

[a]Type 1 pattern, increase of di- and asialotransferrin and decrease of tetra-, penta-, and hexasialotransferrin; °type 2 pattern, increase of tri-, di-, mono-, and/or asialotransferrin and decrease of tetra-, penta-, and hexasialotransferrin

| Disease | Apolipoprotein C-III IEF pattern (S) |
|---|---|
| 68.117–68.124 | Cathodal shift |
| All other CDG | Normal pattern |

## Diagnostic Flowchart

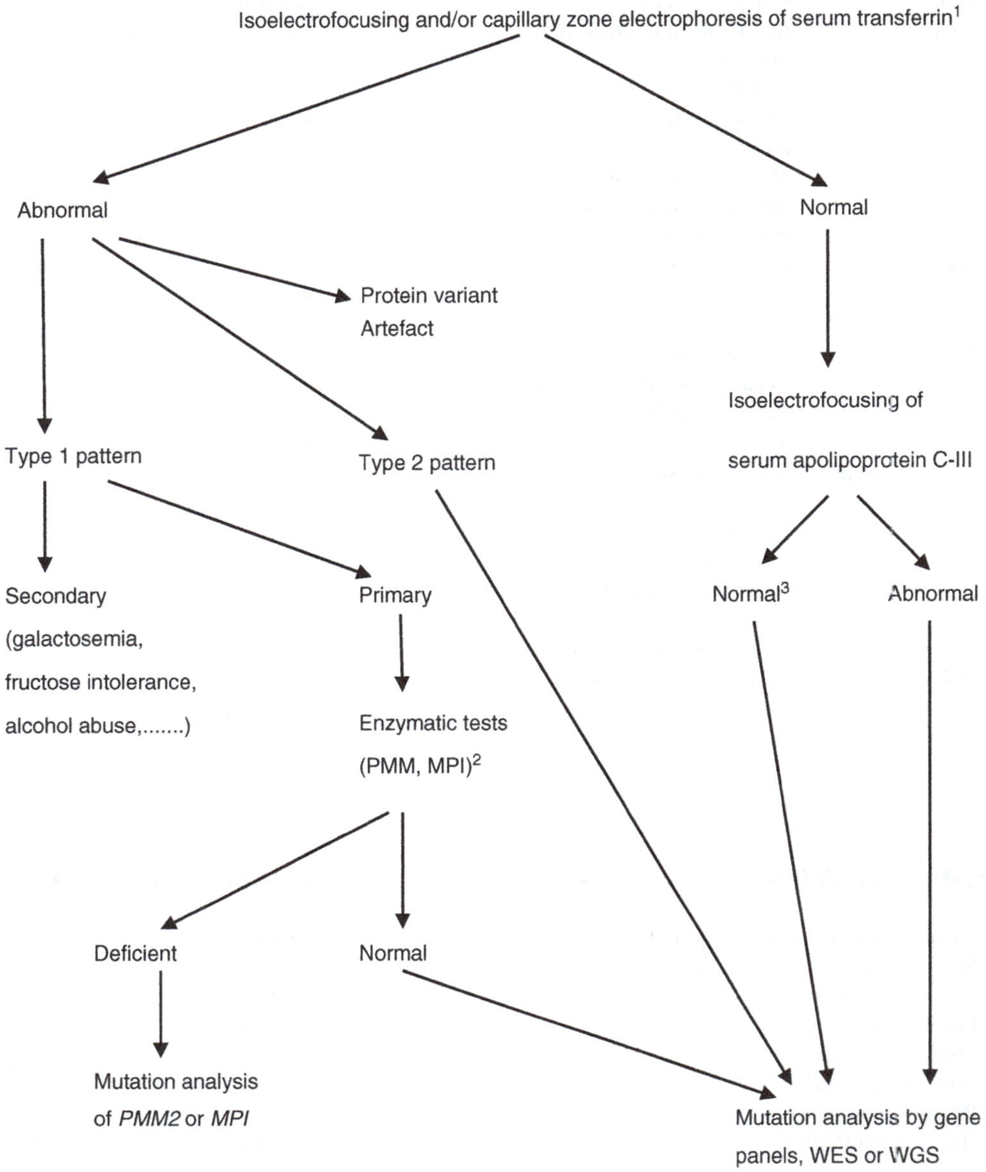


WES: whole exome sequencing (checking first established genes for CDG defects and afterwards candidate genes for CDG defects and/or all other genes).

WGS: whole genome sequencing (checking first established genes for CDG defects and afterwards candidate genes for CDG defects and/or all other genes).

1: In specialized centers for CDG diagnostics, glycomics MS assays have been developed and may be used for initial screening as well (Bakar et al 2018; Ashikov et al 2018).

2: Enzymatic tests may be performed when there is a typical PMM2-CDG or MPI-CDG phenotype.

3: In case of strong clinical suspicion of CDG, genetic testing is advocated.

**Fig. 68.2** Flowchart for the diagnosis of CDG

## Specimen Collection

| Test | Precondition | Material | Handling | Pitfalls |
|---|---|---|---|---|
| Sialotransferrins | | S | Frozen (−20 °C) | No EDTA plasma |
| Apolipoprotein C-III | | S | Frozen (−20 °C) | |
| Phosphomannomutase | | WBC, FB | Frozen (−20 °C) | |
| Phosphomannose isomerase | | WBC, FB | Frozen (−20 °C) | |

## Prenatal Diagnosis

| Disorder | Material | Timing, trimester |
|---|---|---|
| All (68.1–68.125) | CV sampling or cultured AFC | I, II |

Prenatal diagnosis is performed by DNA diagnostics on genomic DNA when the genetic defect has been established in a particular family. Maternal contamination has to be excluded by haplotype (CA repeat) testing of the AFC and maternal blood.

## DNA Testing

| Disorder | Material | Methodology |
|---|---|---|
| All (68.1–68.125) | F, WBC | Direct sequencing of genomic DNA |

## Treatment

Besides the well-established symptomatic and supportive therapies for all CDG, there are very few specific/curative treatments: mannose for MPI-CDG, fucose for some patients with SLC35C1-CDG, benzoate for the neurological symptoms of PIGM-CDG, and uridine for CAD-CDG. Galactose is on trial for several CDG mainly PGM1-CDG, SLC35A2-CDG, and TMEM165-CDG. Also on trial is manganese for SLC39A8-CDG. A minority of patients with PMM2-CDG present recurrent stroke-like episodes, thromboses (probably at least in part due to hyperaggregability of blood platelets), and/or bleeding episodes. Guidelines for the preventive and curative treatment of these features are being established by the Paris MetabERN center. The same center also prepares guidelines for the hormonal treatment of pubertal problems in PMM2-CDG.

## Standard Treatment

- **68.2** *Phosphomannose isomerase deficiency*
- Mannose circumvents the defective step because it can be directly converted to mannose-6-phosphate by hexokinases. Oral mannose, 0.2 g/kg of body weight per 4 h, is recommended. The clinical symptoms usually disappear rapidly, but it takes several months for the serum transferrin isoform pattern to improve or normalize.
- **68.114** *GDP-fucose transporter deficiency*
- Oral fucose, 150 mg/kg of body weight, five times a day, abolishes or prevents infections and normalizes neutrophil counts in some patients (depending on genotype).
- **68.85** *PIGM deficiency*
- Oral sodium phenylbutyrate (a histone deacetylase inhibitor), 20–30 mg/kg body weight, three times a day, has been given to three patients with a clearly beneficial effect on seizures and psychomotor development.

## Dangers/Pitfalls

- **68.2** Higher mannose doses can induce osmotic diarrhea. Some patients develop hemolytic jaundice under mannose therapy. The alternative is then liver transplantation.
- **68.114** Higher fucose doses can induce autoimmune neutropenia.

## Experimental Treatment

- **68.105** *Phosphoglucomutase 1 deficiency*
- In pilot studies, oral galactose administration (1 g/kg per day) caused an improvement of liver transaminases, antithrombin and factor XI, endocrine parameters (to a variable degree), and glycosylation and a decreased frequency of rhabdomyolysis (review in Witters et al. 2017).
- **68.110** *CAD trifunctional protein deficiency*
- Oral uridine administration (100 mg/kg per day) abolished the epilepsy and the anemia, improved psychomotor development, and normalized UDP sugars in fibroblasts (Koch et al. 2017).
- **68.112** *UDP-galactose transporter deficiency*
- On oral galactose, seizures tend to improve. In one patient, glycosylation was nearly completely restored, but serum transaminases remained elevated (review in Witters et al. 2017).
- **68.116** *SLC39A8 deficiency*
- In two patients, oral $MnSO_4$ administration (15 and 20 mg/kg per day) considerably improved motor abilities, hearing, and other neurological functions and completely normalized enzyme dysfunctions (Park et al. 2018).
- **68.124** *Transmembrane protein 165 deficiency*
- In two patients, oral galactose administration caused a substantial improvement of N-glycosylation, endocrine function, and some coagulation parameters (Morelle et al. 2017).

## References


Abu Bakar N, Lefeber DJ, van Scherpenzeel M. Clinical glycomics for the diagnosis of congenital disorders of glycosylation. J Inherit Metab Dis. 2018;41:499–513.

Carchon H, Chevigné R, Falmagne JB, Jaeken J. Diagnosis of congenital disorders of glycosylation by capillary zone electrophoresis of serum transferrin. Clin Chem. 2004;50:101–11.

Coman D, Irving M, Kannu P, Jaeken J, Savarirayan R. The skeletal manifestations of the congenital disorders of glycosylation. Clin Genet. 2008;73:507–15.

Ferreira CR, Altassan R, Marques-Da-Silva D, Francisco R, Jaeken J, Morava E. Recognizable phenotypes in CDG. J Inherit Metab Dis. 2018;41:541–53.

Francisco R, Marques-da-Silva D, Brasil S, et al. The challenge of CDG diagnosis. Mol Genet Metab. 2018a; https://doi.org/10.1016/j.ymgme.2018.11.003.

Francisco R, Pascoal C, Marques-da-Silva D, et al. Keeping an eye on congenital disorders of O-glycosylation: a systematic literature review. J Inherit Metab Dis doi. 2018b; https://doi.org/10.1007/s10545-017-0119-2.

Grünewald S. The clinical spectrum of phosphomannomutase 2 deficiency (CDG-Ia). Biochim Biophys Acta. 2009;1792:827–34.

Jaeken J, Hennet T, Matthijs G, Freeze HH. CDG nomenclature: time for a change! Biochim Biophys Acta. 2009;1792:825–6.

Jaeken J, Lefeber D, Matthijs G. Clinical utility gene card for : phosphomannose isomerase deficiency. Eur J Hum Genet. 2014; https://doi.org/10.1038/ejhg.2014.29.

Jaeken J, Péanne R. What is new in CDG? J Inherit Metab Dis. 2017;40:569–86.

Jaeken J, van Eijk HG, van der Heul C, et al. Sialic acid-deficient serum and cerebrospinal fluid transferrin in a newly recognized syndrome. Clin Chim Acta. 1984;144:245–7.

Jaeken J, Vanderschueren-Lodeweyckx M, Casaer P, et al. Familial psychomotor retardation with markedly fluctuating serum proteins, FSH and GH levels, partial TBG-deficiency, increased serum arylsulphatase a and increased CSF protein: a new syndrome? Pediatr Res. 1980;14:179.

Koch J, Mayr JA, Alhaddad B, et al. CAD mutations and uridine-responsive epileptic encephalopathy. Brain. 2017;140:279–86.

Marques-da-Silva D, Dos Reis Ferreira V, Monticelli M, et al. Liver involvement in congenital disorders of glycosylation (CDG): a systematic review. J Inherit Metab Dis. 2017a;40:195–207.

Marques-da-Silva D, Francisco R, Webster D, Dos Reis Ferreira V, Jaeken J, Pulinilkunnil T. Cardiac complications of congenital disorders of glycosylation (CDG): a systematic literature review. J Inherit Metab Dis. 2017b;40:657–72.

Matthijs G, Schollen E, Pardon E, et al. Mutations in PMM2, a phosphomannomutase gene on chromosome 16p13, in carbohydrate-deficient glycoprotein type I syndrome (Jaeken syndrome). Nat Genet. 1997;16:88–92. (erratum in Nat Genet 1997 Jul; 16(3): 316)

Monticelli M, Ferro T, Jaeken J, Dos Reis Ferreira V, Videira PA. Immunological aspects of congenital disorders of glycosylation (CDG): a review. J Inherit Metab Dis. 2016;39:765–80.

Morava E, Thiemes V, Thiel C, et al. ALG6-CDG: a recognizable phenotype with epilepsy, proximal muscle weakness, ataxia and behavioral and limb anomalies. J Inherit Metab Dis. 2016;39:713–23.

Morava E, Wosik HN, Sykut-Cegielska J, et al. Ophthalmological abnormalities in children with congenital disorders of glycosylation type I. Br J Ophthalmol. 2009;93:350–4.

Morelle W, Potelle S, Witters P, et al. Galactose supplementation in patients with TMEM165-CDG rescues the glycosylation defects. J Clin Endocrinol Metab. 2017;102:1375–86.

Ng BG, Freeze HH. Perspectives on glycosylation and its congenital disorders. Trends Genet. 2018;34:466–76.

Ng BG, Shiryaev SA, Rymen D, et al. ALG1-CDG: clinical and molecular characterization of 39 unreported patients. Hum Mutat. 2016;37:653–60.

Park JH, Hogrebe M, Fobker M, et al. SLC39A8 deficiency: biochemical correction and major clinical improvement by manganese therapy. Genet Med. 2018;20:259–68.

Van Schaftingen E, Jaeken J. Phosphomannomutase deficiency is a cause of carbohydrate-deficient glycoprotein syndrome type I. FEBS Lett. 1995;370:318–20.

Witters P, Cassiman D, Morava E. Nutritional therapies in congenital disorders of glycosylation (CDG). Nutrients. 2017; https://doi.org/10.3390/nu9111222.

Wopereis S, Grünewald S, Morava E, et al. Apolipoprotein C-III isofocusing in the diagnosis of genetic defects in O-glycan biosynthesis. Clin Chem. 2003;49:1839–5.

# Part XI
# Various

# Cerebral Organic Acidurias

# 69

Stefan Kölker

## Contents



**Summary**

A group of organic acidurias, including Canavan disease (*N*-acetylaspartic aciduria), glutaric aciduria type I, L-2-hydroxyglutaric aciduria and D-2-hydroxyglutaric aciduria types I and II, are characterised by a predominantly or even exclusively neurological presentation and have therefore been termed 'cerebral'. The clinical presentation frequently includes developmental delay, cognitive disability, movement disorder and epilepsy, resulting from acute and/or chronic pathological changes in various brain regions including grey matter (cortex, basal ganglia, cerebellum) and white matter (periventricular and subcortical). Unlike 'classic' organic acidurias (e.g. propionic and methylmalonic aciduria), acute metabolic decompensations with hyperammonaemia, metabolic acidosis and elevated concentrations of lactate and ketone bodies are uncommon for cerebral organic acidurias. Biochemically, these diseases are characterised by accumulation of characteristic organic acids, mostly dicarboxylic acids, in body fluids. At high concentrations, some of these may become neurotoxic. Since the blood–brain barrier has a low transport capacity for dicarboxylic acids, cerebral accumulation of dicarboxylic acids is facilitated. Impairment of brain energy metabolism is suggested to play a central role in the pathophysiology of this disease group. Metabolic treatment initiated in neonatally diagnosed patients with glutaric aciduria type I has significantly improved the neurological outcome, whereas current treatment strategies for the other cerebral organic acidurias are ineffective.

S. Kölker (✉)
Division of Pediatric Neurology and Metabolic Medicine, Clinic I, Center for Pediatric and Adolescent Medicine, Heidelberg, Germany
e-mail: stefan.koelker@med.uni-heidelberg.de





N. Blau et al. (eds.), *Physician's Guide to the Diagnosis, Treatment, and Follow-Up of Inherited Metabolic Diseases*, https://doi.org/10.1007/978-3-030-67727-5_69

## Introduction

Canavan disease (Van Bogaert–Bertrand disease, *N*-acetylaspartic aciduria), a debilitating and lethal leukodystrophy, is caused by an autosomal recessively inherited deficiency of aspartoacylase (aminoacylase 2) which is exclusively expressed in oligodendrocytes. Most patients have the infantile form which generally manifests at 2–4 months of age with head lag, muscular hypotonia and macrocephaly, progressing to marked developmental delay, seizures, optic nerve atrophy, progressive spasticity and opisthotonic posturing (Matalon et al. 1995). Death usually occurs in a few years. However, the initial symptoms may already start at or shortly after birth (neonatal form) or after the age of 5 years (juvenile form). Cranial MRI studies show diffuse or exclusively subcortical involvement of the white matter due to spongiform myelinopathy and involvement of the thalamus and globus pallidus. Diagnosis can be made by finding elevated *N*-acetylaspartate concentrations in urine using GC/MS analysis of organic acids. A decreased aspartoacylase activity in cultured skin fibroblasts and/or the identification of two disease-causing mutations in the *ASPA* gene localised on 17p13.2 confirms the diagnosis. *N*-Acetylaspartate is formed in neurons and hydrolysed to L-aspartate and acetate by oligodendrocytes. No effective treatment exists for Canavan disease. Lithium citrate decreases brain *N*-acetylaspartate concentrations (Assadi et al. 2010), and glyceryl triacetate treatment supplies the brain with acetate (Segel et al. 2011). Although this treatment is considered as safe, there is no proof for its therapeutic efficacy. Initial attempts of *ASPA* gene therapy have not met expectations (Leone et al. 2000). Recombinant adeno-associated virus-based gene therapy targeting astrocytes (Gessler et al. 2017), however, achieved complete and sustained rescue of the lethal phenotype in a mouse model of Canavan disease. Translation into clinical studies is pending.

Glutaric aciduria type I (glutaric acidaemia type I) is caused by an autosomal recessively inherited deficiency of glutaryl-CoA dehydrogenase, an FAD-dependent mitochondrial matrix enzyme. This enzyme is involved in the catabolic pathways of lysine, hydroxylysine and tryptophan, catalysing the oxidative decarboxylation of glutaryl-CoA to crotonyl-CoA. Transient muscular hypotonia and macrocephaly are often found in newborns. At this age, cranial MRI of affected individuals reveals temporal hypoplasia, dilated external CSF spaces, subependymal pseudocysts, myelination delay and an immature gyral pattern which all may improve or even resolve in early treated children (Harting et al. 2009). In the time interval between 3 and 36 (−72) months, however, most untreated patients develop a complex movement disorder best described as generalised dystonia superimposed on axial hypotonia (Gitiaux et al. 2008). These symptoms are the consequence of bilateral striatal injury which may occur acutely during acute encephalopathic crises precipitated by catabolism or insidiously without preceding crises (Kölker et al. 2006). Aside from striatal injury, MRI may show additional frontal atrophy and subdural haemorrhage. A few adolescent and adult patients with a late-onset form have been reported presenting with headaches, vertigo, reduced fine motor skills and white matter abnormalities (Harting et al. 2009). Patients can be identified in the first week of life by newborn screening using glutarylcarnitine as a diagnostic parameter. Glutarate and 3-hydroxyglutarate concentrations are increased in urine and other body fluids but may be (intermittently) normal in patients with a low-excreter phenotype. Therefore, a normal organic acid analysis result does not unequivocally exclude the diagnosis. Suspected diagnosis is confirmed by significantly decreased glutaryl-CoA dehydrogenase activity in leucocytes or fibroblasts and/or the identification of two disease-causing mutations in the *GCDH* gene localised on 19p13.13. Glutarate and 3-hydroxyglutarate concentrations are 100–1000-fold higher in the brain than in plasma which is caused by the very low efflux transport of dicarboxylic acids across brain capillary endothelial cells (Sauer et al. 2006). At high concentrations, accumulating dicarboxylic acids may become neurotoxic inhibiting energy metabolism (2-oxoglutarate dehydrogenase, dicarboxylate shuttle between astrocytes and neurons) and activating *N*-methyl-D-aspartate receptors. The development of prognostic relevant striatal injury can be prevented in the majority of children if the diagnosis is made and metabolic treatment is started neonatally (Heringer et al. 2010; Boy et al. 2018). Metabolic treatment according to a recently revised guideline includes a low lysine diet, carnitine supplementation and emergency treatment to counteract catabolism (Kölker et al. 2011; Boy et al. 2017a, b). Patients with a high- and low-excreter phenotype have the same risk of developing striatal injury and thus receive the same treatment (Kölker et al. 2006); however, the neurological long-term risk of individuals with high-excreter phenotype might be increased (Boy et al. 2017a, b). Regardless of therapy, some individuals develop mild to moderate degree chronic kidney disease starting at school age. The prognosis of this renal manifestation needs to be elucidated.

L-2-Hydroxyglutaric aciduria (L2HGA) is an autosomal recessive inborn error of metabolism, caused by mutations in the *L2HG dehydrogenase* (*L2HGDH*) gene. The *L2HGDH* gene product, i.e. L2HGDH, is an FAD-dependent membrane-bound enzyme responsible for the conversion of L-2-hydroxyglutarate (L2HG) into 2-ketoglutaric acid (2KG). The current opinion is that nonspecific mitochondrial formation of L2HG out of 2KG by L-malic dehydrogenase is the sole source of L2HG and that L2HGDH is an enzyme for metabolite repair (Van Schaftingen et al. 2009). L2HGA has an insidious onset starting in childhood with developmental delay, macrocephaly, epilepsy and cerebellar ataxia as clinical signs. In a minority of patients, the diagnosis is established in adulthood, but retrospective evaluation of the clinical course reveals an earlier subtle onset (Steenweg et al. 2010). MRI reveals disease-specific alterations characterised by predominantly subcortical cerebral white matter abnormalities and abnormalities of the dentate nucleus, globus pallidus, putamen and caudate nucleus (Steenweg et al. 2009). Metabolic investigations will reveal increased 2HG in the urinary organic acid screening, and subsequent chiral differentiation shows the increased excretion of exclusively L2HG. Apart from the massive increase of L2HG in all body fluids, a modest increase of CSF lysine is observed, while plasma lysine levels may be normal. Since the massive increase of L2HG is the major biochemical finding, pathology is likely to be explained by the pathologic levels of L2HG; however, lowered (peripheral) 2KG levels might also attribute to the disease. Currently, there is no established treatment protocol for L2HGA apart from two anecdotic reports mentioning positive effects of treatment with riboflavin and/or FAD.

D-2-Hydroxyglutaric aciduria (D2HGA) type I is one of the two subtypes of D2HGA and has an autosomal recessive pattern of inheritance. The disease is caused by mutations in the *D2HG dehydrogenase* (*D2HGDH*) gene, resulting in a deficiency of D-2-hydroxyglutarate (D2HG) dehydrogenase (Struys et al. 2005). This FAD-dependent mitochondrial enzyme converts D2HG, most likely formed by the action of hydroxyacid-oxoacid transhydrogenase (HOT), into 2KG. Although several hypothetical metabolic pathways for D2HG have been proposed, there is strong evidence that D2HG is directly and exclusively formed out of 2KG (Struys et al. 2004). The disease displays a strong clinical heterogeneity from severely affected individuals to asymptomatic individuals. However, frequently reported clinical findings are developmental delay, hypotonia and epilepsy. Usually, patients are first recognised by an increase of 2HG in the urinary organic acid screening. In contrast with L2HGA, these elevations can be modest. The increase of D2HG in all body fluids is the sole biochemical alteration in this disease, and the pathophysiology of the disease is likely to be explained by this. Currently, there is no treatment. However, it can be hypothesised that in individual cases, riboflavin supplementation might be beneficial.

D-2-Hydroxyglutaric aciduria (D2HGA) type II is the second form of D2HGA and is caused by a gain-of-function mutation in the *isocitrate dehydrogenase 2* (*IDH2*) gene (Kranendijk et al. 2010). Heterozygous mutations in IDH2 result in the formation of a neomorph enzyme which is able to efficiently convert 2KG into D2HG. This is in contrast with the normal action of IDH2, i.e. the conversion of isocitrate into 2KG. D2HGA type II has an autosomal dominant trait, and in the vast majority of patients, the mutation arose de novo. The degree of D2HG accumulation in D2HGA type II is higher than in type I, despite properly functioning D2HG dehydrogenase. Patients affected with D2HGA type II suffer from developmental delay, muscular hypotonia and epilepsy, and their clinical presentation is generally more severe than that of patients with D2HGA type I. Cardiomyopathy is frequently observed in D2HGA type II and absent in type I. Specific inhibition of the neomorph enzyme by a small molecule rescued cardiomyopathy and improved survival in a mouse model for D2HGA type II (Wang et al. 2016).

## Nomenclature

| No. | Disorder | Alternative name | Abbreviation | Gene symbol | Chromosomal localisation | Affected protein | OMIM no. |
|---|---|---|---|---|---|---|---|
| 69.1 | Canavan disease | Van Bogaert–Bertrand disease | CD | *ASPA* | 17p13.2 | Aspartoacylase (aminoacylase 2) | 271900 |
| 69.2 | Glutaric aciduria type I | Glutaric acidaemia type I | GA-I | *GCDH* | 19p13.13 | Glutaryl-CoA dehydrogenase | 231670 |
| 69.3 | L-2-Hydroxyglutaric aciduria | L-2-Hydroxyglutarate dehydrogenase deficiency | L2HGA | *L2HGDH* | 14q21.3 | L-2-Hydroxyglutarate dehydrogenase | 236792 |
| 69.4 | D-2-Hydroxyglutaric aciduria type I | D-2-Hydroxyglutarate dehydrogenase deficiency | D2HGA type I | *D2HGDH* | 2q37.3 | D-2-Hydroxyglutarate dehydrogenase | 600721 |
| 69.5 | D-2-Hydroxyglutaric aciduria type II | Isocitrate dehydrogenase 2 deficiency | D2HGA type II | *IDH2* | 15q26.1 | Isocitrate dehydrogenase 2 | 613657 |

## Metabolic Pathways

### Canavan Disease (Aspartoacylase Deficiency)

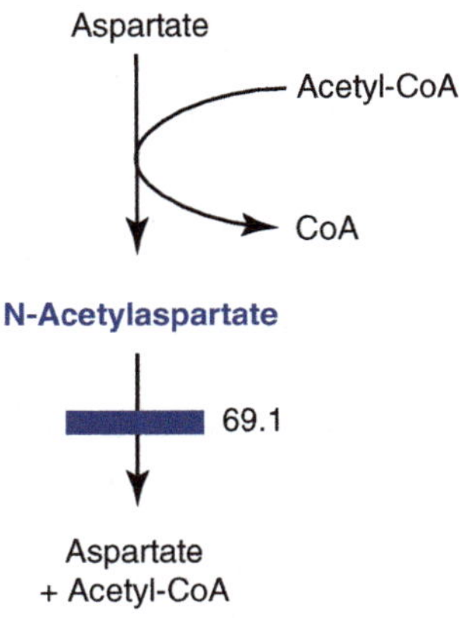


**Fig. 69.1** Metabolic pathway of Canavan disease. *N*-Acetylaspartate is produced in neurons from L-aspartate and acetyl-CoA and is transported to oligodendrocytes where it is hydrolysed to L-aspartate and acetyl-CoA by aspartate aminoacylase 2. Inherited deficiency of this enzyme results in accumulation of *N*-acetylaspartate in patients with Canavan disease

## Glutaric Aciduria Type I (Glutaryl-CoA Dehydrogenase Deficiency)

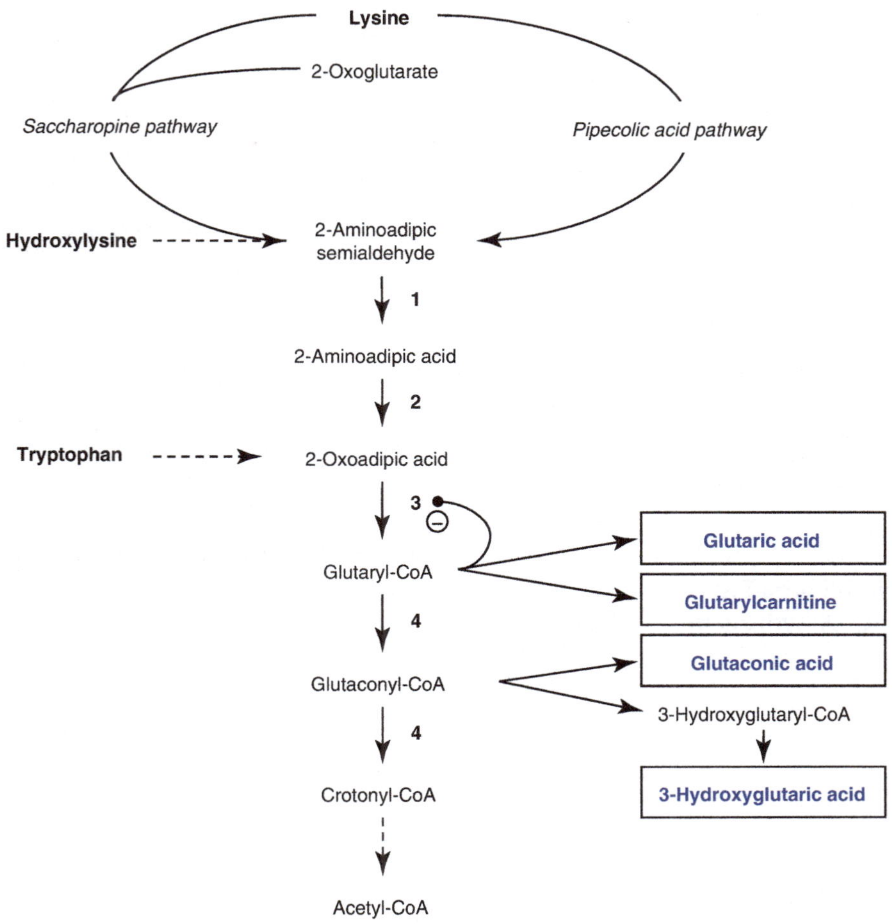


**Fig. 69.2** Metabolic pathway of glutaric aciduria type I. Glutaryl-CoA is formed within the catabolic pathways of lysine, tryptophan and hydroxylysine. The quantitatively major precursor is lysine. Deficient activity of glutaryl-CoA dehydrogenase (4) results in variable accumulation of glutaric, 3-hydroxyglutaric and glutaconic acid as well as glutarylcarnitine, which are important for the diagnosis and can be determined in body fluids. Elevated glutaryl-CoA—similar to homologous succinyl-CoA—results in feedback inhibition of the TCA cycle enzyme 2-oxoglutarate dehydrogenase complex (3). *1*, 2-aminoadipic semialdehyde dehydrogenase (enzyme is deficient in pyridoxine-dependent epilepsy), *2*, 2-aminoadipate aminotransferase, *3*, 2-oxoglutarate dehydrogenase-like complex (enzyme complex contains three subunits: DHTKD1, a E1 component with substrate specificity for 2-oxoadipate, is deficient in 2-aminoadipic/2-oxoadipic aciduria; the E2 subunit is deficient in 2-oxoglutarate dehydrogenase complex deficiency; E3 subunit (lipoamide dehydrogenase), which is shared with pyruvate dehydrogenase and branched-chain oxoacid dehydrogenase complexes, is deficient in E3 deficiency, biochemically resembling maple syrup urine disease, 2-oxoglutarate dehydrogenase complex deficiency and pyruvate dehydrogenase complex deficiency, *4*, glutaryl-CoA dehydrogenase

## L-2-Hydroxyglutaric Aciduria (L-2-Hydroxyglutarate Dehydrogenase Deficiency)

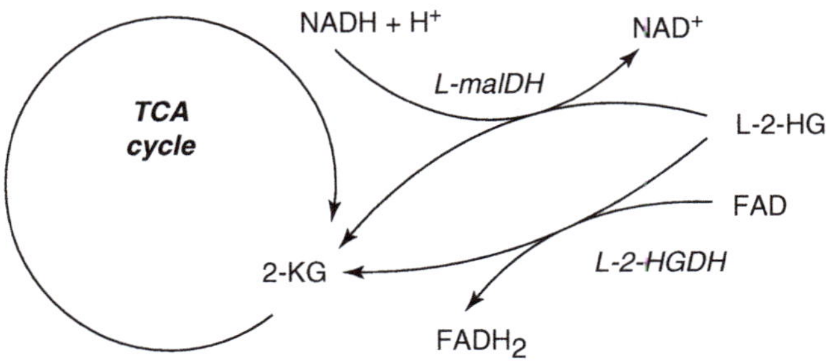


**Fig. 69.3** Metabolic pathway of L-2-hydroxyglutaric aciduria. L-2-Hydroxyglutaric acid is formed by a nonspecific conversion of mitochondrial 2KG into L-2-hydroxyglutaric acid by the action of NADH-dependent l-malic acid dehydrogenase. L2HG dehydrogenase corrects for this metabolic imperfection by reconverting L2HG into 2KG

## D-2-Hydroxyglutaric Aciduria Type I (D-Hydroxyglutarate Dehydrogenase Deficiency)

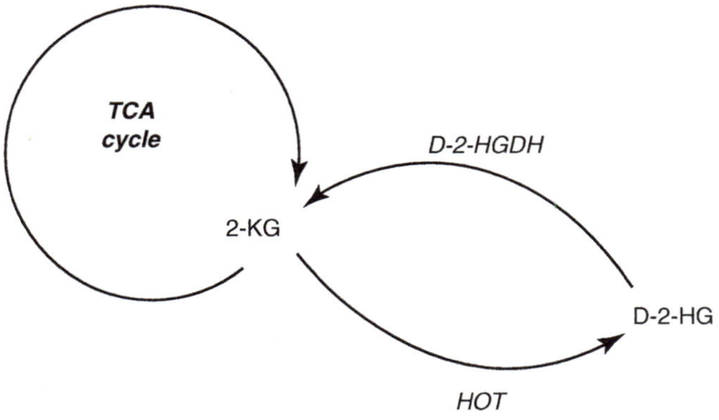


**Fig. 69.4** Metabolic pathway of D-2-hydroxyglutaric aciduria type I. D-2-Hydroxyglutaric acid is formed out of mitochondrial 2KG by the action of hydroxyacid-oxoacid transhydrogenase (*HOT*). D2HG is reconverted into 2KG by D2HG dehydrogenase. This pathway is thought to play a role in GABA/GHB homeostasis

## D-2-Hydroxyglutaric Aciduria Type II (Isocitrate Dehydrogenase 2 Deficiency)

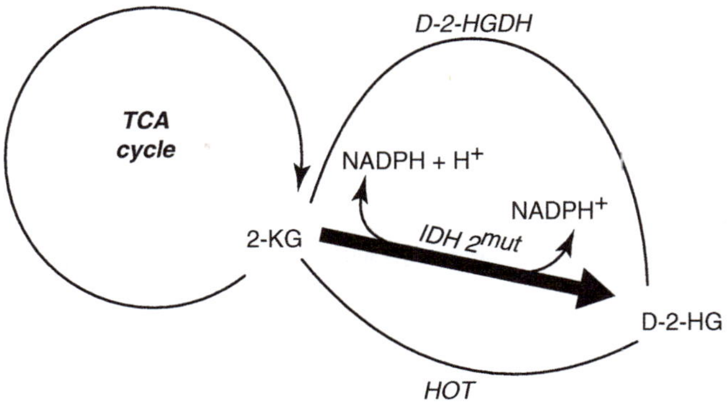


**Fig. 69.5** Metabolic pathway of D-2-hydroxyglutaric aciduria type II. As a consequence of a heterozygous mutation in IDH2, the neomorph IDH2 enzyme produces vast amounts of D2HG, which exceed the capacity of D2HG dehydrogenase, an enzyme with a low $K_m$, and as a net result, D2HG accumulates. The neomorph IDH2 enzyme consumes both 2KG and NADPH, which might lead to their shortages

## Signs and Symptoms

**Table 69.1** Canavan disease

| System | Symptoms and biomarkers | Neonatal (birth–1 month) | Infancy (1–18 months) | Childhood (1.5–11 years) | Adolescence (11–16 years) | Adulthood (>16 years) |
|---|---|---|---|---|---|---|
| CNS | Decerebrate posture | | | ± | ± | ± |
| | Dysarthria | ± | ± | ± | ± | ± |
| | Epilepsy | ± | ± | ± | ± | ± |
| | Extrapyramidal movement disorder | ± | ± | ± | ± | ± |
| | **Loss of very early milestones** | | + | + | + | + |
| | **Mental retardation** | + | + | + | + | + |
| | Motor retardation | + | + | + | + | + |
| | **Muscular hypotonia** | ± | + | + | ± | ± |
| | Opisthotonos | ± | ± | ± | ± | ± |
| | **Spasticity** | | ± | + | + | + |
| Ear | Deafness | ± | ± | ± | ± | ± |
| Eye | Blindness | | + | + | + | + |
| | Nystagmus | ± | ± | ± | ± | ± |
| | Optic atrophy | | + | + | + | + |
| Musculoskeletal | **Macrocephaly** | + | + | + | + | + |
| Laboratory findings | MRI: bilateral subcortical leukodystrophy + involvement of globus pallidus | ± | + | + | + | + |
| | *N*-acetylaspartic acid (CSF, P) | | ↑ | ↑ | ↑ | ↑ |
| | *N*-acetylaspartic acid (U) | | ↑ | ↑ | ↑ | ↑ |

Most patients follow the infantile form which mostly manifests at 2–4 months of age with head lag, muscular hypotonia and macrocephaly, progressing to marked developmental delay, seizures, optic nerve atrophy, progressive spasticity and opisthotonic posturing (Matalon et al. 1995).

**Table 69.2** Glutaric aciduria type I

| System | Symptoms and Biomarkers | Neonatal (birth–1 month) | Infancy (1–18 months) | Childhood (1.5–11 years) | Adolescence (11–16 years) | Adulthood (>16 years) |
|---|---|---|---|---|---|---|
| CNS | Abasia | | ± | ± | ± | ± |
| | Astasia | | | ± | ± | ± |
| | Ataxia | | | ± | ± | ± |
| | Chorea | | ± | ± | ± | ± |
| | **Dysarthria** | | ± | ± | ± | ± |
| | **Dystonia** | | ± | ± | ± | ± |
| | **Encephalopathic crisis, acute** | | ± | ± | | |
| | Headache | | | | ± | ± |
| | Hypokinesia | | ± | ± | ± | ± |
| | Hypotonia, axial | ± | ± | ± | | |
| | Spasticity | | | ± | ± | ± |
| | Swallowing difficulties | | ± | ± | ± | ± |
| | Vertigo | | | | ± | ± |
| Digestive | Feeding difficulties | | ± | ± | ± | ± |
| | Vomiting | | ± | ± | ± | ± |
| Musculoskeletal | **Macrocephaly** | ± | + | ± | ± | ± |
| Respiratory | Pneumonia | | ± | ± | ± | ± |
| Kidney | Chronic kidney disease | | | ± | ± | ± |
| Routine laboratory | ASAT/ALAT (P) | | (↑) | (↑) | (↑) | (↑) |
| | Creatine kinase (P) | | (↑) | (↑) | (↑) | (↑) |
| Laboratory findings | 3-Hydroxyglutaric acid (U) | n-↑ | n-↑ | n-↑ | n-↑ | n-↑ |
| | C5DC glutarylcarnitine (P, B) | n-↑ | n-↑ | n-↑ | n-↑ | n-↑ |
| | Glutaconic acid (U) | n-↑ | n-↑ | n-↑ | n-↑ | n-↑ |
| | Glutaric acid (U) | n-↑ | n-↑ | n-↑ | n-↑ | n-↑ |
| | MRI: periventricular white matter and other extrastriatal MR abnormalities | | ± | ± | + | + |
| | MRI: striatal atrophy | | ± | ± | ± | ± |
| | MRI: temporal hypoplasia, dilated external CSF spaces | + | + | ± | ± | ± |

**Table 69.3** L-2-Hydroxyglutaric aciduria

| System | Symptoms and biomarkers | Neonatal (birth–1 month) | Infancy (1–18 months) | Childhood (1.5–11 years) | Adolescence (11–16 years) | Adulthood (>16 years) |
|---|---|---|---|---|---|---|
| CNS | **Ataxia** | | ± | + | + | + |
| | Choreoathetosis | | | ± | ± | ± |
| | Dysarthria | | ± | ± | ± | ± |
| | Dystonia | | | ± | ± | ± |
| | Hypotonia | ± | ± | ± | ± | ± |
| | **Mental retardation** | | ± | + | + | + |
| | **Seizures** | | ± | ± | ± | ± |
| | **Spasticity** | | | ± | ± | ± |
| | Tremor | | | ± | ± | ± |
| Musculoskeletal | Macrocephaly | | ± | ± | ± | ± |
| Laboratory findings | Ammonia (B) | n-↑ | | | | |
| | L-2-hydroxyglutaric acid (U, P, CSF) | ↑ | ↑ | ↑ | ↑ | ↑ |
| | Lactate (P) | n-↑ | | | | |
| | Lysine (P, CSF) | n | n-↑ | n-↑ | n-↑ | n-↑ |
| | **MRI/CT: white matter abnormalities** | ± | + | + | + | + |
| | **MRI: globus pallidus and dentate nudeus lesions** | ± | + | + | + | + |
| | Protein (CSF) | | ↑ | ↑ | | |

**Table 69.4** D-2-Hydroxyglutaric aciduria type I

| System | Symptoms and Biomarkers | Neonatal (birth–1 month) | Infancy (1–18 months) | Childhood (1.5–11 years) | Adolescence (11–16 years) | Adulthood (>16 years) |
|---|---|---|---|---|---|---|
| Cardiovascular | Cardiomyopathy | n | n | n | n | n |
| CNS | **Developmental delay** | + | + | + | + | + |
| | Epilepsy | ± | ± | ± | ± | ± |
| | **Hypotonia** | + | + | + | ± | ± |
| Laboratory findings | D2HG (U, P, CSF) | ↑ | ↑ | ↑ | ↑ | ↑ |

**Table 69.5** D-2-Hydroxyglutaric aciduria type II

| System | Symptoms and Biomarkers | Neonatal (birth–1 month) | Infancy (1–18 months) | Childhood (1.5–11 years) | Adolescence (11–16 years) | Adulthood (>16 years) |
|---|---|---|---|---|---|---|
| Cardiovascular | **Cardiomyopathy** | ± | ± | ± | ± | ± |
| CNS | **Developmental delay** | + | + | + | + | + |
| | Epilepsy | + | + | + | + | + |
| | **Hypotonia** | + | + | + | ± | ± |
| Laboratory findings | D2HG (U, P, CSF) | ↑ | ↑ | ↑ | ↑ | ↑ |

## Reference Values

*N*-Acetylaspartic acid (NAA)

| Age | NAA (U) mmol/mol creatinine | NAA (P) μmol/L | NAA (CSF) μmol/L |
|---|---|---|---|
| | 6–36 | 0.17–0.84 | 0.25–2.8 |

Gas chromatography/mass spectrometry (preferably with stable isotope dilution assay)

Glutaric acid (GA)

| Age | GA (U) mmol/mol creatinine | GA (P) μmol/L | GA (CSF) μmol/L |
|---|---|---|---|
| | < 10 | 0.5–2.9 | 0.18–0.63 |

Gas chromatography/mass spectrometry (preferably with stable isotope dilution assay)

3-Hydroxyglutaric acid (3-OH-GA)

| Age | 3-OH-GA (U) mmol/mol creatinine | 3-OH-GA (P) μmol/L | 3-OH-GA (CSF) μmol/L |
|---|---|---|---|
| | < 8 | 0.2–1.36 | < 0.2 |

Gas chromatography/mass spectrometry (preferably with stable isotope dilution assay)

Glutarylcarnitine (C5DC)

| Age | C5DC (DBS) mmol/mol creatinine | C5DC (P) μmol/L | C5DC (U) μmol/L |
|---|---|---|---|
| | <cut-off[a] | <cut-off[a] | <cut-off[a] |

Tandem mass spectrometry
[a]Cut-off needs to be set by each lab

L-2-Hydroxyglutaric acid (L2HG)

| Age | L2HG (U) mmol/mol creatinine | L2HG (P) μmol/L | L2HG (CSF) μmol/L |
|---|---|---|---|
| | 1–19 | 0.5–1 | 0.3–2.3 |

Separation and individual quantification of the D- and L-isomer of 2HG by gas chromatography–mass spectrometry or liquid chromatography-tandem mass spectrometry

D-2-Hydroxyglutaric acid (D2HG)

| Age | D2HG (U) mmol/mol creatinine | D2HG (P) μmol/L | D2HG (CSF) μmol/L |
|---|---|---|---|
| | 3–17 | 0.3–0.9 | 0.07–0.3 |

Separation and individual quantification of the D- and L-isomer of 2HG by gas chromatography–mass spectrometry or liquid chromatography-tandem mass spectrometry

## Pathological Values

### *N*-Acetylaspartic Acid (NAA)

*N*-Acetylaspartic acid (NAA)

| Age | NAA (U) mmol/mol creatinine | NAA (P) μmol/L | NAA (CSF) μmol/L |
|---|---|---|---|
| | 60–10,000 | Up to 10 | |

Gas chromatography/mass spectrometry (preferably with stable isotope dilution assay)

### Glutaric Acid (GA), 3-Hydroxyglutaric Acid (3-OH-GA) and Glutarylcarnitine (C5DC)

Glutaric acid (GA)

| Age | GA (U) | GA (P) | GA (CSF) |
|---|---|---|---|
| | mmol/mol creatinine | µmol/L | µmol/L |
| | N–10,000 | N–200 | N–40 |

Gas chromatography/mass spectrometry (preferably with stable isotope dilution assay)

3-Hydroxyglutaric Acid (3-OH-GA)

| Age | 3-OH-GA (U) | 3-OH-GA (P) | 3-OH-GA (CSF) |
|---|---|---|---|
| | mmol/mol creatinine | µmol/L | µmol/L |
| | N–500 | N–30 | N–5 |

Gas chromatography/mass spectrometry (preferably with stable isotope dilution assay)

Glutarylcarnitine (C5DC)

| Age | C5DC (DBS) | C5DC (P) | C5DC (U) |
|---|---|---|---|
| | mmol/mol creatinine | µmol/L | µmol/L |
| | >cut-off[a] | >cut-off[a] | >cut-off[a] |

Tandem mass spectrometry
[a]Cut-off needs to be set by each lab

### L-2-Hydroxyglutaric Aciduria

| Age | L2HG (U) | L2HG (P) | L2HG (CSF) |
|---|---|---|---|
| | mmol/mol creatinine | µmol/L | µmol/L |
| | 226–4299 | 7–84 | 23–474 |

Separation and individual quantification of the D- and L-isomer of 2HG by gas chromatography–mass spectrometry or liquid chromatography-tandem mass spectrometry

### D-2-Hydroxyglutaric Aciduria Type I

| Age | D2HG (U) | D2HG (P) | D2HG (CSF) |
|---|---|---|---|
| | mmol/mol creatinine | µmol/L | µmol/L |
| | 103–2414 | 26–123 | 6–18 |

Separation and individual quantification of the D- and L-isomer of 2HG by gas chromatography–mass spectrometry or liquid chromatography-tandem mass spectrometry

### D-2-Hydroxyglutaric Aciduria Type II

| Age | D2HG (U) | D2HG (P) | D2HG (CSF) |
|---|---|---|---|
| | mmol/mol creatinine | µmol/L | µmol/L |
| | 448–11,305 | 99–757 | 30–172 |

Separation and individual quantification of the D- and L-isomer of 2HG by gas chromatography–mass spectrometry or liquid chromatography-tandem mass spectrometry

## Diagnostic Flowchart(s)

### N-Acetylaspartic Acid (NAA)

If neurological symptoms occur and/or neuroradiological abnormalities are found (→ **69.4** "Signs and Symptoms") which are characteristic for Canavan disease, the diagnostic process should be initiated by analysis of *N*-acetylaspartate (NAA) in urine. If increased NAA concentrations are found, the diagnosis can be confirmed by significantly decreased aspartoacylase activity in cultured skin fibroblasts and/or the identification of two disease-causing mutations in the *ASPA* gene.

## Glutaric Aciduria Type I

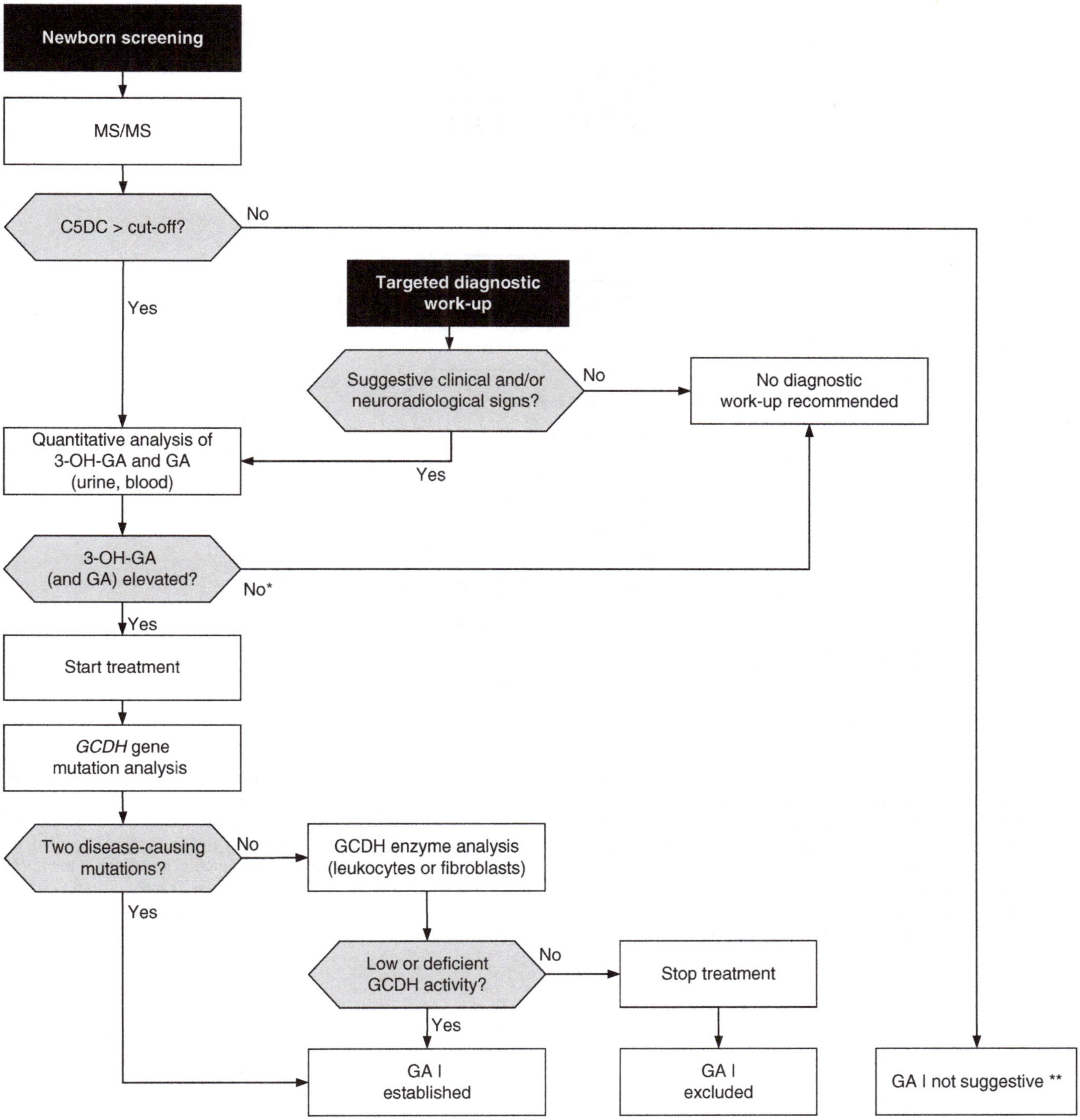


**Fig. 69.6** Diagnostic flowchart for glutaric aciduria type I. (a) *Newborn screening* for glutaric aciduria type I (GA-I) is performed using tandem mass spectrometry (MS/MS). (b) *Targeted diagnostic work-up* should be started if diagnosis of GA-I is suspected or a positive family history is known. Note that a few patients with a low-excreting phenotype may show (intermittently) normal urinary excretion of 3-hydroxyglutaric acid (*3-OH-GA*) and glutaric acid (*GA*) (*). If an individual shows normal 3-OH-GA (and GA) concentrations in urine but presents with highly suspicious signs and symptoms for GA-I, it should be decided individually whether diagnostic work-up is continued (**)

## L-2-Hydroxyglutaric Aciduria, D-2-Hydroxyglutaric Aciduria Type I and D-2-Hydroxyglutaric Aciduria Type II

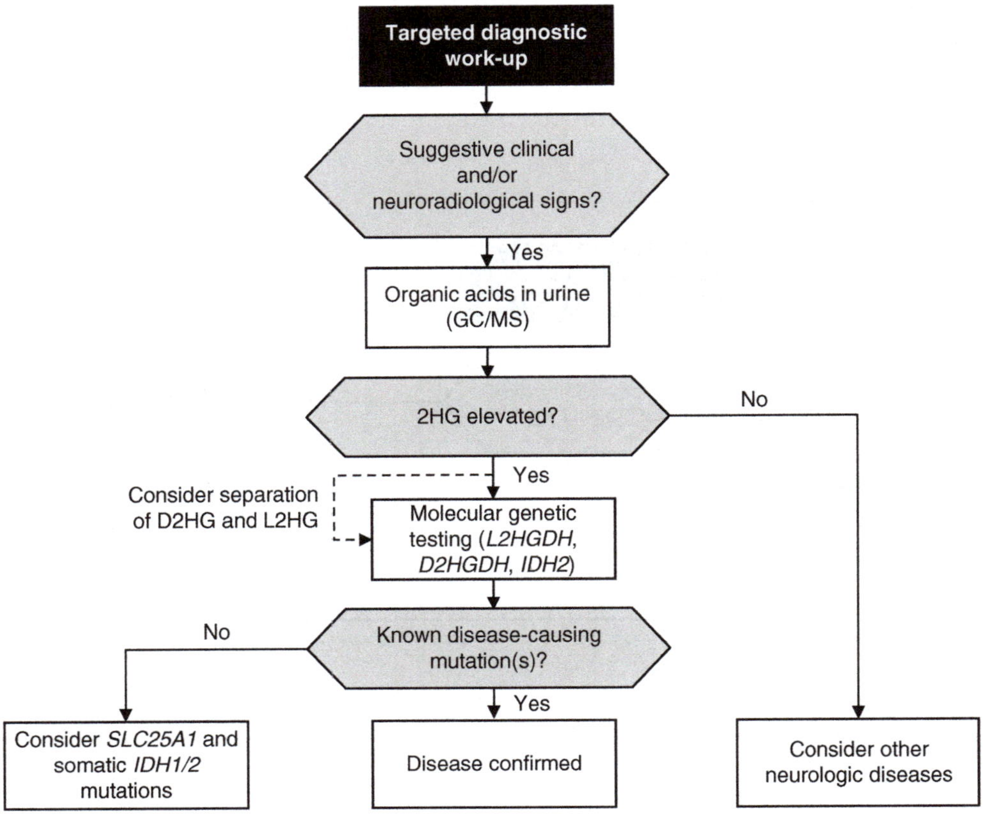


**Fig. 69.7** Flowchart for diseases 69.3, 69.4 and 69.5. Elevated 2HG in GC/MS analysis of urinary organic acids is the biochemical hallmark of these diseases. According to discriminating biochemical (elevated CSF lysine and protein in L-2-hydroxyglutaric aciduria, elevated CSF GABA and elevated urinary 2-ketoglutarate in D-2-hydroxyglutaric aciduria), clinical (cardiomyopathy in D-2-hydroxyglutaric aciduria type II, progressive spasticity in L-2-hydroxyglutaric aciduria) and neuroradiologic parameters (pathognomonic MRI pattern of L-2-hydroxyglutaric aciduria), molecular genetic testing of *L2HGDH*, *D2HGDH* and *IDH2*, respectively, are often the next steps. However, enantiomeric separation and individual quantification of D2HG and L2HG may help to direct diagnostic work-up (dotted line). In case of negative molecular genetic tests, alternative diseases should also be considered including D-2–/L-2-hydroxyglutaric aciduria (caused by SLC25A1 deficiency), somatic gain-of-function mutations of the *IDH1* and *IDH2* genes in adult patients with gliomas or acute myeloid leukaemia or secondary increased D2HG in SSADH deficiency and GA-I

## Specimen Collection

| Disease no. | Symbol | Test | Preconditions | Material | Handling | Pitfalls |
|---|---|---|---|---|---|---|
| 69.1 | CD | Organic acids (NAA) | None | Urine | Keep frozen (–20 °C) | Compound has poor recovery in organic solvent extraction |
| 69.2 | GA-I | Quantitative amino acids | 3.5–4 h postprandially, no dietary changes prior to the test | Plasma | Keep frozen (–20 °C) | |
| | | Tryptophan | 3.5–4 h postprandially, no dietary changes prior to the test | Plasma | Keep frozen (–20 °C) | Losses due to inappropriate deproteinisation |
| | | Organic acids (3-OH-GA, GA) | None | Urine | Keep frozen (–20 °C) | Reliable identification of 3-OH-GA may require the use of a quantitative GC/MS method; differential diagnoses of elevated GA and 3-OH-GA include GA-II and GA-III, SCHAD deficiency and ketosis |
| | | Carnitine status | None, also informs on adherence to carnitine supplementation | Plasma serum | Keep frozen (–20 °C) | |
| | | Acylcarnitine profile (C5DC) | None | Dried blood spots<br>Plasma | Plasma; keep frozen (–20 °C) | C5DC may be also elevated in GA-II, renal insufficiency, MCAD deficiency (pseudoglutarylcarnitinemia) |
| | | Enzyme activity (GCDH) | None | Fibroblasts | RT | |
| | | | | Leucocytes from heparinised blood | Keep frozen (–20 °C) | |
| 69.3 | L2HGA | Organic acids | None | Urine | Keep frozen (–20 °C) | For specific quantification of L2HG, enantiomeric separation, hyphenated to mass spectrometry, is required |
| | L2HGA | L2HG dehydrogenase activity | Isolation of cells according to specific protocol | Fibroblasts, lymphoblasts, lymphocytes | RT, pellets should be frozen | |
| 69.4 | D2HGA type I | Organic acids | None | Urine | Keep frozen (–20 °C) | For specific quantification of D2HG, enantiomeric separation, hyphenated to mass spectrometry, is required |
| | D2HGA type I | D2HG dehydrogenase activity | Isolation of cells according to specific protocol | Fibroblasts, lymphoblasts | RT, pellets should be frozen | |
| 69.5 | D2HGA type II | Organic acids | None | Urine | Keep frozen (–20 °C) | For specific quantification of D2HG, enantiomeric separation, hyphenated to mass spectrometry, is required. D2HG also accumulates GA-I and SSADH |
| | D2HGA type II | IDH2 gain-of-function assay | Isolation of cells according to specific protocol | Lymphoblasts | RT, pellets should be frozen | |

*3-OH-GA* 3-hydroxyglutarate, *C5DC* glutarylcarnitine, *GA* glutarate, *GA-II* glutaric aciduria type II, *GA-III* glutaric aciduria type III, *GCDH* glutaryl-CoA dehydrogenase, *GC/MS* gas chromatography/mass spectrometry, *MCAD* medium-chain acyl-CoA dehydrogenase, *NAA* *N*-acetylaspartate, *SCHAD* short-chain 3-hydroxyacyl-CoA, *SSADH* succinic semialdehyde dehydrogenase deficiency

## Prenatal Diagnosis

| Disease no. | Symbol | Material | Timing trimester | Pitfalls |
|---|---|---|---|---|
| 69.1 | CD | Chorionic villi (accomplished) | I | Assay of aspartoacylase in amniocytes is not reliable. A combination of mutation analysis together with the exact quantitation of *N*-acetylaspartate in the amniotic fluid is recommended |
| | | Amniotic fluid, amniocytes (accomplished) | II | |
| 69.2 | GA-I | Chorionic villi | I | |
| | | Amniocytes, amniotic fluid | II | |
| 69.3 | L2HGA | Chorionic villi | I | |
| | | Amniocytes, amniotic fluid | II | |
| 69.4 | D2HGA type I | Chorionic villi | I | |
| | | Amniocytes, amniotic fluid | II | |
| 69.5 | D2HGA type II | Chorionic villi | I | Disease is usually caused by a heterozygous de novo mutation. Somatic and germline mosaicism in the parents cannot be excluded; thus, the recurrence risk for the parents is not zero. Therefore, prenatal diagnosis should always be offered |
| | | Amniocytes, amniotic fluid | II | |

In case of DNA-based prenatal diagnosis, maternal contamination should be excluded by VNTR marker analysis. Trimester one: only mutation analysis. Trimester two: a combination of metabolite and DNA investigations is recommended

## DNA Testing

| Disease no. | Symbol | Tissue | Methodology |
|---|---|---|---|
| 69.1 | CD | Lymphocytes, fibroblasts | Sequencing |
| 69.2 | GA-I | Lymphocytes, fibroblasts | Sequencing |
| 69.3 | L2HGA | Blood, lymphocytes, fibroblasts, lymphoblasts | Sequencing |
| 69.4 | D2HGA type I | Blood, lymphocytes, fibroblasts, lymphoblasts | Sequencing |
| 69.5 | D2HGA type II | Blood, lymphocytes, fibroblasts, lymphoblasts | Sequencing, targeted mutation analysis |

## Treatment Summary

Effective metabolic treatment has only been described for glutaric aciduria type I (low lysine diet, carnitine supplementation, emergency treatment). Riboflavin should be considered as a treatment option for patients with L-2-hydroxyglutaric aciduria aiming to activate residual enzyme activity. Treatment of patients' Canavan disease with lithium citrate, lowering brain *N*-acetylaspartate concentrations, and glycerol triacetate, supplying the brain with acetate, is considered as safe; however, it is yet unknown whether it improves the clinical outcome. Metabolic treatment for D-2-hydroxyglutaric aciduria types I and II has not yet been described.

Although effective treatment is only known for some cerebral organic acidurias, symptomatic and supportive treatment is important. This includes adequate supply with nutrient, minerals and micronutrients, physiotherapy, occupational therapy and pharmacotherapy of epilepsy and extrapyramidal movement disorder, among others. The therapeutic concept should be implemented after the assessment of individual needs and, subsequently, monitored and evaluated by an interdisciplinary team of specialists.

**Emergency Treatment Table for All Disorders of Your Chapter** (If Applicable) **and Medication Requirements** (A. Including Box After the Table, with Pitfalls and Important Information).

### **Diseases** 69.1 **and** 69.3–69.5

No emergency treatment is available.

### Disease 69.2 (GA-I)

Emergency treatment is thought to be the most effective component of the current treatment strategies to prevent acute striatal injury during infectious disease and for other causes of catabolism in glutaric aciduria type I (Heringer et al. 2010; Boy et al. 2018). It must be initiated before the onset of severe neurological signs, which already indicate the manifestation of neuronal damage. Therefore, during episodes that are likely to induce catabolism (e.g. infectious disease), emergency treatment should start without delay. Treatment should consist of frequent high carbohydrate feeds and increased carnitine supplementation, followed by high-dose intravenous glucose and carnitine (Kölker et al. 2011; Boy et al. 2017a, b). All patients with glutaric aciduria type I should be supplied with an emergency card. This concept should be strictly followed for the first 6 years of life. After this age, emergency treatment is individually adjusted.

Emergency treatment at home

| A. Oral carbohydrates[a] | Maltodextrin | | | |
|---|---|---|---|---|
| Age (years) | % | Kcal/100 mL | KJ/100 mL | Volume (mL) per day orally |
| Up to 0.5 | 10 | 40 | 167 | Min. 150/kg |
| 0.5–1 | 12 | 48 | 202 | 120/kg |
| 1–2 | 15 | 60 | 250 | 100/kg |
| 2–6 | 20 | 80 | 334 | 1200–1500 |
| **B. Protein intake** | | | | |
| Natural protein | Stop for max. 24 (−48) h, and then reintroduce and increase stepwise until the amount of maintenance treatment is reached within 48 (−72) h | | | |
| AAM | If tolerated, AAM should be administered according to maintenance therapy | | | |
| **C. Pharmacotherapy** | | | | |
| l-carnitine | Double oral carnitine supplementations | | | |

According to Kölker et al. 2011; Boy et al. 2017a, b

[a]Solutions should be administered every 2 h day and night. Patients should be reassessed every 2 h. AAM, lysine-free, tryptophan-reduced amino acid mixtures

Emergency treatment in hospital (according to Kölker et al. 2011; Boy et al. 2017a, b).

| **A. Intravenous infusions** | | |
|---|---|---|
| Glucose | Age (years) | Glucose (g/kg per day IV) |
| | 0–1 | (12–)15 |
| | 1–3 | (10–)12 |
| | 3–6 | (8–)10 |
| Insulin | If persistent hyperglycaemia >150 mg/dL (>8 mmol/L) and/or glucosuria occurs, start with 0.05 IE insulin/kg per h IV, and adjust the infusion rate according to serum glucose | |
| **B. Protein intake** | | |
| Natural protein | Stop for max. 24 (−48) h, and then reintroduce and increase stepwise until the amount of maintenance treatment is reached within 48 (−72) h | |
| AAM | If tolerated, AAM should be administered orally or by nasogastric tube according to maintenance therapy | |
| **C. Pharmacotherapy** | | |
| l-carnitine | 100(−200) mg/kg per day IV | |

*AAM* lysine-free, tryptophan-reduced amino acid mixtures.

**Standard Treatment Table for All Disorders of Your Chapter** (If Applicable) **and Medication Requirements** (A. Including Box After the Table, with Pitfalls and Important Information).

## **Diseases** 69.1, 69.3, 69.4 **and** 69.5

No specific treatment is available.

## **Disease** 69.2 **(GA-I)**

| Disorder no. | Symbol | Age | Medication/diet | Dosage | Doses/day (*n*) |
|---|---|---|---|---|---|
| 69.2 | GA-I | <6 years | Carnitine | (50–)100 mg/kg per day | 3 |
| | | >6 years | Carnitine | (30–)50 mg/kg per day | 3 |
| | | | Riboflavin[a] | 100 mg | 2 |
| | | | Treatment of extrapyramidal movement disorders[b] | | |
| | | | Antiepileptic treatment[c] | | |
| | | | Diet (see below) | | |

[a]Riboflavin is not a recommended therapy in glutaric aciduria type I since riboflavin responsiveness seems to be very rare (if at all present) and no standard protocol exists to test it. There is no proven clinical benefit of riboflavin supplementation (Kölker et al. 2006)

[b]The complex movement disorder of symptomatic patients with glutaric aciduria type I is difficult to treat. Baclofen and benzodiazepines as monotherapy or in combination are often used as first-line drug treatment for focal and generalised dystonia. Intrathecal baclofen is used for additional therapy in individuals with generalised dystonia and spasticity. Trihexyphenidyl can be considered as second-line treatment for dystonia, particularly in adolescents and adults, and botulinum toxin A injections as additional therapy for severe focal dystonia (according to Kölker et al. 2011; Boy et al. 2017a, b)

[c]The risk of epilepsy is mildly elevated in glutaric aciduria type I. Dystonic and epileptic movements, however, may be confused with seizures. Indication, prescription and monitoring of antiepileptic treatment should be performed by a child neurologist or neurologist. Valproate is not recommended due to the theoretical risk of mitochondrial dysfunction and secondary carnitine depletion

Dietary treatment (low lysine diet, according to Kölker et al. 2011; Boy et al. 2017a, b).

| Treatment | Dosage | Age 0–6 months | 7–12 months | 1–3 years | 4–6 years | >6 years |
|---|---|---|---|---|---|---|
| Lysine (from natural protein)[a] | mg/kg per day | 100 | 90 | 80–60 | 60–50 | Controlled protein intake using natural protein with a low lysine content and avoiding lysine-rich food |
| Protein from amino acid mixtures[b] | g/kg per day | 1.3–0.8 | 1.0–0.8 | 0.8 | 0.8 | |
| Energy | Kcal/kg per day | 100–80 | 80 | 94–81 | 86–63 | |
| Micronutrients[c] | % | ≥100 | ≥100 | ≥100 | ≥100 | ≥100 |

[a]The lysine/protein ratio (i.e. 2–9 mg lysine/100 mg protein) varies in natural food, and thus natural protein intake in children on a low lysine diet is dependent on the natural protein source

[b]Lysine-free, tryptophan-reduced amino acid mixtures should be supplemented with minerals and micronutrients as required to maintain normal levels. Safe intakes of essential amino acids are provided from natural protein and lysine-free, tryptophan-reduced amino acid supplements

[c]According to dietary recommendations

**Dangers/Pitfalls**

1. Dietary treatment needs to be adapted to the individual needs, in particular in dystonic patients. Overtreatment by protein restriction may result in malnutrition with essential nutrients.
2. Dysphagia is a frequent problem in dystonic patients. Tube feeding (via nasogastric tube or percutaneous gastrostomy) should be considered if oral food intake is inadequate.

## Experimental Treatment

| Disease no. | Symbol | Alternative therapies/experimental trials |
|---|---|---|
| 69.1 | CD | Lithium citrate |
| | | Glycerol triacetate |
| | | rAAV-based gene therapy (translational and preclinical studies) |
| 69.2 | GA-I | Arginine or homoarginine supplementation has yet only been studied in Gcdh-deficient mice, an animal model for GA-I, and in a small number of patients (arginine). The safety and efficacy of arginine supplementation as well as optimal dosage are unknown |
| 69.3 | L2HGA | Riboflavin supplementation |
| 69.4 | D2HGA type I | On the basis that D2HG dehydrogenase is an FAD-dependent enzyme, riboflavin supplementation is a therapeutic option |
| 69.5 | D2HGA type II | AGI-026, a mutant IDH2 protein inhibitor of the human IDH2R140Q-mutant enzyme, suppressed 2HG production, rescued cardiomyopathy and provided a survival benefit in Idh2R140Q mice (translational and preclinical studies) |

## References


Assadi M, Janson C, Wan DJ, et al. Lithium citrate reduces excessive intracerebral N-acetylaspartate in Canavan disease. Eur J Paediatr Neurol. 2010;14:354–9.

Boy N, Heringer J, Brackmann R, et al. Extrastriatal changes in patients with late-onset glutaric aciduria type I highlight the risk of long-term neurotoxicity. Orphanet J Rare Dis. 2017a;12:77. PMID: 28438223

Boy N, Mengler K, Thimm E, et al. Newborn screening: a disease-changing intervention for glutaric aciduria type 1. Ann Neurol. 2018;83:970–9. PMID: 29665094

Boy N, Mühlhausen C, Maier EM, et al. Proposed recommendations for diagnosing and managing individuals with glutaric aciduria type I: second revision. J Inherit Metab Dis. 2017b;40:75–101. PMID: 27853989

Gessler DJ, Li D, Su Q, et al. Redirecting N-acetylaspartate metabolism in the central nervous system normalizes myelination and rescues Canavan disease. JCI Insight. 2017;2:e9087. PMID: 28194442

Gitiaux C, Roze E, Kinugawa K, et al. Spectrum of movement disorders associated with glutaric aciduria type 1: a study of 16 patients. Mov Disord. 2008;23:2392–7.

Harting I, Neumaier-Probst E, Seitz A, et al. Dynamic changes of striatal and extrastriatal abnormalities in glutaric aciduria type I. Brain. 2009;132:1764–82.

Heringer J, Boy SPN, Ensenauer R, et al. Use of guidelines improves the neurological outcome in glutaric aciduria type I. Ann Neurol. 2010;68:743–52.

Kölker S, Christensen E, Leonard JV, et al. Diagnosis and management of glutaric aciduria type I—revised recommendations. J Inherit Metab Dis. 2011;34:677–94.

Kölker S, Garbade S, Greenberg CR, et al. Natural history, outcome, and treatment efficacy in children and adults with glutaryl-CoA dehydrogenase deficiency. Pediatr Res. 2006;59:840–7.

Kranendijk M, Struys EA, Van Schaftingen E, et al. IDH2 mutations in patients with D-2-hydroxyglutaric aciduria. Science. 2010; 330:336.

Leone P, Janson CG, Bilanuk L, et al. Aspartoacylase gene transfer to the mammalian central nervous system with therapeutic implications for Canavan disease. Ann Neurol. 2000;48:27–38.

Matalon R, Michals K, Kaul R. Canavan disease: from spongy degeneration to molecular analysis. J Pediatr. 1995;127:511–7.

Sauer SW, Okun JG, Fricker G, et al. Intracerebral accumulation of glutaric and 3-hydroxyglutaric acids secondary to limited flux across the blood–brain barrier constitutes a biochemical risk factor for neurodegeneration in glutaryl-CoA dehydrogenase deficiency. J Neurochem. 2006;97:899–910.

Segel R, Anikster Y, Zevin S, et al. A safety trial of high glucose triacetate for Canavan disease. Mol Genet Metab. 2011;103:203–6.

Steenweg ME, Jakobs C, Errami A, et al. An overview of L-2-hydroxyglutarate dehydrogenase gene (L2HGDH) variants: a genotype-phenotype study. Hum Mutat. 2010;31:380–90.

Steenweg ME, Salomons GS, Yapici Z, et al. L-2-Hydroxyglutaric aciduria: pattern of MR imaging abnormalities in 56 patients. Radiology. 2009;2009(251):856–65.

Struys EA, Salomons GS, Achouri Y, et al. Mutations in the D-2-hydroxyglutarate dehydrogenase gene cause D-2-hydroxyglutaric aciduria. Am J Hum Genet. 2005;76:358–60.

Struys EA, Verhoeven NM, Brunengraber H, et al. Investigations by mass isotopomer analysis of the formation of D-2-hydroxyglutarate by cultured lymphoblasts from two patients with D-2-hydroxyglutaric aciduria. FEBS Lett. 2004;557(1–3):115–20.

Van Schaftingen E, Rzem R, Veiga-da-Cunha M. L-2-hydroxyglutaric aciduria, a disorder of metabolite repair. J Inherit Metab Dis. 2009;32:135–42.

Wang F, Travins J, Lin Z, et al. A small molecule inhibitor of mutant IDH2 rescues cardiomyopathy in a D-2-hydroxyglutaric aciduria type II mouse model. J Inherit Metab Dis. 2016;39:807–20.

# 3-Methylglutaconic Acidurias

# 70

Saskia B. Wortmann and Johannes A. Mayr

## Contents



**Summary**

Increased urinary 3-methylglutaconic acid excretion is a relatively common finding in inborn errors of metabolism, especially in mitochondrial disorders. In most cases 3-methylglutaconic acid is only slightly elevated and accompanied by other (disease-specific) metabolites.

There is, however, a group of disorders with significantly and consistently increased 3-methylglutaconic acid excretion, where the 3-methylglutaconic aciduria is a hallmark of the phenotype and the key to diagnosis: inborn errors with 3-methylglutaconic aciduria as a discriminative feature (3-MGA-IEM). One should distinguish between "primary 3-methylglutaconic acidurias" formerly known as type I (3-methylglutaconyl-CoA hydratase deficiency, AUH defect) due to defective leucine catabolism and the—currently known— 11 "secondary 3-methylglutaconic acidurias." The latter should be further classified and named by their defective protein or the historical name as follows: TAZ-defect or Barth syndrome, SERAC1-defect or MEGDEL syndrome, AGK-defect or Sengers syndrome, OPA3-defect or Costeff syndrome, TMEM70, MICOS13, DNAJC19, TIMM50, and HTRA2 defect.

S. B. Wortmann (✉)
University Children's Hospital, Paracelsus Medical University, Salzburg, Austria

Institute for Human Genetics, Technische Universität München, Munich, Germany
e-mail: s.wortmann@salk.at

J. A. Mayr
University Children's Hospital, Paracelsus Medical University, Salzburg, Austria
e-mail: h.mayr@salk.at


N. Blau et al. (eds.), *Physician's Guide to the Diagnosis, Treatment, and Follow-Up of Inherited Metabolic Diseases*,
https://doi.org/10.1007/978-3-030-67727-5_70

## Introduction

The branched-chain organic acid 3-methylglutaconic acid (3-MGA) is an intermediate of the mitochondrial leucine catabolism. In the urine of healthy individuals, 3-MGA is found only in traces (<20 mmol/mol creatinine); in young infants it can be higher (up to 30 mmol/mol creatinine) as the creatinine is relatively lower due to lower muscle mass.

In patients with inborn errors with 3-methylglutaconic aciduria as a discriminative feature **(3-MGA-IEM)**, urinary 3-MGA concentrations can (intermittently) rise above 1000 mmol/mol creatinine (Wortmann et al. 2013a, b).

The leucine pathway shows the metabolic pathway of leucine. 3-MGA, 3-methylglutaric acid (3-MG), and 3-hydroxy-isovaleric acid (3-HIVA) accumulate when the conversion of 3-methylglutaconyl-CoA to 3-hydroxy-3-methylglutaryl-CoA by the enzyme 3-methylglutaconyl-CoA hydratase (3-MGH, EC 4.2.1.18 encoded by *AUH*) is disturbed (Fig. 70.1) (Wortmann et al. 2010). This is the primary 3-methylglutaconic aciduria (3-MGA-uria) or AUH-defect, formerly known as 3-MGA-uria type I. **The urinary excretion of 3-MGA is generally higher in primary 3-MGA-IEM, AUH defect, than in all other (secondary) 3-MGA-IEM.** Patients with AUH defect excrete even higher amounts of urinary 3-MGA after a leucine-rich, or in general a protein-rich, meal (Table 70.12) (Wortmann et al. 2014). This is not the case in all other patients with 3-MGA-uria underlining that the excreted 3-MGA does not originate from leucine degradation. Another distinctive feature between primary and secondary 3-MGA-IEM is the elevation of 3-HIVA which is only seen in the AUH defect.

3-MGA-uria can be frequently seen (3% of all urine samples of patients with suspected IEM) in association with several IEM, such as organic acidurias, glycogen storage disorders, fatty acid oxidation disorders, and urea cycle disorders (Fig. 70.1 classification updated from) (Wortmann et al. 2013a, b). Therefore it is important to repeat urinary organic acid analysis in patients with 3-MGA-uria and to carefully interpret the other general clinical chemistry (blood gas analysis, glucose, lactate, ammonia, full blood counts, etc.) and metabolic screening tests (serum amino acids, acylcarnitines in dried blood spot, oligosaccharides in urine). This will allow to confirm that 3-MGA-uria is only an accompanying finding.

In another group of patients, 3-MGA-uria is only slightly and/or intermittently elevated, and 3-MGA-uria is a minor finding. The majority of patients in this group are patients with mitochondrial disorders where it is detected in about 11% of all patients. It is more frequently seen in ATPase-related disorders, with mitochondrial DNA depletion or deletion (e.g., Pearson syndrome), but not in patients with single respiratory chain complex deficiencies with exception of ATPase-related disorders (Wortmann et al. 2013a, b). As 3-MGA-uria is not found in all of these patients with the mentioned specific mitochondrial disorders, these disorders are discussed and not here.

Once 3-MGA-uria has been proven to be an isolated and consistently present finding, 3-MGA-uria as a major finding, the diagnosis of a 3-MGA-IEM can be made. One subgroup is formed by the disorders involving defective phospholipid biosynthesis (*TAZ*, *SERAC1*, *AGK*) (Clarke SL et al. 2013; Thiels C et al. 2016; Mass RR et al. 2017; Roeben B et al. 2018; Wortmann SB et al. 2015; Wortmann SB et al. 2012; Haghighi A et al. 2014; Mayr JA et al. 2012), all other 3-MGA-IEM share mitochondrial (membrane) dysfunction (*OPA3*, *DNAJC19*, *CLPB*, *HTRA2*, *TIMM50*, *TMEM70*, *MIC13*, Fig. 70.2) (Anikster et al. 2006; Ucar SK et al. 2017; Davey KM et al. 2006; Pronicka E et al. 2017; Wortmann SB et al. 2015; Kovacs-Nagy R et al. 2018; Shahrour MA et al. 2017; Magner M et al. 2015; Kishita Y et al. 2020). There are no additional (metabolic) clues that can help to further distinguish between the different types of 3-MGA-IEM with exception of the clinical features (see table on differential diagnosis at the section signs and symptoms). All 3-MGA-IEM show a distinctive pattern of signs and symptoms which allows to distinguish between them; however patients affected by the different 3-MGA-IEM show a spectrum within their subtype (Fig. 70.1).

## Nomenclature

| No. | Disorder_name | Alternative name | Gene symbol | Chromosomal location | Mode of Inheritance | Affected protein | OMIM No. |
|---|---|---|---|---|---|---|---|
| 70.1 | AUH deficiency | 3-methylglutaconic aciduria type 1 | *AUH* | 9q22.31 | AR | 3-methylglutaconyl-CoA hydratase | 600529 |
| 70.2 | TAZ deficiency | Barth syndrome; Taffazin deficiency | *TAZ* | Xq28 | XLR | Taffazin | 300394 |
| 70.3 | SERAC1 deficiency | 3-methylglutaconic aciduria with dystonia, deafness, hepatopathy, encephalopathy, and Leigh-like syndrome (MEGDHEL) | *SERAC1* | 6q25.3 | AR | Serine active site-containing protein 1 | 614725 |
| 70.4 | AGK deficiency | Sengers syndrome | *AGK* | 7q34 | AR | Acylglycerokinase | 212350 |
| 70.5 | OPA3 deficiency | Optic atrophy type 3 (dominant); 3-methylglutaconic aciduria type 3, Costeff syndrome (recessive) | *OPA3* | 19q13.2–13.3 | AD, AR | | 606580 |
| 70.6 | DNAJC19 deficiency | Dilated cardiomyopathy with ataxia (DCMA syndrome); 3-methylglutaconic aciduria type 5 | *DNAJC19* | 3q26.33 | AR | - DNAJ/HSP40 homolog, subfamily C, member 19 | 608977 |
| 70.7 | CLPB deficiency | 3-methylglutaconic aciduria type 7, with cataracts, neurologic involvement and neutropenia | *CLPB* | 11q13.4 | AR | - Caseinolytic peptidase B | 616254 |
| 70.8 | HTRA2 deficiency | 3-methylglutaconic aciduria type 8 | *HTRA2* | 2p13.1 | AR | - HTRA serine peptidase 2 | 606441 |
| 70.9 | TIMM50 deficiency | 3-methylglutaconic aciduria type 9 | *TIMM50* | 19q13.2 | AR | Translocase of inner mitochondrial membrane 50 | 607381 |
| 70.10 | TMEM70 deficiency | Transmembrane protein 70 deficiency | *TMEM70* | 8q21.11 | AR | Complex V assembly protein | 612418 |
| 70.11 | MICOS13 deficiency | MICOS complex subunit MIC13 deficiency | *MICOS13* | 19p13.3 | AR | MICOS complex, 13-KD subunit | 618329 |

## Metabolic Pathways

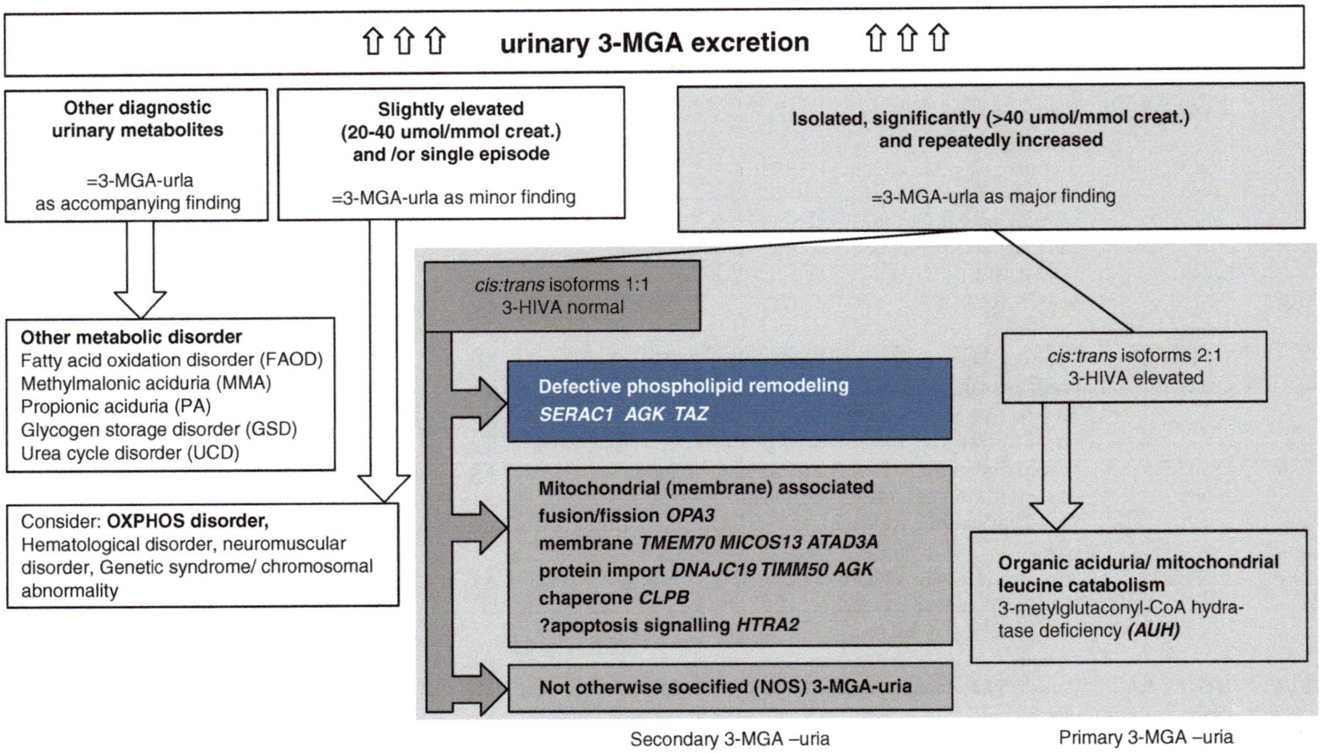


**Fig. 70.1** Inborn errors with 3-methylglutaconic aciduria as discriminative feature (3-MGA-IEM). (Updated from Wortmann et al. 2013a, b)

**Fig. 70.2** Leucine metabolism (Updated from Wortmann et al. 2013a, b)

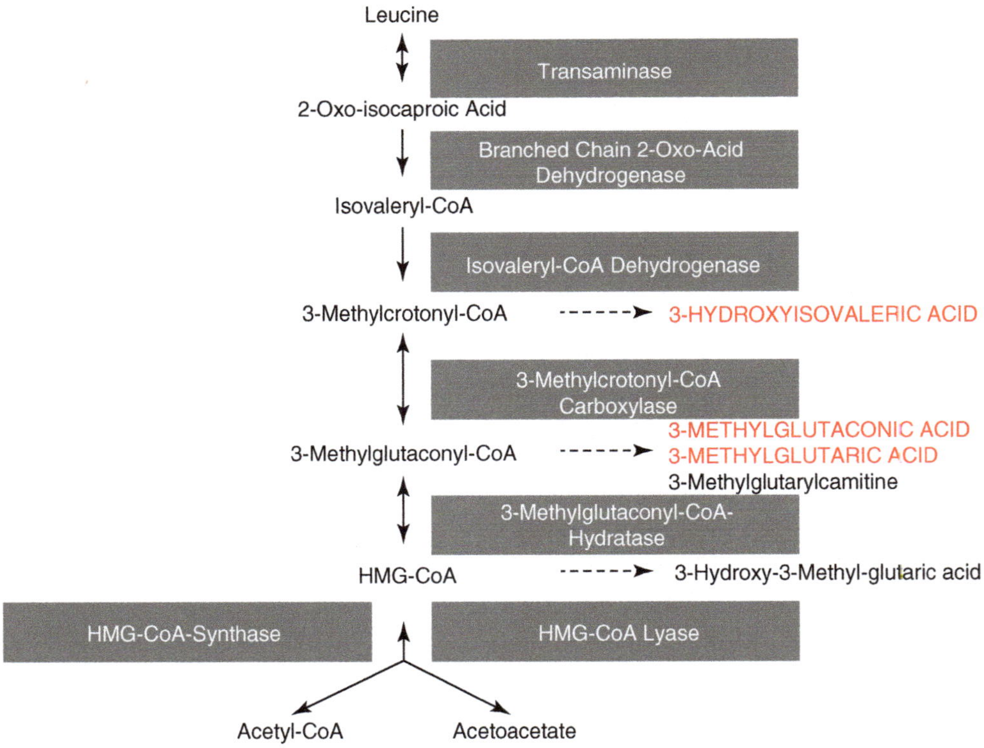

## Signs and Symptoms

| | AUH-def. | TAZ-def. | SERAC1-def. | AGK-def. | OPA3-def. | DNAJC19-def | CLPB-def. | HTRA2-def. | TIMM50-def. | TMEM70-def. | MIC13-defect |
|---|---|---|---|---|---|---|---|---|---|---|---|
| MIM # | 250950 | 302060 | 614739 | 212350 | 258501 | 610198 | 616271 | 617248 | 617698 | 614052 | 618329 |
| Gene | *AUH* | *TAZ* | *SERAC1* | *AGK* | *OPA3* | *DNAJC19* | *CLPB* | *HTRA2* | *TIMM50* | *TMEM70* | *MIC13* |
| 3-MGA-uria | x | x | x | x | x | x | x | x | x | x | x |
| Mode of inheritence | AR | XLR | AR | AR | AR | AR | AR | AR | AR | AR | AR |
| Typical age at onset | 4-5th decade | Neonatal | Neonatal-first year | Childhood | Childhood | Childhood | Neonatal | Neonatal | Neonatal | Neonatal | Neonatal |
| Developmental delay | | (x) | x | (x) | x | x | x | x | x | x | x |
| Intellectual disability | | | x | | | x | x | x | x | x | x |
| Movement disorder | x | | x | | x | x | x | x | | | x |
| Central hypopnea | | | | | | | x | x | | | |
| Optic atrophy | | | (x) | | x | | | | | | |
| Deafness | | | x | | | | | | | | |
| Epilepsy | | | (x) | | | | (x) | | x | | x |
| Cataracts | | | | x | | | x | x | | | |
| Cardiomyopathy | | x | | x | | x | | | | x | |
| Neutropenia | | x | | | | | x | x | | | |
| Growth failure | | x | x | x | x | x | x | x | x | x | x |
| Liver involvement | | | x | | | | | | | | x |

**Table 70.1** AUH deficiency

| System | Symptoms and Bbomarkers | Neonatal (birth-1 month) | Infancy (1–18 months) | Childhood (1.5–11 years) | Adolescence (11–16 years) | Adulthood (>16 years) |
|---|---|---|---|---|---|---|
| CNS | **Ataxia** | ± | ± | ± | + | + |
| | Athetosis | ± | ± | ± | ± | ± |
| | Basal ganglia lesions (MRI) | ± | ± | ± | ± | ± |
| | Cerebellar abnormalities | ± | ± | ± | ± | ± |
| | Cerebellar abnormalities | ± | ± | ± | ± | ± |
| | Cerebral atrophy (MRI) | ± | ± | ± | ± | ± |
| | Dementia | ± | ± | ± | ± | ± |
| | Fits | ± | ± | ± | | |
| | **Leukoencephalopathy** | ± | ± | + | + | + |
| | **Regression** | + | + | + | + | + |
| | **Retardation** | + | + | + | + | + |
| | **Retardation, psychomotor** | ± | + | + | ± | ± |
| | Seizures, febrile | ± | ± | ± | | |
| | Spasticity, limbs | ± | ± | ± | ± | + |
| | White matter changes (MRI) | ± | ± | ± | ± | ± |
| Digestive | Hepatomegaly | ± | ± | ± | ± | ± |
| | Liver dysfunction | ± | ± | ± | ± | ± |
| Eye | Nystagmus | ± | ± | ± | ± | ± |
| | Optic atrophy | ± | ± | ± | ± | ± |

(continued)

**Table 70.1** (continued)

| System | Symptoms and Bbomarkers | Neonatal (birth-1 month) | Infancy (1–18 months) | Childhood (1.5–11 years) | Adolescence (11–16 years) | Adulthood (>16 years) |
|---|---|---|---|---|---|---|
| Hematological | Thrombocytopenia | ± | ± | ± | | |
| Metabolic | Metabolic acidosis | ± | ± | ± | | |
| | Hypoglycemia | ± | ± | ± | | |
| Laboratory findings | 3-Hydroxyisovaleric acid (MRS) | n-↑ | n-↑ | n-↑ | n-↑ | n-↑ |
| | 3-Hydroxyisovaleric acid (urine) | ↑-↑↑↑ | ↑-↑↑↑ | ↑-↑↑↑ | ↑-↑↑↑ | ↑-↑↑↑ |
| | 3-Methylglutaconic acid (urine) | ↑-↑↑↑ | ↑-↑↑↑ | ↑-↑↑↑ | ↑-↑↑↑ | ↑-↑↑↑ |
| | 3-Methylglutaconyl-CoA hydratase (fibroblasts) | ↓ | ↓ | ↓ | ↓ | ↓ |
| | 3-Methylglutaric acid (urine) | ↑-↑↑ | ↑-↑↑ | ↑-↑↑ | ↑-↑↑ | ↑-↑↑ |
| | Ammonia (blood) | n-↑ | n-↑ | n-↑ | n-↑ | n-↑ |
| | ASAT/ALAT (plasma) | n-↑ | n-↑ | n-↑ | n-↑ | n-↑ |
| | C5-OH Acylcarnitine (dried blood spot) | ↑-↑↑↑ | ↑-↑↑↑ | ↑-↑↑↑ | ↑-↑↑↑ | ↑-↑↑↑ |
| | C5-OH Acylcarnitine (plasma) | ↑-↑↑↑ | ↑-↑↑↑ | ↑-↑↑↑ | ↑-↑↑↑ | ↑-↑↑↑ |
| | C6-unsaturated acylcarnitine (blood) | ↑-↑↑ | ↑-↑↑ | ↑-↑↑ | ↑-↑↑ | ↑-↑↑ |
| | C6-unsaturated acylcarnitine (plasma) | ↑-↑↑ | ↑-↑↑ | ↑-↑↑ | ↑-↑↑ | ↑-↑↑ |
| | Carnitine, esterified (plasma) | n-↑ | n-↑ | n-↑ | n-↑ | n-↑ |
| | Carnitine, free (dried blood spot) | ↓-n | ↓-n | ↓-n | ↓-n | ↓-n |
| | Carnitine, free (plasma) | ↓-n | ↓-n | ↓-n | ↓-n | ↓-n |
| | Creatine kinase (plasma) | n-↑ | n-↑ | n-↑ | | |
| | Glucose (plasma) | ↓-n | ↓-n | ↓-n | | |
| | N-acetylaspartate (MRS) | ↓-n | ↓-n | ↓-n | ↓-n | ↓-n |

**Table 70.2** TAZ deficiency

| System | Symptoms and biomarkers | Neonatal (birth–1 month) | Infancy (1–18 months) | Childhood (1.5–11 years) | Adolescence (11–16 years) | Adulthood (>16 years) |
|---|---|---|---|---|---|---|
| Cardiovascular | Cardiac arrhythmia | ± | ± | ± | ± | ± |
| | **Cardiomyopathy** | + | + | + | + | + |
| | Cardiomyopathy, dilated | ± | ± | ± | ± | ± |
| | Heart failure | ± | ± | ± | ± | ± |
| | **Left ventricular non-compaction** | ± | ± | ± | ± | ± |
| Dermatological | Chronic aphthous ulceration | ± | ± | ± | ± | ± |
| Digestive | Feeding difficulties | ± | ± | ± | ± | ± |
| Hematological | **Neutropenia** | + | + | + | + | + |
| | Sepsis | ± | ± | ± | ± | ± |
| Musculoskeletal | Exercise intolerance | ± | ± | ± | ± | ± |
| | **Growth retardation** | + | + | + | + | + |
| | Hypotonia, muscular-axial | ± | ± | ± | ± | ± |
| | **Myopathy** | ± | ± | ± | ± | ± |
| Respiratory | Respiratory distress | ± | ± | ± | ± | ± |
| Other | Mild dysmorphic features | ± | ± | ± | ± | ± |
| Laboratory findings | 2-Ethylhydracrylic acid (urine) | n-↑ | n-↑ | n-↑ | n-↑ | n-↑ |
| | 3-Hydroxyisovaleric acid (urine) | n | n | n | n | n |
| | 3-Methylglutaconic acid (urine) | ↑-↑↑ | ↑-↑↑ | ↑-↑↑ | ↑-↑↑ | ↑-↑↑ |
| | 3-Methylglutaric acid (urine) | ↑ | ↑ | ↑ | ↑ | ↑ |
| | Abnormal cardiolipin profile (DBS) | + | + | + | + | + |
| | Cholesterol (serum) | ↓-n | ↓-n | ↓-n | ↓-n | ↓-n |

**Table 70.3** SERAC1 deficiency

| System | Symptoms and biomarkers | Neonatal (birth–1 month) | Infancy (1-18 months) | Childhood (1.5–11 years) | Adolescence (11–16 years) | Adulthood (>16 years) |
|---|---|---|---|---|---|---|
| CNS | **Bilateral sensory hearing loss** | + | + | + | + | + |
| | **Cerebellar atrophy (MRI)** | + | + | + | + | + |
| | **Cerebral atrophy (MRI)** | + | + | + | + | + |
| | **Dystonia** | + | + | + | + | + |
| | **Encephalopathy** | + | + | + | + | + |
| | Epilepsy | ± | ± | ± | ± | ± |
| | Extrapyramidal signs | ± | ± | ± | ± | ± |
| | Hypotonia | ± | ± | + | + | + |
| | **Leigh-like lesions (MRI)** | + | + | + | + | + |
| | Regression | + | + | + | + | + |
| | Retardation | + | + | + | + | + |
| | **Spasticity** | ± | + | + | + | + |
| Digestive | Feeding difficulties | ± | ± | ± | ± | ± |
| | Jaundice | ± | ± | | | |
| | **Liver dysfunction** | ± | | | | |
| Laboratory findings | ASAT/ALAT (plasma) | n-↑↑ | n-↑↑ | n-↑↑ | n-↑↑ | n-↑↑ |
| Metabolic | Hypoglycemia | ± | ± | ± | ± | ± |
| Other | Failure to thrive | ± | ± | ± | ± | ± |
| Laboratory findings | 3-Hydroxyisovaleric acid (urine) | n | n | n | n | n |
| | 3-Methylglutaconic acid (urine) | ↑↑ | ↑↑ | ↑↑ | ↑↑ | ↑↑ |
| | 3-Methylglutaric acid (urine) | ↑ | ↑ | ↑ | ↑ | ↑ |
| | Cholestasis | n-↑↑↑ | n-↑↑↑ | n | n | n |
| | Filipin test | n-↑ | n-↑ | n-↑ | n-↑ | n-↑ |
| | Glucose (plasma) | ↓-n | n | n | n | n |
| | Lactate (cerebrospinal fluid) | n-↑↑ | n-↑↑ | n-↑↑ | n-↑↑ | n-↑↑ |
| | Lactate (plasma) | n-↑↑↑ | n-↑↑↑ | n-↑↑↑ | n-↑↑↑ | n-↑↑↑ |

**Table 70.4** AGK deficiency

| System | Symptoms and biomarkers | Neonatal (birth–1 month) | Infancy (1–18 months) | Childhood (1.5–11 years) | Adolescence (11–16 years) | Adulthood (>16 years) |
|---|---|---|---|---|---|---|
| Cardiovascular | **Cardiomyopathy, hypertrophic** | + | + | + | + | + |
| Eye | **Cataract** | ± | ± | ± | ± | ± |
| Metabolic | Lactic acidosis | + | + | ± | ± | ± |
| | Metabolic acidosis | + | + | + | + | ± |
| Musculoskeletal | **Hypotonia, muscular-axial** | + | + | + | + | + |
| Laboratory findings | 3-Hydroxyisovaleric acid (urine) | n | n | n | n | n |
| | 3-Methylglutaconic acid (urine) | ↑↑ | ↑↑ | ↑↑ | ↑↑ | ↑↑ |
| | 3-Methylglutaric acid (urine) | ↑ | ↑ | ↑ | ↑ | ↑ |
| | Lactate (plasma) | ↑-↑↑↑ | ↑-↑↑↑ | ↑-↑↑↑ | ↑-↑↑↑ | ↑-↑↑↑ |

**Table 70.5** OPA3 deficiency

| System | Symptoms and biomarkers | Neonatal (birth–1 month) | Infancy (1–18 months) | Childhood (1.5–11 years) | Adolescence (11–16 years) | Adulthood (>16 years) |
|---|---|---|---|---|---|---|
| CNS | **Ataxia** | | ± | + | + | + |
| | Cerebral atrophy (MRI) | ± | ± | ± | ± | ± |
| | **Extrapyramidal movement disorder** | | ± | + | + | + |
| | **No intellectual disability** | + | + | + | + | + |
| | **Spastic paraplegia** | | ± | + | + | + |
| | **Spasticity** | | ± | + | + | + |
| Eye | Nystagmus | ± | + | + | + | + |
| | **Optic atrophy** | ± | + | + | + | + |
| Laboratory findings | 3-Hydroxyisovaleric acid (urine) | n | n | n | n | n |
| | 3-Methylglutaconic acid (urine) | ↑ | ↑ | ↑ | ↑ | ↑ |
| | 3-Methylglutaric acid (urine) | ↑ | ↑ | ↑ | ↑ | ↑ |

**Table 70.6** DNAJC19 deficiency

| System | Symptoms and biomarkers | Neonatal (birth–1 month) | Infancy (1–18 months) | Childhood (1.5–11 years) | Adolescence (11–16 years) | Adulthood (>16 years) |
|---|---|---|---|---|---|---|
| Cardiovascular | **Cardiomyopathy, dilated** | + | + | + | + | + |
| | Cardiac conduction defect/ long QT | + | + | + | + | + |
| CNS | **Ataxia** | ± | + | + | + | + |
| | Intellectual disability | ± | ± | ± | ± | ± |
| | Seizures | ± | ± | ± | ± | ± |
| Digestive | Liver steatosis | ± | ± | ± | ± | ± |
| Ear | Hearing loss | ± | ± | ± | ± | ± |
| Eye | Optic atrophy | ± | ± | ± | ± | ± |
| Genitourinary | **Genitourital anomalies** | ± | ± | ± | ± | ± |
| | Testicular dysgenesis | ± | ± | ± | ± | ± |
| Hematological | **Anemia, microcytic** | + | + | + | + | + |
| Musculoskeletal | **Growth retardation** | + | + | + | + | + |
| Laboratory findings | 3-Hydroxyisovaleric acid (urine) | n | n | n | n | n |
| | 3-Methylglutaconic acid (urine) | ↑↑ | ↑↑ | ↑↑ | ↑↑ | ↑↑ |
| | 3-Methylglutaric acid (urine) | ↑ | ↑ | ↑ | ↑ | ↑ |
| | Lactate (cerebrospinal fluid) | n-↑↑ | n-↑↑ | n-↑↑ | n-↑↑ | n-↑↑ |
| | Lactate (plasma) | ↑-↑↑↑ | ↑-↑↑↑ | ↑-↑↑↑ | ↑-↑↑↑ | ↑-↑↑↑ |

**Table 70.7** CLPB deficiency

| System | Symptoms and biomarkers | Neonatal (birth–1 month) | Infancy (1–18 months) | Childhood (1.5–11 years) | Adolescence (11–16 years) | Adulthood (>16 years) |
|---|---|---|---|---|---|---|
| CNS | Ataxia | ± | ± | ± | ± | ± |
| | Cerebellar atrophy (MRI) | + | + | + | + | + |
| | Cerebral atrophy (MRI) | + | + | + | + | + |
| | Dystonia | ± | ± | ± | ± | ± |
| | Hyperekplexia | ± | | | | |
| | Hypertonia, extremities | ± | ± | + | + | + |
| | Hypotonia, muscular | + | + | ± | ± | ± |
| | Intellectual disability | + | + | + | + | + |
| | Retardation | + | + | + | + | + |
| | Seizures | ± | ± | ± | ± | ± |
| | Seizures, intrauterine | ± | | | | |
| | Spasticity | | | | | |
| | Stiffness | ± | | | | |
| Endocrine | Endocrine abnormalities | ± | ± | ± | ± | ± |
| Eye | **Cataract** | + | + | + | + | + |
| Hematological | **Neutropenia** | + | + | + | + | + |
| Other | Death | ± | | | | |
| | Intrauterine growth retardation | ± | | | | |
| | Ulcerations, oral, genital | ± | ± | ± | ± | ± |
| Laboratory findings | 3-Methylglutaconic acid (urine) | ↑↑ | ↑↑ | ↑↑ | ↑↑ | ↑↑ |
| | 3-Methylglutaric acid (urine) | ↑ | ↑ | ↑ | ↑ | ↑ |
| | 3-Hydroxyisovaleric acid (urine) | n | n | n | n | n |

**Table 70.8** HTRA2 deficiency

| System | Symptoms and Biomarkers | Neonatal (birth–1 month) | Infancy (1–18 months) | Childhood (1.5–11 years) | Adolescence (11–16 years) | Adulthood (>16 years) |
|---|---|---|---|---|---|---|
| CNS | **Apnea** | + | + | | | |
| | Brain atrophy (MRI) | + | + | | | |
| | **Central hypopnea** | + | + | | | |
| | Developmental delay | + | + | | | |
| | Hypertonia, extremities | + | + | | | |
| | Hypotonia, muscular | + | + | | | |
| | Intellectual disability | + | + | | | |
| | **Jitteriness** | + | + | | | |
| | **Neurodegeneration** | + | + | | | |
| | Seizures | + | + | | | |
| | **Tremor** | + | + | | | |
| Digestive | **Dysphagia** | + | + | | | |
| Hematological | **Neutropenia** | + | + | | | |
| Other | **Death** | + | + | | | |
| | Loss of skills | + | + | | | |
| | Intrauterine growth retardation | + | + | | | |
| Laboratory findings | Lactate (plasma) | ↑-↑↑↑ | ↑-↑↑↑ | ↑-↑↑↑ | ↑-↑↑↑ | ↑-↑↑↑ |
| | Lactate (cerebrospinal fluid) | n-↑↑ | n-↑↑ | n-↑↑ | n-↑↑ | n-↑↑ |
| | 3-Methylglutaconic acid (urine) | ↑↑ | ↑↑ | ↑↑ | ↑↑ | ↑↑ |
| | 3-Methylglutaric acid (urine) | ↑ | ↑ | ↑ | ↑ | ↑ |
| | 3-Hydroxyisovaleric acid (urine) | n | n | n | n | n |

**Table 70.9** TMEM70 deficiency

| System | Symptoms and Biomarkers | Neonatal (birth–1 month) | Infancy (1–18 months) | Childhood (1.5–11 years) | Adolescence (11–16 years) | Adulthood (>16 years) |
|---|---|---|---|---|---|---|
| Cardiovascular | **Cardiomyopathy, hypertrophic** | + | + | + | + | + |
| | Wolf-Parkinson-white syndrome | ± | ± | ± | ± | ± |
| CNS | Apnea | ± | ± | ± | ± | ± |
| | Basal ganglia lesions (MRI) | ± | ± | ± | ± | ± |
| | Cerebellar hypoplasia, mild | ± | ± | ± | ± | ± |
| | Cortical atrophy (MRI) | ± | ± | ± | ± | ± |
| | **Encephalopathy** | + | + | + | + | + |
| | **Hypotonia, muscular-axial** | + | + | + | + | + |
| | Microcephaly | ± | ± | ± | ± | ± |
| | **Retardation, psychomotor** | ± | + | + | + | + |
| | Subcortical atrophy (MRI) | ± | ± | ± | ± | ± |
| Digestive | Gastrointestinal dysmotility | ± | ± | ± | ± | ± |
| | Hepatomegaly | + | + | ± | ± | ± |
| | Liver dysfunction | ± | ± | ± | ± | ± |
| Eye | Cataract | ± | ± | ± | ± | ± |
| Genitourinary | Cryptorchidism | ± | ± | ± | ± | ± |
| | Hypospadias | ± | ± | ± | ± | ± |
| Metabolic | **Hyperammonemia, during crisis** | + | + | + | + | ± |
| | **Hyperuricemia, during crisis** | + | + | + | + | ± |
| | **Ketonuria, pronounced during crisis** | + | + | + | + | + |
| | **Lactic acidosis** | + | + | ± | ± | ± |
| | **Metabolic acidosis** | + | + | + | + | ± |
| Musculoskeletal | Contractures | ± | ± | ± | ± | ± |
| | Facial dysmorphism | ± | ± | ± | ± | ± |
| Renal | Renal tubulopathy | ± | ± | ± | ± | ± |
| Respiratory | **Persistent pulmonary hypertension of the newborn** | ± | | | | |
| | Respiratory insufficiency | ± | ± | ± | ± | ± |
| Other | Failure to thrive | + | + | + | + | + |
| | Growth retardation, postnatal | ± | ± | ± | ± | ± |
| | Low birth weight | ± | | | | |
| Laboratory findings | Alanine (plasma) | ↑-↑↑ | ↑-↑↑ | ↑-↑↑ | ↑-↑↑ | ↑-↑↑ |
| | Ammonia (blood and plasma) | n-↑↑ | n-↑↑ | n-↑↑ | n-↑↑ | n-↑↑ |
| | Anion gap | ↑ | ↑ | ↑ | ↑ | ↑ |
| | Uric acid | n-↑↑ | n-↑↑ | n-↑↑ | n-↑↑ | n-↑↑ |
| | Citrulline (plasma) | n-↑ | n-↑ | n-↑ | n-↑ | n-↑ |
| | Complex V activity (skeletal muscle) | ↓ | ↓ | ↓ | ↓ | ↓ |
| | Creatine kinase (plasma) | n-↑↑ | n-↑↑ | n-↑↑ | n-↑↑ | n-↑↑ |
| | Glutamine (plasma) | n-↑ | n-↑ | n-↑ | n-↑ | n-↑ |
| | Lactate (cerebrospinal fluid) | n-↑↑ | n-↑↑ | n-↑↑ | n-↑↑ | n-↑↑ |
| | Lactate (plasma) | ↑-↑↑↑ | ↑-↑↑↑ | ↑-↑↑↑ | ↑-↑↑↑ | ↑-↑↑↑ |
| | Orotate (urine) | n-↑ | n-↑ | n-↑ | n-↑ | n-↑ |
| | 3-Methylglutaconic acid (urine) | ↑-↑↑ | ↑-↑↑ | ↑-↑↑ | ↑-↑↑ | ↑-↑↑ |

**Table 70.10** TIMM50 deficiency

| System | Symptoms and biomarkers | Neonatal (birth–1 month) | Infancy (1–18 months) | Childhood (1.5–11 years) | Adolescence (11–16 years) | Adulthood (>16 years) |
|---|---|---|---|---|---|---|
| CNS | Behavior, aggressive | ± | ± | ± | ± | ± |
| | Bilateral symmetric lesions globus pallidus and brain stem (MRI) | ± | ± | ± | ± | ± |
| | Brain atrophy (MRI) | ± | ± | ± | ± | ± |
| | Developmental delay | + | + | + | + | + |
| | **Epilepsy** | + | + | + | + | + |
| | Hypotonia | + | + | + | + | + |
| | Hypsarrhythmia (EEG) | + | + | + | + | + |
| Eye | **Optic atrophy** | + | + | + | + | + |
| Other | Failure to thrive | + | + | + | + | + |
| Laboratory findings | 3-Hydroxyisovaleric acid (urine) | n | n | n | n | n |
| | 3-Methylglutaconic acid (urine) | ↑↑ | ↑↑ | ↑↑ | ↑↑ | ↑↑ |
| | 3-Methylglutaric acid (urine) | ↑ | ↑ | ↑ | ↑ | ↑ |
| | Lactate (cerebrospinal fluid) | n-↑↑ | n-↑↑ | n-↑↑ | n-↑↑ | n-↑↑ |
| | Lactate (plasma) | ↑-↑↑↑ | ↑-↑↑↑ | ↑-↑↑↑ | ↑-↑↑↑ | ↑-↑↑↑ |

**Table 70.11** MICOS13 deficiency

| System | Symptoms and biomarkers | Neonatal (birth–1 month) | Infancy (1–18 months) | Childhood (1.5–11 years) | Adolescence (11–16 years) | Adulthood (>16 years) |
|---|---|---|---|---|---|---|
| CNS | Cortical atrophy (MRI) | ± | ± | | | |
| | **Epilepsy** | ± | ± | | | |
| | Hypotonia, muscular | ± | ± | | | |
| | Microcephaly | ± | ± | | | |
| | Regression | ± | ± | | | |
| | Retardation, psychomotor | ± | ± | | | |
| | Subcortical atrophy (MRI) | ± | ± | | | |
| | White matter abnormalities (MRI) | ± | ± | | | |
| Digestive | **Liver failure, acute** | + | + | | | |
| | **Liver dysfunction** | + | + | | | |
| Metabolic | Hypoglycemia | ± | ± | | | |
| Other | **Death** | + | + | | | |
| | Failure to thrive | ± | ± | | | |
| Laboratory findings | 3-Hydroxyisovaleric acid (urine) | n | n | | | |
| | 3-Methylglutaconic acid (urine) | ↑↑ | ↑↑ | | | |
| | 3-Methylglutaric acid (urine) | ↑ | ↑ | | | |
| | Ammonia (blood) | n | n | | | |
| | ASAT/ALAT (plasma) | ↑ | ↑ | | | |
| | Bilirubin, conjugated (plasma) | ↑ | ↑ | | | |
| | Disturbed clotting | ↑ | ↑ | | | |
| | Glucose (plasma) | ↓-n | ↓-n | | | |
| | Lactate (plasma) | ↑ | ↑ | | | |

[a]All patients died (maximum age 13 months)

## Reference Values

| Metabolite | Reference value |
|---|---|
| 3-Hydroxyisovaleric acid (U) | 0–25 mmol/mol creatinine (0–2 month)<br>0–50 mmol/mol creatinine (2 months–2 years)<br>0–45 mmol/mol creatinine (2–10 years)<br>0–15 mmol/mol creatinine (10–18 years)<br>0–20 mmol/mol creatinine (> 18 years)<br>(GCMS, TML laboratory, Radboud university, Nijmegen, NL) |
| 3-Methylglutaconic acid (U) | 0–20 mmol/mol creatinine (0–2 month)<br>0–15 mmol/mol creatinine (2 months–2 years)<br>0–10 mmol/mol creatinine (>2 years)<br>(GCMS, TML laboratory, Radboud university, Nijmegen, NL) |
| 3-Methylglutaric acid (U) | Absent, if present not quantified (GCMS, TML lab, Radboud University, Nijmegen, NL) |

## Pathological Values

| Metabolite | Pathological value |
|---|---|
| 3-Methylglutaconic acid (U) | 20–40 mmol/mol creatinine: Suggestive for mitochondrial dysfunction as it can be seen in numerous inborn errors of metabolism<br>> 40 mmol/mol creatinine: Suggestive for inborn error of metabolism with 3-methylglutaconic aciduria as discriminative feature |

## Leucine Loading Test

Indication: To distinguish between primary and secondary 3-methylglutaconic aciduria.

Procedure: Collect a urine portion for urinary organic acid analysis and a venous blood sample for serum amino acids. Give 100 mg/kg (max. 6 g) leucine powder orally, and repeat listed investigations 1 h after the leucine gift. Collect a 24-h urine sample for another urinary organic acid analysis.

Interpretation: Table below lists the typical findings before and after leucine loading in several 3-methylglutaconic acidurias. Only in primary 3-MGA_uria due to AU deficiency a clear increase in urinary 3-MGA occurs.

Results of the leucine loading tests in different 3-methylglutaconic acidurias

| Defect | Elevated urinary 3-HIVA | Lowest urinary 3-MGA before loading (Ref < 20 mmol/mol creatinine) | Peak urinary 3-MGA after loading (Ref < 20 mmol/mol creatinine) | Ratio *cis:trans* isoforms of 3-MGA | Mean ratio (range, N patients) |
|---|---|---|---|---|---|
| *AUH* | + | 400 | 2982 | 2:1 | 4.1 (3.9–4.5; *N* = 3) |
| *TAZ* | – | 32 | 192 | 1:1 | 1.8 (1.1–5.3; *N* = 9) |
| *OPA3* | – | 29 | 26 | 1:1 | 0.9 (*N* = 1) |
| *SERAC1* | – | 60 | 234 | 1:1 | 1.3 (1.3–1.3; *N* = 2) |
| *CLPB* | – | 52 | 53 | 1:1 | 1.0 (*N* = 1) |
| NOS | – | 21 | 410 | 1:1 | 1 (0.5–1.1; *N* = 5) |

*3-HIVA* 3-hydroxyisovaeleric acid, *3-MGA* 3-methylglutaconic acid

## Specimen Collection

Urine for organic acid analysis should be analyzed immediately or frozen at −20 °C.

## DNA Testing

All 3-MGA-IEM show a distinctive pattern of signs and symptoms which justifies single gene testing. In less clear presentations, the whole exome or genome sequencing (WES/WGS) is the method of choice. As both point mutations and deletion(s) in the mitochondrial DNA can cause disorders with unspecific 3-methylglutaconic aciduria, one should inquire at the genetic lab and make sure that the genetic test chosen covers these. Leucocyte-derived DNA from 3–5 ml EDTA blood (children, adults) will be enough for all mentioned genetic tests, and WGS can be performed in much less blood even from a dried blood spot.

## Treatment Summary

AUH defect is a disorder of leucine catabolism. Acute deteriorations in relation to catabolism as in other intoxication-type IEM has not been described. The clinical manifestation is an adult-onset (fourth decade onwards) slowly progressive leukoencephalopathy with ataxia and spasticity (Wortmann et al. 2010). A leucine-restricted diet or a protein-defined (vegetarian) diet could be considered; data on this are lacking and will be difficult to obtain. In general, only a supportive treatment is available for all 3-MGA-IEM.

## References


Anikster Y. 2006 Jul 28 [updated 2020 Apr 30]. In: Adam MP, Ardinger HH, Pagon RA, Wallace SE, Bean LJH, Mirzaa G, Amemiya A, editors. GeneReviews® [Internet]. Seattle (WA): Costeff Syndrome. University of Washington, Seattle; 1993–2021. PMID: 20301646.

Clarke SL, Bowron A, Gonzalez IL, Groves SJ, Newbury-Ecob R, Clayton N, Martin RP, Tsai-Goodman B, Garratt V, Ashworth M, Bowen VM, McCurdy KR, Damin MK, Spencer CT, Toth MJ, Kelley RI, Steward CG. Barth syndrome. Orphanet J Rare Dis. 2013;8:23.

Davey KM, Parboosingh JS, McLeod DR, Chan A, Casey R, Ferreira P, Snyder FF, Bridge PJ, Bernier FP. Mutation of DNAJC19, a human homologue of yeast inner mitochondrial membrane co-chaperones, causes DCMA syndrome, a novel autosomal recessive Barth syndrome-like condition. J Med Genet. 2006;43(5):385–93.

Haghighi A, Haack TB, Atiq M, Mottaghi H, Haghighi-Kakhki H, Bashir RA, Ahting U, Feichtinger RG, Mayr JA, Rötig A, Lebre AS, Klopstock T, Dworschak A, Pulido N, Saeed MA, Saleh-Gohari N, Holzerova E, Chinnery PF, Taylor RW, Prokisch H. Sengers syndrome: six novel AGK mutations in seven new families and review of the phenotypic and mutational spectrum of 29 patients. Orphanet J Rare Dis. 2014;9:119.

Kishita Y, Shimura M, Kohda M, Akita M, Imai-Okazaki A, Yatsuka Y, Nakajima Y, Ito T, Ohtake A, Murayama K, Okazaki Y. A novel homozygous variant in MICOS13/QIL1 causes hepato-encephalopathy with mitochondrial DNA depletion syndrome. Mol Genet Genomic Med. 2020;8(10):e1427.

Kovacs-Nagy R, Morin G, Nouri MA, Brandau O, Saadi NW, Nouri MA, van den Broek F, Prokisch H, Mayr JA, Wortmann SB. HTRA2 Defect: A Recognizable Inborn Error of Metabolism with 3-Methylglutaconic Aciduria as Discriminating Feature Characterized by Neonatal Movement Disorder and Epilepsy-Report of 11 Patients. Neuropediatrics. 2018;49(6):373–8. https://doi.org/10.1055/s-0038-1667345. Epub 2018 Aug 16. PMID: 301147.

Maas RR, Iwanicka-Pronicka K, Kalkan Ucar S, Alhaddad B, AlSayed M, Al-Owain MA, Al-Zaidan HI, Balasubramaniam S, Barić I, Bubshait DK, Burlina A, Christodoulou J, Chung WK, Colombo R, Darin N, Freisinger P, Garcia Silva MT, Grunewald S, Haack TB, van Hasselt PM, Hikmat O, Hörster F, Isohanni P, Ramzan K, Kovacs-Nagy R, Krumina Z, Martin-Hernandez E, Mayr JA, McClean P, De Meirleir L, Naess K, Ngu LH, Pajdowska M, Rahman S, Riordan G, Riley L, Roeben B, Rutsch F, Santer R, Schiff M, Seders M, Sequeira S, Sperl W, Staufner C, Synofzik M, Taylor RW, Trubicka J, Tsiakas K, Unal O, Wassmer E, Wedatilake Y, Wolff T, Prokisch H, Morava E, Pronicka E, Wevers RA, de Brouwer AP, Wortmann SB. Progressive deafness-dystonia due to SERAC1 mutations: A study of 67 cases. Ann Neurol. 2017;82(6):1004–15.

Magner M, Dvorakova V, Tesarova M, Mazurova S, Hansikova H, Zahorec M, Brennerova K, Bzduch V, Spiegel R, Horovitz Y, Mandel H, Eminoğlu FT, Mayr JA, Koch J, Martinelli D, Bertini E, Konstantopoulou V, Smet J, Rahman S, Broomfield A, Stojanović V, Dionisi-Vici C, van Coster R, Morava E, Sperl W, Zeman J, Honzik T. TMEM70 deficiency: long-term outcome of 48 patients. J Inherit Metab Dis. 2015;38(3):417–26.

Mayr JA, Haack TB, Graf E, Zimmermann FA, Wieland T, Haberberger B, Superti-Furga A, Kirschner J, Steinmann B, Baumgartner MR, Moroni I, Lamantea E, Zeviani M, Rodenburg RJ, Smeitink J, Strom TM, Meitinger T, Sperl W, Prokisch H. Lack of the mitochondrial protein acylglycerol kinase causes Sengers syndrome. Am J Hum Genet. 2012;90(2):314–20.

Pronicka E, Ropacka-Lesiak M, Trubicka J, Pajdowska M, Linke M, Ostergaard E, Saunders C, Horsch S, van Karnebeek C, Yaplito-Lee J, Distelmaier F, Õunap K, Rahman S, Castelle M, Kelleher J, Baris S, Iwanicka-Pronicka K, Steward CG, Ciara E, Wortmann SB; Additional individual contributors. A scoring system predicting the clinical course of CLPB defect based on the foetal and neonatal presentation of 31 patients. J Inherit Metab Dis. 2017;40(6):853–60.

Roeben B, Schüle R, Ruf S, Bender B, Alhaddad B, Benkert T, Meitinger T, Reich S, Böhringer J, Langhans CD, Vaz FM, Wortmann SB, Marquardt T, Haack TB, Krägeloh-Mann I, Schöls L, Synofzik M. SERAC1 deficiency causes complicated HSP: evidence from a novel splice mutation in a large family. J Med Genet. 2018;55(1):39–47.

Shahrour MA, Staretz-Chacham O, Dayan D, Stephen J, Weech A, Damseh N, Pri Chen H, Edvardson S, Mazaheri S, Saada A; NISC Intramural Sequencing, Hershkovitz E, Shaag A, Huizing M, Abu-Libdeh B, Gahl WA, Azem A, Anikster Y, Vilboux T, Elpeleg O, Malicdan MC. Clin Genet. 2017;91(5):690–6.

https://doi.org/10.1111/cge.12855. Epub 2016 Oct 12. PMID: 27573165.

Thiels C, Fleger M, Huemer M, Rodenburg RJ, Vaz FM, Houtkooper RH, Haack TB, Prokisch H, Feichtinger RG, Lücke T, Mayr JA, Wortmann SB. Atypical Clinical Presentations of TAZ Mutations: An Underdiagnosed Cause of Growth Retardation?. JIMD Rep. 2016;29:89–93. https://doi.org/10.1007/8904_2015_525. Epub 2016 Jan 3. PMID: 26724946.

Ucar SK, Mayr JA, Feichtinger RG, Canda E, Çoker M, Wortmann SB. Previously Unreported Biallelic Mutation in DNAJC19: Are Sensorineural Hearing Loss and Basal Ganglia Lesions Additional Features of Dilated Cardiomyopathy and Ataxia (DCMA) Syndrome?. JIMD Rep. 2017;35:39–45.

Wortmann SB, Duran M, Anikster Y, et al. Inborn errors of metabolism with 3-methylglutaconic aciduria as discriminative feature: proper classification and nomenclature. J Inherit Metab Dis. 2013a;36:923–8.

Wortmann SB, Kluijtmans LA, Rodenburg RJ, et al. 3-Methylglutaconic aciduria--lessons from 50 genes and 977 patients. J Inherit Metab Dis. 2013b;36:913–21.

Wortmann SB, Kluijtmans LA, Sequeira S, Wevers RA, Morava E. Leucine loading test is only discriminative for 3-methylglutaconic aciduria due to AUH defect. JIMD Rep. 2014;16:1–6.

Wortmann SB, Kremer BH, Graham A, et al. 3-Methylglutaconic aciduria type I redefined: a syndrome with late-onset leukoencephalopathy. Neurology. 2010;75:1079–83.

Wortmann SB, van Hasselt PM, Barić I, Burlina A, Darin N, Hörster F, Coker M, Ucar SK, Krumina Z, Naess K, Ngu LH, Pronicka E, Riordan G, Santer R, Wassmer E, Zschocke J, Schiff M, de Meirleir L, Alowain MA, Smeitink JA, Morava E, Kozicz T, Wevers RA, Wolf NI, Willemsen MA. Eyes on MEGDEL: distinctive basal ganglia involvement in dystonia deafness syndrome. Neuropediatrics. 2015;46(2):98–103.

Wortmann SB, Vaz FM, Gardeitchik T, Vissers LE, Renkema GH, Schuurs-Hoeijmakers JH, Kulik W, Lammens M, Christin C, Kluijtmans LA, Rodenburg RJ, Nijtmans LG, Grünewald A, Klein C, Gerhold JM, Kozicz T, van Hasselt PM, Harakalova M, Kloosterman W, Barić I, Pronicka E, Ucar SK, Naess K, Singhal KK, Krumina Z, Gilissen C, van Bokhoven H, Veltman JA, Smeitink JA, Lefeber DJ, Spelbrink JN, Wevers RA, Morava E, de Brouwer AP. Mutations in the phospholipid remodeling gene SERAC1 impair mitochondrial function and intracellular cholesterol trafficking and cause dystonia and deafness. Nat Genet. 2012;44(7):797–802.

Wortmann SB, Ziętkiewicz S, Kousi M, Szklarczyk R, Haack TB, Gersting SW, Muntau AC, Rakovic A, Renkema GH, Rodenburg RJ, Strom TM, Meitinger T, Rubio-Gozalbo ME, Chrusciel E, Distelmaier F, Golzio C, Jansen JH, van Karnebeek C, Lillquist Y, Lücke T, Õunap K, Zordania R, Yaplito-Lee J, van Bokhoven H, Spelbrink JN, Vaz FM, Pras-Raves M, Ploski R, Pronicka E, Klein C, Willemsen MA, de Brouwer AP, Prokisch H, Katsanis N, Wevers RA. CLPB mutations cause 3-methylglutaconic aciduria, progressive brain atrophy, intellectual disability, congenital neutropenia, cataracts, movement disorder. Am J Hum Genet. 2015;96(2):245–57.

# Biochemical Phenotypes of Questionable Clinical Significance

71

Stephen I. Goodman

## Contents



**Abstract**

Most of the many known inherited metabolic defects are associated with clinical disease; a few, however, are not—or their association with clinical disease is tenuous at best.

The latter include iminoglycinuria, hyperprolinemia type I, hydroxyprolinemia, histidinemia, urocanic aciduria, FIGLU-uria, trimethylaminuria, dimethylglycinuria, sarcosinemia, hyperlysinemia and saccharopinuria, 2-aminoadipic and 2-ketoadipic aciduria, glutaric aciduria type 3, hydroxykynureninuria, cystathioninuria, 3-methylcrotonylglycinuria and 2-methylglycinuria, as well as deficiencies of carnosinase, oxoprolinase, glycerol kinase, methionine adenosyltransferase, methylmalonyl-CoA epimerase, and short-chain acyl-CoA dehydrogenase (SCAD).

Only time will tell us if some of the disorders now considered pathogenic are not and if some of the former indeed cause clinical disease—perhaps in adulthood.

Stephen I. Goodman was deceased on October 30, 2020.

S. I. Goodman (✉)
University of Colorado Denver School of Medicine,
Aurora, CO, USA

## Introduction

It is noteworthy that one of the four inborn errors that comprise Garrod's tetrad is pentosuria, a biochemical abnormality whose primary clinical importance is its occasional misdiagnosis as diabetes mellitus. Several other inborn errors have little if any clinical relevance. In many of them, however, this realization has followed a lengthy period during which they were thought to cause disease, and in most cases, the problem has been one of sampling bias.

The first subject to be described with a novel inborn error is almost invariably screened because of clinical disease, and any biochemical abnormality that is detected may initially be thought of as linked to the clinical phenotype. In some cases, the perceived association is strengthened or weakened by studying other family members, particularly siblings, but in most cases the link between biochemical and clinical phenotype remains an open issue until, with the passage of time, more individuals with the defect are recognized. And this can take a long time. Biochemical phenotypes such as hydroxylysinemia (Goodman et al. 1972), phosphohydroxylysinuria (Dorland et al. 1990), and beta-mercapto-


N. Blau et al. (eds.), *Physician's Guide to the Diagnosis, Treatment, and Follow-Up of Inherited Metabolic Diseases*,
https://doi.org/10.1007/978-3-030-67727-5_71

cysteine-lactate disulfiduria (Crawhall et al. 1968), despite their initial descriptions more than 20 years ago, are too infrequently reported to allow firm conclusions about pathogenicity.

Newborn screening programs have compressed the timeline considerably, and it is now possible to detect a biochemical defect in infancy and to follow its effect, if any, on clinical phenotype. Such programs have also identified many enzyme-deficient subjects who would likely not have come to clinical attention, such as the clinically unaffected females with 3-methylcrotonylglycinuria and glutaric acidemia type 1 whose infants tested positive for hydroxy-C5 carnitine ester and low carnitine, respectively.

This chapter will attempt to describe the biochemical phenotypes of some inborn errors whose clinical relevance is in question. Some, like hydroxykynureninuria, are primarily of historical importance, although recognition of an abnormal compound in amino or organic acid analysis can cause consternation to patient and physician alike. Much of what we write reflects the authors' personal views of what is now known about these conditions, and it may well be that a condition that we now think is of questionable clinical significance will on more intense and detailed study revert. An excellent example of the latter is hyperprolinemia type II, in which an early impression that patients tended to have seizures was confirmed and shown to be due to sequestering of vitamin $B_6$ by accumulated $\Delta^1$-pyrroline-5-carboxylic acid. A continuing discussion of the topics will almost certainly keep the field alive and fascinating.

## Disorders

### Iminoglycinuria

Iminoglycinuria, i.e., increased amounts of proline, hydroxyproline, and glycine in urine, is most commonly seen in (premature) infants, when it is due to the immaturity of a shared renal tubular transporter for these amino acids. Iminoglycinuria due to tubular immaturity usually disappears by 1 year of age. It can also be seen in hyperprolinemia types I and II, when elevated proline in the glomerular filtrate saturates a transporter and competitively inhibits tubular reabsorption of glycine and hydroxyproline and when a transporter fails to operate properly due to mutation. The latter is called familial iminoglycinuria and is inherited as an autosomal recessive trait. Depending on which transporter is involved, the defect may also be expressed in the small intestine. Heterozygotes sometimes have hyperglycinuria without hyperglycinemia. While occasionally found in symptomatic individuals, familial iminoglycinuria is probably without clinical significance.

The condition is easily recognized on urine amino acid analysis by the increases in proline, hydroxyproline, and glycine, accompanied by a normal concentration of proline in blood. Hyperprolinemia type I (see below) and iminoglycinuria of the newborn are clinically benign, so the only clinically relevant condition that must be excluded in an individual with iminoglycinuria is hyperprolinemia type II. This is usually quite simple, as plasma proline is very high in hyperprolinemia type II, and $\Delta^1$-pyrroline-5-carboxylic acid (P5C) and $\Delta^1$-pyrroline-3-hydroxy-5-carboxylic acid (hydroxy-P5C) are increased in urine.

P5C and hydroxy-P5C in the urine appear as discrete peaks on amino acid analysis and also cause the urine to react positively with *o*-aminobenzaldehyde (Efron 1965). When using sodium citrate buffers, hydroxy-P5C elutes just after hydroxyproline, and P5C elutes just before proline (Goodman et al. 1974). The urine organic acid analysis of hyperprolinemia patients will reveal the presence of pyrrole-5-carboxylglycine, possibly the most accessible characteristic metabolite.

### Hyperprolinemia Type I

Hyperprolinemia type I (HPI) is due to a defect in proline oxidase, a FAD-containing mitochondrial protein found mainly in the liver, kidney, and brain that converts proline to $\Delta^1$-pyrroline-5-carboxylic acid (P5C). The condition was initially described in a patient with Alport-like renal disease (Schafer et al. 1962) and was subsequently reported in patients with a wide variety of renal and nonrenal manifestations, including eye abnormalities, developmental delay, and other neurologic manifestations. Evidence from subjects identified by newborn screening shows that HPI is usually benign (e.g., Fontaine et al. 1970), and the early association with clinical phenotypes is now thought to have been due to sampling bias although the reports about the association of this defect with various clinical problems such as epilepsia and schizophrenia are still appearing. The condition's primary importance is that it must be differentiated from hyperprolinemia type II, in which a defect in P5C dehydrogenase is often associated with intellectual disability and/or seizures.

The condition is easily recognized by finding increased proline (500–2000 μM; normal <420) on amino acid analysis of plasma, usually accompanied by increased proline, hydroxyproline, and glycine in urine. Iminoglycinuria is due to the saturation of the renal transporter for proline, hydroxyproline, and glycine by the increased proline in the glomerular filtrate.

Plasma proline concentrations in hyperprolinemia type II are often higher (>1300 μM), and the urine contains P5C, hydroxy-P5C, and pyrrole-5-carboxylglycine (see above).

## Hydroxyprolinemia

Hydroxyprolinemia was described in 1962 (Efron et al. 1962) in association with intellectual disability and has since been described in several additional subjects with a variety of clinical manifestations and in several healthy hydroxyprolinemic siblings (Kim et al. 1997). In addition, one hydroxyprolinemic baby has been detected by newborn screening and continues to be clinically normal. It is now thought that, as with hyperprolinemia type I, deficiency of hydroxyproline oxidase does not cause clinical disease and that the early association with the disease was due to sampling bias.

As in proline oxidation, hydroxyproline is normally oxidized first to $\Delta^1$-pyrroline-3-hydroxy-5-carboxylic acid by hydroxyproline oxidase and then to hydroxyglutamic semialdehyde by $\Delta^1$-pyrroline-5-carboxylic dehydrogenase, the enzyme in the proline pathway that is deficient in hyperprolinemia type II.

Hydroxyprolinemia, which is inherited as an autosomal recessive trait, causes elevations of hydroxyproline in plasma and urine, without iminoglycinuria and with a normal excretion of peptide-bound hydroxyproline. Its diagnosis is relatively simple and depends on demonstrating high hydroxyproline in plasma (200–500 μM; normal <50) and urine.

## Histidinemia

Histidinemia, first described in two siblings by Ghadimi et al. (1961), was thought in the past to cause speech defects as an almost specific clinical phenotype. As more subjects with the condition have been found, however, many of them by newborn screening programs, it has been learned that most enzyme-deficient individuals have normal intelligence and speech (Ishikawa 1987), and it is now thought that the condition is benign in most instances.

Histidine is deaminated to *trans*-urocanic acid by histidase (histidine ammonia-lyase), an enzyme found mainly in the liver and in the stratum corneum of the skin, but further metabolism of urocanic acid to 5-formyl-tetrahydrofolate and glutamate via imidazolone propionic acid and formiminoglutamic acid (FIGLU) appears to occur only in the liver. Histidinemia is caused by histidase deficiency. The enzyme defect is transmitted as an autosomal recessive trait.

Biochemical findings in histidinemia, which is the most common inborn error in Japan, include increased histidine in plasma, urine and cerebrospinal fluid, low concentrations of urocanic acid in blood and sweat, and increased concentrations of histidine metabolites such as imidazole pyruvic acid in urine. Enzyme-deficient subjects differ widely in their plasma histidine levels and tolerance to oral histidine loads, and this may well be due to differences in mutations and residual enzyme activity.

Histidine can be as high as 1500 μM (normal <150). The increased imidazole pyruvic acid in urine can usually be detected by the ferric chloride test or the Phenistix reagent strip. Diagnosis can be confirmed, if necessary, by demonstrating histidase deficiency in the skin and by mutation analysis (Kawai et al. 2005). Treatment with a histidine-restricted diet normalizes the biochemical phenotype but is not indicated for what is most likely a harmless condition.

## Urocanic Aciduria

Urocanic aciduria, which is caused by a deficiency of urocanase, is characterized by increased urocanic acid in urine, with normal or slightly increased concentrations of histidine in plasma and urine. Said to be very rare, the condition is probably underdiagnosed because the increased urocanic acid cannot be detected by the usual methods used to screen for amino and organic acids in blood and urine. Older methods used thin-layer chromatography and staining with the Pauly reagent, but more specific HPLC methods have also been developed (e.g., Kuracka et al. 1996). Urocanic acid can appear in the HPLC analysis of urine purines and pyrimidines using UV detection. Alternatively, NMR analysis of a urine sample will readily detect an increased urocanic acid (UF Engelke, SSIEM-symposium Istanbul 2010). While initially diagnosed in retarded individuals, several children identified by newborn screening have developed normally without therapy, and the enzyme defect is now thought to be benign in most instances.

The condition is apt to be detected during the investigation of increased histidine in blood and/or urine, when increased urocanic acid is found in urine instead of the decrease expected in histidinemia, which is much more common. Diagnosis can be confirmed by demonstrating reduced enzyme activity in the liver or by molecular analysis of the *UROC1* gene (Espinós et al. 2009).

## Glutamate Formiminotransferase-Cyclodeaminase Deficiency (FIGLU-Uria)

Increased excretion of formimino-L-glutamic acid (FIGLU), an intermediate in the oxidation of histidine, was first noted to result from an inherited deficiency of formiminotransferase-cyclodeaminase (FTCD) when amino acid analysis became routine when evaluating children with developmental disabilities. The compound does not react with ninhydrin but quickly breaks down to glutamate during many analytic procedures. FIGLU excretion is also increased in folic acid and $B_{12}$ deficiency and in cblC disease (see Chaps. 21 and 29).

FTCD deficiency is a relatively common recessively inherited defect of histidine metabolism and has both severe and mild phenotypes, with the former characterized by megaloblastic anemia, intellectual disability, and elevated urine FIGLU following a histidine load. The mild phenotype includes high FIGLU in blood and urine without loading, and, if developmental delay is present, it is mild.

Elevated FIGLU is now most frequently encountered during analysis of plasma acylcarnitine esters (Malvagia et al. 2006). If folic acid deficiency and cblC disease are eliminated by appropriate studies, confirmation of the defect can be by enzyme analysis in the liver or by molecular analysis of the *FTCD* gene (Hilton et al. 2003). An additional diagnostic marker is urine hydantoin-5-propionic acid, a metabolite of imidazolone-propionic acid which is easily detected by urine organic acid analysis.

## Carnosinase Deficiency and Homocarnosinosis

Formerly thought to be two conditions, carnosinase deficiency and homocarnosinosis are now thought to be variants of the same disorder. Carnosine is a dipeptide of β-alanine and histidine and is present in several human tissues, including the skeletal muscle and brain. Homocarnosine (γ-aminobutyryl-L-histidine) exists only in the brain and in amounts much larger than those of carnosine. Both dipeptides can be hydrolyzed by carnosinase (EC 3.4.13.20), an enzyme that is present in plasma and several tissues, including the brain, and encoded by the *CN1* gene on human chromosome 18. A closely related *CN2* gene is located near CN1 and encodes a much less specific dipeptidase that hydrolyzes carnosine only under non-physiological conditions (Teufel et al. 2003).

Carnosinemia and carnosinuria due to recessively inherited deficiency of carnosinase were initially described in patients with neurological disease (Perry et al. 1967) but have since been observed repeatedly in normal subjects. It is now thought that any relationship to clinical symptoms is fortuitous. Homocarnosinosis, which may be caused by a more severe deficiency of the same enzyme, is much less common and is characterized by increased homocarnosine (the major form of bound GABA) in the cerebrospinal fluid and increased carnosine in urine. It has been described only once, in a healthy 72-year-old woman and in three of her four children. All three children, but not their mother, had recessively inherited hereditary spastic paraplegia due to mutations in the *SPG11* gene (Sjaastad et al. 2018); the specific cause of the elevated CSF homocarnosine, however, remains obscure.

Persistent carnosinemia (0.005–0.03 μM; normal = not detected) and carnosinuria on a meat- (and therefore carnosine-) free diet strongly suggest a diagnosis of carnosinase deficiency, which is easily confirmed by enzyme assay. CSF homocarnosine in such individuals is normal, i.e., less than 15 μM. Because serum carnosinase also hydrolyzes anserine, a dipeptide of β-alanine and 1-methyl-L-histidine found in the skeletal muscle of birds and some mammals, normal subjects excrete 1-methylhistidine in urine after eating fowl. Carnosinase-deficient subjects do not, however, and instead excrete intact anserine. Because enzyme activity is low in infancy and increases gradually to achieve adult levels in adolescence, it is important to compare enzyme activity with appropriate age-matched control data.

A diagnosis of homocarnosinosis will initially be suggested by increased carnosine in urine, even on a meat-free diet, accompanied by elevated homocarnosine in cerebrospinal fluid (50–75 μM; normal <15). As in serum carnosinase deficiency, anserine is excreted intact after eating anserine-containing foods.

## Trimethylaminuria

Trimethylaminuria is a recessively inherited condition in which absorbed trimethylamine (TMA), formed by gut bacteria from dietary precursors such as lecithin and choline, accumulates behind a defect in flavin-containing monooxygenase 3 (FMO3), the enzyme that oxidizes TMA to TMA N-oxide (TMAO). TMA is not toxic to tissues but is highly volatile, and FMO3-deficient subjects develop a pungent odor similar to that of rotting fish. Sometimes called "fish odor syndrome," the condition causes severe social stigmatization and psychological distress to the affected individuals and to their families.

Usually suspected because of the odor, diagnosis is made by demonstrating an abnormal ratio of TMA:TMAO in urine at rest or after a choline load; the latter is particularly useful when the odor is intermittent or mild and can consist most simply of a marine fish meal. The analysis of TMA and TMAO in urine can be quite cumbersome but a recently described method using tandem mass spectrometry (Johnson 2008) appears to be simple, quick, and accurate. Alternatively, an in vitro NMR analysis of the urine will unequally demonstrate the presence of TMA (see below). There is normally much more TMAO in urine than TMA, so the TMAO:TMA + TMAO ratio in normal subjects exceeds 0.92. The ratio in severely enzyme-deficient subjects can be as low as 0.04.

Several polymorphisms as well as severe and mild mutations have been described in the *FMO3* gene, and the latter usually correlate with the severity of the metabolic block (Hernandez et al. 2003). Treatment is by restricting the intake of high choline- and lecithin-containing foods, in particular fish, dairy products, eggs, and chocolate, and eliminating bacterial TMA production by gut sterilization.

## Dimethylglycinuria

Dimethylglycine (DMG) is formed by the transfer of a methyl group from betaine, a choline metabolite, to homocysteine, forming methionine. DMG is then converted to sarcosine by oxidative demethylation catalyzed by DMG dehydrogenase, a flavin-containing enzyme that requires folate as a cofactor. Sarcosine is converted to glycine by a similar and related enzyme. Electrons from the flavins of DMG and sarcosine dehydrogenase enter the respiratory chain via electron transfer flavoprotein (ETF) and ETF-ubiquinone oxidoreductase. Increased excretion of DMG has been observed in folate deficiency and in subjects receiving large doses of betaine as a therapeutic agent. Theoretically one should expect DMG to accumulate in the multiple acyl-CoA dehydrogenation defect (MADD, glutaric aciduria type II), but this has not been confirmed so far.

Dimethylglycinemia and -uria due to deficiency of dimethylglycine dehydrogenase has been observed only once, in an adult (Moolenaar et al. 1999) with a fishlike odor, chronic muscle fatigue, and increased serum creatine kinase. A search for trimethylamine in urine by $^1$H-NMR spectroscopy instead detected an approximately 20-fold increase of DMG (450 mmol/mol creatinine; normal <26) and was confirmed by GC-MS of the trimethylsilyl derivative. DMG was increased 100-fold in plasma (221 μM; normal <5), and molecular analysis showed homozygosity for an inactivating mutation in the *DMGDH* gene (Binzak et al. 2001).

Except for the "fish odor," which is characteristic of dimethylglycine, the relationship between the enzyme deficiency and the rest of the clinical phenotype is not clear and may well be fortuitous. The diagnosis should probably be considered in the many patients with a fishlike odor who do not have trimethylamine oxidase deficiency.

## Sarcosinemia

Sarcosine (monomethylglycine) is converted to glycine, with the oxidation of its methyl group to "active" formaldehyde by sarcosine dehydrogenase, a mitochondrial flavoprotein from which electrons enter the respiratory chain through electron chain flavoprotein (ETF) and ETF:ubiquinone oxidoreductase (ETF:QO). Like dimethylglycine dehydrogenase, the enzyme requires folate as a cofactor.

Sarcosinemia, a biochemical phenotype characterized by increased sarcosine in blood and urine, was first described in a 10-month-old child (Gerritsen and Waisman 1966) with intellectual disability and hypertonia and was subsequently reported in association with a variety of clinical phenotypes and a variable association with developmental issues. More recently it has been identified by newborn screening in developmentally normal subjects (Levy et al. 1984), and it is now thought that the biochemical phenotype is without clinical effect in most instances. The enzyme defect has not been demonstrated in affected individuals, but several pathogenic mutations have now been demonstrated in the *SARDH* gene (Bar-Joseph et al. 2012).

Increased sarcosine is also occasionally found in the multiple acyl-CoA dehydrogenation defect (MADD, glutaric aciduria type II), and it is important that the finding of increased sarcosine in blood and/or urine be followed by a careful search for the organic acids and/or acylcarnitine esters characteristic of GA2.

Not normally detectable in plasma or urine, plasma sarcosine levels in sarcosinemia range from 50 to 700 μM, and urine excretion ranges from 170 to 5080 mmol/mol creatinine.

## Hyperlysinemia and Saccharopinuria

The initial steps in the mitochondrial oxidation of lysine in the liver and kidney are catalyzed by a single bifunctional enzyme, i.e., 2-aminoadipic semialdehyde synthase. The first reaction is a condensation of lysine with 2-ketoglutarate, carried out by lysine-2-ketoglutarate reductase, to form saccharopine, and the second, catalyzed by saccharopine dehydrogenase, releases glutamate and 2-aminoadipic semialdehyde. Recessively inherited mutations in the bifunctional enzyme cause familial hyperlysinemia when the first or both activities are deficient and saccharopinuria when appreciable residual activity is retained only in the first.

Although hyperlysinemia with and without saccharopinuria were initially recognized in mentally retarded children (Woody 1964; Carson et al. 1968), it soon became apparent that many patients with hyperlysinemia who were diagnosed subsequently, some of whom were ascertained through newborn screening programs, were clinically normal and that the initial association of hyperlysinemia with neurodevelopmental abnormalities may well have been due to ascertainment bias (Dancis et al. 1983). This may also be true of saccharopinuria, in which the added metabolite is rapidly cleared by the kidney, but we do not know of a large study that has demonstrated this conclusively.

Plasma lysine in hyperlysinemia often exceeds 1000 μM (normal <250) and is accompanied by impressive lysinuria together with increased levels of the two N-acetyllysines and homocitrulline, sometimes with minimal saccharopinuria. While only two patients have been described with saccharopinuria, plasma lysine is lower than in familial hyperlysinemia, and urine saccharopine is much higher. The relationship of the enzyme defect to clinical manifestations is questionable in both disorders.

While saccharopinuria is difficult to miss—the compound runs as a 570 nm absorbing peak in the area of cystine on an amino acid analyzer—isolated hyperlysinemia and/or hyperlysinuria can represent a difficult diagnostic challenge. If elevated lysine is first detected in urine, plasma should be examined to ensure that it is due to overflow and not to the defects in renal transport that cause cystinuria and lysinuric protein intolerance. Hyperlysinemia must be distinguished from the secondary hyperlysinemia that occurs in infantile pyruvate carboxylase deficiency, where it is accompanied by hyperammonemia, lactic acidemia, and citrullinemia. A rarer cause of hyperlysinemia is mitochondrial NADP(H) deficiency due to *NADK2* mutations, which causes severe neurological disease and laboratory findings of mitochondrial dysfunction and dienoyl-CoA reductase deficiency (Houten et al. 2014).

## 2-Aminoadipic and 2-Ketoadipic Aciduria

2-Aminoadipic acid, an intermediate in lysine oxidation, is transaminated to 2-ketoadipic acid, which is then oxidatively decarboxylated to glutaryl-CoA by 2-ketoglutarate dehydrogenase (Hirashima et al. 1967) or by another enzyme similar to the dehydrogenases for pyruvate, branched-chain ketoacids, and 2-ketoglutarate.

Several subjects with recessively inherited 2-aminoadipic and/or 2-ketoadipic acidemia and aciduria have been described, most of them initially ascertained because of developmental delay and a variety of neurological manifestations. Because several siblings of these patients have been developmentally normal, and because a family is known in which all three biochemically affected subjects are clinically normal, it is now thought that clinical manifestations in these individuals are due to sampling bias and that the condition is benign. The condition is due to a variety of missense and nonsense mutations in *DHTKD1*, which encodes a peptide analogous to the $E_1$ subunits of pyruvate and 2-ketoglutarate dehydrogenases (Danhauser et al. 2012; Hagen et al. 2015; Stiles et al. 2016).

While a few individuals with 2-aminoadipic acidemia without 2-ketoadipic aciduria have been thought to be deficient in a 2-aminoadipic acid transaminase, one of them has also been shown to have mutations in *DHTKD1* (Hagen et al. 2015).

2-Aminoadipic acid concentrations in serum and urine have been 34–120 μM (normal <5) and 66–350 mmol/mol creatinine (normal <17), respectively. The urine concentration of 2-ketoadipic in one patient was 133 mmol/gm creatinine. Because similar amino and organic acid profiles have been observed in Reye-like episodes associated with various organic acidemias and other familial disorders (Elpeleg et al. 1990), diagnostic samples should be taken when the patients are not acutely ill.

The notion that 2-aminoadipic/2-ketoadipic (2AA/2KA) aciduria is harmless is hard to reconcile with the observation that Charcot-Marie-Tooth disease type 2 tracks with, and presumably caused by, heterozygosity for a nonsense mutation (pY485X) in *DHTKD1* in a large Chinese family (Xu et al. 2012), unless this mutation confers a new function on the *DHTKD1* gene product. Several other nonsense mutations have been described in individuals with 2-aminoadipic/2-ketoadipic aciduria, and to our knowledge, none of them (or their parents) have had similar neurological diseases. It is interesting to note that knockout mice homozygous for *DHTKD1* deficiency have 2-aminoadipic and 2-ketoadipic aciduria as well as a neurological phenotype not unlike human Charcot-Marie Tooth disease (Xu et al. 2018).

## Glutaric Aciduria Type 3

Clinically significant disorders in the pathway of lysine (and tryptophan) oxidation include glutaric aciduria types 1 and 2 and pyridoxine dependent seizures and are discussed in Chaps. 32, 34 and 69. A condition in which glutaric acid is increased in blood and urine, but without accumulation of other organic acids and carnitine esters typical of glutaric aciduria types 1 and 2, has been called glutaric aciduria type 3.

This condition was first described in a child with β-thalassemia and attributed to the deficiency of peroxisomal glutaryl-CoA oxidase (Bennett et al. 1991) but has since been described in several clinically diverse situations and in normal subjects, and the view has developed that, whatever the primary defect, the condition is benign.

The defect was mapped in three subjects in the Pennsylvania Old Order Amish, and homozygosity demonstrated for a missense mutation in *C7orf10*, which appears to encode a mitochondrial enzyme with a coenzyme A transferase domain (Sherman et al. 2008). Mutations in this gene were also present in several additional patients, and *these* included homozygosity for a chain-terminating mutation in the child whose defect had been thought initially to be in a peroxisomal oxidase. Because the enzyme product may esterify glutaric acid, it was suggested that the product of 2-ketoadipic dehydrogenase in the pathway of lysine oxidation is free glutaric acid, and not glutaryl-CoA. This seems unlikely in view of the relatively low glutaric acid excretion produced even by chain-terminating mutations in *C7orf10*, and it seems equally possible that the enzyme's primary function is to esterify free glutaric acid from other sources, such as gut bacteria.

Diagnosis, which is suspected by finding increased glutaric acid in blood and/or urine without the abnormal organic acids and carnitine esters found in glutaric aciduria types 1 and 2, can be confirmed by molecular analysis of *C7orf10*.

## Hydroxykynureninuria

The oxidation of tryptophan in the liver proceeds through kynurenine, 3-hydroxykynurenine, and 3-hydroxyanthranilic acid to a branch point; most of the carbon skeleton is then oxidized to acetyl-CoA via 2-ketoadipic acid and glutaryl-CoA, but some is instead diverted to the biosynthesis of nicotinic acid and nicotinamide.

The conversion of 3-hydroxykynurenine to 3-hydroxyanthranilic acid by kynureninase is $B_6$ dependent, and renewed interest in vitamin deficiency and dependency states in the mid-1960s prompted an examination of tryptophan metabolites in patients with $B_6$-sensitive disorders and/or symptoms reminiscent of pellagra. Hydroxykynureninuria was first described (Komrower et al. 1964) in a mildly retarded 4-year-old girl with what had been thought to be a nicotinic acid deficiency in infancy. Xanthurenic acid, kynurenine, and 3-hydroxykynurenine were increased in urine and were increased by oral loading with L-tryptophan. A few children with similar metabolite excretion patterns have since been described without symptoms or with only mild pellagra-like findings, and it is now thought that the enzyme block is clinically relevant only if niacin intake is limited.

The cumbersome paper and thin-layer chromatography methods once used to investigate the disorder are no longer necessary. Diagnosis is now possible by detecting increased urine xanthurenic acid on organic acid analysis; increased xanthurenic acid, kynurenine and 3-hydroxykynurenine in urine and plasma by HPLC; and/or mutations in the *KYNU* gene, which encodes kynureninase (Christensen et al. 2007).

## Cystathioninuria

Even when first described in a 64-year-old mentally retarded woman (Harris et al. 1959) and attributed to a probable recessively inherited deficiency of γ-cystathionase, the $B_6$-requiring enzyme that cleaves cystathionine to 2-ketobutyrate and cysteine, the suspicion was that the metabolic abnormality was related only by chance to the clinical presentation. Large reviews suggest that the latter is indeed the case; a review of patients ascertained in a bias-free manner found very few with symptoms, and even fewer whose symptoms could not be attributed to another cause (Mudd et al. 2001).

Cystathionine is efficiently cleared by the kidney, and accumulation is much more easily detected in urine than in blood. Urine concentrations in enzyme-deficient individuals are up to 2200 mmol/mol creatinine (normal <0.5). Urine cystathionine is often increased in newborns (probably because liver γ-cystathionase appears late in fetal life), in $B_6$ deficiency, and in patients with functional neural tumors and hepatoblastomas, presumably because of an imbalance between production by cystathionine β-synthase and hydrolysis, and remethylation defects (Chap. 28).

Although rarely necessary, an inherited enzyme deficiency may be confirmed by molecular analysis of the *CTH* gene (Wang and Hegele 2003).

## 3-Methylcrotonylglycinuria

3-Methylcrotonyl-CoA is formed by oxidation of isovaleryl-CoA, an intermediate in leucine metabolism, and is normally converted to 3-methylglutaconyl-CoA by a biotin-requiring holocarboxylase. Deficiency of 3-methylcrotonyl-CoA carboxylase (3MCC) can be isolated or, in biotin deficiency, biotinidase deficiency and holocarboxylase synthase deficiency, combined with the deficiency of carboxylases specific for acetyl-CoA, propionyl-CoA, and pyruvate (see Chap. 30). 3MCC is probably an $\alpha_6\beta_6$ dodecamer (Huang et al. 2010), and 3MCC deficiency can be due to mutations in either subunit.

Most early descriptions of isolated enzyme deficiency were in infants and children with acute disease in infancy and in children with Reye-like symptoms, and there was little doubt about the relevance of the biochemical defect to clinical disease until newborn screening by tandem mass spectrometry detected increased hydroxy-C5 carnitine in several infants whose mothers had asymptomatic enzyme deficiency. It is not yet clear how many individuals with isolated carboxylase deficiency develop symptoms, but none of the affected subjects picked up by newborn screening developed any symptoms (Arnold et al. 2008). Kindreds with multiple "healthy" affected sibs had been reported before (Mourmans et al. 1995).

Though an occasional patient with 3MCC deficiency has isolated 3-hydroxyisovaleric aciduria (Wolfe et al. 2007), most also have an easily detected peak of 3-methylcrotonylglycine, and the abnormal organic acid pattern is easily recognized, be it in an ill child or an asymptomatic female. While it appears that the defect can sometimes cause clinical disease, there is considerable disagreement about the management of the asymptomatic mother and/or newborn (Arnold et al. 2008).

## 2-Methylbutyrylglycinuria (2-Methylbutyryl-CoA Dehydrogenase Deficiency)

2-Methylbutyryl-CoA is an intermediate in the oxidation of isoleucine. It is produced by oxidative decarboxylation of 2-keto-3-methylvaleric acid and is normally oxidized to tiglyl-CoA by methylbutyryl-CoA dehydrogenase (SBCAD), one of the several mitochondrial flavin-containing dehydrogenases that pass electrons into the respiratory chain via ETF and ETF:ubiquinone oxidoreductase.

Deficiency of SBCAD was first observed in a 3-year-old boy with hypotonia and developmental delay and in his asymptomatic mother (Andresen et al. 2000). The parents were first cousins, and both mother and child were homozygous for the same missense mutation in the *SBCAD* gene. Subjects that were subsequently described have had a variety of clinical presentations, and many in fact have been completely normal. The enzyme deficiency is quite common in the Hmong population in the Midwest USA. A recent review of 12 non-Hmong enzyme-deficient subjects found that all 11 that had been detected by newborn screening were well; the oldest of them was 4 years of age (Alfardan et al. 2010). These findings suggest that the association between the biochemical phenotype and clinical disease is fortuitous.

The diagnosis in newborns is usually suspected when an elevated C5 acylcarnitine is found on screening by tandem mass spectrometry and is confirmed on urine organic acid analysis by finding a (usually) small peak of 2-methylbutyrylglycine (MBG), often with small amounts of isobutyrylglycine and ethylhydracrylic acid and without isovalerylglycine. It is important to note that the amount of MBG in urine in this condition is often 10- to 50-fold less than the amount of isovalerylglycine excreted in isovaleric acidemia. Inherited defects of *ETHE1* (ethylmalonic acid encephalopathy) may be accompanied by modestly elevated branched-chain acylglycines and should therefore be ruled out. While available, enzyme and molecular analysis is seldom indicated.

## Oxoprolinase Deficiency

Excretion of large amounts of pyroglutamic acid (5-oxoproline) can be due to deficiency of glutathione synthetase, when it is invariably associated with clinical disease (Chap. 16). Rarely, however, it is due to the inherited deficiency of oxoprolinase, a condition with a much more benign clinical course. Oxoprolinase deficiency was first described in two siblings whose symptoms seemed unrelated to their enzyme block (Larsson et al. 1981) and has since been reported in six additional patients, many of whom have been entirely normal.

As in glutathione synthetase deficiency, a large peak of pyroglutamic acid (>2 mol/mol creatinine; normal <0.05) is seen on organic acid analysis. If not due to deficiency of glutathione synthetase, the diagnosis of oxoprolinase deficiency can be made by demonstrating enzyme deficiency in white blood cells or cultured fibroblasts or by molecular analysis of the *OPLAH* gene (Almaghlouth et al. 2011).

## Glycerol Kinase Deficiency

Glycerol kinase phosphorylates glycerol to glycerol-3-phosphate. X-linked deficiency of this enzyme (GKD) was first described in two male siblings with increased glycerol in blood and urine, psychomotor retardation, osteoporosis, myopathy, and adrenal hypoplasia (Guggenheim et al. 1980). Subsequent evaluation of many additional patients has shown that glycerol kinase deficiency by itself is important only in its ability to give a falsely elevated estimation of serum triglyceride if the latter is measured by glycerol release after lipolysis, but not before. Clinical phenotypes associated with GKD deficiency are most often due to the fact that the GKD gene is closely linked to genes encoding ornithine transcarbamylase, congenital adrenal hypoplasia, and Duchenne muscular dystrophy, and the disease is often caused by deletions of several contiguous genes (McCabe 2001). Isolated GKD may be associated with mild fasting intolerance and hyperketonemia in childhood, but causes no symptoms at all in adults (Sjarif et al. 2000).

GKD deficiency is usually diagnosed when organic acid analysis detects a large peak of glycerol in a patient being investigated for signs and symptoms due to deficiency of one of the adjacent genes or during evaluation for pseudohypertriglycerolemia. Subsequent investigations will vary depending on how and why it was detected. The enzyme defect is easily demonstrated in many tissues, including leukocytes and cultured fibroblasts, and molecular analysis of the *GKD* gene is also available.

Plasma glycerol in GKD deficiency is 1.8–8.3 mmol/L (normal <0.27), and in urine is 90–193 mmol/mmol creat (normal = not detected); the latter is sufficiently high to be seen on organic acid analysis despite its being poorly extracted into organic solvents. Increased urine glycerol may not be detected in the acidic fraction prepared by ion-exchange chromatography but will be seen instead in the neutral fraction. Further, glyceroluria due to GKD deficiency must be distinguished from that due to glycerol in a variety of oral, rectal, and intravenously administered medications, as well as direct glycerol contamination of blood and urine specimens.

## Methionine Adenosyltransferase Deficiency

The initial reaction in the transsulfuration pathway through which methionine is converted to homocysteine and cysteine is the formation of S-adenosylmethionine (AdoMet) by methionine adenosyltransferase. Over 60 patients with inherited deficiency of this enzyme are known, many of them detected by high serum methionine on newborn screening. Most of these patients have remained free of symptoms, and the condition has long been thought to be benign (Gaull et al. 1981). The latter may not be true in all instances, as a few patients with more severe enzyme deficiencies have developed demyelinating disorders.

Plasma methionine in methionine adenosyltransferase deficiency can be as high as 2500 μM (normal <50), and, when detected, other causes of hypermethioninemia such as metabolic liver disease, tyrosinemia type I, cystathionine β-synthase deficiency, glycine N-methyltransferase deficiency, and citrin deficiency must be excluded (Mudd 2011).

Although the diagnosis is usually arrived at by exclusion, diagnosis can be confirmed by enzyme assay on the liver or by molecular analysis of *MAT1A*, which encodes the catalytic subunit of the two isoenzymes of methionine adenosyltransferase in the mammalian liver. Most of the mutations identified to date are transmitted as autosomal recessives, but one, p.Arg264His, causes reduced activity even when heterozygous and can cause the occasional situation in which hypermethioninemia is transmitted as an autosomal dominant (Blom et al. 1992).

## Methylmalonyl-CoA Epimerase Deficiency

Inherited methylmalonic acidemia is usually due to decreased conversion of L-methylmalonyl-CoA to succinyl-CoA by methylmalonyl-CoA mutase; in some cases this is due to mutations of the *MUT* gene, which encodes the mutase, and in others it is due to defects in the biosynthesis of adenosylcobalamin, the mutase cofactor (Chap. 28). Very rarely, however, methylmalonic acidemia is due to deficiency of the epimerase (or racemase) responsible for the interconversion of D- and L-methylmalonyl-CoA.

Three individuals in two families have been reported with mild methylmalonic acidemia(uria) due to homozygosity for a nonsense mutation (p.Arg47Ter) in the *MCEE* gene (Bikker et al. 2006; Dobson et al. 2006). The lone patient in one family was a girl who at age 2 years had retarded motor development and signs of spasticity, possibly because she also had sepiapterin reductase deficiency (Bikker et al. 2006). There were two siblings in the other family: a girl who presented at 1 year of age with a single episode of severe ketoacidosis and who then remained symptom-free on daily hydroxycobalamin (1 mg po) and an older sister with congenital hydrocephalus, normal development, and no symptoms of metabolic disease.

Urine methylmalonic acid in these patients has been as high as 1500 mmol/mol creatinine (normal <10) but decreased considerably with age to approx. 50 mmol/mol creatinine. Suppression of gene expression in HeLa cells led only to a small reduction in pathway activity, suggesting that nonenzymatic conversion of D- to L- isomer contributes to flux through the pathway and perhaps explaining the relatively mild organic aciduria and symptoms even with a truncating mutation.

It now appears that epimerase deficiency is a relatively rare cause of methylmalonic aciduria and, since the diagnosis might have prognostic significance, molecular analysis of the *MMCE* gene may well become more widely used when evaluating patients detected in newborn screening programs.

## SCAD Deficiency

Short-chain acyl-CoA dehydrogenase (SCAD) is one of the four chain length-specific acyl-CoA dehydrogenases involved in mitochondrial β-oxidation of fatty acids. Hexanoyl- and butyryl-CoA are its preferred substrates, and, like other members of the enzyme family, electrons from the enzyme flavin enter the respiratory chain at the level of coenzyme Q, and secondary SCAD deficiency therefore occurs in multiple acyl-CoA dehydrogenase deficiency. Like most of the other acyl-CoA dehydrogenases, the mature enzyme is in the mitochondrial matrix and exists as a tetramer of four identical subunits.

While inherited deficiencies of medium- and very long-chain acyl-CoA dehydrogenase cause clinical disease in most instances, it now appears that SCAD deficiency rarely if ever causes symptoms.

SCAD deficiency was initially identified in patients with carnitine deficiency and a variety of neurological or skeletal muscle problems (Roe and Ding 2001). Urine organic acid analysis often showed increased ethylmalonic acid, methylsuccinic acid and/or butyrylglycine, and acylcarnitine analysis an increase in the C4 ester. The diagnosis could be confirmed by enzyme assays on muscle or cultured fibroblasts, followed by identifying pathogenic mutations in the *ACADS* gene, and, while pathogenesis defied easy explanation, it was generally thought that SCAD deficiency caused disease in most instances but that the clinical phenotype was very diverse.

Follow-up of patients identified by newborn screening with tandem mass spectrometry has provided a quite different perspective. Newborn screening programs in Australia (Wilcken et al. 2009) and Massachusetts (Waisbren et al. 2008) have followed SCAD-deficient infants detected on the basis of an elevated C4 acylcarnitine in newborn blood spots and have found that most of them grow and develop normally. And in those that do not, a clinical disease can often be attributed to another cause. These data, which suggest that SCAD deficiency does not cause disease in the great majority of cases, have led several programs to stop screening for the disorder.

A diagnosis should not be made unless ethylmalonic encephalopathy and multiple acyl-CoA dehydrogenation defect (glutaric acidemia type II) have been excluded. While patients with the latter conditions often have additional organic acids, glycine esters, and carnitine esters in blood and urine, a molecular analysis of the relevant genes may be necessary to arrive at the proper diagnosis.

## Signs and Symptoms

**Table 71.1** Iminoglycinuria

| System | Symptoms and biomarkers | Neonatal (birth–1 month) | Infancy (1–18 months) | Childhood (1.5–11 years) | Adolescence (11–16 years) | Adulthood (>16 years) |
|---|---|---|---|---|---|---|
| Other | No clinical significance | + | + | + | + | + |
| Laboratory findings | Glycine (urine) | ↑ | ↑ | ↑ | ↑ | ↑ |
| | Hydroxyproline (urine) | ↑ | ↑ | ↑ | ↑ | ↑ |
| | Proline (urine) | ↑ | ↑ | ↑ | ↑ | ↑ |

**Table 71.2** Hyperprolinemia type I

| System | Symptoms and biomarkers | Neonatal (birth–1 month) | Infancy (1–18 months) | Childhood (1.5–11 years) | Adolescence (11–16 years) | Adulthood (>16 years) |
|---|---|---|---|---|---|---|
| Other | No clinical significance | + | + | + | + | + |
| Laboratory findings | Glycine (urine) | n-↑ | n-↑ | n-↑ | n-↑ | n-↑ |
| | Hydroxyproline (urine) | n-↑ | n-↑ | n-↑ | n-↑ | n-↑ |
| | Proline (urine) | n-↑ | n-↑ | n-↑ | n-↑ | n-↑ |
| | Proline (plasma) | ↑↑ | ↑↑ | ↑↑ | ↑↑ | ↑↑ |

**Table 71.3** Hydroxyproline dehydrogenase deficiency

| System | Symptoms and biomarkers | Neonatal (birth–1 month) | Infancy (1–18 months) | Childhood (1.5–11 years) | Adolescence (11–16 years) | Adulthood (>16 years) |
|---|---|---|---|---|---|---|
| Other | No clinical significance | + | + | + | + | + |
| Laboratory findings | Hydroxyproline (plasma) | ↑ | ↑ | ↑ | ↑ | ↑ |
| | Hydroxyproline (urine) | ↑ | ↑ | ↑ | ↑ | ↑ |

**Table 71.4** Histidinemia

| System | Symptoms and biomarkers | Neonatal (birth–1 month) | Infancy (1–18 months) | Childhood (1.5–11 years) | Adolescence (11–16 years) | Adulthood (>16 years) |
|---|---|---|---|---|---|---|
| Other | No clinical significance | + | + | + | + | + |
| Laboratory findings | Histidase (fibroblasts) | ↓ | ↓ | ↓ | ↓ | ↓ |
| | Histidine (plasma) | ↑ | ↑ | ↑ | ↑ | ↑ |
| | Histidine (urine) | ↑ | ↑ | ↑ | ↑ | ↑ |
| | Histidine (cerebrospinal fluid) | ↑ | ↑ | ↑ | ↑ | ↑ |
| | Imidazole pyruvic acid (urine) | ↑ | ↑ | ↑ | ↑ | ↑ |
| | Ketones (urine) | | + | + | + | + |

**Table 71.5** Urocanase deficiency

| System | Symptoms and biomarkers | Neonatal (birth–1 month) | Infancy (1–18 months) | Childhood (1.5–11 years) | Adolescence (11–16 years) | Adulthood (>16 years) |
|---|---|---|---|---|---|---|
| Other | No clinical significance | + | + | + | + | + |
| Laboratory findings | Urocanic acid (urine) | ↑ | ↑ | ↑ | ↑ | ↑ |
| | Urocanoylglycine (urine) | ↑ | ↑ | ↑ | ↑ | ↑ |

**Table 71.6** Glutamate formimino transferase deficiency

| System | Symptoms and biomarkers | Neonatal (birth–1 month) | Infancy (1–18 months) | Childhood (1.5–11 years) | Adolescence (11–16 years) | Adulthood (>16 years) |
|---|---|---|---|---|---|---|
| Other | No clinical significance | + | + | + | + | + |
| Laboratory findings | Formiminoglutamic acid, FIGLU (urine) | ↑ | ↑ | ↑ | ↑ | ↑ |
| | Hydantoin-5-propionic acid (urine) | ↑ | ↑ | ↑ | ↑ | ↑ |

**Table 71.7** Carnosinemia and homocarnosinosis

| System | Symptoms and biomarkers | Neonatal (birth–1 month) | Infancy (1–18 months) | Childhood (1.5–11 years) | Adolescence (11–16 years) | Adulthood (>16 years) |
|---|---|---|---|---|---|---|
| Other | No clinical significance | + | + | + | + | + |
| Laboratory findings | Anserine (urine) | ↑ | ↑ | ↑ | ↑ | ↑ |
| | Carnosine (plasma) | ↑ | ↑ | ↑ | ↑ | ↑ |
| | Carnosine (urine) | ↑ | ↑ | ↑ | ↑ | ↑ |
| | Homocarnosine (cerebrospinal fluid) | ↑ | ↑ | ↑ | ↑ | ↑ |

**Table 71.8** Trimethylaminuria

| System | Symptoms and biomarkers | Neonatal (birth–1 month) | Infancy (1–18 months) | Childhood (1.5–11 years) | Adolescence (11–16 years) | Adulthood (>16 years) |
|---|---|---|---|---|---|---|
| Other | **Fish odor (urine)** | + | + | + | + | + |
| | No clinical significance | + | + | + | + | + |
| Laboratory findings | Trimethylamine (urine) | ↑ | ↑ | ↑ | ↑ | ↑ |
| | TMAO/TMA ratio (urine) | ↓ | ↓ | ↓ | ↓ | ↓ |

**Table 71.9** Dimethylglycinuria

| System | Symptoms and biomarkers | Neonatal (birth–1 month) | Infancy (1–18 months) | Childhood (1.5–11 years) | Adolescence (11–16 years) | Adulthood (>16 years) |
|---|---|---|---|---|---|---|
| Other | **Fish odor (urine)** | | | | | + |
| | No clinical significance | + | + | + | + | |
| Laboratory findings | Dimethylglycine (urine) | | | | | ↑ |
| | Dimethylglycine (plasma) | | | | | ↑ |

**Table 71.10** Sarcosinemia

| System | Symptoms and biomarkers | Neonatal (birth–1 month) | Infancy (1–18 months) | Childhood (1.5–11 years) | Adolescence (11–16 years) | Adulthood (>16 years) |
|---|---|---|---|---|---|---|
| Other | **No clinical significance** | + | + | + | + | + |
| Laboratory findings | Sarcosine (plasma) | ↑ | ↑ | ↑ | ↑ | ↑ |
| | Sarcosine (urine) | ↑ | ↑ | ↑ | ↑ | ↑ |

**Table 71.11** Hyperlysinemia and saccharopinuria

| System | Symptoms and biomarkers | Neonatal (birth–1 month) | Infancy (1–18 months) | Childhood (1.5–11 years) | Adolescence (11–16 years) | Adulthood (>16 years) |
|---|---|---|---|---|---|---|
| Other | **No clinical significance** | + | + | + | + | + |
| Laboratory findings | Homocitrulline (urine) | n-↑ | n-↑ | n-↑ | n-↑ | n-↑ |
| | Lysine (cerebrospinal fluid) | ↑ | ↑ | ↑ | ↑ | ↑ |
| | Lysine (plasma) | ↑ | ↑ | ↑ | ↑ | ↑ |
| | Lysine (urine) | ↑ | ↑ | ↑ | ↑ | ↑ |
| | N-acetyl-lysine (urine) | n-↑ | n-↑ | n-↑ | n-↑ | n-↑ |
| | Saccharopine (cerebrospinal fluid) | ↑ | ↑ | ↑ | ↑ | ↑ |
| | Saccharopine (plasma) | ↑ | ↑ | ↑ | ↑ | ↑ |
| | Saccharopine (urine) | ↑ | ↑ | ↑ | ↑ | ↑ |

**Table 71.12** 2-Ketoadipic aciduria

| System | Symptoms and biomarkers | Neonatal (birth–1 month) | Infancy (1–18 months) | Childhood (1.5–11 years) | Adolescence (11–16 years) | Adulthood (>16 years) |
|---|---|---|---|---|---|---|
| Other | No clinical significance | ± | ± | ± | ± | ± |
| CNS | Developmental delay | | ± | ± | | |
| | Seizures | | ± | ± | | |
| Metabolic | Metabolic acidosis | | ± | ± | | |
| Laboratory findings | 2-Aminoadipate (urine) | | ↑ | ↑ | | |
| | 2-Hydroxyadipate (urine) | | ↑ | ↑ | | |
| | 2-Ketoadipate (urine) | | ↑ | ↑ | | |
| | 3-Hydroxyglutaric acid (urine) | | ↑ | ↑ | | |
| | 3-Hydroxyisovaleric acid (urine) | | ↑ | ↑ | | |
| | 3-Methylglutaconic acid (urine) | | ↑ | ↑ | | |
| | Dicarboxylic acids (urine) | | ↑ | ↑ | | |
| | Ethylmalonic acid (urine) | | n-↑ | n-↑ | | |
| | Ketones, during hypoglycemia | | + | + | | |

**Table 71.13** Glutaric aciduria type 3

| System | Symptoms and biomarkers | Neonatal (birth–1 month) | Infancy (1–18 months) | Childhood (1.5–11 years) | Adolescence (11–16 years) | Adulthood (>16 years) |
|---|---|---|---|---|---|---|
| Other | No clinical significance | + | + | + | + | + |
| Laboratory findings | 3-Hydroxyglutaric acid (urine) | n | n | n | n | n |
| | Glutaric acid (plasma) | ↑ | ↑ | ↑ | ↑ | ↑ |
| | Glutaric acid (urine) | ↑ | ↑ | ↑ | ↑ | ↑ |

**Table 71.14** 3-Hydroxykynureninase deficiency

| System | Symptoms and biomarkers | Neonatal (birth–1 month) | Infancy (1–18 months) | Childhood (1.5–11 years) | Adolescence (11–16 years) | Adulthood (>16 years) |
|---|---|---|---|---|---|---|
| Other | No clinical significance | ± | ± | ± | ± | ± |
| Laboratory findings | 3-Hydroxykynurenine (urine) | | ↑ | ↑ | ↑ | |
| | 3-Hydroxykynurenine; 3HK (plasma) | ↑ | ↑ | | | |
| | Kynurenine (urine) | | ↑ | ↑ | ↑ | |
| | NAD+ (plasma) | ↓ | ↓ | | | |
| | Xanthurenic acid (urine) | | ↑ | ↑ | ↑ | |

**Table 71.15** Cystathionase deficiency

| System | Symptoms and biomarkers | Neonatal (birth–1 month) | Infancy (1–18 months) | Childhood (1.5–11 years) | Adolescence (11–16 years) | Adulthood (>16 years) |
|---|---|---|---|---|---|---|
| Other | No clinical significance | + | + | + | + | + |
| Laboratory findings | Cystathionine (plasma) | ↑↑↑ | ↑↑↑ | ↑↑↑ | ↑↑↑ | ↑↑↑ |
| | Cystathionine (urine) | ↑↑↑ | ↑↑↑ | ↑↑↑ | ↑↑↑ | ↑↑↑ |
| | Cysteine (plasma) | n | n | n | n | n |
| | Homocysteine, total (plasma) | n-↑ | n-↑ | n-↑ | n-↑ | n-↑ |
| | Methionine-to-cystathionine ratio (plasma) | ↓↓ | ↓↓ | ↓↓ | ↓↓ | ↓↓ |

**Table 71.16** 3-Methylcrotonylglycinuria

| System | Symptoms and biomarkers | Neonatal (birth–1 month) | Infancy (1–18 months) | Childhood (1.5–11 years) | Adolescence (11–16 years) | Adulthood (>16 years) |
|---|---|---|---|---|---|---|
| Other | No clinical significance | + | + | + | + | |
| Laboratory findings | 3-Hydroxyisovaleric acid (urine) | ↑-↑↑↑ | ↑-↑↑↑ | ↑-↑↑↑ | ↑-↑↑↑ | ↑-↑↑↑ |
| | 3-Methylcrotonylcarnitine | n-↑↑ | n-↑↑ | n-↑↑ | n-↑↑ | n-↑↑ |
| | 3-Methylcrotonylglycine (urine) | ↑-↑↑↑ | ↑-↑↑↑ | ↑-↑↑↑ | ↑-↑↑↑ | ↑-↑↑↑ |
| | Ammonia (blood) | n-↑ | n-↑ | n-↑ | n-↑ | n-↑ |
| | Anion gap | ± | ± | ± | ± | ± |
| | ASAT/ALAT (plasma) | n-↑ | n-↑ | n-↑ | n-↑ | n-↑ |
| | Base excess | ± | ± | ± | ± | ± |
| | C5-OH Acylcarnitine (dried blood spot) | ↑-↑↑↑ | ↑-↑↑↑ | ↑-↑↑↑ | ↑-↑↑↑ | ↑-↑↑↑ |
| | C5-OH Acylcarnitine (plasma) | ↑-↑↑↑ | ↑-↑↑↑ | ↑-↑↑↑ | ↑-↑↑↑ | ↑-↑↑↑ |
| | Carnitine, esterified (plasma) | n-↑ | n-↑ | n-↑ | n-↑ | n-↑ |
| | Carnitine, free (dried blood spot) | ↓-n | ↓-n | ↓-n | ↓-n | ↓-n |
| | Carnitine, free (plasma) | ↓-n | ↓-n | ↓-n | ↓-n | ↓-n |
| | Glucose (plasma) | ↓-n | ↓-n | ↓-n | ↓-n | ↓-n |
| | Methylcrotonyl-CoA carboxylase (fibroblasts) | ↓ | ↓ | ↓ | ↓ | ↓ |
| | Uric acid (plasma) | n-↑ | n-↑ | n-↑ | n-↑ | n-↑ |

**Table 71.17** 2-Methylbutyrylglycinuria

| System | Symptoms and biomarkers | Neonatal (birth–1 month) | Infancy (1–18 months) | Childhood (1.5–11 years) | Adolescence (11–16 years) | Adulthood (>16 years) |
|---|---|---|---|---|---|---|
| Other | No clinical significance | ± | ± | ± | ± | ± |
| Laboratory findings | 2-Ethylhydracrylic acid (blood) | n-↑ | n-↑ | n-↑ | n-↑ | n-↑ |
| | 2-Ethylhydracrylic acid (plasma) | n-↑ | n-↑ | n-↑ | n-↑ | n-↑ |
| | 2-Methylbutyric acid (urine) | ↑↑ | ↑↑ | ↑↑ | ↑↑ | ↑↑ |
| | 2-Methylbutyryl-CoA dehydrogenase (fibroblasts) | ↓ | ↓ | ↓ | ↓ | ↓ |
| | 2-Methylbutyrylglycine (urine) | ↑↑ | ↑↑ | ↑↑ | ↑↑ | ↑↑ |
| | Anion gap | ± | ± | ± | ± | ± |
| | C5 2-Methylbutyrylcarnitine (blood) | ↑-↑↑ | ↑-↑↑ | ↑-↑↑ | ↑-↑↑ | ↑-↑↑ |
| | C5 2-Methylbutyrylcarnitine (plasma) | ↑-↑↑ | ↑-↑↑ | ↑-↑↑ | ↑-↑↑ | ↑-↑↑ |
| | C5/C2 Acylcarnitines ratio | ↑ | ↑ | ↑ | ↑ | ↑ |
| | Glucose (plasma) | ↓-n | ↓-n | ↓-n | | |
| | Isobutyrylglycine (urine) | n-↑ | n-↑ | n-↑ | n-↑ | n-↑ |

**Table 71.18** Oxoprolinuria

| System | Symptoms and biomarkers | Neonatal (birth–1 month) | Infancy (1–18 months) | Childhood (1.5–11 years) | Adolescence (11–16 years) | Adulthood (>16 years) |
|---|---|---|---|---|---|---|
| Other | No clinical significance | + | + | + | + | |
| CNS | Retardation, psychomotor | ± | ± | ± | ± | ± |
| Laboratory findings | 5-Oxoproline (urine) | ↑ | ↑ | ↑ | ↑ | ↑ |
| | 5-Oxoprolinase (fibroblasts) | ↓ | ↓ | ↓ | ↓ | ↓ |
| | 5-Oxoprolinase (white blood cells) | ↓ | ↓ | ↓ | ↓ | ↓ |

**Table 71.19** Glycerol kinase deficiency

| System | Symptoms and biomarkers | Neonatal (birth–1 month) | Infancy (1–18 months) | Childhood (1.5–11 years) | Adolescence (11–16 years) | Adulthood (>16 years) |
|---|---|---|---|---|---|---|
| Other | No clinical significance | + | + | + | + | |
| Laboratory findings | Glucose (plasma) | ↓-n | ↓-n | ↓-n | ↓-n | ↓-n |
| | Glycerol (plasma) | ↑ | ↑ | ↑ | ↑ | ↑ |
| | Glycerol (urine) | ↑ | ↑ | ↑ | ↑ | ↑ |
| | Triglyceride, pseudo (plasma) | ↑ | ↑ | ↑ | ↑ | ↑ |

**Table 71.20** Methionine adenosyltransferase deficiency

| System | Symptoms and biomarkers | Neonatal (birth–1 month) | Infancy (1–18 months) | Childhood (1.5–11 years) | Adolescence (11–16 years) | Adulthood (>16 years) |
|---|---|---|---|---|---|---|
| Other | No clinical significance | + | + | + | + | |
| Laboratory findings | Methionine (plasma) | ↑ | ↑ | ↑ | ↑ | |

**Table 71.21** Methylmalonyl-CoA epimerase deficiency

| System | Symptoms and biomarkers | Neonatal (birth–1 month) | Infancy (1–18 months) | Childhood (1.5–11 years) | Adolescence (11–16 years) | Adulthood (>16 years) |
|---|---|---|---|---|---|---|
| Other | No clinical significance | + | + | + | + | |
| Laboratory findings | Methylmalonic acid (urine) | ↑ | ↑ | ↑ | ↑ | |

**Table 71.22** Short-chain acyl CoA dehydrogenase deficiency

| System | Symptoms and biomarkers | Neonatal (birth–1 month) | Infancy (1–18 months) | Childhood (1.5–11 years) | Adolescence (11–16 years) | Adulthood (>16 years) |
|---|---|---|---|---|---|---|
| Other | No clinical significance | + | + | + | + | |
| | Predisposition for symptomatic disease | + | + | + | + | + |
| | Second mitochondrial affection | + | + | + | + | + |
| Laboratory findings | Butyrylglycine (urine) | n-↑ | n-↑ | n-↑ | n-↑ | n-↑ |
| | C4 Butyrylcarnitine (blood) | ↑ | ↑ | ↑ | ↑ | ↑ |
| | C4 Butyrylcarnitine (plasma) | ↑ | ↑ | ↑ | ↑ | ↑ |
| | C4-Acylcarnitine (dried blood spot) | ↑ | ↑ | ↑ | ↑ | ↑ |
| | C4-Acylcarnitine (plasma) | ↑ | ↑ | ↑ | ↑ | ↑ |
| | Ethylmalonic acid (urine) | ↑↑ | ↑↑ | ↑↑ | ↑ | n-↑ |
| | Glucose (plasma) | ↓-n | ↓-n | ↓-n | | |
| | Methylsuccinic acid (urine) | ↑ | ↑ | ↑ | ↑ | ↑ |
| | Short-chain acyl-CoA dehydrogenase (fibroblasts) | ↓ | ↓ | ↓ | ↓ | ↓ |

## Concluding Remarks

The list of inborn errors of questionable clinical significance provided is almost certainly incomplete, as future clinical studies of patients detected by selective or newborn screening will show that some disorders do in fact cause disease in some patients, and that others do not. Further, newer diagnostic methods like whole genome analysis or exome sequencing will add novel disorders to the mix, and these too will have to undergo intensive analysis to decide if they are indeed clinically relevant.

## References


Alfardan J, Al-Walid M, Copeland S, et al. Characterization of new ACADSB gene sequence mutations and clinical implications in patients with 2-methylbutyrylglycinuria identified by newborn screening. Mol Genet Metab. 2010;100:333–8.

Almaghlouth IA, Mohamed JY, Al-Amoudi M, et al. 5-Oxoprolinase deficiency: report of the first human *OPLAH* mutation. Clin Genet. 2011; https://doi.org/10.1111/j.1399-0004.2011.01728.x.

Andresen BS, Christensen E, Corydon TJ, et al. Isolated 2-methylbutyrylglycinuria caused by short/branched chain acyl-CoA dehydrogenase deficiency: identification of a new enzyme defect, resolution of its molecular basis, and evidence for distinct acyl-CoA dehydrogenases in isoleucine and valine metabolism. Am J Hum Genet. 2000;67:1095–103.

Arnold GL, Koeberl DD, Matern D, et al. A Delphi-based consensus clinical practice protocol for the diagnosis and management of 3-methylcrotonyl CoA carboxylase deficiency. Mol Genet Metab. 2008;93:363–70.

Bar-Joseph I, Pras E, Reznik-Wolf H, et al. Mutations in the sarcosine dehydrogenase gene in patients with sarcosinemia. Hum Genet. 2012;131:1805–10.

Bennett MJ, Pollitt RJ, Goodman SI, et al. Atypical riboflavin-responsive glutaric aciduria, and deficient peroxisomal glutaryl-CoA oxidase activity: a new peroxisomal disorder. J Inherit Metab Dis. 1991;14:165–73.

Bikker H, Bakker HD, Abeling NGGM, et al. A homozygous nonsense mutation in the methylmalonyl-CoA epimerase gene (MCEE) results in mild methylmalonic aciduria. Hum Mutat. 2006;27:640–3.

Binzak BA, Wevers RA, Moolenaar SH, et al. Cloning of dimethylglycine dehydrogenase and a new human inborn error of metabolism, dimethylglycine dehydrogenase deficiency. Am J Hum Genet. 2001;68:839–47.

Blom HJ, Davidson AJ, Finkelstein JD, et al. Persistent hypermethioninemia with dominant inheritance. J Inherit Metab Dis. 1992;15:188–97.

Carson NAJ, Scally BG, Neill DW, Carre IJ. Saccharopinuria—a new inborn error of lysine metabolism. Nature. 1968;218:679.

Christensen M, Duno M, Lund AM, et al. Xanthurenic aciduria due to a mutation in *KYNU* encoding kynureninase. J Inherit Metab Dis. 2007;30:248–55.

Crawhall JC, Parker R, Sneddon W, et al. Beta mercaptolactate-cysteine disulfide: Analog of cystine in the urine of a mentally retarded patient. Science. 1968;160:419–20.

Dancis J, Hutzler J, Ampola MG, et al. The prognosis of hyperlysinemia: an interim report. Am J Hum Genet. 1983;35:438–42.

Danhauser K, Sauer SW, Haack TB, et al. *DHTKD1* mutations cause 2-aminoadipic and 2-oxoadipic aciduria. Am J Hum Genet. 2012;91:1082–7.

Dobson CM, Gradinger A, Longo N, et al. Homozygous nonsense mutation in the MCEE gene and sRNA suppression of methylmalonyl-CoA epimerase expression: a novel cause of methylmalonic aciduria. Mol Genet Metab. 2006;88:327–33.

Dorland L, Duran M, de Bree PK, et al. O-Phosphohydroxylysinuria: a new inborn error of metabolism. Clin Chim Acta. 1990;188:221–6.

Efron ML. Familial hyperprolinemia: report of a second case associated with congenital renal malformations, hereditary hematuria, and mild mental retardation, with demonstration of an enzyme defect. N Engl J Med. 1965;272:1243–54.

Efron ML, Bixby EM, Palattao LG, Pryles CV. Hydroxyprolinemia associated with mental deficiency. N Engl J Med. 1962;267:1193–4.

Elpeleg ON, Christensen E, Hurvitz H, Branski D. Recurrent, familial Reye-like syndrome with a new complex amino and organic aciduria. Eur J Pediatr. 1990;149:709–12.

Espinós C, Pineda M, Martinez-Rubio D, et al. Mutations in the urocanase gene (UROC1) are associated with urocanic aciduria. J Med Genet. 2009;46:407–11.

Fontaine G, Farriaux JP, Dautrevaux M. Type I hyperprolinemia. Study of a familial case. Helv Paediatr Acta. 1970;25:165–75.

Gaull GE, Tallan HH, Lonsdale D, et al. Hypermethioninemia associated with methionine adenosyltransferase deficiency: clinical, morphologic, and biochemical obervations on four patients. J Pediatr. 1981;98:734–41.

Gerritsen T, Waisman HA. Hypersarcosinemia: an inborn error of metabolism. N Engl J Med. 1966;275:66–9.

Ghadimi H, Partington W, Hunter A. A familial disturbance of histidine metabolism. N Engl J Med. 1961;265:221–4.

Goodman SI, Browder JA, Hiles RA, Miles BS. Hydroxylysinemia, a disorder due to a defect in the metabolism of free hydroxylysine. Biochem Med. 1972;6:344–54.

Goodman SI, Mace JW, Miles BS, et al. Defective hydroxyproline metabolism in type II hyperprolinemia. Biochem Med. 1974;10:329–36.

Guggenheim MA, McCabe ERB, Roig M, et al. Glycerol kinase deficiency with neuromuscular, skeletal, and adrenal abnormalities. Ann Neurol. 1980;7:441–9.

Hagen J, te Brink H, Wanders RJ, et al. Genetic basis of alpha-aminoadipic and alpha-ketoadipic aciduria. J Inherit Metab Dis. 2015;38:873–9.

Harris H, Penrose LS, Thomas DHH. Cystathioninuria. Ann Hum Genet. 1959;23:442–53.

Hernandez D, Addou S, Lee D, et al. Trimethylaminuria and a human FMO3 mutation database. Hum Mutat. 2003;22:209–13.

Hilton JF, Christensen KE, Watkins D, et al. The molecular basis of glutamate formiminotransferase deficiency. Hum Mutat. 2003;22:67–73.

Hirashima M, Hayakawa T, Koike M. Mammalian alpha-keto acid dehydrogenase complexes. II. An improved procedure for the preparation of 2-oxoglutarate dehydrogenase complex from pig heart muscle. J Biol Chem. 1967;242(5):902–7.

Houten SM, Denis S, Te Brinke H, Jongejan A, van Kampen AH, Bradley EJ, Baas F, Hennekam RC, Millington DS, Young SP, Frazier DM, Gucsavas-Calikoglu M, Wanders R. Mitochondrial NADP(H) deficiency due to a mutation in NADK2 causes dienoyl-CoA reductase deficiency with hyperlysinemia. Hum Mol Genet. 2014;23(18):5009–16.

Huang CS, Sadre-Bazzaz K, Shen Y, et al. Crystal structure of the alpha(6)beta(6) holoenzyme of propionyl-coenzyme a carboxylase. Nature. 2010;466:1001–5.

Ishikawa M. Developmental disorders in histidinemia: follow-up study of language development in histidinemia. Acta Paediatr Jpn. 1987;29:224–8.

Johnson DW. A flow injection electrospray ionization tandem mass spectrometric method for the simultaneous measurement of trimethylamine and trimethylamine N-oxide in urine. J Mass Spectrom. 2008;43:495–9.

Kawai Y, Moriyama A, Asai K, et al. Molecular characterization of histidinemia: identification of four missense mutations. Hum Genet. 2005;116:340–6.

Kim SZ, Varvogli L, Waisbren SE, Levy HL. Hydroxyprolinemia: comparison of a patient and her unaffected twin sister. J Pediatr. 1997;130:437–41.

Komrower GM, Wilson V, Clamp JR, Westall RG. Hydroxykynureninuria, a case of abnormal tryptophan metabolism probably due to a deficiency of kynureninase. Arch Dis Child. 1964;39:250–6.

Kuracka L, Kalnovicova T, Liska B, Turcani P. HPLC method for measurement of purine nucleotide degradation products in cerebrospinal fluid. Clin Chem. 1996;42:756–60.

Larsson A, Mattsson B, Wauters EA, et al. 5-Oxoprolinuria due to hereditary 5-oxoprolinase deficiency in two brothers—a new inborn error of the gamma-glutamyl cycle. Acta Paediatr Scand. 1981;70:301–8.

Levy HL, Coulombe JT, Benjamin R. Massachusetts metabolic disorders screening program: III. Sarcosinemia. Pediatrics. 1984;74:509–13.

Malvagia S, La Marca G, Casetta B, et al. Falsely elevated C4-carnitine as expression of glutamate formiminotransferase deficiency in tandem mass spectrometry newborn screening. J Mass Spectrom. 2006;41:263–5.

McCabe ERB. Disorders of glycerol metabolism. In: Scriver CR, Beaudet AL, Sly WS, Valle D, editors. The metabolic and molecular bases of inherited disease. 8th ed. New York: McGraw-Hill; 2001. p. 2217–37.

Moolenaar SH, Poggi-Bach J, Engelke UF, et al. Defect in dimethylglycine dehydrogenase, a new inborn error of metabolism: NMR spectroscopy study. Clin Chem. 1999;45:459–64.

Mourmans J, Bakkeren J, de Jong J, et al. Isolated (biotin-resistant) 3-methylcrotonyl-CoA carboxylase deficiency: four sibs devoid of pathology. J Inherit Metab Dis. 1995;18:643–5.

Mudd SH. Hypermethioninemias of genetic and non-genetic origin: a review. Am J Med Genet C Semin Med Genet. 2011;157:3–32.

Mudd SH, Levy HL, Kraus JP. Disorders of transsulfuration. In: Scriver CR, Beaudet AL, Valle D, Sly WS, editors. The metabolic and molecular bases of inherited disease. 8th ed. New York: McGraw-Hill; 2001. p. 2007–56.

Perry TL, Hansen S, Tischler B, et al. Carnosinemia: a new metabolic disorder associated with neurologic disease and mental defect. N Engl J Med. 1967;277:1219–27.

Roe CR, Ding J. Mitochondrial fatty acid oxidation disorders. In: Scriver CR, Beaudet AL, Sly WS, Valle D, editors. The metabolic and molecular bases of inherited disease. 8th ed. New York: McGraw-Hill; 2001. p. 2297–326.

Schafer IA, Scriver CR, Efron ML. Familial hyperprolinemia, cerebral dysfunction and renal anomalies occurring in a family with hereditary nephritis and deafness. N Engl J Med. 1962;267:51–60.

Sherman EA, Strauss KA, Tortorelli S, et al. Genetic mapping of glutaric aciduria, type 3, to chromosome 7 and identification of mutations in C7orf10. Am J Hum Genet. 2008;83:604–9.

Sjaastad O, Blau N, Rydning SL, et al. Homocarnosinosis: a historical update and findings in the *SPG11* gene. Acta Neurol Scand. 2018;138:245–50.

Sjarif D, Dorland L, Sperl W, et al. Hyperketonaemia in glycerol kinase deficiency. J Inherit Metab Dis. 2000;23:760–4.

Stiles AR, Venturoni L, Mucci G, et al. New cases of *DHTKD1* mutations in patients with 2-ketoadipic aciduria. JIMD Rep. 2016;25:15–9.

Teufel M, Saudek V, Ledig J-P, et al. Sequence identification and characterization of human carnosinase and a closely related non-specific dipeptidase. J Biol Chem. 2003;278:6521–31.

Waisbren SE, Levy HL, Noble M, et al. Short-chain acyl-CoA dehydrogenase (SCAD) deficiency: an examination of the medical and neurodevelopmental characteristics of 14 cases identified through newborn screening or clinical symptoms. Mol Genet Metab. 2008;95:39–45.

Wang J, Hegele RA. Genomic basis of cystathioninuria (MIM 219500) revealed by multiple mutations in cystathionine gamma-lyase (CTH). Hum Genet. 2003;112:404–8.

Wilcken B, Haas M, Joy P, et al. Expanded newborn screening: outcome in screened and unscreened patients at age 6 years. Pediatrics. 2009;124:e241–8.

Wolfe LA, Finegold DN, Vockley J, et al. Potential misdiagnosis of 3-methylcrotonyl-coenzyme a carboxylase deficiency associated with absent or trace urinary 3-methylcrotonylglycine. Pediatrics. 2007;120:e1335–40.

Woody NC. Hyperlysinemia. Am J Dis Child. 1964;108:543–53.

Xu WY, Gu MM, Sun LH, et al. A nonsense mutation in *DHTKD1* causes Charcot-Marie-tooth disease type 2 in a large Chinese pedigree. Am J Hum Genet. 2012;91:1088–94.

Xu WY, Zhu H, Shen Y, et al. DHTKD1 deficiency causes Charcot-Marie-tooth disease in mice. Mol Cell Biol. 2018;38:e00085–18.

# Knowledge Base of Inborn Errors of Metabolism (IEMbase): A Practical Approach

# 72

Tamar V. Av-Shalom, Jessica J. Y. Lee, Carlos R. Ferreira, Nenad Blau, Clara D. M. van Karnebeek, and Wyeth W. Wasserman

## Contents




### Summary

Here we give an overview of the inborn errors of metabolism knowledge base, or IEMbase, a comprehensive electronic repository of the IEMs described in this book. Developed as a companion application to this textbook, IEMbase provides two key functions: first, it is a free and openly available repository of the features characterizing the different IEMs; second, it has an artificial intelligence (AI) search tool to aid the diagnosis of IEMs. Given the highly specialized knowledge necessary to accurately diagnose IEMs and the necessity for timely diagnosis, it is essential that all clinicians involved in IEM diagnoses have quick access to the disease-characterizing features of known IEMs. IEMbase fills this gap by providing a highly accessible tool to aid clinicians in overcoming the barriers to IEM diagnosis.



T. V. Av-Shalom · J. J. Y. Lee · W. W. Wasserman (✉)
Department of Medical Genetics, Centre for Molecular Medicine and Therapeutics, BC Children's Hospital Research Institute, University of British Columbia, Vancouver, BC, Canada
e-mail: wyeth@cmmt.ubc.ca

C. R. Ferreira
Division of Genetics and Metabolism, Children's National Health System, Washington, DC, USA
e-mail: carlos121180@gmail.com

N. Blau
Division of Metabolism, University Children's Hospital, Zürich, Switzerland
e-mail: nenad.blau@kispi.uzh.ch

C. D. M. van Karnebeek
Department of Pediatrics, Emma Children's Hospital, Amsterdam University Medical Centres, Amsterdam, The Netherlands


## Introduction

Inborn errors of metabolism (IEMs) represent a large class of rare genetic disorders that result from congenital defects in metabolic pathways. While individually rare, as a group IEMs have a collective incidence rate higher than 1:1000. Early timely diagnosis is crucial for these disorders as early intervention has proven to be effective in improving the quality of life and preventing serious sequelae that if left untreated, can lead to end-organ damage and death. Technological advances




N. Blau et al. (eds.), *Physician's Guide to the Diagnosis, Treatment, and Follow-Up of Inherited Metabolic Diseases*,
https://doi.org/10.1007/978-3-030-67727-5_72

in DNA sequencing and metabolomics have greatly improved our ability to detect, diagnose, and manage IEMs in recent years (Vernon 2015). However, with the large number of these disorders as well as the associated genetic and phenotypic heterogeneity, timely diagnosis can often be delayed (Hawkes et al. 2011). Nonspecialists often have challenges with the diagnosis and management of these disorders due to the large amount of specialist knowledge required (Hawkes et al. 2011).

IEMbase was created as an accessible digital application to store standardized information about IEMs taken from the IEM community knowledge base (Lee et al. 2018). The system is implemented as two complementary parts: a digital knowledge base of IEMs and a mini-expert AI to aid diagnosis. The regularly updated knowledge base is compiled by experts from the IEM community consisting of clinicians, geneticists, and scientists. It houses over 1000 disorders and their associated profiles, including information on relevant genomic, biochemical, and clinical markers. The mini-expert AI is designed to help with the diagnosis of IEMs. It allows users to input lists of biochemical and clinical phenotypes and to compare them quickly with the database of disorder profiles.

## Knowledge Base

The specific steps regarding compilation and assembly of IEMbase have been previously described (Lee et al. 2018). For the purpose of this chapter, we will describe the components and content making up IEMbase, with a focus on the facilitating use of the system by potential users.

In its essence, IEMbase is a collection of disorder characterizing profiles for known IEMs. Each disorder profile stores known disorder names, causal gene information, and links to external databases. The links to external databases include OMIM (OMIM 2020), UniProt (UniProt Consortium 2019), NCBI Gene (Brown et al. 2015), GeneCards (Stelzer et al. 2016), Kyoto Encyclopedia of Genes and Genomes (KEGG 2020), National Institutes of Health Genetic Testing Registry (NIH 2020), and GeneReviews (Adam et al. 1993). Each disorder profile also contains a list of associated symptoms and biomarkers, information regarding the age of onset and severity of symptoms, as well as the pathological level(s) of associated biomarkers (Lee et al. 2018). Onset information is organized into five developmental categories: neonatal, infancy, childhood, adolescence, and adulthood. Severities of symptoms are denoted by plus signs, and pathological levels of biochemical markers are denoted by up/down arrows.

In the "backend" of the system, the disorder profiles and associated symptoms/biochemical markers are stored in a PostgreSQL database as three tables: disorders, biochemical/clinical phenotypes, and disorder-phenotype associations. As of April 2020, there are 1342 disorders, 3424 biochemical/clinical phenotypes, and 18,672 disorder-phenotype associations.

IEMbase is actively updated to reflect new information in the field. The first version of IEMbase was compiled as version 1.0.0. Regular updates have yielded new versions of the database, with the latest version at the time of writing (April 2020) being 1.4.3. Mobile Apps for Android and iOS are available in corresponding stores.

## Mini-Expert

With over 1000 distinct IEMs in our database, several of which have overlapping symptoms and/or biochemical marker profiles, IEMbase includes an AI tool for diagnosing IEMs called the mini-expert. The mini-expert takes as input, a list of biochemical and clinical phenotypes. The system then uses a two-step algorithm to identify IEMs with matching profiles and presents them in ranked order (Fig. 72.1). Specific information regarding the algorithm for the mini-expert system is previously published (Lee et al. 2018).

## Application Walkthrough

The IEMbase application is made of three parts: a search feature, a browsing feature, and the mini-expert. When the user enters the site at http://iembase.org they are presented a disclaimer. Once the user agrees, they are then redirected to the main page (Fig. 72.2); this page features a search bar and three buttons: browse, search, and mini-expert. This main page is identical to the search page.

### Search

The search bar feature is found both on the main page and the search page. Using the search bar, the user can enter a disorder name, symptom, or gene name. The search feature will bring up a results page with all disorders that have a partial match with the search term entered (Fig. 72.3). Clicking the "more" button on a disorder from the results list will bring the user to the disorder view page, which will be discussed later in this walkthrough.

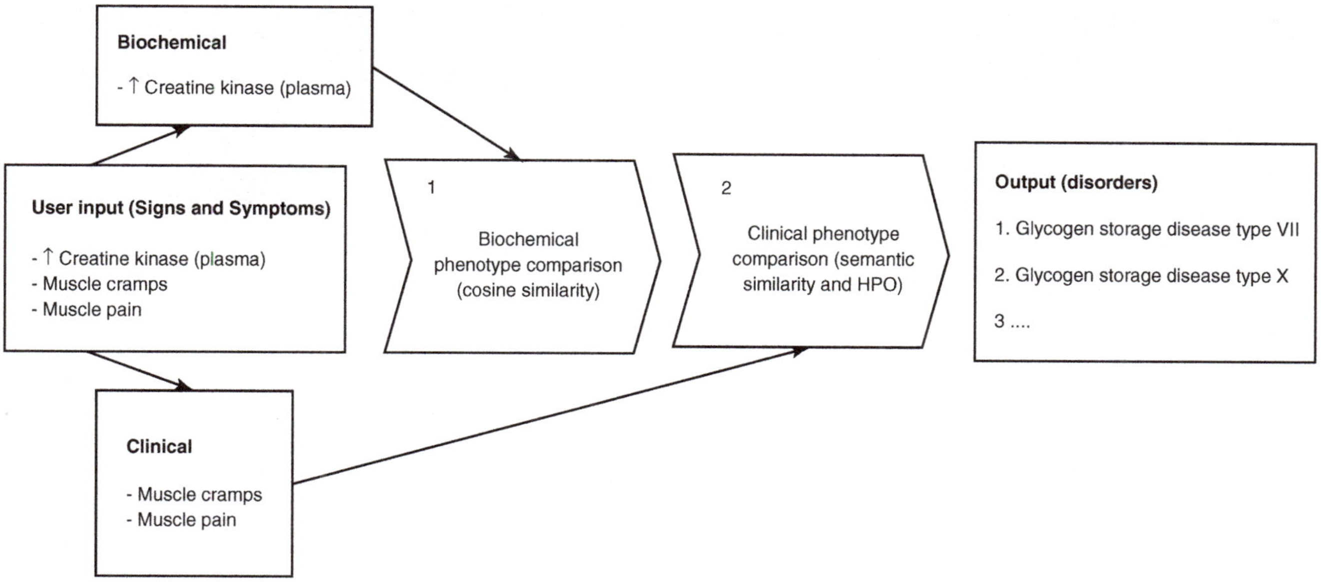


**Fig. 72.1** Mini-expert algorithm flowchart. The user enters a list of signs and symptoms into the mini-expert. The biochemical signs entered are used in step 1 for comparison with the disorder profiles in the system using a cosine similarity measurement, while the clinical symptoms are compared in step 2 using a semantic similarity measurement. The mini-expert then outputs a ranked list of disorders matching the user input

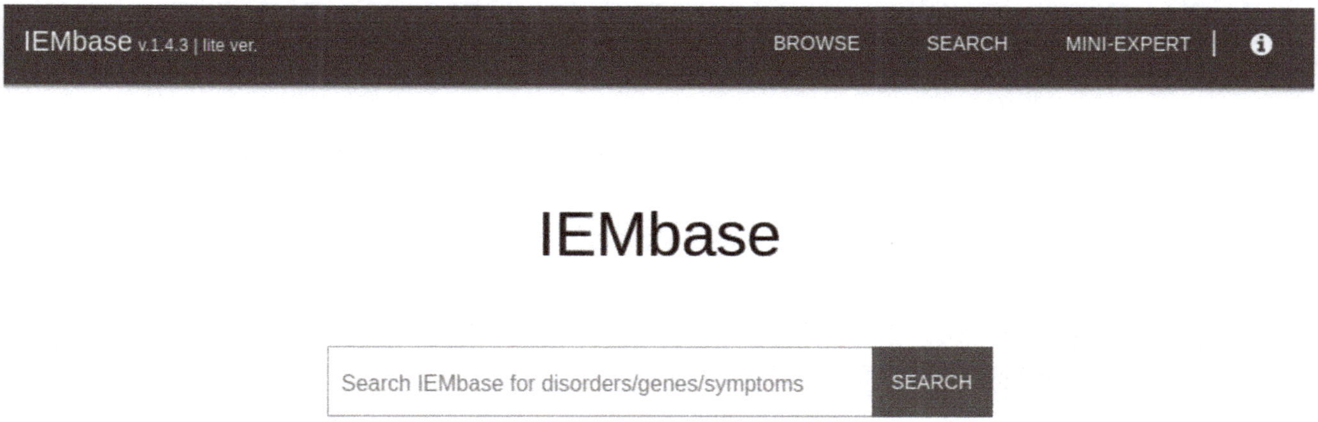


**Fig. 72.2** Main page and search page. This page allows users to search IEMbase for a disorder but entering a partial name, gene symbol, or symptom

## Browse

By clicking the browse button, the user navigates to the browsing page (Fig. 72.4). This page displays a dropdown list of all the IEMs stored in IEMbase organized by the disorder group, where the groupings are consistent with the textbook chapters. The user can expand different disorder groups and subgroups to look for specific disorders. By clicking a specific disorder, the user is redirected to that disorder's view page, which will be discussed in the next section.

The browse section also contains a search bar, which connects to a simplified search that only looks for substrings of a specific disorder name or disorder group name.

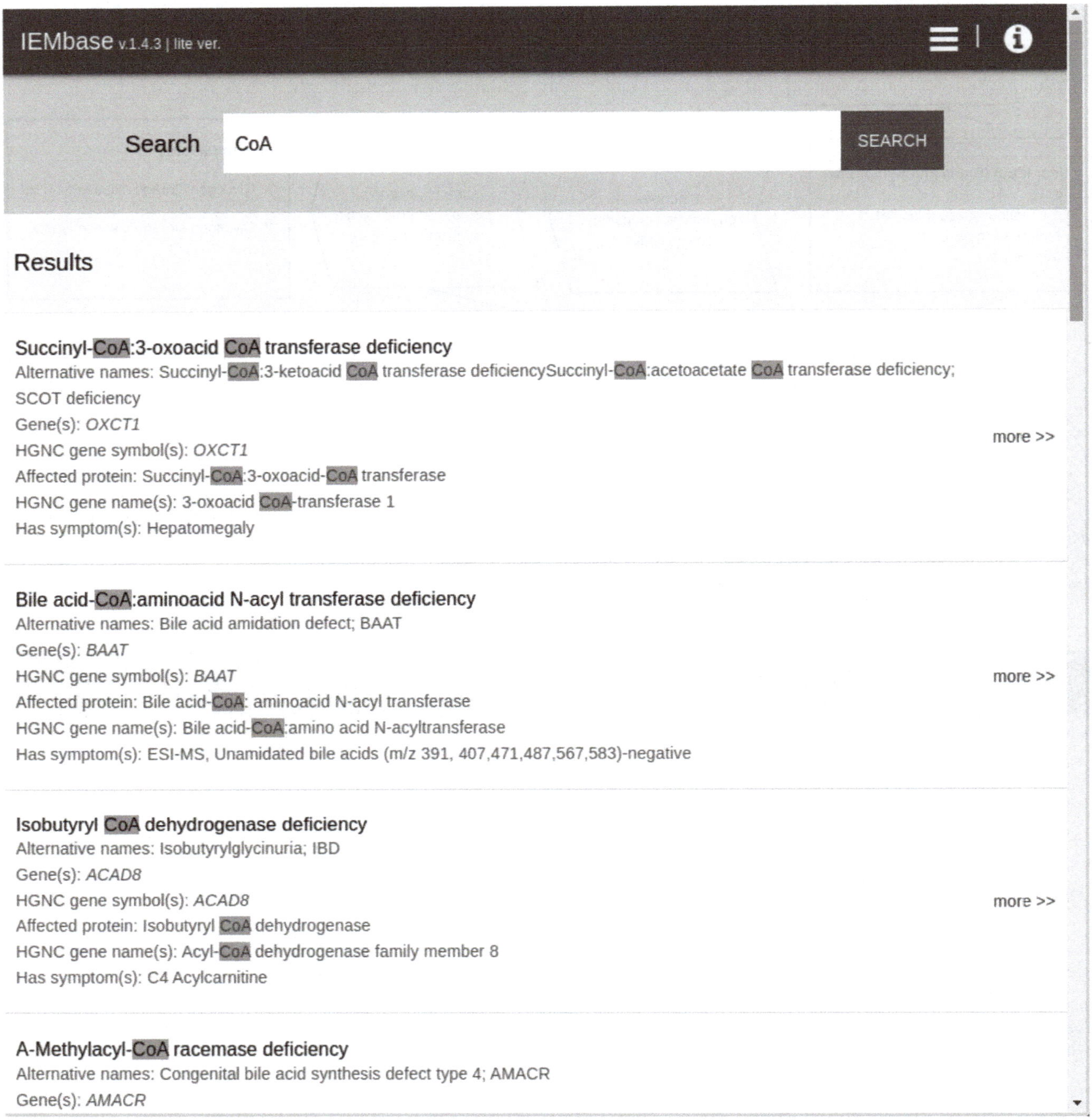


**Fig. 72.3** Search results. After users enter a search term, the results returned include all disorders that have that search term in their summary. The summary consists of the disorder name and alternate names, associated gene(s), affected protein, and associated symptoms

## Disorder View

When a user selects a disorder, either through the search or browse functions, they are redirected to that disorder's view page. This page has four sections: disorder information, clinical symptoms, biochemical markers, and gene information. The user can expand or hide each of these individual sections. Some parts of these sections have clickable features, such as the OMIM number, which redirect the user to relevant external databases.

## Mini-Expert

When the user clicks on the mini-expert button, they are redirected to the mini-expert AI. The first page prompts the user to enter biochemical markers of clinical symptoms (Fig. 72.5). For biochemical markers the user can also specify the relative level by clicking on the up or down arrows. The user can then press the match button, which runs the AI and returns a ranked list of disorders that match the inputted features. The match-

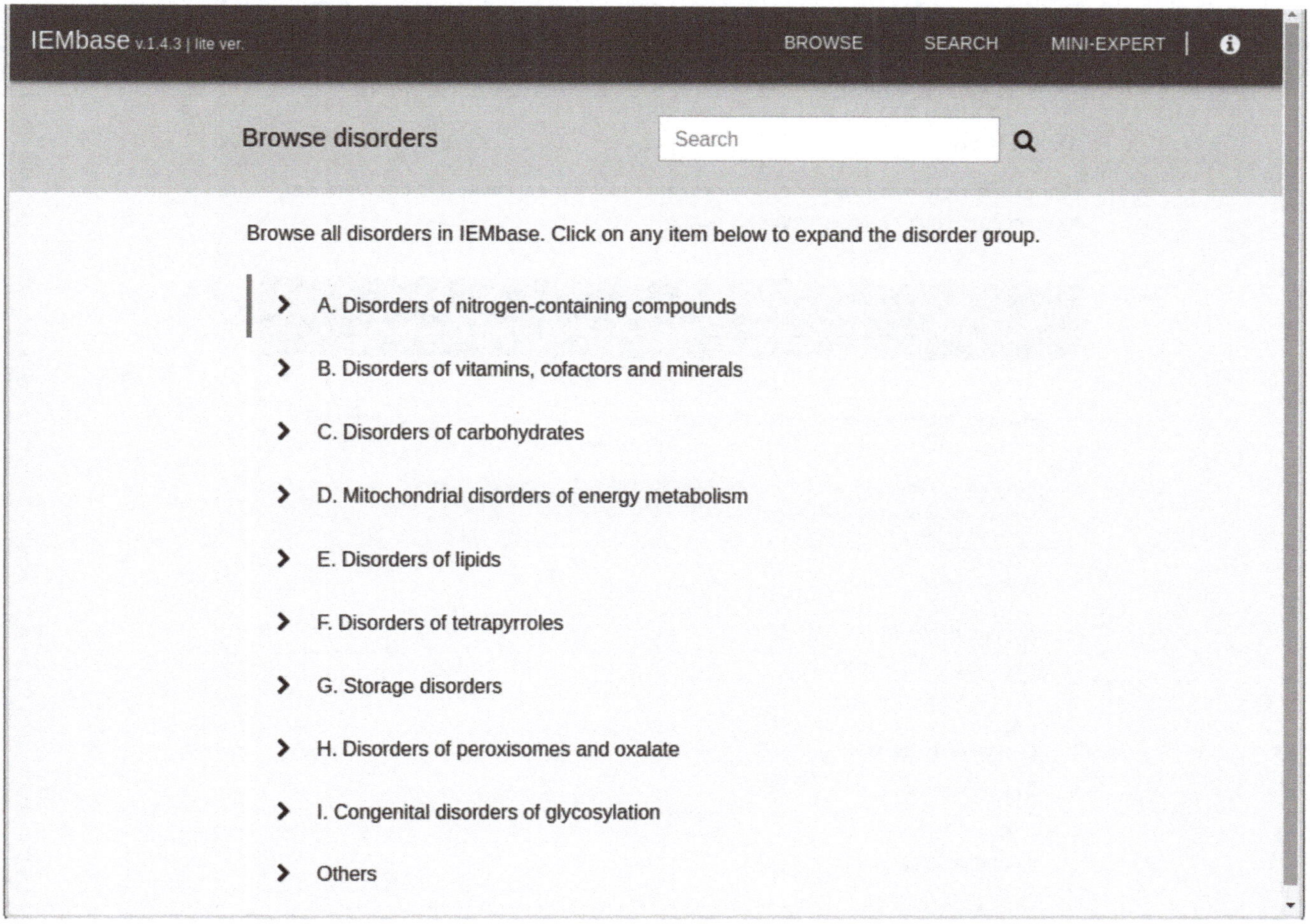


**Fig. 72.4** Browse feature. The user is presented with a dropdown list of disorder groups. Clicking on any of these groups will expand them to show the specific subgroups and disorders under that category

ing algorithm prioritizes biochemical markers and will only work if at least one biochemical marker is input.

The result page (Fig. 72.6) has on the top a summary of the query and then panel options: results, differential diagnosis (DDX), biochemical tests, and gene panel. The DDX, biochemical tests, and gene panel options allow the user to select any subset of disorders from the results of the mini-expert, and it will then create a summary of the selected disorders depending on the option.

## Future Directions

Over the long-term, IEMbase benefits most from the continuous effort of editors and experts to maintain the currency of the disorder characterizing profiles, and we are committed to continuous renewal.

Excluding technical updates, which are necessary for any informatics resource, we are exploring several innovations that may enhance the utility of IEMbase for users. We are attempting to incorporate the embedded display of information from external resources, such as the display within IEMbase of pathway diagrams from pathway databases. The system has largely focused on aiding diagnosis, but we are exploring how we could display information that is useful for clinicians planning treatment of patients. Finally, we are exploring improved AI and search functions that would allow results to be generated based on either verbal description of patient characteristics or submission of a transcribed medical record note.

Users are encouraged to provide feedback, particularly if there are features that would improve the utility of the IEMbase system.

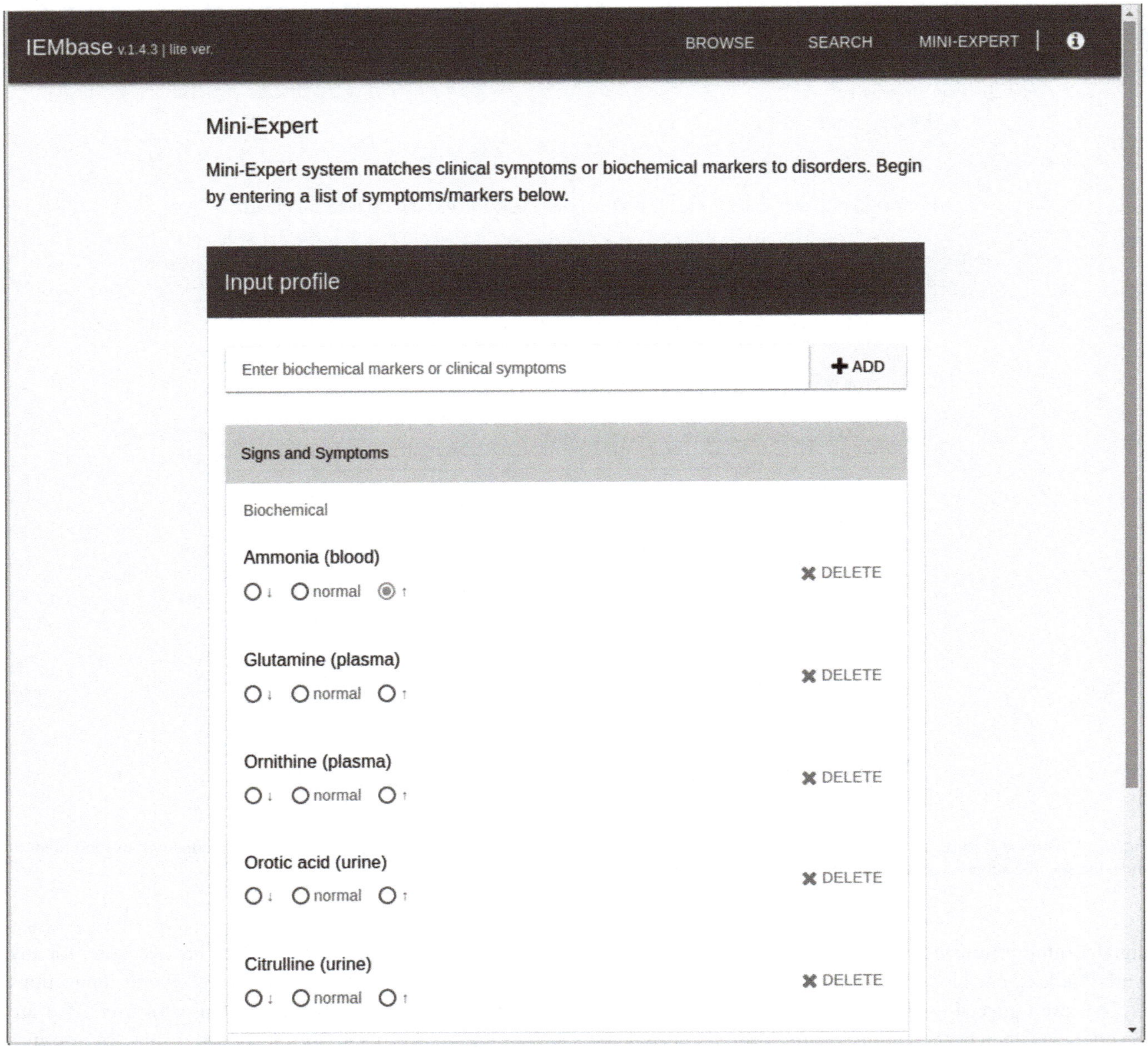


**Fig. 72.5** Mini-expert input. The user can search for biochemical markers or clinical symptoms and can add them to the search query. For biochemical markers, the user can specify a level by selecting the up/down arrow or normal

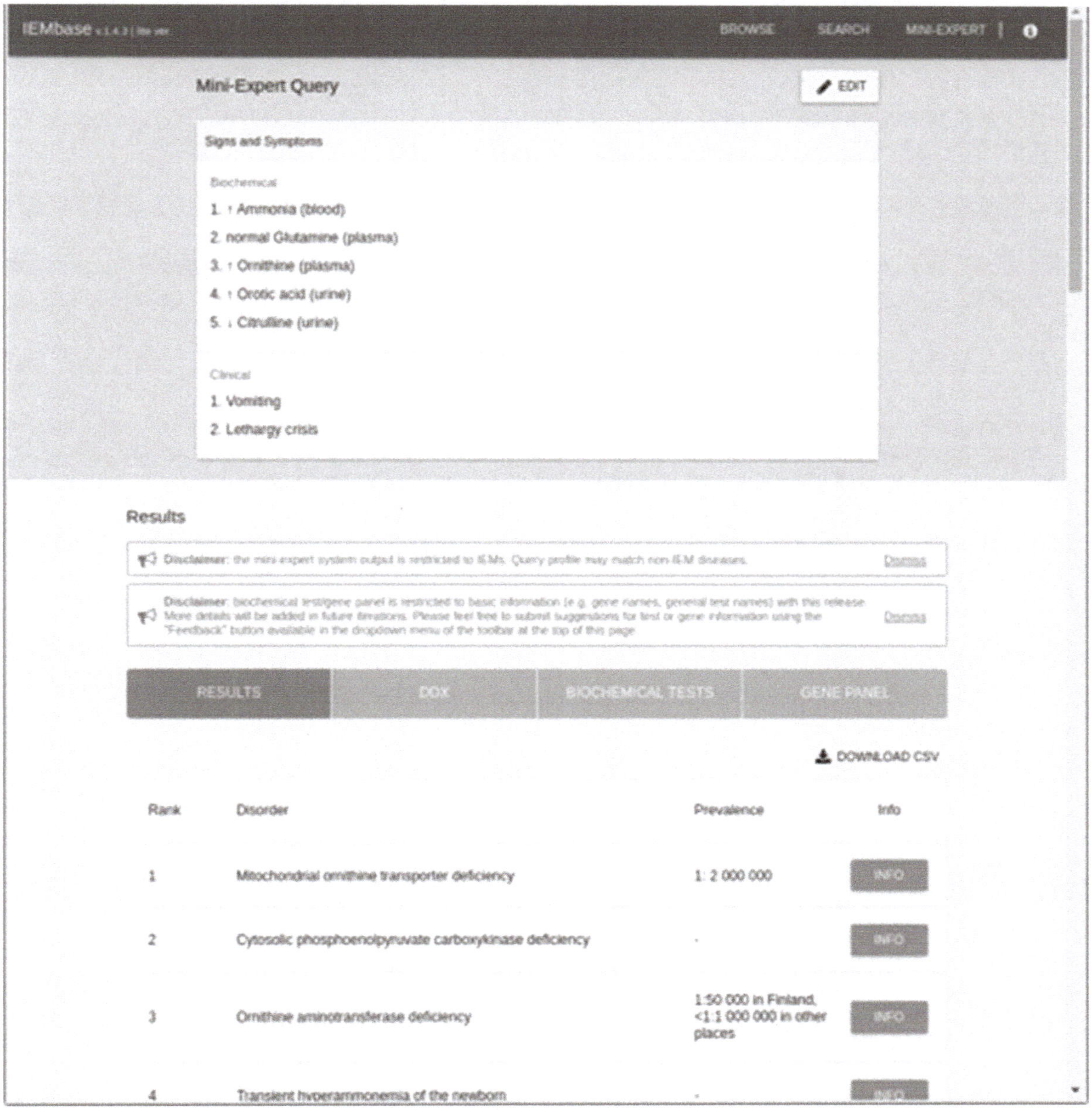


**Fig. 72.6** Mini-expert results. The results from the mini-expert query consist of a summary of the query and a ranked list of matching disorders. There are three additional tabs, DDX, biochemical tests, and gene panel, which allow the user to create summary tables from the ranked results

## References


Adam MP, Ardinger HH, Pagon RA, Wallace SE, Bean LJ, Stephens K, Amemiya A, editors. GeneReviews®. Seattle, WA: University of Washington, Seattle; 1993.

Brown GR, Hem V, Katz KS, et al. Gene: a gene-centered information resource at NCBI. Nucleic Acids Res. 2015;43:D36–42.

Hawkes CP, Walsh A, O'Sullivan S, Crushell E. Doctors' knowledge of the acute management of inborn errors of metabolism. Acta Paediatr 1992. 2011;100:461–3.

KEGG as a reference resource for gene and protein annotation. – PubMed – NCBI. https://www.ncbi.nlm.nih.gov/pubmed/26476454. Accessed 21 Apr 2020.

Lee JJY, Wasserman WW, Hoffmann GF, van Karnebeek CDM, Blau N. Knowledge base and mini-expert platform for the diagnosis of inborn errors of metabolism. Genet Med. 2018;20:151–8.

OMIM - Online Mendelian Inheritance in Man. https://omim.org/. Accessed 21 Apr 2020.

Stelzer G, Rosen N, Plaschkes I, et al. The GeneCards suite: from gene data mining to disease genome sequence analyses. Curr Protoc Bioinformatics. 2016;54:1.30.1–1.30.33.

The NIH genetic testing registry: a new, centralized database of genetic tests to enable access to comprehensive information and improve transparency. https://www.ncbi.nlm.nih.gov/pmc/articles/PMC3531155/. Accessed 21 Apr 2020.

UniProt Consortium. UniProt: a worldwide hub of protein knowledge. Nucleic Acids Res. 2019;47:D506–15.

Vernon HJ. Inborn errors of metabolism: advances in diagnosis and therapy. JAMA Pediatr. 2015;169:778–82.

# WikiPathways: Integrating Pathway Knowledge with Clinical Data

# 73

Denise N. Slenter, Martina Kutmon, and Egon L. Willighagen

## Contents



**Summary**

Throughout the chapters in this book, pathways are used to visualize how genetically inheritable metabolic disorders are related. These pathways provide common conceptual models which explain groups of chemical reactions within their biological context. Visual representations of the reactions in biological pathway diagrams provide intuitive ways to study the complex metabolic processes. In order to link (clinical) data to these pathways, they have to be understood by computers. Understanding how to move from a regular pathway drawing to its machine-readable counterpart is pertinent for creating proper models. This chapter outlines the various aspects of the digital counterparts of the pathway diagrams in this book, connecting them to databases and using them in data integration and analysis. This is followed by three examples of bioinformatics applications including a pathway enrichment analysis, a biological network extension, and a final example that integrates pathways with clinical biomarker data.

The original version of this chapter was previously published non-open access. A Correction to this chapter is available at https://doi.org/10.1007/978-3-030-67727-5_74

D. N. Slenter (✉) · E. L. Willighagen
Department of Bioinformatics - BiGCaT, NUTRIM, Maastricht University, Maastricht, The Netherlands
e-mail: denise.slenter@maastrichtuniversity.nl; egon.willighagen@maastrichtuniversity.nl

M. Kutmon
Department of Bioinformatics - BiGCaT, NUTRIM, Maastricht University, Maastricht, The Netherlands

Maastricht Centre for Systems Biology – MaCSBio, Maastricht University, Maastricht, The Netherlands
e-mail: martina.kutmon@maastrichtuniversity.nl



N. Blau et al. (eds.), *Physician's Guide to the Diagnosis, Treatment, and Follow-Up of Inherited Metabolic Diseases*, https://doi.org/10.1007/978-3-030-67727-5_73

## Introduction

The metabolic pathways in this book are common conceptual models which help us understand groups of chemical reactions within their biological context. These conversion reactions are catalyzed by enzymes and triggered by receptors or transporters, causing a wide variety of metabolites to be present in bodily fluids and tissues. Visual representations of the reactions in biological pathway diagrams provide intuitive ways to study complex metabolic processes. If we want to link clinical data to these pathways, we need pathways that can be understood by computers. By creating machine-readable versions of the pathways relevant for (rare) disorders, clinical data can be processed and analyzed in an automated fashion, allowing fast and visual interpretation (Kutmon et al. 2014a; Villaveces et al. 2015). However, modeling these pathways for data analysis comes with some challenges and limitations (Howe et al. 2008; Khare et al. 2016), which are discussed in this chapter in more detail.

Even though there is still a substantial amount of unexplored territory in human molecular biology, data on biological mechanisms, pathways, and related diseases has increasingly become available due to improvements in measurement and computational techniques. A crucial step to enable advanced data analysis is structuring and sharing the knowledge obtained from biological experiments. This chapter provides some examples of what types of data analysis can be performed with machine-readable pathways and related knowledge. More examples are available in literature, e.g., visualization of drug metabolism related expression changes (Jennen et al. 2010), integrating molecular interaction data (Herwig et al. 2016), and fully automatable processing steps of metabolomics data (Stanstrup et al. 2019). We hope to inspire the metabolic rare disease community to aid our quest in transforming, structuring, and collecting knowledge about molecular processes in machine-readable pathway models and databases. Finally, all these data acquisition and modeling steps will lead to a better understanding of the phenotype of a patient.

## IEMBase and WikiPathways

The knowledge captured in the chapters of this book holds vital information on genetically inheritable metabolic diseases, genes, and proteins involved, metabolic biomarkers, pathways, relevant literature, diagnosis, and treatment. A great effort has been done digitizing most of this information in the IEMBase (www.iembase.org) (Lee et al. 2018), but one key element missing were machine-readable pathways, which are being added through a collaboration with the WikiPathways pathway database (www.wikipathways.org) (Kelder et al. 2012; Kutmon et al. 2016; Slenter et al. 2018). This database allows researchers to add machine-readable pathways, including literature references, and creates a traceable history of edits. The results are freely accessible and reusable by everyone in the world. Furthermore, adding a pathway to WikiPathways exposes the biological knowledge captured in the model via various other data formats (http://help.wikipathways.org) and tools (http://tools.wikipathways.org), allowing researchers to directly integrating the new knowledge within their tool of choice.

We aim to provide all pathways in the chapters of this book as machine-readable pathway models in WikiPathways. You can find the currently available pathways on http://iem.wikipathways.org.

## Machine-Readable Metabolic Pathway Models

Researchers can use different tools to model machine-readable pathways from schematic drawings in publications. WikiPathways stores all pathways in the graphical pathway markup language (GPML), which can be drawn in PathVisio (www.pathvisio.org) (Kutmon et al. 2015). This format is flexible enough to allow modeling of detailed biological phenomena, while relying on a machine-readable structured backbone for automated data analysis. In the following subsections, we highlight relevant topics for creating pathways on genetically inheritable metabolic rare diseases. This information is complemented with an online step-by-step tutorial (academy.wikipathways.org).

### Modeling Biological Entities

The biological entities in GPML-encoded pathways (e.g., gene products, proteins, and metabolites) are captured as *DataNodes* (Fig. 73.1a). These nodes have a textual label and biological type and can contain the following additional information: literature references, free text comments, and a unique database identifier (Fig. 73.1b). The textual label is the visible name of the entity while the type represents which biological entity is modeled: genes are modeled as *GeneProducts*, proteins and enzymes as *Proteins* and chemicals as *Metabolites* (Fig. 73.1a). Additional modeling options include *Complexes*, *Groups*, *RNAs*, (full) *Pathways*, and *States* such as posttranslational modifications (Fig. 73.1c). *DataNodes* can be connected to literature, ideally using PubMed identifiers. Another section allows users to add free text in the comment field, to explain additional details relevant for the pathway. Finally, a database identifier and the accompanying database (Fig. 73.1b) provides the framework required for data integration later (Figs. 73.4

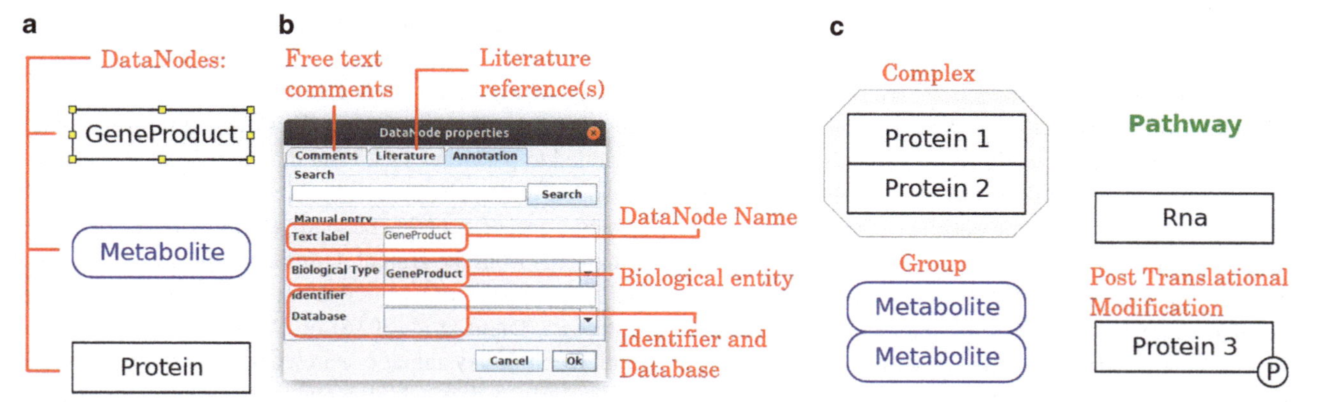


**Fig. 73.1** Visualization of modeling properties for biological entities in PathVisio. (**a**) Main *DataNodes*, where the *GeneProduct* is selected (indicated with small yellow blocks). (**b**) Pop-up menu allowing connecting a *DataNode* to literature, identifier, and database. (**c**) Additional modeling options, where multiple *DataNodes* can be used to form *Complexes* and *Groups*. Nodes can also be used to point to other *Pathways* (including identifier) and *RNA*. *DataNodes* can also be extended with a *State* like posttranslational modifications

and 73.5). An online database identifier allows the retrieval of additional facts about the entity in the pathway. PathVisio makes use of the BridgeDb identifier mapping framework (www.bridgedb.org) (van Iersel et al. 2010) and can therefore support a variety of databases and mappings between them. Since these identifiers are crucial for data analysis, the next two sections discuss them in more detail.

## Identifiers for Pathway Entities

There are many online resources storing information about the proteins, molecules, and interactions in pathways. Ideally, each element in the pathway is annotated with a specific identifier from one of the online databases. Because there are many different databases to choose from, we provide some general guidelines for the annotations of *DataNodes* and interactions in pathways.

Genes and proteins can be annotated with over 60 different databases. However, there are some subtle differences between what type of information is modeled in these databases. Ensembl (Cunningham et al. 2019) and NCBI (Entrez) Gene (Agarwala et al. 2018) focus on gene and transcript identifiers, while UniProt (UniProt Consortium 2019) models their data at a protein level. Therefore, one gene identifier in Ensembl could point to multiple UniProt entries. Enzyme commission numbers (EC-codes) (McDonald and Tipton 2014) can be very useful to annotate a group of enzymes which serve a similar biological function or to classify a chemical conversion to a specific reaction mechanism, without knowing the actual protein structure or gene involved. However, since this classification is not specific for one gene or protein, numerous mappings can be created which complicates data analysis. Thus, regarding identification of biological entities, the more specifically the identifier points to one entity, the more straightforward data can be connected to *GeneProduct* (Ensembl, NCBI Gene) and *Protein* (UniProt) *DataNodes*. For *Complexes* with multiple enzymes, each individual enzyme should receive a unique identifier from UniProt. In addition, distinctive isoforms could also have unique identifiers and be drawn as separate *DataNodes*.

Metabolites can be annotated with over 25 databases, where most of these databases have their own focus (nutrition, toxicology, human metabolism, medication) and possess different levels of chemical detail. These different levels can be quite relevant for the biological implications of these compounds and corresponding interactions, such as stereochemistry (e.g., chirality, isomers), protonation state, (de) phosphorylation, and tautomerization. For several pathways and reactions, the specific level can also be unknown, which is particularly the case for lipid pathways. These are more often considered to behave biologically similar when the head and tail of the lipid are comparable; however a small difference in number of double bonds or location thereof could lead to distinct biological behavior. Identifiers exist to be able to add groups of compounds as *Metabolite DataNodes* in pathways. Nevertheless, this does not solve the issue of straightforward data analysis as discussed for genes and proteins. We would therefore advise to use chemical identifiers which correspond to the known level of chemical detail, e.g., ChEBI (Hastings et al. 2016) for metabolites, DrugBank (Wishart et al. 2018) for drugs, and LIPID MAPS (Fahy et al. 2009) for lipids.

Interactions can currently be annotated with 14 databases, for which some allow easy integration with other resources. A good coverage of metabolic conversions between metabolites is provided by the Rhea database (Lombardot et al. 2019).

### Interaction Types

As mentioned previously, interactions are separate elements within the pathway model. An interaction clearly connects two or more biological entities to depict a relationship between them. Understanding the biological meaning of a connection between different entities is needed to create accurate machine-readable models. PathVisio supports several types of interaction (standards): basic interactions, molecular interaction map (MIM) interactions (Luna et al. 2011), and the interaction types described in the systems biology graphical notation (SBGN) (van Iersel et al. 2012).

For the pathways in this book, we advise the application of MIM interactions, which include conversion and catalysis for reactions between metabolites and related enzyme(s) (Fig. 73.2a); stimulation and inhibition for signaling functions (Fig. 73.2b); transcription/translation for *GeneProduct* to *Protein* (Fig. 73.2c); modification for posttranslational or other modifications and binding for complex formation (Fig. 73.2d); and translocation for transport of metabolites between different cellular compartments (Fig. 73.2e).

### Modeling Diseases and Interactions

Most pathways in this book clearly indicate which step(s) in a pathway are disease causing. This disease information can be added to pathways in several manners. First, diseases can be added to a pathway as text labels and connected to the related gene or protein. Second, a pathway can be tagged with terms from the Human Disease Ontology (Köhler et al. 2019) Pathway Ontology (Petri et al. 2014) and Cell Type Ontology (Diehl et al. 2016) on WikiPathways. The information enables systematic search and browse functionalities with clearly defined child-parent relationships; for example find all pathways, which are linked to the term "inborn error of metabolism pathway" (purl.bioontology.org/ontology/PW/PW:0001589) or all pathways linked to possible child terms. Third, genes and proteins are often linked to OMIM gene entries (Amberger et al. 2015) through BridgeDb, allowing navigation from a specific pathway to disease databases. Finally, including the disease name or class in the title of the pathway or description also helps searching for relevant pathways.

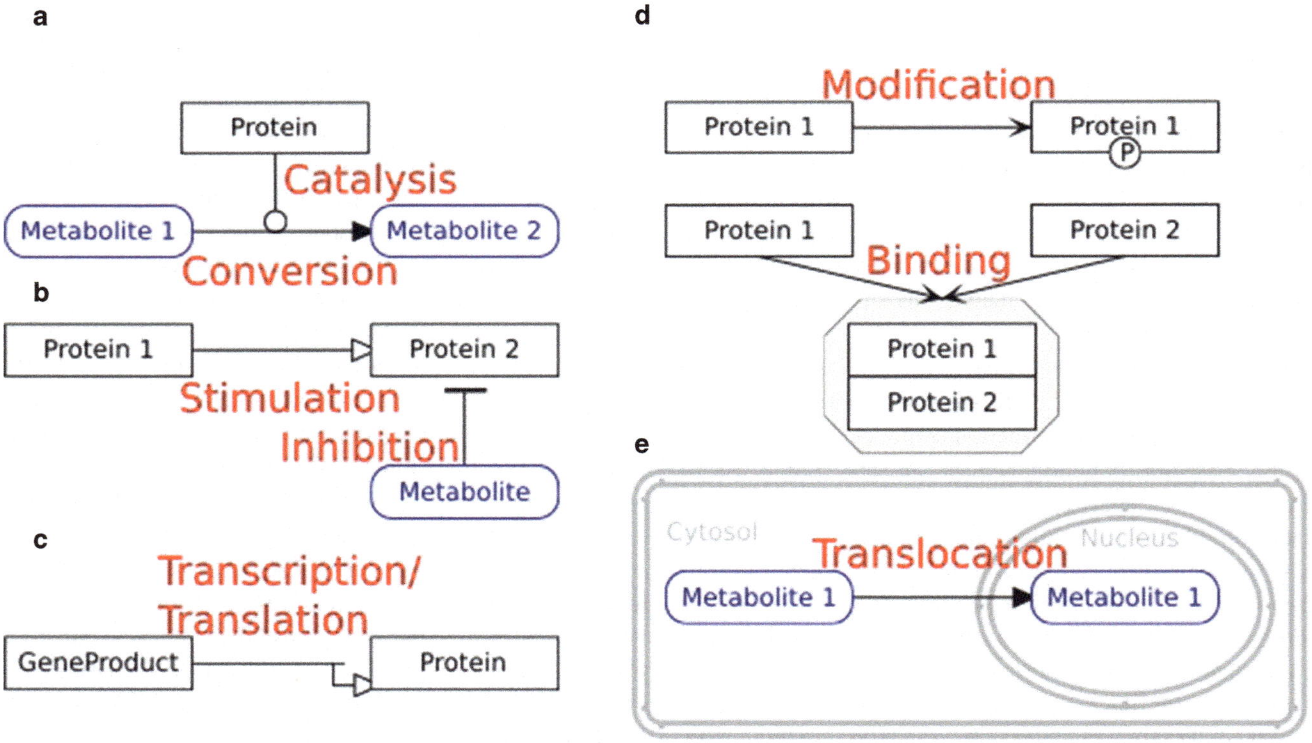


**Fig. 73.2** Overview of MIM interaction types and how these can be used to connect biological entities in PathVisio. (**a**) *Metabolite* 1 is enzymatically converted to *Metabolite* 2, which is catalysed by a *Protein*. (**b**) *Protein* 1 stimulates *Protein* 2; *Protein* 2 is inhibited by a *Metabolite*. (**c**) A *GeneProduct* is transcribed and/or translated to a *Protein*. (**d**) top: A *Protein* undergoing a phosphorylation (P) Post-Translational-Modification (PTM); bottom: two *Proteins* binding together to form a complex. (**e**) A translocation from cytosol to nucleus for a *Metabolite*

## Genetically Inheritable Metabolic Disorder Pathways on WikiPathways

A majority of the pathways in the chapters of this book are already available on WikiPathways (iem.wikipathways.org). As an example, Fig. 73.3 visualizes a complete example of a machine-readable version of the purine pathway (Chap. 13, WikiPathways:WP4792, www.wikipathways.org/instance/WP4792), which is linked to over 20 genetically inheritable diseases (available at WikiPathways:WP4224). Even though at first glance, this figure resembles the original drawing quite closely, all the individual metabolites, proteins, and biomarkers are annotated with identifiers and linked to databases, all interactions connect these elements together and have the appropriate MIM types. The following sections provide several examples on how these pathways can now be used for data analysis.

## Using Pathway Models to Analyze Clinical Data

Pathways can be used to analyze various types of clinical data including whole exome sequencing (WES), transcriptomics and proteomics, genome-wide association studies (GWAS), metabolomics, or targeted chemical assay data. In this section, we provide several examples on how the created pathway models can be used for data analysis. Scripts and instructions for performing these analyses can be found online (bigcat-um.github.io/IEMPathwayAnalysis).

### Pathway Analysis

The availability of pathways as machine-readable models enables us to visualize molecular data on the elements in the pathways and to perform advanced computational analysis including gene set enrichment and network analysis. While whole-genome sequencing is already well established in clinical practice, transcriptome analysis seems promising for diagnosing rare disease patients (Gonorazky et al. 2019).

Pathway analysis for transcriptomics data is a powerful tool to put the data into a biological context. As an example, we selected a publicly available transcriptomic dataset of patients with Lesch-Nyhan disease (LND) (geo:GSE24345, omim:300322) (Kang et al. 2011). The disease is caused by mutations in the *HPRT1* gene (ensembl:ENSG00000165704), producing the hypoxanthine phos-

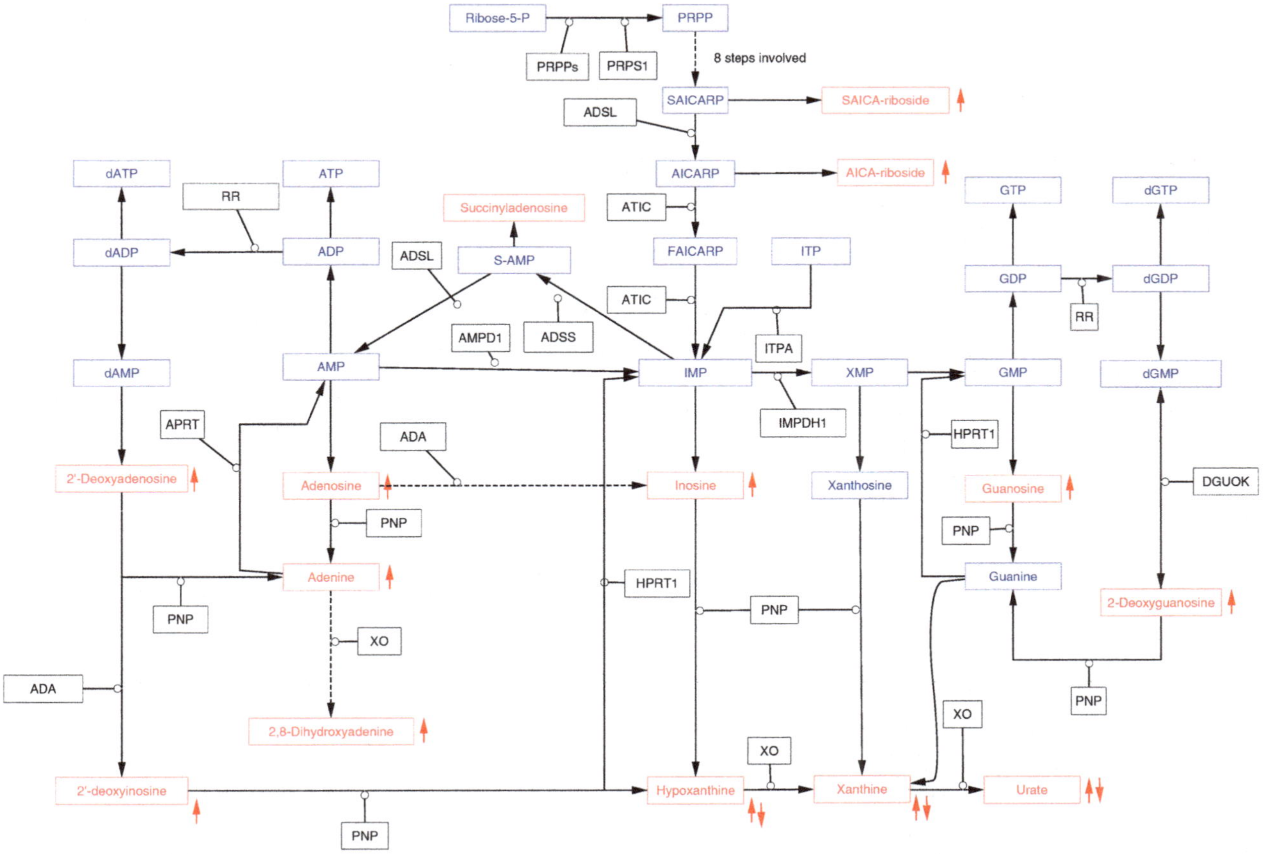


**Fig. 73.3** Machine-readable version of the purine pathway, with metabolites in blue, proteins in black, and biomarker molecules in red (WikiPathways:WP4792)

phoribosyltransferase 1 enzyme (uniprot:P00492) which enables cells to recycle purines. After statistical analysis with GEO2R (Davis and Meltzer 2007), the differential gene expression data was visualized on the previously described purine pathway (Fig. 73.3) using the WikiPathways app in Cytoscape (apps.cytoscape.org/apps/wikipathways) (Kutmon et al. 2014b); see Fig. 73.4. Cytoscape (www.cytoscape.org) (Shannon et al. 2003) is a widely adopted network analysis and visualization software tool, and the WikiPathways app provides direct access to the WikiPathways pathway content. The log2 fold changes (difference in gene expression between patients and control group) are visualized as a gradient from blue (less expressed) over white (not changed) to red (more expressed). A strong downregulation of the *HPRT1* gene is immediately visible by the corresponding blue gene boxes. Based on this dataset, it seems that several of the other enzymes in the pathway (*PNP*, *APRT*, *PRPS1*) attempt to compensate for the lower transcript availability of HPRT1 and are upregulated in LND patients. Other enzymes, which are up- or downstream from the affected purine pathway, could also show changes relevant for the phenotype of the patient. Therefore, enrichment analysis on other pathway models can be used to assess the relevance of these pathways and find interesting affected processes in a certain dataset. Enrichment analysis showed several immune-related processes including the complement system as well as the Wnt signaling pathway affected in LND patients. Reimand et al. published a protocol that provides a description of pathway enrichment analysis and a practical step-by-step guide (Reimand et al. 2019).

Tutorial videos and R scripts for the data visualization (1A, Fig. 73.4) and pathway enrichment analysis (1B) can be found in the PathwayAnalysis folder on GitHub (bigcat-um.github.io/IEMPathwayAnalysis).

## Pathways as a Source for Network Biology

Well-annotated pathway models are also an immensely useful source for network biology approaches. They can be used to extend biological pathways and networks (combinations of pathways) with additional knowledge, such as drug targets.

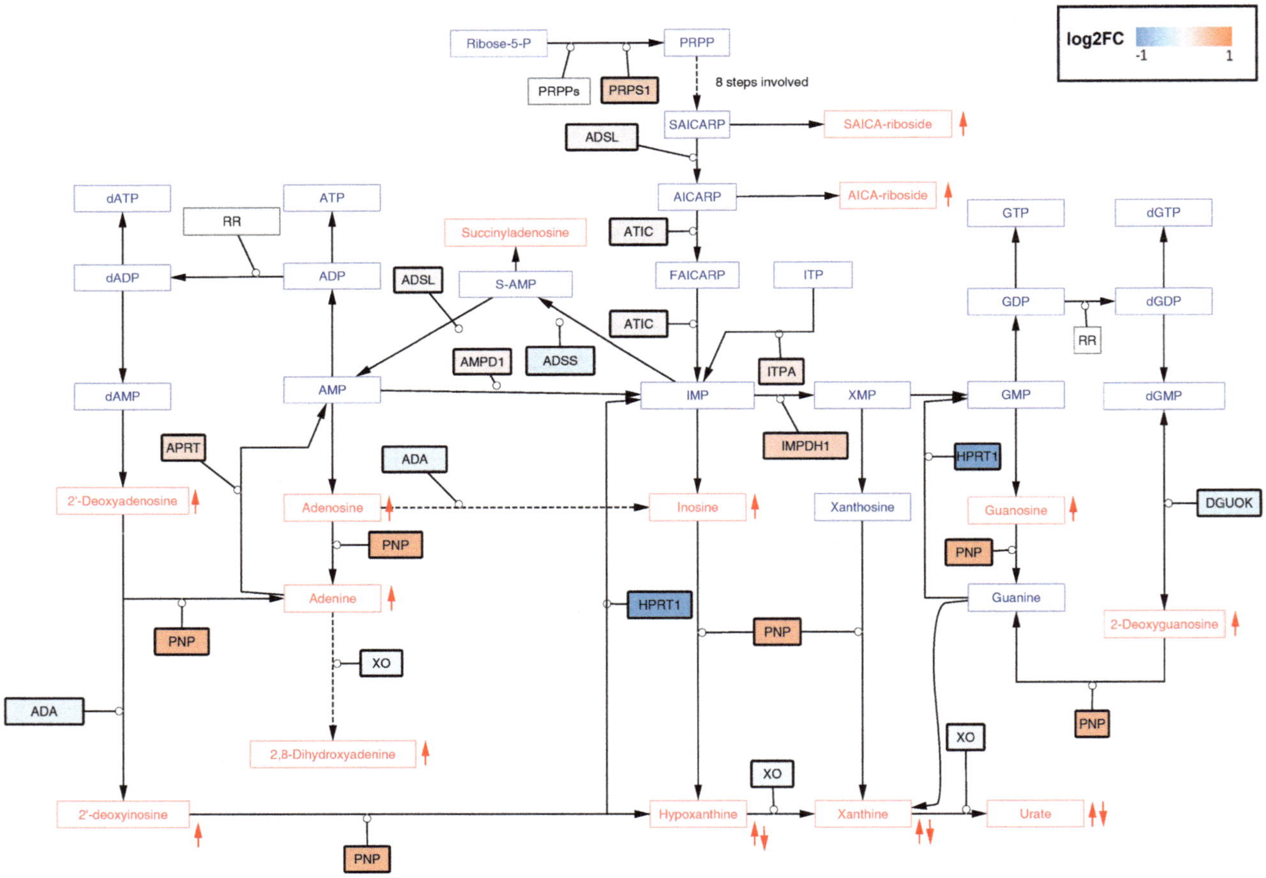


**Fig. 73.4** Visualization of changes in gene expression in patients with Lesch-Nyhan disease in the purine metabolism pathway (WikiPathways: WP4792)

Using the WikiPathways app in Cytoscape, pathways can be visualized in two different views: the pathway view and the network view. The network view retains the existing biological interactions in the pathway only and applies an automatic layout allowing the pathways to be used for network analysis. Pathways can then be automatically enriched with additional information, e.g., regulatory mechanisms, known drugs, or disease annotations. The CyTargetLinker app for Cytoscape was specifically designed for this purpose (cytargetlinker.github.io) (Kutmon et al. 2019). In the following example, we will extend the purine metabolism pathway with approved drugs from DrugBank; see Fig. 73.5. The pathway contains fifteen enzymes, shown as rounded rectangles. In DrugBank, 21 drugs (shown as green diamonds) are reported to target one or more of these enzymes. Nine of the 15 enzymes are targeted by at least one drug, as shown in orange. The LND-causing gene *HPRT1* (highlighted with the red rectangle) is targeted by three drugs, azathioprine, mercaptopurine, and α-phosphoribosyl pyrophosphoric acid. The first two are immunosuppressants and inhibit *HPRT1*. The last molecule is a key substance in the biosynthesis of histidine, tryptophan, purine, and pyrimidine nucleotides and has unknown pharmacological action on *HPRT1*.

Tutorial videos and R scripts for the following example can be found in the Network Analysis folder on GitHub (bigcat-um.github.io/IEMPathwayAnalysis).

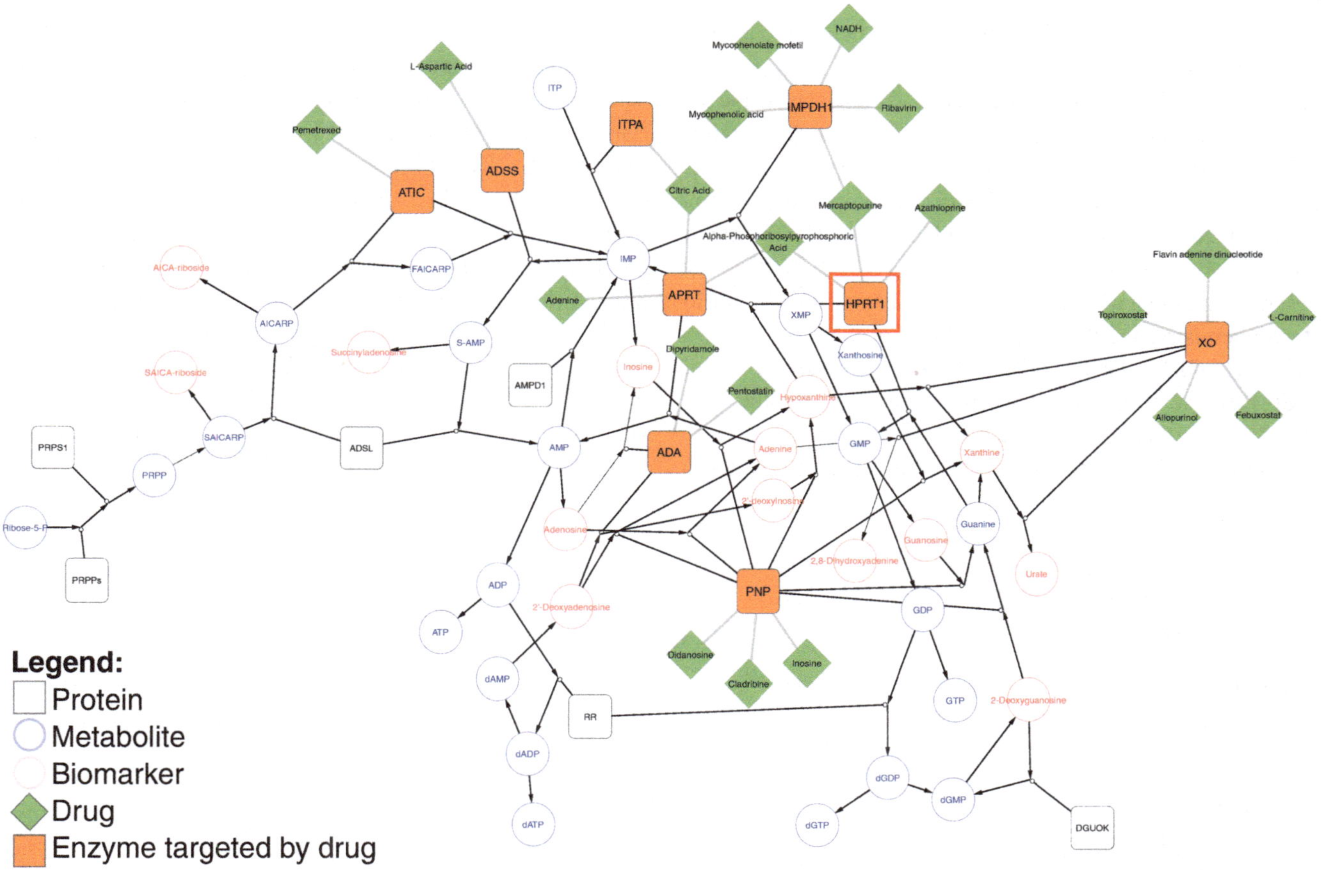


**Fig. 73.5** Known drug-target interactions (from DrugBank) for the purine metabolism pathway

## Linking Chemical (Biomarker) Data with RDF

The two examples in the previous sections work well for transcriptomics data. However, connecting metabolomics or chemical biomarker data to pathways can be challenging with the methods presented above, since the amount of data is significantly lower. Furthermore, as previously mentioned in Sect. 73.3.2, various levels of chemical detail exist within pathway models. To overcome these problems, we want to highlight another method to connect biomarkers data with pathways using an automated approach. The workflow for this example is visualized in Fig. 73.6a. One starts with chemical data from targeted (clinically validated) assays or with (un) targeted metabolomics data from mass spectrometry (MS) and/or nuclear magnetic resonance (NMR). After preprocessing of this data, for example, in R (Stanstrup et al. 2019), and annotation of relevant peaks with the corresponding chemical structure, one can also add an identifier from a (supported) database to the data. For subsequent data analysis steps, we used BridgeDb to link these identifiers to their corresponding InChIKey (a shortened version of the InChI) (Heller et al. 2015), which links the chemical structure to the original compound identifier in a machine-readable manner. The InChIKey consists of three parts (separated by a bar "-"); the first describes the general structure of a molecule, the second its stereochemistry, and the third the charge of the molecule. For example, "CKLJMWTZIZZHCS-REOHCLBHSA-M" is the InChIKey for L-aspartic acid monoanion, where the "M" stands for a –1 charge. In order to link these compounds to (metabolic) pathways, we will use a SPARQL query (Galgonek et al. 2016). This query is a structured method to ask questions to a database such as WikiPathways, which has been converted to the Resource Description Framework (RDF) format (Waagmeester et al. 2016). This RDF format unifies and harmonizes pathway data over all models, with several filtering and search options; data can be queried for specific species, *DataNodes*, literature, and more. Figure 73.6b provides an example of a SPARQL query where we investigated the occurrence of five compounds within the pathway models of WikiPathways. More details on the structure of the WikiPathways RDF and example queries are available on the Semantic Web portal: rdf.wikipathways.org. We also provide a beginners' tutorial on how to write SPARQL queries in the SPARQL folder on GitHub (bigcat-um.github.io/IEMPathwayAnalysis).

To visualize the concepts of SPARQL and data mapping, we chose the five naturally charged proteinogenic amino acids (positive charge: aspartic acid (Asp, D) and glutamic acid (Glu, E); negative charge: arginine (Arg, R), histidine (His, H), and lysine (Lys, K)). Lines 6–10 in Fig. 73.6b provide the InChIKeys for these compounds, which we will link to pathway data in line 15 (wp:bdbInChIKey ?inchikey). The results of the example query reveal in which pathways these compounds can be found, which are listed from lowest to highest (line 22) occurrence counts (line 4) in pathways, to find the most relevant pathways for further analysis. This results in 15 pathways, which all have one of these compounds present (RDF data release 2021-03-10). However, since pathways can be annotated with the uncharged form of these amino acids as well, we can also query all compounds

**a**

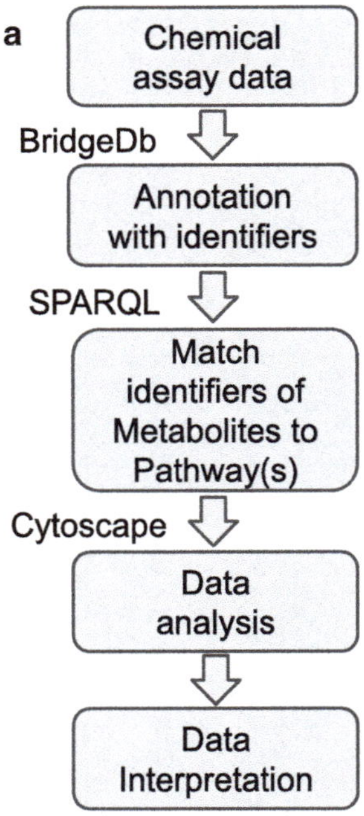


**b**

```
1 prefix ik:      <https://identifiers.org/inchikey/>
2 prefix purl:    <http://purl.obolibrary.org/obo/>
3
4 select distinct ?pathwayRes ?wpid ?title (count(distinct ?inchikey) AS ?MetabolitesInPWs)
5 where {
6 VALUES ?inchikey {ik:CKLJMWTZIZZHCS-REOHCLBHSA-M     # L-aspartic acid monoanion
7                    ik:ZDXPYRJPNDTMRX-VKHMYHEASA-M     # L-glutamine anion
8                    ik:KDXKERNSBIXSRK-UHFFFAOYSA-O     # Lysine monocation
9                    ik:ODKSFYDXXFIFQN-UHFFFAOYSA-O     # Arginine monocation
10                   ik:HNDVDQJCIGZPNO-UHFFFAOYSA-O }   # Histidine monocation
11
12     ?metabolite a wp:Metabolite ;
13                 dcterms:identifier ?id ;
14                 dcterms:isPartOf ?pathwayRes ;
15                 wp:bdbInChIKey ?inchikey .
16
17     ?pathwayRes a wp:Pathway ;
18                 wp:organism purl:NCBITaxon_9606 ; #Homo sapiens Taxon ID.
19                 dcterms:identifier ?wpid ;
20                 dc:title ?title .
21 } GROUP BY ?pathwayRes ?wpid ?title
22 ORDER BY DESC(?MetabolitesInPWs)
```

**Fig. 73.6** Proposed workflow for data analysis of metabolic biomarkers with semantic web technologies. (**a**) Moving from chemical assay data to data interpretation using BridgeDb, SPARQL and Cytoscape. (**b**) Example of a SPARQL query on metabolic data in the WikiPathways RDF

with the same stereochemistry independent of change status, obtaining a more complete result. By changing the end of each compounds InChIKey to their neutral counterpart ("CKLJMWTZIZZHCS-REOHCLBHSA-M" becomes "CKLJMWTZIZZHCS-REOHCLBHSA-N") and changing line 15 to "rdfs:seeAlso ?inchikey," we obtain a total of 38 pathways, with 15 pathways containing 2 of the 5 amino acids (either in their neutral or charged form). This example is explained in more detail in the SPARQL folder on GitHub (bigcat-um.github.io/IEMPathwayAnalysis).

The next step in this workflow downloads the relevant pathways from WikiPathways in Cytoscape; see Sect. 73.4.1 and 73.4.2 for further details. When moving to a network tool, more advanced analysis approaches can be used. The chemical data can be visualized on the nodes in the network, while the edges (interactions between nodes) can be used to visualize fluxomic data (if available). After the data has been added, interpretation can be facilitated by additional features in Cytoscape, such as visualizing the chemical structure of the compounds, connecting several pathways (as networks) to obtain a more complete overview, adding other experimental data (e.g., transcriptomics; see Sect. 73.4.1), or expanding the network with biological knowledge from other databases (see Sect. 73.4.2).

## Limitations

Every type of data analysis comes with its own set of limitations. For pathway analysis, the results depend on the coverage of the selected database (s), the mappings between identifiers from the dataset to the pathway knowledge, the statistics, and cut-off value used for the fold change to discover significant findings. Especially regarding this first issue, WikiPathways is a useful resource, since users can add missing information on pathways and interaction themselves, allowing them and others to use them directly in data analysis. Furthermore, the machine-readable model behind this database is flexible enough to accommodate the needs of researchers from the genetic inheritable metabolic disease research area. We hope that this chapter, as well as the created examples of machine-readable pathways from the figures in this book, provides other users inspiration to add more biological knowledge to databases. For more information on how to model these pathways, please visit help.wikipathways.org.

## Conclusions

While regular pathway drawings are a great resource to visualize relevant biological interactions, these figures are not interactive and not directly reusable for data analysis. Understanding how to move from a regular pathway drawing to its machine-readable counterpart is pertinent for creating proper models. As shown in this chapter, having a digital pathway can link to reference databases and allows us to preform data integration and analysis. This will require some time and effort from the side of the user; however once these skills are mastered, adding new information is relatively easy, will decrease other research time needed for data analysis, and aid the research community as a whole.

## References


Agarwala R, Barrett T, Beck J, et al. Database resources of the National Center for Biotechnology Information. Nucleic Acids Res. 2018;46:D8–D13.

Amberger JS, Bocchini CA, Schiettecatte F, Scott AF, Hamosh A. OMIM.org: online Mendelian Inheritance in Man (OMIM®), an online catalog of human genes and genetic disorders. Nucleic Acids Res. 2015;43:D789–98.

Cunningham F, Achuthan P, Akanni W, et al. Ensembl 2019. Nucleic Acids Res. 2019;47:D745–51.

Davis S, Meltzer PS. GEOquery: a bridge between the gene expression omnibus (GEO) and BioConductor. Bioinformatics. 2007;23:1846–7.

Diehl AD, Meehan TF, Bradford YM, Brush MH, Dahdul WM, Dougall DS. et al. The Cell Ontology 2016: Enhanced content, modularization, and ontology interoperability. J Biomed Semantics. 2016;7(1):44.

Fahy E, Subramaniam S, Murphy RC, Nishijima M, Raetz CRH, Shimizu T, Spener F, van Meer G, Wakelam MJO, Dennis EA. Update of the LIPID MAPS comprehensive classification system for lipids. J Lipid Res. 2009;50:S9–S14.

Galgonek J, Hurt T, Michlíková V, Onderka P, Schwarz J, Vondrášek J. Advanced SPARQL querying in small molecule databases. J Cheminform. 2016;8:31.

Gonorazky HD, Naumenko S, Ramani AK, et al. Expanding the boundaries of RNA sequencing as a diagnostic tool for rare Mendelian disease. Am J Hum Genet. 2019;104:466–83.

Hastings J, Owen G, Dekker A, Ennis M, Kale N, Muthukrishnan V, Turner S, Swainston N, Mendes P, Steinbeck C. ChEBI in 2016: improved services and an expanding collection of metabolites. Nucleic Acids Res. 2016;44:D1214–9.

Heller SR, McNaught A, Pletnev I, Stein S, Tchekhovskoi D. InChI, the IUPAC international chemical identifier. J Cheminform. 2015;7:23.

Herwig R, Hardt C, Lienhard M, Kamburov A. Analyzing and interpreting genome data at the network level with ConsensusPathDB. Nat Protoc. 2016;11:1889–907.

Howe D, Costanzo M, Fey P, et al. The future of biocuration. Nature. 2008;455:47–50.

Jennen DGJ, Gaj S, Giesbertz PJ, van Delft JHM, Evelo CT, Kleinjans JCS. Biotransformation pathway maps in WikiPathways enable direct visualization of drug metabolism related expression changes. Drug Discov Today. 2010;15:851–8.

Kang TH, Guibinga G-H, Friedmann T, Friedmann T. HPRT deficiency coordinately dysregulates canonical Wnt and Presenilin-1 Signaling: a neuro-developmental regulatory role for a housekeeping gene? PLoS One. 2011;6:e16572.

Kelder T, van Iersel MP, Hanspers K, Kutmon M, Conklin BR, Evelo CT, Pico AR. WikiPathways: building research communities on biological pathways. Nucleic Acids Res. 2012;40: D1301–7.

Khare R, Good BM, Leaman R, Su AI, Lu Z. Crowdsourcing in biomedicine: challenges and opportunities. Brief Bioinform. 2016;17:23–32.

Köhler S, Carmody L, Vasilevsky N, et al. Expansion of the human phenotype ontology (HPO) knowledge base and resources. Nucleic Acids Res. 2019;47:D1018–27.

Kutmon M, Ehrhart F, Willighagen EL, Evelo CT, Coort SL. CyTargetLinker app update: a flexible solution for network extension in Cytoscape. F1000Res. 2019;7:743.

Kutmon M, Evelo CT, Coort SL. A network biology workflow to study transcriptomics data of the diabetic liver. BMC Genomics. 2014a;15:971.

Kutmon M, Lotia S, Evelo CT, Pico AR. WikiPathways app for Cytoscape: making biological pathways amenable to network analysis and visualization. F1000Res. 2014b;3:152.

Kutmon M, Riutta A, Nunes N, et al. WikiPathways: capturing the full diversity of pathway knowledge. Nucleic Acids Res. 2016;44:D488–94.

Kutmon M, van Iersel MP, Bohler A, Kelder T, Nunes N, Pico AR, Evelo CT. PathVisio 3: an extendable pathway analysis toolbox. PLoS Comput Biol. 2015;11:e1004085.

Lee JJY, Wasserman WW, Hoffmann GF, van Karnebeek CDM, Blau N. Knowledge base and mini-expert platform for the diagnosis of inborn errors of metabolism. Genet Med. 2018;20:151–8.

Lombardot T, Morgat A, Axelsen KB, et al. Updates in Rhea: SPARQLing biochemical reaction data. Nucleic Acids Res. 2019;47:D596–600.

Luna A, Sunshine ML, van Iersel MP, Aladjem MI, Kohn KW. PathVisio-MIM: PathVisio plugin for creating and editing molecular interaction maps (MIMs). Bioinformatics. 2011;27:2165–6.

McDonald AG, Tipton KF. Fifty-five years of enzyme classification: advances and difficulties. FEBS J. 2014;281:583–92.

Petri V, Jayaraman P, Tutaj M, et al. The pathway ontology—updates and applications. J Biomed Semantics. 2014;5:7.

Reimand J, Isserlin R, Voisin V, et al. Pathway enrichment analysis and visualization of omics data using g:profiler, GSEA, Cytoscape and EnrichmentMap. Nat Protoc. 2019;14:482–517.

Shannon P, Markiel A, Ozier O, Baliga NS, Wang JT, Ramage D, Amin N, Schwikowski B, Ideker T. Cytoscape: a software environment for integrated models of biomolecular interaction networks. Genome Res. 2003;13:2498–504.

Slenter DN, Kutmon M, Hanspers K, et al. WikiPathways: a multi-faceted pathway database bridging metabolomics to other omics research. Nucleic Acids Res. 2018;46:D661–7.

Stanstrup J, Broeckling C, Helmus R, et al. The metaRbolomics toolbox in Bioconductor and beyond. Metabolites. 2019;9:200.

UniProt Consortium. UniProt: a worldwide hub of protein knowledge. Nucleic Acids Res. 2019;47:D506–15.

van Iersel MP, Pico AR, Kelder T, Gao J, Ho I, Hanspers K, Conklin BR, Evelo CT. The BridgeDb framework: standardized access to gene, protein and metabolite identifier mapping services. BMC Bioinform. 2010;11:5.

van Iersel MP, Villeger AC, Czauderna T, et al. Software support for SBGN maps: SBGN-ML and LibSBGN. Bioinformatics. 2012;28:2016–21.

Villaveces J, Koti P, Habermann B. Tools for visualization and analysis of molecular networks, pathways, and -omics data. Adv Appl Bioinforma Chem. 2015;11

Waagmeester A, Kutmon M, Riutta A, Miller R, Willighagen EL, Evelo CT, Pico AR. Using the semantic web for rapid integration of WikiPathways with other biological online data resources. PLoS Comput Biol. 2016;12:e1004989.

Wishart DS, Feunang YD, Guo AC, et al. DrugBank 5.0: a major update to the DrugBank database for 2018. Nucleic Acids Res. 2018;46:D1074–82.

# Correction to: Physician's Guide to the Diagnosis, Treatment, and Follow-Up of Inherited Metabolic Diseases

**Correction to:**

N. Blau et al. (eds.), *Physician's Guide to the Diagnosis, Treatment, and Follow-Up of Inherited Metabolic Diseases*, https://doi.org/10.1007/978-3-030-67727-5
The original version of the book was published with errors and was updated with the following corrections:

1. Chapter 73, WikiPathways: Integrating Pathway Knowledge with Clinical Data was previously published non-open access. It has now been changed to open access under a CC BY 4.0 license and the copyright holder updated to 'The Author(s)'. The book has also been updated with this change.
2. The affiliation of the fifth editor Dr. Clara D. M. van Karnebeek was updated to 'Departments of Pediatrics and Human Genetics, Emma Children's Hospital, Amsterdam University Medical Centers, Amsterdam, The Netherlands'.

The updated version of this book can be found at https://doi.org/10.1007/978-3-030-67727-5



N. Blau et al. (eds.), *Physician's Guide to the Diagnosis, Treatment, and Follow-Up of Inherited Metabolic Diseases*,
https://doi.org/10.1007/978-3-030-67727-5_74

# Disorder Index




N. Blau et al. (eds.), *Physician's Guide to the Diagnosis, Treatment, and Follow-Up of Inherited Metabolic Diseases*,
https://doi.org/10.1007/978-3-030-67727-5

## B

**D**

**H**

## N

**Q**



**R**

## S

**U**



**V**



**W**



**X**

**Y**



**Z**

# Test and Medication Index: Strange Association




N. Blau et al. (eds.), *Physician's Guide to the Diagnosis, Treatment, and Follow-Up of Inherited Metabolic Diseases*, https://doi.org/10.1007/978-3-030-67727-5

**D**

## H

## I

**M**

## Q



## R



## S

**T**



**U**

## V



## X



## Z

# Sign and Symptoms Index





N. Blau et al. (eds.), *Physician's Guide to the Diagnosis, Treatment, and Follow-Up of Inherited Metabolic Diseases*,
https://doi.org/10.1007/978-3-030-67727-5

## B

## C

**D**

## H

## I

## M

## T

U



V

## W



## X



## Y



## Z

GPSR Compliance

*The European Union's (EU) General Product Safety Regulation (GPSR) is a set of rules that requires consumer products to be safe and our obligations to ensure this.*

*If you have any concerns about our products, you can contact us on ProductSafety@springernature.com*

In case Publisher is established outside the EU, the EU authorized representative is:

Springer Nature Customer Service Center GmbH
Europaplatz 3
69115 Heidelberg, Germany

**Batch number: 10777741**

Printed by Printforce, the Netherlands